MW00846233

BRADDOM'S
PHYSICAL MEDICINE & REHABILITATION

Edited by

DAVID X. CIFU, MD
Professor and Chairman
Physical Medicine and Rehabilitation
Virginia Commonwealth University
Richmond, Virginia

National Director for Physical Medicine and Rehabilitation Services
Office of Rehabilitation and Prosthetic Services
U.S. Department of Veterans Affairs
Washington, District of Columbia

Associate Editors

DARRYL L. KAELIN, MD
University of Louisville Endowed Chair of Stroke and Brain Injury Rehabilitation
Chief, Division of Physical Medicine and Rehabilitation
Director, Physical Medicine and Rehabilitation Residency Program
Department of Neurological Surgery
University of Louisville School of Medicine
Frazier Rehab Institute/Jewish Hospital
Neuroscience Collaborative Center
Louisville, Kentucky

KAREN J. KOWALSKE, MD, PhD
Professor
Physical Medicine and Rehabilitation
University of Texas Southwestern Medical Center
Dallas, Texas

HENRY L. LEW, MD, PhD
Professor
Physical Medicine and Rehabilitation
Virginia Commonwealth University School of Medicine
Richmond, Virginia

Professor
Communication Sciences and Disorders
University of Hawaii School of Medicine
Honolulu, Hawaii

MICHELLE A. MILLER, MD
Clinical Assistant Professor
Departments of Physical Medicine and Rehabilitation
The Ohio State University Wexner Medical Center
Section Chief, Pediatric Physical Medicine and Rehabilitation
Medical Director, Inpatient Pediatric Rehabilitation Services
Nationwide Children's Hospital
Columbus, Ohio

KRISTJAN T. RAGNARSSON, MD
Lucy G. Moses Professor and Chairman
Department of Rehabilitation Medicine
Icahn School of Medicine at Mount Sinai
New York, New York

GREGORY M. WORSOWICZ, MD, MBA
Professor of Clinical Physical Medicine and Rehabilitation
Chairman, Department of Physical Medicine and Rehabilitation
University of Missouri HealthSouth Endowed Chair of Physical Medicine and Rehabilitation
University of Missouri School of Medicine
Columbia, Missouri

BRADDOM'S PHYSICAL MEDICINE & REHABILITATION

FIFTH EDITION

ELSEVIER

ELSEVIER

1600 John F. Kennedy Blvd.
Ste 1800
Philadelphia, PA 19103-2899

BRADDOM'S PHYSICAL MEDICINE AND REHABILITATION, FIFTH EDITION

ISBN: 978-0-323-28046-4

Library of Congress Cataloging-in-Publication Data

Braddom's physical medicine & rehabilitation / edited by David X. Cifu; associate editors, Darryl L. Kaelin, Karen J. Kowalske, Henry L. Lew, Michelle A. Miller, Kristjan T. Ragnarsson, Gregory Worsowicz.—Fifth edition.
p.; cm.
Braddom's physical medicine and rehabilitation
Physical medicine & rehabilitation
Preceded by: Physical medicine and rehabilitation / [edited by] Randall L. Braddom. 4th ed. C2011.
Includes bibliographical references and index.
ISBN: 978-0-323-28046-4 (hardcover: alk. paper)
I. Cifu, David X., editor. II. Title: Braddom's physical medicine and rehabilitation. III. Title: Physical medicine & rehabilitation.
[DNLM: 1. Physical Therapy Modalities. 2. Rehabilitation—methods. WB 460]
RM700
615.8'2—dc23

2015025018

Content Strategist: Helene Caprari
Senior Content Development Specialist: Ann Ruzycka Anderson
Publishing Services Manager: Patricia Tannian
Senior Project Manager: Claire Kramer
Design Direction: Amy Buxton

Printed in Canada

Last digit is the print number: 9 8 7 6 5 4

This book is dedicated to the memory of my parents, John and Rosa, who made me all that I am and to the vision of my children, Brie and Belle, who continue to make me even better.

A special thank you to Randy Braddom for his years of hard work and cheerleading that established this foundational textbook and for his confidence in me to continue to carry the torch.

Thank you to my amazingly supportive faculty, staff, and trainees in the Virginia Commonwealth University Department of Physical Medicine and Rehabilitation for their mentorship, their friendship, and the time to complete this project.

Thank you to the wonderful members of the Office of Rehabilitation and Prosthetic Services in the U.S Department of Veterans Affairs for all they do for America's Veterans and Service Members and for allowing me the time to complete this project.

Thank you to the thousands of patients and their family members who allowed me to participate in their care over the years; you have taught me so much.

Thank you to my family, friends, and other loved ones for your ongoing support that allows me to pursue my work and career.

CONTRIBUTORS

J. Dennis Alfonso, MD
Department of Rehabilitation Medicine
University of Texas Health Science Center at San Antonio
San Antonio, Texas
28 Chronic Medical Conditions: Pulmonary Disease, Organ Transplantation, and Diabetes

Derrick B. Allred, MD
Polytrauma Rehabilitation Center
South Texas Veterans Health Care System
San Antonio, Texas
Department of Rehabilitation Medicine
University of Texas Health Science Center at San Antonio
San Antonio, Texas
28 Chronic Medical Conditions: Pulmonary Disease, Organ Transplantation, and Diabetes

Michael Andary, MD, MS
Professor
Physical Medicine and Rehabilitation
Michigan State University College of Osteopathic Medicine
East Lansing, Michigan
8 Electrodiagnostic Medicine

Karen L. Andrews, MD
Physical Medicine and Rehabilitation
Mayo Clinic
Rochester, Minnesota
25 Vascular Diseases

Thiru M. Annaswamy, MD, MA
Section Chief
Spine and Electrodiagnostic Sections
Physical Medicine and Rehabilitation Service
Veterans Affairs North Texas Health Care System
Dallas, Texas
Associate Professor
Department of Physical Medicine and Rehabilitation
University of Texas Southwestern Medical Center
Dallas, Texas
7 Quality and Outcome Measures for Medical Rehabilitation
17 Physical Agent Modalities

Patricia M. Arenth, PhD
Assistant Professor
Physical Medicine and Rehabilitation
University of Pittsburgh
Pittsburgh, Pennsylvania
43 Traumatic Brain Injury

W. David Arnold, MD
Associate Professor
Division of Neuromuscular Disorders
Department of Neurology
Department of Physical Medicine and Rehabilitation
Department of Neuroscience
The Ohio State University
Columbus, Ohio
40 Motor Neuron Diseases

Rita Ayyangar, MD, MBBS
Associate Professor
Department of Physical Medicine and Rehabilitation
Program Director
Pediatric Rehabilitation Medicine Program
University of Michigan
Ann Arbor, Michigan
41 Rehabilitation of Patients with Neuropathies
48 Myelomeningocele and Other Spinal Dysraphisms

Steven M. Barlow, PhD
Corwin Moore Professor
Department of Special Education and Communication Disorders
Center for Brain, Biology, and Behavior
Professor (affiliate)
Department of Biological Systems Engineering
Director
Communication Neuroscience Laboratories
Barkley Memorial Center
University of Nebraska
Lincoln, Nebraska
3 Adult Neurogenic Communication and Swallowing Disorders

Karen P. Barr, MD
Associate Professor
Rehabilitation Medicine
Residency Program Director
Rehabilitation Medicine
University of Washington
Seattle, Washington
33 Low Back Pain

Matthew Bartels, MD, MPH
Chairman
Rehabilitation Medicine
Albert Einstein College of Medicine/Montefiore Medical Center
Bronx, New York
27 Acute Medical Conditions

Theresa Berner, MOT, OTR/L, ATP
Instructor
Occupational Therapy Division
The Ohio State University
Columbus, Ohio
Rehabilitation Clinic Manager
Assistive Technology Center
The Ohio State University Wexner Medical Center
Columbus, Ohio
14 Wheelchairs and Seating Systems

Cathy Bodine, PhD, CCC-SLP
Associate Professor
Departments of Bioengineering and Pediatrics
Executive Director
Assistive Technology Partners
Anschutz Medical Campus
University of Colorado
Denver, Colorado
19 Computer Assistive Devices and Environmental Controls

Jaclyn Bonder, MD
Assistant Professor
Physical Medicine and Rehabilitation
Weill Cornell Medical College
New York, New York
38 Pelvic Floor Disorders

Susan Brady, MS, CCC-SKP
Research Coordinator and Clinical Educator
Speech Language Pathology
Marianjoy Rehabilitation Hospital
Wheaton, Illinois
3 Adult Neurogenic Communication and Swallowing Disorders

Jeffrey S. Brault, DO
Consultant
Physical Medicine and Rehabilitation
Mayo Clinic
Rochester, Minnesota
16 Manipulation, Traction, and Massage

Thomas N. Bryce, MD
Professor
Department of Rehabilitation Medicine
Icahn School of Medicine at Mount Sinai
New York, New York
49 Spinal Cord Injury

Diana D. Cardenas, MD, MHA
Professor and Chair
Department of Physical Medicine and Rehabilitation
University of Miami Miller School of Medicine
Miami, Florida
Chief of Service
Jackson Rehabilitation Hospital
Miami, Florida
20 Bladder Dysfunction

William Carne, PhD
Associate Professor
Department of Physical Medicine and Rehabilitation
Virginia Commonwealth University
Richmond, Virginia
Clinical Psychologist
Parkinson's Disease Research, Education and Clinical Center (PADRECC)
Hunter Holmes McGuire Veterans Affairs Medical Center
Richmond, Virginia
45 Degenerative Movement Disorders of the Central Nervous System

Priya Chandan, MD, MPH
Health Services Organization and Research Doctoral Program
Department of Health Administration
Department of Physical Medicine and Rehabilitation
Virginia Commonwealth University
Richmond, Virginia
45 Degenerative Movement Disorders of the Central Nervous System

Wen-Shiang Chen, MD, PhD
Professor
Physical Medicine and Rehabilitation
National Taiwan University
Taipei, Taiwan
Attending Physician
Physical Medicine and Rehabilitation
National Taiwan University Hospital
Taipei, Taiwan
17 Physical Agent Modalities

Andrea L. Cheville, MD, MSCE
Professor
Physical Medicine and Rehabilitation
Mayo Clinic
Rochester, Minnesota
29 Cancer Rehabilitation

George C. Christolias, MD
Assistant Professor of Rehabilitation Medicine and Regenerative Medicine
Columbia University College of Physicians and Surgeons
New York, New York
1 The Physiatric History and Physical Examination

Allison N. Clark, PhD
Assistant Professor
Physical Medicine and Rehabilitation
Baylor College of Medicine
Houston, Texas
Research Scientist
Brain Injury Research Center
TIRR Memorial Hermann
Texas Medical Center
Houston, Texas
4 Psychological Assessment and Intervention in Rehabilitation

Leah G. Concannon, MD
Clinical Assistant Professor
Rehabilitation Medicine
University of Washington
Seattle, Washington
33 Low Back Pain

Anita Craig, DO
Assistant Professor
Physical Medicine and Rehabilitation
University of Michigan
Ann Arbor, Michigan
41 Rehabilitation of Patients with Neuropathies

Deborah Daimaru, BS
Registered Kinesiotherapist/Integrative Medicine Program Coordinator
Physical Medicine and Rehabilitation
Hunter Holmes McGuire Veterans Affairs Medical Center
Richmond, Virginia
18 Integrative Medicine in Rehabilitation

R. Drew Davis, MD
Associate Professor and Division Director
Division of Pediatric Rehabilitation Medicine
Departments of Pediatrics and Physical Medicine and Rehabilitation
University of Alabama at Birmingham/Children's of Alabama
Birmingham, Alabama
48 Myelomeningocele and Other Spinal Dysraphisms

Jean M. de Leon, MD
Professor and Director of University Hospital Wound Care Clinic
Department of Physical Medicine and Rehabilitation
University of Texas Southwestern Medical Center
Dallas, Texas
24 Chronic Wounds

Arthur J. De Luigi, DO
Associate Professor of Rehabilitation Medicine
Georgetown University School of Medicine
Director of Sports Medicine
MedStar NRH/Georgetown University Hospital
Washington, District of Columbia
39 Sports Medicine and Adaptive Sports

George W. Deimel, MD
Northwest Sports, Spine, and Physical Medicine
Northwest Health System
Springdale, Arkansas
36 Musculoskeletal Disorders of the Lower Limb

Ana Delgado, MD
Medical Director
Stroke Rehabilitation
Madonna Rehabilitation Hospital
Lincoln, Nebraska
3 Adult Neurogenic Communication and Swallowing Disorders

Michael J. DePalma, MD
President and Medical Director
Director of Interventional Spine Care Fellowship
Virginia iSpine Physicians, PC
President and Director of Research
Virginia Spine Research Institute, Inc.
Richmond, Virginia
32 Common Neck Problems

Carmen P. DiGiovine, PhD, ATP/SMS, RET
Associate Professor
Occupational Therapy Division
The Ohio State University
Columbus, Ohio
Program Director
Assistive Technology Center
The Ohio State University Wexner Medical Center
Columbus, Ohio
14 Wheelchairs and Seating Systems

Timothy Dillingham, MD, MS
The William J. Erdman II, Professor and Chair
Department of Physical Medicine and Rehabilitation
Chief Medical Officer
Pennsylvania Institute for Rehabilitation Medicine
The University of Pennsylvania
Philadelphia, Pennsylvania
8 Electrodiagnostic Medicine

Carole V. Dodge, OTR/L, CHT
Supervisor/Clinical Specialist
Occupational Therapy
University of Michigan Hospital and Health System
Ann Arbor, Michigan
11 Upper Limb Orthoses

David F. Drake, MD
Director
Interventional and Integrative Pain Medicine
Physical Medicine and Rehabilitation
Hunter Holmes McGuire Veterans Affairs Medical Center
Richmond, Virginia
Associate Professor
Physical Medicine and Rehabilitation
Virginia Commonweath University
Richmond, Virginia
18 Integrative Medicine in Rehabilitation

Daniel Dumitru, MD, PhD
Professor
Department of Rehabilitation Medicine
University of Texas Health Science Center at San Antonio
San Antonio, Texas
8 Electrodiagnostic Medicine

Blessen C. Eapen, MD
Traumatic Brain Injury/Polytrauma Fellowship Program Director
Section Chief
Polytrauma Rehabilitation Center
South Texas Veterans Health Care System
San Antonio, Texas
Adjunct Assistant Professor
Department of Rehabilitation Medicine
University of Texas Health Science Center
San Antonio, Texas
28 Chronic Medical Conditions: Pulmonary Disease, Organ Transplantation, and Diabetes

Sarah M. Eickmeyer, MD
Assistant Professor
Rehabilitation Medicine
University of Kansas Medical Center
Kansas City, Kansas
38 Pelvic Floor Disorders

Susan Koch Fager, PhD, CCC-SLP
Director, Communication Center
Institute for Rehabilitation Science and Engineering
Madonna Rehabilitation Hospital
Lincoln, Nebraska
3 Adult Neurogenic Communication and Swallowing Disorders

Jonathan T. Finnoff, DO
Consultant
Department of Physical Medicine and Rehabilitation
Mayo Clinic
Rochester, Minnesota
Clinical Professor
Department of Physical Medicine and Rehabilitation
University of California Davis School of Medicine
Sacramento, California
35 Upper Limb Pain and Dysfunction

Colleen Fitzgerald, MD, MS
Associate Professor
Obstetrics and Gynecology
Physical Medicine and Rehabilitation
Division of Female Pelvic Medicine and Reconstructive Surgery
Loyola University Chicago Medical Center
Chicago, Illinois
38 Pelvic Floor Disorders

Angela Flores, MD
Assistant Professor
Department of Neurology and Neurotherapeutics
University of Texas Southwestern Medical Center
Dallas, Texas
46 Multiple Sclerosis

Gerard E. Francisco, MD
Department of Physical Medicine and Rehabilitation
University of Texas Health Science Center (UTHealth)
Houston, Texas
NeuroRecovery Research Center
TIRR Memorial Hermann
Houston, Texas
23 Spasticity

Vincent Gabriel, MD, MSc, BSc, FRCPC
Clinical Associate
Clinical Neurosciences, Pediatrics, and Surgery
University of Calgary
Calgary, Alberta, Canada
26 Burns

Justin J. Gasper, DO
Interventional Spine Care Fellow
Virginia iSpine Physicians, PC
Richmond, Virginia
32 Common Neck Problems

Carl D. Gelfius, MD
Assistant Professor—Clinical
Physical Medicine and Rehabilitation
The Ohio State University
Columbus, Ohio
Pediatric Physiatrist
Pediatric Physical Medicine and Rehabilitation
Nationwide Children's Hospital
Columbus, Ohio
Assistant Professor
Physical Medicine and Rehabilitation
Baylor College of Medicine
Houston, Texas
Pediatric Physiatrist
Pediatric Physical Medicine and Rehabilitation
Texas Children's Hospital
Houston, Texas
42 Myopathy

Lance L. Goetz, MD
Associate Professor
Physical Medicine and Rehabilitation
Virginia Commonwealth University
Richmond, Virginia
Staff Physician
Spinal Cord Injury and Disorders
Hunter Holmes McGuire Veterans Affairs Medical Center
Richmond, Virginia
20 Bladder Dysfunction

Robert J. Goldman, MD, ABPMR, ABPM-UHM, CWS
Medical Director
Fort HealthCare Wound and Edema Center
Fort Atkinson, Wisconsin
24 Chronic Wounds

Jennifer Gomez, MD
Chief Resident
Department of Physical Medicine and Rehabilitation
Albert Einstein College of Medicine/Montefiore Medical Center
Bronx, New York
6 Employment of People with Disabilities

Gregory L. Goodrich, PhD
Supervisory Research Psychologist
Psychology Service and Western Blind Rehabilitation Center
Veterans Affairs Palo Alto Health Care System
Menlo Park, California
50 Auditory, Vestibular, and Visual Impairments

Mark Hakel, PhD, CCC-SLP
Director, Workforce Management System
Workforce Retention and Development
Madonna Rehabilitation Hospital
Lincoln, Nebraska
3 Adult Neurogenic Communication and Swallowing Disorders

Pamela A. Hansen, MD
Associate Professor
Physical Medicine and Rehabilitation
University of Utah
Salt Lake City, Utah
36 Musculoskeletal Disorders of the Lower Limb

R. Norman Harden, MD
Professor Emeritus
Departments of Physical Medicine and Rehabilitation and Physical Therapy and Human Movement Sciences
Northwestern University
Feinberg School of Medicine
Chicago, Illinois
37 Chronic Pain

Mark A. Harrast, MD
Medical Director
Sports Medicine Center at Husky Stadium
Clinical Professor of Rehabilitation Medicine, Orthopaedics, and Sports Medicine
University of Washington
Seattle, Washington
33 Low Back Pain
39 Sports Medicine and Adaptive Sports

Richard L. Harvey, MD
Associate Professor
Department of Physical Medicine and Rehabilitation
Northwestern University Feinberg School of Medicine
Wesley and Suzanne Dixon Stroke Chair and Medical Director
Stroke Rehabilitation
The Rehabilitation Institute of Chicago
Chicago, Illinois
44 Stroke Syndromes

William J. Hennessey, MD
President
PA Physical Medicine, Inc.
Greensburg, Pennsylvania
12 Lower Limb Orthoses

A. Michael Henrie, DO
Assistant Professor
Division of Physical Medicine and Rehabilitation
University of Utah
Salt Lake City, Utah
36 Musculoskeletal Disorders of the Lower Limb

Edson Hirohata, AuD, CCC-A
Assistant Professor
Communication Sciences and Disorders
University of Hawaii School of Medicine
Honolulu, Hawaii
50 Auditory, Vestibular, and Visual Impairments

Radha Holavanahalli, PhD
Associate Professor
Physical Medicine and Rehabilitation
University of Texas Southwestern Medical Center
Dallas, Texas
26 Burns

Amy Houtrow, MD, PhD, MPH
Associate Professor
Physical Medicine and Rehabilitation and Pediatrics
University of Pittsburgh
Pittsburgh, Pennsylvania
7 Quality and Outcome Measures for Medical Rehabilitation

Lin-Fen Hsieh, MD
Associate Professor
School of Medicine
Fu Jen Catholic University
New Taipei City, Taiwan
Director
Department of Physical Medicine and Rehabilitation
Shin Kong Wu Ho-Su Memorial Hospital
Taipei, Taiwan
31 Rheumatologic Rehabilitation

Sarah Hwang, MD
Assistant Professor
Clinical Physical Medicine and Rehabilitation
University of Missouri
Columbia, Missouri
38 Pelvic Floor Disorders

Carlos Anthony Jaramillo, MD, PhD
Staff Physician
Polytrauma Rehabilitation Center
South Texas Veterans Health Care System
San Antonio,Texas
Clinical and Research Faculty
Geriatric Research, Education and Clinical Center (GRECC)
South Texas Veterans Health Care System
San Antonio, Texas
Adjunct Assistant Professor
Department of Rehabilitation Medicine
University of Texas Health Science Center San Antonio
San Antonio, Texas
30 The Geriatric Patient

Jeffrey G. Jenkins, MD
Associate Professor of Clinical Physical Medicine and Rehabilitation
University of Virginia School of Medicine
Charlottesville, Virginia
15 Therapeutic Exercise

Shawn Jorgensen, MD
Clinical Associate Professor
Physical Medicine and Rehabilitation
Albany Medical Center
Albany, New York
40 Motor Neuron Diseases

Brian M. Kelly, DO
Professor
Physical Medicine and Rehabilitation
Medical Director
Division of Orthotics and Prosthetics
University of Michigan
Ann Arbor, Michigan
11 Upper Limb Orthoses

Daniel J. Kim, MD
Clinical Instructor
Department of Physical Medicine and Rehabilitation
The Ohio State University
Columbus, Ohio
Medical Director
Wheelchair Seating and Mobility Clinic
The Ohio State University Wexner Medical Center
Columbus, Ohio
14 Wheelchairs and Seating Systems

Adam P. Klausner, MD
Associate Professor/Warren Koontz Professor of Urologic Research
Division of Urology
Department of Surgery
Virginia Commonwealth University
Richmond, Virginia
Staff Physician
Surgery Service
Hunter Holmes McGuire Veterans Affairs Medical Center
Richmond, Virginia
20 Bladder Dysfunction

Heidi Klingbeil, MD
Chief of Physical Medicine and Rehabilitation
James J. Peters Veterans Affairs Medical Center
Bronx, New York
Associate Professor of Rehabilitation Medicine
Columbia University
New York, New York
6 Employment of People with Disabilities

Alicia Koontz, PhD
Research Biomedical Engineer
Human Engineering Research Laboratories
Veterans Affairs Pittsburgh HealthCare System
Pittsburgh, Pennsylvania
Associate Professor
Department of Rehabilitation Science and Technology
University of Pittsburgh
Pittsburgh, Pennsylvania
14 Wheelchairs and Seating Systems

Christina Kwasnica, MD
Medical Director Neurorehabilitation
Barrow Neurological Institute
Phoenix, Arizona
Faculty, Creighton University College of Medicine
Omaha, Nebraska
43 Traumatic Brain Injury

Scott R. Laker, MD, BS
Assistant Professor
Department of Physical Medicine and Rehabilitation
University of Colorado School of Medicine
Denver, Colorado
39 Sports Medicine and Adaptive Sports

Charles Law, MD
Medical Director
United Cerebral Palsy of Greater Birmingham
Birmingham, Alabama
48 Myelomeningocele and Other Spinal Dysraphisms

Henry L. Lew, MD, PhD
Professor
Physical Medicine and Rehabilitation
Virginia Commonwealth University School of Medicine
Richmond, Virginia
Professor
Communication Sciences and Disorders
University of Hawaii School of Medicine
Honolulu, Hawaii
50 Auditory, Vestibular, and Visual Impairments

Sheng Li, MD, PhD
Department of Physical Medicine and Rehabilitation
University of Texas Health Science Center (UTHealth)
Houston, Texas
NeuroRecovery Research Center
TIRR Memorial Hermann
Houston, Texas
23 Spasticity

C. David Lin, MD
Associate Professor of Clinical Rehabilitation Medicine
New York–Presbyterian/Weill Cornell Medical Center
New York, New York
1 The Physiatric History and Physical Examination

William Lovegreen, MS,CPO
Prosthetist-Orthotist Regional Clinical Director
Physical Medicine and Rehabilitation
Veterans Administration
Richmond, Virginia
10 Lower Limb Amputation and Gait

Hui-Fen Mao, MS
Assistant Professor
School of Occupational Therapy
College of Medicine
National Taiwan University
Taipei, Taiwan
31 Rheumatologic Rehabilitation

Erin Maslowski, MD
Departments of Physical Medicine and Rehabilitation and Sports Medicine
Gundersen Health System
La Crosse, Wisconsin
39 Sports Medicine and Adaptive Sports

Emily H. McCullough, MPH, PA-C
University of Pittsburgh Medical Center
Pittsburgh, Pennsylvania
43 Traumatic Brain Injury

Michelle A. Miller, MD
Clinical Assistant Professor
Departments of Physical Medicine and Rehabilitation
The Ohio State University Wexner Medical Center
Section Chief, Pediatric Physical Medicine and Rehabilitation
Medical Director, Inpatient Pediatric Rehabilitation Services
Nationwide Children's Hospital
Columbus, Ohio
2 History and Examination of the Pediatric Patient

Daniel P. Moore, MD
Chairman and Professor
Department of Physical Medicine and Rehabilitation/ Pediatrics
East Carolina University
Greenville, North Carolina
13 Spinal Orthoses

Douglas P. Murphy, MD
Associate Professor of Physical Medicine and Rehabilitation
Virginia Commonwealth University College of Medicine
Richmond, Virginia
10 Lower Limb Amputation and Gait

Christian M. Niedzwecki, DO, MS
Assistant Professor
Physical Medicine and Rehabilitation
Baylor College of Medicine
Houston, Texas
47 Cerebral Palsy

John W. Norbury, MD
Clinical Assistant Professor
Department of Physical Medicine and Rehabilitation
Brody School of Medicine at East Carolina University
Greenville, North Carolina
13 Spinal Orthoses

Amy Nordness, PhD, CCC-SLP
Director of Speech
Munroe-Meyer Institute
University of Nebraska Medical Center
Omaha, Nebraska
3 Adult Neurogenic Communication and Swallowing Disorders

Bardia Nourbakhsh, MD
Department of Neurology
University of California San Francisco
San Francisco, California
46 Multiple Sclerosis

Michael W. O'Dell, MD
Chief of Clinical Services and Professor of Clinical Rehabilitation Medicine
Department of Rehabilitation Medicine at New York–Presbyterian Hospital/Weill Cornell Medical Center
Medical Director
Inpatient Rehabilitation Medicine Center
New York, New York
1 The Physiatric History and Physical Examination

Jeffrey B. Palmer, MD
Lawrence Cardinal Shehan Professor and Chair
Department of Physical Medicine and Rehabilitation
Johns Hopkins University
Baltimore, Maryland
3 Adult Neurogenic Communication and Swallowing Disorders

Preeti Panchang, MD
Resident Physician
Department of Physical Medicine and Rehabilitation
University of Louisville School of Medicine
Louisville, Kentucky
15 Therapeutic Exercise

Nicholas J. Pastorek, PhD, ABPP
Clinical Neuropsychologist
Rehabilitation and Extended Care Line
Michael E. DeBakey Veterans Affairs Medical Center
Houston, Texas
Assistant Professor
Physical Medicine and Rehabilitation
Baylor College of Medicine
Houston, Texas
4 Psychological Assessment and Intervention in Rehabilitation

Atul T. Patel, MD, MHSA
Director of Rehabilitation Services
Kansas City Bone and Joint Clinic
Overland Park
Kansas City, Kansas
11 Upper Limb Orthoses

Adrian Popescu, MD
Assistant Professor of Clinical Physical Medicine and Rehabilitation
Assistant Professor of Anesthesiology and Critical Care
University of Pennsylvania
Philadelphia, Pennsylvania
24 Chronic Wounds

David Z. Prince, MD
Director, Cardiac Rehabilitation
Rehabilitation Medicine
Albert Einstein College of Medicine/Montefiore Medical Center
Bronx, New York
27 Acute Medical Conditions

Daniel A. Proto, PhD
Clinical Neuropsychologist
Joint Ambulatory Care Center
Veterans Affairs Gulf Coast Veterans Healthcare System
Pensacola, Florida
4 Psychological Assessment and Intervention in Rehabilitation

Abu A. Qutubuddin, MD, MB, BS
Assistant Professor
Department of Physical Medicine and Rehabilitation and Neurology
Virginia Commonwealth University
Richmond, Virginia
Director of Rehabilitation
Parkinson's Disease Research, Education, and Clinical Center (PADRECC)
Hunter Holmes McGuire Veterans Affairs Medical Center
Richmond, Virginia
45 Degenerative Movement Disorders of the Central Nervous System

Mohammed I. Ranavaya, MD, JD, MS, FRCPI, CIME
Professor and Chief
Division of Occupational Medicine
Joan C. Edwards School of Medicine at Marshall University
Huntington, West Virginia
President
American Board of Independent Medical Examiners
Huntington, West Virginia
Medical Director
Appalachian Institute of Occupational and Environmental Medicine
Huntington, West Viriginia
5 Practical Aspects of Impairment Rating and Disability Determination

James K. Richardson, MD
Professor
Physical Medicine and Rehabilitation
University of Michigan
Ann Arbor, Michigan
41 Rehabilitation of Patients with Neuropathies

Gianna Rodriguez, MD
Assistant Professor
Physical Medicine and Rehabilitation
University of Michigan
Ann Arbor, Michigan
21 Neurogenic Bowel: Dysfunction and Rehabilitation

Desiree L. Roge, MD
Assistant Professor
Physical Medicine and Rehabilitation
Baylor College of Medicine
Houston, Texas
47 Cerebral Palsy

Robert D. Rondinelli, MD, PhD, MS, MA, CIME
Medical Director Rehabilitation Services
Physical Medicine and Rehabilitation
UnityPoint Health Des Moines
Des Moines, Iowa
5 Practical Aspects of Impairment Rating and Disability Determination

Richard (Sal) Salcido, MD, EdD
Professor
The William Erdman Professor of Physical Medicine and Rehabilitation Senior Fellow
Institute on Aging
Associate
Institute for Medical Bioengineering
University of Pennsylvania
Philadelphia, Pennsylvania
24 Chronic Wounds

Angelle M. Sander, PhD
Associate Professor
Physical Medicine and Rehabilitation
Baylor College of Medicine and Harris Health System
Houston, Texas
Senior Scientist and Director
Brain Injury Research Center
TIRR Memorial Hermann
Texas Medical Center
Houston, Texas
4 Psychological Assessment and Intervention in Rehabilitation

Deepthi Saxena, MD, FAAPMR
Attending Physician
Physical Medicine and Rehabilitation
Clinical Assistant Professor
Department of Internal Medicine
University of Nevada School of Medicine
Las Vegas, Nevada
Adjunct Instructor
Touro University
College of Osteopathic Medicine
Henderson, Nevada
Director
Affiliated Medical Rehabiliation
Avant-Garde Medicine, Illinois, Indiana, Michigan, & Nevada
Chicago, Illinois
7 Quality and Outcome Measures for Medical Rehabilitation

Mark Schmeler, PhD, OTR/L, ATP
Assistant Professor
Department of Rehabilitation Science and Technology
School of Health and Rehabilitation Sciences
University of Pittsburgh
Pittsburgh, Pennsylvania
14 Wheelchairs and Seating Systems

Robert A. Schulman, MD
Director
West County Integrative Medicine,
Freestone, California
18 Integrative Medicine in Rehabilitation

Aloysia L. Schwabe, MD
Associate Professor
Physical Medicine and Rehabilitation
Baylor College of Medicine
Houston, Texas
47 Cerebral Palsy

Kelly M. Scott, MD
Associate Professor
Physical Medicine and Rehabilitation
University of Texas Southwestern Medical Center
Dallas, Texas
22 Sexual Dysfunction and Disability
38 Pelvic Floor Disorders

Anjali Shah, MD
Associate Professor
Department of Physical Medical and Rehabilitation
University of Texas Southwestern Medical Center
Dallas, Texas
46 Multiple Sclerosis

Terrence P. Sheehan, MD
Chief Medical Officer
Adventist Rehabilitation Hospital of Maryland
Rockville, Maryland
The George Washington University School of Medicine
Associate Professor in Department of Neurology
Division Director of Rehabilitation Medicine
Washington, District of Colubmia
Medical Director
Amputee Coalition of America
Manassas, Virginia
9 Rehabilitation and Prosthetic Restoration in Upper Limb Amputation

Mehrsheed Sinaki, MD, MS
Professor
Department of Physical Medicine and Rehabilitation
Mayo Medical School
Rochester, Minnesota
34 Osteoporosis

J. Ricky Singh, MD
Assistant Professor of Rehabilitation Medicine
New York–Presbyterian/Weill Cornell Medical Center
New York, New York
1 The Physiatric History and Physical Examination

Curtis W. Slipman, MD
Director
The Penn Spine Center
University of Pennsylvania Medical Center
Philadelphia, Pennsylvania
32 Common Neck Problems

William K. Smith, MD
President
Center for International Rehabilitation
Washington, District of Columbia
10 Lower Limb Amputation and Gait

Kevin T. Sperber, MD
Vice Chairman
Department of Physical Medicine and Rehabilitation
New York City Health and Hospitals Corporation
North Bronx Healthcare Network
Bronx, New York
6 Employment of People with Disabilities

Steven P. Stanos, DO
Swedish Pain Services
Swedish Health System
Seattle, Washington
37 Chronic Pain

Siobhan Statuta, MD
Assistant Professor
Department of Family Medicine
University of Virginia School of Medicine
Charlottesville, Virginia
15 Therapeutic Exercise

Phillip Stevens, MED, CPO
Hanger Clinic
Salt Lake City, Utah
Assistant Adjunct Professor
Division of Physical Medicine and Rehabilitation
University of Utah
Salt Lake City, Utah
10 Lower Limb Amputation and Gait

Steven A. Stiens, MD, MS
Associate Professor
University of Washington
Department of Rehabilitation Medicine
Seattle, Washington
Attending Physician
Veterans Affairs Puget Sound Health Care System
Spinal Cord Injury Unit
Seattle, Washington
21 Neurogenic Bowel: Dysfunction and Rehabilitation

Olaf Stüve, MD, PhD
Associate Professor
Department of Neurology and Neurotherapeutics
University of Texas Southwestern Medical Center at Dallas
Dallas, Texas
46 Multiple Sclerosis

Rahki Garg Sutaria, MD
Chief Resident
Department of Physical Medicine and Rehabilitation
Albert Einstein College of Medicine/Montefiore Medical Center
Bronx, New York
6 Employment of People with Disabilities

Chiemi Tanaka, PhD, CCC-A
Assistant Professor
Department of Communication Sciences and Disorders
John A. Burns School of Medicine
University of Hawai'i at Mānoa
Honolulu, Hawaii
50 Auditory, Vestibular, and Visual Impairments

Kate E. Temme, MD
Assistant Professor
Department of Physical Medicine and Rehabilitation and Department of Orthopaedic Surgery
University of Pennsylvania
Philadelphia, Pennsylvania
22 Sexual Dysfunction and Disability

Edward Tilley, Certified Orthotist
Manager
Orthotic Services
Vidant Medical Center
Greenville, North Carolina
13 Spinal Orthoses

Mark D. Tyburski, MD
Assistant Chief
Department of Physical Medicine and Rehabilitation
The Permanente Medical Group, Inc.
Sacramento/Roseville, California
37 Chronic Pain

Heikki Uustal, MD
Medical Director, Prosthetic/Orthotic Team
Physical Medicine and Rehabilitation
JFK Johnson Rehabilitation Institute
Edison, New Jersey
Associate Professor
Physical Medicine and Rehabilitation
Rutgers Robert Wood Johnson Medical School
Piscataway, New Jersey
12 Lower Limb Orthoses

Amy K. Wagner, MD
Associate Professor
Physical Medicine and Rehabilitation
University of Pittsburgh
Pittsburgh, Pennsylvania
43 Traumatic Brain Injury

Tyng-Guey Wang, MD
Professor and Chief
Physical Medicine and Rehabilitation
National Taiwan University Hospital
College of Medicine
National Taiwan University
Taipei, Taiwan
17 Physical Agent Modalities

Carla P. Watson, MD
Subacute Medical Director
Schwab Rehabilitation Hospital
Chicago, Illinois
31 Rheumatologic Rehabilitation

Joseph Webster, MD
Associate Professor of Physical Medicine and Rehabilitation
Virginia Commonwealth University School of Medicine
Richmond, Virginia
10 Lower Limb Amputation and Gait

Robert P. Wilder, MD
Professor and Chair
Department of Physical Medicine and Rehabilitation
University of Virginia School of Medicine
Charlottesville, Virginia
15 Therapeutic Exercise

Stuart E. Willick, MD
Professor
Physical Medicine and Rehabilitation
University of Utah
Salt Lake City, Utah
36 Musculoskeletal Disorders of the Lower Limb

Christopher J. Wolf, DO, BA
Assistant Professor of Clinical Physical Medicine and Rehabilitation
Department of Physical Medicine and Rehabilitation
University of Missouri
Columbia, Missouri
16 Manipulation, Traction, and Massage

Laurie L. Wolf, MD
Acuity Neurology
Wausau, Wisconsin
25 Vascular Diseases

Weibin Yang, MD, MBA
Associate Professor
Department of Physical Medicine and Rehabilitation
University of Texas Southwestern Medical Center
Dallas, Texas
Chief
Physical Medicine and Rehabilitation Service
Veterans Affairs North Texas Health Care System
Dallas, Texas
7 Quality and Outcome Measures for Medical Rehabilitation
17 Physical Agent Modalities

Richard D. Zorowitz, MD
Staff Physician
MedStar National Rehabilitation Network
Georgetown University
Washington, District of Columbia
44 Stroke Syndromes

PREFACE

Braddom's Physical Medicine and Rehabilitation represents the amalgamation of more than 75 years of formal physical medicine and rehabilitation (PM&R) research and practice in the United States, with additional decades of contributions from around the globe. It took the dedicated team of authors, editors, and support staff nearly 2 years to bring this completely updated fifth edition to you, with state of the art technologic links; easy to use tables and videos; practical, evidence-influenced approaches to diagnosis and management; and a strong focus on the application of the core principles of PM&R. The field of PM&R has come a long, long way from its nineteenth century informal roots in the U.S. Civil War and the postbellum modalities craze, as well as from its more formal origins in the world wars of the early twentieth century. Although an interdisciplinary team focus on the needs of individuals with acute and chronic disability has remained at the heart of the field, increasingly, the role of technology and interventional procedures to diagnose, monitor, manage, and deliver virtual care for neurologic, musculoskeletal, and connective tissue disorders and disability has helped to move the field into the twenty-first century. As with the impact of warfare on the informal and formal origins of PM&R, the Persian Gulf wars of the twenty-first century have played a significant influence on the recent advances in the field of PM&R. This textbook helps to serve as a vital bridge between the essential core principles and approaches of PM&R that have allowed the field to become the mainstay of care for individuals with illnesses and injuries that result in neurologic and orthopedic dysfunction, and the cutting edge research and innovative technologies that are expanding the scope of conditions that can be assessed and managed by PM&R professionals and are offering effective new tools for the core conditions that PM&R clinicians see. It also serves as a connection between the long-standing, consensus-based PM&R models of care that have enhanced the lives of millions of individuals living with disabling conditions and the evidence-based research findings that are being disseminated in the scientific literature, introducing new and modified approaches to care that bring together decades of clinical experience and excellence with emerging translational findings. Given the veritable explosion of knowledge translation and dissemination in the field of PM&R, this fifth edition features an easy to access electronic version with additional information, self-assessment questions and videos, as well as Internet linkage to additional resources. Just as the field of PM&R has progressed and expanded exponentially, so too has *Braddom's Textbook of Physical Medicine and Rehabilitation* kept pace with the information explosion. This textbook represents the key, overarching resource for practitioners in the field of PM&R, and its users are fortunate to have the nation's long-time, established academic leaders and its up and coming new generation of educators as its authors. The topical areas have been organized to reflect both the essentials of the field and its emerging trends. Take full advantage of all the textbook has to offer and use it to continue on the traditions of excellence that have made PM&R perhaps the most relevant fields of health care in the twenty-first century.

David X. Cifu, MD
Professor and Chairman
Physical Medicine and Rehabilitation
Virginia Commonwealth University
Richmond, Virginia
National Director for Physical Medicine and Rehabilitation Services
Office of Rehabilitation and Prosthetic Services
U.S. Department of Veterans Affairs
Washington, District of Columbia

ACKNOWLEDGMENTS

This textbook would not have been possible without the tireless effort of so many individuals, all dedicated to producing the highest quality textbook possible. As with all good things in physical medicine and rehabilitation, it took a highly skilled and interdisciplinary team to get the optimal outcome demonstrated in this textbook; the contributions of all members of the team are eagerly acknowledged. Specifically, let me acknowledge the outstanding work of my Associate Editors who cracked the whips and used their laptops into the long hours of the night; thank you Karen, Michelle, Kris, Henry, Greg, and Darryl. All the authors who contributed to this process for little more than a copy of the textbook are to be acknowledged and celebrated. The team at Elsevier, led by Ann Anderson, have been fantastic collaborators who have always been highly flexible and professional throughout. On a more local level, let me acknowledge the patience and organization of my Department office staff, led by my personal assistant, Connie Hawkes, who keeps me on task and track as much as is possible.

CONTENTS

SECTION 4 Issues in Specific Diagnoses

VIDEO CONTENTS

BRADDOM'S
PHYSICAL MEDICINE & REHABILITATION

SECTION I

Evaluation

CHAPTER 1

THE PHYSIATRIC HISTORY AND PHYSICAL EXAMINATION

Michael W. O'Dell, C. David Lin, J. Ricky Singh, George C. Christolias

The physiatric history and physical examination (H&P) serves several purposes. It is the data platform from which a treatment plan is developed. It serves as a written record that communicates to other rehabilitation and nonrehabilitation health care professionals. Finally, the H&P provides the basis for physician billing[17] and serves as a medicolegal document. Physician documentation has become the critical component in inpatient rehabilitation reimbursement under prospective payment (e.g., interdisciplinary plan of care, admission screening) as well as proof for continued coverage by private insurers.[18] The scope of the physiatric H&P varies enormously, depending on the setting, from the focused assessment of an isolated knee injury in an outpatient setting, to the comprehensive evaluation of a patient with traumatic brain or spinal cord injury admitted for inpatient rehabilitation. An initial evaluation is almost always more detailed and comprehensive than subsequent or follow-up evaluations. An exception would be when a patient is seen for a follow-up visit with substantial new signs or symptoms. Physicians in training tend to overassess, but with time the experienced physiatrist develops an intuition for how much detail is needed for each patient, given a particular presentation and setting.

The physiatric H&P resembles the traditional format taught in medical school but with an additional emphasis on history, signs, and symptoms that affect function or performance. The physiatric H&P also identifies those systems *not* affected that might be used for compensation.[27] Familiarity with the 1997 World Health Organization classification is invaluable in grasping the philosophic framework for viewing the evaluation of persons with physical and cognitive disabilities (Table 1-1).[96] Identifying and treating the primary *impairments* to maximize *performance* becomes the primary thrust of physiatric evaluation and treatment.

Because patients cared for in rehabilitation medicine can be extremely complicated, the H&P is constantly a work in progress. Confirmation of historical and functional items by other team members, health care professionals, and family members can take several days. Many of the functional items discussed in this chapter will actually be assessed and explored more fully by other interdisciplinary team members during the course of inpatient or outpatient treatment. It is imperative that the physiatrist stays abreast of additional information and findings as they become available and that lines of verbal or written communication be directed through the medical leadership of the team.

The exact structure of the physiatric assessment is determined in part by personal preference, training background, and institutional requirements (physician billing compliance expectations, proper linkage to resident documentation, forms committees, and regulatory oversight). The use of templates can be invaluable in maximizing the thoroughness of data collection and minimizing documentation time. Pertinent radiologic and laboratory findings should be clearly documented. The essential elements of the physiatric H&P are summarized in Table 1-2. Assessment of some or all of these elements is required for a complete understanding of the patient's state of health and the illness for which he or she is being seen. These elements also form the basis for a treatment plan.

An emergence in the use of the electronic medical record (EMR) has significantly altered the landscape for documentation of the physiatric H&P in both the inpatient and outpatients settings.[28] Tracking of a variety of items to justify "meaningful use" of the EMR and the "quality" of the physician encounter is commonplace.[44] Among the advantages of the EMR are increased legibility, a certain degree of time efficiency afforded by the use of templates and "smart phrases" that can be tailored to individual practitioners or clinical presentations, automated warnings regarding medication interactions or errors, and faster and more accurate billing. Disadvantages include the unacceptable use of the "copy and paste" function, leading to redundancy among consecutive notes and the perpetuation of potentially inaccurate information, automated importation of data not necessarily reviewed by the practitioner at the time of service, and "alarm fatigue." As regulation of hospital and physician practice and billing increases, the EMR will become more important in ensuring the proper, and sometimes convoluted, documentation required for safety initiatives[49] and physician payment.[17]

The Physiatric History

History-taking skills are part of the art of medicine and are required to fully assess a patient's presentation. One of the unique aspects of physiatry is the recognition of functional deficits caused by illness or injury. Identification of these deficits allows for the design of a treatment program to restore performance. In a person with stroke, for example, the most important questions for the physiatrist are not only the etiology or location of the lesion but also "What functional deficits are present as a result of the stroke?" The answer could include deficits in swallowing, communication, mobility, cognition, activities of daily living (ADL), or a combination of these.

Table 1-1 World Health Organization Definitions

Term	Definition
Impairment	Any loss or abnormality of body structure or of a physiologic or psychological function (essentially unchanged from the 1980 definition)
Activity	The nature and extent of functioning at the level of the person
Participation	The nature and extent of a person's involvement in life situations in relationship to impairments, activities, health conditions, and contextual factors

From World Health Organization: International classification of impairments, activities, and participation, Geneva: World Health Organization; 1997, with permission of the World Health Organization.

The time spent in taking a history also allows the patient to become familiar with the physician, establishing rapport and trust. This initial rapport is critical for a constructive and productive doctor–patient–family relationship and can also help the physician learn about sensitive areas, such as sexual history and substance abuse. It can also have an impact on outcome because a trusting patient tends to be a more compliant patient.[80] Assessment of the tone of the patient or family (such as anger, frustration, resolve, and determination), an understanding of the illness, insight into disability, and coping skills are also gleaned during history taking. In most cases, the patient leads the physician to a diagnosis and conclusion. In other cases, such as when the patient is rambling and disorganized, frequent redirection and gentle refocus are required.

Patients are generally the primary source of information. However, patients with cognitive, mood (denial or decreased insight), or communication deficits, as well as small children, might not be able to fully express themselves. In these cases, the history taker might rely on other sources, such as family members; friends; other physicians, nurses, and medical professionals; or previous medical records. This can also have an impact on physician billing. The use of an interpreter to interview patients who are not fluent in the language of the examining physician is mandatory. Caution must be exercised in using previous medical records because inaccuracies are sometimes repeated from provider to provider, sometimes referred to as "chart lore."

Chief Complaint

The chief complaint is the symptom or concern that caused the patient to seek medical treatment. The most common chief complaints seen in an outpatient physiatric practice are pain, weakness, or gait disturbance of various musculoskeletal or neurologic origins. On a physiatric consultation on an inpatient rehabilitation service, the predominant chief complaints are related to mobility, ADL, communication, or cognitive deficits and candidacy for inpatient rehabilitation. Unlike the relatively objective physical examination, the chief complaint is purely subjective and, when possible, the physician should use the patient's own words. A patient can have several related or unrelated complaints, in which case it is helpful to have the patient rank problems from "most bothersome" to "least bothersome" while reinforcing that only one or

Table 1-2 Essential Elements of the Physiatric History and Physical Examination

Component	Examples
Chief Complaint	
History of present illness	Exploring location, onset, quality, context, severity, duration, modifying factors, and associated signs and symptoms
Functional history	Mobility: Bed mobility, transfers, wheelchair mobility, ambulation, driving, and devices required Activities of daily living: Bathing, toileting, dressing, eating, hygiene and grooming, etc. Instrumental activities of daily living: Meal preparation, laundry, telephone use, home maintenance, pet care, etc. Cognition Communication
Medical and surgical history	Specific conditions: Cardiopulmonary, musculoskeletal, neurologic, and rheumatologic Medications
Social history	Home environment and living circumstances, family and friends support system, substance abuse, sexual history, vocational activities, finances, recreational activities, psychosocial history (mood disorders), spirituality, and litigation
Family history	
Review of systems	
General Medical Physical Examination	
	Cardiac Pulmonary Abdominal Other
Neurologic Physical Examination	
	Level of consciousness Attention Orientation Memory General fund of knowledge Abstract thinking Insight and judgment Mood and affect
Communication	
Cranial nerve examination	
Sensation	
Motor control	Strength Coordination Apraxia Involuntary movements Tone
Reflexes	Superficial Deep Primitive
Musculoskeletal Physical Examination	
Inspection	Behavior Physical symmetry, joint deformity, etc.
Palpation	Joint stability Range of motion (active and passive) Strength testing (see above) Painful joints and muscles
Joint-specific provocative maneuvers	

two of those problems will be addressed at the current appointment.

The specific circumstance of a patient offering a chief complaint can also allude to a degree of disability or handicap. For example, knowing that an obese mail carrier has the chief complaint of difficulty in walking because of knee pain could suggest not only the impairment but also an impact on his vocation and role as a provider for his family (participation).

History of the Present Illness

The history of the present illness (HPI) details the chief complaint(s) for which the patient is seeking medical attention, as well as any related or unrelated functional deficits. It should also explore other information relating to the chief complaint, such as recent and past medical or surgical procedures, complications of treatment, and potential restrictions or precautions. The HPI should include some or all of eight components related to the chief complaint: location, time of onset, quality, context, severity, duration, modifying factors, and associated signs and symptoms (see Table 1-2).

In this case example, the patient is a 70-year-old man referred by his neurologist for physical therapy because the patient cannot walk properly (chief complaint). Over the past few months (duration), he has noted slowly progressive weakness of his left leg (location). Subsequent workup by his neurologist suggested amyotrophic lateral sclerosis (context). The patient was active in his life and working up until a few months previously, ambulating without an assistive device (context). Now he uses a straight cane for fear of falling (modifying factor). Besides difficulty with walking, the patient also has some trouble swallowing foods (associated signs and symptoms).

Functional Status

Detailing the patient's current and previous functional status is an essential aspect of the physiatric HPI. This generally entails better understanding of the issues surrounding mobility, ADL, instrumental activities of daily living (I-ADL), communication, cognition, work, and recreation, among others. The data should be as accurate and detailed as possible to guide the physical examination and develop a treatment plan with reasonable short- and long-term goals.

Assessing the potential for functional gain or deterioration requires an understanding of the natural history, cause, and time of onset of the functional problems. For example, most spontaneous motor recovery after stroke occurs within 3 months of the event.[86] For a patient with considerable motor impairments who recently underwent a stroke, there is a greater expectation for significant functional gain than in a patient with minor deficits related to a stroke that occurred 2 years previously.

Mobility

Mobility is the ability to move about in one's environment and is taken for granted by most healthy people. Because it plays such a vital role in society, any impairment related to mobility can have major consequences for a patient's quality of life. A clear understanding of the patient's functional mobility is needed to determine independence and safety, including the use of, or need for, mobility assistive devices. There is a range of mobility assistive devices that patients can use, such as crutches, canes, walkers, orthoses, and manual and electric wheelchairs (Table 1-3).

Table 1-3 Commonly Used Mobility Assistive Devices

Category	Example
Crutches	Axillary crutches Forearm crutches Platform crutches
Canes	Straight cane Wide- or narrow-based quad cane Hemiwalker or pyramid cane
Walkers	Standard or pick-up walker Rolling walker Platform walker
Wheelchairs	
Types	Manual Powered Lightweight
Common modifications or specifications	Folding or solid frame Elevated or removable leg rests Removable armrests Reclining
Off-the-Shelf Ankle/Foot Orthoses	
Common custom orthoses	Plastic ankle-foot orthosis Metal ankle-foot orthosis Knee orthosis Knee-ankle-foot orthosis

Bed mobility includes turning from side to side, going from the prone to supine positions, sitting up, and lying down. A lack of bed mobility places the patient at greater risk for skin ulcers, deep vein thrombosis, and pneumonia. In severe cases, bed mobility can be so poor as to require a caregiver. In other cases, bed rails might be appropriate to facilitate movement. Transfer mobility includes getting in and out of bed, standing from the sitting position (whether from a chair or toilet), and moving between a wheelchair and another seat (car seat or shower seat). Once again, the history taker should assess the level of independence, safety, and any changes in functional ability.

Wheelchair mobility can be assessed by asking whether patients can propel the wheelchair independently, how far or how long they can go without resting, and whether they need assistance with managing the wheelchair parts. It is also important to assess the extent to which they can move about at home, in the community, and up and down ramps. Whether the home is potentially wheelchair-accessible is particularly important in cases of new onset of severe disability.

Ambulation can be assessed by how far or for how long patients can walk, whether they require assistive devices, and if they need rest breaks. It is also important to know whether any symptoms are associated with ambulation, such as chest pain, shortness of breath, pain, or dizziness. Patients should be asked about any history of falling or instability while walking and their ability to navigate uneven surfaces. Stair mobility, along with the number of stairs the patient must routinely climb and descend at home or in the community, and the presence or absence of handrails should also be determined.

Driving is a crucial activity for many people, not only as a means of transportation but also as an indicator and facilitator of independence. For example, older adults who stop driving have an increase in depressive symptoms.[64] It is important to identify factors that might prevent driving, such as decreased cognitive function and safety awareness, and decreased vision or reaction time. Other factors affecting driving can include lower limb weakness, contracture, tone, or incoordination. Some of these conditions might require use of adaptive hand controls for driving. Cognitive impairment sufficient to affect the ability to drive can be due to medications or organic disease (dementia, brain injury, stroke, or severe mood disturbance). Ultimately, the risks of driving are weighed against the consequences of not being able to drive. If the patient is no longer able to drive, alternatives to driving should be explored, such as the use of public or assisted transportation. Laws differ widely from state to state on the return to driving after a neurologic impairment develops.

Activities of Daily Living and Instrumental Activities of Daily Living

ADL encompass activities required for personal care, including feeding, dressing, grooming, bathing, and toileting. I-ADL encompass more complex tasks required for independent living in the immediate environment, such as care of others in the household, telephone use, meal preparation, house cleaning, laundry, and in some cases use of public transportation. In the Occupational Therapy Practice Framework, there are 11 activities for both ADL and I-ADL (Box 1-1).[4]

The clinician should identify and document ADL that the patient can and cannot perform and determine the causes of limitation. For example, a woman with a stroke might state that she cannot put on her pants. This could be due to a combination of factors, such as a visual field cut, balance problems, weakness, pain, contracture, hypertonia, or deficits in motor planning. Some of these factors can be confirmed later in the physical examination. A more detailed follow-up to a positive response to the question is frequently needed. For example, a patient might say "yes" to the question "Can you eat by yourself?" On further questioning, it might be learned that she cannot prepare the food by herself or cut the food independently. The most accurate assessment of ADL and mobility deficits often comes from the hands-on assessment by therapists and nurses on the rehabilitation team or from the patient's family.

BOX 1-1

Activities of Daily Living (ADL) and Instrumental Activities of Daily Living (I-ADL)

ADL

- Bathing and showering
- Bowel and bladder management
- Dressing
- Eating
- Feeding
- Functional mobility
- Personal device care
- Personal hygiene and grooming
- Sexual activity
- Sleep and rest
- Toilet hygiene

I-ADL

- Care of others (including selecting and supervising caregivers)
- Care of pets
- Child rearing
- Communication device use
- Community mobility
- Financial management
- Health management and maintenance
- Home establishment and management
- Meal preparation and cleanup
- Safety procedures and emergency responses
- Shopping

Cognition

Cognition is the mental process of knowing (see Chapters 3 and 4). Although objective assessment of cognition comes under physical examination (memory, orientation, and the ability to assimilate and manipulate information), impairments in cognition can also become apparent during the course of the history taking. Because persons with cognitive deficits often cannot recognize their own impairments (agnosia), it is important to gather information from family members and others familiar with the patient. Cognitive deficits and limited awareness of these deficits are likely to interfere with the patient's rehabilitation program unless specifically addressed. These deficits can pose a safety risk as well. For example, a man with a previous stroke who falls, sustaining a hip fracture requiring replacement, might not be able to follow hip precautions, resulting in possible refracture or hip dislocation. Executive functioning is another aspect of cognition, which includes the mental functions required for planning, problem solving, and self-awareness. Executive functioning correlates with functional outcome because it is required in many real-world situations. Asking the basic questions of the mental status examination (MSE) will not give a complete picture of mental function, particularly for issues such as impulsivity or judgment.[56]

Communication

Communication skills are used to convey information including thoughts, needs, and emotions. Verbal expression deficits can be subtle and might not be noticed in a first encounter. If there is a reason to think that speech or communication has been affected by a recent event, it is advisable to ask family members if they have noticed recent changes. Patients who cannot communicate through speech might or might not be able to communicate through other means, known as augmentative communication, depending on the type of communication dysfunction and other physical and cognitive limitations. This can include writing and physicality (such as sign language, gestures, and body language). They can also use a variety of augmentative communication aids ranging from simple picture, letter, and word boards to electronic devices.

Past Medical and Surgical History

The physiatrist should understand the patient's past medical and surgical history. This knowledge allows the physiatrist to understand how preexisting illnesses affect current status and how to tailor the rehabilitation program for precautions and limitations. The patient's medical history can also have a major impact on rehabilitation outcome.

Cardiopulmonary

Mobility, ADL, I-ADL, work, and leisure can be severely compromised by cardiopulmonary deficits. The patient should be asked about any history of congestive heart failure, recent and distant myocardial infarction, arrhythmias, and coronary artery disease. Past surgical procedures, such as bypass surgery, heart transplantation, stent placement, and recent diagnostic testing (stress test or echocardiogram) should be ascertained. This information is important to ensure that exercise prescriptions do not exceed cardiovascular activity limitations. Patients should also be asked about their activity tolerance, surgery, such as lung volume reduction or lung transplant, and their use of home oxygen. Dyspnea from chronic obstructive pulmonary disease can be a significant contributor to functional limitations. Often, medication adjustment to maximize cardiac and pulmonary function accompanies mobilization. It is also important to identify modifiable risk factors for cardiac disease, such as smoking, hypertension, and obesity.

Musculoskeletal

There can be a wide range of musculoskeletal disorders from acute traumatic injuries to gradual functional decline with chronic osteoarthritis. The patient should be asked about a history of trauma, arthritis, amputation, joint contractures, musculoskeletal pain, congenital or acquired muscular problems, weakness, or instability. It is important to understand the functional impact of such impairments or disabilities. Patients with chronic physical disability often develop overuse musculoskeletal syndromes, such as the development of shoulder pain secondary to chronically propelling a wheelchair.[40]

Neurologic Disorders

Preexisting congenital or acquired neurologic disorders can have a profound impact on the patient's function and recovery from both neurologic and nonneurologic illness. It is helpful to know whether a neurologic disorder is congenital compared with acquired, progressive compared with nonprogressive, central compared with peripheral, demyelinating compared with axonal, or sensory compared with motor. This information can be helpful in understanding the pathophysiology, location, severity, prognosis, and implications for management. The interviewer must assess the premorbid need for assistive devices, orthoses, and the degree of speech, swallowing, and cognitive impairments.

Rheumatologic

The history should include the type of rheumatologic disorder, time of onset, number of joints affected, pain level, current disease activity, and past orthopedic procedures. Discussions with the patient's rheumatologist might address whether medication changes could improve activity tolerance in a rehabilitation program (see Chapter 36).

History of cancer is important because of residual effects of chemotherapy with generalized fatigue or weakness or peripheral neuropathy. Also, a history of cancer may broaden the differential diagnosis to include cancer recurrence or metastatic disease (see Chapter 29).

Medications

All medications should be documented, including prescription and over-the-counter drugs, as well as nutraceuticals, supplements, herbs, and vitamins. Medications should be documented from the last institutional venues (acute care, nursing home) and from home before institutionalization. Decreasing medication errors by means of medication reconciliation is a major thrust of the National Patient Safety Goals initiative.[49] Patients typically do not mention medications that they do not think are relevant to their current problem, unless asked about them in detail. Drug and food allergies should be noted. It is especially important to gather the complete list of medications being used in patients who are seeing multiple physicians. Particular attention should be paid to nonsteroidal antiinflammatory agents because these are commonly prescribed by physiatrists for musculoskeletal disorders and care must be taken not to double-dose the patient or prescribe them for patients with kidney dysfunction.[33,39] The indications, precautions, and side effects of all drugs prescribed should be explained to the patient.

Social History

Home Environment and Living Situation

Understanding the patient's home environment and living situation includes asking if the patient lives in a house or an apartment, if there is elevator access, whether it is wheelchair-accessible, if there are stairs, whether the bathroom is accessible from the bedroom, and whether the bathroom has grab bars or handrails (and on which side). A home visit might be required to gain the best assessment. If there is no caregiver at home, the patient could require a home health aide. These factors help determine many aspects of the discharge plan.

Family and Friends Support

Patients who have lost function might require supervision, emotional support, or actual physical assistance. Family, friends, and neighbors who can provide such assistance should be identified. The clinician should discuss the level of assistance they are willing and able to provide. The assistance provided by caregivers can be limited if they are elderly, have some type of impairment, work, or are not willing to assist with bowel or bladder hygiene.

Substance Abuse

Patients should be asked about their history of smoking, alcohol use or abuse, and drug abuse. Because patients often deny substance abuse, this topic should be discussed in a nonjudgmental manner. Patients frequently feel embarrassment or guilt in admitting substance abuse and also fear the legal consequences of such an admission. Substance abuse can be a direct or indirect cause of disability and is often a contributing factor in traumatic brain injury.[22] It can also have an impact on community reintegration because patients with pain or depression are at risk for further abuse. Patients who are at risk should be referred to social work to explore options for further assistance, either during the acute rehabilitation or later in the community.

Sexual History

Patients and health care practitioners alike are often uncomfortable discussing the topic of sexuality, so developing a good rapport during history taking can be helpful. Discussion of this topic is made easier if the health care practitioner has a basic knowledge of how sexual function can be changed by illness or injury. Sexuality is particularly important to patients in their reproductive years (such as with many spinal cord- and brain-injured persons), but the physician should inquire about sexuality in adolescents and adults, including older adults. Sexual orientation and safer sex practices should be addressed when appropriate.

Vocational Activities

Vocation not only is a source of financial security but also significantly relates to self-confidence and even identity. The history should include the patient's educational level, recent work history, and the ability to fulfill job requirements subsequent to the injury or illness. If an individual cannot fully regain the previous function level, the vocational options available should be explored. It is possible that the work environment can be modified to compensate for a functional loss or minimize musculoskeletal pain complaints. An example of this would be the installation of a wheelchair ramp for an accountant with paraplegia. Vocational planners and referral to state vocational agencies may facilitate work reentry planning.

Finances and Income Maintenance

Patients can have financial concerns that are attributable to or exacerbated by their illness or injury. These concerns can also be addressed by the rehabilitation team social worker. Whether a patient has the financial resources or insurance to pay for adaptive devices, such as a ramp or mobility equipment, can significantly affect discharge planning. If patients cannot safely be discharged home, skilled nursing facility placement might need to be explored, at least on a temporary basis.

Recreation

The ability to engage in hobbies and recreational activities is important to most people, and any loss or limitation of the ability to perform these activities can be stressful. Recreation is a primary outcome in sports medicine. The recreational activity affected can involve physical exercise, such as a sporting activity, or can be more sedentary, such as playing cards. The team recreational therapist can be helpful in helping to restore the patient's favorite recreations and offer new ones.

Psychosocial History

The history taker must recognize the psychosocial impact of impairment. Beyond the loss of function, the patient can also feel a loss of overall health, body image, mobility, or independence. The loss of function, and possibly of income as well, can place great stress on the family unit and caregivers. The treatment plan should recognize the patient's psychosocial context and provide assistance in developing coping strategies, especially for depression and anxiety. This can help accelerate the patient's process of adjusting to a new disability.

Spirituality and Belief

Spirituality is an important part of the lives of many patients, and some preliminary studies indicate that it can have positive effects on rehabilitation, life satisfaction, and quality of life.[13] Health care providers should be sensitive to the patient's spiritual needs, and appropriate referral or counseling should be provided.[19]

Pending Litigation

Patients should be asked in a nonjudgmental manner whether they are involved in litigation related to their illness, injuries, or functional impairment. The answer should not change the treatment plan, but litigation can be a source of anxiety, depression, or guilt. In some cases, the patient's legal representative can play an important role in obtaining needed services and equipment.

Family History

Patients should be asked about the health, or cause and age of death, of parents and siblings. It is always important to know whether any family members have a similar condition, either to assist with diagnosis or to better understand anxieties experienced by the patient. They should also be asked about any family history of heart disease, diabetes, cancer, stroke, arthritis, hypertension, or neurologic illness. This will help to identify genetic disorders within the family. Knowledge of the general health of family members can also provide insight into their ability to provide functional assistance to the patient.

Review of Systems

A detailed review of organ systems should be done to discover any problems or diseases not previously identified during the course of the history taking. Table 1-4 lists some questions that can be asked about each system.[29] Note that this list is not comprehensive, and more detailed questioning might be necessary, particularly as it relates to a patient's primary diagnosis.

The Physiatric Physical Examination

Neurologic Examination

Neurologic problems are common in the setting of inpatient and outpatient rehabilitation, including functional deficits in persons with conditions such as stroke, multiple sclerosis, peripheral neuropathy, spinal cord injury, brain injury, neurologic cancers, and spine disease. The neurologic examination should be conducted in an organized manner to confirm or reconfirm the neurologic disorder

Table 1-4 Sample Questions for the Review of Systems

System	Questions
Systemic	Any general symptoms, such as fever, weight loss, fatigue, nausea, and poor appetite?
Skin	Any skin problems? Sores? Rashes? Growths? Itching? Changes in hair or nails? Dryness?
Eyes	Any changes in vision? Pain? Redness? Double vision? Watery eyes? Dizziness?
Ears	How are the ears and hearing? Running ears? Poor hearing? Ringing ears? Discharge?
Nose	How are your nose and sinuses? Stuffy nose? Discharge? Bleeding? Unusual odors?
Mouth	Any problems with your mouth? Sores? Bad taste? Sore tongue? Gum trouble?
Throat and neck	Any problems with your throat and neck? Sore throat? Hoarseness? Swelling? Swallowing?
Breasts	Any problems with your breasts? Lumps? Nipple discharge? Bleeding? Swelling? Tenderness?
Pulmonary	Any problems with your lungs or breathing? Cough? Sputum? Bloody sputum? Pain in the chest on taking a deep breath? Shortness of breath?
Cardiovascular	Do you have any problems with your heart? Chest pain? Shortness of breath? Palpitations? Cough? Swelling of your ankles? Trouble lying flat in bed at night? Fatigue?
Gastrointestinal	How is your digestion? Any changes in your appetite? Nausea? Vomiting? Diarrhea? Constipation? Changes in your bowel habits? Bleeding from the rectum? Hemorrhoids?
Genitourinary	Male: Any problems with your kidneys or urination? Painful urination? Frequency? Urgency? Nocturia? Bloody or cloudy urine? Trouble starting or stopping? Female: Number of pregnancies? Abortions? Miscarriages? Any menstrual problems? Last menstrual period? Vaginal bleeding? Vaginal discharge? Cessation of periods? Hot flashes? Vaginal itching? Sexual dysfunction?
Endocrine	Any problems with your endocrine glands? Feeling hot or cold? Fatigue? Changes in skin or hair? Frequent urination? Fatigue?
Musculoskeletal	Do you have any problems with your bones or joints? Joint or muscle pain? Stiffness? Limitation of motion?
Nervous system	Numbness? Weakness? Pins and needles sensation?

From Enelow AJ, Forde DL, Brummel-Smith K: *Interviewing and patient care*, ed 4, New York: Oxford University Press; 1996, with permission of Oxford University Press.

and subsequently to identify which components of the nervous system are the most and the least affected.[15, 93] The precise location of the lesion should be identified, if possible, and the impact of the neurologic deficits on the overall function and mobility of the patient should be noted. If a cause of the patient's condition has not been identified at presentation to the rehabilitation provider, a differential diagnosis list should be developed, the neurologic examination tailored appropriately, and consultations garnered, if indicated. An accurate and efficient neurologic examination requires that the examiner have a thorough knowledge of both central and peripheral neuroanatomy *before* the examination.

Weakness is a primary sign in neurologic disorders and is seen in both upper motor neuron (UMN) and lower motor neuron (LMN) disorders. UMN lesions involving the central nervous system (CNS) are typically characterized by hypertonia, weakness, and hyperreflexia without significant muscle atrophy, fasciculation, or fibrillation (on electromyography). They *tend* to occur in a hemiparetic, paraparetic, and tetraparetic pattern. UMN causes include stroke, multiple sclerosis, traumatic and nontraumatic brain and spinal cord injuries, and neurologic cancers, among others. LMN defects are characterized by hypotonia, weakness, hyporeflexia, significant muscle atrophy, fasciculations, and electromyographic changes. They occur in the distribution of the affected nerve root, peripheral nerve, or muscle. UMN and LMN lesions often coexist; however, the LMN system is the final common pathway of the nervous system. An example of this is an upper trunk brachial plexus injury on the same side as spastic hemiparesis in a person with traumatic brain injury.[65]

Similar to physical examination in other organ systems, testing of one neurologic system is often predicated by the normal functioning of other systems. For example, severe visual impairment can be confused with cerebellar dysfunction, as many cerebellar tests have a visual component. The integrated functions of all organ systems should be considered to provide an accurate clinical assessment, and potential limitations of the examination should be considered. Unusual findings, such as sensory changes that split the midline or inconsistent muscle strength, may suggest conversion or malingering but these diagnoses can only be made when underlying disease is thoroughly excluded.

Mental Status Examination

The MSE should be performed in a comfortable setting where the patient is not likely to be disturbed by external stimuli, such as televisions, telephones, pagers, conversation, or medical alarms. The bedside MSE is often limited secondary to distractions from within the room. Having a familiar person, such as a spouse or relative, in the room can often help reassure the patient. The bedside MSE might need to be supplemented by observations in therapy and in a far more detailed and standardized evaluation performed by neuropsychologists, especially in cases of vocational and educational reintegration. General observation should include grooming (clean, disheveled), posture, tracking (with severe disorders of consciousness), interactions with family members present, and environmental clues (carrying a book, ability to prepare for the examination independently). Language is the gateway for assessment of cognition and is therefore limited in persons with significant aphasia (see Chapter 3).

Level of Consciousness. Consciousness is the state of awareness of one's surroundings. A functioning pontine reticular activating system is necessary for normal conscious functioning. The conscious patient is awake and responds directly and appropriately to varying stimuli. Decreased consciousness can significantly limit the MSE and the general physical examination.

The examiner should understand the various levels of consciousness. Lethargy is the general slowing of motor processes (such as speech and movement) in which the patient can easily fall asleep if not stimulated but is easily aroused. Obtundation is a dulled or blunted sensitivity in which the patient is difficult to arouse, and once aroused is still confused. Stupor is a state of semiconsciousness characterized by arousal only by intense stimuli, such as sharp pressure over a bony prominence (e.g., sternal rub), and the patient has few or even no voluntary motor responses.[72] The Aspen Neurobehavioral Conference proposed, and several leading medical organizations have endorsed, three terms to describe severe alterations in consciousness.[35] In *coma,* the eyes are closed with absence of sleep-wake cycles and no evidence of a contingent relationship between the patient's behavior and the environment.[35] *Vegetative state* is characterized by the presence of sleep-wake cycles but still no contingent relationship. *Minimally conscious state* indicates a patient who remains severely disabled but demonstrates sleep-wake cycles and even inconsistent, nonreflexive, contingent behaviors in response to a specific environmental stimulation. In acute settings, the Glasgow Coma Scale is the most often used objective measure to document level of consciousness, assessing eye opening, motor response, and verbal response (Table 1-5).[48]

Attention. Attention is the ability to address a specific stimulus for a short period without being distracted by internal or external stimuli.[83] Vigilance is the ability to hold attention over longer periods. For example, with inadequate vigilance a patient can begin a complex task but be unable to sustain performance to completion. Attention is tested by digit recall, where the examiner reads a list of random numbers and the patient is asked to repeat those numbers. The patient should repeat digits both forward and backward. A normal performance is repeating seven numbers in the forward direction, with fewer than five indicating significant attention deficits.[67,83]

Table 1-5 Glasgow Coma Scale

Function	Rating
Eye Opening	**E**
Spontaneous	4
To speech	3
To pain	2
Nil	1
Best Motor Response	**M**
Obeys	6
Localizes	5
Withdraws	4
Abnormal flexion	3
Extensor response	2
Nil	1
Verbal Response	**V**
Oriented	5
Confused conversation	4
Inappropriate words	3
Incomprehensible sounds	2
Nil	1
Coma score (E + M + V)	3-15

From Jennett B, Teasdale G: Assessment of impaired consciousness, *Contemp Neurosurg* 20:78, 1981, with permission.

Orientation. Orientation is necessary for basic cognition. Orientation is composed of four parts: person, place, time, and situation. After asking the patient's name, place can be determined by asking the location the patient is currently in or her or his home address. Time is assessed by asking the patient the time of day, the date, the day of the week, or the year. Situation refers to why the patient is in the hospital or clinic. Time sense is usually the first component lost, and person is typically the last to be lost. Temporary stress can account for a minor loss of orientation; however, major disorientation usually suggests an organic brain syndrome.[87]

Memory. The components of memory include learning, retention, and recall. During the bedside examination, the patient is typically asked to remember three or four objects or words. The patient is then asked to repeat the items immediately to assess immediate acquisition (encoding) of the information. Retention is assessed by recall after a delayed interval, usually 5 to 10 minutes. If the patient is unable to recall the words or objects, the examiner can provide a prompt (e.g., "It is a type of flower" for the word "tulip"). If the patient still cannot recall the words or objects, the examiner can provide a list from which the patient can choose (e.g., "Was it a rose, a tulip, or a daisy?"). Although abnormal scores must be interpreted within the context of the remaining neurologic examination, normal individuals younger than 60 years should recall three of four items.[83]

Recent memory can also be tested by asking questions about the past 24 hours, such as "How did you travel here?" or "What did you eat for breakfast this morning?" Assuming the information can be confirmed, remote memory is tested by asking where the patient was born or the school or college attended.[58] Visual memory can be tested by having the patient identify (after a few minutes) four or five objects hidden in clear view.

General Fundamentals of Knowledge. Intelligence is a global function derived from the general tone and content of the examination and encompasses both basic intellect and remote memory. The examiner should note the patient's educational level and highest grade completed during the history. Examples of questions that can be asked include names of important elected officials, such as the current president of the United States or recent past presidents. It can be difficult to identify when a patient with a very high intelligence premorbidly drops to a more average level after injury or illness. The history of memory or intellectual decline from a family member or close friend should prompt further evaluation of the patient.

Abstract Thinking. Abstraction is a higher cortical function and can be tested by the interpretation of common proverbs such as "a stitch in time saves nine" or "when the cat's away the mice will play," or by asking similarities, such as "How are an apple and an orange alike?" A concrete explanation for the first proverb would be "You should sew a rip before it becomes bigger," whereas an abstract explanation would be "Quick attention to a given problem would prevent bigger troubles later." An abstract response to the similarity would be "They are both kinds of fruit," and a concrete response would be "They are both round" or "You can eat them both." Most normal individuals should be able to provide abstract responses. A patient also demonstrates abstraction when he or she understands a humorous phrase or situation. Concrete responses are given by persons with dementia, mental retardation, or limited education. Abstract thinking should always be considered in the context of intelligence and cultural differences.[87]

Insight and Judgment. Insight has been conceptualized into three components: awareness of impairment, need for treatment, and attribution of symptoms. Insight can be ascertained by asking what brought the patient into the hospital or clinic.[11] Recognizing that one has an impairment is the initial step for recovery. A lack of insight can severely hamper a patient's progress in rehabilitation and is a major consideration in developing a safe discharge plan. Insight can be difficult to distinguish from psychological denial.

Judgment is an estimate of a person's ability to solve real-life problems. The best indicator is usually simply observing the patient's behavior. Judgment can also be assessed by noting the patient's responses to hypothetical situations in relation to family, employment, or personal life. Hypothetical examples of judgment that reflect societal norms include "What should you do if you find a stamped, addressed envelope?" or "How are you going to get around the house if you have trouble walking?" Judgment is a complex function that is part of the maturational process and is consequently unreliable in children and variable in the adolescent years.[87] Assessment of judgment is important to assess the patient's capacity for independent functioning.

Mood and Affect. Mood can be assessed by asking: "Do you often feel sad or depressed?"[91] Establishing accurate information pertaining to the length of a particular mood is important. The examiner should document if the mood has been reactive (e.g., sadness in response to a recent disabling event or loss of independence) and whether the mood has been stable or unstable. Mood can be described in terms of being, including happy, sad, euphoric, blue, depressed, angry, or anxious.

Affect describes how a patient feels at a given moment, which can be described by terms such as blunted, flat, inappropriate, labile, optimistic, or pessimistic. It can be difficult to accurately assess mood in the setting of moderate to severe acquired brain injury. A patient's affect is determined by the observations made by the examiner during the interview.[12]

General Mental Status Assessment. The Folstein Mini-Mental Status Examination is a brief and convenient tool to test general cognitive function. It is useful for screening patients for dementia and brain injuries. Of a maximum 30 points, a score of 24 or above is considered within the normal range.[31] Also available is the easily administered Montreal Cognitive Assessment.[69] The clock-drawing test is another quick test sensitive to cognitive impairment. The patient is instructed as follows: "Without looking at your watch, draw the face of a clock, and mark the hands to show 10 minutes to 11 o'clock." This task uses memory, visual spatial skills, and executive functioning. The drawing is scored on the basis of whether the clock numbers are generally intact or not intact out of a maximum score of 10.[84] The use of the three-word recall test in addition to the clock-drawing test, which is known collectively as the Mini-Cog Test, has recently gained popularity in screening for dementia. The Mini-Cog Test can usually be completed within 2 to 3 minutes.[77] The reader is referred to other excellent descriptions of the MSE for further reading.[83]

Communication

Aphasia. Aphasia involves the *loss of production or comprehension of language*. The cortical center for language resides in the dominant hemisphere. Naming, repetition, comprehension, and fluency are the key components of the physician's bedside language assessment. The examiner should listen to the content and fluency of speech. Testing of comprehension of spoken language should begin with single words, progress to sentences that require only yes/no responses, and then progress to complex commands. The examiner should also assess visual naming, repetition of single words and sentences, word-finding abilities, and reading and writing from dictation and then spontaneous reading and writing. Circumlocutions are phrases or sentences substituted for a word the person cannot express, such as responding "What you tell time with on your wrist" when asked to name a watch. Alexia without agraphia is seen in dominant occipital lobe injury. Here the patient is able to write letters and words from a spoken command but is unable to read the information after dictation.[14] Some commonly used standardized aphasia measures include the Boston Diagnostic Aphasia Examination and the Western Aphasia Battery (see Chapter 3).[85]

Dysarthria. Dysarthria refers to *defective articulation* but with the content of speech unaffected. The examiner should listen to spontaneous speech and then ask the patient to read aloud. Key sounds that can be tested include "ta ta ta," which is made by the tongue (lingual consonants); "mm mm mm," which is made by the lips (labial consonants); and "ga ga ga," which is made by the larynx, pharynx, and palate.[58] There are several subtypes of dysarthria, including spastic, ataxic, hypokinetic, hyperkinetic, and flaccid.[67]

Dysphonia. Dysphonia is a deficit in sound production and can be secondary to respiratory disease, fatigue, or vocal cord paralysis. The best method to examine the vocal cords is by indirect laryngoscopy. Asking the patient to say "ah" while viewing the vocal cords is used to assess vocal cord abduction. When the patient says "e," the vocal cords will adduct. Patients with weakness of both vocal cords will speak in whispers with the presence of inspiratory stridors.[58]

Verbal Apraxia. Apraxia of speech involves a deficit in motor planning (i.e., awkward and imprecise articulation in the *absence* of impaired strength or coordination of the motor system). It is characterized by inconsistent errors when speaking. A difficult word might be spoken correctly, but trouble is experienced when repeating it. People with verbal apraxia of speech often appear to be "groping" for the right sound or word, and might try to speak a word several times before saying it correctly. Apraxia is tested by asking the patient to repeat words with an increasing number of syllables. Oromotor apraxia is seen in patients with difficulty organizing nonspeech oral motor activity. This can adversely impact swallowing. Tests for oromotor apraxia include asking patients to stick out their tongue, show their teeth, blow out their cheeks, or pretend to blow out a match (see Chapter 3).[1]

Cognitive Linguistic Deficits. Cognitive linguistic deficits involve the pragmatics and context of communication. Examples can include confabulation after a ruptured aneurysm of the anterior communicating artery or disinhibited or sexually inappropriate comments from a patient with frontal lobe damage after a traumatic brain injury. Cognitive linguistic deficits are distinguished from fluent aphasias (Wernicke aphasia) by the presence of relatively normal syntax and grammar.

Cranial Nerve Examination

Cranial Nerve I: Olfactory Nerve. The examiner should test both perception and identification of smell with aromatic nonirritating materials that avoid stimulation of the trigeminal nerve fibers in the nasal mucosa. Irritant substances such as ammonia should be avoided. The patient is asked to close the eyes while the opposite nostril is compressed separately. The patient should identify the smell in a test tube containing a common substance with a characteristic odor, such as coffee, peppermint, or soap. The olfactory nerve is the most commonly injured cranial nerve (CN) in head trauma, resulting from shearing injuries that can be associated with fractures of the cribriform plate making testing in this population an essential part of the physical examination.[5]

Cranial Nerve II: Optic Nerve. The optic nerve is assessed by testing for visual acuity and visual fields, and by performing an ophthalmologic examination. Visual acuity refers to central vision, whereas visual field testing assesses the integrity of the optic pathway as it travels from the retina to the primary visual cortex. Testing visual fields by confrontation is most commonly performed. The patient faces the examiner while covering one eye so the other eye fixates on the opposite eye of the examiner directly in front. The examiner wiggles a finger at the outer boundaries of the four quadrants of vision while the patient points to the quadrant where he or she senses movement. More accurately, a red 5-mm pin can be used to map out the visual field.[5] For patients with visual field and extraocular movement deficits (see following discussion), further assessment by a neuro-optometrist or a visually trained occupational therapist can be helpful.

Cranial Nerves III, IV, and VI: Oculomotor, Trochlear, and Abducens Nerves. These three CNs are best tested together because they are all involved in ocular motility. The oculomotor nerve (III) provides innervation to all the extraocular muscles except the superior oblique and lateral rectus, which are innervated by the trochlear (IV) and abducens nerves (VI), respectively. The oculomotor nerve also innervates the levator palpebrae muscle, which elevates the eyelid, the pupilloconstrictor muscle that constricts the pupil, and the ciliary muscle that controls the thickness of the lens in visual accommodation.

The primary action of the medial rectus is adduction (looking in) and that of the lateral rectus is abduction (looking out). The superior rectus and inferior oblique primarily elevate the eye, whereas the inferior rectus and superior oblique depress the eye. The superior oblique muscle controls gaze looking down, especially in adduction.[58]

Examination of the extraocular muscles involves assessing the alignment of the patient's eyes while the eyes are at rest and when the eyes are following an object or finger held at an arm's length. The examiner should observe the full range of horizontal and vertical eye movements in the six cardinal directions.[5] The optic (afferent) and oculomotor (efferent) nerves are involved with the pupillary light reflex. A normal pupillary light reflex (CNs II and III) should result in constriction of *both* pupils when a light stimulus is presented to either eye separately. A characteristic head tilt when looking down is sometimes seen in CN IV lesions.[95]

Cranial Nerve V: Trigeminal Nerve. The trigeminal nerve provides sensation to the face and mucous membranes of the nose, mouth, and tongue. There are three sensory divisions of the trigeminal nerve: the ophthalmic, maxillary, and mandibular branches. These branches can be tested by pinprick sensation, light touch, or temperature along the forehead, cheeks, and jaw on each side of the face. The motor branch of the trigeminal nerve also innervates the muscles of mastication, which include the masseters, the pterygoids, and the temporalis. The patient is asked to clamp the jaws together, and then the examiner will try to open the patient's jaw by pulling down on the lower mandible. Observe and palpate for contraction of both the temporalis and the masseter muscles. The pterygoids are tested by asking the patient to open the mouth. If one side is weak, the intact pterygoid muscles will push the weak muscles, resulting in a deviation toward the weak side. The corneal reflex tests the ophthalmic division of the trigeminal nerve (afferent) and the facial nerve (efferent).

Cranial Nerve VII: Facial Nerve. The facial nerve provides motor innervation to all muscles of facial expression; provides sensation to the anterior two thirds of the tongue and the external acoustic meatus; innervates the stapedius muscle, which helps dampen loud sounds by decreasing excessive movements of the ossicles in the inner ear; and provides secretomotor fibers to the lacrimal and salivary glands.

The facial nerve is first examined by watching the patient as she or he talks and smiles, watching specifically for eye closure, flattening of the nasolabial fold, and asymmetric elevation of one corner of the mouth. The patient is then asked to wrinkle the forehead (frontalis), close the eyes while the examiner attempts to open them (orbicularis oculi), puff out both cheeks while the examiner presses on the cheeks (buccinator), and show the teeth (orbicularis oris). A peripheral injury to the facial nerve, such as occurs in Bell palsy, affects both the upper and the lower face, whereas a central lesion typically affects mainly the lower face.

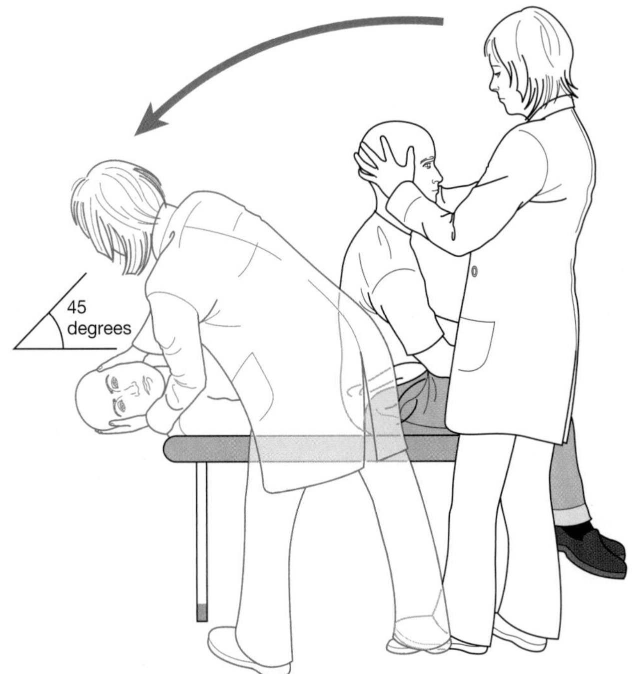

FIGURE 1-1 The Dix-Hallpike maneuver is performed with the patient initially seated upright. The patient is asked to fall backward so that the head is below the plane of his or her trunk. The examiner then turns the patient's head to one side and asks the patient to look in the direction to which the head is turned.

Cranial Nerve VIII: Vestibulocochlear Nerve. The vestibulocochlear nerve, also known as the auditory nerve, comprises two divisions. The cochlear nerve is the part of the auditory nerve responsible for hearing, whereas the vestibular nerve is related to balance. The cochlear division can be tested by checking gross hearing. A rapid screen can be done if the examiner rubs the thumb and index fingers near each ear of the patient. Patients with normal hearing usually have no difficulty hearing this.

The vestibular division is seldom included in the routine neurologic examination. Patients with dizziness or vertigo associated with changes in head position or suspected of having benign paroxysmal positional vertigo should be assessed with the Dix-Hallpike maneuver (Figure 1-1). The absence of nystagmus indicates normal vestibular nerve function. With peripheral vestibular nerve dysfunction, however, the patient complains of vertigo, and rotary nystagmus appears after an approximately 2- to 5-second latency, toward the direction in which the eyes are deviated. With repetition of maneuvers, the nystagmus and sensation of vertigo fatigue and ultimately disappear. In central vestibular disease, such as from a stroke, the nystagmus has latency and is nonfatigable.[32] Rehabilitation therapists with training in vestibular rehabilitation can also provide invaluable data for developing a differential diagnosis of and a treatment plan for balance deficits.

Cranial Nerves IX and X: Glossopharyngeal Nerve and Vagus Nerve. The glossopharyngeal nerve supplies taste to the posterior one third of the tongue, along with sensation to the pharynx and the middle ear. The glossopharyngeal nerve and vagus nerve are usually examined together. The patient's voice quality should be noted because hoarseness is usually associated with a lesion of the recurrent laryngeal nerve, a branch of the vagus nerve. The patient is asked to open the mouth and say "ah." The examiner should inspect the soft palate, which should elevate symmetrically with the uvula in midline. In an LMN vagus nerve lesion, the uvula will deviate to the side that is contralateral to the lesion. A UMN lesion presents with the uvula deviating toward the side of the lesion.[38]

The gag reflex can be tested by depressing the patient's tongue with a tongue depressor and touching the pharyngeal wall with a cotton tip applicator until the patient gags. The examiner should compare the sensitivity of each side (afferent: glossopharyngeal nerve) and observe the symmetry of the palatal contraction (efferent: vagus nerve). The absence of a gag reflex indicates loss of sensation and/or loss of motor contraction. The presence of a gag reflex does *not* imply the ability to swallow without risk of aspiration.[73]

Cranial Nerve XI: Accessory Nerve. The accessory nerve innervates the trapezius and sternocleidomastoid muscles. While standing behind the patient, the examiner should look for atrophy or spasm in the trapezius and compare the symmetry of both sides. Atrophy of the trapezius can be observed by a loss of the C-shaped contour with more of an L-shaped contour. The scapula will also migrate laterally and have an "open door" winging pattern. Traditionally, the strength of the trapezius is tested by asking the patient to shrug the shoulders and hold them in this position against resistance. Unfortunately, this may be inaccurate because of substitution by other shoulder elevators, and assessing for atrophy may prove more reliable. For the strength of the sternocleidomastoid muscle to be tested, the patient should be asked to rotate the head against resistance. The ipsilateral sternocleidomastoid muscle turns the head to the contralateral side. The ipsilateral muscle brings the ear to the shoulder.

Cranial Nerve XII: Hypoglossal Nerve. The hypoglossal nerve is a pure motor nerve innervating the muscles of the tongue. It is tested by asking the patient to protrude the tongue, noting evidence of atrophy, fasciculation, or deviation. Fibrillations in the tongue are common in patients with amyotrophic lateral sclerosis.[37] The tongue typically points to the side of the lesion in peripheral hypoglossal nerve lesions but toward the opposite side of the lesion in UMN lesions such as stroke.

Sensory Examination

The examiner should be familiar with the normal dermatomal and peripheral nerve sensory distribution (Figure 1-2). Evaluation of the sensory system requires testing of both superficial sensation (light touch, pain, and temperature) and deep sensation (involves the perception of position and vibration from deep structures, such as muscle, ligaments, and bone).

Light touch can be assessed with a fine wisp of cotton or a cotton tip applicator. The examiner should touch the skin lightly, avoiding excessive pressure. The patient is asked to respond when a touch is felt and to say whether there is a difference between the two sides. Pain and temperature both travel via the spinothalamic tracts and are assessed

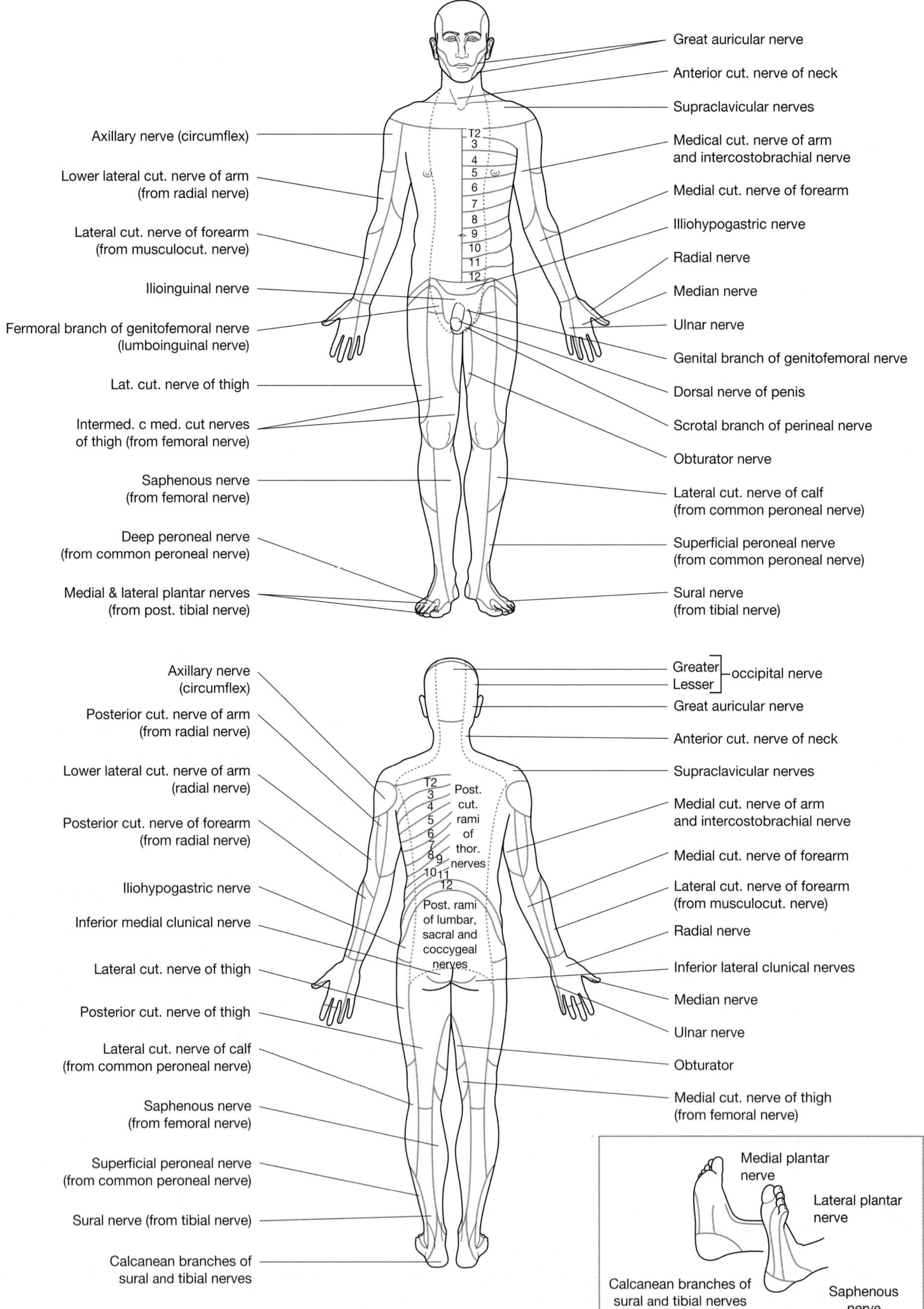

FIGURE 1-2 **Distribution of peripheral nerves and dermatomes.** (Redrawn from Haymaker W, Woodhall B: *Peripheral nerve injuries,* Philadelphia, : Saunders, 1953, with permission.)

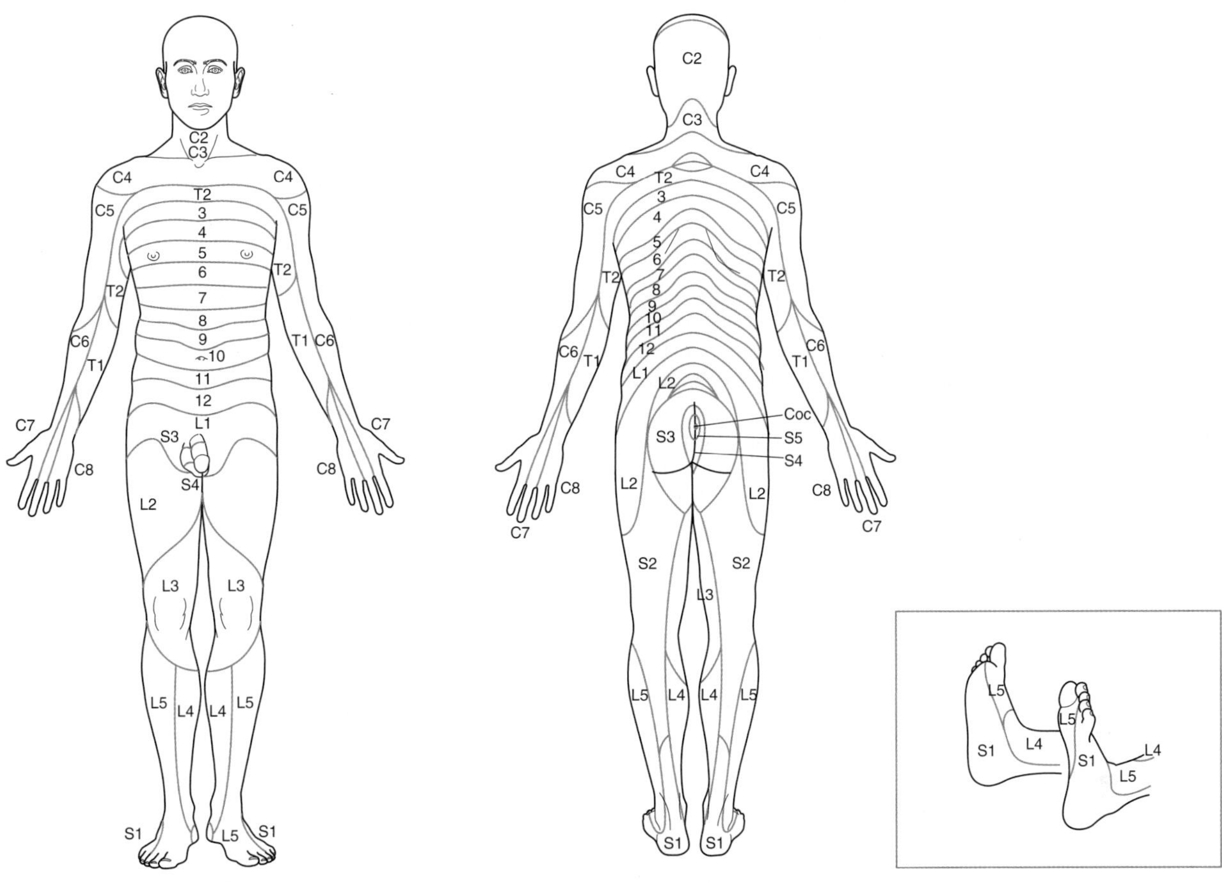

FIGURE 1-2, cont'd

with a safety pin or other sharp sanitary objects, while occasionally interspersing the examination with a blunt object. Patients with peripheral neuropathy might have a delayed pain appreciation and often change their minds a few seconds after the initial stimuli. Some examiners use the single or double pinprick of brief duration to test for pain, whereas others use a continuous sustained pinprick to better test for delayed pain.[64] Temperature testing is not often used and rarely provides additional information, but it is sometimes easier for patients to delineate insensate areas. Thermal sensation can be checked by using two different cups, one filled with hot water (not hot enough to burn) and one filled with cold water and ice chips.

Joint position sense or proprioception travel via the dorsal columns along with vibration sense. Proprioception is tested by vertical passive movement of the toes or fingers. The examiner holds the sides of the patient's fingers or toes and with the patient's eyes closed, asks the patient if the digits are in the upward or downward direction. It is important to grasp the sides of the digits rather than the nailbed because the patient might be able to perceive pressure in these areas, reducing the accuracy of the examination. Most normal persons make no errors on these maneuvers.

Vibration is tested in the limbs with a 128-Hz tuning fork. The tuning fork is placed on a bony prominence, such as the dorsal aspect of the terminal phalange of the great toe or finger, the malleoli, or the olecranon. The patient is asked to indicate when the vibration ceases. The vibration stimulus can be controlled by changing the force used to set the tuning fork in motion or by noting the amount of time that a vibration is felt as the stimulus dissipates. If the examiner has normal sensation, both patient and examiner should feel the vibration cease at approximately the same time.

Two-point discrimination is most commonly tested using calipers with blunt ends. The patient is asked to close the eyes and indicate whether one or two stimulation points are felt. The normal distance of separation that can be felt as two distinct points depends on the area of body being tested. For example, the lips are sensitive to a point separation of 2 to 3 mm, normally identified as two points. Commonly tested normal two-point discrimination areas include the fingertips (3 to 5 mm), the dorsum of the hand (20 to 30 mm), and the palms (8 to 15 mm).[58]

Graphesthesia is the ability to recognize numbers, letters, or symbols traced onto the palm. It is performed by writing recognizable numbers on the patient's palm with his or her eyes closed. Stereognosis is the ability to recognize common objects placed in the hand, such as keys or coins. This requires normal peripheral sensation as well as cortical interpretation.

Motor Control

Strength. Manual muscle testing provides an important method of quantifying strength and is outlined in the later section about musculoskeletal examination.

Coordination. The cerebellum controls movement by comparing the intended activity with actual activity that is achieved. The cerebellum enables smooth motor movements and is intimately involved with coordination. Ataxia or motor coordination can be secondary to deficits of sensory, motor, or cerebellar connections. Patients with ataxia who have intact function of the sensory and motor pathways usually have cerebellar compromise.

The cerebellum is divided into three areas: the midline, the anterior lobe, and the lateral hemisphere. Lesions affecting the midline usually produce truncal ataxia in which the patient cannot sit or stand unsupported. This can be tested by asking the patient to sit at the edge of the bed with the arms folded so they cannot be used for support. Lesions that affect the anterior lobe usually result in gait ataxia. In this case, the patient is able to sit or stand unsupported but has noticeable balance deficits on walking. Lateral hemisphere lesions produce loss of ability to coordinate movement, which can be described as limb ataxia. The affected limb usually has diminished ability to correct and change direction rapidly. Tests that are typically used to test for limb coordination include the finger-to-nose test and the heel-to-shin test.[65]

Rapid alternating movements can be tested by observing the amplitude, rhythm, and precision of movement. The patient is asked to place the hands on the thighs and then rapidly turn the hands over and lift them off the thighs for 10 seconds. Normal individuals can do this without difficulty. Dysdiadochokinesis is the clinical term for an inability to perform rapidly alternating movements.

The Romberg test can be used to differentiate a cerebellar deficit from a proprioceptive one. The patient is asked to stand with the heels together. The examiner notes any excessive postural swaying or loss of balance. If loss of balance is present when the eyes are open and closed, the examination is consistent with cerebellar ataxia. If the loss of balance occurs only when the eyes are closed, this is classically known as a positive Romberg sign indicating a proprioceptive (sensory) deficit.[58]

Apraxia. Apraxia is the loss of the ability to carry out programmed or planned movements despite adequate understanding of the tasks. This deficit is present even though the patient has no weakness or sensory loss. For a complex act to be accomplished, there first must be an idea or a formulation of a plan. The formulation of the plan then must be transferred into the motor system where it is executed. The examiner should watch the patient for motor-planning problems during the physical examination. For example, a patient might be unable to perform transfers and other mobility tasks but has adequate strength on formal manual muscle testing.[88]

Ideomotor apraxia associated with a lesion of the dominant parietal lobe occurs when a patient cannot carry out motor commands but can perform the required movements under different circumstances. These patients usually can perform many complex acts automatically but cannot carry out the same acts on command. Ideational apraxia refers to the inability to carry out sequences of acts, although each component can be performed separately. Other forms of apraxia are constructional, dressing, oculomotor, oromotor, verbal, and gait apraxia. Dressing and constructional apraxia are often related to impairments of the nondominant parietal lobe, which typically are the result of neglect rather than actual deficit in motor planning.[58]

Involuntary Movements. Documenting involuntary movements is important in the overall neurologic examination. A careful survey of the patient usually shows the presence or absence of voluntary motor control. Tremor is the most common type of involuntary movement and is a rhythmic movement of a body part. Myoclonus, a quick jerking movement of a muscle or body part, can be seen with a variety of cerebral and spinal cord lesions and as a side effect of medication. Lesions in the basal ganglia produce characteristic movement disorders. Chorea describes movements that consist of brief, random, nonrepetitive movements in a fidgety patient unable to sit still. Athetosis consists of twisting and writhing movements and is commonly seen in cerebral palsy. Dystonia is a sustained posturing that can affect small or large muscle groups. An example is torticollis, in which dystonic neck muscles pull the head to one side. Hemiballismus occurs when there are repetitive violent flailing movements that are usually caused by deficits in the subthalamic nucleus.[67]

Tone. Tone is the resistance of muscle to stretch or passive elongation (see Chapter 23). Spasticity is a velocity-dependent increase in the stretch reflex, whereas rigidity is the resistance of the limb to passive movement in the relaxed state (non–velocity-dependent). Variability in tone is common because patients with spasticity can vary in their presentation throughout the day and with positional changes or mood. Some patients will demonstrate little tone at rest (static tone) but experience a surge of tone when they attempt to move the muscle during a functional activity (dynamic tone). Accurate assessment of tone might require repeated examinations.[72]

Initial observation of the patient usually shows abnormal posturing of the limbs or trunk. Palpation of the muscle also provides clues, because hypotonic muscles feel soft and flaccid on palpation, whereas hypertonic muscles feel firm and tight. Passive range of motion (ROM) provides information about the muscle in response to stretch. The examiner provides firm and constant contact while moving the limbs in all directions. The limb should move easily and without resistance when altering the direction and speed of movement. Hypertonic limbs feel stiff and resist movement, whereas flaccid limbs are unresponsive. The patient should be told to relax because these responses should be examined without any voluntary control. Clonus is a cyclic alternation of muscular contraction in response to a sustained stretch, and is assessed with a quick stretch stimulus that is then maintained. Myoclonus refers to sudden, involuntary jerking of a muscle or group of muscles. Myoclonic jerks can be normal because they occasionally happen in normal individuals and are typically part of the normal sleep cycle. Myoclonus can result from hypoxia, drug toxicity, and metabolic disturbances. Other causes include degenerative disorders affecting the basal ganglia and certain dementias.[79]

Tone can be quantified by the Modified Ashworth Scale, a six-point ordinal scale. A pendulum test can also be used to quantify spasticity. While in the supine position, the patient is asked to fully extend the knee and then allow the leg to drop and swing like a pendulum. A normal limb swings freely for several cycles, whereas a hypertonic limb quickly returns to the initial dependent starting position.[85]

Table 1-6 Important Normal Superficial Reflexes

Reflex	Elicited By	Response	Segmental Level
Corneal	Touching cornea with hair	Contraction of orbicularis oculi	Pons
Pharyngeal	Touching posterior wall of pharynx	Contraction of pharynx	Medulla
Palatal	Touching soft palate	Elevation of palate	Medulla
Scapular	Stroking skin between scapulae	Contraction of scapular muscles	C5-T1
Epigastric	Stroking downward from nipples	Dimpling of epigastrium ipsilaterally	T7-T9
Abdominal	Stroking beneath costal margins and above inguinal ligament	Contraction of abdominal muscles in quadrant stimulated	T8-T12
Cremasteric	Stroking medial surface of upper thigh	Ipsilateral elevation of testicle	L1, L2
Gluteal	Stroking skin of buttock	Contraction of glutei	L4, L5
Bulbocavernosus (male)	Pinching dorsum of glans	Insert gloved finger to palpate anal contraction	S3, S4
Clitorocavernosus (female)	Pinching clitoris	Insert gloved finger to palpate anal contraction	S3, S4
Superficial anal	Pricking perineum	Contraction of rectal sphincters	S5, coccygeal

Modified from Mancall EL, editor: Examination of the nervous system. In *Alpers and Mancall's essentials of the neurologic examination*, ed 2, Philadelphia, 1981, with permission of FA Davis.

The Tardieu Scale has been suggested to be a more appropriate clinical measure of spasticity than the Modified Ashworth Scale. It involves assessment of resistance to passive movement at both slow and fast speeds. Measurements are usually taken at three velocities (V1, V2, and V3). V1 is taken as slow as possible, slower than the natural drop of the limb segment under gravity. V2 is taken at the speed of the limb falling under gravity. V3 is taken with the limb moving as fast as possible, faster than the natural drop of the limb under gravity. Responses are recorded at each velocity and the degrees of angle at which the muscle reaction occurs.[41]

Table 1-7 Muscle Stretch Reflexes

Muscle	Peripheral Nerve	Root Level
Biceps	Musculocutaneous nerve	C5, C6
Brachioradialis	Radial nerve	C5, C6
Triceps	Radial nerve	C7, C8
Pronator teres	Median nerve	C6, C7
Patella (quadriceps)	Femoral nerve	L2-L4
Medial hamstrings	Sciatic (tibial portion) nerve	L5-S1
Achilles	Tibial nerve	S1, S2

Reflexes

Superficial Reflexes. The plantar reflex is the most common superficial reflex examined. A stimulus (usually by the handle end of a reflex hammer) is applied on the sole of the foot from the lateral border up and across the ball of the foot. A normal reaction consists of flexion of the great toe or no response. An abnormal response consists of dorsiflexion of the great toe with an associated fanning of the other toes. This response is the Babinski sign and indicates dysfunction of the corticospinal tract but no further localization. Stroking from the lateral ankle to the lateral dorsal foot can also produce dorsiflexion of the great toe (Chaddock sign). Flipping the little toe outward can produce the upgoing great toe also and is called the Stransky sign. Other superficial reflexes include the abdominal, cremasteric, bulbocavernosus, and superficial anal reflexes (Table 1-6).[67]

Muscle Stretch Reflexes. Muscle stretch reflexes (which in the past were called deep tendon reflexes) are assessed by tapping over the muscle tendon with a reflex hammer (Table 1-7). o For a response to be elicited, the patient is positioned into the midrange of the arc of joint motion and instructed to relax. Tapping of the tendon results in visible movement of the joint. The response is assessed as 0, no response; 1+, diminished but present and might require facilitation; 2+, usual response; 3+, more brisk than usual; and 4+, hyperactive with clonus. If muscle stretch reflexes are difficult to elicit, the response can be enhanced by reinforcement maneuvers, such as hooking together the fingers of both hands while attempting to pull them apart (Jendrassik maneuver). While pressure is still maintained, the lower limb reflexes can be tested. Squeezing the knees together and clenching the teeth can reinforce responses to the upper limbs.[58]

Primitive Reflexes. Primitive reflexes are abnormal adult reflexes that represent a regression to a more infantile level of reflex activity. Redevelopment of an infantile reflex in an adult suggests significant neurologic abnormalities. Examples of primitive reflexes include the sucking reflex, in which the patient makes sucking movements when the lips are lightly touched. The rooting reflex is elicited by stroking the cheek, resulting in the patient turning toward that side and making sucking motions with the mouth. The grasp reflex occurs when the examiner places a finger on the patient's open palm. Attempting to remove the finger causes the grip to tighten. Many times families mistake this response as a volitional action. The snout reflex occurs when a lip-pursing movement happens when there is a tap just above or below the mouth. The palmomental response is elicited by quickly scratching the palm of the hand. A positive reflex is indicated by sudden contraction of the mentalis (chin) muscle. It arises from unilateral damage of the prefrontal area of the brain.[68]

Gait

Gait evaluation is an important and often neglected part of the neurologic evaluation. Gait is described as a series of rhythmic, alternating movements of the limbs and trunks that result in the forward progression of the center of gravity.[10] Gait is dependent on input from several systems, including the visual, vestibular, cerebellar, motor, and sensory systems. The cause of dysfunction can be determined by understanding the aspects of gait involved. One example is difficulty getting up, which is consistent with Parkinson disease, or a lack of balance and wide-based gait, which is suggestive of cerebellar dysfunction.

The examination starts by asking the patient to walk across the room in a straight line. This can also be assessed by observing the patient walking from the waiting area into the examination room. The patient is then asked to stand from a chair, walk across the room, and come back toward the examiner. The examiner should pay particular attention to the following:

1. *Ease of arising from a seated position.* Can the patient easily arise from a sitting position? Difficulty with a sit-to-stand task may indicate proximal muscle weakness, movement disorders with difficulty initiating movements, or a balance problem.
2. *Balance.* Does the patient lean or veer off to one side, which is an indication of cerebellar dysfunction? Patients with medullary lesions and cerebellar lesions tend to push to the side of the lesion. Diffuse disease affecting both cerebellar hemispheres can cause a generalized loss of balance. Patients with cerebellar disorders usually have balance issues *with or without* their eyes open. Patients with proprioceptive dysfunction can use their visual input to compensate for their sensory deficit.
3. *Walking speed.* Does the patient start off slow and then accelerate uncontrollably? Patients with Parkinson disease will have problems initiating movements, but then lose their balance once they are in motion. Patients with pain, such as knee or hip arthritis, often have limitations of ROM affecting gait speed. It has been shown that a self-selected gait speed of less than 0.8 m/sec is a risk factor for falls in the stroke population.[76] The speed of walking remains stable until about age 70 years when there is a 15% decline per decade. Gait speed is lower because elderly people take shorter steps.[7]
4. *Stride and step length.* Does the patient take a small step or shuffle while walking? Patients with normal pressure hydrocephalus and Parkinson disease usually take small steps or shuffle (decreasing their step and stride length). Stride length is the linear distance between successive corresponding points of heel contact of the same foot, whereas step length is the distance between corresponding successive contact points of opposite feet.[9] An antalgic gait is characterized with the patient spending more time in stance phase on one leg and is usually due to pain in the other leg. An average step length is approximately 2 feet for women and 2.5 feet for men.[92]
5. *Attitude of arms and legs.* How does the patient hold his or her arms and legs? Loss of movement as in a spastic or contracted patient should be assessed. Patients with knee extension weakness might swing their knees into terminal extension, thereby locking their knee (genu recurvatum). The patient is then asked to also walk heel to toe in a straight line. Ask the patient to walk in a straight line by putting one heel of one foot directly in front of the toe of the other. This is also called tandem gait and is a test of higher balance. Tandem gait can be difficult for older patients and in some other medical conditions (even without neurologic disease). Other tests to assess gait function include observing patients walk on their toes and heels. Patients with a Trendelenburg gait tend to sway toward the leg in stance phase because of abductor weakness. Balance can also be assessed by asking patients to hop in place and to do a shallow knee bend. Gait disorders have stereotypical patterns that reflect injury to various aspects of the neurologic system (Table 1-8).

Musculoskeletal Examination

Caveats

The musculoskeletal (MSK) examination confirms the diagnostic impression and lays the foundation for the physiatric treatment plan. It incorporates inspection, palpation, passive and active ROM, assessment of joint stability, manual muscle testing, joint-specific provocative maneuvers, and special tests (Table 1-9).[34,42,61] The functional unit of the musculoskeletal system is the joint, and its comprehensive examination includes related structures, such as muscles, ligaments, and the synovial capsule.[63] The MSK examination also indirectly tests coordination, sensation, and endurance.[34,54] There is overlap between the examination (and clinical presentation) of the neurologic and musculoskeletal systems. Neurologic disease may lead to secondary musculoskeletal complications of immobility and suboptimal movement. The MSK examination should be performed in a routine sequence for efficiency and consistency and must be approached with a solid knowledge of anatomy. The reader is referred to several references that provide in-depth reviews of the MSK examination.*

Inspection

Inspection of the musculoskeletal system begins during the history. Attention to subtle cues and behaviors can guide the approach to the examination. Inspection includes observing mood, signs of pain or discomfort, functional impairments, or evidence of malingering (Waddell signs). The spine should be inspected for scoliosis, kyphosis, and lordosis, whereas limbs should be examined for symmetry, circumference, and contour. In persons with amputation, the level, length, and shape of the residual limb should be appreciated. Depending on the clinical situation, it can be important to assess for muscle atrophy, masses, edema, scars, skin breakdown, and fasciculations.[81] Joints should be inspected for deformity, visible swelling, and erythema.

Recognition of the kinetic chain is fundamental to a comprehensive MSK examination. *Kinetic chain* refers to

*References 3, 21, 34, 45, 46, 56, 74.

Table 1-8 Common Gait Disturbances

Gait Type	Disease or Anatomic Location	Gait Characteristics
Hemiplegic	Unilateral upper motor neuron lesions with spastic hemiplegia	The affected lower limb is difficult to move, and knee is held in extension. With ambulation, the leg swings away from the center of the body, and the hip hikes upward to prevent the toes and foot from striking the floor. This is known as "circumduction." If the upper limb is involved, there may be decreased arm swing with ambulation.[30] The upper limb has a flexor synergy pattern resulting in shoulder adduction, elbow and wrist flexion, and a clinched fist.
Scissoring	Bilateral corticospinal tract lesions often seen in patients with cerebral palsy, incomplete spinal cord injury, and multiple sclerosis	Hypertonia in the legs and hips results in flexion and the appearance of a crouched stance. The hip adductors are overactive causing the knees and thighs to touch or cross in a "scissor-like" movement. In cerebral palsy, there can be associated ankle plantar flexion forcing the patient to tiptoe walk. The step length is shortened by the severe adduction or scissoring of the hip muscles.[30]
Ataxic	Cerebellar dysfunction or severe sensory loss (such as tabes dorsalis)	Ataxic gait is characterized by a broad-based stance and irregular step and stride length. In ataxic gait from proprioceptive dysfunction (tabes dorsalis), gait will markedly worsen with the eyes closed. There is a tendency to sway, whereas watching the floor usually helps guide the uncertain steps. Ataxic gait from cerebellar dysfunction will not worsen with eyes closed. Movement of the advancing limb starts slowly, and then there is an erratic movement forward or laterally. The patient will try to correct the error but usually overcompensates. Tandem gait exacerbates cerebellar ataxia.[74]
Myopathic	Myopathies cause weakness of the proximal leg muscles.	Myopathies result in a broad-based gait and a "waddling-type" appearance as the patient tries to compensate for pelvic instability. Patients will have problems with climbing stairs or rising from a chair without using their arms. When going from floor to standing, the patient will use their arms and hands to climb up their legs—known as Gowers sign.[13]
Trendelenburg	Caused by weakness of the abductor muscles (gluteus medius and gluteus minimus) as in superior gluteal nerve injury, poliomyelitis, or myopathy	During the stance phase, the abductor muscle allows the pelvis to tilt down on the opposite side. To compensate, the trunk lurches to the weakened side to maintain the pelvis level during the gait cycle. This results in a waddling-type gait with an exaggerated compensatory sway of the trunk toward the weight-bearing side. It is important to understand that the pelvis sags on the *opposite side* of the weakened abductor muscle.[13]
Parkinsonian	Seen in Parkinson disease and other disorders of the basal ganglia	Patients have a stooped posture, narrow base of support, and a shuffling gait with small steps. As the patient starts to walk, the movements of the legs are usually slow with the appearance of the feet sticking to the floor. They might lean forward while walking so the steps become hurried, resulting in shuffling of the feet (festination). Starting, stopping, or changing directions quickly is difficult, and there is a tendency for retropulsion (falling backward when standing). The whole body moves rigidly requiring many short steps and there is loss of normal arm swing. There can be a "pill-rolling" tremor while the patient walks.[74]
Steppage	Diseases of the peripheral nervous system including L5 radiculopathy, lumbar plexopathies, and peroneal nerve palsy	The patient with foot drop has difficulty dorsiflexing the ankle. The patient compensates for the foot drop by lifting the affected extremity higher than normal to avoid dragging the foot. Weak dorsiflexion leads to poor heel strike with the foot slapping on the floor.[30] An ankle-foot orthosis can be helpful.
Apraxic	Gait impairment when there is no evidence of sensory loss, weakness, vestibular dysfunction, or cerebellar deficit; seen in frontal lobe injuries, such as a stroke, and traumatic brain injury	Despite difficulty with ambulation, patients can perform complex coordinated activities with the lower limbs.[70]

the summation of individual joint movements linked in a series leading to the production of a larger functional goal.[50] A change in movement of a single joint may affect the motion of adjacent as well as distant joints in the chain. This may result in asymmetric patterns causing disease at seemingly unrelated sites.

Palpation

Palpation is used to further evaluate initial impressions made through inspection. This may help to identify tender areas over soft tissue or bone. In addition, palpation may facilitate localization of trigger points, muscle guarding, or spasticity.[81] Joints and soft tissues should be assessed for effusion, warmth, masses, tight muscle bands, tone, and crepitus.[45] It is important to palpate the limbs and cranium for evidence of fracture in patients with a change in mental status after a fall or trauma.[67]

Assessment of Joint Stability. The assessment of joint stability judges the capacity of structural elements to resist forces in nonfunctional directions.[67,81] Stability is determined by several factors, including bony congruity, capsular and cartilaginous integrity, and the strength of ligaments and muscles.[67] Bilateral examination is critical because assessment of the "normal" side establishes a patient's unique biomechanics. The examiner should identify areas of pain and resistance in the affected joint, followed by an evaluation of ROM, to determine hypomobility or hypermobility.

Text continued on p. 25

Table 1-9 Musculoskeletal Provocative Maneuvers

Test	Description	Reliability (%)
Cervical Spine Tests		
Spurling/neck compression test	A positive test is reproduction of radicular symptoms distant from the neck with passive lateral flexion and compression of the head.	Sensitivity: 40-60 Specificity: 92-100
Shoulder abduction (relief) sign	A positive test is relief or reduction of ipsilateral cervical radicular symptoms with active abduction of the ipsilateral arm with the hand on the head.	Sensitivity: 43-50 Specificity: 80-100
Neck distraction test	A positive test is relief or reduction of cervical radicular symptoms with an axial traction force applied by the examiner under the occiput and the chin while the patient is supine.	Sensitivity: 40-43 Specificity: 100
Lhermitte sign	A positive test is the presence of electric-like sensations down the extremities with passive cervical forward flexion.	Sensitivity: 27 Specificity: 90
Hoffmann sign	A positive test is flexion-adduction of ipsilateral thumb and index finger with passive snapping flexion of the distal phalanx of the middle finger.	Sensitivity: 58 Specificity: 78
Thoracic Outlet Tests		
Adson test	A positive test is a decrease or obliteration of the ipsilateral radial pulse with inspiration, chin elevation, and head rotation to the ipsilateral side.	Specificity: 18-87 Sensitivity: 94
Wright hyperabduction test	A positive test is obliteration of the palpated radial pulse at the wrist when the ipsilateral arm is elevated to 90 degrees.	Sensitivity: 40[36] Specificity: 84
Roos test	A positive test reproduces the patient's usual upper limb symptoms within 3 minutes of moderate opening and closing of the fist with the arms and elbows flexed to 90 degrees.	Sensitivity: 30[36] Specificity: 84
Costoclavicular test	A positive test is indicated by a reduction in the radial pulse with shoulder retraction and depression as well as chest protrusion for 1 minute.	Sensitivity: 53[36] Specificity: 88
Rotator Cuff/Supraspinatus Tests		
Empty can/supraspinatus test	A positive test is pain or weakness in the ipsilateral shoulder with resisted abduction of the shoulder, which is in internal rotation, with the thumb pointing toward the floor, and a forward angulation of 30 degrees.	Sensitivity: 79 Specificity: 38-50
Drop arm test	A positive test is noted if the patient is unable to return the arm to the side slowly or has severe pain after the examiner abducts the patient's shoulder to 90 degrees and then asks the patient to slowly lower the arm to the side.	Sensitivity: 27[75] Specificity: 88
Rotator Cuff/Infraspinatus and Teres Minor Tests		
Patte test	A positive test is pain or inability to support the arm or rotate the arm laterally with the elbow at 90 degrees and the arm at 90 degrees of forward elevation in the plane of the scapula. This indicates tears of the infraspinatus and/or teres minor muscles.	Sensitivity: 36-71 Specificity: 71-91
Lift-off test	A positive test is the inability to lift the dorsum of the hand off the back with the arm internally rotated behind the back as starting position. This indicates a disorder of the subscapularis.	Sensitivity: 50 Specificity: 84-95
Scapular Tests		
Lateral scapular slide test	This test allows for identification of scapulothoracic motion deficiencies with the contralateral side as an internal control. The reference point used is the nearest spinous process. A scapulothoracic motion abnormality is noted if there is at least a 1-cm difference. The first position of the test is with the arm relaxed at the side. The second is with the hands on the hips with the fingers anterior and the thumb posterior with about 10 degrees of shoulder extension. The third position is with the arms at or below 90 degrees of arm elevation with maximal internal rotation at the glenohumeral joint. These positions offer a graded challenge to the functioning of the shoulder muscles to stabilize the scapula.	Sensitivity: 28-50 Specificity: 48-58
Isometric pinch test	This test is used to evaluate scapular muscle strength. The patient is asked to retract the scapula into an "isometric pinch." Scapular muscle weakness can be noted as a burning pain in less than 15 seconds. Normally, the scapula can be held in this position for 15 to 20 seconds with no discomfort.	Unavailable
Scapular assistance test	A positive test is when symptoms of impingement, clicking, or rotator cuff weakness are improved when assisting the lower trapezius by manually stabilizing the upper medial border (of the scapula) and rotating the inferomedial border as the arm is abducted or adducted.	Unavailable
Scapular retraction test	The test involves manually positioning and stabilizing the entire medial border of the scapula, which indicates trapezius and rhomboid weakness. The test is positive when there is increased muscle strength or decreased pain or signs of impingement with the scapula in the stabilized position.	Sensitivity: 100[94] Specificity: 33
Biceps Tendon Tests		
Yergason test	The test is done with the elbow flexed to 90 degrees, with the forearm in pronation. The examiner holds the patient's wrist to resist supination and then directs active supination be made against his or her resistance. Pain that localizes in the bicipital groove indicates a disorder of the long head of the biceps. It can also be positive in fractures of the lesser tuberosity of the humerus.	Sensitivity: 37 Specificity: 86

Table 1-9 Musculoskeletal Provocative Maneuvers (Continued)

Test	Description	Reliability (%)
Speed test	A positive test is pain in the bicipital groove with resisted anterior flexion of the shoulder with extension of the elbow and forearm supination.	Sensitivity: 68-69 Specificity: 14-55
Shoulder Impingement Tests		
Neer's sign test	The test is positive if pain is reproduced with forward flexion of the arm in internal rotation or in the anatomic position of external rotation. The pain is thought to be caused by impingement of the rotator cuff by the undersurface of the anterior margin of the acromion or coracoacromial ligament.	Sensitivity: 75-88 Specificity: 31-51
Hawkin test	This test is positive if there is pain with forward flexion of the humerus to 90 degrees with forcible internal rotation of the shoulder. This drives the greater tuberosity under the coracoacromial ligament resulting in rotator cuff impingement.	Sensitivity: 83-92 Specificity: 38-56
Yocum test	This test is positive if there is pain with raising the elbow while the ipsilateral hand is on the contralateral shoulder.	Sensitivity: 79[78] Specificity: 40
Shoulder Stability Tests		
Apprehension test	The test is positive if there is pain or apprehension while the shoulder is moved passively into maximal external rotation while in abduction followed by forward pressure applied to the posterior aspect of the humeral head. This test can be done either in the standing or supine position.	Sensitivity: 69 Specificity: 50
Fowler's sign	The examiner performs the apprehension test and at the point where the patient feels pain or apprehension the examiner applies a posteriorly directed force to the humeral head. If the pain persists despite the posteriorly applied force, it is primary impingement. If there is full pain-free external range, it is a result of instability.	Sensitivity: 30-68 Specificity: 44-100
Load and shift test	The scapula is stabilized by securing the coracoid and the spine of the scapula with one hand with the patient in a sitting or supine position. The humeral head is then grasped with the other hand to glide it anteriorly and posteriorly. The degree of glide is graded mild, moderate, or severe.	Sensitivity: 91 Specificity: 93
Labral Disorder Tests		
Active compression test (O'Brien)	The patient is asked to forward flex the affected arm 90 degrees with the elbow in full extension. The patient then adducts the arm 10 degrees to 15 degrees medial to the sagittal plane of the body with the arm internally rotated so the thumb is pointed downward. The examiner then applies downward force to the arm. With the arm in the same position, the palm is then supinated and the maneuver is repeated. The test is considered positive if pain is elicited with the first maneuver and is reduced or eliminated with the second maneuver.	Sensitivity: 32-100 Specificity: 13-98.5
Crank test	With the patient in an upright position, the arm is elevated to 160 degrees in the scapular plane. Joint load is applied along the axis of the humerus with one hand while the other performs humeral rotation. A positive test is when there is pain during the maneuver during external rotation with or without a click, or reproduction of the symptoms. The test should be repeated in the supine position when the muscles are more relaxed.	Sensitivity: 46-91 Specificity: 56-100
Compression-rotation test	With the patient supine, the shoulder is abducted to 90 degrees, and the elbow flexed at 90 degrees. A compression force is applied to the humerus, which is then rotated, in an attempt to trap the torn labrum with reproduction of a snap or catch.	Sensitivity: 80 Specificity: 19-49
Acromioclavicular Joint Tests		
Apley scarf test	A positive test is pain at the acromioclavicular joint with passive adduction of the arm across the sagittal midline attempting to approximate the elbow to the contralateral shoulder.	Sensitivity: 77[23] Specificity: 79
Lateral and Medial Epicondylitis Tests		
Resisted wrist extension	For lateral elbow pain, the test is positive if pain is worsened with extension of the wrist against resistance.	Unavailable
Resisted wrist flexion and pronation	This test is positive if medial epicondylar pain is reproduced with forced wrist extension as the patient maintains the elbow in 90 degrees of flexion, with the forearm supinated with the wrist flexed. A positive test indicates involvement of the flexor carpi radialis tendon. Medial elbow pain is most exacerbated with the elbow flexed.	Unavailable
Elbow Stability Tests		
Posterolateral rotatory instability	This test is used to uncover a dislocated radiohumeral joint, which manifests as an obvious dimpling of the skin, generally at a maximum of 40 degrees of elbow flexion. The test is accomplished starting with the patient's forearm in full supination with the elbow in full extension, the examiner slowly flexes the elbow while applying valgus and supination moments and an axial compression force, producing a rotary subluxation of the ulnohumeral joint.	Unavailable
Varus stress	This test is positive if there is excessive gapping on the lateral aspect of the elbow joint. The arm is placed in 20 degrees of flexion with slight supination beyond neutral. The examiner gently stresses the lateral side of the elbow joint.	Unavailable

Continued on following page

Table 1-9 Musculoskeletal Provocative Maneuvers (Continued)

Test	Description	Reliability (%)
Jobe test (valgus stress)	This test is positive if there is excessive gapping on the medial aspect of the elbow joint. The elbow is placed in 25 degrees of flexion to unlock the olecranon from its fossa. The examiner gently stresses the medial side of the elbow joint.	Unavailable
Moving valgus stress test	The examiner maintains a constant moderate valgus torque to a maximally flexed elbow and then rapidly extends the elbow. A positive test occurs if medial elbow pain is reproduced at the medial collateral ligament and is at maximum between 120 degrees and 70 degrees.	Sensitivity: 100[71] Specificity: 75
Carpal Ligament and Joint Tests		
Reagan test (lunotriquetral ballottement test)	The lunate is fixed with the thumb and index finger of one hand while the other hand displaces the triquetrum and pisiform first dorsally then palmarly.	Sensitivity: 64 Specificity: 44
Watson test (scaphoid shift test)	With the forearm slightly pronated, the examiner grasps the wrist from the radial side, placing his thumb on the palmar prominence of the scaphoid and wrapping his fingers around the distal radius. The examiner's other hand grasps at the metacarpal level, controlling wrist position. Starting in ulnar deviation and slight extension, the wrist is moved radially and slightly flexed, with constant pressure on the scaphoid.	Sensitivity: 69 Specificity: 64
Shear test to assess the lunate triquetral ligament	The examiner's contralateral fingers are placed over the dorsum of the lunate. With the lunate supported, the examiner's ipsilateral thumb loads the pisotriquetral joint from the palmar aspect, creating a shear force at the lunate-triquetral joint.	Unavailable
Ulnocarpal stress	Pronation and supination of the forearm with ulnar deviation of the hand generally evokes the wrist symptoms.	Unavailable
Finkelstein test	This test is positive if there is pain at the styloid process of the radius as the patient places the thumb within the hand, which is held tightly by the fingers, followed by ulnar deviation of the hand.	Sensitivity: 81[2] Specificity: 50
Thumb basilar joint grind test	The basal joint grind test is performed by stabilizing the triquetrum with the thumb and index finger and then dorsally subluxing the thumb metacarpal on the trapezium while providing compressive force with the other hand.	Sensitivity: 30[20] Specificity: 96.7
Median Nerve Tests at the Wrist		
Carpal compression test	This test consists of gentle, sustained, firm pressure to the median nerve of each hand simultaneously. Within a short time (15 seconds to 2 minutes) the patient will complain of reproduction of pain, paresthesia, and/or numbness in the symptomatic wrist(s).	Sensitivity: 87 Specificity: 90
Phalen test (wrist flexion)	This test is positive if there is numbness and paresthesia in the fingers. The patient is asked to hold the forearms vertically and to allow both hands to drop into flexion at the wrist for approximately 1 minute.	Sensitivity: 67-88 Specificity: 20-86
Wrist extension test (reverse Phalen test)	The patient is asked to keep both wrists in complete dorsal extension for 1 minute. If numbness and tingling were produced or exaggerated in the median nerve distribution of the hand within 60 seconds, the test is judged to be positive.	Sensitivity: 43 Specificity: 74
Tinel's sign at the wrist	This test is positive if there is numbness and paresthesia in the fingers. It is done by extending the wrist and tapping in a proximal to distal direction over the median nerve as it passes through the carpal tunnel, from the area of the distal wrist crease, 2 to 3 cm toward the area between the thenar and hypothenar eminences.	Sensitivity: 25-44 Specificity: 94-98
Lumbar Spine Motion Tests		
Schober test	The first sacral spinous process is marked, and a mark is made about 10 cm above this mark. The patient then flexes forward, and the increased distance is measured.	Unavailable
Modified Schober test	A point is drawn with a skin marker at the spinal intersection of a line joining the dimples of Venus (S1). Additional marks are made 10 cm above and 5 cm below S1. Subjects are asked to bend forward, and the distance between the marks 10 cm above and 5 cm below S1 is measured.	Specificity: 95 Sensitivity: 25
Lumbar Disk Herniation Tests		
Straight-leg raise	The supine patient's leg is raised with the knee extended until the patient begins to feel pain and the type and distribution of the pain as well as the angle of elevation are recorded. The test is positive when the angle is between 30 degrees and 70 degrees and pain is reproduced down the posterior thigh below the knee.	Sensitivity: 72-97 Specificity: 11-66
Crossed straight-leg raise	The supine patient's contralateral leg is raised with the knee extended until the patient begins to feel pain in the ipsilateral leg, and the type and distribution of the pain as well as the angle of elevation are recorded. The test is positive when the angle is between 30 degrees and 70 degrees and pain is reproduced down the ipsilateral posterior thigh below the knee.	Sensitivity: 23-29 Specificity: 88-100
Bowstring sign	After a positive straight-leg raise, the knee is slightly flexed while pressure is applied to the tibial nerve in the popliteal fossa. Compression of the sciatic nerve reproduces leg pain.	Sensitivity: 71
Slump test	The patient is seated with legs together and knees against the examining table. The patient slumps forward as far as possible, and the examiner applies firm pressure to bow the patient's back while keeping sacrum vertical. The patient is then asked to flex the head, and pressure is added to the neck flexion. Lastly, the examiner asks the patient to extend the knee, and dorsiflexion at the ankle is added.	Sensitivity: 84[60] Specificity: 83

Table 1-9 Musculoskeletal Provocative Maneuvers (Continued)

Test	Description	Reliability (%)
Ankle dorsiflexion test (Bragard sign)	After a positive straight-leg raise, the leg is dropped to a nonpainful range, and the ipsilateral ankle is dorsiflexed, reproducing the leg pain.	Sensitivity: 78-94
Femoral nerve stretch test	With the patient prone, the knee is dorsiflexed. Pain is produced in the anterior aspect of the thigh and/or back.	Sensitivity: 84-95
Sacroiliac Joint Disorder Tests		
Standing flexion test	This test is performed with the patient standing, facing away from the examiner with the patient's feet approximately 12 inches apart so that the patient's feet are parallel and approximately acetabular distance apart. The examiner's thumbs are then placed on the inferior aspect of each posterior superior iliac spine (PSIS). The patient is asked to bend forward with both knees extended. The extent of the cephalad movement of each PSIS is monitored. Normally, the PSIS should move equally. If one PSIS moves superiorly and anteriorly compared with the other, this is the side of restriction.	Sensitivity: 17[57] Specificity: 79
Seated flexion test	This test is performed with the patient seated with both feet on the floor. The examiner stands or sits behind the patient with the eyes at the level of the iliac crests and the examiner's thumbs are placed on each PSIS; the patient is instructed to flex forward. The test is positive if one PSIS moves unequally cephalad with respect to the other PSIS. The side with the greatest cephalad excursion implies articular restriction and hypomobility. While the patient is seated, the innominates are fixed in place, thus isolating out iliac motion.	Sensitivity: 9[57] Specificity: 93
Gillet test (One-leg Stork test)	This test is performed with the patient standing, facing away from the examiner, with the feet approximately 12 inches apart. The examiner's thumbs are placed on each PSIS. The patient is then asked to stand on one leg while flexing the contralateral hip and knee to the chest.	Sensitivity: 8[57] Specificity: 93
Compression test	The examiner places both hands on the patient's anterior superior iliac spine (ASIS) and exerts a medial force bilaterally to implement the test. The compression test is more frequently performed with the patient in a side-lying position. The examiner stands behind the patient and exerts a downward force at the upper part of the iliac crest.	Sensitivity: 69[55] Specificity: 69
Gapping test (Distraction)	This test is performed with the patient in a supine position. The examiner places the heel of both hands at the same time on each ASIS, pressing downward and laterally.	Sensitivity: 11-21[89] Specificity: 90-100
Patrick (FABERE) test	With the patient supine on a level surface, the thigh is flexed and the ankle is placed above the patella of the opposite extended leg. As the knee is depressed, with the ankle maintaining its position above the opposite knee, the opposite ASIS is pressed, and the patient will complain of pain before the knee reaches the level obtained in normal persons.	Sensitivity: 71[13] Specificity: 100
Gaenslen test	The patient lies supine, flexes the ipsilateral knee and hip against the chest with the aid of both hands clasped about the flexed knee. This brings the lumbar spine firmly in contact with the table and fixes both the pelvis and lumbar spine. The patient is then brought well to the side of the table, and the opposite thigh is slowly hyperextended with gradually increasing force by pressure of the examiner's hand on the top of the knee. With the opposite hand, the examiner assists the patient in fixing the lumbar spine and pelvis by pressure over the patient's clasped hands. The hyperextension of the hip exerts a rotating force on the corresponding half of the pelvis in the sagittal plane through the transverse axis of the sacroiliac joint. The rotating force causes abnormal mobility accompanied by pain, either local or referred on the side of the lesion.	Sensitivity: 50-53[55] Specificity: 71-77
Shear test	This test consists of the patient lying in the prone position, and the examiner applies pressure to the sacrum near the coccygeal end, directly cranially. The ilium is held immobile through the hip joint as the examiner applies counter pressure against legs in the form of traction force directed caudad. The test is considered positive if the maneuver aggravates the patient's typical pain.	Sensitivity: 63[55] Specificity: 75
Fortin finger test	The patient is asked to point to the region of pain with one finger. It is positive if the patient can localize the pain with one finger to an area inferomedial to the PSIS within 1 cm and the patient consistently pointed to the same area over at least two trials.	Unavailable
Hip Tests		
Thomas test	The patient lies supine while the examiner checks for excessive lordosis. The examiner flexes one of the patient's hips, bringing the knee to the chest, flattening out the lumbar spine while the patient holds the flexed hip against the chest. If there is no flexion contracture, the hip being tested (the straight leg) remains on the examining table. If a contracture is present, the patient's leg rises off the table. The angle of the contracture can be measured.	Unavailable
Ely test	The patient lies prone while the examiner passively flexes the patient's knee. Upon flexion of the knee, the patient's hip on the same side spontaneously flexes, indicating that the rectus femoris muscle is tight on that side and that the test is positive. The two sides should be tested and compared.	Sensitivity: 56-59[63] Specificity: 64-85

Continued on following page

Table 1-9 Musculoskeletal Provocative Maneuvers (Continued)

Test	Description	Reliability (%)
Ober test	The patient lies on one side with the thigh next to the table flexed to obliterate any lumbar lordosis. The upper leg is flexed at a right angle at the knee. The examiner grasps the ankle lightly with one hand and steadies the patient's hip with the other. The upper leg is abducted widely and extended so that the thigh is in line with the body. If there is an abduction contracture, the leg will remain more or less passively abducted.	Unavailable
Piriformis test	The patient is placed in the side-lying position with the non–test leg against the table. The patient flexes the test hip to 60 degrees with the knee flexed while the examiner applies downward pressure to the knee. Pain is elicited in the muscle if the piriformis is tight.	Sensitivity: 88[30] Specificity: 83
Trendelenburg test	The patient is observed standing on one limb. The test is felt to be positive if the pelvis on the opposite side drops. A positive Trendelenburg test is suggestive of a weak gluteus muscle or an unstable hip on the affected side.	Sensitivity: 72.7 Specificity: 76.9
Patrick (FABERE) test	See earlier (Sacroiliac Joint Disorder Tests).	See above
Stinchfield test	With the patient supine and the knee extended, the examiner resists the patient's hip flexion at 20 to 30 degrees. Reproduction of groin pain is considered a positive test indicating intraarticular hip dysfunction.	Sensitivity: 59[66] Specificity: 32
Anterior Cruciate Ligament Tests		
Anterior drawer test	The patient is supine, hip flexed to 45 degrees with the knee flexed to 90 degrees. The examiner sits on the patient's foot, with hands behind the proximal tibia and thumbs on the tibial plateau. Anterior force is applied to the proximal tibia. Hamstring tendons are palpated with index fingers to ensure relaxation. Increased tibial displacement compared with the opposite side is indicative of an anterior cruciate ligament tear.	Sensitivity: 22-70 Specificity: 97
Lachman test	The patient lies supine. The knee is held between full extension and 15 degrees of flexion. The femur is stabilized with one hand while firm pressure is applied to the posterior aspect of the proximal tibia in an attempt to translate it anteriorly.	Sensitivity: 85[9] Specificity: 94
Pivot shift test	The leg is picked up at the ankle. The knee is flexed by placing the heel of the hand behind the fibula. As the knee is extended, the tibia is supported on the lateral side with a slight valgus strain. A strong valgus force is placed on the knee by the upper hand. At approximately 30 degrees of flexion, the displaced tibia will suddenly reduce, indicating a positive pivot shift test.	Sensitivity: 35-95 Specificity: 98-100
Posterior Cruciate Ligament Tests		
Posterior sag sign	The patient lies supine with the hip flexed to 45 degrees and the knee flexed to 90 degrees. In this position, the tibia "rocks back," or sags back, on the femur if the posterior cruciate ligament is torn. Normally, the medial tibial plateau extends 1 cm anteriorly beyond the femoral condyle when the knee is flexed 90 degrees.	Sensitivity: 79 Specificity: 100
Posterior drawer test	The patient is supine with the test hip flexed to 45 degrees, knee flexed to 90 degrees, and foot in neutral position. The examiner sits on the patient's foot with both hands behind the patient's proximal tibia and thumbs on the tibial plateau. Posterior force is applied to the proximal tibia. Increased posterior tibial displacement as compared with the uninvolved side is indicative of a partial or complete tear of the posterior cruciate ligament.	Sensitivity: 90 Specificity: 99
Patellofemoral Tests		
Patellar grind test (compression test)	The patient is supine with the knees extended. The examiner stands next to the involved side and places the web space of the thumb on the superior border of the patella. The patient is asked to contract the quadriceps muscle while the examiner applies downward and inferior pressure on the patella. Pain with movement of the patella or an inability to complete the test is indicative of patellofemoral dysfunction.	Unavailable
Knee Meniscal Injury Tests		
Joint line tenderness	The medial joint line is easier to palpate with internal rotation of the tibia, allowing for easier palpation. Alternatively, external rotation allows improved palpation of the lateral meniscus.	Sensitivity: 63 Specificity: 77[43]
McMurray test	With the patient lying flat, the knee is first fully flexed; the foot is held by grasping the heel. The leg is rotated on the thigh with the knee still in full flexion. By altering the position of flexion, the whole of the posterior segment of the cartilages can be examined from the middle to the posterior attachment. The leg is brought from its position of acute flexion to a right angle while the foot is retained first in full internal rotation and then in full external rotation. When the click occurs (in association with a torn meniscus), the patient is able to state that the sensation is the same as experienced when the knee gave way previously.	Sensitivity: 70 Specificity: 71[43]
Apley grind test	With the patient prone, the examiner grasps one foot in each hand and externally rotates as far as possible, then flexes both knees together to their limit. The feet are then rotated inward and knees extended. The examiner's left knee is then applied to the back of the patient's thigh. The foot is grasped in both hands, the knee is bent to a right angle, and powerful external rotation is applied. Next, the patient's leg is strongly pulled up, with the femur being prevented from rising off the couch. In this position of distraction, external rotation is repeated. The examiner leans over the patient and compresses the tibia downward. Again, the examiner rotates powerfully and if addition of compression produces an increase of pain, this grinding test is positive and meniscal damage is diagnosed.	Sensitivity: 60 Specificity: 70[43]

Table 1-9 Musculoskeletal Provocative Maneuvers (Continued)

Test	Description	Reliability (%)
Ankle Stability Tests		
Anterior drawer test	With the patient relaxed, the knee is flexed and the ankle at right angles, the ankle is grasped on the tibial side by one hand, and the index finger is placed on the posteromedial part of the talus and the middle finger lies on the posterior tibial malleolus. The heel of this hand braces the anterior distal leg. On pulling the heel forward with the other hand, relative anteroposterior motion between the two fingers (and thus between talus and tibia) is easily palpated and is also visible to both the patient and examiner.	Sensitivity: 80-95 Specificity: 74-84
Talar tilt	The talar tilt angle is the angle formed by the opposing articular surfaces of the tibia and talus when these surfaces are separated laterally by a supination force applied to the hind part of the foot.	Unavailable
Syndesmosis Tests		
Syndesmosis squeeze test	The squeeze test is performed by manually compressing the fibula to the tibia above the midpoint of the calf. A positive test produces pain over the area of the syndesmotic ligaments.	Sensitivity: 30[26] Specificity 93.5
Achilles Tendon Rupture Tests		
Thompson test	The patient lies in a prone position with the foot extending over the end of the table. The calf muscles are squeezed in the middle one third below the place of the widest girth. Passive plantar movement of the foot is seen in a normal reaction. A positive reaction is seen when there is no plantar movement of the foot and indicates rupture of the Achilles tendon.	Sensitivity: 96 Specificity: 93
Palpation test	The examiner gently palpates the course of the tendon. A gap indicates an Achilles tendon rupture.	Sensitivity: 73 Specificity: 89

Modified from Malanga GA, Nadler SF, editors: *Musculoskeletal physical examination: an evidence-based approach*, Philadelphia, Mosby, 2006.

Table 1-10 Types of "End Feels" in Range-of-Motion Testing

End Feel	Normal	Example(s)	Abnormal	Example(s)
Soft	Soft tissue approximation	Knee flexion	Tissue change occurring sooner or later than expected A change in a joint that normally has a firm or hard end feel	Soft tissue edema Synovitis
Firm	Muscular stretch Capsular stretch Ligamentous stretch	Hip flexion Metacarpophalangeal extension Forearm supination	Tissue change occurring sooner or later than expected A change in a joint that normally has a soft or hard end feel	Increased muscular tonus Contracture of capsular, muscular, or ligamentous structures
Hard	Bone contacting bone	Elbow extension	Tissue change occurring sooner or later than expected A change in a joint that normally has a soft or firm end feel	Osteoarthritis Loose bodies in the joint Fracture
Empty	Abnormal joint end feel	—	No end feel noted as a result of resistance caused by pain	Acute joint inflammation Bursitis Abscess Fracture Psychogenic disorder

Modified from Norkin CC, White J: *Measurement of joint motion: a guide to goniometry*, ed 3, Philadelphia, FA Davis, 2003, with permission of FA Davis.

Joint play or capsular patterns assess the integrity of the capsule in positions of minimal bony contact, sometimes referred to as open-packed position.[74] Active ROM (AROM) or voluntary movement of a joint is insufficient to exploit the full ROM for that joint. More extreme end ROM that is not under voluntary control must be assessed by the examiner through passive ROM (PROM) testing. There are several types of end feels when the terminal feel of a joint is evaluated through the extremes of its ROM (Table 1-10). Soft end feel is commonly associated with tissue compression and is normal in extreme elbow or knee flexion with PROM testing. If the sensation, however, is felt prematurely (before the expected full PROM), the cause may be pathologic, such as from inflammation or edema. If tissue (muscle, capsule, or ligament) is stretched at the end of ROM, the resultant end feel is one that is firm yet slightly forgiving, such as with terminal passive metacarpophalangeal extension and hip flexion. Palpation of a premature firm end feel can be a sign of increased tone or capsular tightening. A hard end feel is felt as a result of bony contact and is felt normally with elbow extension or knee extension. If a hard end feel is felt prematurely or inappropriately, it may indicate an arthritic joint or heterotopic ossification. An "empty" feel does not suggest a mechanical restriction but is rather a limitation in ROM due to muscle contraction generated by the patient to guard against pain.

It is important to identify both hypomobile and hypermobile joints. The former increase the risk for muscle strains, tendonitis, and nerve entrapments, whereas the latter increase the risk for joint sprains and degenerative joint disease.[74] An inflammatory synovitis, for example, can increase joint mobility and weaken the capsule (it tightens the capsule acutely and weakens it chronically). In the setting of decreased muscle strength, the risk of trauma and joint instability is increased.[67] If joint instability is suspected, confirmatory diagnostic testing can be done (e.g., radiography)—for example, flexion-extension spine films to assess vertebral column instability or magnetic resonance imaging to visualize the degree of anterior cruciate ligament rupture.[25,46,51,59]

Assessment of Range of Motion General Principles. ROM testing is used to assess the integrity of a joint, to monitor the efficacy of treatment regimens, and to determine the mechanical cause of an impairment.[51] Limitations not only affect ambulation and mobility but also ADL. Normal ROM varies according to age, gender, conditioning, body habitus, and genetics.[67] Males typically have a more limited range when compared with females, depending on age and specific joint action.[8] Vocational and avocational patterns of activity can also alter ROM. For example, gymnasts generally have increased ROM at the hips and lower trunk.[74] Passive ROM should be performed through all planes of motion (sagittal, coronal, and transverse) by the examiner in a relaxed patient to thoroughly assess end feel.[74] Active ROM is performed by the patient through all planes of motion without assistance from the examiner and evaluates muscle strength, coordination of movement, and functional ability.

Contractures are often visualized during inspection because they affect the true full ROM of a joint via either soft tissue or bony changes. A soft tissue or muscle contracture decreases with a prolonged stretch, whereas a bony limitation does not. It can be difficult or impossible to differentiate a contracture from severe hypertonia in certain CNS diseases. A diagnostic peripheral nerve block can eliminate the hypertonia for a few hours to determine the etiology of the contracture and guide the correct treatment for impaired mobility or ADL.

Assessment Techniques. As previously mentioned, ROM is a function of joint morphology, capsule and ligament integrity, and muscle and tendon strength.[74,81] Range is measured with a universal goniometer, a device that has a pivoting arm attached to a stationary arm divided into 1-degree intervals (Figure 1-3). Regardless of the type of goniometer used, reliability is increased by knowing and using consistent surface landmarks and test positions.[34] Joints are measured in their plane of movement with the stationary arm parallel to the long axis of the proximal body segment or bony landmark.[74] The moving arm of the goniometer should also be aligned with a bony landmark or parallel to the moving body segment. The impaired joint should always be compared with the contralateral unimpaired joint, if possible.

Sagittal, coronal, and transverse planes divide the body into three cardinal planes of motion (Figure 1-4). The sagittal plane divides the body into left and right halves, the coronal (frontal) plane into anterior and posterior halves, and the transverse plane into superior and inferior parts.[34] For sagittal plane measurements, the goniometer is placed on the lateral side of the joint, except for a few joint motions, such as forearm supination and pronation. Coronal planes are measured anteriorly or posteriorly, with the axis coinciding with the axis of the joint.

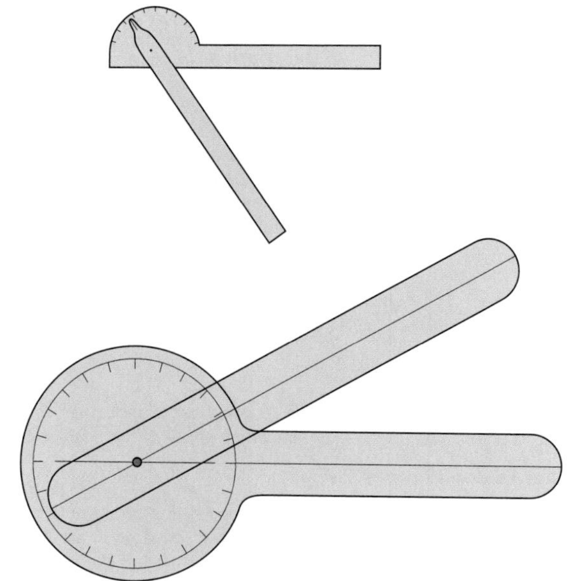

FIGURE 1-3 Universal goniometer. (Redrawn from Kottke FJ, Lehman JF: *Krusen's handbook of physical medicine*, ed 4, Philadelphia, 1990, Saunders; with permission.)

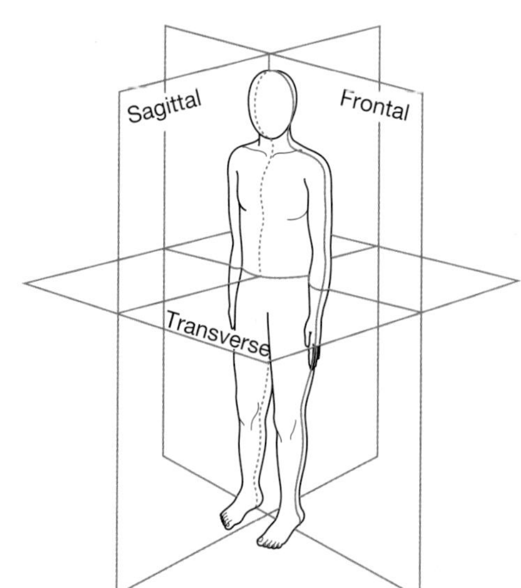

FIGURE 1-4 Cardinal planes of motion.

The 360-degree system was first proposed by Knapp and West[52,53] and denotes 0 degrees directly overhead and 180 degrees at the feet. In the 360-degree system, shoulder forward flexion and extension ranges from 0 to 240 degrees (Figure 1-5, *A*). The American Academy of Orthopedic Surgeons uses a 180-degree system.[70] The standard anatomic position[16] is described as an upright position with the feet facing forward, the arms at the side with the palms facing anterior.[34] A joint at 0 degrees is in the anatomic position, with movement occurring up to 180 degrees away from 0 degrees in either direction.[34] With the use of shoulder forward flexion as an example, the normal range for flexion in the 180-degree system is 0 to 180 degrees, and for extension is 0 to 60 degrees (Figure 1-5, *B*). These standardized techniques have been well described.*

*References 3, 21, 34, 45, 46, 56, 74.

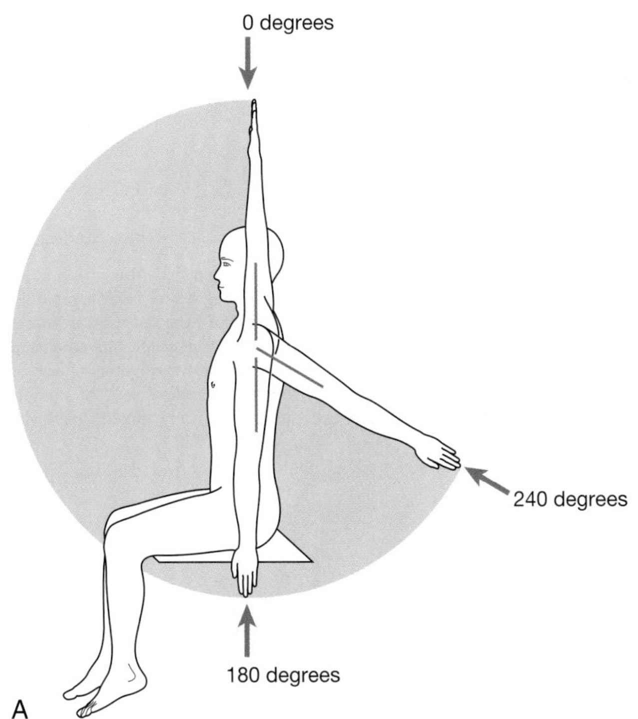

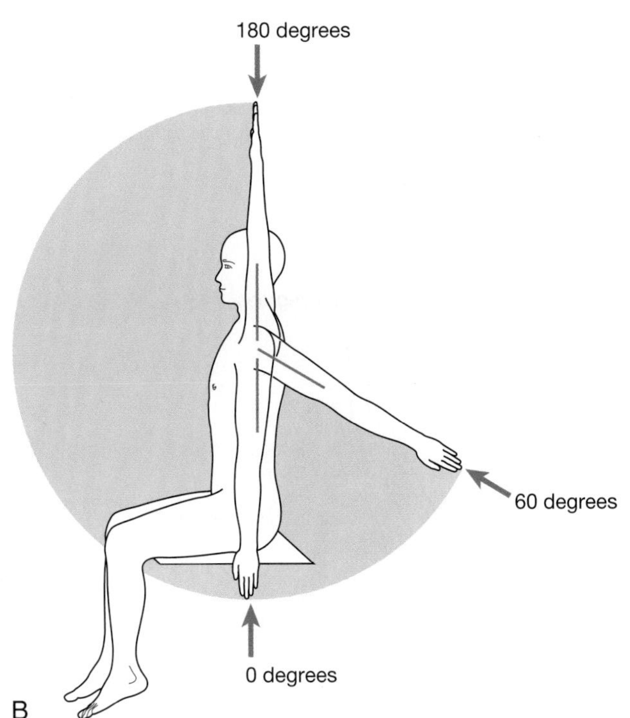

FIGURE 1-5 Comparison of two range-of-motion systems.

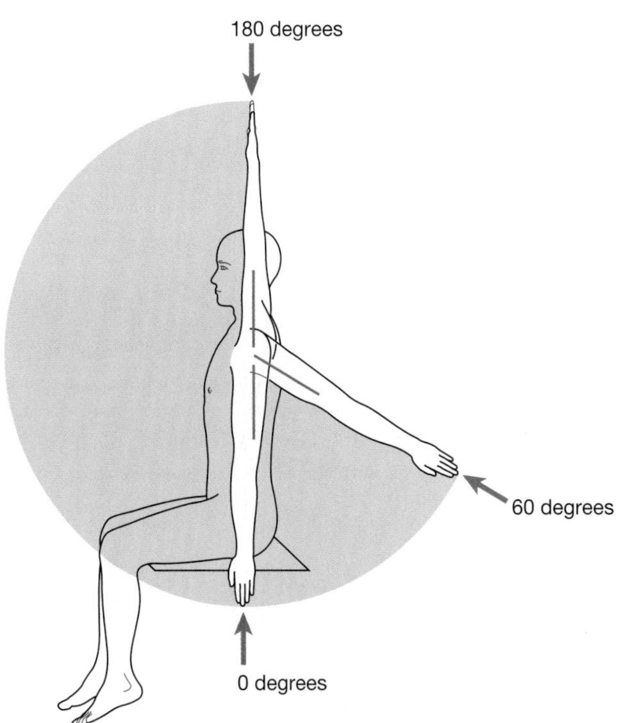

FIGURE 1-6 Shoulder flexion and extension. Patient position: supine or sitting, arm at side, elbow extended. Plane of motion: sagittal. Normal range of motion: flexion, 0 to 180 degrees; extension, 0 to 60 degrees. Movements the patient should avoid: arching back, trunk rotation. Goniometer placement: axis is centered on the lateral shoulder, stationary arm remains at 0 degrees, movement arm remains parallel to humerus.

Figures 1-6 to 1-21 outline the correct patient positioning and plane of motion for the joint and goniometer placement. To increase accuracy, many practitioners recommend taking several measurements and recording a mean value.[74] Measurement inaccuracy can be as high as 10% to 30% in the limbs and can be difficult to quantify in the spine if based on visual assessment alone.[3,90] Spinal ROM is more difficult to measure, and its reliability has been debated.[34,45] The most accurate method of measuring spinal motion is with radiographs; however, this is not practical in most clinical scenarios. In the absence of radiographs, the next best system is based on inclinometers, fluid-filled instruments with a 180- or 360-degree scale.[3,45] The American Medical Association *Guides to the Evaluation of Permanent Impairment*[3] outlines the specific inclinometer techniques for measuring spinal ROM.

Assessment of Muscle Strength

General Principles. Manual muscle testing is used to establish baseline strength, to determine functional ability or the need for adaptive equipment, to confirm a diagnosis, and to suggest a prognosis.[74] Whereas *strength* is a rather generic term and can refer to a wide variety of assessments and testing situations,[6] manual muscle testing specifically measures the ability to voluntarily contract a muscle or muscle group at a specific joint. It is quantified with a system first described by Robert Lovett, M.D., an orthopedic surgeon, in the early twentieth century.[24] Isolated muscles can be difficult to assess. For example, elbow flexion strength depends not only on the biceps muscle but also on the brachialis and brachioradialis muscles. Strength is affected by many factors, including the number of motor units firing, functional excursion, cross-sectional area of the muscle, number of joints crossed, and patient effort.[6,67,74] Pain can result in give-way weakness and should be documented as such. It is important to recognize the presence of substitution when muscles are weak or movement is uncoordinated. Females typically increase strength up to age 20 years, plateau through the 20s, and gradually decline in strength after age 30 years. Males increase strength up

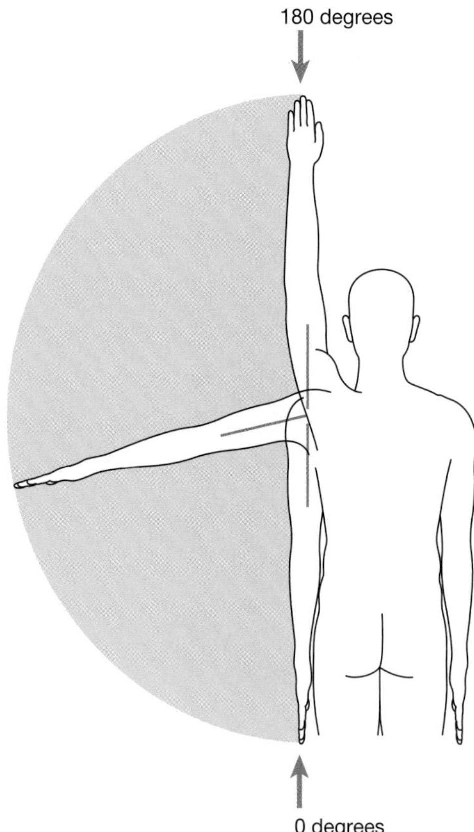

FIGURE 1-7 Shoulder abduction. Patient position: supine or sitting, arm at side, elbow extended. Plane of motion: frontal. Normal range of motion: 0 to 180 degrees. Movements the patient should avoid: trunk rotation or lateral movement. Goniometer placement: axis is centered on posterior or anterior shoulder, stationary arm remains at 0 degrees, movement arm remains parallel to humerus.

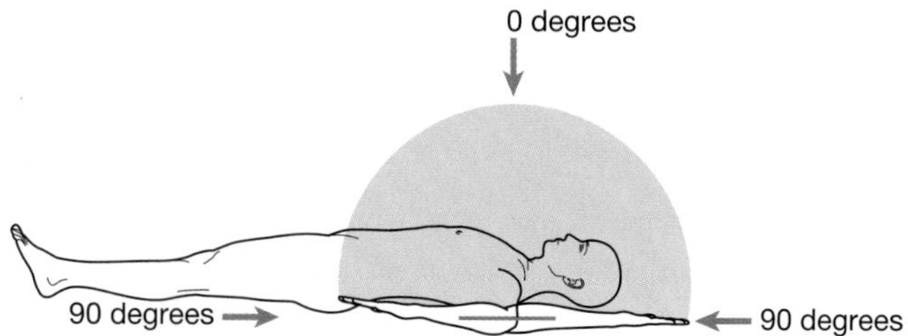

FIGURE 1-8 Shoulder internal and external rotation. Patient position: supine, shoulder at 90 degrees of abduction, elbow at 90 degrees of flexion, radioulnar joint pronated. Plane of motion: transverse. Normal range of motion: internal rotation, 0 to 90 degrees; external rotation, 0 to 90 degrees. Movements the patient should avoid: arching back, trunk rotation, elbow movement. Goniometer placement: axis on elbow joint through longitudinal axis of humerus, stationary arm remains at 0 degrees, movement arm remains parallel to forearm.

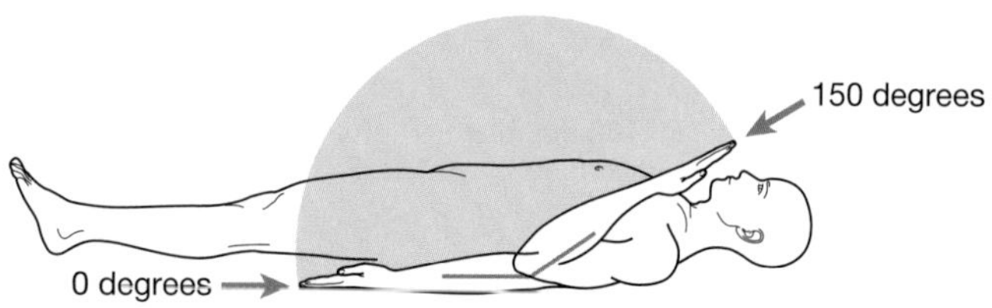

FIGURE 1-9 Elbow flexion. Patient position: supine or sitting, radioulnar joint supinated. Plane of motion: sagittal. Normal range of motion: 0 to 150 degrees. Goniometer placement: axis is centered on lateral elbow, stationary arm remains at 0 degrees, movement arm remains parallel to forearm.

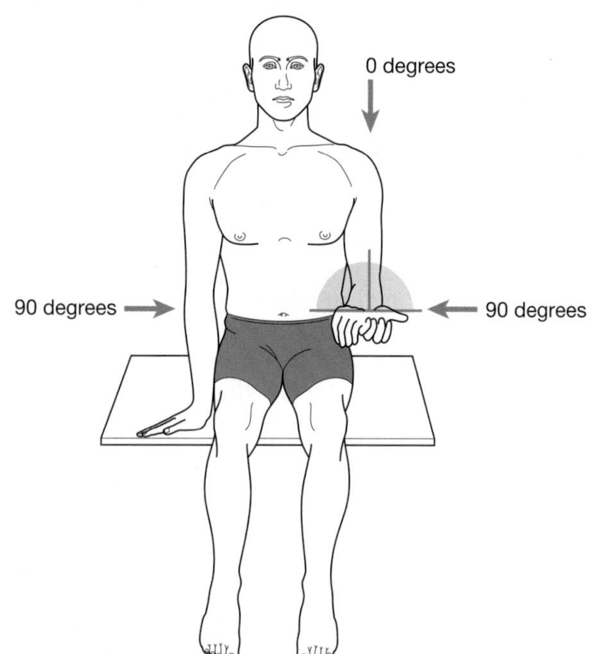

FIGURE 1-10 Radioulnar pronation and supination. Patient position: sitting or standing, elbow at 90 degrees, wrist in neutral, pencil held in palm of hand. Plane of motion: transverse. Normal range of motion: pronation, 0 degrees to 90 degrees; supination, 0 degrees to 90 degrees. Movements the patient should avoid: arm, elbow, and wrist movements. Goniometer placement: axis through longitudinal axis of forearm, stationary arm remains at 0 degrees, movement arm remains parallel to pencil held in patient's hand.

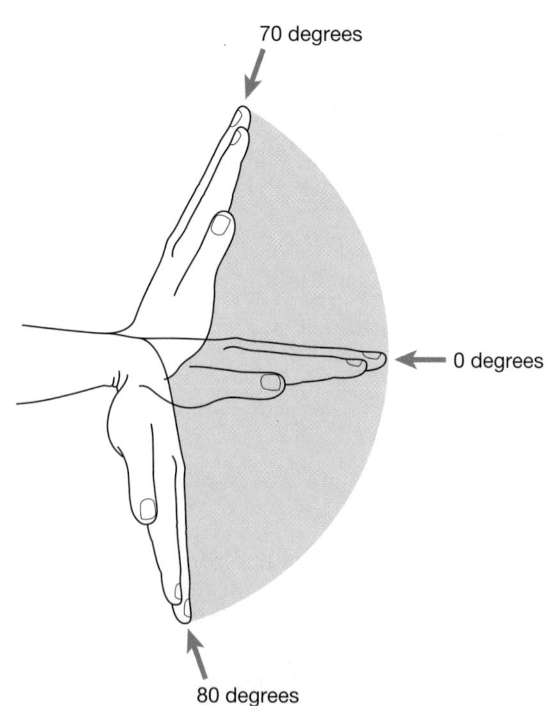

FIGURE 1-11 Wrist flexion and extension. Patient position: elbow flexed, radioulnar pronated. Plane of motion: sagittal. Normal range of motion: flexion, 0 to 80 degrees; extension, 0 to 70 degrees. Goniometer placement: axis is centered on lateral wrist over ulnar styloid, stationary arm remains at 0 degrees, movement arm remains parallel to fifth metacarpal.

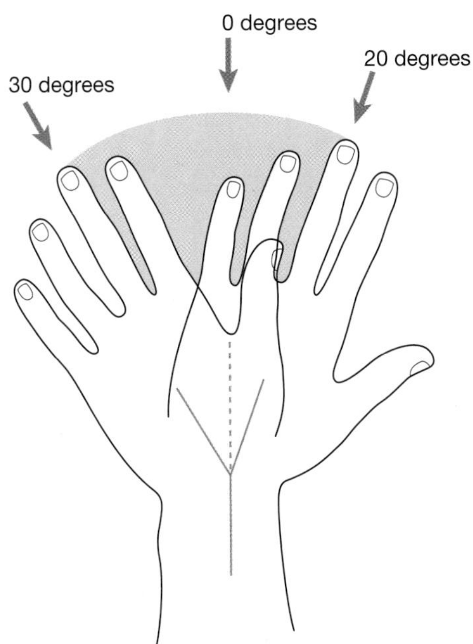

FIGURE 1-12 Wrist radial and ulnar deviation. Patient position: elbow flexed, radioulnar joint pronated, wrist in neutral flexion and extension. Plane of motion: frontal. Normal range of motion: radial, 0 to 20 degrees; ulnar, 0 to 30 degrees. Goniometer placement: axis is centered over dorsal wrist midway between distal radius and ulna, stationary arm remains at 0 degrees, movement arm remains parallel to third metacarpal.

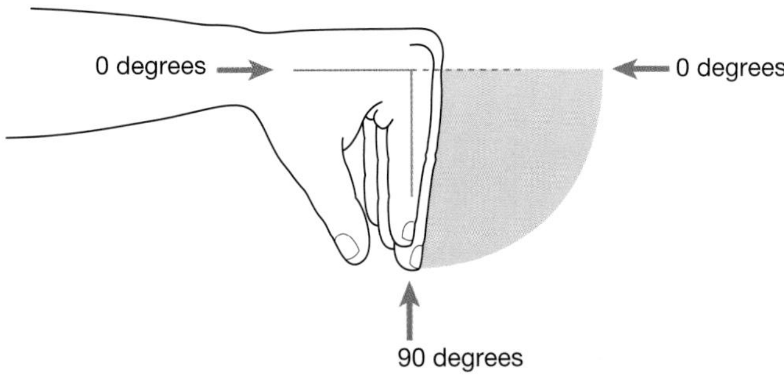

FIGURE 1-13 Second to fifth metacarpophalangeal flexion. Patient position: elbow flexed, radioulnar joint pronated, wrist in neutral, fingers extended. Plane of motion: sagittal. Normal range of motion: 0 to 90 degrees. Goniometer placement: axis on dorsum of each metacarpophalangeal joint, stationary arm remains at 0 degrees, movement arm remains on dorsum of each proximal phalanx.

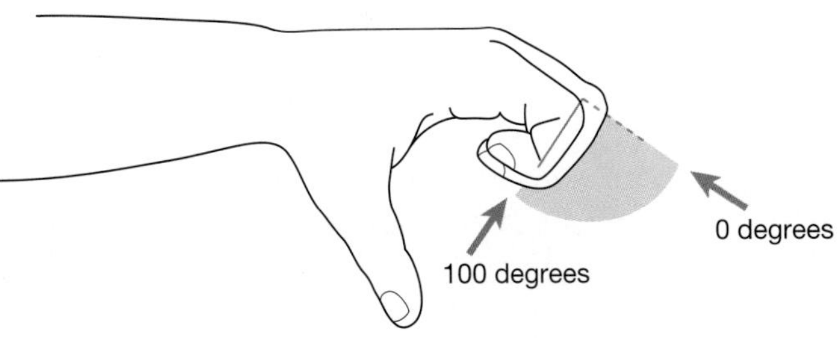

FIGURE 1-14 Second to fifth proximal interphalangeal flexion. Patient position: elbow flexed, radioulnar pronated, wrist in neutral, metacarpophalangeal joints in slight flexion. Plane of motion: sagittal. Normal range of motion: 0 to 100 degrees. Goniometer placement: axis on dorsum of each interphalangeal joint, stationary arm remains at 0 degrees, movement arm remains on dorsum of each middle phalanx.

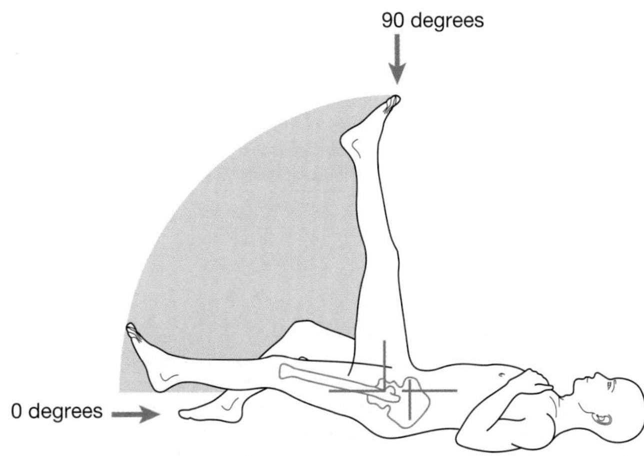

FIGURE 1-15 Hip flexion, knee extension. Patient position: supine or lying on side, knee extended. Plane of motion: sagittal. Normal range of motion: 0 to 90 degrees. Movements the patient should avoid: arching back. Goniometer placement: axis is centered on lateral leg over greater trochanter, stationary arm remains at 0 degrees. (This is found by drawing a line from the anterior superior iliac spine to the posterior superior iliac spine, and then drawing another line, perpendicular to the first, that goes through the greater trochanter. The last line is 0 degrees.) Movement arm remains parallel to lateral femur.

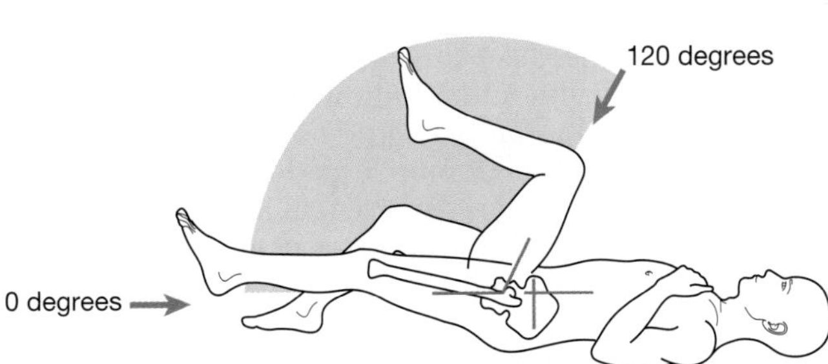

FIGURE 1-16 Hip flexion, knee flexion. Patient position: supine or lying on side, knee flexed. Plane of motion: sagittal. Normal range of motion: 0 degrees to 120 degrees. Movements the patient should avoid: arching back. Goniometer placement: axis centered over greater trochanter, stationary arm is parallel to and below a line on patient drawn through both anterior superior iliac spines (this is perpendicular to 0 degrees), movement arm remains parallel to anterior femur.

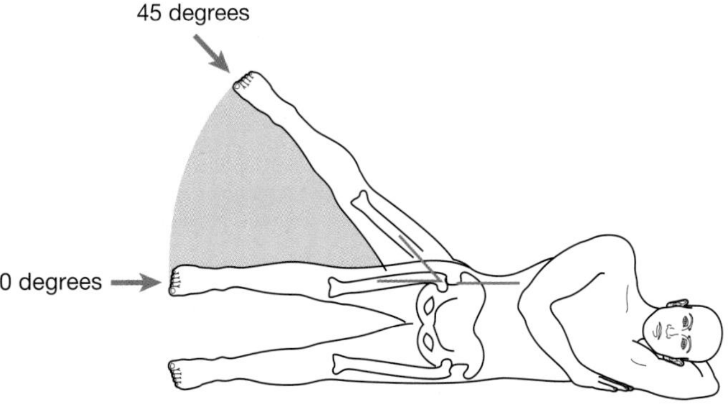

FIGURE 1-17 Hip abduction. Patient position: supine or lying on side, knee extended. Plane of motion: frontal. Normal range of motion: 0 degrees to 45 degrees. Movements the patient should avoid: trunk rotation. Goniometer placement: axis centered over greater trochanter, stationary arm is parallel to and below a line on patient drawn through both anterior superior iliac spines (this is perpendicular to 0 degrees), movement arm remains parallel to anterior femur.

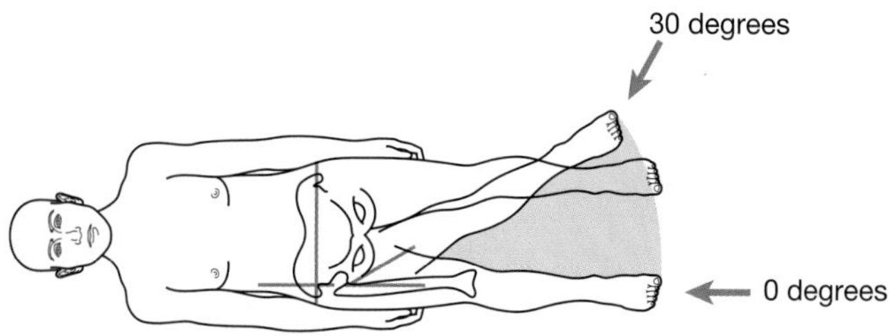

FIGURE 1-18 Hip adduction. Patient position: supine, knee extended. Plane of motion: frontal. Normal range of motion: 0 to 30 degrees. Movements the patient should avoid: trunk rotation. Goniometer placement: axis over knee joint through longitudinal axis of femur, stationary arm remains at 0 degrees, movement arm remains parallel to anterior tibia.

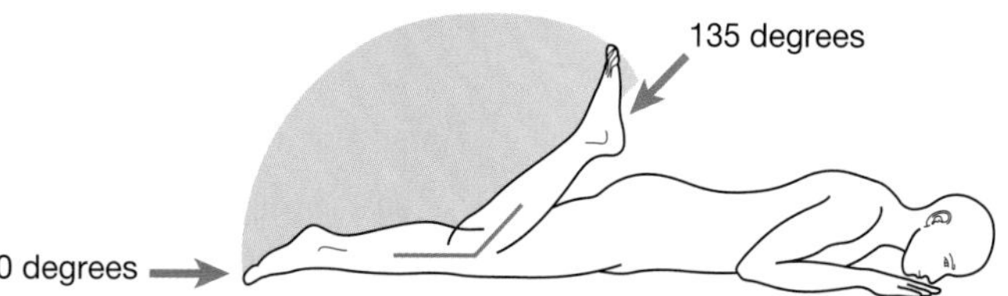

FIGURE 1-19 Knee flexion. Patient position: prone or sitting, hip in neutral. Plane of motion: sagittal. Normal range of motion: 0 to 135 degrees. Goniometer placement: axis on lateral knee joint, stationary arm remains at 0 degrees, movement arm remains parallel to fibula laterally.

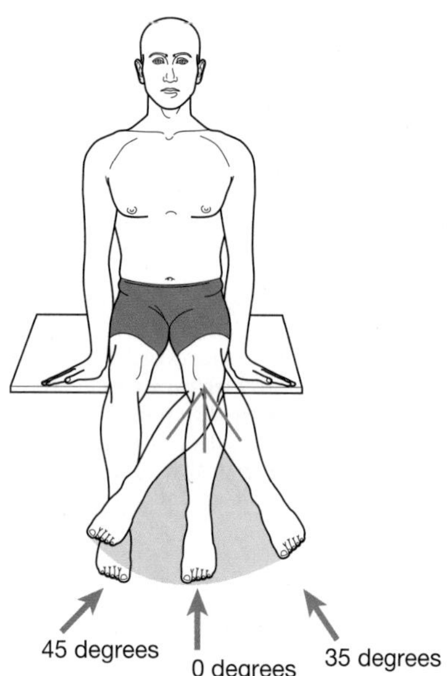

FIGURE 1-20 Hip internal and external rotation. Patient position: supine or sitting, hip at 90 degrees flexion, knee at 90 degrees flexion. Plane of motion: transverse. Normal range of motion: internal, 0 to 35 degrees; external, 0 to 45 degrees. Movements the patient should avoid: hip flexion movement, knee movement. Goniometer placement: axis over knee joint through longitudinal axis of femur, stationary arm remains at 0 degrees, movement arm remains parallel to anterior tibia.

to age 20 years, plateau until older than 30 years before declining.[74] Muscles that are predominantly type 1 or slow-twitch fibers (e.g., soleus muscle) tend to be fatigue resistant and can require extended stress on testing (such as several standing toe raises) to uncover weakness.[74] Type 2 or fast-twitch fibers (e.g., sternocleidomastoid) fatigue quickly, and weakness can be more straightforward to uncover abnormalities. Patients who cannot actively control muscle tension (e.g., those with spasticity from

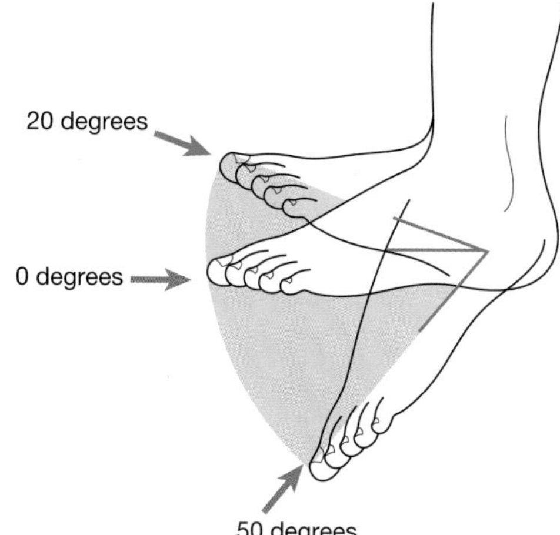

FIGURE 1-21 Ankle dorsiflexion and plantar flexion. Patient position: sitting or supine with knee flexed to 90 degrees. Plane of motion: sagittal. Normal range of motion: dorsiflexion, 0 to 20 degrees; plantar flexion, 0 to 50 degrees. Goniometer placement: axis is on sole of foot below lateral malleolus, stationary arm remains along shaft of fibula (this is perpendicular to 0 degrees), movement arm remains parallel to fifth metatarsal.

Table 1-11 Manual Muscle Testing

Grade	Term	Description
5	Normal	Full available ROM is achieved against gravity and is able to demonstrate maximal resistance.
4	Good	Full available ROM is achieved against gravity and is able to demonstrate moderate resistance.
3	Fair	Full available ROM is achieved against gravity *but* is not able to demonstrate resistance.
2	Poor	Full available ROM is achieved only with gravity eliminated.
1	Trace	A visible or palpable contraction is noted, with no joint movement.
0	Zero	No contraction is identified.

Modified from Cutter NC, Kevorkian CG: *Handbook of manual muscle testing,* New York 1999, :McGraw-Hill, with permission of McGraw-Hill.
ROM, Range of motion.

CNS disease) are not appropriate for standard manual muscle testing methods.[74]

Assessment Techniques. Manual muscle testing takes into account the weight of the limb without gravity, with gravity, and with gravity plus additional manual resistance.[74] Most examiners use the Medical Research Council Scale, where grades of 0 to 2 indicate gravity-minimized positions, and grades 3 to 5 indicate increasing degrees of resistance applied as an isometric hold at the end of the test range (Table 1-11).[74] A muscle grade of 3 is functionally important because antigravity strength implies that a limb can be used for activity, whereas a grade of less than 3 implies that the limb will require external support and is prone to contracture.[81] Interrater reliability is relatively consistent for grades 1 to 3. There is significant variability for muscle grades 4 and 5.[6] Other pitfalls encountered in testing strength are outlined in Table 1-12. For measurement errors to be reduced, one hand should be placed above and one below the joint being tested. As detailed in extended Tables 1-13 and 1-14, the examiner's hands

Text continued on p. 36

Table 1-12 Caveats in Manual Muscle Resting

Caveat	Rationale
Isolation	It is important to isolate individual muscles with similar functions instead of testing the entire muscle group.
Substitution patterns	It is important to be aware of basic substitution patterns (e.g., elbow flexion).
Suboptimal testing conditions	These occur when determining patients' muscle strength when they are under the influence of, for example, sedation, significant pain, positioning, language or cultural barriers, spasticity, and hypertonicity.
Overgrading	This occurs when the examiner applies increased force when the patient is unable to achieve the full available ROM yet is able to demonstrate a muscle grade of 3 or more in a lengthened position.
Undergrading	This occurs when the examiner is not aware of the effects of muscle contracture on ROM and the muscle appears to lack full ROM when it has achieved its full available ROM.

Modified from Cutter NC, Kevorkian CG: *Handbook of manual muscle testing*, New York, 1999, McGraw-Hill, with permission of McGraw-Hill.
ROM, Range of motion.

Table 1-13 Upper Limb Muscle Testing

Upper Limb Chart	Muscle*	Nerve, Roots	Plexus	Manual Muscle Testing Technique	Figure
Shoulder flexion	*Deltoid, anterior portion* Pectoralis major, clavicular portion Biceps brachii Coracobrachialis	Axillary, C5, C6 Medial or lateral pectoral, C5-T1 Musculocutaneous, C5, C6 Musculocutaneous, C5-C7	Posterior cord — Lateral cord	• The shoulder is flexed to 90 degrees with the elbow flexed at 90 degrees. • The practitioner should attempt to force the arm into extension, with force applied over the distal humerus.	
Extension	*Deltoid, posterior portion* Latissimus dorsi Teres major	Axillary, C5, C6 Thoracodorsal, C6-C8 Lower subscapular, C5, C6	Posterior cord	• The shoulder is extended to 45 degrees with the elbow extended. • The practitioner attempts to force the arm into flexion, with force applied over the distal humerus.	
Abduction	*Deltoid, middle portion* Supraspinatus	Axillary, C5, C6 Suprascapular, C5, C6	Posterior cord Upper trunk	• The shoulder is placed in 90 degrees of abduction. • The practitioner attempts to adduct the arm, with force applied over the distal humerus.	
Adduction	*Pectoralis major* Latissimus dorsi Teres major	Medial or lateral pectoral, C5-T1 Thoracodorsal, C6-C8 Lower subscapular, C5, C6	— Posterior cord	• The patient is supine with the shoulder in 120 degrees of abduction and the elbow flexed. • The practitioner resists adduction of the arm.	
Internal rotation	*Subscapularis* Pectoralis major Latissimus dorsi Deltoid, anterior portion Teres major	Upper or lower subscapular, C5, C6 Medial or lateral pectoral, C5-T1 Thoracodorsal, C6-C8 Axillary, C5, C6 Lower subscapular, C5, C6	Posterior cord — Posterior cord	• The patient is prone and the shoulder is abducted to 90 degrees with full internal rotation and the elbow at 90 degrees of flexion. • The practitioner attempts to externally rotate the arm, applying force over the distal forearm.	

Continued on following page

Table 1-13 Upper Limb Muscle Testing (Continued)

Upper Limb Chart	Muscle*	Nerve, Roots	Plexus	Manual Muscle Testing Technique	Figure
External rotation	*Infraspinatus*	Suprascapular, C5, C6	Upper trunk	• The patient is prone and the shoulder is placed in 90 degrees of abduction with full external rotation and the elbow at 90 degrees of flexion. • The practitioner attempts to internally rotate the arm, applying force over the distal forearm.	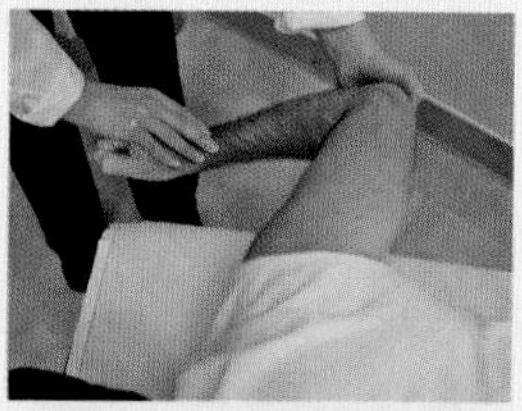
	Teres minor Deltoid, posterior portion	Axillary, C5, C6	Posterior cord		
Elbow flexion	*Biceps brachii* Brachialis	Musculocutaneous, C5, C6	Lateral cord	• The elbow is positioned in 90 degrees of flexion. • The practitioner attempts to extend the elbow, applying force over the distal forearm. • The biceps muscle is the primary elbow flexor, with full forearm supination. • The brachialis is the primary flexor, with full forearm pronation.	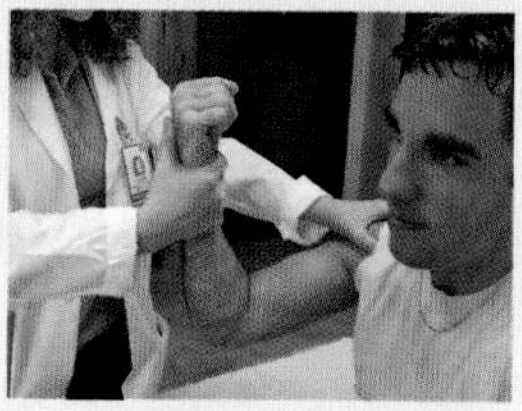
	Brachioradialis	Radial, C5, C6	Posterior cord	• The brachioradialis is the primary elbow flexor when the forearm is in a thumbs-up position.	
Extension	*Triceps*	Radial, C6-C8	Posterior cord	• The elbow is placed into flexion to prevent stabilization and to detect subtle weakness. • The practitioner attempts to flex the elbow, applying force over the distal forearm.	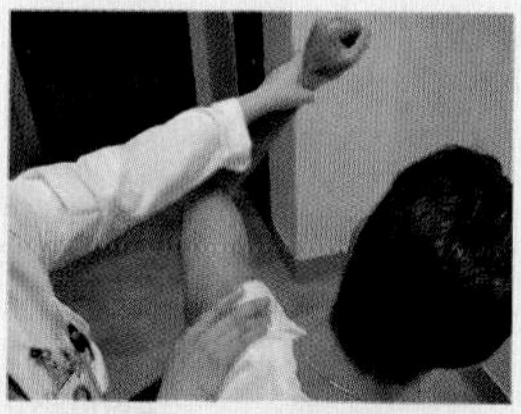
Forearm pronation	*Pronator quadratus*	Anterior interosseus branch of median, C8, T1	—	• The forearm is placed in full pronation. • The practitioner attempts to supinate the forearm, applying force to the distal forearm. • The pronator teres is tested when the elbow is at 90 degrees. • The pronator quadratus is tested when the elbow is in full flexion.	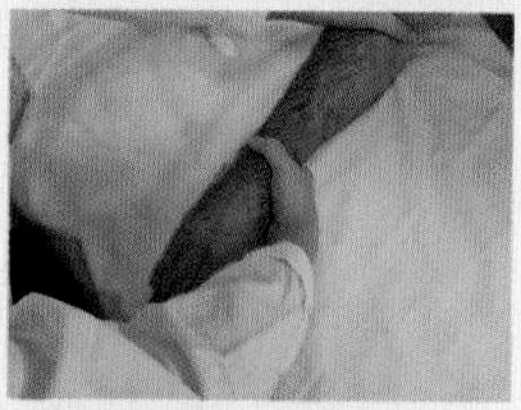
	Pronator teres	Median, C6, C7	Lateral cord		
Forearm supination	*Supinator*	Radial (posterior interosseus nerve), C5, C6	Posterior cord	• The elbow is extended with the forearm in full supination. This position inhibits assistance from the biceps. • The practitioner attempts to pronate the forearm, applying force to the distal forearm.	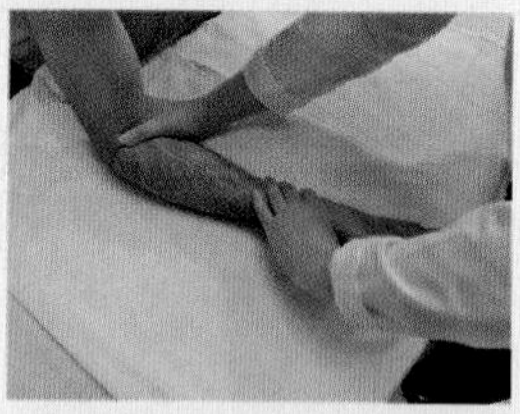
	Biceps brachii	Musculocutaneous, C5, C6	Lateral cord		
Wrist flexion	*Flexor carpi radialis*	Median, C6-C8	Lateral cord	• The wrist is placed in neutral position in full flexion, with the fingers extended. • The practitioner attempts to extend the wrist, applying force at the midpalm level. • The flexor carpi radialis is tested by placing the wrist in radial deviation and full flexion. The practitioner attempts to force the wrist into extension and ulnar deviation.	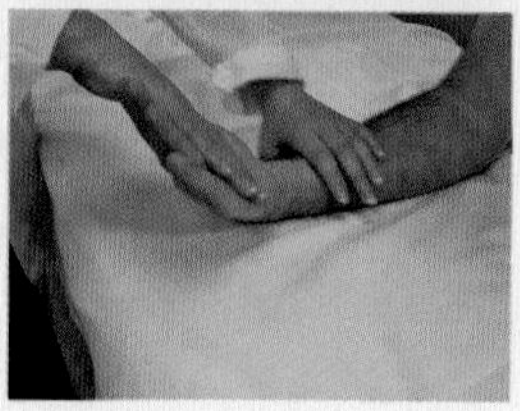
	Flexor carpi ulnaris	Ulnar, C6-C8	Medial cord	• For the flexor carpi ulnaris to be tested, the wrist is placed in ulnar deviation and full flexion. The practitioner attempts to force the wrist into extension and radial deviation.	

Table 1-13 Upper Limb Muscle Testing (Continued)

Upper Limb Chart	Muscle*	Nerve, Roots	Plexus	Manual Muscle Testing Technique	Figure
Wrist extension	*Extensor carpi radialis longus* Extensor carpi radialis brevis Extensor carpi ulnaris	Radial, C6, C7 Radial, C7, C8	Posterior cord	• The wrist is fully extended in a neutral position. • The practitioner attempts to flex the wrist, applying pressure over the dorsum of the hand. • For the extensor carpi radialis longus to be tested, the patient's wrist is placed into radial deviation and full extension. The practitioner attempts to force the wrist into flexion and ulnar deviation. • For the extensor carpi ulnaris to be tested, the wrist is placed in ulnar deviation and full extension. The practitioner attempts to force the wrist into flexion and radial deviation.	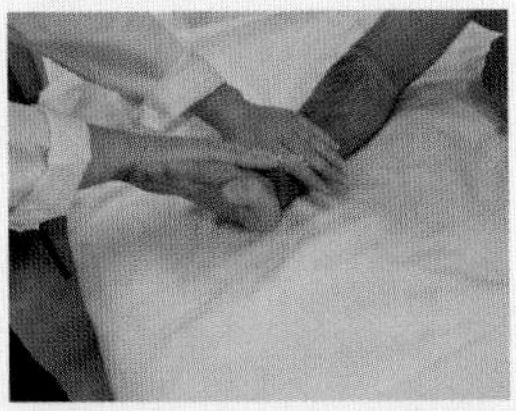
Thumb abduction	*Abductor pollicis brevis* Abductor pollicis longus Extensor pollicis brevis	Median, C8, T1 Radial, C7, C8	Lateral or medial cord Posterior cord	• The thumb is abducted perpendicular to the plane of the palm. • The practitioner attempts to adduct the thumb (toward the palm), applying pressure just above the first metacarpophalangeal joint.	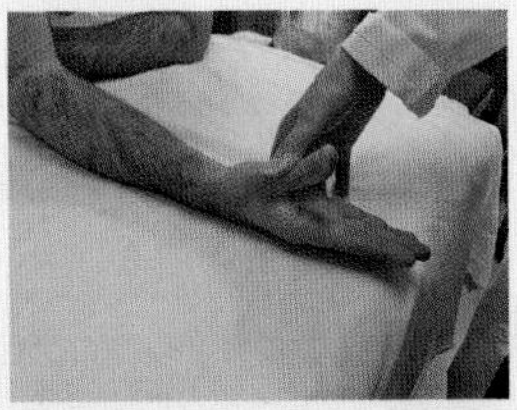
Thumb opposition	*Opponens pollicis* Flexor pollicis brevis Abductor pollicis brevis	Median, C8, T1 Median: superficial head Ulnar: deep head, C8, T1 Median, C8, T1	Lateral or medial cord	• The thumb is placed in opposition. • The practitioner attempts to return the thumb into anatomic position, applying force above the first metacarpophalangeal joint.	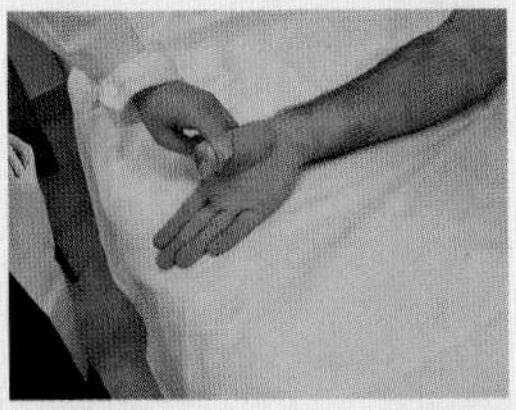
Second to fifth digit flexion	*Flexor digitorum superficialis* Flexor digitorum profundus Lumbricals Interossei	Median, C7, C8, T1 Lateral portion: median Medial portion: ulnar, C7, C8, T1 Lateral two: median Medial two: ulnar, C8, T1 Ulnar, C8, T1	Lateral or medial cord	• The flexor digitorum superficialis extends to the proximal phalanx. • The practitioner attempts to force each proximal phalangeal joint into extension from a position of flexion. • The flexor digitorum profundus extends to the distal phalanx. • The practitioner tests both superficialis and profundus by forcing each middle phalangeal joint into extension from flexion. • The primary flexors of the metacarpophalangeal joints of the second to fourth digits are the lumbricals and the interossei. The practitioner tests these muscles by forcing each metacarpophalangeal joint into extension from a position of flexion. • The primary flexors of the fifth digit metacarpophalangeal joint are the flexor and abductor digiti minimi muscles. • The practitioner can test for fifth digit abduction.	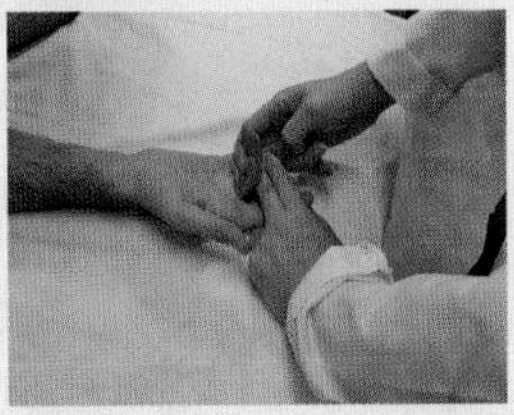 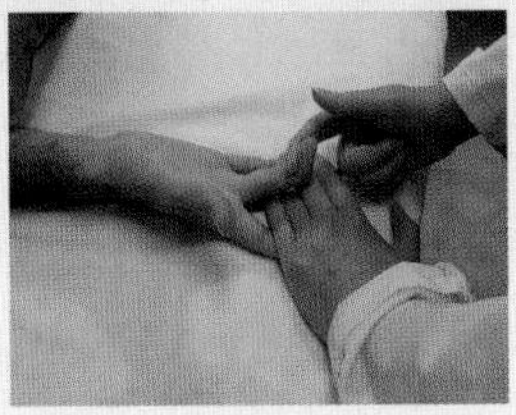
Second to fifth digit extension	*Extensor digitorum communis* Extensor indicis Extensor digiti minimi	Radial, C6-C8 Radial, C7, C8	Posterior cord	• The second to fifth digits are placed in extension with the wrist at neutral position. • The practitioner attempts to force each finger into flexion by applying force over each proximal phalanx.	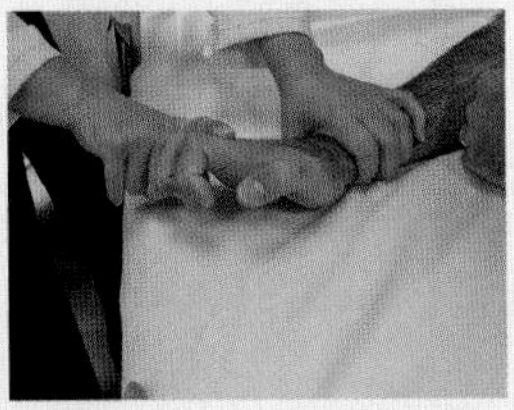

Continued on following page

Table 1-13 Upper Limb Muscle Testing (Continued)

Upper Limb Chart	Muscle*	Nerve, Roots	Plexus	Manual Muscle Testing Technique	Figure
Second to fourth digit abduction, first to fifth digit adduction	*Dorsal* or palmar interossei	Ulnar, C8, T1	Medial cord	• Abduction is tested by placing each digit in abduction and attempting to force the digit into adduction. • The third digit cannot adduct, as movement of this digit to either side is abduction.	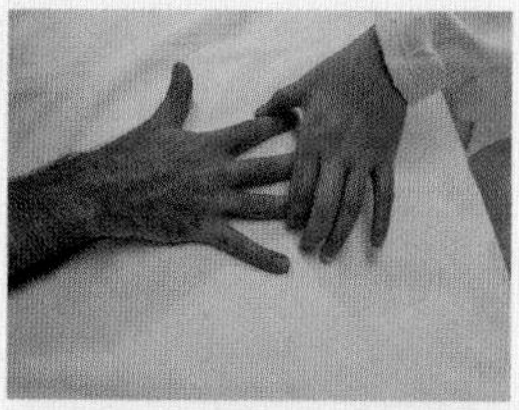
Fifth digit abduction	*Abductor digiti minimi* Flexor digiti minimi			• The patient's fifth digit is placed in abduction. • The practitioner attempts to force the digit into adduction by applying force above the metacarpophalangeal joint.	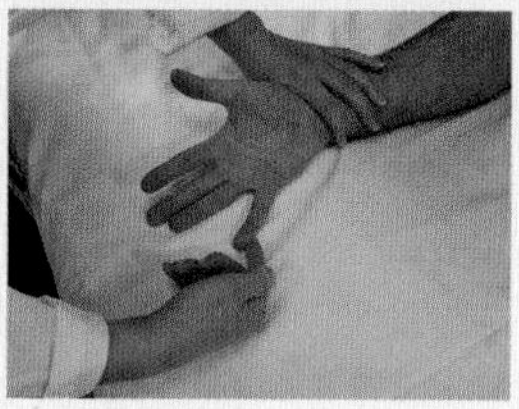

Modified from Jenkins DB: *Hollinshead's functional anatomy of the limbs and back*, ed 7, Philadelphia, 1998, Saunders and Cutter NC, Kevorkian CG: *Handbook of manual muscle testing*, New York, 1999, McGraw-Hill, 1999, with permission of McGraw-Hill.

**The primary muscles tested in the figures are in italics.*

Table 1-14 Lower Limb Muscle Testing

Lower Limb Chart	Muscle(s)*	Nerve, Roots	Testing	Figure
Hip flexion	*Iliacus* *Psoas* Tensor fascia lata Rectus femoris Pectineus Adductor longus, brevis, anterior portion of magnus	Femoral, L2-L4 Lumbar plexus, L1-L4 Superior gluteal, L4, L5, S1 Femoral, L2-L4 Femoral or obturator, L2, L3 Obturator, L2-L4	• Hip flexion can be tested with the patient in a seated or supine position. • With the patient in the supine position, the practitioner forces the hip into extension, applying force over the distal anterior thigh. • With the patient in a sitting position, the hip is flexed while the practitioner attempts to extend the knee.	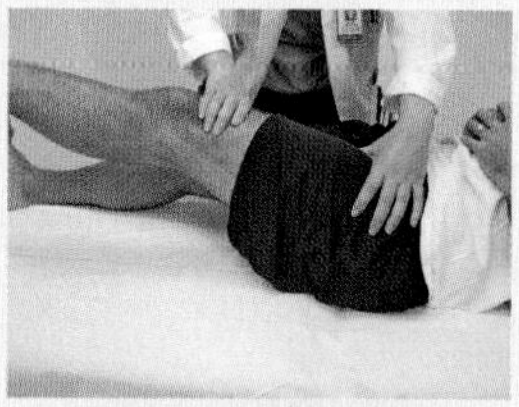
Hip extension	*Gluteus maximus*	Inferior gluteal, L5, S1, S2	• With the patient in a prone position, the hip is extended with the knee flexed to 90 degrees. • The practitioner attempts to flex the hip, applying force over the distal posterior thigh.	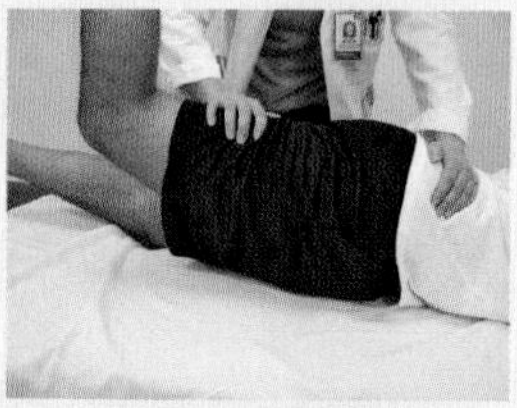
Hip abduction	*Gluteus medius* Gluteus minimus Tensor fascia lata	Superior gluteal, L4, L5, S1	• The patient is placed in a side-lying position with the hip abducted. • The practitioner attempts to adduct the hip, applying force over the distal lateral thigh. • The test can also be performed with the patient seated. With the patient seated, the hips are abducted. The practitioner adducts the hips, applying force over the distal lateral thighs.	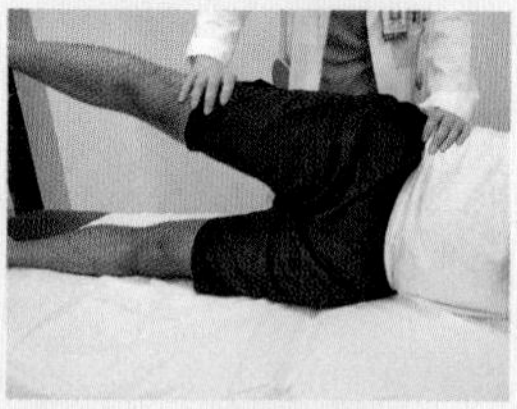
Hip adduction	*Adductor brevis* *Adductor longus* *Adductor magnus, anterior portion* *Pectineus*	Obturator, L2-L4 Obturator, L3, L4 Femoral or obturator, L2, L3	• With the patient in a side-lying position, the practitioner positions the top leg in abduction, and the patient is asked to bring the bottom leg up into adduction to meet the top leg. • The practitioner attempts to abduct the bottom leg, applying pressure over the distal medial thigh. • The test can also be performed with the patient seated. With the patient seated, the hips are adducted. The practitioner abducts the hips, applying force over the distal medial thighs.	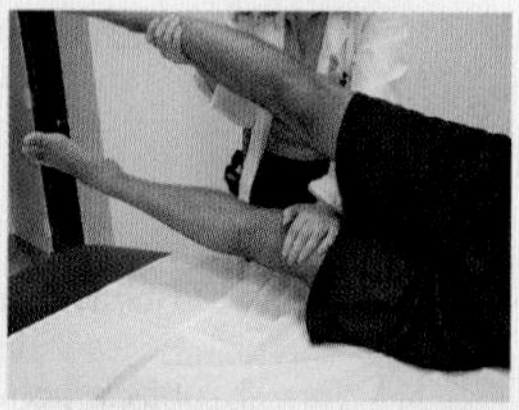 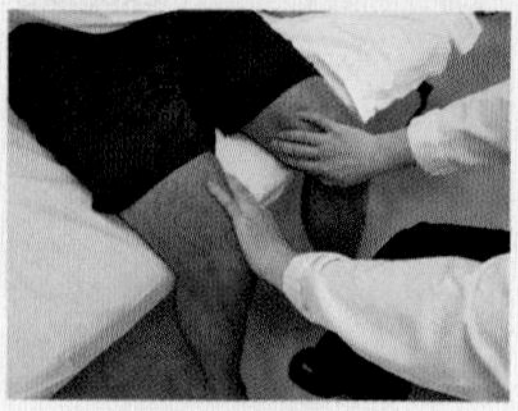

Table 1-14 Lower Limb Muscle Testing (Continued)

Lower Limb Chart	Muscle(s)*	Nerve, Roots	Testing	Figure
Hip internal rotation	*Tensor fascia lata* Pectineus Gluteus minimus, anterior portion	Superior gluteal, L4, L5, S1 Femoral or obturator, L2, L3 Superior gluteal, L4, L5, S1	• The patient is seated with knees flexed at 90 degrees, and the hip is internally rotated. • The practitioner uses one hand to externally rotate the leg, applying lateral force just above the ankle while stabilizing the knee with the other hand.	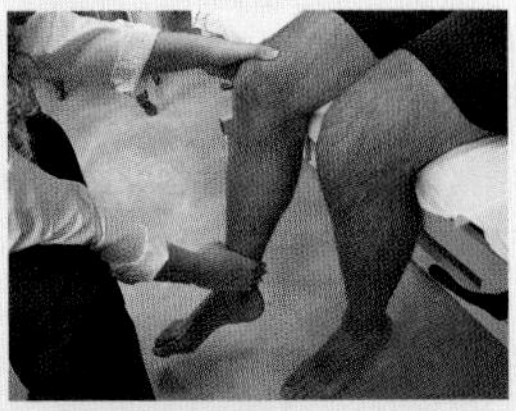
Hip external rotation	*Piriformis* Gluteus maximus Superior gemelli or obturator internus Inferior gemelli or quadratus femoris	Nerve to piriformis, S1, S2 Inferior gluteal, L5, S1, S2 Nerve to obturator internus, L5, S1, S2 Nerve to quadratus femoris, L4, L5, S1	• The patient is seated with knees flexed at 90 degrees, and the hip is externally rotated. • The practitioner uses one hand to internally rotate the leg, applying medial force just above the ankle while stabilizing the knee with the other hand.	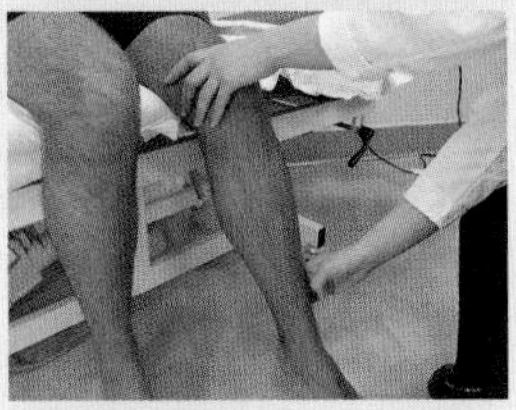
Knee flexion	*Semitendinosus* *Semimembranosus* *Biceps femoris*	Tibial portion of sciatic, L5, S1 Tibial portion of sciatic, L5, S1, S2	• The patient's knee is flexed at 90 degrees while the patient is prone. • The practitioner attempts to force the leg into extension, applying pressure over the posterior tibial surface.	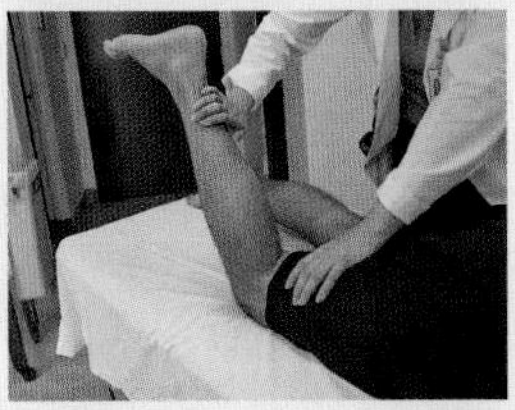
Knee extension	*Quadriceps femoris*	Femoral, L2-L4	• The knee is placed at 30 degrees of flexion while the patient is seated or supine. Try to avoid full knee extension because the patient can stabilize the knee, allowing minor weakness to be missed. • The practitioner attempts to force the leg into flexion, applying pressure over the anterior tibial surface.	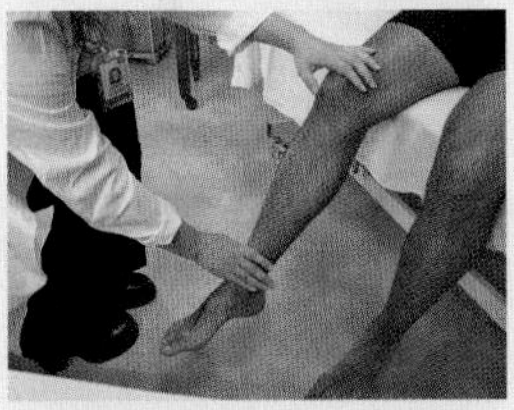
Ankle dorsiflexion	*Tibialis anterior* Extensor digitorum longus Extensor hallucis longus	Deep peroneal, L4, L5, S1	• The ankle is placed in dorsiflexion. • The practitioner attempts to force the ankle into plantar flexion, applying force over the dorsum of the foot. • To test the anterior tibialis, the ankle is inverted and fully dorsiflexed. The practitioner attempts to plantar flex and evert the ankle. • To test the extensor digitorum longus, the ankle is everted and fully dorsiflexed. The practitioner attempts to plantar flex and invert the ankle.	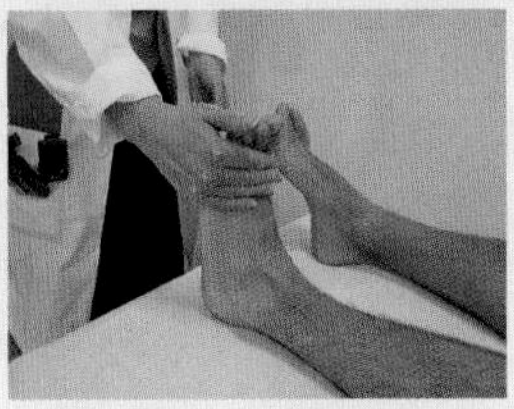
Plantar flexion	*Gastrocnemius* Soleus	Tibial, S1, S2	• The ankle is placed in plantar flexion. • The practitioner attempts to dorsiflex the foot, applying pressure over the plantar surface of the foot. • For the gastrocnemius to be tested, the knee is extended. • For the soleus to be tested, the knee is flexed at 90 degrees. • More functional tests, such as standing or walking on toes, can show weakness missed during manual muscle testing.	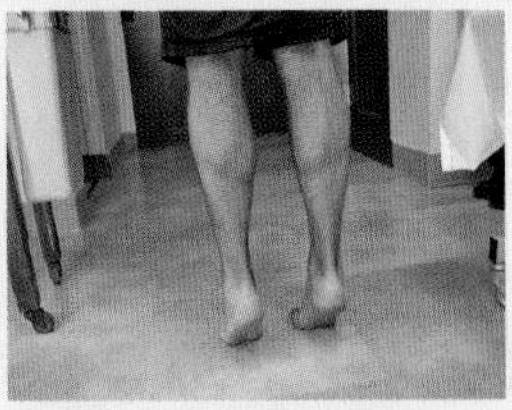
Inversion	Tibialis anterior *Tibialis posterior* Flexor digitorum longus Flexor hallucis longus	Deep peroneal, L4, L5, S1 Tibial, L5, S1 Tibial, L5, S1, S2	• The tibialis anterior is tested in a position of inversion and dorsiflexion. The practitioner attempts to evert and plantar flex the foot, applying pressure on the medial surface of the foot. • The other three muscles produce plantar flexion and inversion. They are more selectively tested with placement of the foot in inversion and plantar flexion. The practitioner attempts to evert and dorsiflex the foot, applying pressure on the medial surface of the foot.	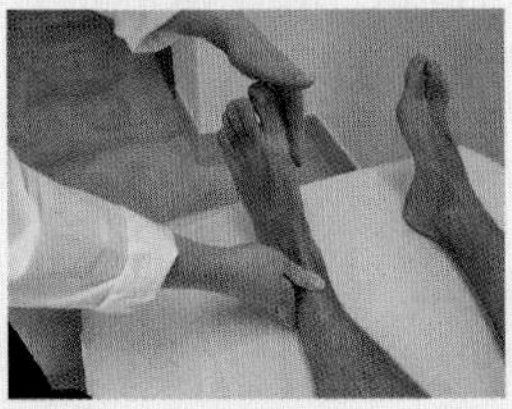

Continued on following page

Table 1-14 Lower Limb Muscle Testing (Continued)

Lower Limb Chart	Muscle(s)*	Nerve, Roots	Testing	Figure
Eversion	Extensor digitorum longus *Peroneus longus* *Peroneus brevis*	Deep peroneal, L4, L5, S1 Superficial peroneal, L4, L5, S1	• The extensor digitorum longus is tested in the position of eversion and dorsiflexion. • The practitioner attempts to invert and plantar flex the foot, applying pressure over the lateral surface of the foot. • The peroneus longus and brevis produce plantar flexion and eversion. They are more selectively tested with the foot everted and plantar flexed. The practitioner attempts to invert and dorsiflex the foot, applying pressure over the lateral surface of the foot.	
First digit extension	Extensor hallucis longus	Deep peroneal, L4, L5, S1	• The first toe is placed in full extension. • The practitioner attempts to flex the toe, applying pressure over the dorsum of the first toe.	
Second to fifth digit extension	*Extensor digitorum longus* Extensor digitorum brevis	Deep peroneal, L4, L5, S1 Deep peroneal, L5, S1	• The second and fifth toes are fully extended. • The practitioner attempts to flex them, applying pressure over the dorsum of the toes.	
First digit flexion	*Flexor hallucis longus* Flexor hallucis brevis	Tibial, L5, S1, S2 Medial plantar, L5, S1	• The first toe is placed in full flexion. • The practitioner attempts to extend the toe, applying pressure over the plantar surface of the first toe.	
Second to fifth digit flexion	*Flexor digitorum longus* Flexor digitorum brevis	Tibial, L5, S1 Medial plantar, L5, S1	• The second to fifth toes are placed in full flexion. • The practitioner attempts to extend them, applying pressure over the plantar surface of the toes.	

Modified from Jenkins DB: *Hollinshead's functional anatomy of the limbs and back*, ed 7, Philadelphia, 1998, Saunders and Cutter NC, Kevorkian CG: *Handbook of manual muscle testing*, New York, 1999, McGraw-Hill, 1999, with permission of McGraw-Hill.

**The primary muscles tested in the figures are in italics.*

should not cross two joints, if possible. Placing a muscle at a mechanical disadvantage, such as flexing the elbow beyond 90 degrees to assess triceps strength, can help demonstrate mild weakness.[45] Extended Tables 1-13 and 1-14 summarize the joint movement, innervation, and manual strength testing techniques for all major upper and lower extremity muscle groups, respectively.

Assessment, Summary, and Plan

Only after completing a thorough H&P is the physiatrist able to develop a comprehensive treatment plan. The organization of the initial treatment plan and goals can vary from setting to setting but should clearly state impairments, performance deficits (activity limitation), community or role dysfunction (participation), medical conditions that can affect achieving the functional goals, and goals for the interdisciplinary rehabilitation team (if other disciplines are involved in the patient's care). Follow-up treatment plans and notes are likely to be shorter and less detailed, but they *must* address important interval changes since the last documentation and any significant changes in treatment or goals. This documentation is often used to justify continued payment for third-party payers. Noting whether problems are new, stable, improving, or worsening can be critical for accurate physician billing compliance documentation. Accurate identification and

BOX 1-2

Inpatient Rehabilitation Plan

Summary Statement

Ms. Jones is a divorced, right-handed, 69-year-old woman with a medical history of hypertension, coronary artery disease, and depression, with recent rupture of a left middle cerebral artery aneurysm, now 9 days postcraniotomy for clipping. She is currently slightly lethargic and has moderately severe right hemiparesis, mild aphasia, right shoulder pain, and possible exacerbation of her underlying depression. She is receiving a regular diet with thickened liquids and is continent of bladder but has experienced some constipation. She is participating well in therapies, walking 15 feet with a wide-based quad cane, transferring with minimal assistance, and requiring moderate assistance in virtually all activities of daily living (ADL). Ms. Jones lives alone in an elevator-accessible apartment building where two of her daughters also live with their families.

Rehabilitation Problem List and Management Plan

- *Ambulatory dysfunction resulting from right hemiparesis:* Initiate neurodevelopmental techniques, forced-use paradigms. Defer ankle-foot orthosis for now, evaluate for best assistive device, narrow-based quad cane, tone not a limitation at present.
- *ADL dysfunction resulting from right hemiparesis:* Use neurodevelopmental techniques and encourage weight-bearing on right upper extremity. Defer nighttime splint unless substantial increase in tone. See shoulder pain later. Tone not a limitation at present.
- *Mild expressive aphasia:* Speech-language disorder to evaluate, focus on higher-level communication, especially in home setting.
- *Dysphagia:* Swallowing evaluation per speech, proceed to modified barium swallow if needed.
- *Shoulder pain:* Use of glass lap tray for constant support of right arm, will speak with physiotherapist regarding use of sling only with ambulation, to consider trial of nonopiate analgesic (watch for sedation), or diagnostic or therapeutic shoulder injection.
- *Bowel and bladder:* Bladder fine; initiate oral stimulant to facilitate regular bowel habits.

Medical Problem List and Management Plan

- *Ruptured left MCA aneurysm:* Discontinue nimodipine 21 days after surgery, check phenytoin level as possible cause of slight lethargy, check with neurosurgery about changing or stopping antiepileptic because she has remained seizure free, consider repeat brain computed tomography to rule out hydrocephalus as cause of lethargy.
- *Hypertension:* Stable in 140/90 mm Hg range, monitor vitals closely in physiotherapy and occupational therapy, continue beta-blocker and diuretic.
- *CAD:* No angina currently; monitor for shortness of breath, chest pain, and lightheadedness in therapies.
- *Depression:* Continue trazodone 150 mg at bedtime, doubt a cause of sleepiness because has been taking this dosage for many years. Monitor for mood disturbance, as a limitation in therapy participation.
- *Precautions:* Cardiac precautions, frequent vital sign monitoring during initial therapy sessions.

Goals

- Independent ambulation for household distances with assistive device (to be determined).
- Independent in all transfers.
- Supervision with assistive device for short-distance community ambulation, even surfaces.
- Independent in ADL, except shoes, with assistive devices (to be determined); minimal assist for shoes.
- Independent in all instrumental ADL (IADL), except meal preparation, supervision for meal preparation.
- Independent in home exercise program, including passive range of motion (ROM) to right hand or wrist and ankle.
- Identify family members to provide supervision after discharge and complete hands-on teaching.
- Maintain mood to participate fully in therapy.

documentation of the cause of the impairment and disability can be required for initial and continuing hospital payment.

A summary statement of no more than a few sentences is helpful to medical consultants and other team members. Although development of a separate medical and functional problems list is acceptable and often recommended, the physiatrist should make very clear how those medical issues alter the approach to treatment (e.g., how brittle diabetes, activity-induced angina, or pain issues might affect mobilization).

With a medical and functional problem list in hand, the management plan can be developed. Considering six broad interventional categories as originally outlined by Stolov and colleagues[82] is very helpful, particularly with complex patients in an inpatient rehabilitation setting. These six categories include prevention or correction of additional disability, enhancement of affected systems, enhancement of unaffected systems, use of adaptive equipment, use of environmental modification, and use of psychological techniques to enhance patient performance and education. The physician should clearly delineate the therapeutic precautions for the other team members. Both short- and longer-term goals should be outlined, as well as estimated time frames for achieving those goals. Boxes 1-2 and 1-3 show examples of rehabilitation plans for an inpatient after subarachnoid hemorrhage and an outpatient with back pain, respectively.

Summary

Physiatrists should pride themselves in their ability to complete a comprehensive rehabilitation H&P. The physiatric H&P begins with the standard medical format but goes beyond that to assess impairment, activity limitation (disability), and participation (handicap). Physiatrists' understanding of the MSK examination and musculoskeletal principles is a primary distinction from neurologists and neurosurgeons. Similarly, physiatrists' understanding of neurology and the neurologic examination is a primary distinction from orthopedists and rheumatologists. The H&P is critical in gathering the information needed to formulate a treatment plan that can help the patient achieve the appropriate goals in the most efficient, least dangerous, and most cost-effective way possible.

BOX 1-3

Outpatient Rehabilitation Plan

Summary Statement

Mr. Smith is a right-handed, 47-year-old man with a medical history of hypertension and depression, who has a recent worsening of lower back pain. He notes a history of primary lower back pain of several years that worsened recently while emptying his office wastepaper basket. The location is primarily in the lumbosacral junction above the posterior superior iliac spine. He notes associated radiation down the posterior right thigh to the calf. The pain is described as a sharp, spasm-like pain, current visual analog scale rating of 8/10 in intensity, although he notes episodes of debilitating 10/10 pain. The pain is improved with rest and supine positioning and worsened with prolonged sitting or standing. He denies specific weakness or numbness but notes tingling in the lateral aspect of his calf. He also denies bowel or bladder symptoms. He has undergone imaging in the past, which demonstrated disk space narrowing at the L5-S1 level. Past treatments have included physical therapy, which at the time consisted of hot packs and massage. He finds Advil is helpful in diminishing the intensity of the pain. Although he notes no difficulties with normal activities, the pain prevents him from working out in the gym, which primarily consisted of weight training and spinning classes. He also notes difficulty sleeping because of the pain. He denies difficulties at work. Also, he reports no need for pharmacologic treatment of his depression for some time. Mr. Smith currently lives in an elevator-accessible apartment building with his wife. He denies history of similar diagnoses within first-degree relatives. Physical examination is pertinent for right greater than left lower lumbar paraspinal and gluteus medius tenderness, positive slump and straight leg raise tests, very tight hamstrings, and weakness at the right extensor hallucis longus.

Rehabilitation Problem List and Management Plan

- Physical therapy: 8 to 12 sessions. Trial extension-based exercises to attempt to centralize the pain. Modalities as needed for pain control. Lower extremity strengthening and stretching with focus on core-strengthening exercises.
- Workstation ergonomics evaluation, biomechanics and posture awareness training.
- Precautions: None.

Medical Problem List and Management Plan

- Review of diagnosis and prognosis with the patient, which includes a review of the natural history of lumbar disc herniations and contribution of depression to pain complaints.
- Medications include an antiinflammatory medication with a muscle relaxant. May also include opioids as needed for severe exacerbations. Consider an epidural steroid injection if pain is refractory to oral medications and movement therapies. Sleep may improve as a side effect of the muscle relaxant and/or opioids.
- Imaging not required at this time because he has a good potential to recover with physical therapy. If no improvement with high-quality physical therapy, may consider lumbar magnetic resonance imaging (MRI) without contrast.
- Depression: Consider adding antidepressant if pain remains refractory to above treatment.

Goals

- Decreased pain.
- Return to workout routine.
- Improved "back hygiene."

ACKNOWLEDGMENT: We thank Nancy Fung, M.D., and Andre Panagos, M.D., who contributed substantially to the writing of this chapter in previous editions.

KEY REFERENCES

3. American Medical Association: *Guides to the evaluation of permanent impairment*, ed 4, Chicago, 1993, American Medical Association.
4. Anonymous: Occupational Therapy Practice Framework: domain and process, *Am J Occup Ther* 56:609–639, 2002. (Erratum in: *Am J Occup Ther* 2003;57:115).
5. Bates BA: *Guide to physical examination and history taking*, ed 7, Philadelphia, 1998, Lippincott.
6. Beasley WC: Quantitative muscle testing: principles and application to research and clinical services, *Arch Phys Med Rehabil* 42:398–425, 1961.
8. Bell BD, Hoshizak TB: Relationships of age and sex with range of motion of seventeen joint actions in humans, *Can J Appl Sport Sci* 6:202–206, 1981.
11. Birchwood M, Smith J, Drury V, et al: A self-report insight scale for psychosis: reliability, validity, and sensitivity to change, *Acta Psychiatr Scand* 89:62–67, 1994.
12. Brannon GE: History and mental status examination, 2002. Available at: <http://www.emedicine.com>.
15. Campbell W, editor: *Dejong's: the neurological examination*, ed 6, Philadelphia, 2005, Lippincott Williams & Wilkins.
17. Centers for Medicare and Medicaid Services: Available at: http://www.cms.gov/Outreach-and-Education/Medicare-Learning-Network-MLN/MLNEd/WebGuide/EMDOC.html.
18. Centers for Medicare and Medicaid Services: Document guidelines. Available at: http://www.cms.gov/Regulations-and-Guidance/Guidance/Manuals/downloads/bp102c01.pdf.
19. Chally PS, Carlson JM: Spirituality, rehabilitation, and aging: a literature review, *Arch Phys Med Rehabil* 85(Suppl 3):S60–S65, 2004.
21. Cole TM, Tobis JS: Measurement of musculoskeletal function. In Kottke FJ, Stillwell GK, Lehmann JF, editors: *Handbook of physical medicine and rehabilitation*, ed 3, Philadelphia, 1982, Saunders.
22. Corrigan JD: Substance abuse as a mediating factor in outcome from traumatic brain injury, *Arch Phys Med Rehabil* 76:302–309, 1995.
24. Cutter NC, Kevorkian CG: *Handbook of manual muscle testing*, New York, 1999, McGraw-Hill.
25. DeGowin RL: *DeGowin's diagnostic examination*, ed 6, New York, 1994, McGraw-Hill.
27. DeLisa JA, Currie DM, Martin GM: Rehabilitation medicine: past, present and future. In DeLisa JA, Gans BM, editors: *Rehabilitation medicine: principles and practice*, ed 3, Philadelphia, 1998, Lippincott.
29. Enelow AJ, Forde DL, Brummel-Smith K: *Interviewing and patient care*, ed 4, New York, 1996, Oxford University Press.
31. Folstein MF, Folstein SE, McHugh PR: Mini-Mental State: a practical method for grading the cognitive state of patients for the clinician, *J Psychiatr Res* 12:189–198, 1975.
34. Gerhardt JJ, Rondinelli RD: Goniometric techniques for range-of-motion assessment, *Phys Med Rehabil Clin N Am* 12:507–527, 2001.
35. Giacino JT, Katz DI, Schiff N: Assessment and rehabilitation management of individuals with disorders of consciousness. In Zasler ND, Katz DI, Zafonte RD, editors: *Brain injury medicine: principles and practice*, New York, 2007, Demos.
39. Griffin MR, Yared A, Ray WA: Nonsteroidal anti-inflammatory drugs and acute renal failure in elderly persons, *Am J Epidemiol* 151:488–496, 2000.

40. Groah SL, Lanig IS: Neuromusculoskeletal syndromes in wheelchair athletes, *Semin Neurol* 20:201–208, 2000.
44. Helsey-Grove D, Danehy LN, Consolzio M, et al: A national study of challenges to electronic health record adoption and meaningful use, *Med Care* 52:144–148, 2014.
45. Hislop HJ: *Daniels and Worthingham's muscle testing: techniques of manual examination*, ed 6, Philadelphia, 1995, Saunders.
46. Hoppenfeld S: *Physical examination of the spine and extremities*, Norwalk, 1976, Appleton & Lange.
48. Jennett B, Teasdale G: Assessment of impaired consciousness, *Contemp Neurosurg* 20:78, 1981.
50. Karandikar N, Vargas OO: Kinetic chains: a review of the concept and its clinical applications, *PM R* 3:739–745, 2011.
51. Kendall FP, McCreary EK, Provance PG: *Muscles: testing and function*, Baltimore, 1993, Williams & Wilkins.
52. Knapp ME: Measuring range of motion, *Postgrad Med* 42:A123–A127, 1967.
53. Knapp ME, West CC: Measurement of joint motion, *Univ Minn Med Bull* 15:405–412, 1944.
56. Lezak MD, Howieson DB, Loring DW: *Neurological assessment*, ed 4, New York, 2004, Oxford University Press.
58. Lindsay KW, Bone I, Callander R: *Neurology and neurosurgery illustrated*, ed 3, New York, 1997, Churchill Livingstone.
67. Members of the Department of Neurology: *Mayo Clinic examinations in neurology*, ed 7, Rochester, 1998, Mayo Clinic and Cano Foundation.
72. O'Sullivan SB: Assessment of motor function. In O'Sullivan SB, Schmitz TJ, editors: *Physical rehabilitation: assessment and treatment*, ed 4, Philadelphia, 2001, FA Davis.
73. Palmer JB, Drennan JC, Baba M: Evaluation and treatment of swallowing impairments, *Am Fam Physician* 61:2453–2462, 2000.
74. Palmer ML, Epler ME: *Fundamentals of musculoskeletal assessment techniques*, ed 2, New York, 1998, Lippincott.
77. Scalan J, Borson S: The Mini-Cog: receiver operating characteristics with expert and naive raters, *Int J Geriatr Psychiatry* 16(2):216–222, 2001.
80. Stewart MA: Effective physician-patient communication and health outcomes: a review, *CMAJ* 152:1423–1433, 1995.
81. Stolov WC: Evaluation of the patient. In Kottke FJ, Stillwell GK, Lehmann JF, editors: *Handbook of physical medicine and rehabilitation*, ed 3, Philadelphia, 1982, Saunders.
82. Stolov WC, Hayes RM, Kraft GH, editors: *Treatment strategies in chronic disease and disability: a contemporary approach to medical practice*, New York, 1994, Demos.
83. Strub RL, Black FW: *The mental status examination in neurology*, ed 4, Philadelphia, 2000, FA Davis.
85. Tan JC: *Practical manual of physical medicine and rehabilitation*, St Louis, 1998, Mosby.
86. Teasell R, Nestor NA, Bitensky J: Plasticity and reorganization of the brain post stroke, *Top Stroke Rehabil* 12:11–26, 2005.
87. Tomb D: *House officer series: psychiatry*, ed 5, Baltimore, 1995, Williams & Wilkins.
95. Woo BH, Nesathurai S: *The rehabilitation of people with traumatic brain injury*, Malden, 2000, Blackwell Science.
96. World Health Organization: *International classification of impairments, activities, and participation*, Geneva, 1997, World Health Organization.

The full reference list for this chapter is available online.

CHAPTER 2

HISTORY AND EXAMINATION OF THE PEDIATRIC PATIENT*

Michelle A. Miller

History

The approach to obtaining the history on a pediatric patient will vary based on their age and developmental level. As much as possible, the child should be included in the discussion of his or her health. With very young children, the history is typically obtained from the parent or caregiver. However, a parent's perception of a child's function and health is often inconsistent with the child's perception. With adolescents, it is beneficial to have the parent or caregiver leave the examination area briefly to allow the child to provide additional history or ask questions that they may be uncomfortable doing in the presence of their family.

On the initial visit, it is helpful to the patient and family to summarize the reason for the referral. Often, families do not know why their child has been referred. They have limited understanding of what a pediatric physiatrist is and what they can expect from the visit. A brief description of what the evaluation will entail, the focus on functional assessment, and what the physiatrist can offer the child and family helps to set the tone and alleviate anxiety. Asking the child and family what they feel is the underlying diagnosis or problem also assists in evaluating the family's current understanding of the child's medical condition and what concerns are important to the family.

Birth History

A thorough history should include any issues during the pregnancy as well as during labor and delivery. Maternal complications during pregnancy, such as seizures, febrile illnesses, hypertension, or hyperglycemia, should be evaluated. Any medications or drugs that the mother took during the pregnancy should be reviewed for potential impact on the fetus. Infants exposed to alcohol or cocaine, for example, often have significant cognitive, behavioral, and motoric impairments. The duration of gestation, presence of multiples, and presentation at birth are also important factors. Premature delivery and multiples are known risk factors for cerebral palsy.[1,35] The examiner should ask if the mother received prenatal care. If a mother did not receive prenatal care, she may not have taken additional folate to decrease the risk for spinal dysraphisms.[25] The family should be asked if there was a decrease in fetal movements noted at any time during the pregnancy that could indicate a neuromuscular problem such as spinal muscular atrophy.

The child's birth weight and length as well as the Apgar scores should be noted. Higher birth weights with a vaginal delivery may lead to a fractured clavicle and brachial plexus injury. The Apgar score consists of five components: activity, pulse, grimace, appearance, and respiration. Each component is scored from 0 to 2 and recorded at 1 minute, 5 minutes, and 9 minutes. A score of 7 to 10 is considered normal. Postnatal complications such as hyperbilirubinemia, retinopathy of prematurity, respiratory difficulties, feeding difficulties, and duration of respiratory support may provide clues to underlying pathology and functional impact. Complications with previous pregnancies such as stillbirth, miscarriages, or fetal anomalies should be recorded.

History of Presenting Problem

The physician should determine the onset of the current problem and any associated factors. It should be noted if the symptoms are worsening, static, or improving. It is important to determine which diagnostic tests have been performed as well as any treatments that have been initiated. Questions regarding the child's temperament and personality can provide insight into their readiness to participate in therapies as well as which approaches may be most helpful. The child's medical history should be reviewed for any similar problems as well as any significant illnesses, hospitalizations, surgeries, procedures, or previous trauma. Medications should be reviewed for any possible side effects on the nervous and/or muscular systems. Allergies should also be reviewed, including any feeding intolerances. A history of early allergies with different formulas may indicate a feeding difficulty rather than a true allergy. Immunization status is important to determine because of the risk for disorders such as tetanus.

Developmental History

This is one of the most important aspects of the pediatric history. Illnesses, injuries, and different disease processes can have a profound impact on the attainment of developmental milestones. Delays may be noted in gross motor, fine motor, speech and language, and/or psychosocial areas. A thorough understanding of the developmental milestones (Table 2-1) and the age at which the child attained them can assist with diagnosis and treatment protocols. If the delays are primarily motoric in nature, then

*The contributions of Pamela E. Wilson and Susan D. Apkon, who wrote on this topic in the previous edition, are acknowledged.

Table 2-1 Developmental Milestones

Age	Gross Motor	Language	Fine Motor	Social
3 mo	Good head control in sitting Rolls back to side	Cries Coos	Grasps toy Object to mouth Hands to midline	Smiles at face
6 mo	Ability to sit Rolls both ways	Babbles Makes vowels sounds	Thumb opposition emerging Reaches with one hand	Recognizes family members
9 mo	Crawls Pulls to stand and cruises	Uses gestures Understands "no"	Can release voluntarily Pincer grasp (crude) Can point	Plays patty cake Plays peek-a-boo
12 mo	Walks with hand held or independently Can squat (stand to sit)	Mama/dada specific Has at least two other words Responds to name	Bangs two blocks together Grossly turns pages in a book Puts objects in a container Pincer grasp (mature)	Waves bye-bye
18 mo	Can run Walks stairs	Four to 20 words Follows simple instructions One or more body parts	Builds tower of two to four cubes Throws ball Scribbles	Feeds self Takes off simple clothes
24 mo	Kicks ball Runs better	Two-word sentences Body parts Intelligible most of the time (70%) 200 words	Builds tower of six or seven cubes Turns a door knob Can draw a vertical line	Can put on some clothes
3 yr	Balances on one foot Rides a tricycle	First and last name Knows age and sex Three-word sentences Can count three objects	Builds tower of 9 to 10 cubes Holds crayon with fingers Copies circle	Dresses Potty trained Separates easily
4 yr	Hops on one foot Stands on one foot for 5 seconds	Four- to five-word sentences Counts to four Knows colors	Throws ball overhead Uses scissors Draws circle and square Draws person of two to four parts	Tries to be independent Imaginary play
5 yr	Skipping Stands on one foot for 10 seconds Mature gait Walks backward heel-toe	Counts 10 or more objects Six- to eight-word sentences Knows coins Knows address	Catches a ball Copies triangle Draws person with a body	Ties shoelaces Sings and dances

a neuromuscular disorder is more likely. If the delays are noted in speech and language skills, then further assessment of the child's hearing is warranted. Infants with hearing loss start to fall behind after 6 to 8 months of age and may present with decreased babbling. Parents should be asked if there is a history of recurrent ear infections.

A discussion of the developmental milestones is also helpful in educating the family regarding what the child should be doing and what skills they should be working on. Often families are focused on their child walking when they need to take a step back and work on their child sitting independently or working on standing balance, for example. It should also be emphasized that there is a wide age range of normal for the attainment of certain skills, and families may notice that their child progresses at different rates within the different areas.

Family History

The family history should include any history of early stroke, early myocardial infarction, peripheral neuropathy, joint or tissue abnormalities, myopathies, or bony abnormalities. Gait abnormalities or developmental delays should be investigated through multiple generations. Certain disease processes such as myotonic dystrophy will present in milder forms in previous generations and may be missed until a more severely affected family member presents for medical evaluation. If a genetic disorder is suspected, the child and family should be referred for genetic testing. This can help with planning for future pregnancies and to provide counseling to the extended family.

Social and Educational History

The examiner should inquire about the child's environment including who lives with them in the home, who the primary and secondary caregivers are, and the layout of the home. Accessibility is assessed by determining the number of stairs to enter the home, the levels of the home, and where the child's bedroom and bathroom are located. It is important to also evaluate the child's peer group and their interactions with their peers. Extracurricular activities can give insight into a child's social skills and personality. The child's current educational history should include the grade they are in, the presence of an individualized education plan or 504 plan for additional education supports, any failed or repeat grade levels, and if the child ever received early intervention services.

Physical Examination

There is not a standardized approach to the examination of the pediatric patient.[2,21] It should be tailored to the age and developmental level of the child. The examination commences with the first introductions. As the examiner is obtaining the history, observation of the child can provide a great deal of information about social skills, language, motor movements, and personality. Before touching the child, it is helpful to develop a rapport by playing or talking with him/her. A pen light, a badge on a retractable holder, or bubbles are easy tools to engage a child and test visual fixation, reach, grasp, and release at the same time. Knowledge of popular cartoon or movie characters, popular athletes/teams, or singers can be very helpful in engaging children.

Very young children are typically most comfortable on their parent's lap during the examination, where they feel safe. The infant is usually very tolerant of gentle physical handling by a stranger until about 9 months of age, when stranger anxiety develops. Older children and adolescents can easily be evaluated on the examination table.

Growth

Height and weight should be plotted and monitored as the child grows. The average full-term newborn measures 50 cm in length. Height increases 50% by age 1 and doubles by 4 years of age.[18] A child's adult height can be estimated by doubling their height at age 2 years. Short stature may be seen with Turner syndrome and Down syndrome. Growth may be arrested early as a result of precocious puberty with premature closure of the growth plates. Precocious puberty is defined as the onset of puberty in girls younger than 8 years and boys younger than 9 years of age.[41] Precocious puberty is commonly seen in cerebral palsy and other brain injuries, as well as spina bifida.

The average full-term newborn in the United States weighs 3400 g. It is normal for the infant to initially lose weight, but this is regained quickly and by 5 months of age should have doubled. By a year, the child should have tripled his/her birth weight. Any deviation off of the child's expected growth curve should be evaluated closely. Decreases in height velocity or weight loss may be associated with poor nutrition or malabsorption. Significant increases may indicate a pituitary tumor, metabolic disorder, or poor diet. Childhood obesity has now reached epidemic proportions in the United States and is considered a health care emergency. There are growth charts available for specific genetic syndromes such as Turner syndrome and Down syndrome, as well as the cerebral palsy population, based on their gross motor functional classification, and the myelomeningocele population.

In evaluating the infant, a head circumference should be checked and monitored serially for the first several years. The average head circumference at birth is 35 cm and increases to 47 cm by 1 year of age.[18] If the child has macrocephaly, defined as a head circumference greater than 2 standard deviations above the mean, a quick inspection of the parents' head sizes may help to differentiate between a familial trait and hydrocephalus or some type of mass. Hydrocephalus may be present at birth or develop over time. It is commonly seen after closure of a myelomeningocele defect. Microcephaly is a head circumference greater than 2 standard deviations below the mean. This indicates that the brain has not fully formed, as in anencephaly, or that growth has been arrested as a result of some sort of insult such as anoxia or infection. It may also be seen in certain neurodegenerative disorders.

Inspection

On evaluating the child, initial inspection should assess the child's general appearance, movements, engagement, and overall health. Close observations of any facial anomalies, joint abnormalities, or asymmetry of stature or sides should be noted. The presence of certain physical abnormalities is linked with some common syndromes, as noted in Table 2-2.

Skin examination may be significant for birth marks such as port wine stains, hyperpigmented areas such as café-au-lait spots (Figure 2-1), axillary freckling, or acute changes such as the scalded skin appearance of Stevens-Johnson syndrome or the purpura of meningococcal infections. Port wine stains in the distribution of the first branch of the trigeminal nerve are associated with Sturge-Weber syndrome. A sacral dimple, skin lesions over the spine, and/or a hairy tuft over the lumbar or sacral spine may indicate spina bifida occulta.[33] In children with ataxia, telangiectasias are typically present over the flexor surfaces

Table 2-2 Common Syndromes and the Associated Abnormal Features

Syndrome	Abnormalities
Angelman syndrome	Severe mental retardation, delay in attainment of motor milestones, microbrachycephaly, maxillary hypoplasia, deep-set eyes, blond hair (65%), ataxia, jerky arm movements resembling those of a marionette (100%), seizures
Hunter syndrome	Growth deficiency, coarsening of facial features, full lips, macrocephaly, macroglossia, contractures of joints, broadening of bones, hepatosplenomegaly, delayed tooth eruption
Marfan syndrome	Tall stature with long slim limbs, little subcutaneous fat, arachnodactyly, joint laxity, scoliosis (60%), retinal detachment, upward lens subluxation, dilatation of ascending aorta
Neurofibromatosis syndrome	Areas of hyperpigmentation or hypopigmentation with café-au-lait spots (94%); "freckling" of axilla, inguinal folds, and perineum; cutaneous neurofibromas that are small, soft, pigmented nodules; plexiform neurofibromas; Lisch nodules

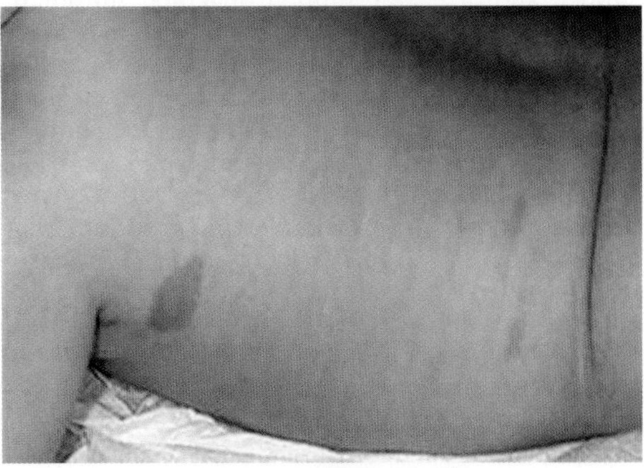

FIGURE 2-1 Café-au-lait spots.

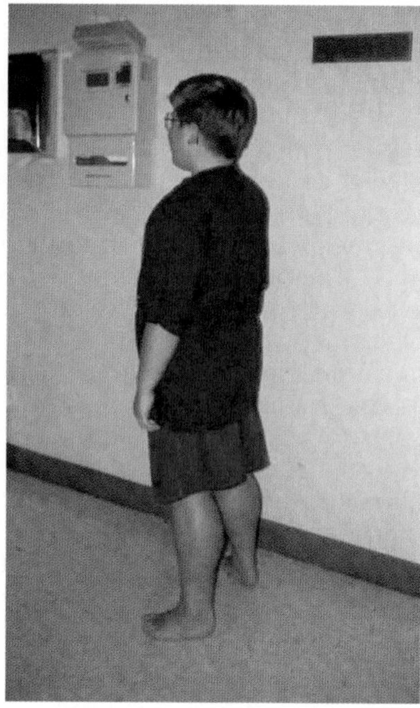

FIGURE 2-2 Calf pseudohypertrophy.

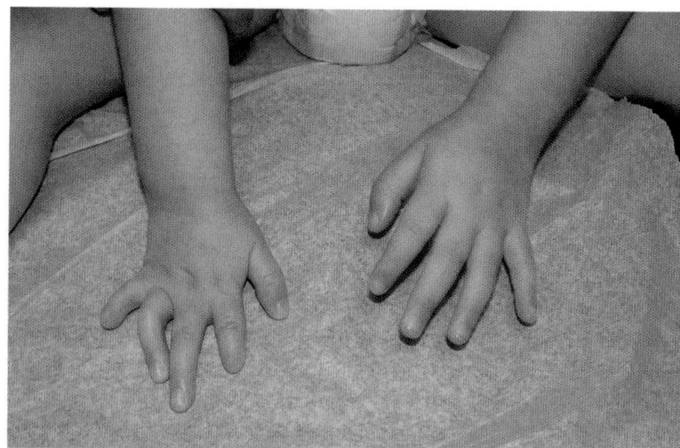

FIGURE 2-3 The absence of the pectoral muscle and ipsilateral hand deformities with brachydactyly or syndactyly is described in Poland syndrome.

of the elbows and knees. The ash leaf spot in association with seizures and hemiplegia is present in tuberous sclerosis.

Evaluation of the head and neck should note cranial deformities, facial dysmorphisms, and asymmetries. With the institution of the Back to Sleep program in 1992, many children now present to their pediatricians with flattening of the occiput, brachycephaly, or plagiocephaly, which usually resolves when the child begins to sit independently.[29] Epicanthal folds and palmar simian creases are well-known hallmarks of Down syndrome. Other conditions present with anomalies such as low-set ears, hypertelorism, wide-set eyes, and micrognathia. If the sclera of the eyes has a bluish tinge, the examiner should consider osteogenesis imperfecta.

Musculoskeletal Assessment

The musculoskeletal assessment includes inspection and palpation of the bones, joints, and muscles. Any asymmetries in muscle mass or limb size should be noted. Lymphedema may present as swelling and increased growth in an upper and/or lower limb. Congenital amputations associated with amniotic band syndrome may include digital, transhumeral, transradial, or transtibial amputations. Apparent calf hypertrophy with a doughy feeling on palpation of the muscles is consistent with Duchenne muscular dystrophy (Figure 2-2). The absence of the pectoral muscle and ipsilateral hand deformities with brachydactyly or syndactyly is described in Poland syndrome (Figure 2-3). Palpation of the joints evaluates for tenderness, swelling, warmth, and synovial thickening.

Both passive and active range of motion of all joints should be evaluated. Joint mobility will change during growth.[27,36] A full-term infant may lack as much as 25 degrees of elbow extension and 30 degrees of hip extension. A preterm infant, conversely, tends to have increased range of motion as a result of lower muscle tone.

Loss of range of motion may be attributable to joint contracture from arthrogryposis, orthopedic conditions such as Klippel-Feil syndrome, spasticity, pain, inflammatory disorders such as juvenile inflammatory arthritis, or trauma. Connective tissue disorders such as Marfan syndrome will result in joint hypermobility as well as an increase in skin elasticity. An anxious child may not be as easy to examine, and the examiner will need to determine whether there is a volitional component affecting the range of motion.

The back and spine examination should focus on any bony abnormalities as well as any muscular asymmetries. The child should be examined in both sitting and standing positions because any leg length discrepancy may impact the spine and pelvis examination. Shoulder height, the position of the scapulae, the space between the trunk and the upper limbs, and the height of the pelvis should be evaluated. A rib hump and increased space between the trunk and upper limbs is noted in children with scoliosis (Figure 2-4). The curve should be evaluated by serial radiographs to determine the severity, flexibility, and progression of the curve over time. Idiopathic scoliosis in adolescent girls is the most common type of scoliosis, with a right thoracic curve noted.[12] The rib hump can be further accentuated by having the child bend forward. Other spinal abnormalities are listed in Table 2-3. A congenital elevation of the scapula or a Sprengel deformity (Figure 2-5) is often seen in association with Klippel-Feil syndrome and cervical spine abnormalities.

The lower limb examination may demonstrate range of motion and bony abnormalities. Evaluating gait is a common referral for the physiatrist. In addition to evaluating the child, the child's shoes should be assessed for abnormal wear patterns. Parents are often concerned about the position of their child's foot while walking, whether intoeing or outtoeing. The most common foot deformity that will appear as intoeing is metatarsus adductus (Figure 2-6). The metatarsals are medially deviated. If the foot is flexible, this can often be corrected by a straight-last shoe or wearing the wrong shoe on the affected foot. Inflexible feet will probably require surgical intervention.

The most common cause of intoeing in the toddler is tibial torsion. The distal tibia twists in relation to the proximal tibia.[24] This can be assessed with the child in prone, measuring the thigh foot angle (Figure 2-7). The foot progression angle is assessed with the knee flexed to 90 degrees and then compared with the foot progression angle with the knee fully extended. The angle should range from −10 to +10 degrees. In the older child, the most common cause for intoeing is femoral anteversion. The femur twists between the femoral neck and the femoral condyles, bringing the femoral neck more anterior and causing increased internal rotation at the hip. The normal range of motion for internal rotation is 15 to 25 degrees. Children with femoral anteversion are often W-sitters, and in walking the patella is noted to be medially deviated.

In addition to the evaluation of hip rotation, hip abduction should be evaluated (Figure 2-8). If there is significantly reduced range of motion at the hip or a leg length discrepancy is noted, the hip may be subluxed or dislocated. A Galeazzi sign is present when a thigh length discrepancy is noted with the hips flexed. As the femoral head is pulled superiorly and posteriorly with subluxation or dislocation, the thigh appears shorter in comparison with

Table 2-3 Spinal Abnormalities

Spine Abnormality	Clinical Findings
Scoliosis (idiopathic, congenital, neuromuscular)	Curvature of spine on forward bending Rib humping Shoulder asymmetry Pelvic obliquity
Kyphosis (congenital, Scheuermann, neuromuscular)	Abnormal posture increases with flexion
Spondylolisthesis	Loss of lordosis, reduced range of motion Step-off back deformity Gait abnormalities Transverse abdominal creases

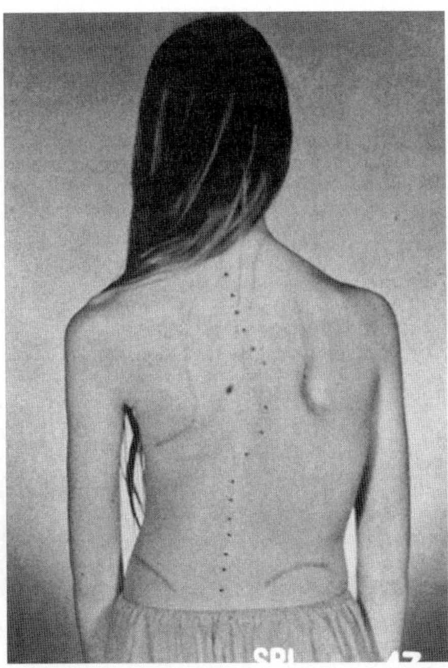

FIGURE 2-4 The evaluation of scoliosis includes an assessment of the spine with the child sitting or standing. This adolescent girl has an obvious curve in the standing position. She also has a rotational component.

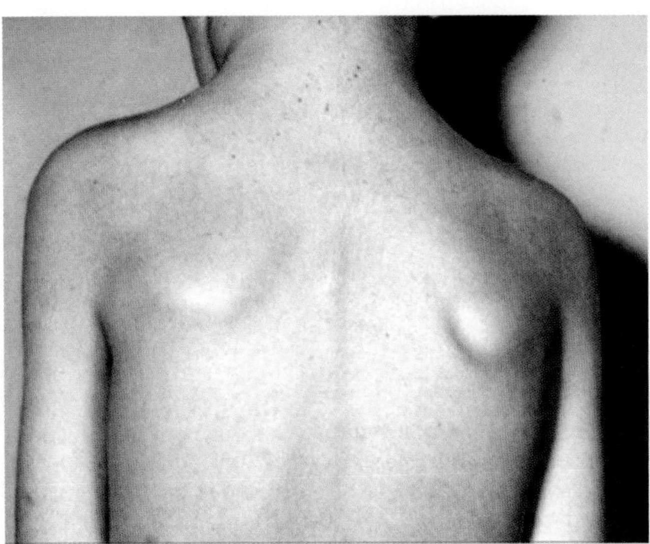

FIGURE 2-5 Sprengel deformity, a congenital elevation of the scapula, is often seen in association with Klippel-Feil syndrome and cervical spine abnormalities.

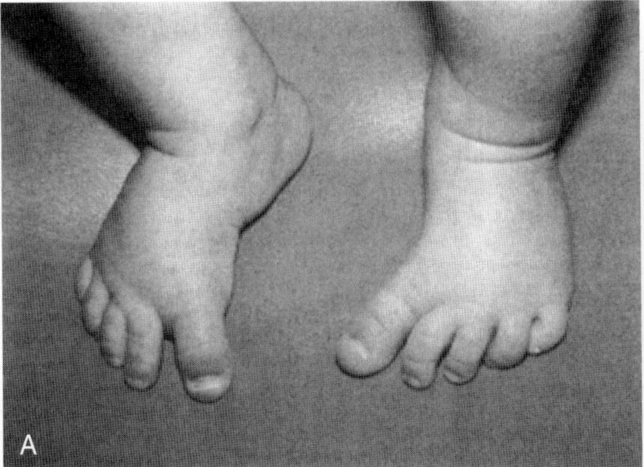

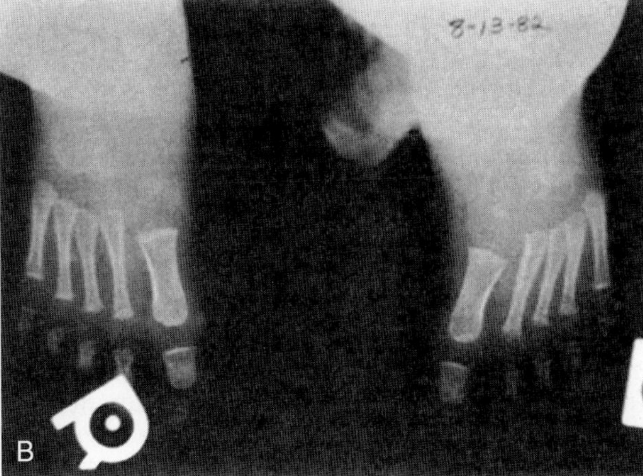

FIGURE 2-6 **A,** A child with bilateral metatarsus adductus. **B,** Radiograph showing medial deviation of the metatarsal bones.

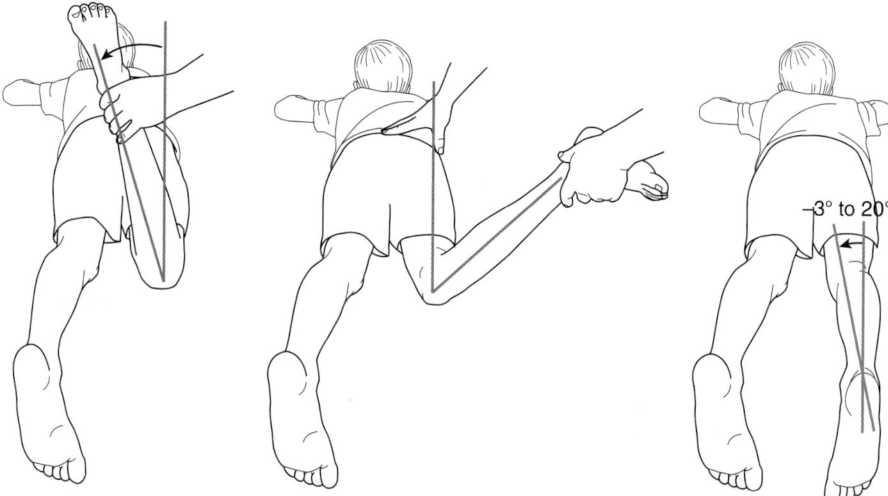

FIGURE 2-7 Evaluation of a child in the prone position allows assessment of the thigh-foot angle and internal and external rotation of the hip. The thigh-foot angle is demonstrated in the right diagram and ranges from −3 degrees to +20 degrees.

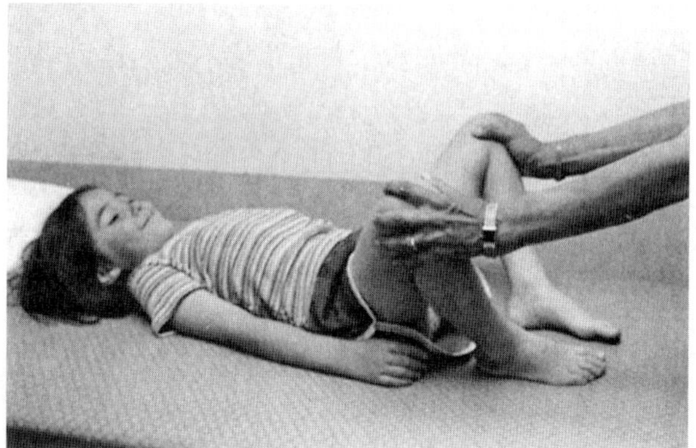

FIGURE 2-8 Examination of the hips should include passive range of motion, such as hip abduction, along with assessment of tone and spasticity.

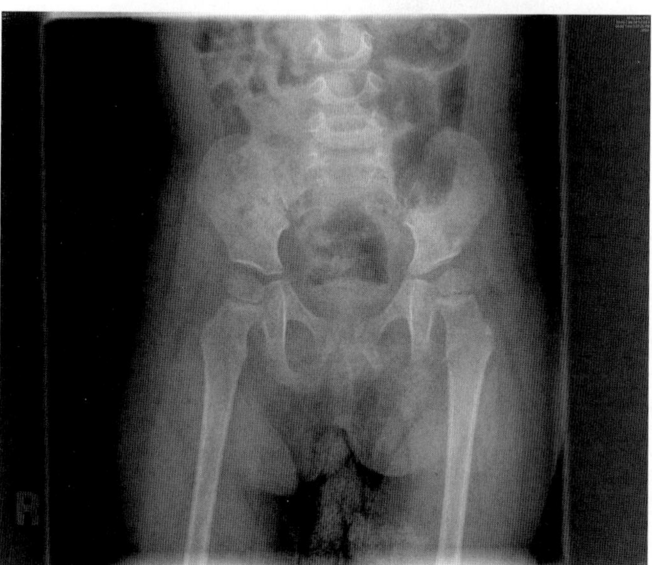

FIGURE 2-9 An anteroposterior pelvis film delineating the degree of subluxation in hip dislocation.

the normal hip. An anteroposterior pelvis film will delineate the degree of subluxation (Figure 2-9).

The child's knee should be evaluated for stability, mobility, and positioning. When a child presents as bowlegged (genu varus position), this may indicate rickets or Blount disease (Figure 2-10). However, children have normal, physiologic bowing up to age 2 years. Rickets is caused by vitamin D deficiency and results in the softening of the growth plates of a child's bones. The legs will appear bowed and the ankles thickened (Figure 2-11). Blount disease is more common in the African-American population and has also been associated with obesity and early walking. It is typically progressive and may need surgical intervention.

A child's foot can be normally flat (pes planus) until 3 to 5 years of age.[27] A flexible flat foot can be a normal variant into adulthood and does not need intervention. However, if the foot is rigid or painful, this may be the result of a tarsal coalition. The most commonly involved joints are the talocalcaneal and the calcaneonavicular. A rigid flat foot with a rocker bottom appearance is caused by a congenital vertical talus with dorsal dislocation of the navicular on the talus and has been associated with myelodysplasia and arthrogryposis (Figure 2-12).

Pes cavus is a high arched foot (Figure 2-13). When associated with sensory loss, foot intrinsic muscle wasting, weakness in the ankle dorsiflexors, and clawing of the toes, further investigation for a sensorimotor neuropathy such as Charcot-Marie-Tooth disease or other neuromuscular disorders should be initiated.

Neurologic Assessment

The neurologic assessment evaluates cranial nerve function, sensory function, strength, movement, reflexes, coordination, balance, gait, and cognitive function. Sensory function may be difficult to evaluate in the very young child and a complete examination including an assessment of light touch, proprioception, vibratory, pain, and temperature sensation may only be possible in older children.[7] When assessing infants and young children, the examiner should use the child's nonverbal cues such as looking at a light touch stimulus or pulling the limb away when touched. Vibratory toys may be helpful in the evaluation.

Responses to visual stimuli may be attempted with a bright light or an interesting object. Infants will track an object to midline at 1 month of age and from side to side

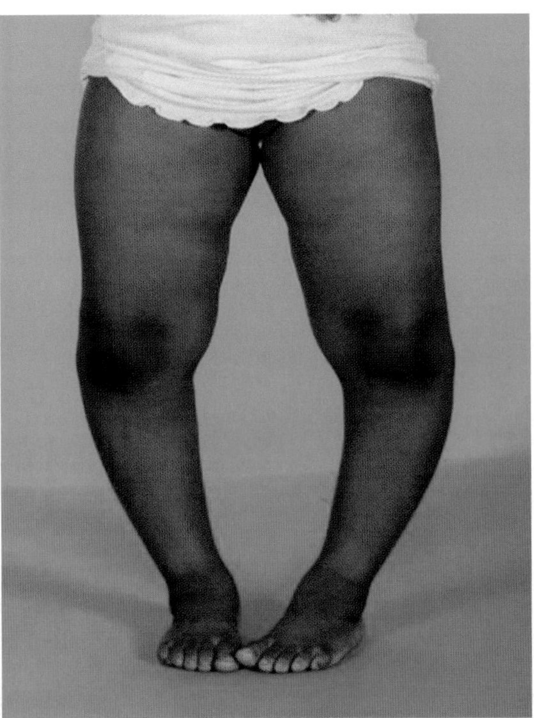

FIGURE 2-10 Bowlegged (genu varus position) presentation may indicate Blount disease.

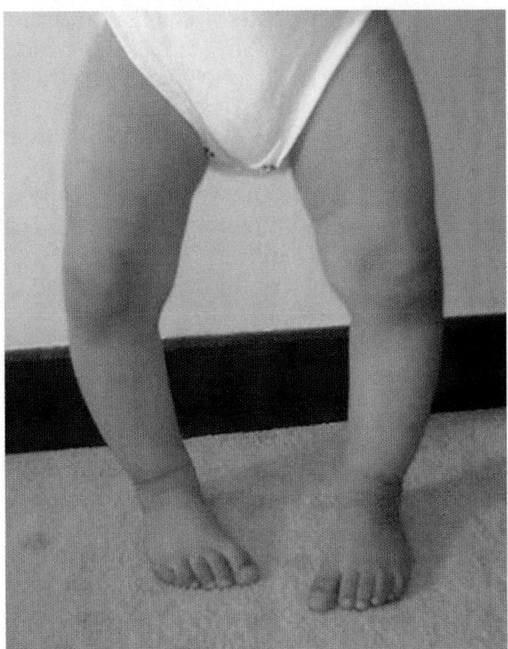

FIGURE 2-11 Softening of the growth plates of a child's bones causes the bowed legs and the thickened ankles seen in rickets.

at 3 months of age. Perception of color develops by 8 weeks of age and depth perception by 3 to 5 months of age. The child should be evaluated for any obvious ocular imbalance. Strabismus is a common finding in children with cerebral palsy. Patching, corrective lenses, and/or surgery is necessary at an early age to improve visual function.[23]

Auditory evaluation is a part of routine newborn screening. It should be reassessed with any child who demonstrates speech and language delays, articulation errors, inattentiveness to sound, a history of recurrent ear infections or history of brain injury.[6,26] In the infant, hearing can be evaluated by clapping or making a loud noise and watching for a startle (Moro) or blink response. Older children should respond to rubbing fingers close to their ears or toys that make sounds. If abnormalities are noted, the ears should be checked for impaction or infection. If the canals are clear and there are no signs of infection, then a comprehensive auditory evaluation is warranted.

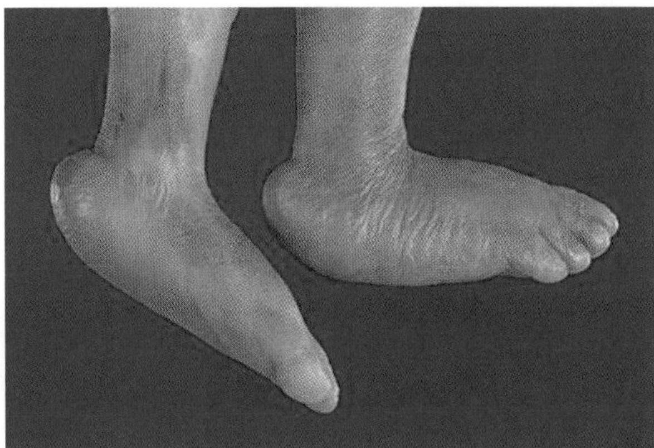

FIGURE 2-12 Rigid flat foot with a rocker bottom caused by a congenital vertical talus with dorsal dislocation of the navicular on the talus associated with myelodysplasia and arthrogryposis.

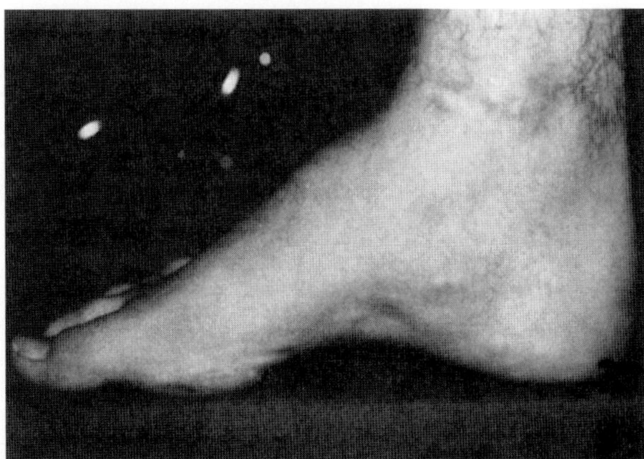

FIGURE 2-13 High-arched foot, or pes cavus, is seen in neuromuscular disorders.

Evaluation of primitive reflexes and postural responses is a helpful tool in evaluating the infant's motor responses. These reflexes (Table 2-4) are controlled at the level of the brainstem and spinal cord.[13] While the central nervous system matures, the reflexes are integrated and suppressed between 3 and 6 months of age. Obligatory primitive reflexes, a reflex that a child cannot move out of, are never normal and indicate a central nervous system problem. Any asymmetry of reflexes may reflect an underlying stroke or peripheral nerve disorder such as a brachial plexus injury. Primitive reflexes are replaced by postural reactions (Table 2-5) starting at approximately 2 months of age. These responses allow the child to progress with motor development. Asymmetry in these responses is considered abnormal and could indicate hemiplegia or a peripheral nerve injury.

Table 2-4 Gait Abnormalities

Gait	Characteristic(s)	Clinical Association
Spastic	Adducted hips Internal rotation of hips Toe walking	Cerebral palsy
Crouched	Weak quadriceps Weak hip extensors Excessive dorsiflexion Hip or knee contractures	Neuromuscular disease Cerebral palsy
Hemiparetic	Posturing of upper limb Circumduction of hip Inversion of foot	Cerebral palsy Cerebral vascular accident
Waddling (Trendelenburg)	Weakness of hip girdle Wide-based gait	Neuromuscular disease
Ataxic	Coordination problems Poor tandem walking	Cerebellar ataxia Friedreich ataxia

Table 2-5 Common Primitive Reflexes and the Period They Typically Disappear

Reflex	Stimulus	Response	Disappears by (mo)
Moro	Sudden neck extension	Shoulder abduction, elbow and finger extension followed by shoulder adduction and elbow flexion	4 to 6
Rooting	Stroking area around mouth	Head and mouth move toward stimulus	4
Asymmetrical tonic neck	Head turned to side	Arm or leg extend on face side and flex on occipital side	6 to 7
Symmetrical tonic neck	Neck flexion, neck extension	Arms flex, legs extend; arms extend, legs flex	6 to 7
Palmar grasp	Touch palm	Flexion of all fingers	5 to 6

A true manual muscle examination is not very accurate before the age of 5 years, but the child should show at least antigravity strength. Strength can be qualitatively assessed by evaluating the child's ability to hold their head in midline, sit without support, reach for objects overhead, hold on to objects, creep, stand, and walk. The strength examination is affected by tone and must be interpreted carefully in children with hypertonia resulting from the inability to differentiate between voluntary and involuntary muscle activation.

When evaluating a child's muscle tone, remember that the tone will change during development. Premature infants often have lower muscle tone that should improve with time. If the child is still hypotonic as a toddler or demonstrates motoric delays, then there is likely an underlying neuromuscular abnormality. Hypertonia may be subdivided into spasticity, dystonia, and rigidity.[32] This is never normal and indicates a central nervous system disorder. Children with cerebral palsy are often hypotonic as infants and then develop hypertonia within the first year of life. Hypotonia with associated areflexia in a newborn is consistent with spinal muscular atrophy. Acute onset hypotonia and areflexia in a previously healthy child is suggestive of botulism or acute inflammatory demyelinating polyneuropathy.

Table 2-6 Postural Reactions and the Period They Typically Occur

Postural Reaction	Stimulus	Response	Age of Emergence
Head righting	Vestibular or visual	Head and face aligned vertical and mouth aligned horizontal	Prone, 2 mo; supine, 3 to 4 mo
Protective extension	Center of gravity displaced outside base of support in sitting	Abduction of upper limb toward displacement to prevent falling	Sitting anterior, 5 to 7 mo; lateral, 6 to 8 mo; posterior, 7 to 8 mo
Parachute reaction	Center of gravity displaced	Extension of upper limbs outside base of support in standing	Standing, 12 to 14 mo toward displacement to prevent falling

Gait assessment requires an understanding of the impact of joint mobility, bony alignment, weakness, and tonal abnormalities on gait. Interventions such as bracing, surgery, and medications will be based on both the examination of muscles at rest and during the functional activity of walking. A child's gait pattern changes and progresses from the age of 1 to approximately 7 years old.[20] As a child's balance and coordination improve, the base of support narrows during the gait cycle. The arms progress from a high guard position to a mature arm swing. The stance phase progresses from a foot flat pattern with an increased foot progression angle to a heel-to-toe progression with the foot in more neutral alignment. The stride length increases and the cadence decreases. Common gait deviations are listed in Table 2-6.

Functional Assessment

There are many evaluation tools to evaluate and quantify functional status in the pediatric population. The commonly used Functional Independence Measure (FIM) for adults has been adapted to children (weeFIM) by adjusting for developmental stages. The levels of assistance are the same between the two scales, but the expected FIM level for age differs based on developmental level, for example, a 12-month-old baby would be expected to be a weeFIM level 1 (complete dependence) for toileting. This tool has been used successfully to measure progress and outcome for pediatric inpatient rehabilitation services as well as in the outpatient setting.

Developmental skills can be formally assessed with a variety of tools (Table 2-7). The Denver Developmental Screening Test (DDST-II) is useful as a quick screen to determine whether a child is achieving developmental milestones in the areas of gross motor, fine motor, language, and personal-social skills.[16] It can be used with children ages birth to 6 years old. The DDST-II is both an observational assessment and an assessment based on parental report. If a child fails the Denver screening, then a more formalized assessment with the Bayley Scales of

Table 2-7 Developmental Evaluation and Screening Tests

Test	Age Range	Scope and Value
Denver Developmental Screening Test[14]	Birth to 6 years	Quick screen for deviations from normal development of normal and near-normal children; pattern of functional deviations guides further evaluation
Bayley Scale of Infant Development[3]	Birth to 30 months	Separate mental and motor scales; well standardized; heavily weighted with motor-based items, which limits predictive value in physically handicapped children
Gesell Developmental Schedule[16]	4 weeks to 6 years	Indicator of current developmental level

Table 2-8 Intellectual Evaluations

Test	Age Range (years)	Scope and Value
Stanford-Binet Intelligence Scale[37]	2 to adult	Detailed diagnostic assessment (mental age and IQ); guidelines for hearing, visual, and motor handicaps
Wechsler Preschool and Primary Scale of Intelligence-Revised (WPPSI-R)[40]	3 to 6.5	Verbal, performance, and full-scale scores; delineates strengths and weaknesses; not appropriate for children with severe developmental delays
Wechsler Intelligence Scale for Children-Revised (WISC-R)[39]	6 to 16	Verbal, performance, and full-scale scores; subtests point to specific areas of strength or dysfunction
Kaufman Assessment Battery for Children[19]	2.5 to 12	Measures mental processes independent of the content of acquired knowledge; useful for children from disadvantaged backgrounds

IQ, Intelligence quotient.

Infant Development[3] or the Gesell Developmental Schedule[14] is recommended. These tests are typically given by therapists. The Bayley test is appropriate for children ages birth to 30 months, and the Gesell test is for children ages 4 weeks to 6 years. These tests are based on direct observation of the child's skills. The major drawback of these tests is that cognitive ability is estimated based on motoric performance. For children with significant physical impairment, the tests often underestimate their cognitive abilities.

Cognition and potential for academic achievement can be assessed in the preschool and school-age child with several different tests (Table 2-8). These tests evaluate both intellectual and physical abilities. They are very much motorically and language based. For children with physical limitations or language impairments, alternative nonverbal and motor-eliminated tests are available (Table 2-9). Interestingly, vocabulary tests have the highest correlation with school success and overall intellectual ability.

Table 2-9 Alternative Nonverbal and Motor-Eliminated Tests

Test	Age Range (yr)	Scope and Value
Peabody Picture Vocabulary Test (PPVT)[11]	2.5 to 18	Effective test of language, especially in children with speech and motor impairments
Leiter International Performance Scale[22]	2 to 18	Measures nonverbal problem-solving abilities in deaf and in speech- and motor-handicapped children
Pictorial Test of Intelligence[15]	3 to 8	Measures intellectual ability of multiply handicapped children; requires receptive language
Raven's Progressive Matrices[30]	6 to adult	Measures nonverbal intelligence and concept formation

Table 2-10 Perceptual Evaluations

Test	Age Range (y)	Scope and Value
Beery-Buktenica Development Test of Visual Motor Integration[4]	2 to 16	Assesses visual motor performance, ability to copy geometric shapes, age equivalence
Bender Visual Motor Gestalt Test[5]	5 to adult	Assesses visual motor performance; easy to administer; nine geometric designs

Table 2-11 Academic Achievement Tests

Test	Grade Level or Age Range	Scope and Value
Wide Range Achievement Test-Revised (WRAT)[17]	Kindergarten to twelfth grade	Yields academic achievement level in reading, spelling, arithmetic; can measure progress
Woodcock-Johnson Psychoeducational Battery: Test of Achievement[42]	3 yr to adult	Yields age and grade level, percentiles, and standard scores in reading, mathematics, written language, and general tasks
Peabody Individual Achievement Test[10]	Kindergarten to twelfth grade	Only pointing response for overview of achievement; useful for handicapped

To evaluate visual motor abilities, the Beery-Buktenica Developmental Test of Visual Motor Integration[4] and the Bender Visual Motor Gestalt Test[5] were developed (Table 2-10). These tests can detect delays in visual perceptual skills and eye-hand coordination in children ages 2 years old through adult. The Rey-Osterrieth Complex Figure Test[8] can further test visual organization and visual memory. It entails the copying of a complex figure followed by delayed recall of the figure. The test may also assist with discerning visual field cuts or areas of visual neglect. The test is appropriate for children ages 6 years old to adult. There are additional evaluation tools to assess perceptual motor, auditory processing, and tactile functioning.

Academic achievement tests measure a child's proficiency in school subject areas such as reading and mathematics. Table 2-11 lists some of the more commonly used

Table 2-12 Social and Adaptive Skills

Test	Age Range	Scope and Value
Vineland Adaptive Behavior Scale[34]	1 mo to adult	Questionnaire of social competence in communication, socialization, daily living skills, and motor skills; adjusted for handicapped
American Association of Mental Deficiency Adaptive Behavior Scale[28]	3 yr to adult	Activities of daily living; adaptive and maladaptive behaviors; assists in program planning

Table 2-13 Quality-of-Life Measures

Test	Age Range (yr)	Scope and Value
Pediatric Quality of Life Inventory (PedsQL) self-report and parent-proxy questionnaire	2 to 18	Measures health-related quality of life
Child Health Questionnaire (CHQ) self-report and parent-proxy questionnaire	5 to 18	Measures 14 unique physical and psychosocial concepts

tests. The scores are reported as a grade equivalent. Subsets of these tests can be administered on the inpatient unit to assess a child's current academic level. It is particularly helpful for children who have sustained a brain injury. The information assists with reintegration back into the school setting by setting a baseline of knowledge from which to proceed.

In addition to physical, perceptual, and cognitive skills, it is important to evaluate a child's social and adaptive skills and their perceived quality of life (Tables 2-12 and 2-13). The Vineland Adaptive Behavioral Scale[34] is appropriate for children with and without disabilities. It measures a child's ability to use skills to function in everyday settings. It is composed of four components: communication, daily living, socialization, and motor skills. It also has a scale for maladaptive behaviors that surveys inappropriate social or behavioral displays. Information is collected from the child, the parent or caregiver, and the school. The Pediatric Quality of Life Inventory (PedsQL) evaluates a child's opinion regarding satisfaction with personal health and wellness.[38] It measures the child's perceived quality of life in physical, emotional, social, and school functioning.

Disability-specific assessment tools include the Gross Motor Function Measure (GMFM-66),[31] the Manual Abilities Classification Scale (MACS), and the Quality of Upper Extremity Skills Test (QUEST) for cerebral palsy. The GMFM-66 is a subset of the original GMFM-88 that evaluates gross motor functions such as lying, rolling, sitting, crawling, standing, walking, running, and jumping. Individual items are scored on a 4-point scale ranging from 0 (no initiation) to 4 (completion of the task). The MACS and the QUEST both evaluate fine motor skills and hand manipulation. The MACS categorizes children into one of five levels of function. These levels range from level 1 (handles objects well and easily) to level 5 (unable to handle objects). The QUEST evaluates movement patterns and hand function.[9]

Summary

The pediatric history and physical examination should be tailored to each child and family. The developmental level of the child must be evaluated and rehabilitation approaches selected and instituted based on that developmental level and the goals for continued development. There are a wide range of assessment tools available to assist with determining the child's strengths and weaknesses in all domains.

REFERENCES

1. Aicardi J: Diseases of the nervous system in childhood, *Clin Dev Med* 11:118, 1992.
2. Barness CA: *Principles and practice of pediatrics*, Philadelphia, 1994, Lippincott.
3. Bayley N: *Bayley scale of infant development*, New York, 1969, Psychological Corp.
4. Beery K, Buktenica N: *Developmental test of visual-motor integration*, Chicago, 1967, Follett.
5. Bender L: *Bender visual-motor Gestalt test*, New York, 1946, American Orthopsychiatric Association.
6. Brown SB: Neurologic examination during the first 2 years of life. In Swaiman YF, Wright FS, editors: *The practice of pediatric neurology*, St Louis, 1982, Mosby, pp 9–21.
7. Brown SB: Neurologic examination of the older child. In Swaiman YF, Wright FS, editors: *The practice of pediatric neurology*, St Louis, 1982, Mosby, pp 35–50.
8. Corwin J, Bylsma FW: Translations of excerpts from Andre Rey's psychological examination of traumatic encephalopathy and P.A. Osterrieth's the complex figure copy test, *Clin Neuropsychol* 7:3–15, 1993.
9. DeMatteo C, Law M, Russell D, et al: *QUEST: quality of upper extremity skills test*, Hamilton, 1992, McMaster University.
10. Dunn L, Markwardt F: *Manual: peabody individual achievement test*, Circle Pines, 1970, American Guidance Service.
11. Dunn LM: *Peabody picture vocabulary test-revised*, Circle Pines, 1970, American Guidance Service.
12. El-Hawary R, Chukwunyerenwa C: Update on evaluation and treatment of scoliosis, *Pediatr Clin North Am* 61:1223–1241, 2014.
13. Fiorentino MR: *Normal and abnormal development*, Springfield, 1972, Charles C Thomas.
14. Frakenburg WC, Dodds J, Archer P: *Denver II technical manual*, Denver, 1990, Denver Developmental Materials.
15. French J: *Manual: pictorial test of intelligence*, Boston, 1964, Houghton Mifflin.
16. Gesell A: *Gesell developmental schedule*, New York, 1979, Psychological Corp.
17. Jastak S, Wilkinson GS: *The wide range achievement tests-revised*, Wilmington, 1984, Jastak Associates.
18. Johnson CP, Blasco PA: Infant growth and development, *Pediatr Rev* 18:224–242, 1997.
19. Kaufman A, Kaufman N: *Kaufman assessment battery for children*, Circle Pines, 1983, American Guidance Service.
20. Keen M: Early development and attainment of normal mature gait, *J Prosthet Orthot* 5:35–38, 1993.
21. Kliegman RM, Nelson WE, editors: *Nelson's textbook of pediatrics*, Philadelphia, 2007, Saunders Elsevier.
22. Leiter R: *The Leiter international performance scale*, Chicago, 1969, Stoelting.
23. Lewis M, Taft LT, editors: *Developmental disabilities. Theory, assessment and intervention*, New York, 1982, SP Medical and Scientific Books.
24. Lincoln TL, Suen PW: Common rotational variations in children, *J Am Acad Orthop Surg* 11:312–320, 2003.
25. Medical Research Council Vitamin Study Research Group: Prevention of neural tube defects: results of the Medical Research Council Vitamin Study, *Lancet* 338:131–137, 1991.
26. Milstein JM: Abnormalities of hearing. In Swaiman YF, Wright FS, editors: *The practice of pediatric neurology*, St Louis, 1982, Mosby.
27. Morrisy RT, Weinstein SL, editors: *Lovell and Winter's pediatric orthopaedics*, ed 4, Philadelphia, 1996, Lippincott.

28. Nihira K, Foster R, Shellhaas M, Leland H: *AAMD adaptive behavior scale*, 1975 revision: manual, Washington, DC, 1975, American Association on Mental Deficiency.
29. Persing J, James H, Swanson J, et al: Prevention and management of positional skull deformities in infants. American Academy of Pediatrics Committee on Practice and Ambulatory Medicine, Section on Plastic Surgery and Section on Neurological Surgery, *Pediatrics* 112(Pt 1):199–202, 2003.
30. Raven J: *Raven's progressive matrices*, Dumfries, 1958, Crichton Royal.
31. Russell DJ, Rosenbaum PL, Cadman DT, et al: The Gross Motor Function Measure: a means to evaluate the effects of physical therapy, *Dev Med Child Neurol* 31:341–352, 1989.
32. Sanger TD, Delgado MR, Gaebler-Spira D, et al: Classification and definition of disorders causing hypertonia in childhood, *Pediatrics* 111:e89–e97, 2003.
33. Shurtleff DB, editor: *Myelodysplasias and extrophies: significance, prevention and treatment*, New York, 1986, Grune and Stratton.
34. Sparrow SS, Balla DA, Ciccheti DV: *Vineland adaptive behavior scale*, Circle Pines, 1984, American Guidance Service.
35. Stanley F, Blair E, Alberman E: *Cerebral palsies: epidemiology and causal pathways*, London, 2000, Mac Keith Press.
36. Steindler A: *Kinesiology of the human body*, Springfield, 1955, Charles C Thomas.
37. Thorndike RL, Hagen EP, Sattler JM: *The Stanford-Binet intelligence scale*, ed 4, Chicago, 1986, Riverside.
38. Varni JW, Seid M, Rode CA: The PedsQL: measurement model for the pediatric quality of life inventory, *Med Care* 37:126–139, 1999.
39. Wechsler D: *Wechsler intelligence scale for children-revised*, New York, 1974, Psychological Corp.
40. Wechsler D: *Wechsler preschool and primary scales of intelligence-revised*, San Antonio, 1989, Psychological Corp.
41. Wheeler MD, Styne DM: Diagnosis and management of precocious puberty, *Pediatr Clin North Am* 37:1255–1271, 1990.
42. Woodcock R, Johnson MD: *Woodcock-Johnson psychoeducational battery: tests of achievement*, Allen, 1989, DLM Teaching Resources.

CHAPTER 3

ADULT NEUROGENIC COMMUNICATION AND SWALLOWING DISORDERS

Susan Koch Fager, Mark Hakel, Susan Brady, Steven M. Barlow, Amy Nordness, Ana Delgado, Jeffrey B. Palmer

A wide range of communication and swallowing disorders result from neurologic injury. This chapter provides the physiatrist with a broad overview of some of the impairments that result from acquired neurologic conditions and how they are assessed and treated by a speech-language pathologist. In addition to providing an understanding the underlying impairment, this chapter describes the impact these impairments have on the activity and participation levels of individuals undergoing rehabilitation.

Rehabilitation of Patients with Communication Disorders

Aphasia

Aphasia is a communication disorder typically resulting from damage to the language-dominant hemisphere in the brain. Stroke is the most common cause of aphasia with approximately 20% to 40% of patients with stroke having aphasia.[152,158] Aphasia, however, can occur in traumatic brain injury or dementia and other progressive neurologic disorders.

Aphasia affects an individual's ability to express and understand language. Aphasia types include Broca, Wernicke, conduction, global, transcortical motor, transcortical sensory, anomic, and crossed and primary progressive Aphasia (Table 3-1). Some individuals may have relatively intact receptive language capabilities but demonstrate significant challenges with expression, whereas others may have significant deficits in both areas. Speech-language pathologists play a primary role in teasing out these deficits and identifying strengths to capitalize on during recovery.[56] Apraxia of speech is a common co-occurring deficit and differential diagnosis is key to appropriate intervention.[56,114]

Assessment by the speech-language pathologist involves identification of the specific areas of language deficit, including spoken language, auditory comprehension, reading and writing, and the severity of these deficits. Standardized assessments, such as the Western Aphasia Battery–Revised[85] and the Boston Naming Test,[80] are often used to identify specific areas of deficit to guide treatment planning.

Intervention with adults with aphasia is unique in that these are individuals who typically were literate before injury and have a lifetime of experiences to communicate and share.[86] However, the language deficits associated with aphasia make it difficult for these individuals to not only communicate basic wants and needs but also to be able to maintain their previous life roles. Many become isolated, and their social networks significantly diminish after injury.[32,38,150] Although the exact rate and extent of recovery varies, many are left with substantial communication impairments. Therefore speech-language pathologists focus their interventions on *restorative* as well as *compensatory* strategies and techniques to supplement language deficits and to facilitate participation with the greatest level of independence possible.

Early in recovery in the acute rehabilitation setting, patients may be struggling to not only express what their wants, needs, and ideas are but to also understand what is being said to them. Language deficits related to aphasia can make it challenging for the patient to fully participate in rehabilitation with all disciplines; therefore the speech-language pathologist's intervention will focus on developing and implementing compensatory strategies and techniques and training/supporting therapy, nursing, and family in these strategies and techniques. Compensatory strategies and techniques for individuals with aphasia are also referred to as augmentative and alternative communication (AAC). AAC can take the form of low-tech (pictures, communication boards, talking photo albums, augmented input such as writing) to high-tech (computerized communication devices and software that the patient can use to communicate) options.[14,15] The specific content (pictures compared with words), the complexity of the content (e.g., low tech compared with high tech, amount of communicative content represented) is determined through careful assessment and trials with the patient as well as specific feedback from the rehabilitation staff and family. For example, a patient with auditory receptive deficits may benefit from adding written words on a dry-erase board or pictures of content in addition to the auditory cues given in therapy. In another example, a patient with severe expressive deficits may benefit from photographic images presented in a communication device to communicate basic requests to staff and family as well as to support communication of biographic information (e.g., home, family, vocation, interests). These compensatory AAC strategies and techniques help the patient communicate their current needs and in the contexts in which they need to participate to the fullest extent possible.[93,138] In addition, the speech therapist will often focus on attempting to

Table 3-1 Aphasia Types

Aphasia Type	Lesion	Expressive and Receptive Language Impairments
Broca aphasia	Left posterior inferior frontal cortex and underlying structures	Expressive: Nonfluent aphasia with effortful speech, anomia, and reduced utterance length. Receptive: Impaired but typically better than expressive language.
Wernicke aphasia	Left superior temporal region or inferior parietal cortex involving angular gyri	Expressive: Fluent with normal prosody but significant paraphasias, neologisms, and empty content. They appear unaware of these deficits. Receptive: Often severely impaired with inability to understand spoken language.
Conduction aphasia	Left superior temporal area or the supramarginal gyrus of the parietal lobe	Expressive: Fluent with considerable anomia, paraphasias, self-correcting behavior, and difficulty with repetition. Receptive: Relatively intact auditory comprehension of spoken language.
Global aphasia	Frontotemporoparietal	Expressive: Limited speech output but may exhibit ability to produce repetitive perseverative utterances. Receptive: Severely impaired ability to understand spoken and written language.
Transcortical motor aphasia	Occlusion of anterior cerebral artery with damage to the border zone areas in the frontal lobe superior or anterior to Broca area	Expressive: Similar to Broca aphasia, nonfluent, limited speech with dysarthric component. Receptive: Generally intact.
Transcortical sensory aphasia	Posterior or inferior to Wernicke area	Expressive: Similar to Wernicke aphasia but able to repeat and can exhibit echolalia. Receptive: Significant impairment understanding spoken and written language.
Anomic aphasia	Focal damage to the left temporal and parietal areas	Expressive: Primary challenge is word finding and naming. Speech includes pauses and circumlocutions and they typically have a good prognosis for recovery. Receptive: Generally intact.
Crossed aphasia	Rare incidence of right hemisphere lesion resulting in aphasia	Expressive and receptive: Mirrors aphasias of left hemisphere. Some may also have co-occurring visual-spatial deficits consistent with right hemisphere lesion.
Primary progressive aphasia	Insidious onset	Initial symptoms include word finding deficits similar to acute aphasia but later expands to greater difficulty with expressive and receptive language along with dementia and other cognitive communication deficits.

restore deficit areas to a more functional level (e.g., naming, conversation, reading, writing). This combined approach is essential, particularly for those with severe impairments because their recovery of expressive and receptive language abilities may be an ongoing process. These individuals may plateau at a level where they will require compensatory tools for the long term.

There is evidence that currently supports the intensity of treatment offered to the patient with aphasia. In general, shorter bouts of intense treatment have been shown to improve communication outcomes compared with less intense treatment over longer periods.[10,16,26,68] However, extended periods of therapy that include a strict regimen of intervention (2 to 4 hours daily) can also result in substantial improvements in communication.[10] Constraint-induced aphasia therapy has been compared with multimodal aphasia therapy with comparable results.[25,128,129]

The impact of new interventions with repetitive transcranial magnetic stimulation (rTMS) is being explored,[5,28,45,145] along with the development of computerized treatment options to augment and supplement speech treatment.[24,67,81,92] In addition, pharmacologic therapy modulating the activity of several neurotransmitter systems with medications, such as levodopa, donepezil, galantamine, and memantine, have been used along with language therapy for treatment of aphasia with moderate success.[11,12,51]

Education is a key component of treatment because it is often difficult for family and friends to understand the difference between cognitive and language deficits. Family and friends must understand that individuals with aphasia are aware of what is occurring around them and that they remember who people are but that they cannot access the "language" to communicate this information. In addition, they may need to rely on modalities other than spoken language to understand what is being said to them (e.g., writing key words down may facilitate comprehension of the topic of conversation). The long-term nature of some deficits can be difficult to accept for patients and family because they have a significant impact on the patient's ability to return to preferred life roles (e.g., work, family, and social roles). Providing education about the existing deficits and providing training on the use of compensatory strategies and techniques to facilitate full participation are essential as the patient and family begin to adjust to changes in life roles.[4,137]

Special Considerations: Handedness and Language Dominance

Since the description of left hemisphere language regions in right-handed patients by Paul Broca in the nineteenth century, it has been speculated that the reverse, that is, right hemisphere language dominance, should be true of those who are left-handed. This claim has been widely accepted as the Broca rule, although Broca never explicitly postulated such a rule.[61] Luria was among the first to point out that such an association could not be universally true because even in those who are left-handed, aphasia usually occurs after a lesion to the left hemisphere.[104] Ninety-three percent of the population is right handed, with the left hemisphere being dominant for language in 99% of right-handed individuals.[39] In left-handed individuals, 70% have language control in the left hemisphere, with only 15% having it in the right hemisphere, and 15% in both hemispheres,[117] localizing the language control in the left hemisphere in approximately 97% of the population.

Even now, our knowledge about the suspected association between handedness and language dominance rests almost exclusively on studies of neurologic patients. In this population, however, there is an increased incidence of pathologic left-handedness and right language dominance because the control of both dexterity and language can shift to the right hemisphere after long-standing left hemisphere lesions.[100,124,148,156]

Cognitive Communication Disorders

Cognitive communication disorders is a term used to describe a cluster of deficits that impair the processes of memory, new learning, awareness, problem solving, organizing, planning and execution, and all areas of executive function. The causes of these impairments vary as does the approach to intervention. In addition, whether the condition is severe and whether the condition is recovering or degenerative affect the exact focus of treatment. The following sections describe the management of cognitive communication disorders that result mostly from right hemisphere stroke, traumatic and nontraumatic brain injury, and Alzheimer disease and other dementia.

Right Hemisphere Stroke

Cognitive communication disorders that result from right hemisphere strokes include a range of deficits, including memory, attention, problem solving, decreased awareness/insight into severity of deficits, processing and expressing higher level/abstract language concepts, decreased or flat affect, organizing, planning, and other executive functions. Visuospatial neglect is often a co-occurring deficit and affects scanning and attention for reading, writing, and functioning safely in all environments. The most commonly reported cognitive communication deficits in patients who have had right hemisphere damage include attention, neglect, perception, and learning/memory.[17] Speech-language pathologists formally assess these deficits with a variety of standardized tests, including the Ross Information Processing Assessment (RIPA),[131] the Cognitive Linguistic Quick Test (CLQT),[63] or the Scales of Cognitive Assessment Test Battery (SCATBI).[1]

Specific treatment goals and intervention strategies vary on the basis of severity of deficits. However, increasing insight into deficits can be a particularly challenging barrier in rehabilitation. Coupled with a common left neglect, more severely affected patients require significant cues and support to safely navigate and participate in all environments. Research has indicated that those without neglect tend to have reduced cognitive communication deficits compared with patients with left visual field neglect.[23] Education of family on how to manage these deficits and provide the level of cueing and supervision necessary for the patient is essential.

Intervention with the speech-language pathologist might focus on activities related to home, community, and work reentry. Taking the specific deficits into account and how these deficits affect reintegration back into these environments is essential. For example, if a patient is expected to return to work, the ability to perform daily work functions (e.g., reading, writing, problem solving, time management) is assessed, and specific interventions are designed to compensate for deficits and to restore certain areas that were affected by the stroke.

Traumatic and Nontraumatic Brain Injury

Individuals who have sustained a brain injury demonstrate a range of neurobehavioral and cognitive disorders. Brain injuries are typically classified as traumatic (e.g., resulting from impact, translational pressure, or rotational forces to the brain) or nontraumatic (e.g., tumor, anoxia, aneurysm). Traumatic injuries include penetrating (open) head injury that often causes focal damage and closed head injuries that often result in diffuse axonal damage. Brain injury recovery typically occurs in stages, and speech-language intervention goals and objectives vary by stage.

The cognitive communication disorders associated with brain injury are often described with the Rancho Los Amigos Levels of Cognitive Functioning (Table 3-2).[55] For clinical intervention, these levels are often grouped into stages and treatment goals focus on supporting and optimizing the progressions through these stages. The stages of recovery include early (Rancho Levels I-III), middle (Rancho Levels IV-V), and late (Rancho Levels VI-VIII).[159]

Early Stage of Recovery: At this level, the speech-language pathologist focuses on stimulating and shaping responses for basic communication and will look for consistency of ability to respond, follow basic commands, and helping the team identify when the patient is transitioning from generalized to localized responses. Most patients at this level are nonspeaking and in the early stages of demonstrating consciousness.

Middle Stage of Recovery: As the patient transitions from early to the middle stage of recovery, they may be very agitated and treatment generally focuses on structuring the environment to reduce agitation so that the patient can continue to participate as fully as possible in rehabilitation. The patient transitions from an agitated to a nonagitated state, but confusion and disorientation are still evident. Evidence has shown that this stage of recovery is particularly important with regard to speech recovery. As a patient begins to cognitively "clear" at this stage, many will become verbal communicators.[41] For those who remain nonspeaking through this middle phase of recovery, it is a long-term disability attributable to either significant motor speech impairment/or aphasia/apraxia. If a patient remains nonspeaking at this level, AAC will be implemented by the speech-language pathologist. Because of the significant cognitive challenges that are still apparent at this stage, a variety of AAC systems will likely be developed and implemented over time. Some examples may include the use of a single message switch that has recorded messages to

Table 3-2 Rancho Los Amigos Levels of Cognitive Functioning

Rancho Level	Communication/Behaviors
I. No response	Unresponsive to any stimuli and there is no evidence of language processing.
II. Generalized response	Reacts inconsistently and unpurposefully to stimuli in nonspecific manner. Receptively and expressively there is no evidence of processing or verbal or gestural expression.
III. Localized response	Reacts specifically, but inconsistently, to stimuli. May follow simple commands in an inconsistent, delayed manner. Language begins to emerge (e.g., automatic verbal and gestural responses, yes/no head nodding, single words, limited reading).
IV. Confused, agitated	Behavior may appear bizarre and outbursts may be common. Attention to environment is very short and recall is limited. Disinhibition is common with inability to self-monitor behavior. Literal paraphasia may be present and incomplete expression of thoughts. Marked disruptions in auditory and visual processing may be apparent.
V. Confused, inappropriate, nonagitated	Able to respond to simple commands with consistency. Disoriented/confused with limited short-term recall. May be able to sustain short bursts of appropriate automatic social behavior. Verbalizations may be bizarre with many confabulatory statements. Semantic and syntactic confusion may be impaired.
VI. Confused, appropriate	Shows goal-directed behavior, follows simple commands, and demonstrates some increases in short-term memory. Processing of receptive language is delayed with some difficulty in retaining and synthesizing information. Difficulty with new learning is evident. Speech may be characterized by monopitch, monostress, and monoloudness.
VII. Automatic, appropriate	Appropriate and oriented to immediate environment, able to follow daily routine with structure/support. Ability to process and retain receptive language improves for simple/concrete information. Expressive language may be tangential, concrete, and self-oriented. Judgment remains impaired.
VIII. Purposeful and appropriate	Increasing memory/recall and ability to learn and retain new information. May demonstrate higher level cognitive-language deficits that become more apparent under new or stressful situations.

Adapted from Hagen C: Language disorders in head trauma. In Holland A, editor: *Language disorders in adults*, Austin, 1984, Taylor & Francis, pp 257-258.

make basic requests, eye-gaze boards to communicate yes/no, or simple digitized message devices with a small number of messages to communicate basic needs or personally relevant information. The particular device, access method, and types of messages to be communicated are individualized per patient and dependent on the physical capabilities of the patient, his or her cognitive and language status, and the needs of the family and rehabilitation team. If AAC is a long-term recommendation for a patient with a brain injury, it may evolve and gradually change into consistent use of a more sophisticated computerized communication device once the patient has reached the late stages of recovery.

For patients who regain their ability to speak at this stage, the focus of intervention is to increase orientation and insight, short-term and prospective memory, new learning, processing auditory and visual information, managing language of confusion and confabulations, and ability to learn new information, following directions, and processing and increasing functional participation in rehabilitation.

Late Stage of Recovery: At this level, speech intervention focuses on increasing orientation, memory, carryover of new learning, and eventually higher-level executive functions for home, school, and community reintegration.

Mild Brain Injury. Some individuals sustain mild brain injuries that are not easily detectable through brain imaging, and many may bypass an acute inpatient hospital stay. However, high-level cognitive communication disorders associated with these injuries can affect work, home, and community reintegration.[136] Impairments of executive function (e.g., planning, organization, attention, self-monitoring, prospective memory, insight) are common.[146] Many of these individuals receive therapy on an outpatient basis. Intervention focuses on increasing awareness of deficits, education, and the development and application of a range of compensatory strategies (e.g., organizational systems, memory logs, planners, specific recall strategies, electronic reminders, reorganization of work environment to facilitate recall and organization). Some may be struggling to maintain their employment and driving given the deficits they are experiencing; therefore intervention focuses on compensating for these losses so that the individual can maintain employment and life roles. Over time, many report a lessoning or resolution of impairments. For those with lasting deficits, compensatory strategies developed during intervention become lifelong habits that enable these individuals to fully participate in work and life roles as independently as possible.

Alzheimer Disease and Other Dementia

The pathophysiologic features of dementia can vary by person and can be caused by neurodegenerative changes in the brain, vascular in origin, the result of toxic reactions, infections, or repeated head injury. Diagnosis is based on extensive patient history and excludes other associated issues, cognitive and neuropsychological testing, psychiatric evaluation, and brain scanning. Definitive diagnosis hinges on evidence of short- and long-term memory impairment in addition to at least the presence of aphasia, apraxia, agnosia, or impaired executive functioning.[2] Speech-language pathologists can assist in identifying specific cognitive communication disorders, the severity of these disorders, and the presence of other conditions.

Treatment focuses primarily on patient, family, and caregiver education and compensatory strategy implementation. Some direct intervention strategies have been identified as potentially beneficial, such as spaced retrieval (specific memory intervention where recall is systematically lengthened).[27] In the early stages, when impairments are mild/moderate, treatment may focus on developing strategies to compensate for memory loss to maintain the greatest level of independence possible. If co-occurring expressive language deficits exist, strategies to supplement communication would be addressed. Actively engaging family and caregivers in treatment is necessary to provide them with the skills to support the patient over time as the dementia progresses and the patient becomes more dependent on others for daily needs. Treatment often occurs in bouts at crucial times during the patient's disease progression to develop new strategies and provide education for the patient and caregivers.

Motor Speech Disorders

Dysarthria

Dysarthria is a motor speech disorder resulting from a wide range of acquired injuries, including (but not limited to) stroke, brain injury, and neurodegenerative conditions (e.g., amyotrophic lateral sclerosis, Parkinson disease, multiple sclerosis). Dysarthria, present in many disorders, is a major source of disability because of its impact on communication. Dysarthria can be categorized into types based upon the Darley, Aronson, and Brown[36,37] dysarthria classification system and include the following: flaccid, spastic, ataxic, hypokinetic, hyperkinetic, and mixed (Table 3-3). Dysarthria involves all or some of the speech subsystems, including respiration, phonation (laryngeal), resonance (velopharyngeal), and articulation (tongue, lips).

In addition to determining the dysarthria type and the specific subsystems involved resulting in speech impairment, the speech-language pathologist has a range of tools to quantify the impairment to guide treatment planning. Objective intelligibility testing can be accomplished with a range of possible measures, including the *Word Intelligibility Test*[83] or the *Speech Intelligibility Test*.[161] These assessments quantify the impact of the dysarthria on phoneme production and serve as a general measure of how the dysarthria affects the patient's ability to be understood in day-to-day environments. Computerized aerodynamic assessment allows for quantification of intraoral pressure (centimeters of water) and the amount of nasal airflow (cubic centimeters per second) present, with identification of potential timing of soft palate closure. Endoscopy can also assist in visualization of the velopharyngeal function. Computerized voice analysis programs, such as the Visi-Pitch IV,[151] also assist in quantifying specific vocal characteristics that may be impaired, including pitch, shimmer, and jitter. Along with bedside assessment and initial motor speech examination, these tools can provide a comprehensive analysis of the type, severity, and functional impact of the dysarthria and guide the speech-language pathologist in the specific targets for remediation.

Management of dysarthria depends on subsystem involvement and severity. For example, poor respiratory support may be managed with specific exercises, binders, abdominal paddles, biofeedback tools, such as respiratory induction plethysmography (Respitrac),[125] and voice amplification devices. If velopharyngeal dysfunction is a prominent feature, immediate management of hypernasality is warranted because it affects respiratory drive for speech. A nasal obturator and palatal lift prosthesis are common interventions in cases of velopharyngeal incompetence. Opportunities for extensive practice are necessary to make functional changes in speech.

Some types of dysarthria have been documented to respond particularly well to specific treatments. For example, the Lee Silverman Voice Treatment program has been shown to be a highly effective treatment for those with hypokinetic dysarthria common in Parkinson disease.[122,132,162] New treatments, including the SpeechVive,[140] have had promising results for even those with significant cognitive impairment along with hypokinetic dysarthria. Other strategies, such as alphabet supplementation, have been documented as effective interventions for some that greatly increase functional intelligibility.[60,74,75]

For those with moderate to severe dysarthria or for those who have degenerative conditions, such as amyotrophic lateral sclerosis, AAC is often a warranted intervention. Evidence supports the assessment for and implementation of a high-tech AAC system for individuals with amyotrophic lateral sclerosis once their speaking rate reaches 120 words per minute.[6,13] Ball and colleagues[6] have found that although intelligibility may be relatively high (90% or above), once a patient's speaking rate reaches 120 words per minute, or half of the normal speaking rate, there is a precipitous drop in intelligibility that typically follows shortly thereafter. Using this guideline in intervention helps speech-language pathologists make timely decisions for ordering and implementing high-tech devices to ensure that these patients can continue to communicate

Table 3-3 Dysarthria Types

Type of Dysarthria	Site of Lesion	Neuromuscular Symptoms	Speech Characteristics
Flaccid	Peripheral nervous system or lower motor neuron system	Weakness, decreased muscle tone	Hypernasal, imprecise articulation, slurred speech, breathiness
Spastic	Pyramidal and extrapyramidal systems	Weakness, increased muscle tone	Harsh voice quality, imprecise articulation, strain-strangled voice quality, hypernasality
Ataxic	Cerebellum	Slow and inaccurate movement	Prolonged speech, slow rate, imprecise articulation, irregular articulatory breakdowns
Hypokinetic	Basal ganglia and subcortical structures	Slow movements, limited range of movements	Rapid speech, low volume, reduced articulatory movements
Hyperkinetic	Basal ganglia and subcortical structures	Quick, unsustained, involuntary movements	Harsh and/or strain-strangled vocal quality, voice stoppages associated with dystonia, involuntary speech movements
Mixed	Upper and lower motor neuron	Varies depending on level of motor neuron involvement	Variable, example: harsh but breathy vocal quality

effectively throughout their course of illness. AAC devices and strategies can be semitemporary or long-term communication tools used by individuals with dysarthria even as they continue to work on regaining speech. Studies have shown that some individuals can make functional improvements in speech production many years after injury,[78,157] demonstrating the need for ongoing speech practice support and the need for technologies and strategies to supplement or augment speech over time.

Apraxia

Apraxia of speech (AOS) is a motor speech disorder that is caused by a disturbance in the planning and programming of movements for speech despite normal muscle functioning. AOS can occur simultaneously with aphasia and dysarthria or, although infrequently, can occur as a "pure" apraxia.[153] The neurologic insult resulting in AOS has been suggested to be in the left cerebral hemispheres in the premotor and motor cortices, although Broca area and the insula have also been implicated.[53] In addition to AOS, other ideomotor apraxias can include limb apraxia and nonverbal oral motor apraxia. In all ideomotor apraxia, individuals know what they need to do but cannot sequence the movements. This typically affects voluntary movements, with automatic movements remaining intact. The primary clinical characteristics of acquired AOS include slow speaking rate, lengthened sounds and durations between sounds, sound distortions, consistent errors, and abnormal prosody.[114,153] Although not discriminatory of AOS, other characteristics may include articulatory groping, perseverative errors, increased errors with increased word length, difficulty initiating speech, and a preference for automatic speech instead of novel speech.[114,153] In those with a severe AOS, their speech may be limited to only a few words. A speech-language pathologist typically assesses for AOS by completing an oral mechanism examination, which includes a physical examination to look at the structure and function of the speech mechanism, as well as a motor speech examination to assess performance across various speech tasks, including single word repetitions, repetitions of words of increasing length, alternating motion rates (single syllable repetitions), sequential motion rates (syllable sequence repetitions), a comparison of automatic and volitional speech, and assessment of speech in reading and conversation. A formal assessment that may be used for adults includes the *Apraxia Battery for Adults*, second edition (ABA-2).[33] Formal assessments used with children include the Kauffman Speech Praxis Test,[82] the Verbal Motor Production Assessment for Children,[62] as well as the Dynamic Evaluation of Motor Speech Skills (DEMSS) (in development).[142] Therapy typically involves intense, repetitive behavioral therapy, most frequently an articulatory-kinematic approach that focuses on the position or movement of the articulators,[153] and is based on principles of motor learning.[133] Articulatory-kinematic approaches use integral stimulation (i.e., "watch me, listen to me, say it with me") for cueing and work through a hierarchy of steps to increase accuracy of speech production, such as Sound Production Treatment.[154] Individuals with AOS need intensive practice and benefit from blocked, consistent practice and immediate, frequent feedback early on to lead to initial success, while progressing to random, variable practice and delayed, infrequent feedback later to lead to greater generalization.[105] Treatment approaches may use visual feedback, such as watching video self-recordings or using the VAST[149] application developed for the iPad. Other treatment approaches, such as script training, work on personalized, core phrases and sentences to develop automaticity.[163] Treatment approaches that focus on rate and rhythm control are also being explored. Progression through therapy for AOS can be lengthy; therefore it is vital to ensure that the individual with AOS has a means of communication while working on improving speech. Low-tech and high-tech AAC should be established early to provide an effective means of communication.

Rehabilitation of Patients with Swallowing Disorders

Oropharyngeal swallowing is a complex sensorimotor behavior involving the precise selection and sequencing of many paired muscle systems, which are regulated by the central and peripheral nervous systems, and modified by sensory mechanisms.[72] The safe and efficient passage of food items allows nutritional and hydration needs to be met without the risk of airway compromise. Swallowing disorders, or dysphagia, affect more than 6 million individuals with acquired and congenital disorders and 22% of individuals older than 55 years.[69] The successful management of swallowing disorders is best accomplished through evaluation and treatment with an interdisciplinary team of professionals who are involved with the delivery of clinical services for patients with dysphagia. The most effective teams typically involve a speech-language pathologist, occupational therapist, physiatrist, dietician, and psychologist. In most clinical situations, the speech-language pathologist is typically the principal provider of dysphagia diagnostic and treatment services. A physiatrist requires a strong working knowledge of all rehabilitation modalities (e.g., physical therapy, occupational therapy, and speech-language pathology) and, more specifically, swallowing disorders to guide dysphagia services as the physician assumes ultimate responsibility for directing the overall care of a patient.[22] This section of the chapter provides an overview of neurophysiology, an overview of common assessment tools, and a brief overview of disorders and treatment.

Physiology

The normal swallow is typically divided into four stages: oral preparatory, oral transit, pharyngeal transit, and esophageal. During the oral preparatory stage, liquids and solids are prepared for transport to the pharyngeal cavity. Sucking is one of the very first motor behaviors a human infant will perform in life. There are several muscles that converge lateral to the oral angle to form a semitendinosus node known as the modiolus.[29] The movements of the modiolus are central to the actions of lip rounding and spreading, as well as sucking and swallowing.[91]

The mammalian suck is primarily generated by a neuronal network called the suck central pattern generator (sCPG). Central pattern generators (CPGs) are bilateral networks of premotor interneurons that direct output to lower motoneurons to activate and sequence rhythmic, patterned motor outputs.[9] Although CPGs can generate motor patterns in the absence of descending or sensory inputs, these inputs play a highly significant role in modulating and shaping the motor output of CPGs. The sCPG is located within the brainstem pontine and medullary reticular formation, is highly responsive to peripheral inputs, and adapts its patterned motor output to changes in task dynamics and manipulations in the local environment.[7,8]

From a clinical perspective, the ability to safely feed depends on a coordinated suck, swallow, and breathe pattern regulated by a swallow central pattern generator (swCPG) consisting of a network of pontomedullary premotor internuncial circuits, which influence the firing patterns among trigeminal, facial, glossopharyngeal, ambiguous, and hypoglossal lower motor neurons. In mammals, fluids are transported through the oral cavity by consecutive cycles of rhythmic oral activity, which accumulates as a bolus primarily in the valleculae of the oropharynx and periodically empties into the esophagus. The process of emptying the valleculae corresponds to the pharyngeal stage of the classical swallow, and this action is periodically integrated into one of the fluid transporting cycles to form a combined transport/swallow cycle.[50,64] After liquids enter the oral cavity, the bolus is collected by the tongue and positioned between the surface of the tongue and the palate in a "swallow-ready" position. The lips maintain a seal to prevent anterior spillage. Premature leakage of food from the oral cavity to the pharynx is prevented by tongue-palate contact behind the bolus.

For solids, when food enters the mouth, it is positioned to allow for mastication. As with many other vital life functions, such as breathing, sucking, and swallowing, mastication is a rhythmic movement. It is characterized by cyclic jaw movements that vary among animal species and the types of food they consume[103] and in humans requires coordination of more than 20 orofacial muscles, in concert with breathing and swallowing.[88] Similar to sucking, rhythmic mastication is primarily under the control of internuncial circuits within the brainstem and is modulated by descending inputs from a putative cortical masticatory area. In fact, it is still unclear whether the masticatory CPG (mCPG) is an evolution of the sCPG that transforms its intrinsic properties and network connectivity during development or whether the mCPG emerges as its own separate network during weaning.[9,88,115]

The natural masticatory sequence has been divided into three functionally different, consecutive series based on the jaw movement trajectory and jaw muscle activity: (1) *the preparatory series*, where the food in the anterior portion of the mouth is transported back between the molar teeth; (2) *the reduction series*, where the food is broken down between the teeth; and (3) *the preswallowing series*, where the food is transported posteriorly toward the pharyngeal region for the swallow to occur. During rhythmic mastication, there is a disproportionately high level of jaw-closing activity relative to jaw-opening activity. This is necessary for the breakdown of food, and it is common across many species (including humans) that mastication often occurs on one favored side.[64] During mastication, the lips are sealed, and the tongue mixes the food particles with saliva to form a bolus for transportation to the pharynx. The cheeks or buccal walls are also compressed to prevent the bolus from pocketing in the lateral sulcus. Similar to liquids, the bolus is placed in the swallow-ready position immediately posterior to the tongue tip. The lips and cheeks remain compressed, as the tongue flattens anteriorly to posteriorly along the roof of the mouth propelling the bolus into the pharynx.

The pharyngeal stage involves multiple simultaneous muscular events to prevent airway compromise and allow safe passage of the bolus to the esophagus. The soft palate elevates and retracts, with the pharyngeal wall compressing along the soft palate to achieve a velopharyngeal seal. As the bolus passes into the pharynx, the base of tongue retracts posteriorly to contact the posterior pharyngeal wall, which has stiffened and shortened. The pharyngeal wall contracts superiorly to inferiorly, compressing the bolus toward the esophagus. The upper esophageal segment (UES) opens to allow the bolus to pass into the esophagus. As the bolus passes through the pharynx, multiple events occur to protect the airway. The true vocal folds adduct, the arytenoids tilt to the base of the epiglottis, and the hyolaryngeal mechanism is pulled upward and forward by contraction of the suprahyoid and thyrohyoid muscles.

The cricopharyngeus muscle is typically contracted between swallows, opening briefly during the swallow. The opening is influenced by hyolaryngeal elevation, relaxation of the cricopharyngeus muscle, and pressure of the bolus against the UES.

The esophagus is quite different from the pharynx because it is primarily composed of striated muscle in its cervical portion and smooth muscle in its thoracic portion. Because the thoracic esophagus is a largely smooth muscle, it has intrinsic contractile activity that can be increased or inhibited by autonomic nerves. Once the bolus has passed through the UES, it is propelled down the esophagus by peristalsis (defined as a wave of inhibition followed by a wave of excitation that propels material down a hollow viscus).[66] In the upright position, gravity assists peristalsis. The lower esophageal sphincter (LES) is held closed by tonic muscle contraction between swallows. It relaxes during a swallow and is pushed open by the pressure of the descending bolus.

Central "Cortical" Representation of Swallowing

Recent evidence on deglutition and swallowing supports the notion of reciprocal or heterarchical control among cerebral cortex, forebrain, cerebellum, and brainstem loci.[76,116] Functional neuroimaging in humans indicates an elaborate network of cortical areas participating in the volitional swallow. The blood oxygen level–dependent (BOLD) response associated with the functional magnetic resonance imaging (fMRI) technique during *reflexive swallows* reveals a cerebral network localized bilaterally to the lateral primary somatosensory and motor cortex. *Voluntary swallows* produced by healthy young adults show a more elaborate bilateral activation in the insula, prefrontal (Brodmann area [BA] 24, 32, 33), anterior cingulate, parietooccipital (BA 7, 17, 18, 19, 26, 30, 31), and primary somatosensory and motor cortices (BA 1, 2, 3, 4) with an asymmetry favoring the right brain.[57,84] This pattern of asymmetry is reversed during reflexive swallows. The expanded representation during volitional swallows is likely to be related to motor planning and the urge to swallow when presented a small water bolus. Transcortical magnetic stimulation studies in humans indicate the presence of multiple cortical areas, including oral motor, pharyngeal motor, and esophageal motor cortex, in BA 4. The face sensorimotor cortex, cortical masticatory area (CMA), and cortical swallowing area (CSA) are active during deglutition in awake primates with intracortical microstimulation.[109,134] Swallowing can be evoked by electrical stimulation of face primary motor cortex (M1), face primary somatosensory cortex (S1), CMA, and an area deep to CMA.[108]

Pathophysiology

Dysphagia can lead to malnutrition, dehydration, inability to safely protect the airway resulting in respiratory compromise, and a decrease in quality of life. Swallowing disorders are frequently described in terms of stage affected: oral, pharyngeal, or esophageal. Regardless of site, it is useful to consider whether a given impairment of swallowing affects food transport (preparation and propulsion of the bolus), airway protection (prevention of laryngeal aspiration), or both, because these have implications for treatment.

During the oral preparatory and transit stages, the lips, tongue, cheeks, and jaw are active in completing mastication, bolus preparation, and transportation from the oral to the pharyngeal cavity. Weak or uncoordinated oral movements may result in retention of the bolus in the oral cavity. An impaired labial seal can result in spillage anteriorly. Pocketing in the lateral sulcus can occur as a result of buccal weakness or lingual incoordination resulting in difficulty with forming a cohesive bolus. Posterior spillage from the mouth to the throat can occur secondary to posterior lingual weakness or incoordination with the bolus falling prematurely into the pharynx during mastication.

Pharyngeal disorders are difficult to visualize during the clinical assessment and should be evaluated through instrumentation. There are many signs and symptoms that can be observed during a meal, such as coughing, choking, multiple swallows, but the cause of these behaviors is unknown until instrumental assessment is completed. Disorders at this stage may include impaired swallow initiation, ineffective bolus propulsion, retention of a portion of the bolus in the pharynx after swallowing, and aspiration of the bolus. Nasal regurgitation may be noted when the soft palate does not elevate and the pharyngeal wall contraction is incomplete around the soft palate. When tongue base retraction is weak, pharyngeal propulsive force can be inadequate, resulting in retention of all or part of the bolus in the pharyngeal recesses after swallowing. Similar findings can be produced by weakness of the pharyngeal constrictor musculature. Epiglottic inversion is a passive movement reliant on bolus pressures, base of tongue retraction, and hyolaryngeal elevation. If the epiglottis does not invert during swallowing, it might act as a physical barrier, resulting in retention of part of the bolus in the valleculae after swallowing.

Another cause of food retention in the pharynx after swallowing is impaired opening of the UES. This can be caused by increased stiffness of the UES, as in fibrosis or inflammation, or failure to relax the closing muscle of the sphincter (primarily the cricopharyngeus muscle). Because UES opening is an active process, failure of opening can also be caused by weakness of the muscles of sphincter opening, particularly the anterior suprahyoid musculature. Dyscoordination of the swallow can also lead to failure of UES opening. Because the UES is ordinarily closed between swallows, its opening is obligatory for swallowing to occur. This means that failure of UES relaxation and opening can produce obstruction of the food pathway.

Airway protection is a critical function of swallowing; however, airway protection mechanisms are not always effective. Failure of laryngeal protective mechanisms can reflect reduced laryngeal elevation, incomplete closure of the laryngeal vestibule, or inadequate vocal fold closure caused by weakness, paralysis, or anatomic fixation. For the purpose of dysphagia rehabilitation, *laryngeal penetration* is defined as passage of material into the larynx but not through the vocal folds. *Aspiration* is defined as passage of material through the vocal folds. Laryngeal penetration can be observed in healthy individuals. Aspiration of microscopic quantities occurs in healthy individuals, but aspiration that is visible on fluoroscopy or endoscopy is pathologic and is associated with an increased risk of aspiration pneumonia or airway obstruction.[106] The normal response to aspiration is a strong reflex coughing or throat clearing. Laryngeal sensation is often abnormal, however, in individuals with severe dysphagia.[48] Silent aspiration, or aspiration in the absence of visible response, has been reported in 25% to 30% of patients referred for dysphagia evaluations.[48] The effects of aspiration are highly variable, and some individuals tolerate small amounts of aspiration without apparent ill effects.[48] Several factors determine the effect of aspiration in a given individual, including the quantity of the aspirate, the depth of the aspiration material in the airway, the physical properties of the aspirate (acidic material is most damaging to the lung), and the individual's pulmonary clearance mechanism.[118] Predictors of aspiration pneumonia risk include diagnoses of chronic obstructive pulmonary disease and congestive heart failure, presence of a feeding tube, oral/dental status, bedbound status, and presence of dysphagia.[135]

Dysphagia can result from a wide variety of disorders. A major cause of dysphagia is stroke. Dysphagia is found in approximately half of individuals with a recent stroke. Most recover within the first 2 weeks, but dysphagia can be severe and persistent. Brainstem lesions can result in particularly severe dysphagia, given their proximity to the major swallow centers.[77,144]

Reduced laryngeal elevation, insufficient UES opening, vocal fold weakness, and severe weakness of oropharyngeal muscles are common in patients with stroke. Cerebral lesions can result in dyscoordination of the swallow, with impaired oropharyngeal bolus propulsion and airway protection. Swallow dysfunction is typically more severe in bilateral cerebral lesions because there is bilateral cortical representation for swallow function. By contrast, the brainstem motor nuclei innervate only ipsilateral muscles, so lesions of cranial nerves or their nuclei can result in unilateral sensory or lower motor neuron dysfunction.[21]

In neurodegenerative disorders, dysphagia can be the first symptom.[43] Oral-stage dysphagia is common in Parkinson disease, characterized by tremor, dyskinesia, and bradykinesia in lips, tongue, jaw, and larynx, which hamper oral and pharyngeal food transport. Medication for Parkinson disease does not improve swallowing, even when it is effective for improving other aspects of motor function. Alzheimer disease can result in agnosia for food within the oral cavity, characterized by oral holding and incoordination of swallowing. In motor neuron disease, progressive degeneration of motor neurons in the brain and spinal cord results in weakness in the muscles of mastication, respiration, and swallowing. Inflammatory muscle diseases, including dermatomyositis and polymyositis, commonly affect striated muscles, resulting in weakness of the pharynx. By contrast, progressive systemic sclerosis affects smooth muscle and commonly produces esophageal dysfunction, including reduced peristalsis, dilatation of the lower esophagus, and gastroesophageal reflux disease (GERD).

Tumors of the oral cavity, pharynx, and larynx can be treated with surgical excision, deletion of anatomic structures, chemotherapy, or radiation therapy. Dysphagia occurs from tissue loss or dysfunction. Oral cavity cancer often requires partial or complete glossectomy and mandibulectomy, which can limit lingual and mandibular function for bolus formation and propulsion, and significantly increase aspiration risk. Pharyngeal tumor excision can require removal of structures critical for swallowing, including the faucial arches, hyoid bone, epiglottis, and pharyngeal constrictors. Ineffective laryngeal protection and reduced pharyngeal transport are common. Supraglottic laryngectomy, a common cancer surgery, spares the true vocal cords but eliminates the epiglottis, laryngeal vestibule, and false vocal folds. Without these laryngeal protective mechanisms, individuals are at increased aspiration risk. Pharyngeal transport problems are also common. Total laryngectomy separates the airway from the pharynx with a permanent tracheostomy. Although there is no risk for aspiration, pharyngeal transport problems resulting from weakness, tissue fixation, and cricopharyngeal dysfunction are common.

Radiation therapy can cause fibrosis of the oral cavity, pharynx, and larynx immediately after radiation or, in some cases, years later. Xerostomia (dry mouth) and edema are common when salivary glands are within the radiation field, hampering bolus formation and timing of oral and pharyngeal transport. The salivary changes are often permanent. Fibrosis can result in delayed swallow initiation, decreased pharyngeal transport, and ineffective laryngeal protection.[89]

Structural abnormalities, whether congenital or acquired, can impair swallow function. Birth defects, such as clefts of the lip and palate often produce inadequate labial control for sucking and bolus control, or velopharyngeal insufficiency with nasal regurgitation. The resulting dysphagia can lead to malnutrition, requiring surgical repair of the defect during infancy.

Structural abnormalities can impair pharyngeal transport and airway protection. Cervical osteophytes are common in the elderly and can impinge on the pharynx. This can also be seen with edema or hematoma after anterior cervical fusion. Webs and strictures can obstruct the food pathway. Diverticula can form along the pharyngeal or esophageal walls. The Zenker diverticulum is a pulsion diverticulum of the hypopharynx. Its mouth is located just above the cricopharyngeus muscle, but the body of the pouch can extend much lower. Food or liquid collects in the diverticulum and can be regurgitated to the mouth or result in aspiration.

Esophageal dysfunction is common and is often asymptomatic. Webs, rings, or strictures of the esophagus can obstruct the lumen and might require dilatation. Esophageal motor disorders include conditions of either hyperactivity (e.g., esophageal spasm) or hypoactivity (e.g., weakness) of the esophageal musculature. Either of these can lead to ineffective peristalsis with retention of material in the esophagus after swallowing. Retention can result in regurgitation of material from the esophagus back into the pharynx, with aspiration of the regurgitated material. Patients who complain of discomfort or the food sticking in the chest almost always have an esophageal problem.

Patients suspected of having esophageal dysphagia should be referred to a gastroenterologist because there may be structural disorders, including strictures or even cancer. Persistent pain on swallowing (odynophagia) is suggestive of esophageal cancer. In esophageal cancer, early detection and treatment can save lives. Another possibility is achalasia of the esophagus; this also requires prompt evaluation and treatment. When there is structural narrowing of the esophagus, dilatation is often effective but generally must be repeated periodically because narrowing can recur. Esophageal dysphagia can also be due to physiologic disorders, even when the anatomy is normal. These include spasm and ineffective peristalsis and may be amenable to pharmacotherapy.

GERD can affect swallowing indirectly. In GERD, the LES has insufficient tone, rendering it ineffective for preventing gastric contents from passing back through the LES into the esophagus. Because the esophageal lining is not resistant to acid (as is the stomach lining), reflux of highly acidic stomach contents can result in inflammation (esophagitis) or scarring (stricture) of the esophagus. This can lead to pain or obstructive symptoms. In severe cases, the refluxate can pass all the way up the esophagus and into the pharynx, passing through the UES. The individual with severe GERD is particularly vulnerable at night, when protective reflexes are less effective. Under these conditions the refluxate can be aspirated, causing inflammation or scarring of these vital airway structures. Although GERD is not a swallowing disorder per se, it can be an underlying cause of dysphagia or aspiration pneumonia.

Dysphagia is often iatrogenic. Several drugs can impair swallowing, including anticholinergic drugs and benzodiazepines. Neuroleptic agents, also called antipsychotic drugs, can cause movement disorders affecting the face and mouth, such as tardive dyskinesia, especially after long-term use. These can impair eating and swallowing. Any medication that causes sedation can have an adverse effect on swallowing and potentially impair airway clearance (e.g., cough) in response to aspiration.

Postoperative dysphagia is a common complication of anterior cervical fusion, occurring in approximately half of patients.[139] Individuals with multiple cervical surgical levels demonstrate a higher risk of having dysphagia when compared with those undergoing survey at one level.[35] The mechanism is unclear, but it might be related to injury of the pharyngeal constrictor muscles or their innervation. Most patients recover within the first 2 months. Compromised and altered respiratory function increases the risk for dysphagia. Chronic obstructive pulmonary disease alters the coordination of respiration and deglutition.[135] Patients who have undergone lung transplantation may demonstrate dysphagia, with a high risk of silent aspiration.[3]

Exacerbations can lead to aspiration. Endotracheal intubation and ventilator dependency can cause decreased laryngeal sensation, pooling of secretions in the pharynx and larynx, impaired swallow initiation, and aspiration. The presence of a tracheostomy tube alters normal pharyngeal aerodynamics, eliminating the positive subglottic pressure normally associated with swallowing and hampering laryngeal protective reflexes. An inflated cuff does not fully eliminate aspiration,[54,90] because secretions can still leak around the cuff into the trachea. A cuffless tracheostomy tube is often better tolerated. A unidirectional tracheostomy speaking valve prevents expiratory airflow through the tracheostomy tube, providing expiratory flow through the larynx and upper airway, and restoring positive subglottic air pressure thereby reducing laryngeal penetration and aspiration.[54]

Evaluation

To effectively treat swallowing disorders (i.e., providing appropriate dietary recommendations, behavior management strategies, and rehabilitation exercises) and decrease risk for dysphagia-associated medical complications, the health care team first needs to correctly identify the specific biomechanical aspects of the swallowing function through the appropriate use and interpretation of a diagnostic swallow procedure.[20,96] The purpose of the swallowing evaluation is to assess dysphagia and, when appropriate, make recommendations for diet, swallow safety strategies, and rehabilitation interventions. Swallowing evaluations can be divided into two main categories of bedside/clinical assessments and instrumental assessments.

Instrumental swallowing assessments include evaluation procedures, such as the videofluoroscopic swallow study (VFSS), the fiberoptic endoscopic examination of the swallow (FEES), high-resolution manometry (HRM), and ultrasonography. Regardless of the type of assessment used to evaluate the swallow, the examiner should recognize that the results represent only a snapshot picture of a patient's swallow function at any moment in time.[98] Many variables, such as the underlying medical condition, medication timing, distractions, or even unknown factors potentially influence swallow function in either a positive or negative manner.[98] Furthermore, it is not unusual for a person with dysphagia to demonstrate variable swallowing performance depending on the time of day because of fatigue or timing of medications. The variability of swallowing performance throughout the day may be especially prominent in patients with progressive neurologic diseases or with elderly patients. Therefore it is imperative to interpret the results of the swallowing assessment in conjunction with the overall clinical picture of the patient.

Bedside/Clinical Swallow Assessments

Swallow Screenings. The swallow screening is usually the first step to identify the risk of dysphagia and is often completed by the nurse or the physician. The screening protocols may take on a variety of forms, and although the most valid screening protocol remains to be determined, it is generally agreed that the screening protocol should be quick and minimally invasive. The purpose of the swallow screen is to accurately identify individuals who present a risk of dysphagia and to expedite a referral to speech-language pathologist for further evaluation.[34] The swallow screening may identify risk factors for dysphagia by means of self-report, by clinical history, or by direct clinical observation.

One type of swallow screen available is the Yale Swallow Protocol, or as it is more commonly known, the 3-ounce water challenge.[95] The Yale Swallow Protocol has three components: a brief cognitive screen, an oral mechanism examination, and the 3-ounce water challenge. To pass the Yale Swallow Protocol, the individual must consume the 3 ounces of water uninterrupted without any overt signs of aspiration (e.g., cough, wet voice quality). If a person is unable to drink the entire amount uninterrupted or demonstrates coughing during or immediately after consuming the water, then this is considered a fail on the Yale Swallow Protocol.

Other swallow screenings reported in the literature also use water with volumes ranging from 5 to 90 mL and with different criteria for pass/fail.[34] Direct assessment of the swallow by having the individual actually swallow something has been associated with higher quality screenings.[34] Furthermore, the use of water as part of a screening makes the screening relatively easy to administer. Questions regarding the safety of allowing a patient to self-administer 3 ounces of water during the screening remain, and further research is required to determine which water-screening protocol is the most valid along with defining the most appropriate algorithm to identify dysphagia risk factors.[34]

Clinical Swallow Examination. The clinical swallow examination (CSE) is often conducted after the individual fails the swallow screening and is usually completed by a speech-language pathologist. Although the CSE does not allow for any direct observation of the physiology of the swallow, other pertinent information can be obtained related to swallow function. The CSE is used in settings, such as nursing homes, and in home health where access to an instrumental assessment of the swallow (e.g., VFSS or FEES) may not be readily available.[113]

The CSE has five basic components: (1) medical history and current medical status; (2) cognitive/mental status function; (3) oral motor function; (4) laryngeal and pulmonary function; and (5) trial swallows.[98,113] Medical history and current medical status include a review of the individual's nutritional status, hospital treatments, laboratory values, medications, and respiratory status. The cognitive/mental status evaluation may include an assessment of alertness, orientation, memory (i.e., long-term, immediate, delayed), ability to follow directions, and reasoning/problem-solving skills. The oral motor assessment includes primarily an evaluation of the lips, tongue, dentition, and hard/soft palatal structures. The oral mechanism structures are evaluated for abnormalities with strength, tone, symmetry, or movement (e.g., apraxia) of the structures, as well as any structural deviations related to surgical/acquired condition or congenital factors. Preliminary studies are beginning to emerge demonstrating potential objective measures of oral strength and range, which may be beneficial during the initial evaluation for predictors of swallowing outcomes.[94,95] Dentition and condition of the oral mucosa are also evaluated during the oral motor assessment. Laryngeal function is indirectly assessed by evaluating strength of the cough and vocal quality. Pulmonary status is assessed by the observation of the individual's respiratory rate at rest.

Depending on the results for the cognitive/mental status function, oral motor function, and laryngeal/pulmonary function, the clinician may then attempt trial swallows. Usually the clinician will have the individual attempt a saliva swallow, followed by an ice chip, and then other bolus sizes and consistencies as deemed appropriate. The clinician can observe for oral phase deficits as evident by labial spillage, buccal pocketing, or prolonged mastication. It is also helpful for the clinician to place his or her fingers gently on the patient's neck to assess submandibular movement, hyoid bone movement, and laryngeal movement during the swallow trials.[98] The correct placement of the fingers will further assist the clinician with making additional observations related to the timeliness and strength of the swallow response. Furthermore, the clinician observes for any overt signs of aspiration with the presence of a cough, throat clear, or "wet" vocal quality either during or immediately after the swallow. If the patient demonstrates any clinical signs of aspiration during the swallow trails, this usually triggers a referral for an instrumental assessment of the swallow.

Blue Dye Clinical Swallow Examination. When a CSE is conducted with an individual with a tracheostomy tube, the use of food coloring (e.g., FD&C Blue Dye No. 1) mixed with the food and liquid is done to enhance the visualization of the bolus to assist the examiner with the detection of tracheal aspiration. If blue-tinged secretions are present in or around the tracheostomy tube or suctioned through the tracheostomy tube after the swallow trials, then the examination result is considered positive for aspiration. The amount of blue dye added to the food and liquid during the blue dye clinical swallow examination (BDCSE) is relatively small (1 to 2 mL). There has been some reported potential risks related to the use of blue dye or food coloring with patients with increased gastrointestinal permeability (e.g., sepsis, burns, trauma, shock, renal failure, celiac sprue, and inflammatory bowel disease), and caution may be warranted with these patient populations.[19]

The usefulness of the BDCSE has been questioned by many researchers. Several studies with rehabilitation patients who had a tracheotomy revealed that the BDCSE had sensitivity rates ranging from 38% to 79% for the detection of aspiration by the BDCSE as compared with the VFSS.[21,121] The accuracy of aspiration detection of the BDCSE has also been compared with the FEES procedure. During simultaneous BDCSE and FEES, the BDCSE again only had a 50% sensitivity rate for the detection of aspiration when compared with the FEES.[43]

Given the relatively poor sensitivity of the BDCSE to detect aspiration in patients with a tracheostomy tube, it is recommended in cases where the patient has a negative BDCSE (i.e., no aspiration detected) that further workup either by means of a VFSS or an FEES be conducted to confirm the results before the initiation of oral feedings. In cases where the BDCSE result is positive for aspiration, the examiner may then want to defer the instrumental swallow assessment of either the VFSS or FEES until the BDCSE is negative. The BDCSE is designed to only detect the presence or absence of tracheal aspiration in patients with a tracheostomy tube (with only a 50% false-negative error rate), and the BDCSE cannot determine why the patient is aspirating or whether strategies may be used to eliminate or reduce the aspiration. Therefore in some cases where the patient has a positive BDCSE result, a VFSS or FEES may be indicated if it is suspected that the instrumental examination at that time would provide additional diagnostic information that would allow the individual to successfully advance to oral feedings.

Cervical Auscultation. Cervical auscultation is a noninvasive technique used during a CSE and involves a listening device (i.e., stethoscope) usually placed at the lateral aspect of the neck above the cricoid cartilage to evaluate swallow and airway sounds during the pharyngeal phase of swallow.[18] On the basis of the sounds the examiner hears, judgments are made as to whether the "swallowing sounds" were considered normal or abnormal. An abnormal swallowing sound would suggest the presence of aspiration. The clinical efficacy of using cervical auscultation during a CSE to detect aspiration has been mixed. Criticism of this technique include limited interrater reliability related to how the swallowing sounds correlate with various physiologic events during the swallow and the presence or absence of aspiration.[97,143]

Instrumental Swallow Assessment

Videofluoroscopic Swallow Study. The VFSS is the most commonly performed instrumental swallow assessment and is known by several different names, such as the "modified barium swallow," the "cookie swallow," or the "pharyngogram with video recording."[49,110] The arrival of cinefluorography (i.e., motion picture x-ray film) in the 1950s allowed for the examination of the swallow as a dynamic process. As technology advanced, the use of video recordings for the fluoroscopic images began to replace the cine recordings as radiation exposure were less for the video recordings as compared with the cine recordings and thus lead to the introduction of the VFSS.[127]

The VFSS involves the use of a fluoroscopic x-ray image along with various consistencies of barium sulfate to evaluate the physiology of the swallow function during the oral, pharyngeal, and esophageal phases.[49] The VFSS allows the examiner to identify normal and abnormal anatomy and physiology; evaluate the integrity of airway protection before, during, and after the swallow; and evaluate the effectiveness of bolus modifications, postural changes, and swallowing maneuvers used to improve swallow safety and efficiency.[20] The VFSS is recorded to allow further analysis with a frame-by-frame review of the film. At most facilities, the VFSS is completed in the radiology department with a radiologist, radiology technologist, and a swallowing clinician (usually a speech-language pathologist); however, at some facilities, the VFSS is completed with a physiatrist or other physician specialist with an interest in swallowing disorders instead of a radiologist.[126] For members of the health care team conducting the VFSS, they should receive additional training and education regarding radiation protection, wear protective lead shielding (e.g., thyroid collar, full lead apron, protective eye goggles), and/or stand behind a glass lead shield or barrier during the examination.[49]

There are several standardized VFSS protocols available in the literature, and in clinical practice there are even additional variations to these standard VFSS protocols. The basic components of most VFSS protocols involve assessing various bolus consistencies (e.g., thin liquids, nectar-thick liquids, honey-thick liquids, puree, semisolids, and solids), bolus sizes (e.g., 1 mL, 3 mL, 5 mL, uncontrolled large bolus), and presentation methods (e.g., cup sip, straw sip, patient-administered, clinician-administered). Further, most VFSS protocols involve the introduction of compensatory strategies (e.g., positioning, swallowing maneuvers, and bolus modifications) to identify the most optimal conditions for swallowing performance. The challenge when performing a VFSS is to determine when it is necessary to perform a standardized protocol versus performing a tailor-made study designed to match typical eating behaviors. Additionally, when conducting the VFSS protocol for clinical practice, the examiner must take into account how to obtain as much information about the swallow function with the minimum amount of radiation exposure.[20,141] Finally, a particular bolus consistency or size should be deferred during the VFSS protocol if it is judged that advancing the patient to test the item would be unsafe.[20]

Assessment of the esophageal phase is not a major component of the VFSS protocol; however, some examiners may choose to scan the esophagus when clinical indications (e.g., globus) are present. Patients who complain of discomfort or the food sticking in the throat or neck may have a problem in either the pharynx or the esophagus (including the thoracic esophagus). For this reason and others, it is wise to image esophageal swallowing as well as oral and pharyngeal when performing a VFSS. This is one of the advantages of fluoroscopy over FEES. Currently, there are no practice guidelines available on the proper performance of an esophageal screen. The patient's position (e.g., upright versus supine), viewing position (lateral versus anteroposterior view), bolus size, and bolus consistency may all influence the esophageal screen.[44]

FEES Procedure. The FEES is the second most common instrumental assessment of the swallow and allows for an evaluation of the anatomic structures of the larynx and pharynx, accumulated oropharyngeal secretion levels, swallowing ability, and sensory ability with a flexible laryngoscope with a halogen or xenon light source.[20] During the FEES, the oral phase and the height of the swallow during the pharyngeal phase cannot be directly observed, and the examiner must make inferences based on the preswallow and postswallow components of the FEES. The examiner (i.e., endoscopist) visualizes the images of the pharynx directly through the eyepiece or with a chip camera attached to the laryngoscope. The use of a chip camera allows viewing of the images on a monitor and can be recorded for further analysis.

The FEES protocol includes an assessment of the anatomic structures of the larynx at rest and in movement, the accumulated oropharyngeal secretion level, and bolus flow of various foods and liquids while swallowing. If difficulty with swallowing is observed during the FEES, then similar to the VFSS protocol, compensatory swallow safety strategies (e.g., positioning, swallowing maneuvers, and bolus modifications) may be introduced to identify the most optimal conditions for swallowing performance.

The main advantage of the FEES not only includes the ability to identify the signs and symptoms of dysphagia but also provides a view of the anatomy and physiology of the swallow and accumulated oropharyngeal secretion levels. A common physiologic abnormality observed during the FEES is the presence of reduced vocal fold mobility, which has been associated with increased risk of aspiration.[96] Before any bolus presentation, the FEES clinical protocol involves an observation of secretions including describing the amount and location.[20] The evaluation of secretion levels is important because the examiner uses this information to quickly differentiate between safe levels of accumulated secretions and those that are dangerously high because the presence of endolaryngeal secretions are highly predictive of subsequent aspiration on the FEES.[42]

Another important clinical component of the FEES protocol is identifying the relationship among sensory input, airway protection, and swallowing ability. With the FEES protocol, sensation as it relates to swallow function may be either directly assessed with light touching of the endoscope to the pharyngeal/laryngeal structures or indirectly assessed on the basis of the patient's response to the presence of pharyngeal residue, laryngeal penetration, or aspiration. The FEES protocol may also be enhanced with a specialized endoscope with a side instrument channel that allows for the delivery of calibrated puffs of air to the mucosa of the larynx.[59] The calibrated puffs of air during the FEES protocol is known as the fiberoptic endoscopic evaluation of swallowing with sensory testing (FEESST). During the FEESST protocol, laryngeal sensation is inferred through observation of the laryngeal adductor reflex elicited after the delivery of the puffs of air. The degree of sensory deficit is inferred by the amount of calibrated puffs of air required to elicit the laryngeal adductor reflex during the FEESST. The inclusion of the calibrated puffs of air during the FEESST is not a required element for the FEES.[20]

Comparison of VFSS and FEES. Many authors have stated that the VFSS is the "gold standard" to evaluate swallow function; however, evidence in the literature supports that both the VFSS and FEES are valuable procedures to evaluate the swallow.[20] During simultaneous VFSS and FEES, findings related to laryngeal penetration, tracheal aspiration, and pharyngeal residue between the two procedures have demonstrated excellent agreement.[123] Furthermore, recommendations for diet level and compensatory swallow safety strategies have been reported as similar between the two examinations.[123] The selection of either the VFSS or FEES procedure is usually driven by specific patient characteristics (i.e., the field of view necessary to best identify the pathophysiologic condition of the swallowing dysfunction) or availability of equipment and personnel at the facility to perform the procedure.[20,96]

High-Resolution Manometry. HRM is a relatively new procedure and uses 36 circumferential sensors placed 1 cm apart to measure pressure events during the pharyngeal and esophageal phases of the swallow.[65,112] HRM accurately captures the complex pressure events along the entire length of the pharynx and esophagus that provides a more comprehensive picture of how bolus volumes may affect swallow physiologic function.[65] HRM is promising as an emerging technology because its use may reveal subtle findings that perhaps were not detectable with traditional manometry.[112]

Ultrasonography. Ultrasonography has been used to evaluate swallowing physiologic function for a long time; however, the clinical efficacy of this procedure in standard clinical practice has been inconclusive. When ultrasonography is used to evaluate swallow function, a submental placement is often used to visualize bolus transport during the oral phase of swallow and to also measure hyoid bone displacement in the pharyngeal phase of the swallow.[70] The advantages of ultrasonography include no exposure to radiation, noninvasiveness, and portability. The limitations of ultrasonography are the limited use in clinical practice and training opportunities available. Finally, further studies are required to evaluate the reliability of aspiration detection with ultrasonography.[70]

Electromyography. Electromyography (EMG) of the muscles of the pharynx and larynx is a reliable method for detecting lower motor neuron dysfunction and aberrant central motor patterning.[118] EMG is not a sufficient test for demonstration of swallow physiologic function, however, and should be used only as an adjunct to other instrumental assessments. EMG can be used in biofeedback as an adjunct to dysphagia therapy.

Treatment of Dysphagia

Similar to the earlier description of treatment for communication disorders, treatment approaches are described in terms of restorative (exercise) or compensatory (posture, diet modification, swallowing maneuvers, surgery). Early treatment of dysphagia has been shown to reduce the patient's risk for aspiration pneumonia, to reduce medical complications related to malnutrition and dehydration, and to reduce the length of the hospital stay.[30] Equally important is the amelioration of barriers that decrease an individual's ability to participate in and enjoy the pleasures of eating orally. Small physiologic improvements in swallowing that do not result in an increase in quality of life miss the true goal of rehabilitation.[8]

Restorative: Exercise Training and Plasticity Considerations

The oropharyngeal system exhibits considerable plasticity in the adaptation of new tasks or sensory experiences in health and disease. For example, during daily tongue training, the proportion of neurons in the primary somatosensory cortex (S1) and the primary motor cortex (M1) correlated with tongue protrusion increased with training. Additional studies have shown the importance of task-related specificity among tongue motor representations and the CMA.[134] The specificity in orofacial gestures and swallowing for targeted neuroplasticity interventions suggest that consideration be given for stimulus salience (nonswallow task training compared with swallow-specific task training) to affect beneficial behavioral change and adaptive plasticity for swallowing and oral motor behaviors.[107]

The strength training principles of overloading and specificity have been successfully applied to swallowing training. Following the principle of specificity, it is best to select exercises that are similar to the target behavior.[30] The Mendelsohn and Masako exercises apply this principle as the individual is attempting swallowing function during these exercises. Overloading involves competing exercises at resistance levels higher than typically used. During the Mendelsohn maneuver, the swallow is prolonged longer than the normal duration. For Masako, the anterior tongue is anchored, resulting in increased pharyngeal constrictor activity. Examples of exercise training that incorporate increased intensity of resistance are the isometric lingual exercise, expiratory muscle strength training (EMST), effortful swallow, Mendelsohn maneuver, Masako maneuver, and Shaker exercise.

Pharyngeal and esophageal motor cortical representations undergo expansion and suppression, respectively, following brief periods (approximately10 minutes) of 10-Hz electrical pharyngeal sensory stimulation in healthy adult participants.[58] The swallowing motor cortex can be altered for a sustained period of time after sensory stimulation of the pharynx. Pharyngeal stimulation appears to produce a larger effect on potentiation of the swallowing network compared with voluntary swallowing in adult patients with dysphagia; thus peripheral stimulation is favored over volitional exercises.[46] Sensory interventions are logical targets of neuroplasticity research. Pulse trains or repetitive peripheral stimulation is more effective than single pulse stimulation.[73,101] Low-frequency (<1 Hz) stimulation induces inhibition, whereas high-frequency stimulation (>5 Hz) generally results in excitatory effects.[119] rTMS at 5 Hz positioned over the swallowing motor cortex increases the excitability of the corticobulbar projection to the pharyngeal musculature.[52] The suppression of the pharyngeal motor representation with rTMS is both intensity dependent and frequency dependent in the control of swallowing. The feature of transference is demonstrated by the finding that pharyngeal stimulation can lead to a suppression and decrease in the central representation of the esophageal motor cortex. It logically follows that peripheral sensory stimulation represents an important neurotherapeutic intervention in swallowing rehabilitation.[107]

The application of electrical stimulation to improve muscle function is not new in rehabilitative medicine and is biologically plausible in theory for dysphagia treatment. In a neuromuscular electrical stimulation typical treatment session, surface electrodes are taped to the skin overlying the submental or anterior cervical strap muscles. With a commercial device marketed specifically for dysphagia therapy, pulsed electrical stimulation is delivered in a controlled, structured manner (59 seconds on, 1 second off, for 60 continuous minutes daily).[47]

Studies have demonstrated that electrical stimulation results in depression of the hyolaryngeal complex.[102] Electrical stimulation can put patients with severe dysphagia at risk for penetration as the hyolaryngeal complex descends. Electrical stimulation should only be used with patients who can overcome the hyolaryngeal lowering.

Compensatory Strategies in Swallowing Rehabilitation

Compensatory strategies are designed to increase safe swallowing in the presence of abnormal physiology. These can be divided into posture, maneuvers, and diet modification. They are to be performed with every swallow or just before a meal, as in the case of a novel approach pioneered by Japanese physiatrists. Patients are taught to perform self-dilatation of the UES when the sphincter does not relax satisfactorily during a swallow. This is accomplished by patients inserting a balloon catheter into their UES before each meal.[66] Another compensatory strategy that is performed before eating is thermal tactile stimulation. This strategy is recommended when delayed pharyngeal swallow is observed. A chilled laryngeal mirror is used to stroke the anterior faucial pillars five to six times before a meal and intermittently throughout the meal.[79] Improved timing of swallow initiation has been demonstrated to occur for up to three swallows after application, but long-term benefits of thermal tactile stimulation have not been observed.[130] This treatment should be viewed as a short-term compensatory strategy.

Postural strategies have been reported to successfully address 80% of all swallowing disorders.[99] These strategies involve use of gravity or changes in anatomy to assist in propelling bolus of improving airway protection. Examples include collapsing pharyngeal space by turning the patient's head toward the impaired side, having the patient do a chin tuck to widen the vallecula, and positioning the epiglottis in a more protective position posteriorly to prevent laryngeal penetration or aspiration. For a description of compensatory interventions and purpose, refer to Table 3-4.

Modification of food and liquid properties (in terms of texture and viscosity) and presentation (volume and temperature) is one of the most common strategies, although most clinicians are in agreement that these should be the treatments of last resort.[71] The *National Dysphagia Diet*, published by the American Dietetic Association, proposes standardized terminology for liquid viscosities and food

Table 3-4 Postural and Compensatory Strategies

Postural/Compensatory Strategy	Clinical Rationale	Clinical Indication for Use
Chin tuck posture	Widens the valleculae; positions base of tongue closer to posterior pharyngeal wall	Premature spillage; laryngeal penetration; pharyngeal residue in valleculae; aspiration attributable to delayed swallow response
Head turn posture (one side only)	Head turn to weaker side to redirect bolus flow to stronger side of pharynx	Unilateral pharyngeal residue
Head rotation (to both sides)	Enhances opening of UES	Pharyngeal residue at level of UES
Head tilt posture	Tilt head to stronger side (ear to shoulder) to use gravity to divert bolus down the stronger side of the pharynx	Unilateral pharyngeal residue
Throat clear	Voluntary throat clear to expel airway invasion	Laryngeal penetration; aspiration
Mendelsohn maneuver	To increase vertical and anterior laryngeal motion for improved laryngeal closure and to increase UES opening	Reduced laryngeal elevation and closure resulting in laryngeal penetration or aspiration; pharyngeal residue at the UES
Effortful swallow	To improve base of tongue retraction; to improve pharyngeal constrictor strength contraction	Pharyngeal residue
Breath-holding (i.e., supraglottic and super-supraglottic swallow)	To improve voluntary airway closure before the swallow	Laryngeal penetration; aspiration
Multiple swallows	Cued or spontaneous "dry" swallow to clear residue after primary bolus swallow	Oral residue; pharyngeal residue
Liquid wash; alternating liquids and solids	Used to clear oral and pharyngeal solid bolus residue	Oral residue; pharyngeal residue
Oral hold	Voluntary oral hold used with liquid boluses to reduce premature spillage and reduce swallow response delay	Laryngeal penetration or aspiration before the swallow secondary to premature spillage or delayed swallow response
Bolus modification	May include viscosity (e.g., thickened liquids), volume (e.g., small sips), and sensory modifications (e.g., sour bolus) to improve the safety and efficiency of the swallow	Laryngeal penetration; aspiration; pharyngeal residue

UES, Upper esophageal sphincter.

texture diets to increase the reliability of diet modification across facilities and practitioners. For patients who have decreased oral strength or coordination, soft solid foods, such as chopped or pureed food, might increase the safety and ease of consumption. In patients with neurogenic dysphagia, thin liquids can be aspirated because of poor bolus control, reduced lingual propulsion, delayed pharyngeal swallow, or a combination of these factors. Imaging of the swallow is necessary to determine the appropriate viscosity. Other food properties, such as taste and chemesthesis, appear to increase oral and pharyngeal transit in patients with dysphagia.[120] Chemesthesis is oral irritation mediated by the trigeminal nerve and is responsible for the perception of the hotness of chili peppers and the coolness of menthol and carbonation. To date, only a very sour taste that also has chemesthetic properties has been shown to elicit normative swallowing behaviors in patients with neurogenic dysphagia. A palatable sweet-sour taste (similar to the lemon products sold commercially) was not found to elicit any positive change in swallowing in one small pilot study.[120]

Surgery for Dysphagia

Surgery is rarely indicated for treatment of oropharyngeal dysphagia. Dilatation can be indicated in cases of UES stenosis when rehabilitation has been unsuccessful. Surgery is often performed for Zenker diverticulum when the diverticulum is large enough to interfere significantly with eating and drinking.[155] Cricopharyngeal myotomy is a procedure that disrupts the cricopharyngeus muscle for the purpose of reducing UES pressure, thereby decreasing resistance to flow from the pharynx to the esophagus. However, evidence of its effectiveness is limited.[31] Botulinum toxin injections are sometimes used to treat dysphagia, especially in cases of oromandibular or lingual dystonia, trismus, or cricopharyngeal dysfunction with failure of UES relaxation.[164] In severe and chronic aspiration, surgery can be necessary to separate the airway from the food way. This can be accomplished by combining a permanent tracheostomy with a laryngectomy or another procedure to close the larynx.[147] Although this definitively prevents aspiration, it has the serious consequence of preventing phonation and can result in significant dysphagia.

Pharyngeal Bypass

When adequate and safe oral intake is not possible, pharyngeal bypass procedures eliminate the need for swallowing and provide alternative means for achieving nutrition and hydration (Table 3-5).[87] Short-term feeding options include nasogastric and orogastric tubes, whereas jejunostomy and gastrostomy tubes are medium- and long-term feeding options. Nasogastric feeding tubes should be used when alternative nutrition will be required for 6 weeks or less. Gastrostomy tube feeding is used safely by thousands of individuals with severe dysphagia. However, the use of feeding tubes does not necessarily prevent aspiration, and tube feeding might in fact promote gastroesophageal reflux with secondary aspiration of stomach contents. In one study, pneumonia developed in up to 44% of patients with acute stroke who were fed with gastrostomy. Furthermore, 66% of these patients continued to aspirate chronically, with mortality rates greater than 50% after 1 year.[40] Measures to minimize aspiration include head elevation, good hygiene with bag and line handling, use of slow, continuous feeding rather than bolus, and monitoring for gastric residue.

Prevention of Aspiration Pneumonia

Aspiration pneumonia is one of the serious complications that can occur in patients with dysphagia. Preventing aspiration pneumonia is essential to a dysphagia rehabilitation program. Physicians should be aware that neither tube feeding nor tracheostomy tubes prevent aspiration pneumonia. Patients might aspirate food or saliva from the mouth or materials from the stomach (especially in the recumbent position). With tube feeding, food is not aspirated from the mouth because nutrition goes directly to the stomach. Saliva can be aspirated continuously, however, in patients receiving tube feedings. Airway protective reflexes are less effective during sleep, so patients are more likely to aspirate saliva while sleeping. If oral hygiene is poorly controlled, bacteria in the oral cavity can be aspirated with saliva, which increases the risk for aspiration pneumonia. Proper oral care reduces potentially pathogenic bacterial colonization, thereby reducing the risk for aspiration pneumonia.[160] Upright positioning during and after meals is also critical to reduce the aspiration risk from food, as well as refluxed material, and to maximize the effectiveness of rehabilitation techniques.

The duration of a meal should be considered to avoid aspiration pneumonia. A meal that lasts too long can fatigue the patient with dysphagia, increasing the risk for aspiration. Alternatively, if the patient eats too quickly and impulsively, these behaviors can also increase the risk for aspiration. These factors are often assessed during the clinical swallowing evaluation and follow-up treatment. It is important that family and staff caregivers be educated

Table 3-5 Alternative Feeding Options

Feeding Tube	Insertion	Indication	Possible Complications
Nasogastric	Inserted transnasally at bedside; confirmed via stethoscope or x-ray film	Short-term feeding	Easily dislodged; can lead to ulceration and stricture
Orogastric	Inserted transorally at bedside	Short-term feeding; unable to use nasal passage	—
Gastrostomy	Generally inserted endoscopically	Long-term nutrition and hydration	Infection, bleeding, perforation, clogging, and aspiration
Jejunostomy	Inserted surgically into small intestine	Absence of or inability to use the stomach; severe reflux aspiration	Clogging, diarrhea; questionable benefit for reducing aspiration

about these risk factors and trained to help prevent aspiration or aspiration pneumonia.

Psychological Considerations

Research by Martino and colleagues[111] compared the perceptions that clinicians, caregivers, and patients have about the medical consequences of dysphagia and found that patients do not hold the same views as clinicians. Although clinicians and caregivers think that poor nutrition and physical health are the most serious consequences of dysphagia, individuals with dysphagia of recent onset worry most about choking to death, believing that their nutrition and overall health status will be monitored and effectively maintained by the medical staff. For the patient with dysphagia undergoing short-term care, the most reassuring information might be to provide education and reassurance regarding the risk for airway obstruction. People with dysphagia and their families/caregivers should be taught the Heimlich maneuver. It is the responsibility of the swallowing therapist to make sure this happens. It can make the difference between life and death in cases of solid food aspiration with airway obstruction. If their dysphagia becomes chronic, however, their focus of concern changes, and they no longer focus on fear of choking to death because they have learned effective strategies that have kept them safe over time. Instead, they focus on the debilitating social embarrassment and loss of enjoyment in sharing a meal with friends and family. These results have important implications for medical personnel who work with patients in acute care settings as opposed to outpatient clinics. In the outpatient setting, patients need help with social and community reintegration in the face of severe dysphagia. These issues are integral to the rehabilitation process in dysphagia and should not be ignored.

Severe dysphagia causes significant disruption of social and psychological function. This disruption can lead to an affective disorder and significantly affect participation in therapy. It can exacerbate social isolation, with a negative impact on family and social relationships. Clinicians should be attentive to the mental health of individuals with dysphagia, and psychological consultation should be requested when appropriate. Cognitive problems can also occur in individuals with dysphagia because of the nature of the underlying disease. Cognitive impairment can make it difficult for patients to participate effectively in therapy programs and to use strategies for safe swallowing.

Given the variety of disorders that can cause dysphagia, and the serious complications that can result, a comprehensive understanding of normal and abnormal swallow function and prognosis is essential. A team approach to addressing the medical, cognitive, physical, and psychosocial aspects of swallowing facilitates as near a return to independence as possible.

ACKNOWLEDGMENTS: The authors wish to acknowledge Cathy A. Pelletier and Koichiro Matsuo for original publication because their content is used in the revisions for this chapter. In addition, the authors wish to thank Susanne Butte for her assistance in the completion of this chapter.

KEY REFERENCES

2. American Psychiatric Association: *Diagnostic and statistical manual of mental disorders*, ed 4, Washington, DC, 1994, American Psychiatric Association.
4. Avent J, Aventa J, Glista S, et al: Family information needs about aphasia, *Aphasiology* 19:365–375, 2005.
6. Ball L, Beukelman D, Pattee G: A protocol for identification of early bulbar signs in ALS, *J Neurol Sci* 191:43–53, 2001.
8. Barlow S, Lee J, Wang J, et al: Frequency-modulated orocutaneous stimulation promotes non-nutritive suck development in preterm infants with respiratory distress syndrome or chronic lung disease, *J Perinatol* 34:136–142, 2014.
9. Barlow S, Lund J, Estep M, Kolta A: Central pattern generators for speech and orofacial activity. In Brudzynski S, editor: *Handbook of mammalian vocalization*, Oxford, 2011, Elsevier, pp 351–370.
11. Berthier M, Green C, Lana P, et al: Memantine and constraint-induced aphasia therapy in chronic poststroke aphasia, *Ann Neurol* 65:577–585, 2009.
12. Berthier ML, Pulvermüller F, Dávila G, et al: Drug therapy of post-stroke aphasia: a review of current evidence, *Neuropsychol Rev* 21:302–317, 2011.
15. Beukelman DR, Yorkston KM, Garrett KL, editors: An introduction to AAC services for adults with chronic medical conditions. In *Augmentative communication strategies for adults with acute or chronic medical conditions*, Baltimore, 2007, Brookes Publishing Co, pp 1–15.
17. Blake ML, Duffy JR, Myers PS, Tompkins CA: Prevalence and patterns of right hemisphere cognitive/communicative deficits: retrospective data from an inpatient rehabilitation unit, *Aphasiology* 16:537–547, 2002.
18. Borr C, Hielscher-Fastabend M, Lücking A: Reliability and validity of cervical auscultation, *Dysphagia* 22:225–234, 2007.
19. Brady S: The use of blue dye and glucose oxidase reagent strips for detection of pulmonary aspiration: efficacy and safety updates, *Dysphagia* 14:8–13, 2005.
20. Brady S, Donzelli J: The modified barium swallow and the functional endoscopic evaluation of swallowing, *Otolaryngol Clin North Am* 46:1009–1022, 2013.
21. Brady S, Hildner C, Hutchins B: Simultaneous videofluoroscopic swallow study and modified Evans blue dye procedure: an evaluation of blue dye visualization in cases of known aspiration, *Dysphagia* 14:146–149, 1999.
23. Cherney L, Halper A, Kwasnica C, et al: Recovery of functional status after right hemisphere stroke: relationship with unilateral neglect, *Arch Phys Med Rehabil* 82:322–328, 2001.
24. Cherney LR, Halper AS, Kaye RC: Computer-based script training for aphasia: emerging themes from post-treatment interviews, *J Commun Disord* 44:493–501, 2011.
25. Cherney LR, Patterson JP, Raymer A, et al: Evidence-based systematic review: effects of intensity of treatment and constraint-induced language therapy for individuals with stroke-induced aphasia, *J Speech Lang Hear Res* 51:1282–1299, 2008.
26. Cherney LR, Patterson JP, Raymer AM: Intensity of aphasia therapy: evidence and efficacy, *Curr Neurol Neurosci Rep* 11:560–569, 2011.
37. Darley FL, Aronson AE, Brown JR: Differential diagnostic patterns of dysarthria, *J Speech Hear Res* 12:249–269, 1969.
40. Dharmarajan T, Unnikrishnan D: Tube feeding in the elderly. The technique, complications, and outcome, *Postgrad Med* 115:51–54, 58-61, 2004.
41. Dongilli PA, Hakel ME, Beukelman DR: Recovery of functional speech following traumatic brain injury, *J Head Trauma Rehabil* 7:91–101, 1992.
42. Donzelli J, Brady S, Wesling M, Craney M: Predictive value of accumulated oropharyngeal secretions for aspiration during video nasal endoscopic evaluation of the swallow, *Ann Otol Rhinol Laryngol* 112:469–475, 2003.
43. Donzelli J, Brady S, Wesling M, Craney M: Simultaneous modified Evans blue dye procedure and video nasal endoscopic evaluation of the swallow, *Laryngoscope* 111:1746–1750, 2001.
46. Fraser C, Rothwell J, Power M, et al: Differential changes in human pharyngoesophageal motor excitability induced by swallowing, pharyngeal stimulation, and anesthesia, *Am J Physiol Gastrointest Liver Physiol* 285:G137–G144, 2003.
47. Freed M, Freed L, Chatburn R: Electrical stimulation for swallowing disorders caused by stroke, *Respir Care* 46:466–474, 2001.
49. Gayler B: Fluoroscopic equipment for video swallowing studies: current state of technology and future trends, *Perspectives on Swallowing and Swallowing Disorders (Dysphagia)* 16:2–7, 2007.
50. German R, Crompton A, Thexton A: Integration of the reflex pharyngeal swallow into rhythmic oral activity in a neurologically intact pig model, *J Neurophysiol* 102:1017–1025, 2009.

51. Gill SK, Leff AP: Dopaminergic therapy in aphasia, *Aphasiology* 28:155–170, 2014.
52. Gow D, Rothwell J, Hobson A, et al: Induction of long-term plasticity in human swallowing motor cortex following repetitive cortical stimulation, *Clin Neurophysiol* 115:1044–1051, 2004.
53. Graff-Radford J, Jones DT, Strand EA, et al: The neuroanatomy of pure apraxia of speech in stroke, *Brain Lang* 129:43–46, 2014.
54. Gross R, Mahlmann J, Grayhack J: Physiologic effects of open and closed tracheostomy tubes on the pharyngeal swallow, *Ann Otol Rhinol Laryngol* 112:143–152, 2003.
55. Hagan C, Malkmus D, Durham P: Levels of cognitive functioning. In Rancho Los Amigos Hospital: *Rehabilitation of the head injured adult: comprehensive physical management*, Downey, 1979, Professional Staff Association of Rancho Los Amigos Hospital.
56. Hallowell B, Chapey R: Introduction to language intervention strategies in adult aphasia. In Chapey R, editor: *Language intervention strategies in aphasia and related neurogenic communication disorders*, ed 5, Baltimore, 1978, Lippincott Williams & Wilkins, pp 3–8.
65. Hoffman M, Ciucci M, Mielens JJ, et al: Pharyngeal swallow adaptations to bolus volume measured with high-resolution manometry, *Laryngoscope* 120:2367–2373, 2010.
70. Hsiao M, Chang Y, Chen W, et al: Applications of ultrasonography in assessing oropharyngeal dysphagia in stroke patients, *Ultrasound Med Biol* 8:1522–1528, 2012.
72. Humbert I, German R: New directions for understanding neural control in swallowing: the potential and promise of motor learning, *Dysphagia* 28:1–10, 2013.
86. King JM, Simmons-Mackie N, Beukelman DR, editors: Supporting communication: improving the experience of living with aphasia. In *Supporting communication for adults with acute and chronic aphasia*, Baltimore, 2013, Paul H. Brookes Publishing Co, pp 1–10.
87. Klose J, Heldwein W, Rafferzeder M: Nutritional status and quality of life in patients with percutaneous endoscopic gastrostomy (PEG) in practice: prospective one-year follow-up, *Dig Dis Sci* 48:2057–2063, 2003.
95. Leder S, Suiter D: *The Yale swallow protocol: an evidence-based approach to decision making*, Cham, 2014, Springer International Publishing.
97. Leslie P, Drinnan M, Zammit-Maempel I, et al: Cervical auscultation synchronized with images from endoscopy swallow evaluations, *Dysphagia* 22:290–298, 2007.
98. Logemann J: *Evaluation and treatment of swallowing disorders*, ed 2, Austin, 1998, Pro-Ed.
99. Logemann J: Non-imaging techniques for the study of swallowing, *Acta Otorhinolaryngol Belg* 48:139–142, 1994.
100. Loring DW, Meador KJ, Lee GP, et al: Cerebral language lateralization: evidence from intracarotid amobarbital testing, *Neuropsychologia* 28:831–838, 1990.
105. Maas E, Robin DA, Austermann Hula SN, et al: Principles of motor learning in treatment of motor speech disorders, *Am J Speech Lang Pathol* 17:277–298, 2008.
118. Palmer J, Drennan J, Baba M: Evaluation and treatment of swallowing impairments, *Am Fam Physician* 61:2453–2462, 2000.
120. Pelletier C, Lawless HH: Effect of citric acid and citric acid-sucrose mixtures on swallowing in neurogenic oropharyngeal dysphagia, *Dysphagia* 18:231–241, 2003.
123. Rao N, Brady S, Chaudhuri G, et al: Analysis of the videofluoroscopic and fiberoptic endoscopic swallow examinations, *J Appl Res* 3:89–96, 2003.
131. Ross-Swain D: *Ross information processing assessment*, Austin, 1986, Pro-Ed.
132. Sapir S, Ramig LO, Fox CM: Intensive voice treatment in Parkinson's disease: Lee Silverman Voice Treatment, *Expert Rev Neurother* 11:815–830, 2011.
133. Schmidt RA, Lee TD: *Motor learning and performance. From principles to application*, ed 5, Champaign, IL, 2013, Human Kinetics.
134. Sessle BJ, Yao D, Nishiura H, et al: Properties and plasticity of the primate somatosensory and motor cortex related to orofacial sensorimotor function, *Clin Exp Pharmacol Physiol* 32:109–114, 2005.
136. Shames J, Treger I, Ring H, Giaquinto S: Return to work following traumatic brain injury: trends and challenges, *Disabil Rehabil* 29:1387–1395, 2007.
138. Simmons-Mackie N, King JM, Beukelman DR: *Supporting communication for adults with acute and chronic aphasia*, Baltimore, 2013, Paul H. Brookes Publishing Co.
139. Smith-Hammond C, New K, Pietrobon R: Prospective analysis of incidence and risk factors of dysphagia in spine surgery patients: comparison of anterior cervical, posterior cervical, and lumbar procedures, *Spine* 29:1441–1446, 2004.
140. Stathopoulosa E, Huberb J, Richardson K, et al: Increased vocal intensity due to the Lombard effect in speakers with Parkinson's disease: simultaneous laryngeal and respiratory strategies, *J Commun Disord* 48:1–17, 2014.
145. Thiel A, Hartmann A, Rubi-Fessen I, et al: Effects of noninvasive brain stimulation on language networks and recovery in early post-stroke aphasia, *Stroke* 44:2240–2246, 2013.
146. Thomas K: Neuropsychological treatment of mild traumatic brain injury, *J Head Trauma Rehabil* 8:74–85, 1993.
148. Vargha-Khadem F, O'Gorman AM, Watters GV: Aphasia and handedness in relation to hemispheric side, age at injury and severity of cerebral lesion during childhood, *Brain* 108:677–696, 1985.
153. Wambaugh J, Duffy JR, McNeil MR, et al: Treatment guidelines for acquired apraxia of speech: treatment descriptions and recommendations, *J Med Speech Lang Pathol* 14:xxxv–xvii, 2006.
158. Yavuzer G, Kucukdeveci A, Arasil T, Elhan A: Rehabilitation of stroke patients: clinical profile and functional outcome, *Am J Phys Med Rehabil* 80:250–255, 2001.
159. Ylvisaker M, Szekeres SF: A framework for cognitive rehabilitation. In Ylvisaker M, editor: *Traumatic brain injury rehabilitation: children and adolescents*, Boston, 1998, Butterworth-Heinemann, pp 125–158.

The full reference list for this chapter is available online.

CHAPTER 4

PSYCHOLOGICAL ASSESSMENT AND INTERVENTION IN REHABILITATION

Nicholas J. Pastorek, Daniel A. Proto, Angelle M. Sander, Allison N. Clark

Rehabilitation has been defined as a process of assessment, goal setting, intervention, and reassessment.[100] This iterative rehabilitative process is consistent with the World Health Organization's framework for measuring health and disability, which defines disablement as the manifestation of bidirectional influences between health conditions and contextual factors.[106] Embedded within this model is the implication that health is a complex interaction between three components: body structures and functions, activities and participation, and environmental and personal factors (i.e., contextual factors). As it were, psychologists with specialty training in rehabilitation are well equipped to provide assessment and intervention within all three health-related components. Depending on the goal of the individual, a psychologist working in rehabilitation can provide direct cognitive remediation (i.e., body structure and function), can increase social participation through the application of behavioral management principles (i.e., activities and participation), and can provide psychotherapeutic services to family members (i.e., contextual factors). The critical role that psychologists play at each stage of the rehabilitation process is reflected in the standards of the Commission on Accreditation of Rehabilitation Facilities, which necessitate the availability of psychological services across many rehabilitation contexts.[17] The role of psychologists in the management of specific rehabilitation populations, such as military veterans or athletes with a history of traumatic brain injury (TBI), has also been formally established.[24,60]

This chapter is broadly divided into two sections that represent the most common roles of psychologists in rehabilitation settings: assessment and intervention. The section on assessment is organized in such a way as to mirror the changing role of the psychologist across acute care, inpatient, and postacute rehabilitation settings, which is largely dictated by the evolving needs of clients, caregivers, and the rehabilitation team. Psychologists have advanced training in the assessment and treatment of cognitive, emotional, and behavioral problems. As such, both sections focus largely on the psychologist's role in managing these aspects of health.

Psychological Assessment in Rehabilitation

With regard to assessment, one of the core competencies of a psychologist working in rehabilitation is the capability to select and interpret psychometric tests and measures.[41] As such, psychologists are well prepared to explicate the complex relation between health conditions and contextual factors associated with disablement. Psychological assessment in rehabilitation serves many specific purposes including identification of cognitive, behavioral, and psychological strengths and weaknesses; quantification of adjustment to disability by the individual and family; information about treatment planning; prognostication; clinical auditing; and research. Whenever possible, rehabilitation psychologists use measures of impairment, activities, and participation with standardized administration procedures, known psychometric properties, and normative data sets. When administered by a trained professional, such measures can be applied in a straightforward manner to highlight areas of impairment, activity limitations, and participation restrictions. Psychologists can combine such data with their knowledge of medical and psychological rehabilitation principles to identify the greatest environmental or personal barrier to successful community reintegration, determine the extent to which an individual has benefited from care, evaluate the effectiveness of a rehabilitation program, and determine which administrative elements or clinical processes might best account for treatment gains.

Measurement of individualized and sometimes abstract (e.g., health-related satisfaction with life) treatment goals in rehabilitation requires a critical review of existing scales to select instruments that are most appropriate to assess the progress or success of individuals, specific treatments, or entire programs. In some cases, the development of new measures or scales may be necessary to adequately quantify progress toward a particularly unique set of goals.[55] Psychologists' understanding of scale development allows them to critically evaluate the psychometric quality of performance-based (e.g., cognitive) and report-based (e.g., self-, caregiver-, or clinician-rated) measures. Psychologists are well suited to weigh various test characteristics, such as reliability, validity, floor and ceiling effects, and sensitivity to change, when selecting measures for various clinical, research, or administrative purposes in rehabilitation. Generalizability is also an important consideration in test selection, especially when an individual's performance will be used to inform real-world decisions, such as a return to driving. In addition to the high psychometric standards of many of the assessment tools used by psychologists, most of these measures allow for normative comparison so that treatment team members can better appreciate the magnitude of strengths and weaknesses identified by the psychologists. The use of such standardized measures is also thought to enhance communication among team members.[47]

Assessment in the Acute Care Setting

In the acute care setting, the focus is typically on sustaining life through the management of emergency medical issues. Although physical, or in the case of brain injury, cognitive impairments at this stage of recovery may preclude the individual from completing most standardized psychological assessment tools, psychologists in this setting can assist in collecting information to formulate important prognostications regarding likely eventual outcome. Indeed, injury characteristics, such as duration of loss of consciousness, Glasgow Coma Scale score, and duration of posttraumatic amnesia (PTA), and premorbid demographic information, such as preinjury levels of education, socioeconomic status, and intellectual functioning, are often some of the only empirically supported data points available for use in predicting long-term outcomes of short-term inpatients.[46,101] However, even small amounts of additional data obtained from simple bedside measures administered during the short-term recovery period can be of use, and psychologists and neuropsychologists can assist in obtaining this information. The ability to freely recall three words after a 24-hour delay, for example, is predictive of numerous long-term (i.e., 4 years postinjury) outcome variables, including return to productivity, quality of life, and psychosocial distress.[21] Additionally, Dawson et al.[21] found in their sample that of those persons with moderate or severe brain injuries whose 24-hour three word free recall ability had not returned in fewer than 3 weeks postinjury, none had returned to work at the 4-year follow-up point. Furthermore, routine monitoring for the resolution PTA during the short-term recovery period is also important because such resolution is often considered a prerequisite to inclusion in neuropsychological research and assessment.[7]

Beyond formal cognitive testing, psychologists can assist in working with family members, friends, or caregivers to provide information and support services. Also, given their formal training in research methods, psychologists can also participate in study design and implementation involving short-term inpatients, which is particularly important given the unique opportunity and continued need for prospective rather than retrospective research paradigms in this setting. Even if formal academic output (e.g., scientific journal publications, conference presentations) is not the end goal of these research-related activities, the obtained information can be useful in tracking patient progress and outcome, treatment efficacy, and various provider-related variables at the individual and clinic- or department-wide levels.

Assessment in the Inpatient Rehabilitation Setting

As individuals with significant physical and neurologic injuries progress from the short-term to inpatient rehabilitation settings, the role of psychologists in collecting information about the individual's emotional, behavioral, and cognitive functioning begins to expand considerably. At this stage, psychologists can use a range of methods to collect meaningful information about individuals including interviews, behavioral observation, review of historical records, and standardized testing. All of these methods are brought to bear in the important task of assessing behavioral and emotional functioning. Careful assessment of preinjury and current psychological functioning is necessary to identify facilitators and barriers to recovery that can be addressed through individual and family interventions. As has been previously noted, success in adapting to health conditions requires that the individual can cope with stress and adapt to new demands.[26] As discussed later, the role of the psychologist in evaluating emotional functioning in particular continues to expand in the postacute setting as individuals gain a greater appreciation for activity limitations and participation restrictions and the resulting changes in roles that may arise from their injury.

As with the acute care setting, neuropsychologists in particular typically focus their inpatient rehabilitation evaluations on individuals with known or suspected neurologic insult. Also as mentioned earlier, previous neuropsychological research has often excluded individuals from testing until they are able to demonstrate resolution of PTA, such as by obtaining scores of 76 or higher on the Galveston Orientation and Administration Test[50] across two consecutive administrations[7,85] or exhibiting the ability to freely recall three words after a 24-hour delay.[21] Still, neuropsychologists can provide useful information in patients still experiencing PTA, which is particularly important in light of decreasing inpatient stay lengths and the concomitant increasing potential for discharge before PTA resolution. For example, the ability to simply complete a neuropsychological testing battery at 1 month after injury is associated with Disability Rating Scale and Glasgow Outcome Scale scores at 6 months after injury [68] and was predictive of employment status at 1- and 2-year follow-up points.[22] In addition, although individuals with PTA may perform more poorly on most neuropsychological measures, research indicates that these individuals are nonetheless often able to participate in some testing, particularly if the administered measures are relatively simple and assess a range of cognitive abilities.[45,77] Although there exists some debate as to the optimal postinjury time point(s) at which to conduct a full neuropsychological evaluation,[31,84] the predictive value and treatment planning utility of these assessments is significant, as is described later.

Perhaps one of the greatest strengths of neuropsychological data, owing to its psychometrically based and normatively derived status, is the ability to track statistical and clinically significant change over time. Through initiation of serial assessments of the same individual, such as at resolution of PTA and then at the 3- and 6-month and 1- and 2-year postinjury marks,[84] the patient is able to serve as his or her own baseline. Then, by gathering a few test-related pieces of information (e.g., the pretest and posttest group means and standard deviations, the pretest and posttest score correlation coefficient), the psychologist is able to determine what a standardized measure of the size of any observed changes is, whether the changes are likely to be attributable to chance or practice effects, and in what proportion of the population as a whole or a select illness-specific subpopulation such a change is likely to occur.[18] Indeed, brief measures of orientation and cognition (e.g., O-Log,[43] Cog-Log[1]) have been developed and validated specifically for serial bedside assessment, with these instruments correlating both with later performance on formal neuropsychological assessment and Mini Mental State Examination scores.[69] Such definitive information about change can then be used to track an individual's recovery, to monitor for any unexpected declines in functioning or cognitive performance, and to evaluate the potential efficacy of initiated treatments. This definitive information about recovery and treatment effects is critical for the individuals, their family, treatment providers, researchers, and third-party payers.

In addition to tracking the progress of the individual over time, early neuropsychological assessment is useful in predicting long-term patient outcomes above and beyond demographic- and injury-related information. Sherer et al.[84] reviewed a number of studies evaluating the outcome prediction potential of neuropsychological testing, finding that there was strong support for the use of early neuropsychological testing in particular (i.e., at resolution of PTA or by 1-month after injury) to predict employment status at 1 or more years after injury. Green et al.[31] came to a somewhat similar conclusion, stating that performance on untimed neuropsychological measures (i.e., memory and executive functioning) but not timed measures at 5 months after injury was predictive of return to productivity. Particularly promising is the finding that lengthy (e.g., full-day or multiday) assessments are not always necessary because even brief neuropsychological batteries are predictive of various outcome variables, such as select scores on the Functional Independence Measure, Disability Rating Scale, and Glasgow Outcome Scale-Extended.[36]

Along with the distinctive predictive characteristics of global neuropsychological performance regarding cognitive and functional outcome, neuropsychological assessment can also uniquely identify and quantify current cognitive functioning and potential impairment in a variety of specific domains.[81] Depending on the type and location of neurologic insult/injury, cognitive deficits may be global or circumscribed, and neuropsychological assessment can assist in delineating the affected cognitive areas. In addition, objective cognitive testing can reveal subtle deficits in domains that may not have been expected on the basis of injury characteristics or that may not be evident without such formal assessment. In the inpatient setting, assessment of expressive and receptive language functions, basic attention, and verbal memory as a result of the potential influence of these cognitive areas on individuals' participation in rehabilitative therapies tends to be of particular importance. Evaluation of these and other cognitive domains can also assist in determining which types of services may be most beneficial or appropriate. Occasionally, neuropsychologists may need to alter their choice of assessment instruments or adapt the administration procedures to account for the individuals' physical and cognitive limitations (e.g., mobility difficulties, hemiparesis, visual disturbances). Such alterations can affect the interpretability of results obtained by means of these standardized measures, and, as such, the expertise of the neuropsychologist in test construction and design plays a key role in these situations in allowing them to glean what and how information gathered in nontraditional testing situations should be interpreted (see Brooks et al.[10] for a review of neuropsychological test interpretation and related concepts). Ultimately, the testing data, combined with observational information obtained from treatment sessions with other providers, may then be useful in identifying specific areas of expected difficulty and potential supports that might most effectively remediate these challenges, alleviate disability, and allow for a smoother and more complete reintegration into the family and community on discharge.

Beyond the assessment of performance in individual cognitive domains, psychologists are often also versed in the use of instruments designed specifically to inform questions regarding capacity (e.g., medical decision-making capacity, financial capacity). Comprehensive measures, such as the Independent Living Scales,[54] allow clinicians to compare the performances of individual patients to normative sample data stratified by level of supervision needed in various instrumental activities of daily living to determine how much day-to-day assistance may be required in these areas. Neuropsychologists have also developed domain-specific tests, such as the Financial Capacity Instrument,[58] that allow for in-depth assessment of specific capacities and that have subsequently resulted in covalidation of rating scales that can be administered and interpreted by other health care providers (e.g., the Semi-Structured Clinical Interview for Financial Capacity[57]). In these ways, psychologists, particularly on educating themselves on the capacity-related laws in their state of practice, can use their skills in psychometric instrument selection and interpretation and clinical interviewing to aid physicians in making capacity-related decisions. The American Psychological Association, in a joint effort with the American Bar Association, has also released material to aid psychologists in this endeavor on a national level.[2] As patients near the end of their inpatient stay, psychologists can combine assessment data, interview information, and capacity-related concepts to assist physiatrists and other treatment team members in determining the appropriate discharge destination level of supervision.

Assessment in the Postacute Rehabilitation Setting

As with the acute and inpatient care settings, psychological assessment in the postacute rehabilitation setting is dictated by the purpose of the evaluation and the condition of the individual. Although still important, assessment of the presence and severity of impairments starts to give way to the evaluation of the individual's activity and participation and their overall health-related quality of life as they prepare to transition back to the home and community.[11,93] The focus of this stage of recovery is typically on maximizing community reintegration through the identification of personal and environmental assets that can be used to overcome residual activity limitations and participation restrictions. Individuals at this stage of recovery are often living in the community and participating in outpatient care. In the case of brain injury, this outpatient care is ideally delivered through an interdisciplinary, milieu-based approach. These consumers are expected to become increasingly involved in managing their instrumental activities of daily living. Mirroring the increasingly complex demands placed on persons with injury who are transitioning back to their homes and communities, there are vast numbers of standardized psychological assessment tools available to assess the emotional, behavioral, and cognitive functioning of these higher-functioning persons. Psychological assessment tools for outpatients typically provide a much greater depth of information than brief, broad measurement tools more appropriate for assessment of inpatients who may have very significant impairments in their body functions or structures that preclude them from participating in lengthy assessments. The length of these assessment tools makes them more sensitive to subtle changes that might otherwise go unnoticed on briefer measures, which then makes them ideal for tracking changes in functioning in the postacute setting.

As individuals begin to spend less time in the treatment setting and more time living in the community, the evaluation of the quality of their social and civic life takes on greater importance. The Craig Handicap Assessment and Reporting Technique[103] (CHART) was an attempt to create a measure of community participation that conformed to an earlier version of the International Classification of Functioning, Disability, and Health (ICF).[106] More recently, the Participation Assessment with Recombined Tools-Objective was developed by combining items from the CHART and two other commonly used participation measures.[105] Although these instruments provide important information about the frequency of participation in various community-based activities, broader measures of community participation and health-related quality of life incorporating the perspective of the patient are now considered to be an essential component of assessment.[98] Patient reported outcomes are subjective in nature and inherently allow for individuals to consider their personal and cultural values when rating their overall health-related quality of life. The inclusion of the perspective of the person with injury reflects patient-centered care and may help to focus assessment and treatment on the individual's desired outcomes.[25]

Careful assessment of potential environmental facilitators and inhibitors is essential to optimize successful reintegration into the community.[79] Despite the long-standing appreciation of the influence of environment on disability and participation in the field of rehabilitation, psychologists and other rehabilitation professionals have made relatively little headway in operationalizing environmental factors important to rehabilitation and developing psychometrically sound measures in this area.[104] Recently, the ICF defined five categories of environment including products and technology; natural environment and human-made changes to environment; support and relationships; attitudes; and services, systems, and policies. Although much work remains in quantifying environment and understanding exactly how these variables influence outcome, psychologists possess a sound knowledge base regarding the influence of environmental factors on health status and tools to assist in the measurement of environment factors, such as family structure and support.

Emotional adjustment to changes in body structures and functions, activity limitations, and participation restrictions after injury can present a major challenge in inpatient and postacute rehabilitation settings. In the case of brain injury, emotional and behavioral problems may be a direct result of the injury. Although it is not entirely clear whether major psychiatric disorders are generally a response to disability following injury or whether psychiatric disorders lead to greater functional limitations following injury,[82] the rate of psychiatric comorbidities is known to be high in rehabilitation settings. This is especially true in rehabilitation populations where the injury itself, or the context within which it occurs, is associated with psychological trauma, as is often the case in military service members.[94]

Owing to the overlap of symptoms secondary to brain injury and psychiatric disorders, psychologists and other qualified rehabilitation specialists must carefully consider differential diagnoses when emotional and behavioral problems are evident in the rehabilitation setting. For example, depression must be distinguished from symptoms possibly related to the brain injury (e.g., apathy, irritability, pseudobulbar affect), and from other psychiatric conditions, such as adjustment disorder, normal sadness, and grief, over changes in physical or social functioning (see Dafer et al.[20] for a review). To accomplish this, the psychologist takes into account multiple sources of information to determine if the person meets criteria for a clinical disorder, including the clinical presentation, information obtained from the clinical interview, responses to questionnaires, knowledge of brain-behavior relationships, review of medical and psychosocial history, and cultural background. Psychologists also have appropriate training and tools to assess for the presence of personality traits and psychiatric factors that may influence recovery in the inpatient and postacute settings. Recently, psychologists have also started focusing on positive psychological factors that are associated with adaptive adjustment and coping in persons recovering from physical illness. Psychologists can contribute to the rehabilitation process by assessing and monitoring negative and positive psychological factors that can affect outcome and life satisfaction in those persons participating in rehabilitation.

Assessment or reassessment of cognitive functioning also remains important in the postacute rehabilitation setting. In the inpatient care context, one of the primary applications of neuropsychological testing is the prediction of various long-term outcome-related variables such as return to work in individuals with acquired neurologic insult/injury. Conversely, as individuals transition to outpatient rehabilitation services care, somewhat less emphasis is traditionally placed on predicting outcome, in no small part because initial predictions have probably already occurred. One key exception to this shift, however, would be individuals who did not undergo neuropsychological assessment while admitted to an inpatient unit, whether as a result of lack of service availability, scheduling difficulties, incomplete resolution of PTA, or any of a host of other reasons. In these instances, neuropsychological testing retains its utility to inform long-term prognosis estimates. In addition, there are some other specific instances when predictive utility is still retained in the postacute, outpatient environment. For example, neuropsychological testing performance at 1 year after injury predicts or is associated with cognitive and functional change at up to 5 years after injury.[34,35,63] Outside of such situations, greater emphasis is often placed on the following areas, many of which are identified by neuropsychologists as key assessment goals: monitoring progress and, relatedly, evaluating treatment response and efficacy; informing treatment plans; aiding in the assessment of capacity to return to various life activities (e.g., independent living and decision-making, work, school); providing updated feedback to individuals and family members/caregivers; and detecting novel complications or unexpected declines in functioning.[84]

As individuals proceed through outpatient treatment, regular reassessment of their neuropsychological status is a useful tool for measuring cognitive recovery and comparing it with expected recovery trajectories. The 3- and 6-month postinjury marks in particular can be important periods for formal cognitive evaluation as a result of the relatively rapid early spontaneous recovery that may occur and represent assessment points specifically recommended by neuropsychologists following moderate-to-severe TBI.[84] Such testing allows for updated information to be provided to treatment team members, family/caregivers, and the individuals themselves regarding cognitive strengths and persisting impairments. In addition, if recovery does not go as expected (e.g., if regression is observed), neuropsychological assessment allows for delineation of the nature of the decline and can thereby aid in identifying its potential cause. Neuropsychological reassessment, then, allows for continued monitoring of cognitive status and ongoing refinement of prognosis, which can be particularly important given that data can indicate that persisting impairments may change in both severity and type over the extended recovery period, such as from global dysfunction to disruption of specific cognitive domains.[23,35]

In a related manner, by virtue of its objective and norm-referenced nature, neuropsychological reassessment also allows for evaluation of treatment efficacy through single-case design methods, such as A-B-A-B, or multiple baseline designs (see Levine and Downey-Lamb[51] for a review). Treatments not resulting in the anticipated improvements can then be identified, and possible patient-related factors contributing to these situations (e.g., previously unidentified cognitive or emotional difficulties) can be targeted for intervention. Neuropsychological reassessment also allows for adjustments in treatment goals on the basis of the individual's true recovery relative to that which may have initially been predicted. Even in the case of mild TBI, neuropsychological testing can be beneficial to treatment planning: research tentatively suggests that results from a screening of executive functioning are predictive of patient-reported cognitive functioning and ability after participation in an outpatient treatment program.[49] Because early intervention by means of provision of education can be useful in decreasing postconcussive symptoms in this population,[64,71] identification of individuals at risk for greater perceived long-term cognitive dysfunction may be useful in detecting patients who require more in-depth early intervention efforts.

With interventions often targeting increased independence and participation in meaningful activities as goals, neuropsychological assessment can specifically assist in making progress toward these end points. As discussed earlier, acute neuropsychological data have been shown to provide additional predictive ability in returning to work above and beyond patient demographics and injury characteristics.[31,84] Neuropsychological assessment has also been shown to differentiate between individuals who have returned to work and those who have not,[84] and in that way potentially identifies those cognitive abilities that are highly important as individuals pursue reemployment. In addition, eligibility for work-related programs such as vocational rehabilitation may require in-depth documentation of cognitive status, and receipt of academic accommodations for those individuals wishing to return to school or to receive technical training may also necessitate such formal assessment. In this way, outpatient neuropsychological evaluations directly assist in helping individuals to qualify for such services and can inform these programs as to particular supports that may be necessary (e.g., extra time to complete tasks and access to reduced-distraction environments for individuals exhibiting attention and processing speed impairments). Similarly, for individuals initially determined to be incapable of living independently or managing medical and financial decisions, neuropsychological reassessment allows for continued monitoring of status in these respects. As cognitive abilities improve, testing can aid in determining when it is appropriate and safe for individuals to assume increased responsibilities in these life domains. Finally, although there are more directly ecologically valid means of assessing or predicting an individual's driving ability, neuropsychological assessment has some utility in this regard[70,86] and, at the least, can provide additional information to accompany a formal driving evaluation.

Another unique aspect of outpatient evaluations is that as emphasis shifts from critical to rehabilitative care, there exists increased potential for involvement in litigation. In such instances, rehabilitation professionals can be asked to fill dual roles, such as care provider and fact or expert witness; it is thus of paramount importance in the outpatient setting that physicians, psychologists, and other providers clarify their role as being of clinical or litigation-related service delivery. Patient involvement in litigation presents numerous challenges to care providers, such as a heightened risk for and vulnerability to feigning or exaggerating cognitive and physiological impairments. Indeed, estimates of the proportion of individuals seen for assessment in medicolegal or disability claims-related contexts suspected of exhibiting disingenuous symptom reports or suboptimal effort range from approximately 30% to upward of 70%, which is substantially higher than that observed in general medical contexts.[32,65] As such, neuropsychologists have developed numerous measures of effort and engagement that are supported by significant amounts of research indicating their accuracy and appropriateness for use in various populations, and thereby resulting in multiple professional organizations recommending their use in all neuropsychological evaluations.[12,39] Thus, neuropsychologists can fill a unique role by providing objectively informed statements regarding the validity or invalidity of testing data.

Although psychologists play an essential role in selecting and administering appropriate measures of cognition, emotion, and behavior based on characteristics of the individual and the purpose of the assessment, their most important role may be the translation of information obtained by these measures into actionable plans to address specific concerns regarding community reintegration and health-related quality of life. Malec[55] describes a process for collaborating with individuals to create measurable, achievable goals that take into account the values of the client. The process essentially involves working with the individual to identify goals and the intermediate steps necessary to attain each goal. Given their expertise in promoting positive change in behavior, psychologists are well positioned to assist individuals in progressing toward their goals, especially where the modification of contextual factors of the person (e.g., coping style) and environment (e.g., supports and relationships) are essential to the attainment of the individual's goals.

Psychological Management of Cognitive, Emotional, and Behavioral Problems

The role of psychologists in the rehabilitation setting goes beyond simply assessing and reporting results. One of the greatest values of psychologists in a rehabilitation setting is their expertise with interventions for cognitive, emotional, and behavioral problems. The following sections describe the evidence base with respect to treatment of cognitive, emotional, and behavioral problems in the rehabilitation setting. When available, existing evidence-based recommendations for specific interventions are provided. Intensity of services varies by type of rehabilitation setting, and this is addressed for each of the interventions discussed. The goal of this section is not to enable the reader to carry out interventions but to be an educated consumer of psychological and neuropsychological intervention services to make appropriate referral of patients.

Interventions for Cognitive Problems

Impaired Awareness

Impaired awareness can be one of the most challenging consequences of brain injury for rehabilitation staff, as well as for family members and other caregivers. Impaired awareness refers to the lack of ability to recognize deficits resulting from injury to the brain.[73] In contrast to denial, which is a psychological defense, impaired awareness is a neurologically based problem, resulting directly from damage to the brain; however, denial and impaired awareness can coexist because persons with brain injury can have awareness of some deficits and not others or may be partially aware of specific deficits. Persons with impaired awareness may seem to have no understanding of limitations, which may affect their motivation to participate in therapies and to follow through with medical recommendations. Despite this, their impaired awareness cannot be interpreted as lack of motivation because this implies an intentional component that is not present. Conflicts with staff and family members often occur when they interpret the individual's behavior as representing poor motivation or denial, when it is in fact as a result of impaired awareness. Research has shown that persons with TBI are more likely to have impaired awareness for cognitive and emotional problems as opposed to physical problems.[72,83]

Impaired awareness is not an all-or-nothing phenomenon. Persons can have more or less awareness of deficits. Crosson et al.[19] described a hierarchy of awareness levels that has implications for the level of intervention needed. Intellectual awareness refers to the basic understanding that abilities are reduced relative to preinjury and that this reduction in abilities may affect everyday functional activities. Emergent awareness refers to the ability to recognize a problem in real time—when it is happening. For example, persons with brain injury may be able to tell you that they have a problem getting off the topic when speaking (intellectual awareness) but may have difficulty recognizing when they are actually doing it (emergent awareness). Anticipatory awareness refers to the ability to predict that a particular problem may occur in specific situations and settings. For example, persons with intact anticipatory awareness would predict that they are likely to get off the topic when speaking with others at a party and could think through and plan strategies to help reduce the problem. Emergent and anticipatory awareness are task dependent and context dependent, meaning that they can be affected by demands of tasks and the environment.[97]

Because impaired awareness can represent a safety risk, the most basic level of neuropsychological intervention, particularly during inpatient rehabilitation, is to assess the impact on everyday safety and to modify the environment to reduce the risk. For more specific interventions in impaired awareness, neuropsychological treatments should be tailored to the individual needs and level of awareness exhibited by the person with injury. Fleming and Ownsworth[29] recommend selecting performance tasks that will demonstrate the problem to the person with injury and providing an opportunity for feedback and education. Persons with impaired awareness can still benefit from experience and from procedural learning, and thus they may be asked to perform tasks a certain way or to use a specific compensatory strategy, even though they may not understand the reason for this. Therapeutic alliance plays an important role in their willingness to do so, and staff should not underestimate the importance of developing good rapport in the rehabilitation environment. Having the person with injury predict his or her own performance on tasks and then chart the predictions against the actual performance is also a powerful therapeutic tool. The neuropsychologist can then assist the person in developing strategies to improve performance. This performance-based focus can eliminate the need for arguing with the person about whether he or she has a "memory problem" or some other "problem."

In the outpatient setting, impairments in emergent or anticipatory awareness are most typical. Holistic, milieu-oriented therapy environments, including both group and individual therapies, are a way to address impaired awareness. In group therapies, persons with impaired awareness can learn by observing the behavior of others and providing feedback that could then be used to monitor their own behavior. Because intervention in impaired awareness is an underlying component of nearly all rehabilitation therapies, conducting randomized controlled trials to demonstrate the effectiveness of awareness interventions is difficult. In their systematic review of cognitive rehabilitation effectiveness, Cicerone et al.[14] recommended the use of metacognitive strategies to improve executive functioning, including awareness as a practice standard for persons with TBI and stroke. Metacognition refers to the ability to be aware of one's own cognitive functions, and metacognitive strategies are those that improve one's ability to self-monitor and alter cognitive functions. Awareness has been shown to improve following training that combines therapist feedback with experiential learning in which clients predict, monitor, and evaluate their own performance.[13] Similar training has been shown to improve cognitive aspects of instrumental activities of daily living performance, as well as ability to self-regulate behavior.[30] Neuropsychologists working to improve awareness in persons with brain injury will typically use these empirically based metacognitive strategies.

Attention

Impaired attention is an almost universal consequence of brain injury, regardless of type and severity. Attention is a multidimensional concept, and different aspects of attention can be affected after injury. When intervention is determined, viewing attention as a hierarchical construct is helpful.[88] The most basic level of attention is focused attention, which is the ability to respond discretely to specific sensory stimuli. For example, the ability to observe a bird against a backdrop of trees would be focused attention. Sustained attention is the ability to maintain a consistent behavioral response during continuous, repetitive activity. Examples of everyday sustained attention are maintaining attention during a therapy exercise or playing a board game. A higher level of attention is selective attention, which is the ability to maintain cognitive or behavioral set in the face of competing or distracting stimuli. An example is being able to attend to a conversation at a party while other conversations can be heard in the background. Alternating attention refers to the ability to shift focus between tasks that have different cognitive or behavioral requirements. This ability is otherwise known as cognitive flexibility. An example is being able to shift between cooking a meal and helping a child with homework. The highest level on the attention hierarchy is divided attention. This refers to the ability to respond spontaneously to multiple task demands. Examples are driving while carrying on a phone conversation or taking care of a baby while working on the computer. A person who has impairments at one of the lower levels of attention will necessarily have impairment at all of the higher levels as well.

In the rehabilitation setting, a person with impaired focused attention will be unable to attend to therapies, regardless of circumstances. A patient with intact focused attention and impaired sustained attention may be able to attend to therapy for very short intervals but be unable to maintain attention for an entire 30-minute therapy session. The individual with intact sustained attention and impaired selective attention will be able to sustain attention for the duration of a therapy session, provided that there are minimal distractions. If the individual is working in a noisy or crowded environment, attention is likely to be diverted. Impairments in alternating or divided attention are usually the most difficult to detect in an everyday setting. These impairments can be subtle and only manifest in cognitively challenging contexts. The structured rehabilitation setting will often not create the necessary challenges for these deficits to emerge, yet persons with brain injury may notice these problems when they return to their homes and communities and attempt to resume preinjury activities.

In their systematic reviews of the research on interventions to improve attention, Cicerone et al.[14] concluded that there is insufficient evidence to recommend direct attention training during the acute recovery period, including inpatient rehabilitation. Although direct attention training may not be effective during inpatient rehabilitation, environmental modifications can help to decrease the impact of impaired attention on functional activities. For persons with impaired sustained attention, therapy sessions should be broken down into shorter sessions or a break should be allowed partway through a standard session. When returning to a task following a break, it is usually necessary to remind the individual of what was being worked on and to repeat instructions. If a person has impairment in selective attention, distractibility can be partly reduced by conducting therapy or providing medical/nursing education in a quiet room that is apart from the distractions of the inpatient unit or therapy gym. It is important to note that persons with impaired selective attention are distracted by internal thoughts and feelings as well as by external stimuli. Therefore, even in a quiet environment, they may be distracted by bodily sensations or competing thoughts. In these cases, redirection to the task at hand, with repetition of instructions as needed, is usually the best action. If impairments in alternating or divided attention become apparent in the rehabilitation environment, they can be managed by having patients work on only one task at a time. It is best to keep the materials for other tasks out of their working space. It is also helpful to ensure that procedures and education sessions are not occurring in parallel. For example, if the physician is providing education, it is best not to have a nurse or resident checking their blood pressure or dressing a wound while the physician is talking.

More direct forms of attention intervention are most successful in the postacute, outpatient setting. On the basis of the existing research evidence, Cicerone et al.[14] recommend direct attention training in the postacute period as a practice standard. Attention Process Training is a form of attention training in which clients complete a series of hierarchical computer tasks to improve attention. The levels of task complexity parallel the levels of attention (e.g., focused, sustained). The person with injury must master tasks at one level before moving on to the next level. This type of hierarchical attention training has demonstrated effectiveness for improving performance on cognitive tasks of attention in persons with TBI[90,96] and stroke.[102] The computer tasks that have shown effectiveness have involved systematic, hierarchical training. There is no evidence for the effectiveness of nonhierarchical computer training in improving attention. Therefore simply playing computer games or working on simple computer tasks may have no direct benefit on attention.

It should also be noted that although attention training improves performance on cognitive tasks of attention, generalization to real-world activities may be limited. Cicerone et al.[14] recommend supplementing direct attention training with training in compensatory strategies (such as use of checklists or memory notebooks) and metacognitive strategies (such as self-monitoring, self-verbalization, and problem-solving) to improve generalization to real-world activities. Direct therapist contact is necessary for all of these types of training. As stated by Cicerone et al.,[14] reliance on computer tasks without the assistance or guidance of a therapist is not recommended for improving attention following brain injury.

Memory

Memory problems are among the most frequent complaints of persons with brain injury. Memory problems in everyday life may be caused by deficits in attention and processing speed, as well as directly by memory impairment. The most typical manifestations of memory problems in everyday life include difficulty keeping track of belongings, forgetting what needs to be done (e.g., appointments, chores, questions to ask a doctor), forgetting how to get to places, forgetting what people have told them or what they have learned, and forgetting how to do something (i.e., procedures).[78] Assessing self-report of everyday memory functioning is an important supplement to formal neuropsychological assessment. Persons who perform well on memory assessment conducted in a structured setting may still experience difficulties in everyday situations outside of testing. Similarly, persons who perform poorly on formal memory tests may not report functional memory problems because they have learned to use compensatory strategies that reduce the impact of memory impairments in their everyday lives. In addition to formal memory assessment, a comprehensive interview about memory functioning in everyday life will provide the foundation for treatment planning to address memory impairments.

Interventions targeting memory can be classified into two broad areas: restorative and compensatory.[88] Restorative treatments are based on the idea that memory abilities can be restored through practice, and they typically include systematic training and repetitive drills. Computer exercises focused on improving memory are often used. Unfortunately, there is minimal empirical evidence for the effectiveness of restorative treatments targeting memory. According to recent systematic reviews, they are not recommended in either the inpatient or outpatient settings for persons with TBI or stroke because their effectiveness has not been demonstrated.[14]

Training in use of compensatory memory strategies has demonstrated effectiveness for improving memory performance and everyday memory functioning following TBI and stroke.[14] The goal of compensatory memory strategy training is to help persons with injury develop ways to "get around" memory impairment so that they can accomplish functional goals. The premise is that functional memory can improve with strategy use, even if the person continues to exhibit memory impairment on formal testing. Compensatory strategies can be classified as internal or external. Internal strategies rely on internal processes to learn and remember information. Examples include visual imagery, rehearsal, and organization (e.g., trying to remember information by forming an acronym). Research has shown that internal memory strategies are effective for improving performance on neuropsychological tests of memory[62,95]; however, generalization to real-world memory tasks has not been demonstrated. A further limitation of these strategies is their reliance on cognitive abilities of the person with injury, including attention and organization. Use of these strategies may tax an already compromised cognitive capacity in persons with moderate to severe memory impairment and therefore may be more appropriate for persons with mild memory impairment.

In contrast to internal strategies, external memory strategies rely on cues outside of persons to remind them of important information. External memory strategies can be paper based or electronic. Examples of paper-based aids are memory notebooks, planners/organizers, and checklists. Electronic aids include mobile phones and portable digital voice recorders. Memory notebooks and daily journals have demonstrated effectiveness for reducing everyday memory failures.[80,110] Several small studies and case studies have demonstrated the potential of electronic memory aids for improving performance on a variety of everyday memory tasks, including remembering to take medications and keeping track of tasks to complete.[37,92,107]

On the basis of their systematic review of the literature, Cicerone et al.[14] recommended memory strategy training, using either internal or external strategies, as standard practice for persons with mild to moderate memory impairment. Persons with more severe memory impairment are likely to have difficulty learning and applying these strategies. Therefore Cicerone et al.[14] recommended training in the use of external memory strategies with direct application to functional activities as a practice guideline for persons with severe memory impairment.

The recommendations of Cicerone et al.[14] have direct applicability for intervening in memory within both inpatient and outpatient settings. During inpatient rehabilitation, many persons will have memory impairment that is severe enough to preclude them from benefitting from memory strategy training. Providing these patients with a memory notebook or other memory aid may have minimal impact unless they participate in intensive training sessions with a therapist to help them learn to use it. Researchers have found that it can take persons with severe TBI months to learn to use a memory notebook adequately.[89] Understandably, therapists feel responsible for providing assistance to persons with memory impairment while they are in the inpatient unit, which should be encouraged; however, assistance should be given in accordance with the individual's capacity to benefit from the intervention. For persons who are still exhibiting PTA, meaning that they have not begun to form day-to-day memories, rehabilitation staff should consistently provide them with orienting information (e.g., place, time, and what happened/why they are in the hospital) throughout the day. Maintaining a white board in the room with information on the names of their therapists, physician, and nurse, and the times of their therapies, is also recommended. If rehabilitation staff think that a memory notebook should be given to all patients, it is important that a family member or significant other be trained in how to use the strategy and in how to prompt the person with injury to use it regularly. Without the assistance of a family member or other caregiver, persons with injury are unlikely to learn to use the notebook and apply it in their home and community environments.

In the outpatient setting, neuropsychologists are more likely to assist persons with injury in developing compensatory strategies to reduce the impact of memory impairment on their daily lives. Because one compensatory strategy may not work for everyone, it is best to present different choices (e.g., memory notebook, checklist, phone calendar, and reminders) and have the persons with injury select the one that best fits their needs and preferences. Training with real-world memory tasks, such as remembering questions to ask a physician or remembering when to get their prescriptions refilled, is more likely to result in generalizability to their home and community environments. If possible, training should occur in their everyday environment. If this is not possible, simulated real-world tasks can be used. Involvement of family members/caregivers in training helps to ensure success.

Problem-Solving

Problem-solving deficits have long been noted as a problem for persons with brain injury.[99] Impairments can manifest at any level of problem-solving, including analyzing problem situations, generating potential solutions, evaluating alternatives, choosing a solution, and evaluating the real-world consequences of solutions. Researchers have shown that problem-solving is a multidimensional ability and is related to speed of processing.[74,76] Brain injury results in slowed processing of information so that the normal demands of everyday life cannot be adequately processed, leading to difficulty with analyzing information and solving problems. Problem-solving deficits can have a negative impact on almost every aspect of daily functioning and social roles, affecting abilities such as how to prioritize financial commitments, how to decide between two possible medical treatments, how to care for a sick child, and how to make new friends or deal with conflict between family members.

Interventions to improve problem-solving have generally been grouped under the heading of executive function interventions because problem-solving is an aspect of executive functioning. Relative to other executive functions (such as goal planning and organization), there has been a substantial amount of research on cognitive rehabilitation interventions to improve problem-solving skills. On the basis of the existing research evidence, Cicerone et al.[14] have recommended training in formal problem-solving strategies as a practice guideline for persons with TBI in the outpatient, postacute setting.[14] The best evidence is for interventions that combine the use of self-monitoring and emotional regulation for effective problem-solving orientation with training in systematic analysis and solution of problems.[75] Some neuropsychologists may address problem-solving by training people to self-monitor periodic progress toward goals, otherwise known as goal management training.[52] This type of intervention actually addresses multiple aspects of executive function, including problem-solving. Cicerone et al.[14] recommend that the problem-solving training be conducted with direct application to real-word situations and functional activities. Therefore neuropsychologists should individualize the problem-solving training so that it is directly applicable to the everyday problem situations that clients encounter.

Interventions for Emotional and Behavioral Problems

Emotional Problems

Psychotherapeutic interventions in civilian rehabilitation settings often focus on treating depression and anxiety disorders because these are the most common emotional problems experienced by rehabilitation populations. Numerous studies have documented high rates of depression and anxiety disorders among rehabilitation populations, including TBI,[8] stroke,[4] and spinal cord injury.[27] Posttraumatic stress disorder is an especially common psychiatric comorbidity in service members and veterans with a history of combat-related mild TBI.[16] Emotional problems are important targets of interventions in rehabilitation settings because they can have a negative impact on participation in therapy[56] and are associated with poorer functional outcomes.[38] The relation between emotional problems and functional outcomes is somewhat complicated. For example, postinjury depression may contribute to reduced participation as a result of an individual's withdrawal from activities and interests, or an inability to participate in activities and interest as a result of injury-related deficits may contribute to the development and maintenance of depression. Longitudinal studies in persons with TBI suggest that the experience of functional limitations precedes the development of later depression.[67] Despite the frequency and impact of emotional changes after brain injury, there is relatively limited evidence regarding the effectiveness of psychological and pharmacologic interventions for mental health conditions following acquired brain injury, such as TBI and stroke.[28,33] Pharmacologic interventions for poststroke depression have some support in the literature, although prescribers must also weigh the risk of increased adverse events.[33] Although definitive practice guidelines are not available regarding the use of pharmacologic interventions for emotional problems secondary to acquired brain injury, recommendations based on current standards of practice have been published (see Jorge and Arciniegas[44] for an example).

This section focuses on three types of psychological interventions that may be used in rehabilitation settings: cognitive behavioral, behavioral, and supportive. Cognitive-behavioral therapies (CBTs) are based on the theory that thoughts, emotions, and behaviors are founded on an underlying belief system and that emotional symptoms arise from negative, maladaptive, underlying beliefs. Cognitive aspects of these interventions include increasing awareness of cognitive distortions and their impact on one's emotional and interpersonal functioning. Persons are trained to identify and evaluate the validity of maladaptive beliefs so that they can challenge such dysfunctional belief structures and generate more adaptive beliefs. Behavioral components of CBT include monitoring of one's mood and its relation to activity levels, behavioral activation strategies such as activity scheduling, and behavioral experiments aimed at testing beliefs and developing new learning experiences that will produce more adaptive and prosocial behaviors.[5]

Behavioral interventions do not attempt to identify and modify maladaptive beliefs and thoughts, which is one of the key components of CBT. Instead, behavioral therapies focus on helping patients identify current patterns of coping and how they may exacerbate emotional symptoms, and develop improved coping patterns and greater access to reinforcing and pleasant life events. Specific life situations and how they serve to maintain emotional distress are discussed, as well as "new" behaviors that could potentially improve mood. Some of the behavioral strategies frequently used in this type of therapy are similar to those discussed earlier, including activity scheduling to increase the number of reinforcing events. Functional activities that are associated with feelings of accomplishment, pleasure, or both are examples of reinforcing events. Graded task assignments, in which actions are broken down into smaller, more manageable steps, and therapist-client role play are other techniques that may be used.[59]

Supportive psychotherapy is another type of intervention that may be used in rehabilitation settings. The focus of this intervention, similar to all psychotherapeutic interventions, is on improving psychological functioning and reducing distress and dysfunction in the context of a positive therapeutic relationship. Frequently used techniques include communicating acceptance and empathy, providing opportunities to share thoughts and feelings in a secure environment, validating experiences, offering reassurance and suggestions when appropriate, encouraging use of supports, and providing psychoeducation. Behavioral and cognitive-behavioral techniques may also be used.[6] Finally, another technique that may be incorporated in psychotherapy to help alleviate anxiety is progressive relaxation, which involves focused attention to breathing, visualization of a pleasant and relaxing image, and tightening and relaxing of different muscle groups.

There is a growing body of literature investigating CBTs and behavioral interventions in rehabilitation populations with some promising findings, especially for CBT for psychosocial issues in persons with spinal cord injury.[61] Researchers have urged caution when implementing CBT in persons with cognitive impairment, however, including persons with stroke or TBI because those impairments can negatively affect their ability to learn and apply cognitive-behavioral techniques.[53] For example, there is insufficient evidence to support practice recommendations regarding specific psychological treatments for individuals with a history of brain injury.[28,91] As a result, adaptations to the structure and content of psychological interventions, such as provision of supplementary written materials, built-in repetition of key concepts, focus on concrete goals, and decreased emphasis on self-directed, higher-level reasoning skills play an important role in the development and implementation of these treatments in individuals receiving rehabilitative care. Findings to date suggest that persons with cognitive deficits can participate in and show benefit from these adapted interventions.[9,42,87]

There are several factors that are taken into account when psychotherapeutic services are implemented in acute rehabilitation settings, including the nature and severity of the emotional problem, the presence and severity of cognitive deficits, previous experience with psychotherapy, and the length of stay. For example, with respect to length of stay, initiation of brief, focused supportive psychotherapy may be more appropriate for persons admitted for a relatively short period of time, with referrals for additional psychotherapy made at discharge. In this example, a CBT intervention may not be appropriate because there may not be sufficient time for appropriate implementation. With respect to cognition, CBT will likely be more effective for persons with intact cognition, whereas supportive psychotherapy may be more appropriate for persons with severe cognitive deficits.

Psychological treatment for emotional problems is also a key component of postacute rehabilitation programs, and there is evidence that participation in these programs is associated with improved outcomes including community integration, life satisfaction, self-efficacy, and emotional functioning.[15,96] The factors that affect treatment planning in the acute phase noted earlier also affect planning in postacute rehabilitation settings. These programs often offer group interventions in addition to individual interventions; thus treatment planning must also take these different formats into account. There are several advantages to group interventions, including increased opportunities for imitative behaviors, interpersonal learning, altruism, and decreased sense of social isolation,[108] as well as cost-effectiveness. However, the individual's strengths and weaknesses will be important to consider when readiness to participate in a group intervention is determined. For example, persons with significant behavioral control issues or cognitive deficits may benefit from individual interventions initially. As cognition and behavioral control improve, they may then benefit from participation in a group intervention.

Emotional problems do not occur in a vacuum. In other words, they can have a significant impact on an individual's compliance and motivation with rehabilitation in both acute and postacute settings, which can negatively affect outcomes. In cases in which a client's anxiety or depression is interfering with participation in therapy, the psychologist may provide cotreatment with physical and occupational therapists to address the emotional issues that may be serving as a barrier to engagement or participation in the therapy.

Behavioral Problems

Behavioral problems arising in rehabilitation settings, such as agitation, disinhibition, aggression, and impulsivity, can be frustrating and distressing for family members and rehabilitation care providers and may contribute to poor compliance and cooperation with therapies. A combination of pharmacologic and nonpharmacologic interventions may be required for treatment of these issues.[3] However, medication side effects such as increased sleepiness could also interfere with participation in therapies. The use of physical restraints may lead to injuries and contribute to increased agitation.[40,48] This section focuses on behavioral interventions implemented by psychologists as part of a collaborative, multidisciplinary approach to treating behavioral problems following brain injury. Numerous studies have demonstrated the effectiveness of these interventions, and they have been proposed as a treatment guideline for certain rehabilitation populations, such as adults with behavior disorders following TBI.[109]

The first step in planning and executing an effective behavioral intervention to treat a problem behavior is the completion of an individualized functional behavioral analysis. This analysis establishes the function of a behavior through careful observation of the actual problem behavior and examination of the antecedents to and the consequences of the behavior via direct patient observation and interviews with rehabilitation care providers, family, and patients, if appropriate. The problem behavior should be described in terms of its nature (e.g., yelling, throwing objects), frequency, severity, and duration. Observation of potential antecedents entails attention to both the individual's "internal" experience (e.g., pain, poor comprehension) and characteristics of the external environment (e.g., places, events, time of day, people) that occur before the problem behavior. Observation of consequences involves attention to events that occur immediately after the problem behavior, including events, the reactions of others, gains, and losses.

Consequences that increase the probability of a behavior are referred to as *reinforcements* and are described as "positive" (e.g., receiving something the individual finds meaningful or important) or "negative" (e.g., removal or withdrawal from an aversive environment). Consequences that decrease the probability of a behavior are referred to as *punishments*. Contextual factors, such as diagnosis, stage of recovery, medications, nature and severity of cognitive deficits, and sleep cycle, should also be considered when an analysis of problem behaviors in persons with brain injury is completed.[66]

Information obtained from the functional behavioral analysis will contribute to the development of hypotheses regarding the situations or events that predict the behavior and the consequences that maintain the behavior. The problem behavior can then be addressed through manipulation of the antecedents to prevent the problem behavior from occurring or through contingency management, which is the systematic and planned manipulation of consequences that are designed to increase or decrease specific behaviors. Some examples of response prevention and contingency management techniques are presented in Tables 4-1 and 4-2.

Behavioral interventions often include management of both antecedents and consequences. In general, these interventions require continued monitoring of the individual's behavior to determine if the intervention is effective. Additional observation and modification of the underlying hypothesis and intervention plan is required if the individual's behavior is not improving. Behavioral interventions that focus on prevention/manipulation of antecedents have been recommended for use with persons with brain injury in the inpatient rehabilitation unit because these strategies are often less time consuming and stressful than those that focus on manipulation of consequences.[66]

Table 4-1 Contingency Management of Problem Behaviors

Contingency Management Technique	Example
Withdrawal of reinforcement	Ignore inappropriate behavior Time out on the spot
Reward for positive behavior	Token economy procedures: receive token that can be traded for a later reward
Differential reinforcement of incompatible behavior	Reinforce behaviors that are incompatible with problem behavior
Differential reinforcement of low rates of responding	Reinforce low rates of problem behavior during a specified time period
Response-cost procedures	Lose points for negative behaviors

Table 4-2 Antecedent Management of Problem Behaviors

Antecedent of Problem Behavior	Management Technique
Overstimulating environment	Minimize noise Limit visitors to one or two at a time
Decreased comprehension	Use positive nonverbal communication skills, including tone of voice, gestures, and facial expressions
Pain	Use distraction techniques Introduce strategies to increase patient control in situations in which pain may be experienced (e.g., physical therapy)
Difficulty communicating	Allow additional time for patient to communicate Do not interrupt patient Do not finish patient's thoughts

Education of the family and rehabilitation care providers regarding the functional behavioral analysis is a key component of these treatment plans. Family members as well as rehabilitation staff may be unaware of the triggers that lead to the problem behavior or may be unaware of how a response to a problem behavior may be reinforcing the behavior. For example, some people may laugh in response to an "inappropriate" behavior because they feel uncomfortable or nervous. This laughter may actually reinforce a problem behavior because the individual perceives that he or she did something funny that caused the other person to laugh; he or she could not discern that the laughter expressed discomfort rather than joy. As a result, the client may repeat the behavior to make others laugh. The behavioral intervention may include education to family and other providers regarding the importance of not laughing when the client exhibits the problem behavior and making a nonreinforcing response instead. Cotreatment with other therapists may be necessary for some individuals with behavior problems to successfully implement the intervention.

Other Considerations

Patients in rehabilitation settings are more than their injury. In other words, they are admitted to rehabilitation with unique lifetime experiences, strengths, and weaknesses, including academic and vocational history, psychiatric history, substance use, coping skills, family functioning, economic resources, and home environments. Psychologists also take such factors into consideration when making treatment and referral recommendations. For example, the role of the individual's family and support system is an important focus in rehabilitation because their involvement and support will facilitate translation of rehabilitation strategies to home and community settings and the psychologist often plays an important role in providing family with education and support. For some individuals, their relatively limited time in rehabilitation may be their only opportunity to receive specialized medical management and information related to their injury; thus an inclusive approach to psychoeducation may be beneficial for both clients and families. For example, in the acute recovery period following mild TBI, psychologists are expected to play an integral role in the delivery of empirically supported, psychoeducational interventions known to reduce the occurrence of postconcussion syndrome and enhance functional outcome.[60] Finally, psychologists not only focus on treatments to reduce distress and dysfunction but also capitalize on opportunities to promote well-being and positive emotional adjustment following injury.

ACKNOWLEDGMENTS: Preparation of this chapter was partially supported by U.S. Department of Education National Institute on Disability and Rehabilitation Research (NIDRR) grants H133A070043, H133B090023, and H133A120020 to TIRR Memorial Hermann.

KEY REFERENCES

2. American Bar Association/American Psychological Association: *Assessment of older adults with diminished capacity: a handbook for psychologists*, Washington, 2008, American Bar Association/American Psychological Association.
3. Arciniegas DB, Wortzel HS: Emotional and behavioral dyscontrol after traumatic brain injury, *Psychiatr Clin North Am* 37:31–53, 2014.
4. Ayerbe L, Avis S, Rudd AG, et al: Natural history, predictors, and associations of depression 5 years after stroke: the South London Stroke Register, *Stroke* 42:1907–1911, 2011.
7. Boake C, Millis SR, High WM, Jr, et al: Using early neuropsychologic testing to predict long-term productivity outcome from traumatic brain injury, *Arch Phys Med Rehabil* 82:761–768, 2001.
8. Bombardier CH, Fann JR, Temkin NR, et al: Rates of major depressive disorder and clinical outcomes following traumatic brain injury, *JAMA* 303:1938–1945, 2010.
9. Bradbury CL, Christensen BK, Lau MA, et al: The efficacy of cognitive behavior therapy in the treatment of emotional distress after acquired brain injury, *Arch Phys Med Rehabil* 89:S61–S68, 2008.
10. Brooks BL, Sherman EM, Iverson GL, et al: Psychometric foundations for the interpretation of neuropsychological test results. In Schoenberg MR, Scott JG, editors: *The little black book of neuropsychology: a syndrome-based approach*, New York, 2011, Springer, pp 893–922.
11. Bullinger M, Azouvi P, Brooks N, et al: Quality of life in patients with traumatic brain injury—basic issues, assessment, and recommendations, *Restor Neurol Neurosci* 23:111–124, 2002.
13. Cheng SK, Man DW: Management of impaired self-awareness in persons with traumatic brain injury, *Brain Inj* 20:621–628, 2006.
14. Cicerone KD, Langenbahn DM, Braden C, et al: Evidence-based cognitive rehabilitation: updated review of the literature from 2003 through 2008, *Arch Phys Med Rehabil* 92:519–530, 2011.
15. Cicerone KD, Mott T, Azulay J, et al: A randomized controlled trial of holistic neuropsychologic rehabilitation after traumatic brain injury, *Arch Phys Med Rehabil* 89:2239–2249, 2008.
16. Collins RL, Pastorek NJ, Tharp AT, et al: Behavioral and psychiatric comorbidities of TBI. In Tsao JW, editor: *Traumatic brain injury*, New York, 2012, Springer.
18. Crawford JR, Garthwaite PH: Comparing patients' predicted test scores from a regression equation with their obtained scores: a significance test and point estimate of abnormality with accompanying confidence limits, *Neuropsychology* 20:259–271, 2006.
19. Crosson B, Barco PP, Velozo CA, et al: Awareness and compensation in postacute head injury rehabilitation, *J Head Trauma Rehabil* 4:46–54, 1989.
20. Dafer RM, Rao M, Shareef A, Sharma A: Poststroke depression, *Top Stroke Rehabil* 15:13–21, 2008.
21. Dawson DR, Levine B, Schwartz ML, et al: Acute predictors of real-word outcomes following traumatic brain injury: a prospective study, *Brain Inj* 18:221–238, 2004.
22. Dikmen SS, Temkin NR, Machamer JE, et al: Employment following traumatic head injuries, *Arch Neurol* 51:177–186, 1994.
23. Dikmen SS, Machamer JE, Powel JM, et al: Outcome 3 to 5 years after moderate to severe traumatic brain injury, *Arch Phys Med Rehabil* 84:1449–1457, 2003.
24. Echemendia RJ, Iverson GL, McCrea M, et al: Role of neuropsychologists in the evaluation and management of sport-related concussion: an inter-organizational position statement, *Arch Clin Neuropsychol* 27:119–122, 2012.
27. Fann JR, Bombardier CH, Richards JS, et al: Depression after spinal cord injury: comorbidities, mental health service use, and adequacy of treatment, *Arch Phys Med Rehabil* 92:352–360, 2011.
28. Fann JR, Hart T, Schomer KG: Treatment for depression after traumatic brain injury: a systematic review, *J Neurotrauma* 26:2383–2402, 2009.
29. Fleming J, Ownsworth T: A review of awareness interventions in brain injury rehabilitation, *Neuropsychol Rehabil* 16:474–500, 2006.
31. Green RE, Colella B, Hebert DA, et al: Prediction of return to productivity after severe traumatic brain injury: investigations of optimal neuropsychological tests and timing of assessments, *Arch Phys Med Rehabil* 89(Suppl 12):S51–S60, 2008.
33. Hackett ML, Anderson CS, House A, Xia J: Interventions for treating depression after stroke, *Cochrane Database Syst Rev* (8):CD003437, 2008.
34. Hammond FM, Grattan KD, Sasser H, et al: Five years after traumatic brain injury: a study of individual outcomes and predictors of change in function, *NeuroRehabilitation* 19:25–36, 2004.
35. Hammond FM, Hart T, Bushnik T, et al: Change and predictors of change in communication, cognition, and social function between 1 and 5 years after traumatic brain injury, *J Head Trauma Rehabil* 19:314–328, 2004.
39. Heilbronner RL, Sweet JJ, Morgan JE, et al: American Academy of Clinical Neuropsychology consensus conference statement on the neuropsychological assessment of effort, response bias, and malingering, *Clin Neuropsychol* 23:1093–1129, 2009.
41. Hibbard MR, Cox DR: Competencies of a rehabilitation psychologist. In Frank RG, Rosenthal M, Caplan B, editors: *Handbook of rehabilitation psychology*, ed 2, Washington, 2010, American Psychological Association, pp 467–475.
44. Jorge RE, Arciniegas DB: Mood disorders after TBI, *Psychiatr Clin North Am* 37:13–29, 2014.
51. Levine B, Downey-Lamb MM: Design and evaluation of rehabilitation experiments. In Eslinger PJ, editor: *Neuropsychological interventions*, New York, 2002, Guilford Press.
53. Lincoln NB, Flannaghan T: Cognitive behavioral psychotherapy for depression following stroke: a randomized controlled trial, *Stroke* 34:111–115, 2003.
55. Malec J: Goal attainment scaling in rehabilitation, *Neuropsychol Rehabil* 9:253–275, 1999.
56. Malec JF, Moessner AM: Self-awareness, distress and post-acute rehabilitation outcome, *Rehabil Psychol* 45:227–241, 2000.
60. McCrea M, Pliskin N, Barth J, et al: Official position of the Military TBI Task Force on the role of neuropsychology and rehabilitation psychology in the evaluation, management, and research of military veterans with traumatic brain injury, *Clin Neuropsychol* 22:10–26, 2008.
61. Mehta S, Orenczuk S, Hansen KT, et al: An evidence-based review of the effectiveness of cognitive behavioral therapy for psychosocial issues post-spinal cord injury, *Rehabil Psychol* 56:15–25, 2011.
63. Millis SR, Rosenthal M, Novack TA, et al: Long-term neuropsychological outcome after traumatic brain injury, *J Head Trauma Rehabil* 16:343–355, 2001.
64. Mittenberg W, Canyock EM, Condit D, et al: Treatment of post-concussion syndrome following mild head injury, *J Clin Exp Neuropsychol* 26:829–836, 2001.

66. Nakase-Richardson R, Evans CC: Behavioral assessment of acute neurobehavioral syndromes to inform treatment. In Sherer M, Sander AM, editors: *Handbook on the neuropsychology of traumatic brain injury*, New York, 2014, Springer, pp 157–172.
78. Sander AM, Van Veldhoven LM: Rehabilitation of memory problems associated with traumatic brain injury. In Sherer M, Sander AM, editors: *Handbook of the neuropsychology of traumatic brain injury*, New York, 2014, Springer, pp 173–190.
82. Schönberger M, Ponsford J, Gould KR, et al: The temporal relationship between depression, anxiety, and functional traumatic brain injury: a cross-lagged analysis, *J Int Neuropsychol Soc* 17:781–787, 2011.
84. Sherer M, Novack TA, Sander AM, et al: Neuropsychological assessment and employment outcome after traumatic brain injury: a review, *Clin Neuropsychol* 16:157–178, 2002.
85. Sherer M, Sander AM, Nick TG, et al: Early cognitive status and productivity outcome after traumatic brain injury: findings from the TBI model systems, *Arch Phys Med Rehabil* 83:183–192, 2002.
87. Simpson GK, Tate RL, Whiting DL, et al: Suicide prevention after traumatic brain injury: a randomized controlled trial of a program for the psychological treatment of hopelessness, *J Head Trauma Rehabil* 26:290–300, 2011.
88. Sohlberg MM, Mateer CA: *Cognitive rehabilitation: an integrated neuropsychological approach*, New York, 2001, Guilford Publications.
91. Soo C, Tate R: Psychological treatment for anxiety in people with traumatic brain injury, *Cochrane Database Syst Rev* (18):CD005239, 2007.
94. Tanielian T, Jaycox LH: *Invisible wounds of war: psychological and cognitive injuries, their consequences, and services to assist recovery*, Santa Monica, 2008, RAND Corporation.
98. Tulsky DS, Carlozzi NE, Cella D: Advances in outcomes measurement in rehabilitation medicine: current initiatives from the National Institute of Health and the National Institute on Disability and Rehabilitation Research, *Arch Phys Med Rehabil* 92(Suppl):S1–S6, 2011.
100. Wade D: Describing rehabilitation interventions, *Clin Rehabil* 19:811–818, 2005.
104. Whiteneck G, Dijkers MP: Difficult to measure constructs: conceptual and methodological issues concerning participation and environmental factors, *Arch Phys Med Rehabil* 90(Suppl):S22–S35, 2009.
105. Whiteneck GG, Dijkers MP, Heinemann AW, et al: Development of the Participation Assessment with Recombined Tools-Objective for use after traumatic brain injury, *Arch Phys Med Rehabil* 92:542–551, 2011.
109. Ylvisaker M, Turkstra L, Coehlo C, et al: Behavioural interventions for children and adults with behaviour disorders after TBI: a systematic review of the evidence, *Brain Inj* 21:769–805, 2007.
110. Zencius A, Wesolowski MD, Burke WH: A comparison of four memory strategies with traumatically brain-injured clients, *Brain Inj* 4:33–38, 1990.

The full reference list for this chapter is available online.

CHAPTER 5

PRACTICAL ASPECTS OF IMPAIRMENT RATING AND DISABILITY DETERMINATION

Robert D. Rondinelli, Mohammed I. Ranavaya

The field of physical medicine and rehabilitation (PM&R) is primarily devoted to the clinical evaluation and treatment of disabling consequences to those individuals who have illness, injury, infirmity, or deformity at some point in their lives. As such, PM&R physicians can expect, from time to time, to be called on to make formal assessment of the disability to their patients. Furthermore, the face of medicine continues to undergo changes brought about by the aging Baby Boomer generation; by advances in medical and surgical technology, as well as health awareness that help people live longer and survive even after catastrophic trauma or illnesses; and by continuing casualties of global conflict and other cataclysmic events. According to recent estimates, approximately 57 million Americans are currently living with disabilities,[49] and these numbers can be expected to continually increase during the coming decade. By 2030, an estimated 37 million Baby Boomers will have more than one chronic condition.[5] This impending shift in demographics affords additional opportunities for PM&R specialists to adapt their practice to optimally address the health care needs of patients, through acquisition of a greater understanding of the conceptual foundation and terminology of disablement and application of the same to the practices of impairment rating and disability determination.

This chapter is intended to provide the reader with a brief historical perspective of disability evaluation; a conceptual foundation for understanding the current models of disablement; a descriptive overview of key features and nuances of the various U.S. disability systems; a working vocabulary and practical application of tools available and procedures to follow for proper and valid performance of impairment ratings and disability determinations, including use of the most relevant physician guides; and a heightened awareness of the medicolegal framework, pitfalls, and ramifications of such undertakings.

Terminology and Conceptualization of Disablement

During much of the nineteenth and twentieth centuries, disability was conceptualized in terms of a "medical model" of disease, whereby causation was viewed as directly linked to some underlying pathologic condition potentially identifiable at a histologic and physiologic level and arising out of illness or trauma. Because the diagnosis and treatment of disease was the purview of physicians, diagnosis and treatment of the resulting disability also fell within their expected domain of expertise.[22,33] With the advent of the stethoscope, microscope, x-ray, and other technologies, the physician was armed with instruments of precision and objectivity with which to rate severity of impairment (at an organ system level) and hence objectify the associated disability. The model worked well for disease entities that were relatively devoid of diagnostic ambiguity and where the disease was well understood, as well as for treatment goals and expected therapeutic end points.[42,53] Today, the medical model still serves as the fundamental basis for Social Security disability determinations and for physician-rating schedules that remain largely anatomically and diagnostically based.

A "social model" of disability grew out of the advocacy movement of the 1970s and 1980s, making society accountable for disability in the face of disease through its failure to accommodate the special needs of individuals with disability in terms of environmental access, availability of adaptive equipment, discrimination, prejudicial thinking, and other attitudinal barriers at the time.[33] A better documentation and understanding of the role of social barriers to functioning has helped foster strategies and tactics to neutralize the same and to enable and empower the members of our society with disability.[17]

A "biopsychosocial model" of disability[15] is now the preferred model and has gained wide acceptance when disability is conceptualized. The *biological* component refers to the physical or mental aspects, or both, of an individual with a given health condition; the *psychological* component recognizes personal beliefs, coping strategies, emotional, and other psychological factors that may affect functioning; and the *social* component recognizes contextual, infrastructural, and other environmental factors that may also affect functioning in any given case.[52,53]

From Classification of Causes of Death to International Classification of Functioning, Disability, and Health

The World Health Organization (WHO) has created an international classification system of diseases and of disablement whose origins can be traced directly to the publication of Bertillon's *Classification of Causes of Death* (1893) and, subsequently, the *International Statistical Classification of Diseases, Injuries, and Causes of Death.*[56] By 1948 the WHO began leading this effort and ultimately created the *International Classification of Impairments, Disabilities, and Handicaps (ICIDH),*[54] which is reproduced in simplified form in Figure 5-1.

This system was an attempt to relate the pathologic features of a specific disease or trauma to the resulting impairment (physiologic consequences in terms of signs and symptoms of dysfunction at an organ system level), disability (functional consequences of impairment in terms of abilities lost in one's personal sphere), and handicap (social and societal consequences, freedoms lost in terms of role fulfillment). The relationship lends itself to being depicted in a simplified linear manner, which implies unidirectional nature and causation, and fails to adequately account for confounders of a personal and environmental nature. More recently, the ICIDH has been replaced by the *International Classification of Functioning, Disability, and Health (ICF),*[55] reproduced in modified form in Figure 5-2.

The ICF system more aptly displays the interactive (i.e., nonlinear) relationships between the impairment that an individual afflicted with a particular health condition might face; the potential functional consequences of impairment with respect to that individual's personal and social sphere; and the contextual factors that may mitigate or amplify these consequences, including environmental factors, personal experiences, and choices. By taking environmental and personal factors into account, the ICF has adopted the biopsychosocial model of disablement discussed earlier. The components of disablement according to the ICF classification system include the following:

- *Body functions and body structures:* Physiologic functions and body parts, respectively
- *Activity:* Execution of a task or action by an individual (typically functioning within their own personal sphere)
- *Participation:* Involvement in a life situation (typically within one's social sphere)
- *Impairments:* Problems in body function or structure, such as a significant deviation or loss
- *Activity limitations:* Difficulties that an individual may have in executing activities
- *Participation restrictions:* Problems that an individual may experience in involvement in life situations

The ICF offers a conceptual platform for identifying the disabling consequences of impairment to an individual with a health condition (disorder or disease), whereby the modifying influence (in a positive or negative sense) of environmental and personal factors can also be recognized and more properly accounted for.

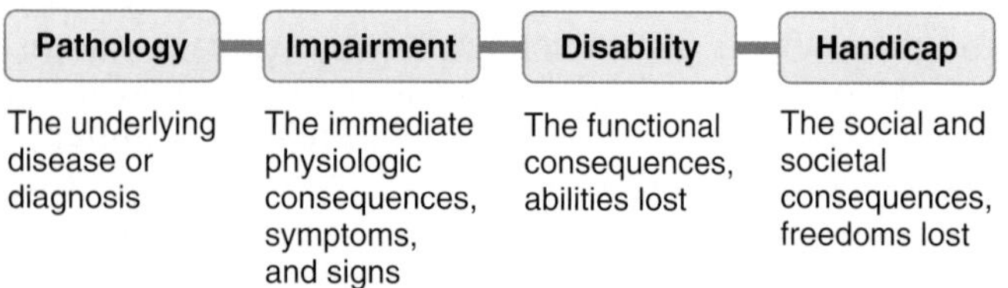

FIGURE 5-1 The World Health Organization International Classification of Illness.

Americans with Disabilities Act and Implications

With the passage of the Americans with Disabilities Act (ADA) in 1990, Americans with disabilities were guaranteed equal rights to employment opportunities, transportation, and public access. The ADA has its own key terminology and defines disability as "a physical or mental impairment that substantially limits one or more of the major life activities of such individual, a record of such impairment or being regarded as such impairment."[9] Although it is broad and somewhat imprecise, this definition is narrowed under "Title 1" of the ADA (Employment) to recognize employment as a major life activity and views disability within the context of performance of the

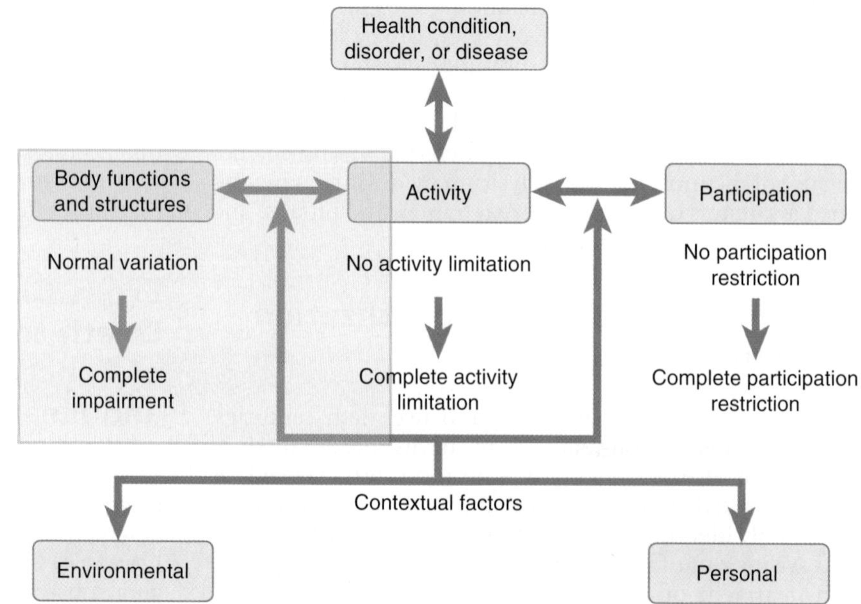

FIGURE 5-2 International Classification of Functioning, Disability, and Health (ICF) model of disablement. (From Rondinelli R, Eskay-Averbach M, Ranavaya M, Brigham C: AMA guides to the evaluation of permanent impairment, sixth edition: a response to the NCCI study, *AMA Guides Newsletter* November/December, 2012. Copyright 2012 American Medical Association.)

essential functions of an employment position with or without *reasonable accommodation*. Reasonable accommodation can include structural modifications of the work site to improve accessibility; availability of modified duty options; and acquisition of adaptive equipment or devices to enable an otherwise qualified worker with a disability to perform the essential functions of the job. Accommodations exempted under ADA include those that pose "undue hardship" to the employer in terms of cost or feasibility of implementation or those that would pose a "direct threat" to the health and safety of the individual with a disability and/or co-workers.[9]

As can be seen from the preceding ICF discussion, accommodation under the ADA is a fundamental social environmental modifier mandated by statutes to mitigate the disabling consequences of impairment in the workplace, in terms of accessibility with respect to activity limitations and participation restrictions. The ADA perspective can be further conceptually integrated with this broader ICF terminology and definitions by viewing impairment, reasonable accommodation, activity limitations, and participation restrictions in relation to a major life activity (work functioning), according to Tables 5-1 and 5-2. According to Table 5-1, if the impairment potentially interferes with activities of daily living (ADLs) in the context of one's workplace that requires accommodation and if that accommodation is provided, no disability in terms of activity limitations need exist. If accommodation is not judged reasonable or otherwise cannot be provided, then disability in terms of activity limitations exists. According to Table 5-2, if the impairment potentially interferes with the ability to safely and efficiently perform the essential functions required of the job and for which specific accommodation is required and can be provided, no disability in terms of participation restrictions need exist relative to that job. If the accommodation required is not reasonable (poses undue hardship or direct threat) and is thereby denied, then disability in terms of participation restrictions exists relative to that job. Although participation restrictions in the workplace can arise out of impairment, they may not be determined solely (or for that matter, primarily) by the impairment itself because other contextual factors might be the primary determinant of disability in any particular case. Consider, for example, the vastly differing work-related consequences of a partial foot (e.g., first digital ray transmetatarsal) amputation to a ballerina who must perform "on point" and to a construction worker who habitually wears steel-toed work boots on the job. The former amputee might face career-ending changes, whereas the construction worker could arguably experience minimal participation restrictions for the same level of impairment by using minor footwear modifications.

Table 5-1 Relationship of Impairment, Accommodation, and Activity Limitations in the Workplace When Impairment is Present

Impairment Potentially Interferes with Activities of Daily Living	Accommodation Needed	Accommodation Provided	Participation Restrictions
Yes	Yes	Yes	No
Yes	Yes	No	Yes
No	No	No	No

Table 5-2 Relationship of Impairment, Reasonable Accommodation, and Participation Restrictions in the Workplace When Impairment is Present

Impairment Potentially Interferes with Essential Functions	Accommodation Needed	Accommodation Provided	Participation Restrictions
Yes	Yes	Yes	No
Yes	Yes	No	Yes
No	No	No	No

Although the ADA helps to ensure that individuals with disabilities cannot be discriminated against in the workplace and that reasonable accommodation in terms of access must be provided to avoid such discrimination, the workers' compensation system is not presently directly accountable to this legislative mandate. However, the physician examiner seeking to return an injured worker safely to the workplace is well served to review the worker's formal job description and to tailor the ensuing therapy treatment plan to the specific material handling and activity requirements listed according to the essential functions therein; in addition, return-to-work decisions can be driven by the claimant's observed performance in therapy according to these essential functions, thereby releasing the claimant to return to work when the worker's physical performance meets or exceeds these requirements, or by recommending restricted duty and suggesting accommodations when they do not.[43] However, the employer is ultimately responsible for determining reasonable accommodation. It is not the responsibility of the disability-evaluating physician to determine the essential functions of a job, to devise accommodation, or to determine reasonableness of any accommodation proposed by the employer.[24]

Relating Impairment to Disability and Compensation Formulas

Although the major current disability systems of the United States and elsewhere exhibit significant differences from each other (discussed later), they all share a common mandate according to their design and intent to compensate individuals financially for losses due to their qualifying disablement. The challenge becomes one of providing fair and equitable compensation for losses that typically can be expected to occur in three major domains: work disability, nonwork disability, and quality of life (QOL), as depicted in Figure 5-3.[30]

An impairment rating provides an objective measure of severity of disability in terms of organ system disease and associated loss of structure and function. As such, it is a keystone to any disability determination but not the sole or necessarily adequate determinant of losses to the affected

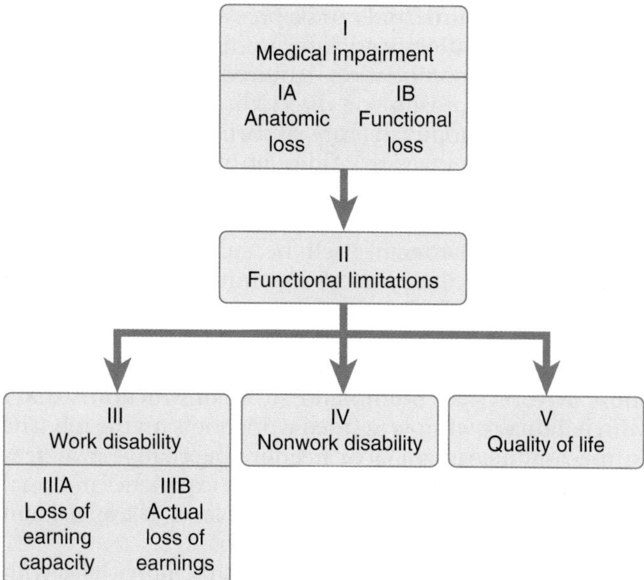

FIGURE 5-3 Disabling consequences of illness or injury. (From Rondinelli R, Eskay-Averbach M, Ranavaya M, Brigham C: AMA guides to the evaluation of permanent impairment, sixth edition: a response to the NCCI study, *AMA Guides Newsletter* November/December, 2012. Copyright 2012 American Medical Association.)

individual. Metrics also exist to calculate losses to the impaired individual in terms of work disability (loss of earnings or earning capacity) and are commonly applied when actuarial analysis takes place. Less obvious, and perhaps less accessible, are metrics to assess *avocational* (e.g., nonwork) disability, such as losses in ability to pursue hobbies and recreational activities, and *QOL* disability, such as losses in terms of medical burden of care and overall life satisfaction. In reality, these more complex domains of disability are typically overlooked for the sake of expediency, simplicity, and practicality, and are often gratuitously (rather than empirically) accounted for. A procedural short-cutting typically takes place whereby the impairment rating becomes a surrogate for the disability rating according to a predetermined formula whereby the impairment percentage is multiplied times a number of weeks arbitrarily established as the "worth" of the whole person times a percentage (usually two thirds to three quarters) of the average weekly wage (up to a cap) to generate a lump sum payout.[42]

In summary, impairment rating is important to the categorization of disablement for the following several reasons:

- It serves as a standard reference point in terms of linking a specific diagnosis to an associated percentage of physical and functional loss in compensable injury claims.
- It enables the impaired individual to exit the system of temporary disablement (e.g., temporary total or permanent partial disablement under workers' compensation) at. maximum medical improvement (MMI).
- It provides a diagnosis-based classification of severity to segue to alternative systems management of long-term disablement.[42]

Major U.S. Disability Systems Compared with Attention to the Role of the Examining Physician

The physician who deals with claims of impairment and disability and issues regarding return to work or staying at work should become familiar with the multiple U.S. compensation systems, which exist both at the federal and state levels, to provide economic and other benefits to claimants experiencing work incapacity because of injury, illness, or aging. Chief among these are the Social Security Administration (SSA), federal and state workers' compensation systems, the Veterans Benefits Administration (VBA), personal injury claims, and others. A physician working within the jurisdictional boundaries of any of these systems plays a critical role and is expected to diagnose the problem, opine as to the causation of an injury or illness (particularly in a workers' compensation setting), provide care, and assess the work fitness of the injured claimant for "modified" duty or return to full duty during recovery. Therefore the physician must also become familiar with the definitions, eligibility requirements, and rating criteria of each particular system and must follow the system-specific rules and procedures prescribed in each particular case.

Social Security Disability Insurance and Supplemental Security Income

The SSA is the largest U.S. disability system, providing assistance to approximately 33% and 50% of all persons who qualify as disabled. The SSA offers two separate disability programs: the first, Social Security Disability Insurance (SSDI), provides benefits to those individuals who have worked in a qualified job for a requisite period, paid into the Social Security system, and subsequently become disabled before age 65 years. SSDI is funded by payroll deductions that, in combination with deductions for old age insurance, comprise the Federal Insurance Contribution Act (FICA) tax, with matching contributions from the employer.[36]

Eligibility for SSDI requires that a "medically determinable impairment" be established whose resulting incapacitation is so severe that it prevents the affected individual from engaging "in any substantial gainful activity (SGA) by reason of any medically determinable physical or medical impairment that can be expected to result in death or that has lasted or can be expected to last for a continuous period of not less than 12 months." SSDI also requires that the individual has worked in a qualified job for at least 5 of the 10 years before onset of disability.[36,48]

SSDI benefits are provided to those considered totally incapacitated and extend to their surviving spouse and children. Benefits are paid as a monthly stipend, and beneficiaries may receive payments until age 65 years, after which they are eligible for Social Security retirement benefits.[41]

The second program, Supplemental Security Income (SSI), provides income for medically indigent persons who are blind, are disabled, or are older (>65 years of age). SSI also provides assistance to children if they have "medically determinable impairments of comparable severity" to an adult's and if the impairment "limits the child's ability to function independently, appropriately, and effectively in an age-appropriate manner." SSI operates as a federal-state partnership that is jointly funded through general revenue (federal and state income tax). Eligibility is determined according to a means test and does not require a work history. SSI also requires that a "medically determinable impairment" be established.[36,41]

When an applicant submits an SSA application and nonmedical eligibility has been established, the application is forwarded to their state Disability Determination Service (DDS) for further medical review. The SSA has its own set of medical criteria, the "listing of impairments," which, if met or equaled, will result in an automatic award of benefits. There are separate listings for adults and children arranged by body system. Each listing typically contains a diagnosis and some clinical markers of severity. If listing criteria are not met, the applicant can appeal on the basis of "residual functional capacity."[41]

Physicians, including the patient's treating physician, who assist applicants when filing for SSDI or SSI disability should be familiar with the "five-step" appeals process and the listings themselves.[48] They may be asked to provide the DDS evaluating team with a statement about the patient's ability to do work-related activities and backed by objective evidence. They may also be asked to comment on an applicant's physical and psychological capacities and limitations and, in the event that the condition in question does not meet or equal the listings, to assist the DDS evaluating team in estimating the claimant's "residual functional capacities."[41]

Federal Workers' Compensation Systems

In the United States, the workers' compensation laws originated both at the federal and state levels at the beginning of the twentieth century and have evolved over the past 100 years into the current programs to provide no-fault–based compulsory broad coverage of injuries and illnesses arising out of and in the course of employment.[36]

The major federal workers' compensation programs are administered by the Office of Workers' Compensation Programs; an agency within the U.S. Department of Labor. One of the major federal programs, the Federal Employee's Compensation Act covers 2.9 million federal employees in more than 70 different agencies along with a number of other worker groups adopted by Congress in various acts of expansion of the federal authority.[29] In addition, the Longshore and Harbor Workers' Compensation Act, Energy Employees Occupational Illness Compensation Act, and Federal Black Lung Program (coal mine workers' compensation) are other federally mandated compensation acts administered by the Office of Workers' Compensation Programs. The U.S. Department of Labor maintains exclusive jurisdiction over these programs subject to judicial review. These four major federal workers' compensation programs provide wage replacement benefits, medical treatment, vocational rehabilitation, and other benefits to injured workers that experience work-related injury or occupational disease, or their dependents.[36]

Other federally mandated workers' compensation programs include the Federal Employers Liability Act commonly known as the railroad worker act; the Jones Act (Merchant Marine Act); and the Defense Based Act (DBA). The DBA provides workers' compensation protection to civilian employees working outside the United States on U.S. military bases or under a contract with the U.S. government for public works or for national defense.[36]

State Workers' Compensation Systems

At the individual state level in the United States, each state has enacted a workers' compensation law that protects the injured worker for injuries arising out of and in the course of employment. Each jurisdiction has its own nuances; however, the following fundamental features are common to all of these statutory schemes[45]:

- Compulsory insurance is required for employers with very few exceptions.
- A no-fault system exists for injuries arising out of and in the course of employment.
- Expedited benefits are included for medical and rehabilitation treatment and for wage replacement.
- Benefits also include compensation for permanent partial and permanent total disability.
- The law ensures access to an exclusive source of remedy for employees for work-related injuries/illnesses with few exceptions.
- The injured worker retains the right to sue any third party liable for injury.
- Disputes are usually resolved through administrative law adjudication with less rigorous rules of procedure and evidence.
- Administration is through a state agency designated to oversee workers' compensation law.

Workers' compensation benefits include survivor benefits (in the event of death); coverage of medical and rehabilitative expenses; and wage-loss benefits (which typically provide two thirds of weekly wages up to a cap) during the healing period of temporary disablement. Disability under workers' compensation can be determined to be temporary or permanent, partial or total. Many states have also enacted a *second injury fund*, whereby employment of individuals with preexisting work-related disabilities is encouraged. Such funds can reduce employer risk (e.g., cost of insurance) for additional compensation and medical expenses in such cases.[31]

The physician examiner can play a variety of roles in the work-related injuries associated with workers' compensation claims. There are four possible phases of involvement, including (1) initial evaluation and treatment of injury either as an approved and designated attending physician or as an authorized consultant; (2) overseeing rehabilitation, including return-to-work or staying-at-work issues; (3) determination of any residual impairment (permanent) or disability (work restrictions); and (4) estimating long-term care needs in catastrophic injuries (e.g., limb amputations, spinal cord injuries, major multiple trauma), including participation in life care planning.[28] The PM&R physician can be particularly successful in meeting the needs of the workers' compensation system by maintaining functionality as his or her key focus when setting treatment goals and monitoring progress toward the same; by enabling a return-to-work treatment focus that holds both patient and employer accountable; and by exercising appropriate control over the duration of treatment before an MMI determination is made (discussed later) to help ensure optimal results for both the patient and the system. The physician may choose to participate only in the selected phase, such as impairment and disability evaluation, which requires an understanding of the process of an independent medical examination (IME), as well as application of the appropriate impairment rating guidelines that may vary by jurisdiction.

Compensation and Pensioning Under the Veterans Benefits Administration

In 1953, the VBA was created within the Veterans Health Administration (VHA) to administer the GI Bill and the U.S. Department of Veterans Affairs (VA) Compensation and Pension Service (C&P) and Programs.

Eligibility for VA disability benefit is based on discharge from active military service (full-time service to the Army, Navy, Air Force, Marines, or Coast Guard, or as a commissioned officer of the Public Health Service, the Environmental Services Administration, or the National Oceanic and Atmospheric Administration.) Only *honorable* and *general* discharges (as opposed to *dishonorable* or *bad-conduct* discharges) qualify. Entitlement to compensation is determined by the Adjudication Division of the C&P Service within the VBA and is classified as *service connected* if the disability relates directly to injury or disease incurred while on active duty or as a direct result of VA care or as *nonservice connected* if determined to have not been incurred while on active duty. *Presumptive service connection* applies to various conditions, such as chronic diseases (e.g., hypertension, diabetes mellitus) or tropical diseases (e.g., malaria), and qualifies for compensation if such conditions manifest themselves within 1 year of discharge from active duty.[32]

Disability compensation is paid as a monthly stipend to veterans who are disabled because of service-connected injury or disease. The amount of compensation received depends on the amount of impairment caused by the injury or disease where the rating percentages themselves are expressed according to "the average impairment in earning capacity resulting from such disease and injuries and their residual conditions in civil occupations." Disability compensation is not subject to federal or state income tax, it varies according to number of dependents, and it is regularly adjusted to reflect changes in cost of living. Benefits may also include disability pensions for veterans of low income according to a means test, who are permanently and totally disabled, and who have experienced 90 days or more of active duty, at least 1 day of which was during wartime. Other benefits include insurance benefits, specially adapted housing, motor vehicle modifications, and durable medical equipment.[32]

VA C&P examinations may be performed by physicians, nurse practitioners, physician assistants, psychologists, optometrists, audiologists, and "other qualified" clinical personnel. The VHA oversees and ensures that C&P examiners are adequately qualified, and all C&P examination reports must be assigned by a physician or psychologist. The physician examiner is asked to render an opinion as to diagnosis of the ratable condition, to address permanency of the condition, and to opine as to whether the individual with the condition is considered totally disabled (fails to meet minimal employability criteria), which is defined as physical inability to be employable at a sedentary level, or psychiatric or psychological inability to be employed in a loosely supervised situation with minimal exposure to the public.[32]

Physician disability evaluations are generally performed at VHA facilities with the Automated Medical Information Exchange (AMIE) data processing system and associated Disability Examination Worksheets and the VA's Schedule of Rating Disabilities.[50]

Personal Injury Claims

American law recognizes physical or psychological injury as a personal injury for which monetary damages can be awarded under the law of torts. A claim is usually made against the defendant for personal injury arising out of negligence and in some instances an intentional act. Common examples include those claims arising out of motor vehicle accidents, slip and fall claims against property owners (both private and business), defective products, medical negligence, hospital and nursing home negligence, assault claims, as well as work-related injuries outside of the aegis of workers' compensation. Plaintiffs are entitled to monetary awards for both actual and general damages (e.g., pain and suffering, nonpecuniary damages). The severity of the injury is the main driver for the compensation and physician-independent medical examiners (as expert witnesses) are retained by both sides to evaluate the plaintiff's claims of personal injury. The physician typically is required to evaluate the causation, the nature, and the severity of the injury, the exacerbation or aggravation of the preexisting pathologic condition, if any, as well as apportionment. In some instances, the physician may also be called on to comment on the necessity of the treatment previously provided or future treatment proposed for the condition under question.

Impairment Rating Guides for Physicians with Attention to Guides, Sixth Edition

As described in the previous sections, there is a high degree of variability among and within the various U.S. disability systems and significant nuances that distinguish them from one another. Nevertheless, the process whereby a disability determination is made uniformly requires an initial medical determination of an impairment rating based on the schedule recognized by the particular jurisdiction and according to specific medical criteria. Historically, the physician is charged and empowered to render impairment ratings. In response, the American Medical Association (AMA) has produced a rating manual to assist physicians in measuring and rating medical impairments according to a commonly accepted method and scale for assigning impairment percentages to the "whole person" unit. The AMA *Guides to the Evaluation of Permanent Impairment* (AMA

Guides)[7] is a standardized and objective reference and reporting guide for physicians, other health care providers, and other professional stakeholders including attorneys, adjudicators, insurance adjustors, and the like. The AMA Guides was originally published in 1971 and has been periodically revised and updated to the present sixth edition. Each revision incorporates the latest scientific evidence and input from a panel of contributors who are recognized experts in their respective medical or surgical fields and represents a consensus view developed through a modified Delphi process to reflect the prevailing medical opinions on organ system impairment ratings. The AMA Guides has gained widespread recognition both nationally and globally. For most jurisdictions within the U.S. state and federal workers' compensation systems, various editions are either mandated or else recommended by statute as the standard reference for impairment ratings. It is the preferred reference for the U.S. Department of Labor and for many domestic personal injury claims. It is gaining widespread international adoption as the preferred reference for disability claims in Canada, The Netherlands, South Africa, Australia, New Zealand, Korea, and Hong Kong.[37,44]

The sixth edition of the AMA Guides has adopted the ICF terminology, definitions, and conceptual framework of disablement discussed earlier. They define impairment rating as a "consensus-derived percentage estimate of loss of activity reflecting severity of a given health condition and the degree of associated limitations in terms of activities of daily living." As such, they have adopted metrics sensitive and specific to medical (i.e., anatomic and physiologic) aspects of organ system disease, as well as functional aspects (mobility and self-care) of losses that can occur (see shaded area on the left side of Figure 5-2). These subject areas are considered well within the sphere of physician expertise expected for physicians who typically evaluate and treat patients with disabilities. At the same time, they have avoided metrics that focus on the participation restrictions domain of disablement (e.g., "burden of care" compliance, losses in terms of advanced or "instrumental" ADLs, work loss) because measuring these requires a level of evaluative skills and training typically outside of the sphere of knowledge of most physicians.[44]

The sixth edition also maintains an important focus on and inclusion of four essential elements of physician evaluation and reporting about patients, as follows:

- What is the clinical diagnosis?
- What difficulty does the patient report (symptoms, functional loss)?
- What are the examination findings?
- What are the results of clinical studies?

To more properly address functional aspects of the impairment rating, the sixth edition has adopted an ADL-based functional history and ordinal measures of ADL assessment to serve as important modifiers of the final impairment rating where applicable. This is particularly important to any impairment rating of the musculoskeletal system (discussed later).

Despite the common assumption that physicians by their training are skilled in evaluating impairment or disability resulting from work-related injury or illness, the reality is that physicians in general never receive any formal training in impairment or disability assessment during their medical education or postdoctoral residency training.[35] In response, a number of continuing medical educational venues now exist to provide ongoing training in the use of the impairment rating guides and other aspects of disability medicine. These can be readily accessed through the following organizations and entities: the American Medical Association,[6] the American Academy of Orthopedic Surgeons,[2] the American Academy of Disability Evaluating Physicians,[1] the American Board of Independent Medical Examiners,[3] and the American College of Occupational and Environmental Medicine.[4]

Application of the AMA Guides, Sixth Edition, to Musculoskeletal Impairments

The following brief overview is intended to orient the reader conceptually to the musculoskeletal section of the AMA Guides sixth edition. The reader is encouraged to consult the AMA Guides directly for greater detail and discussion than space permits here.

Qualitative Impairments

Qualitative impairments are anatomically based and belong to discrete, mutually exclusive categories that can only be measured in descriptive terms. Nominal or ordinal scales of measurement can apply to such groupings to yield a hierarchical assembly, but the actual magnitude of such difference between groupings is nonuniform and lacks true proportionality to assigned numerical value. Examples of qualitative impairments recognized for the musculoskeletal system include amputation, joint ankylosis, sensory changes (present compared with absent), and disfigurement or deformity (present compared with absent).

Quantitative Impairments

Quantitative impairments are also anatomically based. They are measured according to continuous scales (interval or ratio) whose units represent fixed values, the ordering of which reflects a uniform and consistent increase in magnitude. The AMA Guides recognizes loss of motion (in degrees) in each cardinal plane of function for a given joint as representing quantitative impairment relative to the normally accepted range of motion (ROM) for that joint. Although ROM has intuitive appeal as a standardized, objective, and quantitative measure of joint function, its practical application remains problematic and has been subject to much criticism for its lack of reliability, reproducibility, validity, and feasibility in a typical impairment rating clinical setting.[7,44] Consequently, ROM has been abandoned as a separate rating criterion for the spine. However, ROM still serves as an impairment class (IC) differentiator for some of the "diagnosis-based impairments" (DBIs; discussed later) of the upper and lower extremities, and as a grade modifier within ICs for others; it has also been retained as part of a "stand-alone" rating for the joints of the upper and lower extremities when the DBI method cannot be readily applied (e.g., burn injuries with multiple contractures) or does not fully capture the impairment (e.g., combining proximal losses in joint ROM in the presence of more distal limb amputations.)

Diagnosis-Based Impairment Method

The AMA Guides sixth edition has adopted a DBI method as an outgrowth of an earlier "diagnosis-related estimate" approach; there are important additions and changes that are designed to overcome weaknesses of earlier approaches and that are most evident in the musculoskeletal organ system. For example, a uniform platform has been adopted that applies a template (grid) with five columns for mutually exclusive functionally based ICs of incremental severity (classes 0 to 4) patterned after the ICF classification scheme. Whereas all accepted diagnoses for musculoskeletal conditions affecting the spine or extremities can potentially be viewed within such an ordinal hierarchy, not all conditions will qualify for the higher class ratings. Accordingly, accepted conditions are hierarchically arranged as a succession or rows beginning with the least severe ratable conditions (by convention, typically soft-tissue injuries, sprains, and strains) at the top, and ending with the more severe conditions (muscle and tendon traumas, followed by ligament, bone, and joint conditions) at the bottom.[44]

To use this rating system properly, the rating physician must initially determine an accepted diagnosis for the condition being rated and establish permanency in terms of MMI (discussed later). The first step of the DBI method is to select the most appropriate IC within the most appropriate DBI grid. For the musculoskeletal system, the DBI grids are regionally defined. The spine is divided into four respective regional grids: cervical spine, thoracic spine, lumbar spine, and pelvis. The upper extremity (limb) is also divided into four respective regional grids: digit, wrist, elbow, and shoulder; and the lower extremity (limb) is divided into three respective regional grids: foot and ankle, knee, and hip. Once the diagnosis has been established and linked to the most appropriate regional DBI grid, the IC assignment can be made. Each IC will have an available range of five discrete impairment rating scores, with the middle score being the "default" value for the class. The second step follows whereby three separate grade modifiers are independently used to determine the level of severity within the IC (i.e., grade on a scale of 0 to 4) according to functional history (GMFH), physical examination findings (GMPE), and clinical study results (GMCS), respectively. A final step is to calculate the sum of the differences in numerical severity of the impairment grade modifiers minus the IC numeric and summate. It is then possible to triangulate the final impairment score within the IC according to the formula: (GMFH – IC) + (GMPE – IC) + (GMCS – IC). If the sum is zero the final impairment rating remains at the middle (default) value; if the sum is +1 or –1 the impairment rating moves one position to the right or left, respectively; if it is +2 or –2 it moves two positions to the right or left, respectively, as illustrated in Figure 5-4.

The DBI method has multiple advantages over earlier approaches. It enables the rater to capture important and useful information on clinical severity and functional disability for a given individual and ratable condition and to weigh the same according to precise criteria of severity rather than solely relying upon "clinical judgment." It plays to the strength of the physician rater as a diagnostician and offers greater precision and resolution for a broad array of diagnostic choices than was previously possible. Finally, it offers methodological uniformity, transparency, and ease of application within and between the organ systems of interest in all cases.[42,44]

Spine and Extremities as Regional Units

The *spine* is divided into four discrete regional anatomic units: the cervical, thoracic, lumbar, and pelvis. Qualitative impairments include DBI listings as separate "grids" for each unit. Quantitative impairments of the spine do not apply because the ROM method has been removed for this section of the AMA Guides.

Diagnosis-based impairment

	Grid	Class 0	Class 1	Class 2	Class 3	Class 4
Diagnosis / criteria	Table 17–6	No problem	Mild problem	Moderate problem	Severe problem	Very severe problem

Adjustment factors – grade modifiers

Non-key factor	Grid	Grade modifier 0	Grade modifier 1	Grade modifier 2	Grade modifier 3	Grade modifier 4
Functional history	Table 17–6	No problem	Mild problem	Moderate problem	Severe problem	Very severe problem
Physical exam	Table 17–7	No problem	Mild problem	Moderate problem	Severe problem	Very severe problem
Clinical studies	Table 17–8	No problem	Mild problem	Moderate problem	Severe problem	Very severe problem

FIGURE 5-4 Diagnosis-based impairment (DBI) method used in determining DBI in disorders of the spine and extremities. (From Rondinelli R, Eskay-Averbach M, Ranavaya M, Brigham C: AMA guides to the evaluation of permanent impairment, sixth edition: a response to the NCCI study, *AMA Guides Newsletter* November/December, 2012. Copyright 2012 American Medical Association.)

The *upper extremity** is divided into four discrete regional anatomic units: the digits and hand, wrist, elbow, and shoulder. Qualitative impairments include DBI listings as separate "grids" for each unit, as well as separate sections for peripheral nerve injuries, including causalgia (i.e., complex regional pain syndrome type 2 or CRPS2), complex regional pain syndrome type 1 (CRPS1), and amputations. Quantitative impairments include ROM as a stand-alone. Ankylosis is a qualitative modification to the ROM tables, which are otherwise organized into discrete ranges to which specific impairment numbers are assigned.

The *lower extremity** is divided into three discrete regional anatomic units: the ankle and foot, knee, and hip. Similar to the upper limb, qualitative impairments include DBI listings as separate "grids" for each unit, as well as separate sections for peripheral nerve injuries, including causalgia (i.e., CRPS2), CRPS1, and amputations. Quantitative impairments include ROM as a stand-alone. Ankylosis is a qualitative modification to the ROM tables, which are otherwise organized into discrete ranges to which specific impairment numbers are assigned.

Combining Impairments to Whole Person Impairment Ratings

When dealing with multiple impairments in a single claim, the AMA Guides provide a method for *combining* impairment rather than adding to avoid 100% plus final number. Combining is accomplished with the combined values chart provided in the appendix of the AMA Guides and is based on the principle that if two or more values are to be combined, the largest one comes out of the 100% first and the subsequent values come out of the remaining percentage of the "whole person." The values are derived from the formula A + B (1 − A) = combined value of A and B, where A and B are the decimal equivalents of the impairment ratings to the same anatomic unit.

The general rule is that all impairments are combined with few exceptions (listed later). Combining must occur at the same hierarchal level; for example, upper extremity impairment can only be combined with another upper extremity impairment from the same limb, and whole person impairment can only be combined with another whole person impairment. In the case of impairments from different limbs (either from both upper or lower limbs), even though expressed at the same hierarchal limb level, they should only be combined at the whole person impairment level after each individual limb is fully rated and the final impairments for each limb are expressed at whole person impairment level.

Exceptions to the "combine rule" include the following:

- Impairments from ROM loss at the same joint are always added.
- All hand impairments for multiple digits as expressed at hand unit level are added.
- Impairments from ROM loss from all thumb joints are added.
- Palmar digital sensory losses from radial and ulnar digital sides are added.[38]

*Note that *limb* and *extremity* are used interchangeably in the AMA Guides, sixth edition; *limb* is technically the anatomically correct term because the extremity is the terminal portion of the limb.

Independent Medical Examination: Elements and Reporting Requirements

An IME is (typically) a one-time evaluation performed by a physician who is not directly involved in treating the claimant for the express purpose of answering a series of interrogatory questions posed by the referring party to proceed toward resolution of medical ambiguities and achieve claim settlement. The information gathered by an IME can be used as evidence in litigation claims and other legal proceedings. It may help to untangle the often complex interrelationship between a pathologic condition that may be attributable to a compensable injury and resulting impairment, activity limitations, and participation restrictions in a given case. The opinions set forth by the independent medical examiner must be expressed in terms of medical possibility versus probability according to the definitions and conventions described in the following sections.

Diagnosis and Medical Necessity

The physician examiner is expected to provide the specific diagnosis for each and all allowed (and potentially relatable) conditions relevant to a specific claim. They must also address the medical necessity and appropriateness of diagnostic testing and medical, surgical, and rehabilitative treatment undertaken to date in relation to each of the relevant diagnoses.

Causation and Allowable Conditions

Of the various key questions asked of a physician when serving as an independent medical examiner or expert witness is the issue of causation. This is an important question because of its significant economic implications to the parties involved. The term *causation* may have different contextual meanings in law compared with medicine, and the physician needs to understand this difference.

Medical causation is biological in nature and is established through scientific analysis[21] of sufficient rigor to demonstrate a cause and effect relationship with a high degree of certainty, for example, with a statistical probability (or *P* value) of .05 or less (or the probability of being wrong 5% or less). For example, a physician can reasonably conclude, within medical probability, that asbestos can cause mesothelioma in an individual exposed to asbestos on the basis of a review of the credible medical evidence in the peer-reviewed scientific literature that has established a causal relationship in this case.

Legal causation, as defined in civil litigation, generally has two prongs. First, an act (e.g., a tort) must be the cause in fact of a particular injury, which means that an act or omission was a necessary antecedent to the personal injury.

Legally, this issue is analyzed by determining whether the injury would have occurred "but for" the act alleged to be the cause. If an injury would have occurred independent of the alleged act or omission, cause in fact has not been established, and no tort has been committed. When multiple acts/factors have led to a particular injury, the alleged act or omission is determined to be the cause in fact only if the evidence demonstrates this to have played a substantial role in causing the injury. Second, it must also be established simultaneously that the alleged act was the proximate cause of an injury before the legal liability will be imposed. The concept of *proximate cause* is very critical because it limits the scope of liability to those injuries that bear some reasonable relationship to the risk created by the wrongdoer. Proximate cause is evaluated in terms of whether a reasonable person should have foreseen the injury resulting from the act. If a given risk could not have been reasonably anticipated, proximate cause has not been established, and no liability will be attached.

In summary, legal causation is mainly a question of "foreseeability." An actor is liable for the foreseeable but not the unforeseeable consequences of his or her act. For example, it is foreseeable that someone who is left alone on a beach in a drunken stupor at low tide may die from drowning in the rising tide rather than from the excessive alcohol or drugs he or she has ingested. However, it is not foreseeable that such an individual will be struck by lightning and killed by that event. In such case, the liability for drowning could have a proximate cause in law (for causing death) for anyone who is found responsible for contributing directly to someone's drunken stupor and leaving that person exposed to risk of death by drowning but not to risk of death from being struck by lightning because of its remoteness in probability.

Two important concepts and terms pertaining to causation in relation to a preexisting and underlying condition are aggravation and exacerbation. *Aggravation* refers to a permanent worsening of a preexisting condition that occurs when a physical, chemical, biological, or other factor results in an increase in symptoms, signs, or impairment that never returns to baseline, or what it would have been except for the aggravation. *Exacerbation* refers to a temporary worsening of a preexisting condition after which the individual recovers to his or her baseline functional status, or what it would have been had the exacerbation never occurred. The differences between these two contingencies are illustrated in Figure 5-5.

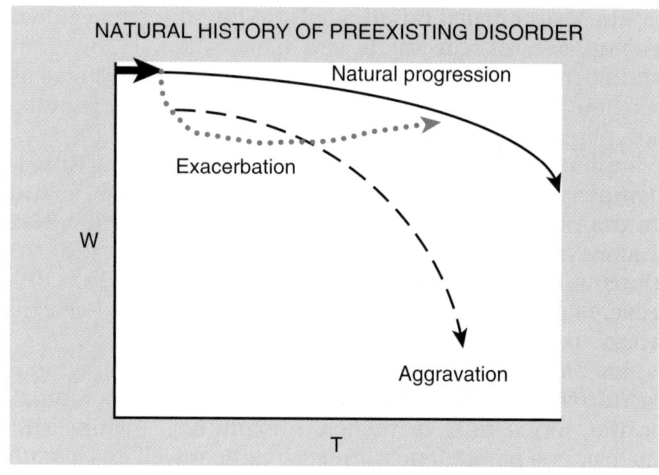

FIGURE 5-5 Exacerbation compared with aggravation.

The workers' compensation systems vary from state to state in terms of their causation and work-relatedness rules. The physician must understand these rules and be proficient in following the same to be successful. In some workers' compensation claims, certain conditions may have been administratively approved to have been caused by the workplace. These include *allowed conditions* in the claim. Certain legislation creates special presumptions for causation for certain workgroups establishing rights for workers and liabilities for employers even in the absence of scientific evidence (and thus medical causation). For instance, many states have laws establishing presumption that cardiovascular diseases, such as hypertension and myocardial infarction, are work related if they occur in firefighters or law enforcement workers as a result of the presumption of the stressful work environment causing these conditions. A law enforcement officer who may have worked all his life in administration and may have never actually been in the highly stressful situations of the job may still find that his naturally occurring cardiovascular disease, as adjudicated by the workers' compensation system, is considered to be work related. Physicians confronted with these realities of the modern workers' compensation legislation need not be frustrated, because these are societal decisions for distribution and redistribution of resources based on prevailing social values and political influences at each jurisdictional level.

Maximum Medical Improvement Determination

The physician examiner is typically required to complete an initial assessment and report, supplemental interim reports, and a final statement at the time of case disposition addressing MMI. Reporting requirements vary by state, but they are generally similar and must include an estimate of when MMI occurred or is expected to occur. The decision of MMI must be rendered before case closure can be achieved. From a rehabilitative perspective, a claimant should not be considered at MMI as long as expectations for continuing functional improvement are being met by demonstrable and ongoing performance gains. The distinction between functional and pain-oriented goal setting must be maintained during treatment so that progress toward goal achievement can be measured and monitored objectively. When functional progress is no longer evident or tenable and a sufficient (typically 6 months) healing period has transpired, MMI is generally thought to have occurred.[43]

The physician examiner is also required to determine the exact date of MMI and to address issues of medical stability from that point forward. Deterioration that might normally be expected with the passage of time (e.g., progression of an osteoarthritic condition) does not preclude MMI determination. The physician should also address issues of future medical management and follow-up anticipated to be necessary to maintain MMI for a given condition.

Future Medical Needs

The scope and content of life care planning according to future medical needs is an extensive topic (see, for example, Lacerte and Johnson[28]), with clinical and actuarial implications well beyond the scope of what can be meaningfully covered here, and is adequately addressed elsewhere in this textbook. However, the physician is typically asked to opine on future aspects of medical care needed to maintain MMI that may include scheduled physician visits, laboratory tests, routine medications, therapy reassessment, equipment maintenance, and excused leaves of absence from work.

Disability as Return-To-Work Restrictions

During the initial evaluation, interim treatment, and MMI phases of reporting, the treating physician or disability examiner will be asked to complete a patient status report and a return-to-work/fitness-for-duty form, examples of which are provided in Figures 5-6 and 5-7.

If treatment is ongoing and transitional work is available, the physician might recommend modified duty in terms of restrictions on the number of hours of work allowed and the permissible activities in terms of frequency or degree of material handling tolerated during the healing period. If no modified duty options are available or apply, the physician may be required to render a temporary total disability determination until MMI is reached. Because the probability of returning to work decreases precipitously as time out of work increases,[11,51] the physician should make every effort to return the claimant safely to a transitional work setting as soon as possible. In cases where transitional return-to-work options are not available, *work conditioning* and *work hardening* may be a preferable and viable alternative to forced inactivity and should be considered where feasible and medically necessary.[43] At the point of MMI, the physician must also render a final opinion on permanent restrictions applicable going forward.

A number of standardized assessment tools are available to assist physicians in determining valid and reliable physical performance expectations for an injured worker. The *functional capacity evaluation (FCE)* is a comprehensive and standardized therapy assessment of an injured individual's strength, flexibility, endurance, and safety in performing job-specific activities, and related material-handling functions.[23] It can provide potentially useful functional metrics to help establish a performance baseline and treatment goals for the injured worker, to monitor recovery as demonstrated by rate of progress toward achieving functional goals during treatment, and to establish a new performance baseline when treatment has been completed for purposes of recommending return-to-work restrictions and accommodation, if needed.[43] The impaired individual's performance during testing can be assessed in terms of degree of effort, consistency, and reliability. In cases where there is a demonstrated lack of consistency or incomplete effort on the part of a claimant, the validity of test results remains suspect and therefore must be interpreted with caution if not dismissed outright.[43] As mentioned earlier, a *job description* is frequently available from the employer and can provide a useful list of the essential functions of the job in question for purposes of identifying required material-handling capacities and addressing specific restrictions that may apply. A job site evaluation (JSE) can be carried out by a specially trained therapist to validate the essential functions listed in the job description with respect to critical physical demands and relative amounts of time spent performing specific activities within each function. In some cases, ergonomic analysis can be useful to help quantify the job physical demands and enable accommodation in terms of job redesign or workplace modification. In addition, employer and claimant willingness and ability to comply with recommended accommodations can also be addressed.

Physician examiners should avail themselves to these assessment tools to ensure that the prognostic inferences derived and sanctions imposed are founded on valid, empirical, and functionally based data to the fullest extent possible.

Legal and Ethical Considerations

Expert Witness Testimony

Physiatrists appear uniquely qualified among medical specialists to perform impairment ratings and disability evaluations because the scientific and medical foundation essential to PM&R maintains a focus on human functioning. The knowledge, skills, and abilities of any physiatrist can be naturally extended to become a routine practitioner within the emerging field of disability medicine, which has been described as a subspecialty of clinical medicine encompassing the identification, prediction, prevention, assessment, evaluation, and management of impairment and disability, both in individuals and populations.[34] Thus far, a major thrust of this field has been the physician's role in providing expert witness testimony regarding personal injury claims within a medicolegal context.

The underlying principle of common law (both law of tort and contracts) is to provide a venue for a person who has suffered damage as a result of an action or inaction by others to seek redress for his or her grievance in the courtroom. Tort law has been described as a great equalizer because it gives the individual seeking redress the ability to bring any offending employer or company (referred to in legal parlance as a *tortfeasor*) before the bar on a more equal footing for alleged wrongdoings. Obviously, the law cannot make tortfeasors undo their injury or harm but makes them accountable through monetary compensation for both intentional wrongs (e.g., defamation, assault, and battery) and unintentional wrongs (e.g., negligence). The law of tort not only shifts the burden of the cost of the injury or damages to the responsible party but also serves to prevent similar harm to other members of society through enforced accountability. The idea is to make the

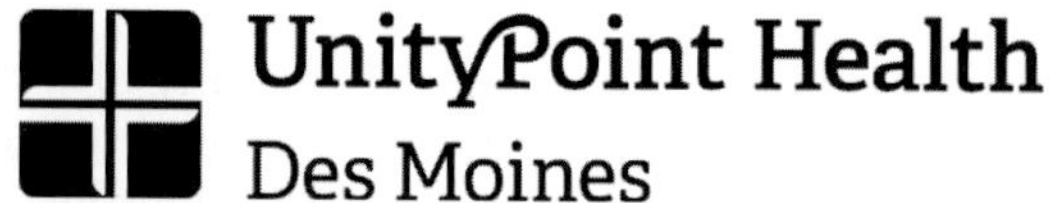

PATIENT STATUS REPORT

Methodist Occupational Medicine
1301 Pennsylvania Ave, Ste 416 P:(515) 262-7619
Des Moines, IA 50316-2367 F:(515) 262-8554

Patient: ______________________ Appt Time: __________
Employer: ______________________ Time In: __________
Date of Injury: __________ Date of Appt. __________ Time Out: __________

Provider Opinion:	Work Status:		Diagnosis:
☐ Work Related	☐ Full Duty	Effective: ________	
☐ Non Work Related	☐ Modified Duty	Effective: ________	
☐ Undetermined	☐ Off Work	Effective: ________	

Restrictions checked are for work and nonwork activities.

- ☐ No / Limit lifting to: __________
- ☐ No / Limit pushing - pulling to: __________
- ☐ No / Limit repetitive bending and twisting to: ______
- ☐ No / Limit / Vary sitting - standing - walking to: ______
- ☐ Sedentary work only
- ☐ No / Limit overhead work to: __________
- ☐ No / Limit ______ arm - hand use to: __________
- ☐ No / Limit grasping - pinching to: __________
- ☐ No / Limit repetitive wrist motions to: __________
- ☐ No / Limit climbing to: __________
- ☐ No / Limit crawling - kneeling – squatting to: ______
- ☐ Limit work to ____ hours per day ___ no overtime
- ☐ Limit driving __to/from work only ______no CMV
- ☐ No driving or operating hazardous machinery
- ☐ Avoid exposure to / skin contact with __________
- ☐ Keep wound clean and dry
- ☐ Splint / Brace / Crutch use required
- ☐ __________________

Treatment

Diagnostic Testing

☐ Results of x-rays / MRI / CT / EMG: ______________________

Treatment – Medications

☐ OTC Medications: ☐ Ibuprofen ☐ Tylenol ☐ Naproxen _____tablets_____times daily with food

☐ Prescriptions: ☐ Given ☐ Reviewed: ______________________

☐ Injections / medications given: ______________________

Treatment – Other

☐ Ice / Heat: ______ minutes per hour ______ times daily

☐ Exercises: ☐ Given ☐ Reviewed: ______________________

☐ Patient education: ☐ Wound Care ☐ Signs of Infection ☐ Head Injury ☐ Other: __________

☐ Medical supplies given: ______________________

☐ Physical Therapy ☐ 3 times a week / 6 visits ☐ Continue PT for _____further visits ☐ Stop PT

Follow-up

☐ Referral: ☐ MRI ☐ EMG ☐ CT ☐ Ortho ☐ Other: ______________________

☐ Discharged from treatment on __________ ☐ Return as needed ☐ MMI ☐ PPI ____%

☐ Return to clinic in __________ days – weeks – months Next appt: __________ Time: __________

Comments: ____
____

Physician Name ______________________
Provider Signature

FIGURE 5-6 Example of a patient status report.

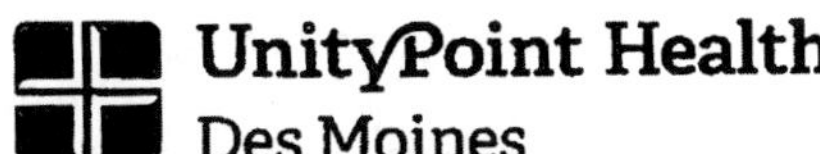

RETURN TO WORK/FITNESS FOR DUTY

Section A - To be completed by Employee
(Form to be submitted to manager 2 working days prior to return to work)

Employee Name (printed)____________ Date leave began ________

Date expect to return to work ________ Dept________ Supervisor________

Employee Signature____________ Date________

Section B - To be Completed by Health Care Provider:

PATIENT NAME____________ Date of Exam________

WORK STATUS: ____Return to regular work without restrictions DATE________
____Return to modified work/reduced hours DATE________

LIMITATIONS (If restrictions apply, please complete the following; if needed, call 241-4418 for a job description)

A. In a normal day, the patient may: 1. Stand/Walk: None____ 1 – 4 hrs____ 4 – 6 hrs ____ 6 – 10 hrs____
2. Sit: 1 – 3 hrs ____ 3 – 5 hrs____ 5 – 10 hrs ____
3. Drive: 1 – 3 hrs ____ 3 – 5 hrs____ 5 – 10 hrs ____

B. Patient may use hands for repetitive actions:

	Simple Grasping	Firm Grasping	Fine Manipulating
Right:	Yes__ No__	Yes__ No__	Yes__ No__
Left:	Yes__ No__	Yes__ No__	Yes__ No__

C. Patient may use feet for repetitive movement, as in operating foot controls: Yes____ No____

D.

Individual is able to:	Maximum pound/effort	0%	1-33%	34-66%	67-100%	Comments
Lift						
Push/Pull						
Bend	N/A					
Squat	N/A					
Climb	N/A					
Kneel/Crawl	N/A					
Grasp	N/A					
Reach	N/A					

E. If employee is to work reduced hours, how many hours per day____, per week____ other________

F. Duration of Restrictions________

G. Date for next evaluation________

H. Remarks____________

Name of attending health care provider			Degree/Specialty
Street Address	City	State	Zip Code
Telephone number	Fax number		
Attending HCP Signature			Date

Also submit copy to: **UnityPoint Health – Des Moines**
Disability Coordinator, Human Resources
1200 Pleasant Street
Des Moines, Iowa 50309-3119

FIGURE 5-7 Example of a return-to-work/fitness-for-duty form.

offensive and undesirable behavior costly to the tortfeasor and, in principle, serves to deter others from engaging in such future offenses.[27]

The opinions set forth in an IME and the resulting formal report comprise expert witness testimony that must validate or refute the presence and severity of injury toward, and resulting disability to, any claimant. This occurs within a legal infrastructure from which that claimant maintains certain legal rights and entitlements and may derive significant monetary gain. The independent medical examiner, in many instances acting as an agent for the consulting party rather than solely as a patient advocate, typically faces the risk of targeted allegations of wrongdoing leveled by any disgruntled claimant, who may view the physician's opinion as adversarial to their claim. Serious allegations of financial,[18] physical,[40,47] or psychological injury[19] to patients in this context are a matter of record, and expert witness physicians are being held accountable when those injuries are proven in a court of law.

Box 5-1 enumerates various legal theories of liability against the IME and expert witness physicians.

Traditionally, courts in all jurisdictions have held that physician expert witness testimony and IMEs are essential to the efficient functioning of workers' compensation and personal injury claim systems and are at once beneficial to employers, insurers, and claimants alike. Such testimony provides a clinical foundation for medicolegal decisions that helps set the standard for society's definition of health and illness and the legal implications that flow from that standard. As a consequence, the U.S. legal system has tended to grant relative immunity to physicians in such court decisions, when acting in an expert witness capacity. Recent court actions in this area raise concerns that such legal shelter no longer applies.

It is noteworthy that until recently, an expert witness enjoyed essentially the same type of immunity as any other witness in the judicial process. This immunity from civil liability dates back to sixteenth century English common law; it was very broad and included protection from claims of defamation and negligence.[14] The principal rationale for witness immunity was to ensure that the witness would speak freely when giving testimony.[20] The argument for such immunity has been that expert witnesses are an important part of the legal system and that in the interest of justice, expert witnesses also need to be protected from liability. The U.S. courts up until very recently have regarded this issue of expert witness immunity to be so important that it was maintained even in cases when there might be negligence.[12]

The judicial philosophy of the nineteenth and twentieth century American jurisprudence emphasized that the object of immunity is not to protect those whose conduct is open to criticism but to protect those who would be subject to unjustified and vexatious claims by disgruntled litigants. The courts generally have affirmed the concept of expert witness immunity for reasons of public policy, because without immunity there would be loss of objectivity. The fear of infinite vexation could also have a chilling effect on any witness resulting in reluctance to testify.[10] However, there has been an erosion in expert witness immunity from civil actions during the past two decades in some U.S. state jurisdictions. Legal commentators have attributed this, in part, to growth and proliferation of the litigation/expert witness industry, as well as to the courts' perception that there is insufficient protection of the injured party from unscrupulous witnesses and inadequacy of traditional safeguards against witness malfeasance through perjury and inadequate cross-examination.

Medical malpractice actions against IME physicians as expert witnesses failed up until recently because of lack of a defined physician-patient relationship with the examinee or plaintiff.[39] Within the context of any IME, the contention was maintained that the physician neither offered nor intended nor was authorized to actively treat the individual examinee; hence there was no established physician-patient relationship to sustain the medical malpractice cause of action.[25,26] Many such cases were either not filed because of a prevailing notion among the legal community based on the previous case law or, when filed, were dismissed on pretrial motions from the defendants.[13,16,46] This has, however, changed significantly in the past two decades, with increasing case law from various jurisdictions holding independent medical examiners and expert witnesses accountable for the alleged harm endured by the plaintiff/examinee. This was initially done under the cause of action of simple negligence and outside the law of torts for medical malpractice.[18]

BOX 5-1

Legal Theories of Causes of Action against Independent Medical Examiner Physicians and Expert Witnesses

A. Intentional torts
   1. Assault
   2. Battery
   3. Intentional infliction of emotional distress
   4. False imprisonment
   5. Defamation
   6. Invasion of privacy
   7. Fraud and misrepresentation
   8. Conspiracy
   9. Bad faith
   10. Deceptive trade practices
B. Unintentional torts
   1. Ordinary negligence
   2. Professional malpractice
   3. Failure to warn
   4. Wrongful death
   5. Loss of chance of recovery or survival
   6. Vicarious liability for the acts of others
   7. Negligent referral
   8. Failure to diagnose
   9. Failure to inform
C. Actions under the law of contract
   1. Breach of contract
   2. Breach of warranty
   3. Abandonment
D. Miscellaneous causes of action
   1. Deceptive trade practices
   2. Violation of a statute or regulation

However, during the past decade, supreme courts in at least two states have allowed civil action against IME physicians to proceed under the traditional medical malpractice theory. The duty of care to the patient despite the absence of a formal physician-patient relationship is the underlying new cause of action against IME physicians and expert witnesses. The Arizona Supreme Court in *Ritchie v Krasner*[40] even allowed medical malpractice to go forward despite no physician-patient relationship by essentially stating that the court can envision no public benefit in not holding a physician accountable to a duty to conform to the legal standard of reasonable care.

In summary, physiatrists and other practitioners in the field of disability medicine performing IMEs and giving expert testimony should be aware of not only the legal liabilities in the overall practice of their subspecialty but also the additional malpractice and civil liabilities entailed with exposure to the practice constraints under which IMEs and expert witness work is performed. It should be emphasized that even though the recent case law in some jurisdictions has significantly removed the traditional malpractice immunity of providers who have no clearly defined physician-patient relationship established with their examinees, considerable demand for expert medical witness services remains. Physicians attracted to disability assessment and inclined to serve as independent medical examiners are encouraged to attend several of the high-quality training programs offered in the United States to independent medical examiners and expert witnesses with the goal of empowering them with greater knowledge, skills, and abilities necessary to practice as an independent medical examiner or expert witness in the field of disability medicine.

IME physicians or expert witnesses can be successful despite these challenges if they remember several key principles including intellectual honesty, professionalism, and respect of the judicial process at all times. An ethical and objective examiner who performs a thorough evaluation, deals with the plaintiff/claimant in an empathetic, unbiased manner, and avoids advocacy has a lesser risk of getting entangled in the allegations of wrongdoing.

The physician examiner should be judicious in gathering all the facts and available objective data and base opinions on evidence rather than subjective anecdotal experiences. The American judicial process is typically carried out in an adversarial arena where challenges to one's expert opinion are likely to arise no matter which side is being represented. Opinions based on scientific evidence and sound judgment are, therefore, much more likely to withstand the adversarial scrutiny and challenge of even the most skilled cross-examiner. The following list of *do'* s and *don't*s hopefully can serve as a guideline for the physician examiner providing expert witness testimony:

- Present a positive image; be respectful of the judicial process and take it seriously.
- When appearing in court arrive on time or early, dress conservatively, and be relaxed.
- Prepare yourself; review all of the facts.
- Know both the strengths and weaknesses of your case.
- Always tell the truth.
- Listen carefully; understand the question.
- Limit your response to the specific question.
- State opinions only when called for.
- Keep it brief by stating a single fact, without going into long needless discussions.
- Do concede to the opponents point when reasonable or appropriate.
- Do not lose your temper even though you may be provoked.
- Do not go beyond your expertise or specialty.
- Avoid arrogance and sarcasm.
- Do not guess; do not assume.
- Never compromise your integrity.
- Do not be an advocate.
- Do not argue with the opposing counsel.
- Do not answer if you are told not to.
- Do not volunteer information or answers.
- Do not discuss the case in public areas.

Ethical Considerations

The physician examiner must also confront the ethical challenges posed by the patient as a claimant. As has been discussed earlier, there is increasing ambiguity regarding the moral imperative of the traditional physician-patient relationship in these cases. In the arena of workers' compensation, the physician is at once accountable to their client (referral party) whose interests may conflict with those of the patient and their opposing counsel. In addition, the PM&R physician, by nature of the interdisciplinary approach, must remain committed to preserving patient autonomy as a member of the treatment team and also to maximizing functional recovery (thereby minimizing disability) and reducing or eliminating dependency to the fullest extent possible on the treating system and caregivers, including the disability system itself. The patient, as a claimant, is often represented by legal counsel and may be coached and instructed, or may otherwise choose to behave in a manner that is counterproductive to these goals and thereby appear as noncompliant.

The physician must also remain cognizant of the paradox of compensable injury—that financial compensation can discourage return to work and thereby promotes the disability. Undue prolongation of an open claim (through inappropriate and excessive diagnostic or therapeutic endeavors, however well intended) might further serve to legitimize disability in the claimant's mind and can inhibit the likelihood of functional recovery and return to work. Decisions to terminate treatment of compensable injuries and to reach MMI might not always be mutually agreeable to claimant and examiner and in most cases are likely to rest on the final authority of the physician rather than that of the patient. Perhaps the most useful beacon to guide decision making when treating compensable injuries is to promote functional recovery to the fullest extent possible, to terminate treatment when functional recovery is no longer tenable, and to render impairment ratings and return-to-work decisions that enable patients to use their residual abilities (through accommodation if necessary) as soon as possible and to the fullest extent possible. (A list of glossary terms is given in Box 5-2.)

BOX 5-2

Glossary of Terms

Apportionment: A determination of percentage of impairment directly attributable to preexisting or resulting conditions and directly contributing to the total impairment rating derived.[8]

Disability: An umbrella term for activity limitations or participation restrictions in an individual with a health condition, disorder, or disease.

Functional capacity evaluation (FCE): A comprehensive assessment of an individual's strength, flexibility, endurance, and job-specific functional abilities. An FCE includes a feasibility assessment of the individual's ability to perform the essential functions of a specific job and, when validated, may be useful to help predict return-to-work potential and appropriate restrictions in a particular case.[23]

Impairment: A significant deviation, loss, or loss of use of any body structure or function in an individual with a health condition, disorder, or disease.

Impairment rating: A consensus-derived percentage estimate of loss of activity, which reflects severity of impairment for a given health condition, and the degree of associated limitations in terms of activities of daily living.

Job description: A formal listing of the essential functions constituting a particular job in terms of the specific physical performance requirements.

Job site evaluation (JSE): An on-site analysis of the workplace to determine optimal ergonomic design and validate specific physical performance requirements of the job. A JSE can be useful in concert with an FCE to determine applicable return-to-work restrictions and to help ensure employer/employee compliance when necessary.[23]

Maximum medical improvement (MMI): The point at which a condition has stabilized and is unlikely to change (improve or worsen) substantially in the next 12 months, either with or without treatment.

Medical possibility: Something could occur as a result of a particular cause (probability of occurrence is as likely as not and equals or is less than 50%).

Medical probability: Something is more likely to occur than not (probability of occurrence is greater than 50%).

Permanency: Permanency and MMI are related concepts and simply mean that a person with an injury, after having received adequate medical, surgical, and rehabilitative treatment and achieved clinical and functional stability, is now as good as he or she is going to get. Other synonymous terms in use according to jurisdictional preference include fixed and stable, maximum medical recovery, maximum medical stability, and medically stationary. In workers' compensation jurisdictions (listed in the text) these terms are useful to enable the injured person to exit the temporary disablement stage of recovery thereby facilitating claim settlement and case closure.

Scheduled loss: Allocation of a specified value for purposes of indemnification to a regional anatomic or functional unit to which an impairment rating can be assigned. The specified value allowed for a given unit can be expressed in terms of weeks or months of lost wages.[8]

Unscheduled loss: Estimated functional loss to the "whole person" for purposes of indemnification and according to a physiologic system rather than to a regional anatomic or functional unit. The cardiopulmonary, gastrointestinal, and central nervous systems are examples of systems to which an unscheduled loss can apply.[8]

Work hardening: A work-oriented treatment program, delivered in a highly structured environment that simulates the workplace, and designed to improve job productivity of an injured or deconditioned worker. Productivity goals can pertain to work tolerance, job proficiency, or job efficiency.[23]

REFERENCES

1. American Academy of Disability Evaluating Physicians: www.aadep.org.
2. American Academy of Orthopedic Surgeons: www.aaos.org.
3. American Board of Independent Medical Examiners: www.abime.org.
4. American College of Occupational and Environmental Medicine: www.acoem.org.
5. American Hospital Association: *First Consulting Group: when I'm 64: how Boomers will change health care,* Chicago, 2007, American Hospital Association.
6. American Medical Association: www.ama-assn.org.
7. American Medical Association: *Guides to the evaluation of permanent impairment,* ed 6, Chicago, 2008, American Medical Association.
8. American Medical Association: *Guides to the evaluation of permanent impairment,* ed 4, Chicago, 1993, American Medical Association.
9. Americans with Disabilities Act: Part 1. Employment (29 CFR part 1630). *Federal Register,* 1991, pp 35726–35756.
10. *Bruce v Byrne-Stevens & Assoc Engineers Inc,* 776 P2d 666, 667 (Wash 1989).
11. Christian J, Martin D, Brown D, et al: Preventing needless work disability by helping people stay employed. A white paper on the stay-at-work/return-to-work process. Available at www.webility.md/pdfs/SAW-RTW-White-Paper-2006-04-12.pdf.
12. *Clark v Grigson,* 579 SW 2d 263 (Tex 1978).
13. *Craddock v Gross,* 504 A 2d 1300, 1302 (Pa Super Ct 1986).
14. *Cutler v Dixon,* 76 Eng Rep 886 (QB 1585).
15. Engle GL: The need for a new medical model: a challenge for biomedicine, *Science* 196:129–136, 1977.
16. *Ervin v American Guardian Life Insurance Company,* 545 A2d 354 (Pa Super 1988).
17. Fougeyrollas P: Documenting environmental factors for preventing the handicap creation process: Quebec contributions relating to ICIDH and social participation of people with functional differences, *Disabil Rehabil* 17:145–153, 1995.
18. *Greenberg v Perkins,* 845 P.2d 530, 538 (Colo 1993).
19. *Harris v Kreutzer,* 624 S.E. 2d 24, 27 (Va. 2006).
20. *Henderson v Broomhead,* 157 Eng Rep 964, 967-968 (Ex 1859).
21. Hill AB: The environment and disease: association or causation? *Proc R Soc Med* 58:295–300, 1965.
22. Iezzoni LI, Freedman VA: Turning the disability tide: the importance of definitions, *JAMA* 299:332–334, 2008.
23. Isernhagen SJ: Functional capacity evaluation. In Isernhagen SJ, editor: *Work injury: management and prevention,* Rockville, 1988, Aspen Publishers, pp 139–194.
24. Johns RE, Jr, Colledge AL, Holmes EB: Introduction to fitness for duty. In Demeter SL, Andersson GB, editors: *Disability evaluation,* ed 2, St Louis, 2003, Mosby/AMA, pp 709–738.
25. *Johnston v Sibley,* 588 SW 2d 135 (Tex Civ App 1977).
26. *Keene v Wiggins,* 138 Cal Rep 3 (Cal App 1977).
27. Keeton WP, Dobbs DB, Keeton RE, et al: *Prosser and Keeton on the law of torts,* ed 5, St Paul, 1984, West Group Publisher.
28. Lacerte M, Johnson CB: Life care planning, *Phys Med Rehabil Clin N Am* 24:3, 2013.
29. Ladou J: The European influence on workers' compensation reform in the United States, *Environ Health* 10:103, 2011.
30. McGeary M, Ford M, McCutchen SR, editors: *IOM Committee on medical evaluation of veterans for disability compensation: a 21st century system for evaluating veterans for disability benefits. The rating schedule,* Washington, 2007, The National Academies Press.

31. Novick AK, Rondinelli RD: Impairment and disability under workers' compensation. In Rondinelli RD, Katz RT, editors: *Impairment rating and disability evaluation*, Philadelphia, 2000, WB Saunders Company, pp 141–156.
32. Oboler S: Disability evaluation under the Department of Veterans Affairs. In Rondinelli RD, Katz RT, editors: *Impairment rating and disability evaluation*, Philadelphia, 2000, WB Saunders Company, pp 187–211.
33. Oliver M, editor: *Understanding disability: from theory to practice*, New York, 1996, St Martin's Press.
34. Ranavaya MI: *Presidential address*, American Academy of Disability Evaluating Physicians, 1997.
35. Ranavaya MI: Impairment and disability evaluation training in US medical education: a survey of family medicine residency curricula and attitudes, *Disabil Med* 6:3–7, 2008.
36. Ranavaya MI, Rondinelli RD: Review of major disability and compensation systems in the USA, *Disabil Med* 7:2–10, 2009.
37. Ranavaya MI, Brigham C: International use of the AMA Guides to the evaluation of permanent impairment, *AMA Guides Newsletter* 2011.
38. Ranavaya MI, Rondinelli RD: To combine, or not to combine? *AMA Guides Newsletter* 2013.
39. *Rand v Miller*, 408 SE 2d 655 (WVa 1991).
40. *Ritchie v Krasner et al.*, 211 P.3d 1272 (Ariz. Ct. App. 2009).
41. Robinson JP, Wolfe CV: Social Security Disability Insurance and Supplemental Security Income. In Rondinelli RD, Katz RT, editors: *Impairment rating and disability evaluation*, Philadelphia, 2000, WB Saunders Company, pp 159–176.
42. Rondinelli RD: Changes for the new AMA Guides to impairment ratings, 6th edition: implications and applications for physician disability evaluations, *PM R* 1:643–656, 2008.
43. Rondinelli RD, Robinson JP, Scheer SJ, Weinstein SM: Industrial rehabilitation medicine. 4. Strategies for disability management, *Arch Phys Med Rehabil* 78:S21–S28, 1997.
44. Rondinelli R, Eskay-Auerbach M, Ranavaya M, et al: Commentary on NCCI report, *AMA Guides Newsletter* 2012.
45. Rondinelli R, Ranavaya M: Disability assessment. In Benzon HT, Rathmell JP, Wu CL, et al, editors: *Practical management of pain*, ed 5, Philadelphia, 2013, Elsevier-Mosby.
46. *Ryans v Lovell*, 482 A. 2d 1253 (N.J. Super. 1984).
47. *Smith v Welch*, 265 Kan. 881P.2d 727 (1998).
48. Social Security Administration: *Disability evaluation under Social Security*, Washington, 1999, Office of Disability, SSA Pub No 64-039.
49. United States Census Bureau: *Nearly 1 in 5 people have a disability in the U.S. report released to coincide with 22nd anniversary of the ADA, July 2012*, Washington, 2012, United States Census Bureau.
50. Veterans Benefits Administration: *Schedule for rating disabilities. Section 1155, Title 38 CFR, pensions, bonuses, and veterans' relief.*
51. Waddell G, Burton AK: Occupational health guidelines for the management of low back pain at work: evidence review, *Occup Med* 51:124–135, 2001.
52. Waddell G, Burton AK: *Concepts of rehabilitation for the management of common health problems*, London, 2004, The Stationary Office.
53. Waddell G, Burton AK, Aylward M: A bio psychosocial model of sickness and disability, *AMA Guides Newsletter* 2008.
54. World Health Organization: *International classification of impairments, disabilities and handicaps: a manual of classification relating to the consequences of disease*, Geneva, 1980, World Health Organization.
55. World Health Organization: *International classification of functioning, disability, and health (ICF)*, Geneva, 2001, World Health Organization.
56. World Health Organization: *History of the development of the ICD*, Geneva, World Health Organization. Available at: http://www.who.int/entity/classifications/icd/en/HistoryOfICD.pdf.

CHAPTER 6

EMPLOYMENT OF PEOPLE WITH DISABILITIES

Heidi Klingbeil, Kevin T. Sperber, Rahki Garg Sutaria, Jennifer Gomez

Disability is a significant public health and social issue in the United States. The number of Americans who experience disability, activity limitations secondary to chronic illnesses, or impairments has increased, whereas mortality has decreased. A U.S. Census Bureau report found in 2010 that of a total population of 303.9 million, approximately 56.7 million (18.7%) individuals reported some degree of mental or physical disability.[42] Although this represents an increase from the 54.4 million who reported a disability in 2005, the percentage remained statistically unchanged.[42] In the 2010 report, 38.3 million people—or 12.6% of U.S. residents—were classified as severely disabled.[42] Given these findings, disability ranks as the largest public health problem in the United States.

The growing numbers of Americans with disabilities present new medical, social, and political challenges. The major activity limitations found in those with disabilities include an inability to manage personal care, the inability to work and be financially self-supporting, and the inability to integrate socially and enjoy leisure.[40] These limitations have medical, behavioral, social, and economic implications. To help those with disabilities restore functional capacity, prevent further deterioration in functioning, and maintain or improve their quality of life, programs of any type should emphasize rehabilitation and prevention of secondary conditions.[30] These programs must respect disability as multifaceted and foster an interdisciplinary approach to treatment.

Within the medical arena, the specialty of physical medicine and rehabilitation has been concerned with the establishment of physiologic, psychological, and social equilibrium for people with disabilities.[17] According to Rusk,[33] "a rehabilitation program is designed to take a disabled person from his bed back to his job, fitting him for the best life possible commensurate with his disability and more importantly with his ability." To help all people with disabilities achieve their maximum level of independence, avert further deterioration in functioning, and maintain or improve their quality of life, the physiatrist and the medical rehabilitation team must appreciate the multifaceted character of disability. The physiatrist and the medical rehabilitation team must accept the responsibility to initiate appropriate referrals to other collaborating programs that can support these goals beyond the medical arena. One such program is vocational rehabilitation.

This chapter describes the employment of people with disabilities. Specifically, we

- Discuss the concept of disability
- Review national data on disability and employment
- Consider the economic impact of disability
- Review policies supporting employment of people with disabilities
- Discuss economic assistance strategies
- Discuss vocational rehabilitation strategies
- Enumerate the incentives and disincentives for returning to work
- Postulate that vocational rehabilitation serves as a rehabilitation treatment and disability prevention strategy for people with disabilities

Concept of Disability

Disability itself is not always quantifiable. In the Americans with Disabilities Act (ADA) of 1990, an individual with a disability is defined as a person who has a physical or mental impairment that substantially limits one or more major life activities.[42] The concept of disability differs among people who consider themselves to have a disability, professionals who study disability, and the general public.[20] This lack of agreement is an obstacle to all studies of disability, as well as to the equitable and effective administration of programs and policies intended for people with disabilities.[11,12,20,27,30]

The World Health Organization (WHO) has a mandate to develop a global common health language, one that is understood to include physical, mental, and social well-being. The International Classification of Impairments, Disabilities, and Handicaps (ICIDH-2) was developed by the WHO as a tool for classification of the "consequences of disease." The ICIDH-2 reflects the biopsychosocial model of disablement, viewing disablement and functioning as outcomes of an interaction between a person's physical or mental condition and the social and physical environment. Human functioning is characterized at three levels: the body or body part, the whole person, and the whole person in social context. Disablements are the dimensions of dysfunctioning that result for an individual at these three levels; these include impairment, losses or abnormalities of bodily function and structure, limitations of activities, and restrictions of participation.

This biopsychosocial model regards functioning and disablement as outcomes of interactions between health conditions (disorders or diseases) and conceptual factors such as social and physical environmental factors and personal factors. The interactions in this paradigm are dynamic, complex, and bidirectional (Figure 6-1).

Dimensions of dysfunctioning are defined as follows:

- *Impairment* is the loss or abnormality of body structure or of a physiologic or psychological function.

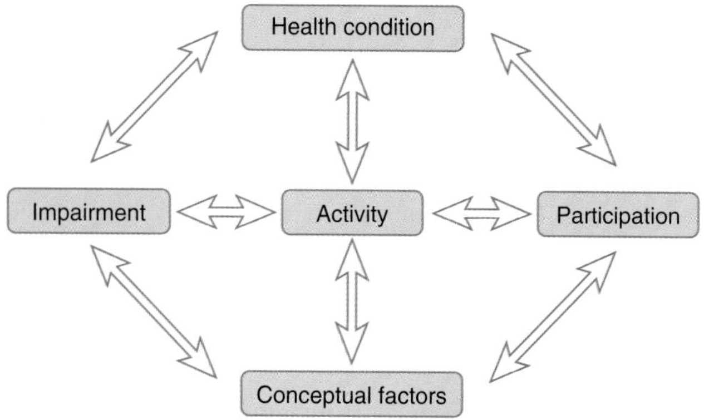

FIGURE 6-1 Biopsychosocial model of disablement.

- *Activity* is the nature and extent of functioning at the level of the person.
- *Participation* is the nature and extent of a person's involvement in life situations in relation to impairment, activities, health conditions, and contextual factors, and can be restricted in nature, duration, and quality.[48]

The concept of disability or disablement continues to be one about which there are many interpretations and opinions. This lack of agreement about the concept of disablement affects epidemiologic studies of disablement and the development of effective treatment and prevention strategies. The biopsychosocial model and the common language of the ICIDH-2 helped to define the need for health care and related services; to define health outcomes in terms of body, person, and social functioning; to provide a common framework for research, clinical work, and social policy; to ensure the cost-effective provision and management of health care and related services; and to characterize physical, mental, social, economic, and environmental interventions that would improve lives and levels of functioning.[53]

The 2001 World Health Assembly subsequently endorsed a revised system, the International Classification of Functioning, Disability, and Health (ICF). This is a classification of health and health-related domains, which are classified from body, individual, and societal perspectives with a list of body functions and structure, as well as a list of domains of activity and participation. The ICF also includes a list of environmental factors to provide context for the disability.[55] The ICF provides a common transcultural language across health care systems and is intended to allow comparison of international data and the measurement of health outcomes, quality, and cost, as well as health disparities.

Table 6-1 Conditions with the Highest Prevalence of Activity Limitation

	Percentage
Main Cause	
Orthopedic impairments	16.0
Arthritis	12.3
Heart disease	22.5
Visual impairments	4.4
Intervertebral disk disorders	4.4
Asthma	4.3
Nervous disorders	4.0
Mental disorders	3.9
Hypertension	3.8
Mental retardation	2.9
Diabetes	2.7
Hearing impairments	2.5
Emphysema	2.0
Cerebrovascular disease	1.9
Osteomyelitis or bone disorders	1.1
All Causes	
Orthopedic impairments	21.5
Arthritis	18.8
Heart disease	17.1
Hypertension	10.8
Visual impairments	8.9
Diabetes	6.5
Mental disorders	5.6
Asthma	5.5
Intervertebral disk disorders	5.2
Nervous disorders	4.9
Hearing impairments	4.3
Mental retardation	3.2
Emphysema	3.1
Cerebrovascular disease	2.9
Abdominal hernia	1.8

From La Plante MP: The demographics of disability, *Milbank Q* 69:55-77, 1991, with permission.

Data: Impairment and Disability

The U.S. Census Bureau provides extensive information on the number and characteristics of people with disabilities. Data from the Americans with Disabilities Report of 2010 indicate that 56.7 million people, or 18.7% of the U.S. population,[42] have some level of disability. Among those 6 years or older, 12.3 million individuals or 4.4% needed assistance with one or more activities of daily living without an assistive device.[42] This represents an increase in both the number and percentage that needed assistance in 2005.[42]

Impairments resulting from chronic disease have become increasingly significant risk factors of disability.[9,20] Table 6-1 lists the 15 conditions with the highest prevalence of functional compromise or disability.[20] The prevalence of disability with these conditions appears to be attributable to the prevalence of the condition itself and the chance that the condition will cause a disability. Table 6-2 shows the ranking of people, by percentage of specific conditions, who have functional limitations secondary

Table 6-2 Conditions with the Highest Risk for Disability

Chronic Condition	Number of Conditions (in 1000s)	Causes Activity Limitation (%)	Rank	Causes Major Activity Limitation (%)	Rank	Causes Need for Help in Basic Life Activities (%)	Rank
Mental retardation	1202	84.1	1	80.0	1	19.91*	9
Absence of leg(s)*	289	83.3	2	73.1	2	39.0*	2
Lung or bronchial cancer	200	74.8	3	63.5	3	34.5*	4
Multiple sclerosis*	171	70.6	4	63.3	4	40.7*	1
Cerebral palsy*	274	69.7	5	62.2	5	22.8*	8
Blind in both eyes	396	64.5	6	58.8	6	38.1*	3
Partial paralysis in extremity*	578	59.6	7	47.2	7	27.5*	5
Other orthopedic impairments*	316	58.7	8	42.6	8	14.3†	12
Complete paralysis in extremity*	617	52.7	9	45.5	9	26.1*	6
Rheumatoid arthritis*	1223	51.0	10	39.4	12	14.9*	11
Intervertebral disk disorders*	3987	48.7	11	38.2	14	5.3*	—
Paralysis in other sites (complete or partial)*	247	47.8	12	43.7	10	14.1†	13
Other heart disease disorders‡	4708	46.9	13	35.1	15	13.6*	14
Cancer of digestive tract	228	45.3	14	40.3	11	15.9†	15
Emphysema	2074	43.6	15	29.8	—	9.6*	15
Absence of arm(s) or hand(s)*	84	43.1	—	39.0	13	4.1*	—
Cerebrovascular disease*	2599	38.2	—	33.3	—	22.9*	7

From La Plante MP: The demographics of disability, *Milbank Q* 69:55-77, 1991, with permission.
*Conditions frequently managed by physiatrists.
†Figure has low statistical reliability or precision (relative standard error >39%).
‡Heart failure (9.8%), valve disorders (15.3%), congenital disorders (15.0%), other ill-defined heart conditions (59.9%).

to that condition.[20] In general, many of the conditions that are significant risk factors for disability are low in prevalence. For example, multiple sclerosis has a low overall prevalence but is a significant risk factor for disability. Examination of this ranking shows 7 of the top 10 disabling conditions are conditions frequently managed by the physiatrist and the rehabilitation team. These conditions or diseases are typically chronic, requiring a lifetime of rehabilitative management to have an effect on the disabling process, prevent secondary conditions, and maintain quality of life.

Socioeconomic Effect of Disability

Disablement has significant socioeconomic consequences for the individual with disabilities and for society. When a person is unable to participate in her or his social role as a worker or homemaker because of a physical or mental condition, that person is said to have a work disability or a work participation restriction.[8,56] Work participation restriction results in dependency and loss of productivity for that person. Society, in turn, incurs direct and indirect costs.

Direct expenditures include those for medical and personal care, architectural modification, assistive technology, and institutional care, as well as income support for the person with a disability. For the individual, these expenses contribute to impoverishment.[7,51] Society's response to the expenditures related to disablement includes disability-related programs such as Social Security Disability Insurance (SSDI), Supplemental Security Income (SSI), Medicare, and Medicaid. In 2008, federal and federal-state programs for working-aged people with disabilities were estimated to cost $357 billion, or 12% of all federal spending of the United States.[39]

Table 6-3 Employment and Earnings

	Employment Rate of People 21 to 64 Years Old (%)	Median Monthly Earnings 21 to 64 Years Old ($)	Median Monthly Family Income 21 to 64 Years Old ($)
No disability	79.1	2724	4771
Any disability	41.1	—	—
Nonsevere disability	71.2	2402	3959
Severe disability	27.5	1577	2376

From U.S. Census Bureau: *Americans with disabilities: 2010 report*, Washington, 2012, U.S. Census Bureau.

Disablement is costly to the individual and to society because of the loss of productivity. People with disabilities are more likely to be unemployed or underemployed and have lower average salaries than their peers without disabilities (Table 6-3). The indirect monetary costs for the individual are reckoned in terms of losses in earnings and homemaker services.[57] A 2006 study by researchers at the University of California, with 1997 as an example year, found that people with disabilities were estimated to spend an average of 4.5 times as much on medical expenses[57] and that the overall net salary loss associated with disability was $115.3 billion, or 1.4% of the 1997 gross domestic product.[57]

Disablement is associated with poverty. In 2011, 23% of people with disabilities, aged 5 years and older were below the poverty level as opposed to only 15% of those without a disability.[43] In 2010, people 21 to 64 years of age without a disability had median monthly earnings of $2724. Those with a nonsevere disability had $2402 median monthly earnings, and those with a severe disability had $1577 median monthly earnings (Table 6-3).[42] The indirect monetary cost to society is loss from the labor force.[7] For example, in 1996, spinal cord injury alone was estimated to have cost the U.S. economy $9.73 billion, including $2.6 billion in lost productivity.[22]

Disablement imposes indirect nonmonetary costs to the individual and to society. Fifty-seven percent of people with disabilities thought their disability prevented them from reaching their full potential.[13] Restriction in work participation, in particular, places the individual in a position of dependency on insurance payments or government benefits for income support and medical care. Dependency affects people's feelings about themselves and their overall satisfaction with life.

Pressure from various customers, and especially the third-party payers, for accountability in medical care focuses attention on outcome and cost-effectiveness. Interventions directed at disablement should be assessed with measures of both outcome and cost-effectiveness. Disablement is more than a medical phenomenon: It is a complex socioeconomic process. Assessment of the outcome and cost-effectiveness of an intervention should take into consideration the quality of life and indirect monetary costs, as well as direct expenditures.

Vocational rehabilitation is an intervention that can limit restrictions in work participation. In 1993, the Social Security Administration estimated that for every dollar spent on vocational rehabilitation services, five dollars in future direct expenditures was saved.[21] A 2006 analysis of spending by the New Mexico Division of Vocational Rehabilitation found a total benefit/cost ratio of 5.63.[28] Although employment is the expected outcome of vocational rehabilitation, the impact of this intervention goes beyond simple employment and saving of direct expenditures. The positive effects of working are demonstrated when the characteristics of working and nonworking people with disabilities are compared. Those who work are better educated, have more money, are less likely to consider themselves disabled, and in general are more satisfied with life.[13]

Comprehensive rehabilitation of people with disabilities should include strategies that reduce work restrictions, such as vocational rehabilitation. The outcomes include increased independence and increased productivity. The cost-effectiveness of comprehensive rehabilitation should be measured in direct and indirect monetary and nonmonetary costs over the lifetime of the individual.[3]

Treatment of the Injured Worker

Workers' Compensation Medicine

Physiatrists are often the providers of choice for treatment of injured workers, being both well-grounded in musculoskeletal medicine and, generally, conservative in the use of resources, with a preference for nonoperative treatment. Different nations and states vary widely in the rights and responsibilities of both employers and employees after a work-related injury. Obviously knowing the regulations in your practice area is essential. However, the best way to view what can become an adversarial process, particularly when health care is not otherwise provided by the state, is as follows: keep in mind that you are foremost a health care provider and should be devoid of any other interests. If any condition or activity requires any particular treatment, it should be provided. If any particular restrictions or limitations are warranted they should be clearly expressed. However, using your common sense is encouraged. Claims of severe pain following minor events, accompanied by normal diagnostic tests, deserve some scrutiny, particularly if test results, such as the Waddell test , are positive and normal movement about the examination room occurs without difficulty. Many jobs are not that enjoyable and also do not pay particularly well. Not returning to such jobs may not be an altogether unpleasant scenario. In fact, it is well known that the less pleasant the relationship with one's supervisor was before an injury, the longer a return to work will take. In addition, the longer the worker is out, the less likely is an eventual return to work. With this in mind, instituting brief restrictions to sedentary (0 to 10 lb lifting maximum, occasionally) or light duty work (20 lb maximum, occasionally), but not taking the worker off work, should be done if possible. For individuals who have been out of work for some time, returning part-time for a few weeks initially can be reassuring and allow a gradual reacclimatization to the workplace. Overall, the goal of worker's compensation medicine is to provide medically necessary care for the injured worker, as well as to work with the patient and his or her employer to facilitate a safe return to work. In most cases, standard medical examination is sufficient but aggressive evaluation and treatment may be required to prevent prolonged and excessive disability. The Functional Capacity Evaluation, Work Hardening Programs, and Functional Restoration Programs are tools that may be indicated in problematic cases.

Functional Capacity Evaluation

A Functional Capacity Evaluation (FCE) is a series of performance-based tests that evaluates an individual's ability to perform work activities related to his or her participation in employment[39] and a specific job. Capabilities tested can include perception, range of motion, strength, endurance, coordination, ability to lift, assume certain postures, and ability to tolerate standing walking and climbing. Various measures attempt to detect submaximal effort and objectively assess an employee's ability to meet the demands of a work environment. The tests gauge physical demands and the cognitive demands of the job, and for complicated patients, the tests are used to predict an individual's return to work.[19,39]

There is generally no mandate to perform an FCE, and sometimes they are not readily available. The tests are generally not necessary for sedentary workers because there is by definition no lower level of activity. Many workers with only moderately demanding jobs are well aware of their present abilities from simply performing the activities of routine life(i.e., lifting bags of potatoes of set weights). The tests will prove invaluable only when a worker is returning to moderately or heavily strenuous work and the worker is truly uncertain of whether he or she can perform the required activities of their occupation.

Work Hardening Program

Work Hardening is a multidisciplinary "work-oriented treatment program" that consists of work tolerance screening and work capacity evaluation components.[23] It features physical conditioning with job simulation activities combined with psychological treatment to address mild-to-moderate cognitive and behavioral factors accompanying the subacute pain/disability. Patients with complex pain syndromes or psychological comorbidities may benefit from an interdisciplinary pain program. Types of psychological issues commonly addressed include anger at employer, fear of return to work, fear of injury, and interpersonal problems with co-workers. The impact intense physical conditioning for subacute back pain has on the duration of work absence remains unclear owing to conflicting study results.[35]

Functional Restoration Program

Functional Restoration Programs were first described in 1985 by Dr. Tom Mayer and his colleagues at the University of Texas Health Science Center and Productive Rehabilitation Institute of Dallas for Ergonomics (PRIDE) for the treatment of patients with chronic lower back pain.[6,24] The goal of a Functional Restoration Program is to restore the patient's physical, psychosocial, and socioeconomic situation. It is a physician-driven interdisciplinary program requiring, but not limited to, the participation of physical/occupational therapists, social workers, and psychologists. These programs emphasize the importance of function over the elimination of pain, with the key concepts being pain acceptance, pain management, and the creation of active coping strategies.[29] Patients are required to participate in intensive exercise sessions where no passive modalities are included. The sessions are then associated with cognitive-behavioral therapy and may be followed by ergonomic therapy sessions.

In a 2007 systematic review by Poiraudeau et al.,[29] the authors found that despite the favorable claims of various Functional Restoration Program studies reporting of a 65% to 90% return-to-work rate, many of the studies lacked or had inadequate control groups.[29] In spite of the lack of adequate control groups, the reviewers found that Functional Restoration Programs when coupled with Work Hardening Programs were associated with a double increase in their return-to-work rate. These findings are echoed in a more recent 2013 Cochrane review, which found that the number of sick leave was reduced in workers undergoing Work Hardening activities incorporated into their Functional Restoration Programs.[35] Currently, further studies with proper control groups are needed to accurately indicate if Functional Restoration Programs successfully increase and maintain the vocational outcomes of patients.

Disability-Related Programs and Policies

Programs

A plethora of disability-related programs and policies exist. Each program and policy has its own definition of disablement and disability, and differs in the eligibility and application criteria. The programs can be characterized as ameliorative or corrective.[14] Ameliorative programs provide payment for income support and medical care. Corrective programs facilitate the individual's ability to return to work and to reduce or remove the disablement. Whether ameliorative or corrective, all programs influence the biopsychosocial model of disablement.

Disability-related programs can be categorized into three basic types: cash transfers, medical care programs, and direct service programs. Table 6-4 presents specific programs within these three basic types.[7] Estimates of the expenditures of these disability-related programs provide insight into expenditure trends. In 1970, 61.4% of the disability dollar went for cash transfers, 33% for medical care, and 5.4% for direct services. By 1986, the proportion of the disability dollar for direct services had decreased to 2.1%, although the proportion for medical care had increased.[7] In 2008, of the estimated $357 billion spent, 40.6% went to income maintenance, 54.9% went to health care programs, 2.7% went to housing and food, and 1.2% for education training and employment.[39] The trend toward ameliorative programs capturing more of the resources is a concern. Studies of the socioeconomic consequences of disability support the utility of rehabilitating people with disabilities, allowing them to enter the labor market

Table 6-4 Disability-Related Programs

Type of Program	Specific Programs
Cash transfer	Social insurance: Social Security Disability Insurance Private insurance Indemnity compensation Income support: Supplemental Security Income, veterans' pensions, Aid to Families with Dependent Children
Medical care	Medicare Private disability insurance Veterans' programs Workers' compensation Tort settlements Medicaid
Direct services	Rehabilitation and vocational education veterans' programs Services for people with specific impairments General-funded programs (e.g., SNAP, developmental disabilities, blind, mentally ill) Employment assistance programs (e.g., comprehensive employment training program)

From Berkowitz M, Hill MA, eds: Disability and the labor market: an overview. In *Disability and the labor market: economic problems, policies, and programs*, New York, 1989, ILR Press, with permission.

SNAP, Supplemental Nutrition Assistance Program.

and thereby decrease their dependency and loss of productivity.

The physiatrist has an important supportive role in initiating referrals to the corrective programs. These programs are in keeping with the philosophy of rehabilitation, which is to maximize individual functioning and lessen disability.

Public Disability Policies

Public policy in the United States has begun to recognize that many barriers to integration faced by people with disabilities are the result of discriminatory policy and practices. Some also have the view that disability is an interaction between an individual and the environment. This has played a fundamental role in shaping public policy toward disability during the past 20 years. Since the late 1960s, Congress has passed a series of laws aimed at enhancing the quality of life for people with disabilities. These laws have mandated that housing and transportation be accessible, that education for children with disabilities be appropriate, and that employment practices be nondiscriminatory.[1,10,49]

Three legislative actions deserve to be highlighted. The Rehabilitation Act of 1973 extended civil rights protection to people with disabilities. This legislation included antidiscrimination and affirmative action in employment. The Rehabilitation Act Amendments of 1978 broadened the responsibility of the Rehabilitation Services Administration to include independent living programs, and created the National Council of the Handicapped (the National Council of the Handicapped became the National Council on Disability in January 1989). The capstone of this legislative tradition is the ADA of 1990. This legislation established a clear and comprehensive prohibition of discrimination based on disability.[10,47,49,52]

More recent legislation, such as the Workforce Investment Act and the Ticket to Work and Work Incentives Improvement Acts of 1998, continue to attempt to eliminate the barriers that prevent individuals with disabilities from working.

Table 6-5 reviews the prominent federal disability laws.

Vocational Rehabilitation

The objective of vocational rehabilitation is to allow people with physical disabilities to engage in gainful employment. Historically, formal vocational rehabilitation services were instituted to provide returning World War II veterans with disabilities assistance in obtaining suitable occupations.[49]

Before the 1970s, jobs earmarked for people with disabilities were provided through government-subsidized sheltered workshops. The Comprehensive Employment Training Act (CETA) of 1973 provided public service jobs for people with disabilities and for the disadvantaged, along with training programs for this population. At its peak in 1980, CETA and sheltered workshops provided more than 1 million jobs for a broadly defined "disabled" population. The CETA program lasted from 1973 to 1982, when the federal government subsequently returned to state-run vocational rehabilitation agencies for provision of these services to people with disabilities.

The Rehabilitation Act of 1973 authorized federal funding for state rehabilitation agencies to provide a variety of services to qualified people with disabilities. The federal

Table 6-5 Federal Disability Laws

Law	Description
Americans with Disabilities Act of 1990	Prohibits discrimination on the basis of disability in employment, state and local government, public accommodations, commercial facilities, transportation, and telecommunications
Telecommunications Act of 1996	Requires manufacturers of telecommunications equipment and providers of telecommunications services to ensure that such equipment and services are accessible to and usable by people with disabilities, if readily achievable
Fair Housing Amendments Act of 1988	Prohibits housing discrimination on the basis of race, color, religion, sex, disability, familial status, and national origin
Air Carrier Access Act of 1986	Prohibits discrimination in air transportation by domestic and foreign air carriers against individuals with physical or mental impairments
Voting Accessibility for the Elderly and Handicapped Act of 1984	Attempts to ensure polling places across the United States to be physically accessible to people with disabilities for federal elections; this law also requires states to make available registration and voting aids for voters with disabilities and elderly voters
National Voter Registration Act of 1993 (Motor Voter Act)	Attempts to improve the low registration rates of minorities and people with disabilities that have resulted from discrimination; all offices of state-funded programs that are primarily engaged in providing services to people with disabilities are required to provide all program applicants with voter registration forms, assistance in completing the forms, and to transmit completed forms to the appropriate state official
Civil Rights of Institutionalized Persons Act	Authorizes the U.S. attorney general to investigate conditions of confinement at state and local government institutions such as prisons, jails, pretrial detention centers, juvenile correctional facilities, publicly operated nursing homes, and institutions for people with psychiatric or developmental disabilities
Individuals with Disabilities Education Act	Requires public schools to make available to children with disabilities a free appropriate public education in the least restrictive environment appropriate to their individual needs
Rehabilitation Act of 1973	Prohibits discrimination on the basis of disability in programs conducted by federal agencies, in programs receiving federal financial assistance, in federal employment, and in the employment practices of federal contractors
Architectural Barriers Act of 1968	Requires that buildings and facilities that are designed, constructed, or altered with federal funds, or leased by a federal agency, comply with federal standards for physical accessibility

From U.S. Department of Justice, Civil Rights Division: *A guide to disability rights laws*, Washington, 2005, U.S. Department of Justice.[46]

BOX 6-1

Services Provided by Vocational Rehabilitation Specialists

Diagnosis and Evaluation

- Counseling and guidance
- Restoration*
- Transportation
- College or university training
- Income maintenance

Adjustment Training

- Business or vocational training
- Miscellaneous training
- Placement
- Referrals
- On-the-job training

*Includes medical treatment, prosthetic devices, or medically necessary services to correct or modify a physical or mental disorder.

government supplies 80% of the funding for state vocational rehabilitation agencies, whereas the states must provide the remaining 20%. State agencies administer the programs under the Rehabilitation Services Administration in the U.S. Department of Education. The intent of the Rehabilitation Act was to provide services to people with disabilities with emphasis placed on serving those with more severe disabilities (General Accounting Office testimony).[48] State agencies are usually located in the state division or bureau of vocational rehabilitation. The state division provides direct services and also refers individuals to private rehabilitation agencies and training programs when indicated.

Traditional Approaches to Vocational Rehabilitation

A variety of approaches to vocational rehabilitation have been developed over the years. The traditional approach begins with the referral of a person with a disability to a vocational rehabilitation counselor (Box 6-1). This referral can be generated by the person with a disability, a physician, a social worker, or a case manager. The initial referral includes medical records, documentation of disabilities and capabilities, and neuropsychological testing (if available).

The initial interview between the counselor and the client (person with a disability) establishes rapport and provides background information about previous job skills and experiences. The interview also provides information about the individual's educational level, motivation, perceived abilities and disabilities, and areas of interest. If the client was employed before the onset of disability, there is often potential for placement with the former employer. This previous employer should be contacted to learn of employment opportunities for the person with a disability. The vocational rehabilitation counselor also assesses the premorbid skills the person had and the skills needed before placement in a suitable position. If no positions are available, vocational testing is performed.

Aptitude Matching Compared with Work Sample

Vocational testing is performed to assess the client's level of general intelligence, achievement, aptitudes, interests, and work skills. Formal testing consists of administering a battery of paper-and-pencil standardized tests, examples of which are listed in Table 6-6. This type of approach is known as aptitude matching. It determines the client's aptitudes or traits in the areas of general intelligence, visuospatial perception, eye-hand coordination, motor coordination, and dexterity. Performance on the tests is compared against a list of essential aptitudes, grouped by occupation, in the *Dictionary of Occupational Titles* published by the U.S. Department of Labor.[25] When a client's aptitudes match a particular occupation, a job search is undertaken by the counselor.

Table 6-6 Tests Administered by Vocational Rehabilitation Counselors or Neuropsychologists

Test	Type
Wechsler Adult Intelligence Scale—Revised	Intelligence
General Aptitude Test Battery	Aptitude
Differential Aptitude Test	Aptitude
Wide Range Achievement Test	Achievement
Strong-Campbell Interest Inventory	Interest
Career Assessment Inventory	Interest
Minnesota Multiphasic Personality Inventory	Personality
Halstead-Reitan	Cognitive evaluation
Luria-Nebraska	Cognitive evaluation

A work sample approach is often used in conjunction with aptitude batteries. The work sample approach measures general characteristics such as size discrimination, multilevel sorting, eye-hand-foot coordination, and dexterity. The Valpar Component Work Sample Series (VCWSS) is a good example of the work sample approach. The VCWSS uses complex work apparatus to measure almost exclusively motor responses. Less focus is applied to general intelligence, aptitude, and academic performance. Work samples can also evaluate the type of "work group" in which the client is most skilled. This simulated work requires performance of a series of tasks, such as drill press operation or circuit board or bench assembly.[25]

Once the client's skills have been evaluated and interests explored, a vocational goal is developed. The requirements of the potential position must first be determined. This is accomplished by performing a job analysis of the position and then identifying the physical and mental requirements and any necessary job site modifications (e.g., adaptive equipment). If training is proposed, it must be accessible and available to the client. Transportation should be arranged and can be paid for by the vocational rehabilitation agency. Tuition, books, and adaptive equipment to allow performance of the position can also be provided by the agency.

Training programs vary in length depending on the potential vocational goal. They can last from a few weeks to several years. Training can be conducted at a trade school, college, university, or on the job with state vocational rehabilitation agency funding.

On-the-job training requires job development. The counselor or the client explores community business resources to develop suitable positions. Tax incentives for potential employers can help convince industry to offer training. Sliding-scale wages can be arranged to assist in developing positions. For example, the state rehabilitation agency might fund 100% of salary for 3 to 6 months. The employer gradually assumes that responsibility over the next 3 to 6 months as the new employee becomes trained. Many employers want to keep the employees they have trained, but some prefer to act in the capacity of trainers for a series of people with disabilities. In this case, the counselor still has the task of placing the newly trained people.

Once an individual has completed training and has been placed for 60 days, the state vocational rehabilitation agency considers the case a "success" and closes its file. No follow-up evaluation is typically provided.

Sheltered Workshops

One of the problems with the traditional approach of the vocational rehabilitation agency has been its poor record of success, especially for people with severe disabilities. Forty-five percent fewer people were successfully vocationally rehabilitated in 1988 than in 1974, despite increased financial support and larger numbers of people with disabilities.[49] A 1987 General Accounting Office survey found that of SSDI recipients receiving vocational rehabilitation, less than 1% left the SSDI rolls.[38] Although now a bit better, these numbers remain small. A 2007 General Accounting Office report to Congress noted that by 2005 an average of 7% of Social Security Administration beneficiaries had left the roles after vocational rehabilitation. The International Center for the Disabled survey reported that although 60% of people with disabilities knew about vocational rehabilitation services, only 10% took advantage of those services. Of those using the services, more than 50% thought they were not useful in securing gainful employment.[13]

As a result of the poor placement record, alternative strategies have been developed for enabling people with disabilities to obtain gainful employment. These include sheltered workshops, day programs, transitional and supported employment, Projects with Industry, independent living center (ILC)-directed employment, and others. Funding for these programs has come from public, nonprofit, and private industry, state and federal social service programs, religious entities, corporate and foundation contributions, and individual donations.

A sheltered workshop is a "public nonprofit organization certified by the U.S. Department of Labor to pay 'subminimum' wages to persons with diminished earning capacity."[15] More than 5000 of these workshops exist, including Goodwill, Inc., serving approximately 250,000 people with disabilities. This form of employment serves people with severe disabilities, including limited vision, mental illness, mental retardation, and alcoholism. Although sheltered workshops provide job experience and income, critics report that sheltered workshops rarely lead to competitive, integrated employment. People with severe disabilities can be competitively employed in the community through the use of some modern strategies, as outlined later.

Day Programs

Day programs have existed since before the 1970s and are meant to provide supervised vocational activity for people with severe disabilities, usually those with mental retardation or mental illness. These programs are funded by private and corporate sponsors, as well as by state and federal agencies. They are not designed as a transition into competitive employment, nor do they allow community integration. They are geared toward providing supervised day activities while the caretakers of these people work or perform their own daily routines. Activities are performed in facilities that serve only people with disabilities.

Home-Based Programs

Another more traditional method for assisting people with severe disabilities to obtain employment is the home-based program. Home-based programs can be funded by state vocational rehabilitation, insurance carriers, foundations, and societies, or by other agencies. The person with a disability can perform a variety of jobs, including telephone solicitation, typing, or computer-assisted occupations. Some examples include graphics, accounting, or drafting.

Of these programs—sheltered workshops, day programs, and homebound programs—none emphasizes gainful employment in a non–sheltered-integrated setting. It was the failure of these programs to reintegrate their clients into competitive community employment that resulted in the emergence of transitional and supported employment models.

Other Programs for Employment

Projects with Industry

Projects with Industry is a federally sponsored collaborative program established by the Vocational Rehabilitation Act. Employers design and provide training projects for specific job skills in cooperation with rehabilitation agencies. The goal of Projects with Industry is competitive employment for the participants.

Job fairs have been somewhat successful in matching vacant positions with capable individuals with disabilities. Businesses in a community spend 1 day interviewing applicants with disabilities who have been prescreened by a participating placement agency. The placement agency might provide further services, such as transportation for the potential employee, and make recommendations for work accommodations to the potential employer.

Transitional and Supported Employment

Two newer strategies for returning people with disabilities to competitive, integrated gainful employment are transitional and supported employment. Transitional employment consists of providing the job placement, training, and support services necessary to help people move into independent or supported employment.[41] Independent employment provides at least a minimum wage to the employee and requires no job subsidy or ongoing support. Transitional employment is a short-term provision of services for a period not to exceed 18 months and culminates in an independent or supported employment position.

Supported employment has been used as a successful strategy for placing or returning the individuals who are most severely disabled to competitive, integrated community employment. It requires ongoing support after

BOX 6-2

Critical Criteria for Supported Employment

- Interventions provided at the job site
- Assistance long term or permanent
- Programs serve only the severely disabled
- Real pay for real work
- Work performed in an integrated setting

From Wehman P, Sherron P, Kregel J, et al: Return to work for people following severe traumatic brain injury. Supported employment outcomes after five years, *Am J Phys Med Rehabil* 72:355-363, 1993.

placement, including counseling for the employee and co-workers, and assistance with transportation, housing, and other non–work-related activities. It began as an alternative to sheltered workshops and day programs and has grown to have modest federal funding and broad community support. This support comes from groups of people with disabilities, state vocational rehabilitation agencies, and state departments for the developmentally disabled. This concept became a permanent part of the Rehabilitation Act of 1973 with the passage of the 1986 amendments and additional regulations published in June 1992.[53]

Supported employment is meant to provide ongoing support for people with severe disabilities. According to Wehman et al.,[54] it must meet five critical criteria (Box 6-2). The first is that all interventions, including training, placement, and counseling, be provided at the job site rather than in a therapy room or vocational school. Second, the intervention and services are provided on a permanent or long-term basis as the individual requires them. Third, these programs are intended to serve only those individuals with the most severe disabilities who have been unable to enter the competitive labor market with their disability in the past. Fourth, the work provided is real and meaningful for the employee, and compensation is received equal to that of an able-bodied co-worker for the same duties. Fifth, work must occur in an integrated setting allowing interaction with co-workers without disabilities.[53]

The U.S. Department of Education's operational definition of supported employment requires that employees be paid for working an average of at least 20 hours per week in a position that provides interactions with people who are not disabled and are not paid caregivers. There must be eight or fewer people with disabilities working together at the job site, and there must be ongoing public funding for providing intervention directly related to sustaining employment. Supportive employment defines the type and level of support needed by an individual to be employable now, not after a nonintegrated training program.

Four models of supported employment have been developed. The enclave model consists of a small group of people with disabilities working together at an integrated job site. The mobile work crew model uses a small group of workers who travel from job to job and offer contractual services under the direction of a supervisor. The small business or entrepreneurial model creates a new small business that produces goods or services using both workers with disabilities and those without them. The most frequently used model is the job coach with individual placement.[15]

The job coach, or employment specialist, is an employee of the agency providing supported employment services. The coach works with an individual at the job site to provide interpersonal and coping skills, as well as job skills. The coach performs job development before placement. Once placement occurs, job training and ongoing job retention services are provided. Job coaches might initially be required to complete the duties not yet mastered by the worker with a disability.

Depending on the disability, behavior modification or cognitive training might be required to enable learning of vital skills. These become the responsibility of the job coach. The job coach should be able to evaluate the ecology of the job site, including attitudes of co-workers, accessibility of the job site, and the necessity for adaptive equipment. The job coach should then be able to educate co-workers and ensure implementation of appropriate accommodations for the person with a disability.

Job coach intervention time can be very significant (almost 8 hours a day) initially. Wehman et al.[54] conducted a 5-year study of supported employment for people with traumatic brain injury. They documented an average requirement of 249.1 hours per person of job coach time over 6 months. The job coach's intervention time decreased steadily with time on the job to an average of less than 3 hours per week per person after 30 weeks of employment.

Some people require continued significant intervention to assist them in meeting difficulties that arise from changes at the job site, that is, new job duties or changes in personnel or goods produced. Some workers are able to depend on support from employers and co-workers, however, and require little or no further direct job coach support. Supportive employment has been highly successful in allowing people with severe disabilities to participate competitively in the job market and improve their quality of life and economic situation.

Independent Living Centers

The ILC movement has traditionally provided a core of nonvocational services such as housing, independent living skills, advocacy, and peer counseling. Just as supported employment has broadened its scope, so has the ILC movement. Both provide a combination of nonvocational and vocational services to people with severe disabilities. ILCs often employ workers with disabilities as peer counselors and program administrators. The small business approach of supported employment has been successfully implemented by ILCs to place their clients in competitive community employment. As these two philosophies continue to merge and provide similar services to people with severe disabilities, cooperative ventures between them allow people with severe disabilities to fully achieve their maximum level of independence.

Provision of vocational rehabilitation services to people with disabilities requires a diversity of strategies. The more severe the disability, the more intensive the support and services have to be. Full participation in society is a right of all people. This participation includes being employed in a meaningful job that gives satisfaction to the worker and contributes to society as a whole. The methods for returning people with disabilities to work vary, but creative strategies have proved significantly more successful than noncreative strategies.

Disincentives for Vocational Rehabilitation

Public and political opinion has changed in recent years regarding the ability of people with disabilities to work. Both people with disabilities and policymakers have demonstrated a desire to return people with disabilities to gainful employment. Statements of past presidents of the United States reflect the change of opinion. In 1973, Richard M. Nixon spoke concerning the Rehabilitation Act of 1973, saying it "would cruelly raise the hopes of the handicapped [for gainful employment] in a way that we could never hope to fulfill."[15] Advocacy by groups for the rights of people with disabilities has achieved significant policy changes, as reflected by Ronald Reagan's November 1983 proclamation of the Decade of Disabled Persons, in which the economic independence of all people with disabilities was to become a "clear national goal."[41] With the passage of the ADA in July 1990, George H.W. Bush proclaimed the "end to the unjustified segregation and exclusion of people with disabilities from the mainstream of American life."[15]

Despite the obvious changes in public and political policies and attitudes, disincentives to entering "the mainstream" abound for people with disabilities. To become eligible for cash and medical benefits through SSI and SSDI, people with disabilities must prove that they have total and permanent or long-term disability and must meet strict eligibility criteria. Before meeting those criteria, the individual and the family typically must have experienced a series of indignities, including exhausting all personal resources and submitting to significant bureaucratic red tape. "Red tape" means completing substantial paperwork, obtaining medical reports verifying disability, and enduring long waiting periods for commencement of benefits. This is usually a long and arduous process. Once the person with a disability finally achieves a modest degree of security, an "opportunity" to give it all up and enter the workforce is made available. Naturally, the person with a disability is suspicious about the assurance that benefits will be preserved and eligibility will not be taken away because of returning to or entering the job market.

Stereotypes about people with disabilities being unproductive in society are pervasive. Individuals with disabilities often come to view themselves as totally dependent and unable to work. After all, they are placed in a position to prove their dependency and inability to be productive. The government disability entitlement policies state that if you are unable to work, the government will take care of you. In fact, many government policymakers think that the person with a disability cannot and should not be expected to work. Some even think that sending a person with a disability a check is much simpler than implementing the provisions of the ADA.

Employers' attitudes serve as another disincentive. Obstacles to qualified applicants with disabilities who want to participate in the workforce include employers' ignorance about the capabilities of a potential employee with a disability, inaccessible work sites, transportation inaccessibility, and discrimination in hiring. The ADA is instrumental in changing much of this behavior and removing some of these disincentives. As employees with disabilities take their places, employers and co-workers will become educated and attitudes will change.

The physiatrist and other physicians can also provide disincentives for people with disabilities by labeling them as "totally and permanently disabled" or by restricting their activities. Emphasis should be on the capabilities of people with disabilities and documentation of their functional abilities, both mental and physical.

Incentives for Vocational Rehabilitation

In an effort to overcome disincentives, government policymakers have created incentives for people with disabilities and for potential employers. These incentives often have a long list of requirements and are very specific in wording to prevent abuse.

Incentives for the Individual

Since the inception of the SSI program in 1974, only a small number of beneficiaries have been employed. Social Security bulletins note that in 1976 approximately 71,000 beneficiaries were working. By 2006, that number had increased to 349,000. During the same years, the SSI blind and disabled caseload increased from 2 million to 6.1 million. It appears that in 2006 approximately 6% of those who received an SSI payment were employed. Because these low numbers have been thought to reflect actual disincentives built into the current SSI payment system, a number of incentive programs have been implemented.[18]

Incentive programs are applicable depending on whether the person with a disability receives SSDI or SSI benefits, or both. SSDI work incentives are discussed first. Table 6-7 presents a summary of the terminology and abbreviations for easy reference. Additional references are given here for those wanting more detailed information.*

The initial incentive toward return to work involves a trial work period (TWP). The TWP lets people test their ability to work or run a business without affecting their benefits. This TWP maintains cash benefits for 9 months (not necessarily consecutive) of trial work in a 60-month period. During this period, beneficiaries can earn up to $530 per month.[4]

On completion of the TWP and continued employment at or above the substantial gainful activity (SGA) level, benefits continue to be paid for an additional 3 months and are then terminated.[26,44,45] Any earnings from work below the monetary limit of the SGA level described in Table 6-7 are excluded when figuring monthly benefit amounts. The SGA dollar amount was increased in 1999 from $500 to $700, and a formula was adopted to link this amount in the future to the national average wage index.[4] The SGA dollar amount as of 2014 is $1070.

The extended period of eligibility (EPE) is a period of 36 consecutive months during which cash benefits can be reinstated if, during that period, the individual's earnings fall below the SGA level. If the individual is unable to

*References 26, 31, 32, 36, 38, 44, 45.

Table 6-7 Summary of Incentives for the Individual Receiving Benefits to Enter Work Activities

Incentive	Details
Social Security Disability Insurance (SSDI)	Disability benefits program based on medical disability and a worker's earnings covered by Social Security (Title II—Social Security Act)
Supplemental Security Income (SSI)	Disability benefits program based on medical disability and the amount of income a person receives (Title XVI—Social Security Act)
Trial work period (TWP)	Allows trial return to work to test work ability without affecting benefits (SSDI)
Substantial gainful activity (SGA)	Performance of significant and productive physical or mental work for pay or profit (>$700/month for nonblind [SSDI and SSI] and $810/month for blind recipients [SSDI only])
Extended period of eligibility	Allows reinstatement of cash benefits without a waiting period if the worker's earnings fall below SGA level within 36 months after TWP (SSDI)
Impairment-related work expenses	Allows costs for certain items to be deducted from earnings when figuring SGA level (SSI and SSDI)
Earned income exclusion	Allows exclusion of a portion of earned income when figuring an individual's monthly benefit (SSI)
Blind work expenses	Allows work-related expenses when figuring benefits (SSI)

maintain earnings at the SGA level, benefits resume automatically and no waiting periods are required. Benefits cease at the end of the EPE, but Medicare continues for an additional 3 months.[26,44,45] The elimination of a second waiting period for both cash benefits and Medicare benefits is also an incentive to perform a trial of work.

Under certain circumstances, the person might be able to participate in a Medicare "buy-in." The client must have completed both the TWP and the EPE. In addition, the extended 3 months of Medicare benefits must have passed. Once these conditions are met, Medicare A and B coverage can be purchased. This medical coverage is for those who cannot otherwise obtain health insurance because of preexisting conditions.[26] In March 2010, President Obama signed the Affordable Care Act. This law includes the Preexisting Insurance Plan. When implemented, this plan is intended to provide a new coverage option to individuals who have been uninsured for at least 6 months because of a preexisting condition.

Another major incentive program for those receiving SSDI or SSI is for impairment-related work expenses. This allows the cost of certain items and services to be deducted from earnings when determining the SGA level. Examples include attendant care, medical devices, equipment, and prostheses.[26]

For those people with disabilities receiving SSI benefits, a different, but often similar, set of incentives applies. These incentives provide SSI recipients with assurances that working will not disadvantage them. Section 1619 of the Social Security Act was made permanent by the Employment Opportunities for Disabled Americans Act passed in November 1986. The incentive of Section 1619 allows receipt of SSI cash benefits, even though earned income exceeds the SGA level. Cash benefits are calculated with the earned income exclusion (discussed later). Medicaid benefits continue as an additional incentive even after wages become high enough to cause cessation of SSI cash benefits, provided their continuation is needed to allow the recipient to maintain employment.[26,44,45]

The earned income exclusion allows most of a recipient's earned income to be excluded, including pay received from a sheltered workshop or day activity center, when figuring the SSI monthly amount.[38] "Blind" work expenses is an incentive that allows a person who has visual impairment to pay for work expenses, such as visual aids, guide dogs, or Braille translations. These allowable expenses are then excluded when calculating benefit amounts.

In an effort to prevent work disincentives, benefit caps have been implemented to decrease excessively generous benefits. These caps use various formulas to reduce or limit maximum benefits paid by Social Security. These formulas take into account other sources of income, such as workers' compensation benefits, but do not exclude veterans' benefits or disability pensions from government jobs.

Another incentive program, Plans for Achieving Self-Support, allows an SSI recipient to set aside income and resources necessary to achieve a work goal.[31,44,45]

Incentives for Industry

Government policymakers have made various attempts to offer tax incentives to business and industry. These incentives have mainly been directed at making the workplace accessible. Section 190 of the Internal Revenue Code, enacted in 1976 and revised by the Revenue Reconciliation Act of 1990, allows a set amount per year to be deductible for any expenses incurred in barrier removal (making a business or public transportation accessible).[34]

The Revenue Reconciliation Act of 1990 (which was passed 3 months after the ADA) allows an "access" tax credit with Section 44 of the Internal Revenue Code for small businesses. It allows credit against income taxes for eligible expenditures (auxiliary services for the employee with disabilities and aids are covered). This access credit is allowed only for expenses incurred for the purpose of enabling a business to comply with the ADA.[34]

Tax credits have also been used as incentives to encourage hiring of target groups, including the "hard core" unemployed: people with disabilities and the homeless. The Targeted Jobs Tax Credit (TJTC), originally enacted in 1978, is meant to encourage employers to hire members of these groups. It provides a tax credit for targeted people, including those people receiving SSI benefits and vocational rehabilitation referrals (both groups containing large numbers of people with disabilities). This credit only provides benefits to an employer for 1 year per employee. Many employers use the credit as a windfall; that is, hiring anyone they want and later checking to see whether the new employee falls into a targeted group. This practice is called "retroactive certification."[34]

The TJTC has, unfortunately, not been particularly useful in increasing the number of people with disabilities hired. In fact, legislative incentives in general have not been very successful in achieving the goal of vocationally rehabilitating people with disabilities. Ongoing efforts in Congress, however, are being made to improve the incentives for people with disabilities to return to work. For example, the Work Incentives Improvement Act of 1999 (S.331) provides adequate and affordable health insurance when a person receiving SSI or SSDI goes to work by expanding Medicaid options for states and by continuing access to Medicare after returning to work. It encourages SSDI beneficiaries to return to work by ensuring that cash benefits remain available if employment proves unsuccessful. An expedited eligibility process is proposed for SSDI beneficiaries who lose benefits because of work and need reinstatement of benefits later. A "ticket" program would provide a new payment system for SSDI and SSI beneficiaries for employment services. It reimburses vocational rehabilitation, training, and employment service providers a portion of benefit payments saved when the beneficiary earns more than the SGA level, currently $700 per month ($1000 for blind beneficiaries).[4,17] This program originally called for sanctions (deductions against Social Security benefits or suspension of SSI benefits) for refusal of vocational rehabilitation, but this was eliminated as of January 1, 2001.[5]

Approximately 80% of SSI recipients work before applying for SSI, and 20% work after they start receiving payments.[36] Scott Muller of the Social Security Administration performed a retrospective analysis of a cohort of more than 4000 people who were initially entitled to benefits.[26] Approximately 10% worked during the initial period of entitlement. Of those, 84% were granted a TWP, and of that group, more than 70% completed the TWP. More than 50% did not leave the rolls as a result of their efforts. Less than 3% had benefits terminated as a result of return to work.[22]

It is clear from the research conducted by the Social Security Administration that legislating incentives is not the complete answer to rehabilitating people with work disability. Potential employers and people with disabilities alike must take the initiative, but the search for feasible means to return people with disabilities to work is well worth it. The General Accounting Office estimates that removing even 1% of disabled beneficiaries from the SSDI and SSI programs each year would result in estimated lifetime savings of $3 billion.[37]

Disability Prevention

With disability ranking as the largest public health problem in the United States, it seems reasonable to interface the public health model of prevention with the ICIDH-2 model of disablement. The public health model defines three categories of prevention: primary, secondary, and tertiary.

Primary prevention is intended for healthy people, helping them to avoid the onset of a pathologic condition. In people with disabilities, primary prevention comprises efforts toward preventing a worsening of impairments.

Secondary prevention is aimed at early identification and treatment of a pathologic condition and reduction of risk factors for disablement. For people with disabilities, there are many opportunities for preventing impairment from limiting one or more activities. The ameliorative and corrective programs discussed earlier, including vocational rehabilitation strategies, are aimed at reducing activity limitation. These programs have been effective not only in returning the unemployed person to work but also in preventing job loss in those workers with a disability.[2] Interventions in medical rehabilitation focused on the enhancement of activity, such as provision of assistive technology, can be considered secondary prevention.

The General Accounting Office has studied return-to-work strategies used by Germany and Sweden, and recommends that intervention occur as soon as possible after an actual or potentially disabling event to promote and facilitate return to work. Because the current SSI benefit structure in the United States includes a lengthy application process, and then benefits linked to full, permanent disability only, intervention often is only offered long after an applicant has been removed from the workforce—a situation numerous studies have shown to significantly decrease the chance of a successful return to the workforce.[37]

Tertiary prevention focuses on arresting the progression of a pathologic condition and on limiting further disablement. For people with disabilities, tertiary prevention is designed to limit the restriction of a person's participation in some area by the provision of a facilitator or the removal of a barrier.[56] Environmental modifications, provision of services, removal of physical barriers, changes in social attitudes, and reform in legislation and policy are tertiary prevention strategies. Medical rehabilitation is traditionally considered a tertiary prevention strategy. The public disability policies, such as the ADA, are also efforts to reduce environmental and social barriers to participation.[30,50,56]

Considering functioning and disablement as outcomes of interactions between health conditions (disorders or diseases) and conceptual factors (social, environmental, and personal), there are many opportunities for the physiatrist and the medical rehabilitation team to intervene. Rehabilitation interventions aimed at prevention of activity limitation or prevention of participation restriction are secondary and tertiary prevention strategies that push the dynamic model of disablement in the direction of function. Some physiatrists feel a responsibility to be actively involved in therapeutic and public health management of disablement to develop and support policies that encourage improved function.[16]

Conclusion

Comprehensive rehabilitation is an intervention directed at human functioning. The desired outcome is to maximize the physical, mental, social, and economic function of the individual with disabilities. The physiatrist as team leader has the responsibility of encouraging the team to take a holistic approach to the person with disabilities. The holistic approach includes collaboration with professionals outside the traditional medical rehabilitation team, such as those who can facilitate vocational rehabilitation for people with disabilities.

Vocational rehabilitation is an intervention aimed at preventing impairment from limiting activities and limiting participation in work. Limitation in work participation has significant socioeconomic consequences for the individual and for society. Employment of people with disabilities supports a better quality of life and promotes function. Even for people with severe disabilities, vocational rehabilitation strategies have been successful in facilitation of work participation.

Disability is the largest public health problem in the United States. The demands of this public health issue have captured the attention of public policymakers. This has resulted in implementation of significant federal disability laws. The U.S. public policies on disability reflect the policymakers' acceptance of disability as a complex process. Disablement is considered to be the result of a dynamic, complex, and bidirectional interaction between health conditions and conceptual factors for each individual.

The physiatrist is positioned to serve a primary role in the functioning and disablement paradigm. As people with disabilities become a greater segment of society, the opportunities for involvement of physiatrists are expanded. It is the physiatrist's responsibility to be active in disability prevention, in care and advocacy for people with disabilities, and in the development of public policy on disablement.

REFERENCES

1. Adams PF, Benson V: Current estimates for the National Health Interview Survey, 1988, *Vital Health Stat* 10:1–250, 1989.
2. Allaire S, Li W, LaValley M: Reduction of job loss in people with rheumatic diseases receiving vocational rehabilitation: a randomized controlled trial, *Arthritis Rheum* 48:3212–3218, 2003.
3. Anderson TP: Quality of life of the individual with a disability, *Arch Phys Med Rehabil* 63:55, 1982.
4. Anonymous: Rules and regulations, *Fed Regist* 65:82905–82912, 2000.
5. Anonymous: Rules and regulations, *Fed Regist* 68:40119–40125, 2003.
6. Bendix AE, Bendix T, Haestrup C, Busch E: A prospective, randomized 5-year follow-up study of functional restoration in chronic low back pain patients, *Eur Spine J* 7:111–119, 1998.
7. Berkowitz M: The socioeconomic consequences of SCI, *Paraplegic News* 18–23, 1994.
8. Berkowitz M, Hill M, editors: Disability and the labor market: an overview. In *Disability and the labor market: economic problems, policies, and programs*, New York, 1989, ILR Press.
9. Colvez A, Blanche M: Disability trends in the United States population 1966-76: analysis of reported causes, *Am J Public Health* 71:464–471, 1981.
10. DeJong G, Lifchez R: Physical disability and public policy, *Sci Am* 248:40–50, 1983.
11. Haber LD: Identifying the disabled: concepts and methods in the measurement of disability, *Soc Secur Bull* 51:11–28, 1988.
12. Haber LD: Issues in the definition of disability and the use of disability survey data. In Daniel LB, Aitter M, Ingram L, editors: *Disability statistics, an assessment: report of a workshop*, Washington, 1990, National Academy Press.
13. Harris L: *The ICD survey of disabled Americans: bringing disabled Americans into the mainstream*, New York, 1986, Louis Harris and Associates.
14. Haveman RH, Halberstandt V, Burkhauser RV, editors: *Public policy toward disabled workers: cross-national analyses of economic impacts*, New York, 1984, Cornell University Press.
15. Hearne PG: Employment strategies for people with disabilities: a prescription for change, *Milbank Q* 69:111–128, 1991.
16. Joe TC: Professionalism: a new challenge for rehabilitation, *Arch Phys Med Rehabil* 62:245–250, 1981.
17. Kennedy EM, Jeffonds J, Moynahan DP, et al: The Work Incentives Improvement Act of 1999, *Senate Bill* 331, 1999.
18. Kenney L: Earning histories of SSI beneficiaries working in December 1997, *Soc Secur Bull* 63:34–46, 2000.
19. Kuijer PP, Gouttebarge V, Brouwer S, et al: Are performance-based measures predictive of work participation in patients with musculoskeletal disorders? A systematic review, *Int Arch Occup Environ Health* 85:109–123, 2012.
20. La Plante MP: The demographics of disability, *Milbank Q* 69:55–77, 1991.
21. La Plante MP, Kennedy J, Kaye S, et al: Disability and employment, no. 11. In *Disability Statistics Abstract Series*, San Francisco, 1997, University of California.
22. Lin VW, Cardenas DD: *Spinal cord medicine: principles and practice*, New York, 2003, Demos Medical Publishing.
23. Matheson L, Ogden L, Violette K, Schultz K: Work hardening: occupational therapy in industrial rehabilitation, *Am J Occup Ther* 39:314–321, 1985.
24. Mayer TG, Gatchel RJ, Kishino N, et al: Objective assessment of spine function following industrial injury. A prospective study with comparison group and one-year follow-up, *Spine (Phila Pa 1976)* 10:482–493, 1985.
25. Menchetti BM, Flynn CC: Vocational evaluation. In Rusch FR, editor: *Supported employment: models, methods and issues*, Sycamore, 1990, Sycamore Publishing Co, pp 111–130.
26. Muller LS: Disability beneficiaries who work and their experience under program work incentives, *Soc Secur Bull* 55:2–19, 1992.
27. Nagi SZ: Disability concepts revisited: implication to prevention, appendix A. In Pope AM, Tarlov AR, editors: *Disability in America: toward a national agenda for prevention*, Washington, 1991, National Academy Press, pp 309–327.
28. New Mexico Division of Vocational Rehabilitation: *The economic impact of the New Mexico division of vocational rehabilitation*, New Mexico, 2006, New Mexico Division of Vocational Rehabilitation.
29. Poiraudeau S, Rannou F, Revel M: Functional restoration programs for low back pain: a systematic review, *Ann Readapt Med Phys* 50:425–429, 419-424, 2007.
30. Pope AM, Tarlov AR, editors: *Disability in America: toward a national agenda for prevention*, Washington, 1991, National Academy Press.
31. Rigby DE: SSI work incentive participants, *Soc Secur Bull* 54:22–29, 1991.
32. Rocklin SG, Mattson DR: The Employment Opportunities for Disabled Americans Act: legislative history and summary of provisions, *Soc Secur Bull* 50:25–35, 1987.
33. Rusk HA: The growth and development of rehabilitation medicine, *Arch Phys Med Rehabil* 50:463–466, 1969.
34. Schaffer DC: Tax incentives, *Milbank Q* 69:293–312, 1991.
35. Schaafsma FG, Whelan K, Van Der Beek AJ, et al: Physical conditioning as part of a return to work strategy to reduce sickness absence for workers with back pain, *Cochrane Database Syst Rev* (8):CD001822, 2013.
36. Scott CG: Disabled SSI recipients who work, *Soc Secur Bull* 55:26–36, 1992.
37. Sim J: Improving return-to-work strategies in the United States disability programs, with analysis of program practices in Germany and Sweden, *Soc Secur Bull* 59:41–50, 1999.
38. Social Security Administration: Report of Disability Advisory Council: executive summary, *Soc Secur Bull* 51:13–17, 1988.
39. Soer R, van der Schans CP, Groothoff JW, et al: Towards consensus in operational definitions in functional capacity evaluation: a Delphi survey, *J Occup Rehabil* 18:389–400, 2008.
40. Symington DC: The goals of rehabilitation, *Arch Phys Med Rehabil* 65:427–430, 1984.
41. Thornton C, Maynard R: The economics of transitional employment and supported employment. In Berkowitz M, Hill MA, editors: *Disability and the labor market: economic problems, policies, and programs*, New York, 1989, ILR Press.
42. U.S. Census Bureau: *Americans with disabilities: 2010 report*, Washington, 2012, U.S. Census Bureau.
43. U.S. Census Bureau: *Facts for features: anniversary of Americans with Disabilities Act*, Washington, 2012, U.S. Census Bureau.
44. U.S. Department of Health and Human Services, Social Security Administration: *Redbook on work incentives*, Washington, 1992, Government Printing Office.
45. U.S. Department of Health and Human Services, Social Security Administration: *Social Security handbook*, ed 13, Washington, 1997, Government Printing Office.
46. U.S. Department of Justice, Civil Rights Division: *A guide to disability rights laws*, Washington, 2005, U.S. Department of Justice.
47. U.S. Equal Employment Opportunity Commission, U.S. Department of Justice: *Americans with Disabilities Act handbook (EEOC-BK-19)*, Washington, 1991, Government Printing Office.
48. U.S. General Accounting Office, Report to Congressional Requestors: *Vocational rehabilitation: improved information and practices may enhance*

state agency earnings outcomes for SSA beneficiaries, Washington, 2007, Government Printing Office.

49. U.S. General Accounting Office, Testimony before the Subcommittee on Select Education, Committee on Education and Labor, House of Representatives: *Vocational rehabilitation program: client characteristics, services received, and employment outcomes*, Washington, 1991, Government Printing Office.
50. Vachon RA: Employing the disabled, *Issues Sci Technol* winter:44–50, 1989-1990. www.ada.gov/guide.htm.
51. Vachon RA: Employment assistance and vocational rehabilitation for people with HIV or AIDS: policy, practice, and prospects. In O'Dell MW, editor: *HIV-related disability: assessment and management: physical medicine and rehabilitation: state of the art reviews*, Philadelphia, 1993, Hanley & Belfus.
52. Vachon RA: Inventing a future for individuals with work disabilities: the challenge of writing national disability policies. In Woods DE, Vandergoot D, editors: *The changing nature of work, society and disability: the impact on rehabilitation policy*, New York, 1987, World Rehabilitation Fund.
53. Verville R: The rehabilitation amendments of 1978: what do they mean for comprehensive rehabilitation? *Arch Phys Med Rehabil* 60:141–144, 1979.
54. Wehman P, Sherron P, Kregel J, et al: Return to work for people following severe traumatic brain injury: supported employment outcomes after five years, *Am J Phys Med Rehabil* 72:355–363, 1993.
55. Wilson RW: Do health indicators indicate health? *Am J Public Health* 71:461–463, 1981.
56. World Health Organization: *International classification of functioning, disability, and health*, Geneva, 2001, World Health Organization.
57. World Health Organization: *Towards a common language for functioning and disablement: ICIDH-2, the international classification of impairments, activities, and participation*, Geneva, 1998, World Health Organization.

CHAPTER 7

QUALITY AND OUTCOME MEASURES FOR MEDICAL REHABILITATION

Thiru M. Annaswamy, Amy Houtrow, Deepthi Saxena, Weibin Yang

Health care quality can be defined as providing safe and effective care that improves outcomes, optimizes health, and results in high patient satisfaction and quality of life. As such, delivering high quality of care should be a top priority for all rehabilitation professionals. In the past, the focus of practitioner and payer alike has been on efficiency of care and timely and appropriate reimbursement for services provided. However, in the current environment of health care reform in the United States, the focus has shifted from the fee-for-services model, in which volume of health care services rendered was rewarded, to emphasis on quality, safety, and outcomes as top priorities. Thus, the evaluation, measurement, and reporting of quality and outcomes have become the business of not only every health care institution and hospital but also every individual health care provider. This chapter discusses health care quality, evidence-based medicine (EBM), clinical practice guidelines (CPGs), outcome measures, performance measures, practice improvement, patient safety, and accreditation.

Access, affordability, and high quality in health care are the main objectives of the Patient Protection and Affordable Care Act of 2010. To accomplish these goals, the U.S. Department of Health and Human Services (HHS) has outlined a National Quality Strategy (NQS) that was developed through a collaborative and participatory process including input from a wide variety of stakeholders from all over the health care industry. Each agency with the HHS, including the Centers for Medicare and Medicaid Services (CMS), is required to develop a quality strategy and report on its progress and development to the HHS. The quality strategy of the CMS is depicted in Figure 7-1. One of the three key aims of the NQS is "better care," which is about improving quality of care and safety. To achieve these goals, the CMS and other health care insurance providers rely on simple, meaningful, efficient, and accurate measurements of health care quality and safety delivered by providers.

In addition to the CMS, several other governmental and many nongovernmental agencies monitor and oversee health care quality and safety. For example, the National Committee for Quality Assurance (NCQA) is a nonprofit organization focusing on health care quality. Health insurance plans all over the United States seek and obtain the NCQA seal of approval, which is a reflection of their high-quality health care and service. According to the NCQA, accredited plans cover 109 million Americans, or 70.5% of all Americans enrolled in health insurance plans.[24] The quality standards and performance measures used by the NCQA and other similar agencies are tools that individual clinicians and organizations use to self-report the quality and safety of health care they delivered. These measures are then used (1) to compare against local, regional, or national standards; (2) by consumers (patients), media, and other members of the public to compare clinicians, plans, and institutions against each other; and (3) compared with similar scores over time to identify opportunities for improvement, such as designing practice and performance improvement projects.

An important concept in health care quality is the concept of value. Despite a common objective of improving performance in health care delivery, there are several stakeholders in health care, sometimes with conflicting goals. This can lead to divergent approaches to improving health care quality, resulting from a lack of clarity and cohesion among stakeholders, resulting in slow rate of progress. Porter[28] makes a case for achieving high value to be the overarching goal of health care delivery, regardless of your perspective or role. Value, in this instance, was defined as health outcomes achieved per dollar spent. Health care outcomes were divided into three tiers: tier 1, health status achieved or retained; tier 2, process of recovery; and tier 3, sustainability of health. Porter[28] recommended that measuring "valuable" medical outcomes in any medical condition or disease must include at least one measure in each tier.

Quality of care is a measure of the performance on the six Institute of Medicine's (IOM) specified health care aims: (1) safety, (2) timeliness, (3) effectiveness, (4) equity, (5) efficiency, and (6) patient centeredness. Safety refers to "freedom from accidental injury" and it entails reducing errors. An error is the failure of a planned action to be completed as intended or the use of a wrong plan to achieve an aim. Based on performance metrics, providers, individual, organizations, and health plans are incentivized to improve quality through accountability, thereby achieving the IOM's six aims.[16]

Efforts to accurately and efficiently measure quality continue to grow rapidly. These measures are introduced to and adopted by health plans and clinicians based on several factors. Quality measures need to be meaningful and relevant to patients and society, as well as valid and based on sound evidence. The measurement of quality needs to be transparent, fair, and reliable. Reliability prevents accidents by good design and management to reduce conditions that cause errors. Transparency supports safety

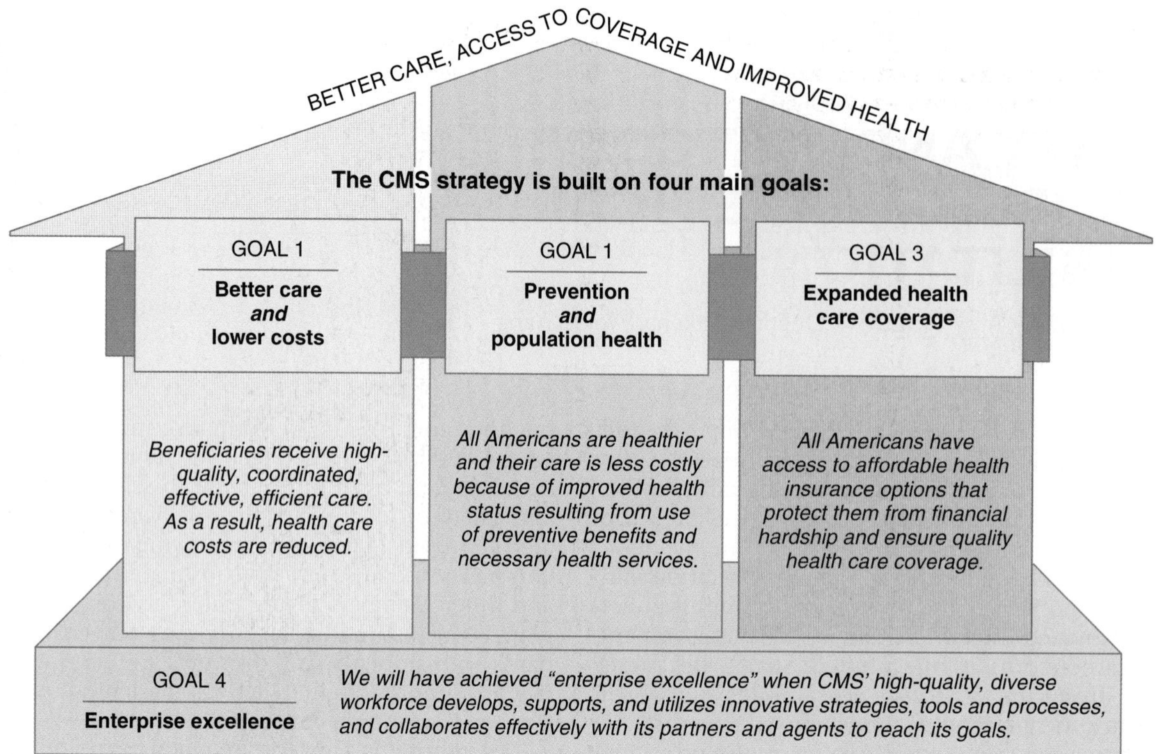

FIGURE 7-1 **Diagram of the Centers for Medicare and Medicaid Services' quality strategy.** (From Centers for Medicare and Medicaid Services: *Quality strategy 2013-beyond*, November 18, 2013. www.cms.gov/Medicare/Quality-Initiatives-Patient-Assessment-Instruments/QualityInitiativesGenInfo/Downloads/CMS-Quality-Strategy.pdf.)

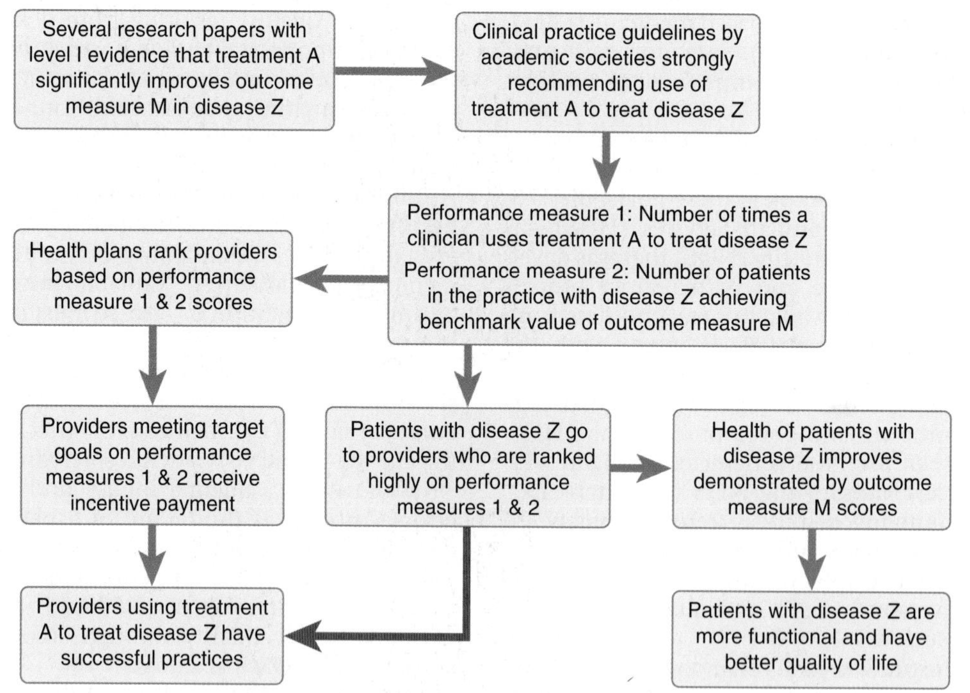

FIGURE 7-2 Schematic illustration of evidence-based quality measures achieving desired health outcomes.

by making the reliability of organizations visible by offering comparisons through public reporting of performance measures. Quality measurement must not place too much additional burden on clinicians, their institutions, or health plans. And, providing high quality and safe care has to be appropriately rewarded and incentivized.

Figure 7-2 illustrates a model of how evidence-based clinical research translates into quality measures that eventually lead to health improvement. Ideally, all quality measures are based on the highest possible quality of scientific evidence but, in reality, some measures are adopted because they are in the best interest of consumers and the society

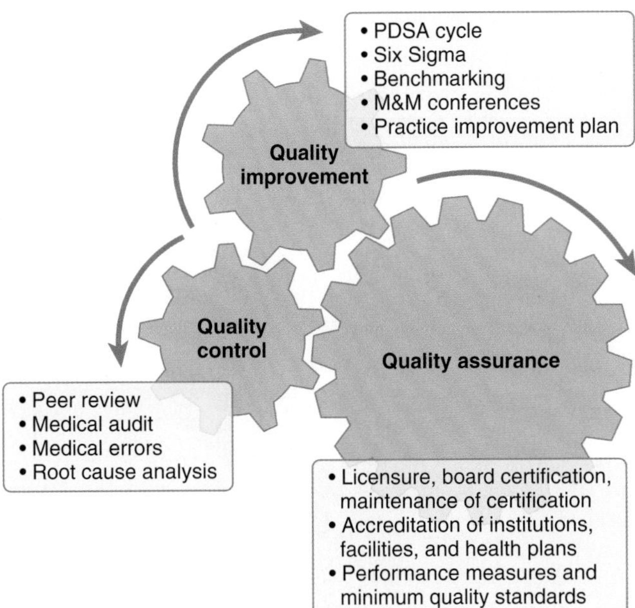

FIGURE 7-3 Health care quality perspectives. *M&M*, Morbidity and mortality; *PDSA*, plan-do-study-act.

at large, even if they are based on best available evidence and not the best possible evidence.

The ultimate objective is to deliver high-quality health care and rehabilitation and to improve the health of the population we serve. What one can do to turn the gears of the quality machine depends on the role they plan in the quality arena. One way to conceptualize the interplay between how efforts at providing high-quality health care can vary depending on one's perspective and role in the health care system is illustrated in Figure 7-3. Each aspect of quality and outcomes pertains to the practice of physical medicine and rehabilitation (PM&R).

Outcome Measures

Broadly speaking, an outcome is the result or end product that follows an activity, intervention, or situation. In health care, an outcome is the health consequence resulting from health care provided. The National Quality Measures Clearinghouse of the Agency of Healthcare Research and Quality (AHRQ) defines a clinical outcome as "a health state of a patient resulting from health care."[3] Thus, an outcome measure is the assessment of clinical outcomes through qualitative or quantitative means. Outcome measurement assesses what is important to the patient, provider, and health system and includes measurement of positive outcomes such as improved function and negative outcomes such as hospital-acquired skin breakdown. There are other outcomes that are the result of health care such as financial burden or family impact that are secondary to the primary clinical outcomes.

Types of Outcome Measures

Outcome measures should be distinguished from process measures. In 1966, Donabedian[12] conceptualized how information regarding health care quality may be gathered and modeled three dimensions of health care: structure, process, and outcome. The structure is the context in which health care is delivered; the buildings, equipment, resource, and the organizational characteristics. The structure of health care is often implicated as an upstream cause of a problem. For example, the current payment structure for health care services rewards interventions (higher payments for injections than regular office visits), which may incentivize providers to recommend and perform interventions. The process of health care is the additive sum of all actions and activities involved in the delivery of health care services. This includes how patients access health care, how patients are assessed and diagnoses made, the way in which treatments are rendered, and the activities involved in counseling, health education, and health promotion. For example, the process of making a diagnosis involves information gathering, conducting an examination, synthesizing data, eliciting additional information in the form of testing or additional consultations, and making an assessment. Finally, from the Donabedian perspective, the outcome is the effect of health care on a patient or a population. Because it is difficult to ascertain if an outcome is the direct result of health care, it is often challenging to accurately measure if, or how much of, an outcome is attributable to an intervention or health care process. Nonetheless, achieving a specific outcome is the reason why specific health care processes take place and therefore is essential to measure. Figure 7-4 illustrates the Donabedian concept with some rehabilitation relevant examples included in each dimension.

When considering the use of outcome measure(s), it is important to determine if the measure has been subject to evaluation of validity (how well the test measures what it intends to measure) and reliability (the degree to which the measure produces consistent and stable results). Consider the following example: a patient with spinal cord injury is diagnosed with a urinary tract infection (UTI) based on the presence of greater than 100,000 colony-forming units (CFU) on urine culture. The patient is prescribed a course of antibiotics and on repeat urine culture 2 weeks later, greater than 100,000 CFU were again found. The goal of the treatment with antibiotics was to eliminate the UTI. Based on the outcome measure of choice in this example, that is, repeat urine culture (a reliable and valid way to measure UTI), the outcome was not achieved. Thus, why was the desired outcome not achieved? It could be because of a deficit in the health care process, such as not prescribing an antibiotic to which the bacteria was susceptible or intending to call in a prescription to a pharmacy but not actually doing it. Alternatively, the patient may have decided to take the prescribed antibiotic for a day and then stop. Or, as is often the case, it is a combination of health care factors and patient factors that impact outcomes. Even in the situation where the patient prematurely stopped taking the prescribed medication, there may have been health care process factors contributing to the poor outcome such as not explaining how to take the medication or not labeling the medication in the patient's native language. Similarly, other health care processes could have been put in place to improve adherence, such as a telephone or a text check-in with the patient. As evidenced by this example, achieving a particular health care outcome,

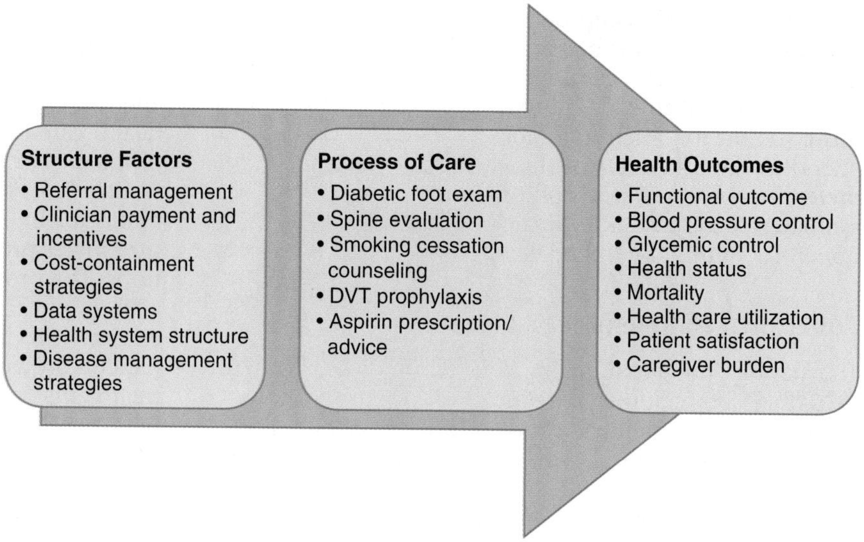

Structure Factors
- Referral management
- Clinician payment and incentives
- Cost-containment strategies
- Data systems
- Health system structure
- Disease management strategies

Process of Care
- Diabetic foot exam
- Spine evaluation
- Smoking cessation counseling
- DVT prophylaxis
- Aspirin prescription/advice

Health Outcomes
- Functional outcome
- Blood pressure control
- Glycemic control
- Health status
- Mortality
- Health care utilization
- Patient satisfaction
- Caregiver burden

FIGURE 7-4 Donabedian concept of health care dimensions and outcomes. *DVT,* Deep vein thrombosis.

even when the management plan is clear and the science behind the treatment is solid, is challenging.

Because attribution of outcomes to particular processes is challenging, many providers and hospitals prefer to measure processes instead of outcomes. Processes are easier to control and often are easier to measure. Often a process measure is used as a proxy for an outcome. Measuring 30-day readmission rates is an assessment of process but tends to be understood as representative of poor health outcomes. Thirty day readmission rates indicate that the health status of the population served was not stable enough and that the hospitalization process did not achieve its intended goal of assuring health. The reasons why patients are readmitted are many, including some that are well outside of the control of the hospital process during the original admission. In addition, readmission may be purposeful. Therefore it is necessary to consider the underlying reasons why patients may return to the hospital when setting process measure goals.

In general, when selecting a process measure it is important to determine that there is strong scientific evidence linking the process to the outcome. As an example, hand washing reduces nosocomial infections and therefore measuring hand hygiene policy adherence is an appropriate process measure. Additionally, there is no contraindication to hand hygiene and thus the process measure goal for achievement would be 100%. This is in contrast to the above example of 30-day readmission rates in which a target goal of 0% would be unrealistic and inappropriate. Another important consideration when picking a process measure is the ease of data collection. In the era of electronic health care records, queries of process are much easier to conduct. Electronic health care records allow for keyword searching, categorization of patients by diagnostic codes to determine if protocols were followed, tracking of orders, and monitoring the compliance of providers. Overall, the use of process measures helps guide quality improvement in a more straightforward manner than focusing on outcome measures.

Adjust for risk factors or stratify the population (risk stratification) when using outcome measures because it is challenging to account for all of the factors that may influence health outcomes. In a large number of patients or cases, it is often necessary to allow for the statistical adjustment of risk. Nonetheless, it is essential to measure outcomes of health care delivery to assure that the system is optimized to promote the health of the population served.

International Classification of Functioning, Disability, and Health

The PM&R community is well versed in outcome measurement, especially as it relates to functional outcomes and pain reduction. The International Classification of Functioning, Disability and Health (ICF) was released in 2001 as an update by the World Health Organization to their International Classification of Impairments, Disabilities and Handicaps.[18] In the ICF, function is understood as occurring at three levels: (1) at the level of the body part or system, (2) at the level of the person (activities), and (3) at the level of the person in society (participation). Function is the result of an interaction between an individual's health conditions and their environment and personal factors. Environmental and personal factors mediate function at each level in positive and negative ways.[20] In PM&R, functional outcomes can be measured at each of the levels described in the ICF and interventions may be geared at any one or more of these levels. The goal of a particular treatment may be to alleviate pain or improve range of motion (body functions and structures), or the goal may be to improve walking (an activity), or to improve the patient's attendance at work so that they do not lose their job (participation); or, as is often the case, the goal is to improve outcomes at all three levels. An intervention such as a joint injection to the knee may directly impact the patient's body function, but hopefully also impacts ambulation and therefore also the ability to participate in work. Prescribing a walker may directly impact ambulation and allow for improved work attendance, but does not impact knee function. Recommending work site adaptations may improve participation but not the patient's body function or their ability to ambulate. There is not a clear linear causal relationship between each level of functioning; therefore there is no guarantee that a prescribed treatment that was successful at impacting one level of functioning will impact another. Thus, when considering the outcome of interest to measure, it is important to attend to the influences of the patient's environment and preferences because an optimal outcome measure will evaluate all the results of health care delivery, which are hopefully minimally influenced by other factors.

Functional Independence Measure

Translating individual patients' outcome measurements to patient populations is relatively straightforward. The aggregation of individual patient outcome measurements allows providers and hospitals to benchmark and can help identify areas for improvement in health care delivery. The most familiar example of this in PM&R is the use of functional assessments for inpatient rehabilitation. Most inpatient rehabilitation programs submit their patients' Functional Independence Measure (FIM) scores to the Uniform Data System (UDS). The FIM instrument (Box 7-1) for adults and the WeeFIM instrument for children measure function in self-care, sphincter control, transfers, locomotion, communication, and social cognition with 18 different items. These items are scored on a 1 to 7 ordinal scale based on how much help is needed from another person to complete the tasks with a score of 1 indicating total assistance needed and a score of 7 indicating complete independence.[21] Tracking functional progress is a key activity in inpatient rehabilitation and aggregate data can speak volumes about how the facility and its providers are doing to promote function. The UDS provides report cards that detail FIM change (discharge FIM–admission FIM) and FIM efficiency (FIM change/length of stay) for patients by impairment grouping. It also tracks the percentage of patients that are successfully discharged to home. Therefore it is possible to track functional outcomes across the population served. With the data submitted to the UDS, it is possible to stratify by impairment type, age, gender, and insurance status. It is important to note that the change in function that a population of patients experience during rehabilitation is attributable to a host of factors outside of the control of the rehabilitation physician. Therefore FIM change and FIM efficiency may better outcome measures for the institution instead of the physician. However, there are statistical methods of controlling for other factors that would allow for the patients' FIM change and efficiency scores of one physician to be compared with other physicians' scores. This would allow for physician level benchmarking, but it requires a large sample size.

BOX 7-1

Functional Independence Measure Instrument

LEVELS		
	Independence 7—Complete independence (no helper, no setup, no device) 6—Modified independence (device, extra time, safety)	NO HELPER
	Modified Dependence 5—Supervision (standby assist, setup) 4—Minimal assist (patient = 75%+) 3—Moderate assist (patient = 50% to 74%)	HELPER NEEDED
	Complete Dependence 2—Maximal assist (patient = 25% to 49%) 1—Total assist (patient = less than 25%)	

DOMAINS

Self-Care
Eating
Grooming
Bathing
Dressing: upper body
Dressing: lower body
Toileting

Sphincter Control
Bladder management
Bowel management

Transfers
Bed, chair, wheelchair
Toilet
Tub, shower

Locomotion
Walk/wheelchair
Stairs

Motor Subtotal Rating

Communication
Comprehension
Expression

Social Cognition
Social interaction
Problem solving
Memory

Cognitive Subtotal Rating

Patient-Reported Outcomes

As described earlier, outcome measures may be classified by level of function. In the rest of medicine most of those measures focus on body function and structures, but in PM&R outcome measures frequently focus on activities with the use of assessment instruments such as the FIM. Additionally, outcome measures can be categorized by whether or not they are reported by the patient. Some outcome measures are self-reported and others require a clinician to administer. For example, health-related quality of life is patient-reported (patient-reported outcome [PRO]), whereas pulmonary function is provider-assessed (provider-based assessment). Both types of measures are important, valuable, and can be rigorously applied.

The Patient-Reported Outcomes Measurement Information System (PROMIS) is a system created by the National Institutes of Health that provides several reliable and precise PRO measures.[29] PROMIS measures are valid and dynamic; can efficiently study the self-reported health status of patients' physical, mental, and social well-being; and are particularly useful in chronic disease states and across a wide range of demographics. PROMIS has a core set of questions to assess common patient-relevant outcomes across a wide range of conditions in addition to specific item banks that focus on areas such as pain, fatigue, physical functioning, etc. The 10-item, 29-item, and 57-item PROMIS instruments are available to choose from depending on the time available and level of detail desired.

However, a particularly attractive feature of PROMIS is that it uses item response theory and computerized adaptive testing (CAT) that allows for statistical modeling to determine the most appropriate follow-up question to ask a patient based on their response to an initial question. Unlike a traditional questionnaire that is the same for all patients, a CAT instrument tailors questions to the specific patient.[19] If a patient's response to an initial question indicates that he/she is able to complete a task with little help, the CAT selects the next question with a more difficult task than the first task. If that response indicates higher difficulty in completing the more difficult task, the CAT selects the following question with an easier task than in the second question. This process continues until the computer identifies that the preprogrammed confidence interval has been met or the patient has answered the maximum number of items used to estimate the score.[19]

When considering outcome measures for children, it is important to keep in mind that outcome measures for adults may not be appropriate for children. Pediatric outcome measures should be age appropriate and ideally acknowledge the life course health perspective. Pediatric PROs should allow for child report and parental report. Note that both the child's and parents' perspectives are valuable and may differ from one another. The measurement of functional outcomes should be developmentally appropriate because the self-care, cognitive, and mobility expectations change substantially over the course of childhood. Because children live within the context of their families, it is also important to consider the measurement of family function, health, and well-being.

The AHRQ has quality indicators[1] for children receiving care in hospitals, a few of which are particularly relevant to rehabilitation care such as the number of stage III or stage IV ulcers as a secondary diagnosis per 1000 discharges or the number of central venous catheter–related bloodstream infections per 1000. Similarly, for the rehabilitation population, the outcome of ventilator-associated pneumonia is an important outcome of interest because hospital complications can lead to worsening debility and a delay in rehabilitative care.

Choosing Outcome Measures

The Rehabilitation Measures Database[31] has numerous measures listed that can be used to track outcomes in a patient population of interest. The database intends to provide clinicians with a list of instruments that can be used to screen and monitor patient progress. Outcome measures from this database can be geared at the individual patient or at groups of patients to assure overall quality of care. Some representative examples of outcome measures in various topic areas within PM&R are shown in Table 7-1.

When determining which outcome measure to use, careful consideration should be given to what group of patients the measure applies, and as described earlier how much of the outcome can be attributed to the intervention (Box 7-2). For example, the use of the 6-Minute Walk Test (6MWT) may be a better indicator of the success of a pulmonary rehabilitation program than the mobility section of the Craig Handicap Assessment and Reporting Technique (CHART), because there are a multitude of factors that impact CHART, whereas pulmonary rehabilitation is very likely to be a major driver of endurance and speed on the 6MWT. If one of the goals of pulmonary rehabilitation is to improve ambulation speed and endurance, testing clients prepulmonary and postpulmonary rehabilitation and calculating the average change on the 6MWT of the whole population would be a good measure of the quality and success of the program.

Assessing the outcomes of a pain management program could include a simple calculation of the average change achieved on the 10-Point Numerical Rating Pain Scale before and after treatment, but if the goal of the pain program is to improve pain control and impact function, then the use of the 10-Point Pain Scale would be inadequate to determine the outcome of the program. In this case, a measure of function would be necessary. It could be a general measure of function or one designed to measure functional status related to back pain, such as the Back Pain Functional Scale.[37,38] In this case, it may also be important to evaluate the feasibility of measuring the outcome.

Evidence and Guidelines

Definitions of Evidence-Based Medicine

In 1992, the Evidence-Based Medicine Working Group published a treatise on EBM calling it a "new paradigm for medical practice."[13] EBM has been defined as "the integration of best research evidence with clinical expertise and patient values."[34] By using EBM, physicians can address clinical questions by assessing the quality of evidence in medical information available in both basic science and clinical research.[40] Sackett and colleagues[33] also explained EBM as the integration of individuals' clinical expertise with the best available external evidence from systematic research and recommended using EBM as "the conscientious, explicit, and judicious use of current best evidence in making decisions about the care of individual patients."

Acknowledging the limitations of making clinical decisions, solely on one's knowledge of pathophysiology of disease processes, clinical intuition, and individual clinical experience, is important. However, with the EBM approach, one can use his or her individual clinical knowledge and acumen, careful history taking, and physical examination skills to then evaluate existing evidence, and combine it with the clinical information thus obtained in a systematic and reproducible manner.[13] The clinical decisions thus made with the EBM approach are more reproducible and free of bias than the traditional approach. Another advantage to this approach is that it allows for a clinician to adapt to and accept new scientific evidence more easily.

Table 7-1 Examples of Outcome Measures in Physical Medicine and Rehabilitation

	Measure and Description	ICF Domain(s)
Inpatient rehabilitation	Functional Independence Measure (FIM): contains 18 items assessing self-care, mobility, bowel and bladder management, cognition, language and social interaction	Activities/participation
Brain injury	Community Integration Questionnaire: contains 15 items assessing home and social integration and productive activity Ashworth Scale/Modified Ashworth Scale: measures spasticity. Can be used to assess responsiveness to medication	Activities/participation Body functions/structures
Spinal cord injury	Spinal Cord Independence Measure: assesses self-care, respiratory and sphincter management, and mobility Spinal Cord Injury Functional Ambulation Inventory: observational gait assessment evaluating parameters of gait, assistive device use, and temporal distance	Body functions/structures Activities/participation Activities/participation
Musculoskeletal medicine/pain	Medical Outcomes Study Short Form 36 (SF-36): physical and mental composite domains Numeric Pain Rating Scale: 10-point scale; 0 = no pain and 10 = the most intense pain imaginable	Activities/participation Body functions/structures
Pediatric rehabilitation	WeeFIM: companion measure to the FIM Glasgow Outcome Scale Extended Pediatric Version (GOS-E Peds): used in pediatric traumatic brain injury and evaluates consciousness, independence in and out of the home, school, social and leisure activities, family and friendships, and return to normal life	Activities/participation Body functions/structures Activities/participation
Stroke	Rivermead Mobility Index: assesses mobility after stroke with 14 self-report measures and one direct observation measure Four Square Step Test: assesses dynamic balance	Activities/participation Activities/participation
Amputation/limb deficiency	10-Meter Walk Test: measures time to walk set distance Medicare K Levels: estimates functional ability and which prosthesis would be most appropriate	Activities/participation Activities/participation
Pulmonary rehabilitation	Saint George's Respiratory Questionnaire: addresses pulmonary symptoms, activities, and impact of disease on daily life 2-Minute or 6-Minute Walk Test: measure of endurance	Body functions/structures Activities/participation Activities/participation
Spine	Oswestry Disability Index: addresses functional disabilities commonly seen in spine patients	Activities/participation

ICF, International Classification of Functioning, Disability, and Health.

With the availability of new research findings challenging traditionally held clinical beliefs, one then does not need to completely reinvent themselves clinically, but rather apply the new evidence at the appropriate point in their clinical decision-making algorithm to make corresponding changes to their clinical practice.

Assessing, Evaluating, and Applying Evidence

Sackett and colleagues[34] recommend the application of EBM with a simple and straightforward approach to answer any clinical question: (1) define a clinical question, (2) find the evidence that will help answer the question, (3) assess whether this evidence is valid and important, and (4) apply the evidence to the patient.

For PM&R clinicians trying to apply available scientific evidence to their practice, this means that, first, they would need to be aware of the existing evidence base in the topic area of their interest. In topic areas where there are few published research articles, this task can be accomplished by performing a basic literature search and assessing the evidence base of the intervention in the articles reviewed. However, as is often the case, several published articles exist in the topic area of interest, frequently, with conflicting results. In such an instance, a review article published in this area often reveals a summary of evidence collated from published research in the area of interest.

BOX 7-2

Important Questions to Ask When Determining Which Outcome Measure to Use

- What is my outcome of interest? And to whom is this outcome important?
- What level of function does the intervention intend to address (body functions and structures, activities, and participation)?
- For whom will the outcome measure be used (individual patients or groups of patients)?
- Who will be assessed by the outcome measure (a hospital, a practice, a program, a provider)?
- What is the validity of my potential measure of choice?
- What is the reliability of my potential measure of choice?
- Is the outcome measure sufficiently responsive to a change? Is there a ceiling or floor effect that may limit the use of the measure?
- What is the feasibility of using my potential measure of choice?
- Is the outcome measure patient-reported or clinician-assessed?
- What are the other factors besides the intervention that could influence the outcome? What number of patients would I need to have to adequately control for those other factors in statistical analyses?

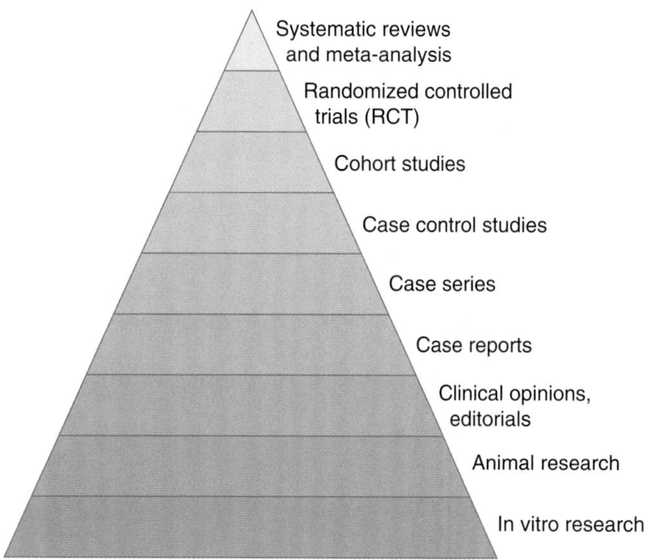

FIGURE 7-5 Evidence-based research pyramid.

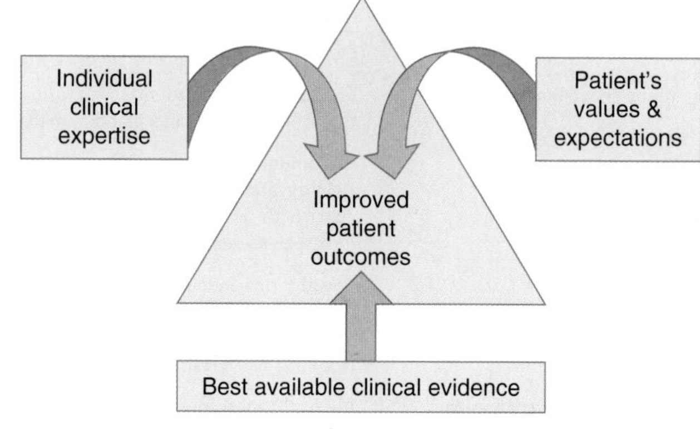

FIGURE 7-6 Evidence-based triad.

In general, the level of evidence provided by a published article can be determined from the level of evidence hierarchy (Figure 7-5). However, one can also appraise the level of evidence of a research article with evidence tables. The Oxford Center for Evidence-Based Medicine has an easy-to-use level of evidence table that can be employed to determine the level of evidence of a published article.[26] It is widely accepted and well regarded in the scientific community. The table adopted by the American Academy of Physical Medicine and Rehabilitation (AAPMR) has five levels, for each of four types of studies: (1) therapeutic, (2) prognostic, (3) diagnostic, and (4) economic or decision modeling.[41] Using either table, one can evaluate the level of evidence of the articles they review to research a clinical question. Once the clinician is aware of the evidence, secondly, he/she would need to then "conscientiously, explicitly, and judiciously" apply such evidence in making clinical decisions about the care of individual patients.

For a PM&R clinician reading an original research article or a review article and wondering how it might alter the management of a specific patient in question, another potentially useful EBM concept is the "evidence-based triad" discussed by Glasziou et al.[15] This concept provides a guide for deciding on the applicability of evidence to individual patients by seeking common ground in the triad of (1) clinical impression based on individual clinical expertise, (2) best available external evidence, and (3) the patient's unique values and expectations (Figure 7-6).

Another EBM concept that has been discussed in the medical literature in the context of patient management is called patient-oriented evidence that matters (POEM).[35,36] The POEM strategy recommends that once a clinician has assessed evidence they then critically appraise the evidence for its validity (do the findings validly approximate the reality?) and clinical applicability (is it relevant to their patient?). Subsequently, the clinician is recommended to discuss whether the evidence found answers to their clinical question and, if so, how it might alter the management of the patient in question. The POEM strategy can direct clinicians whether an intervention or procedure helps patients live better, directly and without the need for extrapolation. This type of information may guide a clinician directly with regard to whether or not the evidence reviewed merits a change in practice pattern.

When it comes to the use of EBM to answer a clinical diagnostic decision-making question, the following stepwise approach has been recommended.[42] Step 1: Define a clinical question and its four components: patient, intervention, comparison, and outcome. Step 2: Find the available evidence that will help answer the question. Step 3: Assess whether this evidence is valid and important. Step 4: Apply the evidence to the patient. This step includes assessing whether the test can be used, determining whether it will help the patient, finding whether the study patients are similar to the patient in question, determining a pretest probability, and deciding if the test will change one's management of the patient (Figure 7-7).

Clinical Practice Guidelines

CPGs are systematically developed written statements, made after a systematic evaluation of available evidence, and intended to assist practitioners and patients make appropriate decisions about health care in specific conditions or circumstances. Broadly speaking, the purpose of CPGs are: (1) to describe the most appropriate care based on the best available evidence; (2) to reduce inappropriate variation in practice for a specified condition; (3) to provide a more rational basis for interventions and referrals; (4) to promote efficient use of health care resources; (5) to act as a point of focus for quality control and audit; (6) to highlight shortcomings of existing literature and suggest appropriate future research; and (7) to provide an impetus for continuing education.

The schematic shown in Figure 7-8 provides a model for how evidence-based guidelines are created. The IOM, in response to a request from the U.S. Congress, came up with a report on the best methods to be used in developing CPGs that are rigorous and trustworthy. The IOM's eight standards for developing CPGs are considered the "gold standard" that every CPG aims to reach.

The National Guideline Clearinghouse (NGC) is a useful website to find relevant CPGs to suit one's needs. It is a public resource published online by the AHRQ.[2] Several rehabilitation relevant guidelines can be found

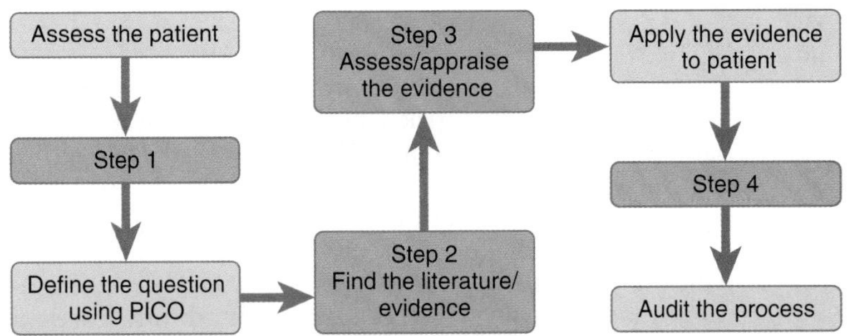

FIGURE 7-7 Incorporating evidence-based medicine into clinical practice. *PICO*, P—Patient, problem, or population; I—intervention; C—comparison, control, or comparator; O—outcomes.

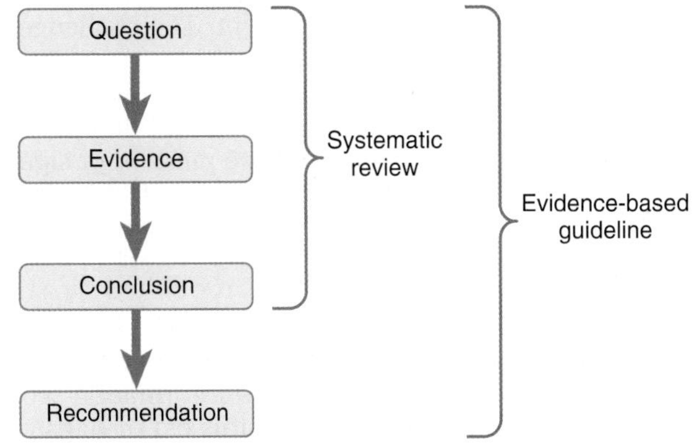

FIGURE 7-8 Model for creation of an evidence-based guideline.

online at NGC. CPGs critical to the field of PM&R that are developed, advocated, or/and endorsed by the AAPMR are also available for review.[5]

CPGs have been used in pediatrics for decades. The American Academy of Pediatrics has published seven since 2011. Perhaps the most relevant one for the rehabilitation physician is the guideline for attention deficit hyperactivity disorder.[11] The American Academy of Neurology[4] also has several guidelines that are relevant to pediatric rehabilitation medicine. For example, they recently developed guidelines for the evaluation and management of sports concussion that were published in 2013.[14] The James M. Anderson Center for Health Systems Excellence at Cincinnati Children's Hospital also provides topic-specific evidence-based care recommendations.[17] At the time of publication, there were several evidence-based care recommendations relevant to *pediatric rehabilitation medicine* including, but not limited to, lower extremity orthoses for children with hemiplegic cerebral palsy, constraint-induced movement therapy, coordination of outpatient rehabilitative care for patients with traumatic brain injury and their families, and serial casing of the lower extremities.

Performance Measures and Metrics

Performance measurement is a way to compute whether and how often the health care system does what it should. The result of a measure is a ratio or a percentage, which helps to compare providers and benchmark local and national performance.

The "measure" formula: Number who had a specific treatment/Number eligible for treatment = %.

Therefore development of performance metrics helps in transforming health care quality by measuring sustained gains obtained with improvement methodologies to create data-driven processes in organizations. To pursue this change objectively, current measurement emphasizes not only collaborative but also a multidisciplinary approach involving physicians, nurses, therapists, pharmacists, and all categories of clinicians and nonclinicians. Stakeholders who support and drive this change by reporting on quality and on the patient safety culture in hospitals include local and regional purchasers, payers, consumer representatives, and communities.

Measure Development

Development of performance metrics needs financial, human, technological, education, and a learning environment over long time lines to reduce variation in care delivery across the United States. The Annual National Healthcare Quality Report (NHQR) released in May of 2014 reported that 70% of recommended quality care is actually received with wide variations among different states. Although the measures used in the report included a wide range of structure, process, and outcome measures, several important dimensions of quality are not currently measured. These dimensions pertaining to rehabilitation medicine that currently need measure development include, but are not limited to (1) pain reduction and functional improvement in patients undergoing back surgery, total joint replacements, and other orthopedic procedures; and (2) rate of decline in the function of patients with multiple sclerosis.

Tracking the rate of change over 4 years of data, the NHQR found that although the quality of hospital care is improving, the quality of ambulatory care is slow to improve. There are not only fewer measures to trend limitations in activity but also fewer showed improvement in activity resulting from the larger standard errors of estimates of people with activity limitations. Not only is the gap between best possible care and what is routinely delivered substantial but also access to health care worsened from 2002 to 2010, leveling off in 2011. These statistics from the NHQR track health care quality and report everyday experiences of patients and their providers across the United States. The number of people with disabilities, which is currently 20% of the adult population, is expected to rise with the increase in life expectancy attributable to the aging of Baby Boomers. This increase in people born with disabilities and those who acquire disabilities, particularly in the context of multiple chronic conditions and disparities in care, requires the continued development of ways to measure performance toward the NQS. Development of new measures becomes particularly critical because these reports retire those measures that reach a 95% threshold. Additionally, the CMS uses different criteria such as lack of applicability across specialties to remove measures, further compelling the development of new performance metrics, which is challenging.

Challenges in Measure Development

The development of performance measures is difficult for several reasons.

Desirable Attributes of a Measure Are Complex

By consensus from the American Medical Association (AMA), The Joint Commission (TJC), and the NCQA, a performance measure must: (1) address a topic area that is of high priority to maximize the health of persons or populations, be financially important, and demonstrate a variation in care and/or potential improvement; (2) have usefulness in improving patient outcomes based on established clinical recommendations and be potentially actionable, meaningful to, and interpretable by the user; (3) have a measure design with well-defined specifications, documented reliability and validity, and allow risk while being feasible, confidential, and publicly available.

Measure Testing That Is Critical to the Process of Its Development Is Elaborate

Measure testing must be conducted in a variety of practice settings. For example, ambulatory measures must be tested in solo to large-sized practices. Measure testing requires the involvement of all stakeholders, patients, and providers including insurers, technology providers, individual or groups of clinicians, and health care organizations.

Measures are Tested by Different Agencies Before They are Vetted

The AMA's Physician's Consortium for Process Improvement[27] is one such organization that recommends that performance measures must be tested in the areas of: (1) needs assessment, (2) feasibility and implementation, (3) reliability, (4) validity, (5) unintended consequences, and (6) applications.

Measure Development Necessitates Extensive Costs Through the Intricate Life Cycle of the Measure

For example, the life cycle of a measure endorsed by the National Quality Forum,[25] which sets priorities for performance measurement entails: (1) studying evidence-based data on disease prevalence; (2) using an assessment tool to study disease severity; (3) applying local initiative to measure improvement with process; (4) leading change toward improvement locally; (5) public reporting on local performance; (6) endorsing the measure as a national consensus standard; (7) retooling the measure for use in electronic health care records; and (8) including the meaningful use program of the CMS so that measure adoption is widespread and leads to improvement in patient care.

Risk Adjustment[22]

Different hospitals and other provider organizations serve patients with varying risk factors. These risk factors are patient characteristics that associate a statistically significant level of variance to allow valid comparisons across providers and organizations. Factors include age, gender, race, admitting diagnoses, socioeconomic status, level of education, social support systems, substance use, community or facility from which the patient is admitted or sent to the provider, comorbidities, interactions between multiple diseases, and organ systems, and so on. Risk adjustment requires several steps with a large reference population to compute the weight of each risk factor that affects the outcome of care of a particular patient. The challenge in this process is further compounded by the need for statistical testing to compare very specific predicted versus actually observed differences in performance and outcomes to determine whether these variations are random or significant. Such a specific level of standardization helps with identifying priorities in performance improvement.

Privacy, Security, and Databases[8]

Because public reporting is done with multiple systems and methods for transparency, with measures collected in databases or registries, to keep patient information secure from external threats, particularly in this era of transition to electronic health care records across providers, training and monitoring of providers is required. This increases in complexity when multiple stakeholders and cross-cutting measures are used, making measuring performance a very necessary but challenging task.

Strategically Improving Health Care Quality with Performance Measurement

Despite the various challenges, performance measurement is imperative because it helps to provide quality at a lesser cost. Performance measurement aligns providers to the NQS' six priorities: (1) safer care by reducing harm in the delivery of care; (2) engaging each person and family in their own care; (3) promoting effective communication and coordination of care; (4) promoting the most effective prevention and treatment of the leading causes of mortality, starting with cardiovascular disease; (5) promoting wide use of best practices to enable healthy living in communities; and (6) developing and spreading new health care delivery models for affordable quality care for individuals, families, employers, and governments.

There is a shift in paradigm from performance improvement being valuable to hospital performance improvement to aligning providers by its evidence-based data, which all clinicians relate to. This is particularly useful in aligning multidisciplinary teams when they jointly review evidence-based data that performance metrics provide to meet their common goal of improving clinical processes.

Performance metrics can be used as "clinical intelligence" with data, information, and technology to provide decision support, particularly in the management of chronic diseases. Enterprise resource planning can for the time being, at least theoretically, integrate databases so that clinical information is available to across points of care, to individuals and communities, and local health care networks, ultimately leading to the evolution of a national network.

In reality, these principles currently being adopted in health care are not new because performance measurement is in the line with the Six Sigma cycle of define, measure, analyze, improve, and control, known to other industries.[9] Although the development of measures and their cycles are similar to this and "lean management," it is necessary that the use of these tools is accompanied by a cultural change across health care. A change in thinking to seek and share organized information for patient safety is imperative as we move toward tying payment with quality.

Performance measures are a source for purchasers and payers to force quality while containing expenditure of health care with value-based purchasing. Since 2008, payers such as WellPoint and Aetna have followed in Medicare's footsteps to differential reimbursement based on measurement and comparison. Performance metrics support pay-for-performance initiatives and accreditation in health plans.

Pediatric-specific performance measures are also generally lacking compared with the plethora of measures available for adults. The patient-centered medical home measures now include the word "family" to acknowledge how optimal care is delivered to children.[30] And the Healthcare Effectiveness Data and Information Set (HEDIS) includes measures on childhood immunization rates, access to primary care providers, height and weight screening with nutritional counseling, and well-child care.

In 2012, results from the National Expert Panel for the Development of Pediatric Rehabilitation Quality Care Indicators were published.[32] The Panel developed process measures for the inpatient rehabilitation management of children with traumatic brain injury. These measures were classified into the following domains: general management; family-centered care; cognitive-communication, speech, language, and swallowing impairments; gross and fine motor skill impairments; neuropsychological, social, and behavioral impairments; school reentry; and community integration.[32]

Safety and Accreditation

Health plan accreditation standards are used to ensure that they are performing on par with industry standards in quality by measuring their performance. Not only do consumers use these data to compare plans and shop but other purchasers such as employers and state and federal regulators use these performance metrics so that they pay for performance. The National Committee for Quality Assurance (NCQA), Utilization Review Accreditation Commission, and TJC are such agencies. These agencies rank insurance plans by using tools such as the Medicare Health Outcomes Survey in which all managed care organizations holding Medicare Advantage contracts are required to enroll in HEDIS. The AHRQ's Consumer Assessment of Health Providers and Systems is another such tool.

The Leapfrog Group advocates for quality and safety in hospitals with transparency in pricing and reports on several performance measures, which compare hospitals, including preventing medication errors, appropriate intensive care unit staffing, steps to avoid harm, managing serious errors, safety-focused scheduling, and hospital-acquired conditions. The peer-reviewed Hospital Safety Score methodology grades hospitals as A, B, C, D, or F based on how safe they are for patients by measuring infections, injuries, and medical and medication errors that frequently cause harm or death during a hospital stay. Performance metrics data from the CMS is available through its Hospital Compare website.[23]

Public reporting by the CMS on nursing homes and measuring the performance of home and community-based services with financial incentives have been steps toward improving health care quality in the long term and in postacute care arenas. Physician performance metrics are gathered through the Physician Quality Reporting System, which are tied into financial incentives and penalties. The public reporting of performance metrics is a driver of health care quality because it encourages transparency and accountability.

Value Equation

Quality measurement dates back to Donabedian's paper in 1966,[12] which categorizes quality into structure, process, and outcomes. Measurement was started to improve quality in 1998 when TJC launched its ORYX initiative, the first national program for the measurement of hospital quality. Subsequently, a study was published in the *Journal of Hospital Medicine*, in 2011, which had studied 4000 hospitals from 2004 to 2008 for performance trends and TJC association. The study showed that TJC-accredited hospitals outperformed nonaccredited hospitals in nationally standardized quality measures such as heart failure and pneumonia. However, because these data were plugged into the value equation, it became necessary to ascertain whether accreditation signifies higher quality and improvement in quality or whether it also helps with performance that increases the value of care provided.

The value of care is now an important consideration because performance measurement is a complex and expensive process. Therefore, the focus of measurement has shifted to "accountability" measures, which achieve the goal of maximizing health benefits to patients.[10] Accountability measures must meet four criteria. (1) Research: There must be randomized controlled trials and more than one study providing scientific evidence to demonstrate that a given process of care improves health care outcomes (either directly or by reducing the risk of adverse outcomes). (2) Proximity: The process being measured must be connected to the outcome it impacts. (3) Accuracy: The measure should be able to assess whether an evidence-based process is effectively delivered for improvement to occur. (4) Adverse Effects: The measure should minimize or eliminate unintended adverse effects.

Measures that meet all four criteria are now used for accreditation, public reporting, and pay-for-performance. Performance measurement with these "accountability" measures has transformed passive payers and consumers into purchasers of efficient high-quality health care, that is, value-based purchasing.

Value = Quality or Outcomes/Cost

Seemingly simple, this equation has a potential to cause confusion if it is not understood that the denominator "cost" refers to the total costs of the full episode of care, not the cost of individual services.[28] Measuring value in the context of improvement in the value of health care by way of performance metrics allows decisions on which services need more spending so that the need for others is reduced.

Today, higher cost of care is also associated with poorer quality of care. However, it is imperative to be aware that improvement in value cannot be done by cost containment alone. A cultural change involving innovation and accountability is critical to improving value in health care delivery. Such an improvement is possible with performance measurement because of the transparency with which performance metrics are reported.

BOX 7-3

American Board of Physical Medicine and Rehabilitation Maintenance of Certification Components and Competencies

Four Components

- Professional standing (license)
- Lifelong learning and self-assessment (Continuing Medical Education)
- Cognitive expertise (examination)
  - Practice performance (Performance in Practice/Practice Improvement Project)

Six Competencies

- Medical knowledge
- Patient care
- Interpersonal and communication skills
- Professionalism
- Practice-based learning and improvement
  - Systems-based practice

Maintenance of Certification and Quality Improvement

The American Board of Physical Medicine and Rehabilitation (ABPMR) is one of the 24 member boards of the American Board of Medical Specialties (ABMS). Since 1993, all certificates issued by the ABPMR have been valid for 10 years, at which point diplomates are required to "recertify." In recent years, the recertification process has been elevated to a more involved process of Maintenance of Certification (MOC). The change has taken place in an effort to assure the public that board-certified specialists have remained current with evolving knowledge, that their practices meet acceptable quality and safety standards, and that they are recognized and respected as specialists by their patients and peers. This ongoing process is designed to verify a diplomate's credentials, licensure, professional standing, and practice performance. MOC is intended to be a quality driver, but its relevance and value to society is often questioned.

The ABPMR MOC program has one primary MOC and three specialty MOCs (Pain Medicine, Pediatric Rehabilitation Medicine, and Spinal Injury Medicine). The program provides a mechanism for measuring, on a continual basis, a diplomate's competencies in the PM&R specialty. To maintain time-limited certification, diplomates are required to complete four components that measure the six competencies (Box 7-3).

The ABPMR states that the standards of certification are distinct from those of licensure. Possession of a board certificate does not indicate total qualification for practice privileges, nor does it imply exclusion of other physicians not thus certified.

Diplomates' MOC participation status, either "Meeting MOC Requirements" or "Not Meeting MOC Requirements," will be available to the public when the searchable "Verify a Physician's Certification" tool on the ABPMR website is used.

Although everyone is in agreement that the public interest is the foremost concern, it is important for physicians to maintain ongoing competence. This has ranged from minor to major controversy on whether or not the competency evaluation should be through the MOC program, how to develop and demonstrate competence, and whether the MOC program is cost-effective.[39] With the development of new technologies in the medical field and the ever-changing complexity of the health care delivery system, there is a need to assure the public of the safety and quality of health care providers. According to the ABPMR, through its MOC program, the ABPMR supports its diplomates' dedication to lifelong learning and assures the public the quality of its diplomates.

Even though the MOC program sounds rational and generally seems well designed to advance medical knowledge and promote quality improvement of the health care providers, the effectiveness, meaningfulness, and cost-effectiveness of the MOC program has not been proven scientifically.[39] The eventual goal is that with greater transparency and accountability, a board-certified diplomate of any specialty will be held to equal standards. Through the MOC program, board-certified physicians are expected to advance the quality and standard of health care nationwide. The ABMS believes that higher standards mean better care and considers the MOC program an essential element of this process.

Quality Improvement and Practice Improvement

One of the six competencies of the ABPMR MOC program is to evaluate practice-based learning and improvement. ABPMR diplomates are encouraged to demonstrate the ability to investigate and evaluate the care of patients, to appraise and assimilate scientific evidence, and to continuously improve patient care based on constant self-evaluation and lifelong learning. Diplomates with time-limited certificates issued before 2012 must complete a minimum of one practice performance project during the 10-year MOC cycle. Diplomates with time-limited certificates issued in 2012 and beyond must complete two ABPMR-approved practice performance projects (one in years 1 to 5 and one in years 6 to 10) during the 10-year MOC cycle (Table 7-2).[7]

Table 7-2 Activities Required to Recertify

Certificate Issue Date	Activities Required to Recertify
Before 2012	• Licensure • Complete and report a minimum of 300 Category I CME credits • Complete at least four ABPMR-approved self-assessment activities • Examination • Complete at least one ABPMR-approved PIP
2012 and beyond	• Licensure • Complete and report 150 Category I CME credits in years 1 to 5 and 6 to 10 of the MOC cycle (for a total of 300 Category I CME credits) • Complete an average of 8 CME credits per year (for a total of 40 CME credits in years 1 to 5 and 40 CME credits in years 6 to 10) involving ABPMR-approved self-assessments • Examination • Complete two ABPMR-approved PIPs (one in years 1 to 5 and one in years 6 to 10)

ABPMR, American Board of Physical Medicine and Rehabilitation; *CME*, Continuing Medical Education; *MOC*, Maintenance of Certification; *PIP*, Performance in Practice/Practice Improvement Project.

The ABPMR has provided three options for fulfilling the practice improvement project (PIP) requirement[6]: the Clinical Care Practice Improvement Project (Clinical Care PIP), the AAPMR Practice Improvement Project (PIP), and the American Association of Neuromuscular and Electrodiagnostic Medicine (AANEM) Performance in Practice: Electrodiagnostic Report Writing. It seems there is confusion regarding the term "PIP," even though it is always used for step IV of MOC. Although most of the members of the ABMS use "PIP" for "Performance in Practice," the ABPMR and AAPMR use the abbreviation "PIP" for "Practice Improvement Process."

Practice Improvement Project Options

Clinical Care Practice Improvement Project (Clinical Care PIP)

The ABPMR has developed a self-guided program to allow the individual diplomate the opportunity to demonstrate clinical care improvement within his/her own practice through the use of a Continuous Quality Improvement (CQI) process. Compared with the other two options, this option is free of charge. The diplomates will however not receive Continuing Medical Education (CME) credit.

Using CQI methodology, the diplomate develops a specific project to improve an element of the practice. The diplomate has the freedom to select an area of performance improvement that impacts the quality of patient care, either directly or indirectly. It follows a process that is very similar to the CQI protocol: plan-do-check-act. The diplomate identifies an area that needs to be improved, sets up measurable outcome, plans the procedures of improvement, implements the changes, and reassesses the outcome data. Baseline data and follow-up data are collected to measure impact of the change. Completion of this project will demonstrate proficiency in practice-based learning/improvement and in systems-based practice. The outcomes of the project should show improvement in practice performance.

Diplomates will report the results of objective measurements taken before and after the implementation of corrective actions. Measurements should be quantifiable, with actual data presented. Completed Clinical Care PIPs will be evaluated according to the ABPMR Clinical Care PIP Criteria by the ABPMR.

AAPMR Practice Improvement Project

The second option of PIP is developed by the AAPMR. The diplomate is guided through an EBM process by answering a series of set questions: self-evaluation of an issue, practice-based assessment of the issue, and self-selection of three areas for improvement from a predetermined list based on answers to the self-evaluation and practice-based assessment questions. The diplomate creates an improvement program specific to his/her practice with a variety of tools and resources available.

The diplomate needs to pay a fee for this service and earns 20 CME credit hours. PIPs are available on limited clinical topics such as low back pain, stroke, deep vein thrombosis, and osteoporosis. The AAPMR is working on developing other topics.

AANEM Performance in Practice: Electrodiagnostic Report Writing

The third option of PIP is provided by the AANEM. It is designed to enhance quality patient care by focusing on providing quality electrodiagnostic services. The PIP was formed from an expert consensus document created by AANEM members. The diplomate needs to pay a fee for this service and earns 20 CME credit hours.

According to the AANEM, the PIP module will help physicians evaluate the quality of their electrodiagnostic reports and identify areas of potential improvement and implement the action for changes. The PIP includes three steps: preimplementation chart review, a toolkit for continued learning in 30 days, and postimplementation chart review. It has a feedback module that allows the diplomate to solicit patient and peer feedback. Diplomates are required to review a minimum of five health care records in both preimplementation and postimplementation chart review sections. Diplomates will grade themselves based on the criteria provided.

The AANEM requires diplomates to maintain confidential files because the ABPMR could request documentation at any time. The PIP can be downloaded from the AANEM website. Both AANEM members and nonmembers will be able to access the PIP activity with different prices.

Although the PIP program is well structured, patient and peer feedback solicitation can be time-intensive.

Summary

We are in a state of turbulent transition from volume-based health care to value-based health care. The two main drivers of this change are increasing costs and decreasing or stagnant quality. For this transition to succeed and eventually lead to efficient, safe, effective, and valuable health care, all rehabilitation professionals including physiatrists must work together with a unified focus on better quality and outcomes for our patients. Practicing safe and evidence-based medicine, with unchanging focus on value and outcomes, can help us get there. A fair, transparent, valid, and objective measurement of quality and safety can be embraced by everyone. Together, we can evolve an accessible, affordable, high-quality health care system that can be valuable and sustainable long term.

REFERENCES

1. Agency for Healthcare Research and Quality: Pediatric quality indicators. www.qualityindicators.ahrq.gov/Modules/pdi_resources.aspx, 2014.
2. Agency of Healthcare Research and Quality: National Guideline Clearinghouse. www.guideline.gov/, 2014.
3. Agency of Healthcare Research and Quality: Selecting health outcome measures for clinical quality measurement. www.qualitymeasures.ahrq.gov/tutorial/HealthOutcomeMeasure.aspx, 2014.
4. American Academy of Neurology: Guidelines. www.aan.com/Guidelines, 2014.
5. American Academy of Physical Medicine and Rehabilitation: PM&R applicable guidelines. www.aapmr.org/research/practice-guidelines/Pages/Applicable-PMR-Guidelines.aspx, 2014.
6. American Board of Physical Medicine and Rehabilitation: MOC part IV practice performance—ABPMR-approved options. www.abpmr.org/diplomates/pp_options_table.html, 2014.
7. American Board of Physical Medicine and Rehabilitation: *Maintenance of certification: booklet of information*, Rochester, 2013, American Board of Physical Medicine and Rehabilitation.
8. Aspden P, Corrigan JM, Wolcott J, Erickson SM, Committee on Data Standards for Patient Safety, and Board on Health Care Services: *Patient safety: achieving a new standard for care (quality chasm)*, ed 1, Washington, 2004, National Academies Press.
9. Chassin MR: Is health care ready for Six Sigma quality?, *Milbank Q* 76:565–591, 1998.
10. Chassin MR, Loeb JM, Schmaltz SP, Wachter RM: Accountability measures–using measurement to promote quality improvement, *N Engl J Med* 363:683–688, 2010.
11. Disorder Subcommittee on Attention-Deficit/Hyperactivity, Improvement Steering Committee on Quality, Management, Wolraich M, Brown L, Brown RT, DuPaul G, et al: ADHD: clinical practice guideline for the diagnosis, evaluation, and treatment of attention-deficit/hyperactivity disorder in children and adolescents, *Pediatrics* 128:1007–1022, 2011.
12. Donabedian A: The quality of care. How can it be assessed?, *JAMA* 260:1743–1748, 1988.
13. Evidence Based Medicine Working Group: Evidence-based medicine: a new approach to teaching the practice of medicine, *JAMA* 268:2420–2425, 1992.
14. Giza CC, Kutcher JS, Ashwal S, et al: Summary of evidence-based guideline update: evaluation and management of concussion in sports: report of the Guideline Development Subcommittee of the American Academy of Neurology, *Neurology* 80:2250–2257, 2013.
15. Glasziou P, Guyatt GH, Dans AL, et al: Applying the results of trials and systematic reviews to individual patients, *ACP J Club* 129:A15–A16, 1998.
16. Institute of Medicine: *Crossing the quality chasm: a new health system for the 21st century*, Washington, 2001, National Academy of Sciences.
17. James M, Anderson Center for Health Systems Excellence: Evidence-based care recommendations. www.cincinnatichildrens.org/service/j/anderson-center/evidence-based-care/recommendations/default, 2014.
18. Jette AM: Toward a common language for function, disability, and health, *Phys Ther* 86:726–734, 2006.
19. Jette AM, Haley SM: Contemporary measurement techniques for rehabilitation outcomes assessment, *J Rehabil Med* 37:339–345, 2005.
20. Jette AM, Tao W, Haley SM: Blending activity and participation subdomains of the ICF, *Disabil Rehabil* 29:1742–1750, 2007.
21. Keith RA, Granger CV, Hamilton BB, Sherwin FS: The Functional Independence Measure: a new tool for rehabilitation, *Adv Clin Rehabil* 1:6–18, 1987.
22. Mainz J: Defining and classifying clinical indicators for quality improvement, *Int J Qual Health Care* 15:523–530, 2003.
23. Medicare: GOV, hospital compare. www.medicare.gov/hospitalcompare/search.html?AspxAutoDetectCookieSupport=1, 2014.
24. National Committee for Quality Assurance: About NCQA. www.ncqa.org/AboutNCQA.aspx, 2014.
25. National Quality Forum: An illustrative example. Lifecycle of a performance measure: depression remission at 6 months. http://public.qualityforum.org/Chart%20Graphics/Lifecycle%20of%20a%20Performance%20Measure%20-%20Depression%20Remission%20at%206%20months.pdf, 2012.
26. Oxford Center for Evidence-Based Medicine (OCEBM) Levels of Evidence Working Group: The Oxford 2011 Levels of Evidence, Oxford Centre for Evidence-Based Medicine. www.cebm.net/index.aspx?o=5653.
27. Physician Consortium for Performance Improvement: Measure testing protocol for Physician Consortium for Performance Improvement (PCPI) performance measures. www.ama-assn.org/resources/doc/cqi/pcpi-testing-protocol.pdf, 2007.
28. Porter ME: What is value in health care?, *N Engl J Med* 363:2477–2481, 2010.
29. Patient-Reported Outcomes Measurement Information System (PROMIS) Network Center: PROMIS: dynamic tools to measure health outcomes from the patient perspective. www.nihpromis.org.
30. Raphael JL, Sadof M, Stille CJ, et al: *Not just little adults: considerations for quality measures of child health care*, Rockville, 2014, National Quality Measures Clearinghouse.
31. Rehabilitation Institute of Chicago, Center for Rehabilitation Outcomes Research, and Northwestern University Feinberg School of Medicine Department of Medical Social Sciences Informatics Group: Rehabilitation measures database. www.rehabmeasures.org/default.aspx, 2014.
32. Rivara FP, Ennis SK, Mangione-Smith R, et al: Indicators National Expert Panel for the Development of Pediatric Rehabilitation Quality Care: quality of care indicators for the rehabilitation of children with traumatic brain injury, *Arch Phys Med Rehabil* 93:381–385, 2012.
33. Sackett DL, Rosenberg WM, Gray JA, et al: Evidence based medicine: what it is and what it isn't, *BMJ* 312:71–72, 1996.
34. Sackett DL, Straus SE, Richardson WS, et al: *Evidence-based medicine: how to practice and teach EBM*, ed 2, London, 2000, Churchill Livingstone.
35. Shaughnessy AF, Slawson DC: POEMs: patient-oriented evidence that matters, *Ann Intern Med* 126:667, 1997.
36. Shaughnessy AF, Slawson DC: What happened to the valid POEMs? A survey of review articles on the treatment of type 2 diabetes, *BMJ* 327:266, 2003.
37. Stratford PW, Binkley JM: A comparison study of the Back Pain Functional Scale and Roland Morris Questionnaire. North American Orthopaedic Rehabilitation Research Network, *J Rheumatol* 27:1928–1936, 2000.
38. Stratford PW, Binkley JM, Riddle DL: Development and initial validation of the Back Pain Functional Scale, *Spine (Phila Pa 1976)* 25:2095–2102, 2000.
39. Van Harrison R, Olson CA: Evolving health care systems and approaches to maintenance of certification, *J Contin Educ Health Prof* 33(Suppl 1):S1–S4, 2013.
40. Welch HG, Lurie JD: Teaching evidence-based medicine: caveats and challenges, *Acad Med* 75:235–240, 2000.
41. Wright JG, Swiontkowski MF, Heckman JD: Introducing levels of evidence to the journal, *J Bone Joint Surg Am* 85:1–3, 2003.
42. Zakowski L, Seibert C, Van Eyck S: Evidence-based medicine: answering questions of diagnosis, *Clin Med Res* 2:63–69, 2004.

CHAPTER 8

ELECTRODIAGNOSTIC MEDICINE

Timothy Dillingham, Michael Andary, Daniel Dumitru

Electrodiagnostic medicine and electrophysiologic testing are an extension of the history and physical examination tailored to the clinical scenario. A wide range of tests are available and it is incumbent on the electrodiagnostician to select those relevant to the clinical circumstances. The testing procedure may change as data are acquired and new findings interpreted. High-quality consultations are rendered by physicians with experience and technical competence coupled with an understanding of the peripheral nervous system. This chapter provides an overview of electrodiagnostic tests, the extent of such testing for different clinical scenarios based on guidelines, and the types of abnormalities one can expect to find with different neuromuscular disorders.

Clinical Assessment: History and Physical Examination

History

A directed history enables the electrodiagnostician to develop a conceptual framework for subsequent testing. The history should include the referral reason, information as to whether symptoms are confined to a single limb or more than one limb, and the characteristic, nature of, the duration and time of onset, of symptoms. Pain and numbness indicate that the sensory system is involved. Motor weakness without pain and numbness indicates primarily involvement of the motor system, motor axons, neuromuscular junction, or muscles. For patients with more generalized symptoms—that is, symptoms in more than one limb—the electrodiagnostician should inquire about other neurologic complaints, such as dyspnea, bladder urgency, dysphagia, dysphonia, and visual changes. Previous cervical or lumbar spine conditions, such as spinal stenosis or surgical interventions, should be noted. Activities that aggravate or relieve a patient's symptoms can often help differentiate musculoskeletal problems from entrapments, plexopathies, and radiculopathies. Hand numbness at night is associated with carpal tunnel syndrome.

Diabetes and alcohol are common causes of polyneuropathy in the United States, and an appropriate history should include questioning about such issues. Any family history of neurologic disorders is important to elicit for persons with generalized or unexplained symptoms. A brief recording of the person's work activities is often helpful to identify persons at risk for overuse syndromes.

Important past medical history includes any history of malignancy, chemotherapy, or radiation, because these conditions and treatments can have peripheral neurologic implications. Previous surgeries for entrapment neuropathies, such as ulnar transposition or carpal tunnel release, should be ascertained. For instance, a transposed ulnar nerve complicates nerve conduction calculations for the segment across the elbow because measurement is less precise, and stimulus sites above and below the elbow can be more difficult to find. Whether a person is thrombocytopenic, has bleeding disorders, or is receiving anticoagulants should also be noted.

Physical Examination

Strength, sensation, and reflex testing are the most important aspects of the physical examination. Motor weakness is often seen in neuromuscular disorders. Subtle motor weakness can be elucidated by comparing sides and examining smaller muscles, such as the extensor hallucis longus or the hand intrinsic muscles. Reduced reflexes indicate peripheral nervous system problems, whereas increased reflexes suggest a central nervous system disorder, particularly when seen in combination with a Babinski sign, spasticity, and increased tone. An important caveat is that in acute spinal cord injury, there can be an initial reduction in reflexes because of spinal shock. Cranial nerve examination should be performed if stroke or another generalized condition is suspected.

An algorithmic approach to using physical examination and symptom information to tailor the electrodiagnostic evaluation is shown in Figure 8-1. In this approach, the patient's sensory complaints and physical examination signs of sensory loss and weakness create a conceptual framework for approaching these sometimes daunting problems. For the purposes of this discussion, generalized findings are defined as being present in two or more limbs. Although helpful, there are many exceptions to this taxonomy. The electrodiagnostician must refocus the diagnostic effort as data are acquired. Sensory loss is a key finding on examination for someone presenting with generalized symptoms, and provides a branch point in the algorithmic approach to tailoring the electrodiagnostic study (see Figure 8-1).

Myopathies, neuromuscular junction disorders, motor neuron disease, and multifocal motor neuropathy are all characterized by preservation of the sensory system. In contrast, polyneuropathies, bilateral radiculopathies, myelopathies, and central nervous system disorders

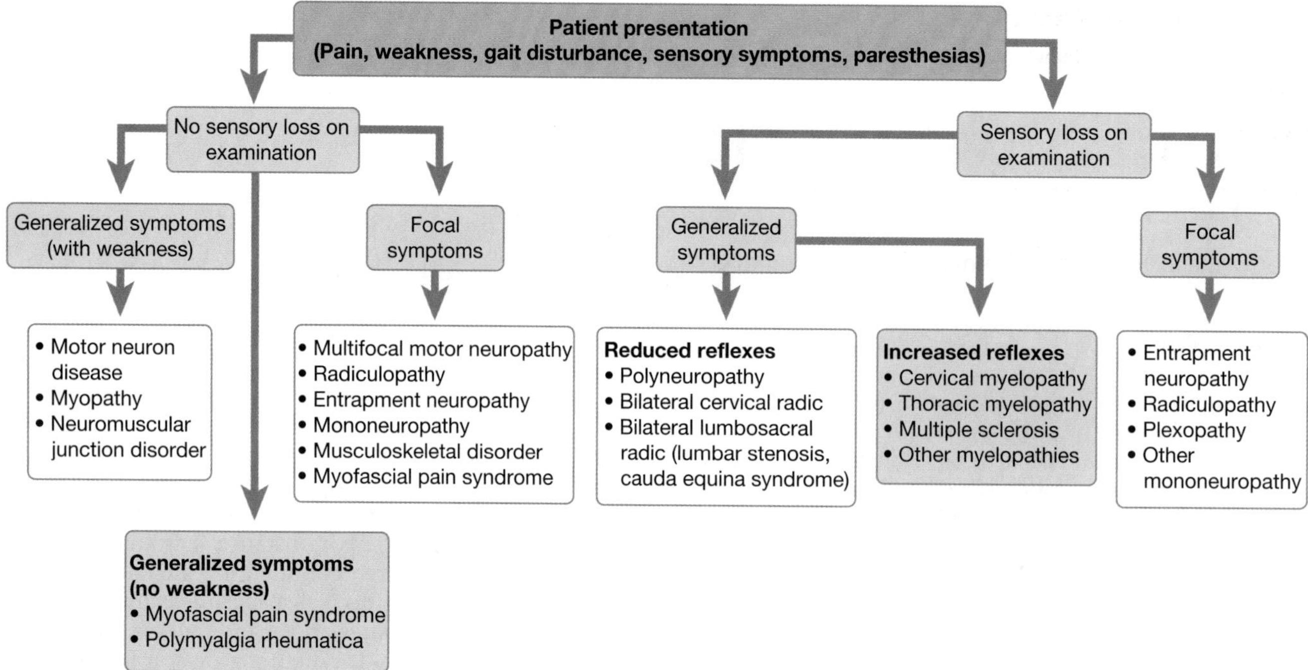

FIGURE 8-1 An algorithmic approach to using physical examination and symptom information to tailor the electrodiagnostic evaluation.

frequently result in reduced sensation. In persons with no sensory loss or weakness on examination and preserved reflexes, the electrodiagnostician should maintain a heightened suspicion for myofascial pain syndrome or fibromyalgia, polymyalgia rheumatica, or other musculoskeletal disorders.[10]

Purpose of Electrodiagnostic Testing

See Appendix 8A of the electronic version for physiologic basis for electrodiagnostic testing.

Electrodiagnostic testing excludes conditions in the differential diagnosis and alters the referring diagnostic impression 42% of the time.[52] Electrodiagnostic testing can also suggest severity or extent of the disorder beyond the clinical symptoms. Finally, there is utility in solidifying a diagnosis. For example, an unequivocal radiculopathy on electromyography (EMG) provides greater diagnostic certainty and identifies avenues of management.

The value of any test depends on the a priori certainty of the diagnosis in question. For a condition or diagnosis for which there is great certainty before additional testing, the results of the subsequent tests are of limited value. For instance, in a patient with acute-onset sciatica while lifting, L5 muscle weakness, a positive straight leg raise, and magnetic resonance imaging (MRI) showing a large extruded L4 to L5 nucleus pulposus, an EMG test will be of limited value in confirming the diagnosis of radiculopathy because the clinical picture is so convincing with or without EMG findings. In contrast, an elderly diabetic patient with sciatica, having limited physical examination findings and equivocal or age-related MRI changes, presents an unclear picture. In this case, electrodiagnostic testing may be of greater value, putting in perspective the imaging findings and identifying diabetic polyneuropathy if present.

Nerve Injury Classification

Peripheral nerve injury is one of the most common types of pathology likely to be encountered during an electrodiagnostic medicine evaluation. It is necessary to be familiar with the various classification systems available to categorize an insult to neural tissue.

Seddon Classification

The degree to which a nerve is damaged has obvious implications with regard to its present function and potential for recovery. There are essentially two general classification systems.[29] In Seddon classification, there are three degrees or stages of injury to consider: neurapraxia, axonotmesis, and neurotmesis (Table 8-1).

Neurapraxia

The term *neurapraxia* is used to designate a mild degree of neural insult that results in blockage of impulse conduction across the affected segment. It is also acceptable to simply designate this type of neural insult as conduction block. The most important aspect of conduction block is its reversibility. Muscle wasting usually does not occur in conduction block because muscle innervation is maintained, and recovery is typically rapid enough to avoid disuse atrophy. Fibrillation potentials should not be observed in conduction block because the axon is not disrupted. Many nerve injuries are mixed lesions in which some fibers have conduction block, some have axonal loss, and others are demyelinated. In this case, it is certainly possible to observe fibrillation potentials.

Axonotmesis

The second degree of neural insult in Seddon classification is axonotmesis, which is a specific type of nerve injury

Table 8-1 Nerve Injury Classification

Type	Function	Pathologic Basis	Prognosis
Lundborg			
Physiologic Conduction Block			
Type a	Focal conduction block	Intraneural ischemia; metabolic (ionic) block; no nerve fiber changes	Excellent; immediately reversible
Type b	Focal conduction block	Intraneural edema; increased endoneurial fluid pressure; metabolic block; little or no fiber changes	Recovery in days or weeks
Seddon-Sunderland			
Neurapraxia			
Type 1	Focal conduction block; primarily motor function and proprioception affected; some sensation and sympathetic function may be present	Local myelin injury, primarily larger fibers; axonal continuity; no Wallerian degeneration	Recovery in weeks to months
Axonotmesis			
Type 2	Loss of nerve conduction at injury site and distally	Disruption of axonal continuity with Wallerian degeneration; endoneurial tubes, perineurium, and epineurium intact	Axonal regeneration required for recovery; good prognosis, because original end organs reached
Type 3	Loss of nerve conduction at injury site and distally	Loss of axonal continuity and endoneurial tubes; perineurium and epineurium preserved	Disruption of endoneurial tubes, hemorrhage, and edema produce scarring; axonal misdirection; poor prognosis; surgery may be required
Type 4	Loss of nerve conduction at injury site and distally	Loss of axonal continuity, endoneurial tubes, and perineurium; epineurium intact	Total disruption of guiding elements; intraneural scarring and axonal misdirection; poor prognosis; surgery necessary
Neurotmesis			
Type 5	Loss of nerve conduction at injury site and distally	Severance of entire nerve	Surgical modification of nerve ends required; prognosis guarded and dependent on nature of injury and local factors

From Lundborg G: *Nerve injury and repair*, Edinburgh, 1988, Churchill Livingstone, with permission.

where only the axon is physically disrupted, with preservation of the enveloping endoneurial and other supporting connective tissue structures (perineurium and epineurium). Compression of a profound nature and traction on the nerve are typical lesion etiologies. Once the axon has been disrupted, the characteristic changes of Wallerian degeneration occur. The fact that the endoneurium remains intact is a very important aspect of this type of injury. A preserved endoneurium implies that once the remnants of the degenerated nerve have been removed by phagocytosis, the regenerating axon simply has to follow its original course directly back to the appropriate end organ. A good prognosis can be expected when neural damage results only in axonotmesis.

Neurotmesis

The greatest degree of nerve disruption is designated in Seddon classification as neurotmesis. This is complete disruption of the axon and all supporting connective tissue structures, whereby the endoneurium, perineurium, and epineurium are no longer in continuity. This lesion has a poor prognosis for complete functional recovery. Surgical reapproximation of the nerve ends, if possible, will probably be required. Surgery does not guarantee proper endoneurial tube alignment, but it improves the chances that axonal growth will occur across the injury site.

Sunderland Classification

A second popular and more detailed classification is that proposed and modified by Sunderland. Sunderland classification is divided into five types of injury, based exclusively on which connective tissue components are disrupted (see Table 8-1). Type 1 injury corresponds to Seddon designation of neurapraxia. Seddon axonotmesis is subdivided by Sunderland into three gradations of neural insult (types 2 to 4). Sunderland type 5 injury corresponds to Seddon neurotmesis (complete neural disruption).

Clinical Testing of Motor and Sensory Nerves

Electrodiagnostic testing consists of EMG and nerve conductions. Standard nerve conduction studies (NCSs) that are used in the evaluation of patients include motor nerve conductions, sensory nerve conductions, F-waves, and H-reflexes. It is important to properly perform these tests and compare the data with well-derived normative values. Enough testing should be performed to properly delineate the conditions being sought and eliminate other conditions in the differential diagnosis.

Although it is important to be aware of individuals who have implanted cardiac devices, in a study involving patients with dual-chamber pacemakers and implanted cardiac defibrillators, NCSs including median motor testing with an Erb point stimulation on the left side of the body resulted in no change in the function of these devices, nor did any stimulation show up on any of the electrocardiogram tracings.[92] These investigators concluded that conventional NCSs have no effects on these implanted devices, and their findings should diminish the anxiety of electrodiagnosticians when working with such patients.[92] These findings further support the safety of performing such testing in persons with implanted cardiac devices and dispel some of the concern expressed in previous recommendations.[5]

Sensory nerve conductions should nearly always be performed when assessing a patient.[6] In the upper limb, multiple sensory nerves are easily accessible and allow assessment for both entrapments and polyneuropathies. In the lower limbs, the most readily accessible sensory nerve is the sural nerve, which has been recommended as an excellent nerve for screening for distal symmetrical polyneuropathy.[45]

Motor NCSs should be performed in almost all situations.[6] Examiners should assess the morphology of the waveform, its latency, amplitude, and conduction velocity. Conduction should be performed across any suspected sites of entrapment or injury.

Despite efforts to minimize variability and enhance quality in the practice of electrodiagnostic medicine, it is well recognized that universal standards for NCSs are not used in the United States. The majority of electrodiagnostic physicians and laboratories, rather than develop their own normative values, have instead relied on the peer-reviewed literature. However, many published studies, compiled in various reference texts, do not meet contemporary standards for statistical and methodological rigor.

What is concerning about the lack of standardization of nerve conduction testing is the poor interrater reliability for identifying abnormal results that lead to differing diagnostic conclusions. A recent study delineated the problems in identifying polyneuropathy that arise when different experts and technologists use their own laboratory standards when evaluating patients with and without diabetic sensorimotor polyneuropathy.[44] In this well-done prospective study they found that "interobserver variability" was attributed to differences in performance of nerve conduction testing.[44]

In a companion study, Litchy et al.[44,73] instituted standard instructions, standard techniques and procedures, and significantly reduced the interobserver differences in nerve conduction. Together, these two investigations underscore the need for standard well-derived reference values for practice across the United States.

H-Reflexes

The commonly used H-reflex is an electrophysiologically recorded Achilles muscle stretch reflex without the use of the muscle spindle. Clinical H-reflexes are generated by recording over the gastrocnemius and soleus muscles and stimulating the tibial nerve in the popliteal fossa. Care must be taken to perform this test correctly. It is a submaximal elicited reflex response. The stimulus duration is 1 ms, and the stimulus should be slowly increased by 3- to 5-mA increments. The patient should be relaxed, and the stimulus frequency should be less than once per second to avoid habituation of the response. The H-reflex is consistent in latency and morphology, and occurs when the motor response over the gastrocnemius and soleus is submaximal. As the stimulus current is gradually increased, the H-reflex reaches its maximum amplitude, and then extinguishes as the motor response becomes maximal. Many researchers have evaluated its sensitivity and specificity with regard to lumbosacral radiculopathies, and generally found a range of sensitivities from 32% to 88%.[70] The specificity, however, has been reported at 91% for H-reflexes in lumbosacral S1 radiculopathy.[76] The H-reflex can also help separate S1 radiculopathy from L5 radiculopathy, the latter being more likely to have a normal reflex.[76]

H-reflexes are useful for assessing for demyelinating polyneuropathy, cauda equina syndrome, and for confirming a sciatic neuropathy. Remember that delay or decreased amplitude in the H-reflex can occur with lesions anywhere along its course, including the sciatic nerve, the lumbosacral plexus, or the S1 root. H-Reflex studies of other nerves are more difficult to elicit and they are not commonly used in clinical practice.

F-Waves

F-waves are late responses involving the motor axons and axonal pool at the spinal cord level. They can be elicited in most upper and lower limb muscles, and are typically tested by stimulating the median, ulnar, peroneal, or tibial nerves when recording from muscles they innervate. In contrast to H-reflexes, they are elicited by maximal stimulation of the nerve. They vary in morphology and latency, although when recording multiple F-waves, they should fall roughly within the same latency period. When responses that look like F-waves are seen across the screen at widely varying latencies, the examiner should turn up the machine volume, discharge the stimulator while it is off the skin, and determine whether background motor unit firing is the cause of these widely varying responses. F-waves demonstrate low sensitivities for radiculopathy and thus have a limited role in such evaluations[91]; however, they are useful in the assessment of suspected polyneuropathy.

Needle Electromyography

One of the most important means of evaluating for neuromuscular diseases is EMG using a monopolar pin or coaxial needle ("needle" is used to mean either pin or needle). Surface EMG has no clinical use over standard needle EMG.[78] EMG testing, a vital part of electrodiagnostic evaluations, provides useful information and, although somewhat uncomfortable, poses minimal risks to the patient. The American Association of Neuromuscular and Electrodiagnostic Medicine (AANEM) supports the Occupational Safety and Health Administration rule that mandates the use of gloves and universal precautions during testing. Disposable needles are now readily available and are sufficiently inexpensive that they should be used. Reusable surface electrodes should be cleaned with a 1 : 10 dilution of household bleach or 70% isopropyl alcohol solution between patients. Disposable surface electrodes are inexpensive, widely available, and easy to use.[5]

Needlestick injuries are reported by the majority of electrodiagnosticians to have occurred at least once during their career.[77] The most common preventable reason for injury was a perceived lack of time.[77] Using a device to clamp the plastic sleeve that holds the needle and replacing the needle with a one-handed technique are recommended to help prevent needle sticks.

In most cases, it makes no difference whether the skin is antiseptically prepared before needle insertion.[5] Some examiners use alcohol as an antiseptic, and certainly if the skin is not clean then alcohol represents a useful skin preparation. With regard to lymphedema one should use caution and sterilize the skin, as well as avoid traversing an infected space or an area of clearly taut skin that could weep serous fluid after the needle insertion. Care should also be used to avoid cellulitis.[7] The needle should not penetrate infected skin or open ulcerations or wounds. Needle EMG is not listed by the American Heart Association as a procedure requiring prophylactic antibiotic treatment to prevent endocarditis.[5]

Hemorrhagic complications from needle EMG are rare and are asymptomatic when they occur.[50] In one case series, minor paraspinal muscle hematomas were noted on MRI performed shortly after needle EMG examination in 4 of 17 patients who were not receiving anticoagulants. These hematomas were small and of no clinical significance.[19] In this report, the authors state that there has never been a case report of paraspinal hematoma compressing the spinal roots or the epidural space.[19] Ultrasound evaluation of over 700 muscles showed only two small subclinical hematomas in patients who were anticoagulated.[14] However, since then, there has been at least one case of threatened compartment syndrome in the anterior tibialis of a patient who was subtherapeutically anticoagulated.[17] Although clinicians should always weigh carefully the risk-to-benefit ratio of testing, a person with appropriate levels of anticoagulation for venous thromboembolism can be safely studied with little risk of neurologic complications. Appropriate pressure should be applied to the area after testing to prevent intramuscular hematoma. The paraspinal muscles are such an important region to study, not only for persons with suspected radiculopathy but also in neuromuscular evaluations that electrodiagnosticians should examine them whenever reasonably possible.

As noted, the electrodes for standard EMG generally fall into two categories. Monopolar needles are those in which the needle is coated with Teflon except for the tip, and the differences in potential from the tip of the electrode to a nearby surface electrode are recorded. Concentric needles are those with a fine wire running through the center of an insulated shaft that is electrically referenced to an outer metal shaft. Concentric needles are useful for quantitative motor unit analysis and are commercially available in disposable form. Background interference is minimized with concentric needles, and the ground electrode can remain in one place for a given limb.

The needle examination consists of assessing four separate aspects of needle EMG. These aspects are (1) insertion activity, (2) spontaneous activity, (3) the morphology and size of motor unit action potentials (MUAPs), and (4) motor unit recruitment.

Needle Insertional Activity

Placing a needle (monopolar or standard concentric) recording electrode into healthy muscle tissue and advancing it in quick but short intervals results in brief bursts of electrical potentials referred to as insertional activity (Figure 8-2, *A*).[15]

The observed electrical activity is believed to result from the needle electrode mechanically depolarizing the muscle fibers surrounding its leading edge as it pierces and deforms the tissue. Insertional activity and spontaneous activity are usually examined with three or four insertions in each of four muscle vectors or quadrants. Smaller muscles, such as the abductor pollicis brevis, can be adequately assessed with fewer needle movements. After brief small movement of the needle, insertional activity usually persists for no more than a few hundred milliseconds. Minimal and localized muscle tissue damage may occur from direct needle trauma and is the basis for the synonymous term of injury potentials. The purpose of including insertional activity analysis as part of the electromyographic examination is that the probing needle might provoke transient and/or sustained abnormal potentials associated with membrane instability before this abnormal activity with the muscle at rest.

Decreased Insertional Activity

Atrophied muscle that has been replaced by fibrous or fatty tissue, or that is otherwise electrically inexcitable, can no longer generate electrical activity. Consequently, the needle electrode is incapable of mechanically depolarizing this tissue. The result is that few, if any, electrical waveforms will be detected after needle movement and usually lasts less than 100 ms. This is usually considered abnormal. Care must be taken to insure that the lack of electrical activity is not caused by placement of the needle into subcutaneous tissue instead of muscle (see Figure 8-2, *B*).

Increased Insertional Activity

Practitioners have noted that insertional activity can appear to persist after needle movement cessation. This finding has led to the term increased insertional activity. In disease states in which the muscle is no longer connected to its nerve or the muscle membrane is inherently unstable from primary muscle pathology or abnormal ion channels, the increased insertional activity completes a temporal continuum from the previously normal insertional activity to the development of sustained membrane instability or positive sharp wave (PSW) fibrillation potentials (see Figure 8-2, *C*). Practitioners differ as to the significant differences if any between increased insertional activity and PSWs. There is no clear conventional cut-off time between the time that persistent increased insertional activity becomes a run of fibrillation potentials. Many practitioners consider this cut-off time between 1 and 3 seconds after the needle has stopped moving. Very few authors

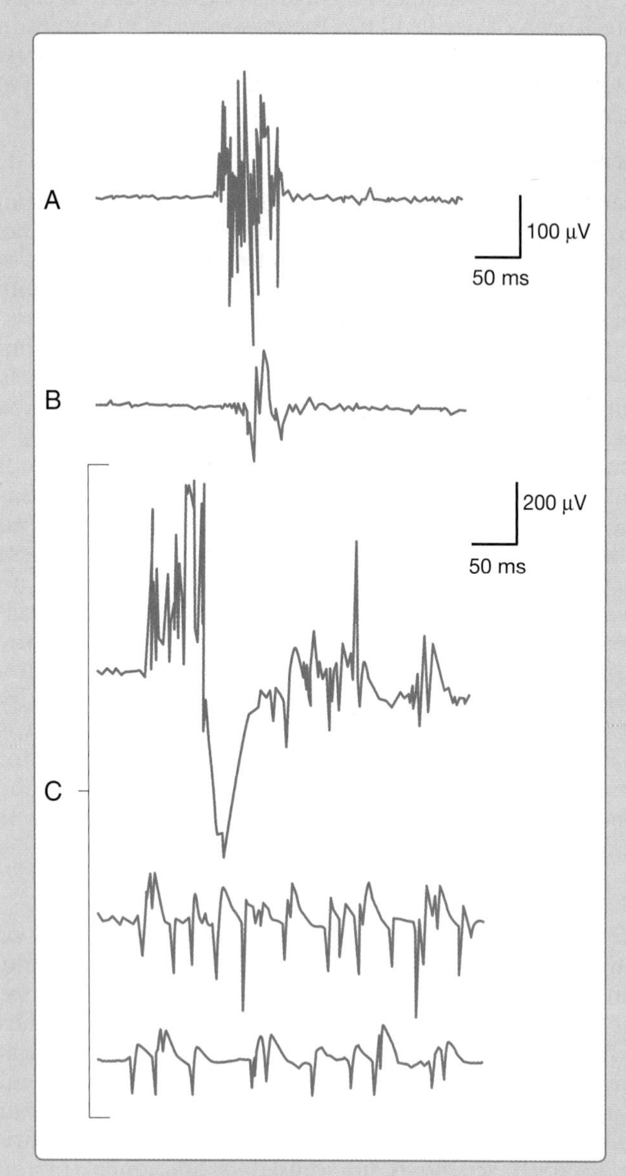

FIGURE 8-2 **A,** Inserting a monopolar needle into healthy muscle tissue results in mechanical depolarization of muscle tissue, which generates a brief burst of electrical activity designated as insertional activity. **B,** Inserting the same needle into fibrotic muscle or subcutaneous fatty tissue results in decreased insertional activity. **C,** Inserting a monopolar needle into denervated muscle tissue produced not only the initial burst of electrical activity but also associated positive sharp waves and fibrillation potentials that abate over several hundred milliseconds. (Redrawn from Dumitru D, Amato AA, Zwarts MJ: *Electrodiagnostic medicine,* ed 2, Philadelphia, 2002, Hanley & Belfus, with permission.)

specifically address this detail.[27] The use of the longer time of 2 or 3 seconds improves the specificity and limits false-positive results but slightly decreases the sensitivity of the needle EMG. Diffuse abnormal insertional activity with prolonged trains of PSWs in essentially every muscle, yet without any symptoms or disability, has been described as "EMG disease." This is a rare condition that is infrequently encountered in clinical practice and is of unclear clinical significance.

Table 8-2 Characteristics of End-Plate Noise

Characteristic	Details
Appearance	Monophasic negative waves
Rhythm	Irregular
Frequency	Usually so frequent and can be superimposed upon each other so that they cannot be individually seen
Amplitude	10 µV or less
Stability	Persist until the needle is moved
Observed in	Normal finding recorded from the end-plate zone

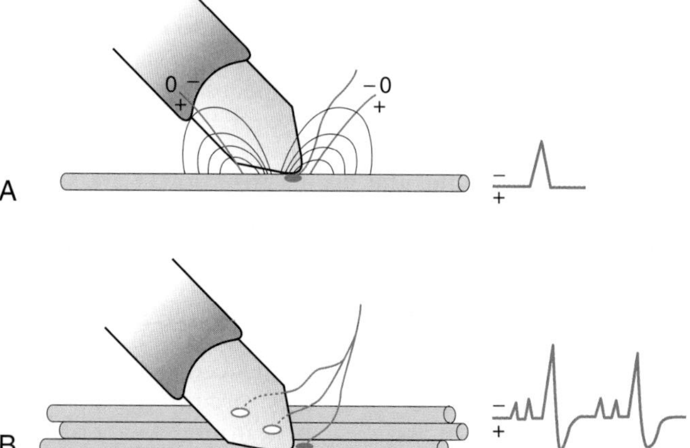

FIGURE 8-3 **A,** Monopolar needle electrode located over the end plate of a muscle records the spontaneous depolarization of a miniature end-plate potential (MEPP). As the electrode is located over the subthreshold central current sink of this potential, and hence does not propagate, a monophasic negative potential is recorded. **B,** The large recording electrode is usually positioned over several end plates, thus recording multiple MEPPs and end-plate spikes (Redrawn from Dumitru D, Amato AA, Zwarts MJ: *Electrodiagnostic medicine,* ed 2, Philadelphia, 2002, Hanley & Belfus, with permission.)

End-Plate Potentials

An active needle electrode located in the end-plate region can record two distinct waveforms: either miniature end-plate potentials (MEPPs) or end-plate spikes.

Miniature End-Plate Potentials

One of the waveforms is a short-duration (0.5 to 2 ms), small (10 to 50 µV), irregularly occurring (once every 5 seconds per axon terminal), monophasic negative waveform.[15,41] These potentials represent the random release of acetylcholine vesicles. Volume conduction theory would suggest that for a potential to be monophasic and negative, the current sink would have to start and finish within the very small recording region of the active electrode (Table 8-2). Clinically, multiple MEPPs are the same as end-plate noise, and the sound is referred to as resembling a "seashell murmur," which sounds like noise generated by a seashell held close to the ear (Figure 8-3).

End-Plate Spikes

A second waveform (end-plate spikes) can be detected with an active needle electrode placed in the end-plate region. These potentials are generated from the actual muscle fiber, similar to fibrillation potentials, and they are relatively short in duration (3 to 4 ms), of moderate amplitude (100 to 200 μV), irregularly firing, and biphasic with an initial negative deflection[15,41] (Table 8-3). End-plate spikes and MEPPs are frequently observed together, because they arise from the same region (Figure 8-4). They can be mistaken for fibrillation potentials, but they fire irregularly, a distinction usually made visually on the display screen as well as by listening carefully. The needle should be moved to a new location after it enters an end-plate region, to reduce pain and enter muscle more conducive to assessment for fibrillation potentials.

Table 8-3 Characteristics of End-Plate Spikes

Characteristic	Details
Appearance	Biphasic or triphasic spikes or positive waves
Rhythm	Irregular
Frequency	Intervals frequently less than 50 ms
Amplitude	50 to 300 μV
Stability	Persists until the needle is moved
Observed in	Is a normal finding

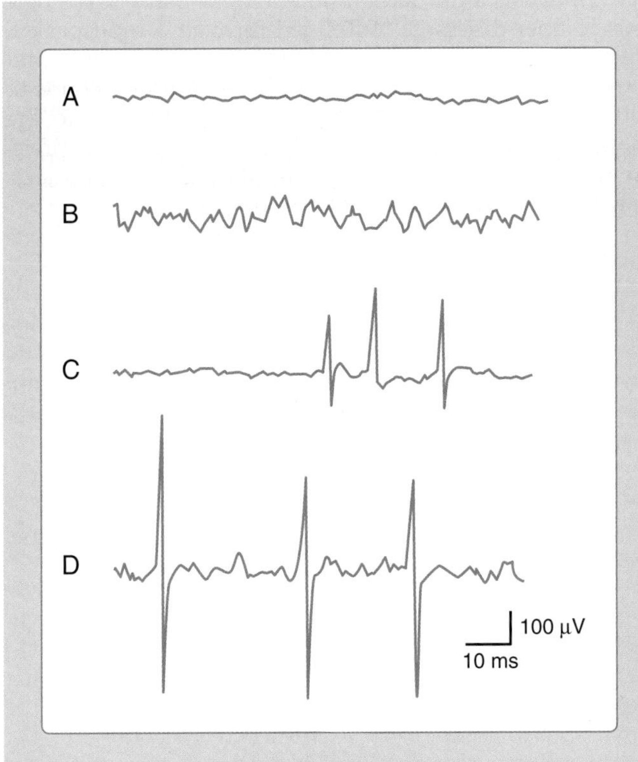

FIGURE 8-4 **A,** Monopolar needle located in a healthy muscle at rest. **B,** Slight needle movement positions the electrode in an end-plate region with the recording of multiple miniature end-plate potentials of a negative spike configuration. **C,** Repositioning the needle electrode to a slightly different region primarily records biphasic, initially negative end-plate spikes. **D,** Advancing the needle electrode slightly permits the simultaneous recording of both potentials noted individually in (**B**) and (**C**). (Redrawn from Dumitru D, Amato AA, Zwarts MJ: *Electrodiagnostic medicine,* ed 2, Philadelphia, 2002, Hanley & Belfus, with permission.)

Single Muscle Fiber

The single muscle fiber generates three waveforms that are at times difficult to separate: end-plate spikes and the two types of fibrillations (PSWs and spike fibrillation potentials). Distant motor units can mimic the shape of the PSW but fire in a semirhythmic manner and by moving the needle closer the positive waveform becomes an MUAP. In contrast, moving the needle electrode 1 to 5 mm will cause fibrillations to disappear. End-plate spikes can have the identical morphology of PSW and fibrillation potentials. The major key to separating them is that PSW and fibrillation potentials have a regular firing rate and can slowly trail off before they disappear. End-plate spikes usually fire irregularly. The extracellular waveform configuration of a single muscle fiber, similar to nerve tissue, depends on the characteristics of the intracellular action potential of a muscle. The action potential of a muscle is approximately 4 to 20 times longer than that of a nerve, because of the prolonged repolarization process.[15] A triphasic waveform with a small terminal phase should be recorded from an extracellular active electrode placed adjacent to a propagating single muscle fiber action potential at some distance from the end-plate region (Figure 8-5).

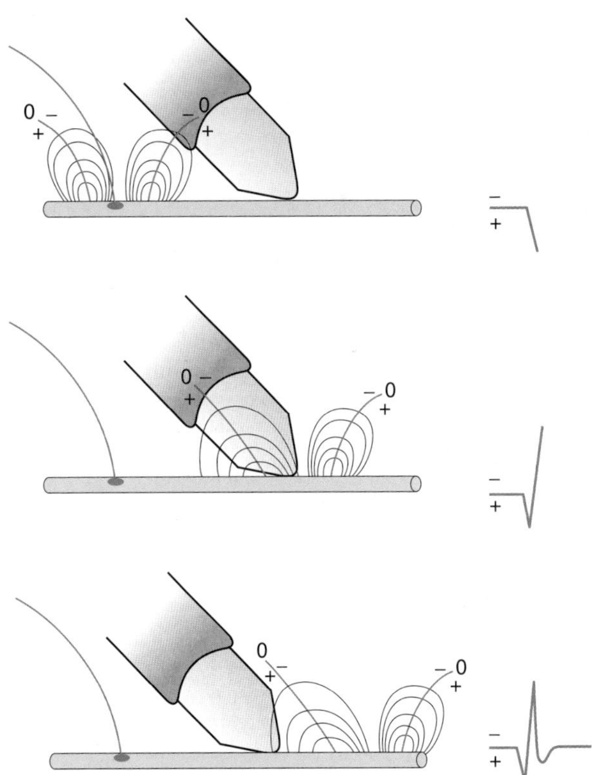

FIGURE 8-5 A single muscle fiber action potential propagating past a needle recording electrode results in a triphasic waveform. This is because the voltage distribution creates an initial and terminal positive voltage source surrounding a negative current sink zone. (Redrawn from Dumitru D, Amato AA, Zwarts MJ: *Electrodiagnostic medicine,* ed 2, Philadelphia, 2002, Hanley & Belfus, with permission.)

Fibrillation Potentials: Spike Form and Positive Sharp Waves

There is debate as to whether fibrillation potentials are distinct from PSWs, and if so, whether or not this has any clinical significance. Fibrillation potentials have been characterized as the spike form or biphasic waveform.[43] Characteristics are shown in Table 8-4. There is strong evidence that the PSW is a fibrillation that has a different shape primarily because the needle electrode is touching the fibrillating muscle cell, altering the muscle membrane, and consequently the shape of the waveform. It is unlikely that there are any clinically significant differences between the two.

Fibrillation potentials are simply spontaneous depolarizations of a single muscle fiber and demonstrate waveform configurations similar to those of single muscle fibers that are voluntarily activated (Figure 8-6). Fibrillation potentials are typically short in duration (less than 5 ms), less than 1 mV in amplitude, and fire at rates between 1 and 15 Hz. They have a typical sound, likened to a high-pitched tick similar to "rain on a tin roof," when amplified through a loudspeaker. When the recording electrode is located in the previous end-plate zone of a denervated muscle, fibrillation potentials can be biphasic with an initial negative deflection. A recording electrode outside the end-plate zone, but far from the tendinous region, will detect fibrillation potentials that are triphasic (positive-negative-positive).

It is possible to generate waveforms with similar configurations to fibrillation potentials while examining healthy muscle tissue. Specifically, inadvertently irritating the terminal axon or end-plate zone with the shaft of an electrode, and evoking end-plate potentials while simultaneously recording at some distance from the end-plate zone, will generate triphasic end-plate spikes that are identical in appearance to fibrillation potentials (Figure 8-7).[15] This is understandable because both waveforms are single muscle fiber discharges. The key to identification is the rapid and irregular discharge of end-plate spikes, whereas fibrillation potentials usually fire slower and very regularly. Irregularly firing fibrillation potentials occur at times, and are less well understood but thought to arise from spontaneous depolarizations within the transverse tubule system.

Table 8-4 Characteristics of Fibrillation Potentials

Characteristic	Details
Appearance	Brief spike or positive sharp wave
Rhythm	Regular, rarely irregular
Frequency	0.5 to 15 Hz
Amplitude	20 to 300 μV
Stability	Gradually taper off
Observed in	Nearly all lower motor neuron disorders, severe myopathies, and occasionally severe neuromuscular junction disorders. Chronic spinal cord injuries and stroke.

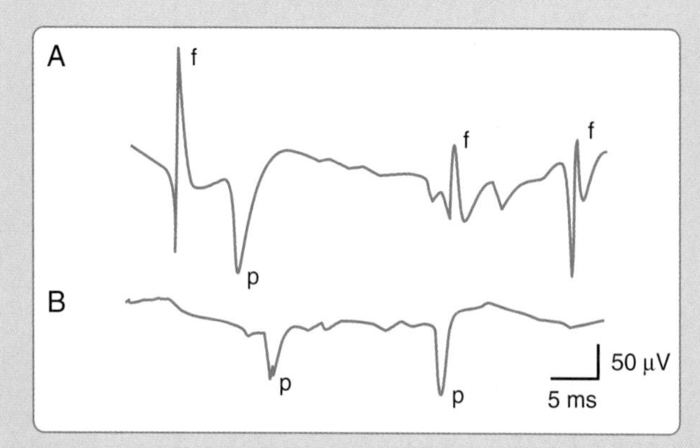

FIGURE 8-6 **A,** Monopolar needle recording of positive sharp waves (PSWs) (*p*) and fibrillation potentials (*f*). **B,** Only PSWs are depicted. (Redrawn from Dumitru D, Amato AA, Zwarts MJ: *Electrodiagnostic medicine*, ed 2, Philadelphia, 2002, Hanley & Belfus, with permission.)

Positive Sharp Waves

PSWs are fibrillation potential waveforms that can be recorded from a single muscle fiber having an unstable resting membrane potential secondary to denervation or intrinsic muscle disease. Typically, they have a large primary sharp positive deflection followed by a small negative potential. These potentials are called PSWs (see Figure 8-6). This waveform is thought to have the same clinical significance as a fibrillation potential, in that it is a single muscle fiber discharge. Amplified through a loudspeaker, PSWs have a regular firing rate (1 to 15 Hz) and a dull thud sound. Their durations range from several milliseconds to 100 ms or longer. Although commonly observed to fire spontaneously, PSWs can be provoked by electrode movement, as can the spike form of fibrillation potentials.

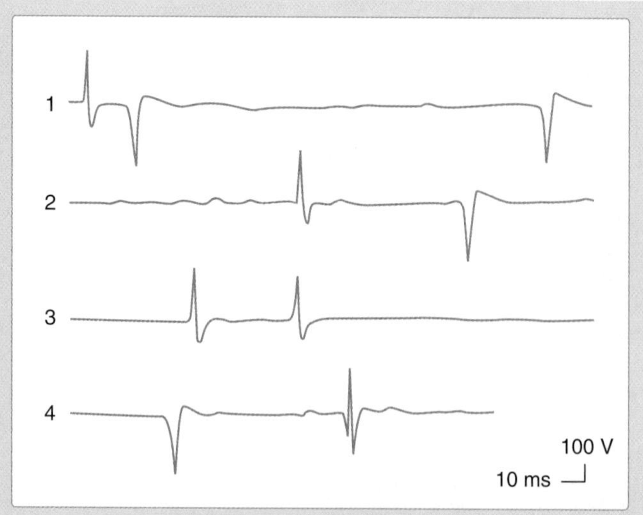

FIGURE 8-7 A needle electrode is purposefully located in an end-plate region where prototypical and atypical end-plate spikes are evoked. Note that end-plate spikes may appear biphasic, initially negative, as anticipated, as well as triphasic and biphasic, initially positive, resembling fibrillation potentials and positive sharp waves, respectively. The important distinction between normal and abnormal waveforms in this case is not waveform configuration but rather firing rate (highly irregular for end-plate spikes). (Redrawn from Dumitru D, Amato AA, Zwarts MJ: *Electrodiagnostic medicine*, ed 2, Philadelphia, 2002, Hanley & Belfus, with permission.)

A number of other waveforms can be observed that have the configurations resembling a PSW. An MUAP recorded from the tendinous region can also have an initial positive deflection followed by a negative potential, because the current sink cannot pass beyond the recording electrode.[41] It is also possible for the recording electrode to damage a number of muscle fibers in close proximity to the recording surface, again preventing an action potential from passing its recording surface, resulting in a primarily positive potential. These two potentials can be distinguished from a PSW in that they are MUAPs and subject to voluntary control, whereas a PSW is not. Asking the individual to contract and relax the muscle under investigation should demonstrate that the waveform has a variable firing rate. A PSW typically fires at a regular rate and is not under voluntary control. If any doubt remains, the electrode should be repositioned until successful recordings are obtained. Similar to end-plate noise and end-plate spikes, PSWs and fibrillations will usually disappear when the needle electrode is moved a small distance such as 1 to 5 mm, whereas a motor unit will usually remain on the screen and change shape. This is because the fibrillation potential is generated by a very small electrical charge from only one muscle fiber, whereas an MUAP is generated by hundreds of muscle fibers covering an area of 1 to 3 cm^2.

Transient runs of "PSW-appearing potentials" can be seen in healthy skeletal muscle, particularly in the paraspinal and hand or foot intrinsic muscles. The "nonpathologic" PSWs are thought to arise because the needle electrode is oriented in such a manner as to irritate the terminal axon of an end-plate, but extend along the muscle fiber while compressing the tissue and preventing action potential conduction.[15] The induced end-plate spike appears similar to a PSW, but it displays a relatively rapid and irregularly firing rate characteristic of end-plate spikes (see Figure 8-7). Sustained PSWs are more significant than unsustained PSWs.

Diffuse abnormal insertional activity with prolonged trains of PSWs in essentially every muscle, yet without any symptoms or disability, has been described as "EMG disease."[104] This is a rare condition that is infrequently encountered in clinical practice.

Fibrillations are seen in any condition causing denervation, including nerve disease, inflammatory myopathies, and direct muscle trauma.[84] In persons with complete spinal cord injury, muscles innervated by roots below the level of the lesion also demonstrate fibrillation potentials.[98] Such prevalence of these findings in the legs of patients with spinal cord injuries can make electrodiagnostic testing for such patients ineffective at identifying radiculopathies or entrapment neuropathies. Similar fibrillations and positive waves can also be seen in the hemiparetic limbs of patients with strokes, and such findings should be interpreted with caution.[57]

Fibrillation potentials as well as PSWs are commonly graded with a 0- to 4-grading scheme. This grading scale is described as follows:

1+: Transient but reproducible trains of discharges (fibrillations or PSWs) after moving the needle in more than one site or quadrant.

2+: Occasional spontaneous potentials in more than two different quadrants.

3+: Spontaneous potentials present in all quadrants.

4+: Abundant spontaneous potentials nearly filling the screen in all four quadrants.

The finding of a fibrillation or PSW in only one area of the muscle that is not easily reproducible is probably of uncertain significance and can represent an end-plate spike as discussed earlier. There is little scientific evidence that there is a difference between the various grades of fibrillations. The density of fibrillation potentials does not necessarily correlate with the degree of nerve damage and loss of axons. The compound muscle action potential (CMAP) gives a better estimate of the proportion of axons remaining. The innervation ratio is the average size of the motor unit expressed as a ratio between the total number of extrafusal muscle fibers and the number of innervating motor axons. For small extraocular muscles, this ratio is 1 to 3. For large muscles such as the gastrocnemius, this ratio increases to approximately 1934 muscle fibers per motor axon. This means that the loss of relatively few motor axons results in many fibrillating muscle fibers in these larger muscles.[62,63] The amplitude of fibrillation potentials can be helpful in determining the time course of a direct nerve injury. Small fibrillation potentials suggest a more chronic problem that has lasted over 6 months.[67]

Complex Repetitive Discharge

A complex repetitive discharge (CRD) is a spontaneously firing group of action potentials (formerly called bizarre high-frequency discharges or pseudomyotonic discharges) and require a needle recording electrode for detection.[15] The configuration of these waveforms is that they are continuous runs of simple or complex spike patterns (fibrillation potentials or PSWs) that regularly repeat at 0.3 to 150 Hz. The repetitive pattern of spike potentials has the same appearance with each firing and bears the same relationship with its neighboring spikes (Table 8-5).

A distinct sound, likened to that of heavy machinery or an idling motorcycle, is produced by the firing of CRDs. In addition to the sound and repetitive pattern, a hallmark of these waveforms is that they start and stop abruptly. CRDs might begin spontaneously or be induced by needle movement, muscle percussion, or muscle contraction. Nerve

Table 8-5 Complex Repetitive Discharge Characteristics

Characteristic	Details
Appearance	May take any form, but this form is constant from one potential complex to the next
Rhythm	Regular
Frequency	10 to 100 Hz
Amplitude	50 to 1000 μV
Stability	Abrupt onset and cessation
Observed in	Myopathies: polymyositis, limb-girdle dystrophy, myxedema, Schwartz-Jampel syndrome. Neuropathies: poliomyelitis, spinal muscular atrophy, amyotrophic lateral sclerosis, hereditary neuropathies, chronic neuropathies, carpal tunnel syndrome. "Normal": iliopsoas, biceps brachii.

Modified from Dumitru D: Needle electromyography. In Dumitru D, editor: *Electrodiagnostic medicine*, Philadelphia, 1995, Hanley & Belfus.

block and curare do not abolish CRDs, suggesting that the origin of these potentials is within the muscle tissue. Single-fiber and standard electromyographic studies suggest that CRDs are generated by an ephaptic activation of adjacent muscle cells.[11,27] Detection of these waveforms usually suggests that a chronic process has resulted in a group of muscle fibers becoming separated from their neuromuscular junctions. They may be associated with a currently active disease or be the residua of a past disorder.

Myotonic Discharges

The phenomenon of delayed muscle relaxation after muscle contraction is referred to as myotonia or action myotonia.[15] The finding of delayed muscle relaxation after reflex activation, or induced by striking the muscle belly with a reflex hammer, is called percussion myotonia. Clinical myotonia is usually accentuated by energetic muscle activity after a rest period. Continued muscle contraction lessens the myotonia and is known as the "warmup." It is thought that cooling the muscle accentuates myotonia, but this finding has only been objectively documented in paramyotonia congenita.

Myotonic discharges can present in one of two waveform types (Table 8-6).

The myotonic potential induced by needle electrode insertion usually assumes a morphology similar to that of a PSW or a fibrillation potential. It is thought that the needle movement induces a repetitive firing of the unstable membranes of multiple single muscle fibers. This is because the recording needle is thought to have damaged that portion of the muscle fiber with which it is in contact. Regardless of the waveform type, the hallmark of myotonia is the waxing and waning in both frequency and amplitude. The myotonic discharge has a characteristic sound, likened to that of a dive bomber. Trains of PSW that trail off and stop but do not restart (wane, but do not wax) can be confused with myotonia. Amplitudes range from 20 to 300 μV, and firing rates from 20 to 100 Hz.[97]

Myotonic discharges can occur with or without clinical myotonia. The observation of these potentials requires needle movement or muscle contraction. These waveforms persist after nerve block, neuromuscular block, or frank denervation. This suggests that their site of origin is the muscle membrane itself, and they appear to be attributable to a channelopathy. Although the exact mechanism of myotonic discharge production remains unclear, myotonia is found in channelopathies of both the sodium and potassium channels.[27] Myotonic discharges are not specific for any one disorder. In addition to the myotonic disorders of muscle, myotonic discharges can also be detected occasionally in acid maltase deficiency, polymyositis, drug-induced myopathies, severe axonal neuropathies, and at times in any nerve or muscle disorder.

Table 8-6 Characteristics of Myotonic Discharges

Characteristic	Details
Appearance	Brief spikes, positive waveform
Rhythm	Wax and wane
Frequency	20 to 100 Hz
Amplitude	Variable (20 to 300 μV)
Stability	Firing rate alterations
Observed in	Myopathies: myotonic dystrophy, myotonia congenita, paramyotonia, polymyositis, acid maltase deficiency, hyperkalemic periodic paralysis. Other: chronic radiculopathy, chronic peripheral neuropathy.

Modified from Dumitru D: Needle electromyography. In Dumitru D, editor: *Electrodiagnostic medicine*, Philadelphia, 1995, Hanley & Belfus.

Fasciculation Potentials

The visible spontaneous contraction of a portion of muscle is referred to as a fasciculation. When these contractions are observed with an intramuscular needle recording electrode, they are called fasciculation potentials.[41] A fasciculation potential is the electrically summated voltage of depolarizing muscle fibers belonging to all or part of one motor unit. Occasionally, fasciculation potentials can be documented only with needle EMG because they lie too deep in muscle to be seen from the skin. Recently, ultrasound has been used to visualize fasciculation potentials in skeletal muscle.

Fasciculation waveforms can be characterized with regard to phasicity, amplitude, and duration (Table 8-7). Their discharge rates (absent or less than 1 per minute to 1 to 2 Hz) are irregular and occur randomly. They are not under voluntary control, nor are they influenced by mild contraction of the agonist or antagonist muscles. The site of origin of fasciculation potentials remains unclear, although it appears that there are three possible sites: the spontaneous discharge might arise from the anterior horn cell, or along the entire peripheral nerve (particularly the terminal portion), or at times within the muscle itself.

Fasciculation potentials occur in almost all normal persons in the foot intrinsic or gastrocsoleus muscles, and in patients with a variety of diseases. Typical diseases in which fasciculation potentials can be found include motor neuron disorders, radiculopathies, entrapment neuropathies, and cervical spondylotic myelopathy. Fasciculation potentials have also been described in metabolic disturbances, including tetany, thyrotoxicosis, and

Table 8-7 Characteristics of Fasciculation Potentials

Characteristic	Details
Appearance	Single motor unit
Rhythm	Irregular and random
Frequency	Variable, absent to 1 to 2 Hz
Amplitude	Variable, similar to motor units, 20 μV to 20 mV depending on needle location and motor unit characteristics.
Stability	Each fasciculation is an individual motor unit and is looks different. If the same unit is fasciculating frequently, it is usually stable unless that motor unit happens to be unstable and thus likely to be pathologic.
Observed in	Nearly all normal people. Is more frequent in nearly any lower motor neuron disorders. If they are accompanied by fibrillations they are much more likely to be abnormal.

anticholinesterase overdoses. Studies have unsuccessfully attempted to distinguish between benign (normal) and pathologic fasciculation potentials. There is no reliable way to categorize whether fasciculation potentials indicate a disease state just by considering their inherent characteristics based on routine needle EMG. Perhaps the best way to evaluate fasciculation potentials is to analyze the "company they keep." A careful analysis of voluntary MUAP morphology, combined with a search for abnormal spontaneous potentials, is required before concluding that fasciculation potentials are either a normal or an abnormal finding. Their frequency can be measured by waiting for 1 minute and documenting the number of fasciculations per minute.

Myokymic Discharge

Myokymia is frequently readily observable as vermicular (bag of live worms) or rippling movement of the skin but can be invisible on the skin. It is usually associated with myokymic discharges.[41] The myokymic discharge consists of bursts of normal-appearing motor units with interburst intervals of electrical silence. Thus, there are two frequencies. Typically, the slow firing rate is 0.1 to 10 Hz in a semirhythmic pattern. Each burst has 2 to 10 potentials within a single burst that can fire at 20 to 150 Hz. These potentials are not affected by voluntary contraction. The sounds associated with these potentials vary and have been described as a type of sputtering often heard with a low-powered motorboat engine, marching soldiers, or bursts of machine gun. The actual discharge may be distinguished from CRDs in that myokymic discharges do not display a regular pattern of spikes from one burst to the next, nor do they typically start and stop abruptly. Myokymic discharges are groups of motor units, whereas CRDs represent groups of single muscle fibers. The groups of motor units within a burst may fire only once or possibly several times. The sputtering bursts of myokymic discharges usually sound very different than the continuous drone of a CRD.

Myokymic potentials are rarely seen in healthy people. They are likely to originate from demyelinated motor axons either spontaneously or through ephaptic transmission.[86] Characteristics of myokymic discharges are seen in Table 8-8.

Cramp Potentials

A sustained and possibly painful muscle contraction of multiple motor units, lasting seconds or minutes, can appear in normal individuals or specific disease states. In healthy individuals, a cramp usually occurs in the calf muscles or other lower limb muscles after exercise, abnormal positioning, or maintaining a fixed position for a prolonged period. Cramps might also be induced by hyponatremia, hypocalcemia, vitamin deficiency, ischemia, early motor neuron disease, and peripheral neuropathies. Familial syndromes have been reported that involve fasciculations and cramps; alopecia, diarrhea, and cramps; and simply an autosomal dominantly inherited cramp syndrome.

A needle recording electrode placed into a cramping muscle shows multiple motor units firing synchronously between 40 and 60 Hz, and occasionally reaching 200 to 300 Hz (Figure 8-8 and Table 8-9). Cramps are believed to arise from a peripheral portion of the motor unit. A cramp that results in a taut muscle with electrical silence is the physiologic contracture seen in McArdle disease.

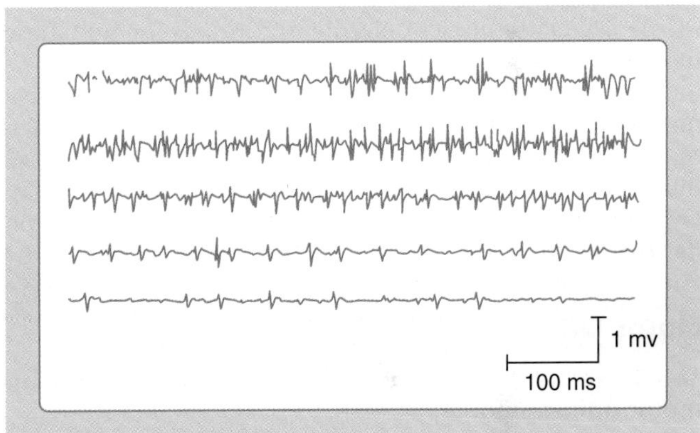

FIGURE 8-8 A characteristic muscle cramp as recorded with an intramuscular needle electrode. There is an initial burst of motor unit activity that eventually subsides as the cramp dissipates. (Redrawn from Daube JA: *AAEM minimonograph 11: needle examination in electromyography,* Rochester, 1979, AAEM. Copyright © 2008 American Association of Neuromuscular and Electrodiagnostic Medicine.)

Table 8-8 Characteristics of Myokymic Discharges

Characteristic	Details
Appearance	Normal motor unit action potentials
Rhythm	Regular
Frequency	0.1 to 10 Hz
Burst frequency	20 to 250 Hz
Stability	Persistent firing or occasional abrupt cessation.
Observed in	Facial: multiple sclerosis, brainstem neoplasm, polyradiculopathy, Bell palsy, normal. Extremity: radiation plexopathy, chronic nerve compression (carpal tunnel syndrome, radiculopathy), rattlesnake venom.

Modified from Dumitru D: Needle electromyography. In Dumitru D, editor: *Electrodiagnostic medicine*, Philadelphia, 1995, Hanley & Belfus.

Table 8-9 Characteristics of Cramp Potentials

Characteristic	Details
Appearance	Single and multiple motor units.
Rhythm	Can fire similar to motor units in groups.
Frequency	Very fast, 40 to 200 Hz.
Amplitude	Variable similar to motor units, 20 μV to 20 mV depending on needle location and motor unit characteristics.
Stability	Variable number of units that fire, but each unit is usually the same morphology.
Observed in	Can be seen in normal people (nocturnal or after exercise). Wide range of neuropathic, endocrinologic, and metabolic conditions.

Table 8-10 Characteristics of Neuromyotonia Potentials

Characteristic	Details
Appearance	Single and multiple motor units that decrease in size over the time of the contraction.
Rhythm	Appear regular.
Frequency	Very fast, 150 to 250 Hz.
Amplitude	Variable similar to motor units but decrease over time, 20 μV to 20 mV depending on needle location and motor unit characteristics.
Stability	Stable and gradually decrease but each unit is usually the same morphology.
Observed in	Isaacs' syndrome, extremely chronic neuropathic diseases, familial neuromyotonia.

Table 8-11 Characteristics of Motor Units

Characteristic	Details
Appearance	Variable can be triphasic or polyphasic.
Rhythm	Semirhythmic or variable regularity. Not randomly irregular.
Frequency	5 to 50 Hz.
Amplitude	Variable, 20 μV to 20 mV depending on needle location and motor unit characteristics.
Stability	Stable if normal, occasional alterations in shape in some diseases.
Observed in	Normal and abnormal patients if they have motor units

Neuromyotonic Discharges

Neuromyotonia is a rare "peripheral" form of continuous muscle fiber activity originating in the peripheral motor axon, usually referred to as Isaac syndrome (Table 8-10). The continuous motor unit activity is eliminated by neuromuscular block but not peripheral nerve block, spinal or general anesthesia, or sleep. The motor unit activity usually begins in the lower limbs in the late teens and progresses to all skeletal muscles. Needle recordings demonstrate motor unit discharges with frequencies up to 300 Hz, including doublets, triplets, and multiplets. Intraoperative mechanical stimulation of a nerve can cause a form of neuromyotonia called neurotonic discharges. These bursts of motor units can alert the surgeon that the nerve is being mechanically disturbed and is at risk of being damaged.[41]

Motor Units

See Appendix 8B of the electronic version for details on motor unit morphology.

Motor unit morphology assessment is generally a qualitative statement and less clear than the presence or absence of fibrillations. Such motor unit changes, however, when clear and profound can be very helpful, particularly in the proper clinical context. The "rule of five" suggests that in normal situations, the ratio of highest firing rate to the number of units seen on a 100-ms display screen is less than five. This means that if the firing rate of the fastest firing motor unit is 20 Hz, approximately four distinct motor units should be seen.[63] In practice this becomes difficult because counting the exact number of motor units can be problematic when there are distant and/or small motor units. When this firing ratio is increased to greater than 10, it indicates a dropout of motor units and is termed reduced recruitment.

Reduced recruitment with a high firing ratio represents one end of a spectrum of recruitment findings, strongly suggestive of motor axonal loss or functional dropout resulting from conduction block. At the other end of a spectrum of recruitment findings is a situation in which many units are recruited to generate a low level of force. This is termed early or myopathic recruitment and is seen in myopathies and neuromuscular junction disorders. Such recruitment is often seen with small, short-duration MUAPs that are characteristic for myopathies. At these two extremes of recruitment, findings are relatively specific for the underlying types of neuromuscular pathology. Beyond this, many recruitment findings are less clear and nearly impossible to reliably differentiate from normal. In the case of pain, poor cooperation, or upper motor neuron disorders, there can be slow firing rates with few units activated (Table 8-11).

Extent of Electrodiagnostic Testing

See Appendix 8C of the electronic version for instrumentation.

Guidelines from the AANEM, published in 1999,[4] provide valuable guidance regarding the extent of appropriate electrodiagnostic testing in 90% of cases. The guidelines and recommendations are summarized in Table 8-12.[4] Guidelines in electrodiagnostic medicine provide recommendations for testing and give clinicians and insurers crucial information regarding how many tests should be conducted in most cases to expeditiously arrive at a diagnosis (e.g., what is enough and what is excessive). These guidelines were developed to improve electrodiagnostic patient care, as well as to combat unscrupulous providers of electrodiagnostic services in the United States who perform excessive studies beyond what is necessary to make a diagnosis, simply for the purpose of increasing the electrodiagnostic fee.

Limitations of Electrodiagnosis

Unfortunately, very few electrodiagnostic findings are clearly specific for any single diagnostic entity. Repetitive nerve stimulation at 2 or 3 Hz can reveal decrements in neuromuscular junction disorders, but also in motor neuron disease, myopathies, peripheral neuropathies, and myotonic disorders.[60] Fibrillations and PSWs are seen in polyneuropathies, motor neuron disease, inflammatory myopathies, radiculopathies, and entrapment neuropathies. Marked facilitation of the CMAP to more than 400% of the baseline amplitude after a brief contraction in persons with Lambert-Eaton myasthenic syndrome (LEMS) is one finding that is unique to this uncommon disease.[89]

The time course over which a disease process progresses and the time at which electrodiagnostic testing is conducted both play major roles in determining whether the

Table 8-12 Recommendations Representing Minimum Study for Addressing a Target Disorder

Suspected Condition	Sensory Testing	Motor Testing	Electromyography	Proximal Conductions	Other Special Tests
Radiculopathy	One sensory NCS to exclude polyneuropathy	One motor NCS to exclude polyneuropathy	Sufficient number of muscles representing all myotomes with paraspinal muscles	None	None
Carpal tunnel syndrome	Median sensory NCS and another for comparison	Median motor NCS and another for comparison	Optional, although useful to determine severity of CTS and exclude concomitant C8 radiculopathy	None	None
Ulnar neuropathy	Ulnar sensory NCS and another for comparison	Ulnar motor NCS and another for comparison; need to examine conduction velocity across elbow	Several ulnar-innervated muscles, always the first dorsal interosseus, as it is most frequently abnormal, plus median muscles for comparison to exclude C8 radiculopathy	None	Inching motor NCS across the elbow
Peroneal NCS neuropathy	Superficial peroneal sensory NCS and another for comparison	Peroneal motor with stimulation below and above the fibular head, assessing for conduction velocity and amplitude changes; test another for comparison	Peroneal nerve–innervated muscles and tibial nerve muscles for comparison; suggest paraspinal and L4-L5 muscles to assess for radiculopathy	None	None
Entrapment neuropathies	Two sensory NCSs, one in the distribution and a comparison	Two motor NCSs, one in the distribution and a comparison	Muscles in the involved distribution and comparison muscles	None	None
Myopathy	One or two sensory NCSs in a clinically involved limb	One or two motor NCSs in a clinically involved limb	Two muscles (proximal and distal) in two limbs, one of which is symptomatic	—	Consider repetitive nerve stimulation
Neuromuscular junction disorders	One sensory NCS in a clinically involved limb	One motor NCS in a clinically involved limb	One proximal and one distal muscle in clinically involved limbs	—	Repetitive nerve stimulation at 2 to 3 Hz in clinically weak muscle and, if normal, other weak muscles; single-fiber electromyography if high suspicion and repetitive nerve stimulation is negative—can be first test in ocular myasthenia gravis
Polyneuropathy	Sensory NCS in at least two extremities: if abnormalities in one limb, study the contralateral limb; four or more may be necessary to classify the polyneuropathy	Motor NCS in at least two extremities: if abnormalities in one limb, study the contralateral limb; four or more may be necessary to classify the polyneuropathy	One distal muscle in both legs and a distal muscle in one arm	Consider proximal NCSs (H-reflexes, F-waves, and blink reflexes) to assess demyelination	—
Motor neuron diseases	One sensory NCS in at least two clinically involved limbs	One motor NCS in at least two clinically involved limbs; proximal stimulation sites to exclude conduction block in the case of multifocal motor neuropathy	Several muscles in three extremities, *or* two extremities and cranial nerve–innervated muscles as well as lumbar or cervical paraspinal muscles; thoracic paraspinal muscles may be considered an extremity; sample distal and proximal muscles	Consider F-waves	Consider repetitive nerve stimulation

Modified from the American Association of Electrodiagnostic Medicine: Guidelines in electrodiagnostic medicine, *Muscle Nerve* 8(Suppl):S1-S300, 1999, with permission.
CTS, Carpal tunnel syndrome; *NCS*, nerve conduction study.

Table 8-13 Probability (%) of Finding False-Positive "Abnormal" Results, on the Basis of Chance, According to the Number of Independent Measurements Made*

No. of Measurements	No. of "Abnormalities"				
	1+	2+	3+	4+	5+
1	2.5				
2	4.9	0.1			
3	7.3	0.2	<0.1		
4	9.6	0.4	<0.1	<0.1	
5	11.9	0.6	<0.1	<0.1	<0
6	14.0	0.9	<0.1	<0.1	<0
7	16.2	1.2	<0.1	<0.1	<0
8	18.3	1.6	0.1	<0.1	<0
9	20.4	2.0	0.1	<0.1	<0
10	22.4	2.5	0.2	<0.1	<0
15	31.5	5.2	0.5	<0.1	<0
20	39.5	8.5	1.3	0.1	<0

Modified from Dorfman LJ, Robinson LR: AAEM minimonograph no. 47: normative data in electrodiagnostic medicine, *Muscle Nerve* 20:4-14, 1997.

*Each measurement has a 2.5% false-positive rate (mean ± 2 standard deviations for a Gaussian distribution).

electrodiagnostic testing can provide a reasonably certain diagnosis. It is frequently necessary to repeat the study if the diagnosis remains in question or if the clinical situation changes. One important issue related to electrodiagnostic medicine is the possibility of false-positive results. In Table 8-13, the probabilities of finding false-positive results on the basis of chance alone are shown according to the number of independent measures.[37]

It is important to realize that if five measurements are performed, there is a 12% chance of having one false-positive result. If nine measurements are made, there is a 20% chance of a spuriously false-positive result. If there are two abnormal results when six tests are conducted, however, the likelihood that they are false-positive findings is very low, less than approximately 1%. This underscores the need for electrodiagnosticians to critically examine their findings and not overdiagnose a disorder based on one subtle abnormality. If one electrodiagnostic parameter is markedly abnormal, far beyond the upper limit of normal, this can be compelling, particularly when that abnormality is consistent with the clinical impression. The study should be repeated to make certain of its validity. Two abnormalities indicating the same diagnosis, however, are far more likely to represent true findings and a clear underlying disorder.

Other common conditions, such as diabetes and its corresponding polyneuropathy, can make electrodiagnostic testing more difficult to interpret. With a diffuse polyneuropathy, the consultant is often unable to identify focal lesions against the backdrop of this disorder. In this scenario, the electrodiagnostician must assess the magnitude of the background polyneuropathy and make a judgment as to whether findings for the nerve in question are out of proportion to the background polyneuropathy. Caution is urged in this scenario to avoid overcalling entrapment neuropathies when a generalized polyneuropathy is present. These issues are another reason why it is critically important that the electrodiagnostician have sufficient training to be able to interpret the findings appropriately in the clinical context of the patient.

Anatomic variations in muscle and nerve pathways can also confound electrodiagnostic interpretation. Two well-described variants are important for the electrodiagnostician. The Martin-Gruber anastomosis is formed by a branch from the median nerve, usually the anterior interosseous nerve, joining the ulnar nerve in the forearm. In this situation, the median CMAP with wrist stimulation is smaller than that with proximal stimulation. The ulnar nerve demonstrates a larger amplitude with wrist stimulation than with below-elbow or above-elbow stimulation. If a suspected conduction block is found in the forearm when testing the ulnar nerve, then median nerve conduction should be performed to exclude a Martin-Gruber anastomosis as the cause of CMAP reduction with proximal stimulation.

An accessory deep peroneal nerve is an anomalous part of the deep peroneal nerve that remains with the superficial peroneal nerve and innervates the extensor digitorum brevis after passing behind the lateral malleolus. It should be suspected if stimulation at the fibular head yields a larger CMAP than ankle stimulation when recorded over the extensor digitorum brevis. Stimulation of the accessory deep peroneal nerve behind the lateral malleolus will confirm the presence of such an anatomic variant.

Standards of Practice for Electrodiagnostic Medicine

The AANEM has addressed the need to set standards for the evaluation and interpretation of studies in response to the burgeoning and disquieting practice of decoupling nerve conductions and needle EMG. It is the contention of the organization that electrodiagnostic studies should be performed by physicians properly trained in electrodiagnostic medicine, that interpretation of NCS data alone, absent face-to-face patient interaction and control over the process provides substandard care, and that performance of NCS without needle EMG has the potential of compromising patient care.[8] Considerable concern exists that there has been a dramatic increase in NCSs without EMG testing.[8] EMG testing is crucial for the assessment of radiculopathies and plexopathies as well as to complement NCSs and give additional information about entrapments and nerve injuries. Interpreting NCS findings without the benefit of a focused history and examination is also inappropriate.[8] Communication of the consultation results to the referring physician and other health care providers is essential. The AANEM recommends that the electrodiagnostic report contain (1) a description of the problem and the reason for referral; (2) a focused history and examination; (3) tabular NCS and EMG information with normative reference values; and (4) temperature and limbs studied.[7] It is recommended that the study results are defined as normal or abnormal, and a probable physiologic diagnosis is presented. Any limitations to the study should be included.[7] An optional section after this summary can be a synthesis of the clinical and electrophysiologic information into clinical recommendations or a stronger set of conclusions.

Such a section should be separate from the electrophysiologic testing. The EMG and NCS data and the conclusions they support should stand alone. Visual depictions of the waveforms, although not required, are an ideal means of documenting the nerve conduction findings and are usually available on modern electrodiagnostic instruments.

Pediatric Electrodiagnosis

The pediatric examination poses challenges for even the most experienced electrodiagnostic physician. Diagnosis of pediatric neuromuscular disorders is a specialized and rapidly evolving area of medicine in which genetic testing plays an ever greater role in diagnosis. Interested readers are encouraged to examine specialized textbooks and recent articles because much of this material is beyond the scope of this chapter.

In terms of equipment required for pediatric electrodiagnosis, a pediatric bipolar stimulating probe is available and is useful for small children.[102] Monopolar needles are generally used because their diameter is smaller and insertional resistance is less, which is attributable to their Teflon coating. It is critically important to maintain a skin surface temperature of 36° C to 37° C to avoid spurious results.[102]

There are strong advocates for and against the use of sedation and analgesia during electrodiagnostic examination.[102] Performance of all conscious sedation and anesthesia should be done by specialists in pediatric anesthesia. When general anesthetic is required, children with possible neuromuscular diseases should not be given halogenated inhalation agents such as halothane because of the risks for malignant hyperthermia.[97] Nerve conduction testing should include both sensory and motor studies. The needle examination, although difficult, should always be part of the diagnostic evaluation. Despite the challenging nature of the needle examination, a complete needle EMG is necessary to reach appropriate conclusions. A single muscle exploration is insufficient for diagnosis in a child.[102]

The conduction velocities in newborns are approximately half of those found in adults. There is a rapid increase in values during the first year of life. Median values for conduction velocities in children and adults are equalized by 5 years of age.[102] Tables 8-14 and 8-15 show values for infants and newborns.[82] Motor conduction velocities in full-term infants should be no less than 20 m/s.[102]

Late responses evaluate an infant's proximal peripheral nervous system. They offer several advantages including reduced problems with temperature control, longer

Table 8-14 Motor Conduction Studies in 155 Children*

	Median Nerve†				*Peroneal Nerve*‡			
Age (*n*)	**Distal Motor Latency (ms)**	**Conduction Velocity (m/s)**	**F-Latency (ms)**	**Amplitude (mV)**	**Distal Motor Latency (ms)**	**Conduction Velocity (m/s)**	**F-Latency (ms)**	**Amplitude (mV)**
7 days to 1 mo (20)	2.23 (0.29)	25.43 (3.84)	16.12 (1.50)	3.00 (0.31)	2.43 (0.48)	22.43 (1.22)	22.07 (1.46)	3.06 (1.26)
1 to 6 mo (23)	2.21 (0.34)	34.35 (6.61)	16.89 (1.65)	7.37 (3.24)	2.25 (0.48)	35.18 (3.96)	23.11 (1.89)	5.23 (2.37)
6 to 12 mo (25)	2.13 (0.19)	43.57 (4.78)	17.31 (1.77)	7.67 (4.45)	2.31 (0.62)	43.55 (3.77)	25.86 (1.35)	5.41 (2.01)
1 to 2 yr (24)	2.04 (0.18)	48.23 (4.58)	17.44 (1.29)	8.90 (3.61)	2.29 (0.43)	51.42 (3.02)	25.98 (1.95)	5.80 (2.48)
2 to 4 yr (22)	2.18 (0.43)	53.59 (5.29)	17.91 (1.11)	9.55 (4.34)	2.62 (0.75)	55.73 (4.45)	29.52 (2.15)	6.10 (2.99)
4 to 6 yr (20)	2.27 (0.45)	56.26 (4.61)	19.44 (1.51)	10.37 (3.66)	3.01 (0.43)	56.14 (4.96)	29.98 (2.68)	7.10 (4.76)
6 to 14 yr (21)	2.73 (0.44)	57.32 (3.35)	23.23 (2.57)	12.37 (4.79)	3.25 (0.51)	57.05 (4.54)	34.27 (4.29)	8.15 (4.19)

Modified from Parano E, Uncini A, DeVivo DC, et al: Electrophysiologic correlates of peripheral nervous system maturation in infancy and childhood, *J Child Neurol* 8:336-338, 1993.
*Mean (standard deviation).
†Median motor recorded from abductor pollicis brevis and stimulated at wrist.
‡Peroneal motor recorded over extensor digitorum brevis and stimulated at ankle.

Table 8-15 Sensory Conduction Studies in 155 Children*

	Median Nerve†		*Sural Nerve*	
Age (*n*)	**Conduction Velocity (m/s)**	**Amplitude (μV)**	**Conduction Velocity (m/s)**	**Amplitude (μV)**
7 days to 1 mo (20)	22.31 (2.16)	6.22 (1.30)	20.26 (1.55)	9.12 (3.02)
1 to 6 mo (23)	35.52 (6.59)	15.86 (5.18)	34.63 (5.43)	11.66 (3.57)
6 to 12 mo (25)	40.31 (5.23)	16.00 (5.18)	38.18 (5.00)	15.10 (8.22)
1 to 2 yr (24)	46.93 (5.03)	24.00 (7.36)	49.73 (5.53)	15.41 (9.98)
2 to 4 yr (22)	49.51 (3.34)	24.28 (5.49)	52.63 (2.96)	23.27 (6.84)
4 to 6 yr (20)	51.71 (5.16)	25.12 (5.22)	53.83 (4.34)	22.66 (5.42)
6 to 14 yr (21)	53.84 (3.26)	26.72 (9.43)	53.85 (4.19)	26.75 (6.59)

Modified from Parano E, Uncini A, DeVivo DC, et al: Electrophysiologic correlates of peripheral nervous system maturation in infancy and childhood, *J Child Neurol* 8:336-338, 1993.
*Mean (standard deviation).
†Median sensory recorded at wrist with stimulation of index fingers.

conduction distance, reduced measurement error, and a single stimulation site. In contrast to adults, the H-reflex can be elicited from any muscle during infancy, but most responses are gradually and variably suppressed by 1 year of age.[102] The tibial nerve, however, retains its electrophysiologic H-reflex throughout life.

The needle EMG examination in infants is challenging and should begin with the muscles of highest diagnostic yield such as those in a weak limb. Needle manipulation and repositioning are often necessary because of the greater relative amount of adipose tissue and reduced muscle activation. Muscle relaxation to examine for spontaneous or normal insertional activities is best obtained by placing the muscle at its shortest length from origin to insertion.[102] The infant's foot and hand intrinsic muscles can best be used to study insertional and spontaneous activity because they are usually not very active.[102] These distal muscles, however, exhibit high levels of end-plate noise because of the relatively larger end-plate regions, which can be confused with fibrillation potentials.[102] Extensor muscles are not activated as often by the neonate and therefore are good choices as well for evaluation of spontaneous and insertional activity.[102]

Assessment of motor unit morphology and recruitment is difficult. Motor unit potentials in the pediatric population differ from those in the adult population. Motor unit potentials in the newborn are usually biphasic or triphasic, their amplitudes range from 100 to 700 μV, and they are shorter in duration at 5 to 9 ms.[61,102] Recruitment of motor units is often difficult to interpret because there is typically no voluntary control. When looking for motor unit morphology and recruitment, it is advisable to examine flexor muscles because there is usually strong flexor tone and muscle activation. It is important to remember that this is a difficult examination and overinterpretation is common for the inexperienced practitioner.

Repetitive nerve stimulation is used to evaluate presynaptic and postsynaptic neuromuscular disorders. Immobilization of the arm or leg and maintenance of warm body and limb temperatures are crucial for optimizing sensitivity for this testing. Use of 20-Hz stimulation to assess for postactivation decrement repair or to look for postexercise facilitation is occasionally necessary. This is painful, and an anesthetized, immobile infant is optimal to derive a meaningful study. Stimulated single-fiber EMG can be performed and is an ideal, sensitive means of testing for neuromuscular junction disorders.[21,25]

The hypotonic infant poses diagnostic challenges, with hypotonia being the most common reason infants are referred for electrodiagnostic examination. Within this category, the most common cause for generalized hypotonia is a central nervous system disorder.[102] In fact, only 10% to 20% of infants and children with hypotonia have a neuromuscular etiology.[102] The most common neuromuscular diagnosis in hypotonic infants is spinal muscular atrophy.

Several peripheral nerve entities occur in the newborn. Partial facial paralysis or asymmetrical faces might occur, and motor NCSs and needle EMG of the facial nerve and its corresponding innervated muscles are useful to clarify the mononeuropathy. Side-to-side comparisons of the CMAPs can give an estimate of the degree of axonal loss and some prognostic information. Brachial plexopathies at birth are uncommon, occurring in 1.5 per 1000 live births.[35] These brachial plexus palsies are difficult to predict and are usually unrelated to identifiable obstetric characteristics such as gestational age, oxytocin augmentation, delivery mode (forceps, spontaneous, breech, or cesarean), or birth weight.[35] However, the duration of labor and presence of shoulder dystocia were significantly related to the occurrence of brachial plexus palsy.[35] Erb palsy involves the upper plexus and C5 or C6 roots. A Klumpke or lower plexus palsy primarily demonstrates C8 or T1, and lower trunk involvement. The needle EMG can help confirm the site of pathology and location of primary involvement.[102] In one series, supracostoclavicular space narrowing caused by anatomic variations such as cervical ribs or fibrous bands was identified as a predisposing factor that rendered the brachial plexus more prone to injury.[9] For situations in which a neurologic deficit is found at the time of delivery, an electrodiagnostic study shortly afterward (within 24 hours) can help elucidate whether such a deficit developed intrauterine or during delivery. Intrauterine onset of a focal neuropathy or plexopathy may demonstrate fibrillation potentials in the weak muscles.[58]

A particularly interesting case report discussed the intrauterine onset of a peroneal neuropathy with fibrillations found within 20 hours of birth in the affected muscles, underscoring the onset before delivery and arguing against obstetric trauma as the cause.[58] In this case report, the authors discuss other cases in which onset predated the delivery, as evidenced by fibrillations in clinically affected muscles shortly after birth. These findings have implications regarding medicolegal issues surrounding brachial plexus palsies and other mononeuropathies in newborns.

Mononeuropathies and Entrapment Neuropathies

Suspected mononeuropathies are the most common reasons for electrodiagnostic laboratory referral. Top among these conditions is median neuropathy at the wrist or carpal tunnel syndrome. Other entrapments include ulnar neuropathy at the elbow, common peroneal neuropathy at the fibular head, and tibial nerve entrapment at the ankle (tarsal tunnel syndrome). In addition to these entrapments, focal nerve injuries can occur with penetrating trauma and fractures. The common entrapments and nerve injuries, their anatomic causes, and their electrodiagnostic correlates are given in Table 8-16.

The approach to assessing for mononeuropathies is to fully test the nerve in question and another nerve in the affected limb for comparison. Stimulation both below and above the suspected site of injury can help assess for conduction block or conduction slowing. EMG of selected muscles innervated by the particular nerve is required. If these muscles are abnormal, the study should be expanded to ensure that these EMG findings are confined to a single peripheral nerve distribution and that they are not attributable to a radiculopathy, plexopathy, or polyneuropathy. The electrodiagnostician should have a low threshold for testing the same nerves in the opposite limb. The examiner must sort out a focal process versus a generalized process such as polyneuropathy.

Table 8-16 Entrapment Neuropathies

Nerve	Causes	Clinical Features	Suggested Electrodiagnostic Evaluation	Potential EMG Findings
Median Neuropathies				
Carpal tunnel syndrome: Median entrapment at wrist	The most common entrapment neuropathy Incidence: 55 to 125 cases/100,000 Causes: Repetitive trauma, obesity, pregnancy, lupus, etc.[41]	Aching pain in forearm and wrist with insidious onset, tingling, paresthesias of thumb, index, and long finger, thenar weakness, nocturnal pain	Sensory NCS across the wrist and another sensory nerve in the affected limb to compare Motor NCS of median nerve and another motor nerve (usually ulnar) Needle EMG is optional[4]	Mild CTS: Prolonged SNAP and/or slightly reduced SNAP amplitude Moderate CTS: Abnormal median SNAP as above, plus prolonged median motor latency[96] Severe CTS: Prolonged motor and sensory distal latencies, plus either an absent SNAP or a low-amplitude or absent CMAP. The EMG often shows fibrillations in thenar (median) muscles if severe[94]
Pronator syndrome: Entrapment of median nerve between heads of the pronator teres and beneath FDS arch at forearm	Trauma from repetitive overuse, tight casting, penetrating injuries such as intravenous catheter, carrying a bag with the arm flexed ("grocery bag neuropathy")[41]	Aching pain in the volar forearm, hand numbness, symptoms worsened by repeated pronation, clumsiness, loss of dexterity, weakness, flexor muscle and thenar muscle wasting if severe, tender pronator muscle	Motor nerve conduction across this area Median sensory study distally EMG of median muscles Evaluation of ulnar nerve for comparison Radiculopathy screen to exclude this condition EMG findings should be confined to median distribution	SNAP: Normal unless axonal loss CMAP: Normal or reduced if motor axonal loss present. NCV slowed across the pronator area or conduction block across this site EMG: Reduced recruitment in median innervated muscles, fibrillations, and motor unit changes if there is motor axonal loss Pronator teres usually spared
Anterior interosseus: Entrapment at forearm (Kiloh-Nevin syndrome)	Direct trauma, inflammation, strenuous exercise, fractures, variant of brachial neuritis, compression by anomalous fibrous bands in this region[41]	Acute pure motor syndrome with pain in forearm and elbow, weak flexor pollicis longus and flexor digitorum profundus of index and long finger, weak pronator quadratus. "OK" sign No sensory complaints	Motor nerve conduction across this area Median sensory study distally EMG of median muscles Evaluation of ulnar nerve for comparison Radiculopathy screen to exclude this condition EMG findings should be confined to anterior interosseous nerve distribution	Median SNAPs are normal Normal median nerve conduction studies to the APB With surface or needle recordings from the pronator quadratus, there can be slowed median NCV On EMG, findings will be limited to FPL, PQ, and FDP (index and long)
Median nerve entrapment beneath the ligament of Struthers	Caused by trauma or inflammation Supracondylar process seen in 0.7% to 2.7% of population[32] Associated with fibrous band from supracondylar process to medial epicondyle (Supracondylar process 5 cm above medial epicondyle on radiograph is noted.)	Weak grip, weakness in flexion of wrist, deep aching pain in forearm, numbness of 1 to 3 digits, weak hand pronation, second and third digit flexion, wasting of APB	Motor nerve conduction across this area Median sensory study distally EMG of median muscles Evaluation of ulnar nerve for comparison Radiculopathy screen to exclude this condition EMG findings should be confined to median distribution Pronator teres often involved	Decreased or absent SNAP amplitude Reduced motor NCV or conduction block across this segment Decreased CMAP from APB EMG findings in median nerve distribution including pronator teres[41]

Continued on following page

Table 8-16 Entrapment Neuropathies (Continued)

Nerve	Causes	Clinical Features	Suggested Electrodiagnostic Evaluation	Potential EMG Findings
Radial Neuropathies				
Radial nerve entrapment at axilla	Improper use of crutches, falling asleep with arm over a sharp chair back or edge	Weakness in all radial nerve–innervated muscles including triceps, decreased sensation in posterior arm and forearm	Superficial radial sensory Radial motor testing with recording from EIP with either surface or needle electrodes. Should stimulate at Erb point Testing at least one additional motor and sensory nerve in the involved limb EMG of radial nerve–innervated muscles EMG screen for radiculopathy (e.g., other muscles not innervated by radial nerve)	Reduced or absent SNAP if axonal loss Normal or reduced motor CMAP if axonal loss occurred Conduction block across the axilla EMG findings in radial nerve–innervated muscles including triceps when motor axonal loss is present
Radial nerve entrapment at spiral groove (Saturday night palsy or honeymooner palsy)	Acute prolonged compression of the nerve in the humeral region caused by a person sleeping on the arm or falling asleep in an improper position Frequently associated with alcohol use Other causes include an injection or compression with a tourniquet	Involves all radial nerve–innervated muscles except triceps brachii and anconeus Wrist extension weakness and finger extension weakness Sensory loss over dorsal hand and posterior forearm	Same as above	Reduced or absent SNAP if axonal loss. Normal or reduced motor CMAP if axonal loss occurred Conduction block across the spiral groove region EMG findings in radial nerve–innervated muscles excluding triceps and anconeus when motor axonal loss is present
Radial nerve with posterior interosseous nerve compression	Radial tunnel syndrome encompasses entrapment by fibrous bands at the radial head, or the sharp tendinous margin of the ECRB Posterior interosseus syndrome or supinator syndrome where the PIN is entrapped at the fibrous band at the origin of supinator muscle, called the arcade of Frohse[41] Other causes include dislocation of elbow, Monteggia fracture, fall on outstretched hand, surgical resection of radial head, mass lesions	Deep pain at elbow Weakness with wrist extension Weakness of MCP extension yet preserved ability to extend IP joints resulting from interossei No loss of sensation	Same as above	Normal superficial radial sensory response Slowed motor conduction across the elbow; low CMAP over EIP EMG findings in PIN-innervated muscles; brachioradialis and ECRL usually spared
Radial nerve entrapment at the wrist (Wartenberg syndrome or handcuff neuropathy)	Bracelets and handcuff neuropathy Ganglions, overuse syndrome	Numbness, paresthesias of dorsoradial aspect of hand and dorsum of first three digits, tender to palpation in this area No motor weakness	Same as above In certain compelling clinical circumstances the examination can be abbreviated and focused on the superficial radial nerve, with another nerve for comparison	Superficial radial sensory response delayed in latency or low in amplitude
Ulnar Neuropathies				
Ulnar nerve compression at Guyon canal at wrist	Chronic pressure from using tools, bicycle riding, ganglion, rheumatoid arthritis	Type 1: Hypothenar and deep ulnar branch Type 2: Deep ulnar branch Type 3: Superficial ulnar sensory branch Numbness, paresthesias, weakness, intrinsic muscle atrophy, nocturnal pain Painless wasting of hand intrinsics	Ulnar sensory testing Ulnar motor testing with recording electrodes over ADM and FDI and conduction across the elbow Dorsal ulnar cutaneous Another motor and sensory nerve in the affected limb for comparison EMG ulnar muscles	Prolonged motor latency Dorsal ulnar cutaneous nerve spared Ulnar sensory response to fifth digit prolonged in latency or normal if mostly motor fibers are involved CMAP decreased if axonal loss present EMG demonstrates fibrillations or motor unit changes in hand intrinsics but not in thenar (median innervated) muscles

Table 8-16 Entrapment Neuropathies (Continued)

Nerve	Causes	Clinical Features	Suggested Electrodiagnostic Evaluation	Potential EMG Findings
Ulnar nerve compression at the elbow	Trauma, cubitus valgus, bony spurs, tumors, overuse, previous fracture Proximal to elbow the nerve may be entrapped by the arcade of Struthers, a fibrous structure associated with the medial triceps muscle Cubital tunnel made of the fibrous entrance to the FCU is the most common site	Vague dull aching forearm, intermittent paresthesia, hypoesthesia on ulnar side of hand, weakness of abduction of little finger, ulnar clawing in severe cases, wasting of first dorsal interosseus and hypothenar eminence, wasting of ulnar border of forearm	Ulnar motor conduction across the elbow and in forearm; if abnormal, additional motor and sensory to exclude diffuse process Consider an inching study across elbows[4,18] Ulnar sensory Dorsal ulnar cutaneous EMG of ulnar muscles	The ulnar sensory nerve may be reduced in amplitude or absent The dorsal ulnar cutaneous nerve may be reduced or absent Ulnar motor amplitude might be reduced Conduction block across the elbow can occur NCV is more than 10 m/s slower across the elbow than in the forearm segment Short segmental inching at 1-cm intervals can reveal greater than 0.4-ms segmental change or a clear discontinuity[18]
Lower Limb Mononeuropathies				
Femoral neuropathy	Trauma, retroperitoneal hematoma caused by anticoagulation, cardiac catheterizations[4]	Weak quadriceps muscle, weakness of knee extension, absent knee jerk, groin pain, and decreased sensation over medial and anterior thigh and lower leg in the saphenous nerve distribution	Motor nerve conduction to quadriceps Saphenous sensory study EMG of quadriceps as well as other L3 and L4 muscles (e.g., the adductor muscles) Consider an EMG screen for radiculopathy	Reduced amplitude or absent saphenous nerve response Reduced CMAP over rectus femoris On EMG, fibrillations in the femoral nerve–innervated muscles
Lateral femoral cutaneous nerve entrapment at thigh (meralgia paresthetica)	Repeated low-grade trauma, obesity, pregnancy, tight clothing most commonly under the lateral end of the ilioinguinal ligament	Pure sensory syndrome at the lateral thigh including unpleasant paresthesias, burning, or a dull ache; no motor symptoms Can be aggravated by prolonged standing or walking	Lateral femoral cutaneous study Femoral evaluation as above should be considered	Reduced amplitude in lateral femoral cutaneous nerve This nerve is technically challenging to study and side-to-side comparisons are useful
Peroneal nerve entrapment at the head of the fibula	Fractures, plaster casts, tight stockings, improper positioning, excessive weight loss, farm work, tumors, crossing legs for a long time	Foot drop, weakness of eversion, numbness on the dorsum of the foot, and pain	SPS testing Motor nerve conduction below and across the fibular head recorded from EDB or tibialis anterior if EDB is atrophied Exclude L5 radiculopathy by EMG Test an additional motor and sensory in the same leg	Reduced or absent SPS response Conduction block across the fibular head Conduction velocity reduced in fibular head segment by greater than 10 m/s compared with leg segment Fibrillations in muscles innervated by peroneal nerve
Tibial nerve entrapment at tarsal tunnel under flexor retinaculum of medial malleolus	Compression from shoes, casting, posttraumatic fibrosis, overuse, ganglion cysts	Pain in foot and ankle, wasting and weakness in feet, sensory impairment at toes and sole of the foot	Plantar sensory (mixed) nerve conductions Tibial motor to AH muscle Another motor and sensory in the same limb to exclude polyneuropathy EMG of intrinsic foot muscles Consider EMG screen for radiculopathy or sciatic neuropathy	Prolonged latencies or low amplitudes in plantar nerves Prolonged tibial motor latency across tarsal tunnel Fibrillations in the flexor digitorum brevis, AH, or other intrinsic foot muscle innervated by the tibial nerve

ADM, Abductor digiti minimi; *AH*, abductor hallucis; *APB*, abductor pollicis brevis; *CMAP*, compound muscle action potential; *CTS*, carpal tunnel syndrome; *ECRB*, extensor carpi radialis brevis; *ECRL*, extensor carpi radialis longus; *EDB*, extensor digitorum brevis; *EIP*, extensor indicis proprius; *EMG*, electromyography; *FCU*, flexor carpi ulnaris; *FDI*, first dorsal interosseus; *FDP*, flexor digitorum profundus; *FDS*, flexor digitorum superficialis; *FPL*, flexor pollicis longus; *IP*, interphalangeal; *MCP*, metacarpophalangeal; *NCS*, nerve conduction study; *NCV*, nerve conduction velocity; *PIN*, posterior interosseous nerve; *PQ*, pronator quadratus; *SNAP*, sensory nerve action potential; *SPS*, superficial peroneal sensory nerve.

Brachial Plexopathies

Brachial plexopathies are important causes of shoulder and neck region pain.[23] The EMG examination is crucial and should be extensive and detailed, particularly for proximal muscles and muscles in which there is clinical weakness.[83] Sensory nerve action potentials (SNAPs) are a key part of the evaluation. SNAPs are readily available for C6 (radial to the thumb), C7 (median to digit 2), and C8 (ulnar to digit 5) root levels in the hand, and L5 (superficial peroneal sensory) and S1 (sural sensory) in the leg. Other SNAPs, such as the lateral antebrachial cutaneous (C5, C6) or the medial antebrachial cutaneous (C8, T1), can provide additional information to the study. SNAPs are generally low in amplitude or absent with postganglionic plexopathies, and help differentiate between radiculopathies and plexopathies. The exception to this rule is in the case of traumatic plexopathy when a root is avulsed. This severe injury with little chance of recovery should be recognized. In this case, the patient's weakness is profound and the CMAPs are low or absent, but the SNAPs are preserved. A myelogram or MRI often reveals a traumatic meningocele associated with such root avulsions.

The amplitudes of CMAPs should be elicited when possible in the weak muscles and compared with the uninvolved side. After Wallerian degeneration has occurred, this gives a rough estimate of the amount of axonal loss. It is thought that CMAPs less than 10% to 20% of the uninvolved side portend poor prognosis; however, the literature supporting this statement is weak and in large measure derived from Bell palsy experience.[28]

Electrodiagnosticians should understand the peripheral neuroanatomy of the lumbosacral and brachial plexuses. A thorough appreciation for muscular anatomy, root innervations, and needle localization is a prerequisite. The consultant should specify, with as much precision as the study will allow, the location of the lesion, the magnitude (severity), and whenever possible rough estimates of probable outcomes. It is important to also appreciate that different parts of the brachial plexus can be involved with differing severities. The electrodiagnostician should determine, when possible, these differential injuries because such information can help surgeons who contemplate tendon transfers and can help guide therapy. Innervated and compensatory muscles should be strengthened. The patient must have a good range-of-motion program to prevent conditions such as adhesive capsulitis that can become a secondary and painful long-term problem.

Radiculopathies

Cervical, thoracic, and lumbosacral radiculopathies are conditions involving a pathologic process affecting the spinal nerve root. There are multiple causes for radiculopathies. One common cause is a herniated nucleus pulposus that anatomically compresses a nerve root within the spinal canal or foramen. Another common etiology for radiculopathy is spinal stenosis, resulting from a combination of degenerative spondylosis, ligament hypertrophy, and/or spondylolisthesis. Inflammatory radiculitis is another pathophysiologic process that can cause radiculopathy. It is important to remember, however, that other more ominous processes, such as malignancy and infection, can manifest the same symptoms and signs of radiculopathy as those of the more common causes.

The dorsal root ganglion lies in the intervertebral foramen. This anatomic arrangement has implications for the clinical electrodiagnosis of radiculopathy, namely that SNAPs are preserved in most radiculopathies. This is because the nerve root is affected proximal to the dorsal root ganglion. A recent study examined the sensory findings in persons with documented herniated disks causing lumbosacral radiculopathy.[81] In this study of 108 patients with lumbosacral radiculopathy, sensory responses in the leg (sural, peroneal, or saphenous) were reduced in amplitude in only 7% of patients. None of these patients had an absent sensory response. This well-designed prospective trial supported the long-held notion that sensory responses are almost always preserved in lumbosacral radiculopathy. An abnormality in the NCS of a sensory nerve should prompt consideration of other causes of a patient's symptoms besides radiculopathy.[81]

In the lumbar spine, the dorsal and ventral lumbar roots exit the spinal cord at about the T11 to L1 bony level and travel in the lumbar canal as a group of nerve roots in the dural sac. This is termed the cauda equina, or "horse's tail." This poses challenges and limitations to the EMG examination. A destructive intramedullary (spinal cord) lesion at T11 can produce EMG findings in muscles innervated by any of the lumbosacral nerve roots and manifest the same findings on needle EMG as those seen with a herniated nucleus pulposus at any of the lumbar disk levels. For this reason, the electromyographer cannot determine with certainty the anatomic location of the lumbar intraspinal lesion producing distal muscle EMG findings in the lower limbs. The needle EMG examination can identify only the root or roots that are physiologically involved but not the precise anatomic site of pathology in the lumbar spinal canal. This is an important limitation requiring correlation with imaging findings to determine which anatomic location is most probably the offending site.

By far the most useful test for confirming the presence of a radiculopathy is needle EMG. Needle EMG testing with a sufficient number of muscles and at least one motor and one sensory NCS should be performed in the involved limb.[6] The NCSs are necessary to exclude polyneuropathy. An EMG study is considered diagnostic for radiculopathy if EMG abnormalities are found in two or more muscles innervated by the same nerve root and different peripheral nerves, yet muscles innervated by adjacent nerve roots are normal.[105] This assumes that other generalized conditions such as polyneuropathy are not present. The need for EMG, particularly in relationship to imaging of the spine, has been highlighted.[88] Needle EMG is particularly helpful given that the false-positive rates for MRI of the lumbar spine are high, with 27% of normal individuals having a disk protrusion.[56] For the cervical spine, the false-positive rate for MRI is lower, with 19% of individuals demonstrating an abnormality, but only 10% showing a herniated or bulging disk.[12] Radiculopathies can occur without structural findings on MRI and likewise without EMG findings. The EMG evaluates only motor axonal loss or motor axon conduction block (reduced recruitment is seen), and for these reasons a radiculopathy affecting the sensory root will not yield abnormalities by EMG. If the rate of denervation is balanced by reinnervation in the muscle, then spontaneous activity is less likely to be seen with EMG. The sensitivity for EMG ranges from 49% to 92%.[101]

The specificity of needle EMG was recently addressed in a group of asymptomatic persons in comparison with a radiculopathy group. When considering the typical distribution of findings to identify a radiculopathy (two abnormal muscles not innervated by the same peripheral nerve), and using six muscle screens and considering only spontaneous activity as abnormal, the needle EMG had 100% specificity. There were no false-positive tests. This is valuable information that supports the usefulness of needle EMG as a confirmatory test that complements spinal imaging.[100]

Cervical and lumbar paraspinal muscles are important to examine with EMG when assessing for radiculopathy. If positive, they localize the site of pathology to the spine or root level. When assessing paraspinal muscles, only fibrillations, PSWs, CRDs, or myotonic discharges have clinical relevance. Recruitment findings and motor unit morphology for these muscles have not been well established. There are no normative data regarding motor unit morphology in either the cervical or lumbar paraspinal muscles to which precise recruitment comparisons can be made. Examiners should not overcall radiculopathies based on reduced "recruitment" or "increased polyphasicity" of the paraspinal muscles. Paraspinal muscles show either spontaneous activity or other abnormal discharges (CRDs), and therefore they localize the lesion to the root, but not to a specific level. There is considerable overlap in paraspinal muscles, with single roots innervating muscle fibers above and below their anatomic levels. For this reason, the level of radiculopathy cannot be delineated by paraspinal EMG alone, but rather is based on the root level that best explains the distribution of limb muscles with EMG abnormalities.

The lumbar paraspinal muscle examination can be easily performed and should be studied in persons with suspected radiculopathies. Haig[51] derived a means of quantifying the degree of findings in the paraspinals by means of an index derived by adding the fibrillations found in a standard set of muscle insertions. Such quantitative assessment distinguishes patients with radiculopathies and spinal stenosis with greater precision. In this miniparaspinal mapping scale, the lumbar paraspinal muscles are identified, and four separate areas in the lumbar paraspinal region are studied.[51] Fibrillations with a score of greater than 3 on the miniparaspinal mapping scale are abnormal. Furthermore, this technique was validated in a group of asymptomatic older adults.[22] The stricter criterion of abnormal spontaneous activity on needle examination, and paraspinal mapping scores greater than 6 being considered abnormal, serve to lower the risk of false-positive EMG testing. These findings, from a well-conducted and blinded study, suggest that EMG is less likely to be abnormal (false positive) in asymptomatic adults than MRI when quantified by paraspinal muscles mapping.[22] Although this technique is rigorous, it is relatively easy to perform and seems to improve the accuracy and reproducibility of paraspinal EMG.

Dumitru et al.[42] examined the lumbosacral paraspinal muscles and intrinsic foot muscles with monopolar EMG. These investigators recorded potentials and found that there were irregularly firing potentials with similar waveform characteristics as fibrillations and PSWs. By excluding irregularly firing potentials (atypical end-plate spikes) and considering only regularly firing potentials with appropriate morphology consistent with fibrillations, they found that only 4% of these individuals had false-positive paraspinal EMG findings. This well-designed quantitative lumbosacral study underscores the need to assess both firing rate and rhythm, as well as discharge morphology, when evaluating for fibrillations and positive waves in the lumbar paraspinal muscles. Fibrillations fire regularly, and this should be confirmed by listening carefully and seeing consistent intervals between fibrillations on the display screen. Electrodiagnosticians should take care not to overcall paraspinal muscle EMG findings by mistaking irregularly firing end-plate spikes for regularly firing fibrillations.

How Many and Which Muscles to Study

A screening EMG study involves determining whether the radiculopathy can be confirmed by EMG. The concept of a screening EMG encompasses identifying the possibility of an electrodiagnostically confirmable radiculopathy. If one of the muscles in the screen is abnormal, the screen must be expanded to exclude other diagnoses and to fully delineate the radiculopathy level. Because of the screening nature of the EMG examination, electrodiagnosticians with experience should look for more subtle signs of denervation and, if present in the screening muscles, then expand the study to determine whether these findings are limited to a single myotome or peripheral nerve distribution. If they are limited to a single muscle, their clinical significance is uncertain.

A prospective multicenter study evaluating patients referred to participating electrodiagnostic laboratories with suspected cervical radiculopathy was conducted to address the issue regarding how many muscles are sufficient to confidently identify an electrodiagnostically confirmable cervical radiculopathy.[30] There were 101 patients with electrodiagnostically confirmed cervical radiculopathies representing all cervical root levels. When paraspinal muscles were one of the screening muscles, five-muscle screens identified 90% to 98% of radiculopathies, six-muscle screens identified 94% to 99%, and seven-muscle screens identified 96% to 100% (Table 8-17). When paraspinal muscles were not part of the screen, eight distal limb muscles recognized 92% to 95% of radiculopathies. Six-muscle screens including paraspinal muscles yielded consistently high identification rates, and studying additional muscles led to marginal increases in identification. Individual screens useful to the electromyographer are listed in Table 8-17. These findings were consistent with those derived from a large retrospective study.[71]

A similar prospective multicenter study was conducted to assess the optimal screening electrodiagnostic assessment for persons with suspected lumbosacral radiculopathy.[29,33] In this study, there were 102 patients with electrodiagnostically confirmed lumbosacral radiculopathies representing all lumbosacral root levels. When paraspinal muscles were one of the screening muscles, four-muscle screens identified 88% to 97%, five-muscle screens identified 94% to 98%, and six-muscle screens identified 98% to 100% (Table 8-18). When paraspinal muscles were not part of the screen, identification rates were lower for all screens, and eight distal muscles were

Table 8-17 Six-Muscle Screen Identifications of Patients with Cervical Radiculopathies

Muscle Screen	Neuropathic* (%)	Spontaneous Activity† (%)
Six Muscles Without Paraspinals		
Deltoid, APB, FCU, triceps, PT, FCR	93	66
Biceps, triceps, FCU, EDC, FCR, FDI	87	55
Deltoid, triceps, EDC, FDI, FCR, PT	89	64
Biceps, triceps, EDC, PT, APB, FCU	94	64
Six Muscles with Paraspinals		
Deltoid, triceps, PT, APB, EDC, PSM	99	83
Biceps, triceps, EDC, FDI, FCU, PSM	96	75
Deltoid, EDC, FDI, PSM, FCU, triceps	94	77
Biceps, FCR, APB, PT, PSM, triceps	98	79

Modified from Dillingham TR, Lauder TD, Andary M, et al: Identification of cervical radiculopathies: optimizing the electromyographic screen, *Am J Phys Med Rehabil* 80:84-91, 2001.

*The "neuropathic" column indicates the identification rates when looking for all types of subtle neuropathic findings.

†The spontaneous activity column indicates identification rates when only fibrillations or positive sharp waves are considered.

APB, Abductor pollicis brevis; *EDC*, extensor digitorum communis; *FCR*, flexor carpi radialis; *FCU*, flexor carpi ulnaris; *FDI*, first dorsal interosseus; *PSM*, cervical paraspinal muscles; *PT*, pronator teres.

Table 8-18 Six-Muscle Screen Identifications of Patients with Lumbosacral Radiculopathies

Muscle Screen	Neuropathic* (%)	Spontaneous Activity† (%)
Six Muscles Without Paraspinals		
ATIB, PTIB, MGAS, RFEM, SHBF, LGAS	89	78
VMED, TFL, LGAS, PTIB, ADD, MGAS	83	70
VLAT, SHBF, LGAS, ADD, TFL, PTIB	79	62
ADD, TFL, MGAS, PTIB, ATIB, LGAS	88	79
Six Muscles with Paraspinals		
ATIB, PTIB, MGAS, PSM, VMED, TFL	99	93
VMED, LGAS, PTIB, PSM, SHBF, MGAS	99	87
VLAT, TFL, LGAS, PSM, ATIB, SHBF	98	87
ADD, MGAS, PTIB, PSM, VLAT, SHBF	99	89
VMED, ATIB, PTIB, PSM, SHBF, MGAS	100	92
VMED, TFL, LGAS, PSM, ATIB, PTIB	99	91
ADD, MGAS, PTIB, PSM, ATIB, SHBF	100	93

Modified from Dillingham TR, Lauder TD, Andary M, et al: Identification of cervical radiculopathies: optimizing the electromyographic screen, *Am J Phys Med Rehabil* 80:84-91, 2001.

*The "neuropathic" column indicates the identification rates when looking for all types of subtle neuropathic findings.

†The spontaneous activity column indicates identification rates when only fibrillations or positive sharp waves are considered.

ADD, Adductor longus; *ATIB*, tibialis anterior; *LGAS*, lateral gastrocnemius; *MGAS*, medial gastrocnemius; *PSM*, lumbar paraspinal muscles; *PTIB*, tibialis posterior; *RFEM*, rectus femoris; *SHBF*, short head of biceps femoris; *TFL*, tensor fascia lata; *VLAT*, vastus lateralis; *VMED*, vastus medialis.

necessary to identify 90%. Other retrospective studies are consistent with these findings.[72]

In summary, for both cervical and lumbosacral radiculopathy screens, the optimal minimum number of muscles appears to be six muscles, which include the paraspinal muscles and muscles that represent all root level innervations. When paraspinal muscles are not reliable, then eight nonparaspinal muscles must be examined. Another way to think of this is as follows: "To minimize harm, six in the leg and six in the arm."

If one of the six muscles studied in the screen is positive, there is the possibility of confirming electrodiagnostically that a radiculopathy is present. In this case, the examiner must study additional muscles to determine the radiculopathy level and to exclude a mononeuropathy. If the findings are found in only a single muscle, they remain inconclusive and of uncertain clinical relevance. If none of the six muscles are abnormal, the examiner can be confident of not missing the opportunity to confirm electrodiagnostically that a radiculopathy is present, and the EMG examination can be stopped. The patient might still have a radiculopathy (purely sensory and not associated with motor axon loss), but other tests such as MRI will be necessary to confirm this clinical suspicion. This logic is illustrated in Figure 8-9.

In the past, a well-defined temporal course of events was thought to occur with radiculopathies, despite the absence of studies supporting such a relationship. It was a commonly held notion that in acute lumbosacral radiculopathies, the paraspinal muscles denervated first, followed by distal muscles, and that reinnervation started with paraspinal muscles and then with distal muscles. This paradigm was addressed with a series of investigations.[33,85] For both lumbosacral and cervical radiculopathies, symptom duration had no significant relationship to the probability of finding spontaneous activity in paraspinal or limb muscles. This simplistic explanation, although widely quoted in the older literature, does not explain the complex pathophysiology of radiculopathies. Electrodiagnosticians should not invoke this relationship to explain the absence or presence of fibrillations in a particular muscle.

When reporting electrodiagnostic conclusions regarding the presence or absence of a radiculopathy, the electrodiagnostician uses the pattern of muscle involvement to identify the minimum number of root levels to explain these EMG findings.

A pattern of unequivocal fibrillations in a myotomal distribution is fairly compelling for radiculopathy. Other softer findings such as reduced recruitment, for instance, should inspire less confidence in the diagnostic conclusions. More subjective findings (reduced recruitment) are open to interpretation and best appreciated by skilled electrodiagnosticians. If the polyphasics are clearly abundant (greater than 30%) and in a myotomal distribution they may indicate radiculopathy but this is a less strong call. In such cases, the contralateral limb should be examined to ensure there is not a generalized process going on.

Traumatic Nerve Injuries

Trauma to the peripheral nervous system often accompanies other traumatic injuries. Electrodiagnosis is a valuable means of identifying the location of a peripheral nerve lesion and can, to some extent, assess the magnitude of the nerve injury.[40] Electrodiagnostic testing has important implications but also clear limitations regarding precise nerve injury classification.[16] Recovery can be expected to be days to weeks in the case of an injury resulting only in

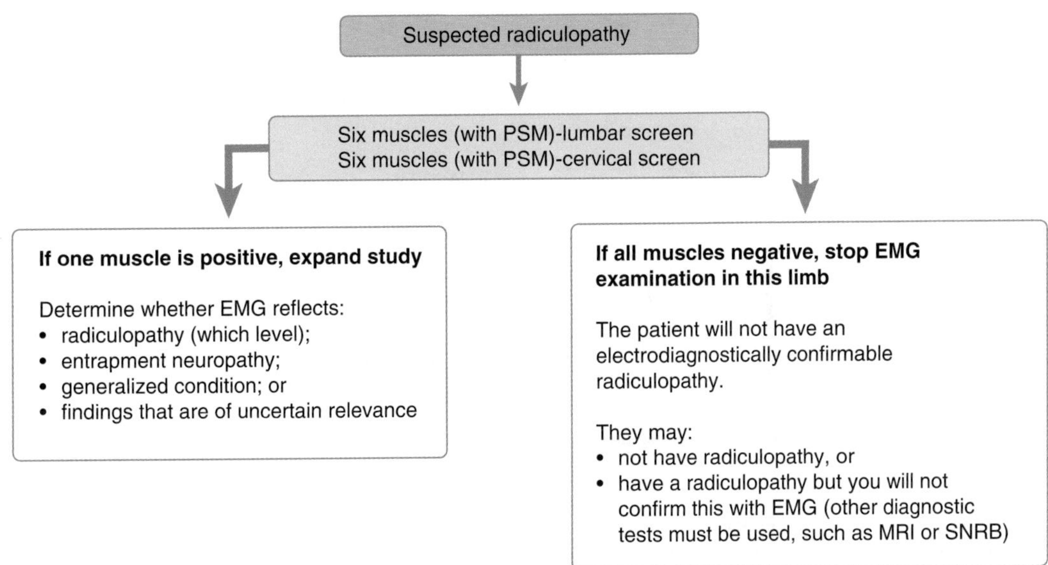

FIGURE 8-9 Algorithm for suspected radiculopathy. *EMG,* Electromyography; *MRI,* magnetic resonance imaging; *PSM,* paraspinal muscle; *SNRB,* sensory nerve root block.

neurapraxia. Months may be required for recovery in peripheral nerve injuries showing substantial axonal loss. NCSs distal to the site of the lesion after Wallerian degeneration has taken place can help delineate the degree of axonal loss. The side-to-side amplitudes can be compared, yielding a semiquantitative means of determining the degree of axonal loss. What must be appreciated is the considerable variability in side-to-side motor and sensory amplitudes. Intraoperative nerve action potential assessment across individual fascicles can further define whether a fascicle has axons in continuity.[59,64-66]

A major use of electrodiagnosis is to identify electrophysiologic evidence of spontaneous regeneration that precedes clinical findings of recovery.[74] In the case of a traumatically injured limb, the electrodiagnostician can usually determine the general location of the lesion and delineate whether axonal loss has occurred. If remaining motor units are firing, the electrodiagnostic examination can determine with certainty that there is not complete neurotmesis (section of the nerve).

After complete nerve section, failure at the neuromuscular junction occurs in 2 to 5 days in animals.[49] In partial nerve injuries, regeneration occurs through axonal sprouting from undamaged axons in proximity to denervated muscle fibers. Axonal sprouting can reinnervate muscle fibers within days. On the other hand, axonal regeneration occurring at the site of injury requires months to reinnervate the denervated muscle fibers.[79]

Chaudhry and Cornblath[20] studied Wallerian degeneration in humans. They found that motor-evoked responses were absent in 9 days, sensory responses were absent by 11 days, and denervation potentials were seen 10 to 14 days after injury. These results indicate that the motor and sensory responses reliably assess the status of the nerve after 11 days. It takes 3 weeks for fibrillations to fully develop and be consistently recorded by needle EMG.

Kraft[67] studied fibrillation potential amplitudes and their relationship to time after injury. The mean fibrillation amplitude in the first 2 months after injury was 612 μV. This important study showed that 1 year after traumatic nerve injury, no population of fibrillation potentials was greater than 100 μV in amplitude. These findings can help determine whether fibrillations are the result of recent or remote denervation.

An informative study regarding fibrillation potential generation resulting from direct muscle injury was reported by Partanen and Danner.[84] They studied 43 patients after muscle biopsy. At 6 to 7 days after biopsy, approximately 50% of the patients showed fibrillations on needle EMG testing. At 16 days, all patients revealed fibrillation potentials in the biopsied muscles, and these fibrillations persisted for up to 8 months. These findings suggest that direct muscle trauma can result in denervation potentials and can occur in the absence of any nerve injury.[84] Such information is important when evaluating traumatically injured limbs. Areas of muscle damage or surgical scars should be avoided because fibrillation potentials in these areas are uninterpretable.

Electrodiagnostic Assessment of Nerve Injuries

The pertinent issues in electrodiagnosis of peripheral nerve injuries are localization of the injury, pathophysiology of the lesion, severity of the dysfunction, and the presence of reinnervation.[30] Frykman et al.[48] presented an algorithmic approach to the assessment and management of traumatic peripheral nerve injuries based on the clinical examination and electrodiagnostic findings (Figure 8-10).

For acute injuries (between 0 and 7 days after injury), the electromyographer can only comment on nerve continuity if there are voluntary motor units, or conduction is found across the area of suspected injury. This suggests that at least some of the nerve is intact and thus the lesion does not reflect complete neurotmesis.

In those patients for whom little or no recovery is evident at 3 weeks by clinical examination, electrodiagnostic studies are performed. If no voluntary motor units and

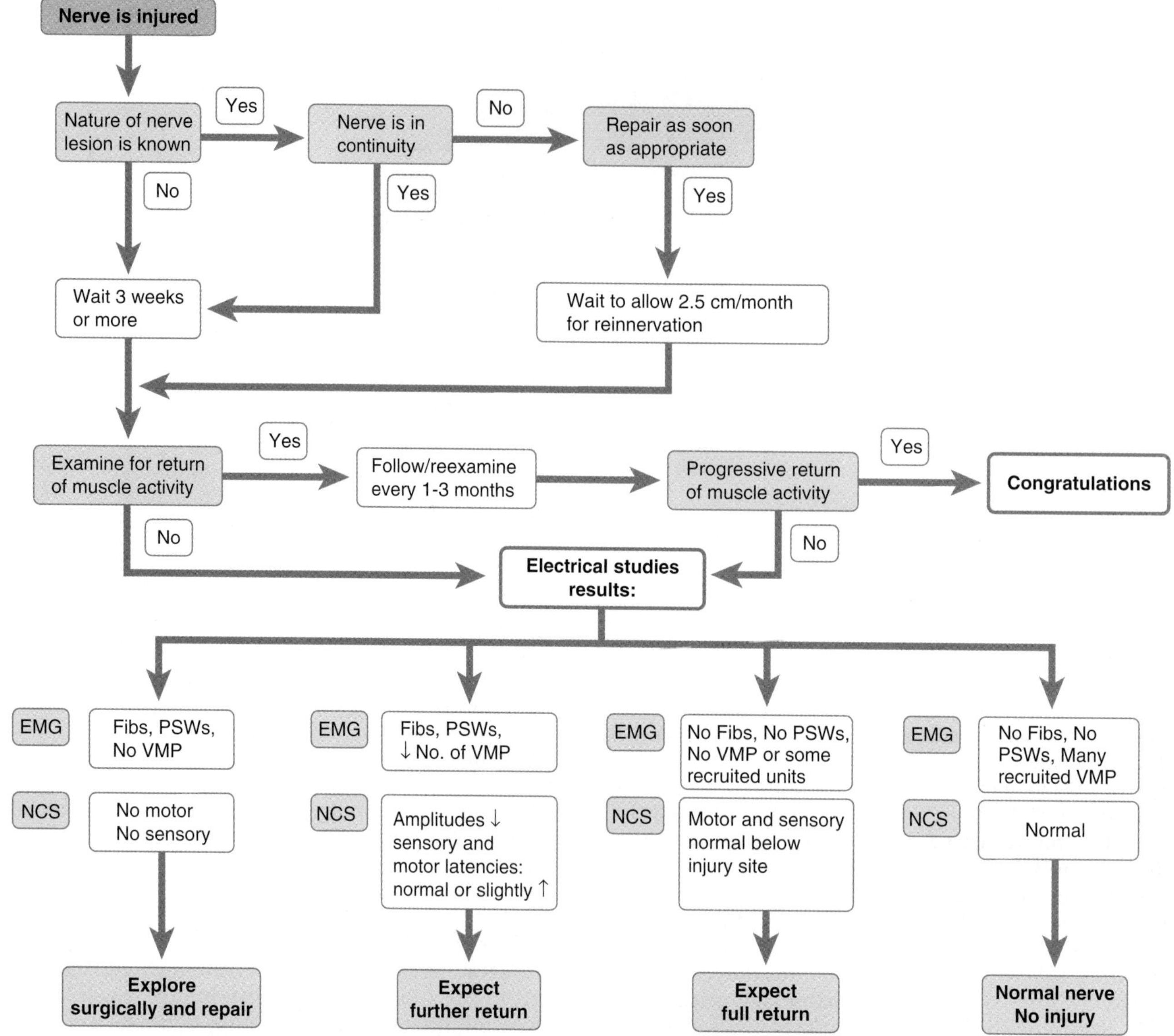

FIGURE 8-10 Algorithm for management of peripheral nerve injuries. *EMG*, Electromyography; *Fibs*, fibrillation potentials; *NCS*, nerve conduction study; *PSWs*, positive sharp waves; *VMP*, voluntary motor unit potentials (interference pattern). (Modified from Frykman GK, Wolf A, Coyle T: An algorithm for management of peripheral nerve injuries, *Orthop Clin North Am* 12:239-244, 1981, with permission.)

no motor or sensory responses are elicited, surgical exploration can be considered. If fibrillations are present, yet some voluntary units are noted along with reduced but present sensory or motor responses, then a partial nerve injury can be diagnosed, and further recovery can be reasonably expected. In a mild or neurapraxic injury with no fibrillations and normal sensory and motor amplitudes, a full recovery can be expected.[48] Although somewhat simplistic, this approach provides a conceptual framework for consolidating electrodiagnostic and clinical information into a treatment plan. The algorithm by Frykman et al.[48] has been updated and slightly modified regarding the presence of voluntary MUAPs. Some newer surgical approaches to peripheral nerve injury are based on intraoperative NCSs. Information derived from peripheral nerve imaging techniques (MRI and ultrasound imaging) might well play an important role. However, the Frykman approach is a reasonable conceptual framework for managing nerve injuries.

During recovery, maintaining joint range of motion and preventing disuse atrophy are important interventions and serve to optimize limb function when the nerve injury finally recovers. Pain management is often another integral part of the care of patients with traumatic nerve injuries.

Generalized Disorders

Electrodiagnostic testing is an extension of the physical examination, and as such should be placed within a conceptual framework of physical findings and patient symptoms. Figure 8-1 provides a conceptual framework for using the clinical scenario and examination findings to address the highest probability disorders. For the purposes of this discussion, generalized disorders are those affecting more than one limb. The guidelines in Table 8-12 provide a framework for structuring the examination to evaluate for these disorders but is by no means a perfect taxonomy.

Polyneuropathy

Evaluation for polyneuropathy involves identifying peripheral nervous system involvement. The electrodiagnostician should also strive to categorize the type of neuropathy based on its electrodiagnostic features. Donofrio and Albers[36] compiled a comprehensive list of polyneuropathies classified by their characteristic electrodiagnostic findings. Determining whether sensory, motor, or both types of nerves are involved, and whether the primary type of pathology is demyelination or axonal loss, allows the electrodiagnostician to narrow the list of potential etiologies for the polyneuropathy (Box 8-1).

The electrodiagnostic changes seen with demyelinating and axonal neuropathies are shown in Table 8-19. Persons with polyneuropathies involving acute or recent motor axonal loss show fibrillations and PSWs in predominantly distal muscles. The distribution of EMG findings in polyneuropathies is such that distal lower limb muscles often demonstrate the greatest involvement. In persons with a more chronic process with either old axonal loss or slow axonal loss that is balanced with reinnervation and reorganization of the motor unit, large-amplitude, long-duration MUAPs can be seen.[68]

Absent SNAPs and CMAPs can reflect either axonal loss or conduction block. EMG can provide supporting information about motor axonal loss. Nerve conduction velocity is an important parameter to measure from multiple nerves. Temporal dispersion suggests an acquired demyelinating polyneuropathy. Care must be taken to study a sufficient number of nerves to confidently determine whether a diffuse process is present rather than a single

BOX 8-1

Classification of Polyneuropathies by Their Electrodiagnostic Characteristics

Uniform, Demyelinating, Mixed Sensorimotor Polyneuropathy

- Hereditary motor sensory neuropathy types 1, 3, and 4
- Metachromatic leukodystrophy
- Krabbe globoid leukodystrophy
- Adrenomyeloneuropathy
- Congenital hypomyelinating neuropathy
- Tangier disease
- Cockayne syndrome
- Cerebrotendinous xanthomatosis

Segmental, Demyelinating, Motor Greater Than Sensory Polyneuropathy

- Acute inflammatory demyelinating polyneuropathy
- Chronic inflammatory demyelinating polyneuropathy
- Multifocal demyelinating neuropathy with persistent conduction block
- Osteosclerotic myeloma
- Waldenström macroglobulinemia
- Monoclonal gammopathy of undetermined significance
- Gamma heavy chain disease
- Angiofollicular lymph node hyperplasia
- Hypothyroidism
- Leprosy
- Diphtheria
- Acute arsenic polyneuropathy
- Pharmaceuticals: amiodarone, perhexiline, high-dose cytarabine (Ara-C)
- Lymphoma
- Carcinoma
- Acquired immune deficiency syndrome (AIDS)
- Lyme disease
- Acromegaly
- Hereditary neuropathy with susceptibility to pressure palsies
- Systemic lupus erythematosus
- Glue-sniffing neuropathy
- Post portacaval anastomosis
- Neuropathy associated with progressive external ophthalmoplegia
- Ulcerative colitis
- Marinesco-Sjögren syndrome
- Cryoglobulinemia

Axon Loss, Motor Greater Than Sensory Polyneuropathy

- Porphyria
- Axonal Guillain-Barré syndrome: acute motor axonal neuropathy
- Hereditary motor sensory neuropathy types 2 and 5
- Lead neuropathy
- Dapsone neuropathy
- Vincristine neuropathy
- Remote effect motor neuronopathy associated with lymphoma
- Remote effect motor neuronopathy associated with carcinoma
- Hypoglycemia or hyperinsulinemia
- West Nile

Axon Loss Sensory Neuronopathy or Neuropathy

- Hereditary sensory neuropathy types 1 to 4
- Friedreich's ataxia
- Spinocerebellar degeneration
- Abetalipoproteinemia (Bassen-Kornzweig disease)
- Primary biliary cirrhosis
- Acute sensory neuronopathy
- Cisplatin toxicity
- Carcinomatous sensory neuronopathy
- Lymphomatous sensory neuronopathy
- Chronic idiopathic ataxic neuropathy
- Sjögren syndrome
- Fisher variant Guillain-Barré syndrome
- Paraproteinemias
- Pyridoxine toxicity
- Idiopathic sensory neuronopathy
- Styrene-induced peripheral neuropathy
- Crohn disease
- Thalidomide toxicity
- Nonsystemic vasculitic neuropathy
- Chronic gluten enteropathy
- Vitamin E deficiency

Axon Loss, Mixed Sensorimotor Polyneuropathy

- Amyloidosis
- Chronic liver disease
- Nutritional disease
- Vitamin B_{12} deficiency

Continued

BOX 8-1

Classification of Polyneuropathies by Their Electrodiagnostic Characteristics—cont'd

- Folate deficiency
- Whipple disease
- Postgastrectomy syndrome
- Gastric restriction surgery for obesity
- Thiamine deficiency
- Alcoholism
- Sarcoidosis
- Connective tissue diseases
- Rheumatoid arthritis
- Periarteritis nodosa
- Systemic lupus erythematosus
- Churg-Strauss vasculitis
- Temporal arteritis
- Scleroderma
- Behçet's disease
- Hypereosinophilia syndrome
- Cryoglobulinemia
- Toxic neuropathy
- Acrylamide
- Carbon disulfide
- Dichlorophenoxyacetic acid
- Ethylene oxide
- Hexacarbons
- Carbon monoxide
- Organophosphorus esters
- Glue sniffing
- Metal neuropathy
- Chronic arsenic intoxication
- Mercury
- Thallium
- Gold
- Pharmaceuticals
- Colchicine
- Phenytoin
- Ethambutol
- Amitriptyline
- Metronidazole
- Misonidazole
- Nitrofurantoin
- Chloroquine
- Disulfiram
- Glutethimide
- Nitrous oxide
- Lithium
- Carcinomatous axonal sensorimotor polyneuropathy
- Chronic obstructive pulmonary disease
- Giant axonal dystrophy
- Olivopontocerebellar atrophy
- Neuropathy of chronic illness
- Acromegaly
- Hypophosphatemia
- Lymphomatous axonal sensorimotor polyneuropathy
- Hypothyroidism
- Myotonic dystrophy
- Necrotizing angiopathy
- Lyme disease
- AIDS
- Jamaican neuropathy
- Tangier disease
- Gouty neuropathy
- Polycythemia vera
- Typical multiple myeloma

Mixed Axon Loss, Demyelinating Sensorimotor Polyneuropathy

- Diabetes mellitus
- Uremia
- AIDS; AIDS-related complex

Table 8-19 Electrodiagnostic Findings in Peripheral Neuropathies

Parameter	Early Demyelinating	Chronic Demyelinating	Acute Axonal	Chronic Axonal
Distal latency	Increased	Increased	Normal or slightly increased	Normal or slightly increased
Nerve conduction velocity	Decreased	Decreased	Normal or slightly decreased	Normal or slightly decreased
F-Latency	Increased or absent	Increased or absent	Normal or absent	Normal or absent
H-Reflex	Increased latency or absent	Increased latency or absent	Absent	Absent
Sensory nerve action potential amplitude	Decreased or absent	Decreased or absent	Decreased or absent	Decreased or absent
Compound motor action potential amplitude	Normal or decreased	Normal or decreased	Decreased	Decreased
Motor unit action potential duration	Normal	Normal (hereditary) or increased (acquired)	Normal	Increased
Motor unit action potential amplitude	Normal	Normal or increased	Normal	Increased
Polyphasics	Normal	Increased	Normal	Increased
Recruitment	Normal or decreased	Decreased, rapid	Decreased, rapid	Decreased, rapid
Abnormal spontaneous activity	None	None, or fibrillations, positive sharp waves, complex repetitive discharges	Fibrillations, positive sharp waves, complex repetitive discharges	None, or fibrillations, positive sharp waves, complex repetitive discharges

Modified from Krivickas L: Electrodiagnosis in neuromuscular diseases, *Phys Med Rehabil Clin N Am* 9:83-114, 1998.

entrapment neuropathy. If one limb is affected, the electrodiagnostician should study the contralateral limb. If this is abnormal, another limb should be examined. For example, a patient with abnormalities in both legs and possible polyneuropathy can be quickly and easily diagnosed by finding fibrillations in the intrinsic hand muscles.

F-waves measure longer neurologic pathways and are important in diagnosing polyneuropathies. They are helpful in identifying diabetic polyneuropathy, acute inflammatory demyelinating polyneuropathy (AIDP), and chronic inflammatory demyelinating polyradiculoneuropathy (CIDP).[47] F-waves and H-reflexes are important tests for assessing proximal segments of the peripheral nervous system and can be helpful for neuropathy evaluations.

Acute inflammatory demyelinating polyneuropathy (AIDP; also known as Guillain-Barré syndrome) is the most common, acute, rapidly progressive polyneuropathy in clinical practice and must be recognized when present.[3] Patients typically present with sensory symptoms and weakness, with disease progression over 2 to 4 weeks. Sensory nerve conduction abnormalities, reduced amplitude, or prolonged distal latency, particularly in the median nerve, are observed but can take 4 to 6 weeks to peak.[41] Motor NCSs reveal prolonged distal latencies, temporal dispersion and conduction block, or slowed velocities in 80% to 90% of these patients. Reduced CMAPs in ulnar nerve (and median nerve) innervated muscles that are 10% to 20% of normal values signify a poorer prognosis and can provide early information to guide clinical management.[80] In severe cases, EMG findings of fibrillations and PSWs can be seen if motor axonal loss has occurred. Facial muscle weakness and bulbar muscle involvement are commonly found in patients with AIDP.[103] Nerve conduction findings of slowed conduction velocity, temporal dispersion, prolonged distal latencies, or late responses should be found in two or more nerves to support a diagnosis of AIDP.[2] In some cases, late responses (F-waves and H-reflexes) are the only findings noted on electrodiagnostic testing early on in persons with AIDP.

CIDP represents a demyelinating polyneuropathy of chronic nature with fluctuating weakness and stepwise progression. Weakness and sensory symptoms similar to those of AIDP are found, but the chronicity is longer. In CIDP, sensory responses are frequently absent in both upper and lower limbs, and the nerve conduction velocities are reduced.[80] EMG findings depend on the rate of disease progression and can reveal reduced recruitment, fibrillation potentials, polyphasic potentials, and reorganized MUAPs with large amplitudes and increased durations. Sensory nerve conduction slowing was recently shown to be a highly specific, yet less sensitive marker for differentiating CIDP from axonal polyneuropathy.[15]

Multifocal motor neuropathy with conduction block is a disorder that is sometimes confused with motor neuron disease. The two have markedly different prognoses. Patients present with asymmetrical weakness in a single body region, frequently the hand, but without sensory symptoms. Progression is slow and spans many years.[99] Sensory nerves are usually normal on electrodiagnostic testing. Motor nerve testing reveals conduction block in multiple nerves at sites not prone to focal entrapments: midforearm, midleg, arm, and brachial plexus. Distal motor latencies and amplitudes are usually normal. Proximal motor nerve stimulations at Erb point are important to exclude conduction block over proximal nerve segments.

Diabetes is on the rise in the United States, with an increasing incidence and prevalence.[53] Diabetes often confounds the accurate diagnosis of radiculopathy and spinal stenosis.[1,24] Inaccurate recognition of sensory polyneuropathy, diabetic amyotrophy, or mononeuropathy can lead to unnecessary surgical interventions. The pattern of involvement can take the form of symmetrical polyneuropathies, or focal and multifocal patterns of mononeuropathies. The proximal lower limb can be involved, with pain and weakness in patients with diabetic amyotrophy. The sensory nerve involvement, particularly in the legs, often results in complaints of numbness, tingling, burning, aching, and pain. Up to 80% of patients with diabetes having clinical polyneuropathies will demonstrate an abnormality of the SNAP.[84] Sensory findings usually precede motor findings. Motor nerve conduction is 15% to 30% below normal. EMG can show fibrillations and motor unit changes along with reduced recruitment.[38]

Accurate assessment for polyneuropathy requires heightened suspicion coupled with sufficient testing. Nonphysicians perform 17% of studies in the United States.[34] In a sample of 6381 patients with diabetes undergoing electrodiagnostic testing in 1998, identification rates for polyneuropathy were highest for physiatrists, osteopathic physicians, and neurologists (12.5%, 12.2%, and 11.9%, respectively).[31] Podiatrists and physical therapists identified 2.4% and 2.1%, respectively, as having polyneuropathy; rates approximately one sixth that of physiatrists and neurologists, despite controlling for case mix differences. Nonphysician providers who did not recognize polyneuropathy in this group of patients with diabetes performed almost exclusively EMG testing (greater than 90%) at the expense of NCSs. These findings underscore the need for high-quality consultations of sufficient scope by well-trained electrodiagnostic physicians to accurately diagnose patients with complex disorders.[31]

Alcoholic polyneuropathy is a common peripheral nerve disease accounting for almost 30% of all cases of generalized polyneuropathy.[93] This clinical entity usually occurs in the setting of long-standing alcoholism and nutritional deficiency. Substantial weight loss often occurs before or concurrent with the development of polyneuropathy. Presenting symptoms typically include pain, dysesthesias, and weakness in the feet and legs. Alcoholic polyneuropathy is an axonal loss disorder affecting both sensory and motor nerves (see Box 8-1).[36] Low SNAP amplitudes are seen in the legs, and EMG often reveals fibrillations and positive waves in distal muscles.

Hereditary sensory and motor neuropathies (HSMNs) are a diverse group of polyneuropathies that are rapidly becoming better characterized through genetic studies, and are reviewed in Chapter 41.[38] From an electrophysiologic standpoint, they are distinctly different from acquired polyneuropathies because of the relative lack of temporal dispersion and conduction block. HSMN type 1 is the hypertrophic variety with onion bulb formation and axonal atrophy.[62] Symptoms begin in the first 2 decades, and markedly reduced nerve conduction velocities are seen but without substantial temporal dispersion. HSMN type

2 presents in adult life or later. Patients have severe distal muscle atrophy and weakness. NCSs show mild-slowing, but EMG reveals large, reorganized MUAPs with fibrillations and PSWs. Dejerine-Sottas (HSMN type 3) is a severe type of neuropathy appearing in infancy with delayed motor development, and reveals the slowest nerve conduction velocities; less than 10 m/s and often as low as 2 to 3 m/s.[66,68]

The AANEM, in conjunction with the American Academy of Neurology and the American Academy of Physical Medicine and Rehabilitation, determined that a formal case definition for polyneuropathy was needed.[45] They described that no single reference standard was most appropriate for distal symmetrical polyneuropathy. The most accurate diagnosis comprised a combination of clinical signs, symptoms, and electrodiagnostic findings. Electrodiagnostic findings should be included as part of the case definition because of their higher level of specificity. Electrodiagnostic studies are sensitive and specific validated measures for the presence of polyneuropathy.

This panel recommended a simplified NCS protocol for screening for the presence of distal symmetrical polyneuropathy.[45] Sural sensory and peroneal motor nerve conductions performed in one lower limb, taken together, were thought by this group to be the most sensitive tests for detecting a distal symmetrical polyneuropathy. If both studies are normal, there is no evidence of typical distal symmetrical polyneuropathy, and in such a situation no further NCSs are necessary. If one of these tests is abnormal, however, then additional NCSs are recommended. This would include at least the ulnar sensory, median sensory, and ulnar motor nerves in one upper limb. A contralateral sural sensory and one tibial motor NCS can also be performed at the discretion of the examiner. These experts recommended caution when interpreting median and ulnar studies, because of the possibility of an abnormality caused by compression at the wrist or elbow.[45] They further recommended that if a response is absent for any of the nerves studied, NCSs of the contralateral nerve should be performed. If a peroneal motor response is absent, an ipsilateral tibial motor nerve conduction should also be performed. These tests (sural sensory and peroneal motor) do not exclude all acquired (e.g., AIDP) or hereditary polyneuropathies; they only exclude distal symmetrical polyneuropathies. The electrodiagnostician should structure evaluation for these other suspected conditions with examination of weak muscles and involved nerve distributions.

Myopathies

Myopathic disorders include acquired inflammatory types such as polymyositis and dermatomyositis, as well as congenital myopathies, metabolic myopathies, muscular dystrophies, and mitochondrial myopathies. A detailed discussion is found in Chapter 42, and the interested reader is directed to other specialized references for a complete description of the rarer forms of myopathy. Unfortunately, the electrodiagnostic examination is less sensitive or specific for detecting myopathies than for any other group of neuromuscular diseases.[68] Myopathies are one of the most challenging disorders to identify and classify by electrodiagnosis because no findings are completely specific for myopathy. There is often patchy involvement of proximal muscles, and the EMG findings can vary depending on the severity and duration of the myopathy. Characteristic findings on EMG can indicate myopathy, yet the precise etiology of the myopathy requires other testing, such as muscle biopsy and genetic testing. The electromyographic findings for myopathies are shown in Table 8-20. NCSs are usually normal except when a muscle is atrophic, and then the CMAP can be reduced. Sensory NCSs are normal unless a concomitant polyneuropathy exists.

Needle EMG is the most helpful part of the examination. In the acute inflammatory myopathies polymyositis and dermatomyositis, the characteristic findings are fibrillations and PSWs, CRDs, and early or increased recruitment of short-duration, polyphasic, low-amplitude MUAPs.[87] Early recruitment or increased recruitment refers to the case in which more motor units are recruited than would be expected to generate a low muscular force. This is because in myopathies, more diseased muscle fibers are necessary to generate force than in the normal situation. This can also result from the motor units having fewer remaining muscle fibers. At low force levels, many units are present on the display screen. Proximal limb girdle and paraspinal muscles are frequently involved. In progressive muscular dystrophies such as Duchenne and Becker, fibrillations and PSWs are widespread, with occasional CRDs and myotonic discharges.[68] Inclusion body myositis accounts for 30% of all inflammatory myopathies and requires muscle biopsy to diagnose the condition. The findings are similar to those seen in polymyositis, with fibrillations and PSWs more widespread and prominent.[68]

Neuromuscular Junction Disorders

Disorders of the neuromuscular junction can be classified as either presynaptic or postsynaptic. The presynaptic disorders are LEMS and botulism. Myasthenia gravis is a postsynaptic disorder.[89] These rare causes of generalized weakness demonstrate characteristic electrodiagnostic features (Table 8-21), making them readily identifiable to the electrodiagnostician with a heightened suspicion for these entities.

Myasthenia gravis is an autoimmune disorder caused by antibodies directed at the acetylcholine receptors of skeletal muscle. Electrodiagnostic techniques most useful for identifying this disorder are repetitive nerve stimulation and single-fiber EMG.[54] Elevated acetylcholine receptor antibodies have been demonstrated in patients with generalized and ocular myasthenia gravis in 81% and 51% of cases, respectively. Elevated acetylcholine receptor antibody levels can be seen in those with penicillamine-induced myasthenia, in some elderly patients with autoimmune diseases, and in first-degree relatives of patients with myasthenia gravis. Decrementing responses in a distal hand muscle on repetitive nerve stimulation at 2 or 3 Hz are seen in 68% of persons with definite generalized myasthenia gravis, and in 31% with mild myasthenia gravis.[60] Repetitive nerve stimulation of a proximal muscle increases the sensitivity to 89% for definite and 68% for mild myasthenia gravis. Single-fiber EMG is the most sensitive test for myasthenia gravis. In persons with generalized myasthenia

Table 8-20 Electrodiagnostic Findings in Myopathies

Parameter	Muscular Dystrophy	Congenital	Mitochondrial	Metabolic	Inflammatory	Channelopathy
Distal latency	Normal	Normal	Normal	Normal	Normal	Normal
Nerve conduction velocity	Normal	Normal	Normal	Normal	Normal	Normal
H-Reflex	Normal or absent	Normal or absent	Normal	Normal	Normal or absent	Normal
Sensory nerve action potential amplitude	Normal	Normal	Normal	Normal	Normal	Normal
Compound motor action potential amplitude	Normal or decreased	Normal or decreased	Normal or decreased	Normal or decreased	Normal or decreased	Normal
Motor unit action potential duration	Decreased and/or increased	Decreased or normal	Decreased or normal	Decreased or normal	Decreased and/or increased (inclusion body myositis)	Decreased or normal
Motor unit action potential amplitude	Decreased and/or increased	Decreased or normal	Decreased or normal	Decreased or normal	Decreased and/or increased (inclusion body myositis)	Decreased or normal
Polyphasics	Increased	Increased or normal	Increased or normal	Increased or normal	Increased	Increased or normal
Recruitment	Increased	Increased or normal	Increased or normal	Increased or normal	Increased	Increased or normal
Fibrillations and positive sharp waves	Yes	Centronuclear myopathy	No	Yes	Yes	Occasionally
Complex repetitive discharges	Yes	Centronuclear myopathy	No	Yes	Yes	Occasionally
Myotonic potentials	Myotonic dystrophy	Centronuclear myopathy	No	Acid maltase deficiency	No	Yes
Electrical silence	No	No	No	Contractures in McArdle disease	No	During attacks of paralysis

Modified from Krivickas L: Electrodiagnosis in neuromuscular diseases, *Phys Med Rehabil Clin N Am* 9:83-114, 1998.

Table 8-21 Electrodiagnostic Findings in Neuromuscular Junction Transmission Disorders

Parameter	Myasthenia Gravis	Lambert-Eaton Myasthenic Syndrome	Botulism
Distal latency	Normal	Normal	Normal
Nerve conduction velocity	Normal	Normal	Normal
Sensory nerve action potential amplitude	Normal	Normal	Normal
Compound motor action potential amplitude	Usually normal	Decreased	Normal or decreased
Slow repetitive stimulation	Decrement	Decrement	± Decrement
Fast repetitive stimulation or brief exercise	± Mild increment	Large increment (lasting 20 to 30 seconds)	Intermediate increment (lasting up to 4 minutes)
Postactivation exhaustion	Yes	Yes	No
Motor unit action potential configuration	Moment-to-moment amplitude variation (weak muscles) ± decreased amplitude and duration	Moment-to-moment amplitude variation (all muscles), decreased amplitude and duration, increased polyphasics	Moment-to-moment amplitude variation (weak muscles), decreased amplitude and duration, increased polyphasics
Recruitment	Normal or increased	Increased	Increased
Spontaneous activity	Fibrillation in severe disease	None	Fibrillation in severe disease
Single-fiber electromyography	Increased jitter and blocking (increases with increased firing rate)	Increased jitter and blocking (decreased with increased firing rate)	Increased jitter and blocking (decreased with increased firing rate)

From Krivickas L: Electrodiagnosis in neuromuscular diseases, *Phys Med Rehabil Clin N Am* 9:83-114, 1998.

gravis, the sensitivity of single-fiber EMG performed on the extensor digitorum communis muscle was 92%. In patients with ocular myasthenia gravis, 78% had abnormal jitter in the extensor digitorum communis, and 92% had increased jitter with a facial muscle study (frontalis). Single-fiber EMG is a nonspecific test unfortunately, and increased jitter can also be seen in amyotrophic lateral sclerosis (ALS), peripheral neuropathies, and some myopathies.

LEMS is a unique condition characterized by weakness and fatigability of proximal limb muscles with sparing of ocular muscles. Dry mouth is often reported, and the patients demonstrate hyporeflexia and normal sensation.[60] There is a strong association with malignancy, most commonly oat cell carcinoma of the lung. There is reduced release of acetylcholine quanta from the presynaptic nerve terminal. A unique feature of this disorder is that with rapid repetitive nerve stimulation (20 Hz) or a brief voluntary maximal contraction, a postactivation increase in CMAP of more than 200% is seen. Although such potentiation can be seen in myasthenia gravis and occasionally botulism, it is usually to a much lesser degree than that seen in LEMS. This profound potentiation is the hallmark electrodiagnostic finding in LEMS. Other features of LEMS that are similar to those found in myasthenia gravis include normal sensory conductions, decrementing response to 2 or 3 Hz stimulation, and increased jitter on single-fiber EMG.[68]

Botulism is a rare disorder caused by the potent toxin of the bacterium *Clostridium botulinum*, through both oral ingestion and wound infection.[60] A rapid-onset paralysis of the eye muscles, followed by rapid spread to other parts of the body, is seen. The toxin irreversibly blocks acetylcholine release from presynaptic nerve terminals. Electrodiagnostic findings reveal low or absent CMAPs, with decrementing responses on 2 or 3 Hz repetitive nerve stimulation. The incremental increase in CMAP amplitude with exercise or rapid frequency stimulation (20 to 50 Hz) is less dramatic than in LEMS but should be greater than 40%.[55] With severe involvement, the neuromuscular junction is completely blocked and no facilitation with rapid stimulation is seen. In these cases, the end plates break down and fibrillation potentials are seen.

In this group of disorders the SNAPs are normal. The CMAPs are normal or of low amplitude, particularly in LEMS and botulism. Needle EMG reveals normal or polyphasic MUAPs with low amplitudes and short durations, similar to those found in myopathies. With EMG, MUAP variation in size can also be seen. Fibrillation potentials are seen only in severe disease with complete disintegration of the neuromuscular junction (see Table 8-21).

Stimulated single-fiber EMG offers advantages over conventional single-fiber EMG. Stimulated single-fiber EMG can be performed in patients who cannot maintain a voluntary contraction or in children and infants.[21] Stimulated single-fiber EMG is less time-consuming and, by controlling the rate of stimulation, better quantification of the neuromuscular junction disorder can be obtained.[21]

Ertas et al.[46] reported the use of concentric needle electrodes for single-fiber EMG. They showed that when the low-frequency filter is set at 2 kHz, concentric needle electrodes are comparable with single-fiber EMG electrodes and yield the same jitter values determined with a single-fiber needle for both normal individuals and for persons with myasthenia gravis. Additional advantages include that they are disposable and thus do not need resterilization. Other investigators have confirmed the usefulness and comparability of single-fiber EMG using a concentric electrode in the evaluation of persons with suspected neuromuscular disorders, and the concentric needle may be even less painful than the conventional single-fiber electrode.[90] Because of a larger recording area, somewhat more single muscle fiber discharges were identified with concentric needle electrodes than with standard single-fiber EMG electrodes.[46]

Motor Neuron Disease

Motor neuron disease will be discussed in the context of the most common type in adults: ALS. This is a progressive motor system disease with upper motor neuron findings from spinal white matter involvement, and lower motor neuron findings on EMG from anterior horn cell loss.[39,69] There are different classifications based on the predominance of these characteristics. From an electrodiagnostic standpoint, EMG is the most helpful part of the study. To electrodiagnostically confirm ALS in the appropriate clinical circumstances, the patient should demonstrate the following findings:

- PSWs and/or fibrillation potentials in three limbs or two limbs and bulbar muscles (El Escorial criteria, discussed later[75]),
- Normal sensory NCSs,
- Normal motor conduction velocities, except if the CMAP is less than 30% of the mean, in which case the conduction velocities may not be less than 70% of normal, and
- Needle examination demonstrates a reduced recruitment, with altered MUAP duration and amplitude.[68]

Motor unit morphology depends on the rate of denervation and reinnervation. Reduced recruitment of MUAPs is the primary EMG finding in ALS (see Chapter 40).[26] In a rapidly progressive ALS, there might be little motor unit remodeling.[75]

Makki and Benatar[75] examined the accuracy of the El Escorial criteria for the diagnosis of ALS. The El Escorial criteria divide the body into four segments: cranial, cervical, thoracic, and lumbosacral. Evidence of lower motor dysfunction in the cervical and lumbosacral segments is defined by the presence of both active denervation (fibrillations and PSWs) and chronic reinnervation (large MUAPs, reduced interference pattern, or unstable motor units) in at least two muscles. Active denervation and chronic denervation in a single cranial or thoracic muscle is sufficient to declare these segments abnormal. If three of the four segments are abnormal by EMG, this is considered supportive evidence of definite ALS. If two segments are abnormal, this suggests possible ALS.[75] Their study was supportive of optimizing the sensitivity and specificity by requiring EMG changes in two muscles in the arm (cervical) or leg (lumbar) segments. These two muscles should demonstrate lower motor neuron findings.[75] There have been modifications to the El Escorial criteria that enhance the sensitivity of identifying correctly persons with ALS.[13] In these modified criteria, neurophysiologic evidence of lower motor neuron involvement is considered equivalent to clinical evidence, and the presence of fasciculation potentials was considered as important as fibrillations and positive sharp waves.

In examining cranial nerves, the trapezius is a high-yield muscle[94] for establishing the presence of cranial segment involvement but can also be involved with spinal cord tumors in the upper cervical region. The thoracic segment can be examined by means of EMG of the thoracic paraspinal muscles or by testing the rectus abdominis.[106]

Accurate identification of persons with ALS is important not only for instituting appropriate counseling and multidisciplinary care but also in minimizing unnecessary surgical interventions. In one retrospective study, 21% of persons with ALS had surgeries within the previous 5 years of diagnosis.[95] It was estimated that 61% of these surgeries were inappropriate and likely to be related to early manifestations of ALS.[95] These included surgeries of the knee and spine despite the absence of pain or paresthesias.[95]

Final Electrodiagnostic Conclusions and Report

The electrodiagnostic report is a crucial document that conveys the findings and conclusions derived from testing. The electrodiagnostic report should include a brief history regarding the presenting complaint, a focused physical examination, the tabulated electrodiagnostic findings, and the final assessment and conclusions. There should be internal consistency within the report, such that the conclusions are supported by the electrophysiologic data. The electrodiagnostician can then comment on how these electrodiagnostic findings correlate with the clinical impression, the limitations of the test, and any other observations. This then gives a more complete clinical picture. In electrodiagnostic reports, the referring question(s) should be addressed. Conditions that were excluded can also be listed. It is best to state that there is "no electrodiagnostic evidence of" a particular disorder if the testing for that disorder was normal. This reflects the fact that electrodiagnostic testing can be normal in persons with the particular condition that the referring physicians suspect. Electrodiagnostic testing is not as sensitive, yet more specific for some conditions (e.g., radiculopathy), and for this reason the findings are very helpful when positive.

It is often useful to the referring physician if the electrodiagnostician comments on other clinical conditions that were identified during the workup, such as shoulder impingement syndrome or lateral epicondylitis. Such observations can reveal other treatment alternatives for the patient that the referring physician can consider.

The limitations of a particular study, as well as confounding issues, should be clearly stated. There are multiple complicating issues. One such issue is pedal edema, which can make it difficult to obtain normal sural and peroneal sensory responses. Morbid obesity can impede adequate stimulus of a peripheral nerve or accurate measurement of conduction distance. Previous surgeries in the spine, carpal tunnel decompression, or ulnar nerve transpositions can complicate interpretation of studies in these areas. Diabetes and aging can confuse interpretation of mild abnormalities. Limited patient tolerance for testing can compromise the completeness of testing. These statements can alert the referring physician or other provider to the limitations of the study and better place into context the strength of the results.

Summary

Electrodiagnostic medicine is a complex consultation that relies on clinical insights, technical skills, solid normative data, and sound clinical judgment. Such consultations can have profound influence on subsequent diagnostic and therapeutic interventions. Only experienced and well-trained physicians should perform such diagnostic procedures. A healthy appreciation for the spectrum of normal values seen in people of different ages and heights should be maintained. Normative values should be well derived and interpreted correctly by electrodiagnosticians to avoid overcalling common disorders. Sufficient testing should be performed to confidently identify the suspected disorder and eliminate from the differential other confounding conditions.

KEY REFERENCES

2. Alan TA, Chaudhry V, Cornblath DR: Electrophysiological studies in the Guillain-Barré syndrome: distinguishing subtypes by published criteria, *Muscle Nerve* 21:1275–1279, 1998.
3. Albers JW, Kelly JJ, Jr: Acquired inflammatory demyelinating polyneuropathies: clinical and electrodiagnostic features, *Muscle Nerve* 12:435–451, 1989.
4. American Association of Electrodiagnostic Medicine: Guidelines in electrodiagnostic medicine, *Muscle Nerve* 8(Suppl):S1–S300, 1999.
5. American Association of Electrodiagnostic Medicine: Guidelines in electrodiagnostic medicine. Risks in electrodiagnostic medicine, *Muscle Nerve* 8(Suppl):S53–S58, 1999.
6. American Association of Electrodiagnostic Medicine: Guidelines in electrodiagnostic medicine: the electrodiagnostic medicine consultation, *Muscle Nerve* 8(Suppl):S73–S90, 1999.
7. American Association of Neuromuscular and Electrodiagnostic Medicine: Needle EMG in certain uncommon clinical contexts, *Muscle Nerve* 31:398–399, 2005.
8. American Association of Neuromuscular and Electrodiagnostic Medicine: Proper performance and interpretation of electrodiagnostic studies, *Muscle Nerve* 33:436–439, 2006.
11. Bird SJ, Brown MJ, Spino C, et al: Value of repeated measures of nerve conduction and quantitative sensory testing in a diabetic neuropathy trial, *Muscle Nerve* 34:214–224, 2006.
12. Boden SD, McCowin PR, Davis DO, et al: Abnormal magnetic-resonance scans of the cervical spine in asymptomatic subjects: a prospective investigation, *J Bone Joint Surg Am* 72:1178–1184, 1990.
15. Bragg JA, Benatar MG: Sensory nerve conduction slowing is a specific marker for CIDP, *Muscle Nerve* 38:1599–1603, 2008.
16. Bralliar F: Electromyography: its use and misuse in peripheral nerve injuries, *Orthop Clin North Am* 12:229–238, 1981.
19. Caress JB, Rutkove SB, Carlin M, et al: Paraspinal muscle hematoma after electromyography, *Neurology* 47:269–272, 1996.
20. Chaudhry V, Cornblath DR: Wallerian degeneration in human nerves: serial electrophysiological studies, *Muscle Nerve* 15:687–693, 1992.
21. Chaudhry V, Crawford TO: Stimulation single-fiber EMG in infant botulism, *Muscle Nerve* 22:1698–1703, 1999.
22. Chiodo A, Haig AJ, Yamakawa KS, et al: Needle EMG has a lower false positive rate than MRI in asymptomatic older adults being evaluated for lumbar spinal stenosis, *Clin Neurophysiol* 118:751–756, 2007.
23. Chuang TY, Chiou-Tan FY, Vennix MJ: Brachial plexopathy in gunshot wounds and motor vehicle accidents: comparison of electrophysiologic findings, *Arch Phys Med Rehabil* 79:201–204, 1998.
24. Cinotti G, Postacchini F, Weinstein JN: Lumbar spinal stenosis and diabetes. Outcome of surgical decompression, *J Bone Joint Surg Br* 76:215–219, 1994.

27. Daube JR, Rubin DI: Needle electromyography, *Muscle Nerve* 39:244–270, 2009.
28. Dillingham TR: *Approach to trauma of the peripheral nerves, American Association of Electrodiagnostic Medicine Course Proceedings*, Orlando, 1998, AAEM Annual Scientific Meeting.
29. Dillingham TR, Lauder TD, Andary M, et al: Identifying lumbosacral radiculopathies: an optimal electromyographic screen, *Am J Phys Med Rehabil* 79:496–503, 2000.
30. Dillingham TR, Lauder TD, Andary M, et al: Identification of cervical radiculopathies: optimizing the electromyographic screen, *Am J Phys Med Rehabil* 80:84–91, 2001.
31. Dillingham TR, Pezzin LE: Under-recognition of polyneuropathy in persons with diabetes by non-physician electrodiagnostic services providers, *Am J Phys Med Rehabil* 84:339–406, 2005.
33. Dillingham TR, Pezzin LE, Lauder TD, et al: Symptom duration and spontaneous activity in lumbosacral radiculopathy, *Am J Phys Med Rehabil* 79:124–132, 2000.
34. Dillingham TR, Pezzin LE, Rice B: Electrodiagnostic services in the United States, *Muscle Nerve* 29:198–204, 2004.
35. Donnelly V, Foran A, Murphy J, et al: Neonatal brachial plexus palsy: an unpredictable injury, *Am J Obstet Gynecol* 187:1209–1212, 2002.
36. Donofrio P, Albers J: AAEM minimonograph #34: polyneuropathy: classification by nerve conduction studies and electromyography, *Muscle Nerve* 13:889–903, 1990.
37. Dorfman LJ, Robinson LR: AAEM minimonograph #47: normative data in electrodiagnostic medicine, *Muscle Nerve* 20:4–14, 1997.
38. Dumitru D: Generalized peripheral neuropathies. In Dumitru D, editor: *Electrodiagnostic medicine*, Philadelphia, 1995, Hanley & Belfus.
40. Dumitru D: Reaction of the peripheral nervous system to injury. In Dumitru D, editor: *Electrodiagnostic medicine*, Philadelphia, 1995, Hanley & Belfus.
41. Dumitru D: Focal peripheral neuropathies. In Dumitru D, editor: *Electrodiagnostic medicine*, ed 2, Philadelphia, 2002, Hanley & Belfus.
42. Dumitru D, Diaz CAJ, King JC: Prevalence of denervation in paraspinal and foot intrinsic musculature, *Am J Phys Med Rehabil* 80:482–490, 2001.
43. Dumitru D, Martinez CT: Propagated insertional activity: a model of positive sharp wave generation, *Muscle Nerve* 34:457–462, 2006.
45. England JD, Gronseth GS, Franklin G, et al: Distal symmetrical polyneuropathy: definition for clinical research, *Muscle Nerve* 31:113–123, 2005.
46. Ertas M, Baslo MB, Yildiz N, et al: Concentric needle electrode for neuromuscular jitter analysis, *Muscle Nerve* 23:715–719, 2000.
48. Frykman GK, Wolf A, Coyle T: An algorithm for management of peripheral nerve injuries, *Orthop Clin North Am* 12:239–244, 1981.
50. Gruis KL, Little AA, Zebarah VA, et al: Survey of electrodiagnostic laboratories regarding hemorrhagic complications from needle electromyography, *Muscle Nerve* 34:356–358, 2006.
51. Haig AJ: Clinical experience with paraspinal mapping. II. A simplified technique that eliminates three-fourths of needle insertions, *Arch Phys Med Rehabil* 78:1185–1190, 1997.
52. Haig AJ, Tzeng HM, LeBreck DB: The value of electrodiagnostic consultation for patients with upper extremity nerve complaints: a prospective comparison with the history and physical examination, *Arch Phys Med Rehabil* 80:1273–1281, 1999.
53. Harris MI: Diabetes in America: epidemiology and scope of the problem, *Diabetes Care* 21(Suppl 3):C11–C14, 1998.
54. Jablecki CK: *AAEM case report #3: myasthenia gravis*, Rochester, 1981, American Association of Electrodiagnostic Medicine.
55. Jablecki CK, Busis NA, Brandstater MA, et al: Reporting the results of needle EMG and nerve conduction studies: an educational report, *Muscle Nerve* 32:682–685, 2005.
57. Johnson EW, Denny ST, Kelley JP: Sequence of electromyographic abnormalities in stroke syndrome, *Arch Phys Med Rehabil* 56:468–473, 1975.
60. Keesey JC: AAEE minimonograph #33: electrodiagnostic approach to defects of neuromuscular transmission, *Muscle Nerve* 12:613–626, 1989.
62. Kimura J: Polyneuropathies. In Kimura J, editor: *Electrodiagnosis in diseases of nerve and muscle: principles and practice*, ed 2, Philadelphia, 1989, FA Davis.
63. Kimura J: Techniques in normal findings. In Kimura J, editor: *Electrodiagnosis in diseases of nerve and muscle: principles and practice*, ed 2, Philadelphia, 1989, FA Davis.
65. Kline DG: Surgical repair of peripheral nerve injury, *Muscle Nerve* 13:843–852, 1990.
66. Kline DG, Hackett ER, Happel LH: Surgery for lesions of the brachial plexus, *Arch Neurol* 43:170–181, 1986.
67. Kraft GH: Fibrillation potential amplitude and muscle atrophy following peripheral nerve injury, *Muscle Nerve* 13:814–821, 1990.
68. Krivickas L: Electrodiagnosis in neuromuscular diseases, *Phys Med Rehabil Clin N Am* 9:83–114, 1998.
69. Kuncl RW, Cornblath DR, Griffin JW: Assessment of thoracic paraspinal muscles in the diagnosis of ALS, *Muscle Nerve* 11:484–492, 1988.
70. Kuruoglu R, Oh SJ, Thompson B: Clinical and electromyographic correlations of lumbosacral radiculopathy, *Muscle Nerve* 17:250–251, 1994.
71. Lauder TD, Dillingham TR: The cervical radiculopathy screen: optimizing the number of muscles studied, *Muscle Nerve* 19:662–665, 1996.
72. Lauder TD, Dillingham TR, Huston CW, et al: Lumbosacral radiculopathy screen. Optimizing the number of muscles studied, *Am J Phys Med Rehabil* 73:394–402, 1994.
74. MacKinnon SE, Dellon AL: *Surgery of the peripheral nerve*, New York, 1988, Thieme Medical Publishers.
75. Makki AA, Benatar M: The electromyographic diagnosis of amyotrophic lateral sclerosis: does the evidence support the El Escorial criteria?, *Muscle Nerve* 35:614–619, 2007.
76. Marin R, Dillingham TR, Chang A, et al: Extensor digitorum brevis reflex in normals and patients with L5 and S1 radiculopathies, *Muscle Nerve* 18:52–59, 1995.
77. Mateen FJ, Grant IA, Sorenson EJ: Needlestick injuries among electromyographers, *Muscle Nerve* 38:1541–1545, 2008.
78. Meekins GD, So Y, Quan D: American Association of Neuromuscular and Electrodiagnostic Medicine evidenced-based review: use of surface electromyography in the diagnosis and study of neuromuscular disorders, *Muscle Nerve* 38:1219–1224, 2008.
79. Miller RG: AAEE minimonograph #28: injury to peripheral motor nerves, *Muscle Nerve* 10:698–710, 1987.
80. Miller RG, Peterson GW, Daube JR, et al: Prognostic value of electrodiagnosis in Guillain-Barré syndrome, *Muscle Nerve* 11:769–774, 1988.
81. Mondelli M, Aretini A, Arrigucci U, et al: Sensory nerve action potential amplitude is rarely reduced in lumbosacral radiculopathy due to herniated disc, *Clin Neurophysiol* 124:405–409, 2013.
83. Parry GJ: Electrodiagnostic studies in the evaluation of peripheral nerve and brachial plexus injuries, *Neurol Clin* 10:921–934, 1992.
84. Partanen JV, Danner R: Fibrillation potentials after muscle injury in humans, *Muscle Nerve* 5(Suppl 9):S70–S73, 1982.
85. Pezzin LE, Dillingham TR, Lauder TD, et al: Cervical radiculopathies: relationship between symptom duration and spontaneous EMG activity, *Muscle Nerve* 22:1412–1418, 1999.
87. Robinson L: AAEM case report #22: polymyositis, *Muscle Nerve* 14:310–315, 1991.
88. Robinson LR: Electromyography, magnetic resonance imaging, and radiculopathy: it's time to focus on specificity, *Muscle Nerve* 22:149–150, 1999.
89. Sanders D, Stalberg E: AAEM minimonograph #25: single fiber electromyography, *Muscle Nerve* 19:1069–1083, 1996.
90. Sarrigiannis PG, Kennett RP, Read S, et al: Single-fiber EMG with a concentric needle electrode: validation in myasthenia gravis, *Muscle Nerve* 33:61–65, 2006.
91. Scelsa SN, Herskovitz S, Berger AR: The diagnostic utility of F waves in L5/S1 radiculopathy, *Muscle Nerve* 18:1496–1497, 1995.
92. Schoeck AP, Mellion ML, Gilchrist JM, et al: Safety of nerve conduction studies in patients with implanted cardiac devices, *Muscle Nerve* 35:521–524, 2007.
93. Shields R: AAEE case report #10: alcoholic polyneuropathy, *Muscle Nerve* 8:183–187, 1985.
94. Sonoo M, Kuwabara S, Shimizu T, et al: Utility of trapezius EMG for diagnosis of amyotrophic lateral sclerosis, *Muscle Nerve* 39:63–70, 2009.
95. Srinivasan J, Scala S, Jones HR, et al: Inappropriate surgeries resulting from misdiagnosis of early amyotrophic lateral sclerosis, *Muscle Nerve* 34:359–360, 2006.
97. Streib EW: AAEM minimonograph #27: differential diagnosis of myotonic syndromes, *Muscle Nerve* 10:603–615, 1987.

98. Taylor BV, Wright RA, Harper CM, et al: Natural history of 46 patients with multifocal motor neuropathy with conduction block, *Muscle Nerve* 23:900–908, 2000.
99. Taylor RG, Kewalramani LS, Fowler WM, Jr: Electromyographic findings in lower extremities of patients with high spinal cord injury, *Arch Phys Med Rehabil* 55:16–23, 1974.
100. Tong HC, Haig AJ, Yamakawa KS, et al: Specificity of needle electromyography for lumbar radiculopathy and plexopathy in 55- to 79-year-old asymptomatic subjects, *Am J Phys Med Rehabil* 85:908–912, quiz 913–915, 934, 2006.
101. Tullberg T, Svanborg E, Isacsson J, et al: A preoperative and postoperative study of the accuracy and value of electrodiagnosis in patients with lumbosacral disc herniation, *Spine* 18:837–842, 1993.
103. Weinberg DH: AAEM case report 4: Guillain-Barré syndrome. American Association of Electrodiagnostic Medicine, *Muscle Nerve* 22:271–281, 1999.
105. Wilbourn AJ, Aminoff MJ: AAEM minimonograph 32: the electrodiagnostic examination in patients with radiculopathies, *Muscle Nerve* 21:1612–1631, 1998.
106. Xu Y, Zheng J, Zhang S, et al: Needle electromyography of the rectus abdominis in patients with amyotrophic lateral sclerosis, *Muscle Nerve* 35:383–385, 2007.

The full reference list for this chapter is available online.

SECTION 2

Treatment Techniques and Special Equipment

CHAPTER 9

REHABILITATION AND PROSTHETIC RESTORATION IN UPPER LIMB AMPUTATION

Terrence P. Sheehan

Limb loss and limb deficiency occur in significant numbers worldwide. Amputations are performed to remove limbs that are no longer functional because of injury or disease. The common reasons for amputation are related to diabetes, peripheral vascular disease, trauma, and malignancy. Genetic variation and mutation are the typical causes for congenital deficiencies. Upper limb loss is more commonly caused by trauma than lower limb loss. Before 1900, war-related injury was the major reason for limb loss in the United States. As America became industrialized, there was a rise in civilian trauma causing upper limb loss as a result of crush injury, laceration, and avulsion. A great deal is owed to our wounded military and manual laborers, then and now, for pushing the development of the technologies and options for those with limb loss today. The evolution of the upper limb prosthesis is founded on the principles of Salisbury and Newton.[35] Prosthetic scientists stood on the shoulders of these giants while building functional tools that assist with performing daily tasks. As technologies advance, we are even more dependent on the training and the technical skill of the upper limb prosthetist. Despite entering the bionic age, the cable-and-hook systems remain the staple of upper limb prostheses because of their relative versatility and simplicity.

Demographics, Incidence, and Prevalence

In the United States an estimated 185,000 persons undergo an amputation of the upper or lower limb each year.[34] In 2008, it was estimated that 1.9 million persons were living with limb loss in the United States (Johns Hopkins Bloomberg School of Public Health, unpublished data). Of this estimate, 500,000 persons were living with minor (fingers, hands) upper limb loss, and 41,000 persons were living with major upper limb amputations.[8] Because of the aging of the population and higher rates of dysvascular disease related to diabetes and obesity, it is projected that the number of people living with lower limb loss in the United States will double by the year 2050.[8]

Trauma accounts for 90% of all upper limb amputations. During the next 50 years, the incidence of amputations secondary to trauma is estimated to remain flat if not decrease.[35] The incidence is hypothesized to decrease because of more successful occupational safety standards.[17] The future is also likely to bring even more aggressive and successful limb reconstruction and replantation. Other causes of upper limb loss include burns, peripheral vascular disease, neurologic disorders, infections, malignancies, contracture, and congenital deformities.[3]

Finger amputation represents the highest percentage (78%) of upper limb amputations reported on hospital discharges.[16] Most amputations involve single digits, with the index, ring, and long fingers accounting for 75% and the thumb 16%.[3] Excluding finger amputation, the most common upper limb amputations are through the forearm (transradial) and humerus (transhumeral), respectively (Table 9-1, Figure 9-1).[47] Most civilian limb injuries that result in amputation occur at work and involve saws or blades (e.g., lawnmowers and snow blowers). Blast-related injuries are rare in the civilian population (8.5%). In the active military, however, amputee injuries are from mortars, gunfire, improvised explosive devices, and rocket-propelled grenades. Because of the extreme forces involved, concomitant injuries, such as traumatic brain injury, visual and hearing impairment, soft tissue loss, and burns, are common. A fifth of all combat-related major amputations involve the upper limb.[14,62] Two thirds of amputations resulting from trauma occur among adolescents and adults younger than 45 years.[8] Males account for greater than 75% of those with upper limb loss, and the more severe the injury, the more likely the victim is male.[3]

An estimated 4.1 per 10,000 babies are born each year with all or part of a limb missing, ranging from a missing part of a finger to the absence of both arms and both legs. Congenital deficiencies in the upper limb are more common (58%), and they occur slightly more often in boys. The most common congenital amputation is at the left short transradial level. Most cases of congenital upper limb deficiency have no hereditary implications. Congenital limb deficiencies occur because of the failure of part or all of a limb bud to form. The first trimester is the critical time for limb formation. The bud appears at 26 days' gestation, and differentiation progresses through the eighth week of gestation. The etiology often is unclear, but teratogenic agents (e.g., medications and radiation exposure) and amniotic band syndrome are two common causes. Maternal ultrasound examination often identifies the limb deficiency before delivery. There have been many descriptions of congenital limb deficiencies (Box 9-1), with the development of the current and preferred system by the International Society for Prosthetic and Orthotics (ISPO; Box 9-2). The ISPO terminology divides the limb amputations into transverse or longitudinal. By definition, a child who has a *transverse deficiency* has no distal remaining

Table 9-1 Upper Limb Amputations by Site: 1993-2006

Procedure	Percentage of Total Upper Limb Amputation Procedures Performed
Amputation through the hand	15
Disarticulation through the wrist	10
Amputation through the forearm (transradial)	31
Disarticulation of the elbow	7
Amputation through the humerus (transhumeral)	28
Shoulder disarticulation	7
Forequarter amputation	2

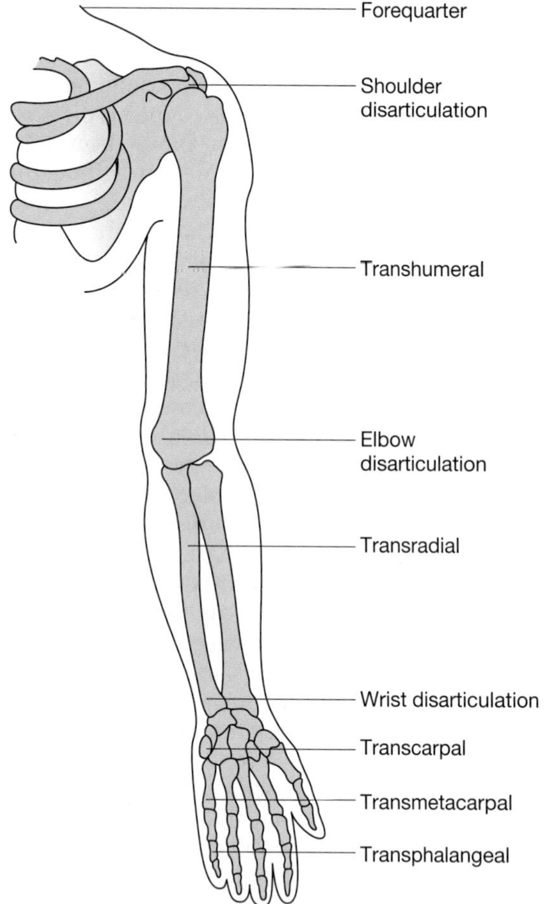

FIGURE 9-1 Types of upper extremity amputations.

BOX 9-1

Original Classification Scheme for Congenital Upper Limb Reductions

- *Amelia:* Absence of a limb
- *Meromelia:* Partial absence of a limb
- *Phocomelia:* Flipperlike appendage attached to the trunk
- *Adactyly:* Absent metacarpal or metatarsal
- *Hemimelia:* Absence of half a limb
- *Acheiria:* Missing hand or foot
- *Aphalangia:* Absent finger or toe

BOX 9-2

ISPO Classification System for Congenital Upper Limb Reductions*

- *Transverse deficiency:* No remaining distal portions. Transverse level is named after the segment beyond which there is no skeletal portion.
- *Longitudinal deficiency:* Some remaining distal portions. Longitudinal deficiencies name the bones that are affected.

*Any bone not named is present and of normal form.
ISPO, International Society for Prosthetic and Orthotics.

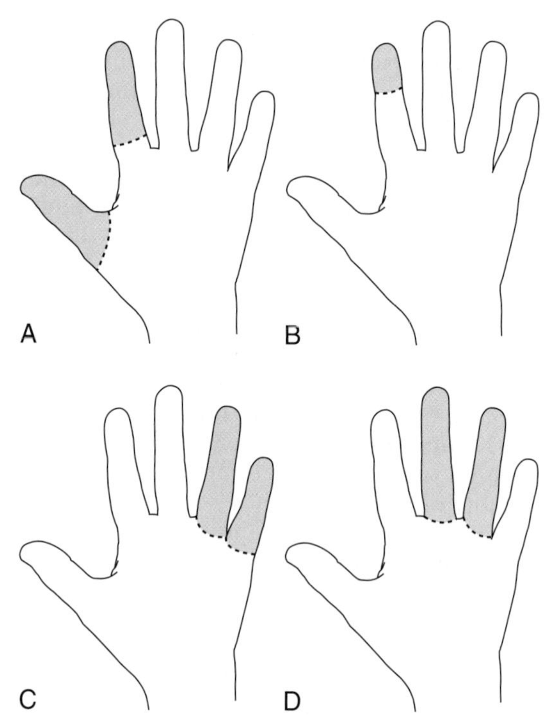

FIGURE 9-2 Types of hand amputations. **A,** Radial. **B,** Fingertip. **C,** Ulnar. **D,** Central.

parts. For example, a child with a transverse radial deficiency has a normal upper arm and a portion of the radius but is missing the hand and fingers. *Longitudinal deficiencies* have distal portions present with a partial or total absence of a specific bone. The most common congenital limb deficiency in the upper limb is a longitudinal partial or complete lack of the radius. Longitudinal hand reductions represent half of all congenital upper limb reductions, and multiple limb reductions are found in less than 20% of live births.[19,56]

Nomenclature and Functional Levels of Amputations

Radial amputations (Figure 9-2, *A*) involve the thumb and index finger and compromise grasp. *Fingertip amputation* (Figure 9-2, *B*) is the most common type of amputation. The thumb is the most functionally critical digit. *Thumb amputation,* partial or complete, results in loss of palmer grip, side-to-side pinch, and tip-to-tip pinch. Amputation of one of the other digits causes less functional loss. *Transverse digit amputations* occur at one or more digits and can be fit with functional finger prostheses. *Ulnar amputations* (Figure 9-2, *C*) involve digits IV and V with resultant loss of hook grasp. The loss of digit V is functionally underestimated because of this powerful grasp. *Central amputation* (Figure 9-2, *D*) involves digits III and IV, and reconstruction is usually not attempted. A cosmetic substitute is used instead. The *residual limb* refers to the remaining part of the amputated limb. The *sound limb* refers to the nonamputated limb. *Wrist disarticulations* are rare, but are preferred over more proximal amputations because maximal pronation and supination are preserved.[12]

Proximal to the hand, amputations are divided into the following categories: *transradial, elbow disarticulation, transhumeral, shoulder disarticulation,* and *forequarter amputation.* Depending on the percentage of the limb remaining compared with the sound side, further categorizations can be made, such as "short" and "long," to define the residual limb. These categorizations have functional implications. For the transradial residual limb, the longer the length, the more pronation (normal, 120 degrees) and supination (normal, 180 degrees) is preserved. Of the pronation and supination preserved, 50% can be transmitted to the prosthesis.[12]

Transradial amputations are based on measurements made from the longest residual bone (ulna or radius) to the medial epicondyle. This is then compared with the measurement of the sound side from the ulnar styloid to the medial epicondyle. The remaining length impacts the ability to pronate and supinate the forearm with the prosthetic device. A *long transradial* amputation preserves 55% to 90% length, allows up to 60 degrees of supination and pronation with a prosthesis, and maintains strong elbow flexion.[57] A *medium transradial* amputation preserves 35% to 55% length, but pronation and supination with a prosthesis are lost. Elbow flexion is reduced because of the inhibiting prosthesis. A *short transradial* amputation is defined as 0% to 35% preservation, which results in difficult prosthetic suspension and the additional loss of full range of motion (ROM) at the elbow.

Elbow disarticulation creates functional and prosthetic fit difficulties related to suspension and elbow joint placement. This level of amputation preserves humeral rotation of the prosthesis and can be accommodated by modern socket fabrication techniques and cosmesis. It is most suitable for the growing child to preserve the epiphysis for growth.[43] Elbow disarticulation is recommended instead of bilateral transhumeral because of functional prosthetic control.

The *transhumeral amputation* can also be classified into three levels. The more humeral length preserved, the more optimal the prosthetic restoration. The *long transhumeral* is defined as preservation of 50% to 90% of length relative to the sound side. Glenohumeral motions are preserved and uninhibited by the prosthetic socket. The *short transhumeral* is defined as preservation of 30% to 50% of length, which results in loss of glenohumeral motion because of the inhibition of the prosthetic socket that encompasses the acromion.[57] The glenohumeral motions of flexion, extension, and abduction are lost with humeral neck level amputation, *shoulder disarticulation,* and *forequarter amputation.* They are usually amputations related to malignancy and severe trauma in which no distal level amputation was possible. These levels of amputation present challenges to achieving adequate suspension and functional use of the prosthesis. Newer myoelectric techniques are gaining ground in achieving the multijoint control that is needed in optimal prosthetic restoration for these very proximal upper limb amputations.

Principles of Limb Salvage and Amputation Surgery

Limb Salvage

Limb-sparing procedures have become possible because of advances in imaging, reconstructive surgery, microsurgery, and cancer treatment. Improved methods of resuscitation and time-sensitive transport have decreased ischemia time. Optimal skin and soft tissue closure with *pedicle flaps* and *microvascular free flaps* allows the surgeon to meet the initial goal of critical limb length and the later goal of skin durability for long-term socket use. Whether it is tumor, trauma, or congenital malformation, the decision to attempt salvage with reconstruction or amputation remains difficult. The best decision is one formed by the consensus of the experienced trauma, oncology, and rehabilitation specialists. Upper and lower limb characteristics are different and must be kept in mind when considering limb salvage or amputation. The upper limb is non–weight bearing. It remains functional with significant sensory impairment, which is different from the lower limb. An upper limb that preserves only assistive function is still often more functional than one with a prosthetic replacement.

Injury scores were developed for severe trauma-related limb injuries, to help determine which vascular injury patients would benefit from primary amputation versus an attempt at limb salvage. Their validity has been questioned. The *mangled extremity syndrome* is defined as significant injury to at least three of the four tissue groups (skin/soft tissue, nerve, vessel, and bone).[24] The *mangled extremity scoring systems* have been shown to be poor predictors of amputation or salvage with regard to functional outcome.[18,44,58] Ly et al.[42] concluded that the available injury severity scores are not predictive of functional recovery of patients who undergo reconstruction surgery. Bosse et al.,[6] using the *Sickness Impact Profile,* presented evidence that the functional outcomes from limb salvage and reconstruction after severe trauma were the same at 2 years for those who underwent amputation. Finally, in this salvage-versus-amputation equation, no significant long-term psychological outcome advantage has been reported for limb salvage surgery compared with amputation.[55] Consequently, objective measures have not functionally supported the natural desires of the patient and the tendency of the trauma team to make all attempts at salvaging the limb.

In severe limb trauma that includes defects from burns and tumor resection, the appropriate soft tissue restoration is an essential component of the overall treatment. This is common both to limb salvage and amputation, especially

BOX 9-3

Skin Flaps

- *Pedicle flap:* A flap in which a local muscle inclusive of the overlying skin is moved over with its own blood supply to fill a large defect.
- *Microvascular free flap:* A flap in which the donor is not local and the microvasculature of the donor muscle is anastomosed to the available vessels at the defect site.

when critical lengths are being preserved. It requires a vascularized flap that can protect the neurovascular and musculotendinous structures (Box 9-3). The *pedicle flap* is a local muscle inclusive of the overlying skin that is moved over with its own blood supply to fill a large defect. A *microvascular free flap* is one in which the donor tissue is taken from a different site and the microvasculature of the donor tissue is anastomosed to the available vessels in the site of the defect. The feasibility of limb salvage is determined partly by the ability to reconstruct the soft tissue defect. In the upper limb, few pedicle flap options are available to repair significant defects. The recent advancement of microvascular reconstruction techniques and free flaps from sites like the rectus abdominis have expanded the option of limb salvage and preserved limb length.

Once it has been decided that amputation is more appropriate than limb salvage, the team must determine the most distal level possible, based on principles of wound healing and functional prosthetic fitting. Skin flaps now afford closures that were not historically possible. The skin closure must be without tension and should be done so that nonadherent, strategically placed, mobile scars are produced. It is the artful surgeon who crafts the distal residual limb with the appropriate muscle padding, rather than producing a bony atrophic limb or one with excessive preservation of soft, redundant tissue that makes it difficult to fit the prosthetic socket. Stable distal muscle padding can be accomplished through *myodesis,* in which the deep layers are sutured directly to the periosteum. It can also be accomplished by *myoplasty,* in which the superficial antagonistic muscles are sutured together and to the deeper muscle layers. These techniques typically produce muscle padding with sufficient balance and tension.

Although these are the conventional surgical techniques to address the residual muscle tissue, myoplasty presents a challenge later when attempting to localize an optimal myoelectrode placement. Because the muscles are sutured together, they tend to contract simultaneously. The ideal distal muscle stabilization occurs with *tenodesis*. If the muscle is preserved with its tendon, the tendon can be sutured to the periosteum.

Neuroma formation is the normal and expected consequence of nerve division. Nerves should be gently withdrawn from the wound, sharply divided, and allowed to retract under cover of soft tissue. The goal is to locate the ends of incised nerves away from areas of external contact, such as the socket interface, so the cicatrix will remain asymptomatic.

For those with *malignant tumors,* 70% to 85% are treated by limb salvage without compromising the oncologic result.[60] The goal of this type of surgery is to preserve function, prevent tumor recurrence, and enable the rapid administration of chemotherapy or radiation therapy. For tumors of the hand, ray resection is done. In the wrist, multiple options are available such as an *endoprosthesis implant* or an *allograft* or *vascularized bone transplant* (e.g., fibula). For the elbow, an endoprosthetic reconstruction is the best possible option. The humerus is similar to the wrist in that an endoprosthesis, or an allograft, or a vascularized bone transplant can be used. For tumors of the scapula or proximal humerus, a forequarter amputation or flail arm is prevented by reconstruction with a combination of an endoprosthesis and allograft. These types of reconstruction would not be possible without major improvements in radiography, chemotherapy, radiotherapy, and staging.[60]

The complication rate is much higher after limb salvage than after amputation in the oncology population. These complications can be divided into early and late. The earliest complications include infection, wound necrosis, and neurapraxia. The late complications include aseptic loosening, prosthetic fracture and dislocation, and graft nonunion.[4] Consequently, additional surgery is often necessary. Advancements in resection techniques, radiation, and chemotherapy have improved both functional limb survival and life expectancy. Serletti et al.,[55] using the *Enneking Outcome Measurement Scale,* reported the functional outcome as "excellent" or "good" in more than 70% of the patients who had reconstruction after resection of limb sarcomas. The Enneking Outcome Measurement Scale is an outcome tool that assesses seven characteristics of upper limb use: ROM, stability, deformity, pain level, strength, functional activity, and emotional acceptance. Limb salvage has cosmetic advantages, but whether the quality of life of these patients is superior to that of those who undergo amputation is unclear.

Hand Replantation

Hand replantation (HR) of traumatically amputated limbs is now possible, especially in children, because of the potential for successful neurologic recovery.[32] Effective treatment of the patient and the ischemic, detached body part requires appropriate early cooling and prompt replantation within the initial 12-hour window. The success of digital replantation is well documented, whereas successful hand and distal forearm replantation is less common.[31] The decision to replant is based on evidence that the function and overall well-being of the patient will be better than with a prosthetic device. All indications for replantation must take into account the patient's general health, the ischemia time and the level, type and extent of tissue damage. It requires prolonged recovery periods, multiple procedures, and motivated patients to achieve optimal outcomes. Predictors of successful replantation include adequate preservation, contraction of the muscle in the amputated limb after stimulation, the level of injury, and no tobacco use. The best predictor of success is the serum potassium level in the amputated segment. If the serum potassium level is higher than 6.5 mmol/L, replantation should be avoided.[61]

Replantation is indicated in levels from the distal forearm to the fingers. The more proximal to the wrist, the greater the amount of ischemic muscle mass and the more

BOX 9-4

Steps in Replantation Surgery

1. Open reduction and internal fixation of the ulna (with six-hole plate) and radius (with eight-hole plate).
2. This was followed by repair of all injured tendons: flexor digitorum profundus (FDP) 2-5, flexor digitorum superficialis (FDS) 2-5, flexor pollicis longus, flexor carpi radialis, flexor carpi ulnaris, palmaris longus, extensor carpi ulnaris, extensor digitorum 2-5, extensor digiti minimi, extensor pollicis longus and brevis, abductor pollicis longus, extensor carpi radialis longus and brevis.
3. The radial and ulnar arteries were repaired.
4. Repair of the median, ulnar, radial, and dorsal ulnar sensory nerves.
5. The basilar vein was repaired, and a 3-cm vein graft repair was made of the cephalic vein.
6. Closure was achieved with advance of skin flap and the use of a skin graft.
7. Total tourniquet time of the surgery was 2 hours and 45 minutes.

complex the metabolic and surgical demands. Approximately 85% of replanted parts remain viable. Sensory recovery with two-point discrimination occurs in 50% of adults.[39] The functional results are more promising in children, but the viability rate is lower because of the technically demanding microvascular surgery. Major limb replantation entails significant metabolic disturbance and risk. It requires scrupulous medical management. Replantation is contraindicated in those with crushed and mangled limbs and those with atherosclerosis. Because nerves transected in the proximal arm must regenerate over a considerable length, only limited motor return is typically seen in the forearm and hand, particularly the intrinsic muscles of the hand. Useful function of the wrist and hand is unusual and limited at best. Function can often be improved by converting these patients to transradial prosthetic wearers. Unfortunately, it means performing a transradial amputation after successful transhumeral replantation. This is known as *segmental replantation,* in which portions of compromised limbs are salvaged that would otherwise have been discarded.

The steps in replantation surgery are given in Box 9-4.

Hand Transplantation

During the past 15 years, collaboration between hand surgeons and immunologists has led to successes in *hand transplantation (HT)*. Advances learned from clinical organ transplant immunosuppression known as composite tissue allograft (CTA) have permitted HT to progress beyond the first operation in the United States in 1997. CTA is the term used to describe transplantation of multiple tissues (skin, muscle, bone, cartilage, nerve, tendon, blood vessels) as a functional unit. The first long-term success was when a team in Louisville, Kentucky performed a transplant on a 24-year-old man who had lost his hand in a firework accident.[33] The Louisville patient is still alive, enjoying a restoration of function and appearance once deemed impossible. Since then, more than 65 hand and upper limb transplantations have been performed around the globe, in the era of immunosuppression.[30] The ultimate goal of HT is to

Table 9-2 Comparison of Hand Transplantation and Hand Replantation

	Hand Transplantation	Hand Replantation
Surgery	Planned and performed electively	Emergency surgery
Donor tissues	Intact	Missing, avulsed, crushed, or contaminated
Modification of donor graft	Tailored to match specific requirements	Limited by type of injury
Recipient site	May be scarred with muscle contracture and reduced tendon excursion	Missing, avulsed, crushed, or contaminated
Warm ischemia time	Minutes	Minutes to hours
Immunosuppression	Long-term antirejection drugs needed	Not necessary

achieve graft survival and useful long-term function. For these goals to be achieved, selection of the appropriate patient, detailed preoperative planning, and precise surgical technique are of paramount importance. Transplantation should be reserved for motivated, consenting adults in good general heath, who are psychologically stable and have failed a trial of prosthetic use.

Although HR and HT are similar with regard to the surgical procedure, differences can exist (Table 9-2) starting with the most obvious: selecting a donor for a HT must involve additional and careful emphasis on matching skin color, skin tone, gender, ethnicity and race, and the size of the hand. Next is a difference in operative sequence. As for HR, the operative sequence of HT varies based on the amount of muscle transplanted. Distal transplantations (distal to the distal one third of the radius) have relatively less muscle mass than more proximal level HTs. The more distal HTs can tolerate a longer period of ischemia. Thus, some groups have delayed the revascularization to later in the surgical sequence. Proximal forearm transplantations, with the concomitant increased muscle bulk, require rapid revascularization to avoid ischemic injury and prevent muscle fibrosis. Ischemia time is one of the main factors influencing the outcome after HT because total ischemia time is often 1.5 to 3 times longer than replantation.[26] Other differences include the fact that HRs are often performed by a single microsurgeon in contrast to HT logistics, which require two surgical teams: the *harvesting team* and the *transplant team,* working in tandem against the clock. In HT, the allograft is harvested according to the specific anatomic needs in the recipient; various structures must be dissected with excess length to facilitate reconstruction and allow vascular and nervous repairs without tension. With HR there is a paucity of tissue, and efforts are made to conserve tissue. Limited bone shortening is done to alleviate tension on the neurovascular and tendon repairs. However, the relative tension and balance between the flexor and extensor tendons is generally left intact. With HT, an excess of tissue is available and one must judge exactly what is needed to suit the recipient's unique requirements. As a result, the relative tension between the flexor and extensor tendons must be reestablished. Barring major traumatic bone loss, forearm length is generally preserved with HR. With HT, the appropriate forearm length must be reconstructed to match the contralateral side. The HT surgery can last from 12 to 16 hours, almost double that of heart and liver transplants. Immunosuppression after CTA is composed of two elements: (1) treatment of the patient with monoclonal antibodies on the day of transplant, followed by (2) a donor bone marrow infusion several days later. Typical postoperative complications include vessel thrombosis, infections, and rejection. *Rejection* can appear as a spotty, patchy, or blotchy rash. It could appear anywhere on the transplant and is usually painless. As rejection appears first in the skin, the clinical team and patients are encouraged to carefully watch for the signs. Unlike internal organ transplants, rejection is easier to detect early.

Rehabilitation After Hand Replantation and Hand Transplantation

Rehabilitation after HR focuses on mobilization of the replanted hand through conventional hand rehabilitation (Box 9-5). Exercises maintain optimal length of ligament and joint capsular structure of the metatarsophalangeal (MP) joints, balancing the tension between flexors and extensors, and, at the same time preventing edema formation in finger joints. After a hand has been lost, much time can pass before a donor is found. Representation of the hand in the individual's brain is lost because of *cortical reorganization* during this time. Researchers have learned through functional magnetic resonance imaging that after transplantation, amputation-induced cortical reorganization is reversed to reestablish the hand "image."[5] Thus, rehabilitation after HT involves cortical reprogramming and reintegration of the transplanted limb, in addition to conventional hand rehabilitation. A rehabilitation protocol should focus on dynamic orthotic intervention, active/passive exercises to improve ROM, grip strengthening, and sensory reeducation over the first year of therapy. Supportive surgeries, interrupting the episodes of therapy, are often needed to treat problems of bone nonunion, tendon transfer, and excessive scar tissue development affecting neural and muscle tissue. Recovery is relatively slow, requiring an extensive program of occupational therapy episodically, for years.

BOX 9-5

Goals of Postoperative Therapy Following Replantation or Transplantation

- Proper hand positioning: wrist extension (15 degrees to 30 degrees) protects extensors for as long as needed to prevent any lag while hand is in intrinsic plus/thumb abducted palmarly and radially.
- Prevent clawing: do not allow full metatarsophalangeal extension until intrinsics have recovered enough function.
- Control edema: elevation and gentle soft tissue massage; no compression.
  - Exercises: early tendon gliding exercises and range of motion.
- Cognitive exercise training with electrostimulation (Perfetti protocol).
- Electromyographic biofeedback training.
- Patient and family education and training of all exercises and orthotic wear.
- Control pain: pain medications (neuropathic), gentle early mobility, and modalities.
- Educate about protection because of sensory precautions.
- Keep limb warm, avoid smoking, caffeine, and cold for at least 3 to 4 weeks.
- Begin dominance retraining when appropriate.

Outcomes

The more proximal level of limb amputation, the lower the chances of regaining satisfactory hand function after transplantation. The major challenge in HT is the long distance between the nerve stumps and their end organs. Experience in "forearm" transplantation suggests that motor function may continue to improve during 5 or more years after transplantation.[53] One of the main hurdles limiting the efficacy of hand rehabilitation is the cortical organization shift that occurs after sensory and motor deprivation in amputees. There is a superiority of reinnervation in HT, including good sensitivity as well as a two-point discrimination. The favorable outcome with regard to nerve regeneration may be related to possible neuroregenerative properties of tacrolimus, which promotes nerve growth in vitro, enhancing regeneration in various peripheral nerve injury models.[49] The functional results achieved after unilateral and bilateral HT worldwide showed that all patients had protective sensitivity, 90% of the recipients had tactile sensitivity, and 84% also had discriminative sensation. Many patients have returned to work. The quality of life scores have improved in 75% of patients after transplant. Patient satisfaction seems to be greater after HT.[48] This may be related to the observation that patients with HT constitute a selected group of highly compliant patients who are well prepared for the surgical procedure and rehabilitation. Their expectations might therefore be more realistic.

In HR, the innervation of intrinsic hand muscles, responsible for precise movements, is limited. A claw hand deformity can occur because of poor positioning and limited and slow nerve regeneration, specifically secondary to decreased ulnar nerve innervations to the intrinsic musculature. This results in functional limitations consisting of poor opposition of the thumb due to lack of innervations to the thenar muscles, diminished fine motor abilities, and lack of sensibility due to lack of ulnar nerve innervation. Traumatic amputations of the hand often result in large cortical areas of the brain being deafferented, which is followed by extensive cortical reorganization so that the adjacent and contralateral cortical areas take over the function of the vacant area. After replantation of the hand, functional return can only occur after the peripheral sensory nerves reclaim their original cortical territory.[5] Thus, after HR, studies have used functional magnetic resonance imaging to map the activation pattern of the motor cortex. Recovery of normal activation pattern varies between patients, but a general consensus of 6 weeks for normal activation pattern is seen. Most patients after HR have fairly good motor function return, although sensory recovery is poor. In addition, they often have severe cold intolerance.[52] It is unclear why these individuals have such an extensive loss of functional sensory recovery. Grip strength was superior after HR, even in cases with extensive bony shortening.

In HR, the severely impaired muscles seem to have greater potential for recovery when compared with inactivated, fibrotic, and atrophic muscles of a HT recipient's stump. Patients undergoing HR are a random group of people undergoing emergency surgery compared with those receiving HT and expect their replanted hand to function as well as before the amputation.

Amputation

Hand function is vital in our competitive and industrialized society. There are many techniques for reconstruction of the hand. It is much better to have a painless hand with some grasp function and sensation preserved than to have a prosthesis. The most important part of the hand is the opposable thumb. The goal is to preserve as much of the sensate thumb as possible. *Phalangization* of the metacarpals is a reconstructive technique in which the web space is deepened between the digits to provide more mobile digits (Figure 9-3). This works well for the thumb, especially if the first metacarpal is adjusted to create opposition to the thumb. *Pollicization* is the process of moving a finger with its nerve and blood supply to the site of the amputated thumb (Figure 9-4). This allows fine and gross grasp through opposition. A prosthesis for a hand amputation is inferior to the functional outcomes achieved with reconstructed hands.[9] In reconstructing the hand, three issues should be considered: (1) preservation of sensitivity to the grasping surface; (2) the consequences of scarring; and (3) cosmetic acceptability.

Wrist disarticulation involves removal of the radius and ulna to the styloid processes, because there is no benefit to retaining the carpal bones. It retains the distal radial-ulnar joint, preserving more forearm rotation. The prosthetic attachment to the bulbous end is enhanced if the distal radial flare is retained for suspension. Burkhalter et al.[10] indicate that it is important that the radial and ulnar styloids be resected slightly to minimize the discomfort the amputee will experience in active supination and pronation within the prosthetic socket. Tenodesis of the major forearm muscles stabilizes these groups and improves functional outcome, including myoelectric performance. Pronation and supination, as well as full elbow motion, are preserved with wrist disarticulation. Some will argue that (1) the wrist disarticulation creates a complicated prosthetic situation with difficult socket fabrication; (2) conventional wrist units are too long and cannot be used; and (3) it is harder to fit with a myoelectric prosthesis because there is no room to conceal the electronics and power supply.

Transradial amputation involves the myodesis of the forearm muscles and equal volar and dorsal skin flaps for closure. It is extremely functional, with forearm rotation and strength that is proportional to the length retained. The shorter the transradial amputation, the more the elbow and humerus are needed for suspension. Preserving the elbow joint is paramount because of the functional outcome possible with prosthetic enhancement. If the amputation must be very proximal, then an ulna 1.5 to 2 inches long is still adequate to preserve the elbow joint. For this very short residual limb to be fit with a prosthesis, it might be helpful to detach the biceps and reattach it to the ulna.[41]

A couple of special situations arise with transradial amputations. First, when one forearm bone is considerably longer than the other and the longer bone can be covered with an adequate soft tissue envelope, it may be preferable to create a one-bone forearm rather than decrease prosthetic function by shortening the longer bone. Second is the Krukenberg amputation, which transforms the residual

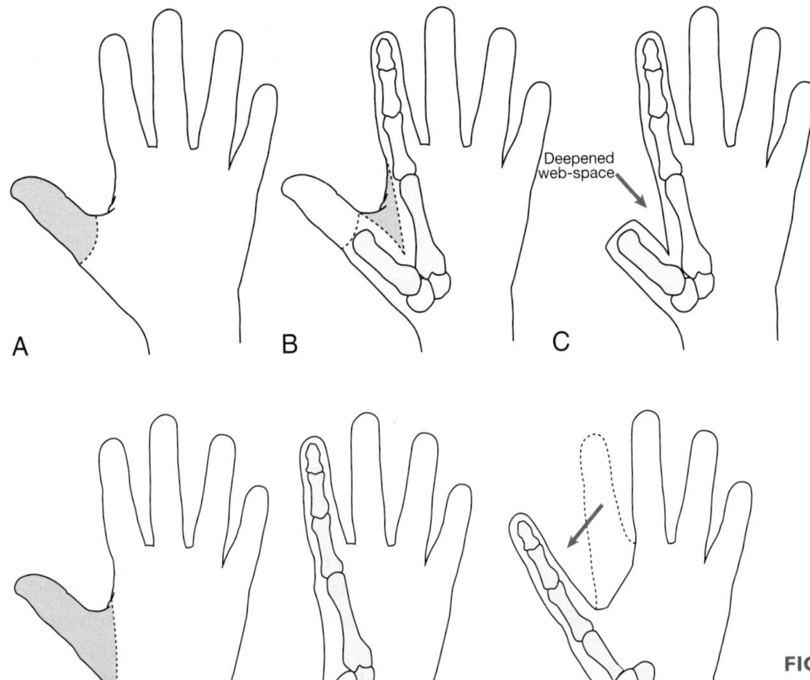

FIGURE 9-3 Phalangization of the metacarpals is a reconstructive technique in which the web space is deepened between the digits, providing more mobile digits. **A,** Amputated thumb. **B,** Web space deepened. **C,** Final web space deepened to provide more mobility.

FIGURE 9-4 Pollicization is the process of moving a finger with its nerve and blood supply to the site of the amputated thumb. **A,** Amputated thumb including metacarpal. **B,** Index finger to be moved. **C,** Final index finger in the thumb's place.

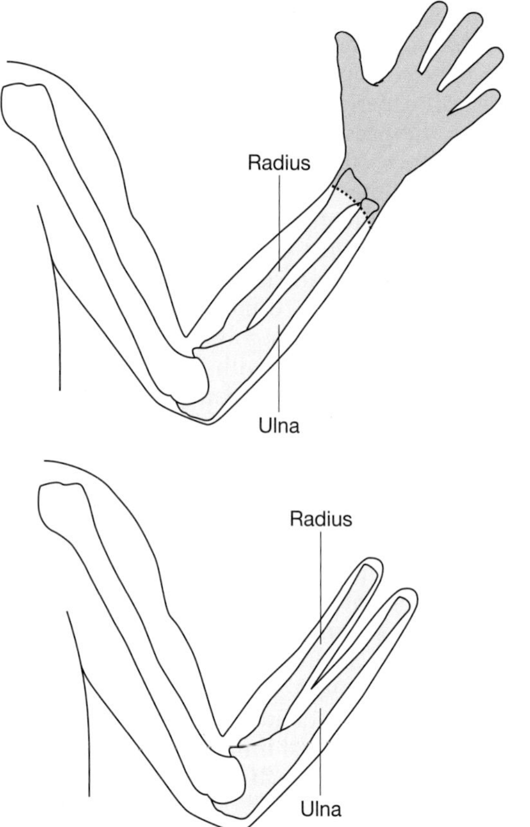

FIGURE 9-5 The Krukenberg amputation transforms the residual ulna and radius into digits that have significant forceful prehension and retained ability to manipulate because of preserved sensation.

ulna and radius into digits that have significant forceful prehension and retained ability to manipulate because of preserved sensation (Figure 9-5). This is an option for patients with at least 4 inches of residual limb, those with bilateral amputation, and those with limited prosthetic facilities. It can be fitted with conventional as well as myoelectric prostheses.

Elbow disarticulation allows the transfer of humeral rotation to the prosthesis, through the myodesis of the biceps and triceps, and it preserves a stronger lever. Although the skin flaps are approximately equal, the posterior muscle flap remains longer than the anterior muscle flap, to wrap around and cushion the end of the humerus. With modern total-contact sockets, the ultimate position of the scar is not critical; however, clinicians should be aware of the vulnerable skin over the medial epicondyle. The full humeral length precludes the use of a myoelectric elbow. Elbow disarticulation causes some prosthetic fitting challenges because the outside "elbow" hinge creates a bulky limb that is longer and asymmetric compared with the opposite limb. Disarticulation is the level of choice for juvenile amputees. The high incidence of residual limb revision because of bony overgrowth is avoided and humeral growth is preserved. It remains controversial who is a good candidate for elbow disarticulation, but modern prosthetic fabrication techniques can overcome the socket and cosmetic difficulties.[12,14]

Transhumeral amputations are performed at or proximal to the supracondylar level. The humerus is sectioned at least 3 cm from the joint to allow for fit of the prosthetic elbow mechanism. Transhumeral amputations should be performed with minimal periosteal stripping to prevent the occurrence of bony spurs. Rough edges should be removed, but beveling of the bone is unnecessary. All possible length should be preserved to transmit glenohumeral motions through the prosthesis. To help preserve humeral length, free flap coverage and skin graft coverage should be considered as possible alternatives for primary closure. The anterior fascia and posterior fascia over the flexor and extensor muscle groups are sutured together to cover the end of the humerus. Biceps and triceps myoplasty preserves strength for prosthetic control and myoelectric signals. Myodesis is rarely needed.[43] Performing a more proximal amputation at the level of the surgical neck, which is the site of insertion of the pectoralis major, results in the same function as if a shoulder disarticulation had been done. This is because independent motion of the humerus is no longer possible. However, because the terminal device is controlled by active shoulder girdle motion, the humeral head should be preserved when amputation has to be done proximally.

Amputations through the glenohumeral and scapulothoracic articulations, *shoulder disarticulation* and *forequarter amputation,* respectively, are rare, and both result in loss of normal shoulder contour. Advances in vascular surgery have made reestablishment of blood flow to severely traumatized limbs effective, but replantation of a limb amputated through the shoulder girdle is seldom feasible. The cosmetic deformity of both of these amputations is significant. When possible, retention of the scapula is far less disfiguring and is of psychological benefit to the patient. Personal concerns of having standard clothing fit supersede more complex concerns of functional restoration. In shoulder disarticulation, the rotator cuff tendons should be sutured together over the glenoid wing. The deltoid is attached to the inferior glenoid and lateral scapular border to fill the subacromial space. In forequarter amputation, the pectoralis major, latissimus dorsi, and trapezius are sutured together to form additional padding and contour over the chest wall. During forequarter amputation, osteotomy of the clavicle should be performed at the lateral margin of the sternocleidomastoid insertion to preserve contour of the neck.

Acute Management: Preamputation Through Early Rehabilitation

Preamputation

The *team approach to amputee rehabilitation* begins in the preamputation phase whenever possible. The surgical team joins forces with the rehabilitation team to educate and counsel each other and the patient. It is important to include family members and other supporting individuals in the counseling. A plan of the surgery must be made that takes into account an understanding of the healing potential and the most realistic and optimal functional prosthetic restoration. This is based on the information flow between the rehabilitation team and the surgical team. Important discussions need to be held with the patient

BOX 9-6

Immediate Postamputation Period Goals

- Promote wound healing
- Control pain
- Control edema
- Prevent contracture
- Initiate remobilization and preprosthetic training
- Manage expectations through supportive counseling
- Continue education, including orientation to prosthetic components

about the planned surgical outcome and postsurgical period. This should include a discussion about the different types of pain that might occur, the prevention of possible complications, and a preview of potential functional outcome. It is important to acknowledge the loss and mitigate the fear with education. A powerful intervention is to have a trained amputee volunteer, a "peer visitor," who has successfully gone through a similar limb loss and can give support to the patient throughout the recovery process.

Acute Postamputation

This phase begins with an understanding that the decision to amputate is emotionally powerful for the patient, family, and clinical team. Amputation is not a failure but rather reconstructive surgery that creates improved functional possibilities and resumption of one's life. The focus of the immediate postamputation period is to control pain and edema, promote wound healing, prevent contractures, initiate remobilization, and continue the supportive counseling and education (Box 9-6). This must be individualized to meet the needs of each patient. *Surgical site infection* needs to be seriously considered when pain, drainage, and edema are increasing despite the reasonable control measures instituted. The earlier an infection is eradicated, the earlier the time-sensitive prosthetic phase can begin. The *goal for rehabilitation* is for patients to acquire the skills and equipment needed to achieve prosthetic acceptance and holistic reintegration back into their own lives. It is imperative that the prosthesis be introduced at the earliest possible time after amputation.

The team has a responsibility to explain and give visualization of the postamputation treatment phases, from the early postoperative phase through rehabilitation and community reentry. Each team member (including the surgeon, physiatrist, prosthetist, and rehabilitation therapist) has specific duties related to physical, educational, and psychological support through these phases. An amputee peer visitor, preferably someone who has been formally trained, is a team member who has a unique perspective because of real-life experience. The Amputee Coalition of America (ACA), which is the national nonprofit limb loss advocacy group in the United States, can serve as a comprehensive source of information to persons with limb loss and their professional team. This includes locating ACA-trained peer visitors and regional support groups.

Pain control requires an early, aggressive approach that considers the multiple potential pain generators in the postsurgical period. The patient-controlled analgesia systems are often the first-line treatment by the surgical team. This is transitioned to regularly scheduled long- and short-acting oral narcotic medications. It is imperative to maintain consistent pain control. Loss of adequate pain control is painful for the patient and disrupts the timely pursuit of the rehabilitation program. The escalation of the doses of opiates needs to be avoided, if possible, by addressing other pain generators. Understanding the characteristics of postsurgical residual limb pain and phantom pain allows the clinical team to choose pain interventions wisely. Residual limb pain is located in the remaining limb and generated from the soft tissue and musculoskeletal components. *Phantom limb pain* is pain in the absent limb and is considered neuropathic.[17] Nonsteroidal antiinflammatory drugs and nonopiate pain relievers are helpful and can diminish the need for higher doses of opiates. Opiates administered at safe doses are often ineffective against phantom pain. Careful attention should be given to the description, timing, and quality of the pain complaint to tease out the central neuropathic pain component inclusive of painful phantom sensations versus peripheral nerve-generated pain. Peripheral nerve pain is more intense at night and is characterized as burning, stabbing, and buzzing. Phantom sensations occur in more than 70% of amputees and do not have to be treated unless painful and disruptive. The use of medications known for controlling neuropathic pain and sensations, such as some anticonvulsants and antidepressants, can also diminish the need for opiates.

The new amputee should be taught how to change the dressings and use desensitization techniques. *Desensitization techniques* help to eliminate the hypersensitivity to touch. They include compression, tapping, massage, and application of different textures. These techniques are performed for 20 to 30 minutes 3 times per day as tolerated by the skin and scar.[22] The use of modalities, such as transcutaneous nerve stimulation, heat, and cold, are also useful adjuvants for pain control and diminish opiate need. Ramachandran and Rogers-Ramachandran[50] have reduced phantom pain using mirrors to visually trick the brain. Because the loss of a limb is emotionally "painful," the team should address and acknowledge this. It should be kept in mind that from the individual's psychological standpoint, it might be more socially acceptable to express the psychological pain in terms of generalized pain complaints. It is important to address the psychological pain early through grief counseling, peer visitation, and education.

Edema control begins once the last suture or staple is placed by the surgeon. If there is no contraindication and the surgeon has the appropriate training, an *immediate postoperative rigid dressing* (IPORD) can be placed in the operating room. This is a special cast placed on the residual limb by the surgeon or certified professional. The control of edema leads to earlier wound healing and improved pain control through the reduction of pain mediators in the accumulated "third-spaced fluid." Typically, additional shrinkage of the residual limb occurs after the initial IPORD placement, necessitating its early replacement. The rigid dressing can be removed in 5 to 7 days and replaced with a fresh cast. The attachment of joints and a terminal device to this rigid dressing creates an *immediate postoperative prosthesis* that can allow early functional use of the residual limb. The IPORD is the preferred treatment approach for the transradial amputation, and if healing progresses without issue, the second cast can be replaced with the first prosthesis.[19]

Traumatic upper limb loss is often accompanied by large tissue defects, burns, and wound contamination from complex infections. These make immediate postoperative techniques impossible. In these cases, once drains and negative pressure dressings are discontinued, a *soft compressive dressing* can be placed to control edema and initiate shaping of the residual limb.

The ideal residual limb shape is cylindrical. The dressing should be placed and replaced by a trained clinician. It should extend beyond the proximal joint to maximize suspension and improve edema control. Those not placed correctly can create problems with distal edema accumulation, skin breakdown, and abnormal shaping (such as a dumbbell shape). The healing surgical and trauma sites frequently have patches of sensory impairment and should be monitored by the team to prevent the development of pressure sores. Once the skin has closed, dressings are replaced with "shrinkers," a silicone liner, or both. Edema control is a lifelong daily management issue for most amputees.

The control of pain and residual limb edema allows for early functional remobilization of the residual limb, which in turn helps *prevent contracture formation*. Contractures are not fully reversible, and it is critical to begin *remobilization* as early as possible. Techniques for prevention of elbow flexion and shoulder adduction contractures should be reinforced with the patient and team. This can be difficult in the setting of uncontrolled pain, burns, and other complex trauma factors, such as fractures, brain or spinal cord injuries, spasticity, and systemic illness.

The *formation of heterotopic bone* impairing joint function and ROM should be considered in these complex trauma cases and can be diagnosed with the help of laboratory testing and triple-phase bone scan. The treatment of *heterotopic ossification* beyond trying to maintain ROM and nonsteroidal antiinflammatory drugs is limited. Surgical intervention is not feasible until the heterotopic bone matures at approximately 12 to 18 months after injury.[23] Proper limb positioning and frequent monitoring of joint mobility are necessary. Any loss of ROM in a joint of the residual limb can have significant effects on functional use of the prosthesis. The loss of ROM needs to be investigated and aggressively managed to maximize range.

Preprosthetic training begins with the early postsurgical therapy visit and continues until prosthetic fitting is completed. Prosthetic fabrication and fitting ideally should be completed within 4 to 8 weeks after surgery. Early prosthetic fitting is important, because prosthetic acceptance declines if fitting is delayed beyond the third postoperative month.[20] Preprosthetic training is critical to maintain motivation and create an easier transition to prosthetic use. Amputation results in a loss of body symmetry. This imbalance results in shoulder elevation and scapula rotation on the affected side, as well as loss of neutral positioning of the residual limb. Close attention must be paid to the individual's awkward or compensatory body motions when approaching an object. The rebalancing begins with observing and correcting static postures in the mirror. The mirror remains an important tool in conscious recognition and correction of the abnormal positioning. The amputee is encouraged to use muscle memory to relearn correct postural and limb positioning control.[22] As remobilization progresses, emphasis is placed on recognizing the abnormal postures and positioning that occur with basic activities of daily living (ADLs).

ADLs are mastered with one hand and, when appropriate, with the use of adaptive equipment. The amputee progresses from independence with basic hygiene to advanced homemaking tasks. Hand dominance is retrained when necessary, especially with handwriting and keyboarding. Repetitive tasks can be used for strengthening. These tasks include fine motor exercises with nuts and bolts or tweezers, as well as gross motor exercises with equipment and mirrors. Proprioceptive neuromuscular facilitation is a particularly effective approach that enables the therapist to work in diagonal planes, vary the amount of resistance, and concentrate on specific areas of weakness. Isometric exercises are effective in creating muscle bulk for stabilization of the arm in the socket of the prosthesis. The stability of the prosthesis depends on both the bulk of the stabilizing musculature and the amputee's ability to voluntarily vary residual limb configuration. Because balance is often disrupted in a new amputee, the goals should include strengthening of the trunk, core, and lower limbs using isometric exercise and aerobic training. Depending on the level of loss, the upper limb amputee should begin to practice several motions that will be needed to control the prosthesis (Box 9-7).

BOX 9-7

Specific Movements Necessary to Control a Prosthesis and Maintenance of Range of Motion

Specific Movements Necessary to Control a Prosthesis

- *Scapular abduction:* Spreading the scapulae apart alone and in combination with humeral flexion will provide the tension needed on the figure-of-eight harness to open the terminal device.
- *Humeral flexion:* The residual limb is raised forward to shoulder level and pushed forward while sliding the scapulae apart as far as possible. This motion also allows the terminal device to open.
- *Shoulder depression, extension, and abduction:* This set of movements operates the body-powered, internal-locking elbow of the transhumeral prosthesis. It is one of the more difficult motor skills to acquire.

Maintenance of Range of Motion

- *Elbow flexion/extension:* Maintaining full elbow range of motion is critical for the transradial amputee for reaching many body locations.
- *Forearm pronation/supination:* Maintaining as much forearm pronation and supination as possible is critical for the amputee to be able to position the terminal device as needed without having to manually preposition the wrist unit.
- *Chest expansion:* This motion should be practiced by deep inhalations that expand the chest amputation. Chest expansion is used by those who have transhumeral, shoulder disarticulation, or forequarter amputation.

Orientation to the planned prosthesis, premyoelectric testing and training, and defining the amputees' *prosthetic expectations* are all important tasks for the team during this period. If a myoelectric prosthesis is being considered, early site testing and training are needed. An emphasis is placed on using specific residual limb muscles efficiently. Electrode site identification is handled by the specially trained occupational therapist to identify the best placement of the electrodes. The occupational therapist needs to work closely with the physician and prosthetist in the design of the socket and optimal electrode site placement. With the use of biofeedback equipment, motor training is done to increase muscle activity at specific sites. These muscles include the elbow flexors used for closing the terminal devices, and extensors used for opening and for supination. Once isolated movements are mastered, proportional control of the muscle is learned. This is necessary for controlling the speed and force of the prosthetic movements. The new amputee needs to have an *orientation to prosthetic component terminology.*

During this time the major components of the prosthesis should be identified, such as the figure-of-eight harness, cable, elbow unit or elbow hinge, wrist unit, terminal device, and hook or hand. It is also important during this time to review the expectations of the person with a new limb loss. The new amputee's initial personal vision of what function the prosthesis will restore is often significantly unrealistic. It is helpful to reinforce the supportive roles the prosthesis will play in cosmesis, gross task and object stabilization, push, and assistive function. Supportive education by the trained peer visitor, therapist, prosthetist, and physician helps to fine-tune a realistic vision of what each type of prosthesis has to offer from a functional standpoint.

Upper Limb Prostheses

Introduction to Upper Limb Prosthetic Systems

Each prosthesis is unique and customized to the individual. Although two prostheses might be alike or very similar, there is no such thing as a "normal" or "standard" prosthesis (especially in the world of upper limb prosthetics). There are four categories of upper limb prosthetic systems: *the passive system, the body-powered system, the externally powered system,* and *the hybrid system.* Selecting among these can be difficult. Each patient's functional and vocational goals, geographic location, anticipated environmental exposures, access to a prosthetist for maintenance, and financial resources all need to be considered (Box 9-8).

BOX 9-8

Four Categories of Upper Limb Prosthetic Systems

- Passive system
- Body-powered system
- Externally powered system
- Hybrid system

A *passive system* is primarily cosmetic but also functions as a stabilizer. A passive system is fabricated if the patient does not have enough strength or movement to control a prosthesis or wears a prosthesis only for cosmesis. Sometimes, young children initially use passive upper limb prostheses for balance and for crawling. A *body-powered system* prosthesis uses the patient's own residual limb or body strength and ROM to control the prosthesis. This includes powering the basic functions of terminal device opening and closing, elbow movement, and shoulder joint mobilization. An *externally powered system* uses an outside power source, such as a battery, to operate the prosthesis. A *hybrid system* uses the patient's own muscle strength and joint movement, as well as an external supply for power. An example of a hybrid system is a body-powered elbow joint with an externally powered terminal device.

The field of prosthetics has a unique vocabulary that is not part of the everyday practice of medicine (Box 9-9).

Socket and Suspension Choices

The *socket* has to have a snug and intimate fit around the residual limb. Although an upper limb prosthesis is not end bearing or weight bearing, it still needs an intimate,

BOX 9-9

Prosthetic Terminology

- *Residual limb:* The remaining portion of the amputated limb.
- *Excursion:* Amount of movement or range of motion that the residual limb can achieve.
- *Component:* A part of the prosthesis.
- *Terminal device:* The prosthetic equivalent of the human hand.
- *Hinge:* A prosthetic component used to assist or replace an anatomic joint.
- *Rigid hinge:* Stiff/solid arrow movement in only one plane, usually flexion and extension.
- *Flexible hinge:* Allows movement in multiple planes (i.e., flexion, extension, pronation, and supination).
- *Socket:* This part of the prosthesis acts as the interface between the residual limb and the prosthetic device as a whole. The socket is designed to distribute forces throughout the residual limb.
- *Prosthetic sock:* A prosthetic component, usually cotton, which fits the residual limb like a sock and is worn between the socket and liner to account for volume changes (size changes) in the residual limb.
- *Laminate:* A plastic composite usually made with carbon fiber and resin.
- *Gel liner:* A prosthetic component made from a silicone gel or similar polymer that rolls onto the residual limb like a sleeve and creates a suction interface between the skin and the socket.
- *Mechanical:* Designates a moving component.
- *Passive:* Describes a prosthesis used only for cosmesis rather than function.
- *Heavy duty:* It connotes a prosthetic designed to withstand strong, repetitive forces and rugged conditions. For example, a heavy-duty prosthetic user could be one who works as an automotive mechanic or construction worker.

secure fit for proper control of the unit. A prosthetic socket can be fabricated from many different materials. The most commonly used are flexible, durable, and lightweight, such as a carbon graphite material or plastic. Upper limb sockets are typically double walled with a second lamination pulled over the first to provide cosmesis and function. They can also contain an inner flexible thermoplastic liner to allow for growth (as in the case of a child) and other fluctuations in size. It is critical that the socket is comfortable and does not irritate or injure the residual limb. During fabrication, the prosthetist properly distributes the pressures around bony prominences, such as the olecranon and distal portion of residual bone. Computer-aided design (CAD system) and computer-aided manufacturing (CAM system) have reduced fabrication time, but whether such techniques are actually improvements over the skilled hands of a seasoned limb maker is debated widely in the field. There is never a single shape for a socket because of the differences in anatomy from user to user. This customization allows for socket designs to adapt to shapes that are the result of congenital or surgical issues. For example, a Krukenberg socket is designed to internally use the unique radial and ulnar branches to pinch grip for the suspension formed from the Krukenberg procedure.

Advances in custom-fitting techniques and *suspension* devices have led to the use of such suspension devices as the "seal-in" liner. This is a system that incorporates a membrane lip placed circumferentially around the distal aspect of the liner to cause a plunger-type negative pressure for suspension. There is also a *pin system* in which the *roll-on gel liner* incorporates a jagged edged pin that locks into a female receptacle in the socket. Such advances in suspension have reduced restriction on elbow flexion, pronation, and supination. The application of roll-on liner suspensions for upper limb prostheses provides not only improved suspension but also more comfort. Conventional transradial self-suspending sockets rely on pressure above the elbow to hold the prosthesis in place, which can lead to discomfort and reduced ROM. With the roll-on suspension design, the liner provides the suspension, whereas the gel protects the skin from pressure and friction. This is different from conventional skin fit suction socket designs that use one-way air valves or external sleeves for suspension and require a stable limb volume to maintain suction.

The shorter the residual limb or the heavier the anticipated workload, the more necessary it is to anchor the prosthesis proximally with single or polycentric hinges, as well as shoulder harness systems. Single pivot hinges do not allow for any pronation or supination and are not recommended for those with bilateral transradial amputations. Flexible hinges allow for some pronation and supination and can replace the single pivot hinges for those with bilateral transradial amputations. Flexible hinges are also recommended for children.

A very heavy-duty user needs a traditional socket with single pivot hinges. A self-suspending socket might not be enough support for the heavy-duty upper limb amputee, regardless of the suspension system used. This amputee might need to wear a traditional transradial socket ("screwdriver" design in cross-section to enhance supination and pronation control) with single pivot elbow hinges that stabilize rotation.

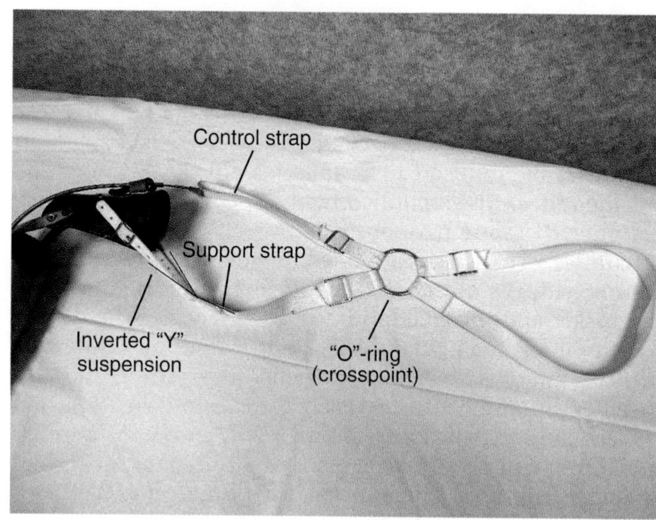

FIGURE 9-6 Components of the figure-of-eight harness: axilla loop, anterior support strap, control attachment strap, and crosspoint.

With a *figure-of-eight harness* for control and suspension, the harness not only operates the terminal device but also functions to keep the socket correctly positioned. There are four main components to the harness: the *axilla loop*, the *anterior support strap*, the *control attachment strap*, and the *crosspoint* (Figure 9-6). While wearing a prosthesis with this harness, the amputee is able to open and control the terminal device with shoulder forward flexion.

Power

- Body-powered prostheses: cable controlled
- Externally powered prostheses: electrically powered
- Myoelectric prostheses
- Switch-controlled prostheses

If amputees are given training on both the myoelectric and the body-powered prostheses, they will self-select their primary choice. It is not uncommon for the amputee to prefer myoelectric for one activity and body powered for another, which then drives whatever terminal device is selected.[24] *Body-powered prostheses* use forces generated by body movements transmitted through cables to operate joints and terminal devices. An example is forward flexing the shoulder to provide tension on the control cable of the prosthesis, resulting in opening the terminal device. Relaxing the shoulder forward flexion results in return of the terminal device to the static closed position. An alternative movement for opening the terminal device is biscapular abduction, which is commonly used when operating the terminal device close to the body. Body-powered prostheses are more durable, give higher sensory feedback, and are less expensive and lighter than myoelectric prostheses.

Externally powered prostheses use muscle contractions or manual switches to activate the prosthesis. Electrical activity from select residual muscles is detected by surface electrodes used to control electric motors. Prostheses powered by electric motors can provide more proximal function and greater grip strength, along with improved cosmesis. They can also be heavy and expensive. Patient-controlled batteries and motors are used to operate these prostheses. Currently available designs generally have less sensory feedback and require more maintenance than do body-powered prostheses.

Externally powered prostheses require a control system. The two types of commonly available *control systems* are myoelectric and switch control. A *myoelectrically controlled* prosthesis uses muscle contractions as a signal to activate the prosthesis. It functions by using surface electrodes to detect electrical activity from select residual limb muscles to control electric motors. Different types of myoelectric control systems exist. The *two-site/two-function (dual-site) system* has separate electrodes for paired prosthetic activity, such as flexion/extension or pronation/supination. This control system is more physiological and easier to control.

When limited control sites (muscles) in a residual limb are available to control all the desired features of the prosthesis, a *one-site/two-function (single-site) system* can be used. This device uses a single electrode to control both functions of a paired activity, such as flexion and extension. The patient uses muscle contractions of different strengths to differentiate between flexion and extension. For example, a strong contraction opens the device, and a weak contraction closes it. When multiple powered components on a single prosthesis must be controlled, sequential or multistate controllers can be used, allowing the same electrode pair to control several by a brief cocontraction of the muscle or by a switch used to cycle between control-mode functions.[27]

Switch-controlled, externally powered prostheses use small switches to operate the electric motors. These switches typically are enclosed inside the socket or incorporated into the suspension harness of the prosthesis, such as the "nudge," which is operated by the chin depressing the switch on the anterior chest strap. A switch can be activated by the movement of a remnant digit or part of a bony prominence against the switch or by a pull on a suspension harness. This can be a suitable option when myoelectric control is otherwise not feasible.[45] A *hybrid system* is one that incorporates both power options.

Level-Specific Upper Limb Amputation Prostheses

Partial hand prostheses are not commonly used. Amputation distal to the wrist is one of the most common upper limb deficiencies, but is difficult to treat successfully with a prosthesis. Poor results are attributable to functional limitations of prosthetic technology, discomfort at the prosthetic interface, unsatisfactory appearance, and absence of tactile sensation.[11] With the advancement of new technologies, the availability of new prostheses has created additional challenges for the prosthetist. Many patients with limb deficiencies distal to the wrist have declined prosthetic intervention in the past, and most limb makers have limited experience with partial hand amputations. Partial hand amputation can involve various levels of longitudinal and transverse loss that dictate different treatment options. The person with a partial hand deficiency has four prosthetic options: (1) no prosthetic intervention, (2) a passive prosthesis, (3) a body-powered prosthesis, and (4) multiple task-specific prostheses. Individuals with passive prostheses actively use their prostheses as frequently as do individuals with functional prostheses.[21] Even though passive prostheses do not offer active grasp and release, they can be used to stabilize objects, to push against items, and to perform other functional tasks. This type of prosthesis usually incorporates a secure socket that is stabilized about the residual limb by means of a total contact suction fit. Body-powered prostheses for partial hand deficiencies can be divided into two categories: cable-driven and wrist- or finger-driven devices. Adequate functional grasp from both system types is limited. Task-specific prostheses are available for both vocational and avocational activities. These prostheses are usually highly customized to effectively meet the functional needs of the individual.

Wrist disarticulation prostheses are suspended using the patient's remaining anatomy, specifically the radial and ulnar styloid processes. The benefit of a wrist disarticulation is that it preserves a longer and more powerful lever arm, as well as maximal preservation of forearm pronation and supination. When fitting someone with a wrist disarticulation prosthesis, preserving symmetric limb length becomes an issue. Wrist units are often not used with wrist disarticulation to conserve length and preserve symmetry. If not using the wrist unit, compensation is gained through maximizing preserved forearm supination and pronation through the socket. Wrist disarticulation is harder to fit with a myoelectric prosthesis because less space is available in which to conceal the electronics and power supply.

There are a number of traditional *transradial socket* options (Figure 9-7). Three traditional styles use anatomic suction suspension so that a harness is not needed. This is known as a "self-suspending" system. These three are each designed to be used with different residual limb lengths and are named the *Muenster, the Northwestern,* and the *TRAC (Transradial Anatomically Contoured)* designs. The Muenster-type socket was introduced in the 1960s for a short transradial level amputation that provided more intimate encapsulation of the residual limb. The elbow is set in a preflexed position (usually 35 degrees) and a channel is provided at the antecubital space for the biceps tendon. This allows for unobstructed flexion. The suspension is achieved through *anterior-posterior compression* around the olecranon. It is not an optimal design for bilateral amputees because it is donned with a pull sock. This led to additional innovations that included the popular Northwestern socket design. Unlike the Muenster socket, the Northwestern uses *medial-lateral compression* of the arm above the epicondyles and less restrictive anterior-posterior compression. It is used primarily in those with long residual limbs. The reduced anterior-posterior compression creates a less snug suspension and can lead to problems with electrode contact and increased forces on the distal residual bone.[36] The socket is known for its ease of donning and is a popular choice for bilateral amputees. The trim lines of the transradial socket are dependent on the length of the residual limb; the shorter the limb, the higher the trim line. For a longer limb, the trim line is lower and there is more allowance for pronation-supination. The patient's ROM will be limited by a transradial prosthesis to approximately 70% of the motion possible without a prosthesis. It might be necessary for the prosthetist to add flexion to the socket so that the end range allows for easy contact with the person's mouth and face. The *TRAC* socket incorporates design elements from both the Muenster and

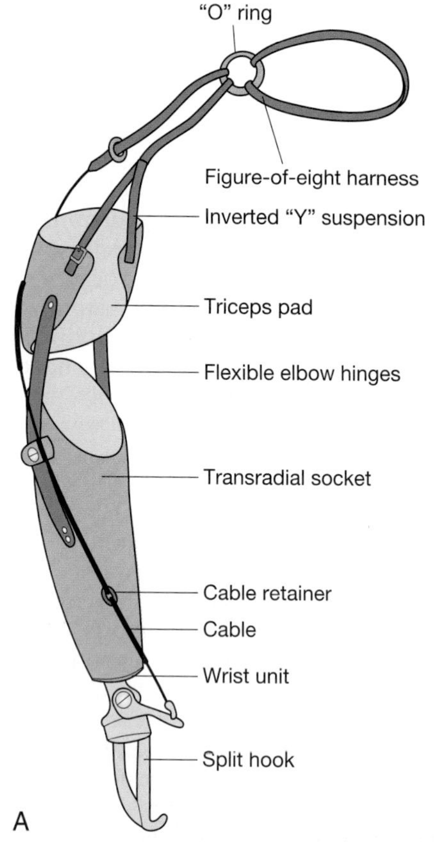

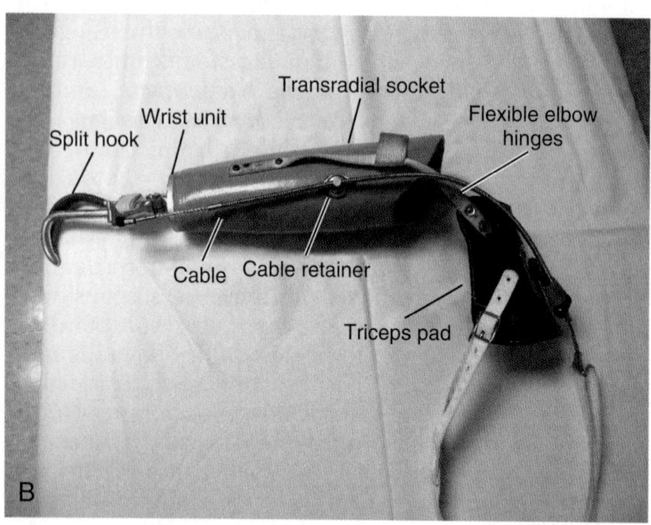

FIGURE 9-7 A, and **B,** Transradial prosthesis.

Northwestern sockets, but with more aggressive contouring of the limb to maximize load-tolerant areas of the residual limb. Similar to the Muenster, the TRAC retains the encapsulation of the olecranon posteriorly and the generous relief of the biceps anteriorly. The TRAC uses *both anterior-posterior and medial-lateral* compression for enhanced stability and comfort. The TRAC socket, through detailed anatomic contouring, transfers the load from the distal end of the radius to the more load-tolerant proximal musculature.

An *elbow disarticulation socket* or a long *transhumeral socket* includes the residual limb and excludes the acromion, the deltopectoral groove, and the lateral border of the scapula (Figure 9-8). At this level of amputation, humeral rotation is captured by the intimate fitting at and above the epicondyles, which creates a well-suspended socket. Elbow disarticulation prostheses require the use of outside locking joints located on either side of the humeral epicondyles and external to the socket. This level might add active rotary control but at the expense of additional bulk to the medial-lateral dimension of the socket. When the elbow joint is stabilized with these hinges, the result is excellent weight-bearing and force dispersion. The elbow disarticulation amputation is least desirable because of the cosmetic asymmetry produced when using the prosthesis, including problems with clothing. Few prosthetic elbows are compatible and amputees typically dislike the appearance. In the bilateral upper limb amputee in whom the transhumeral level is an option, the elbow disarticulation is *more* desirable despite the poor cosmetic appearance of the externally placed elbow. The functional advantages of disarticulation for the bilateral upper limb amputee are in the use of the residual limb for self-care. It is also preferred over the transhumeral level in children because the epiphysis is preserved and bony overgrowth is prevented.

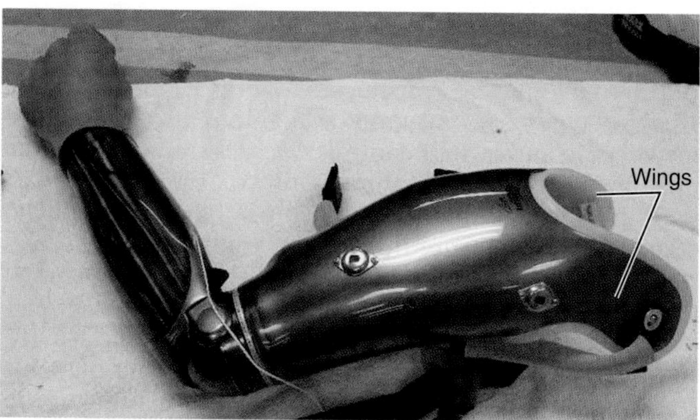

FIGURE 9-8 The transhumeral myoelectronic prosthesis.

With the elbow joint absent, the length of the transhumeral residual limb is a key factor in fitting and successful use of the prosthesis. Prosthetic control varies directly with the length of the humerus. Amputation through the *distal third of the humerus* provides functional control very similar to an elbow disarticulation. However, there is loss of humeral rotary control and epicondylar suspension, which must be provided by the socket design and harnessing. At this level of amputation, control of the prosthesis is by the humerus with additional control from scapular motion. Numerous combinations of body-powered and externally powered components have proved successful. Common examples include using an electric elbow with a body-powered terminal device. Transection of the humerus at least 4 inches above the olecranon allows enough clearance to use all elbow options, including externally powered.

A *medium length transhumeral socket* has trim lines up to the acromion and includes the deltopectoral groove and the lateral border of the scapula. The extra "wings" on this socket are used to stabilize the socket and limit rotation. A *short transhumeral socket* has trim lines that include the acromion and acromioclavicular joint. The trim lines continue medial to the deltopectoral groove and medial to the

BOX 9-10

Cycle of Movements

1. Tension is applied to the cable that flexes the elbow and operates the terminal devices, causing the elbow to flex.
2. The elbow lock cable has tension applied to it and then is released, causing the elbow to lock in this position.
3. Tension is applied to the cable that operates the elbow and terminal devices, causing the terminal device to open.
4. The elbow lock cable is pulled and then released, causing the elbow to unlock.

lateral border of the scapula. These "extended wings" are used to help stabilize the socket and to control rotation.

Amputation at the level of the *proximal third of the humerus* (proximal to the deltoid insertion) is prosthetically challenging. Control is by scapular motion with assistance from the humerus. At this level there is a reduction in strength and leverage, and cable-powered prosthetic control is severely limited. Body-powered systems require up to 5 inches of total excursion of scapular motion to open the terminal device with the elbow in the fully flexed position.[7] A transhumeral prosthesis uses *two control cables,* compared with that of the transradial system in which only *one cable* is used. One of these cables flexes the elbow and operates the terminal device, whereas the remaining cable is used to lock and unlock the elbow. For the system to be fully operated, *a cycle of movements* must take place (Box 9-10). The body motions that typically operate these two cables are shoulder flexion and the simultaneous movement of abduction and slight extension of the shoulder joint. Shoulder flexion is used to apply tension to the cable, causing flexion of the elbow and operating the terminal device. For the elbow to be locked in flexion, the simultaneous movement of abduction and extension of the shoulder joint (similar to the motion of "elbowing" someone standing behind you) is used. The *"figure-of-eight"* body harness can be worn with a transhumeral prosthesis. Often, additional straps and modifications are made to capture as much excursion as possible, especially with higher-level amputations.

The *cables are eliminated with myoelectric prostheses,* which are more comfortable, have a more natural appearance, and provide more precise hand functions with much less effort as compared with body-powered prostheses. Suction suspension is possible for the transhumeral level and allows minimal harnessing. This decreases loading in the contralateral axilla, which can reduce deleterious effects on the sound side brachial plexus and joints, enhance proprioception, and improve myoelectric contact. In some myoelectric prostheses, the harness may be totally eliminated. Suction suspension is usually not possible in transhumeral residual limbs with excessively bulbous distal ends, painfully adherent distal scarring, and those with fresh skin grafts. This is also true for bilateral amputees because they are unable to use a "pull sock."

Shoulder disarticulation (amputation at the glenohumeral joint) involves unique and challenging prosthetic problems. The prosthesis incorporates the greatest number of prosthetic components. There are two commonly used

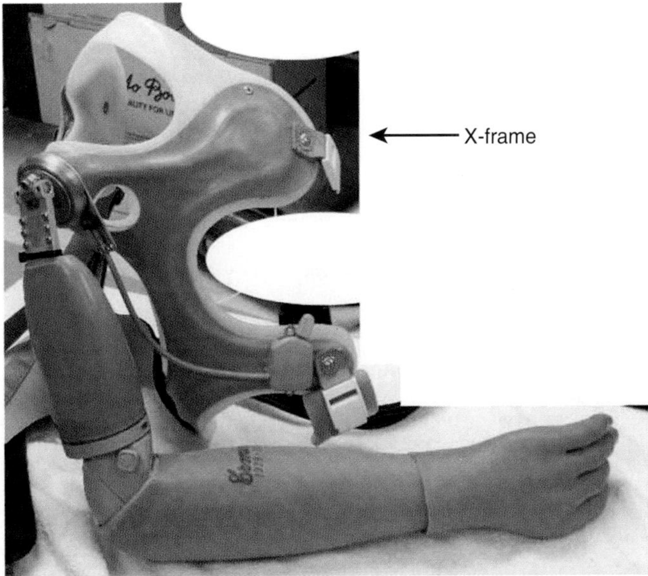

FIGURE 9-9 Shoulder disarticulation and forequarter prosthesis, body-powered elbow, and externally powered wrist and hand.

designs for a shoulder disarticulation socket. The *complete enclosure shoulder socket* encases the shoulder to approximately 5 cm beyond to the middle of the chest. The sockets are difficult to suspend and are often unstable and uncomfortable. The weight of the prosthesis and the ability to dissipate heat (which is important because of the large area of skin covered by plastic) both need to be considered carefully by the rehabilitation team. The second design, the *X-frame shoulder socket,* seeks to reduce these problems and increase the wearing comfort. The X-frame socket uses very rigid materials to maintain a shape that will lock into the wedge-shaped anatomy of the upper torso to provide a secure anchor for the prosthesis (which increases its stability and function). This shape allows the socket to be much smaller and thinner, as well as cooler and lighter, while maintaining secure suspension. With the use of newer carbon composite lamination techniques, the production of thin, lightweight, but very rigid frames is possible for shoulder prostheses. The weight of the prosthesis is usually between 5 and 8 lb.

Forequarter-level amputations present even more of a challenge to fit with a functional prosthesis. Most control options have been removed with the residual limb. The "nudge" control, which is a force-sensitive resistor operated by the chin, can operate the elbow and hand. For those who choose, a lightweight passive prosthesis anchored from the contralateral limb can be fabricated (Figure 9-9). It functions by creating a cosmetically natural appearance. If no prosthetic is used, a cosmetically sculpted insert should be offered for the shoulder symmetry needed for clothing fit.

Advantages and disadvantages of myoelectric and body-powered prostheses are summarized in Table 9-3.

Terminal Devices and Wrist Units

Multitudes of terminal devices are available for upper limb amputees, although the functionality of these terminal

Table 9-3 Advantages and Disadvantages of Myoelectric and Body-Powered Devices

Advantages	Disadvantages
Myoelectric Devices	
• Do not require a harness or cable • Looks like natural-appearing arm • Battery powered, so motor strength and coordinated mobility not as important • Newer batteries have reduced weight • Provides strong grip force	• Higher initial cost • Heavier • Dependence on battery capacity and voltage • Higher repair cost • Dependence on battery life
Body-Powered Devices	
• Lower initial cost • Lighter • Easier to repair • Offer better tension feedback to the body	• Mechanical appearance • Some people have difficulty using them • Dependent on motor strength

BOX 9-11

Types of Terminal Devices

Passive Terminal Devices

- *Functional terminal devices,* such as the child mitt frequently used on an infant's first prosthesis to facilitate crawling, or the ball-handling terminal device used by the older child and adult
- Cosmetic

Active Terminal Devices

- *Hooks,* including prehensors, which are devices that have a thumblike component and a finger component producing a claw or bird's beak type of function
- Artificial hands

devices is limited. Terminal devices generally are broken down into two categories: passive and active (Box 9-11). *Passive terminal devices* fall into two classes: those designed primarily for function and those that provide cosmesis. Examples of the functional passive terminal devices include the child mitt frequently used on an infant's first prosthesis to facilitate crawling, or the ball-handling terminal devices used by older children and adults for ball sports.

Active terminal devices can be broken down into two main categories: *hooks,* including *prehensors* (which are devices that have a thumblike component and a finger component producing a claw or bird's beak type of function), and *artificial hands.* Both device groups can be operated with a cable or by external power. No single device can reproduce the complex functional capability of the human hand. The many terminal devices that have been developed are designed to be quickly switched out to meet the different functional tasks of the amputee. Cable-operated terminal devices (hooks or hands) can be of a voluntary opening design (most commonly used) or a voluntary closing design. With a *voluntary opening mechanism* the terminal device is closed at rest. The patient uses the control-cable motion to open the terminal device against the resistive force of rubber bands (hook) or internal springs or cables (hand). Relaxation of the proximal muscles allows the terminal device to close around the desired object. The number of rubber bands determines the amount of prehensile force that is generated. One rubber band requires 5 lb of force to provide approximately 1 lb of pinch force (pinch force in a nonamputee is typically 15 to 20 lb). For a hook with three rubber bands to operate, the wearer must have at least 2 inches of excursion during shoulder flexion and 15 lb of force to pull on the cable to overcome the tension of the rubber bands. Up to 10 rubber bands can be used. Myoelectrically controlled hooks can typically generate a pinch force greater than that of body-powered controlled hooks (up to 25 lb) and allow for more precise control.

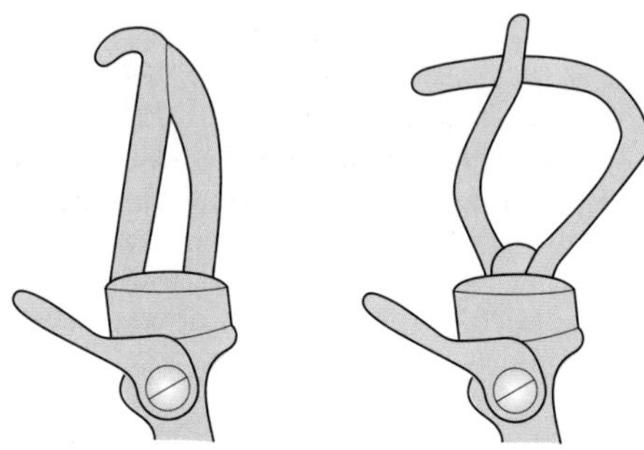

FIGURE 9-10 Hooks.

BOX 9-12

Typical Advantages of Split Hooks

- Basic grasp function
- Efficiency of use
- Ability to grasp small objects, especially when serrations or a neoprene is used for friction
- Durability
- Lower maintenance and repair costs
- Lighter weight
- Better ability of user to see what is being held
- Usually made of metal, so amputees do not have to be as careful around heat, which can melt artificial hands

With a *voluntary closing mechanism* the terminal device is open at rest. The patient uses the control-cable motion to close the terminal device, grasping the desired object. This type of mechanism generates better control of closing pressure (up to 25 lb), but active effort is needed to prevent dropping items.

Hooks have many advantages: they are simple in design, lightweight, enable efficient grasp, are durable, have low maintenance, and permit visual feedback that is unavailable with a mechanical hand (Figure 9-10 and Boxes 9-12 and 9-13). In general, hook-style terminal devices provide the equivalent of active lateral pinch grip, whereas active hands provide a *three-point chuck action.* Many different options are available for terminal devices that address occupations, hobbies, and sports.

The major function of the hand that the prosthesis tries to replicate is grip (Boxes 9-14 and 9-15). Although artificial hands are generally less functional than hooks and prehensors, people often choose them because they look more natural. A *prosthetic hand* usually is bulkier and heavier than a hook. It can be powered by a cable or use external power. With a myoelectrically controlled device, it is possible to initiate palmar fingertip grasp by contracting residual forearm flexors and to release by contracting residual extensors.[38] Many specialized terminal device designs are available or are custom fabricated for individual amputees. Most of the commercially available specialized terminal devices are designed for various vocational and recreational activities. Terminal devices are available for specific activities, such as playing musical instruments, golfing, bowling, swimming, tennis, weightlifting, fishing, skiing, shooting pool, rock climbing, baseball, hunting (bow and rifle), and photography (Figure 9-11).

Various types of electronic hands and terminal devices are available. Some of the current hands on the market have unique grasping characteristics; these include a feature used to eliminate slipping of an item being grasped. A sensor in the second digit senses an item slipping from grasp and tells the hand to grip harder.[46] Just as a real hand would squeeze a cup a little harder when it gets heavier as water is poured into it, this hand automatically monitors grip force and grabs harder when objects get heavier so that they do not fall out of the user's grasp. As a result, users do not have to be as precise with their grip force. Most electronic hands only have motors in the first three digits. This means that the fourth and fifth digit close passively as they are attached to the second and third digits. Not all electronic hands look like natural hands. Hands made for heavy-duty industrial purposes have other, hooklike shapes.

The *wrist unit* provides orientation of the terminal device in space. It can be positioned manually, by cable operation, or with external power (myoelectrically or by switch). Once positioned, the wrist unit is held in place by a friction lock or mechanical lock. Several different designs are available, including a quick-disconnect unit, a locking unit, and a flexion unit (Box 9-16). Friction-control wrist units are easy to position but can slip easily when carrying heavier loads. Wrists and elbows can also be controlled electronically. The electronic wrists can allow for full 360-degree rotation. The elbows flex and extend when sent signals from electrodes, touch pads, or pressure (force) sensors.

BOX 9-13

Advantages and Disadvantages of Prehensors

Typical Advantages

- Do not look as threatening
- Not as likely to scratch objects
- Not as likely to accidentally get caught on things

Typical Disadvantages

- Not as good for picking up and working with small items
- Does not offer as much visual feedback because they are usually bulkier at the end
- Not as good for typing

BOX 9-14

Human Hand Prehensile Patterns

- Cylindrical grasp
- Tip grasp
- Hook grasp
- Palmar grasp
- Spherical grasp
- Lateral grasp

BOX 9-15

Five Types of Grip

- *Precision grip (i.e., pincher grip):* The pad of the thumb and index finger are in opposition to pick up or pinch a small object (e.g., a small bead, pencil, grain of rice).
- *Tripod grip (i.e., palmar grip, three-jaw chuck pinch):* The pad of the thumb is against the pads of the index and middle finger.
- *Lateral grip (i.e., key pinch):* Tips of the fingers and thumb are flexed (e.g., when screwing in a light bulb or turning a doorknob).
- *Hook power grip:* The distal interphalangeal joint and proximal interphalangeal joint are flexed with the thumb extended (as when carrying a briefcase by the handle).
- *Spherical grip*: Tips of the fingers and thumb are flexed (e.g., when screwing in a light bulb or opening a doorknob).

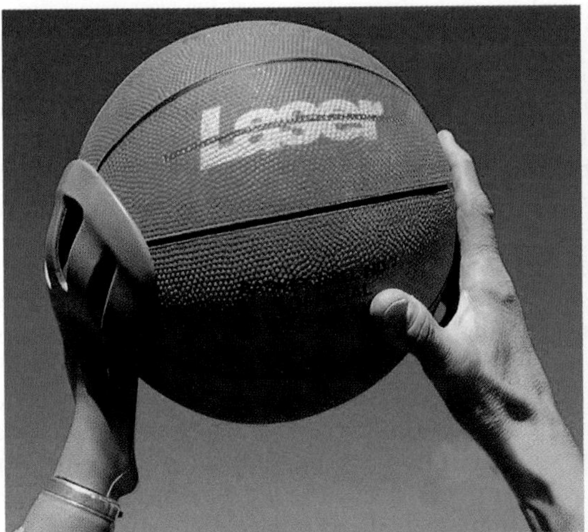
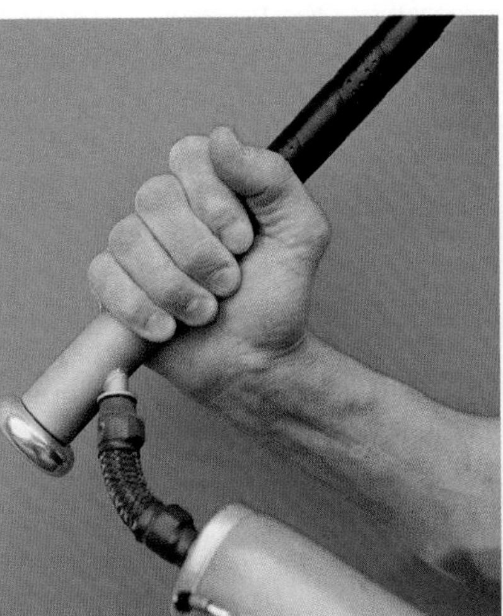
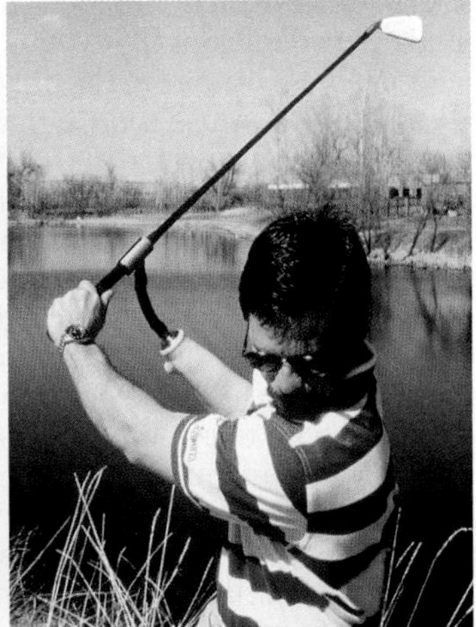

FIGURE 9-11 Terminal devices for specific activities.

BOX 9-16

Wrist Unit Designs

- *Quick-disconnect wrist unit:* This style is configured to allow easy swapping of terminal devices that have specialized functions.
- *Locking wrist unit:* Wrist units with a locking capacity prevent rotation during grasping and lifting.
- *Wrist flexion unit:* A wrist flexion unit can provide an amputee (especially a bilateral upper limb amputee) with improved function for midline activities, such as shaving, manipulating buttons, or performing perineal care. A wrist flexion unit usually is used on only one side, most often the longer of the two residual limbs, but ultimately it should be placed on the side that the amputee prefers. Multifunction wrist units are now available.

These elbows contain microprocessor computer technology that allows for fine-tuned adjustments.[59]

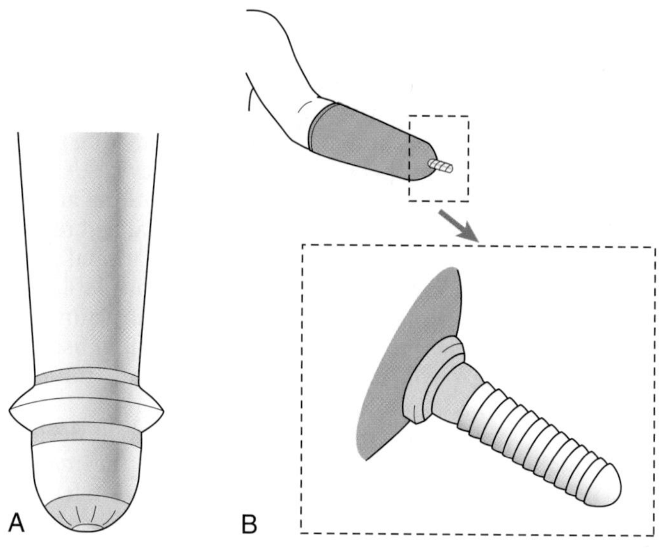

FIGURE 9-12 **A,** Seal-in liner. **B,** Pin system.

Bilateral Upper Limb Amputee

The conceptual framework used for prosthetic fitting and training of the unilateral amputee changes significantly when fitting and training *the bilateral amputee*. The unilateral upper limb amputee uses the prosthesis as an assist, and the sound limb for sensory feedback and fine manipulator activities. The bilateral amputee has no "sound limb" for the prosthetic limb to assist. All activities must be performed with the prostheses. Wear and tear on joints and cables is typically far greater than for the unilateral amputee. The ability to handle complex sensory feedback and fine manipulation is lost. The goal remains, however, to master independent basic ADLs, vocational and avocational tasks. The sockets need to be easily donned and doffed for independence to occur. Bilateral wrist flexion units are mandatory to obtain the positioning necessary to master basic hygiene. The most functional terminal device is the hook. The new amputee rarely appreciates the functional advantages of a prosthetic hook over a prosthetic hand. It must be explained that a prosthetic hook is not an attempt to duplicate the human hand, because it obviously does not look or function like a hand. The prosthetic hook represents an efficient tool that is used for several functions. A major problem unique to the bilateral upper limb amputee is the inability to use sensory feedback once the residual limb skin is covered by the socket. For this reason, the prosthesis should be constructed so it can be partially removed for sensory feedback through the residual limb and then easily reapplied. For example, the socket could have a window or be open ended to expose the distal portion of the residual limb for such maximal sensory purposes (e.g., the Krukenberg prosthesis) (Figure 9-12). With a bilateral upper limb amputee, the *Carlyle formula* is used to determine proper limb length (Box 9-17).

BOX 9-17

Carlyle Formula

- *Bilateral transradial amputee:* The formula for the distance from the apex of the lateral epicondyle to thumb tip (forearm) is the patient's body height × 0.21 (in either English or metric units).
- *Bilateral transhumeral amputee:* The formula for the distance from the acromion to the lateral epicondyle (arm) is the patient's body height × 0.19.

For wrist disarticulation and the long- and medium-length transradial amputation, a conventional socket is indicated with a sufficiently low anterior trim line to permit a full range of elbow flexion. For the more proximal transradial amputee, flexible elbow hinges that are attached to the triceps pad are required for transradial socket stabilization and to permit pronation and supination.[13] The shorter the residual limb, the greater the indication for a polycentric elbow hinge so that prosthetic and anatomic joint congruity can be approached as closely as possible. Polycentric hinges require more maintenance than single pivot hinges. The socket is aligned in such a way that it brings the terminal device closer to the center of the body. The conventional socket design is unchanged in the bilateral transhumeral amputation. The anterior and posterior wings of the socket should extend sufficiently to stabilize the prosthesis against axial rotation. The shorter the amputation level, the higher the socket trim line must extend, particularly the posterior and anterior wings. This is necessary to provide adequate control against longitudinal rotation as well as to provide suspension.[13] Elbow joints with alternating locks and a friction-controlled turntable for internal-external rotation are standard components. It is best to use externally powered prostheses for control of the elbow or terminal device. The alignment needs to be adjusted for wheelchair users. A synergistic, interconnecting harnessing system that interfaces with sockets is needed. Some amputees prefer that each arm be harnessed independently so that they have the option of wearing one prosthesis. Donning and doffing are accomplished by an over-the-head maneuver. Removal is done in a way that places the prostheses in position for redonning.

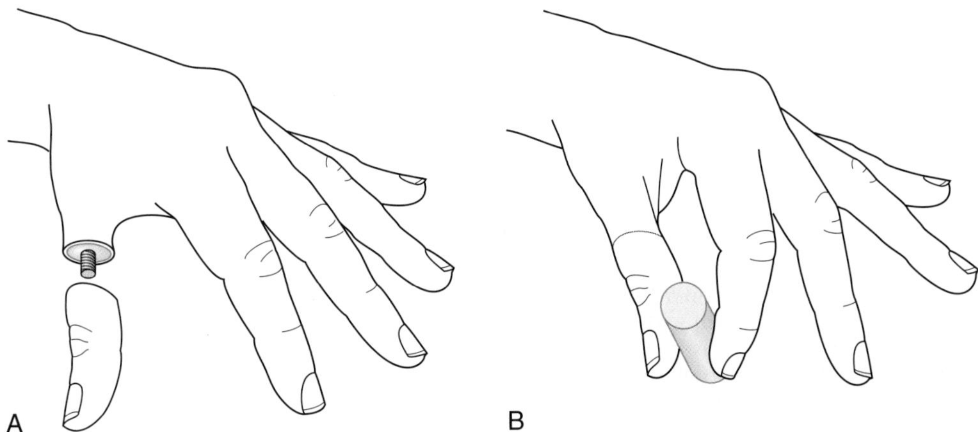

FIGURE 9-13 Osseointegration of a passive thumb prosthesis for a partial amputation showing the device (**A**) and its function when donned (**B**). (Redrawn from Jönsson S, Caine-Winterberger K, Brånemark R: Osseointegration amputation prostheses on the upper limbs: methods, prosthetics and rehabilitation, *Prosthet Orthot Int* 35:190-200, 2011.)

Advances in Prosthetic Technology

Surgical

Osseointegration is an emerging surgical technique for direct skeletal attachment of the prosthesis. It may someday render the "socket" obsolete. The technology of using metallic implants has been around for decades in the dental and maxillofacial fields, and has now progressed to the limb loss world. It entails use of a metal spike (i.e., titanium) inserted into the terminal end of the bone that is eventually connected to the prosthesis after completion of a multistage surgical procedure. The benefits of improved suspension, control, and proprioception have been highlighted. This is in addition to elimination of all problems associated with the use of liners and sockets (e.g., sweating, pain, skin irritation). The major problem has been with infection because of the limited ability to create a bacterial seal at the skin-metal interface similar to the one that naturally forms at the interface of the tooth and gum. Other problems encountered include fracture and loosening[25] (Figure 9-13).

The quest to create a biologically controlled intelligent prosthesis with capacity for sensory feedback has led to an innovative surgical option for the upper extremity amputee. The techniques reroute unused nerves (median nerve, musculocutaneous nerve, radial nerve) to functional muscles. The technique is called *targeted muscle reinnervation (TMR)* and rewires the nerves that no longer have innervation points to the pectoral muscle (Figure 9-14). Myoelectrodes create the interface with the prosthetic arm and the pectoral muscle. The new prosthetic system has built-in feedback loops that allow the user some sensory feedback. Wireless electrodes have been developed that can be implanted into muscle, and brain electrodes have been developed that can sense nerve impulses. Signal processing algorithms known as advance pattern recognition (APR) are used to decipher surface electrode data and associate it with specific desired prosthetic response. The implanted electrodes (both muscle and brain) make the prosthesis easy to wear because of elimination of weight and bulk. To date, the implantable electrodes have been successful and are awaiting clinical trials from the U.S. Food and Drug Administration.

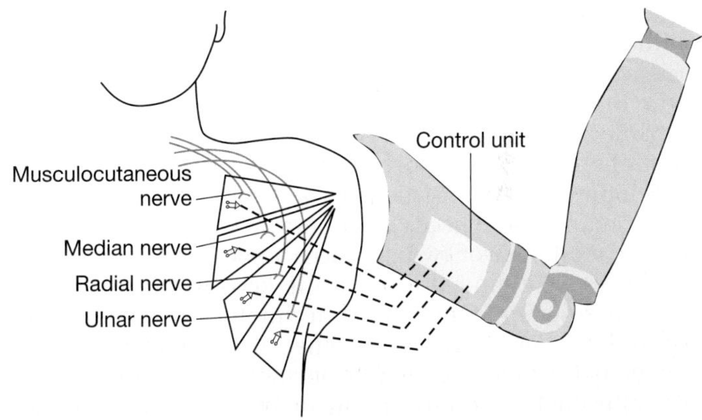

FIGURE 9-14 Targeted reinnervation.

Prosthetic Technology

Many studies show that upper limb amputees are not satisfied with available technology. Many abandon their prostheses or reject using a prosthesis altogether. Numerous factors are related to rejection and abandonment, such as proximal level of amputation, type of device, poor training, late fitting, limited usefulness of devices, and cost of repairs.[51]

Innovations in prosthetics over the past several years have succeeded in improving several critical parameters: control, attachment, functionality, and power. Advances in materials have allowed for the development of devices that are easier to don, retain their charge longer, and offer more versatility and durability (Box 9-18). This has resulted in a prosthesis that offers improved function and satisfaction from wearing it.

In 2005, the United States began funding over $70 million for the advancement of prosthetic technology through the U.S. Defense Advanced Research Projects

BOX 9-18

Advances in Materials and Their Benefits

Mechanical	Multigrasp hands with individually powered digits
Control	Targeted reinnervation with nerves increasing myoelectric sites from 2 to 6
Attachment	Osseointegration
Sensibility	Converting pressure readings from sensors in the terminal device to vibration motors at the end of the residual limb and pressure-generating pneumatically inflated pads
Training	Colocated rehabilitation team with highly specialized and trained personnel to fit and train with the high-tech components
Future	Direct peripheral nerve control via a neuroprosthetic interface or direct brainwave control implantable electrocorticography (ECoG)

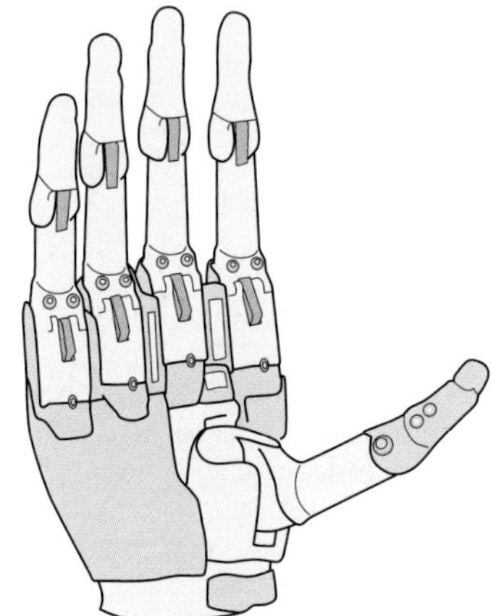

FIGURE 9-15 Bionic hand.

Agency (DARPA). The program has spanned worldwide, with engagement of multiple universities engineering and science laboratories to create the most advanced prosthetic arm that simulates the human arm. A human arm is capable of more than 25 degrees of freedom (independent motions) as well as sensory feedback. Recent work includes development of prosthetic arms with up to 27 degrees of freedom.[40] For the needs of military amputees to be met, the development of two advanced upper limb prosthetic solutions were funded through the Revolutionizing Prosthetics Program. One of the technologies uses neural control (TMR), whereas the other, developed by DEKA Integrated Solutions, uses a "strap and go" system that can be controlled by noninvasive methods (e.g., foot control). The goal of these efforts is to produce a prosthetic arm system that will not require invasive neurosurgery and be accepted by consumers.

Above the elbow amputees and shoulder disarticulation patients are a difficult challenge for prosthetic design because the loss of the elbow or shoulder adds more functional segments to the prosthesis. For these patients, one of the DARPA-funded arms, the *Luke arm,* may soon be available (DEKA Research and Development Corp., Manchester, N.H.). The Luke arm uses both vibratory stimulation and pneumatic pressure pads for sensory feedback. It offers 16 degrees of freedom and weighs less than 9 lb (4 kg) (50th percentile for a female arm). For entire limb replacement, the Johns Hopkins University Applied Physics Laboratory and the University of Pittsburgh are developing the *modular prosthetic limb* (MPL). Funded largely by DARPA as well, the MPL allows 22 degrees of freedom, with individual finger, thumb, wrist, forearm, and elbow control. Because it features brain interface control, the MPL may be useful not only for amputees but also for patients with spinal cord injuries.

A newer type of electronic hand, the "*Bionic hand,*" has motors and sensors in every digit (Figure 9-15). The hand has two unique features. First, a separate motor is in each finger, which means that each finger is independently driven and can articulate. Second, like the human thumb, the electronic thumb can rotate 90 degrees. Two electrodes sit on the skin and record myoelectric signals. They are used by the computer (which sits in the back of the hand) to do two things: interpret those signals and control the hand. This translates into the wearer being able to generate or use myoelectric signals in the arm to control the grabbing function of the hand. The digits do not move separately, although they appear to do so. When gripping, each finger senses contact with the item being gripped. The motors in the first, second, and third digits stall because of contact with the item being held, and the fourth and fifth digits continue to move until they reach a contact point. This creates the illusion of independent, "natural" movement between the digits. Because the fingers are individually powered, a great variety of pinch and grasp patterns is possible. The user may now perform a three-jaw chuck, power grip, tip pinch, key pinch, and many other patterns without the need to switch terminal devices. In addition, the first digit of this electronic hand has the capability of being manually positioned to create multiple grip patterns.[29] The most advanced prosthetic upper limbs on the market are the i-Limb Ultra hand (Touch Bionics, Hilliard, Ohio), the BeBionic V2 hand (RSL Steeper, Leeds, United Kingdom), the Contineo Multi-Grasp hand, and the Michelangelo hand (Otto Bock Healthcare GmbH, Duderstadt, Germany). This has also now allowed improved options for partial hand prosthetics. The advent of self-powered digits also makes it possible to replace as many fingers as necessary for a partial hand amputee. The myoelectric sensors and battery can be placed locally, and concealed by the socket or a bracelet worn at wrist level.

Prosthetic Training

Training for the upper limb amputee should ideally begin before the surgery and continue until advance training is completed. The training is divided into three phases: *preprosthetic training, prosthetic training,* and *advanced prosthetic training*. Each phase is focused on the end goal of maximal functional adaptation and proficiency with the prosthesis. The expectations of the amputee might not match with reality once the prosthesis is delivered and initially worn. It is important to reinforce to the unilateral amputee that the prosthesis will play a nondominant, but important

BOX 9-19

Introduction to the Prosthesis

- *Operational knowledge:* Basic vocabulary and knowledge of components, including the ability to communicate malfunctions.
- *Maintenance and care:* Includes socket inspection, maintenance, cleaning, and adjustments.
- *Residual limb care:* Includes a wearing schedule to progress to full tolerance (~8 hr/day) and learning routine daily inspection of the residual limb for irritation.
- *Controls training:* Includes learning to control the individual components for operation. The five motion elements that are primarily used in hand manipulation are reach, grasp, move, position, and release. The therapist uses many objects, such as wooded blocks, cotton swabs, and a sponge in training the individual.

functional role. It is a "helper." The sound hand will always be dominant for all activities performed. It is understood that the prosthesis is still a poor replacement for the limb that was lost. Progressive attention to the psychological adjustment and changing body image needs to stay at the forefront. Making use of the trained peer visitor is a powerful tool.

The prosthetic training phase begins with the delivery of the prosthesis. Focus is on donning and doffing and wearing the prosthesis for short periods. The goal is integration of the prosthesis into daily activity. Numerous issues arise during this period of rapid change, including maladaptive habits that occur quickly. After the introduction to the prosthesis is completed, training progresses toward mastering basic ADLs (Box 9-19). After ADLs are completed, the amputee is then moved to higher-level homemaking skills and community reentry activities, such as driving, work, and recreation. Protocols for controls training for the body-powered prosthesis and the myoelectric prosthesis have been reported by Ganz et al.[22] A list of activities and a rating guide, designed by Northwestern University, is a helpful tool for the therapist to use to guide activities and assess progress for the unilateral upper limb amputee (Table 9-4).[2] In the case of the bilateral upper limb amputee, the controls training is a more complex and coordinated motor process. The therapist needs to maintain and progress the strength and coordination gained in the preprosthetic training and facilitate the independence of the amputee with this as a daily routine. *Proprioceptive neuromuscular facilitation* enables the therapist to key into specific areas of muscle weakness. *Isotonic exercises* are effective in maintaining muscle bulk for stabilization of the arm in the socket of the prosthesis. The stability of the prosthesis depends on both the bulk of the stabilizing musculature and the amputee's ability to voluntarily vary residual limb configuration. For the transhumeral level, this would be the external rotators and the biceps that stabilize the socket; for the transradial level, it would be the supinators and pronators that stabilize the socket. There is a natural linear flow of these three rehabilitation phases. As the amputee attempts to integrate back into life, prosthetic training advances to mastering more specific and unique tasks (Box 9-20). The prosthetic training phase ends with the proficient use of the prosthesis. Ultimately, successful implementation of advanced prostheses will be largely contingent on the availability of highly specialized and trained clinical personnel to fit and train amputees, and resources to pay for these services.[51]

Table 9-4 Example of a Rating Guide

Criteria	Examples	Grade*
Personal needs	Don/doff pullover shirt Manage zippers and snaps	
Eating procedures	Cut meat Open milk carton	
Desk procedures	Use phone and take notes Sharpen pencil	
General procedures	Operate doorknob Set time on watch	
Housekeeping procedure	Hand wash dishes Dry dishes with a towel	
Use of tools	Hammer Tape measure	
Car procedures	Open and close doors, trunk, and hood Perform steps required to operate vehicles	

*Rating guide grading: 0, not possible; 1, mostly clumsy but accomplished; 2, minimal clumsiness; 3, smooth. (Grading system developed for individualized goals.)

BOX 9-20

Specific Tasks Amputees Should Master

- *Meal preparation:* Full meal process—cook, serve, and clean-up; exposure to adaptive aids.
- *Home repair and maintenance:* Handling groceries, cleaning, minor plumbing.
- *Child and pet care:* Diapering, holding, bathing, feeding.
- *Shopping*: Grocery shopping, checkout process.
- *Driver retraining:* Assessment and training with appropriate modifications made.
- *Yard work:* Shovels, rakes, mower.
- *Recreation and sports:* Know the amputee's history, train with specific terminal devices.
- *Vocational training:* Customize the treatment plan toward specific work-related tasks.

Follow-up

The need for regular lifelong follow-up by the rehabilitation team inclusive of the physiatrist cannot be overemphasized. After discharge from the therapy program, the amputee should be regularly monitored in an outpatient clinic by the rehabilitation team (Box 9-21). Follow-up should be considered the most important aspect of prosthetic rehabilitation and yet might be the most often neglected. Without this consistent communication, the many barriers to successful prosthetic use cannot be addressed, and functional use is sacrificed. Issues such as pain, depression, skin irritation, limb size change, and activity change are all more easily addressed early and

BOX 9-21

Follow-up

- Evaluate new and ongoing medical issues.
- Evaluate pain management.
- Evaluate skin integrity.
- Evaluate emotional adjustment inclusive of family.
- Evaluate prosthetic condition and fit.
- Evaluate progress with functional goals.
- Evaluate family and community reintegration.
- Evaluate recreational and sport adaption.
- Evaluate vocational options.
- Evaluate need for social services.
- Evaluate need for adaptive equipment.

BOX 9-22

Atkins[1] Prosthetic Functional Adaption Rating Scale

100% Wearing all day, using well in bilateral tasks, incorporating well in the body scheme.

75% Wearing all day, using in gross and fine motor tasks.

50% Wearing all day (primarily for cosmetic reasons), incorporating in gross activities (used as a leaning surface [e.g., desk/paper task]).

0% Not wearing or using the prosthesis. This individual is choosing to be essentially unilaterally independent.

Table 9-5 Example of Disability Rating

Disability	Rating (%)
Loss of one upper limb	50
Loss of one hand	45
Thumb amputation	23 (50% of one hand)

thoroughly by "the team" before new behavior patterns start and abandonment of the prosthesis occurs. Many aspects of upper limb prosthetic rehabilitation cannot be addressed until the patient has had reasonable time to become acclimated to the rapid life and functional changes being experienced. The physiatrist is often asked to state the patient's level of disability (Table 9-5).

The team is available to address questions and nurture the newly mastered skills. The fit, comfort, and function of the prosthesis must be maintained and optimized over time as amputees alter and refine their initial goals and aspirations. The successful long-term use of an upper limb prosthesis depends primarily on its comfort and its perceived value to the amputee. Innovative design and careful custom adaptation of socket and harness, careful attention to follow-up adjustments, and prescription revisions based on the amputee's changing needs are the essential factors for successful prosthetic rehabilitation. Atkins devised a rating scale to quantify success of prosthetic functional adaption (Box 9-22).[2]

Box 9-23 lists tips for maintenance and use of the prosthesis.

BOX 9-23

Tips for Prosthetic Maintenance and Use

- The harness should be washed when soiled because perspiration stains the straps. A household cleaner with ammonia works well.
- Do not iron the Velcro closures on straps.
- The elbow lock should be cleaned frequently.
- The cable should be examined frequently for cut or worn areas.
- The neoprene lining of the hook might need to be periodically replaced for a firmer grip. The neoprene is resistant to gasoline, oil, and other petroleum products. It should, however, be protected from hot objects.
- When a rubber band wears out from use, grease exposure, or injury, it should be cut off with scissors and replaced with a new band.
- Take the prosthesis to the prosthetist as soon as damage occurs.
- Never use the terminal device as a hammer, wedge, or lever.
- The prosthesis should be hung up by the harness rather than by the cable or cable strap.
- Detergents should be avoided because they tend to dissolve the lubricating oils in the hook and wrist unit mechanism. When an amputee washes dishes frequently, the stud threads and bearings of the hook should be cleaned and oiled regularly.
- Never reach for a moving object with the hook.
- The cosmetic glove of a mechanical or myoelectric hand is easily stained. The following substances cannot be removed unless *immediately* washed with water or alcohol: ballpoint ink, shoe polish, egg yolk, carbon paper, colored lacquers, brightly dyed fabric, fresh newsprint, tobacco tar, mustard/ketchup, and lipstick.

ACKNOWLEDGMENTS: I would like to thank Jen Aloi, for her prosthetic and orthotics expertise, and Marya Sabalbaro, for her administrative and artistic expertise.

REFERENCES

1. Atkins DJ: Adult upper limb prosthetic training. In Bowker JH, Michael JW, editors: *Atlas of limb prosthetics: surgical, prosthetic, and rehabilitation principles*, ed 2, St Louis, 1992, Mosby.
2. Atkins DJ, Meier RH, editors: *Comprehensive management of the upper limb amputee*, New York, 1989, Springer-Verlag.
3. Atroshi I, Rosberg HE: Epidemiology of amputation and severe injuries of the hand, *Hand Clin* 17:343–350, 2001.
4. Biemer E, Iribacher K, Machertanz J, et al: Reorganization of human motor cortex after hand replantation, *Ann Neurol* 50:240–249, 2001.
5. Blackskin MF, Benevenia J, Patterson FR: Complications after limb salvage surgery, *Curr Probl Diagn Radiol* 33:1–15, 2004.
6. Bosse MJ, MacKenzie EJ, Kellam JF, et al: An analysis of outcomes of reconstruction or amputation after leg threatening injuries, *N Engl J Med* 347:1924–1931, 2002.
7. Bray JJ: *Prosthetic principles: upper extremity amputations (fabrication and fitting principles)*, ed 3, Los Angeles, 1989, Prosthetics Orthotics Education Program, University of California Press.
8. Brookmeyer R, Ephraim PL, MacKenzie EJ, et al: Estimating the prevalence of limb loss in the United States 2005 to 2050, *Arch Phys Med Rehabil* 89:422–429, 2008.
9. Bunnell S: Management of the nonfunctional hand: reconstruction vs. prosthesis. In Callahan AD, Hunter JM, Mackin EJ, editors: *Rehabilitation of the hand*, ed 2, St Louis, 1984, Mosby.
10. Burkhalter WE, Hampton FL, Smeltzer JS: Wrist disarticulation and below-elbow amputation. In Bowker JH, Michael JW, editors: *Atlas of limb prosthetics: surgical and prosthetic principles*, St Louis, 1981, Mosby.

11. Caldwell RR, Sanderson ER, Wedderburn A, et al: A wrist powered prosthesis for the partial hand, *J Assoc Child Prosthet Clin* 21:42–45, 1986.
12. Cook TM, Shurr DG: Upper extremity prosthetics. In Cook TM, Shurr DG, editors: *Prosthetics and orthotics*, East Norwalk, 1990, Appleton and Lange.
13. Dickey R, Lehneis HR: Special considerations: fitting and training the bilateral upper-limb amputee. In Bowker JH, Michael JW, editors: *Atlas of limb prosthetics: surgical, prosthetic, and rehabilitation principles*, ed 2, St Louis, 1992, Mosby.
14. Dillingham TR: Rehabilitation of upper limb amputee. In Dillingham TR, Belandres PV, editors: *Textbook of military medicine. Part IV. Surgical combat casualty care: rehabilitation of the injured combatant*, vol 1, Washington, DC, 1998, Office of the Surgeon General at TMM Publications.
15. Deleted in review.
16. Dillingham TR, MacKenzie EJ, Pezzin LE: Incidence, acute care length of stay, and discharge to rehabilitation of traumatic amputee patients: an epidemiologic study, *Arch Phys Med Rehabil* 79:279–287, 1998.
17. Dillingham TR, MacKenzie EJ, Pezzin LE: Limb amputation and limb deficiency: epidemiology and recent trends in the United States, *South Med J* 95:875–883, 2002.
18. Durham RM, Mazuski JE, Mistry BM, et al: Outcome and utility of scoring systems in the management of the mangled extremity, *Am J Surg* 172:569–573, 1996.
19. Esquenazi A: Upper limb amputee rehabilitation and prosthetic restoration. In Braddom RL, editor: *Physical medicine and rehabilitation*, ed 3, Philadelphia, 2007, Saunders.
20. Fleming LL, Malone JM, Robertson J: Immediate, early and late post surgical management of upper limb amputation, *Prosthet Orthot Int* 23:55–58, 1999.
21. Fraser CM: An evaluation of the use made of cosmetic and functional prosthesis by unilateral upper limb amputees, *Prosthet Orthot Int* 22:216–223, 1998.
22. Ganz O, Gulick K, Smurr LM, et al: Managing the upper extremity amputee: a protocol for success, *J Hand Ther* 21:160–176, 2008.
23. Garrison SJ, Subbar JV: Heterotopic ossification: diagnosis and management, current concepts and controversies, *J Spinal Cord Med* 22:273–283, 1990.
24. Gould RJ, Gregory RT, Peclet M, et al: The mangled extremity syndrome (M.E.S.): a severity grading system for multisystem injury of the extremity, *J Trauma* 25:1147, 1985.
25. Hagberg K, Häggström E, Uden M, Brånemark R: Socket versus bone-anchored trans-femoral prostheses: hip range of motion and sitting comfort, *Prosthet Orthot Int* 29:153–163, 2005.
26. Hartzell TL, Benhaim P, Imbriglia JE, et al: Surgical and technical aspects of hand transplantation: is it just another replant? *Hand Clin* 27:521–530, 2011.
27. Heckathorne CW: Components for electric-powered systems. In Bowker JH, Michael JW, Smith DG, editors: *Atlas of amputation and limb deficiencies*, ed 3, Rosemont, 2004, American Academy Orthopedic Surgeons.
28. Deleted in review.
29. I-Limb brochure: Available at: www.touchbionics.com/i-LIMB.
30. International Registry on Hand and Composite Tissue Transplantation: Available at: www.handregistry.com/page.asp?page.4. Accessed May 5, 2014.
31. Jablecki J, Kaczmarzyk L, Patrzalek D, et al: A detailed comparison of the functional outcome after midforearm replantations versus midforearm transplantation, *Transplant Proc* 41:513–516, 2009.
32. Jaeger SH, Kleinert HE, Tsai T: Upper extremity replantation in children, *Orthop Clin North Am* 12:897, 1981.
33. Jones JW, Gruber SA, Barker JH, et al: Successful hand transplantation. One-year follow-up. Louisville Hand Transplant Team, *N Engl J Med* 343:468–473, 2000.
34. Kozak L, Owings M: Ambulatory and inpatient procedures in the United States, 1996. National Center for Health Statistics, *Vital Health Stat* 13:1–119, 1998.
35. Lake C: The evolution of upper limb prosthetic socket design, *J Prosthet Orthot* 20:83–92, 2008.
36. Lake C, Miguelez JM: The transradial anatomically contoured (TRAC) interface: design principles methodology, *J Prosthet Orthot* 15:148–157, 2003.
37. Deleted in review.
38. Lawrence M, Gross G-P, Lang M, et al: Assessment of finger forces and wrist torques for functional grasp using new multichannel textile neuroprostheses, *Artif Organs* 32:634–638, 2008.
39. Wilhelmi BJ, Lee WP, Pagenstert GI, May JW, Jr: Replantation in the mutilated hand, *Hand Clin* 19:89, 2003.
40. Ling G: DARPA [online], Available at: www.darpa.mil/Our_Work/DSO/Programs/Revolutionizing_Prosthetics.aspx.
41. Louis D: Amputations. In Green DL, editor: *Operative hand surgery*, ed 2, New York, 1988, Churchill Livingstone.
42. Ly TV, Travison TG, Castillo R, et al: The ability of lower-extremity severity scores to predict functional outcome after limb salvage, *J Bone Joint Surg Am* 90:1738–1743, 2008.
43. McAuliffe JA: Elbow disarticulation and transhumeral amputation/shoulder disarticulation and forequarter amputations. In Bowker JH, Michael JW, editors: *Atlas of limb prosthetics: surgical, prosthetic, and rehabilitation principles*, ed 2, St Louis, 1992, Mosby.
44. Mohamed AE: Arterial reconstruction after mangled extremity: injury severity scoring systems are not predictive of limb salvage, *Vascular* 13:114–119, 2005.
45. Muzumdar A: *Powered upper limb prosthesis*, New York, 2004, Springer.
46. Myoelectric upper extremity prosthesis. Otto Bock Healthcare GmbH, 2009. Available at: www.ottobockus.com/cps/rde/xchg/ob_us_en/hs.xsl/6874.html.
47. National Estimates from Healthcare Utilization Project (HCUP), Nationwide Inpatient Sample (NIS), Agency for Healthcare Research and Quality (AHRQ), based on data collected by individual states and provided to AHRQ by the states, Available at: http://www.bing.com/search?q=National+Estimates+from+Healthcare+Utilization+Project+(HCUP),Nationwide+Inpatient+Sample+(NIS),+Agency+for+Healthcare+Researchand+Quality+(AHRQ),+based+on+data+collected+by+individual+statesand+provided+to+AHRQ+by+the+states&src=ie9tr. Accessed June 7, 2014.
48. Ninkovic M, Weissenbacher A, Gabl M, et al: Functional outcome after hand and forearm transplantation: what can be achieved? *Hand Clin* 27(4):455–465, 2011.
49. Owen ER, Dubernard JM, Lanzetta M, et al: Peripheral nerve regeneration in human hand transplantation, *Transplant Proc* 33:1720–1721, 2001.
50. Ramachandran VS, Rogers-Ramachandran D: Synaesthesia in phantom limbs induced with mirrors, *Proc Biol Sci* 263:377–386, 1996.
51. Resnik L, Meucci MR, Lieberman-Klinger S, et al: Advanced upper limb prosthetic devices: implications for upper limb prosthetic rehabilitation supplier, *Arch Phys Med Rehabil* 93:710–717, 2012.
52. Schneeberger S, Zelger B, Ninkovic M, et al: Transplantation of the hand, *Transplant Rev* 19:100–107, 2005.
53. Schuind F, Abramowicz D, Schneeberger S, et al: Hand transplantation: the state-of-the-art, *J Hand Surg Eur* 32:2–17, 2007.
54. Deleted in review.
55. Serletti M, Carras AJ, O'Keefe RJ, et al: Functional outcome for soft tissue reconstruction for limb salvage after sarcoma surgery, *Plast Reconstr Surg* 102(5):1576–1583, 1998.
56. Smith D: Limb loss in children congenital limb deficiencies and acquired amputations. In Motion, Available at: www.amputee-coalition.org/immotion/may./congenital.part3.html.
57. Taylor CL: The biomechanics of control in upper-extremity prosthesis, *Artif Limbs* 2:4–25, 1955.
58. Togawa S, Yamami N, Nakayama H, et al: The validity of the mangled extremity severity score in the assessment of upper limb injuries, *J Bone Joint Surg* 87:1516–1519, 2005.
59. Utah Arm 3. Motion Control, Inc., 2009. Available at: www.utaharm.com/ua3.php. Accessed January 9, 2009.
60. Van Hoesel R, Veth R, Bökkerink JP, et al: Limb salvage in musculoskeletal oncology, *Lancet Oncol* 4:343–350, 2003.
61. Vanadurongwan V, Waikakul S, Sakkarnkosol S, et al: Prognostic factors for major limb re-implantation at both immediate and long term follow-up, *J Bone Joint Surg Br* 80:1024–1030, 1998.
62. Walter Reed Amputee Care Program Database. Military Amputee Care Program, Washington, DC. Available at: http://www.wrnmmc.capmed.mil/Health%20Services/Surgery/Orthopaedics%20and%20Rehabilitation/Amputee%20Care/SitePages/Home.aspx. Accessed June 8, 2014. Updated January 18, 2007.

CHAPTER 10

LOWER LIMB AMPUTATION AND GAIT

William Lovegreen, Douglas P. Murphy, William K. Smith, Phillip Stevens, Joseph Webster

This chapter provides a comprehensive overview of the rehabilitation management for the person with a lower limb amputation. The goal of this chapter is to highlight the principles and concepts that can be applied to the clinical setting across the continuum of care. The chapter also covers epidemiology, amputation terminology, functional classification, and implications of surgical techniques. Management considerations in the areas of medical care and prosthetic restoration are included, with an emphasis on understanding how to ideally match the characteristics of a prosthetic device to the functional needs of each individual with amputation. The chapter additionally includes information on both normal gait and the evaluation and management of prosthetic gait deviations. The chapter concludes with a look into the future of this field.

Advances in medical care, therapy approaches, and prosthetic technology have provided the opportunity for persons with lower limb amputations to achieve enhanced functional abilities and quality of life. To obtain these outcomes, rehabilitation professionals practicing in this field must possess a broad spectrum of knowledge and skills ranging from wound management to observational gait analysis. Progressive developments in the sophistication of prosthetic technology and rehabilitation interventions require providers to maintain a highly specialized understanding of these advances to apply this technology in the clinical setting. The highly technical and specialized nature of amputation care necessitates an interdisciplinary team approach. This team approach can be both a fulfilling style of practice for the rehabilitation professional and the key to optimal patient outcomes.

Lower limb amputation rehabilitation practice includes a broad spectrum of patients, from children with congenital limb deficiencies to elderly individuals with multiple medical conditions and amputations resulting from vascular disease. The challenges with this broad spectrum of patients are two-fold. First, prosthetic restoration and the rehabilitation approach must be individualized for each unique presentation. Second, the different comorbidities associated with the cause of the amputation require incorporating the consideration of these medical conditions and psychosocial issues into the unique treatment plan. For example, children with congenital limb deficiencies may have associated genetic abnormalities. Young adults with traumatic amputations may have associated traumatic brain injury and the elderly with vascular-related amputations may have comorbid cardiovascular and kidney disease.

Epidemiology

Despite advances in surgical interventions and an emphasis on prevention programs, studies have shown a continued increase in the prevalence of people living with limb loss. There were nearly 2 million people living with limb loss in the United States in 2005.[72] One study found that the incidence of dysvascular amputations increased by 27% between 1988 and 1996, although the incidence of civilian traumatic amputations decreased and congenital and cancer-related amputations remained stable.[14] The prevalence of individuals living with limb loss is anticipated to continue to increase in the future as a result of a number of factors, including the aging of the overall population with increased life expectancy and an increase in the incidence of diabetes mellitus (DM). Studies predict a doubling of the elderly dysvascular amputation population by 2030, and that the overall amputation population prevalence will double by 2050.[19,72]

Approximately 185,000 new amputations are performed in U.S. civilian hospitals each year, and in 2009, hospital costs associated with amputation totaled more than $8.3 billion.[26] A large number of amputations are also performed each year in the U.S. Department of Veterans Affairs (VA) medical facilities, with an average of 7669 new amputation procedures performed annually between 2008 and 2013. The total population of veterans with amputations being treated in VA medical centers annually has increased from approximately 25,000 in 2000 to more than 80,000 in 2013.[63] In addition, an increase in amputations of traumatic etiology has been seen in the U.S. Department of Defense (DOD) and VA health care systems as a result of military conflicts in Afghanistan and Iraq. Between 2001 and January 2014, these military conflicts resulted in 1638 U.S. service members who had sustained combat-related amputations, excluding those with amputations of the fingers and toes.[57]

The majority of people with lower limb amputations have acquired their amputations as a result of disease processes, such as DM or peripheral vascular disease. Amputations secondary to vascular conditions and DM have been reported to account for 82% of limb loss related hospital discharges and 97% of vascular-related amputations involve the lower limb.[14] Trauma-related amputations account for approximately 16% of amputations and those resulting from malignancy and congenital deformity are responsible for approximately 1% of amputations each.[14] DM increases the risk of amputation to a greater degree

Table 10-1 Lower Extremity Acquired Amputation Classification Terminology and Description

International Organization for Standardization Terminology	Common Terminology	Description	Major Amputation
Hemipelvectomy	Hemipelvectomy	Removal of the entire lower limb and partial removal of pelvis	Yes
Hip disarticulation	Hip disarticulation	Amputation of the entire lower limb including proximal femur	Yes
Transfemoral	Above knee	Amputation through the shaft of the femur	Yes
Knee disarticulation	Through knee	Amputation through the knee joint with retention of the distal femur	Yes
Transtibial	Below knee	Amputation through the shaft of the tibia	Yes
Ankle disarticulation	Syme	Amputation through the ankle joint	Yes
Partial foot	Chopart, Lisfranc, transmetatarsal, ray	Amputation through the structures of the foot (transverse or longitudinal)	No
Digit(s)	Toe(s)	Removal of one or more toes	No

than either smoking or hypertension. DM is reported to contribute to 67% of all amputations.[50] The age-adjusted amputation rate for persons with DM has been found to be 18 to 28 times greater than that of people without DM.[62] Among people with a lower extremity amputation, smoking cigarettes has been associated with a reamputation risk 25 times that of nonsmokers.[34]

Amputations caused by disease processes generally occur in the aging individual and are associated with numerous comorbidities, such as cardiovascular disease, hypertension, end-stage renal disease, and arthritis. People with amputations caused by trauma, including military-related injuries, are predominantly younger in age and typically require a longer continuum of care following their amputations. These individuals may have more specialized prosthetic and rehabilitation needs secondary to the increased likelihood of returning to work or high-level sports and recreational activities. Individuals with military-related traumatic amputations also require management of commonly associated injuries, such as traumatic brain injury, hearing loss, visual impairment, and posttraumatic stress disorder (PTSD).

The most frequent level of amputation in the lower extremity varies according to the etiology. Toe amputations are the most common level overall when counting both major and minor amputations.[14] With advances in limb salvage techniques, the number of partial foot amputation procedures has shown a significant increase over the past 10 to 15 years.[60] The transtibial level is the most common major amputation level in the lower extremity, with transfemoral being the second most common.

Survival rates after amputation are quite variable depending on the cause of the amputation. The 30-day mortality following a vascular-related amputation ranges from 9% to 21%. More long-term survival has been reported to be 48% to 69% at 1 year, 42% at 3 years, and 35% to 45% at 5 years.[2,49] DM and end-stage renal disease have been shown to negatively affect survival, with 5-year survival rates as low as 31% and 14%, respectively.[2] Individuals with traumatic amputations have been noted to have significant cardiovascular and metabolic issues, which appear to be related to their traumatic amputation and not accounted for by obesity, sedentary lifestyle, or tobacco use. Despite these findings, individuals requiring an amputation secondary to a traumatic injury tend to have relatively normal long-term survival rates.

Amputation Terminology

The International Organization for Standardization (ISO) terminology for the description of both acquired amputations and congenital limb deficiencies has been widely accepted by clinicians, researchers, and professional organizations.[55] Table 10-1 provides a comparison of the ISO terminology and the more traditional, common terminology, and a description of each level of acquired lower limb amputation. Although the common terminology is still used, use of the ISO terminology is recommended to improve the accuracy and consistency of amputation level description. The major and minor classification of amputation levels is also included in Table 10-1. Major amputations have traditionally included amputations that occur at the ankle disarticulation level and more proximal. Although still frequently used, the major and minor amputation terminology can be misleading because amputation levels classified as minor (partial foot and digit amputations) can still have significant functional and quality of life implications for the individual with the amputation.

Rehabilitation Implications of Amputation Level and Surgical Technique

Both the level of amputation and the specific techniques used during surgery can have a profound impact on long-term functional outcomes following lower limb amputation. This impact can be expressed in terms of successful prosthetic mobility, prosthetic socket comfort, and a reduction of skin breakdown complications. Although the primary goal of amputation surgery is removal of the diseased, damaged, or dysfunctional portion of the limb, the surgery must also result in a residual limb that is optimized for motion, motion control, and proprioceptive feedback to achieve the most successful outcomes. Amputation surgery should not be considered to be a procedure of last resort or a failure of care. Instead, amputation surgery should be viewed as a reconstructive procedure that has the potential to improve a person's functional independence, mobility, and quality of life. Although advances in surgical techniques have made limb salvage a more viable option in certain circumstances, delaying definitive amputation with attempts at limb salvage that have a low likelihood of success can create negative consequences.

Several principles should be considered in relation to the impact of amputation surgery level on rehabilitation outcomes. It is generally recommended to preserve as much limb length as possible at the time of amputation surgery. Although this principle holds true in many situations, there are instances in which preserving additional length has no functional benefit and may actually result in a less optimal outcome. For example, performing a transtibial amputation in the distal third of the tibia is typically not recommended because this may limit the use of high-profile prosthetic feet, the lack of soft tissue coverage in the distal third of the tibia can lead to decreased comfort and an increased risk of skin breakdown when wearing a prosthesis. Partial foot amputations provide the potential for short distance ambulation without a device, but these amputation levels are difficult to fit with an adequate prosthesis and also have a high rate of equinovarus deformity secondary to muscular imbalance.

Disarticulation level amputations may provide sparing of additional limb length and can provide the advantage of continued bone growth in those who are skeletally immature at the time of amputation. Knee disarticulation level amputations also provide the potential advantages of distal weight-bearing, self-suspension, and a longer lever arm for greater prosthetic limb control. Amputations at the ankle disarticulation level afford the potential to ambulate short distances without a prosthesis. Disarticulation level amputations may also be favored at times in individuals with spinal cord injury to maintain muscle balance and reduce the risk of contracture formation. However, despite these apparent advantages, disarticulation level amputations are often not recommended because they can result in poorer cosmetic outcomes and may limit the availability of prosthetic component options.

Although the ultimate level of amputation is often dictated by the amount of blood flow and tissue viability in cases of vascular disease or by the extent of soft tissue and bone damage in cases of trauma, it is ideal for rehabilitation providers to provide input regarding the amputation level before the time of surgery when circumstances allow. Prediction of healing requires careful evaluation of multiple variables, including nutritional status and tissue perfusion. As noted, in persons with vascular disease, it is desirable to preserve length; however, performing the amputation at a more proximal level, where the likelihood of timely and successful healing is greater, may be a better option to facilitate rehabilitation and avoid multiple surgical interventions. In cases where there is a need for amputation secondary to cancer, preserving length always has to take lower priority to preserving the person's life. In cases of extremity trauma, advanced surgical techniques with bone growth stimulation and tissue expanders have resulted in greater opportunities for both limb salvage and limb length sparing. The long-term outcomes of limb salvage compared with amputation after extremity trauma remain mixed,[7] although recent studies of U.S. military personnel have shown improved overall functional outcomes, with the Short Musculoskeletal Function Assessment (SMFA) questionnaire, in those with amputations compared with those with limb salvage.[15]

The surgical technique used at the time of amputation can also have a lasting impact on successful prosthetic limb use. Amputation surgery techniques should provide an adequate amount of soft tissue padding for a comfortable interface with the prosthetic socket while avoiding excessive, redundant soft tissues that can make donning the prosthesis difficult and allow excessive motion between the residual limb and the prosthetic socket during ambulation. Preserving skeletal length without adequate soft tissue coverage can lead to recurrent skin breakdown, soft tissue infections, osteomyelitis, and the need for revision surgery. Surgical techniques should also strive to avoid the development of adherent scar tissue over distal bone, which can lead to both pain and recurrent skin breakdown. Surgical technique can also have implications on the development of painful neuromas and heterotopic ossification (HO) in the residual limb.[56]

Surgical management of the remaining muscular structures is also important. Myofascial closure involves closure of the muscle fascial envelope without attachment to the bone. This may provide adequate cushioning over the distal bone, but it provides limited stabilization of the muscle structure and may result in limited muscle power generation. Myoplasty techniques involve suturing of the muscle fibers and fascia. This may enhance muscle stability but can also result in a mobile sling of muscle that creates excess movement and the potential formation of painful bursa. With myodesis techniques, the muscle and fascia are directly sutured to the periosteum of the bone. This provides greater stabilization of the muscles and can enhance the contractile effectiveness and efficiency of the muscle. Adductor myodesis procedures to achieve muscle balance are especially important after transfemoral amputation to avoid excessive femoral abduction both in standing and during ambulation.[56]

Residual Limb and Skin Care

Skin care represents an area of paramount importance that requires a consistent effort on the part of caretakers and the amputee. The latter should form strong, early habits for at least daily inspection of skin of the residual limb and the resolution of skin problems as soon as they develop. No condition should be considered too trivial to treat because a skin disorder, if neglected, has the potential to progress and cause much greater problems, such as sepsis and further surgical revision amputations. Through the use of a prosthesis, the residual limb skin of the amputee is subjected to numerous physical stressors. Friction, excessive pressures, humidity, sweating, and stretching are some of the mechanical ones that can create problems. The suction socket can create both positive and negative pressures, as can some other suspension systems.

General residual limb care recommendations include cleaning the residual limb daily, preferably in the evening, with soap and water. The limb should be pat dry. When the patient is not wearing the prosthesis, a shrinker or an ACE wrap should be applied to minimize or decrease swelling. After prosthetic limb wear, the residual limb should be examined for irritation, breakdown, blistering, or red areas. If any of these exist and a reddened area does not resolve within 20 minutes, the prosthesis should not be worn and a clinical professional should be consulted within 2 days. As the prosthesis is worn throughout the day, socks should be added to assure an appropriate fit is maintained. The amputee should make sure that the anatomic points of the residual limb line up appropriately with relevant points on the prosthesis (e.g., fibular head with the recess for this in the socket and patellar tendon with the patellar tendon bar). Transtibial amputees should keep the knee in full extension when not wearing the prosthesis and transfemoral amputees should not put a pillow under the residual limb or between the legs when in bed to prevent the formation of joint contractures. The skin should be examined once or twice a day, including the use of a mirror, if there are areas, such as the distal end, that are not easily viewed.[41]

This type of close monitoring and care should also be applied to the contralateral extremity and foot. Daily cleansing, drying, and close inspection should occur, particularly for areas difficult to assess, such as between the toes, plantar surfaces of the foot, and the heel. Frequent assessment should also include sensation, pulses, edema, temperature, and examination for any evidence of any trophic or motor changes. Contralateral amputations are common; thus, aggressive preventive measures are warranted. Podiatric care of corns, calluses, and nails is also helpful in the prevention of complications.

In one study of lower extremity prosthetic users,[16] five skin conditions comprised 79.5% of the skin problems in 337 lower extremities with a total of 528 skin lesions. These conditions included irritations, ulcers, inclusion cysts, verrucous hyperplasia, and calluses. In addition to these conditions, other reports [40] indicate the following frequently occurring conditions: allergic contact dermatitis, acroangiodermatitis, epidermal hyperplasia, follicular hyperkeratosis, bullous disease, infections, and malignancies. Allergic contact dermatitis, an erythematous, weeping, and pruritic rash, can represent up to one third of the dermatoses seen in prosthetic wearers,[40] often caused by the prosthetic materials. Patch testing should occur with the first round of testing, including standard allergens, components of the prosthesis, topical medications being used, and locally applied cosmetics and moisturizers. If the first panel is negative, then further testing can extend to adhesives and additional cosmetics. Treatment consists of elimination of the specific allergen and the use of topical and/or oral steroids.

When there is inadequate socket pressure on the distal end of the residual limb, verrucous hyperplasia can develop. This condition has a characteristic appearance consistent with its name "verrucous" or warty. Vascular injury or chronic bacterial infection can also play a role in its development. Shrinker socks and modification of the socket to apply appropriate pressures to the distal end help to resolve this problem. Topical antibacterial agents can be used for bacterial overgrowth.

Other residual limb problems can result from either inadequate socket fit or prosthetic alignment. For the transtibial amputee, bursae can develop. Bursitis from two types of bursae, synovial and adventitious, can develop, with the latter being more common. Synovial bursae develop during intrauterine life, whereas adventitious ones develop after birth. Synovial bursae are fluid-filled sacks that facilitate the movement between muscle and bone, ligaments, and/or tendons, whereas adventitious bursae develop from excessive shearing forces of the skin, particularly over bony surfaces. These shearing forces cause a breakdown of fibrous connective tissue with mucoid and myxomatous degeneration. There is no true synovial, endothelial lining.[20] Bursitis results from either acute or chronic inflammation. On examination, the bursa is a fluctuant, painful swelling, generally over areas such as the fibular head, tibial tubercle, patella, or end of the residual limb.[26] If needed, diagnosis can be confirmed through ultrasound or magnetic resonance imaging. The first line of treatment is usually a modification of the prosthesis. If there is suspicion of an infection, the bursa should be aspirated and the aspirant sent for analysis and culture.

Epidermoid inclusion cysts occur when elements from the epidermis are implanted in the dermis. The cells within the cyst produce keratin and the cyst can drain intermittently. These can be asymptomatic. If they do become symptomatic, they can present as small painful masses, which may also become infected. Treatment consists of excision, incision and drainage, and the use of antibiotics. When asymptomatic and unproblematic, these can be left alone.

Another common problem is hyperhidrosis, or excessive sweating, of the residual limb with use of the prosthesis. This situation can hinder the use of the prosthesis. Approximately 30% to 50% of amputees are affected.[63] This condition has the potential to adversely affect the course of phantom limb pain (PLP) and residual limb pain (RLP). In small, uncontrolled trials, a single set of injections of botulinum toxin type B (1750 units) has been shown to reduce RLP, PLP, and sweating, and improve duration of prosthetic use and overall quality of life for up to 3 months.[31]

HO results from the transformation of pluripotent, mesenchymal cells into osteoblasts that then create abnormal bone formation outside of the normal bone structure. The reasons for this transformation are not currently known. HO can occur weeks to months following amputation. The prevalence in service members with combat-related amputations is estimated to range from 36% to 63%.[47] HO can be asymptomatic or cause symptoms that range in severity from mild to severe. It can also pose significant prosthetic fitting problems resulting in skin breakdown and RLP. In rare circumstances, however, HO can be beneficial and even facilitate fitting.[37] In addition, HO can cause joint range-of-motion limitations and vascular or neurologic compromise that can create problems with mobility and ambulation. The diagnosis of HO occurs through assessment of characteristic symptoms, physical examination, and imaging. Characteristic complaints and examination findings include a change in pain, decreasing joint range of motion (ROM), residual limb swelling or warmth, and a change in socket fit. Imaging options include plain radiographs, computed tomography, magnetic resonance imaging, radionucleotide studies (triple phase bone scan), and ultrasound. Serum alkaline phosphatase levels can be monitored from the active phase into quiescence, but have limited specificity. Measures used to prevent formation or progression of HO include nonsteroidal antiinflammatory medications, bisphosphonates, and radiation therapy.[44] Once the HO has matured, treatment options range from observation to surgical excision. Often, modifications are required to the socket to accommodate this bone growth.

Pain Management

Postamputation pain can range widely in both severity and persistence. The two fundamental types of pain are RLP and PLP. RLP involves pain that is restricted to the anatomic region of the residual limb. PLP involves pain that is perceived in the portion of the limb that is no longer present. This latter type of pain has an estimated prevalence of up to 85%, even years after amputation.[28] Pain from the residual limb can also appear to radiate into the part of the limb that is no longer present. If there is no pain associated with amputated part of the limb, but there still are feelings and sensations in the portion of the limb that is no longer present, then this is called phantom limb sensation (PLS). PLS is nearly universal in the early recovery period postamputation. RLP can further be classified into either neuropathic or somatic origins. Neuropathic origins include neuromas and complex regional pain syndrome (CRPS). On dissection, neuromas demonstrate growths of Schwann cells amidst proliferating axons all encased within scar tissue. The free ends of the axons exist without Schwann cells and the anoxic environment of the scar tissue can create conditions in which the free nerve endings may fire repetitively.[9] Virtually all amputees have neuromas at the site of the amputation, yet only 10% to 15% have pain from these neuromas. Diagnosis is confirmed by the presence of appropriate signs and symptoms. The pain from a neuroma is generally aching, cramping, or shooting with an intermittent, episodic nature. Provocation with pressure at the site of the neuroma helps to confirm the source. Treatment options consist of physical modalities, such as acupuncture, socket modifications, ultrasound, massage, vibration, and percussion.[68] Nonsteroidal antiinflammatory medications, tricyclic antidepressants, and anticonvulsant medications are used with variable effectiveness. Injection with lidocaine, steroid, or phenol can be helpful. Radiofrequency ablation has also been used to treat this condition. Surgical excision can also be performed but runs the risk of creating a new, painful neuroma.

In addition to the development of neuromas, entrapment of nerves within scar tissue at the surgical incision site can occur, with resulting pain. Shear, pressure, and traction forces from the prosthesis can either evoke or worsen this pain. The socket can be modified to decrease pressures in this area or redistribute it. If this is ineffective, then injections into the scar or the use of oral medications are used. Surgical excision of this area is generally not effective.

Somatic pain in the residual limb can originate from a variety of sources, including HO, infection, tumor, ischemia, or arthritic joint changes. Infection may be superficial or occur in deeper tissues with development of osteomyelitis. Poor surgical technique that leaves bone improperly trimmed or muscle and fascia inadequately sutured can result in mechanical residual limb pain that can be exacerbated by wearing the prosthesis. Treatment can include socket or prosthetic modifications or surgical revision of the residual limb. Bony overgrowth can occur in children and more rarely in adults. Growth in the distal end can result in an irregular area of bone that projects into soft tissues, with the potential for causing pain and skin breakdown with prosthetic use. Socket modifications are attempted as a first-line effort to manage this situation, and surgical revision can be done if these efforts fail.

PLP can be perceived in any part of the missing amputated limb. The quality of pain can be variable and described as dull, squeezing, cramping, electrical-like, shooting, or sharp. It commonly manifests in an episodic manner with a severity that ranges from mild to severe and incapacitating. PLP tends to occur within the first few months after amputation and can persist indefinitely. The reported prevalence ranges up to 85% in the first years after surgery.[9] Supraspinal, spinal, and peripheral mechanisms are thought to play a role in the origin of phantom sensations and PLP. Some findings[28] point to a reorganization of the somatosensory cortex around the area representing the amputated part. Treatments can be directed at modulating the activities at any of these levels. Many treatment options have been tried to control PLP (Box 10-1), even though there are few controlled studies to provide guidance in this area. Categories of pharmaceutical interventions include: *N*-methyl-D-aspartate (NMDA) receptor antagonists, opioids, anticonvulsants, antidepressants, local anesthetics, and calcitonin. The NMDA receptor antagonists, such as ketamine, memantine, and dextromethorphan, are thought to exert to their effects at the dorsal horn. Opioids operate at both the spinal and supraspinal levels. Calcitonin exerts its effects centrally. The effectiveness of both calcitonin and anticonvulsants has varied in studies.[28]

Psychological treatments, such as guided imagery, biofeedback, and hypnosis, have aimed at altering negative emotions, increasing adaptation to pain, and adjusting body image. Mirror therapy has some of the strongest research-based support. In this treatment, a mirror is placed adjacent to the intact limb and then moved in exercises designed to promote reorganization of the cortex with this visual input.[28] Virtual reality systems have been used as an alternative to using mirrors.

Multiple electrical stimulation techniques have also been studied. Transcutaneous electrical nerve stimulation has shown promise. There are several studies that indicate effectiveness with placement of the electrodes on the intact limb.[61] More invasive modalities have involved peripheral nerve stimulation, spinal cord stimulation, and deep brain stimulation. Pulse radio frequency energy treatment was reported as successful in one case study.[22]

BOX 10-1

Treatments for Phantom Limb Pain

- Pharmacologic
  - Opioids
    - Oxycodone
    - Hydromorphone
    - Morphine
  - Antidepressants
    - Imipramine
    - Mirtazapine
    - Amitryptyline
    - Nortriptyline
  - Anticonvulsants
    - Gabapentin
    - Carbamazepine
  - *N*-methyl-D-aspartate receptor agonists
    - Dextromethorphan
    - Memantine
    - Ketamine
  - Miscellaneous
    - Clonidine
    - Mexiletine
    - Calcitonin
    - Tramadol
- Injections
  - Lidocaine
  - Corticosteroid
  - Botulinum toxin
- Complementary
  - Transcutaneous electrical nerve stimulation (TENS)
  - Mirror therapy
  - Acupuncture
  - Hypnosis
  - Cognitive behavioral therapy
  - Virtual reality
- Surgical
  - Neuromodulation
  - Peripheral nerve reconstruction

Psychological Support

An amputation and the associated changes in body image and functional capabilities can have a strong emotional impact that requires a period of adjustment and supportive interventions. Naturally, this adjustment involves not just the amputee but also their relationships and roles with regard to family and friends. The amputation of a body part has been compared with the loss of a loved one and the some have described the psychological process in three phases.[44] In phase one, combined feelings of shock, confusion, and numbness lead to a general feeling of emptiness. Daily tasks can be overwhelming. In the second phase, mourning predominates and consumes most of the amputee's energy and focus. Finally, the amputee progresses to the adjustment phase and the amputee finds a sense of self-worth and competency in daily life. Several factors may hamper a progression through the phases to successful adjustment. Such factors include insufficient support from family members[44] and caregivers, negative emotional states, such as a feeling of social isolation, low self-esteem, and a lack of a sense of wholeness, social anxiety, and body image discomfort.

In a study examining the relationship among tenacious goal pursuit (TGP), flexible goal adjustment (FGA), and affective well-being[10] in individuals with lower limb amputation, TGP and FGA had different relationships with subjective well-being. TGP signifies changing one's life situation or behavior to facilitate goals, whereas FGA signifies changing goals to accommodate situational limitations.[10] TGP seemed to foster a positive effect, whereas FGA played a role in reducing negative affect. According to the authors, these two factors could potentially serve two useful functions: identifying amputees who might have negative affective outcomes and providing useful areas of intervention to ameliorate negative affect.

One study evaluated the roles of positive attitudes for amputations, among other diagnoses, and found that hopefulness correlated positively with functional outcomes and participation during the inpatient rehabilitation program. Another study of young traumatic amputees reported that more than half had been given a formal psychological diagnosis. The most frequent included PTSD, anxiety, depression, and substance abuse, with some individuals having two or more. These psychological disorders have the capacity to impair adjustment to physical issues. Almost two thirds of individuals with combat-related amputations have PTSD; anxiety and depression occur in approximately a quarter; and substance abuse is found in approximately 6%. Level of amputation is associated with severity of psychological disorders.

In a study relating spirituality to quality of life[35,45] of predominantly male subjects with traumatic, transtibial amputations, the researchers concluded that "existential spirituality," female gender, and age greater than 50 years had a positive association with increased quality of life. Existential spirituality also correlated positively with satisfaction with life, health, and social integration.

Studies examining return to work after lower limb amputation reveal that, overall, the rate of return to work is around 66%.[6] Although the percentage of amputees keeping their preamputation job ranged from 22% to 67%, the employment achieved after amputation necessitated more education, had greater complexity, and required less physical functional requirements. General parameters that influenced return to work included age, gender, and educational level. Medical factors included level of amputation, number of amputations, comorbidities, the cause for amputation, and continued medical issues with the residual limb. Functional and prosthetic factors that related to return to work were time to fitting of the prosthesis, comfort with wearing the prosthesis, ability to walk distances, and other physical limitations with walking. Vocational factors influencing return to work include support from an employer, salary, who initiated the effort (individual, employer, family, and agency), and a social support network.

Preprosthetic Phase Rehabilitation Considerations

The preprosthetic phase of rehabilitation therapy begins before the surgery and continues until the first fitting and training with a new prosthesis. Most patients fall within a certain timeframe for fitting of the initial or temporary prosthesis and then the subsequent definitive prosthesis.[35] Before the surgery, the rehabilitative team, composed of the physiatrist, physical therapist (potentially including occupational therapy as well), and prosthetist, should provide guidance and information about the rehabilitation process that will unfold after the amputation has been performed. Instruction in proper bed and chair positioning should be provided and an emphasis placed on appropriate exercises to maintain the joint ROM as well as the strength and endurance of important muscle groups. Not all amputees will become prosthetic candidates and this issue must also be approached carefully. Psychological support for the pending "loss" should also be provided.

Where possible, influencing surgical decision on the length of preserved residual limb is critical. Of importance are the lengths of the residual bone (femur or tibia) and the overall limb (proximal mark to the end of the soft tissue). Starting points on the transfemoral limb can be either the ischial tuberosity or greater trochanter, whereas for the transtibial limb the tibial plateau or tibial tubercle can be used. The end point is either the end of the bone or the distal soft tissue. For transtibial amputations, the optimal length of the residual tibia measured from the tibial plateau is 3 to 6 inches.[48] Too short a residual limb (i.e., <3 inches) will compromise control of the prosthesis and too long (i.e., 6 inches) of a residual limb may limit the ability to use the posterior compartment musculature for soft tissue coverage over the distal residual limb. For the transfemoral amputation level, preservation of length must be balanced against displacement of the prosthetic knee center of rotation too far distal compared with the nonamputated limb.

After surgery, the primary emphasis is on wound care and healing, pain management, edema control, maintaining ROM in joints, initiating strength and mobility exercises, overall residual limb and prosthetic use education, and psychological counseling. Edema control of the residual limb can be achieved in multiple ways, including soft dressings, ACE wraps, semirigid dressings, rigid dressings, rigid removable dressings, plaster casts, and immediate postoperative fitting of a prosthesis, all of which not only control edema but also help reduce pain and protect the residual limb and surgical area from trauma. The choice for edema control depends on many factors, including the preference of the surgeon and the familiarity of the staff with the different options. Studies examining efficacy have revealed varying outcomes, but most authors[29,48] have concluded that semirigid and semirigid removable dressings having greater effectiveness for edema control than elastic wraps/garments, but only in the first few weeks.

In addition to edema control, shaping of the residual limb is also important. Ideally, the transfemoral residual limb would evolve into a conical shape, whereas the transtibial one should be more of a cylindrical one. Periodic circumferential measurements of the residual limb should be taken to assess volume and to help determine readiness for fitting. The transtibial residual limb has achieved a more mature shape when the distal end is slightly less in circumference than the proximal area. There is a more marked difference for the transfemoral residual limb.

Educating the preoperative and postoperative patient on appropriate position in bed and wheelchair is critical. In addition to assuring appropriate positioning in the bed and wheelchair to avoid flexion contractures of the hip and knee, monitoring of ROM in these areas should be performed regularly. Careful joint ROM measurements with a goniometer are important, with knee extension measured with the goniometer, the arms are carefully aligned with the femur and tibia, and hip assessment is performed with the Thomas test. Contractures of the hip and knee on the amputated side can hinder the process of fitting a prosthesis or prevent it altogether. A knee flexion contracture can increase the energy, strength, and endurance needed for prosthetic ambulation. A hip flexion contracture greater than 15 degrees makes prosthetic fit difficult, and appropriate alignment modifications to the prosthesis are required.

Preprosthetic mobility after surgery often involves the use of a wheelchair. With the loss of a limb, the center of mass (COM) has changed and balance within a wheelchair can become more precarious if adjustments are not made. Because the COM moves posteriorly, the wheelchair can be made more stable by also moving the axles of the posterior wheels posteriorly. This issue becomes even more significant for individuals with bilateral amputations. For those with very good single limb balance, ambulation with crutches may be a possibility; otherwise, the use of a walker can be useful for negotiating short distances. Practice in the parallel bars may be necessary before sufficient competence has been developed. These skills in ambulation without a prosthesis are not a necessary prerequisite for prosthetic training and ambulation.

Prosthetic Training Phase Considerations

Aside from strengthening, ROM, and endurance exercises, early training for the amputee with a prosthesis involves activities such as maintaining the COM within the base of support, standing and balancing on the prosthetic limb, and simple stepping exercises. Part of the early training in using a prosthesis concerns sock ply management. The patient must consistently apply these principles for as long as the prosthesis is used. The first principle for the amputee to understand is that the residual limb will vary in volume, and this requires an adjustment of prosthetic fit through the addition or deletion of socks. Prosthetic socks commonly come in one, three, five, and six ply. With wear, the socks tend to lose some of their thickness. Factors that affect limb volume include fluid shifts associated with renal failure and dialysis, muscle atrophy, weight gain or loss, and associated medical conditions, such as congestive heart failure. Wearing the prosthesis will create a pumping action that will force fluid out of the residual limb and reduce its size. During the first 3 to 12 months after amputation, the residuum will typically swell if a shrinker is not worn consistently. Socket changes are generally required when the amputee needs 15 ply or more of socks, to accommodate shrinkage of the residual limb. If the residual limb volume is stable for 8 to 12 weeks, then the time is appropriate for fitting of the definitive prosthesis, which usually occurs around 6 to 18 months after surgery.

Close observation of the patient during donning and doffing of the prosthesis can provide valuable information in determining issues with the fit of the socket. For the prosthesis with a pin lock system of suspension, the number of clicks gives some clue as to the level of fit. If the patient is only able to obtain a few clicks into the locking mechanism, the patient may not be fitting down into the socket completely. If the speed of the clicks increases, this could indicate that the residual limb has shrunk and that additional socks should be added. Ease of donning is also a clue. If the prosthesis can be slid onto the residual limb easily and without resistance, then more socks are needed. Red marks on the residual limb also give some indication of the fit. If the distal end of the limb is getting red and sore from too much pressure, then more socks are needed. If after walking with the prosthesis there are reddened areas (reactive hyperemia) that do not resolve after a few minutes, then the socket is creating excessive pressure on the residual limb in these locations, and adjustments have to be made. After the patient understands the importance of sock ply management and how to appropriately adjust this aspect, instruction in donning and doffing the prosthesis can occur. If a liner is being used, the liner must be applied with careful attention to technique. The liner should be turned inside out and the distal end of the residuum should be placed directly against the liner, which should then be rolled upward without any air pockets. An air pocket between the distal end of the residuum and the liner will create suction and will affect the skin accordingly. Liner care should include washing it with soap and water at the end of the day. Drying should occur with the fabric side directed outward. This position will protect the tacky inner area from trapping dirt, dust, and hair that can adversely affect the skin. Spraying the inner part of the liner with diluted rubbing alcohol once or twice a week can reduce the buildup of bacteria on the liner surface and help prevent residual limb infections.[41]

Socks must be donned in a manner that eliminates wrinkles because these will create pressure areas that can cause skin breakdown. Wrinkles can be smoothed away with the tips of fingers. For the wearer of a transtibial prosthesis, the socket must be correctly aligned so that the bony prominences fit into the reliefs that were designed to accommodate them in the socket. The use of too many or too few socks can also prevent the correct seating of the residuum in the socket. In general, the socket should be donned in a consistent manner irrespective of the type of socket.

Once the correct donning technique has been mastered, the amputee can embark on other more advanced pregait activities. These exercises focus on fostering good balance and strength, weight-shifting, and on isolated parts of the gait cycle. Early training involves static weight-bearing, dynamic weight-shifting exercises, reaching activities, repeated stepping actions in all directions, identification, and elimination of gait deviations, and sit-to-stand and stand-to-sit exercises. Tap ups represent one activity that generates skill and confidence in weight-shifting and bearing weight on the prosthesis. Within the parallel bars, the first steps in learning the various parts of the gait cycle can begin. One of the first exercises involves learning the heel/toe pattern with the prosthetic leg. For the transfemoral amputee, this exercise will also initiate the learning process for manipulating the prosthetic knee. Ultimately and according to the patient's capabilities and certainly staying within any safety considerations, the patient may be able to advance to walking on level surfaces in different settings and on uneven terrain. Negotiating environmental obstacles, such as ramps and curbs, will also be important.

Functional Classification

The Centers for Medicare and Medicaid Services (CMS) have published a functional classification system for individuals with amputations to guide prosthetic limb prescription based on the actual or potential functional abilities of the person.[8] The guideline divides functional mobility into five categories and provides recommendations for the prescription of prosthetic components based on the functional mobility category (Table 10-2). These five categories have been referred to as the Medicare Functional Classification Levels (MFCLs), the K-Level Modifiers, or the Functional Index Levels. Although the amputee's functional mobility category determination should, to the extent possible, be based on objective clinical findings, the classification also allows for clinical judgment by the prescribing physician or team in predicting the anticipated functional level of the new amputee once they have been

Table 10-2 Medicare Functional Classification Level (MFCL) Descriptions and Prosthetic Component Recommendations for Each Level

Functional Index Level	Description	Recommended Prosthetic Components
K0	No ability or potential to ambulate or transfer with use of a prosthesis and prosthesis does not enhance the quality of life	None for function Potential for cosmetic prosthesis
K1	Ability or potential to transfer or ambulate with a prosthesis for household distances on level surfaces at a fixed cadence	Feet: solid ankle cushion heel, single axis Knees: manual locking, weight-activated stance control
K2	Ability or potential to ambulate limited community distances and traverse low-level environmental barriers. Ambulation at a fixed cadence	Feet: multiaxial and flexible keel feet Knees: weight-activated stance control
K3	Ability or potential to ambulate unlimited community distances and traverse most environmental barriers. Ambulation with variable cadence	Feet: multiaxial, energy storing Knees: hydraulic, pneumatic, and microprocessor controlled
K4	Ability or potential to exceed normal ambulation activities and use a prosthesis for activities exhibiting high impact, stress, or energy levels	Feet: energy storing or other specialty feet Knees: no specific limitations

fit with the prosthesis. The determination should also take into account the individual's medical conditions and medical comorbidities that could affect the person's ability to function with the use of a prosthetic limb. The patient's goals and desires for prosthetic use must be considered as part of the prescription process, and if the goals of the patient are not realistic with respect to the benefits of a prosthetic limb, education in this regard will be required. It should be emphasized that the final determination of the prosthetic prescription is ideally a team decision involving the physician, prosthetist, therapist, and patient.

Prosthetic Restoration

Essential Elements of the Prosthetic Prescription

The prescription of a lower extremity prosthesis should be approached in an organized manner to assure that the essential elements are included in the prescription. Box 10-2 provides a template that can be used for any level of lower extremity prosthetic prescription. Depending on the level of the amputation and the functional goals of the individual with the amputation, not all elements of the template will be required. Determination of the patient's classification within the MFCL as described is important in the development of the prosthetic prescription, but the unique characteristics and functional goals of each individual need to be considered. With the prosthetic prescription, the emphasis should be on identifying the best-suited class of prosthetic components to achieve the patient's functional goals rather than emphasizing the specific product name for each component of the prescription.

During the prosthetic prescription process, it should be recognized that many factors influence which specific components should be selected for each individual patient. Residual limb length, muscular strength, balance, coordination, vision, and motor control all affect stability during prosthetic ambulation and may require added stability to be incorporated into the prosthesis. The quality of the residual limb skin should be considered in selecting the most appropriate prosthetic suspension and interface system. Hand function, vision, and cognitive abilities need to be considered with regard to donning and doffing the prosthesis. In addition, the amputee's weight can limit the available component options. Lastly, variables such as prosthesis durability, reliability, cosmesis, and cost need to be part of the evaluation to determine the ideal prosthetic prescription. Ultimately, determination of the prosthetic prescription should be a team decision involving the physician, the prosthetist, the therapist, and, most important, the patient. The goal is to educate patients and their families about reasonable, available options and their advantages and disadvantages so that patients can contribute to an informed decision.

BOX 10-2

Prosthetic Prescription Essential Elements

- Socket
- Interface
- Suspension
- Pylon/frame
- Foot and ankle
- Knee unit if knee disarticulation or above
- Hip joint if hip disarticulation or above
- Extras (rotators, covers, etc.)

Socket Designs

The prosthetic socket serves as the platform for connecting the amputated residual limb to the prosthetic limb. In some circumstances, there is direct contact between the residual limb skin and the prosthetic socket, whereas in other circumstances, a liner or other materials are used as the interface between the residual limb and the socket. The socket itself can also function to suspend the prosthesis to the residual limb, but in most instances, the suspension is accomplished through an additional suspension method. For an ideal functional outcome with use of a prosthetic limb to be achieved, the socket must be comfortable and secure, and it must facilitate motion transfer from the residual limb to the prosthetic limb. Having a secure and comfortable connection allows the amputee to effectively weight-bear through the prosthesis and efficiently advance the limb during the swing phase of gait. Prosthetic sockets are made from various materials and there are a variety of socket designs that have been developed for each level of lower limb amputation. The most commonly used prosthetic socket designs are highlighted in the following sections.

Transtibial Socket Design

There are several different transtibial socket designs that are currently being used in the prosthetics field. Some of these designs are considered hybrid designs because they combine the features of one or more traditional designs. Independent of the type of design, the goal is to provide a socket that is well fitting, comfortable, and secure.

Patellar Tendon Bearing. The major weight-bearing area for the residual limb in this design is at the patellar tendon with a counter force in the popliteal region. Current socket technology also provides a total surface contact with specific weight-bearing areas in the soft tissue regions of the residual limb. These would include the anterior muscle compartment, medial tibial flare, shaft of the fibula, gastrocnemius muscle, and the distal end which receives slight pressure. Excessive contact over bony areas is avoided. For the patellar tendon bearing (PTB) socket, the anterior trim line is proximal to the patellar tendon insertion on the patella. The medial-lateral trim line is at the midlevel of the medial condyle. The posterior trim line is at or just below the midpatellar tendon with reliefs for the medial and lateral hamstring tendons (generally at the bend of the knee so that the patient can bring the prosthesis to a 90-degree angle).

Patellar Tendon Bearing and Supracondylar/Suprapatellar. The only difference between the PTB and the PTB-supracondylar/suprapatellar (PTB-SC/SP) socket design is the proximal trim line. By raising the trim line in the medial-lateral dimension to above the medial condyle, additional stabilizing support for the residual limb is provided with added suspension. With the suprapatellar extension, greater anterior/posterior support is provided with a knee hyperextension stop, as well as some additional suspension.

Total Surface Bearing. This socket design creates more equal weight-bearing distribution throughout the socket. Unlike the PTB design, the total surface bearing (TSB) socket is designed to globally apply forces throughout the residual limb. There is very little pressure difference between areas and limited relief for bony areas. Many TSB designs use gel-type interfaces, which also facilitate the more even distribution of forces over a larger surface area. Trim lines are similar to the PTB design. Clinically, the typical transtibial socket design is a combination of both the traditional PTB and the TSB design.

Transfemoral Socket Design

As with transtibial socket designs, there are many versions of the transfemoral socket. Newer socket designs have flexible inner liners with hard external frames that can be fenestrated to allow for bony relief and muscle contraction. The external frames that attach the socket to the distal prosthetic components are laminated with carbon graphite and can be imprinted with a design of the patient's choice. This feature allows for greater incorporation of the prosthesis into the patient's lifestyle and body image.

Quadrilateral Socket (Quad Socket). This type of socket is used only rarely today. As the name implies, this socket is rectangular in shape with the medial-lateral dimension being greater than the anterior-posterior dimension (Figure 10-1) The scarpa's triangle provides a posterior-directed force keeping the ischial tuberosity on a ledge, which is the major weight-bearing area of this design. The distal two thirds of the socket design have the general shape of the residual limb of the patient and is total contact in design with little to no muscle contouring. There is some hydrostatic weight-bearing through this more distal aspect of the socket.

Ischial Containment Socket. The ischial containment socket is the most commonly used transfemoral socket design. The original design for this socket was described by Ivan Long, CP, as a Normal Shape Normal Alignment (NSNA) design. This socket design takes a more anatomic approach to transfemoral socket fitting with the ischial tuberosity now contained inside the proximal trim lines. The principle of this design is to provide a bony lock of the ischium in the prosthetic socket. The inclusion of the ischium along with the lateral femur and pubic ramus prevents excessive abduction of the femur and increases medial-lateral stability during the stance phase of gait. This is especially helpful for individuals with shorter residual limbs and for those with mild hip abductor weakness. The distal two thirds of this design have more muscle contouring compared with the quadrilateral socket.

Subischial Socket Design. The third socket design is the subischial socket. The proximal trim line of this socket falls distal to the ischial tuberosity and relies completely on the thigh musculature for weight-bearing. This socket design usually involves an elevated suction socket and requires a patient that is attentive to their prosthetic care. Figure 10-2 demonstrates the three different transfemoral socket designs.

Prosthetic Limb Suspension

Suspension is the technique by which the prosthesis is connected and held onto a person's residual limb (Figures 10-3 to 10-6). Suspension can be provided through a variety of mechanisms, including the anatomic shape of the limb, a liner, a sleeve, or with suction. Suspension is a critical issue for successful use of lower extremity

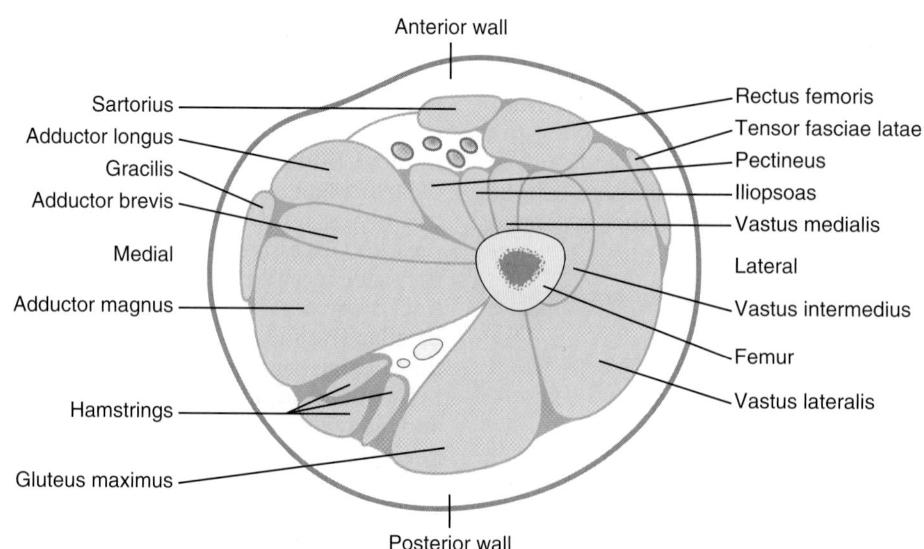

FIGURE 10-1 Transverse cross-section of the proximal aspect of thigh and quadrilateral socket. (From Schuch CM: Transfemoral amputation: prosthetic management. In Bowker JH, Michael JW, editors: *Atlas of limb prosthetics: surgical, prosthetic, and rehabilitation principles*, ed 2, St. Louis, 1992, Mosby-Year Book.)

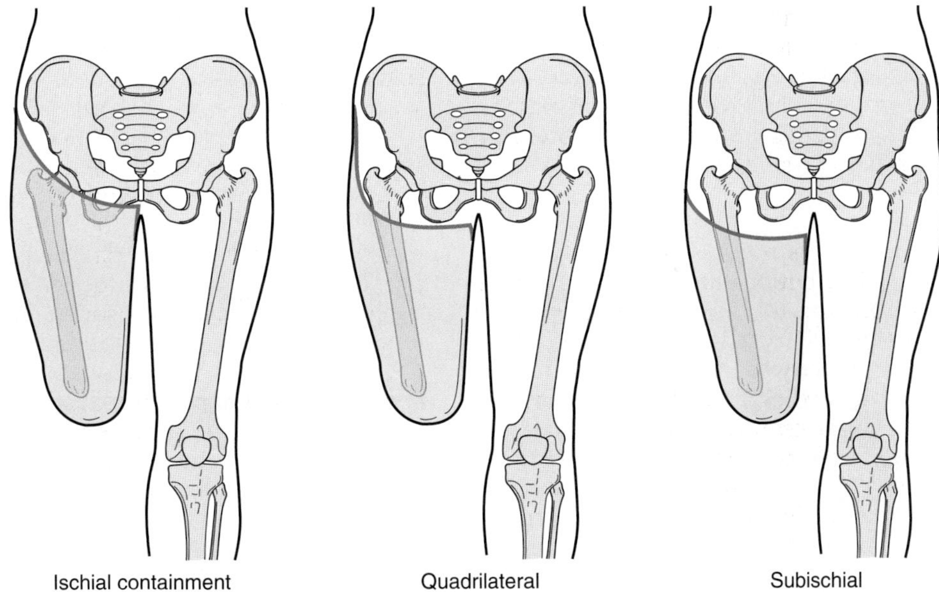

FIGURE 10-2 Transfemoral socket designs. *Left,* Ischial containment. *Center,* Quadrilateral. *Right,* Subischial. (Based on an illustration by Brian Kausek.)

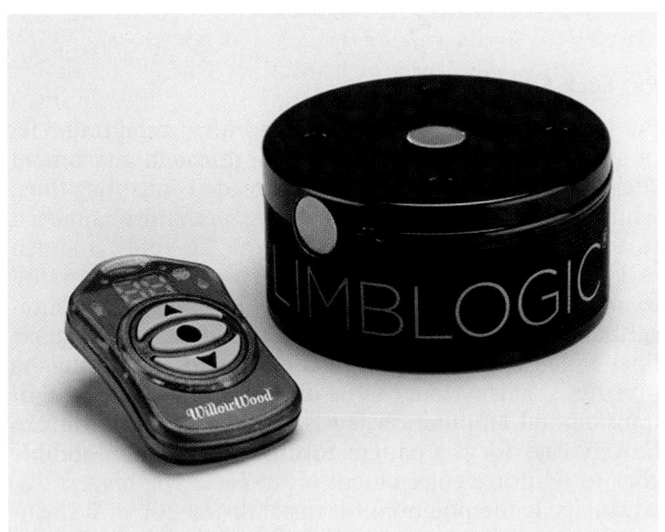

FIGURE 10-3 Electric vacuum pump system with key fob. (LimbLogic, The Ohio Willow Wood Company, Mt Sterling, Ohio.)

prostheses. Without proper suspension, the amputee patient cannot ambulate efficiently and will lack control over their prosthesis. Improper suspension can also increase the risk of falls with ambulation. This lack of suspension will negate the beneficial effects of any newer prosthetic component technology.

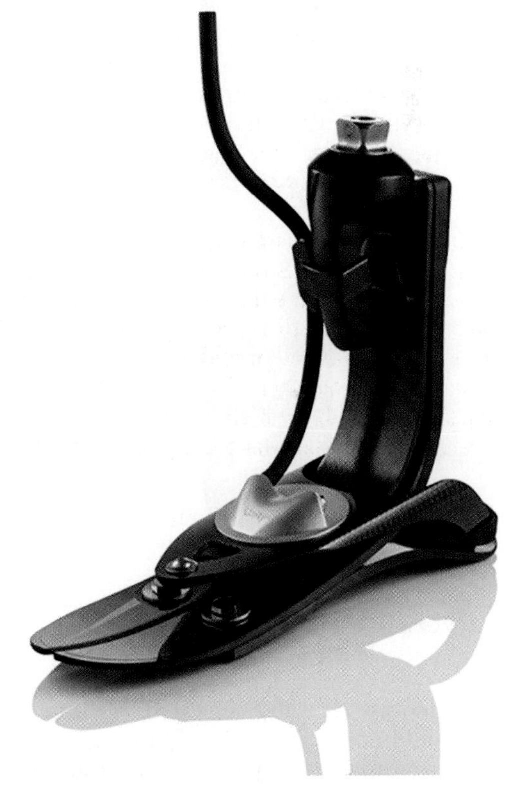

FIGURE 10-4 Mechanical vacuum pump incorporated into prosthetic foot. (Unity, Össur, Reykjavik, Iceland.)

Suction Suspension

By creating a proximal seal within an airtight socket environment, suction sockets create a slight negative pressure to hold the prosthesis on to the residual limb. However, because of this negative pressure, a prosthesis with a lack of distal contact can create skin problems, including verrucous hyperplasia if the lack of distal contact is chronic in nature. Historically, this approach has used a direct skin fit (no socks or liners between the residual limb and socket). The advent of gel liners has enhanced traditional suction suspension methods.

Elevated Vacuum Suspension

Elevated vacuum suspension can be seen as a derivative of suction suspension facilitated in part by the advent of interface liners. In contrast to traditional suction socket systems in which air is passively expelled from the socket

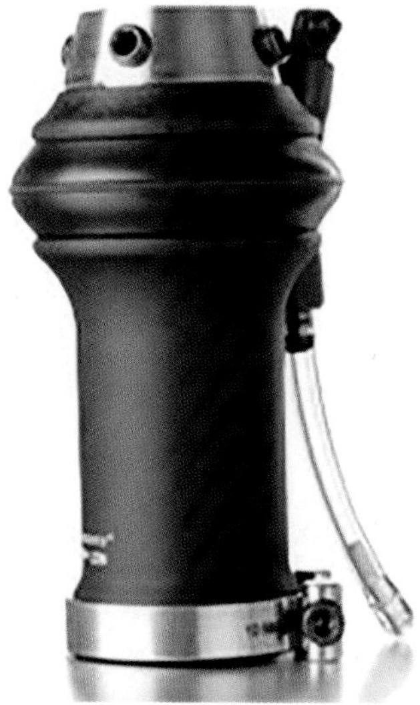

FIGURE 10-5 Mechanical vacuum pump with vertical shock pylon. (Harmony P3, Ottobock, Minneapolis, Minn.)

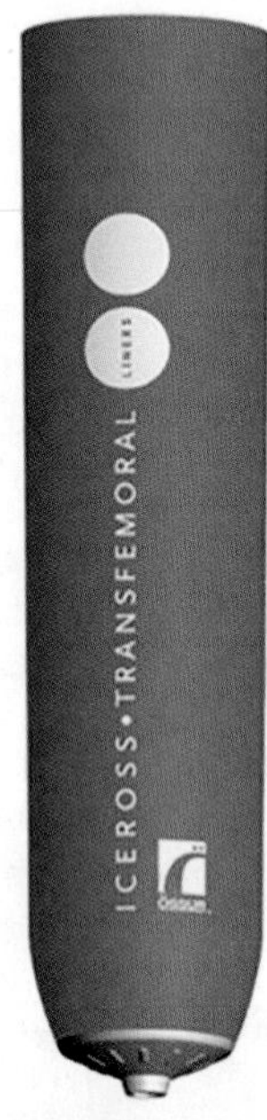

FIGURE 10-6 Transfemoral liner with distal mechanism for pin lock. (Iceross, Össur, Reykjavik, Iceland.)

through a one-way air valve, elevated vacuum systems actively draw additional air from within the socket environment. These designs provide a secure fit and stabilize the prosthesis firmly to the patient's residual limb. There are currently several mechanisms that are used to create an elevated vacuum suspension environment, all of which require a TSB socket. Elevated vacuum systems maintain an enhanced negative pressure between the gel liner and socket wall. This negative pressure provides suspension and may assist with maintaining stability of the patient's residual limb volume. Elevated vacuum requires a pump that draws air out of the prosthetic socket. These pumps can be either manual or powered devices, and this technique can be used for either transtibial or transfemoral levels.

BOX 10-3

Transtibial Suspension Systems

- Supracondylar and suprapatellar cuff/strap
- Supracondylar Pelite liner with compressible or removable wall
- Auxiliary suspension with sleeve
- Liner with pin-locking mechanism
- Suction with or without liner
- Vacuum
- Thigh corset and side joints

BOX 10-4

Transfemoral Suspension Options

- Pin-locking or lanyard system
- Total elastic suspension (TES) belt
- Silesian belt
- Hip joint and waist belt
- Suction or partial suction (dry or wet fit)
- Suction with seal-in liner
- Vacuum

Pin Lock Suspension

Pin lock suspension requires a liner with a distal umbrella of an embedded mesh matrix and a threaded attachment site. A locking pin can then be threaded into that liner, which will then engage into a locking mechanism attached to the prosthetic socket. The lock can be either a clutch mechanism or rotary style. Locks can be either push or pull to unlock. Pin lock suspension provides a secure mechanical link between the amputee and the prosthesis. The gel liner holds onto the patient and the pin locks into the prosthesis. This system can be used for either transtibial or transfemoral amputation levels. Pin lock suspension can be very easy for the patient to use and offers an audible click to reinforce engagement of the lock. The biggest disadvantage is the potential for distal distraction and shearing forces on the tissues of the residual limb.

The lanyard strap suspension is a version of pin lock suspension. Instead of a pin and locking mechanism, a Velcro strap is attached to the gel liner and fed through an opening in the distal portion of a prosthesis by the patient and fastened on the exterior portion of the socket. This system requires that the patient has some manual dexterity but may be simpler than the pin lock to manage.

Alternate Suspension Designs

There are many other methods of suspending a prosthesis. Boxes 10-3 and 10-4 list the most commonly used suspension methods for transtibial and transfemoral level amputations. Sleeves, straps, belts, and buckles have been used in the past and are still being used in some cases either because of patient preference or because of anatomic considerations with the residual limb. These techniques can involve straps to proximal anatomic anchors. With transfemoral amputations, the suspension might involve a hip belt over the contralateral hip (Silesian Belt) or a combination of a hip joint, pelvic band, and waist belt. In

BOX 10-5

Prosthetic Interface Options

- Pelite liner
- Urethane liners
- Thermogel/gel liners
- Silicone liners
- Special feature liners
- Hard interface directly with socket

transtibial level amputations, this could include a cuff suspension strap that is just proximal to femoral condyles.

Prosthetic Interface Options

The contact of the residual limb against the socket can use either a hard or a soft interface (Box 10-5). An example of a hard interface is found in a suction socket where the skin of the residual limb is in direct contact with the hard socket. By contrast, modern prosthetic liners provide protection against both shear and impact forces and can be described as providing a soft interface. Soft interface options are indicated for and used by many amputees. Soft interfaces provide a cushion for the residual limb and allow for adjustment and comfort when the residual limb volume changes. Soft inserts are especially beneficial for patients with significant residual limb soft tissue atrophy with bony prominences or when invaginated, sensitive scar tissue is present. Soft interface materials include Pelite inserts, gel liners, urethane, or silicone liners. The disadvantages of soft inserts are their susceptibility to wear and tear, their added bulkiness, and their ability to absorb odors. Hygiene as well as donning and doffing of these liners can be problematic for some patients. Similar to all the other components of prostheses, there are many different brands and types of liners that are commercially available. Selection of the most appropriate interface system will depend on the individual needs and characteristics of the patient.

Prosthetic Limb Frame Options (Endoskeletal or Exoskeletal)

The prosthetic frame or the method for connecting to the prosthetic components together can be accomplished through either exoskeletal or endoskeletal construction.

Exoskeletal construction uses a rigid exterior lamination from the socket down and has a lightweight filler inside. This construction method is used less frequently, but provides the potential benefit of added strength for heavier patients. Another advantage of this type of frame is that the hard exterior shell is very durable and can help protect the prosthesis in harsh environments. The primary disadvantages of this construction are the added weight, the potential to limit foot and knee options, and the limited ability to adjust alignment or repair components once the construction is complete.

Endoskeletal construction is the most commonly used type of prosthetic frame and this construction uses pipes called pylons to connect the prosthetic components. This construction is lighter weight and more modular. Many endoskeletal systems have pylons made of carbon fiber or titanium, which are even lighter in weight than standard steel pylons. Endoskeletal construction allows for easier prosthetic alignment adjustments, including angular and linear changes in both the sagittal and coronal planes. The height of the prosthesis can also be adjusted if needed. Endoskeletal pylons also allow the ability to finish the prosthesis with a cover that provides a softer and more realistic cosmetic appearance.

BOX 10-6

Categories and Types of Prosthetic Feet

- Nonarticulated
  - Solid ankle cushion heel (SACH) foot
  - Solid ankle flexible endoskeleton (SAFE) foot
- Articulated
  - Single axis foot: plantar flexion/dorsiflexion
  - Multiaxial foot
  - Hydraulic
- Energy storing/dynamic elastic response
  - Low profile
  - High profile
- Microprocessor control
- Microprocessor control with internal power
- Special activity feet

Prosthetic Feet

There are currently a wide variety of prosthetic feet that are commercially available. These feet are made of various materials and are produced by a host of manufacturers. Although each specific foot may have unique properties and specific advantages, this chapter primarily focuses on the different classes of prosthetic feet and the advantages and disadvantages of each class. There are a number of classification schemes that have been proposed for prosthetic feet. The classification system used in this text is included in Box 10-6. With advances in prosthetic designs, the features of one class can be combined with the features of another to produce a foot component that provides several different features.

Nonarticulated Prosthetic Feet

Solid Ankle Cushion Heel Foot. The solid ankle cushion heel (SACH) prosthetic foot is a basic foot that is primarily indicated for individuals in the K1 functional level (Figure 10-7). This foot has no moving parts, which makes it very lightweight, durable, and inexpensive. The foot simulates dorsiflexion and plantar flexion through the cushion heel portion of the foot. Because the keel of the foot provides limited movement, it offers no ability to effectively accommodate to uneven surfaces.

Solid Ankle Flexible Endoskeletal Foot. The solid ankle flexible endoskeletal (SAFE) prosthetic foot is similar to the SACH foot in that it has no joint articulations and is durable and inexpensive. In contrast to the SACH foot, the SAFE foot allows some inversion and eversion motion through the flexible keel of the foot. This provides greater ability to accommodate to uneven terrain, but the motion

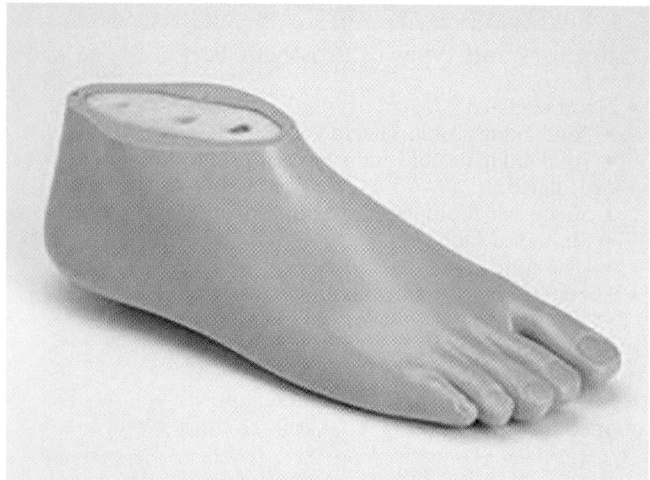

FIGURE 10-7 Solid ankle cushion heel (SACH) prosthetic foot. (Ottobock, Minneapolis, Minn.)

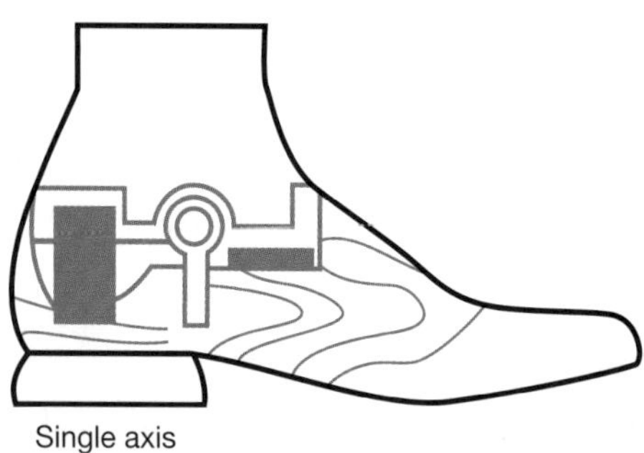

FIGURE 10-8 Single axis prosthetic foot.

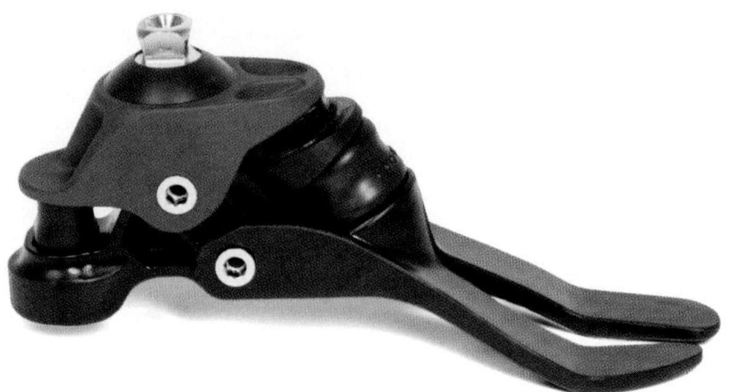

FIGURE 10-9 Multiaxial prosthetic foot. (Trustep, College Park Industries, Warren, Mich.)

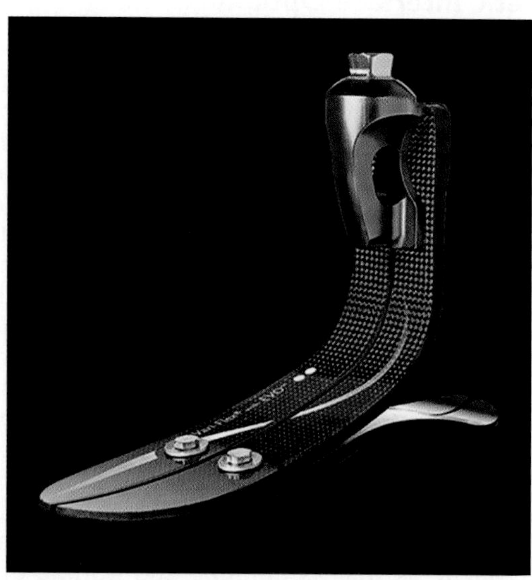

FIGURE 10-10 High-profile energy-storing/dynamic-response prosthetic foot with split keel. (Vari-Flex, Össur, Reykjavik, Iceland.)

is still limited and provides no energy-storing capacity. The SAFE foot is primarily indicated in K1 and low-level K2 level ambulators.

Articulated Prosthetic Feet

Single Axis Feet. Single axis feet allow controlled motion at the ankle in dorsiflexion and plantar flexion (Figure 10-8). Rubber bumpers of various durometers control this motion and the ability of the foot to return to a neutral position. This allows the patient to achieve foot flat more quickly during the loading response phase of gait, which helps maintain stability of the prosthetic knee for individuals with transfemoral level amputations. Single axis feet are typically indicated in individuals who are K1 and K2 level ambulators.

Multiaxial Feet. Multiaxial feet (Figure 10-9) allow motion in multiple planes of movement, including axial rotation depending on the exact type of foot. Multiaxial motion can be obtained through the foot's flexible keel or through true mechanical joints. A flexible keel foot allows the motion to occur within the keel itself as the ground reaction forces cause deformation of the foot. Multiaxial feet that allow motion through mechanical joints can allow motion in all three planes: plantar flexion and dorsiflexion, inversion and eversion, and transverse plane motion. Some multiaxial feet are fabricated with materials for energy storage and also return. A disadvantage to this type of foot is the multiple moving parts, which may require more frequent repairs and maintenance. This type of foot is indicated for K2 and K3 level ambulators.

Specialty Feet

Feet in this category can accommodate various specialty needs. For example, some feet have varying heel height to allow the amputee to wear shoes of different heights. These feet can vary heel height from a flat position to a heel height of 3 inches. Another example of specialty feet are those designed to specifically accommodate running.

Energy-Storing/Dynamic-Response Feet

Energy-storing/dynamic-response feet are generally indicated for more active patients (Figures 10-10 and 10-11). These feet are made of materials (plastic or carbon fiber) that provide the capacity to store energy during weight-bearing and then return energy once the foot is off-loaded. The longer the spring, the more energy that is returned to the patient to provide push-off. Some energy-storing feet also include a shock absorber mechanism to absorb

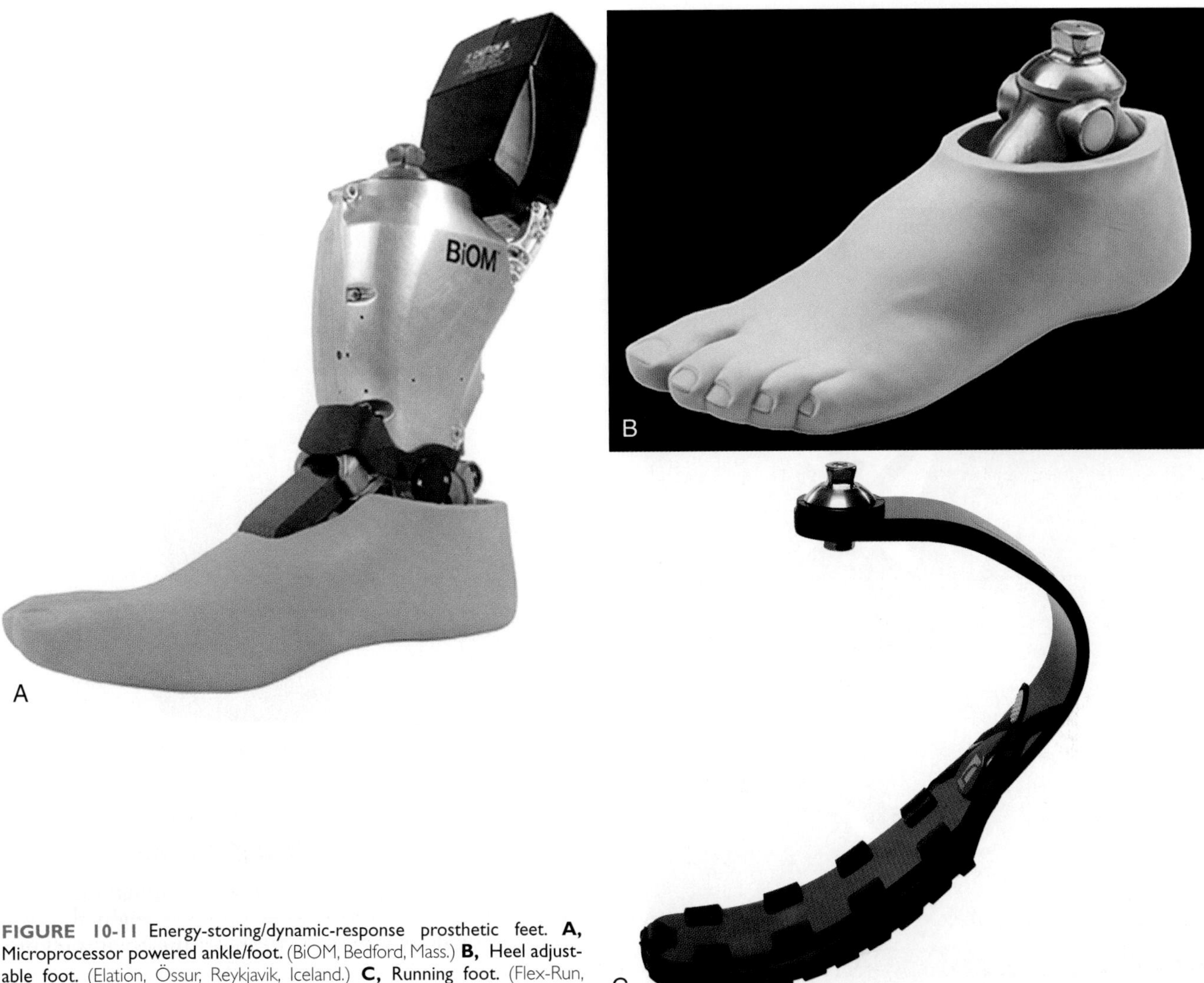

FIGURE 10-11 Energy-storing/dynamic-response prosthetic feet. **A,** Microprocessor powered ankle/foot. (BiOM, Bedford, Mass.) **B,** Heel adjustable foot. (Elation, Össur, Reykjavik, Iceland.) **C,** Running foot. (Flex-Run, Össur, Reykjavik, Iceland.)

vertical forces and reduce the ground reaction forces that are transferred to the patient's residual limb. Depending on style, these feet can also provide similar motion as a multiaxial foot. This type of foot is indicated for K3 and K4 level ambulators.

Microprocessor Feet

Prosthetic feet that are capable of internal power generation are commercially available. Some of these feet provide only active power generation to produce ankle dorsiflexion during the swing phase of gait, whereas others provide both actively powered dorsiflexion and plantar flexion during both stance and swing phase. Powered prosthetic foot and ankle components that provide active plantar flexion can be especially useful for ambulating up inclines or hills, and there is some evidence to suggest that these devices reduce the energy cost of ambulation.[36] Disadvantages to these feet are that they are heavy, cannot get wet, and need to be recharged daily. These feet are useful for a functional level 3 or above, but they are not covered by many insurance companies.

Prosthetic Knees

Prosthetic knees can be classified by use and functional levels. They vary from very simple designs to sophisticated designs with microprocessor control. Selection and fitting of the most appropriate prosthetic knee should take into consideration multiple variables, including the activity level of the patient, residual limb length, as well as proximal muscle strength and control. The internal control mechanism for prosthetic knees can be as simple as mechanical friction which provides constant resistance and works well for a one-speed walker to hydraulic fluid control with or without a microprocessor to allow for varied gait speed. As with prosthetic foot prescription, prosthetic knees should be prescribed based on the patient's current functional needs and future goals as well as upon the environmental conditions during usage of the prosthesis. Box 10-7 lists the most common prosthetic knee design options.

Manual Locking Knee

Manually locking knees positively lock when fully extended and unlock by pulling a lever that is attached to the

BOX 10-7

Prosthetic Knee Design Options

- Manual locking
- Single axis with constant friction
- Weight-activated stance control (safety knee)
- Polycentric
- Hydraulic or pneumatic swing phase control
- Hydraulic swing and stance control
- Microprocessor control (stance or stance and swing phase control)
- Microprocessor with internal power
- Hybrid units with combined features

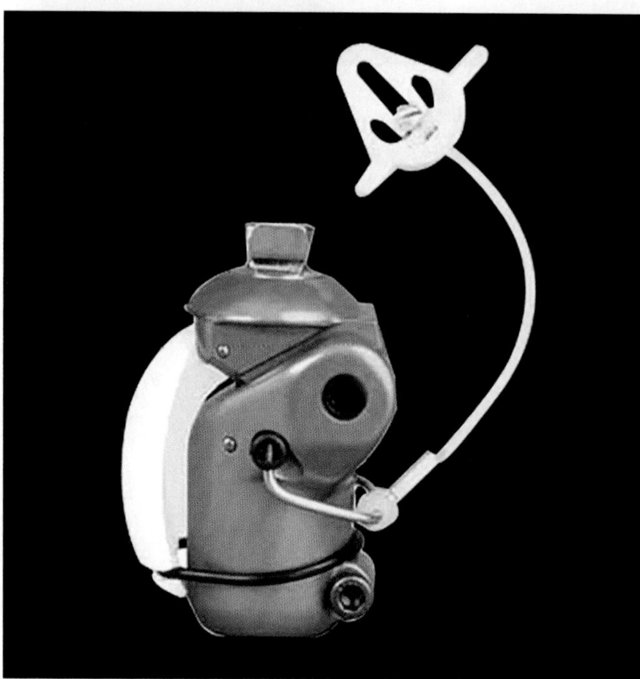

FIGURE 10-12 Manual locking knee. (Ottobock, Minneapolis, Minn.)

proximal portion of the socket (the lever is usually placed laterally or anteriorly) (Figure 10-12). They cannot be flexed until unlocked. Manual locking knees provide the advantage of being the most stable knee designs, whereas the disadvantage of the knee is the compromised gait mechanics that occur because the patient must walk with a straight leg. This knee is used when stability is the primary issue for the patient or sometimes when bilateral fittings are necessary. This knee is relatively durable and inexpensive and is typically indicated for patients in the K1 functional classification category.

Single Axis Knee

A single axis knee is a basic knee joint similar to a hinge. It can have a spring-assisted extension so that the foot can advance more quickly during swing phase and achieve full knee extension sooner. The stability of the knee is based strictly on alignment and voluntary control, so patients need to have good proximal strength and control of the prosthesis to avoid knee instability. This knee is lightweight, durable, and inexpensive. It is typically indicated for patients in the K1 functional classification category.

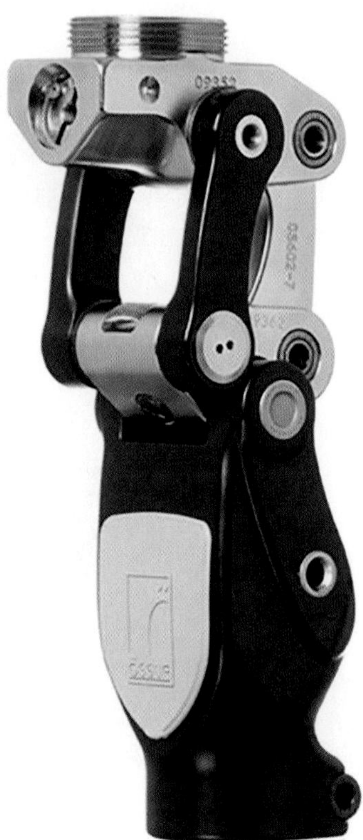

FIGURE 10-13 Polycentric prosthetic knee with six-bar linkage. (Total Knee, Össur, Reykjavik, Iceland.)

Weight-Activated Stance Control (Safety Knee)

A safety knee is a single axis knee with a weight-activated locking mechanism. The patient applies weight through the prosthesis during the stance phase and then the knee locks automatically caused by an internal braking system. For the braking mechanism to function appropriately, the knee cannot be flexed greater than approximately 20 degrees. When the patient's weight shifts off the prosthesis to initiate swing phase, the knee unlocks to allow flexion of the knee during swing phase. This knee can be used for new amputees and allows progressive adjustments from a very safe, locked status during stance phase to just a single axis knee. This knee is generally indicated for amputees who fall into the functional classification K1 and K2 levels.

Polycentric Knees

A polycentric knee has inherent stability because of its construction and multiple points of rotation (Figure 10-13). These multiple joints create an instantaneous center of rotation that shifts as the knee flexes and extends. The instantaneous center of rotation is located more proximally and posteriorly with the knee in an extended position, which provides greater knee stability during the early part of stance phase. As the knee flexes, the instantaneous center of rotation shifts distally and anteriorly, which helps to facilitate knee flexion in late stance phase. These knees are available with hydraulic or pneumatic swing phase control. Because of to the relatively small distance between the knee axis of rotation and the attachment to the socket, this is also an ideal knee for individuals with knee disarticulation level amputations.

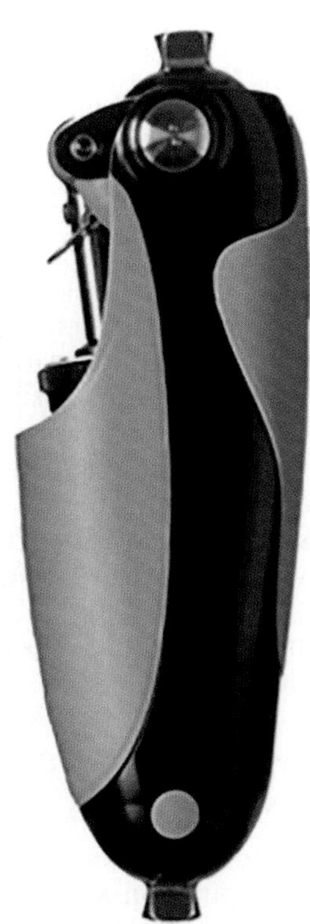

FIGURE 10-14 Hydraulic swing and stance control knee unit. (Mauch SNS Knee, Össur, Reykjavik, Iceland.)

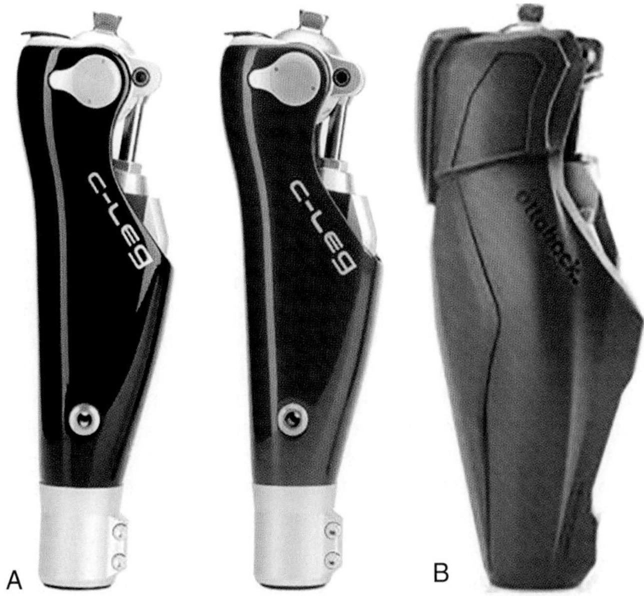

FIGURE 10-15 Microprocessor knees. **A,** C-Leg. **B,** Waterproof X-3. (Ottobock, Minneapolis, Minn.)

Hydraulic or Pneumatic Knees

Hydraulic or pneumatic knees include a cylinder that is either fluid-filled (hydraulic) or air-filled (pneumatic) that provides control during the swing phase of gait with knee extension and flexion (Figure 10-14). Some of these knee designs include mechanical features to also provide stance control. These types of knees are appropriate for active patients who have good control and muscle strength. Because these systems provide the ability to adjust to faster or slower gait speeds, they are indicated for individuals who are able to ambulate with variable cadence (K3 functional classification level).

Microprocessor Knee

Microprocessor knees draw input from various types of sensors that provide input to the microprocessor (Figure 10-15). The types of sensors used include strain gauges, accelerometers, and gyroscopes, which provide detailed information on the knee angle, direction of movement, angular velocity, and weight-bearing status. The microprocessor analyzes this information at rates ranging from 50 to 1000 times per second to control the knee's resistance to flexion. The microprocessor knees have become more durable and reliable over time, but caution is still required with most of these knees when used around water or in other harsh environments. Although microprocessor knees work well for many active patients, most are not designed to be used for running or other high-activity sports. Microprocessor knees are generally indicated for those rated at a functional index level K3. However, there are some microprocessor knees that provide only stance phase microprocessor control, which can be suitable for higher-level K2 ambulators.

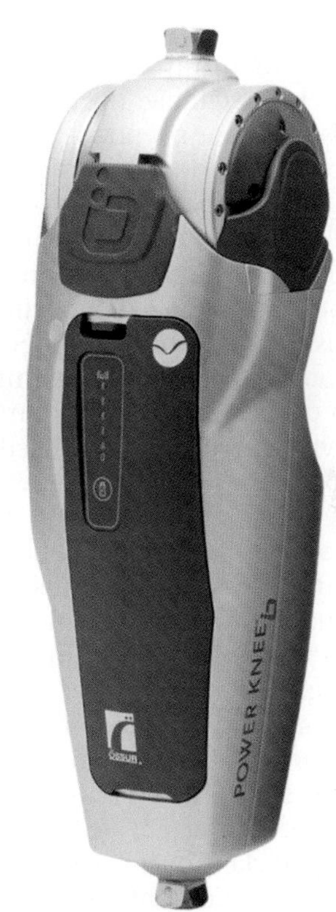

FIGURE 10-16 Microprocessor knee with internal power. (Power Knee, Össur, Reykjavik, Iceland.)

Microprocessor Knees with Internal Power

There is currently one microprocessor knee that is commercially available that also has a motor capable of internal power generation (Figure 10-16). This knee provides active knee flexion and extension, which is particularly useful with sit-to-stand activities and stair ascent.[70] The disadvantages of this knee are greater expense, heavier weight, and limited battery life. The knee is also relatively sensitive to environmental factors such as rain (any type of water) and temperature changes.

Prosthetic Hip Joints

There are two primary styles of hip joints: single axis and multiaxial. The single axis hip with an extension assist has been the most commonly used type of hip in the past. The multiaxial hip joint provides not only flexion and extension but also some rotation, which better simulates the normal motion of the hip. Use of a multiaxial hip joint coupled with a microprocessor knee is generally recommended for the person with a hip disarticulation level amputation who has a strong potential for prosthetic ambulation at the community level.

Additional Componentry Considerations

A multiaxial rotation unit allows for axial rotation in multiple planes. This is commonly called a torque absorber. It allows the foot to be firmly planted on the ground and the rest of the prosthesis to twist. Once the patient unweights the prosthesis it automatically returns to its original position. This unit helps facilitate the twisting movements involved in playing golf. An endoskeletal axial rotation unit allows the patient to manually rotate the knee and foot to cross legs or tie shoes. An alignable system can be realigned during and after definitive fitting. Lightweight refers to materials, such as titanium and carbon, in the components of the prosthesis. A diagnostic or check socket is used by the prosthetist to ensure proper fit and function of the socket before fabricating the definitive socket. It is made from a clear plastic. The length of time it can be worn depends on the type of plastic that is used.

In the past, prosthetic socks were worn against the patient's skin. They provided cushioning, absorbed perspiration, and had some ability to reduce shear forces on the residual limb. Currently, socks are most commonly used as fillers for residual limb volume reduction and are worn over a gel liner. Prosthetic socks come in various thicknesses or plys, ranging from 1 ply to 7 ply. Common sizes are 1, 3, and 5 ply and are used in combination with each other to provide proper fit and function. As a patient's residual limb decreases or increases in size, the number of socks can be added or subtracted. Normally, when a patient is wearing 10 ply of sockets or more over the gel liner, it is time for a prosthetic socket replacement or a whole new prosthesis. Nylon sheaths are used on the patient's residual limb to provide a reduction of shear forces and to allow perspiration to wick away from the residual limb. However, using a sheath under the gel liner also reduces the ability of the liner to stay in place and securely connect to the residual limb.

Cosmetic covers consist of a type of foam (soft or hard) that is placed over the components of the prosthesis making it look and feel like the person's contralateral limb. With the advent of new technology, carbon graphite components and stylized socket designs, many patients prefer no cover. Moreover, when a cosmetic cover gets wet, it acts like a big sponge. However, there are patients who need to see and feel something that looks like the leg that they lost. Prosthetic skins are a synthetic skin material made from silicone or other materials that match the person's skin tone. The two styles of prosthetic skins are custom and noncustom. Noncustom prosthetic skins are semidetailed and the patient and prosthetist pick a color from a swatch that closely resembles the patient's skin. Custom prosthetic skins are an exact match to the patient's contralateral limb and include hair patterns. These are extremely expensive and in some cases can cost as much as the actual prosthesis. Both styles add a measure of water resistance but are not really waterproof for swimming. The prosthetic skin is susceptible to damage and can rip and tear secondary to insult. With a transfemoral prosthesis, a cosmetic skin that is continuous from foot to socket can impede the function of the prosthetic knee. Prosthetic skins that protect a patient's cover from incontinence or extreme conditions need medical justification.

Prosthetic Prescription for Partial Foot Amputations

There are many levels of partial foot amputations ranging from a single ray to amputation at the level of the talonavicular and calcaneocuboid joint (Chopart amputation). One of the concerns with partial foot amputations is the distal end pressure and shear forces placed on the remaining foot. The prosthesis should be designed in such a way that these pressure points and shear forces are reduced. Use of a custom-fabricated, total-contact shoe insert can help to achieve this goal. The insert may include a filler to fill the space in the shoe left from the amputation. Use of a carbon fiber foot plate under the insert or use of rocker bottom shoe modifications can facilitate weight bearing and allow for a more normal gait pattern. For proximal partial foot amputations in the midfoot or hindfoot, incorporation of an ankle-foot orthosis should be considered to enhance the stability of the foot and ankle complex and allow greater functional activity levels. The patient's footwear should also be taken into consideration during the prescription.

Prosthetic Prescription for Ankle Disarticulation (Syme) Amputations

With a disarticulation amputation at the level of the ankle joint (Syme level), the heel pad is kept in place to create a weight-bearing surface. One of the advantages of this surgery is to allow the patient to take limited steps without a prosthesis. However, one disadvantage is that the length of the residual limb precludes the use of most of energy-storing feet. In addition, the heel pad can migrate off the distal end over time and render the distal end non–weight bearing. Because of the bulbous anatomic shape of the distal end, suspension is typically not a problem. However, the bulbous end can create cosmetic problems with the prosthesis. The socket design, specifically the height of the proximal trim line, depends on the distal weight-bearing capacity. If a patient has no weight-bearing ability, then the trim line will need to be brought up to the patellar tendon level. The proximal trim line will move distally to the tibial tubercle if the heel pad is in place and tolerates weight-bearing. The liner can be a custom gel liner or use traditional padding, such as Pelite. The suspension can be built into the liner (extra gel or padding above the malleoli) or can be a window and door configuration medially or posteriorly. Prosthetic foot options include a low profile Syme SACH foot or carbon composite foot. The carbon foot allows some energy storing and also provides better accommodation over uneven surfaces.

Prosthetic Prescription Algorithms for Transtibial Amputees

The choice of components for the transtibial prosthesis prescription depends on the individual's current or potential functional abilities and the patient's goals for prosthetic use. The following recommendations for each functional level are for consideration and it is important to develop a prescription that is individualized. The essential elements for a transtibial prosthesis that need to be included for every functional level are socket, interface, suspension, pylon/frame, and type of foot and ankle. Items included in all prescriptions for a prosthesis are a clear diagnostic socket and socks (single ply and multiple ply, six each). The patient can select a custom-shaped cover and/or prosthetic skin to help address cosmetic concerns.

Functional Level One (K1)

Patients in this functional category have the ability to use a prosthesis for transfers or ambulate over level surfaces for short household distances. Safety is the greatest priority for this population. The socket design should be total contact style with special considerations for comfort during sitting. The type of interface and suspension system used should take into consideration the patient's ability to don and doff the prosthesis and manage his or her hygiene independently. The frame should be lightweight and endoskeletal (with or without alignment ability) in design. Recommended foot and ankle components include a nonarticulated foot, such as the SACH or SAFE foot, or a simple articulated foot, such as the single-axis foot. Also included in this prescription will be a clear diagnostic socket, prosthetic socks, and cosmetic cover.

Functional Level Two (K2)

Patients in this functional category have the ability to perform limited community distance ambulation and traverse some environmental barriers. The major changes in the prosthetic prescription will be that the components should be alignable and the prosthetic foot can be a multiaxial or a flexible keel-type foot to allow for accommodation over uneven terrain. Suspension for this group can use a pin lock, sleeve suspension, or suction suspension with a sleeve and one-way expulsion valve in the socket.

Functional Level Three (K3)

Functional level K3 amputees are community distance ambulators who have the ability to traverse most environmental barriers and ambulate with variable cadence. Special considerations for this group will be the type of prosthetic foot. This will be some type of energy-storing (dynamic-response) foot and, depending on the activities that they are doing, can include a dynamic pylon or features that allow greater accommodation over uneven terrain. Foot and ankle components that incorporate hydraulic units with or without microprocessor control can also be considered in this population. A foot and ankle component with both microprocessor control and internal power may also be indicated in this class of patients. An additional consideration for prosthetic suspension is the use of an elevated vacuum technology.

Functional Level Four (K4)

Patients in this classification level have the ability or potential ability for ambulation that exceeds normal requirements. This may include sports or recreational activities that require high impact, stress, or energy levels that are typical of the prosthetic demands of a child, high-activity adult, or athlete. At this level, specialty components are running feet, waterproof foot and ankle components, and components with heel height adjustability. Suspension is also key for this group to avoid catastrophic value of the prosthetic connection during the activity. This may include use of a backup or secondary suspension method. Special considerations are also needed for the pediatric population because of growth and the wearing out of components secondary to the high use.

Knee Disarticulation

A knee disarticulation level amputation leaves the femur intact and creates a distal weight-bearing surface with retained thigh musculature. This long lever provides for potentially better control of the prosthetic limb and maintains the distal growth plate of the femur, which is important for individuals who are skeletally immature at the time of amputation. The disadvantages to this level of amputation are the discrepancy between the height of the prosthetic knee center and the height of the contralateral anatomic knee, as well as the decreased cosmetic appearance. As for the ankle disarticulation level, the prosthesis proximal trim line will depend on the patient's ability to weight bear on the distal end of the residual limb. If true, full weight-bearing occurs, then the proximal trim can be lowered to the subischial level. If there is no distal end weight bearing, then the residual limb is treated as a transfemoral amputation with use of a more traditional ischial containment socket.

Prescription Criteria

Socket design for this level typically includes an anatomically shaped socket with a flexible inner socket. The proximal trim lines of the socket will be determined based on distal weight-bearing tolerance as noted earlier. Interface and suspension options are generally the same as those for the transfemoral level, but there is also the possibility of creating suspension of the prosthesis with use of the femoral condyles. Polycentric knee units are commonly recommended to reduce the difference in knee centers from the prosthetic limb side to the intact limb side. Depending on the functional goals of the patient, additional features, such as a hydraulic mechanism, may be indicated and beneficial.

Prosthetic Prescription Algorithms for Transfemoral Amputees

The transfemoral prosthesis prescription is also based on the individual's current or potential functional abilities as well as their goals for prosthetic use. In addition to the components included in the transtibial prosthesis prescription, the transfemoral prescription will include the prosthetic knee. Other unique considerations for the prosthetic prescription at the transfemoral level include the greater need for safety and stability compared with the transtibial level. The provider should also take into consideration the greater metabolic cost of ambulation with a transfemoral prosthesis, the greater challenges associated with donning and doffing, and the concerns regarding sitting comfort with a transfemoral prosthesis.

Functional Level One (K1)

When evaluating the person in this functional category, it should be remembered that the goal is limited household walking on level surfaces and the ability to perform transfers. Primary prosthetic considerations are for safety and ease of prosthetic use. During stance phase, the knee needs to remain stable or locked, so the use of knee components, such as a weight-activated stance control knee or manual locking knee, are appropriate. Choosing a prosthetic foot, such as a SACH foot with a soft heel or a single axis foot, can also assist in maintaining knee stability by allowing or simulating ankle plantar flexion during the loading response phase of gait. This helps to keep the ground reaction force anterior to the knee center, thus creating a knee extension moment. The type of socket can be an ischial containment or quadrilateral style and should have a flexible inner liner and a flexible proximal brim with cutouts in the posterior portion to allow for sitting comfort. The socket material can either be a laminate or plastic. A gel liner with pin lock or lanyard can be used for suspension. A hip joint and waist belt method of suspension can be used if there are concerns about safety or if needed from a stability standpoint.

Functional Level Two (K2)

Transfemoral amputees who fall in this functional category typically still benefit from knee components that provide enhanced levels of stance phase stability while allowing greater swing phase motion and function for longer distances and a more normal gait pattern. Examples of prosthetic knees that provide these features include weight-activated stance control knees and polycentric knee units. Some high-level K2 ambulators may benefit from knee units that offer microprocessor stance phase control. Knee units that offer hydraulic or pneumatic swing phase control are not indicated for the K2 level transfemoral amputee, because these individuals do not have the ability or potential to ambulate with variable cadence. Components should be adjustable for alignment. The prosthetic foot can be a multiaxial type or a flexible keel style for better accommodation over uneven terrain.

Functional Level Three (K3)

Patients in this category should have the ability to perform full community ambulation and ambulate with variable cadence. The type of socket selected can be ischial containment or subischial. The socket should have a flexible inner liner with cutouts in the posterior portion to allow for sitting comfort and also a flexible proximal brim. Besides all the previous choices for suspension, elevated vacuum is a consideration at this level. Although stability and safety are still important, these individuals also require prosthetic knees that provide enhanced levels of function. Knee units with pneumatic or hydraulic swing phase control allow for variable cadence ambulation. Polycentric and microprocessor features provide for positive stance stability and a more natural and symmetrical gait pattern. An internally powered knee may be indicated in circumstance where stair and incline ascent are essential. At this level, multiaxial feet and energy-storing feet with or without a dynamic pylon can be considered.

Functional Level Four (K4)

Patients who achieve this level of classification have the ability to use their prosthesis for activities outside of normal ambulation. Because of this, they may benefit from a prosthesis that is used for their regular day-to-day activities as well as a prosthesis that is used for participation in specific athletic or recreational activities (Figure 10-17). The need for a specialty prosthesis may also depend on the frequency and intensity of the recreational or sport activity. If an entirely separate prosthesis is not required for participation in their desired activity, the patient may benefit from components with features that can serve multiple purposes. There is also the possibility of using a coupler or other quick disconnection devices that allow for the exchange of specific components for different activities. There are many varieties of prosthetic components to allow the amputee

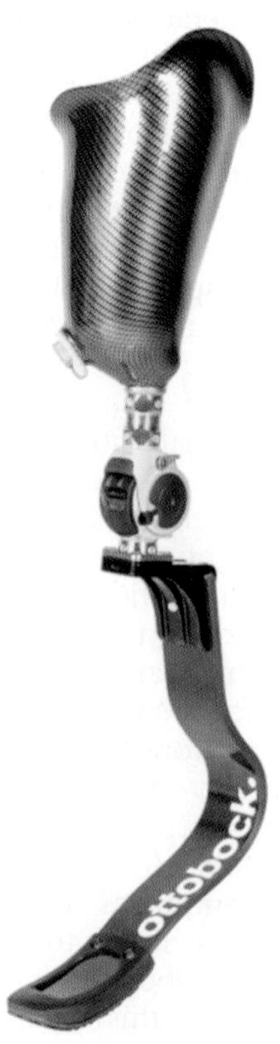

FIGURE 10-17 Specialty transfemoral prosthesis designed for running activities. (Fitness Prosthesis, Ottobock, Minneapolis, Minn.)

to participate in a full range of activities. For example, some components facilitate running and others can help the amputee to participate in scuba diving. Socket fit and suspension are particularly critical for these types of prostheses. The environment in which the prosthesis will be used for the desired activity also needs to be taken into consideration. In general, these require the use of components that are relatively simple and durable; however, some advanced microprocessor knees have now been designed to allow running, be waterproof, and perform in various environments. One of the biggest challenges is obtaining the funding for this type of prosthesis.

Hip Disarticulation and Hemipelvectomy Levels of Amputation

There are several challenges associated with prosthetic fitting and use with these more proximal levels of amputation, including the need to replace three anatomic joints and the significant increase in metabolic cost of ambulation.[43] Because there is a lack of a residual limb with these amputation levels, socket fit, prosthesis suspension, and alignment are also major considerations. Although newer lightweight components are available, the weight of the prosthesis is also a factor.

Prescription Criteria

Once called a "bucket socket," the socket needs to be total contact and extend superiorly to the iliac crest into the waistline and to the level of the thoracic spine for hemipelvectomy levels. It is essential to capture all motions inside this socket, because the patient uses trunk flexion and extension to produce and control motion in the prosthesis. The patient's functional ability and goals help to determine whether a single axis or multiaxial hip joint is used. For the knee joint, either a weight-activated stance control (safety knee) with extension assist or a microprocessor knee are typically recommended to provide enhanced stance phase stability of the prosthesis. Prosthetic foot recommendations include single axis feet for those who will primarily use the prosthesis over level surfaces to multiaxial or dynamic response feet for those with the potential for more community ambulation. To satisfy cosmetic needs, a custom-shaped cover or even a prosthetic skin that protects a patient's cover from incontinence or extreme conditions can be added.

Prosthetic Limb Fitting and Replacement Considerations

The length of time from amputation surgery to the clinic visit for prescription of a prosthesis will determine what type of prosthesis is used. With an initial prosthesis, basic components are used to allow for a quicker fitting. However, with current components and insurance reimbursement rates, it is usually better to prescribe the definitive prosthesis and have the prosthetist perform a socket replacement when the patient has a significant anatomic change to their residual limb.

A prosthesis will typically last for 3 to 5 years, depending on the activity of the patient and anatomic changes in their residual limb. Supplies such as gel liners and socks require replacement over a shorter period of time. They usually need to be ordered every 6 months to a year. A change in the residual limb (reduction or increase in size), a surgical revision of the residual limb, growth (children), and broken components all may require a new prosthetic prescription. The age of the prosthesis and how well the patient is doing with the prosthetic components will determine whether an entirely new prosthesis is required or whether only a socket replacement is needed. The other factor for consideration of a socket replacement versus providing a new prosthesis will be insurance guidelines and reimbursement. The typical wearing schedule for a new amputee is outlined in Table 10-3.

The patient should follow skin care guidelines and do frequent skin checks. Follow-up appointments should be made for the patient to see a physician and prosthetist during week 1.

Energy Consumption

When adults choose a walking speed that is comfortable and customary to them, their rate of oxygen consumption is fairly consistent and not significantly different during aging up to the age of 80 years.[5,39,46] When ambulating with a prosthesis and without assistive devices, the customary walking speed (CWS) also generates an oxygen consumption rate that closely mirrors the one for individuals without amputation or pathology affecting their gait. However, the amputee's gait is less efficient than that in individuals without an amputation, which results in greater levels of energy consumption for a given distance (metabolic cost). The metabolic cost of ambulation increases with more proximal levels of amputation. Thus, the increase in energy consumption for a given distance (metabolic cost) for a traumatic transtibial amputee walking with a prosthesis is around 25% and for a transfemoral amputee 63%.

Table 10-3 Typical Wearing Schedule for New Amputee

Day	Morning	Afternoon
	Week 1	
1	1 hour (20 minutes on, 20 minutes off)	0
2	1.5 hours (20 minutes on, 20 minutes off)	0
3	1 hour	1 hour
4	1.5 hours	1.5 hours
5	1.5 hours	1.5 hours
6	2 hours	1.5 hours
7	2 hours	2 hours
	Week 2	
8	2.5 hours	2 hours
9	2.5 hours	2.5 hours
10	2.5 hours	2.5 hours
11	3 hours	2.5 hours
12	3 hours	3 hours
13	3 hours	3 hours
14	3.5 hours	3 hours
Increase time to full time		

Values for dysvascular amputees at the same levels are 40% and 120%.[5]

Interestingly, ambulation with crutches with a swing through gait and without a prosthesis shows higher values for energy expenditure compared with prosthetic ambulation. Ambulation with a prosthesis thus shows improved energy conservation for these individuals in all cases except for the dysvascular transfemoral amputee who is often required to use crutches even with the prosthesis.

In general, dysvascular amputees have a slower CWS and a higher oxygen consumption rate than traumatic amputees with comparable amputation levels. In studies of residual limb length in transtibial amputees with respect to these parameters, no correlation could be found. However, transtibial amputees with short residual limbs showed a faster CWS and a lower oxygen cost than amputees with knee disarticulations or transfemoral amputations. This finding underscores the importance of preserving a knee joint if possible. For bilateral amputees, energy expenditure is greater than for unilateral amputees. Again, a distinction is found between dysvascular and traumatic bilateral amputees. The latter walk faster and with lower oxygen costs than their counterparts with comparable amputation levels.

Until recently, most studies on energy consumption and gait in amputees have been done on amputees using components with passive systems. In the emerging era of powered knees and foot/ankles, gait parameters can change. For example, an improvement of 10% in self-selected walking speed occurred when a powered foot/ankle was used compared with one without power.[23] In another study, the energy cost of walking was reduced when a bionic foot/ankle was used compared with walking with a dynamic carbon fiber foot.[13]

Bilateral Amputee Considerations

Amputees affected on both limbs, such as bilateral transfemoral amputations, bilateral transtibial amputations, or transfemoral amputation on one side and a transtibial amputation on the other side, face additional challenges. Bilateral amputations can be a result of disease processes, such as peripheral vascular disease, or traumatic injury. Up to 50% of unilateral dysvascular amputees will become bilateral amputees over a 5-year period.[48] Trauma from transportation or industrial accidents, electrocution, and war-related incidents, such as roadside bombs or land mines, are generally responsible for bilateral amputations that occur simultaneously.

Success as a unilateral amputee can be a helpful predictor of success in ambulation as a bilateral amputee. Energy consumption increases during prosthetic ambulation with bilateral amputations. The more proximal the amputations the more energy that is required. Energy requirements increase for unilateral amputees at a certain level and then increase further if there is another amputation on the contralateral limb at the same level. Because of these increased needs, there must be sufficient cardiac capacity and strength capacity to bear these extra burdens. Flexion contractures of the hips or knees can restrict or inhibit prosthetic ambulation in amputees in general but pose even greater issues for the bilateral amputee. The early intervention of the rehabilitation team is therefore paramount in the prevention of contractures.

In general, training with bilateral prostheses requires more time and effort. Because there is loss of proprioceptive sensation from both lower extremities with bilateral amputation, use of bilateral prostheses can cause a greater sense of insecurity that may result in a wider stance, slower pace, and the use of an assistive device. The bilateral amputee faces a greater challenge when negotiating ramps, curbs, stairs, uneven terrain, and other environmental barriers. Important skills would also include sitting and standing from a chair, as well as falling in a controlled manner and recovering from a fall.

In bilateral amputation, preservation of length can have a dramatic impact on the success of prosthetic ambulation. This is especially true if the knee can be preserved.[41] The proportion of amputees with bilateral transfemoral amputations secondary to peripheral vascular disease who will successfully ambulate with bilateral prostheses is small. If the bilateral transfemoral amputations are trauma related and peripheral vascular disease is not present, successful ambulation is more likely. Preservation of one or both knee joints will also contribute to successful ambulation.

The same pool of components used for unilateral amputees are used for bilateral amputees. Most of the same principles for selection apply. In a majority of cases the same ankle-foot complex should be used on both sides. However, this is not an absolute rule and a given individual may have requirements that cause a deviation from this guideline.

Although somewhat controversial, stubbies can provide a useful initial phase in the training of bilateral transfemoral amputees to ambulate.[16] Stubbies consist of an ischial containment socket, a pylon, and specially designed feet to give more stability when leaning backward. The pylons are adjusted to a length that facilitates sitting down in chairs. The feet are of two types. One version is triangular. The pylon inserts at the apex, which is anterior, and thus the base is posterior. The other version is a bean shape and the pylon attaches one third of the longitudinal distance. The longer arm of the foot is positioned posteriorly. Once the amputee has acquired balance and competence in ambulation, the stubbies are advanced first by increasing the pylon length, then by using standard prosthetic feet, and finally by inserting prosthetic knees.

Land Mine–Related Amputation Considerations

A *mine* is defined as "any munition placed under, on or near the ground or other surface area and designed to be detonated or exploded by the presence, proximity or contact of a person or vehicle." Land mines can remain active for decades after conflicts end, and antipersonnel land mines are a significant cause of injuries and amputation in many postconflict areas around the world. Although the production, sale, transfer, stockpiling, and use of antipersonnel mines have been banned by the Mine Ban Treaty, which opened for signature in 1997, a global total of 3628 mine casualties were still recorded in 2012.

Antipersonnel land mine design falls into one of three categories: blast mines, fragmentation mines, and bounding mines. Blast mines are activated when the victim treads directly on the mine, and these mines often drive fragments of casing, dirt, and footwear up into the tissue of the leg. Fragmentation mines are deployed above ground and are usually activated by a tripwire. Finally, bounding mines, sometimes referred to as "bouncing betty," are buried below ground and, when activated by pressure, explode a charge that drives each mine to a height of 1 m, where it detonates.

Land mines are specifically engineered to cause disability rather than death. Land mine injuries can be divided into three types. Type 1 injuries are caused by stepping or standing on a buried mine, resulting in traumatic leg amputation and loss of blood. Type 2 injuries, which consist of random penetrating injuries to the lower limbs, abdomen, and thorax, are caused by being within the maim radius of an exploding fragmentation mine. Type 3 injuries, which are more common in children and deminers, occur when victims are handling mines that explode. The results are most frequently severe upper limb injuries, blindness, hearing loss, and facial injury.

Although every mine victim will need emergency services, type 1 victims typically will be candidates for lower limb surgeries and a below-knee prosthesis. Not surprisingly, upper extremity amputation is most common with type 3 victims. Because upper extremity prosthetic services are often unavailable in mine-affected countries, survivors typically learn to function without a prosthesis or in some cases with a nonfunctional prosthetic cover.

The sustainable delivery of prosthetic and rehabilitation services in most mine-affected areas is challenging and must take into account the relatively low wages of local workers and the high cost of materials. An exhaustive review of state-of-the-art sustainable prosthetic services is beyond the scope of this chapter, but notable global efforts have been undertaken by a number of international nongovernmental and intergovernmental organizations. In the area of care delivery, these include the International Committee of the Red Cross and Handicapped International, although impressive education efforts targeting local workers have been launched and managed by the German GTZ organization and the U.S.-based Center for International Rehabilitation, among others.

Pediatric Lower Limb Loss

The epidemiology and outcomes of limb absence in the pediatric population is very different when compared with the adult population. In this population, congenital limb deficiencies outnumber acquired amputations by more than 2 to 1.[51,64] In contrast to the older adult population where prosthetic usage and benefit are sometimes uncertain, usage rates of prostheses in the pediatric amputee population are very high.[4,64] A study of 258 children with limb deficiencies between the ages of 2 and 21 years suggests that prostheses are often worn for more than 12 hours a day and are commonly used in activities, such as swimming, running, bicycling, and basketball.[64] Similar findings with regard to cycling, swimming, and sports activities have been reported elsewhere.[4] Health-related quality of life (HRQL) for children and adolescents with limb reduction deficiencies have been noted to be higher than those observed in a cohort of their peers with other chronic health conditions, including asthma, arthritis, diabetes, cystic fibrosis, cerebral palsy, and epilepsy[71] and HRQL findings are similar to able-bodied peers.[38] This last statement appears to be unaffected by the degree of lower limb deficiency, the presence of bilateral lower limb deficiency, or a concomitant upper limb deficiency. Only a slight decrease in both the diversity and frequency of social and skill-based activities among adolescents with lower limb deficiencies has been noted.[38]

Prevalence, Classification, and Epidemiology: Congenital Lower Limb Deficiencies

The prevalence of congenital limb *defects* has been reported at 21 cases per 10,000 births.[65] However, figures on limb defects include the prevalence rates of both syndactyly and polydactyly as well as upper limb reduction deficiencies, which are generally reported to be at least twice as common as lower limb reduction deficiencies (LLRDs). The prevalence of LLRD is much lower, with recent observations suggesting 1.6 to 3.0 cases per 10,000 live births in datasets drawn from New York State and the northern Netherlands, respectively.[32,65] These figures are consistent with the rates identified in other studies, which ranged from 1.0 to 6.8 per 10,000 births.[17] Bilateral LLRD appears to be common, reported among 37% of those with LLRDs[51]; similarly, upper limb reduction deficiencies have been reported in 40% of those with LLR.[51]

Several different mechanisms have been developed for the classification of LLRDs. Although formally replaced, the traditional classification system of Frantz and O'Rahilly is still in use in some practice environments, and an overview of this classification system is included in Table 10-4. Within this system, LLRDs are defined as either "terminal," with a complete loss of the distal extremity, or

Table 10-4 Frantz and O'Rahilly Traditional Classification System of Congenital Skeletal Lower Leg Deficiencies

Terminal Deficiencies		Intercalary Deficiencies	
No unaffected parts distal to the deficient portion		Immediate parts are deficient with proximal and distal elements present	
Transverse	**Paraxial**	**Paraxial**	**Phocomelia**
Complete absence distal to the level of loss	Complete longitudinal absence	Absence of preaxial or postaxial elements	Absence of central elements with foreshortening of the limb
Amelia Hemimelia	Hemimelia (tibial or fibular)	Hemimelia (tibial or fibular)	Phocomelia (femoral)

"intercalary," in which an intermediate portion of the limb is deficient, with intact elements of the limb both proximal and distal to the deficiency. Terminal LLRDs include both "transverse," in which there is complete absence of the limb at the level of the loss, and "paraxial," in which there is complete longitudinal absence of either the preaxial element (tibia) or postaxial element (fibula). Intercalary deficiencies include both "paraxial" events, suggesting the localized absence of elements of the tibia or fibula with preserved proximal and distal elements, or "phocomelia," in which there is an absence of central elements of the femur with foreshortening of the otherwise preserved lower limb. Within this structure, the terms "amelia" and "hemimelia" are also used to denote the complete or partial absence of the limb, respectively. Terms such as "fibular hemimelia" and "proximal femoral phocomelia" have persisted despite the formal replacement of this classification system.

The current standard in the classification of LLRDs was introduced in 1989 by the ISO, and identified as ISO 8545-1, Method of Describing Limb Deficiencies Present at Birth[59] (Table 10-5). Within the ISO classification, LLRDs are categorized as either "transverse" or "longitudinal." Transverse deficiencies suggest the absence of any skeletal elements distal to a certain level of the limb. The full description of a transverse deficiency requires the naming of the affected limb segment and the approximate location. Thus, transverse deficiencies of the thigh or leg should be qualified as being "complete," "upper third," "middle third," or "lower third."

According to the ISO system, any LLRD that is not "transverse" is considered "longitudinal," suggesting a reduction or absence of an element within the long axis of the limb. The naming of such deficiencies is done from proximal to distal, listing the bones or segments and whether these segments are totally or partially absent. Within this nomenclature, a hypothetical deficiency formally described as paraxial tibial hemimelia might be described as "longitudinal deficiencies of the tibia total, tarsus partial, ray 1 total." Similarly, proximal femoral focal deficiencies or PFFDs as they have long been called are now formally described as "longitudinal deficiencies of the femur, partial."

More recently, a 2011 publication by the Active Malformations Surveillance Program at the Brigham and Women's Hospital in Boston, Massachusetts suggested that the full classification of congenital limb deficiencies should also include the apparent etiology.[24] These include the categories of chromosomal abnormalities, known syndromes, Mendelian inheritance, familiar inheritance, presumed vascular disruption defects, teratogenic exposure, and unknown causes.

Table 10-5 International Organization for Standardization Classification System of Congenital Skeletal Lower Limb Deficiencies

Transverse Deficiencies	Longitudinal Deficiencies	
No unaffected parts distal to the deficient portion	Any deficiency that is not transverse, named from proximal to distal	
Thigh	**Femur**	
Complete	Total	
Upper third	Partial	
Middle third		
Lower third		
Leg	**Tibia**	**Fibula**
Complete	Total	Total
Upper third	Partial	Partial
Middle third		
Lower third		
Tarsal	**Tarsus**	
Complete	Total	
Partial	Partial	
Metatarsal	**Metatarsals (1-5)**	
Complete	Total	
Partial	Partial	
Phalangeal	**Phalanges (1-5)**	
Complete	Total	
Partial	Partial	

Classification and Etiology: Acquired Amputation

Pediatric-acquired amputations should be described with the same ISO system and classification system that is used in the adult population with acquired limb loss. (Refer to Table 10-1 for the details of this classification system.)

The leading cause of acquired amputation in the pediatric population is trauma with U.S. national statistics estimating roughly 1000 new cases each year.[11] Within this category, the most commonly encountered mechanisms of injury are those in which a body part is caught in or between objects (21%), followed by power tools and/or other cutting instruments (16%), lawn mower injuries (14%), other machinery (14%), and motor vehicle accidents (9%).[55] The ages of the children at the time of amputation vary greatly with roughly equal prevalence figures for children aged 0 to 4, 5 to 9, 10 to 14, and 15 to 17 years.[11] The incidence of pediatric-acquired amputation is much higher in males than females with national statistics suggesting a 3 to 1 ratio.[11] Children living in poverty, those identified as racial or ethnic minorities, or living in single parent homes also appear to be at elevated risks for amputation as a result of injury.[69]

With respect to disease, malignant tumor remains the most common cause of amputation, accounting for over half of these events with the highest incidence occurring in the second decade of life.[69] Commonly encountered tumors include osteogenic sarcoma, and Ewing sarcoma. The orthopedic management of such tumors often involves a choice between limb salvage and amputation. Research findings suggest no difference among the quality of life, body image, self-esteem, and social support between the two approaches in the pediatric population.[33,52] However, patients with more functional lower limbs appear to have better quality of life than their peers, irrespective of whether they underwent amputation or limb salvage surgery.[52]

Fibular Deficiencies, Syme, and Transtibial Amputations

Congenital fibular deficiencies are generally managed with elective amputation, orthopedic lengthening procedures, or aggressive accommodative shoe lifts. This decision is largely based on the viability of the ipsilateral foot for structural weight bearing and the extent of the limb shortening relative to the contralateral limb.[3] Long-term follow-up studies in adults have failed to observe appreciable differences in HRQL or physical function between the two orthopedic pathways of elective amputation and lengthening procedures.[66]

In the presence of a complete or partially absent fibula, a compromised ipsilateral foot, or severe overall limb shortening, an elective Syme amputation is often performed. Because of the absence of the distal fibular condyle, the characteristic bulbous distal end of the residual limb is less pronounced. The remaining tibia often bows anteriorly and presents with a sharply defined, prominent tibial crest. As the child ages, a progressive leg length discrepancy becomes more apparent. However, this is often beneficial as it allows more space for more dynamic, higher profile prosthetic foot and ankle mechanisms.

Among both transtibial and ankle disarticulation level amputations, several authors have observed a tendency in both congenital and pediatric-acquired cases for the tibia to develop angular deformities. In cases in which these deformities become pronounced enough to affect prosthetic function, they can be corrected via surgical osteotomy or hemiepiphysiodesis.[25]

Tibial Deficiencies and Knee Disarticulation Amputation

The management of congenital tibial deficiencies is largely dependent upon the extent of the tibial deficit and the viability of the knee extensors. In cases in which the proximal tibia is well formed and functional knee extensors are present, orthopedic management includes proximal tibial-fibular synostosis and ablation of a typically unsound residual foot with a resultant ankle disarticulation amputation, in which the fibula generally serves as the long bone.[54,58] In the absence of a proximal tibial segment and functional knee extensors, an elective knee disarticulation is generally recommended.[54,58]

Whenever possible, knee disarticulation amputations are preferred over transfemoral amputations in the pediatric population as this spares the distal growth plate of the femur and ultimately permits a longer, more functional residual limb through adolescence and adulthood. In addition, this amputation level retains the balance of the hip musculature, generally enables distal load-bearing, and avoids the potential for postamputation terminal bony overgrowth. The greatest disadvantage associated with adult-acquired knee disarticulation amputations, the inability to match the prosthetic knee center height to the contralateral anatomic knee center, can be readily addressed in pediatric cases by correctly timing a distal femoral epiphysiodesis. This shortens the residual femur creating sufficient space to use a broader range of prosthetic knee mechanisms.

Longitudinal Deficiency of the Femur, Partial

Historically referred to as proximal femoral focal deficiency or PFFD, the management of partial longitudinal deficiencies of the femur, partial (LDFP) can be fairly variable. The Aitken[1] classification, initially proposed in 1969, is still used to categorize the instability present in the hips of these limbs according to the presence and development of the femoral head and acetabulum.[1] Thus, in addition to the inherent leg length inequality, these cases present with varying degrees of femoral malrotation, instability of the proximal joints and inadequacy of proximal musculature. The more commonly encountered orthopedic management strategies include an elective ankle disarticulation amputation combined with knee fusion or a rotationplasty. In the case of the former, the combination of the fused knee and the ablated foot creates a functional residual limb similar to that seen in a knee disarticulation amputation. Thus, it is generally capable of some level of distal end bearing and distal anatomic suspension of the prosthesis. Unlike an acquired knee disarticulation, the functionality of this limb type is often affected by the variable instability at the hip joint that characterizes this limb deficiency.

In rotationplasty the child's foot is turned 180 degrees, allowing the intact ankle joint to mimic the function of the knee. This approach has also been advocated in cases of limb salvage following tumor resection. The acceptability of this approach to individual patients has been mixed. The functionality of this procedure in response to both LDFP and tumor resection is very high,[64] including a frequent return to sports activities in the latter group.[27] However, individuals have identified difficulties in psychological and emotional adjustments to the appearance of the modified limb, particularly during adolescence.[21] These negative affects must be balanced against the reality that similar challenges have also been identified with other possible orthopedic approaches.

Amputation Level and Energy Expenditure in Congenital and Acquired Pediatric Lower Limb Deficiencies

It has generally been established that in the adult population the energy costs of walking following lower limb amputation increases as the amputation level ascends proximally up the lower limb and that amputees adopt slower self-selected walking speeds.[67] However, this principle does not appear to apply to all pediatric cases.[30] As expected, among the most proximal amputation levels of transfemoral and hip disarticulation, there is a 20% to 30% reduction in self-selected walking speed coupled with an increase in metabolic energy costs approximating 150% of normal.[30] Similarly, children with bilateral lower limb amputations walk at a slightly reduced self-selected walking speed with a slightly elevated heart rate.[30] However, children with ankle disarticulations, transtibial amputations, and knee disarticulations appear to walk at essentially the same self-selected walking speeds and oxygen costs as their nonaffected peers.[30]

Financial and Vocational Impacts of Pediatric Limb Loss

The cost of pediatric limb loss to individual families has only recently been addressed in the academic literature.[69] Survey data suggest that approximately 40% of these families have borne out-of-pocket expenses for prostheses with an average annual cost of $1321. Approximately a quarter of the surveyed families indicated that they have had an insurance claim for a new prosthesis denied. Investments of time in procuring and maintaining a prosthesis are also high. Travel times to and from prosthetic providers were reported to be as high as 16 hours and the time spent in the office as high as 9 hours. Cumulatively, the average time spent in transit or on site for prosthetic appointments was 5 hours per visit and 30 hours per year.[69] Additional time investments were made in the form of physical and occupational therapy, related and unrelated hospitalizations, and emergency room visits, in which 25% of surveyed families reported at least one visit in the past year and 10% reported multiple visits.[69] Because of these time requirements, the majority of the parents of these children will make some type of work adjustment as a result of their child's limb loss, including changing their work hours, taking days off, taking extended leaves of absence, or making a job change.[69]

It has generally been established that in the adult population the energy costs of walking following lower limb amputation increases as the amputation level ascends proximally up the lower limb and that amputees adopt slower self-selected walking speeds.[67] However, this principle does not appear to apply to all pediatric cases.[30] As expected, among the most proximal amputation levels of transfemoral and hip disarticulation, there is a 20% to 30% reduction in self-selected walking speed coupled with an increase in metabolic energy costs approximating 150% of normal.[30] Similarly, children with bilateral lower limb amputations walk at a slightly reduced self-selected walking speed with a slightly elevated heart rate.[30] However, children with Syme, transtibial, and through knee amputations appear to walk at essentially the same self-selected walking speeds and oxygen costs as their nonaffected peers.[30]

Future Considerations

Artificial limb technology and amputation rehabilitation have experienced great advances over the past 20 years. These advances include surgical techniques that have made limb salvage and limb sparing more viable options in cases of extremity trauma. These new surgical techniques have complicated early decision making in cases of extremity trauma when both limb salvage and amputation are being considered. Additional advances include the development of artificial limb components with sophisticated microprocessor control and active power systems as well as the development of virtual reality rehabilitation training environments. These developments have improved outcomes for individuals with amputations, but they are also typically associated with increased financial costs and have created new challenges for rehabilitation providers. The appropriate application of these advances in the clinical setting requires highly specialized knowledge and skills. The prosthetic component option with the most sophisticated technology is not always the most appropriate option and issues of insurance reimbursement and potential financial burden on the patient also need to be taken into consideration.

New developments in regenerative medicine, transplant immunology, brain-computer interfaces, and robotics are on the horizon. These advances have the potential to further revolutionize the treatment and outcomes of individuals with amputations. For clinicians to provide the highest quality care to individuals with amputations in the future, they must maintain the most up-to-date training and clinical experience with new technology and procedures. The provision of clinical services is likely to become more and more specialized over time and require provider teams with greater involvement from disciplines, such as biomechanical engineering. With these advances and future opportunities, it is anticipated that the field of amputee rehabilitation will continue to be an exciting, challenging, and rewarding area of practice.

Normal Human Gait

Introduction

Normal human gait can appear simple and effortless to the casual observer. However, it is actually a complex phenomenon and understanding human gait requires a solid knowledge of biomechanical principles. Appreciation of normal gait is essential to the evaluation and management of the gait deviations seen in individuals with amputations who ambulate with the use of prosthetic limbs.

Gait Terminology

Stride: The basic unit of gait which includes all activity between initial contact of a limb (reference limb) and the subsequent initial contact of that same limb.

Stride Length: The distance traveled during one gait cycle or stride.

Step Length: The distance traveled during one step (initial contact to end of preswing on same limb).

Step Width: The distance between the center of the feet during the double limb support portion of the gait cycle when both feet are in contact with the ground. This distance is normally 7 to 8 cm.

Cadence: The number of steps taken in a given period of time (commonly expressed as steps per minute). Average cadence during normal human ambulation is 80 to 110 steps per minute. This corresponds to an average walking speed of 60 to 80 m/min.

Stance Phase: The portion of the gait cycle during which the reference limb is in contact with the ground. During normal walking, this portion accounts for approximately 60% of the gait cycle. Stance phase includes initial contact, loading response, midstance, terminal stance, and preswing.

Swing Phase: The portion of the gait cycle during which the reference limb in NOT in contact with the ground. During normal walking, this portion accounts for approximately 40% of the gait cycle. Swing phase includes initial swing, midswing, and terminal swing.

Single Limb Support: The portion of the gait cycle during which only ONE limb is in contact with the ground. During normal gait, this segment accounts for 40% of the total gait cycle. Single limb support includes midstance and terminal stance.

Double Limb Support: The portion of the gait cycle during which TWO limbs are in contact with the ground. During normal gait, this portion accounts for 20% of the gait cycle. Double limb support includes three different components of the gait cycle: initial contact, loading response, and preswing.

Functional Tasks of Normal Gait: The functional tasks of normal human gait are typically described as: weight acceptance, single limb support, and limb advancement.

Traditional Gait Terminology: This terminology is no longer the preferred terminology used in the description of gait. This terminology generally describes isolated points in time during the gait cycle, such as "heel strike" and "foot flat," rather than periods of time during ambulation. This terminology primarily serves as a historical reference, but is occasionally still used in the clinical setting.

Rancho Los Amigos Gait Terminology: The Rancho Los Amigos Terminology is the preferred terminology to be used in the description of gait (Figure 10-18).

Stance Phase

- *Initial Contact:* Point in time when foot comes in contact with the ground.
- *Loading Response (LR):* Initial contact to the time when the contralateral foot leaves the ground.
- *Midstance (MSt):* From the time the contralateral foot leaves the ground to the time that the ipsilateral heel leaves the ground.
- *Terminal Stance (TSt):* From the time that the ipsilateral heel leaves the ground to the time of contralateral foot initial contact with the ground.
- *Preswing (PSw):* From the time of contralateral foot initial contact with the ground to the time that the ipsilateral foot leaves the ground.

Swing Phase

- *Initial Swing (ISw):* The time from when the foot leaves the ground to ipsilateral foot alignment with the contralateral ankle.
- *Midswing (MSw):* The time from ankle and foot alignment to the swing leg tibia becoming vertical.
- *Terminal Swing (TSw):* The time from the tibia reaching a vertical position to initial contact of the swing foot with the ground.

Determinants of Gait

The six determinants of gait were originally described by Saunders and Inman in 1953.[53] These determinants were used to describe strategies for achieving the most efficient gait through minimizing the movement of the center of gravity (COG). As a person ambulates with a normal gait pattern, the COG follows a smooth, sinusoidal path in the frontal, transverse, and sagittal planes. The actual COG

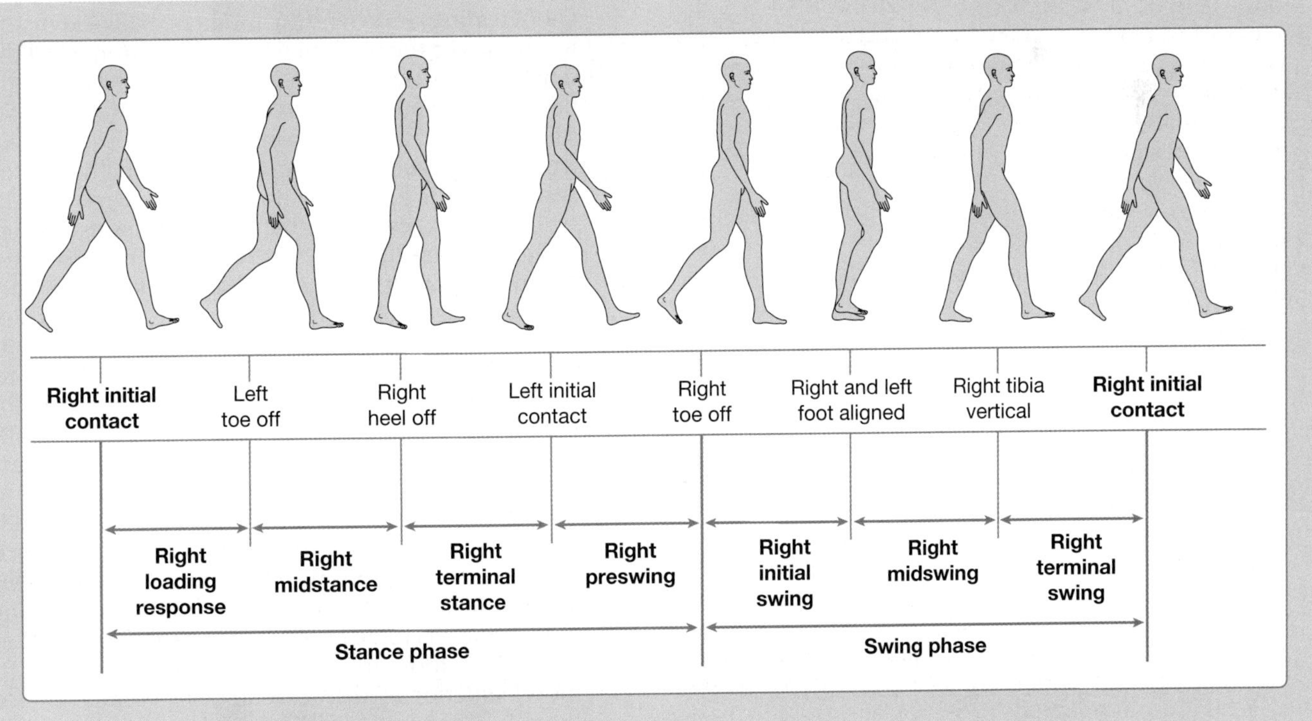

FIGURE 10-18 Gait cycle and phases of gait. (From Esquinazi E, Talaty M: Gait analysis: technology and clinical applications. In Braddom RL, editor: *Physical medicine and rehabilitation,* ed 4, Philadelphia, 2011, Elsevier/Saunders, pp 99-116.)

displacement is approximately 5 cm (2 inches) in each plane during normal gait. Descriptions of the determinants of gait vary in different references and have been revised over time.[12,46,67] The determinants can be divided into three that occur at the level of the pelvis and three that occur in the knee, foot, and ankle mechanisms. The six determinants can be described as pelvic rotation in the horizontal plane, pelvic tilt in the frontal plane, lateral displacement of the pelvis, early knee flexion, foot and ankle mechanisms, and late knee flexion.

Kinematics

Sagittal Plane Kinematics. Sagittal plane kinematics describe the motion that occurs at the hip, knee, and ankle during normal human gait in the sagittal plane[18,42,46,67] (Figure 10-19).

Hip: The hip begins the gait cycle in approximately 30 degrees of flexion at the time of initial contact. The hip undergoes gradual extension throughout stance phase. The hip reaches maximum extension of 10 degrees at the end of terminal stance. At the beginning of preswing, the hip begins to flex before the foot leaves contact with the ground. The hip gradually flexes during the swing phase reaching peak flexion of just over 30 degrees just before initial contact.

Knee: The knee begins the gait cycle with approximately 5 degrees of flexion at initial contact. The knee flexes slightly during loading response to 10 to 15 degrees. Once the limb is in single limb support at the beginning of midstance, the knee begins to extend and it reaches −5 degrees of full extension before beginning a period of rapid knee flexion at the end of stance phase and into initial swing phase. During swing phase, the knee reaches maximum flexion of approximately 60 degrees during midswing before moving into a period of knee extension. The knee reaches full extension at the end of swing phase and begins to flex slightly just before initial contact.

Ankle: The ankle begins the gait cycle in a neutral position at the time of initial contact. There is rapid plantar flexion to approximately 10 degrees of plantar flexion that occurs during the loading response. This period of plantar flexion is followed by a time of gradual dorsiflexion that continues through midstance and terminal stance. Peak dorsiflexion of 10 degrees occurs just before preswing. During preswing, the ankle begins to plantar flex rapidly before the foot leaving contact with the floor. This plantar flexion continues into early swing and reaches a maximum of 20 degrees before the ankle moves back into a neutral position during the remainder of the swing phase.

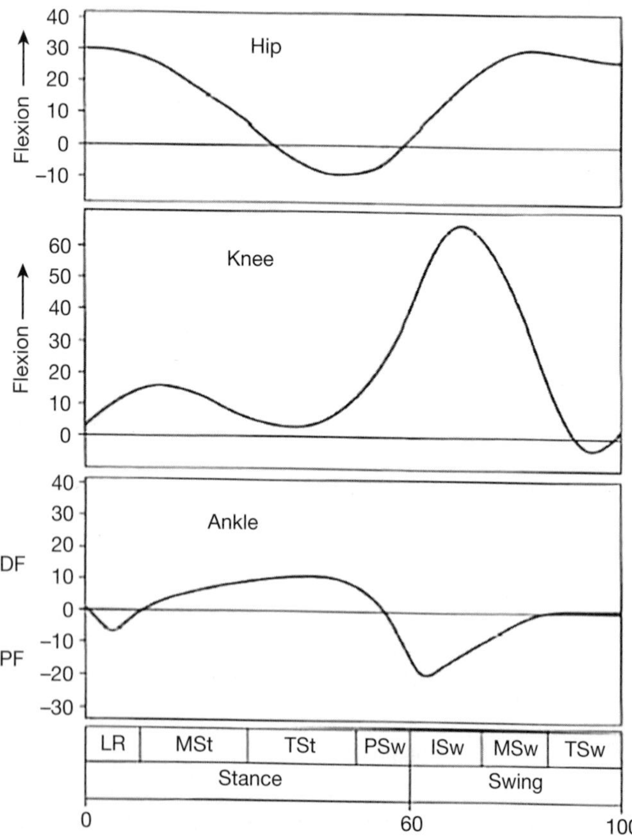

FIGURE 10-19 Sagittal plane kinematics for the hip, knee, and ankle during each phase of the normal gait cycle.

Kinetics

Sagittal Plane Kinetics. Sagittal plane kinetics describe the forces that occur across the hip, knee, and ankle joints during gait. Because these forces are created when the limb is in contact with the ground, they are described only during the stance phase of the gait cycle (Figure 10-20).

Hip: The ground reaction force (GRF) is initially anterior to the hip point of rotation, which creates a flexion moment on the hip at initial contact and during the loading response. During midstance, as the tibia rotates forward, the hip moves anterior to the GRF creating an extension moment. This extension torque across the hip remains in place throughout the remainder of stance phase and activation of the hip flexors is required to overcome this moment in late stance to initiate hip flexion.

Knee: At initial contact, the GRF is normally located anterior to the knee, but the GRF quickly moves posterior to the knee during the loading response, which creates a flexion moment at the knee. This force must be opposed by the knee extensors to keep the knee from collapsing. The knee flexion moment remains in place until terminal stance at which time the GRF moves back anterior to the knee. At the end of preswing, just before the foot is leaving the ground, the period of rapid knee flexion begins and once the GRF moves posterior to the knee, the knee flexion moment that is created helps to facilitate this motion.

Ankle: The GRF is initially located posterior to the ankle at the time of initial contact, which creates a plantar flexion moment. During the loading response, the plantar flexion moment continues at the ankle and this torque has to be resisted by the ankle dorsiflexors to prevent foot drop. During midstance, the GRF moves anterior to the ankle and in terminal stance, there is a strong dorsiflexion moment at the ankle, which must be opposed by the ankle plantar flexors to limit forward progression of the tibia. In preswing,

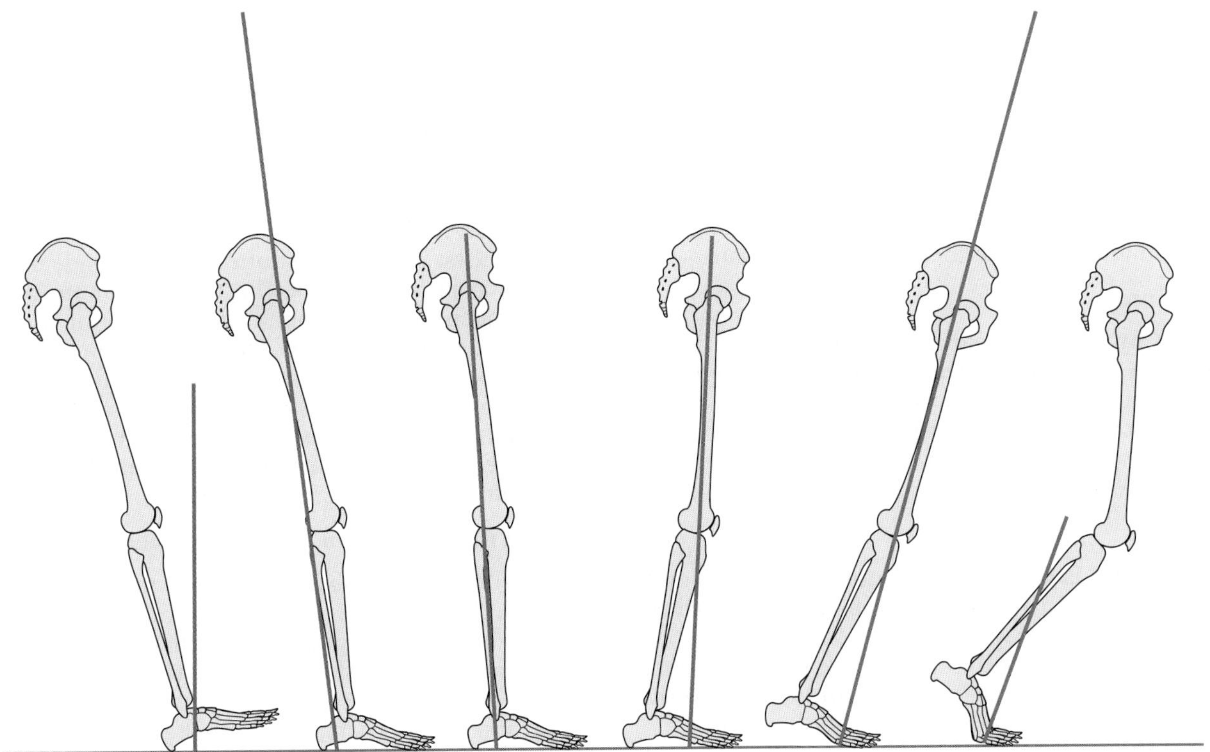

FIGURE 10-20 Location and relative magnitude of the ground reaction force vector (GRFV) in relation to the lower limb during stance phase of gait.

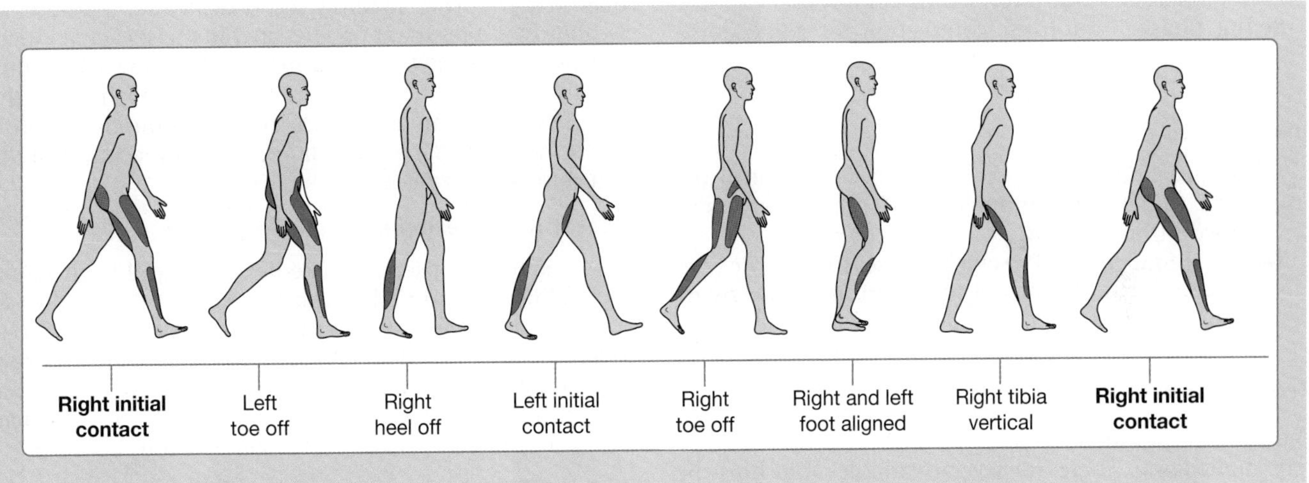

FIGURE 10-21 Normal gait cycle terminology with selected limb electromyography representation. Human figures in the different phases of gait with superimposed primary muscle activity. Muscle shade intensity is roughly proportional to strength of muscle contraction. (From Esquinazi E, Talaty M: Gait analysis: technology and clinical applications. In Braddom RL, editor: *Physical medicine and rehabilitation*, ed 4, Philadelphia, 2011, Elsevier/Saunders, pp 99-116.)

a dorsiflexion moment remains at the ankle. Thus, ankle plantar flexion motion is created by concentric contraction of the ankle plantar flexors and this helps to propel the stance limb forward.

Muscle Activity

Muscle Activity during Gait. Pelvic and lower extremity muscles generate forces to produce movement, resist ground reaction forces, and maintain stability. The timing and extent of these muscle contractions as reported in the literature varies in different references. The information included here is meant to provide a general description of the muscle activity that is occurring in the lower extremity to either produce or inhibit motion in the sagittal plane during dynamic gait. The muscle groups listed in the following sections are either active or inactive during different phases of the gait cycle. For the purpose of this text, only the gait cycle phase in which the muscle group is active is listed (Figure 10-21).

Hip Extensors

Late Swing: Concentric contraction to rotate the thigh posteriorly and to stabilize the limb in preparation for weight-bearing in stance phase.

Early Stance: Concentric or isometric contraction to control hip and knee flexion and stabilize the limb.

Hip Flexors

Late Stance Phase: Eccentric contraction to slow and control posterior rotation (extension) of the thigh.

Swing Phase: Concentric contraction to initiate hip flexion and accelerate the swing limb forward.

Knee Extensors

Initial Contact and Loading Response: Eccentric contraction to control knee flexion and prevent knee buckling.

Late Stance and Early Swing Phase: Eccentric contraction to control collapse of the knee and prevent early heel rise.

Knee Flexors

Early and Midswing Phase: Concentric contraction in swing phase to produce knee flexion and facilitate foot clearance in swing phase.

Late Swing Phase and Early Stance Phase: Eccentric and isometric contraction to control knee extension and stabilize the limb before weight bearing.

Ankle Dorsiflexors

Early Stance Phase: Eccentric contraction to control ankle plantar flexion in loading response.

Swing Phase: Concentric contraction for ankle dorsiflexion and to facilitate foot clearance during swing phase.

Ankle Plantar Flexors

Midstance Phase: Eccentric contraction to control the ankle dorsiflexion moment and prevent excessive forward tibia rotation.

Terminal Stance and Preswing Phase: Concentric contraction for push-off and acceleration of the swing limb.

Prosthetic Gait Deviations

The proper alignment of a lower limb prosthesis can be very challenging. There are several variables that must be considered. These include the choice of prosthetic componentry that has been selected for the individual patient, the position of these prosthetic knee and foot mechanisms relative to the prosthetic socket, and the extent to which each individual has learned to walk effectively with their prosthesis. In light of these considerations, it is unsurprising to note that there are a number of commonly observed gait deviations and that these may result from shortcomings in any of the considerations listed earlier, namely component selection, alignment, and patient training and walking ability. Given these complexities, many clinicians have found value in approaching prosthetic gait analysis in a systematic way. This includes analyzing gait in both the sagittal and coronal planes with consideration of each of the major joint segments across the various phases of the gait cycle. Commonly observed deviations, along with their potential causes, will be discussed.

Transtibial Gait Deviations

Although less dramatic than those seen with transfemoral prostheses, there are a number of gait deviations that are commonly observed in patients using transtibial prostheses.

Uneven Stride Length

Best observed in the sagittal plane, uneven stride lengths can manifest as either a shortened sound side step or a shortened prosthetic step. The former is more common and frequently results from a patient's lack of confidence in their prosthesis. This is especially common in newer amputees that have not yet developed confidence in their prosthesis and can improve with training and experience. By contrast, a shortened prosthetic step is frequently caused by a knee flexion contracture that prevents full extension of the knee joint in terminal swing.

Abrupt Knee Flexion in Loading Response

During loading response, a slight, smooth knee flexion is desired. There are several variables that may create a more abrupt knee flexion event. This will result if the foot is excessively dorsiflexed or if the socket is excessively flexed above the prosthetic foot. This deviation can present suddenly if a patient changes their shoe to one with a higher heel, effectively dorsiflexing the angle between the plantar surface of the shoe and the patient's knee. This will also be seen in patients who fail to eccentrically contract their quadriceps during loading response, either because of weakness or a resultant pain created in the socket. As such, this deviation may be seen more frequently in shorter limb lengths. Finally, the relative stiffness of the heel of the prosthetic foot can also affect this deviation. Stiffer prosthetic heel mechanisms will increase the abruptness of stance phase knee flexion.

Absent Knee Flexion in Loading Response

Less frequently observed, knee flexion may also be absent in loading response. Although this may be the product of a socket that is excessively extended, a foot that is excessively plantar flexed or a prosthetic foot with excessive stiffness in the toe, it may also be a voluntary compensation by patients with weak quadriceps who are apprehensive about allowing this normal gait event to occur.

Visible "Pistoning"

Pistoning is a term often used to describe a problematic movement of the residual limb in the socket. This is often best seen in the coronal plane as the limb reseats into the bottom of the socket during full weight acceptance. Depending on the type of suspension used by the patient, some degree of pistoning may be expected. For example, a visible amount of pistoning is likely to be seen with both anatomic and strap suspension systems. Pistoning may result from compromised suspension, such as a torn sealing sleeve in a suction suspension system, or in a poorly fitting socket in which the volume of the socket and the limb do not match.

Coronal Knee Instability

During midstance a modest varus moment is generally accepted at the knee. Variations are generally a product of prosthetic alignment. A prosthetic foot positioned relatively outset underneath the socket will create a valgus moment. When a prosthetic foot is positioned with an excessively inset alignment, the resultant varus moment can be excessive.

Lateral Trunk Bending

Although more commonly observed in the transfemoral population, a lateral trunk bend over the side of the prosthesis will sometimes be seen in patients using a transtibial prosthesis. This generally suggests a failure to fully load the prosthesis, either because of socket discomfort or inadequate training. This deviation can become a fixed habit if not addressed early in prosthetic gait training.

Early/Late Heel Rise

Deviations to the timing of heel rise can occur at either extreme. An early heel rise is generally the product of excessive ankle dorsiflexion or an excessively posterior position of the foot beneath the socket. Either misalignment effectively shortens the toe lever of the prosthesis and can result in an abrupt loading of the sound side limb. An excessively flexible prosthetic toe or keel will have the same effect. A late heel rise may be a product of an excessively plantar flexed foot, a foot that has been placed anteriorly beneath the prosthesis, or a prosthetic foot with a very rigid keel. All three scenarios will lengthen the prosthetic toe lever, making it difficult for the patient to get over their prosthetic toes during terminal stance.

Abrupt Sound Side Loading

An excessively short or flexible prosthetic toe lever will cause a patient to roll-over to the toe of the prosthesis and "drop-off" on to the sound side limb. This abrupt loading has been linked to elevated risks for osteoarthritis of the knee and hip. Evidence has consistently demonstrated that the dynamic resistances that characterized energy-storing and release prosthetic feet reduce the magnitude of this prosthetic "drop-off" and reduce the abruptness of sound side limb loading.

Sound Side Vaulting

When patients are concerned about clearing the toe of their prosthesis during swing phase, they may adapt a "vaulting" strategy in which a concentric burst of the sound side plantar flexors raises them up on their toes, functionally lengthening the stance limb and ensuring swing phase clearance. Seen in both transtibial and transfemoral gait patterns, this deviation may suggest that the prosthesis is too long or has inadequate suspension, allowing it to functionally lengthen during swing phase. It may also be either a gait habit or preference.

Transfemoral Gait Deviations

Gait deviations at the transfemoral level are both more common and more pronounced. In contrast to the bony anatomy that characterizes most transtibial limbs, transfemoral limbs are relatively fleshy, compromising the ability of patients at this amputation level to control their prostheses through their sockets. In addition, irrespective of the various design approaches, there is always some level of instability associated with prosthetic knee mechanisms that will ultimately affect gait mechanics.

Asymmetrical Step Lengths

At the transfemoral level, step symmetry is often characterized by a long prosthetic step followed by a shorter sound side step. Particularly for the novice walker, apprehension of prosthetic knee instability creates a reluctance to fully load the prosthesis in midstance and terminal stance. As a result, patients tend to take shorter steps with their sound side. This habit is often formed early in rehabilitation and can persist in the absence of corrective gait training. Additionally, many patients at this level develop some level of hip flexor tightness. If this is not adequately accommodated in the alignment of the prosthesis, limitation in hip extensor mobility can also prevent patients from taking a suitable sound side step.

Knee Instability During Loading Response

The same variables that can create abrupt knee flexion during loading response in transtibial walkers can create knee instability for transfemoral walkers. In the absence of an anatomic knee joint, knee extension on the prosthetic side is a product of active hip extension and the mechanical stability properties of the knee. As a result, any factors increasing the knee flexion moment represent a threat to patient stability. Accordingly, at this amputation level many patients prefer prosthetic feet with softer heels safely aligned in relative plantar flexion. This is especially relevant for patients with shorter limbs or weaker hip extensors.

External Foot Rotation

The fleshy nature of the transfemoral limb makes this amputation level more prone to rotational instabilities. This tendency can be exacerbated by any of the alignment characteristics identified earlier that will increase the knee flexion moment during loading response or by an improperly fitting socket. Among newer patients, this deviation may occur when the prosthesis is donned incorrectly in excessive external rotation. Less frequently, the prosthesis may simply be misaligned.

Lateral Trunk Bending

Lateral trunk bending is one of the more commonly observed deviations among transfemoral amputees. In able-bodied walkers, the hip abductors activate in midstance to maintain a level pelvis in single limb support. Following transfemoral amputation, the ability of the prosthetic socket to stabilize the residual femur in the coronal plane is variable, generally decreasing with shorter limb lengths. In the absence of traditional coronal hip stabilization, it is very common for amputees at this level to perform a compensatory lateral trunk bend ipsilateral to the prosthesis during single limb support to bring their weight over the prosthesis. With proper training and practice, this pattern can be altered such that the lateral shift occurs at the hips rather than at the shoulders, thereby reducing the trunk compensations. However, in shorter transfemoral limbs, because of the difficulty in stabilizing the residual femur, some amount of compensatory trunk bend is to be expected.

Excessive Lumbar Lordosis

As stated earlier, hip flexor tightness is common at this amputation level. If the alignment of the prosthesis fails to accommodate this tightness, the patient is forced to stand with excessive lumbar lordosis. Increasing the flexion angle of the socket and sliding the prosthetic knee joint posteriorly underneath the socket will accommodate hip flexor tightness and reduce the need for compensatory lordosis.

Excessive Heel Rise

The amount of heel rise seen in the transfemoral prosthesis should generally match that observed on the sound side. However, the ability to regulate this variable will depend upon the knee joint mechanism. In nonhydraulic knee joints, the friction settings of the knee can only be optimized to a single walking speed. Settings that limit heel rise at higher walking speeds will be perceived as too stiff at lower walking velocities. Conversely, friction settings that allow an appropriate amount of heel rise during self-selected speeds will allow excessive heel rise at elevated speeds. As a result, nonhydraulic knee mechanisms are generally not used for patients capable of variable speed ambulation. Hydraulic knee joints provide variable resistance to knee motion, with increasing resistance at elevated speeds. Excessive heel rise occurring with a hydraulic knee mechanism can often be addressed by altering the resistance settings of the knee.

Swing Phase Whips

The rotation of the prosthetic knee joint underneath the socket will determine the tracking of the knee joint during gait. When the prosthetic knee is set in excessive internal rotation, a lateral "whip" is observed as the heel deviates laterally with prosthetic knee flexion. Conversely, a knee joint set in excessive external rotation will create a medial "whip" as the heel of the prosthesis deviates medially with knee flexion. In many instances, whips can be reduced or eliminated by adjusting the rotational position of the knee beneath the socket. However, some patients generate rotational movements in their hips during limb advancement, creating whips that cannot be aligned out of the prosthesis.

Circumduction

Circumduction describes a pattern of hip motion in which swing phase flexion is coupled with abduction to ensure clearance of a swing leg. This compensation can occur for several reasons. Patients who are apprehensive about sagittal knee instability may employ this strategy to reduce the need for physiologic knee flexion in swing phase. Alternately, the various extension assist mechanisms of the knee joints may be set too high. Prostheses with a very safe alignment, in which the knee joint is positioned relatively posteriorly under the socket, can make it difficult for patients to create knee flexion in swing. Alternately, the prosthesis may simply be too long. Any of these scenarios might create a situation in which circumduction is employed by the patient to ensure swing phase clearance of an inadequately shortened swing phase limb. Initially employed as a compensatory strategy, circumduction can become persistent in the absence of corrective adjustments to the prosthesis or gait training.

Vaulting

Circumduction represents one technique of facilitating swing phase clearance. Vaulting represents another. As described in the transtibial section, a rapid contraction of the sound side plantar flexors during midstance lengthens the stance limb to enable swing phase clearance. The absence of a physiologic knee joint and associated proprioceptive input is such that vaulting is observed more frequently in transfemoral gait than transtibial gait.

Excessive Terminal Impact

Terminal impact of the above-knee prosthesis can be viewed as complementary to excessive heel rise. Just as the resistance to the rising heel in initial swing can be adjusted within many prosthetic knee mechanisms, the amount of terminal impact experienced at the end of terminal swing can often be manipulated by making adjustments to the frictional or hydraulic settings of the knee. Many patients prefer to "feel" the terminal impact of the extending prosthetic knee at the end of each step as this increases their confidence in the sagittal stability of the prosthetic knee. Thus, the amount of terminal impact preferred by individual patients can be relatively variable. Emerging evidence has suggested that the latency period between the moments when the knee reaches full extension and the heel strikes the ground is reduced among patients using the enhanced safety features associated with microprocessor-regulated knee mechanisms.

KEY REFERENCES

1. Aitken GT: Proximal femoral focal deficiency—definition, classification and management. In Aitken GT, editor: *Proximal femoral focal deficiency: a congenital anomaly*, Washington, DC, 1969, National Academy of Sciences.
2. Aulivola B, Hile CN, Hamdan AD, et al: Major lower limb amputation: outcome of a modern series, *Arch Surg* 139(4):395–399, 2004.
3. Birch JG, Lincoln TL, Mack PW, Birch CM: Congenital fibular deficiency: a review of thirty years' experience at one institution and a proposed classification system based on clinical deformity, *J Bone Joint Surg Am* 93(12):1144–1151, 2001.
4. Boonstra AM, Rijnders LJ, Groothoff JW, Eisma WH: Children with congenital deficiencies or acquired amputations of the lower limbs: functional aspects, *Prosthet Orthot Int* 24(1):19–27, 2000.
5. Braddom RL: *Physical medicine and rehabilitation*, ed 4, Philadelphia, 2011, Elsevier/Saunders.
6. Burger H, Marincek C: Return to work after lower limb amputation, *Disabil Rehabil* 29(17):1323–1329, 2007.
7. Busse JW, Jacobs CL, Swiontkowski MF, et al: Complex limb salvage or early amputation for severe lower-limb injury: a meta-analysis of observational studies, *J Orthop Trauma* 21(1):70–76, 2007.
8. Centers for Medicare and Medicaid Services, U.S. Department of Health and Human Services: *HCFA common procedure coding system (HCPCS)*, Springfield, 2001, U.S. Department of Commerce, National Technical Information Service.
10. Coffey L, Gallagher P, Desmond D, Ryall N: Goal pursuit, goal adjustment, and affective well-being following lower limb amputation, *Br J Health Psychol* 19(2):409–424, 2013.
11. Conner KA, McKenzie LB, Xiang H, Smith GA: Pediatric traumatic amputations and hospital resource utilization in the United States, 2003, *J Trauma* 68:131–137, 2010.
12. Della Croce U, Riley PO, Lelas JL, Kerrigan DC: A refined view of the determinants of gait, *Gait Posture* 14(2):79–84, 2001.
13. Delussu AS, Brunelli S, Paradisi F, et al: Assessment of the effects of carbon fiber and bionic foot during overground and treadmill walking in transtibial amputees, *Gait Posture* 38(4):876–882, 2013.

14. Dillingham TR, Pezzin LE, MacKenzie EJ: Limb amputation and limb deficiency: epidemiology and recent trends in the United States, *South Med J* 95(8):875–883, 2002.
15. Doukas WC, Hayda RA, Frisch HM, et al: The Military Extremity Trauma Amputation/Limb Salvage (METALS) study: outcomes of amputation versus limb salvage following major lower-extremity trauma, *J Bone Joint Surg Am* 95(2):138–145, 2013.
16. Dudek NL, Marks MB, Marshall SC: Skin problems in an amputee clinic, *Am J Phys Med Rehabil* 85(5):424–429, 2006.
17. Ephraim PL, Dillingham TR, Sector M, et al: Epidemiology of limb loss and congenital limb deficiency: a review of the literature, *Arch Phys Med Rehabil* 84:747–761, 2003.
19. Fletcher DD, Andrews KL, Hallett JW, Jr, et al: Trends in rehabilitation after amputation for geriatric patients with vascular disease: implications for future health resource allocation, *Arch Phys Med Rehabil* 83(10):1389–1393, 2002.
20. Foisneau-Lottin A, Martinet N, Henrot P, et al: Bursitis, adventitious bursa, localized soft-tissue inflammation, and bone marrow edema in tibial stumps: the contribution of magnetic resonance imaging to the diagnosis and management of mechanical stress complications, *Arch Phys Med Rehabil* 84(5):770–777, 2003.
21. Forni C, Gaudenzi N, Zoli M, et al: Living with rotationplasty—quality of life in rotationplasty patients from childhood to adulthood, *J Surg Oncol* 105:331–336, 2012.
23. Gates DH, Aldridge JM, Wilken JM: Kinematic comparison of walking on uneven ground using powered and unpowered prostheses, *Clin Biomech (Bristol, Avon)* 28(4):467–472, 2013.
27. Hillmann A, Weist R, Fromme A, et al: Sports activities and endurance capacity of bone tumor patients after rotationplasty, *Arch Phys Med Rehabil* 88(7):885–890, 2007.
28. Hsu E, Cohen SP: Postamputation pain: epidemiology, mechanisms, and treatment, *J Pain Res* 6:121–136, 2013.
30. Jeans KA, Browne RH, Karol LA: Effect of amputation level on energy expenditure during overground walking by children with an amputation, *J Bone Joint Surg Am* 93:49–56, 2011.
31. Kern KU, Kohl M, Seifert U, Schlereth T: [Effect of botulinum toxin type B on residual limb sweating and pain. Is there a chance for indirect phantom pain reduction by improved prosthesis use?], *Schmerz* 26(2):176–184, 2012 [in German].
33. Kreshak JL, Fabbri N, Manfrini M, et al: Rotationplasty for sarcomas of the distal femur: long-term survival, function and quality of life, *J Bone Joint Surg Br* 94-B(Suppl XXXVIII):143, 2012.
35. Lusardi MM, Nielsen CC: *Orthotics and prosthetics in rehabilitation*, St Louis, 2007, Elsevier/Saunders.
36. Mancinelli C, Patritti BL, Tropea P, et al: Comparing a passive-elastic and a powered prosthesis in transtibial amputees, *Conf Proc IEEE Eng Med Biol Soc* 8255–8258, 2011.
40. Munoz CA, Gaspari A, Goldner R: Contact dermatitis from a prosthesis, *Dermatitis* 19(2):109–111, 2008.
41. Murphy D: Fundamentals of amputation care and prosthetics, Demos Medical, *New York* 2013.
43. Nowroozi F, Salvanelli ML, Gerber LH: Energy expenditure in hip disarticulation and hemipelvectomy amputees, *Arch Phys Med Rehabil* 64(7):300–303, 1983.
44. Pasquina PF, Cooper RA: *Care of the combat amputee*, Washington, DC, 2009, Borden Institute, Walter Reed Army Medical Center.
45. Peirano AH, Franz RW: Spirituality and quality of life in limb amputees, *Int J Angiol* 21(1):47–52, 2012.
46. Perry J, Burnfield JM: *Gait analysis: normal and pathologic function*, ed 2, Thorofare, 2010, SLACK Incorporated.
47. Potter BK, Burns TC, Lacap AP, et al: Heterotopic ossification following traumatic and combat-related amputations. Prevalence, risk factors, and preliminary results of excision, *J Bone Joint Surg Am* 89(3):476–486, 2007.
49. Remes L, Isoaho R, Vahlberg T, et al: Major lower extremity amputation in elderly patients with peripheral arterial disease: incidence and survival rates, *Aging Clin Exp Res* 20(5):385–393, 2008.
50. Resnick HE, Valsania P, Phillips CL: Diabetes mellitus and nontraumatic lower limb amputation in black and white Americans: the National Health and Nutrition Examination Survey Epidemiologic Follow-up Study, 1971–1992, *Arch Intern Med* 159(20):2470–2475, 1999.
51. Rijnders LJ, Boonstra AM, Groothoff JW, et al: Lower limb deficient children in the Netherlands: epidemiological aspects, *Prosthet Orthot Int* 24:13–18, 2000.
52. Robert RS, Ottaviani G, Huh WW, et al: Psychosocial and functional outcomes in long-term survivors of osteosarcoma: a comparison of limb-salvage surgery and amputation, *Pediatr Blood Cancer* 54(7):990–999, 2010.
53. Saunders JB, Inman VT, Eberhart HD: The major determinants in normal and pathological gait, *J Bone Joint Surg Am* 35-A(3):543–558, 1953.
55. Schuch CM, Pritham CH: International Standards Organization terminology: application to prosthetics and orthotics, *J Prosthet Orthot* 6(1):29–33, 1994.
58. Spiegel DA, Loder RT, Crandall RC: Congenital longitudinal deficiency of the tibial, *Int Orthop* 27:338–342, 2003.
59. International Organization for Standardization: *ISO 8545-1: prosthetics and orthotics—limb deficiencies, part 1: method of describing limb deficiencies present at birth*, Geneva, 1989, International Organization for Standardization.
60. Stone PA, Back MR, Armstrong PA, et al: Midfoot amputations expand limb salvage rates for diabetic foot infections, *Ann Vasc Surg* 19(6):805–811, 2005.
62. Trautner C, Haastert B, Giani G, et al: Amputations and diabetes: a case-control study, *Diabet Med* 19(1):35–40, 2002.
64. Vannah WM, Davids JR, Drvaric DM, et al: A survey of function in children with lower limb deficiencies, *Prosthet Orthot Int* 23:239–244, 1999.
65. Vasluian E, van der Sluis CK, van Essen AJ, et al: Birth prevalence for congenital limb defects in the northern Netherlands: a 30-year population-based study, *BMC Musculoskelet Disord* 14:323, 2013.
67. Waters RL, Mulroy S: The energy expenditure of normal and pathologic gait, *Gait Posture* 9(3):207–231, 1999.
68. Weeks SR, Anderson-Barnes VC, Tsao JW: Phantom limb pain theories and therapies, *Neurologist* 16(5):277–286, 2010.
70. Wolf EJ, Everding VQ, Linberg AA, et al: Comparison of the power knee and C-leg during step-up and sit-to-stand tasks, *Gait Posture* 38(3):397–402, 2013.
72. Ziegler-Graham K, MacKenzie EJ, Ephraim PL, et al: Estimating the prevalence of limb loss in the United States: 2005 to 2050, *Arch Phys Med Rehabil* 89(3):422–429, 2008.

The full reference list for this chapter is available online.

CHAPTER 11

UPPER LIMB ORTHOSES

Brian M. Kelly, Atul T. Patel, Carole V. Dodge

Orthosis (derived from the Greek *orthos*, meaning to correct or make straight) encompasses the full spectrum of devices currently fabricated by therapists and orthotists.[14] As defined by the International Standards Organization of the International Society for Prosthetics and Orthotics, an orthosis is any externally applied device used to modify structural and functional characteristics of the neuromuscular skeletal system.[33] *Orthosis*—or alternatively, *orthotic device*—is the preferred term.[19] The terms *splint* and *brace* are less preferred because they imply only immobilization and do not suggest either improved function or restoration of mobility. The terms *orthotic device* and *splint* will be used interchangeably in this chapter.

Principles and Indications

The objectives of upper limb orthotic applications can be classified into three major areas: protection, correction, and assistance with function.

- *Protection:* Orthotic devices can provide compressive forces and traction in a controlled manner to protect the impaired joint or body part. Restricting or preventing joint motion may correct alignment and prevent progressive deformity. Protective orthoses can also stabilize unstable bony components and promote healing of soft tissues and bones.
- *Correction:* Orthoses help in correcting joint contractures and subluxation of joints or tendons. They assist in the prevention and reduction of joint deformities.
- *Assistance with function:* Orthoses can assist function by compensating for deformity, muscle weakness, or increased muscle tone.

Physicians should prescribe orthotic devices based on their knowledge of the diagnosis, anatomy, and optimal clinical outcomes. Other health professionals, including occupational therapists and orthotists, are involved in the design and application of these devices.

Classification

Many different terms are used to describe upper limb orthotic devices. They are named by the joint(s) they cross, the function they provide (e.g., immobilization), or the condition they treat. Some are named by their appearance (e.g., banjo or sugar tong), and still others bear the name of the person who designed them (e.g., Kleinert).[27]

Most splints are known by their common names (Table 11-1). However, such names are not fully informative, systematic, or universally accepted. This causes a communication barrier between the physician and other health professionals. Consequently, more systematic naming systems have been developed that classify orthotic devices according to anatomic region or to purpose and function. Table 11-1 compares the common names of several orthotic devices with those in three other naming systems.

The simplest naming system was developed by the International Organization for Standards. It uses the anatomic region the orthotic device encompasses. A wrist-hand orthosis, for example, is called a WHO.[35] This system, however, fails to define the purpose or function of the orthosis.

In 1991, the American Society of Hand Therapists (ASHT) published the ASHT *Splint Classification System*.[1] This system provides standard nomenclature for splints based on function. It classifies splints by characteristics (e.g., articular or nonarticular) and location of the body part covered. A humeral fracture brace, for example, is identified as a nonarticular splint–humerus. It also identifies what the direction of the applied force is and whether the splint is for mobilization, immobilization, or restriction. In this system, a long arm splint (Figure 11-1) is characterized as a 45-degree elbow flexion immobilization orthosis. A weakness of this system is that one splint design can provide many different functions.[8]

Biomechanical and Anatomic Considerations

Health care personnel involved in the fabrication and application of orthotic devices must have a good understanding of the biomechanics, anatomy, and physiologic response to tissue healing. Technical and creative skills are needed to design and fabricate orthotic devices that patients will use and satisfy the treatment goals. In the United States, upper limb splinting is performed by occupational therapists, certified hand therapists, orthotists, and some physical therapists. Physicians ordering these devices must understand the biomechanical factors involved in fabrication and fitting. Some of these are listed here.

- The wrist acts as the base for hand positioning and splinting except isolated digital splinting. The weight of the immobile hand, gravity, and resting muscle tension tend to pull the wrist into flexion. This increases tension in the extrinsic extensor tendons, pulling the metacarpophalangeal (MCP) joints into hyperextension. Concurrently, the tension of the extrinsic flexor tendons is maintained and forces the interphalangeal (IP) joints (which include the proximal interphalangeal [PIP] and distal interphalangeal [DIP] joints) into flexion. The metacarpal arch of the

Table 11-1 Nomenclature Systems in Current Use

Common Name	American Society of Hand Therapists *Splint Classification System*[1]	International Organization for Standards[35]	McKee[27]
Humeral fracture brace	Nonarticular splint—humerus	Not applicable	Circumferential nonarticular humerus-stabilizing
Tennis elbow splint or brace	Nonarticular splint—proximal forearm	Elbow orthosis	Circumferential nonarticular proximal forearm strap
Long arm splint	45-degree elbow flexion immobilization; type 16	SEWHO	Posterior static elbow-wrist orthosis
Resting hand splint	Index through small finger PIP extension, thumb CMC palmar abduction mobilization; type 326	WHO	Volar forearm-based static (or serial static) wrist-hand orthosis
Ulnar deviation splint	Index through small finger MCP extension-radial deviation mobilization; type 028	Hand orthosis	Circumferential hand-based dynamic traction D2-D5 MCP corrective radial deviation orthosis
Kleinert splint, modified Kleinert splint, postoperative flexor tendon splint	Wrist, MCP, PIP, DIP flexion immobilization-extension restriction; type 019	WHO	Dorsal forearm-based dynamic MCP-IP protective flexion and MCP extension-blocking orthosis
Duran splint, postoperative flexor tendon splint	Wrist and finger flexion immobilization; type 028	WHO	Dorsal forearm-based static MCP-IP protective flexion and MCP extension-blocking orthosis
Postoperative dynamic extensor tendon splint	Wrist, MCP, PIP, DIP extension immobilization-flexion restriction; type 019	WHO	Volar-dorsal forearm-based dynamic MCP-IP protective extension and flexion-blocking orthosis
Swan neck splint	Index finger PIP extension restriction; type 016	FO	Finger-based static PIP extension-blocking orthosis
Postoperative MCP arthroplasty splint, Swanson splint	Index through small finger MCP extension-radial deviation mobilization; type 132	WHFO	Dorsal forearm-based dynamic D2-D5 MCP assisted extension-radial deviation orthosis
Radial nerve palsy splint	Wrist extension, MCP flexion mobilization or MCP flexion, wrist extension mobilization; type 032	WHFO	Dorsal forearm-based dynamic low-profile wrist and D1-D5 MCP assistive extension orthosis
Ulnar nerve palsy splint	Ring though small finger MCP extension restriction; type 030	HFO	Circumferential hand-based dynamic joint-aligned coil spring D4-D5 MCP assistive flexion orthosis
Median nerve palsy splint	Index through small finger MCP flexion mobilization and thumb CMC opposition mobilization; type 032	HFO	Circumferential hand-based dynamic joint-aligned coil spring D2-D5 MCP assistive flexion and thumb assistive opposition orthosis
Flail arm splint	Not classified	SEWHO	Not classified
Dynamic finger flexion splint, forearm-based	Index through small finger MCP flexion mobilization; type 310	WHFO	Volar hand-based dynamic MCP corrective-flexion orthosis
Dynamic finger final flexion splint, hand-based	Index through small finger flexion mobilization; type 015	WHFO	Volar forearm-based dynamic MCP, PIP, DIP corrective-flexion orthosis
Dynamic finger extension splint, forearm-based	Index through small PIP and DIP extension mobilization; type 219	WHFO	Volar forearm-based dynamic MCP, PIP, DIP corrective-extension orthosis
Dynamic finger extension splint, hand-based	Index through small finger extension mobilization; type 014	WHFO	Circumferential hand-based dynamic D4-D5 MCP, PIP, DIP assistive flexion orthosis
Static progressive splint	Index finger MCP flexion mobilization; type 128	WHFO	Volar forearm-based static progressive MERiT screw MCP flexion orthosis
Dynamic wrist flexion splint	Wrist flexion mobilization; type 016	WHO	Dorsal forearm-based dynamic joint-aligned wrist assistive flexion orthosis
Dynamic wrist extension splint	Wrist extension mobilization; type 016	WHO	Dorsal forearm-based dynamic joint-aligned wrist assistive extension orthosis
Rehabilitation Institute of Chicago tenodesis splint	Not classified	Functional orthosis	Volar forearm-based tenodesis WHO
Elbow flexion splint	Elbow flexion mobilization; type 016	EWO	Posterior dynamic elbow corrective flexion orthosis
Elbow extension splint	Elbow extension mobilization; type 016	EWO	Anterior serial static elbow corrective extension orthosis
Dynamic pronation-supination splint	Forearm pronation-supination mobilization; type 221	Elbow-wrist-hand orthosis	Posterior forearm-based dynamic radius-ulna corrective pronation-supination orthosis

Table 11-1 Nomenclature Systems in Current Use—cont'd

Common Name	American Society of Hand Therapists *Splint Classification System*[1]	International Organization for Standards[35]	McKee[27]
Wrist splint, carpal tunnel splint	Wrist extension immobilization; type 016	Wrist orthosis	Volar forearm-based static wrist orthosis
Thumb spica splint	Thumb MCP extension immobilization; type 221	Wrist-thumb orthosis	Volar forearm-based static wrist-thumb orthosis
Mallet finger splint, DIP extension splint, Stax splint	Index finger DIP extension immobilization; type 021	FO	Volar finger-based static DIP flexion-blocking orthosis
Capener splint, LMB finger extension splint	PIP extension mobilization; type 016	FO	Three-point finger-based dynamic joint-aligned coil spring PIP corrective extension orthosis
Figure-of-eight harness	Nonarticular splint—axilla	Shoulder orthosis	Figure-of-eight nonarticular axilla orthosis
Airplane splint, gunslinger splint	Shoulder abduction immobilization; type 328	SEWHO	Lateral trunk-based static shoulder-elbow-wrist orthosis
Mobile arm support	Not classified	SEWHO	Not classified
Orthosis sugar tong	Elbow extension immobilization; type 328	SEWHO	Bivalved static elbow orthosis

CMC, Carpometacarpal; *D*, digit; *DIP*, distal interphalangeal; *EWO*, elbow-wrist orthosis; *FO*, finger orthosis; *HFO*, hand-finger orthosis; *IP*, interphalangeal; *MCP*, metacarpophalangeal; *PIP*, proximal interphalangeal; *SEWHO*, shoulder-elbow-wrist-hand orthosis; *WHFO*, wrist-hand-finger orthosis; *WHO*, wrist-hand orthosis.

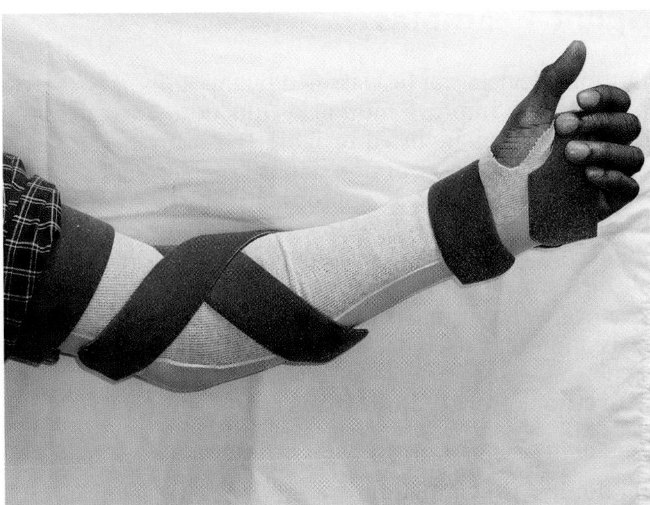

FIGURE 11-1 Long arm splint used for cubital tunnel syndrome.

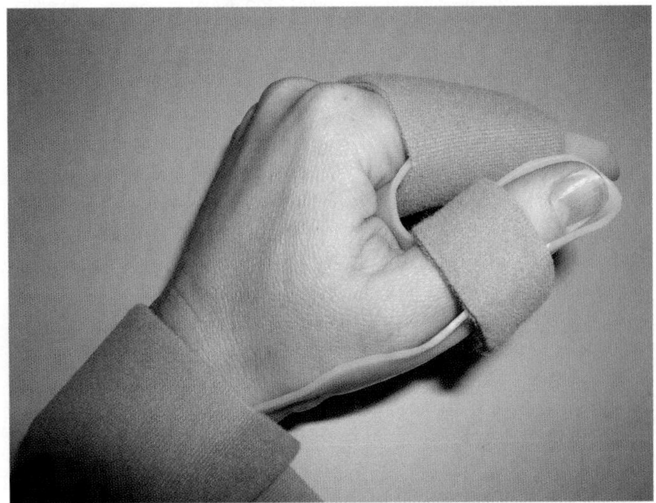

FIGURE 11-2 Hand and wrist are positioned to keep the metacarpophalangeal joints flexed and the interphalangeal joint extended with the wrist in slight extension. This is the "safe" or "intrinsic plus" position.

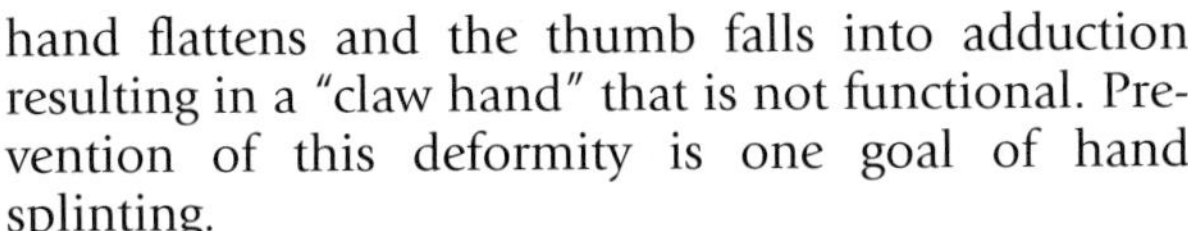

hand flattens and the thumb falls into adduction resulting in a "claw hand" that is not functional. Prevention of this deformity is one goal of hand splinting.

- Bone configuration of the hand and the tension of the muscles and ligaments in this region contribute to the creation of an arch system composed of the proximal transverse and longitudinal distal metacarpal arches. This arch system is vital for positioning the hand for normal function related to grasp and prehension. Incorporating these arches within the orthosis is essential to allow maximum function and comfort.[4]
- The MCP (or MP) joint is the key for finger function. When MCP joints are hyperextended, the IP joints flex because of the tension of the flexors and the delicate balance between the finger extensors and flexors. Extension stability of the wrist is important for optimal function of the hand. The wrist should be placed in slight extension to maintain flexor tendon length and to improve hand function (Figure 11-2). This position will place the MCP collateral ligaments on maximum stretch, preserve the anatomic arches of the hand, and thus oppose the development of a "claw hand" deformity. This position is also referred to as "safe" or "intrinsic plus."[8] This position facilitates the weaker intrinsic motions of MCP flexion and IP extension that are difficult to obtain.
- The hand is used during functional activities through basic prehension patterns: to pinch, to grasp, or to hook objects. There are two basic types of hand grips: power and precision (Figures 11-3 and 11-4). For power grip, the wrist is held in dorsiflexion with the fingers wrapped around an object held in the palm (such as holding a screwdriver with a cylindrical grip). The spherical grip is useful for holding a ball. The

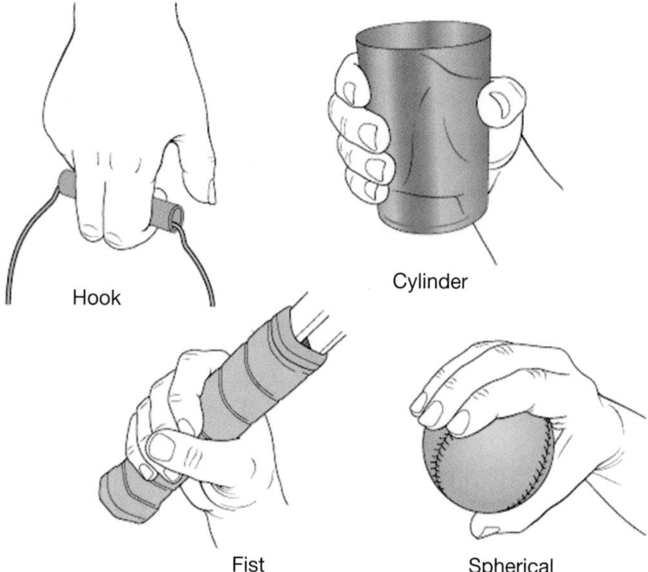

FIGURE 11-3 During power grip the wrist is held in dorsiflexion, allowing the long flexors to press the object against the palm. Lack of mobility or weakness of the fourth and fifth rays may interfere with maximal power grip. (Redrawn from Magee DJ: Forearm, wrist, and hand. In Magee DJ, editor: *Orthopedic physical assessment*, ed 4, Philadelphia, 2002, Elsevier/Saunders, pp 378–379.)

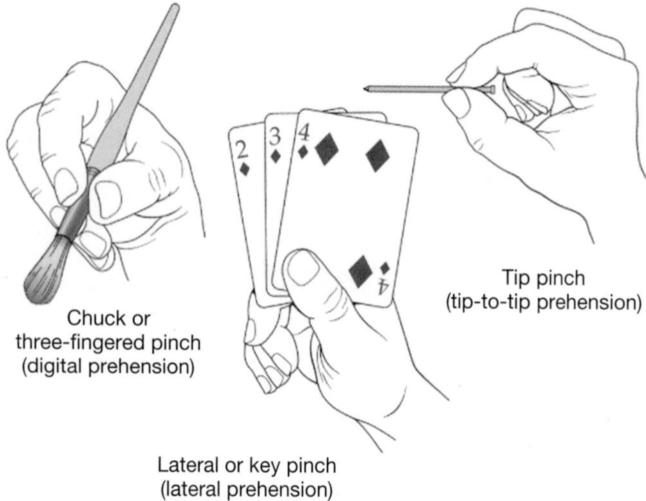

FIGURE 11-4 Precision grip is limited mainly to the metacarpophalangeal joints and primarily involves the radial side of the hand. The intrinsic muscles are more important in precision than with power grip. The thumb is essential for precision grip because it provides stability and control of direction and can provide power to the grip. (Redrawn from Magee DJ: Forearm, wrist, and hand. In Magee DJ, ed: *Orthopedic physical assessment*, ed 4, Philadelphia, 2002, Elsevier/Saunders, pp 378–379.)

hook pattern is useful for carrying heavy objects. For precision grip, the thumb is held against the tip of the index and middle finger. Functional hand splinting is typically aimed at improving pinch. There are three types of pinch: (1) oppositional pinch (three-jaw chuck), (2) precision pinch, and (3) lateral key pinch.[25] It is best to splint toward oppositional pinch. This allows the best compromise between fine precision pinch and strong lateral pinch. No practical orthosis can substitute for or improve thumb adduction.[8] When making a splint, the therapist should fabricate it in a position that enhances prehension and does not force the thumb into a position of extension and radial abduction. This position causes the rest of the arm to have to compensate for poor thumb positioning.[8]

- When increasing joint range of motion (ROM) with splinting, the angle of pull needs to be perpendicular to the bony axis that is being mobilized.[3] Otherwise, the forces on the skin and underlying structures may cause injury through excessive pressure on the skin and deforming stresses on the underlying healing structures.
- The improvement in ROM is directly proportional to the length of time a joint is held at its end range.[16] This is the total end range time (TERT) principle and is used with static progressive splinting. The load should be low and the application time long. The clinically safe degree of force covers a very narrow range.

Diagnostic Categories and Splint Examples

Orthotic devices can be classified by the support (or forces provided) to improve motion or function. The categories of splint design are listed in Table 11-2.[38]

There are many common clinical conditions for which orthotic intervention is appropriate. This section gives a brief overview of the features of specific diagnoses and their commonly indicated type of splint. This is not an all-inclusive list and the reader is referred to comprehensive overviews of upper limb orthotic devices in splinting texts and other references.*

Musculoskeletal Conditions

Tendonitis, Tenosynovitis, and Enthesopathy

Tendonitis (inflammation of the tendon), tenosynovitis (inflammation of the tendon sheaths), and enthesopathy (inflammation at a muscle or tendon origin or insertion) can all result from excessive repetitive movement or external stressors. The upper limb tendons most commonly involved are the wrist extensors and the abductor pollicis longus and extensor pollicis brevis muscles of the thumb. The goal of splinting for these conditions is to immobilize the affected structures to facilitate healing and decrease inflammation. The forearm-based thumb spica splint immobilizes the wrist, the carpometacarpal (CMC) joint, and the MCP joint of the thumb. The IP joint of the thumb does not need fixation because the affected tendons do not move this joint (Figure 11-21).

Lateral epicondylitis is a common enthesopathy of the upper limb[38], which can be treated by a tennis elbow orthosis (Figure 11-22). This is a forearm band that changes the lever arm against which the wrist extensors pull. In essence, it puts the origin of the extensor muscles at rest

*References 1, 4, 8, 9, 12, 17, 19-21.

Text continued on p. 238

Table 11-2 Upper Limb Orthotic Splint Design Categories

Category and Characteristics	Variations	Distinctive Features	Clinical Applications	Notes
Nonarticular Provides support to a body part without crossing any joints and provides protection			Humeral fracture Sarmiento splint	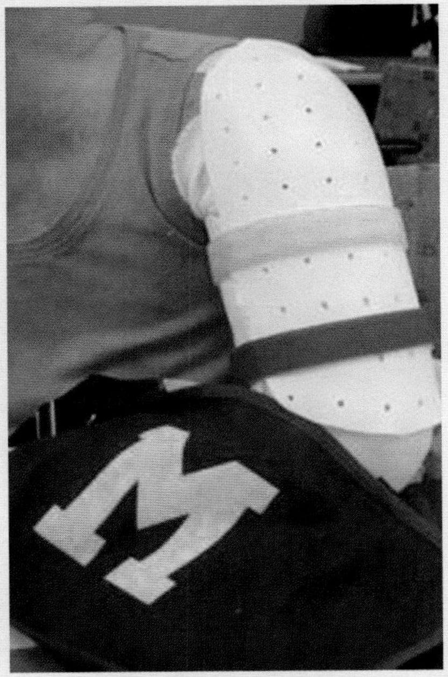 **FIGURE 11-5** A nonarticular Sarmiento brace used to immobilize the humerus after a fracture allows full range of motion of all the joints involved in the injured extremity. (Courtesy Kurt Hiser, OTR/L, CHT.)
			Sugar tong splint to immobilize a proximal radius fracture	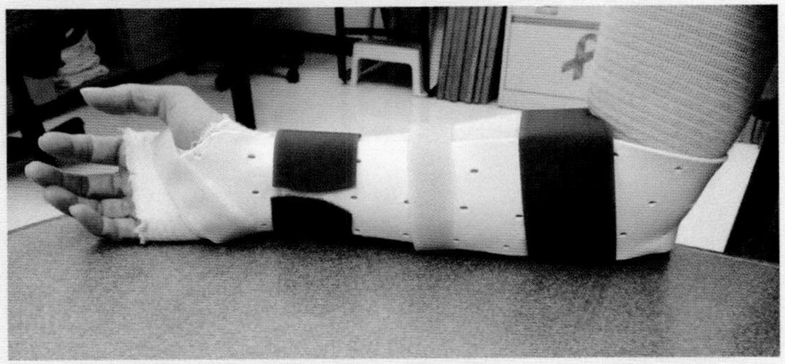 **FIGURE 11-6** A sugar tong splint is ideal for splinting fractures of the radius, ulna, or wrist. It prevents flexion and extension at the wrist, limits flexion and extension at the elbow, and prevents supination and pronation.

Continued on following page

Table 11-2 Upper Limb Orthotic Splint Design Categories—cont'd

Category and Characteristics	Variations	Distinctive Features	Clinical Applications	Notes
			Gel shell splint to exert pressure over a healing scar to prevent hypertrophic scarring	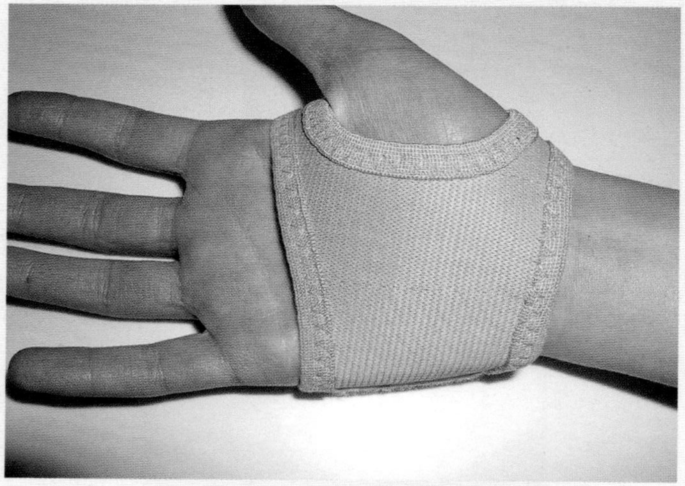 FIGURE 11-7 Gel shell splint.
Static Have a rigid base and immobilize the joints they transverse	Static		Volar wrist splint for acute carpal tunnel syndrome reduces motion and rests injured tissues	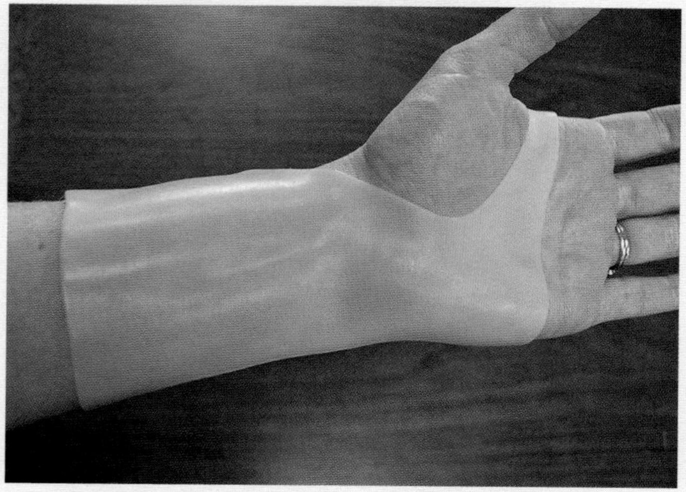 FIGURE 11-8 Wrist splint for carpal tunnel syndrome, with the wrist in a position of 0 degrees to 5 degrees of extension; distal palmar crease free to allow for full metacarpophalangeal motion.

			Protect healing structures, decrease or prevent deformity, and reduce tone in spastic muscles	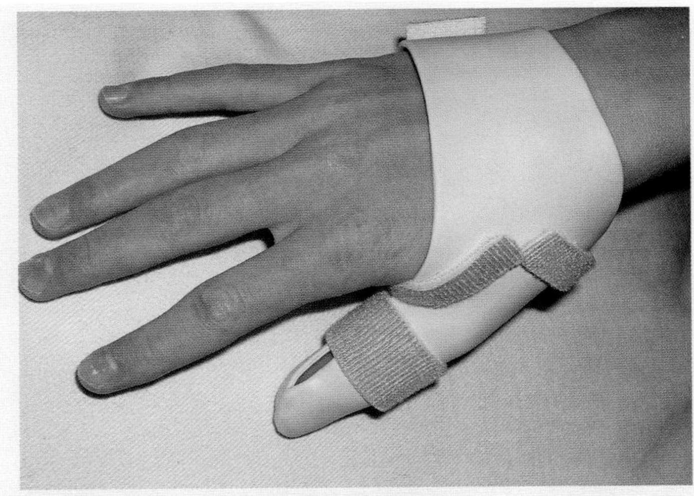 FIGURE 11-9 Hand-based static thumb splint with interphalangeal joint included for immobilization of a distal phalanx fracture.
	Serial static	A static splint that is periodically changed to alter the joint angle	The splints are applied with the tissue at its near maximum length. For example, a wrist splint can be changed periodically to increase extension in a wrist with a flexion contracture after a wrist fracture Provides a prolonged gentle stretch to involved structures, helping a stiff joint regain motion	This serial repositioning provides a prolonged gentle stretch to involved structures, helping a stiff joint regain motion 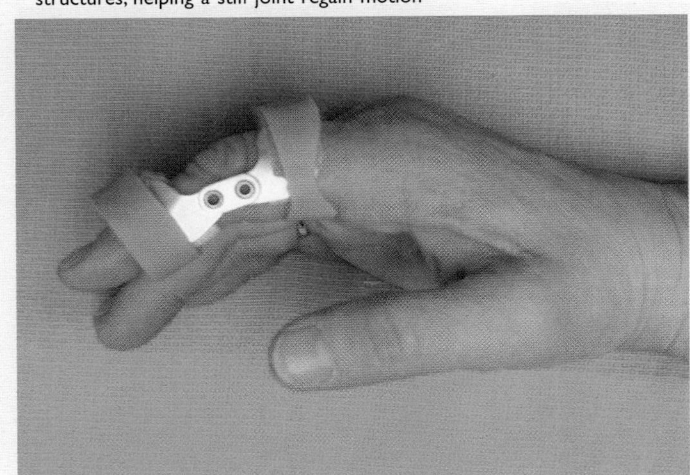 FIGURE 11-10 Serial static prefabricated hinged proximal interphalangeal splint that can adjust the joint angle in time.

Continued on following page

Table 11-2 Upper Limb Orthotic Splint Design Categories—cont'd

Category and Characteristics	Variations	Distinctive Features	Clinical Applications	Notes
	Static motion-blocking	The static motion-blocking splint permits motion in one direction but blocks motion in another	A swan neck splint is designed to allow flexion but block hyperextension of the PIP joint	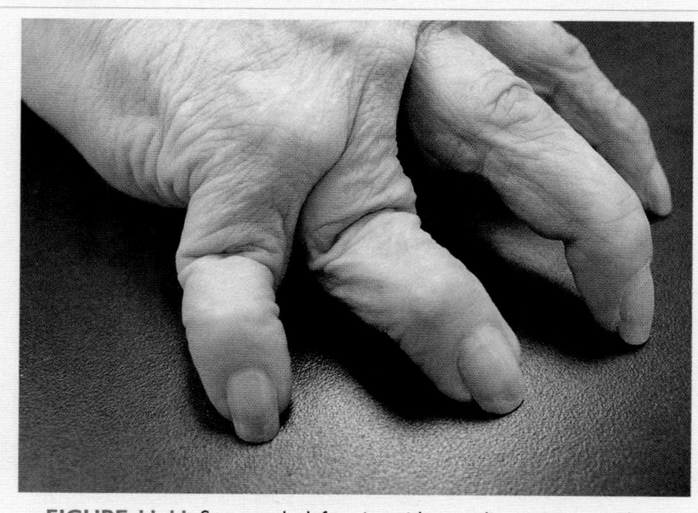 **FIGURE 11-11** Swan neck deformity with no splint support in place. 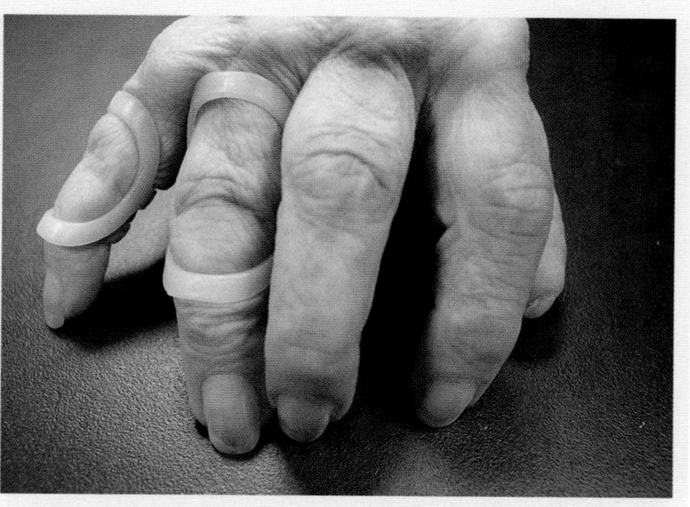 **FIGURE 11-12** Swan neck splint: Oval-8 product of 3-Point Products; note that the deformity is reduced.

	Static progressive	Unlike the serial static splint, the orthosis is not remolded to increase joint motion Differ from serial splints by using nonelastic components, such as static lines, hinges, screws, and turnbuckles to place a force on a joint to induce progressive change	The MERiT static progressive component[3] (available commercially) decreases the static line length as it is turned, thereby increasing the range of joint motion	Most commonly used splint for regaining joint motion Some patients may tolerate static progressive over dynamic orthosis, possibly due to the joint position constant while the tissue accommodates gently and gradually to the tension, without the influence of gravity or motion[26] 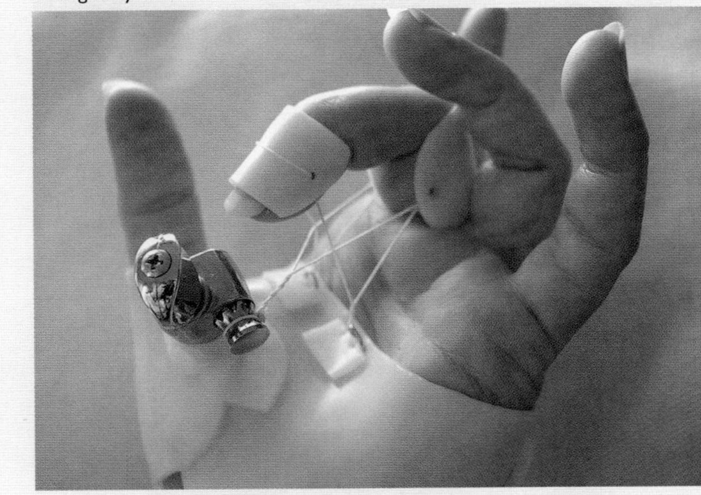 **FIGURE 11-13** Static progressive flexion splint with a MERiT component.
Dynamic Provides an elastic force to help regain joint motion	Dynamic	Finger extension splint, which uses a spring coil or wire tension assist	Designed to increase extension in a PIP joint with a mild contracture	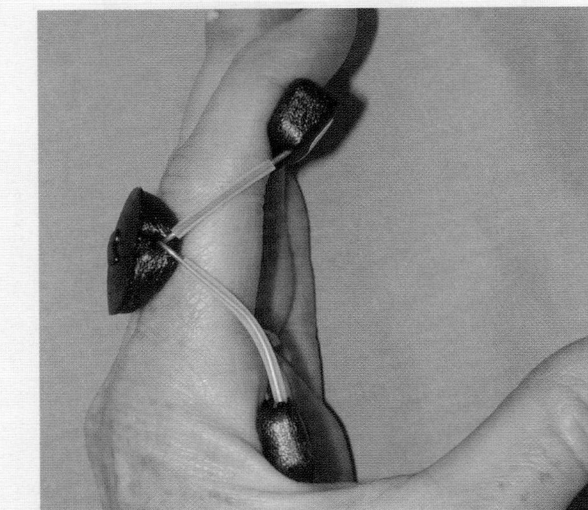 **FIGURE 11-14** LMB extension type of finger splint produces extension of the proximal interphalangeal or distal interphalangeal joints of the fingers or thumb.

Continued on following page

Table 11-2 Upper Limb Orthotic Splint Design Categories—cont'd

Category and Characteristics	Variations	Distinctive Features	Clinical Applications	Notes
	Dynamic motion-blocking	Allows certain motions but blocks others. It uses a passive, elastic line of pull in the desired direction, but permits active motion in the opposite direction	A Kleinert postoperative splint is designed for flexor tendon repairs It passively pulls the finger into flexion with an elastic thread or rubber band	It allows active digital extension, although parts of the splint block full extension of the MCP joint and the wrist 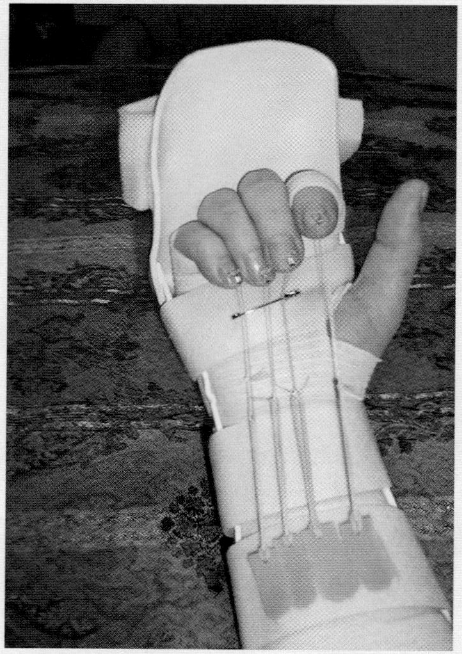 **FIGURE 11-15** Kleinert splint used for postoperative care for patients with flexor tendon injuries. It allows for passive flexion, holding digits flexed at rest.
	Dynamic traction	Offers traction to a joint although allowing controlled motion	Splint for an intraarticular fracture, such as a hand-based PIP extension splint with an outrigger, which gives constant longitudinal traction although the joint is gently moved	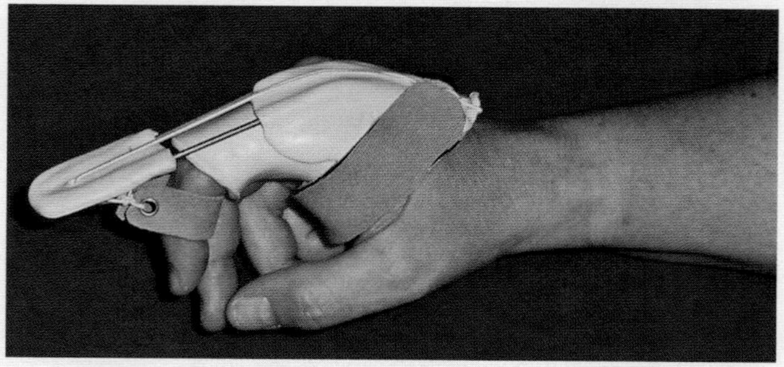 **FIGURE 11-16** Hand-based proximal interphalangeal extension splint with low-profile outrigger placing dynamic traction on the digit while allowing for passive range of motion. (Courtesy Jeanne Riggs, OTR/L, CHT.)

Wrist-driven prehension (tenodesis)	Facilitates function in a hand that has lost motion because of nervous system injury Active extension of the wrist produces controlled passive flexion of the fingers against a static thumb post through a tenodesis action	The Rehabilitation Institute of Chicago tenodesis splint, which assists the patient with a C6 level of spinal cord injury to achieve a functional pinch

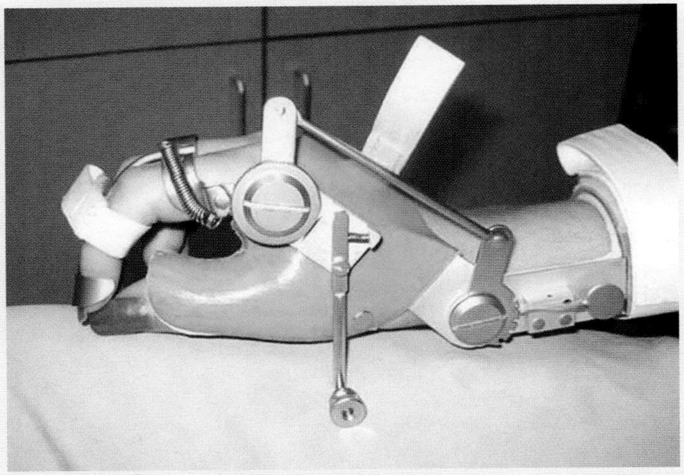

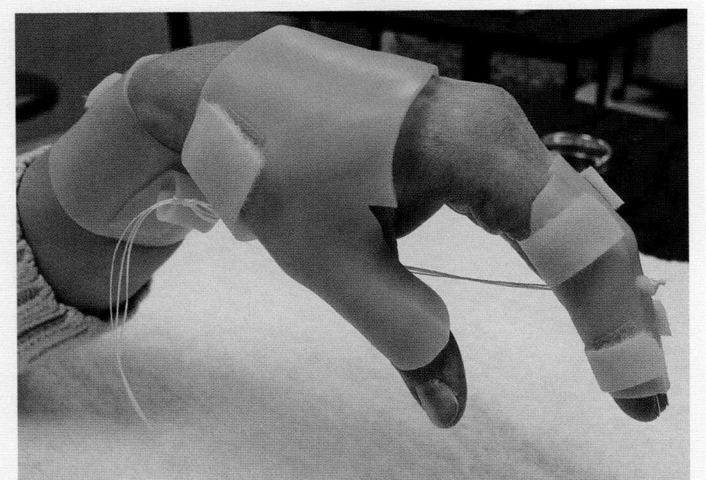

FIGURE 11-17 A functional carbon tenodesis orthosis with wrist ratchet control to adjust for tension. This splint is used for functional pinch during activities of daily living; pinching to thumb post.

FIGURE 11-18 Another example of a tenodesis splint, which uses a cord or string running from the wrist piece, across the palm, and up between the index and ring fingers. The string is lax when the wrist is released and tightens with wrist extension, bringing the fingers closer to the immobilized thumb, creating three-jaw chuck prehension.

Continued on following page

Table 11-2 Upper Limb Orthotic Splint Design Categories—cont'd

Category and Characteristics	Variations	Distinctive Features	Clinical Applications	Notes
	Continuous passive motion	Electrically powered devices that mechanically move joints through a desired range of motion	Keeps the joints supple and maintains articular, ligamentous, and tendinous structure mobility during the healing phases after injury or surgery	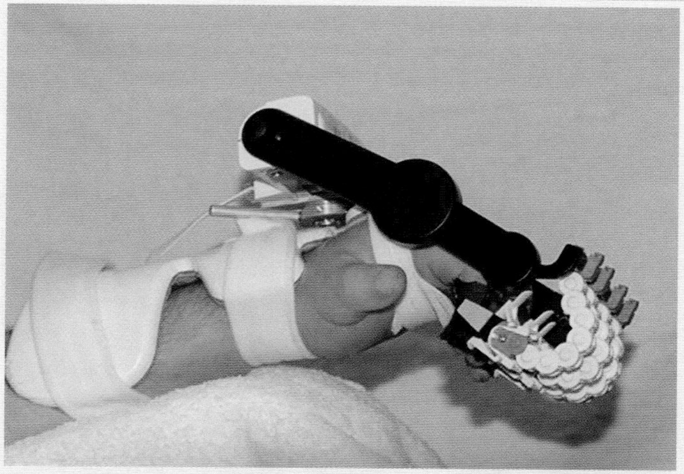 **FIGURE 11-19** Electrically powered orthosis that moves the joints through a desired range of motion. (Courtesy Jeanne Riggs, OTR/L, CHT.)

	Adaptive or functional use	Adaptive or functional usage devices promote functional use of the upper limb with impairment resulting from weakness, paralysis, or loss of a body part	The universal cuff encompasses the hand and holds various small items such as a fork, a pen, or a toothbrush	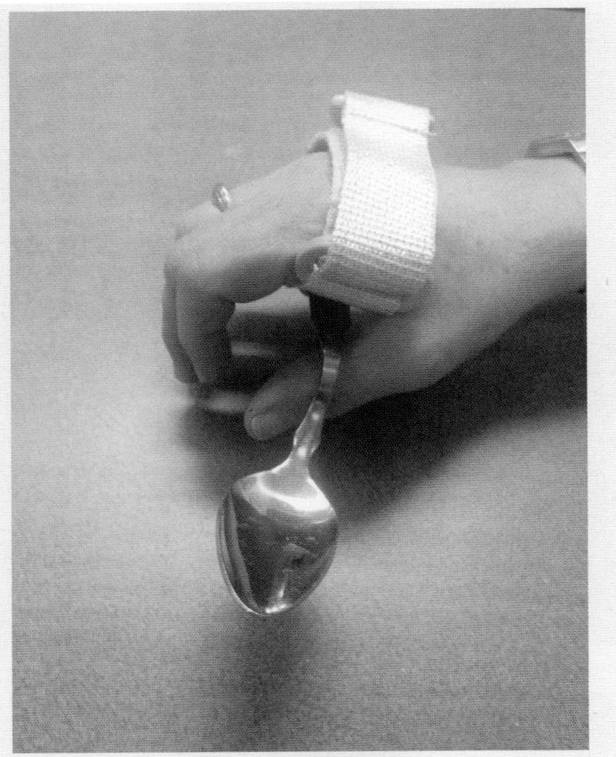 **FIGURE 11-20** A strap that encompasses the hand and holds various small items to enhance independence.

MCP, Metacarpophalangeal; *PIP*, proximal interphalangeal.

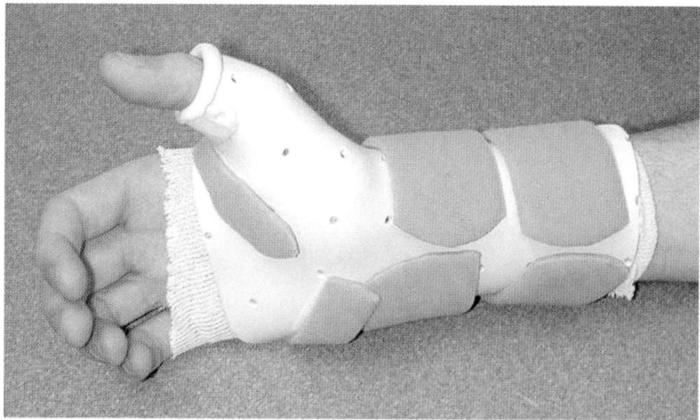

FIGURE 11-21 Forearm-based thumb spica splint used for de Quervain stenosing tenosynovitis. (Courtesy Jeanne Riggs, OTR/L, CHT.)

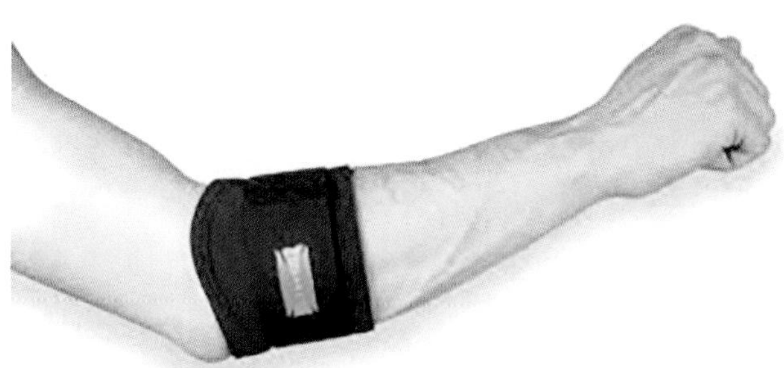

FIGURE 11-22 An elbow strap used for lateral epicondylitis.

and decreases the microtrauma from overuse. This orthotic device is a firm strap against which the extensors press against when contracting and is placed approximately two fingerbreadths distal to the lateral epicondyle. A similar brace is used for medial epicondylitis (also known as golfer's elbow) (see Chapter 35).

Trigger finger causes a snapping sensation in the volar surface of the digits on release of grasp. It is usually a result of trauma to the flexor tendon sheath of the fingers or thumb, producing thickened tendinous sheaths and restriction of motion. In advanced trigger finger, the digit can become "locked" in flexion. The goal in this condition is to halt the repetitive motion temporarily to allow for healing. Functional use of the hand should be maintained although the affected digit is immobilized (Figure 11-23). The splint for trigger finger covers the proximal phalanx and the MCP joint of the involved digit. It decreases the tendinous excursion through the first annular pulley, at the base of the MCP joint, and allows the inflamed structures to rest.

Sprains

Sprains are defined as momentary subluxations with spontaneous reduction that result in torn ligamentous structures. Patients experience pain, swelling, and decreased function. Sprains require joint immobilization in a position of function to allow for healing as well as functional use. Common sprains include dislocation of the IP and MCP joints caused by hyperextension and are often seen in sports injuries (see Chapters 31 and 35). For a first- or second-degree ligamentous tear, the goal is to protect and rest the area by applying functional splinting. The goal for a third-degree tear is to fully immobilize and approximate the ligaments.

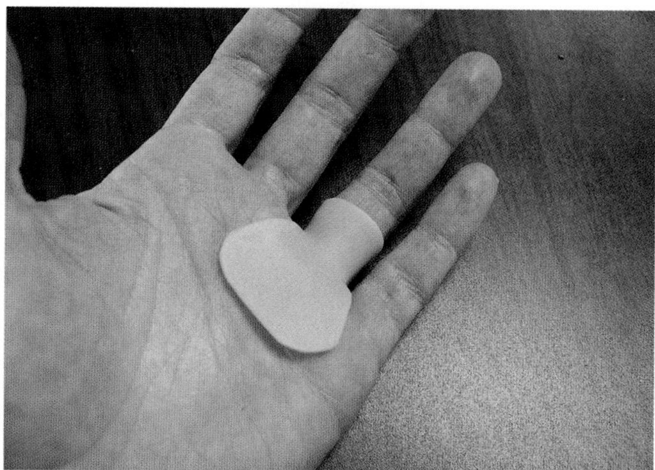

FIGURE 11-23 Trigger finger splint used for conservative treatment.

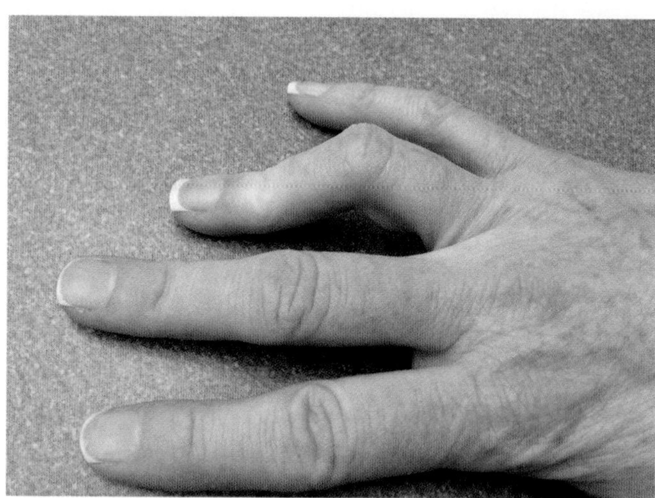

FIGURE 11-24 A boutonnière deformity in the finger is caused by deformity or disruption of the central slip, which is a key component of the extensor mechanism at the proximal interphalangeal joint.

Common splints used for digital sprains are finger extension splints that hold the PIP joint in extension but allow flexion of the DIP joint. This action keeps the oblique retinacular ligament and the terminal extensor tendon lengthened, preventing boutonnière deformities (Figure 11-24) during healing. Ulnar collateral ligamentous injuries at the MCP joint of the thumb are treated with a hand-based thumb spica splint to immobilize the joint during the healing phase (Figure 11-25). Wrist splints that place the wrist in slight extension are used for wrist sprains. For mild sprains, splints with no spline (metal bar insert) permit some motion but avoid creating significant stiffness. They also limit available range to approximately 40 degrees of total motion. Elbow neoprene sleeves are helpful for mild sprains at the elbow because they limit the extremes of range but allow some functional ROM.

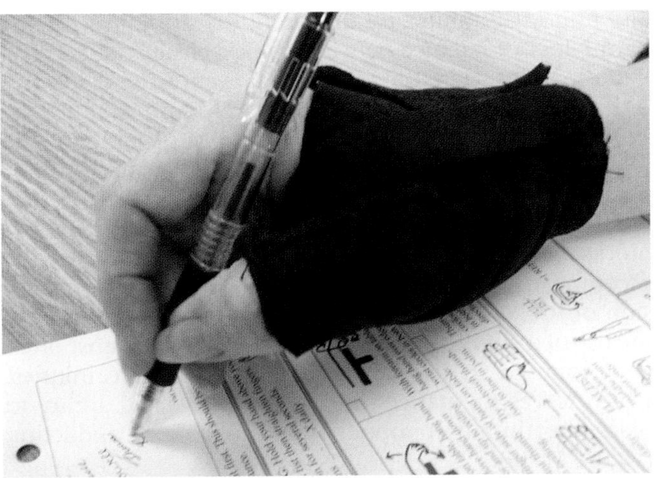

FIGURE 11-25 Comfort Cool splint made of perforated neoprene and terry cloth material is used to limit motion in the metacarpophalangeal and carpometacarpal joint of the thumb.

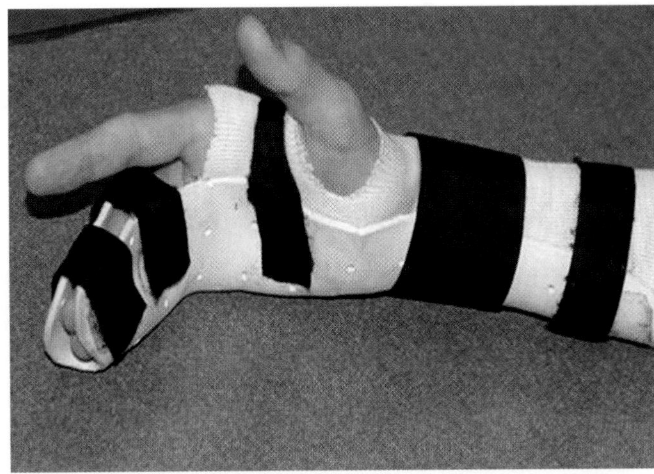

FIGURE 11-27 Ulnar gutter splint to immobilize the fourth and fifth metacarpal (boxer) fracture. The term *gutter* describes a splint that includes only the radial or ulnar portion of the limb. (Courtesy Jeanne Riggs, OTR/L, CHT.)

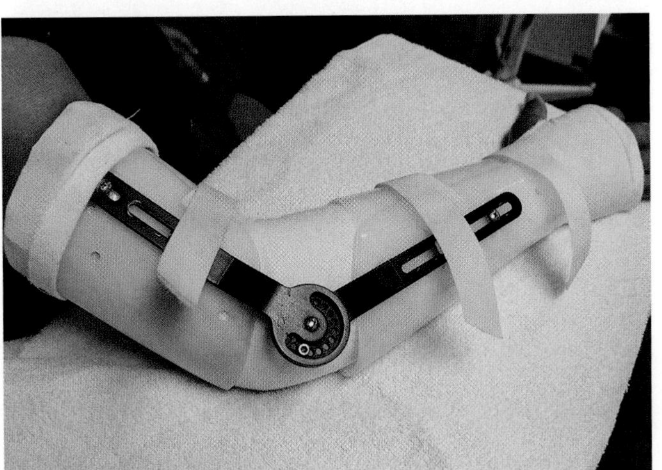

FIGURE 11-26 Hinged elbow splint with stops to limit extremes of motion during the rehabilitation phase after a fracture.

Fractures

Most major fractures need total immobilization by casting, surgical intervention, or both. Some fractures, however, do not need total limb immobilization and can be treated with orthotic devices (Figure 11-26). These devices should immobilize the body part or the joint sufficiently to promote healing while also optimizing function. An example of such an orthotic device is the humeral fracture brace, which has a circumferential design to hold healing bony parts in alignment. This orthosis permits motion of the elbow, forearm, and hand, which helps decrease the development of edema and resultant joint stiffness. A gutter splint is used primarily for phalangeal and metacarpal fractures. These splints extend from the proximal forearm to beyond the DIP joint and can be radial (immobilizing the index and long fingers) or ulnar (immobilizing the ring and little fingers, also called the boxer splint). The splint should be wide enough to surround both fingers and the wrist (Figure 11-27). Other examples include the traction-type splints that allow for very controlled motion during the healing phase of intraarticular finger fractures treated with pinning. Joint movement has been credited with enhancing cartilage nutrition and preventing intraarticular adhesions (see Figure 11-9).[15]

Arthritis

Osteoarthritis is the most common disease affecting the joints in the upper limb. Joint diseases of the hand and wrist have the most significant impact on function. Chronic inflammation often exposes these digital joints to further risk of deformity and injury. Orthotic devices can provide functional positioning to prevent further deformity and loss of use in arthritic diseases as well as protect the joints from further injury.[1]

Rheumatoid arthritis is a chronic inflammatory disease that primarily affects synovial joints. The most frequently affected joints in the upper limb are the wrist, MCP joint, and PIP joint. Deformities include subluxation and ulnar deviation at the MCP joints, subluxation and radial deviation at the wrist, and swan neck and boutonnière deformities of the fingers. These deformities usually progress, especially if no attempt is made to rest and protect the affected joints from overuse (see Chapter 31).

Several options are available for splinting the rheumatoid hand. Ulnar deviation splints that pull the MCP joints toward radial deviation and increase the functional use of the hand are now lightweight and permit full MCP joint motion in flexion and extension. Wrist splints that provide light support for the wrist are usually well tolerated (see Figure 11-25).[7] Swan neck and boutonnière splints can be made from thermoplastics but are often bulky and cosmetically unpleasing. The swan neck splint allows for flexion of the digit but blocks hyperextension (see Figures 11-11 and 11-12). The boutonnière splint holds the DIP or PIP joint in extension.

Osteoarthritis, the most common form of arthritis, is primarily a disease of cartilage. It most commonly involves the CMC joint of the thumb. A hand-based (see Figure 11-25) or forearm-based (see Figure 11-16) thumb spica splint can be prescribed for CMC joint osteoarthritis. By limiting motion at the base of the thumb, the splint decreases pain, especially with pinching-type activities.

Neuromuscular Conditions

Nerve Injuries

When a peripheral nerve is injured, the level and completeness of the injury determines the extent of the deficit incurred. For example, in a distal median nerve injury, a simian hand deformity may occur, and the function most affected is thumb palmar abduction and opposition (Figure 11-28). The goal of an orthotic device is to help restore this function. The splint usually has a spring coil design holding the MCP joints in slight flexion but permitting MCP extension. This splint also has a portion to position the thumb in palmar abduction.

With radial nerve injuries distal to the humeral spiral groove, the common presenting condition is wrist drop and finger drop. The goal in this case is to enhance wrist and finger extension. A radial nerve palsy splint (Figure 11-29) is forearm-based with an outrigger that holds the wrist, fingers, and thumb in extension and allows for flexion of the digits.[19]

With a proximal ulnar nerve injury, the patient has a "benediction hand," that is, hyperextension of the fourth and fifth MCP joints and flexion of the PIP joints caused by the loss of balance between the extrinsic and intrinsic hand muscles. Here the goal is to prevent fixed deformity of the fourth and fifth MCP joints and improve function. An ulnar nerve palsy splint holds the MCP joints of the fourth and fifth fingers in slight flexion by a spring coil or figure-of-eight splint design. The spring coil design assists MCP flexion and permits extension of the MCP joints but blocks hyperextension (Figure 11-30). This can also be accomplished with a static splint that prevents hyperextension of the MCP joints of the fourth and fifth digits with the use of a "lumbrical bar." Thumb position is most often compromised in low median and ulnar nerve injuries, which leaves the patient with no or weakened ability to place the thumb in opposition and palmar abduction (Figure 11-31).

Incomplete nerve injuries can be caused by compression without producing complete paralysis as, for example, in

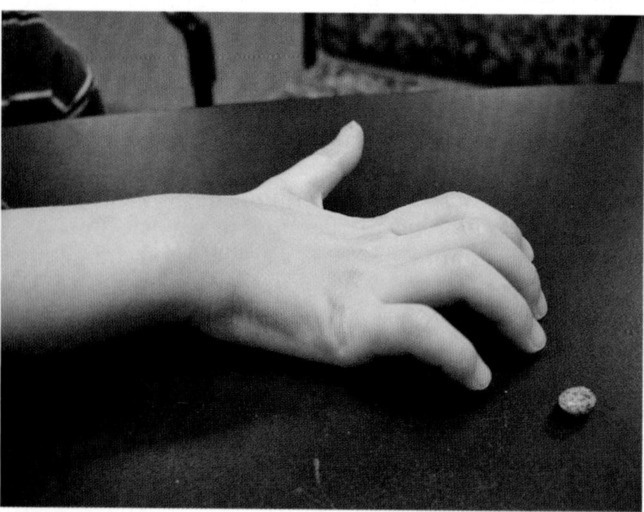

FIGURE 11-28 Simian hand, as seen in low median and ulnar nerve injuries (also called the intrinsic minus hand).

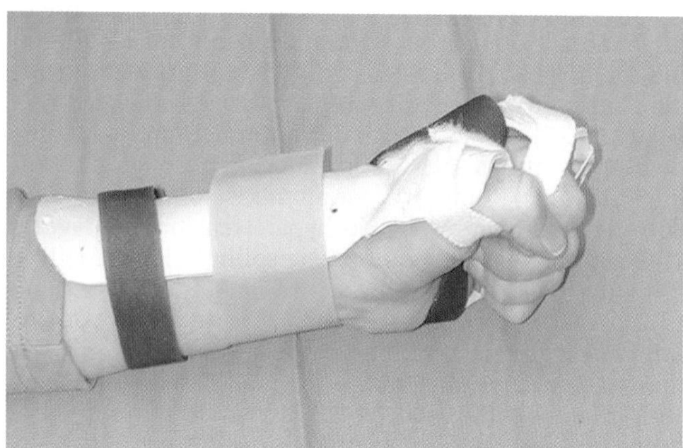

FIGURE 11-29 The radial nerve palsy orthosis assists with wrist and digit extension to improve functional use of the hand.

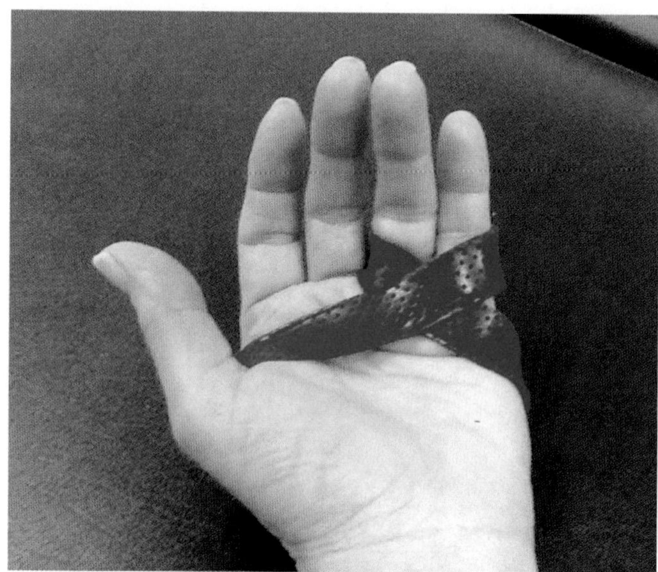

FIGURE 11-30 Ulnar palsy orthosis: allows extension but blocks hyperextension of the metacarpophalangeal joints of the ring and small fingers.

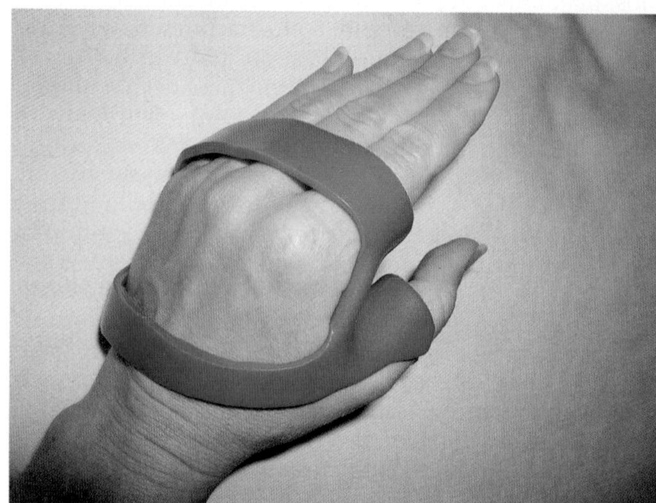

FIGURE 11-31 Combined median and ulnar nerve palsy orthosis blocking the metacarpophalangeal joint into slight flexion.

median nerve injury from carpal tunnel syndrome. One cause of this is an overuse syndrome that produces an inflammatory response in the synovium surrounding the flexor tendons at the wrist, causing decreased blood supply to the median nerve. The purpose of the splint is to immobilize the wrist to minimize swelling from overuse of the tendons. Complete resolution of this syndrome can occur if wrist orthoses are applied early, when symptoms first appear. The splint is molded to the patient from a thermoplastic that offers excellent conformity to hold the wrist in 0 degrees to 5 degrees of extension. Its common name, wrist cock-up splint, is misleading and should be avoided because this name implies that the wrist should be placed in extension (see Figure 11-8). The patient should be instructed to reduce stresses at the wrist and to wear the splint all night.

A word of caution is in order with prefabricated wrist splints for carpal tunnel syndrome. Many of these splints have an angled metal bar to hold the wrist in 45 degrees of extension (Figure 11-32). This angle far exceeds the recommended 0 degrees to 5 degrees of extension needed to decrease pressure in the carpal tunnel. Patients need to be instructed to remove the metal spline, flatten it, and then replace it in the fabric sleeve. Usually, this splint should be worn for 4 to 6 weeks, with gradual weaning from the splint and return to activity with workstation modifications.

Cubital tunnel syndrome (compression of the ulnar nerve at the elbow) can be treated with long arm splints (see Figure 11-1) that hold the elbow in 45 degrees of flexion, the forearm in neutral, and the wrist in 0 degrees to 5 degrees of extension with thumb and fingers free.

In patients with multiple nerve injuries or brachial plexopathy with essentially a flail arm, the goal for orthotic devices is to provide some functional use. One type of orthosis is an exoskeleton on the arm, similar to a prosthesis. This device uses a shoulder harness with scapular activation to produce elbow function that is similar to scapular action in an above-elbow prosthesis.[21]

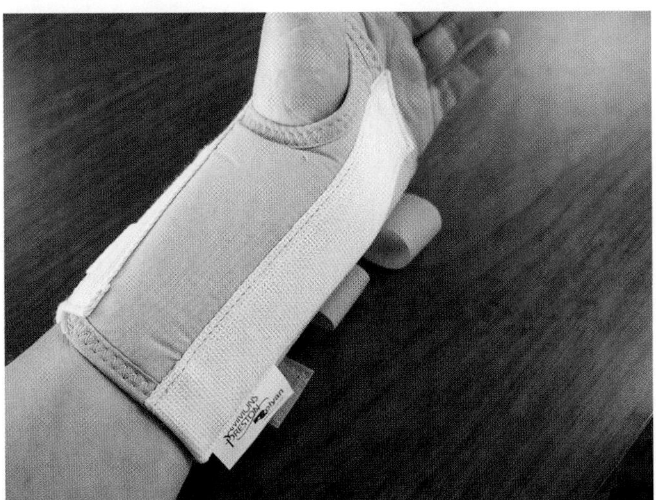

FIGURE 11-32 Commercially available wrist splint. The preset angle, which can be appropriate in some patients with wrist sprains, far exceeds that recommended for the treatment of acute carpal tunnel syndrome.

Brain Injury and Stroke

Depending on the area of brain injury and ensuing deficits, particularly if there is a change in muscle tone, orthotic devices should be designed to prevent deformities and to help adjust muscle tone. Resting and positioning orthotic devices are also necessary to help prevent complications, such as distal edema, joint subluxation, and contracture formation. In upper limb paralysis, a resting hand splint is commonly used to position the wrist in slight extension, the MCP joints in slight flexion, and the IP joints in extension. The thumb is supported in a position between palmar and radial abduction. Full support of the first CMC joint prevents ligamentous stresses on the thumb, especially in the insensate hand. This thumb position uses the reflex-inhibiting posture to decrease tone in the hand (Figure 11-33). Botulinum toxin is commonly used to decrease the tone in patients with focal spasticity, followed by serial or dynamic splinting to regain normal posture or position (Figure 11-34).[10,20,23] The Ball antispasticity splint places the fingers and hand in a reflex-inhibiting position and serves to reduce tone (Figure 11-35)[39] (see Chapters 23, 43, and 44).

Spasticity may be useful and might augment neuroplasticity for motor recovery.[31] The SaeboFlex[34] is a dynamic orthosis with functional electrical stimulation that is most appropriate for patients who have some shoulder and elbow movement but no hand function (i.e., lack of active finger extension). The SaeboFlex positions the wrist and fingers into extension in preparation for functional

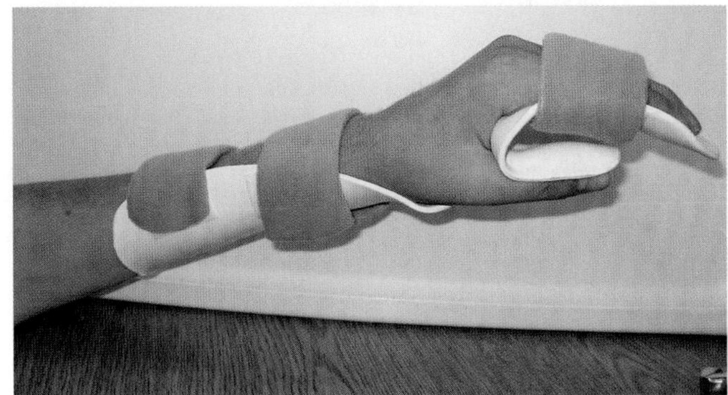

FIGURE 11-33 Resting hand splint.

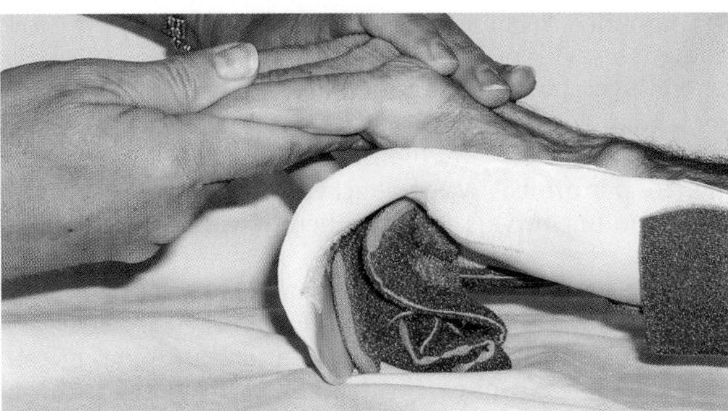

FIGURE 11-34 Improved passive range of motion after botulinum toxin injection to reduce spasticity; splint is preinjection level for passive range of motion.

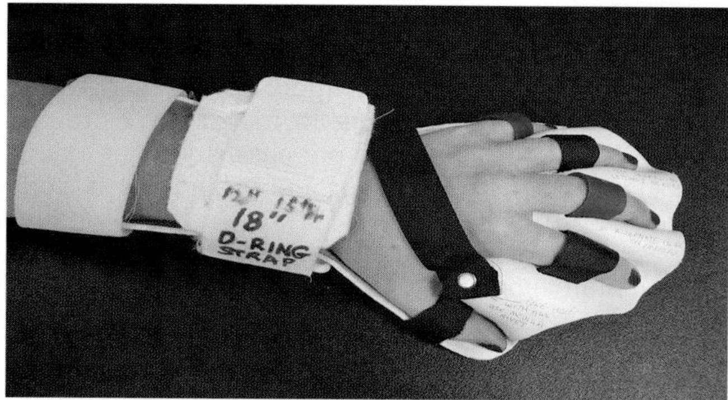

FIGURE 11-35 Ball antispasticity splint to maintain hand and fingers in reflex-inhibiting position and wrist in neutral position to reduce spasticity. (Courtesy Linda Miner, OTR/L.)

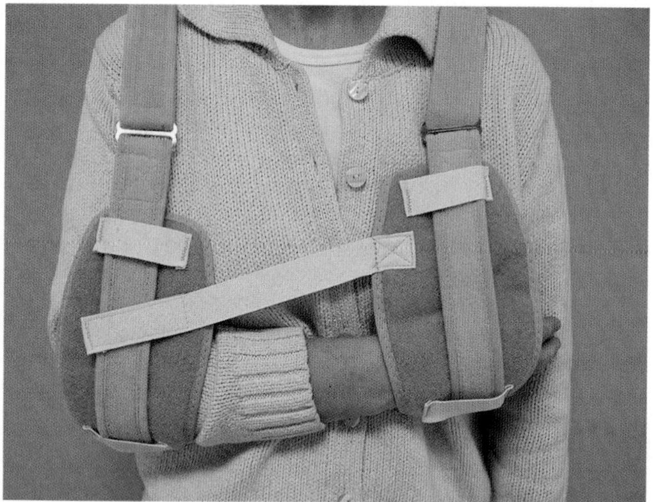

FIGURE 11-36 Rolyan figure-of-eight sling used for arm support and comfort of the shoulder joint in a patient with hemiplegia.

activities. Users are able to grasp an object by voluntarily flexing their fingers after some motor recovery and may be aided by increased muscle tone. The extension spring system assists in reopening the hand to release the object. Phase I trials are promising, with individuals demonstrating improvements in movement at the shoulder and elbow. Wrist extension also improved, but wrist flexion and finger movement did not.[13]

A mobile arm support can be used to enhance function for patients with proximal upper limb weakness, especially when the weakness is profound and the outlook for recovery is guarded. A mobile arm support is particularly helpful when activities of daily living, such as eating and grooming, are performed. When attached to a wheelchair with a swivel joint, this is often called a balanced forearm orthosis.

Many types of slings are available for patients with decreased tone of the upper limb (Figure 11-36). Decreased tone can result in shoulder subluxation, and a sling can decrease this deformity. These slings restrict active motion of the shoulder by keeping the humerus in adduction and internal rotation and placing the elbow in flexion.[37] They are designed to unload the weight of the arm on the shoulder but do not approximate the humeral head back into the glenoid fossa.[16] Slings or half arm trays have not been found to correct shoulder subluxation completely.[17] A sling should not create new problems, such as edema in the hand.[18] The arm trough or half lap board is often preferred because it will not restrict use of the limb and the humerus is more naturally approximated into the glenoid fossa.

Spinal Cord Injury

In patients with spinal cord injury, orthotic devices are needed to enhance function, help with positioning, or both. The type of device depends on the level of injury and the extent of neurologic compromise. With spinal cord injury at the C1-C3 level, the goal is to prevent contractures and to hold the wrist and digits in a position of function with a resting hand splint (see Figure 11-33). In a C4-level injury, the goal is to use the available shoulder strength by providing a mobile arm support to enhance function as previously described. In a C5-level injury, the goal is to statically position the wrist in extension with a ratchet-type hinged orthotic device to hold devices and use the shoulder musculature for function. An orthotic device for a C6 tetraplegia patient can enhance finger flexion with a tenodesis flexion effect from wrist extension. For example, a Rehabilitation Institute of Chicago tenodesis splint molded from thermoplastic materials has several positioning components (see Figures 11-17 and 11-18). A thumb post component positions the thumb in palmar abduction. A dorsal finger piece component, which is attached with a static line to a volar forearm component, holds the PIP joints of the index and long fingers in slight flexion. When the patient extends the wrist, the static line pulls the fingers toward the thumb post. This produces a three-point pinch, allowing the patient to grasp an object. When the patient relaxes the wrist, the fingers extend passively, releasing the object. The degree of pinch varies depending on the strength of the wrist extensors and the degree of finger flexion, extension, and opposition. This custom-made thermoplastic tenodesis device is mainly used in training and practice. If a patient finds the device useful, a light metal custom-made tenodesis orthosis achieves better functional restoration (see Chapter 49). An adaptive or functional use orthosis promotes functional use of the upper limb with impairment resulting from weakness, paralysis, or loss of a body part. An example is the universal cuff (see Figure 11-20), which encompasses the hand and holds various small items such as a fork, a pen, or a toothbrush to enhance independence.

Orthoses for Other Injuries

Postsurgical and Postinjury Orthoses

Many types of splints have been developed to help regain motion in stiff joints. Examples of such splints include dynamic elbow flexion and extension splints after upper arm or elbow fracture (see Figure 11-22), dynamic wrist flexion and extension splints after a Colles fracture, and dynamic finger flexion (Figure 11-37) and extension splints for stiffness after crush injuries to the hand. Similar splints can be fabricated with a static progressive approach. Joints that have a soft end feel do well with dynamic splints. Those with a rigid end feel typically respond better to a

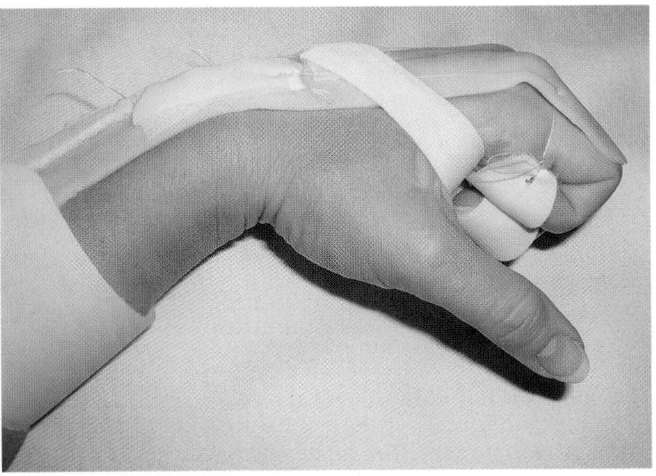

FIGURE 11-37 Extrinsic extensor stretching splint to increase finger flexion in combination with increasing increments of wrist flexion.

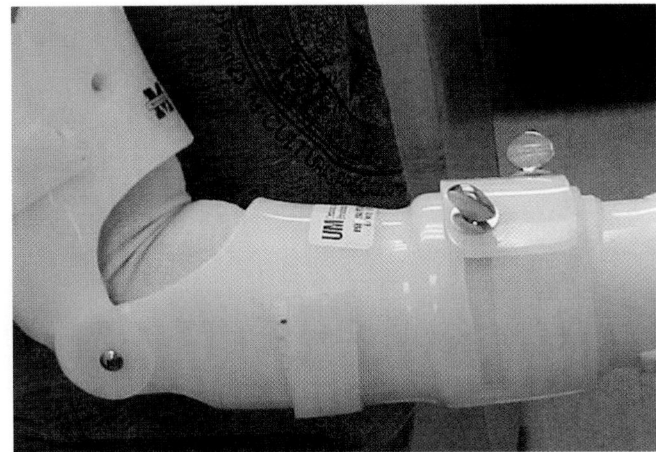

FIGURE 11-39 Static progressive pronation-supination splint used to increase motion in the forearm. (Courtesy Nicole M. Weiss, CO, OTR.)

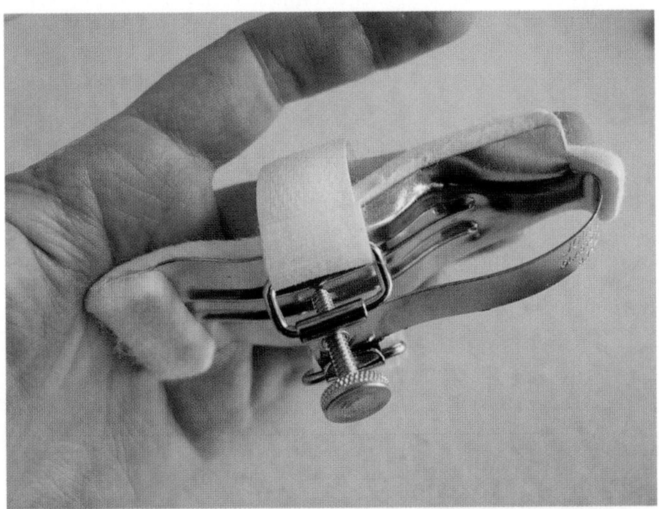

FIGURE 11-38 Joint Jack is a static progressive splint used to increase extension in the proximal interphalangeal joint.

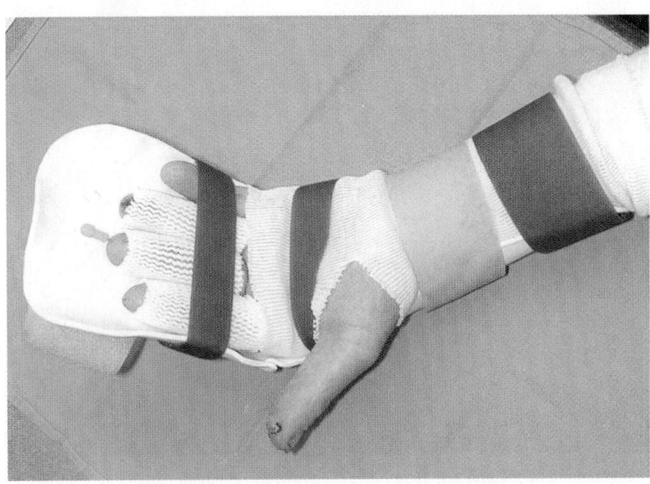

FIGURE 11-40 Duran flexor tendon repair splint used for postoperative care. (Courtesy Jeanne Riggs, OTR/L, CHT.)

static progressive approach that will maintain a constant joint position while the tissue accommodates gently to the tension, without the influence of gravity or motion.[4] Examples of static progressive splints are the Joint Jack (Figure 11-38) or cinch straps and splints for PIP and DIP joint contractures with the MERiT components (see Figure 11-13).[5] Selection of forearm-based or hand-based splints is determined by the need for stabilization. In general, the goal is to immobilize as few joints as feasible. Forearm pronation-supination splints with both dynamic and static features (Figure 11-39) are very helpful in regaining motion after fractures of the radius and ulna.[24]

Several splint designs are currently used after repair of tendon injuries. The type of surgical procedure or injury level often dictates the type of splint used so that the splints cannot be used interchangeably. For flexor tendon repair the Kleinert and Duran splints are commonly used. The Kleinert splint (see Figure 11-15) features dynamic traction into flexion but allows active digit extension within the constraints of the splint. The Duran splint statically positions the wrist and MCP joints in flexion and the IP joints in extension (Figure 11-40). The Indiana Protocol splint can also be used (Figures 11-41 and 11-42). This splint adds a tenodesis-type action splint to the Kleinert componentry for specific, active-assisted range-of-motion exercises. It can be used only if a specific surgical suture technique has been used.

The form of extensor tendon repair splints depends on the level of injury. A mallet finger injury can require only a Stax splint, which is a static splint holding the DIP joint in full extension. A more proximal injury, however, needs a splint that holds the wrist statically in extension with dynamic extension of MCP and IP joints (Figure 11-43). Such a splint permits active flexion of the MCP joints within the constraints of the splint to an angle of approximately 30 degrees. Injuries to the thumb flexor or extensor tendons require more specific splinting (Figure 11-44) and depend on the level of the injury.

Postoperative joint replacements for the PIP, DIP, or MCP joints of the hand require specific splints that promote healing or encapsulation of the joints while preserving ROM during the healing phases (Figure 11-45).

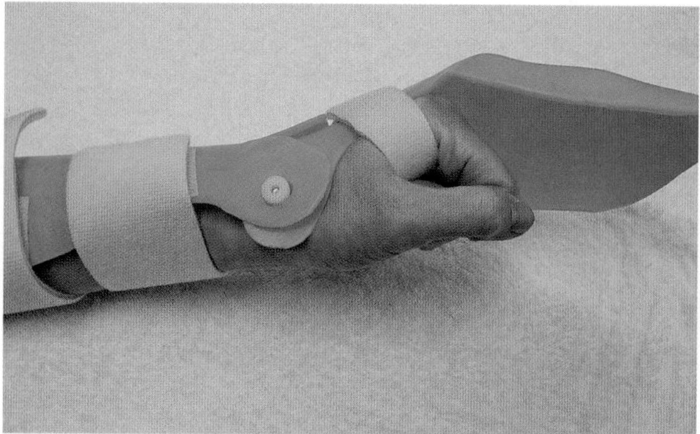

FIGURE 11-41 Indiana Protocol postoperative flexor tendon splint: tenodesis flexion exercises.

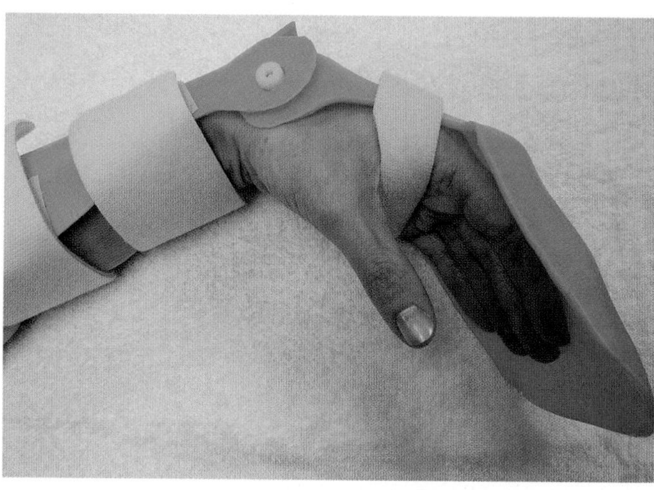

FIGURE 11-42 Indiana Protocol postoperative flexor tendon splint: tenodesis extension exercises.

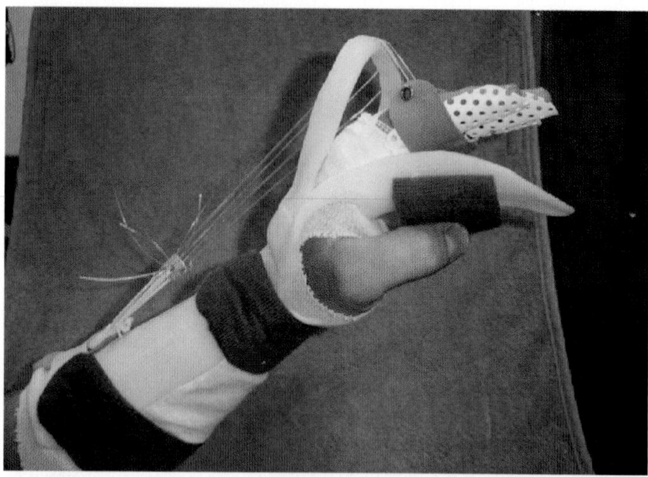

FIGURE 11-43 Extensor tendon splint used for postoperative care, allowing protected motion during the healing phase. (Courtesy Kelly Mikle, OTR/L, CHT.)

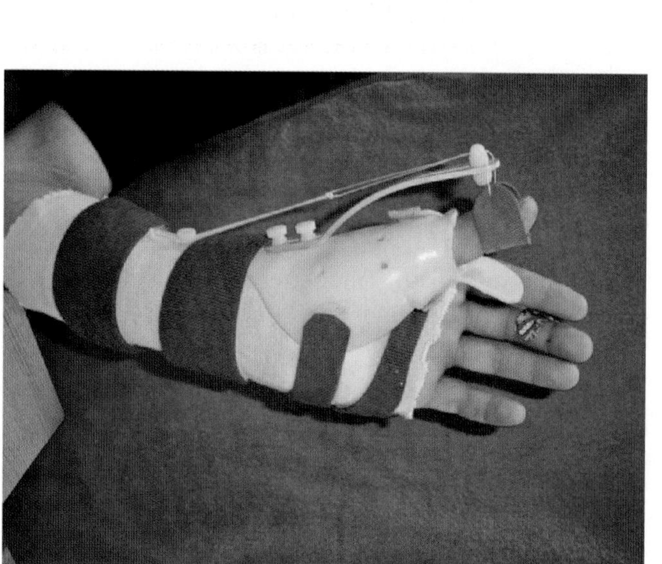

FIGURE 11-44 Postoperative splint for a patient with an extensor tendon pollicis longus repair. (Courtesy Kelly Mikle, OTR/L, CHT.)

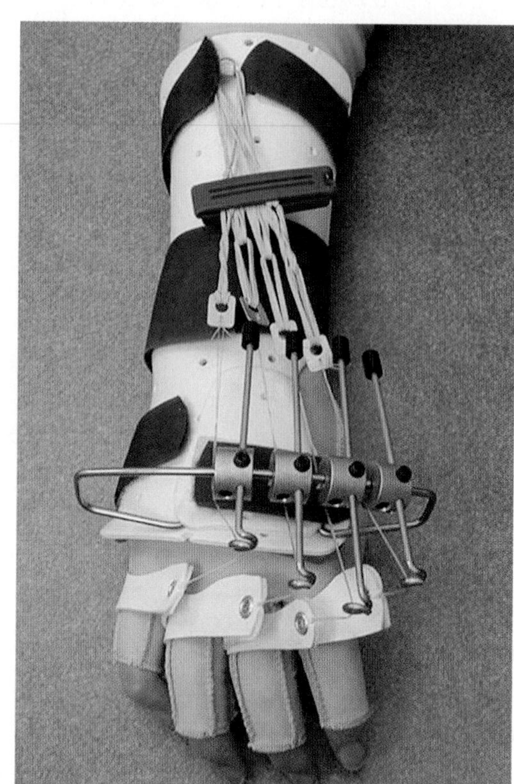

FIGURE 11-45 The metacarpophalangeal arthroplasty postoperative splint positions fingers in extension with slight radial pull. (Courtesy Jeanne Riggs, OTR/L, CHT.)

Orthoses for Burns

Patients with burns typically prefer an adducted and flexed position of the upper limbs to maintain comfort, but this preference can lead to loss of functional ROM. In this case, the splint acts to prevent contractures and deformities from developing. This is especially important when the patient cannot voluntarily maintain the range or when soft tissues underlying the skin are exposed. With tendon exposure, the splint plays a more protective role. It is important to monitor these patients frequently and reassess the needs for splinting.

After burn injuries, body parts should be positioned to prevent the development of expected deformities. For example, in burns of the dorsal surface of the hand, the wrist is placed in 15 degrees to 20 degrees of extension, the MCP joints in 60 degrees to 70 degrees of flexion, the PIP and DIP joints in full extension, and the thumb between radial abduction and palmar abduction (see Figure 11-2). If tendons are exposed then the flexion of the MCP joints should be decreased to 30 degrees to 40 degrees to keep some slack in the tendons until there is wound closure.[22] Palmar hand burns require maximum stretching to prevent the contracting forces of the healing burn.[22] The antideformity position of a palmar burn consists of 15 degrees to 20 degrees of wrist extension, extension of the MCP and IP joints, digital abduction, and thumb abduction and extension. This has been referred to as an "open palm" or "pancake position."[22] For prevention of shoulder adduction deformity after axillary burns, the shoulder should be held in abduction with an airplane splint. The tendency toward hypertrophic scarring after a burn is addressed with a selection of compression garments, elastomer molds, facial splints, gel shell splints, and silicone gel sheeting (see Chapter 26).

Pediatric Applications

Major reasons for use of orthoses in the pediatric population include functional positioning (Figure 11-46), normalizing muscle tone (Figure 11-47), postoperative protection, and positioning after surgery for a congenital deformity (Figure 11-48). Orthotic management of the child must consider the child's age, developmental status, growth, and functional status. Orthoses are expected to last at least a year, so the material must be durable, safe, and accommodate for some growth, for example, in young children who often chew on their hand braces. Parents should be educated on how to apply the orthotic and to watch for any skin injury related to the orthotic.

Children with abnormal tone or progressive neuromuscular disorders (NMDs) are at higher risk for contracture development. A contracture is defined as lack of full active or passive ROM. Contractures are inevitable in some NMD conditions, such as Duchenne muscular dystrophy. A

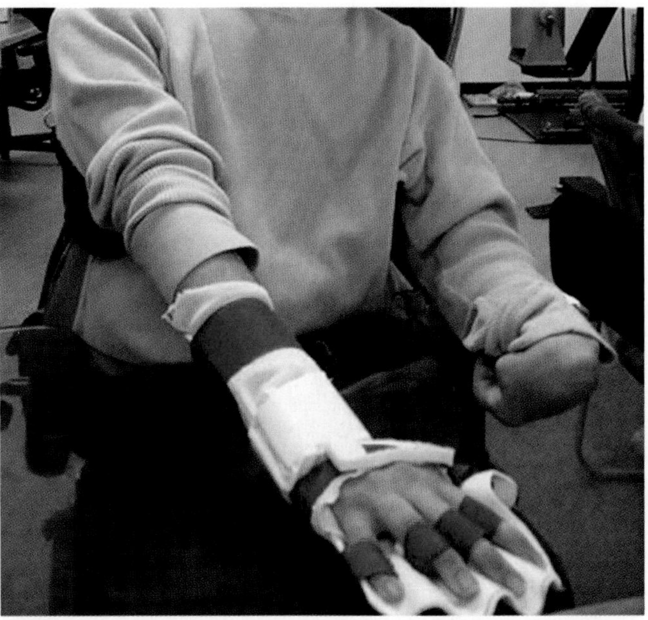

FIGURE 11-47 A ball splint orthosis used to reduce tone in a child with cerebral palsy.

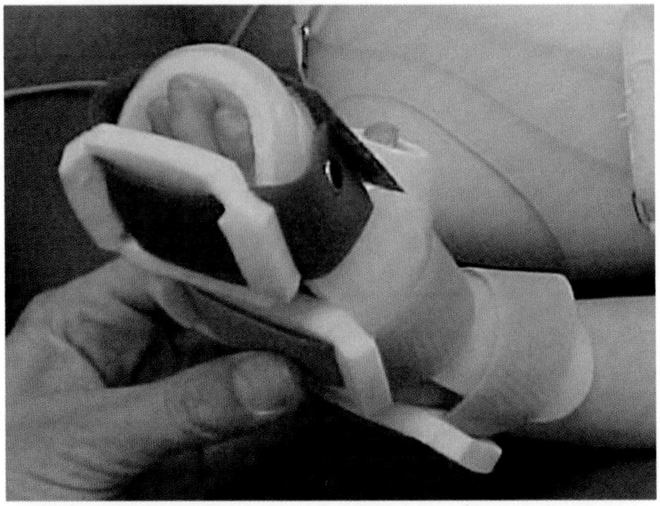

FIGURE 11-46 A soft Benik-type orthosis to position the thumb away (abduction) from the palm.

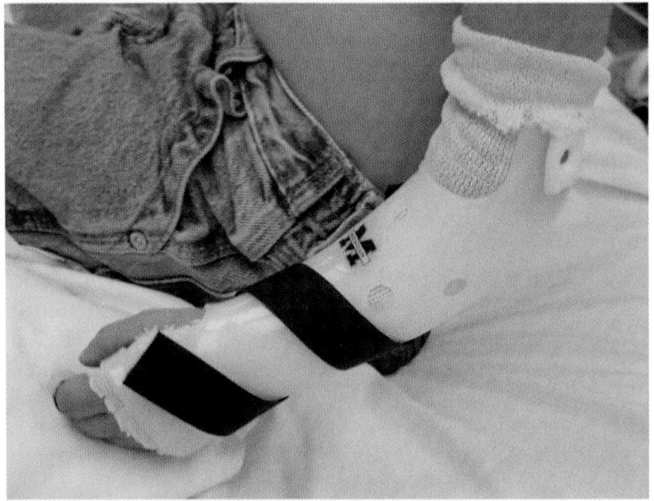

FIGURE 11-48 Custom pediatric Muenster splint restricts forearm rotation and wrist motion after reconstruction while allowing motion at the elbow.

major rationale for controlling the degree of contracture development is to minimize the adverse effects of contractures on function. It is important to acknowledge that static positioning of the limbs in patients with weak musculature is the most important cause of contracture development. Upper limb contractures may not negatively affect function if they are mild. Stretching and ROM are mainstays to preserve function.[29]

Children can have devastating injuries through motor vehicle crashes, sports injury, and accidents. C5-C8 lesions are the most common cervical cord injury for pediatrics. This injury affects the upper limbs, and orthoses can be used to prevent deformity and assist with functional tasks. Static wrist-hand orthoses are commonly used with children to improve hand position for functional activities and to maintain ROM. Dynamic wrist/hand orthoses are much less commonly used because children are often reluctant to use them for functional activities, in part because of decreased sensory feedback caused by the orthosis.[26,28]

Special Considerations

Cosmesis is often a problem for patients because they care about the way splints look and what it means. To ensure patient compliance, the splint has to be as cosmetically acceptable as possible. Patients should have every opportunity to assist in choosing the design and appearance. Patients often have very good ideas about the design of a splint and can suggest good ways to strap it into place (as long as the splint mechanics are not altered).

Comfort is also important. The thinner the materials used and the more care the therapist takes in making a close and comfortable fit, the better the acceptance of the splint. For example, areas around bony prominences need to be relieved to prevent pressure, whereas edges and joints frequently need to be padded to reduce skin irritation. Patients with arthritis who have been taking corticosteroids for long periods often have fragile skin, so their splints should be padded throughout. Stockinette worn under splints also helps, particularly with perspiration in warmer weather.

Splints can be perfectly designed and skillfully fabricated but are useless if not worn. The more choice and input patients have in splint design, the more compliant they are likely to be with splint wear. The wearing schedule depends on the goals for the splint and the patient's tolerance for wear. For example, a patient with a brain injury who is "storming" (i.e., sweating excessively and posturing) may tolerate a resting hand splint for positioning for just 30 minutes on and 3 hours off. By contrast, a patient with stroke and with mild spasticity could wear a resting hand splint 2 hours on and 2 hours off during the day and keep it on all night. Static progressive splint wear depends on the tissue response to gentle stretching. The stretch should be perceived as mild, and it should never awaken the patient at night. In a patient with both flexion and extension splinting needs, the flexion splint can be worn 1 hour on, 2 hours off during the day, and the extension splint can be worn at night.

A resting hand splint for positioning is often indicated when edema is present (see Figure 11-33). However, a splint can also induce edema because of an inflammatory response caused by an overly aggressive stretch, particularly in a patient with increased tone. Special strapping techniques can often lessen the response. Other tissue responses are also possible. Blueness or redness of the digits when wearing a splint tells the observer that an overly aggressive stretch is being applied to the shortened neurovascular bundles. These structures sometimes shorten because of the joint contracture, in which case splint tension must be decreased and the contracture stretch should be less aggressive.[18] Skin checks should be performed after a splint is removed. More frequent checks should occur, especially if the splint is new or recently changed. Complaints of pain or tenderness may signal where to examine closely. The skin is examined for abrasions and erythema. A blanchable lesion will lose its redness when pressed and is not as serious as nonblanchable lesions, which reflect underlying tissue injury.

Splint prescriptions should explain the diagnosis or problem to be addressed. A description of the function or motion desired helps to alleviate confusion. It can also facilitate discussion with the therapist, physician, and patient regarding the best design to meet mutually agreed goals. A good description can also help clarify misunderstandings arising from conflicting naming systems (see Table 11-1).

Orthotic Materials

Most splinting materials are low-temperature thermoplastics. Many are known by their trademark names, such as Orthoplast, Aquaplast, and Orfit.[30,36] Low-temperature thermoplastics become soft and pliable when exposed to relatively low temperatures and can be shaped in a water bath at 150° F to 180° F (66° C to 82° C). High-temperature thermoplastics are more durable but require oven heating (up to 350° F or 177° C) and placement over a mold to achieve the desired shape.[6] All splinting materials have certain characteristics determined by the temperature and material properties. Some, such as Ezeform, are very rigid when cool.[32] Others, such as Polyform, are very drapable when warm.[32] Firm materials may be desirable for patients with increased tone, whereas drapable materials may be desirable when conformability is needed, as when splinting a finger. Some plastic materials have a great deal of "memory." This means they return to their original shape when reheated. This characteristic can help control costs, especially those incurred when providing serial static splinting.[30]

International Considerations

People with a disability are often caught in a vicious cycle of poverty and disability.[2] The World Health Organization estimates that only 5% to 15% of people with disabilities in Third World countries have access to assistive devices.[3] Low-income countries deliver assistive technology (including orthotic devices) differently because of cost, availability, materials, required skilled craftsmanship, health care access, and infrastructure issues. These factors represent the biggest and most difficult challenges to delivering orthotic devices to people in need. Training and retaining professionals in current orthotic principles, materials, and fabrication techniques is challenging. The goal is to fabricate a "universal" splint that has broad applicability and requires minimal adaptations. This same device can go on to benefit another person at another time. The availability of materials can be a challenge for many with limited resources. This can call for ingenuity on behalf of the fabricator to use local materials that might reduce cost, time of fabrication, or withstand the environment better than traditional plastics common to our appliances in the developed world. Donations of resources and old orthotic appliances are critical, although not all places have the infrastructure to deliver the donated items to the people in need. Recognizing the need for recycled orthotics throughout the world, many charity or orthotic and prosthetic programs will donate old or unwanted assistive devices. These devices will find a second life helping individuals with limited access to care or resources.

Community-based rehabilitation is a strategy developed by the World Health Organization for improving disability services in low-income countries.[11] This program empowers local people to serve the disabled in their community, and includes teaching fabrication techniques for orthotic appliances.

Summary

This chapter has provided guidelines concerning the principles for upper limb orthotic devices, as well as various classification systems and descriptions of design categories. For an orthosis to be fabricated, a sound understanding of the anatomy, biomechanics, and tissue physiology of the upper limb is required. Persons prescribing upper limb orthotic devices should have a thorough knowledge of the musculoskeletal and neurologic conditions amenable to treatment by orthoses. They must also understand other avenues of treatment, such as exercise therapy, and be alert to surgical indications.

The most important principle in the prescription of orthotic devices is gaining the cooperation of the patient. Through the attention and concern of the physician and therapist, the patient must be able to see the benefit of the orthosis. It must also fit comfortably and be cosmetically appealing. Everyone involved must have the same goals and purpose for the device, or it will end up being abandoned soon after it has been fitted.

As we continue to learn more about the biomechanics of the hand, we better understand how to redress externally the internal imbalance caused by disease and injury. Keeping the internal dynamics of the hand in mind, splinting is often the most efficient and effective way to redress this mechanical imbalance.[21]

REFERENCES

1. American Society of Hand Therapists, Splint Nomenclature Task Force: *Splint classification system*, Garner, 1991, American Society of Hand Therapists.
2. [Anonymous]: Disability, poverty and development, *World Hosp Health Serv* 38(1):21–33, 2002.
3. Austin GP, Slamet M, Cameron D, et al: A comparison of high-profile and low-profile dynamic mobilization splint designs, *J Hand Ther* 17(3):335–343, 2004.
4. Austin NM, Jacobs M: Orthoses in the management of hand dysfunction. In Lusardi M, Jorge M, Nielsen C, editors: *Orthotics and prosthetics in rehabilitation*, St Louis, 2013, Elsevier/Saunders, pp 392–411.
5. Bash DS, Spur ME: An alternative to turnbuckle splinting for elbow flexion, *J Hand Ther* 13(3):237–240, 2000.
6. Breger-Lee DE, Buford WL, Jr: Update in splinting materials and methods, *Hand Clin* 7(3):569–585, 1991.
7. Callinan NJ, Mathiowetz V: Soft versus hard resting hand splints in rheumatoid arthritis: pain relief, preference, and compliance, *Am J Occup Ther* 50(5):347–353, 1996.
8. Colditz J, editor: Principles of splinting and splint prescription. In *Surgery of the hand and upper extremity*, New York, 1996, McGraw Hill, pp 2389–2410.
9. Coppard B, Lohman H: *Introduction to splinting: a critical-thinking and problem-solving approach*, ed 2, St Louis, 2001, Mosby.
10. Elovic EP, Brashear A, Kaelin D, et al: Repeated treatments with botulinum toxin type A produce sustained decreases in the limitations associated with focal upper-limb poststroke spasticity for caregivers and patients, *Arch Phys Med Rehabil* 89(5):799–806, 2008.
11. Evans PJ, Zinkin P, Harpham T, et al: Evaluation of medical rehabilitation in community based rehabilitation, *Soc Sci Med* 53(3):333–348, 2001.
12. Falkenstein N, Weiss S: *Hand rehabilitation: a quick reference guide and review*, St Louis, 2004, Mosby.
13. Farrell JF, Hoffman HB, Snyder JL, et al: Orthotic aided training of the paretic upper limb in chronic stroke: results of a phase 1 trial, *Neurorehabilitation* 22(2):99–103, 2007.
14. Fess EE: A history of splinting: to understand the present, view the past, *J Hand Ther* 15(2):97–132, 2002.
15. Flowers KRLaStayo P: LaStayo P: Effect of total end range time on improving passive range of motion, *J Hand Ther* 7(3):150–157, 1994.
16. Gilmore PE, Spaulding SJ, Vandervoort AA: Hemiplegic shoulder pain: implications for occupational therapy treatment, *Can J Occup Ther* 71(1):36–46, 2004.
17. Glasgow C, Wilton J, Tooth L: Optimal daily total end range time for contracture: resolution in hand splinting, *J Hand Ther* 16(3):207–218, 2003.
18. Halanski M, Noonan KJ: Cast and splint immobilization: complications, *J Am Acad Orthop Surg* 16(1):30–40, 2008.
19. Hannah SD, Hudak PL: Splinting and radial nerve palsy: a single-subject experiment, *J Hand Ther* 11(3):195–201, 2001.
20. Hesse S, Brandi-Hesse B, Bardeleben A, et al: Botulinum toxin A treatment of adult upper and lower limb spasticity, *Drugs Aging* 18(4):255–262, 2001.
21. Hunter J, Mackin E, Callahan A: *Rehabilitation of the hand: surgery and therapy*, ed 4, St Louis, 1995, Mosby.
22. Kwan MW, Ha KW: Splinting programme for patients with burnt hand, *Hand Surg* 7(2):231–241, 2002.
23. Lai JM, Francisco GE, Willis FB: Dynamic splinting after treatment with botulinum toxin type-A: a randomized controlled pilot study, *Adv Ther* 26(2):241–248, 2009.
24. Mackin E, Callahan A, Skirven T: *Rehabilitation of the hand and upper extremity*, ed 5, St Louis, 2002, Mosby.
25. Magee DJ: Forearm, wrist, and hand. In Magee DJ, editor: *Orthopedic physical assessment*, ed 4, Philadelphia, 2002, Elsevier/Saunders, pp 378–379.
26. McDonald CM: Limb contractures in progressive neuromuscular disease and the role of stretching, orthotics, and surgery, *Phys Med Rehabil Clin N Am* 9(1):187–211, 1998.
27. McKee P: *Orthotics in rehabilitation, splinting the hand and body*, Philadelphia, 2010, FA Davis.
28. McMahon M, Pruitt D, Vargus-Adams J: Cerebral palsy. In Alexander MA, Matthews DJ, editors: *Pediatric rehabilitation: principles and practice*, ed 4, New York, 2010, Demos Medical Publishing, pp 165–197.
29. Nelson VS, Hornyak J: Spinal cord injuries. In Alexander MA, Matthews DJ, editors: *Pediatric rehabilitation: principles and practice*, ed 4, New York, 2010, Demos Medical Publishing, pp 261–276.
30. *North Coast Medical Company hand therapy catalog*, Morgan Hill, Calif., 2014, North Coast Medical Company. www.ncmedical.com/categories/Upper-Extremity24.html.

31. Prange GB, Jannink MJ, Groothuis-Oudshoorn CG, et al: Systematic review of the effect of robot-aided therapy on recovery of the hemiparetic arm after stroke, *J Rehabil Res Dev* 43(2):171–184, 2006.
32. *Preston medical/MERiT final finger flexion kit.* http://pattersonmedical.com.
33. Redford J, Basmajian J, Trautman P: *Orthotics: clinical practice and rehabilitation technology*, New York, 1995, Churchill Livingstone.
34. SaeboFlex. www.saebo.com/.
35. Schuch C, Pritham C: International Standards Organization terminology: application to prosthetics and orthotics, *J Prosthet Orthot* 6(1):29–48, 1994.
36. *Smith & Nephew Inc. rehabilitation division catalog.* http://smith-nephew.com.
37. Sullivan BE, Rogers SL: Modified Bobath sling with distal support, *Am J Occup Ther* 43(1):47–49, 1989.
38. Walker-Bone K, Palmer KT, Reading I, et al: Prevalence and impact of musculoskeletal disorders of the upper limb in the general population, *Arthritis Rheum* 51(4):642–651, 2004.
39. Zafonte R, Elovic EP, Lombard L: Acute care management of post-TBI spasticity, *J Head Trauma Rehabil* 19(2):89–100, 2004.

CHAPTER 12

LOWER LIMB ORTHOSES

William J. Hennessey, Heikki Uustal

An orthosis is defined as a device attached or applied to the external surface of the body to improve function, restrict or enforce motion, or support a body segment.[38] Lower limb orthoses are indicated to assist gait, reduce pain, decrease weight bearing, control movement, and minimize progression of a deformity. Lower limb orthoses assist nonambulatory patients with transfer and mobility skills and assist ambulatory patients in becoming safe walkers. Ambulation aids can be used in combination with lower limb orthoses to help patients ambulate more safely. Ambulation aids represent extensions of the upper limb but are discussed in this chapter because of their importance in gait.

Principles of Lower Limb Orthoses

Orthoses should be used for the specific management of selected disorders. As in all fields of medicine, specific treatment should be based on a specific medical diagnosis, with an established goal of treatment.[56] Placement of orthotic joints should approximate anatomic joints. Box 12-1 outlines this principle as well as other common lower limb orthotic principles. Most orthoses use a three-point system to ensure proper positioning of the limb within the orthosis.[27] For example, a knee that has a tendency to hyperextend, or "back knee," can be treated with a knee orthosis (KO) that applies force posterior to the knee but also applies forces anteriorly along the leg and the thigh. Such an orthosis ensures adequate control of the knee by exerting these forces proximal to, distal to, and at the knee joint.

Terminology for Lower Limb Orthoses

Orthoses are frequently and incorrectly referred to as orthotics. *Orthotic* is the adjective derived from the noun *orthosis*. An orthosis can be referred to as an orthotic device. An orthosis is also made in an orthotic laboratory.

Terminology pertinent to the anatomy of the lower limb is also frequently used incorrectly. The term *extremity* specifically refers to the foot. The term *leg* should be used to refer to the portion of the lower limb between the knee and ankle joints. The thigh is located between the hip and knee joints. Lower limb refers to the thigh, leg, and foot.

Pathologic abnormalities regarding angulation have also been referred to incorrectly as varus and valgus deformities at the knee and hip. Correct use of the Latin-derived terminology for these deformities requires the suffix *-us* at the ankle, *-um* at the knee, and *-a* at the hip. Varus and valgus deformities of the foot are described for both the hindfoot and forefoot (i.e., hindfoot valgus or forefoot varus). A bow-legged condition is correctly referred to as genu varum. Deformity at the hip is referred to as coxa valga and coxa vara.

Lower limb orthoses are frequently referred to with abbreviations. Standard orthotic nomenclature uses the first letter of each joint the orthosis crosses from proximal to distal. It then lists the first letter of the limb to which it is affixed (i.e., "F" for foot). Lastly, the letter "O" is used to signify it is an orthosis. Thus, AFO designates an ankle-foot orthosis. KAFO means knee-ankle-foot orthosis. HKAFO means hip-knee-ankle-foot orthosis.

The orthotic literature uses variable medical terminology. The calcaneus is frequently referred to as the os calcis. A plantar flexion deformity is referred to as an equinus deformity. Torsion and rotation have incorrectly been used interchangeably. Torsion refers to twisting of a portion of a limb. Rotation of a limb occurs only at a joint. Pronation has been referred to as inrolling, whereas supination has been referred to as outrolling. An orthosis is not put on and taken off but rather is donned and doffed. Checkout means an examination of the patient after the orthosis is fitted.

Shoes

The purpose of wearing shoes is to protect the feet. The normal foot does not require support from shoes. The sole should be pliable so as not to interfere with the normal biomechanics of the foot. A practical way of ensuring that a shoe is of adequate length is to determine whether the index finger can be placed between the tip of the great toe and the toe box.[58] The presence of calluses indicates areas of friction from poorly fitting (loose) shoes. The presence of corns indicates areas of friction over bony prominences, most often caused by tight-fitting shoes. Leather shoes are good choices for all types of activity. They are durable, allow ventilation, and mold to the feet with time. A good pair of shoes can often eliminate the need for foot orthoses and should be considered before orthotic prescription.

Shoe Parts

Two types of dress shoes are commonly worn, the Blucher and the Bal (Figure 12-1). The tongue is part of the vamp in the Blucher shoe. The quarters overlap the vamp. A Blucher shoe is recommended for patients requiring an orthosis because there is more room to don and doff the shoe and the orthosis because of the open throat.[63] In the Bal shoe style, the quarters meet at the throat. The vamp

BOX 12-1

Principles of Lower Limb Orthoses

- Use only as indicated and for as long as necessary.
- Allow joint movement wherever possible and appropriate.
- Orthoses should be functional throughout all phases of gait.
- Orthotic ankle joint should be centered over tip of medial malleolus.
- Orthotic knee joint should be centered over prominence of medial femoral condyle.
- Orthotic hip joint should be in a position that allows patient to sit upright at 90 degrees.
- Patient compliance will be enhanced if orthosis is comfortable, cosmetic, and functional.

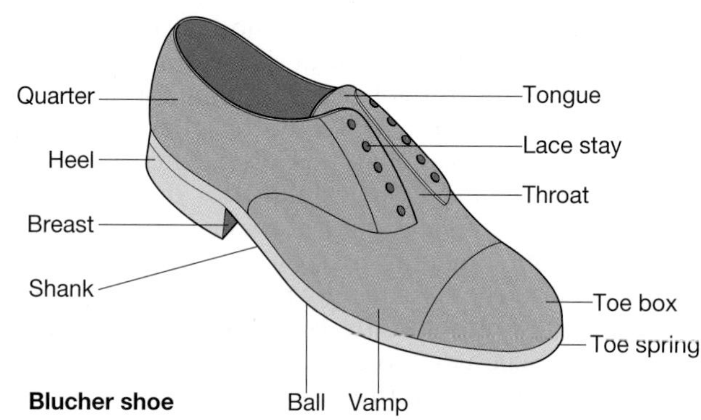

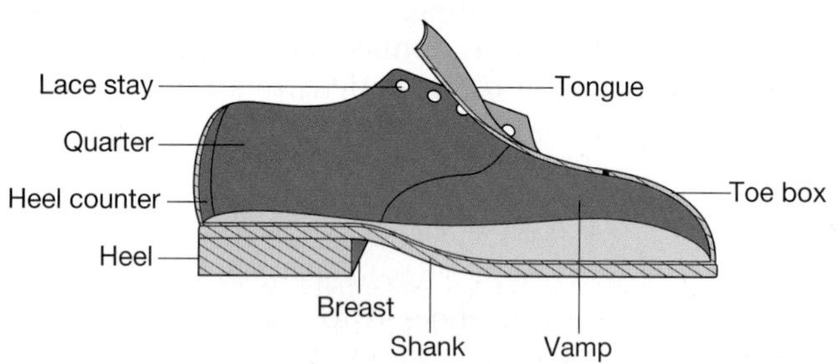

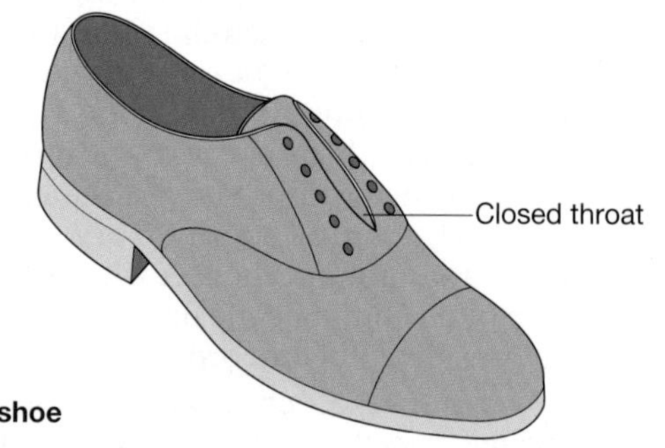

FIGURE 12-1 Shoe types and components. The open throat of the Blucher shoe accommodates an orthosis better than the Bal shoe.

is stitched over the quarters at the throat, thereby limiting the ability of the shoe to open and accommodate an orthosis. The heel counter is the support in the back of the shoe to control the rearfoot. A strong heel counter is critical to control the entire foot.

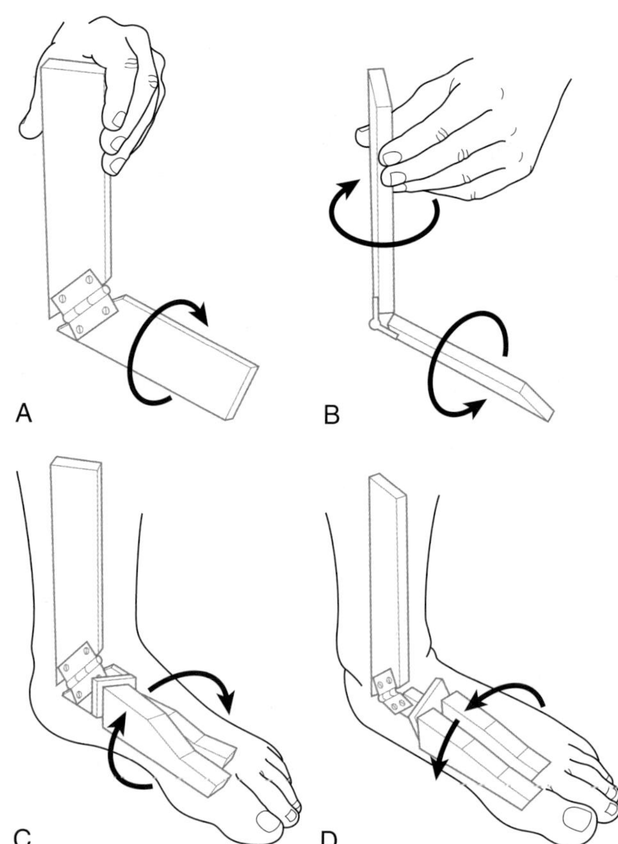

FIGURE 12-2 Analogy of subtalar axes to an oblique hinge. **A** and **C,** Outward rotation of the upper stick (tibia) results in inward rotation of the lower stick (calcaneus). This results in elevation of the medial border of the foot and depression of the lateral border. **B** and **D,** Inward rotation of the upper stick (tibia) results in outward rotation of the lower stick (calcaneus). This results in depression of the medial side of the foot with elevation of the lateral side. (Modified from Mann RA: Biomechanics of the foot. In American Academy of Orthopaedic Surgeons, editors: *Atlas of orthotics,* St Louis, 1985, Mosby–Year Book, p 118.)

Foot Orthoses

Foot orthoses range from arch supports found at a local pharmacy or athletic store to customized orthoses fabricated by an orthotist. The effectiveness of an orthosis depends on proper diagnosis of the foot condition, the appropriate selection of orthotic material, and proper molding. Foot orthoses affect the ground reactive forces acting on the joints of the lower limb. They also have an effect on rotational components of gait (Figure 12-2).

Mild conditions can be treated with over-the-counter orthoses. More severe problems and chronic medical conditions require customized orthoses.[61] These are available in three types. A soft type is most commonly used in over-the-counter orthoses. Orthotists usually provide semirigid orthoses, which provide more support than the soft type but are still shock absorbing. A rigid orthosis is indicated only for a problem that requires aggressive bracing to control a deformity.

For a custom foot orthosis to be made, the subtalar joint should be placed in a neutral position before casting. This position minimizes abnormalities related to foot and ankle rotation, such as hyperpronation, and it is also the position in which the foot functions best.[41] The subtalar neutral position is used to treat conditions associated with hyperpronation, including pes planus, patellofemoral pain, and even patients with painful rheumatoid arthritis affecting the first metatarsophalangeal.[9,48] The foot is then covered with a parting agent, such as stockinette or a clear plastic wrap. The foot is then wrapped in either plaster of Paris strips or fiberglass tape and allowed to harden. Fiberglass casting is also used for difficult orthotic cases in which the fiberglass casting itself can be used as a temporary orthosis to determine whether the mold properly controls the deformity. This negative mold is then removed to allow a positive mold to be made from the negative mold. The positive mold can be modified to increase the effectiveness of the orthosis. The custom orthosis is obtained by heating and form-fitting (often by use of a vacuum) the plastic to the positive mold.

It should be noted that research has not determined the length of time an orthosis remains effective. The orthosis should be examined at each follow-up visit to determine when a new one is necessary.

Common Foot Conditions

Pes Planus (Flat Foot)

Symptomatic relief of pain is obtained by controlling excess pronation of the foot. Pronation of the foot can be defined as a rotation of the foot in the longitudinal axis resulting in a lowering of the medial aspect of the foot. Pronation occurs at the subtalar joint and it is also referred to as inrolling. Foot pronation is a component of eversion. Eversion involves pronation at the subtalar joint, dorsiflexion at the ankle joint, and abduction of the forefoot at the tarsometatarsal joints. The key to controlling excess pronation is controlling the calcaneus to keep the subtalar joint in a neutral position.

Pes planus can be due to abnormalities, such as excessive internal torsion of the tibia (which results in pronation of the foot) or malalignment of the calcaneus. It is the interaction between the tibia and the foot at the subtalar joint that allows disease outside the foot to cause inrolling of the foot (see Figure 12-2).

The reduction of pronation is accomplished by maintaining the calcaneus and the subtalar joint in correct alignment. The subtalar joint should be in a neutral position during the custom-molding process. The subtalar joint neutral position prevents rotational deformities associated with excessive pronation or supination from occurring (see Figure 12-2, *C* and *D*). Elevation of the anteromedial calcaneus exerts an upward thrust against the sustentaculum tali to help prevent inrolling.[6] The orthosis should extend beyond the metatarsal heads to provide better leverage for control of the deformity. A custom-made foot orthosis designed to prevent hyperpronation is also referred to as a UCBL orthosis (or UCB), denoting the University of California Biomechanics Laboratory, where original work regarding this type of orthosis was performed in the 1940s. There are two common mistakes noted in custom foot orthoses. First, some are not made by orthotists who represent the profession best capable of making a proper foot orthosis. Second, some custom foot orthoses do not cup the calcaneus but rather merely serve as a platform to stand on. The orthosis must extend proximally enough on the calcaneus to cup and control the subtalar joint during gait.

Some cases of pes planus are due to ligamentous laxity within the foot. For these cases, a medial longitudinal arch support can be helpful for alleviating pain. Initial use of an arch that is too high can cause discomfort. The height of the arch can be increased as necessary as the foot develops a tolerance for the inlay. A Thomas heel extension (term for increased medial length to heel) can also offer medial support, particularly for heavier individuals. A most practical piece of advice for runners who have hyperpronation/pes planus is to purchase a pair of running shoes with a firm medial heel counter as well as shoes with a wide last at the shank (see Figure 12-1). Each of these applications helps prevent pronation at the subtalar joint.

Pes Cavus (High-Arched Foot)

A typical complication of pes cavus is excess pressure along the heel and metatarsal head areas, which can lead to pain. This can be prevented by making the height of the longitudinal support just high enough to fill in the space between the shank of the shoe and the arch of the foot to distribute weight more effectively. Weight should also be evenly distributed over the metatarsal heads. The lift is extended just to the metatarsal head area to help distribute and alleviate pressure over the metatarsal weight-bearing area. Because there is no tendency to pronate as in pes planus, the high point of the arch is located at the talonavicular joint. If the tibia is externally rotated (see Figure 12-2), this can give the appearance of an elevated arch as the foot supinates and the lateral aspect of the foot assumes additional weight-bearing responsibility. In these cases, a foot orthosis is custom molded with the subtalar joint in a neutral position to prevent excess supination from occurring.

Forefoot Pain (Metatarsalgia)

Relief of pain in the forefoot is accomplished by distributing the weight-bearing forces to an area proximal to the metatarsal heads. This can be done by either internal or external modification. A metatarsal pad (also referred to as a "cookie") can be placed inside the shoe just proximal to the second, third, and fourth metatarsal heads. It should also be just proximal to the lateral aspect of the first metatarsal head and medial to the fifth metatarsal head (Figure 12-3). A metatarsal bar is recommended for cases in which the foot is too sensitive to tolerate a pad inside the shoe. The metatarsal bar is typically a quarter of an inch thick and tapers distally. The distal edge should be proximal to the metatarsal heads. It is often applied to a leather or neoprene sole.[35] The metatarsal bar can also be used for forefoot pain associated with pes cavus. A rocker bottom (Figure 12-4) can also be used for metatarsalgia to decrease the force on the metatarsal pad region at push-off.

Prevention of forefoot pain should also be emphasized to patients. Patients should avoid shoes with high heels or pointed toes, which place excess stress on the metatarsal heads.[4]

Heel Pain

The painful area can be alleviated with an orthosis to help distribute weight. Rubber heel pads can be applied inside the shoe to offer relief in cases of minor discomfort. A calcaneal bar is recommended for cases in which the foot is too sensitive to tolerate a pad inside the shoe and the heel pain is associated with a chronic condition. The calcaneal bar is placed distal to the painful area to prevent the calcaneus from assuming full weight-bearing status. The same can be accomplished with a shoe that has a spring for the heel set on the anterior calcaneus (see Figure 12-4, *A*). The application of a rocker bottom shoe can also be used to help initiate heel strike anterior and the ground reaction force anterior to the painful calcaneus (see Figure 12-4, *B*). Both of these shoe types are now commercially available.A common cause of heel pain along the anteromedial calcaneus is plantar fasciitis. Pain occurs at the attachment site of the fascia along the medial aspect of the heel.[39] Point tenderness is located over the anteromedial calcaneus. It is common in people who hyperpronate their feet, thereby placing excess stress on the medial longitudinal arch. A custom-made orthosis with the subtalar joint in a neutral position (such as that described for pes planus) helps prevent excessive inrolling from occurring and reduces the stress placed along the proximal arch. A custom-made UCB orthosis is indicated for cases in which conservative treatment has failed. From an orthotic standpoint, conservative treatment should include the use of a pair of shoes with a firm medial heel counter and a wide shank.

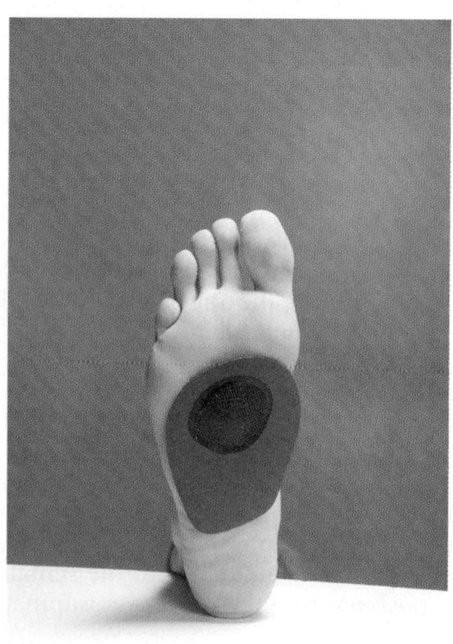

FIGURE 12-3 Metatarsal pad for forefoot pain. This should be placed *proximal* to the metatarsal heads to reduce weight distribution on the metatarsal heads.

An additional orthotic intervention for plantar fasciitis is the application of a plantar fascia night splint, which is a prefabricated AFO placed in a few degrees of dorsiflexion.[16,42] This helps provide the plantar fascia and plantar flexors a therapeutic stretch during sleep hours, assuring the patient several hours of passive stretching daily. Such a device is recommended for as long as is necessary until the patient is asymptomatic (Figure 12-5).

Plantar fasciitis is also common in patients with high arches. For these patients, the medial longitudinal arch undergoes marked stress during weight-bearing. This can be treated with either an elevated arch support or a heel well that helps distribute pressure along the medial longitudinal arch.

Heel spurs are frequently mistaken as the source of heel pain. Heel spurs related to plantar fasciitis are the result of mechanical stress acting through the plantar fascia onto its origin at the calcaneus and are not the source of the pain.[34] Inferior heel spurs are related to advancing age and are not painful in nature.

Heel lifts help some causes of Achilles pain by decreasing the amount of stretch placed on the Achilles tendon (by keeping the ankle joint plantar flexed). A heel lift can be used to treat the pain associated with Achilles enthesitis, an inflammatory reaction at the insertion of the tendon

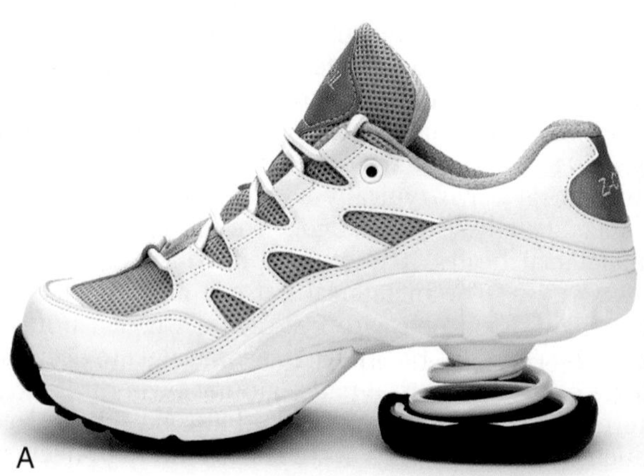

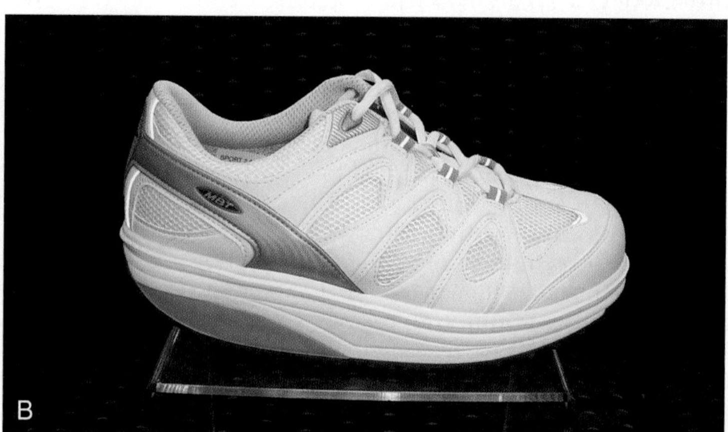

FIGURE 12-4 **A,** A spring coil in this shoe located at the anterior heel can alleviate heel pain by moving the ground reaction force anterior to the painful portion of the calcaneus in addition to lessening impact at heel strike. This can help with knee stability also. The forefoot is also designed as a rocker bottom for forefoot comfort. (Courtesy Z-CoiL Footwear, Albuquerque, N.M.) **B,** Rocker bottom shoe. This is prescribed for patients with ankle fusions to help normalize their gait pattern by simulating plantar flexion. A rocker bottom can also be prescribed for heel pain because it helps move the contact point at heel strike anterior to the painful calcaneus. Hence, the ground reaction force is also moved anterior to the painful heel. For metatarsalgia, it decreases force across the metatarsal heads at push-off. This type of shoe can now be purchased in some shoe stores in addition to being custom built into an existing regular pair of shoes.

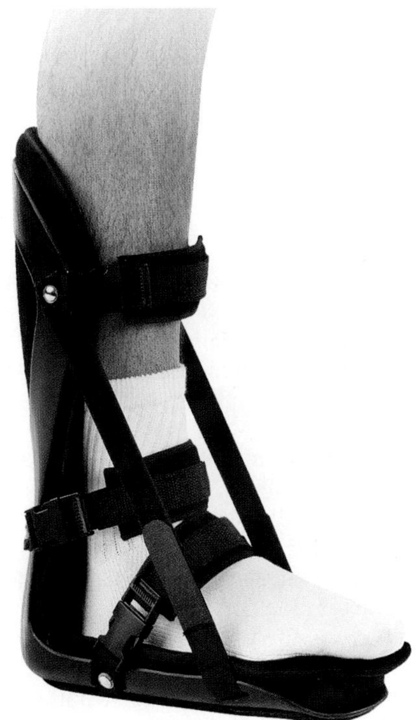

FIGURE 12-5 Plantar fascia night splint. This prefabricated ankle-foot orthosis provides a therapeutic stretch to the plantar fascia and plantar flexors nightly to help alleviate anteromedial heel pain and facilitate a recovery. (Courtesy BREG, Inc., Carlsbad, Calif, and Elizur Corp, Pittsburgh, Pa.)

into the periosteum of the calcaneus. For Achilles enthesitis, a heel lift is meant to be used for weeks, not months, to prevent the development of a plantar flexion contracture. A heel lift can also be helpful for treating plantar flexion spasticity or contracture by increasing the total heel height to help ensure that the patient has a heel strike before toe touch during gait.

Toe Pain

The goal of orthotic intervention in toe pain is to decrease pain by immobilization. This is done by incorporating a full-length carbon insert along the sole of the shoe. Alternatively, a steel shank can be extended forward to reduce the mobility of the distal joints, particularly if metal AFO componentry is being used. Common conditions associated with toe pain include hallux rigidus, gout, and arthritis.

Leg Length Discrepancy

A symptomatic leg length discrepancy should first be evaluated with proper measurement. True leg length is measured from the distal tip of the anterior superior iliac spine to the distal tip of the medial malleolus. Apparent leg length is measured from a midline point, such as the pubic symphysis or umbilicus, to the distal tip of each malleolus. This can be abnormal in cases in which the true leg length is normal but pelvic obliquity is present secondary to conditions, such as scoliosis, pelvic fracture, or muscle imbalance. There is no support in the medical literature for treating low back pain associated with an alleged leg length discrepancy. It is not advised unless there is a traumatic event, such as a femur fracture, resulting in a significant acute onset "leg" (lower limb) length discrepancy.

Leg length discrepancies less than half of an inch do not need correction. The total discrepancy is never corrected. At most, 75% of the leg length discrepancy should be corrected. The first half of an inch of the discrepancy can be managed with a heel pad. Additional correction requires the heel to be built up externally. The sole should also be built up proportionally when the heel is built up externally to provide a comfortable, stable gait.

Osteoarthritis of the Knee

Although osteoarthritis of the knee is not a foot condition, it is mentioned here because pain related to it can be alleviated with foot orthoses. Foot orthoses alter the ground reaction forces affecting the more proximal joints, such as the knee, and this relationship should be considered when prescribing a foot orthosis. Lateral heel wedges can be used for conservative treatment of osteoarthritis when medial compartment narrowing is present. The heel wedges used are a quarter of an inch thick along the lateral border and taper medially. Relief was obtained with heel wedges in 74 of 121 knees from 85 patients in one study.[15] Relief of pain was most frequently obtained in patients with mild osteoarthritis, but it was also documented in some patients with complete obliteration of the medial joint space. Wedge use widened the gait pattern. This orthosis has not been studied in patients with medial meniscus injuries, but it may afford some pain relief with medial compartment unloading.

Pediatric Shoes

Children's shoes should have a simple design. To facilitate gait, a heel should not be present. Soft soles are recommended to permit the natural development of feet. Tennis shoes are adequate for most children. A high quarter or three-quarter shoe will stay on a child's foot better than a low-cut shoe and is recommended during the first few years of life.

It is a common misconception that all flat feet need to be treated in children. Flat feet are usual in infants, common in children, and occur occasionally in adults.[50] Flat feet improve over time, in part because of the loss of subcutaneous fat and the reduction of laxity of the joints that occur with growth[50] and the maturation of the gait pattern. Intensive treatment with corrective shoes or inserts for a 3-year period did not alter the natural history of flat feet in 129 children who were 1 to 6 years of age.[58] One cannot make the symptom-free person feel any better. Frequent shoe size change is necessary in the first few years of life.[59]

Ankle-Foot Orthoses

Ankle-foot orthoses (AFOs) are the most commonly prescribed lower limb orthoses. They were formerly known decades ago as short leg braces. Metal or plastic AFOs can be used effectively to control ankle motion. Metal AFOs are relatively contraindicated in children because the weight of the brace can cause external tibial rotation. Plastic AFOs are now most common in all age groups.

AFOs should provide mediolateral stability as a safety feature.[17] Although much emphasis with AFOs is placed on controlling the amount of dorsiflexion and plantar flexion, movements at the subtalar joint also significantly influence the biomechanics of gait. Inversion includes supination at the subtalar joint, adduction at the tarsometatarsal joints, and plantar flexion at the ankle joint, which results in the foot being in an equinovarus position. Eversion includes pronation at the subtalar joint, abduction of the forefoot at the tarsometatarsal joints, and dorsiflexion at the ankle joint resulting in the foot being in a valgus position. Rotation at the subtalar joint is also accompanied by rotation of the tibia (see Figure 12-2).

AFOs can also stabilize the knee during gait.[23] They are prescribed for conditions affecting knee stability, such as genu recurvatum. An AFO should be considered for conditions affecting the knee, particularly when a concurrent problem exists at the ankle or subtalar joints. A proper AFO prescription considers the biomechanical influence of the orthosis at the foot, ankle, and knee in all planes of movement. *Remember that plantar flexion creates a knee extension moment and dorsiflexion creates a knee flexion moment.*

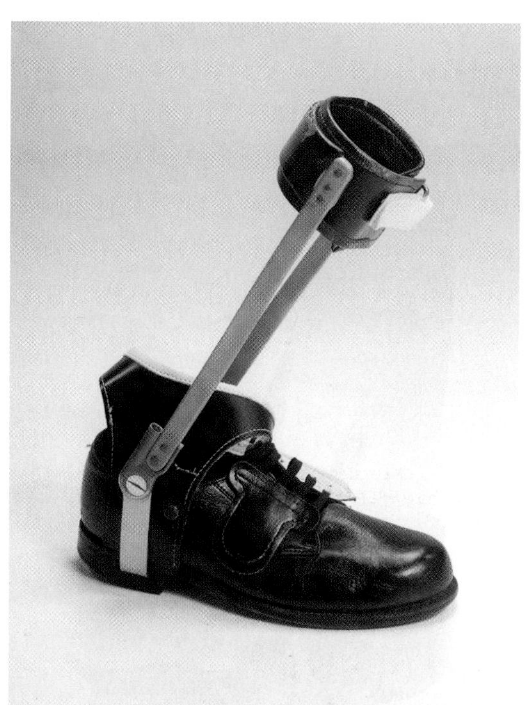

FIGURE 12-6 Metal double-upright dorsiflexion assist ankle-foot orthosis on right shoe with lateral T strap for control of varus deformity. The metal dorsiflexion assist ankle joint has also been referred to in the distant past as a *Klenzak ankle joint.* Note the split stirrup in the heel that allows the wearing of the orthosis with other shoes.

Metal Ankle-Foot Orthoses

Metal AFOs are now used much less commonly than the plastic type. They are discussed for the following four reasons: (1) Much of the research regarding the biomechanical influence of AFOs on gait was performed with metal AFOs. These principles also apply to plastic orthoses. (2) Metal components (especially joints) are frequently used in combination with plastic orthoses. (3) Some older patients wish to continue to use the metal orthoses to which they have become accustomed. (4) Morbidly obese patients may require more if not all-metal componentry for durability and subtalar joint stability. Recent research has offered support that metal AFOs provide better stabilization of the ankle during the gait cycle.[8]

The metal AFO consists of a proximal calf band, two uprights, ankle joints, and an attachment to the shoe to anchor the AFO (Figure 12-6). The posterior metal portion of the calf band should be 1.5 to 3 inches wide to adequately distribute pressure.[11] The calf band should be 1 inch below the fibular neck to prevent a compressive common peroneal nerve palsy. A leather strap with Velcro is used to close the calf band because it provides ease of closure for patients with only one functional upper limb.

Ankle joint motion is controlled by pins or springs inserted into channels (Figures 12-7 to 12-10). The pins are adjusted with a screwdriver to set the desired amount of plantar flexion and dorsiflexion. The spring is also adjusted with a screwdriver to provide the proper amount of tension necessary to aid motion at the ankle joint (used to assist dorsiflexion). Longer channels help prevent the spring mechanism from "bottoming out" and provide for more precise control of ankle motion.

A solid stirrup is a U-shaped metal piece permanently attached to the shoe. Its two ends are bent upward to articulate with the medial and lateral ankle joints (see Figure 12-7). The proximal stirrup attachment sites are shaped to enforce the desired movements at the ankle joint (see Figure 12-8). The sole plate can be extended beyond the metatarsal head area for conditions requiring a longer lever arm for better control of plantar flexion (e.g., plantar spasticity).

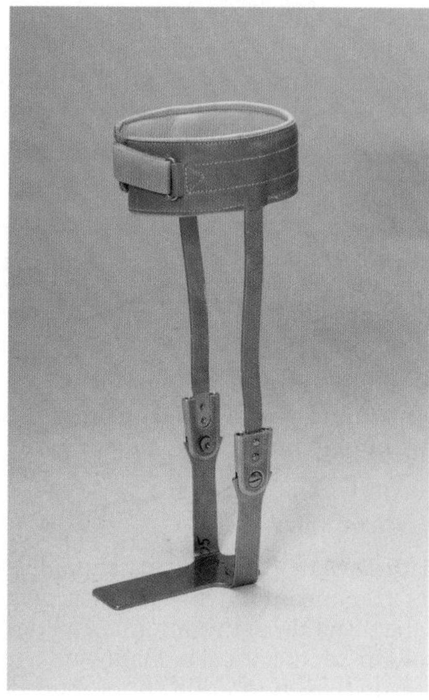

FIGURE 12-7 Double-action metal ankle joint with solid stirrup.

A split stirrup can be used instead of a solid stirrup (see Figures 12-6 and 12-9). The split stirrup has a sole plate with two flat channels for insertion of the uprights. The two uprights are now called calipers because they can open and close distally to allow donning and doffing of the AFO. A split stirrup allows removal of the uprights from the

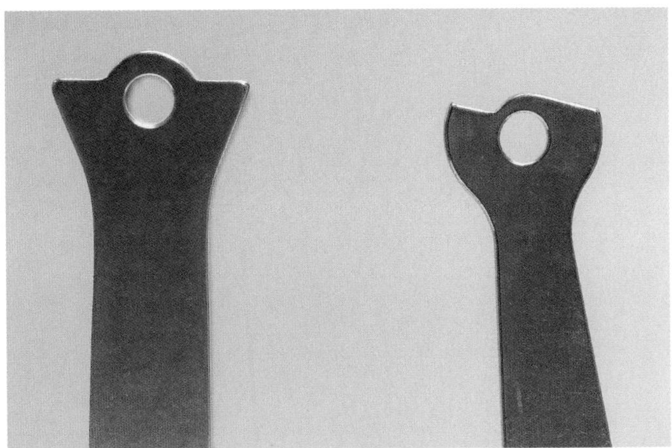

FIGURE 12-8 Double-action stirrup (*left*) and dorsiflexion assist stirrup (*right*), used with the ankle joints shown in Figures 12-7 and 12-6, respectively. (Courtesy USMC, Pasadena, Calif.)

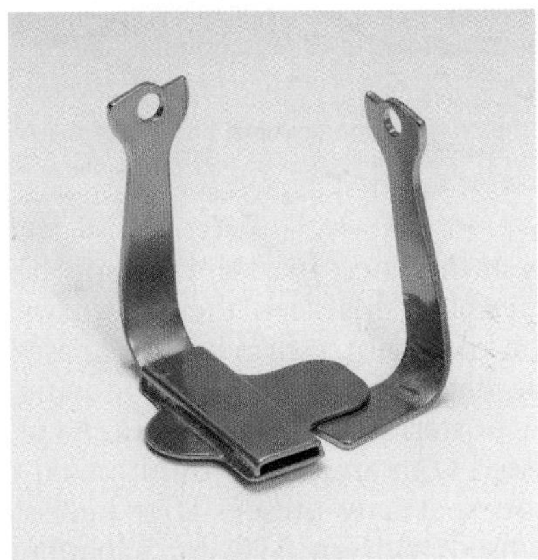

FIGURE 12-9 Split stirrup. The stirrup extends anteriorly to attach at the shank area of a shoe for stability. This stirrup is for dorsiflexion assist.

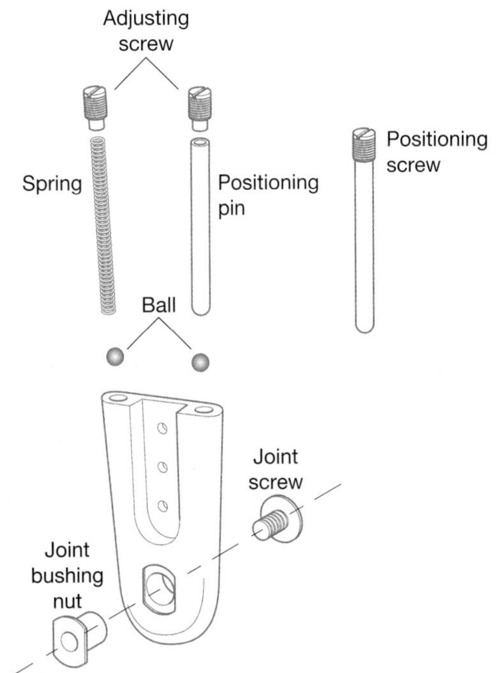

FIGURE 12-10 Schematic drawing of metal ankle joint components. This type of ankle joint is most commonly referred to as a *double-action ankle joint*. It has also been referred to in the distant past as a *double Klenzak ankle joint* or a *BiCAAL* (bichannel adjustable ankle locking) joint. (Courtesy USMC, Pasadena, Calif.)

shoes so that the AFO can be worn with other shoes (see Figure 12-6). Other pairs of shoes should also have the sole plate with channels for calipers incorporated into the heel area. The split stirrup is not as stable as the solid stirrup and the metal uprights can pop out, which is the main reason this is infrequently used.

Ankle Stops and Assists

The ankle joint can be positioned so that it is in a neutral, dorsiflexed, or plantar—flexed position, depending on the gait disturbance. It can be set to permit a partial range of motion or to eliminate a certain motion. An understanding of the effect on the placement of pins and screws into the two channels of an ankle joint (see Figure 12-10) facilitates the proper orthotic prescription for the patient. This section reviews the common uses of the posterior stop (via pin), anterior stop (via pin), and the posterior dorsiflexion assist (via spring) of the orthotic metal ankle joint. A spring in the anterior channel has not been demonstrated to be of clinical value.

Plantar Stop (Posterior Stop). The plantar stop is used to control plantar spasticity or help incrementally stretch plantar contractures. The plantar stop is most commonly set at 90 degrees. A pin is inserted into the posterior channel of an ankle joint, such as that in Figure 12-10, to limit plantar flexion. An AFO with a plantar stop at 90 degrees produces a flexion moment at the knee during heel strike. Because the dorsiflexors cannot eccentrically activate to permit the foot to make contact with the ground, the ground reactive force remains posterior to the knee after heel strike, which creates a flexion moment at the knee (and possibly an unstable gait via buckling). The proximal portion of the AFO also has an effect on knee stability. The posterior portion of the proximal AFO exerts a forward push on the proximal leg to increase the knee flexion moment after heel strike (Figure 12-11). The opposite occurs at toe-off, with an extension moment created at the knee. This concept has been used to develop what has been referred to as a plastic ground reaction AFO, with a solid proximal anterior tibial closing that provides a greater influence on the knee. This device will be discussed in more detail later. The greater the plantar flexion resistance, the greater the flexion moment at the knee at heel strike, and the greater the need for active hip extensors to prevent the body from collapsing forward on a buckling knee.

Also, a solid ankle cushioned heel (SACH) heel wedge can be used to reduce the flexion moment at the knee. The term *SACH* is a misnomer borrowed from the prosthetic literature. The "SA" (solid ankle) refers to the type of prosthetic ankle joint. The SACH heel wedge in this case should be referred to only as a cushioned heel. A cushioned heel serves as a shock absorber at heel strike, and is able to partially substitute for the dorsiflexors, which cannot be eccentrically activated when 'ankle plantar stops of an AFO are set at 90 degrees. A cushioned heel also helps move the ground reactive force more anteriorly at the foot and

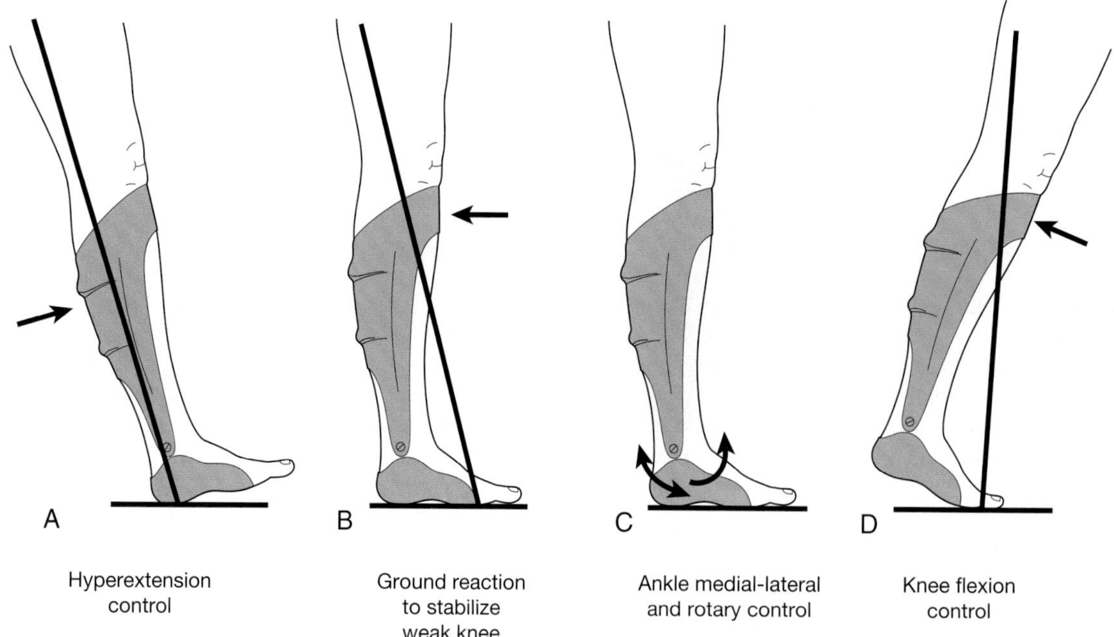

FIGURE 12-11 **A** to **D**, Ground reaction ankle-foot orthosis (AFO) dynamic illustration. Note the effect of the proximal portion of the AFO on the knee throughout gait. (Courtesy Oregon Orthotic System, Albany, Ore.)

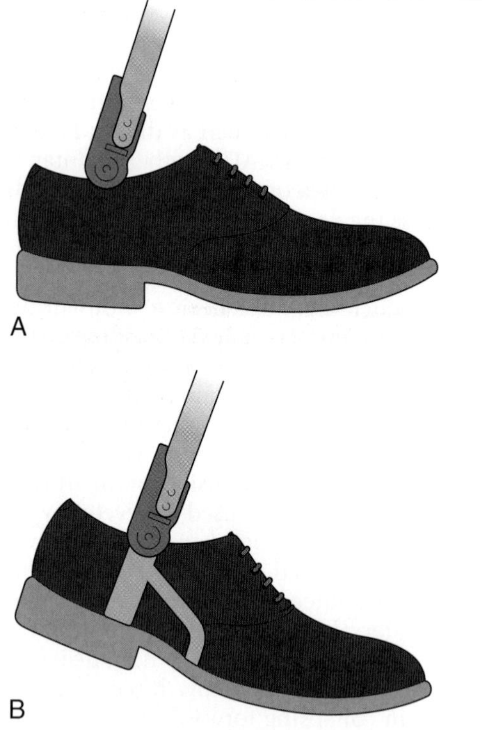

FIGURE 12-12 Schematic drawing of anterior pin stop simulating plantar flexion. **A,** Anterior channels of ankle-foot orthosis component of a knee-ankle-foot orthosis left open in a patient with spinal cord injury. Note that the heel does not lift up (i.e., no plantar flexion). **B,** Anterior channels of same orthosis with anterior pins in place set at 5 degrees of dorsiflexion and with metal sole plate. Note that the heel does lift up (i.e., plantar flexion) as momentum causes the lower limb to "pole vault" over the anterior pin setting.

subsequently at the knee. In essence, a soft heel helps stabilize the knee. It helps keep the ground reaction force anterior to the knee joint. A firm heel decreases knee stability via a knee flexion moment while moving the ground reaction force posterior to the knee joint. A cushioned heel can also be used with an AFO to minimize the amount of plantar flexion spasticity present after heel strike. A firm heel can be used with an AFO for a patient with genu recurvatum.

The posterior stop should be set at the minimal amount of plantar flexion required to clear the foot during swing-through.[18] Remember, *plantar flexion creates a knee extension moment at the knee after heel strike*. This provides a more stable knee during gait than when the ankle plantar stops are set in any degree of dorsiflexion.

A balanced decision should be made between providing resistance to plantar flexion to clear the foot during the swing phase of gait and the amount of instability at the knee during the stance phase of gait. No AFO is effective in reducing the amount of knee flexion to "normal" levels during the stance phase of gait.[20]

Dorsiflexion Stop (Anterior Stop). An anterior stop is used to substitute for the function of the gastrocnemius/soleus complex (Figure 12-12). It is used in conditions with weak calf muscles or weak quadriceps (because of its effect on the knee). Weak calf musculature allows the ankle to enter dorsiflexion and *dorsiflexion creates a knee flexion moment after heel strike*. The anterior stop set at 5 degrees of dorsiflexion best substitutes for gastrocnemius/soleus function.[18,20] Please note that three muscle groups help stabilize the knee during the gait cycle, including the quadriceps, hamstrings, and gastrocnemius/soleus complex. All three of these muscle groups cross the knee joint and should be clinically evaluated and considered when prescribing a lower limb orthosis.

The anterior stop assists with push-off and assists the knee joint into extension. It should be used in combination with a stirrup, with a sole extension to the metatarsal heads, to simulate the action of the calf muscles. The dorsiflexion stop simulates the gastrocnemius/soleus function by causing the heel to rise during the latter part of stance rather than remaining flat on the ground. The shoe pivots over the metatarsal heads, creating an extension moment at the knee that helps stabilize the knee from midstance to toe-off.

The earlier the dorsiflexion stop occurs during the stance phase, the greater the extension moment at the knee. This is useful in clinical situations where quadriceps weakness is also present. If the extension moment at the knee is too great for too long, then genu recurvatum ("back knee") can occur. A balance should be obtained such that the extension at the knee is sufficient to stabilize the knee in extension yet prevent genu recurvatum. If too much dorsiflexion is permitted by the anterior stop, there will be too much knee flexion during gait from midstance to toe-off.

Dorsiflexion Assist (Posterior Spring). The posterior spring (see Figure 12-6) serves two purposes. It substitutes for concentric contraction of dorsiflexors to prevent flaccid foot drop after toe-off. It also substitutes (inadequately) for the eccentric activation of the dorsiflexors after heel strike.

The posterior spring prevents rapid plantar flexion at heel strike during its compression in the posterior channel. The posterior spring is again compressed during plantar flexion during late stance before toe-off. The posterior spring assists with toe clearance during the swing phase of gait by providing a downward thrust posterior to the ankle joint at toe-off, which results in dorsiflexion anterior to the ankle joint. The longer the channel, the greater the ability to control dorsiflexion.

A summary of some of the common indications for the various channel components is found in Table 12-1.

Metal Ankle-Foot Orthoses Varus-Valgus Control. Varus and valgus deformities are associated with rotation at the subtalar joint. A T strap is attached along the side of the shoe distal to the subtalar joint to help minimize the deformity (see Figure 12-6). T straps are also used to help prevent worsening of the deformity. T straps also help distribute pressure properly along the foot during weight-bearing.

T straps are referred to as being either medial or lateral. A lateral T strap is sown to the lateral aspect of the shoe and the belt is cinched around the medial upright of the AFO (see Figure 12-6). A lateral T strap is used to control a varus deformity. The belt is secured with a buckle around the medial upright. This helps create a force directing the subtalar joint outward, which counteracts the supination and adduction tendency that would result in excess varus. The opposite is true for a valgus deformity with the T strap being medially located. A pressure ulcer can develop over the malleolus if the T strap is buckled too tightly.

The T strap inadequately substitutes for the foot pronators, supinators, abductors, and adductors because it does not have an attachment on the plantar surface of the foot to create the mechanical advantage offered by the plantar-attached tendons.

Table 12-1 Clinical Indications for Various Metal Ankle Channel Components

Channel	Pin or Spring	Function	Clinical Indications
Posterior	Pin	Limits plantar flexion	Plantar spasticity, toe drag, pain with ankle motion
Posterior	Spring	Assists dorsiflexion	Flaccid foot drop, knee hyperextension
Anterior*	Pin	Limits dorsiflexion	Weak plantar flexors, weak knee extensors, pain with ankle motion
Anterior	Spring	Assists plantar flexion	None

*Used in combination with an extended sole plate to metatarsal head area to help compensate for weak plantar flexors.

Plastic Ankle-Foot Orthoses

Plastic AFOs are the most commonly used AFOs because of their cost, cosmesis, light weight, interchangeability with shoes, ability to control varus and valgus deformities, provision of better foot support with the customized foot portion, and ability to achieve what is offered by the metal AFO (Figure 12-13). Energy consumption is equal with a plastic solid AFO or a metal double-upright AFO.[2,3] Although a plastic orthosis weighs less than its metal counterpart, the weight of the orthosis is not as important as the influence of the ground reactive force created by the presence of the orthosis. The same orthotic principles apply to orthoses made of plastic or metal. The plastic AFO' effect on knee stability should be recognized. The

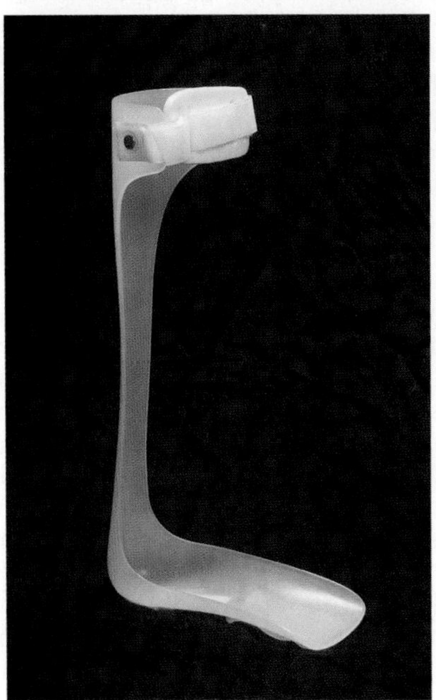

FIGURE 12-13 Custom plastic solid (means no ankle joint although still flexible) ankle-foot orthosis (AFO) with posterior trim line to allow some flexibility with plantar flexion. This is the most commonly prescribed AFO for foot drop. It is also referred to as a posterior leaf spring (PLS) AFO and it is usually set in a few degrees of dorsiflexion.

plastic AFO prescribed for toe clearance should be just rigid enough to provide resistance for toe clearance. Excessive resistance to plantar flexion can make the knee unstable (create a flexion moment) after heel strike.[21]

Plastic AFOs can be prefabricated or custom made. The reasons for prescribing a custom-molded orthosis include long-term need, conformed molding for comfort or insensate feet, placement of the orthosis in a fixed amount of plantar flexion or dorsiflexion, better control of rotational deformities, and further reduction of weight bearing for a tibial fracture or diabetic plantar ulcer. The custom process is similar to that previously described in this chapter for foot orthoses, with the positive mold serving as the model for the orthosis.

Some practical advice should be offered to the patient regarding the use of a plastic AFO. If changing shoes, it is best to have another pair with a similar heel height, to prevent altering the biomechanical effects at the foot, ankle, and knee. Tennis shoes are most accommodating for donning and doffing of the AFO. However, if dress shoes are to be worn, patients should also be told that their shoe size might need to be a half size larger and the next width larger to accommodate the orthosis. A Blucher-style dress shoe with its open tongue helps accommodate the orthosis (see Figure 12-1). If there is a removable insole in the shoe, this should be removed when a plastic AFO is used, to minimize the increase in leg length and provide more space in the shoe.

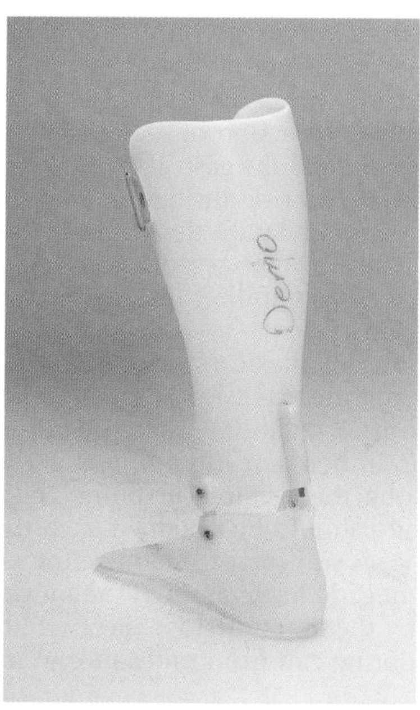

FIGURE 12-14 Midline posterior stop articulated ankle-foot orthosis. Note the use of a plastic ankle joint to further decrease weight. Plastic ankle joints are more common in children (lightweight individuals). The use of a plantar stop with ankle joints is recommended for an active lightweight patient with plantar spasticity (e.g., a child with cerebral palsy).

Plastic Ankle-Foot Orthoses Components

The foot component of the AFO should extend beyond the metatarsal heads. The footplate can be extended beyond the toes to reduce spasticity aggravated by toe flexion. The shape and molding of the foot portion influence the biomechanics of more proximal joints.

The ankle and subtalar joints can be made more stable under four circumstances: (1) extend the trim line more anteriorly at the ankle level (a trim line is the anterior border of the plastic AFO); (2) make the plastic material thicker; (3) place carbon inserts along the medial and lateral aspects of the ankle joint; and (4) incorporate corrugations within the posterior leaf of the AFO. The strength of the AFO should be matched to the patient"s weight and activity level.

Plastic AFOs can also be hinged at the ankle. Ankle hinges allow full or partial ankle motion, which can permit a more natural gait. They should be considered when complete restriction of ankle motion is not required. Plastic ankle joints are light and are a good choice for children. Metal ankle joints are preferred for adults, particularly heavy adults. Newer designs have a single midline posterior pin/spring mechanism (Figure 12-14). This midline spring functions like the more traditional medial and lateral dual posterior spring assist mechanism (see Figures 12-8 and 12-9). This makes the AFO narrower in the mediolateral direction and slightly longer in the anterior-posterior direction, which better conforms to the design of most pants. *Hinging an AFO adds mediolateral stability.* Consider prescribing a hinged AFO for a patient with spasticity with a tendency toward inversion or for a patient with multiplanar ankle and subtalar flaccidity accompanying a foot drop with a history of twisting the ankle.

The leg component should encompass three quarters of the leg and should be padded along its internal surface.[11] The proximal extent should end 1 inch below the fibular neck to prevent a compressive common peroneal nerve palsy.

Solid Plastic Ankle-Foot Orthoses. The solid plastic AFO is the most commonly prescribed plastic AFO (see Figure 12-13). It can be made to serve several purposes. The term *solid* refers to an AFO that is made of a single piece of plastic. It does not have ankle joints. However, the trim line of the AFO will determine the level of flexibility and control at the ankle. Anterior trim lines (anterior to the medial malleolus) are the most rigid, whereas posterior trim lines (behind the medial malleolus) provide some flexibility. The most flexible design has only a thin band of plastic in the posterior aspect, but provides little or no mediolateral control. A solid AFO can still be flexible enough to allow some ankle motion, and it should be flexible with a posterior trim line for the treatment of foot drop without mediolateral instability. A solid AFO with anterior trim lines should be truly solid (not flexible) for the treatment of some cases of plantar spasticity.

Solid AFOs set at 90 degrees are commonly used for foot drop. Less obvious but equally important is 'the ability of the solid AFO to treat conditions affecting the knee. *Again, remember that plantar flexion creates knee extension and dorsiflexion creates knee flexion at heel strike.* The AFO can be fixed in a few degrees of plantar flexion to provide stability at the knee during the stance phase of gait. Genu recurvatum can also be treated with a solid AFO. The more rigid the AFO, the greater the flexion moment at the knee at heel strike, which helps reverse the extension moment at the knee associated with genu recurvatum. The flexion moment at the knee also becomes even greater during midstance if

Table 12-2 Orthotic Componentry with Knee Flexion and Extension Moments

Knee Extension Moment/ Stability	Knee Flexion Moment/ Instability
Cushioned heel	Solid heel
AFO fixed in plantar flexion	AFO fixed in dorsiflexion
Posterior trim line on AFO (flexible)	Anterior trim line on AFO
Posterior offset knee joint	—

AFO, Ankle-foot orthosis.

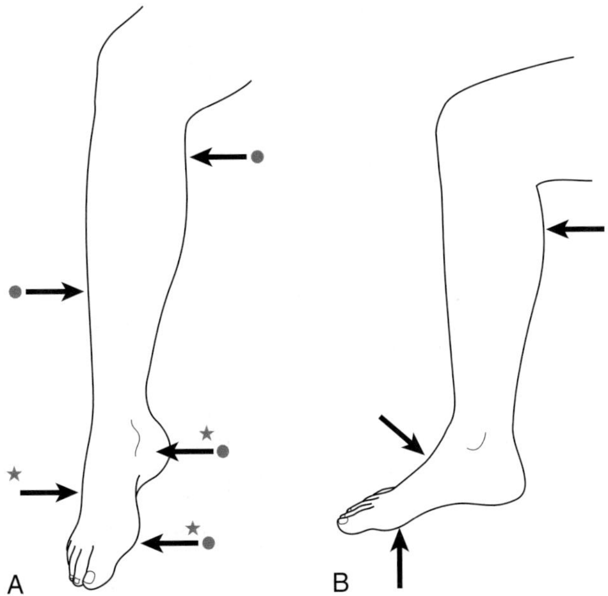

FIGURE 12-15 Three-point system control of equinovarus deformity. **A,** Control of varus rotational component at the foot (*stars*) and subtalar joint (dots). **B,** Control of equinus deformity. (Modified from Marx HW: Lower limb orthotic designs for the spastic hemiplegic patient, *Orthot Prosthet* 28:14, 1974.)

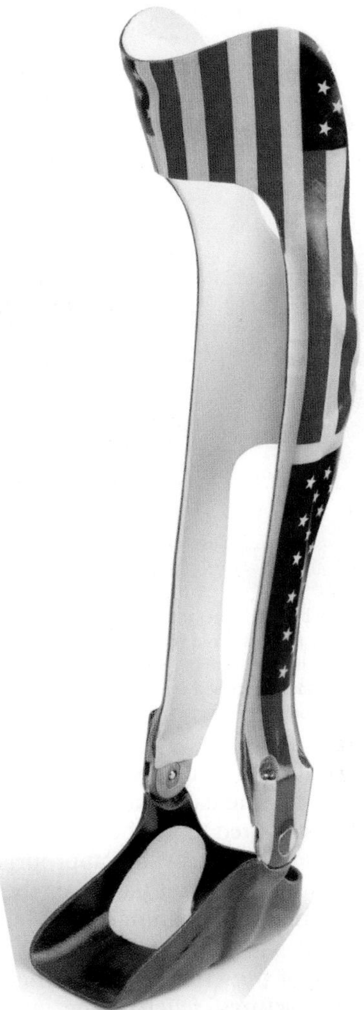

FIGURE 12-16 Oregon Orthotic System rotational control ankle-foot orthosis. Note the corrugations that add strength to the orthosis. Also note the metal ankle joint that is similar to those in Figure 12-10. (Courtesy Oregon Orthotic System, Albany, Ore.)

the ankle is placed in a few degrees of dorsiflexion. Table 12-2 summarizes the important orthotic factors involved in creating knee flexion and extension moments throughout the gait cycle.

Plastic Ankle-Foot Orthoses Varus-Valgus Control. The goal of orthotic intervention is to alter the ground reactive forces with custom molding to help maintain proper alignment of the lower limb by "building up" selected portions of the AFO. A three-point system is used to provide the counter forces necessary to oppose the forces of the deformity (Figure 12-15).[27,30] Some orthotists believe that an orthosis should be firm ("not conforming") to control a deformity. Pressure points should be present in expected areas at follow-up visits if the orthosis is serving its purpose. A custom ground reaction orthosis provides appropriate foot support that influences the rotation of more proximal joints (Figure 12-16). The anterior tibial shell closing helps stabilize the knee during gait (see Figure 12-11).

An equinovarus (or inversion) deformity is controlled by applying forces medially at the metatarsal head area and calcaneus. The next force is applied more proximally along the lateral aspect of the distal fibula using a padded lateral flange. This helps prevent inversion at the subtalar and ankle joints. A more proximal medial tibial force is applied to provide stabilization of the leg portion of the plastic AFO by providing an opposing force to the fibular area (see Figure 12-15). A three-point system also exists at the foot level to help prevent supination of the foot related to the equinovarus deformity (see Figure 12-15). A three-point system is again applied to control the plantar flexion deformity associated with equinovarus (see Figure 12-15).

The reverse of the previously described three-point system to control varus can be used to control valgus at the foot. Movements in all joints should be considered when prescribing an orthosis.

Patellar Tendon Bearing Ankle-Foot Orthoses

A patellar tendon bearing (PTB) AFO uses the patellar tendon and the tibial condyles to partially relieve weight-bearing stress on skeletal structures distally with more weight bearing distributed along the medial tibial condyle.[25] PTB is a misnomer for this orthosis because only

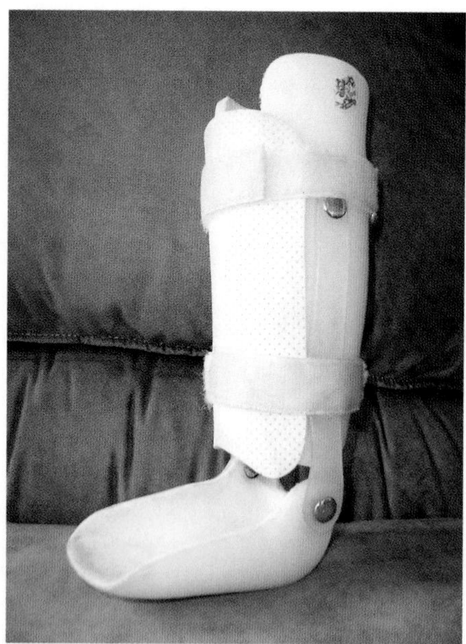

FIGURE 12-17 Custom bivalved patellar tendon bearing ankle-foot orthosis. Ten percent of the weight is transferred to the patellar tendon. Fifty percent weight-bearing reduction is achieved by custom-fitted contact distributed throughout the leg. This was prescribed for a young girl after a large benign left leg tibia tumor resection.

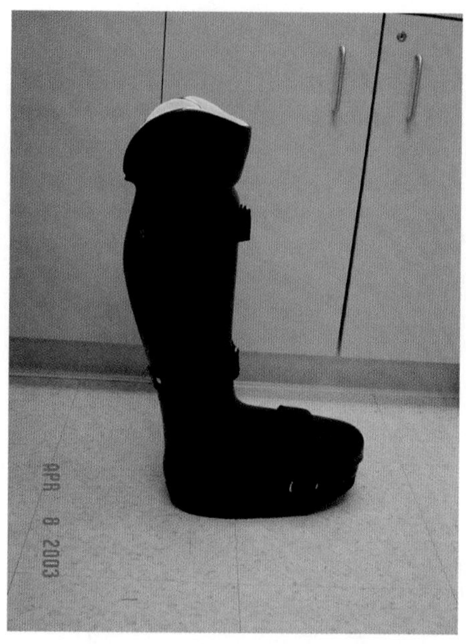

FIGURE 12-18 The Charcot Relief Orthotic Walker (CROW) Boot is a custom-molded bivalve plastic ankle-foot orthosis that is fully padded on the inside with total contact of the foot, ankle, and leg. The purpose of this brace is to off-load a plantar ulcer or stabilize the progressive deformity from Charcot joint of the foot and ankle.

approximately 10% of the weight is distributed along the patellar tendon and the medial tibial condyle. Most of the weight bearing is distributed throughout the soft tissues of the leg that are compressed by an appropriately fitted orthosis. Compression of the soft tissues of the leg is also responsible for maintaining alignment and length of the tibia after a fracture.[45,46]

PTB AFOs are often prescribed for diabetic ulcerations of the foot, tibial fractures, relief of the weight-bearing surface in painful heel conditions, such as calcaneal fractures, postoperative ankle fusions, Charcot joint, and avascular necrosis of the foot or ankle. The orthoses are made of plastic and are bivalved. They fit snugly with the use of Velcro straps (Figure 12-17) or buckles similar to those of ski boots. A custom-molded PTB AFO can reduce weight bearing in the affected foot by up to 50%. A similar design with a laced calf corset design suspended within a metal AFO can also be used to stabilize and off-load the foot and ankle.

Custom-made PTB AFOs are indicated when maximum weight-bearing reduction is necessary to ensure proper healing (such as in a debrided diabetic heel ulcer) and reduction of pain. It should first be determined that the painful condition is associated with weight bearing rather than with range of motion. If pain occurs with range of motion, then the pain-producing range of motion should be eliminated.

The solid plastic orthosis makes contact with the ground before the reactive force is absorbed significantly by the foot and then distributes this force more proximally along the leg. Compared with a prefabricated AFO, a custom-made PTB AFO more effectively distributes pressure over a greater surface contact area for maximal weight-bearing reduction. Additional weight-bearing reduction is obtained by eliminating ankle movement via carbon graphite inserts and/or the use of a rocker bottom (see Figure 12-5), which eliminates active push-off.[26] A rocker bottom is directly incorporated into the plastic orthosis.

Charcot Relief Orthotic Walker Boot

The Charcot Relief Orthotic Walker (CROW) Boot (Figure 12-18) is a custom-molded bivalve plastic AFO that captures the entire foot and leg up to the knee for the purpose of off-loading a plantar ulcer or stabilizing the progressive deformity from Charcot joint of the foot and ankle. The device is fully padded on the inside with total contact of the foot, ankle, and leg. The device has a rocker bottom and rubber sole for indoor and outdoor ambulation. This device is often used instead of total contact casting of diabetic foot ulcers. The CROW Boot is indicated temporarily for wound healing, but may be needed permanently for Charcot joint management.

Pressure Relief Ankle-Foot Orthoses

A pressure relief AFO is also known by its acronym, a PRAFO (Figure 12-19). This type of AFO has different brand names depending on the company who furnished it, including PRAFO, Multi Podus AFO, and Lennard AFO. This orthosis serves two purposes, including pressure relief and contracture prevention. Pressure relief is achieved at the heel by completely eliminating weight bearing with the heel cut out and also by using a hinged lever arm posteriorly that can be adjusted medially or laterally to prevent medial or lateral malleolar pressure sore development. This should be applied on the immobilized or motionless affected lower limb at all times while in bed. A pressure relief AFO is frequently used in demented patients with hip fractures who do not have much lower limb mobility as well as patients with a stroke with dense hemiplegia. Plantar flexion contracture prevention occurs by keeping the ankle joint in a neutral position while the AFO is donned.

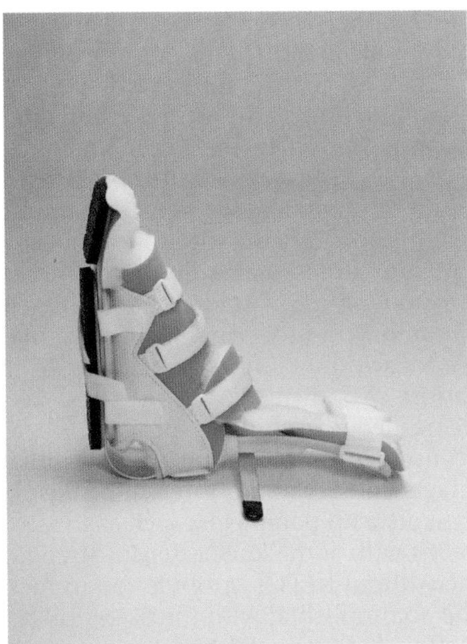

FIGURE 12-19 Pressure relief ankle-foot orthosis. The heel cut out provides complete heel pressure relief and the hinged posterior lever arm prevents ankle pressure sore development either medially or laterally and can be adjusted like a windshield wiper as necessary to prevent medial or lateral malleolar pressure.

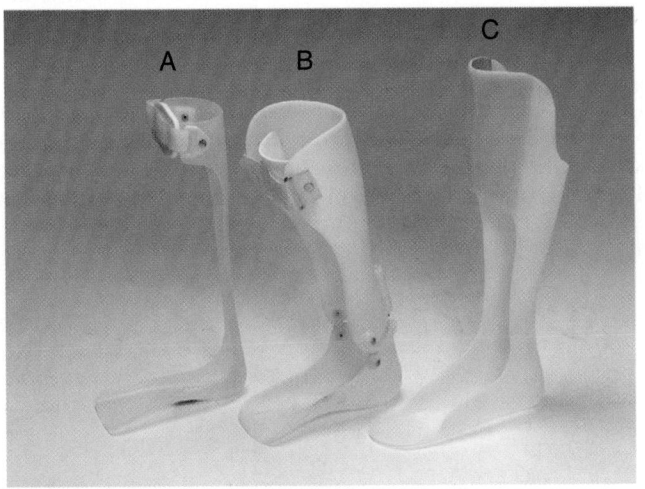

FIGURE 12-20 Common ankle-foot orthosis (AFO) prescriptions. **A,** Foot drop AFO. **B,** Plantar spasticity AFO. **C,** Lumbar spinal cord injury AFO.

Common Ankle-Foot Orthoses Prescriptions

The three most common physiatric AFO prescriptions include those for foot drop, plantar spasticity, and lumbar spinal cord injury (Figure 12-20). The most common AFO prescription for foot drop is a custom nonhinged plastic AFO set in a few degrees of dorsiflexion with a posterior trim line. This is also referred to as a posterior leaf spring AFO. The few degrees of dorsiflexion ensures foot clearance during the swing phase of gait. It also helps the ankle "spring" into dorsiflexion after the foot is lifted off the ground in a plantar-flexed position from push-off. The minimal weight and bulk of this AFO are highly desired by the patient with foot drop. Not only does the avoidance of hinging minimize bulk, but from a practical standpoint it keeps the mediolateral dimension of the AFO narrow to best accommodate a variety of shoes and pants. If there is significant subtalar joint instability (e.g., a patient with a history of inversion injuries and falling), a hinged plastic AFO with metal double-action ankle joints (see Figure 12-10) with springs in the posterior channels (dorsiassist) would provide mediolateral stability, yet also permit plantar flexion. A variety of plastic or polymer insert joints are now available to provide dorsiflexion assist. Alternatively, a hinged midline posterior stop AFO that is spring-loaded (see Figure 12-14) can also provide mediolateral stability for the patient with foot drop.

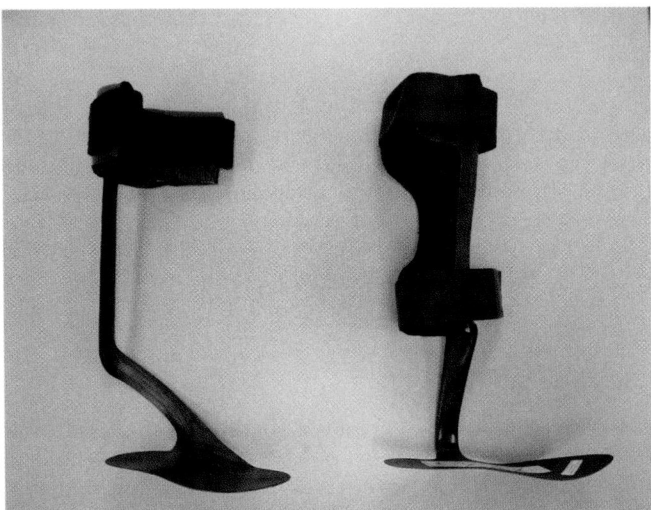

FIGURE 12-21 Prefabricated carbon graphite ankle-foot orthoses. Their advantages include lighter weight, lower profile footplate, the ability to provide some dynamic response/propulsion to substitute for weak plantar flexors, and patient trial before purchase.

The most common AFO prescription for plantar spasticity is either a hinged custom plastic AFO with a single midline posterior stop or a hinged custom plastic AFO with pins in the posterior channels to provide plantar stop at 90 degrees. The former is more likely to be considered in milder cases of spasticity without a significant inversion deformity. The latter is more likely to be considered if there is a significant inversion deformity still present after all other medical treatment measures to manage the spasticity have been exhausted. Metal ankle joints with posterior pins in this case would provide better mediolateral support yet still permit some dorsiflexion with the anterior channels left open. Permitting dorsiflexion allows a more normalized gait and provides a therapeutic stretch to the plantar flexors from midstance to toe-off during gait. Recent research studies support the use of hinged AFOs with plantar stops at neutral (90 degrees) as a preferred AFO for an active pediatric population with lower limb spasticity.[37,40,49,53,54]

There are several variations of prefabricated carbon fiber AFOs (Figure 12-21) now available. The advantages of carbon fiber AFOs are lighter weight, lower profile footplate, and the ability to provide some dynamic response/propulsion to substitute for weak plantar flexors. The disadvantages include poor mediolateral control and the lack of adjustability. Carbon fiber AFOs fit easily into many shoe styles and come with anterior or posterior calf shells.

Unlike custom plastic AFOs, most carbon fiber AFOs are prefabricated, and therefore the patient can have a trial walk with the brace before fit and delivery.

The most common lumbar spinal cord injury AFO prescription is bilateral custom plastic ground reaction (anterior tibial shell closing) AFOs fixed in 10 degrees of plantar flexion. The anterior tibial shell closing and 10 degrees of plantar flexion help create knee extension moments with weight bearing to add stability to the knees during ambulation. A walker or bilateral Lofstrand forearm orthoses are still needed to permit ambulation.

Checkout

The patient should be examined after fitting and use of the orthosis. The first and most obvious form of a checkout is to verify that the gait pattern is improved with the orthosis compared with the gait pattern without the orthosis. The orthotic ankle joint should coincide with the tip of the medial malleolus. The patient is to be checked for ease of donning and doffing the orthosis, and while it is off, observed for areas of skin breakdown. If the AFO was prescribed to control spasticity, the orthotic evaluation should include determining its effectiveness in a dynamic setting because spasticity can worsen with ambulation. In cases in which significant deformity is being addressed with orthotic intervention, some redness can and should be present if the orthosis is doing its job. Some redness is acceptable as long as it is dispersed in as large an area as possible and as long as there is no skin breakdown.

Knee—Ankle-Foot Orthoses

Knee-ankle-foot orthoses (KAFOs) were formerly referred to decades ago as long leg braces. The components are the same as those of an AFO but also include knee joints, thigh uprights, and a proximal thigh band. Various knee joints and knee locks are available for a variety of conditions. KAFOs are used in patients with severe knee extensor and hamstring weakness, structural knee instability, and knee flexion spasticity. The purpose of the KAFO is to provide stability at the knee, ankle, and subtalar joints during ambulation. They are most commonly prescribed bilaterally for patients with spinal cord injuries and unilaterally for patients with polio. There is a common misconception that patients with a complete femoral neuropathy (i.e., no quadriceps function) should have their knees braced. *From a functional anatomic standpoint, it should be kept in mind that there are three stabilizers to the knee: the quadriceps, the hamstrings (via eccentric activation at heel strike), and the plantar flexors (plantar flexion creates a knee extension moment).* These stabilizers should all be evaluated carefully by physical examination before a KAFO is prescribed.

KAFOs can be prescribed for functional ambulation or exercise (or both). The benefits of exercise to the patient requiring bilateral KAFOs include preventing lower limb contractures, enhancing cardiovascular fitness, maintaining upper body strength for activities of daily living, delaying the development of osteoporosis, and fewer medical complications, such as deep venous thromboses.

The use of KAFOs often complements the use of a wheelchair for ambulation. The proprioceptive level is a reliable indicator of which spinal cord—injured patients can achieve ambulation status.[57] It is helpful to have sensation and proprioception in the lower limbs to ambulate safely with KAFOs. The level of the spinal cord injury is also important in predicting the ability to ambulate. Adult spinal cord—injured patients with lesions at or above T12 generally are not functional ambulators because of the metabolic cost involved.[33] Children have a higher center of gravity and can have a functional gait with a higher spinal cord lesion. Muscle function is a predictor of the quality of ambulation. Good trunk control and upper body strength are needed to ambulate with KAFOs because these devices are used in combination with ambulation aids, such as walkers and Lofstrand forearm orthoses.

Some patients with paraplegia, such as those with lower lumbar lesions with some knee extensor strength, are able to ambulate without KAFOs. Ambulation in these patients can often be accomplished with the use of bilateral plastic ground reaction AFOs (see Figures 12-11 and 12-16) with the ankles fixed in 10 degrees to 15 degrees of plantar flexion. The plantar flexion provides an extension moment at the knee during gait for stability with ambulation. The proximal anterior tibial shell closing provides further stability at the knee from midstance to toe-off (see Figure 12-11, *D*). A walker or two Lofstrand forearm orthoses can be used for additional support and balance.

Knee Joints

There are three basic types of knee joints. The straight set knee joint provides rotation about a single axis (Figure 12-22). It allows free flexion but prevents hyperextension.

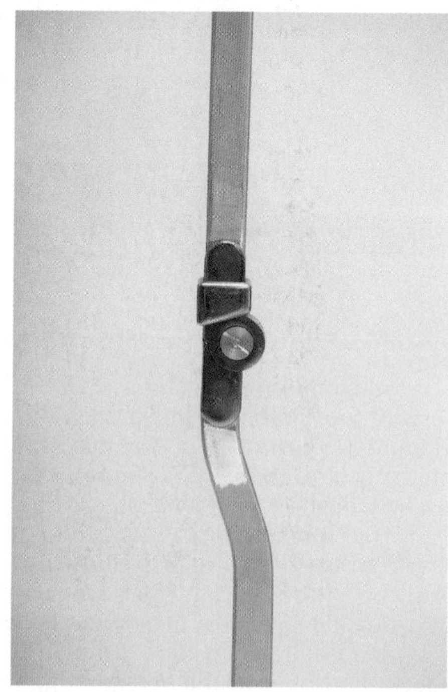

FIGURE 12-22 Straight set knee with drop lock.

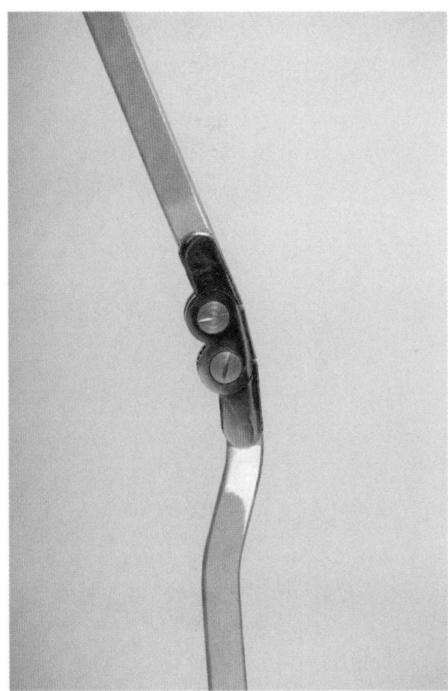

FIGURE 12-23 Polycentric knee joint.

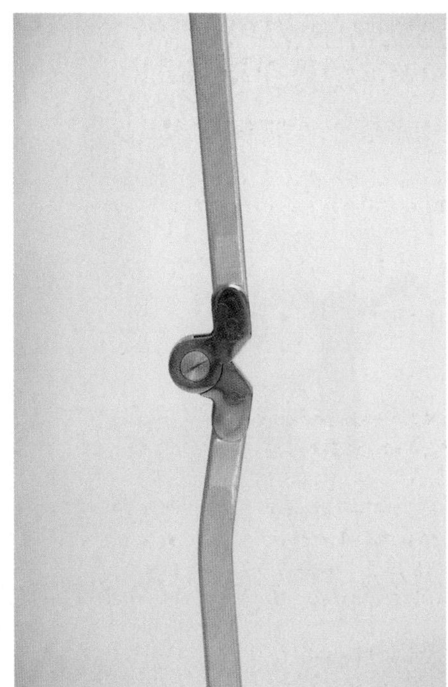

FIGURE 12-24 Posterior offset knee joint.

It is often used in combination with a drop lock, which keeps the knee in extension throughout all phases of gait for further stability.

The polycentric knee joint uses a double-axis system to simulate the flexion-extension movements of the femur and tibia at the knee joint (Figure 12-23). Although this concept is theoretically sound, the polycentric knee joint has not proved to be advantageous over the straight set knee joint, and it is less commonly used. It also adds bulk to the orthosis. It is most frequently used in sport knee orthoses.

The third type of knee joint is the posterior offset knee joint (Figures 12-24 and 12-25; see Table 12-2). It is prescribed for patients with weak knee extensors and some hip extensor strength. It allows free flexion and extension of the knee during the swing phase of gait and helps keep the *orthotic* ground reactive force in front of the knee axis for stability during stance. The center of gravity is normally posterior to the knee at heel strike, creating a flexion moment at the knee, which requires quadriceps and hamstring muscle contraction to counteract this force. The posterior offset knee joint component of the KAFO helps place the ground reactive force anterior to the orthotic knee joint, creating an extension moment at the knee during stance to compensate for the weak knee extensors. The posterior offset knee joint should have a hyperextension stop to help prevent genu recurvatum.

Occasionally, the offset knee joint does not provide adequate stability at the knee. The ankle component of the KAFO can then be set in 10 to 15 degrees of plantar flexion to further help create an extension moment at the knee for stability. Lastly, if these measures are insufficient at providing knee stability, the posterior offset knee joints can be locked in extension with drop locks (see Figure 12-22).

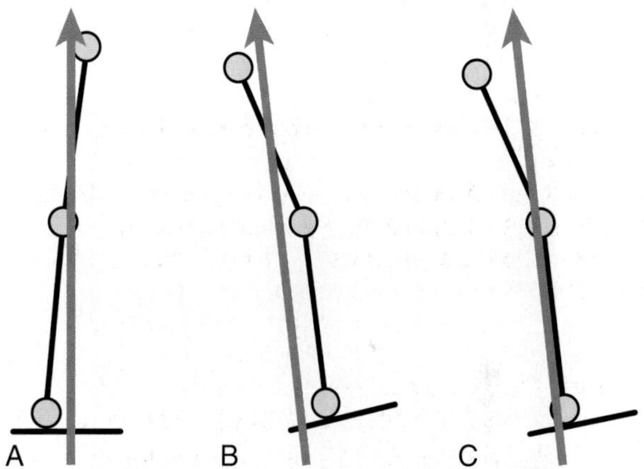

FIGURE 12-25 Ground reaction force (GRF) schematic drawing. The line depicted pointed upward from the ground is representative of the GRF. The knee joint remains extended (e.g., stable) if the GRF is anterior to the knee. A knee flexion moment is created if the GRF is posterior to the knee. **A,** GRF at stance. **B,** GRF at heel strike. **C,** Orthotic GRF at heel strike with posterior offset orthotic knee joint. A solid heel also moves the GRF posteriorly (i.e., knee flexion moment/instability), and a soft heel moves the GRF anteriorly (i.e., knee extension moment/stability).

Knee Locks

Knee locks are used to provide complete stability at the knee. There are four common types of knee locks; these are discussed in order of their frequency of use, beginning with the most commonly used.

The ratchet lock has recently become the most commonly prescribed knee lock (Figure 12-26). The ratchet lock has a catching mechanism that operates in 12-degree increments. As the user rises from a seated to a standing position, if there is a tendency for the knee to become unstable and flex, the ratchet lock prevents that movement

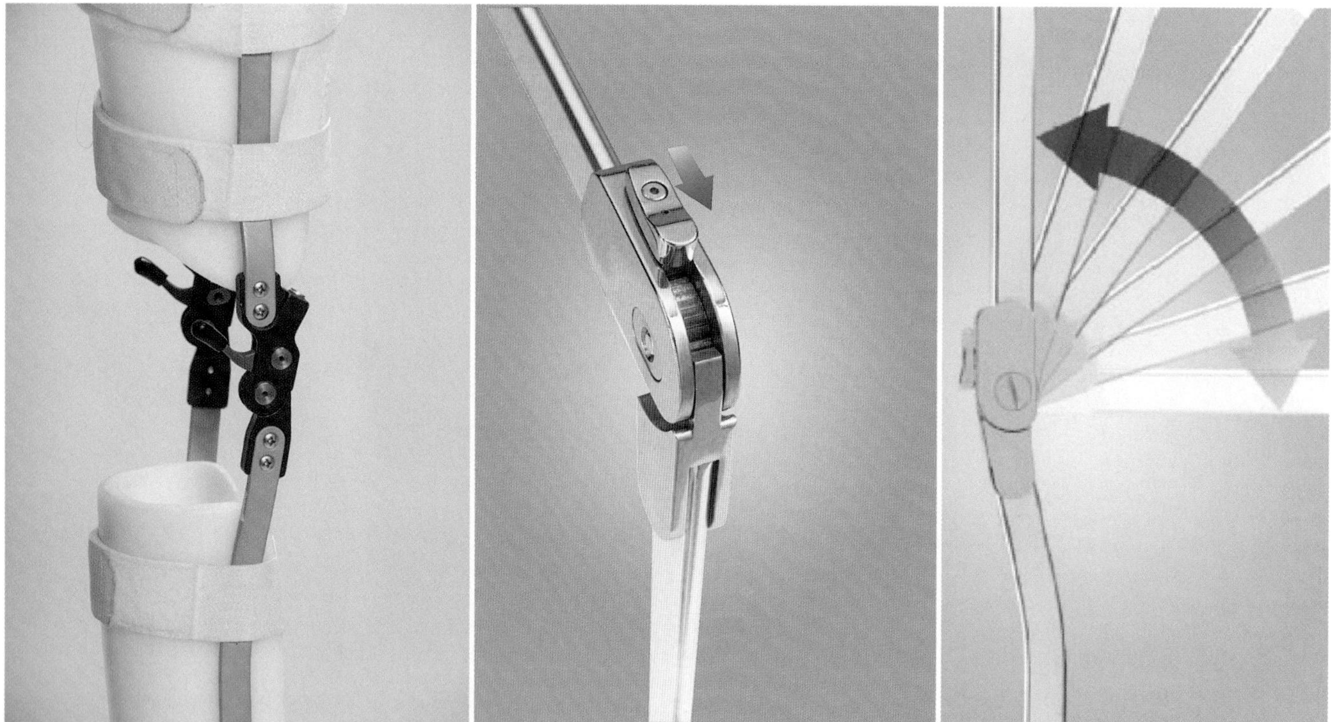

FIGURE 12-26 Ratchet lock. The 12-degree increments gained with knee extension prevent the knee from going into flexion and thereby add stability and a safety factor as one rises from a seated to a standing position. The mechanism is released with the lever arm to allow one to resume a seated position.

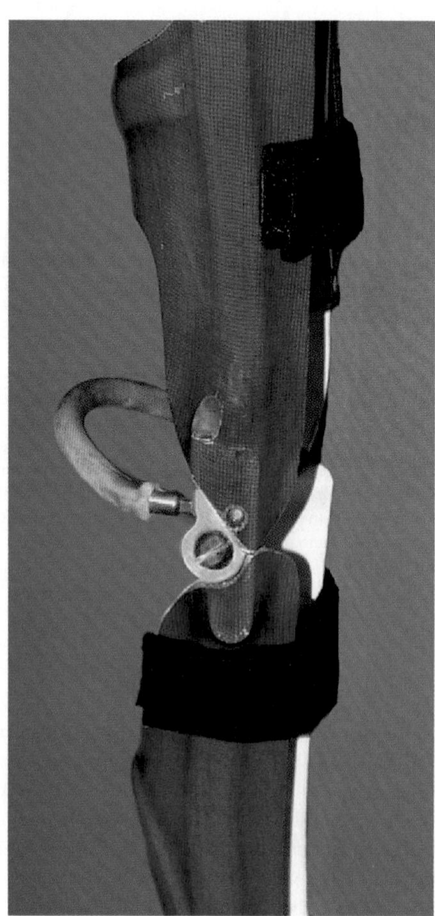

FIGURE 12-27 Padded spring-loaded bail lock. (Courtesy Becker Orthopedic Co, Troy, Mich.)

and keeps the gains made toward extension. Once the patient is standing with the knees extended, knee flexion is achieved either by pressing down on a release lever or by sliding the locking mechanism.

Before the development of the ratchet lock, the drop lock (ring lock) was used most commonly in both the medial and lateral uprights of the KAFO (see Figure 12-22). Its advantage is simplicity of design without bulk. However, fine motor coordination skills are needed to lock the knee in complete extension. In addition, there are two locks per side yet only two hands. The drop lock can also "settle" after ambulation and might be difficult to pull up to unlock the knee. The disadvantage of the drop lock in comparison with the ratchet lock is that there is no locking mechanism until full knee extension is obtained. Consequently, a patient's knee can collapse into flexion when it is not sufficiently extended to activate the drop lock. A collapse into flexion does not occur with the ratchet lock, and thus the patient is less likely to fall. A drop lock can be used unilaterally along the lateral upright if the patient is relatively lightweight and has a low activity level.

The bail lock (also known as the Swiss, French, Schweitzer, or pawl lock) provides the easiest method of simultaneously unlocking the medial and lateral knee joints of a KAFO (Figures 12-27 and 12-28). Two hands can be used for two bail locks, whereas there are a total of four ratchet locks or four drop locks with other bilateral KAFOs. Lifting up the bail posteriorly releases the knee joint to permit flexion, allowing the patient to sit down. The patient can also alternatively catch the bail on the edge of a chair by leaning back to release the lock mechanism to permit sitting. The locking mechanism is spring-loaded to assist locking the knee into extension (see Figure 12-28).

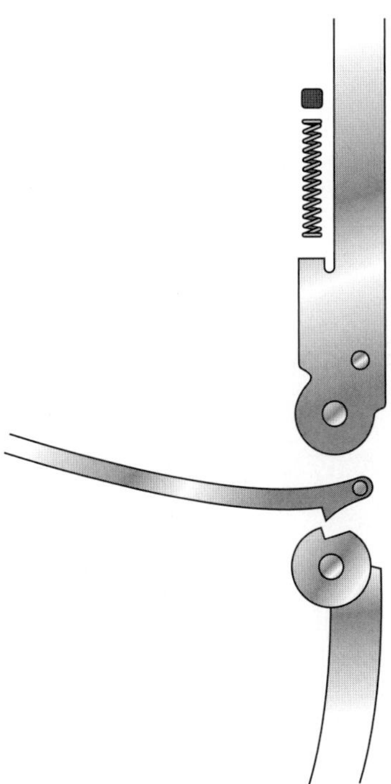

FIGURE 12-28 Spring-loaded bail lock mechanism. Lifting the bail permits free flexion for sitting and the spring mechanism helps lock the knee joint into extension.

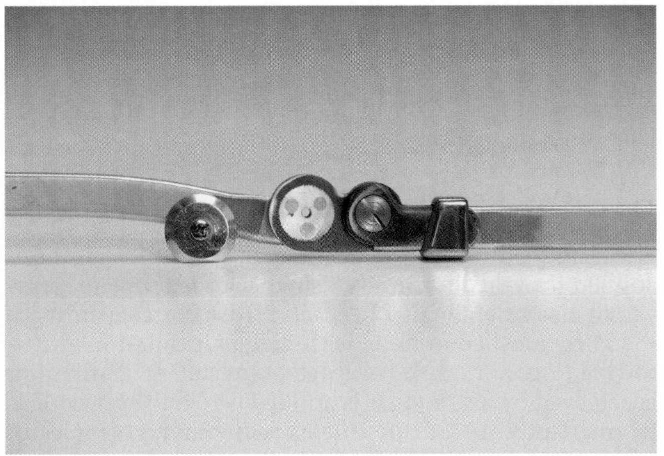

FIGURE 12-29 The dial lock may be adjusted every 6 degrees for precise control of knee flexion.

The bail is often padded with rubber to protect the clothing from being torn or soiled. The KAFO with a bail lock can be worn over or under clothes, depending on the size of the bail lock and the size of the clothing. On its downside, child cruelty can lead to one child kneeing the handicapped child's knee from behind and, with this type of lock, causing him or her to fall—not a good practical joke.

The dial lock (formerly known as a turn buckle) is used to stabilize the knee in varying amounts of flexion (Figure 12-29). It can be adjusted in 6-degree increments and is more precise for the management of a knee with a flexion contracture than a KAFO with ratchet locks. Its uses include helping prevent progression of a flexion contracture or assisting with the gradual reduction of a flexion contracture.

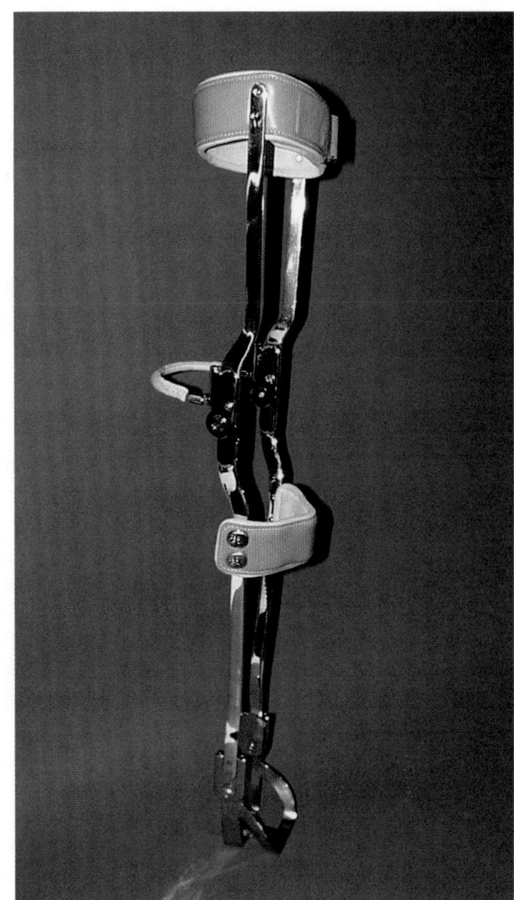

FIGURE 12-30 Scott-Craig knee-ankle-foot orthosis. (Courtesy Becker Orthopedic Co, Troy, Mich.)

When control of knee buckling is the primary goal of the KAFO, then applying an anterior force (extension) at the knee is necessary. This can be accomplished with a leather knee cap or an infrapatellar strap.

Thigh and Calf Components of a Knee-Ankle-Foot Orthosis

The thigh band needs to be wide enough to adequately distribute the pressure of the ground reactive force transmitted through the knee axis. A partial plastic thigh shell can provide a greater contact area and decrease high-pressure areas if properly fitted. Plastic-metal combination KAFOs also decrease the weight of the KAFO, which can increase patient comfort and usage. A low thigh band is used to prevent genu recurvatum. In a similar manner, the calf component of the KAFO can consist of a padded metal calf band or a molded plastic calf shell.

Scott-Craig Orthosis

The Scott-Craig orthosis (Figure 12-30) was designed to provide the patient with paraplegia who has a complete lesion at L1 or higher, with a more functional and comfortable gait.[47] It was also designed to reduce unnecessary hardware, to be a KAFO of lighter weight, and to be easy to don and doff. This orthosis was named after an orthotist, Bruce Scott, who worked at Craig Hospital, Englewood, Colorado.

The orthotic design consists of an ankle joint with anterior (permits 5 degrees of dorsiflexion to simulate plantar flexion) and posterior (set at 90 degrees to prevent toe drag) pin stops, a sole plate extending to the metatarsal heads, a crossbar added to the metatarsal head area for mediolateral stabilization, and an offset knee joint with a bail lock.[47] A rigid anterior tibial band is positioned directly below the tibial tubercle. A rigid proximal thigh band is positioned posteriorly and is closed anteriorly with a soft strap secured with Velcro. These two bands should be shallow enough to hold the knee in extension. A three-point system helps keep the knee in extension by applying pressure at the proximal thigh posteriorly, the proximal tibia anteriorly, and at the calcaneus posteriorly.[22] The ankle joint functions with a dorsiflexion stop used to simulate the triceps surae function as previously described, and with a posterior stop set at 90 degrees to prevent toe drag.

A group headed by Lehmann[24] analyzed the Scott-Craig orthosis and found that it was the easiest of the KAFOs tested to don and doff. The original design of this orthosis is still being prescribed for patients with paraplegia.

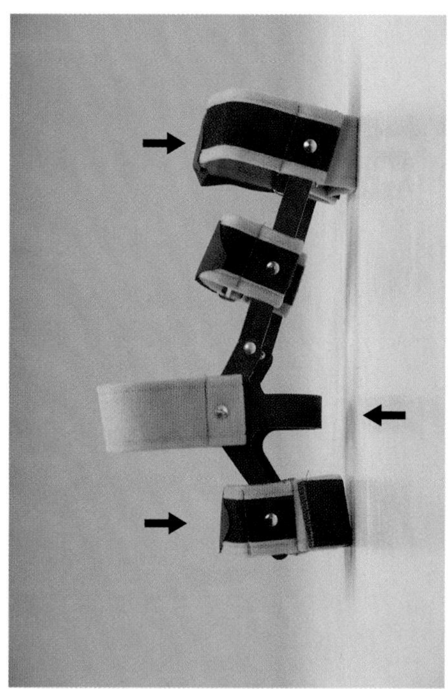

FIGURE 12-31 The articulated Swedish knee cage, which uses a three-point system to control genu recurvatum.

Stance Control Orthosis

The stance control KAFO is designed to lock the knee in stance phase and allow knee flexion in swing phase of gait. This category of KAFOs is still evolving, but currently there are several orthotic manufacturers offering stance control knee joints in centrally fabricated KAFOs. The mechanism to lock and unlock the knee with every step depends on a reciprocal gait pattern. The knee joint relies on a pendulum, a cable to the ankle joint, or electronic controllers to detect stance phase. Proper gait training is necessary to learn to use these devices safely and properly.

Knee Orthoses

Swedish Knee Cage

The KO known as a Swedish knee cage (Figure 12-31) is used to control minor to moderate genu recurvatum caused by ligamentous or capsular laxity. This articulated KO permits full knee flexion and prevents hyperextension. The Swedish knee cage uses a classic three-point orthotic system with two bands placed anterior to the knee axis (one above and one below the knee) and a third band posterior to the knee joint in the popliteal area. It also has an additional thigh band with longer uprights to obtain better leverage at the knee joint. Severe genu recurvatum might need to be controlled with longer lever arms, such as that offered by a KAFO.

Genu recurvatum can also be controlled through additional orthotic measures including a solid plastic AFO that resists plantar flexion. This can be used in cases in which disease also affects the ankle or subtalar joints. The more rigid the AFO, the greater the flexion moment at the knee during heel strike (which counters the extension moment of a knee with recurvatum). A shoe with a solid heel also helps create a greater knee flexion moment, preferred in this case over a shoe with a cushioned heel, which would facilitate a knee flexion moment. An additional flexion moment at the knee during midstance can be obtained by fixing the AFO in a few degrees of dorsiflexion.

Osteoarthritis Knee Orthoses

The same orthotic three-point principle that has been applied for years in the Swedish knee cage for genu recurvatum has recently also been applied to osteoarthritis of the knee, most commonly with medial compartment narrowing (Figure 12-32). The three-point system distribution is achieved by a strap that is applied across the knee joint. In one study, 19 of 20 patients with varying degrees of osteoarthritis experienced significant relief of knee pain.[27] Radiographic improvement in joint alignment was also noted. The limiting factor regarding this knee orthotic prescription is the patient's weight. A morbidly obese patient with an abundance of fatty tissue around the knee will not support the KO adequately. In such cases in which this KO and surgery are precluded, the foot orthoses with lateral buildup (as described earlier in this chapter) should be considered. The foot orthosis with a lateral buildup is considered the preferred first-line orthotic treatment for osteoarthritis of the knee. (See the section on osteoarthritis of the knee in common foot conditions in this chapter.)

Sport Knee Orthoses

There is an increasing abundance of sport orthoses on the market. There is also a lack of definitive research regarding their role in sports. This can lead to much confusion regarding their prescription, unless the KO is reviewed

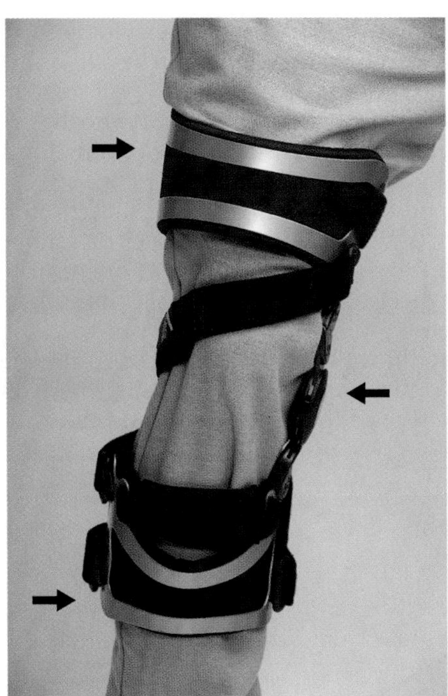

FIGURE 12-32 The Generation II knee orthosis for tricompartmental osteoarthritis of the knee. This uses the standard orthotic three-point distribution system in a mediolateral distribution rather than in an anteroposterior distribution as was noted with the Swedish knee cage (see Figure 12-31).

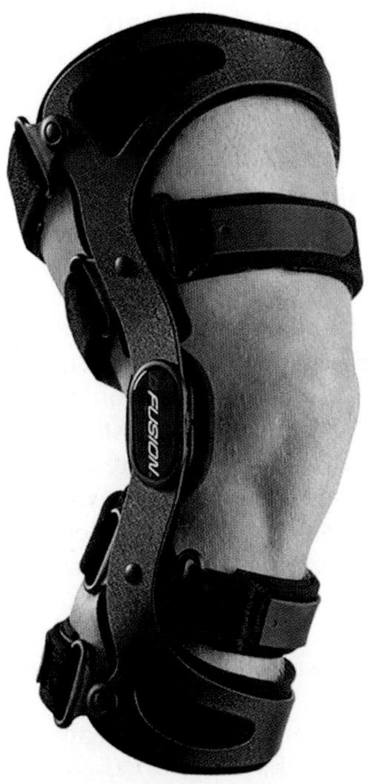

FIGURE 12-33 Fusion anterior cruciate ligament knee orthosis. This type of lightweight knee orthosis is designed to prevent hyperextension and also offer mediolateral stability at the knee. It may also offer some proprioceptive feedback. (Courtesy BREG, Inc., Carlsbad, Calif, and Elizur Corp, Pittsburgh, Pa.)

systematically. Sport KOs can be divided into prophylactic, rehabilitative, and functional categories.[31]

Prophylactic knee bracing attempts to prevent or reduce the severity of knee injuries. There is currently no evidence to support the use or cost benefit of these orthoses. Some studies have found that the use of these orthoses actually increased the number of athletes with knee injuries.[44,52] It is theorized that knee-braced players can put themselves in compromising positions because of overreliance on the orthosis and that this can contribute directly to the increasing injury rates observed. The use of prophylactic knee bracing has also been associated with increased energy consumption, which can impair athletic performance.[13]

Rehabilitative knee bracing is used to allow protected motion within defined limits.[36] It is useful for postoperative and conservative management of knee injuries and most commonly applied postoperatively for anterior cruciate ligament–reconstructed knees (Figure 12-33) and patellofemoral pain syndrome.*

Functional knee bracing is designed to assist or provide stability for the unstable knee. Functional knee bracing does not replace the need for rehabilitation of the knee. Knee braces are used most commonly to stabilize a laterally subluxing patella[7,28] or an anterior cruciate ligament–deficient knee.[2,32,51] Their use has been shown to be effective only at loads much lower than those placed on the knee during athletic participation. In summary, functional knee bracing can possibly play a role in the treatment of pathologic laxity by possibly decreasing the frequency of unstable episodes.[36]

*References 2, 7, 28, 32, 51, 62.

Pediatric Orthoses

Caster Cart

The disabled child should identify early with motion so that ambulatory skills can progress naturally.[1] Without familiarity with motion, disabled children lack the desire to ambulate once placed in a parapodium or reciprocating gait orthosis.

The caster cart (Figure 12-34) is used for children with a developmental delay in ambulatory skills, and it serves as an initial mobility aid. It is most often prescribed for children with spina bifida. Most children are upright and cruising by 10 months.[14] Children with paraplegia should be fitted for a caster cart once they have obtained enough upper limb strength and trunk balance to propel themselves. If balance is a problem for the child, a deep seat bucket can be prescribed to help provide balance so that the child can use the upper limbs for propulsion.

The caster wheel at the back of the cart facilitates multidirectional movement. Initially, the child can be pushed around in the cart with a handle attached posteriorly so that the cart serves as a stroller.

Standing Frame

The use of a standing frame (Figure 12-35) typically follows successful use of a caster cart. The age range for initial use is usually 8 to 15 months. Children can continue to use their caster carts during this time. Children who are pulling themselves up along furniture are typically ready for a standing frame. This is the first sign that they are interested in standing and moving.[14]

The standing frame helps balance the body in space and allows free use of the upper limbs for participation in activities. Children with thoracic level lesions need AFOs to provide good ankle and foot support in the standing frame or parapodium. Initial gait training can occur with the use of the standing frame via a swing-through gait with the assistance of parallel bars.

Parapodium

The parapodium was also referred to in the past as a swivel orthosis (Figure 12-36). Before children are given a parapodium, they should first demonstrate adequate use of a standing frame and exhibit a desire to ambulate. A child's standing frame can be evaluated for wear and tear to determine whether it has been used sufficiently so that the child can advance to a parapodium. A frequently used standing frame (or any orthosis) will show evidence of wear and tear that includes soiling and scratches. It is important to note this because parents frequently set expectations too high for the disabled child. A child who has not used a standing frame will likely be unable or unwilling to ambulate with a parapodium.

A parapodium is an appropriate prescription for children who are unlikely to become functional walkers because of the severity of their impairment. It often complements wheelchair use.[26] It is most commonly prescribed for children between 2.5 and 5 years of age.

A parapodium allows crutchless gait. Ambulation occurs by the child pivoting the hips and using "body English" to swivel one side of the oval-based stand forward and then

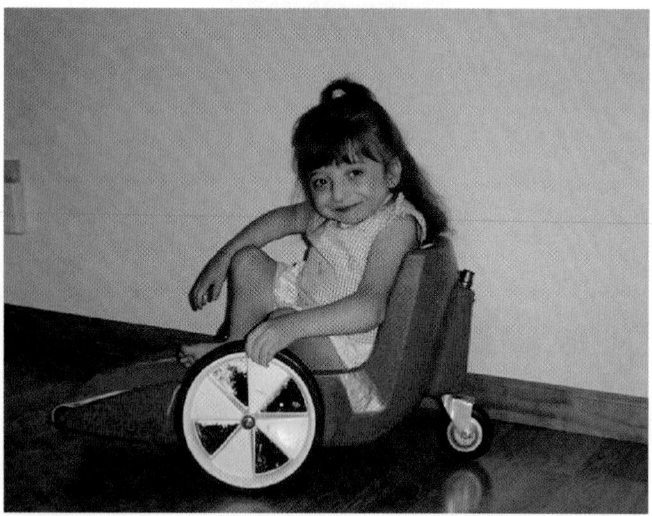

FIGURE 12-34 Caster cart. This is an initial mobility aid for the disabled child. The child uses it as a "prewheelchair device" for mobility.

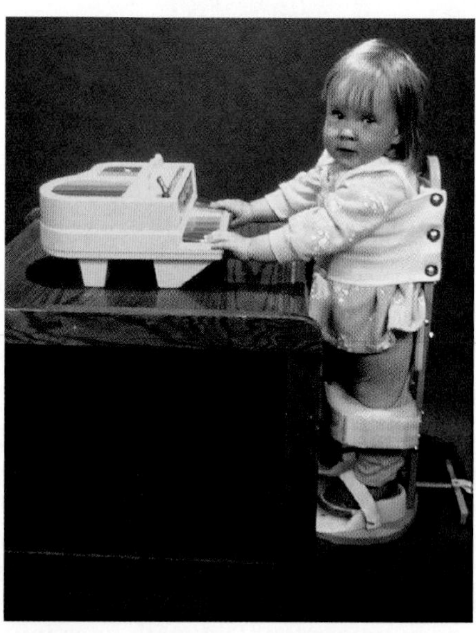

FIGURE 12-35 A standing frame for initial upright activities, which is used by children who desire to stand, as determined by attempts to pull themselves upright.

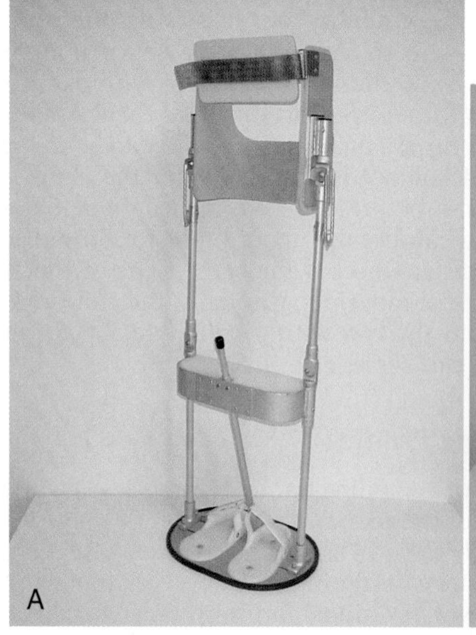

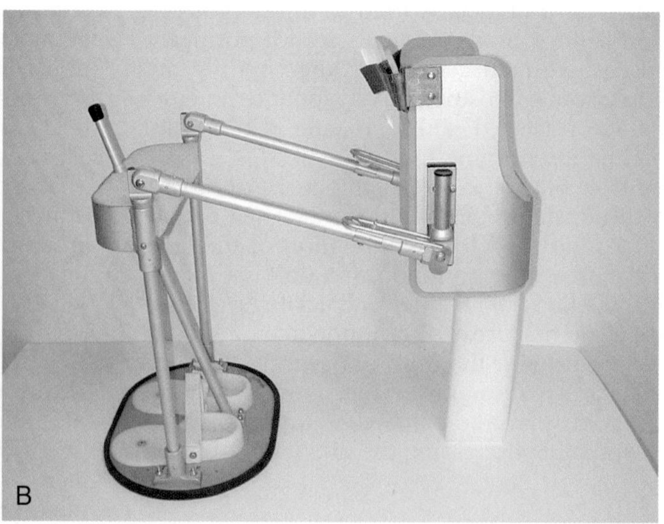

FIGURE 12-36 **A,** Parapodium with hip and knee joints locked in extension. **B,** Parapodium with hip and knee joints unlocked and in a flexed position. (Courtesy Variety Ability Systems, Inc., Toronto, Ontario, Canada.)

repeating the same event for the other side. Its design is similar to the standing frame, but it has hip and knee joints. The hip and knee joints remain locked in extension to permit ambulation in the upright position but can be unlocked (simultaneously in some models) to permit sitting. The difficulties experienced with the use of this orthosis include donning and doffing and rising from a seated position to a standing position.

Reciprocating Gait Orthosis

The reciprocating gait orthosis (RGO) was formerly known as a hip-guided orthosis (HGO) (Figure 12-37). It can also be referred to as a bilateral hip-knee-ankle-foot orthosis (HKAFO). The purpose of the RGO is to provide contralateral hip extension with ipsilateral hip flexion. The RGO is appropriate for children who have used the standing frame, developed good trunk control and coordination, can safely stand, and are mentally prepared for ambulation. Good upper limb strength, trunk balance, and active hip flexion are important positive variables for ambulation.[10,12] Obesity, advanced age, lack of patient or family motivation, scoliosis, spasticity,[8] and contractures are significant negative factors in the long-term use of the RGO. This type of orthosis clearly only complements the use of a wheelchair for mobility purposes and serves therapeutic purposes of exercise and upright activities. One newer type of spinal cord injury orthosis is the Walkabout, which has a scissoring mechanism in the groin area attaching two KAFOs via a hinge. The trade-off with this device is a lack of contralateral hip extension with ipsilateral hip flexion for a less bulky orthosis to don and doff.[34]

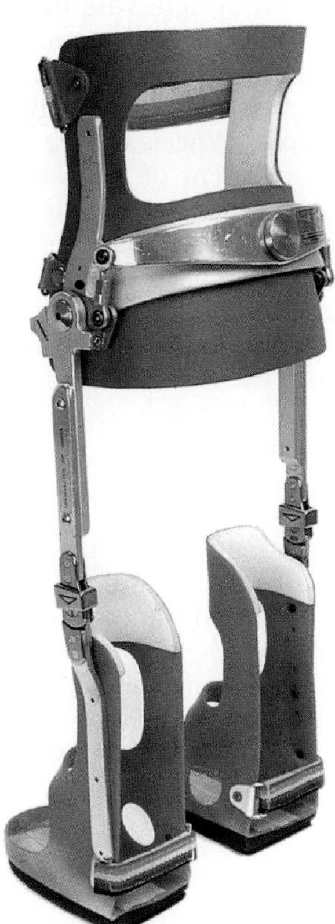

FIGURE 12-37 Isocentric reciprocating gait orthosis (RGO). (Courtesy Center for Orthotic Design, Redwood City, Calif., and Fillauer Companies, Inc., Chattanooga, Tenn.)

Spinal cord injury level is not a very reliable predictor of ambulation capability for children. As children with spinal cord injuries grow taller, they might experience more difficulty walking as their center of gravity becomes lower.

The RGO is prescribed most commonly for children ages 3 to 6 years. The concept of the RGO was developed by researchers working with a patient who had active hip flexion and no hip extension. Gait is initiated with unilateral hip flexion and can be assisted by swaying the trunk when hip flexion is inadequate. This type of gait pattern can also be considered to be a form of physical therapy because hip extension occurs passively with each step, helping to reduce flexion contractures. Cables were initially used to provide the necessary hip motion, but newer mechanical methods of reciprocal gait use a "teeter-totter" concept (see Figure 12-37). This type of RGO has been reported to be more energy efficient than an RGO with cables.[60]

Crutches are used with the RGO to provide a control mechanism, taking advantage of the forward momentum to produce small propulsive forces when needed.[29] This also is a disadvantage of this orthosis (compared with the parapodium) because the upper limbs are not free for other activities. The patient with an RGO is able to negotiate a greater variety of surfaces than would be possible with the parapodium.[43]

The hip joints of the RGO have hip flexion and abduction capabilities on release of the locking mechanisms. It is recommended that one hip joint should have abduction capability to permit catheterization and to allow sitting in a hip-flexed and abducted position.

Ambulation Aids

The purpose of using ambulation aids (Figures 12-38 and 12-39) is to increase the area of support for patients who

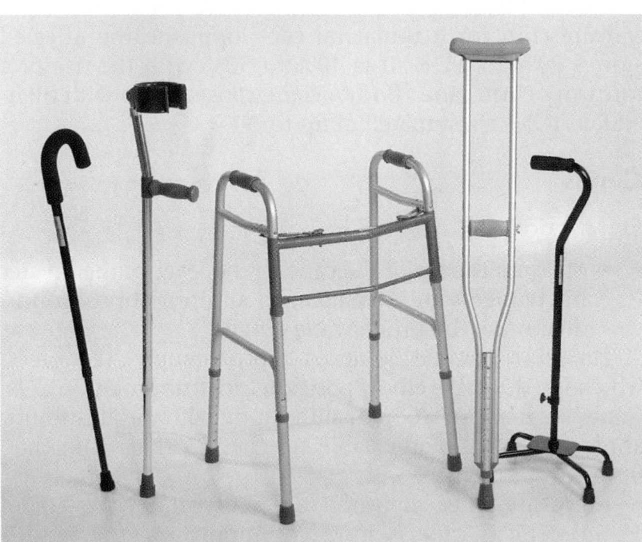

FIGURE 12-38 Ambulation aids. *Left to right,* C cane, Lofstrand forearm orthosis, walker, crutch, and quad cane.

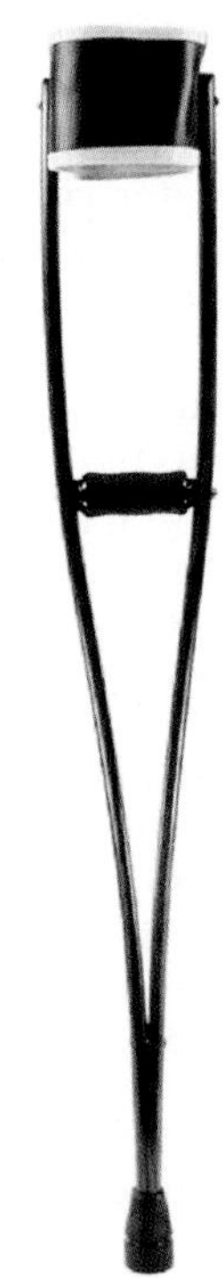

FIGURE 12-39 Wooden forearm orthosis (Kenny stick). The leather band encloses the proximal forearm. (Courtesy Thomas Fetterman, Inc., Southampton, Pa.)

have difficulty maintaining their center of gravity safely over their own support area. A variety of aids are available for the individual needs of patients. Ambulation aids improve balance, redistribute and extend the weight-bearing area, reduce lower limb pain, provide small propulsive forces, and provide sensory feedback. They should be considered an extension of the upper limb. Their proper use requires adequate upper limb strength and coordination. An exercise program for the upper limbs is useful and can complement ambulation with the aid by increasing endurance and stability. A supervised period of training is recommended after prescription of an aid.

The type of aid needed depends on how much balance and weight-bearing assistance is needed. The body weight transmission for a unilateral cane opposite the affected side is 20% to 25%.[4] It is 40% to 50% with the use of a forearm or arm cane.[4] Body weight transmission with bilateral crutches is estimated at up to 80%.[5]

Canes

Prescription

- Measure the tip of the cane to the level of the greater trochanter with the patient in an upright position to determine the proper cane length.[55]

The elbow should be flexed approximately 20 degrees, which is a desirable elbow position for all ambulation aids. Canes are made of wood or aluminum, with the aluminum alloy cane having adjustable notches so that "one cane fits all."

There are three common types of canes (see Figure 12-38). The C cane is most commonly used. It is also known as a crook top cane or a J cane. A functional grip cane offers the patient a grip that can be more comfortable than with the C cane. A quad cane provides an increased area of support compared with the other canes. Quad canes also come in narrow- and wide-based forms for different degrees of support. The lateral two legs are directed away from the body. Only the narrow base quad cane fits safely on a stair tread.

A cane is used on the side opposite the supporting lower limb. It is advanced with the opposite lower limb. It is usually held on the patient's unaffected side. This can be done to lessen the force exerted on a hip with disease. The load is increased by four times the body weight on the stance side during gait because of the gravitational forces and the gluteus medius-minimus force exerted across the weight-bearing hip.[5] The cane helps decrease the force generated across the affected hip joint by decreasing the work of the gluteus medius-minimus complex. This occurs when the upper limb exerts force on the cane to help minimize pelvic drop on the side opposite the weight-bearing lower limb.

Patients should be instructed on how to ascend and descend stairs. The pneumonic "up with the good and down with the bad" serves as an easy reminder. The patient should always have the "good" lower limb assume the first full weight-bearing step on level surfaces.

Walker

Prescription

- Place the front of the walker 12 inches in front of the patient (the walker should partially surround the patient).
- Determine the proper height of the walker by having the patient stand upright with the shoulders relaxed and the elbows flexed 20 degrees.[55]

A walker provides maximum support for the patient but also necessitates a slow gait. It is useful for patients with hemiplegia and ataxia. Wheels can be added to the front legs to facilitate movement of the walker for those who lack coordination in the upper limbs. Patients using wheeled models should be supervised initially to ensure safety. Some walkers also have a front U-shaped extension with extra supports to provide stability for stair climbing. A patient needs to be motivated and have good strength and coordination to use this model of walker.

Visual Impairment Cane

Prescription

- Instruct the patient to flex the shoulder until the upper limb is parallel with the floor.
- Measure the distance from the hand to the floor. That is the proper length.

A visual impairment cane should be lightweight, flexible, and easily collapsible. The distal inches of the cane are red. Please also note the additional physiatric visual impairment pearl for elevator rides: two dings is "down" and one ding is "up."

Crutches

Prescription

- *Crutch length:* Measure the distance from the anterior axillary fold to a point 6 inches lateral to the fifth toe with the patient standing with the shoulders relaxed.

- *Handpiece:* Measure with the 'patient's elbow flexed 30 degrees, the wrist in maximal extension, and the fingers forming a fist. This is measured *after* the total crutch height is determined with the crutch 3 inches lateral to the foot.[55]

A crutch is defined as a device that provides support from the axilla to the floor. Although there are different types of crutches and canes, they can all be referred to as orthoses because they are applied to the external surface of the body to improve function.

The patient should be able to raise the body 1 to 2 inches by complete elbow extension. Despite the popularity of padding the axillary area of the crutch, this should not be done. It needs to be emphasized to the patient that crutches are not designed to be rests for body support. This point should be made to the patient to reduce the incidence of compressive radial neuropathies or plexopathies.

Nonaxillary Crutches

Nonaxillary crutches are more appropriately called forearm or arm canes, or forearm or arm orthoses. The Lofstrand forearm orthosis, Kenny sticks, the Everett or Warm Spring orthosis, the Canadian crutch, and the platform forearm orthosis are discussed in the following sections (see Figures 12-38 and 12-39).

Forearm Orthoses

Lofstrand Forearm Orthosis

Prescription

- Measure the handpiece as described above for crutches, with the patient standing upright and the elbow in 20 degrees of flexion.

The proximal portion of the orthosis is also angled at 20 degrees to provide for a comfortable, stable fit. It is often made of tubular aluminum. It provides less support than crutches for ambulation, but is sufficient for many patients. Lofstrand forearm orthoses are most often used bilaterally. The open end of the cuff is placed on the lateral aspect of the forearm to permit elbow flexion and grasping without dropping the orthoses. The advantages of this orthosis are that it is shorter than an axillary crutch, and the forearm cuff pivots to allow the patient to lean on the crutch for hand activities.

Wooden Forearm Orthosis (Kenny Stick)

Another forearm orthosis option is the Kenny stick (see Figure 12-39). It was named after Sister Kenny, who sawed off the top half of wooden crutches and placed a leather band around the proximal portion of the forearm. It was designed for patients with polio who had satisfactory proximal upper limb musculature but were weak distally and unable to effectively hold and control the orthosis. Its advantage over the Lofstrand orthosis is the presence of a closed leather band. This assures the patient (more so than the Lofstrand forearm orthosis does) that he or she will not drop the ambulation aid.

Platform Forearm Orthosis

Prescription

- Have the patient stand upright with the shoulders relaxed and the elbows flexed 90 degrees. The distance from the ground to the forearm rest is the proper length.

This orthosis is helpful for patients with painful wrist and hand conditions as well as for those with elbow contractures. Velcro straps are applied around the forearm, especially for patients with weak hand grips.

Triceps Weakness Orthoses (Arm Orthoses)

These orthoses, also known as triceps weakness crutches, were originally developed for patients with poliomyelitis. The metal version is known as a Warm Spring crutch or Everett crutch. The wooden version is known as a Canadian crutch. These crutches resemble the "axillary" crutches in style but end proximally with a cuff at the midarm level. These ambulation aids help prevent flexion (buckling) of the elbow during gait.

Crutch Tips and Hand Grips

The purpose of crutch tips is to absorb shock and prevent slippage. Crutches are only as safe as the quality of their crutch tips. Special crutch tips are available for rainy and icy conditions (Figure 12-40). At each checkup, the physician should make sure that the crutch tips are not worn out. Hand grips are used to reduce pressure on the hands and are also safety features because they help prevent slippage.

Prescription

A medical diagnosis with delineation of the impairment and any resulting disability should be made before an orthotic prescription is written. The orthotic goals should be documented for the orthotist. An AFO prescription should include the type of ankle (rigid, flexible, or jointed) and the position of the ankle (neutral, dorsiflexed, or plantar flexed). If the ankle is jointed, the range of motion should be specified. In the case of a compressive peroneal nerve palsy, for example, the physical impairment would be a flaccid foot drop. The ankle should be flexible and held in a neutral position with a plastic AFO set in a few

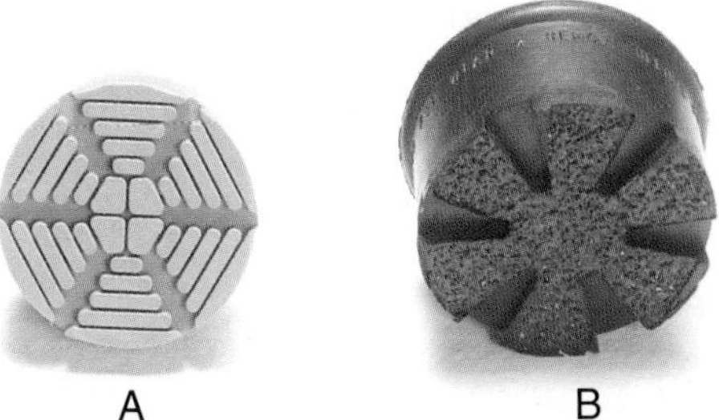

FIGURE 12-40 A, Snow Boot crutch tip for use in snowy and icy conditions. **B,** Rain Guard crutch tip for use in wet conditions. (Courtesy Hi-Trac Industries, Holley, Mich.)

degrees of dorsiflexion. The goals include toe clearance during swing-through and prevention of foot slap during early stance.[19]

From an orthotic prescription standpoint, most of this chapter is concisely summarized in Figure 12-41, a full-size prescription pad with convenient checkboxes and room at the top of the page to copy this onto letterhead for clinical use. Adjacent to this sheet is a quick summary reference that can be copied onto the back of the prescription sheets (Box 12-2).

Summary

An appropriate lower limb orthotic prescription requires a thorough biomechanical analysis of gait and knowledge of

Lower limb orthotic prescription

Name: ______ Age ______

Diagnosis: ______

Orthotic goals: ______

Justification: ______

Orthotic company: ______

Referring physician: ______

☐ FO ☐ AFO ☐ KAFO ☐ HKAFO ☐ KO

☐ Right ☐ Left ☐ Bilateral

☐ Custom

☐ Plastic ☐ Metal ☐ Combination

Ankle type: ☐ Solid (flexible) ☐ Solid (rigid) ☐ Hinged: __ dorsi-assist
__ dorsi-stop
__ plantar stop

Ankle ROM: ☐ Plantar flexion __ degrees
☐ Dorsiflexion __ degrees
☐ Neutral (90°)

Knee type: ☐ Straight set ☐ Posterior offset ☐ Polycentric

Knee locks: ☐ Two per knee joint ☐ One per knee joint

Knee lock type: ☐ Ratchet lock ☐ Drop lock ☐ Bail lock ☐ Dial lock

Hip joints with drop locks ☐ Standard ☐ Abduction

Miscellaneous ______

Physician name ______ **Date** ______

FIGURE 12-41 Lower limb orthotic prescription sheet.

BOX 12-2

Summary Reference for Prescription Pad

Foot Orthosis

- *UCBL (University of California Biomechanics Laboratory):* Hyperpronating "flat" foot
- *Metatarsal pad:* Temporary mild to moderate metatarsalgia
- *Metatarsal bar to shoe:* Severe metatarsalgia (cannot stand something in shoe) or permanent metatarsalgia (e.g., arthritis)
- *Heel lift:* Temporary use for Achilles tendinitis or plantar fasciitis
- *Heel cup:* Fat pad syndrome (heel bruise)
- *Lateral heel wedge:* Osteoarthritis with medial compartment narrowing

Ankle-Foot Orthosis

- *Over the counter:* For a trial basis only
- *Custom:* For long-term use
- *Plastic:* For almost everyone
- *Metal:* For the patient >250 lb with a hinged ankle-foot orthosis

Common Types

- *Custom solid (flexible) ankle-foot orthosis set at 90 degrees:* Foot drop
- *Custom solid (rigid) ankle-foot orthosis set at 90 degrees:* Plantar spasticity

Hinge Indications

- Significant mediolateral instability at subtalar joint but patient with ankle dorsiflexion and plantar flexion (rare)
- Tight plantar flexors in patients with spasticity with improving lower limb function (they can take advantage of a more "normal" gait via dorsiflexion from midstance to toe-off, and plantar stretching is therapeutic over this part of the gait cycle)
- An active patient with foot drop or plantar flexor spasticity can take advantage of the hinged feature during stair climbing, rising from sit to stand, frequent walking, etc.

Knee-Ankle-Foot Orthosis

Knee Type

- *Straight set:* Most common; always used unless posterior offset is indicated
- *Posterior offset:* Patient with weak knee extensor triad (quads, plantar flexors, and hamstrings)
- *Polycentric:* A two-joint system that theoretically simulates femur-tibia translation
  - Standard on most sport orthoses for the above marketing purpose
  - No clear-cut indications

Knee Locks

- *Ratchet lock:* Most common.
- *Drop lock:* Can be difficult to pull up after "settling in" from walking
- *Bail lock:* Bulkier and less desirable than the drop locks for most patients but necessary for those without fine hand control
- *Dial lock:* Used to lock an unstable knee in extension but they are adjusted to account for knee flexion contractures

Hip Joints (common to prescribe one of each of the following)

- *Standard:* Allows flexion and extension
- *Abduction:* Permits flexion and extension but also permits abduction to allow self-catheterization of the urinary bladder and seating in a hip-flexed and abducted position

the available orthotic components available to treat specific conditions. The prescribing physician should maintain a close working relationship with the certified orthotist to make certain that the patient is receiving the best orthotic options available.

Patient complaints about orthoses usually are related to cosmesis, comfort, clothing soiling or damage, weight, and difficulty with donning and doffing. All practitioners should work toward the goal of achieving the ideal orthosis for the patient that enhances comfort, cosmesis, and function. Accomplishing this will in turn enhance compliance. The ideal orthosis would be weightless, invisible, without cost, maintenance free, comfortable, and strong, and would normalize the gait pattern while simultaneously reducing energy consumption to within normal limits.

ACKNOWLEDGMENTS: A special thanks to Kurt Kuhlman, DO, and Richard Kozakiewicz, MD, for reviewing this chapter. We also thank Al Gallegos of Z-coiL Footwear, R. Douglas Turner of Becker Orthopedic, Wally Motloch, CO, Carla David of Fillauer Companies Inc., Robert Evans of High-Trac Industries Inc., Martin Mifsud of Variety Ability Systems Inc., Thomas Fetterman Inc., and BREG Inc for providing photographs of their products for this chapter. We thank Dennis Pushkar, owner, Impressions Studio, Jeannette, Pennsylvania, for his time, expertise, and assistance with many of the high-quality color orthotic images. Lastly, we must thank Ernest Johnson, MD, and Randy Braddom, MD, for teaching us about lower limb orthoses and entertaining us with their grammatical banter that will forever affect (not impact) our writing skills! May Dr. Johnson's soul rest with God in physiatric heaven.

REFERENCES

1. Bleck EE: Developmental orthopaedics: III. Toddlers, *Dev Med Child Neurol* 24:533–555, 1982.
2. Chew KY, Lew HL, Date E, et al: Current evidence and clinical applications of therapeutic knee braces, *Am J Phys Med Rehabil* 86(8):678–686, 2007.
3. Corcoran PJ, Jebsen RH, Brengelmann GL, et al: Effects of plastic and metal leg braces on speed and energy cost of hemiparetic ambulation, *Arch Phys Med Rehabil* 51:69–77, 1970.
4. D'Ambrosia RD: Conservative management of metatarsal and heel pain in the adult foot, *Orthopedics* 10:137–142, 1987.
5. Deathe AB, Hayes KC, Winter DA: The biomechanics of canes, crutches, and walkers, *Crit Rev Phys Rehab Med* 5:15–29, 1993.
6. Diveley RL: Foot appliances and alterations. In American Academy of Orthopaedic Surgeons, editor: *Orthopaedic appliances atlas*, vol 1, Ann Arbor, 1952, JW Edwards, pp 463–464.
7. Draper CE, Bsier TF, Santos JM, et al: Using real-time MRI to quantify altered joint kinematics in subjects with patellofemoral pain and to evaluate the effects of a patellar brace or sleeve on joint motion, *J Orthop Res* 27:571–577, 2009.
8. Gok H, Kucukdeveci A, Yavuzer G, et al: Effects of ankle-foot orthoses on hemiparetic gait, *Clin Rehabil* 17:137–139, 2003.
9. Gross MT, Foxworth JL: The role of foot orthoses as an intervention for patellofemoral pain, *J Orthop Sports Phys Ther* 33:661–670, 2003.
10. Guidera KJ, Smith S, Raney E, et al: Use of the reciprocating gait orthosis in myelodysplasia, *J Pediatr Orthop* 13:341–348, 1993.
11. Halar E, Cardenas D: Ankle-foot orthoses: clinical implications, *Phys Med Rehabil State Art Rev* 1:45–66, 1987.
12. Harvey LA, Smith MB, Davis GM, et al: Functional outcomes attained by T9-12 paraplegic patients with the Walkabout and the isocentric reciprocal gait orthoses, *Arch Phys Med Rehabil* 78:706–711, 1997.

13. Houston ME, Goemans PH: Leg muscle performance of athletes with and without knee support braces, *Arch Phys Med Rehabil* 63:431–432, 1982.
14. Johnson EW, Spiegel MH: Ambulation problems in very young children, *JAMA* 175:858–863, 1961.
15. Keating EM, Faris PM, Ritter MA, et al: Use of lateral heel and sole wedges in the treatment of medial osteoarthritis of the knee, *Orthop Rev* 22:921–924, 1993.
16. Lee SY, McKeon P, Hertel J: Does the use of orthoses improve self-reported pain and function measures in patients with plantar fasciitis? A meta-analysis, *Phys Ther Sport* 10(1):8–12, 2009.
17. Lehmann JF: The biomechanics of ankle foot orthoses: prescription and design, *Arch Phys Med Rehabil* 60:200–207, 1979.
18. Lehmann JF, Condon SM, de Lateur BJ, et al: Ankle-foot orthoses: effect on gait abnormalities in tibial nerve paralysis, *Arch Phys Med Rehabil* 66:212–218, 1985.
19. Lehmann JF, Condon SM, de Lateur BJ, et al: Gait abnormalities in peroneal nerve paralysis and their correlation by orthoses: a biomechanical study, *Arch Phys Med Rehabil* 67:380–386, 1986.
20. Lehmann JF, de Lateur BJ, Warren CG, et al: Biomechanical evaluation of braces for paraplegics, *Arch Phys Med Rehabil* 50:179–188, 1969.
21. Lehmann JF, Esselman P, Ko MJ, et al: Plastic ankle foot orthoses: evaluation of function, *Arch Phys Med Rehabil* 64:402–407, 1983.
22. Lehmann JF, Warren CG: Restraining forces in various designs of knee ankle orthoses: their placement and effect on anatomical knee joint, *Arch Phys Med Rehabil* 57:430–437, 1976.
23. Lehmann JF, Warren CG, de Lateur BJ: A biomechanical evaluation of knee stability in below knee braces, *Arch Phys Med Rehabil* 51:687–695, 1970.
24. Lehmann JF, Warren CG, Hertling D, et al: Craig-Scott orthosis: a biomechanical and functional evaluation, *Arch Phys Med Rehabil* 57:438–442, 1976.
25. Lehmann JF, Warren CG, Pemberton DR, et al: Load bearing function of patellar tendon bearing braces of various designs, *Arch Phys Med Rehabil* 52:367–370, 1971.
26. Liptak GS, Shurtleff DB, Bloss JW, et al: Mobility aids for children with high-level myelomeningocele: parapodium versus wheelchair, *Dev Med Child Neurol* 34:787–796, 1992.
27. Loke M: New concepts in lower limb orthotics, *Phys Med Rehabil Clin North Am* 11:477–496, 2000.
28. Lun VM, Wiley JP, Meeuwisse WH, et al: Effectiveness of patellar bracing for treatment of patellofemoral pain syndrome, *Clin J Sport Med* 15(4):235–240, 2005.
29. Major RE, Stallard J, Rose GK: The dynamics of walking using the hip guidance orthosis (HGO) with crutches, *Prosthet Orthot Int* 5:19–22, 1981.
30. Marx HW: Lower limb orthotic designs for the spastic hemiplegic patient, *Orthot Prosthet* 28:14–20, 1974.
31. Matsuno H, Kadowaki KM, Tsjui H: Generation II knee bracing for severe medial compartment osteoarthritis of the knee, *Arch Phys Med Rehabil* 78:745–749, 1997.
32. McDevitt ER, Taylor DC, Miller MD, et al: Functional bracing after anterior cruciate ligament reconstruction: a prospective, randomized, multicenter study, *J Bone Joint Surg Am* 32:1887–1892, 2004.
33. Merritt JL: Knee-ankle-foot orthotics: long leg braces and their practical applications, *Phys Med Rehabil State Art Rev* 1:67–82, 1987.
34. Middleton JW, Yeo JD, Blanch L, et al: Clinical evaluation of a new orthosis, the 'Walkabout', for restoration of functional standing and short distance mobility in spinal paralysed individuals, *Spinal Cord* 35:574–579, 1997.
35. Milgram JE, Jacobson MA: Footgear: therapeutic modifications of sole and heel, *Orthop Rev* 7:57–61, 1978.
36. Millet C, Drez D, Jr: Knee braces, *Orthopedics* 10:1777–1780, 1987.
37. Radtka SA, Skinner SR, Dixon DM, et al: A comparison of gait with solid, dynamic and no ankle-foot orthoses in children with spastic cerebral palsy, *Phys Ther* 77:395–409, 1997.
38. Redford JB: Orthoses. In Basmajian JV, Kirby RL, editors: *Medical rehabilitation*, Baltimore, 1984, Williams & Wilkins, p 101.
39. Reid DC: Heel pain and problems of the hindfoot. In Reid DC, editor: *Sports injury assessment and rehabilitation*, ed 1, New York, 1992, Churchill Livingstone, pp 196–212.
40. Rethlefsen S, Kay R, Dennis S, et al: The effects of fixed and articulated ankle-foot orthoses on gait patterns in subjects with cerebral palsy, *J Pediatr Orthop* 19:470–474, 1999.
41. Riegler HF: Orthotic devices for the foot, *Orthop Rev* 16:293–303, 1987.
42. Roos E, Engstrom M, Soderberg B: Foot orthoses for the treatment of plantar fasciitis, *Foot Ankle Int* 27(8):606–611, 2006.
43. Rose GK, Stallard J, Sankarankutty M: Clinical evaluation of spina bifida patients using hip guidance orthoses, *Dev Med Child Neurol* 23:30–40, 1981.
44. Rovere GD, Haupt HA, Yates CS: Prophylactic knee bracing in college football, *Am J Sports Med* 15:111–116, 1987.
45. Sarmiento A: A functional below the knee brace for tibial fractures: a report of its use in 135 cases, *J Bone Joint Surg Am* 52:295–311, 1970.
46. Sarmiento A, Gersten LM, Sobol JA, et al: Tibial shaft fractures treated with functional braces: experience with 780 fractures, *J Bone Joint Surg Br* 71:602–609, 1989.
47. Scott BA: Engineering principles and fabrication techniques for Scott-Craig: long leg brace for paraplegics, *Orthop Prosthet* 28:14–19, 1974.
48. Shrader JA, Siegel KL: Nonoperative management of functional hallux limitus in a patient with rheumatoid arthritis, *Phys Ther* 83:831–843, 2003.
49. Smiley SJ, Jacobsen FS, Mielke C, et al: A comparison of the effects of solid, articulated, and posterior leaf-spring ankle-foot orthoses and shoes alone on gait and energy expenditure in children with spastic diplegic cerebral palsy, *Orthopedics* 25:411–415, 2002.
50. Staheli LT, Chew DE, Corbett M: The longitudinal arch, *J Bone Joint Surg Am* 69:426–428, 1987.
51. Sterett WI, Briggs KK, Farley T, et al: Effect of functional bracing on knee injury in skiers with anterior cruciate ligament reconstruction: a prospective cohort study, *Am J Sports Med* 34:1581–1585, 2006.
52. Teitz CC, Hermanson B, Kronmal RA, et al: Evaluation of the use of braces to prevent injury to the knee in collegiate football players, *J Bone Joint Surg Am* 69:2–9, 1987.
53. Thomas SS, Buckon CE, Jakobson-Huston SJ, et al: Stair locomotion in children with spastic hemiplegia: the impact of three different ankle foot orthosis (AFOs) configurations, *Gait Posture* 16:180–187, 2002.
54. Thomas SS, Buckon CE, Jakobson-Huston SJ, et al: Comparison of three ankle-foot orthosis configurations for children with spastic hemiplegia, *Dev Med Child Neurol* 43:371–378, 2001.
55. Varghese G: Crutches, canes, and walkers. In Redford JB, editor: *Orthotics etcetera*, ed 2, Baltimore, 1980, Williams & Wilkins, pp 453–463.
56. Von Werssowetz OF: Basic principles of lower extremity bracing, *Orthot Prosthet Appl J* 41:323–350, 1962.
57. Waters RL, Miller L: A physiologic rationale for orthotic prescription in paraplegia, *Clin Prosthet Orthot* 11:66–73, 1987.
58. Wenger DR, Mauldin D, Morgan D, et al: Foot growth rate in children age one to six years, *Foot Ankle* 3:207–210, 1983.
59. Wenger DR, Mauldin D, Speck G, et al: Corrective shoes and inserts as treatment for flexible flatfoot in infants and children, *J Bone Joint Surg Am* 71:800–810, 1989.
60. Winchester PK, Carollo JJ, Parekh RN, et al: A comparison of paraplegic gait performance using two types of reciprocating gait orthoses, *Prosthet Orthot Int* 17:101–106, 1993.
61. Woodburn J, Barker S, Helliwell PS: A randomized control trial of foot orthoses in rheumatoid arthritis, *J Rheumatol* 29:1377–1383, 2002.
62. Wright RW, Fetzer GB: Bracing after ACL reconstruction: a systematic review, *Clin Orthop Relat Res* 455:162–168, 2007.
63. Zamosky I, Redford JB: Shoes and their modifications. In Redford JB, editor: *Orthotics etcetera*, ed 2, Baltimore, 1980, Williams & Wilkins, pp 388–452.

CHAPTER 13

SPINAL ORTHOSES

John W. Norbury, Edward Tilley, Daniel P. Moore

History of Spinal Orthotic Management

The first evidence of the use of spinal orthoses can be traced back to Galen (c. 131-201 AD). Primitive orthotic devices were made of items that were readily available during this period (Figure 13-1). These items included leather, whalebone, and tree bark. The word *orthosis* is Greek and means "to make straight."[3] Ambroise Paré (1510-1590) wrote about bracing and spinal supports, and Nicolas Andry (1658-1742) coined the term *orthopaedia*, pertaining to the straightening of children.[5] Unstable areas, such as fractures, were often held in a corrected position with an orthosis for healing to occur. Orthopaedia was the predecessor to the field of orthotics.[2]

In the past there were no organized training programs in the fabrication and application of orthoses, and an orthotist began as an apprentice, much like the village blacksmith. The training process for orthotists is now well defined and rigorous, with a certification process in the United States. Orthotists are now required to have extensive knowledge of pathologic conditions and the proper fabrication and use of orthotic devices. Technology has revamped the field of orthotics, with new stronger and lighter materials. Although materials available for orthotic construction have changed, the types of pathologic conditions treated have remained virtually constant for years.

The primary goal of modern orthoses is to aid a weakened muscle group or correct a deformed body part. The orthosis can protect a body part to prevent further injury, or can correct the position (immediate term or long term) of the body part. The same approach is true for spinal orthoses. The clinician's priority should be to determine which spinal motion to control. Good clinical outcomes can be maximized through the proper selection, use, and application of the orthosis. (See Chapters 11 and 12 for further information on orthoses.)

Terminology

Terminology is currently often misused in the field of orthotics. Definitions of some terms commonly used in the field are listed as follows:

- *Orthosis:* A singular device used to aid or align a weakened body part.
- *Orthoses:* Two or more devices used to aid or align a weakened body part(s).
- *Orthotics:* The field of study of orthoses and their management.
- *Orthotic:* An adjective used to describe a device (e.g., an orthotic knee immobilizer); this term is improperly used as a noun (e.g., "the patient was fitted with a foot orthotic").
- *Orthotist:* A person trained in the proper fit and fabrication of orthoses.
- *Certified orthotist (e.g., American Board for Certification in Prosthetics and Orthotics):* For a person to become a certified orthotist, extensive training in the proper fit and fabrication of orthoses is required. After the education and residency is completed, a national examination for certification can be taken in the United States, supplied by the American Board for Certification in Prosthetics and Orthotics.

Acronyms are frequently used to describe orthoses. They are named for the parts of the body where they are located and have some influence on the motion in that body region. Some examples of spinal orthoses are as follows:

- *CO:* Cervical orthosis
- *CTO:* Cervicothoracic orthosis
- *CTLSO:* Cervicothoracolumbosacral orthosis
- *TLSO:* Thoracolumbosacral orthosis
- *LSO:* Lumbosacral orthosis
- *SO:* Sacral orthosis

Prefabricated or Custom Orthoses

The availability of prefabricated orthoses today presents the rehabilitation team with a variety of choices and some challenges. Many of the prefabricated orthoses come in various sizes and can be fitted to patients often with little or no adjustment. Although this can be a benefit to the patient and the team in terms of time, care should be taken to ensure that the design and function of these orthoses are appropriate for the patient's condition and not used purely for convenience. Custom orthoses, in most cases, provide a more comfortable fit with a higher degree of control, and can be designed to accommodate a patient's unique body shape or deformities. Recognition of the time needed to fabricate the orthosis, the experience of the fabricator, the patient's specific condition, and the expectations of the patient are all factors that should be considered when ordering a custom orthosis.

Orthotic Prescription

The orthotic prescription allows for improved communication between clinicians, and it serves as a justification of the funding of the orthosis. Insurer-requested justification for the orthosis is becoming more common as medical costs have increased. Insurer approval of the prescription is more likely if the orthosis clearly increases independence

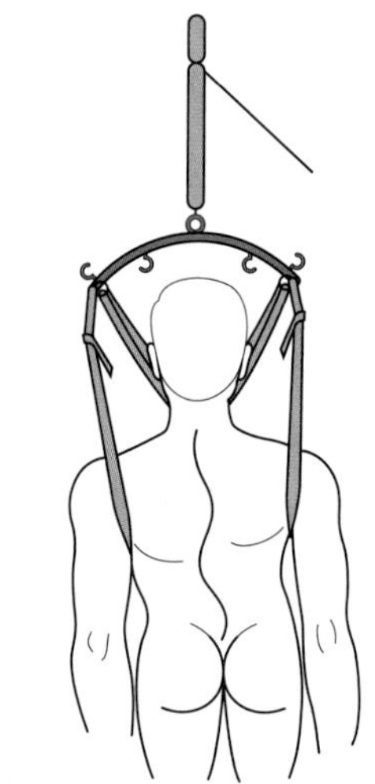

FIGURE 13-1 Traction device, 1889.

or helps prevent detrimental outcomes, such as a fall. The prescribing rehabilitation physician is responsible for the final order. The prescription should be accurate and descriptive but not so descriptive as to limit the orthotic team's independent ability to maximize functionality and patient acceptance.

Prescriptions should include the following items: patient identifiers, date, date the orthosis is needed, diagnosis, functional goal, orthosis description, and precautions. Prescriptions should include a justification, such as the correction of alignment, to decrease pain, or to improve function. Brand names and eponyms for the orthosis should be avoided. Established acronyms are acceptable (e.g., TLSO). Detailed descriptions of the orthosis, the joints involved, and the functional goals are important. Before the prescription is finalized, input from the patient, physician, therapist, and orthotist is needed. It is especially important for physicians to review the use, or lack of use, of past orthoses, because this will help guide their new prescription. If a patient discontinues the use of an orthosis prematurely, the reason why this occurred should be investigated by the provider before additional resources are expended. Knowledge of the patient's medical condition(s) is essential for a number of reasons. For example, the condition might be progressive, with further expected functional loss. By contrast, the condition might be expected to improve partially or completely in the future.

Spinal Anatomy

The vertebral column is composed of 33 vertebrae, including 7 cervical, 12 thoracic, 5 lumbar, 5 inferiorly fused vertebrae that form the sacrum, and 5 coccygeal. The spinal column not only bears the weight of the body but it also allows motion between body parts and serves to protect the spinal cord from injury. Before birth, there is a single C-shaped concave curve anteriorly. At birth, infants have only a small angle at the lumbosacral junction. As a child learns to stand and walk, lordotic curves develop in the cervical and lumbar regions (age 2 years). These changes can be attributed to the increase in weight-bearing and differences in the depth of the anterior and posterior regions of the vertebrae and disks.[30,35]

The cervical vertebrae are small and quadrangular, except for C1 and C2, which have some unique features. The cervical articular processes face upward and backward, or downward and forward. The orientation of the facet joints is important to note, as it relates to limitations of movement of the vertebral column. The thoracic vertebrae have heart-shaped bodies. The thoracic vertebrae are intermittent in size but increase in size caudally. This is related to the increased weight-bearing requirements. The dorsal length of the thoracic vertebrae is approximately 2 mm more than the ventral side, which could account for the thoracic curve. Their superior articular processes face backward and outward, and the inferior ones face forward and inward. The lumbar vertebrae have a large, kidney-shaped body. Their upper articular processes face medially and slightly posteriorly, and the lower ones face laterally and slightly anteriorly. The five sacral vertebrae are fused in a solid mass and do not contain intervertebral disks. The sacral bony structure acts as a keystone, and weight-bearing increases the forces that maintain the sacrum as an integral part of the spinal pelvic complex.

The intervertebral disk is composed of a nucleus pulposus, annulus fibrosus, and cartilaginous end plate. Disks make up approximately one third of the entire height of the vertebral column. The nucleus contains a matrix of collagen fibers, mucoprotein, and mucopolysaccharides. They have hydrophilic properties, with a very high water content (90%) that decreases with age.[29] The nucleus is centrally located in the cervical thoracic spine, but more posteriorly located in the lumbar spine. The annulus fibrosus has bands of fibrous laminated tissue in concentric directions, and the vertebral end plate is composed of hyaline cartilage.[12]

Normal Spine Biomechanics

Movement of the vertebral column occurs as a combination of small movements between vertebrae. The mobility occurs between the cartilaginous joints at the vertebral bodies and between the articular facets on the vertebral arches. Range of motion is determined by muscle location, tendon insertion, ligamentous limitations, and bony prominences. In the cervical region, axial rotation occurs at the specialized atlantoaxial joint. At the lower cervical levels, flexion, extension, and lateral flexion occur freely. In these areas, however, the articular processes, which face anteriorly or posteriorly, limit rotation. In the thoracic region, movement in all planes is possible, although to a lesser degree. In the lumbar region, flexion, extension, and lateral flexion occur, but rotation is limited because of the inwardly facing articular facets.[15] An understanding of the three-column concept of spine stability/instability is helpful to ensure that the proper orthosis is prescribed. The anterior column consists of the anterior longitudinal ligament, annulus fibrosus, and the anterior half of the vertebral body. The middle column consists of the posterior longitudinal ligament, annulus fibrosus, and the posterior half of the vertebral body. The posterior column consists of the interspinous and supraspinous ligaments, the facet

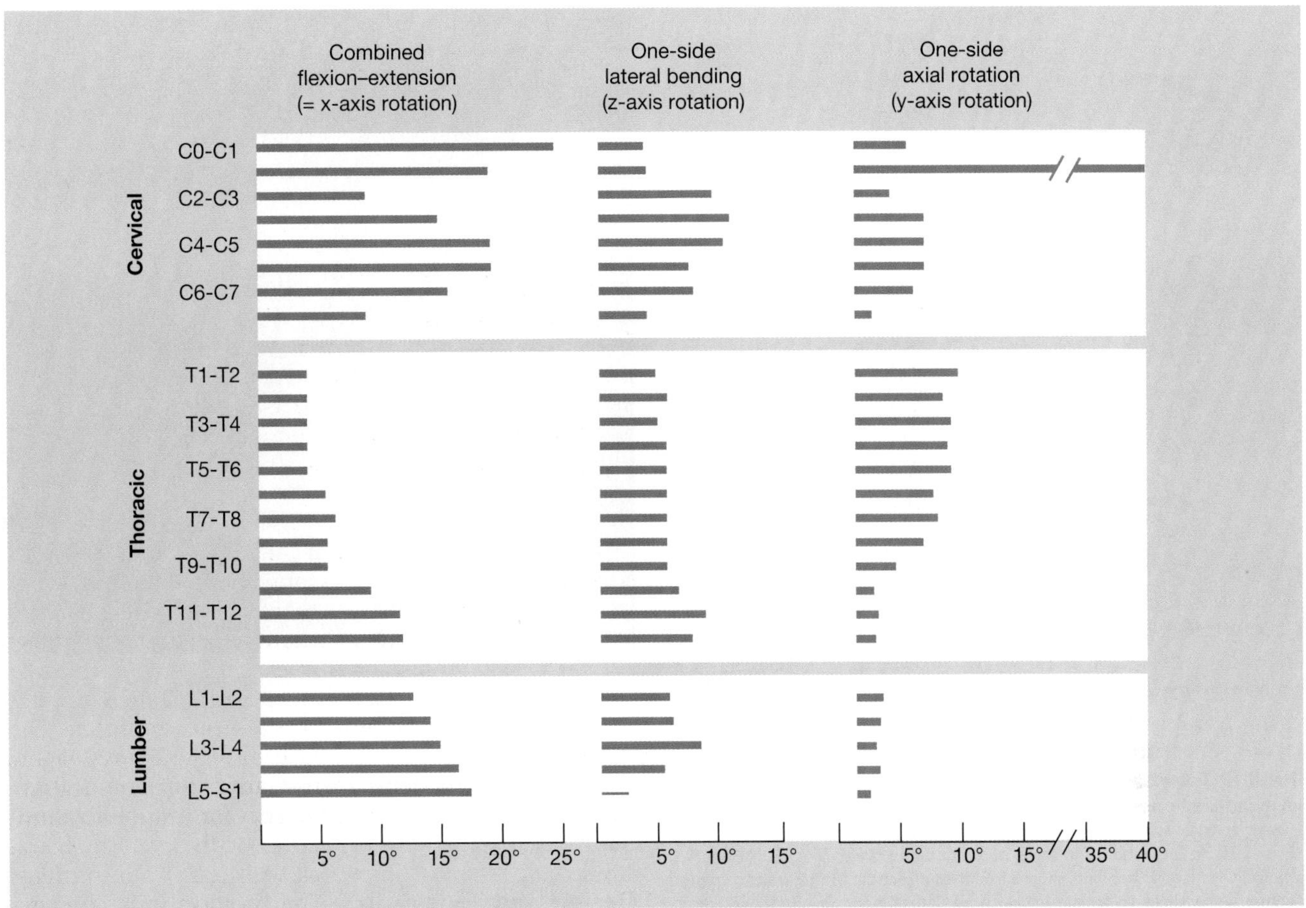

FIGURE 13-2 Representative values for range of motion of the cervical, thoracic, and lumbar spine as summarized from the literature. (Data from White AA, Panjabi MM: The lumbar spine. In White AA, Panjabi MM, editors: *Clinical biomechanics of the spine*, ed 2, Philadelphia, 1990, Lippincott.)

joints, lamina, pedicles, and the spinous processes. When the middle column and either the anterior or posterior column are compromised, the spine may be unstable.[8,9]

Spine motion can be classified with reference to the horizontal, frontal, and sagittal planes. Spinal motion can shift the center of gravity, which is normally located approximately 2 to 3 cm anterior to the S1 vertebral body. White and Panjabi[37] have provided a summary of the current literature, revealing motion in flexion and extension, laterally, and axially (Figure 13-2). In the cervical spine, extension occurs predominantly at the occipital C1 junction. Lateral bending occurs mainly at the C3-C4 and C4-C5 levels. Axial rotation occurs mostly at the C1-C2 levels. In the thoracic spine, flexion and extension occur primarily at the T11-T12 and T12-L1 levels. Lateral bending is fairly evenly distributed throughout the thoracic levels. Axial rotation occurs mostly at the T1-T2 level, with a gradual decrease toward the lumbar spine. The thoracic spine is the least mobile because of the restrictive nature of the rib cage. In the lumbar spinal segment, movement in the sagittal plane occurs more at the distal segment, with lateral bending predominantly at the L3-L4 level. There is insignificant axial rotation in the lumbar spinal segment.

Knowledge of the normal spinal range of motion helps in understanding how the various cervical orthoses can limit that range (Table 13-1). Soft collars provide very little restriction in any plane. The Philadelphia-type collar mostly limits flexion and extension. The four-poster brace has better restriction, especially with flexion-extension and rotation. The halo brace and Minerva body jacket have the most restriction in all planes of motion.

Table 13-1 Normal Cervical Motion from Occiput to First Thoracic Vertebra and the Effects of Cervical Orthoses

	Mean of Normal Motion (%)		
Orthosis	**Flexion or Extension**	**Lateral Bending**	**Rotation**
Normal*	100.0	100.0	100.0
Soft collar*	74.2	92.3	82.6
Philadelphia collar	28.9	66.4	43.7
Sternal occipital mandibular immobilizer orthosis	27.7	65.6	33.6
Four-poster brace	20.6	45.9	27.1
Yale cervicothoracic brace	12.8	50.5	18.2
Halo device*	4.0	4.0	1.0
Halo device†	11.7	8.4	2.4
Minerva body jacket‡	14.0	15.5	0

*Data from Johnson et al.[17]
†Data from Lysell.[22]
‡Data from Maiman et al.[23]

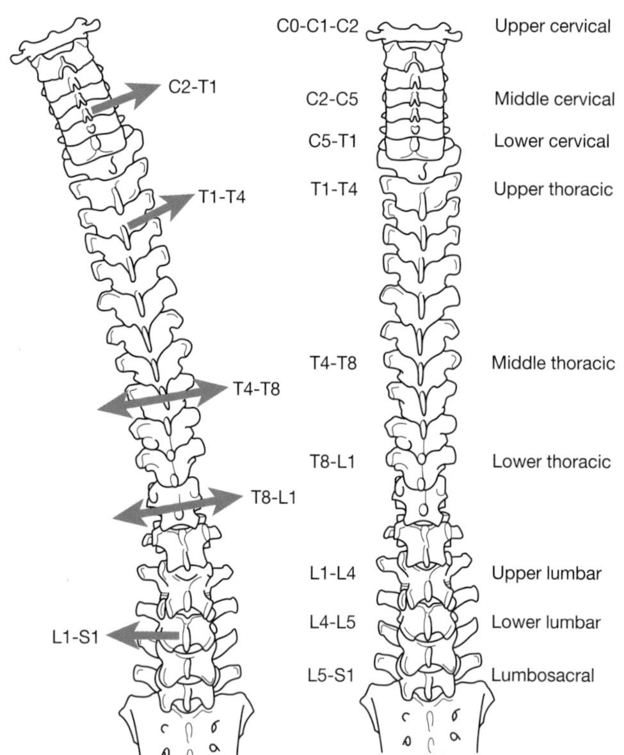

FIGURE 13-3 Regional coupling patterns. Summary of the coupling of lateral bending and axial rotation in various subdivisions of the spine. In the middle and lower cervical spine, as well as the upper thoracic spine, the same coupling pattern exists. In the middle and lower thoracic spine, the axial rotation, which is coupled with lateral bending, can be in either direction. In the lumbar spine, the spinous processes go to the left with left lateral bending. (Redrawn from White AA, Panjabi MM: The lumbar spine. In White AA, Panjabi MM, editors: *Clinical biomechanics of the spine*, ed 2, Philadelphia, 1990, Lippincott.)

An interesting phenomenon related to movement in the spine occurs during motion. If the movement along one axis is consistently associated with movement around another axis, *coupling* is occurring. For example, if a patient performs left *lateral movement* (frontal plane) motion, the middle and lower cervical and upper thoracic spine rotate to the left in the *axial* plane (Figure 13-3). This causes the spinous processes (posterior side of the body) to move to the *right*. In the lower thoracic spinal segment, left lateral movement in the frontal plane can cause rotation in the axial plane, with the spinal processes moving in either direction. The lumbar area has a contradictory movement pattern when compared with the cervical spine. With left lateral bending of the lumbar spine, the spinous processes move to the *left*. A three-dimensional perspective is important to maintain during examination. Patients with scoliosis and patients who undergo radiologic testing would benefit from an evaluation for the normal coupling patterns noted.

Description of Orthoses

Head Cervicothoracic Orthoses

Type: Halo Orthosis

Biomechanics. The halo orthosis (Figure 13-4) provides flexion, extension, and rotational control of the cervical region. Pressure systems are used for control of motion, as well as to provide slight distraction for immobilization of the cervical spine.

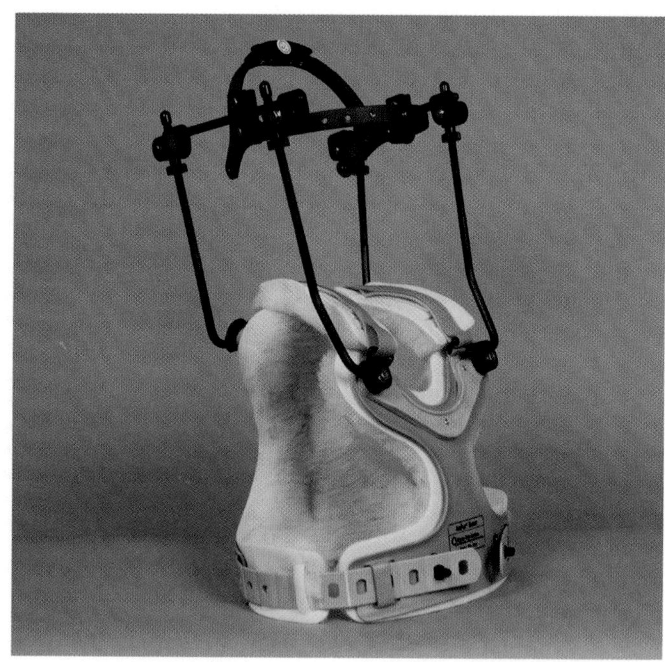

FIGURE 13-4 Halo orthosis.

Design and Fabrication. The halo orthosis consists of prefabricated components, such as a halo ring, pins, uprights (or superstructure), and vest. The halo ring is fixed to the outer table of the skull bones with generally four or more metal pins. On the typical adult patient, the pins are optimally placed with the patient under local anesthesia, less than 1 inch above the lateral third of each eyebrow (to avoid sinuses) and less than 1 inch above and just posterior to the top of each ear. Upright bars or superstructure connects the ring to a rigid plastic thoracic vest, which is lined with lamb's wool.

The halo is adjustable for flexion, extension, anterior and posterior translation, rotation, and distraction. The vest wraps around the thoracic region of the spine and is fastened laterally, usually by buckles. The design is used to effectively immobilize the cervical spine.

This orthosis provides maximum restriction in motion of all the cervical orthoses. It is the most stable orthosis, especially in the superior cervical spine segment. A halo is used for approximately 3 months (10 to 12 weeks) to ensure healing of a fracture or of a spinal fusion. Usually, a cervical collar is indicated after the halo is removed because the muscles and ligaments supporting the head become weak after disuse. All pins on the halo ring should be checked to ensure tightness 24 to 48 hours after application, and retorqued if necessary.

Indications. The halo is generally used for unstable cervical fractures or postoperative management.

Contraindications. This orthosis is not indicated for stable fractures or when less invasive management could

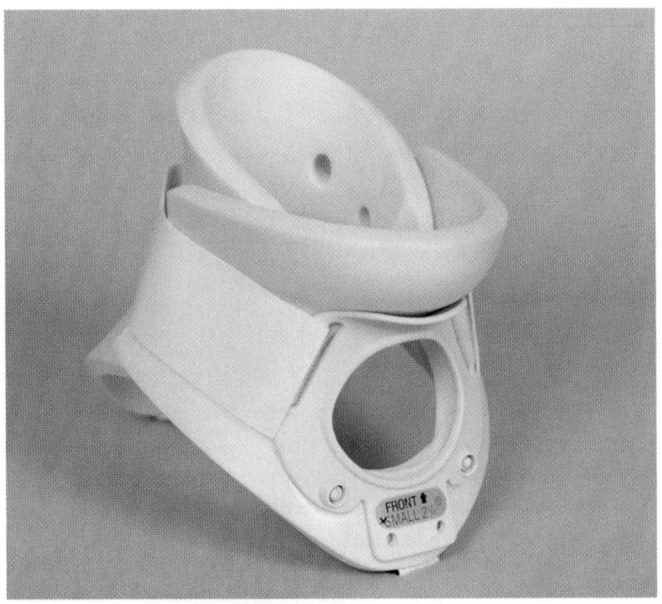

FIGURE 13-5 Philadelphia orthosis.

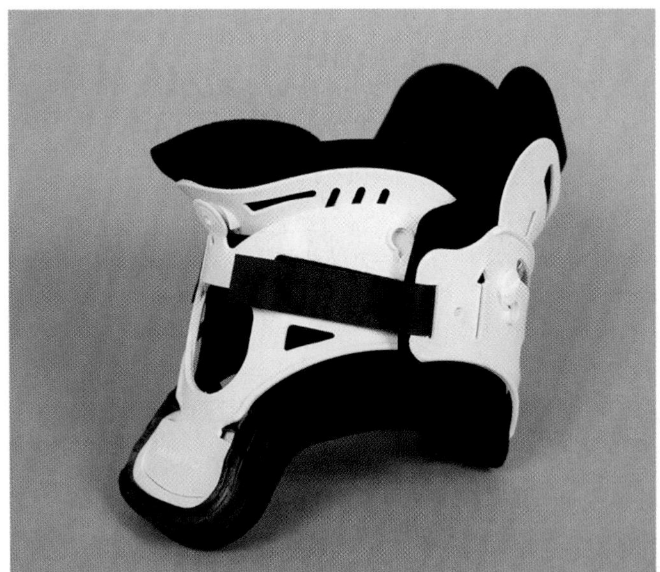

FIGURE 13-6 Miami J orthosis.

be used. Patients with an extremely soft skull might not tolerate the pin placement.

Special Considerations. Skull density determines halo pin placement as well as the number of halo pins to be used. Although four pins are used on average, more can be necessary in soft skulls (e.g., osteoporotic, fractured, or in an infant) to distribute the force over a broader area of the skull. The use of halo devices in older patients has become more controversial because the halo orthosis has been associated with respiratory compromise, aspiration, and an 8% mortality in this population.[33]

Cervical Orthoses

Type: Philadelphia, Miami J, and Aspen Collar

Biomechanics. The Philadelphia (Figure 13-5), Miami J (Figure 13-6), and Aspen cervical orthoses provide some control of flexion, extension, and lateral bending, and minimal rotational control of the cervical region. Pressure systems are used for control of motion, as well as to provide slight distraction for immobilization of the cervical spine. Circumferential pressure is also intended to provide warmth and as a kinesthetic reminder for the patient.

Design and Fabrication. These orthoses are prefabricated, consisting of one or two pieces that are usually attached with Velcro straps. Two-piece designs have an anterior and posterior section. The anterior section supports the mandible and rests on the superior edge of the sternum. The posterior aspect of the collar supports the head at the occipital level.

Indications. They are used primarily for cervical sprains, strains, or stable fractures. They can also be used for protection and for limited mobility after surgery to allow healing.

Contraindications. In cadaver models, these orthoses have been found to be insufficient for immobilizing the unstable spine.[16] The cervical orthoses tend to lose effectiveness at higher and lower cervical levels (occiput-C2 and C6-C7) and thus a more restrictive device may be appropriate in this population.[1]

Type: Soft Cervical Collar

This orthosis is usually used as a kinesthetic reminder for patients to limit their neck motion. Because it is not stabilized against the upper trunk or occiput, it does not provide any mechanical restriction of the head motion. It can provide some warmth and comfort for patients with muscle strain. The collar is usually made from a block of foam rubber material that may be contoured around the chin. The foam is covered with a stockinette material, and Velcro is added to the ends to provide closure.

Cervicothoracic Orthoses

Type: Sternal Occipital Mandibular Immobilizer

Biomechanics. The sternal occipital mandibular immobilizer (SOMI; Figure 13-7) provides control of flexion, extension, lateral bending, and rotation of the cervical spine. Pressure systems are used for control of motion, as well as to provide slight distraction for immobilization of the spine. A benefit of the SOMI orthosis is that it can be donned while the patient is in the supine position. The SOMI is a good choice for patients who are restricted to bed because there are no posterior rods to interfere with the comfort of the patient. A headband can be added so that the chin piece can be removed. This maintains stability but improves accessibility for daily hygiene and eating.

Design and Fabrication. The SOMI is prefabricated, consisting of a cervical portion with removable chin piece and bars that curve over the shoulders. Also used are posts that fixate the cervical portion to the sternal portion of the orthosis. The anterior section supports the mandible and rests on the superior edge of the sternum, with the inferior anterior edge terminating at the level of the xiphoid. The

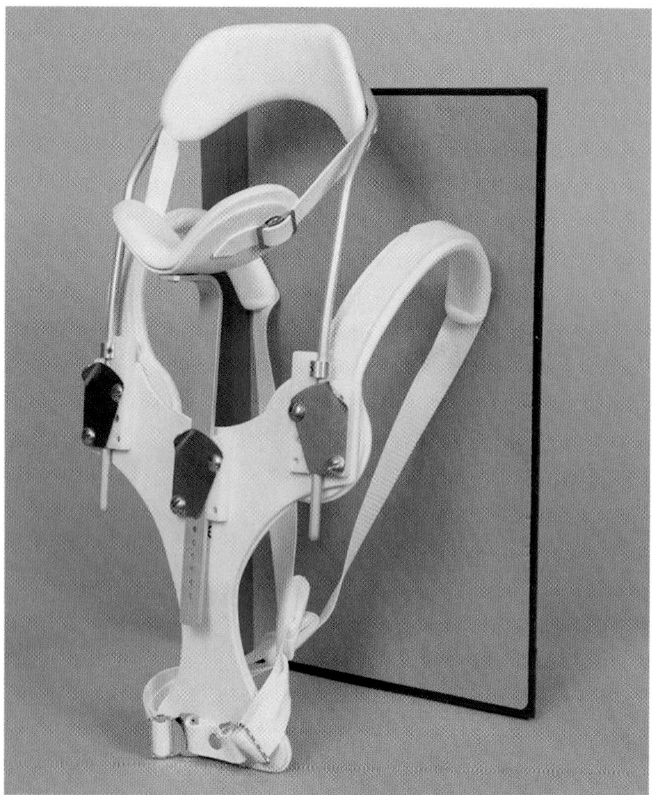

FIGURE 13-7 Sternal occipital mandibular immobilizer.

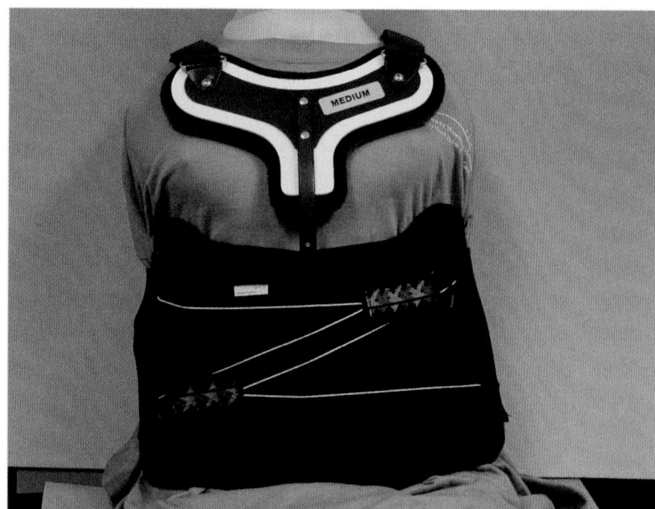

FIGURE 13-8 Thoracolumbosacral orthosis (prefabricated).

posterior aspect of the orthosis supports the head at the occipital level.

Indications. The SOMI is used primarily for cervical sprains, strains, or stable fractures with intact ligaments. It can also be used for protection and for limited mobility during the healing process in the postoperative patient.

Contraindications. This orthosis is not indicated for unstable fractures with ligament instability.

Four-Poster

The four-poster is a rigid cervical orthosis with anterior and posterior sections consisting of pads that lie on the chest and are connected by leather straps. The struts on the anterior and posterior sections are adjustable in height. Straps are used to connect the occipital and mandibular support pieces by way of the over-the-shoulder method.

Also note that some cervical orthoses can also incorporate a sternal extension addition, which converts them from a cervical orthosis to a cervicothoracic orthosis (e.g., Aspen, Philadelphia, Miami J).

Cervicothoracolumbosacral Orthoses

Type: Milwaukee Orthosis

Biomechanics. The Milwaukee orthosis is used for scoliosis management (scoliosis is discussed later in this chapter). The Milwaukee provides control of flexion, extension, and lateral bending of the cervical, thoracic, and lumbar spine. It also provides some rotational control of the thoracic and lumbar spine. Pressure systems are used for control of motion, as well as to provide correction for the spine. The Milwaukee is a good choice for patients who need correction in the higher thoracic region of the spine.

Design and Fabrication. The Milwaukee is custom made, consisting of a cervical portion with the option of a removable cervical ring. Also used is the thoracolumbar section of the orthosis in which the correction of the lower thoracic and lumbar spines is achieved.

Indications. The Milwaukee brace is used primarily for scoliotic management of the high thoracic curves along with thoracic and lumbar curves of the spine.

Contraindications. This orthosis is not indicated for lower thoracic and lumbar curves only. With lower thoracic and lumbar curves, a thoracolumbar orthosis could be used without the use of the cervical component.

Thoracolumbosacral Orthoses

Type: Thoracolumbosacral Orthosis (Prefabricated)

Biomechanics. The thoracolumbosacral orthosis (TLSO; prefabricated) (Figure 13-8) provides control of flexion, extension, lateral bending, and rotation using three-point pressure systems and circumferential compression.

Design and Fabrication. This orthosis can be designed in modular forms, with anterior and posterior sections connected by padded lateral panels and fastened with Velcro straps or pulley systems. Many of these are covered in breathable fabric and have a variety of different shapes and options, such as sternal pads or shoulder straps.

Indications. This orthosis can be used for treatment of traumatic or pathologic spinal fractures in the mid to lower thoracic region or lumbar region.

Contraindications. These include a body habitus that is obese with a pendulous abdomen, excessive lordosis, or a need for increased lateral stability.

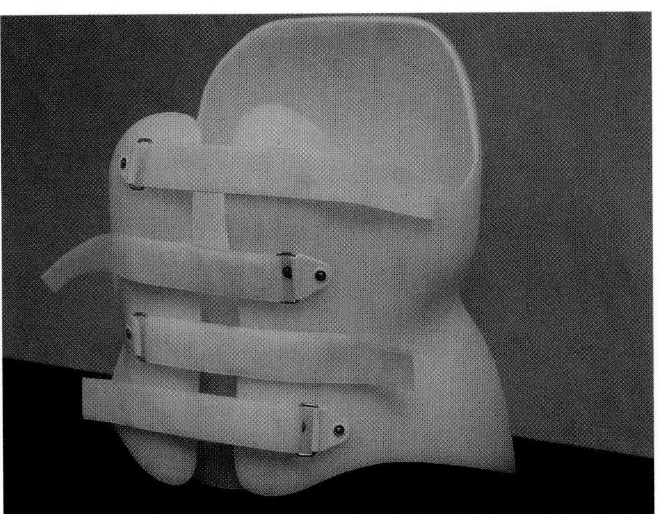

FIGURE 13-9 Thoracolumbosacral orthosis (custom-fabricated body jacket).

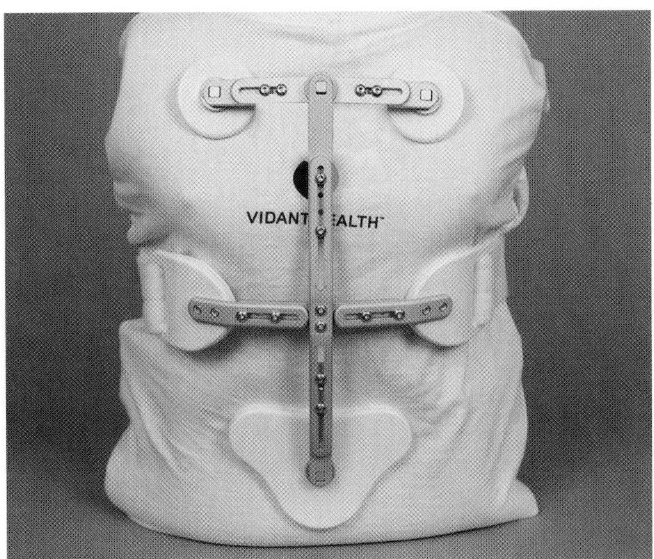

FIGURE 13-10 Cruciform anterior spinal hyperextension thoracolumbosacral orthosis.

Special Considerations. Cost is reduced in some models because of the mass production of prefabricated modules. The use of breathable material can increase compliance with wearing.

Type: Thoracolumbosacral Orthosis (Custom-Fabricated Body Jacket)

Biomechanics. The body jacket (Figure 13-9) provides control of flexion, extension, lateral bending, and rotation. It uses three-point pressure systems and circumferential compression.

Design and Fabrication. It is molded to fit the patient and designed for patient needs. Anterior trim lines are usually located inferior to the sternal notch and superior to the pubic symphysis. The posterior trim lines have a superior border at the spine of the scapula and an inferior border at the level of the coccyx. These trim lines are adjusted during fitting to allow patients to sit comfortably and to use their arms as much as possible without compromising the function of the orthosis.

Indications. This orthosis can be used for treatment of traumatic or pathologic spinal fractures in the mid to lower thoracic region or lumbar region. Most are used for postsurgical management of fractures, such as compression, chance, or burst. The brace is also used after surgical correction spondylolisthesis, scoliosis, spinal stenosis, herniated disks, and disk infections.

Contraindications. These include application of the orthosis over a chest tube, colostomy, or large dressings.

Special Considerations. Care must be taken to ensure that contact is maximized to decrease the pressure in any one area. Changes in the trim line must be made in small increments to prevent loss of control in terms of both leverage and tissue control. Ventilating holes are often made to improve airflow. Other factors to be considered when making the design include patients who might attempt to remove the orthosis when out of bed. The orthosis can be made with a posterior opening to reduce the risk.

Type: Cruciform Anterior Spinal Hyperextension Thoracolumbosacral Orthosis

Biomechanics. The cruciform anterior spinal hyperextension (CASH) TLSO (Figure 13-10) provides flexion control for the lower thoracic and lumbar regions. It accomplishes this by way of a three-point pressure system. The system consists of posteriorly directed forces through a sternal and suprapubic pad and an anteriorly directed force applied through a thoracolumbar pad attached to a strap that extends to the horizontal anterior bar.

Design and Fabrication. The CASH is prefabricated, consisting of an anterior frame in the form of a cross, from which pads are attached laterally on a horizontal bar and at the sternal and suprapubic areas. A thoracolumbar pad is attached to a strap that extends to the lateral sections of the horizontal bar and adjusts the tension on the body. When properly fitted, the sternal pad is half an inch below the sternal notch, and the suprapubic pad is half an inch above the symphysis pubis.

Indications. This orthosis is used primarily for the treatment of mild compression fracture of the lower thoracic and thoracolumbar regions.

Contraindications. The CASH is not indicated for unstable fractures or burst fractures.

Special Considerations. Excessive pressure on the sternum can result in poor compliance with wearing schedule. Subclavicular pads may be added to help distribute this pressure.

Type: Jewett Hyperextension Thoracolumbosacral Orthosis

Biomechanics. The Jewett hyperextension TLSO (Figure 13-11) provides flexion control for the lower thoracic and

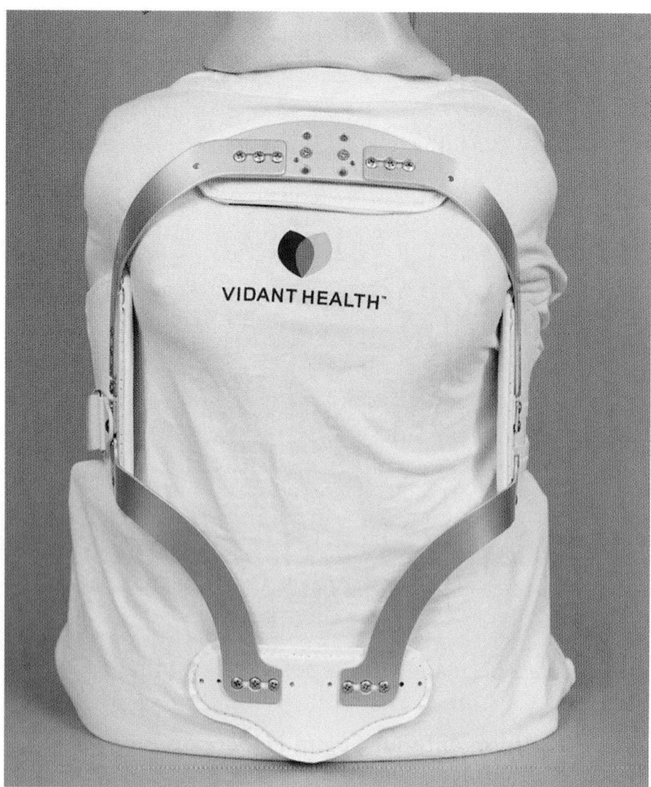

FIGURE 13-11 Jewett hyperextension thoracolumbosacral orthosis.

lumbar regions. This is done with a three-point pressure system consisting of posteriorly directed forces through a sternal and suprapubic pad and an anteriorly directed force applied through a thoracolumbar pad attached to a strap that extends to the lateral uprights.

Design and Fabrication. It is prefabricated, consisting of an anterior and lateral frame to which pads are attached laterally on and at the sternal and suprapubic areas. A thoracolumbar pad is attached to a strap that extends to the lateral uprights and adjusts the tension on the body. When properly fitted, the sternal pad is half an inch below the sternal notch, and the suprapubic pad is half an inch above the symphysis pubis.

Indications. The Jewett hyperextension TLSO is used primarily for the treatment of mild compression fractures of the lower thoracic and thoracolumbar regions. The Jewett has more lateral support than the CASH.

Contraindications. It is not indicated for unstable fractures or burst fractures.

Special Considerations. Excessive pressure on the sternum might result in poor compliance with wearing schedule. Subclavicular pads can be added to help distribute this pressure.

Type: Taylor and Knight-Taylor

Biomechanics. The Taylor and Knight-Taylor orthoses provide control of flexion, extension, and a minimal amount of axial rotation by means of the three-point pressure systems for each direction of motion. For example, flexion is controlled by the posteriorly directed forces applied through the axillary straps and the abdominal apron and an anteriorly directed force through the paraspinal uprights.

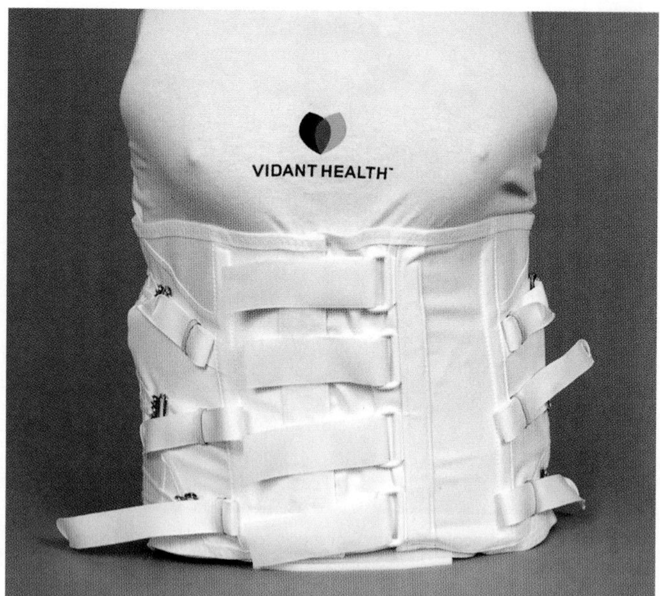

FIGURE 13-12 Lumbosacral corset.

Design and Fabrication. The design of the Taylor consists of a posterior pelvic band extending past the midsagittal plane and across the sacral area. Two paraspinal uprights extend to the spine of the scapula. An apron front extends from the xiphoid to just above the pubic area. There are straps extending from the top of the posterior uprights around the posterior axillary to the scapular bar and forward to the apron. Other straps extend from the paraspinal uprights to the apron.

The Knight-Taylor has an additional thoracic band that extends from the uprights just below the inferior angle of the scapula to the midsagittal plane and a lateral upright on each side that connects the pelvic band and the thoracic band. These bands provide additional lateral support and motion control to the trunk.

Indications. These orthoses have been used for years for postsurgical support of traumatic fractures, spondylolisthesis, scoliosis, spinal stenosis, herniated disks, and disk infections. However, clinicians typically now prefer the custom-molded TLSO body jackets because better control of position is obtained.

Contraindications. These are unstable fractures that require maximum stabilization.

Special Considerations. Pressure per square inch is higher because of the width of the bands and uprights.

Lumbosacral Orthoses

Type: Lumbosacral Corset

Biomechanics. The lumbosacral corset (Figure 13-12) provides anterior and lateral trunk containment, and assists in the elevation of intraabdominal pressure.

Restriction of flexion and extension can be achieved with the addition of steel stays posteriorly.

Design and Fabrication. This orthosis is usually made from cloth that wraps around the torso and hips. Adjustments are done with laces on the sides, back, or front. Closure can be with hook and loop (Velcro) or hook and eye fasteners or snaps. Many different styles are available in prefabricated sizes, usually in 2-inch increments, and are designed to fit the body circumference at the level of the hips. The orthosis can be adjusted for body type and proper fit by taking tucks in the cloth, as needed. Steel stays must be contoured to the body shape to encourage a reduction of lordosis or to accommodate a deformity. Custom corsets can be fabricated based on careful measurements of the individual patient.

Indications. This orthosis is the most frequently prescribed support for patients with low back pain.[31] It has been used for herniated disks and lumbar muscle strain and for the control of gross trunk motion for pain control after single-column compression fractures with one-third or less anterior height loss.[38]

Contraindications. The orthosis should not be used for unstable fractures and for fractures or conditions above the lower lumbar region.

Special Considerations. Long-term use of a lumbosacral corset can cause an increase in motion in the segments above or below the area controlled by the orthosis.[28] Muscle atrophy can also potentially occur after long-term use, causing an increased risk of reinjury. Patients can also have a psychological dependence on the support after injury.[21]

Type: Lumbosacral Chairback Orthoses

Biomechanics. This brace (Figure 13-13) provides limitation of flexion, extension, and lateral flexion. It also provides elevation of intraabdominal pressure.

Design and Fabrication. This orthosis has a pelvic band that lies posteriorly and extends laterally to just anterior to the midsagittal line. Laterally, the ends fall midway between the iliac crest and the greater trochanter. The superior edge of the thoracic band is at the level of T9-T10 or just distal to the inferior angle of the scapulae. The pelvic and thoracic bands are connected by two paraspinal uprights posteriorly and a lateral upright on each side at the midsagittal line. Orthoses can be fabricated from a traditional aluminum frame covered in leather or thermoplastic material molded into the same shape. Straps are connected in a variety of ways to the frame, providing attachment to the anterior apron front.

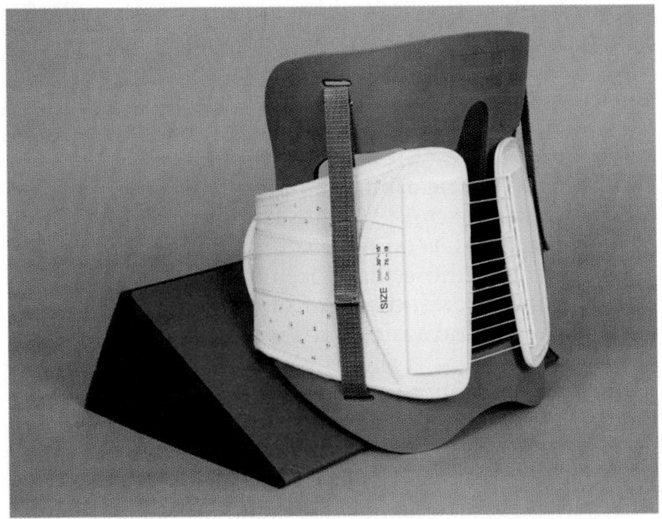

FIGURE 13-13 Lumbosacral orthosis chairback brace.

Indications. This brace is often used for lower lumbar pathologic conditions, including degenerative disk disease, herniated disk, spondylolisthesis, and mechanical low back pain, and for postsurgical supports for lumbar laminectomies, fusions, or diskectomies.[27]

Contraindications. These are unstable fractures or conditions in the upper lumbar or thoracic area.

Special Considerations. Adequate clearance of the paraspinal uprights is required to allow for some reduction of lumbar lordosis when the anterior apron is tightened and while the patient is sitting. Clearance on the lateral uprights over the iliac crests is also an area to be monitored.

Sacroiliac Orthoses

Type: Sacroiliac Orthosis or Sacral Orthosis

Biomechanics. The sacroiliac orthosis provides anterior and lateral trunk containment and assists in the restriction of some pelvic flexion and extension. It also aids in compression of the pelvis.

Design and Fabrication. This orthosis is usually made from cloth that wraps around the pelvis and hips. Some models include laces on the side by which adjustments can be made, whereas others use straps for adjusting. Closure can be with hook and loop (Velcro) or hook and eye fasteners or snaps. Many different styles are available in prefabricated sizes, usually in 2-inch increments, and are designed to fit the circumference of the body at the level of the hips. The orthosis can be adjusted for body type and proper fit by taking tucks in the cloth, as needed. Custom orthoses can be fabricated based on careful measurements of the individual patient.

Indications. This orthosis is the most frequently prescribed as a support for patients with pelvic fractures or symphysis pubis fractures or strains. It is useful to control motion and for pain control.

Contraindications. The orthosis should not be used for unstable fractures and for fractures or conditions in the lumbar region.

Scoliosis

Idiopathic (infantile, juvenile, adolescent), congenital, and neuromuscular scolioses have different etiologies, treatment approaches, and outcomes. Idiopathic scoliosis is the most common form.[32] Idiopathic infantile scoliosis is typically described from birth to 3 years of age, juvenile is from 4 years until the onset of puberty, and the adolescent type from puberty to closure of the facets.

With idiopathic scoliosis the evaluation should reveal no anomalous vertebrae, spinal tumors, or other neurologic abnormalities. Most cases remain stable for a long period and progress late in life when osteoporosis and degenerative spinal conditions normally have their onset. Progressive curves need to be treated, but there is not adequate evidence that scoliosis can be treated by electrical stimulation, nutritional supplementation, exercise, or chiropractic treatment. There is strong evidence to indicate that an orthosis can slow the progression of idiopathic scoliosis, and therefore it is the nonoperative treatment of choice.[36]

Juvenile idiopathic scoliosis is more likely to be associated with adult cor pulmonale and death. Treatment should begin when curves reach approximately 25 degrees. Because thoracic curves predominate, the Milwaukee brace might be more effective than the TLSO. The Milwaukee (CTLSO) brace has a pelvic section with close contact with the iliac crest and lumbar spine. Three uprights (one anterior and two posterior) typically connect to a neck ring, throat mold, and occipital pad. The Boston brace is a TLSO that uses symmetrical standardized modules, eliminating the need for casting. It extends from below the breast to the beginning of the pelvic area and below the scapulae posteriorly. It maintains flexion of the lumbar area by increasing pressure on the abdomen and is a popular TLSO brace.

Adolescent idiopathic scoliosis is the most common type for which an orthosis is indicated, usually for curves between 25 degrees and 45 degrees. Curves with an apex at T9 or lower can be managed with a TLSO. Curves with a higher apex require a Milwaukee brace. Single lumbar curves are treated with a lumbosacral orthosis.[11]

Congenital scoliosis is secondary to a vertebral anomaly that is present at birth. Failure of part of the vertebrae to form (e.g., hemivertebrae) or failure of the vertebrae to properly segment (block vertebrae), or a combination of both, can occur. Congenital scoliosis is associated with abnormal development in the embryo, and associated developmental abnormalities in other organ systems should be considered, especially in the renal, urinary, and cardiac systems.[25]

Neuromuscular diseases are also associated with scoliosis. The prevalence of scoliosis in this population is much higher than with idiopathic scoliosis, from 25% to 100%. In pediatric patients with a spinal cord injury, almost 100% have scoliosis. In general, there is a significant chance of progression in the presence of severe neurologic disease. In adults, however, scoliosis curvatures tend to be relatively benign and of the C-type appearance and are less likely to progress to the extent that they cause clinical cardiopulmonary problems. Progression of the curve can occur in adulthood, which is typical for scoliosis in general. Spasticity or flaccidity can be present, depending on whether there is upper or lower motor neuron involvement. Multisystem involvement is more common in this group because these diseases are not isolated to the spinal column. Consideration should also be made for the presence of contractures, hip dislocations, sensory abnormalities, mental retardation, and pressure ulcers.[20]

Scoliosis can continue to progress despite the proper use of an orthosis, and in these cases appropriate surgical referrals should be made. An important factor to consider before surgery is the pulmonary function in a patient with neuromuscular disease. Before surgery is considered, the forced vital capacity and forced expiratory volume in 1 second should be at least 40% of that predicted for the patient's age. Fusions are delayed as long as possible in an attempt to achieve maximal spinal growth (>10 years of age). Declining pulmonary function, however, is a consideration for performing surgery earlier.[26]

Duval-Beaupere[10] followed the long-term progression of idiopathic scoliosis and noted that curve progression accelerated during growth spurts. He noted that the younger the child, the higher the risk of curve progression because of a greater amount of growth that remained. It has also been shown that the greater the curve, the more likely the curve would increase.[19] Curves measured from 5 degrees to 29 degrees and the curves from 20 degrees to 29 degrees progressed in almost 100% of the patients. Approximately 50% of the curves from 5 degrees to 19 degrees appeared to progress.

Curve progression has been explained with the Euler theory of elastic buckling of a slender column.[34] Axial compressive forces evidently cause a column to buckle. This is associated with height growth and weight gain, especially because of increased upper limb weight during growth spurts. An increase in height and weight commonly occur together and might synergistically promote curve progression. It has been noted by us and others that the condition of a child with a large curve is more likely to progress than that of a child with a small curve.

The timing for surgery in a child with scoliosis is controversial. A child who has a curve greater than 45 degrees, a child who is still growing, or a child who cannot or does not wear a brace is at a greater risk of curve progression and may be considered for surgery.

Type: Thoracolumbosacral Low-Profile Scoliosis Orthoses

Boston Brace, Miami Orthosis, Wilmington Brace

Biomechanics. The TLSO low-profile scoliosis orthoses (Figure 13-14) provide dynamic action using three principles (end-point control, transverse loading, and curve correction) to prevent curve progression and to stabilize the spine.

Design and Fabrication. The use of orthoses or other devices to halt the curve progression of structural scoliosis has been reported as far back as Hippocrates.[24] Many different types of orthoses have been described in the literature. The one that stands out as being the most successful is the Milwaukee orthosis, which is described earlier in the chapter.

The effective nonoperative treatment of idiopathic scoliosis with a low-profile TLSO has been demonstrated over the past 30 years. The most common of these orthoses is the Boston brace, introduced by Hall and Miller[14] in 1975.[4] This system is available in prefabricated modules that are

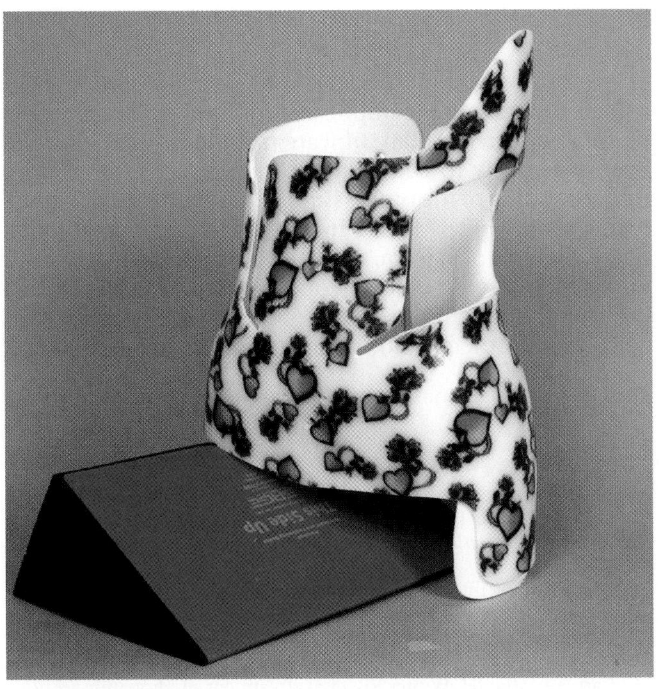

FIGURE 13-14 Thoracolumbosacral low-profile scoliosis orthosis.

available in 30 sizes and can be ordered by measurement; they are then custom-fit to the patient. Modules can be used to fit approximately 85% of patients. Six of these sizes will fit approximately 60% of patients requiring an orthosis.[13] The orthosis can also be custom-fabricated from a mold of the patient's body. Trim lines are established on the basis of the patient's curve; they are designed to provide pressure in specified areas to maximize corrective forces and at the same time be less visible under the patient's clothing.

Indications. This orthosis is indicated in patients with an immature skeleton and documented progression of a thoracic or thoracolumbar idiopathic scoliosis that measures 25 degrees to 35 degrees (measured by the Cobb method) and has an apex of T7 or lower.[6]

Contraindications. The orthosis is contraindicated in patients who have curves that measure more than 40 degrees and who are skeletally immature or who have curves in excess of 50 degrees after the end of growth. Both of these types of patients are typically candidates for surgery.[7]

Special Considerations. Idiopathic scoliosis occurs mostly in adolescent females. Treatment regimens, both nonoperative and operative, are major events for the patients and their families. To be successful, the treatment team must be sensitive, supportive, honest, and communicate accurate information to patients and their families.

The effectiveness of any orthotic system depends on compliance with the wearing schedule. Most patients should wear the orthosis 23 to 24 hours per day for it to be effective. Some physicians allow time out of the orthosis to participate in athletic activities or swimming and some special occasions, and this seems to improve acceptance and compliance.

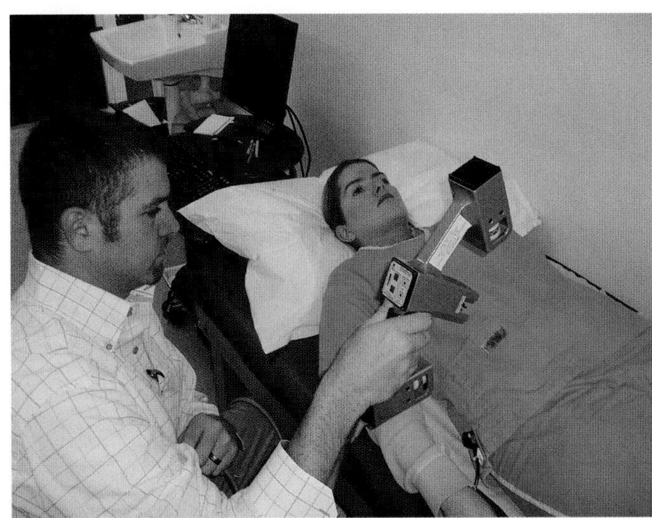

FIGURE 13-15 BioScanner handheld laser scanner system.

Emerging Technology

Computer-Aided Design and Computer-Aided Manufacturing

Technology is available to help the practitioner improve efficiency in design and fabrication, as well as reduce the invasiveness of orthotic measurement of the patients. The development of computer-aided design (CAD) and computer-aided manufacturing (CAM) has allowed the fabrication of orthoses today in less time than it took only a few years ago. The BioScanner BioSculptor is one of the CAD-CAM systems available (Figure 13-15). (BioScanner BioSculptor information is available online at www.biosculptor.com.) It combines CAD, laser scanning, three-dimensional imagery, and motion-tracking technology to design orthotic and prosthetic devices. This is an alternative to traditional casting methods. The body part involved is scanned with a handheld scanning wand, which uses a motion-tracking device embedded in the scanner. The wand is passed over the body part. A three-dimensional image of the body part is transmitted to the computer, and the software interprets the data. A miniature transmitter is placed on the body to accommodate for any movement. The BioScanner is able to image negative and positive models, allowing the clinician to use the clinical techniques required for each patient. With scan-through-glass technology that the company provides for use with its scanner, the clinician can position the body horizontally for a TLSO. The BioScanner automatically corrects the refraction. The precision of the BioScanner captures shapes to an accuracy of 0.178 mm. It provides the clinician with detailed and accurate three-dimensional measurements. Patients can be scanned for spinal jackets without movement from supine to prone positions. An option in the computer software allows one hemisphere to be scanned, and then the computer develops the other hemisphere to

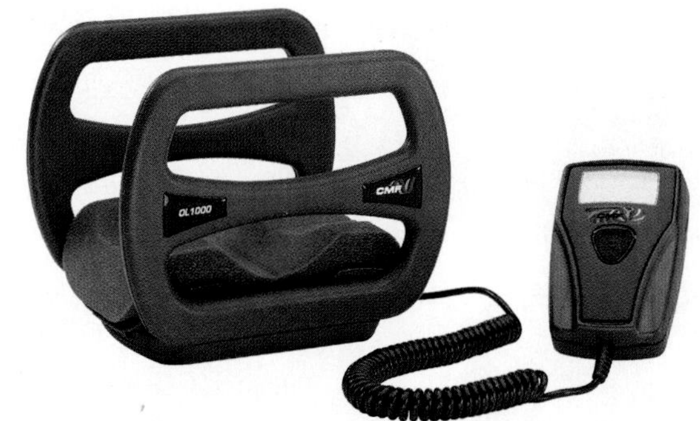

FIGURE 13-16 CMF SpinaLogic bone stimulator. (Courtesy DJO Global, Inc, Vista, Calif.)

form a complete image. The older plaster cast methods are becoming obsolete because of the following advantages of the scanning system: it is not messy, can be done quickly, minimizes pain for the patient, and is more accurate. Modifications to these scanned computerized models can then be made before fabrication of the device begins.

Accuracy of measurement gives detailed surface information often lost with a cast or mechanical digitizer. The patient's scan is maintained in the computer database, allowing for rapid refitting and medical justification of new devices by showing volumetric changes.

Bone Stimulation

The CMF SpinaLogic bone growth stimulator is a portable, battery-powered, microcontrolled, noninvasive bone growth stimulator indicated for adjunct electromagnetic treatment to primary lumbar spinal fusion surgery for one or two levels (Figure 13-16). (Information about the CMF SpinaLogic is available at the website of DJO Global, Inc: www.djortho.com.)

There are different bone stimulators on the market in use today. Some are used in conjunction with spinal orthoses and do not interfere with the control that the orthosis provides or the treatment protocol set by the physician. Some of the benefits of these bone stimulators are as follows: (1) they are lightweight, comfortable, and easy to use; (2) they can be used after an anterior or posterior approach in surgery; and (3) they are noninvasive.

This treatment has been shown to give a 21% point increase in healing over those who did not use the stimulator. It also helps the body's own healing process to begin working.

Three-Dimensional Clinical Ultrasound

Recent advances in three-dimensional clinical ultrasound have allowed estimation of the spinous process angle (SPA) in patients with adolescent idiopathic scoliosis. This in turn has been able to provide orthotists a fast and safe method to assess the SPA in real time and determine the optimal placement of pressure pads to maximize the effectiveness of the orthotic in correcting the spinal deformity.[18]

Summary

The proper prescription, construction, and fitting of a spinal orthosis are complicated processes. A complete, clear, and agreed plan of care should be constructed. Success is likely to be limited if there is no agreement or understanding of the process and goals. The typical orthotic team in the United States includes the patient, orthotist, rehabilitation physician, and therapist. Experienced and knowledgeable providers working in a team approach provide the maximum likelihood that the orthosis will contribute to the overall therapeutic goals for the patient.

REFERENCES

1. Agabegi SS, Asghar FA, Herkowitz HN: Spinal orthoses, *J Am Acad Orthop Surg* 18:657–667, 2010.
2. Andry N: *Orthopaedia [facsimile reproduction of the first edition in English, London, 1743]*, Philadelphia, 1961, Lippincott.
3. Anonymous: *Dorland's medical dictionary*, ed 24, Philadelphia, 1989, Saunders.
4. Boston Brace International, Available at: <www.bostonbrace.com>. Accessed January 2014.
5. Bunch WH, Keagy R: *Principles of orthotic treatment*, St Louis, 1975, Mosby.
6. Carr WA, Moe JH, Winter RB, et al: Treatment of idiopathic scoliosis in the Milwaukee brace: long term results, *J Bone Joint Surg Am* 62:599–612, 1980.
7. Cassella MC, Hall JE: Current treatment approaches in the nonoperative and operative management of adolescent idiopathic scoliosis, *Phys Ther* 71:897–909, 1991.
8. Denis F: The three column spine and its significance in the classification of acute thoracolumbar spinal injuries, *Spine* 8:817–831, 1983.
9. Denis F: Spinal instability as defined by the three-column spine concept in acute spinal trauma, *Clin Orthop* 189:65–76, 1984.
10. Duval-Beaupere G: Pathogenic relationship between scoliosis and growth. In Zorab BA, editor: *Proceedings of the third symposiums on scoliosis and growth*, Edinburgh, 1971, Churchill Livingstone.
11. Fisher SV, Winter RB: Spinal orthosis in rehabilitation. In Braddom RL, editor: *Physical medicine and rehabilitation*, Philadelphia, 1996, Saunders.
12. Gavin TM, Carandang G, Havey R, et al: Biomechanical analysis of cervical orthoses in flexion and extension: a comparison of cervical collars and cervical thoracic orthoses, *J Rehabil Res Dev* 40:527–537, 2003.
13. Hall JE, Miller ME, Cassella MC, et al: *Manual for the Boston brace workshop*, Boston, 1976, Children's Hospital.
14. Hall JE, Miller W, Shuman W, et al: A refined concept in the orthotic management of idiopathic scoliosis, *Prosthet Orthot Int* 29:7–13, 1975.
15. Hall-Craggs EC: The back and spinal cord. In Tyler NC, editor: *Anatomy as a basis for clinical medicine*, Baltimore, 1985, Urban & Schwarzenberg.
16. Horodyski M, DiPaola CP, Conrad BP, Rechtine GR: Cervical collars are insufficient for immobilizing an unstable cervical spine injury, *J Emerg Med* 41:513–519, 2011.
17. Johnson RM, Hart DL, Simmons EF, et al: Cervical orthoses: a study comparing their effectiveness in restricting cervical motion in normal subjects, *J Bone Joint Surg Am* 59:332, 1977.
18. Li M, Cheng J, Ying M, et al: Could clinical ultrasound improve the fitting of spinal orthosis for the patients with AIS?, *Eur Spine J* 21:1926–1935, 2012.
19. Lonstein JE: Orthoses for spinal deformities. In Goldberg B, Hsu JD, editors: *Atlas of orthotics: biomechanical principles and application*, ed 2, St Louis, 1985, Mosby-Year Book.
20. Lonstein JE, Carlson M: The prediction of curve progression in untreated idiopathic scoliosis during growth, *J Bone Joint Surg Am* 66:1061–1071, 1984.
21. Luskin R, Berger N: *Atlas of orthotics: biomechanical principles and application: American Academy of Orthopaedic Surgeons*, St Louis, 1975, Mosby.
22. Lysell E: Motion in the cervical spine, thesis, *Acta Orthop Scand* (Suppl 123):1, 1969.

23. Maiman D, Millington P, Novak S, et al: The effects of the thermoplastic Minerva body jacket on cervical spine motion, *Neurosurgery* 25:363–368, 1989.
24. Moe JH, Bradford DS, Winter RB, et al: *Scoliosis and other spinal deformities*, Philadelphia, 1978, Saunders.
25. Monstein JK: Orthosis for spinal deformities. In Goldberg B, Hsu JD, editors: *Atlas of orthoses and assistive devices*, ed 3, St Louis, 1997, Mosby.
26. Murphy KP, Steele BM: Musculoskeletal conditions and trauma in children. In Molnar DE, Alexander MA, editors: *Pediatric rehabilitation*, ed 3, Philadelphia, 1999, Hanley & Belfus.
27. Nachemson A: Orthotic treatment for injuries and diseases of the spinal column, *Phys Med Rehabil Clin North Am* 1:22–24, 1987.
28. Norton P, Brown T: The immobilization efficiency of back braces: the effect on the posture and motion of the lumbosacral spine, *J Bone Joint Surg Am* 39:111–130, 1957.
29. Panagiotacopulos ND, Pope MH, Bloch R, et al: Water content in human intervertebral discs: part II. Viscoelastic behavior, *Spine* 12:918–924, 1987.
30. Panjabi MM, Takata K, Goel V, et al: Thoracic human vertebrae, quantitative three-dimensional anatomy, *Spine* 16:888–901, 1991.
31. Perry J: The use of external support in the treatment of low back pain, *J Bone Joint Surg Am* 52:1440–1442, 1970.
32. Tachdejian MO: *Pediatric orthopedics*, ed 2, Philadelphia, 1990, Saunders.
33. Taitsman LA, Altman DT, Hecht AC, Pedlow FX: Complications of cervical halo-vest orthoses in elderly patients, *Orthopedics* 31:446, 2008.
34. Timoshenko S, Gere J: *Theory of elastic stability*, ed 2, New York, 1961, McGraw-Hill.
35. Wambolt A, Spencer DL: A segmental analysis of the distribution of lumbar lordosis in the normal spine, *Orthop Trans* 11:92–93, 1987.
36. Weinstein SL, Dolan LA, Wright JC, Dobbs MB: Effects of bracing in adolescents with idiopathic scoliosis, *N Engl J Med* 369:1512–1521, 2013.
37. White AA, Panjabi MM: The lumbar spine. In White AA, Panjabi MM, editors: *Clinical biomechanics of the spine*, ed 2, Philadelphia, 1990, Lippincott.
38. White AA, Panjabi MM: Extension injuries. In White AA, Panjabi MM, editors: *Clinical biomechanics of the spine*, ed 2, Philadelphia, 1990, Lippincott.

CHAPTER 14

WHEELCHAIRS AND SEATING SYSTEMS

Carmen P. DiGiovine, Alicia Koontz, Theresa Berner, Daniel J. Kim, Mark Schmeler

Wheelchairs and Seating Systems

Wheelchairs and seating systems allow individuals with mobility impairments to actively participate at home, work, school, and the community. The quality of life of an individual is reflective of the overall effectiveness of the wheelchair and seating system when considering activities of daily living (ADLs). Therefore, it is imperative that the multidisciplinary team of rehabilitation professionals considers not only the individual and the wheelchair but also the activities, context, policies, and personal assistance associated with the technology.[16] Historically, rehabilitation professionals have focused on functional mobility at the time of implementation of the wheelchair and seating system. Now, as a result of changes in the overall health care environment, driven by a need for increased value, rehabilitation professionals must integrate a more holistic approach to manage costs while improving outcomes at the time of implementation and throughout the life of the wheelchair and seating systems.[49] To better understand the long-term effects of the wheelchair and seating system, and to maximize the functional outcomes of the individual, rehabilitation professionals across the multidisciplinary health care team must understand the advances in current technology, as well as best practices in the service delivery process. The value of the wheelchair and seating system within the context of health care now extends beyond the four walls of a traditional clinic to the community in which the individual uses the wheelchair and seating system.

The term *wheelchair* is ubiquitous throughout the mobility literature and has different meanings for different stakeholders. Therefore, for the purpose of this text, we will use the terms as described in the *Glossary of Wheelchair Terms and Definitions*.[60] For example, the most generic term for a wheelchair is a *wheeled mobility device* (WMD), and the most generic term for a seating system is a *seating support system*. Refer to Box 14-1 for a list of the terms that are commonly used in this chapter.

As of 2005, over 3.3 million adults in the United States use some form of manual wheelchair, power wheelchair, or scooter. Given the annualized rate of increase of 4.6% from 1990 to 2005,[41] the number of individuals using wheelchairs and scooters is expected to increase significantly. Not surprisingly, the rate of WMD use increases with age.[41] As the number of individuals using a WMD has increased, so has the rate of breakdowns, repairs, and adverse consequences related to WMDs. Historically, the number of repairs and consequences (e.g., stranded, injured, or missed work, school, or appointment) has also increased.[61] Examining a cohort of individuals with spinal cord injury who use their power wheelchair at least 40 hours per week, Worobey et al.[62] found the rate of repairs and associated consequences were high across all manufacturers. Not surprisingly, the number of repairs for power wheelchairs is significantly higher than that for manual wheelchairs.[44,61] The increased number of individuals that require a WMD and the negative consequences of increased repairs for WMDs have put greater demand on clinicians and physicians throughout the health care system. Therefore, the multidisciplinary team must understand the features that are currently available on WMDs and the indications/contraindications for use among multiple patient populations. The purpose of this chapter is to identify the key features of WMDs, the indications/contraindications for use, and the rehabilitation technology that is available for the proper selection of WMDs.

Delivery Process

The wheelchair and seating system service delivery process is crucial to the ultimate success of the individual who uses a wheelchair and seating system. The wheelchair and seating system service delivery process has numerous steps, each with a crucial role in the ultimate success of the client's mobility.[1,2,28] A breakdown in the service delivery process can lead to poor outcomes ranging from limited mobility to the development of pressure ulcers, postural deformities, or upper extremity injuries. Therefore, to ensure a successful outcome, the wheelchair service delivery process is an iterative process that requires a multidisciplinary team.

The key steps of the service delivery process are the same regardless of the location: for example, an academic medical center, community clinic, or a less-resourced setting. The key steps include the following: the referral; assessment; equipment recommendation and selection; funding and procurement; fitting; training; follow-up, maintenance, and repairs; and outcome measurement.[1,2,28] This process is repeated iteratively for individuals who are lifelong wheelchair users to ensure better health and quality of life in the community. The participants, locations, and resources may change, but the final outcome is effective mobility within the community.

Professionals and Participants

Active participation by the consumer, the family, and/or caregivers in all stages of the seating and mobility assessment is crucial. A proper assessment begins with listening to the needs, concerns, and goals for a device.

BOX 14-1

Glossary of Terms Used in This Chapter

Wheeled mobility device	Mobility-related assistive technology device that provides wheeled mobility in a sitting, lying, or standing position for people with impaired mobility. Includes manual and power wheelchairs, scooters (power-operated vehicles), toilet and shower wheelchairs, prone mobility carts, and other unique mobility devices.
Manual wheeled mobility device	Wheeled mobility device used by an individual with mobility limitations that relies on an occupant or attendant to provide manual power for its operation. Includes manual wheelchairs, adapted stretchers, or prone carts.
Power wheeled mobility device	Wheeled mobility device used by an individual with mobility limitations that relies on power control for its operation. Includes power wheelchairs, scooters (power-operated vehicles), and other devices such as powered prone carts.
Wheelchair	Wheeled mobility device with a seating support system for a person with impaired mobility, intended to provide mobility in a seated position as its primary function. Includes manual and power wheelchairs.
Manual wheelchair	Wheelchair that relies on an occupant or an assistant for manual propulsion.
Power wheelchair	Wheelchair in which the motor power is derived from an integral source of electric power.
Scooter (power-operated vehicle)	A power mobility device designed to provide mobility in a sitting position, with a platform style base that serves as both the foot support and the structural support for the wheels, seating system, and steering mechanism. These devices have a captain style seat and/or back support without attached foot support, and a tiller to control movement and steering functions. Includes three-wheeled scooters and four-wheeled scooters.
Seating support system (seating system)	Body support system used in a device intended to support the occupant in a sitting position, specifically those parts of a wheelchair, positioning chair, or other seated mobility device that are intended to directly contact, support, or contain the body of the occupant, including the seat, back support, arm support, lower leg support, and foot support.
Postural support device	Structure, which is a component of a body support system, that has a surface intended to contact a part of the occupant's body and is used to perform one or more functions including modifying or accommodating the occupant's posture, managing tissue integrity, and/or providing sensory input. Examples of postural support devices used in a seating support system are the back support, head support, medial knee support, or lateral trunk support.

Refer to Waugh K: *Glossary of wheelchair terms and definitions,* Denver, 2013, University of Colorado, for a complete list of terms.

Optimal wheelchair prescription occurs when performed by an interdisciplinary team that includes a physiatrist and an occupational therapist or physical therapist with specialty training or certification and a good working knowledge of wheelchair seating and mobility needs. A rehabilitation engineer also plays an important role in understanding and assessing the capabilities and application of various technologies. A qualified equipment supplier is another important team member to include early in the process because the supplier is well versed in available devices and how they can be applied to solve problems and address needs. The supplier is also the team member who, in most service delivery models, orders, assembles, and delivers the equipment, and consults with the team regarding securing funding. The Rehabilitation Engineering and Assistive Technology Society of North America (RESNA) offers the certifications for Assistive Technology Professional, Seating and Mobility Specialist, and Rehabilitation Engineering Technologist. These certifications are for clinicians, engineers, and suppliers who meet certain qualifications and who pass an examination to demonstrate generalist knowledge in the area of assistive technology. The RESNA provides a directory of certified professionals (www.resna.org).

Referral

The referral process begins with the identification of the need for a wheelchair. This may occur through the traditional medical model, as is the case for an individual with a traumatic spinal cord injury, or through self-referral, as is the case for an individual who is aging into a disability. Either way, once the need is established, an individual should be referred to a multidisciplinary team that can properly assess the individual and help the individual, and her/his family/caregivers when appropriate, select the appropriate seating and mobility system.

Assessment

Initial Interview

Selecting the most appropriate wheelchair and seating system for a patient requires obtaining information about his or her specific mobility impairment(s), history of present illness, past medical and surgical history, current medications, prognosis, rehabilitation history, physical capacity and limitations, involvement in work or related activities, physical and social environment, and means of transportation. Inquiring about the patient's history with wheelchair and seating technology can also provide an indication of what has and has not worked for the person in the past.

Medical Variables

The physiatrist's role includes assessing, documenting, and sharing with the team the underlying medical conditions that require a prescription for a wheelchair. The prognoses for certain conditions need to be considered in the prescription decision, especially if a condition is progressive or has a highly variable presentation. Equipment should ideally address current and future needs based on the anticipated natural progression or projected variability of a disease or condition. In addition to age, other factors that need to be taken into account include pain, obesity, cardiopulmonary or musculoskeletal problems, genitourinary or gastrointestinal issues, alterations in mental status, overall cognitive capacity, and risk for falls. Potential risks and secondary injuries, such as pressure ulcers, postural deformities, or upper limb repetitive strain injuries, associated with the use of equipment must also be assessed and considered.

Physical and Functional Variables

Obtaining a basic understanding of the wheelchair user's capacities is an important step in considering equipment needs. This includes a physical-motor assessment of strength, range of motion, coordination, balance, posture, tone, contractures, endurance, sitting posture, trunk stability, cognition, perception, and use of external orthoses. Clinic-based capacity assessments do not necessarily indicate conclusively whether a person will be able to safely and effectively use mobility equipment. This is often best assessed by giving the user an opportunity to try the equipment to determine how they perform. For example, people with low vision are often capable of using powered mobility devices under appropriate circumstances and interventions, just as people with low vision are able to ambulate with the use of a navigation cane.

Physical assessments should be followed by observed performance of ADLs that are reported as essential by the patient or his/her family or caregiver. These include self-care, reaching, accessing surfaces at various heights, transferring to various surfaces, and functional mobility. Functional mobility should be assessed in the user's home and community. Ambulation should be assessed from the perspective of the surfaces and distances encountered in a routine day and whether walking or pushing a manual wheelchair is safe and efficient. When considering the use of a manual wheelchair for a patient, the amount of stress applied to the upper limbs must be taken into account, as it can lead to repetitive strain injuries. There is no evidence that upper limb strength correlates with the ability to propel manual wheelchairs, especially in the context of patients with cardiac or pulmonary impairments, arthritis, multiple sclerosis, or cerebral palsy.

Obtaining proper positioning while seated and determining the necessary componentry to ensure such positioning requires observation of a patient's posture both while seated and while on a therapy mat table, to assess postural alignment and joint range of motion. This can determine what limitations are present, the degree to which they are present, and whether they are fixed or flexible. Assessment of pelvic alignment is crucial because the pelvis serves as the base of all seating support. An obliquity of the pelvis to one side needs to be accommodated or corrected (if possible) to prevent leaning of the trunk or development of spinal deformities superiorly. Likewise, spinal deformities need to be accommodated in the design of the backrest, to allow the user to tolerate sitting. The amount of hip flexion available at the user's pelvis determines the tolerated seat-to-back angle. Inferiorly, the degree of knee extension available while the user's hips are flexed is an important indicator of hamstring mobility, as they cross both the knee and hip joints. Tight hamstrings, which are common in many wheelchair users, can therefore significantly affect foot positioning. It is important that excessive tension not be placed on the hamstrings as this can be painful and pull the pelvis into a posterior tilt. It is also necessary to respect a person's preference for different seated postures, even if they do not appear to be technically correct. Many patients may become accustomed to seemingly unorthodox seating positions that they have found to be comfortable, functional, and stable.

After the physical motor assessment, measurements of the body are taken (see the section on Basic Wheelchair Dimensions later). The various seating system options can then be considered. As described in the sections on wheelchair seating and back supports, there are a wide variety of cushions, back supports, and custom seating systems available.

Environmental Variables

It is important to assess both the physical and social environments in which a patient spends most of his or her time. Physical accessibility within the home, work, school, or other areas in the community often has a major impact on the feasibility of wheelchair and seating system options. A thorough assessment and survey of the home is almost always warranted when determining which mobility equipment options are most appropriate to the user. A home assessment is often needed to ensure that the device will be usable, especially when there are stairs, narrow doorways, and hallways, or other tight spaces to be negotiated. The assessment involves taking mobility devices to the home, surveying the environment for accessibility, and having the user get into the device to maneuver within the spaces he or she uses in a typical day. The home assessment should also involve having the wheelchair user complete specific mobility-related tasks such as transferring to and from various surfaces, including those used for bathing and toileting; reaching for objects, which may be necessary for activities such as dressing and grooming; and pulling up to tables or work surfaces, which may be necessary for feeding and meal preparation. The surfaces, terrains, and distances the user will encounter on a daily basis also need to be factored into the prescription and decision-making process.

The social environmental assessment includes the roles, interests, responsibilities, and occupation important to the user. These roles may include being a parent, spouse, worker, homemaker, student, or community volunteer. The level of available assistance that the user has from others needs to be assessed from the perspective of the user's ability to maintain and troubleshoot potentially complex equipment. The physical capacity and health of the user's caregivers also need to be assessed in this context. It is important to recognize that an individual's family, social, and cultural values can be either barriers or facilitators to a person's inclusion in the community.

Aesthetics

Aesthetics can be an extremely important factor in the wheelchair prescription, depending on the user. Wheelchairs are extremely personal and intimate devices for children and adults alike and act as an extension of one's own body. For many users, a wheelchair can also be a vehicle for self-expression. The stock appearance of a wheelchair is mainly a function of its frame design and materials. For example, titanium metal has a satin, polished finish and maintains a new, fresh look. Some users may choose to customize various components of their wheelchairs, such as the tires or casters, in a multitude of different colors and finishes. It is important that the user is pleased with the appearance of his or her wheelchair because it is an extension of his or her body. An aesthetically pleasing wheelchair is more likely to be used and gains positive attention from peers and from the community as a whole.

Transportation Variables

The modularity of powered mobility devices now permits greater transportability of scooters and portable power wheelchairs within a standard motor vehicle. The feasibility of equipment assembly and disassembly by the user or the user's caregiver, however, needs to be carefully assessed. It should be noted that portability can come at the cost of durability and may compromise the capabilities of a device to negotiate uneven or soft surfaces. If transporting the wheelchair and seating system is an essential goal, the person who will be responsible for stowing the device should get an opportunity to attempt to do so before the final mobility equipment prescription is written.

If wheelchair users plan to be transported by an accessible vehicle, such as a van with a lift or ramp, they should try driving their device into such a vehicle, maneuvering it into an appropriate position for securement or transfer to another seat, and exiting the vehicle. It is crucial to make certain that both the wheelchair and the vehicle that will be transporting the wheelchair have the appropriate and compliant (such as American National Standards Institute [ANSI]/RESNA WC-19 Standards) attachment points to ensure optimal safety during transportation.

Equipment Recommendation and Selection (Prescription)

The mobility assessment should lead directly into the equipment recommendation and selection process. The assessment and recommendation steps will often overlap. The user should take an active role in the equipment selection process to ensure his or her buy-in with the final recommendation and maximize the likelihood of a positive outcome. If possible, the user should first trial the wheelchair and seating system under the supervision of a trained mobility equipment expert, such as a physician or specialized therapist. The advantages/disadvantages of the system being trialed should be well documented, including the use of appropriate assessment tools. This information will be crucial in the final selection process and in the implementation of the system at the time of the fitting. Finally, the consumer should participate in selecting the components on the system and any compromises that are necessary, given the competing goals (e.g., mobility, posture, transportation) of the process, should be identified and reviewed. The equipment recommendation and selection process is a collaborative process among all of its participants and is crucial to the final outcome.

Seating Principles

What is traditionally defined as an ideal sitting position (knees at 90 degrees of flexion, hips at 90 degrees of flexion, and elbows at 90 degrees of flexion) may not be comfortable, functional, or even possible for some users because of musculoskeletal deformity or other physical limitations. Proper positioning of the pelvis and trunk provides a stable base for the upper limbs. An unstable base may lead to upper limb overuse and injury. Without proper base positioning, the head and neck will not be well aligned with the spine. The pelvis should be stabilized on a cushion that provides postural support as well as optimal pressure distribution. The cushion should be mounted onto a hard surface that maintains its position, as opposed to placing it directly onto a sling upholstery seat (unless otherwise preferred by the user). Solid seat inserts (thin wood boards) are often inserted into the cushion cover to provide a solid base for sitting. For flexible deformities, the pelvis should sit in as neutral a position as possible, with the trunk maintaining a normal degree of lumbar and cervical lordosis. The seating system needs to accommodate the pelvis and trunk in positions other than neutral. Proper positioning and support of the head and neck facilitates proper breathing and swallowing, and can prevent excessive strain of the head and neck stabilizer muscles. Tilt and recline systems should always be equipped with a headrest to support the head when adjusting seat orientation and back angles.

Additional seating considerations are needed for patients with sensory loss, paralysis and paresis, contractures, or spasticity and high tone, as discussed later.

Sensory Loss

When people who are unimpaired sit on hard or irregular surfaces, they rapidly feel discomfort and alter their position to provide adequate pressure relief. Alternatively, they may simply stand up to relieve pressure completely. If sensation is impaired, however, the individual may be unaware that a particular contact area is being injured. An inadequate pressure-relieving seating system or technique can ultimately lead to pressure ulcer formation.

Paralysis and Paresis

Paralysis and paresis may prevent an individual from easily changing positions and limit circulation normally increased by movement and voluntary muscle contraction. It can destabilize body segments (trunk, legs, arms, and head). Unless these segments are adequately supported and protected, they can collapse into a "gravity position." This may cause increased areas of pressure over bony prominences, joint subluxations, and other secondary skeletal and joint deformities. Pressure ulcers may also develop in areas where the skin is vulnerable to sheering forces, such as along skin folds, at the sacrum, or any areas that are continuously exposed to moisture. Finally, paretic limbs may become entangled in the components of the wheelchair.

Contractures

Contractures often represent a significant challenge to properly positioning a patient in his or her wheelchair. Contractures represent a static shortening of muscle and are therefore best supported by adjustable hardware that can be arranged to accommodate the fixed joint positions of a patient. Examples of this type of hardware include adjustable-angle leg rests to support knee flexion contractures and seating systems that recline to open up the seat-to-back angle for those with hip extension contractures.

Spasticity and Hypertonicity

Patients with spasticity and high tone usually require very aggressive and sturdy seating systems to obtain optimal positioning and pressure distribution. Unlike contractures, spasticity and high tone are categorized as dynamic muscle dysfunctions, which do not always lend themselves to support in any single joint position. It is not uncommon for the high forces generated during extensor thrusts (as a result of knee extensor, hip extensor, and plantar flexor spasticity) to damage the seat back or leg rests of a wheelchair, which even when highly adjustable cannot often provide the level of true dynamic support that is necessary to accommodate spasticity or high tone. In some cases, it is possible to manage spasticity and high tone with custom-contoured seating systems. These types of systems provide total contact support, and can include dynamic seating components such as back support attachments that "give" and bounce back into place during and after an extensor thrust.

Funding

Wheelchairs and seating systems are reimbursed in a variety of ways within the United States, with health insurance being the most common means of funding. The Medicare program is the largest payer of this equipment and sets the standard for coverage policies. These policies have recently been significantly changed because of increased use of these benefits associated with an aging population as well as direct-to-consumer advertising by certain suppliers.

Wheelchairs and seating systems are considered a durable medical equipment benefit and require documentation as being medically necessary as defined by the Social Security Act of 1965, section 1862(a)(1)(A). It is important for the physiatrist and clinician to clearly document the need for wheelchair and seating system interventions in clinic notes and in letters of medical necessity. A few basic strategies to follow when writing letters of medical necessity are to describe in detail the person's medical condition and contextual situation, why the equipment is needed to compensate for functional deficits or address medical needs, and why lower cost alternatives are not appropriate. A description of the potential ramifications of equipment denial (e.g., loss of further function and the onset of secondary medical problems) helps to justify funding by third-party payers. Under more recent Centers for Medicare and Medicaid Services (CMS) policy, a wheeled mobility and seating device, referred by the CMS as mobility-assistive equipment, is covered if users have a mobility limitation that significantly impairs their ability to participate in one or more mobility-related ADLs (MRADLs) in the home. A mobility limitation is one that (1) prevents the individual from accomplishing the MRADLs entirely (independence); (2) places the individual at reasonably determined heightened risk of morbidity or mortality secondary to the attempts to participate in MRADLs (safety); or (3) prevents the individual from completing the MRADLs within a reasonable time frame (quality).

Other payers, such as the Veterans Administration, Vocational Rehabilitation, or Workers' Compensation, might not be as restrictive and might consider the user's needs beyond home-based ADLs, such as the need for community mobility for work, school, or recreational pursuits.

Fitting, Delivery, and Training

When the wheelchair is delivered and is ready for use by the patient, the fitting should ideally take place in the presence of the multidisciplinary team that was present at the time of the assessment. At a minimum, this should include the therapist and supplier. During the fitting session, the goals established during the initial assessment should be reviewed because a significant amount of time might have lapsed. The fitting process may take multiple appointments, especially for complex situations. The person using the equipment needs to feel comfortable, knowing adjustments can be made to optimize fit and address functional needs. The equipment will often need to go back to the supplier's shop for alteration before the final delivery.

During the final fitting, the person and any caregivers need to be fully trained and return-demonstrate the proper use and maintenance of the equipment. The wheelchair skills program is an excellent method for demonstrating the proper use of the equipment (www.wheelchairskills program.ca).[4,37,51] The person should be advised of parties to contact in case of equipment failure. Training by a therapist might be necessary to ensure the safe and effective operation of a device. The fitting and training portions of this step of the service delivery process is often minimized or dismissed altogether. However, this often leads to poor functional, health, and satisfaction outcomes because the patient is unable to fully use the features built into the wheelchair and seating system. Therefore, the fitting, delivery, and training process is crucial for better health and quality of life. Follow-up appointments should be scheduled on a regular basis to ensure the equipment is meeting the person's needs and to identify any need for modification, preventive maintenance, or replacement.

Follow-Up, Maintenance, and Repair

Follow-up appointments with the clinicians and supplier provide the patient an opportunity to further fine-tune the wheelchair and seating system to meet his or her unique needs. Once the patient has had an opportunity to use the system in the community for 2 to 6 weeks, he or she often identifies opportunities for further customization of the system. Current wheelchairs and seating systems offer numerous adjustments that can improve the postural support of the seating system and the performance of the wheelchair.

The wheelchair user must take a vested interest in the long-term performance of the system. He or she should initiate the maintenance schedule that was discussed during the delivery process. Furthermore, as the patient identifies issues with the wheelchair and seating system, he or she should contact the clinician and/or supplier, as appropriate. The sooner the issue is resolved, the sooner the patient will be able to resume normal activities in the community. Given that the wheelchair and seating system is prone to parts failures over time, just as any other mechanical system, it is important to watch for these issues. Timely resolution of these problems helps to prevent medical complications (e.g., postural deformities, pressure ulcers, or upper extremity injuries) or a reduction in overall quality of life.

Outcome Measures

As with most services in health care, the effectiveness of seating and mobility interventions needs to be demonstrated. To meet this need, standardized outcome measures related to these interventions are evolving. These range from simple but validated self-report questionnaires, such as the Functioning Mobility Assessment,[38,46] to more involved capacity and performance measures, such as the Wheelchair Skills Test.[51] The tools can be administered before the provision of an intervention, yielding a numeric score, which can be compared with scores that are determined after the provision of the intervention.

Considerations for Select Populations

Pediatric Patients

Children with mobility deficits have unique mobility equipment needs. Early disability during a child's formative years, when they are growing and acquiring a positive self-image, can affect multiple spheres of living (i.e., attending school, accessing learning materials, and interacting with peers). Early use of powered mobility if medically appropriate is of paramount importance to promote psychosocial development, reduce learned helplessness, and facilitate social and educational integration and independence.[50] Therefore, several factors that are unique to this patient population must be taken into account during selection of wheelchair and seating componentry.

Wheeled mobility for pediatric patients must have a high degree of adjustability to accommodate future growth. Pediatric mobility equipment must also have the ability to be cared for and transported by a parent or guardian (i.e., a wheelchair that disassembles to facilitate transport within a vehicle). Pediatric patients may require specialized technology to facilitate the completion of school assignments, such as augmentative communication aids, alternative computer access devices, or sensory aids. Such devices are often mounted directly to the child's wheelchair to accommodate travel with them to and from school. Features that facilitate interaction with other children are also of great importance. For example, a power wheelchair that is able to lower its seating surface to the floor can allow a child to be at eye level with his or her peers and participate in the same activities that they carry out while seated on the floor (Figure 14-1).

Progressive Disorders

Progressive disorders such as amyotrophic lateral sclerosis, multiple sclerosis, or Parkinson disease require special consideration when prescribing a wheelchair and seating system. Although many individuals with these disorders begin with manual wheelchairs, they may begin to struggle over time with independent propulsion because of increased fatigue, tremors, ataxia, or weakness. Power wheelchairs with programmable functions are good choices for those with progressive disorders because they can be tailored to an individual's driving abilities as his or her disease progresses and can accept multiple inputs (e.g., joystick, head array, sip-and-puff switch). From a seating perspective, these patients will need periodic seating updates as their disease progresses. Interchangeable seating and positioning hardware as well as tilt and/or recline options are available for indoor-outdoor power wheelchairs. It is important to think about power wheelchair use

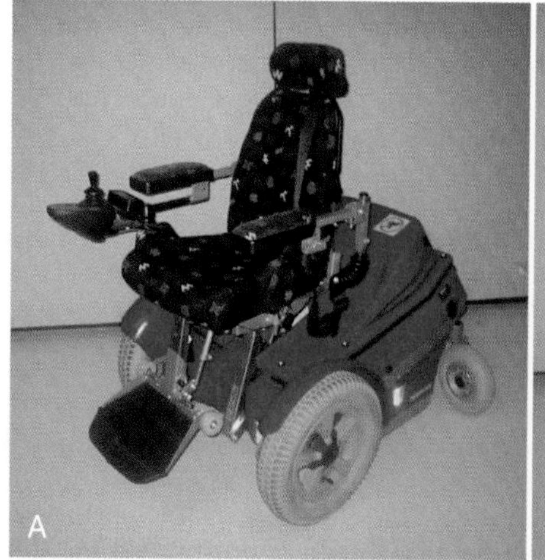

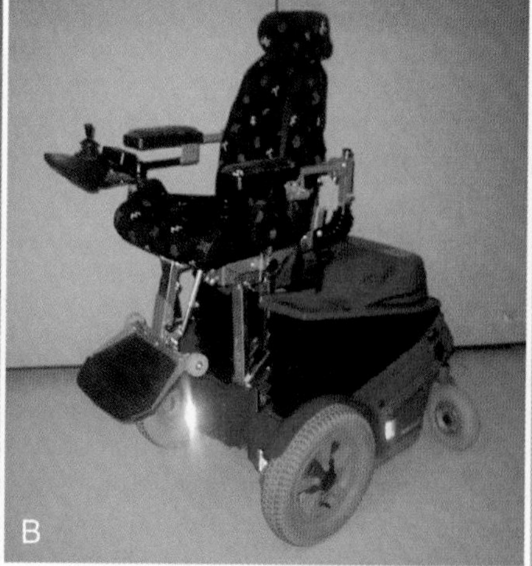

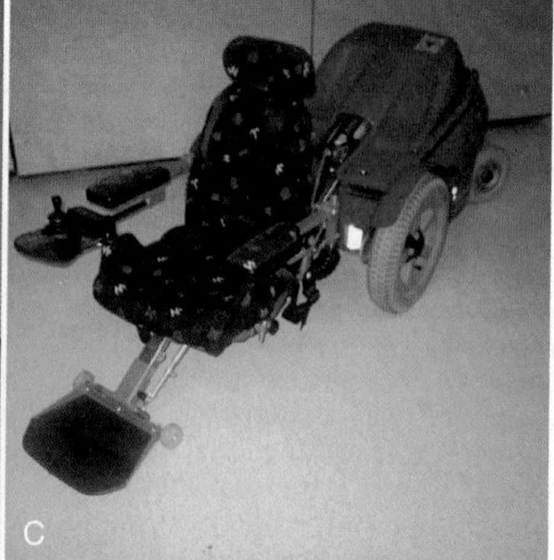

FIGURE 14-1 **A** to **C,** Pediatric power wheelchair with a seat that can be lowered to the floor for play.

early on in the course of a progressive disorder and to consider the patient's source of funding. It may take several months before some patients receive their wheelchairs as a result of the approval and review processes set forth by their funding sources.

Impaired Vision

Individuals with low vision have an additional challenge when using wheeled mobility. When individuals with low vision walk, they typically use their upper limbs, either with hands outstretched or with a long cane, to provide them with haptic feedback of their surroundings and warn them of potential hazards. When using wheeled mobility, a patient's arms can no longer explore ahead of their body and may be occupied either with propulsion or operation of a joystick to drive. Driving safety with wheeled mobility must be assessed on a case-by-case basis because of the high variability of visual impairments and adaptive abilities of patients that have them.

Weight Disparity

Many patients with impaired mobility are also chronically under or over their ideal body weight. Individuals with cerebral palsy who have athetoid movements and difficulty with mastication, for example, may become chronically underweight as a result of malnutrition. Special attention must be paid to patients who are underweight or malnourished when prescribing mobility equipment because of their increased risk for developing pressure sores over bony prominences and poor wound healing capacity secondary to nutritional deficits. Alternatively, the sedentary lifestyle of patients with wheeled mobility can result in poor overall fitness and obesity. In addition to the common health risks associated with obesity, being overweight has a unique impact on the use of wheeled mobility equipment. A wider, heavier, and more durable wheelchair is required for the obese patient. Such devices can be more difficult to maneuver and have accessibility limitations, especially through narrow doorways and within small rooms. Propulsion of a manual wheelchair may be more difficult for the obese patient resulting from range-of-motion and positioning limitations caused by body habitus and increased energy expenditure because more force is required to overcome increased rolling resistance. Transfers, pressure relief, and personal hygiene are also often more difficult for the obese patient to perform, which may increase the risk for skin breakdown and pressure ulcers. Finally, third-party funding for mobility equipment may be delayed in some instances if the funding source considers obesity a preventable health complication.

Older Adults

Aging can be thought of as a collection of progressive disorders and can further complicate wheelchair prescription and seating selection. Effects of aging vary widely, but common problems that are pertinent to mobility equipment selection span a wide array of systems within the body. A higher incidence of osteoporosis, stress fractures, and arthritis, for example, may cause increased pain, limited range-of-motion and weight-bearing capacity, and reduced sitting tolerance. Impaired circulation resulting from coronary artery disease, peripheral vascular disease, or diabetes may increase the risk of pressure ulcers in older adults. A more sedentary lifestyle, with associated weight gain and reduced muscular strength may lead to limitations in endurance and overall maximum energy expenditure. Furthermore, a higher incidence of cognitive impairment and depression can profoundly affect a user's ability to safely and effectively use mobility equipment. Many older adult patients rely on a caretaker or family member to perform ADLs. This type of reliance can be further complicated if the caretaker or family member is also an older adult or has ongoing medical issues. Care of the patient in this instance can result in injury to the caregiver during a strenuous procedure such as transferring. Finally, older adult patients are often on a fixed income and may not be able to absorb the cost of mobility-related accessories that are not covered by Medicare.

In general, most older adult patients are frailer and therefore require greater diligence by the clinician in prescribing the appropriate mobility equipment. The older adult patient's caretaker(s) and loved ones should be included in the clinical decision-making process if they have direct involvement in the patient's day-to-day care and activities. It is often necessary to complete a home assessment to determine if any additional hazards are present or if any additional accommodations are necessary within a patient's everyday environment.

Assessment Tools

Anthropometrics

Anthropometric measurements play a crucial role in customizing a wheelchair to match the unique dimensions and angles of the human body. Rehabilitation professionals use calipers, rigid and soft tape measures, goniometers, scales, and digital cameras.[21] These measurements are then translated into the specific dimensions of the wheelchair and seating system. The measurements document physical changes in the individual, which is necessary when adjusting the wheelchair and seating system, or recommending new equipment.

Propulsion Analysis

The analysis of an individual's propulsion characteristics is used to set up the wheelchair, train individuals on proper propulsion techniques, and document the change in propulsion characteristics over time. Propulsion analyses are crucial for minimizing the development of upper limb pain and injury and for maximizing function within the community. Multiple tools are available for analyzing manual wheelchair propulsion, ranging from the wheelchair propulsion test[4] that uses a stop watch, tape measure, and clinical observation to the SmartWheel protocol[20] that uses a force, torque, and distance-measuring pushrim, along with clinical observation. Ideally, propulsion analyses should be performed during the assessment process, with the individual's current wheelchair (if applicable), when comparing wheelchairs during the selection process, and during the fitting and training process to ensure that the goals identified during the assessment process are met. Propulsion analyses are crucial for maintaining the long-term health of the individual by minimizing the likelihood for the development of upper limb pain and injury.

Pressure Analysis

Similar to propulsion analysis, pressure analysis is used to set up the seating system, train individuals on proper pressure-relieving techniques as a biofeedback mechanism, compare seating systems, and document the change in sitting tolerance over time. A pressure-mapping system is used in addition to clinical observations and impressions. This is a thin mat with pressure sensors that can be placed over a surface where the person sits to determine interface pressures. The mat is connected to a computer that produces the topography of pressure that can be displayed on a monitor (Figure 14-2).[22] Pressure-mapping systems are used to measure the peak pressure index, dispersion index, and gradient.[55] Pressure mapping alone should not be the sole determinant for selecting a specific cushion because there are performance trade-offs with different seating system designs and materials. For example, the durability and maintenance of the system and the ease of transfers from one surface to another should be considered. Consumer input on the overall effectiveness of the cushion is essential. Pressure analyses provide a quantitative mechanism for measuring the pressure-relieving properties of the seating system to minimize the likelihood for the development of pressure ulcers and postural deformities.

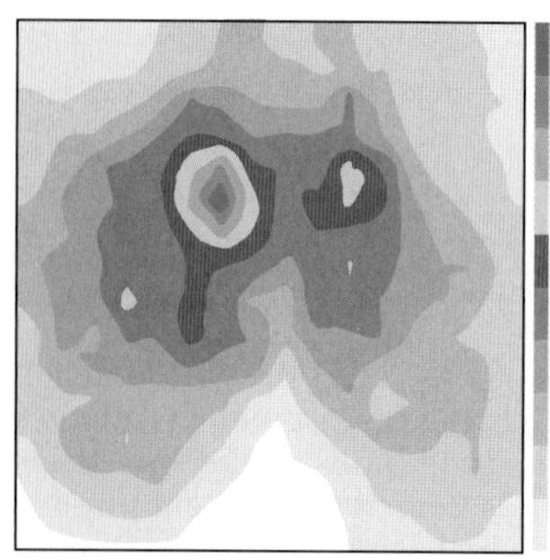
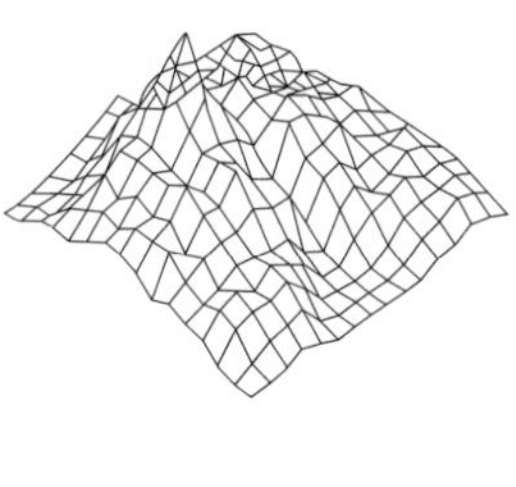

A

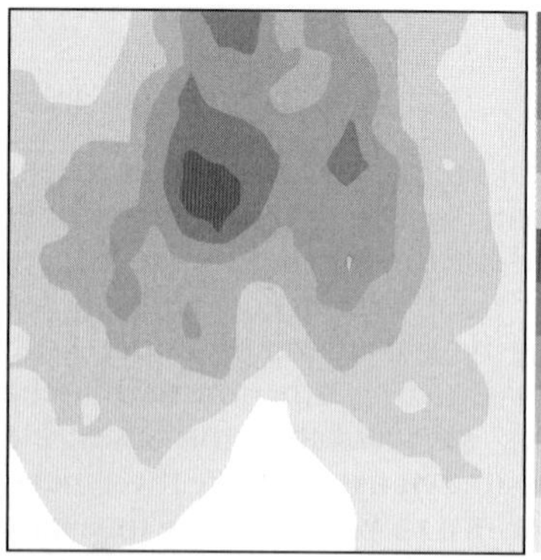
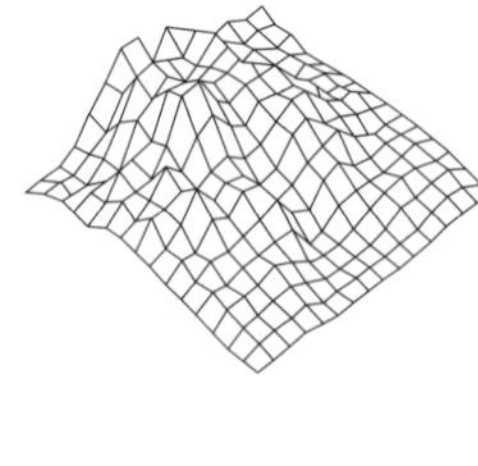

B

FIGURE 14-2 Pressure mapping of the wheelchair seat–buttocks interface. **A,** The backrest is in an upright position. **B,** The backrest is reclined 24 degrees. Areas of high pressure are denoted as varying shades of blue. The higher the pressure, the darker the shade of blue. Areas of low pressure are denoted as varying shades of gray. The lower the pressure, the lighter the shade of gray.

Wheelchair Skills

Wheelchair skills assessment is important in determining if a person has the physical and cognitive capacity to use a wheelchair, the appropriate type of mobility, and for training on the proper use of the wheelchair and seating system. The wheelchair skills program uses a broad-based assessment that addresses both the individual with a disability and her or his caregiver.[33,37,51] The wheelchair skills test includes approximately 30 activities for both power wheelchair users and manual wheelchair users. The activities range from traveling in a straight line and turns to accessing ramps and curbs. Furthermore, the assessment also examines mobility-related tasks such as transfers and charging a power wheelchair. The wheelchair skills test provides a quantitative method for assessing the ability of an individual to use a wheelchair and provides a mechanism for documenting change in overall mobility function.

Wheelchairs

Manual Wheelchairs

People with good upper body function and stamina might well be able to use a manual wheelchair for mobility. Manual wheelchairs for daily use are often categorized by their design features and costs. Table 14-1 provides an overview of each adult wheelchair category as defined by the CMS, which is the leading third-party payer for wheelchairs. These categories are outdated and are being revised to reflect the actual composition of manual wheelchairs on the market.

The standard wheelchair (Figure 14-3) is designed for short-term hospital or institutional use and is not recommended as a primary mode of mobility. It folds for storage and transportability. As noted in Table 14-1, it can be rather heavy with limited sizes available. Figure 14-3 illustrates the basic components of a wheelchair. A "hemi" wheelchair is essentially a standard wheelchair with a lower seat-to-floor height for people of shorter stature or who use one or both feet for propulsion. A lightweight wheelchair is slightly lighter in weight but with limited sizes. The first three models have few adjustable parts (some models have no adjustable parts) and generally have sling-type upholstery for the seat and back support. Sling upholstery has no capacity to provide pressure relief, and the hammock effect that occurs from wear causes uncomfortable and unstable inward rotation of the hips. However, many users have been sitting in a sling seating system for years and have become accustomed to the hammock effect for comfort. Making the switch to a seating system that better supports their posture can be both frustrating and uncomfortable.

The high-strength lightweight and ultralight wheelchairs are designed for long-term use by individuals who spend

Table 14-1 Types of Adult Manual Wheelchairs for Daily Mobility

Class*	Weight (lb)	Seat Widths (inches)	Seat Heights (inches)	Seat Depth (inches)	Back Height (inches)
Standard	>36	16, 18	>19 and <21	16	16, 17
Standard hemi	>36	16, 18	>15 and <17	16	16, 17
Lightweight	<36	16, 18	>17 and <21	16	16-17
High-strength lightweight	<34	14, 16, 18	>17 and <21	14, 16	15-19
Ultralightweight	<30	14, 16, 18	>17 and ≤21	12-20	>8 and <21
Heavy duty	Supports person weighing >250 lb	≥18	>19 and <21	16, 17	16, 17
Extra–heavy duty	Supports person weighing >300 lb	≥18	>19 and <21	16, 17	16, 17

*Manual wheelchair classes as defined by the Centers for Medicare and Medicaid Services (http://www.cignamedicare.com/dmerc/lmrp_lcd/index.html).

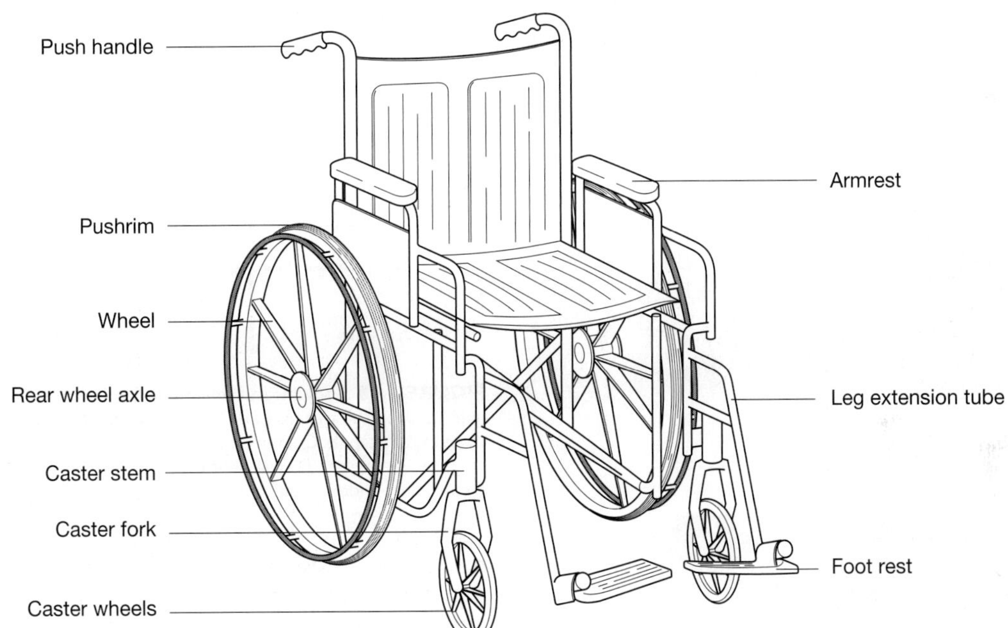

FIGURE 14-3 Standard manual wheelchair and components.

more than a couple of hours each day in a wheelchair. They have adjustable features, especially the ultralight manual wheelchairs. There are many advantages to using ultralight wheelchairs over the other wheelchair types. These are highlighted in the following sections that discuss selecting the appropriate seat dimensions, setting up the wheelchair, propulsion mechanics, and transportability. An ultralight wheelchair is depicted in Figure 14-4.

The last two classes of manual wheelchairs listed in Table 14-1 pertain to people who weigh more than 250 lb. These wheelchairs are heavier than the wheelchairs in the other classes to support more body weight. These categories are also outdated because of the increasing number of people with disabilities who are overweight or obese and need wheelchairs. This trend has resulted in an expanded class of "extra–heavy-duty" wheelchairs, referred to as bariatric wheelchairs, which are built to support individuals who weigh between 300 and 1000 lb.

Pediatric manual wheelchairs are similar to the adult wheelchairs but are smaller (seat width or depth less than 14 inches). Many of these wheelchairs have adjustable frames or kits for accommodating the growth of the child (Figure 14-5). If the child is unable to self-propel the chair, a powered mobility device might provide independent mobility.[50] Strollers equipped with a wide range of seating options (Figure 14-6) can also be used to transport children with orthopedic deformities.

Sports and recreation wheelchairs are designed specifically for participating in such athletic, fitness, and recreational endeavors as racing, cycling, rugby, tennis, and

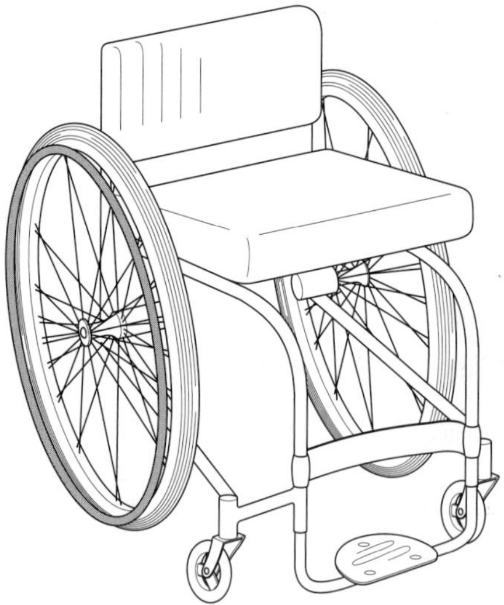

FIGURE 14-4 Ultralight manual wheelchair.

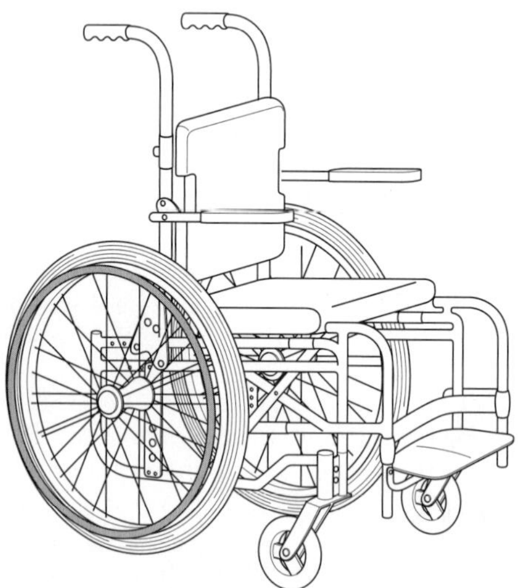

FIGURE 14-5 Pediatric manual wheelchair.

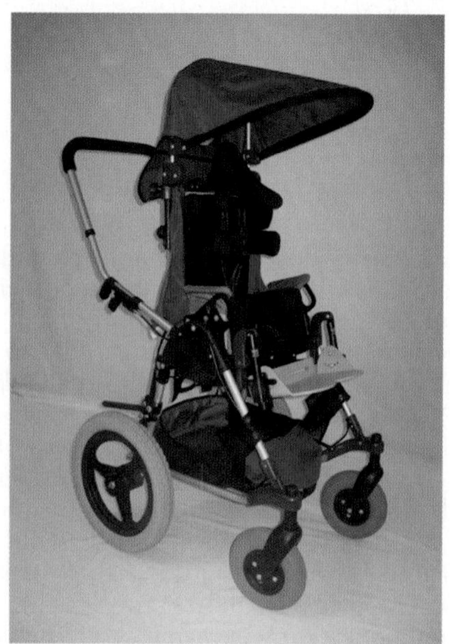

FIGURE 14-6 Pediatric adaptive stroller. (Courtesy Sunrise Medical, Longmont, Calif.)

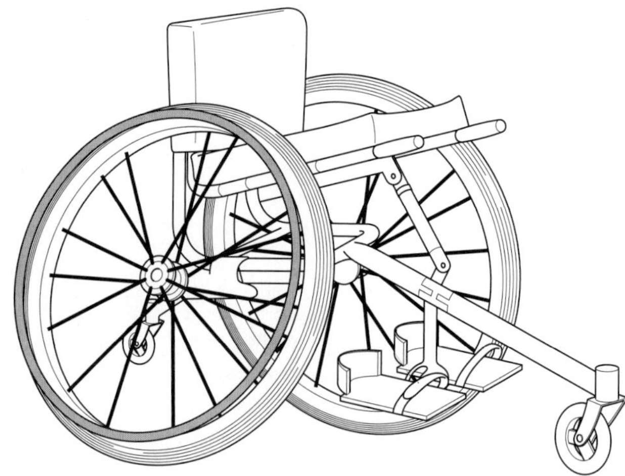

FIGURE 14-7 Tennis sport wheelchair.

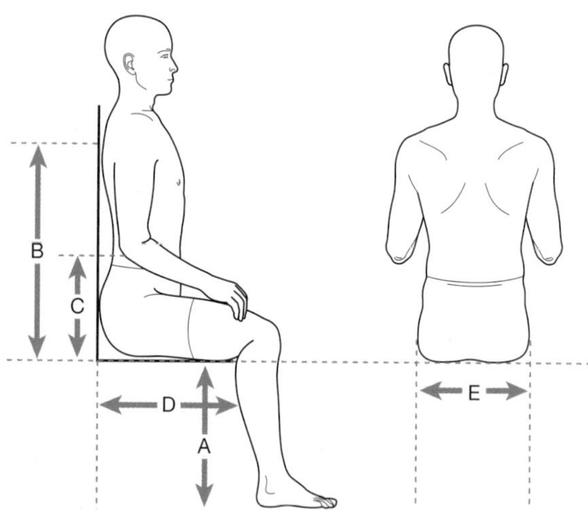

FIGURE 14-8 Body measurements. *A*, Leg length: distance from bottom of heel to popliteal area. *B*, Back height: distance from buttocks to the inferior angle of the scapula. *C*, Armrest height: distance from buttocks to forearm with elbow at 90 degrees. *D*, Seat depth: distance from back of buttocks to popliteal area. *E*, Seat width: distance between the widest parts of the buttocks.

basketball. These wheelchairs are made of lightweight materials, and usually have very aggressive axle positions and camber. Some of the sport wheelchairs have only one wheel in the front, which allows quick turns and enhanced maneuverability (Figure 14-7). Wheelchairs equipped with arm crank mechanisms (called hand cycles) for exercise are available from many manufacturers. Arm crank exercise can help improve cardiovascular fitness, with research showing that arm cranking is more efficient and less of a physical strain than conventional wheelchair propulsion.[47]

Basic Wheelchair Dimensions

The anatomic measurements of an individual are used to specify the size of the manual or power wheelchair, and the seating system (e.g., seat cushion, back support, leg rest). The typical anatomic measurements are shown in Figure 14-8. Each measure has a direct impact on the overall function and comfort of each component in the system.[12] Maximizing the mobility of an individual while he or she is using the wheelchair and seating system is dependent on properly matching the anatomic dimensions of the person to the wheelchair dimensions.

Seat Height

The seat should be just high enough to accommodate leg length while leaving enough space under the footrests (approximately 2 inches or so) to clear obstacles.[12] People with longer legs often need angled or elevating leg rests that extend the legs slightly outward instead of straight down (knee angle of 90 degrees). This allows individuals to get their knees underneath tables. It is more difficult to do if the individual has tight hamstrings. The height of the seat should be adjusted so that the person has enough knee clearance to fit under tables, counters, and sinks at home, work, school, and in the community (the Americans with Disabilities Act mandates at least 27-inch-high knee clearance under tables and surfaces). Seat height is also an important consideration for people who drive an automobile while seated in the wheelchair and need to be able to access the steering wheel or hand controls.

Seat Depth

The depth of the seat provides support for the thighs. A 1- to 2-inch gap between the popliteal area and front edge of the cushion is recommended, but might need to be more if the person propels with the feet.[12] A seat that is too shallow causes higher sitting pressures because less of the seat is in contact with the thighs. A seat that is too deep can cause excess pressure behind the knees and calves. There can also be a tendency for the pelvis to slide into a posterior tilt so that the back is no longer supported by the backrest.

Seat Width

The wheelchair seat width should be approximately 1 inch wider than the width of the widest part of the buttocks. When sitting on the seat, the individual's hips should be at or close to the edge of the cushion. If the seat is too narrow, the individual might develop pressure sores on the pelvic bony prominences. If the seat is too wide, the individual is forced to abduct their shoulders excessively, making it more difficult to propel the chair.

Back Height

The height of the back is determined by the amount of postural support the person needs. The backrest should be low enough to provide adequate support, but still allow the upper limbs access to as much of the pushrims as possible. Many practitioners use the inferior angle of the scapula as a basis for determining backrest height. The backrest height should be below the inferior angle so that it does not impede arm movements. There are various types of back supports (Table 14-2), and some have a tapered area that allows for greater freedom of scapular movement. Typically, the high-strength lightweight and ultralight wheelchairs permit the attachment of different types of back supports.

Armrest Height

The armrest height is determined by measuring the distance between the forearm and the seated surface. The forearm should be parallel to the ground when positioned on the armrest. If the armrests are too high, then the person will continually elevate her/his shoulders, and it will be difficult to access the pushrims. If it is too low, then the armrest will not properly support the upper limbs, including the shoulder complex.

Manual Wheelchair Setup

Ultralight wheelchairs provide the highest degree of adjustability and customization. This makes it possible to optimize the fit of the wheelchair to the user, which is likely to have a positive impact on propulsion biomechanics.[45] In addition to the basic adjustments on most other wheelchairs (e.g., footrests, armrests), ultralight wheelchairs have adjustable seat and back angles, rear wheel camber, and rear axle position.

Seat and Back Angle Adjustments

The seat angle, which is defined as the angle that the seat makes relative to the horizontal plane, and the back angle, which is defined as the angle the back makes relative to the vertical plane, are both adjustable and configurable on ultralight manual wheelchairs. The adjustments, separately or together, optimize the postural support and comfort for the individual. Adjusting the seat so that it slopes downward toward the rear of the wheelchair (also referred to as seat dump) can assist people with limited trunk control by stabilizing their pelvis and spine, making it easier to propel the wheelchair. It can decrease extensor tone and posturing. Too much dump, however, can cause the pelvis to rotate backward and the lumbar spine to flatten. This increases pressure on the sacrum, increases the risk of skin breakdown, and makes it more difficult to transfer into and out of the wheelchair. An increased back angle or reclined back might be needed when the person's hips do not flex well or gravity is needed to assist with balancing the trunk. Using a combination of seat and back angle adjustments increases the number of possible postural accommodations.

Rear Wheel Camber

Camber is the angle of rear wheel rotation about an axis in the fore-aft direction. Zero degree of camber implies that the rear wheels line up vertically with the side of the wheelchair. Angling the rear wheels so the top is tilted inward and the bottom outward (see Figure 14-7) results in increased camber and distance between the bottoms of the rear wheels. Most wheelchairs generally do not have more than 8 degrees of camber. Although more camber is possible, it can impede the ability to enter and exit doors and openings. Box 14-2 lists the advantages and disadvantages of camber.

Rear Axle Position

Ultralight manual wheelchairs have adjustable rear axles that allow for optimal positioning of the rear wheels in the vertical and fore-aft directions. The placement of the rear wheels relative to the individual's upper limbs directly affects propulsion biomechanics and therefore the likelihood of upper limb pain and injury.

Table 14-2 Back Supports

Back Support Type	Image	Application	Benefits	Limitations
Basic upholstery fabric (vinyl or nylon) sling back found on standard wheelchairs		Casual transport for multiple patient	Inexpensive Easy to fold	Nonadjustable in either height or width "Hammock"-quality support
Fabric back with tension ties		For consumers needing moderate customization	Relatively inexpensive Easy to adjust without tools and readjust as needed	Limited support; still a suspension back
Firm back, minimum contour		Consumers with moderate trunk support needs	Remains firm longer than suspension systems Option to choose height Provides added support for propulsion and activities of daily living	More cost and weight than suspension support
Contour-molded foam over hard back		For people with unstable trunks or back curvatures needing support	Provides lateral trunk as well as back support Different size options	Higher cost and weight Cannot be resized More effort to break down chair for travel
Hardback with softer foam or gel central region		For consumers with asymmetries or prone to pain	Higher comfort Option to remove foam to obtain custom fit	Higher cost and more skill required of the practitioner Thicker foam requires a larger size and a wider seat frame

Horizontal Axle Position

Moving the axle forward moves the seat back relative to the rear wheels. This results in a shift of the user's weight to over or slightly behind the rear axles.[11] A more forward axle position requires less muscle effort because rolling resistance is lowered when more weight is distributed over the larger rear wheels than the smaller front casters.[43] This position also facilitates "popping a wheelie," negotiating obstacles, and ascending or descending curbs. However, moving the axle forward can make the wheelchair more "tippy" and difficult to push up a ramp because of the tendency to tip backward. For this reason, wheelchairs are usually delivered with the axle in the most rearward position possible. This position usually needs to be changed, based on input from the consumer and the rehabilitation professional. An antitipper (Figure 14-9) can help prevent rearward falls, but might also make it more difficult to negotiate a curb and perform a wheelie. Because of the effects on stability, the axle should be moved forward incrementally with input from the wheelchair user. Adding weight to the chair can also affect stability and maneuverability of the wheelchair.[36] Therefore, packages or backpacks ideally should be located underneath the seat of the wheelchair.

Vertical Axle Position

Raising the axle has the effect of lowering the seat, whereas lowering the axle raises the seat. A lower seat position can improve propulsion biomechanics by increasing hand contact with the pushrim lowering stroke frequency, and increasing mechanical efficiency.[6,8] Lowering the seat height also increases the stability of the wheelchair. If the seat height is too low, however, the patient has to push with the shoulder abducted. This can increase the risk of shoulder impingement, an upper limb injury common among manual wheelchair users. The ideal seat height is the point at which the angle between the upper arm and forearm is between 100 and 120 degrees when the hand is resting on the top and center of the pushrim (Figure 14-10, *A*).[6,58] An alternative method that can be used to approximate the same position and angle is to have the individual rest with their arms hanging at the side. The fingertips should be at the same level as the axle of the wheel. If the seat height is too high, less of the pushrim can be accessed and more strokes are needed to go the desired speed (Figure 14-10, *B*).

Amputee Axle

People with lower limb amputations might need to have their axles adjusted farther back than those without amputations to increase the stability of the wheelchair. This is due to the loss of the counterbalancing weight of the lower limbs. Amputee axle adapters can be attached to the wheelchair frame to add additional rearward axle positions. However, a rearward axle position can have serious negative effects on shoulder biomechanics.

BOX 14-2

Advantages and Disadvantages of Camber

Advantages

- Brings wheels inward and closer to the body, which enables the arms to access more of the pushrim
- Reduces shoulder abduction because the wheels are closer to the body
- Increases lateral stability

Disadvantages

- Wider wheelchair, which can be problematic in tight areas
- Diminished traction and uneven tire wear on a conventional tire (some tires have offset treads that accommodate for camber)

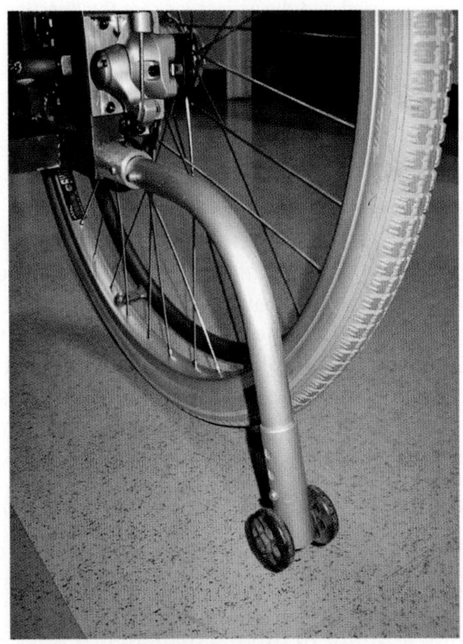

FIGURE 14-9 Antitipper.

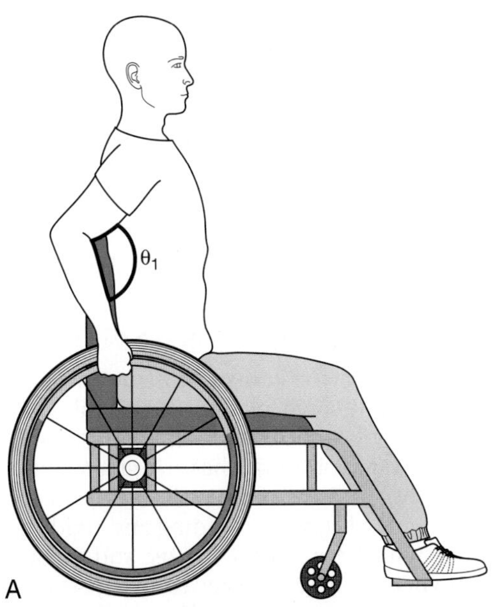

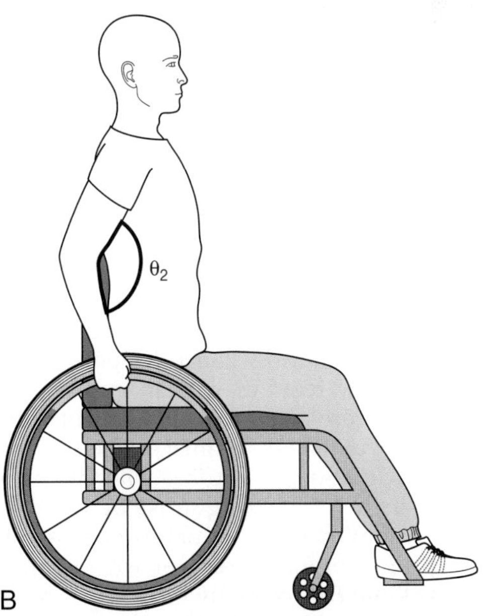

FIGURE 14-10 The differences in the elbow flexion angle (θ) and hand contact with the pushrim are shown after adjusting the height of the axle. **A,** The recommended elbow angle (θ_1 = 100 to 120 degrees). **B,** Angle θ_2 is larger because the seat is too high (axle too low), resulting in less hand contact with the pushrim.

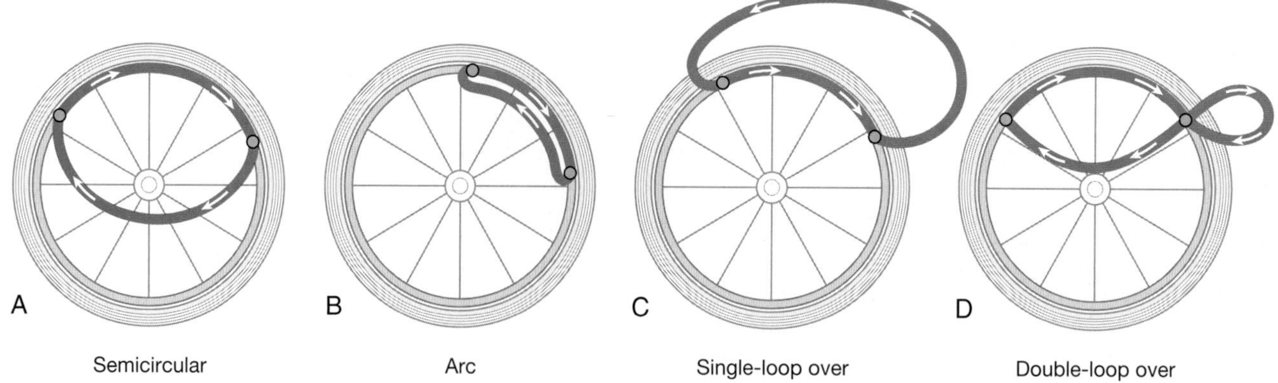

FIGURE 14-11 **A** to **D**, The four propulsion patterns identified from the hand motions of manual wheelchair users. The thick blue line on the wheel is the path followed by the hand, and the arrows indicate the direction the hand moves. The circles indicate hand-pushrim contact and hand release.

Wheelchair Propulsion

The ability to effectively propel the wheelchair depends on the physical capabilities of the individual (e.g., strength, stamina, spasticity, fatigue), the weight of the wheelchair, the quality of the wheelchair and setup, and the propulsion technique. The previously described service delivery process drives the assessment of the individual, the selection and setup of the wheelchair, and propulsion training. Effective propulsion is dependent on the services delivery model and the multidisciplinary team to maximize function while minimizing pain and injury.

Wheelchair Weight

The weight of the wheelchair is an important consideration, especially when recommending manual wheelchairs. Less propulsive force is needed to push a lighter wheelchair. Ultralight manual wheelchair frames and components are manufactured with materials having high strength-to-weight ratios, such as aluminum, titanium, and carbon fiber. One study, directly comparing ultralight and standard wheelchairs, found that ultralight wheelchair users pushed at faster speeds, traveled farther, and used less energy.[5] The reduction of force is even more prominent on inclines where gravitational forces increase the rolling resistance. The *Clinical Practice Guide*[9] recommends selecting the lightest wheelchair possible to minimize propulsive forces and maximize efficiency.

Quality of the Wheelchair and Setup

Ultralight wheelchairs have stronger, more durable components that are less likely to become misaligned with use, which helps minimize rolling resistance. Keeping the chair in good working order requires regular inspection for wheel lock, caster and tire alignment, as well as tire pressure.[15] Furthermore, ultralight manual wheelchairs are more durable than lightweight manual wheelchairs and standard wheelchairs.[17,18,31] Lowering stroke frequency and forces through a combination of propulsion training, wheelchair setup, and proper choice of wheelchair can protect the median nerve from injury.[9] The ability to configure an ultralight manual wheelchair to the unique characteristics of the individual and the improved durability of the ultralight manual wheelchair decrease the force necessary to propel the wheelchair, increase the maneuverability, and improve access to the community.

Propulsion Technique

The propulsion techniques of manual wheelchair users have been examined in detail.[8,9] Propulsive strokes are generally described in two phases: when the hand is in contact with the pushrim applying forces (contact phase), and when the hand is off the rim and preparing for the next stroke (recovery phase).[40] Four distinct propulsion patterns have been identified, which are defined by the path the hand takes during the recovery phase: arc, semicircular, single-looping over, and double-looping over (Figure 14-11). The single-looping over form of propulsion, which consists of having the hand above the pushrim during recovery, is the most prevalent pattern in individuals with paraplegia.[7] However, the semicircular pattern, in which the user's hand drops below the pushrim during recovery, has better biomechanics (see Figure 14-11, *A*). The semicircular pattern has been associated with lower stroke frequency and greater time spent in the push phase relative to the recovery phase.[7] The semicircular pattern is preferred because the hand follows an elliptical pattern, with no abrupt changes in direction and no extraneous hand movements. For example, a long stroke (see Figure 14-11, *A*), as opposed to a short stroke (see Figure 14-11, *B*), is likely to minimize the number of strokes needed to push at a desired speed. By applying forces to the pushrim in smooth, long strokes, the same amount of energy is imparted to the rim without high peak forces or a high rate of force loading.

Manual Wheelchair Transfers in Automobiles

For individuals who transfer to/from an automobile seat and use a manual wheelchair, the overall weight and compactness of the wheelchair is crucial for safe and effective transfers. Transportability has the greatest impact on individuals who use a two-door or four-door sedan as opposed to a van with a lift/ramp. Folding and rigid frame ultralight manual wheelchairs have assets and liabilities. Folding frame wheelchairs are easier to collapse for stowage, but are heavier and more cumbersome. Alternatively, the rigid frame wheelchair back supports fold down for increased compactness and quick-release axles allow for easy removal of the wheels. Therefore the rigid wheelchair is lighter and easier to stow. Although both wheelchairs are transportable, the decreased weight of the rigid ultralight manual wheelchair makes it a better option for many individuals.

Manual Wheelchair Components and Accessories

Components and accessories on wheelchairs allow the wheelchair to be individualized to the user's needs. Both power and manual wheelchairs have similar components, but some frame styles have standard options. The type of wheelchair frame dictates which components can be safely attached to the wheelchair. The components described in this section are listed from proximal to distal to illustrate how the components can affect the user's position in terms of proximal stability and distal function. Although seat cushions and back supports are often purchased separate from the wheelchair frame, they are essential for the overall function of the wheelchair system. Therefore, they are included in this section.

Wheelchair Seating

Wheelchairs can come with a seat pan or sling seat. There are times when this interface makes a difference in the seating comfort and/or pressure distribution. Most power wheelchairs come with a solid seat pan and most manual wheelchairs come with a sling seat. Some manual wheelchairs come with a solid seat pan that facilitates the long-term performance of the seat cushion.

Cushions are divided into five categories depending on the function of the cushion. The category of wheelchair cushions are: (1) general use, (2) skin protection, (3) positioning, (4) skin protection and positioning, and (5) custom-molded cushions. An algorithm is used to justify the classification of each cushion. The cushions themselves can consist of various mediums and properties such as foam, air, gel, foam, and various composites (Table 14-3).

Numerous components can be added directly to the wheelchair cushion or to the wheelchair frame to provide increased postural support. These include adductor pads, abductor pads, hip guides, positioning belts, and transfer handles. It is best to understand the user's range-of-motion and positioning needs so that the components can offer guidance and support to the user rather than trying to correct deficits in range of motion. Unnecessary components can be a source of pressure if used incorrectly and the chair should never be used to stretch a person. Careful attention to the seating assessment will prevent unnecessary use of these components.

Adductor pads prevent the thighs from abduction or lying to the side. Hip guides provide the same functionality. Hip guides can be used without adductor pads for increased proximal control. Both of these can be removed for transfers. Abductors pads (also known as pummels), by contrast, are used to control extensive adduction and offer more aggressive positioning than offered in a seat cushion. Careful attention to the amount of pressure on the thighs will prevent skin concerns. These should be removable or flip down, also, for transfers. These pads should never be used to prevent an individual from sliding out of the wheelchair.

Positioning belts can help keep the buttocks back in the seat and keep the individual from sliding forward. Positioning belts can be two-point or four-point positioning. Two-point positioning belts are traditionally applied anterior and inferior to the anterior superior iliac spine for best placement. Some individuals benefit from the seat belt being placed across the thighs. Options for attachment points are important to maximize this option. A four-point positioning offers more stability for the individual that does not maintain position with a two-point positioning belt. The belts can be padded, if necessary. Padding prevents skin breakdown over the pelvis for individuals who are thin and bony. Positioning belt releases come in options such as push button or airplane release.

Back Supports

Manual chairs come with sling backs, and most power chairs come with seat canes for attachment of an aftermarket back support. Similar to seat cushions, back supports are characterized by their function. The four categories of back supports are: (1) general use, (2) positioning, (3) skin protection and positioning, and (4) custom-molded backs. An algorithm for proper use of the back supports is necessary to properly justify the selection of back support. Back supports are typically planar, contour, or custom. Properties of back supports are typically limited to foam and combinations of foam/gel or foam/air (see Table 14-2). There are numerous contours and heights available in off-the-shelf back supports to match the unique characteristics of the individual.

Armrests

Armrests can assist the stability of the individual if they are positioned close to the individual and at the correct height. Some frame styles allow the armrests to be adjusted closer to the trunk for this increased stability. Armrests function as upper limb supports if positioned properly. The armrests themselves can be selected based on length of the armrest, height adjustment, materials of the arm pad, and styles. How the armrests are attached also plays a factor in the style of the device. Armrest lengths may be full length or desk length. Full-length armrests allow greater surface for the forearm and offer more assistance for sit-to-stand activities. Desk-length armrests are shorter than full-length armrests so that one can get closer to tables. Armrest pads can be standard leather, breathable materials, or gel pads. The wear and tear of the material should be taken into consideration because this is a surface that has a lot of interface with the user.

The attachment points of armrests include single post, dual post, and cantilever. Dual-post armrests can be swing away, whereas most single-post armrests must be removed. Cantilever armrests attach to the back of the chair and can swing behind the wheelchair. Stability and durability of the armrests should be investigated to match the needs of an individual.

Laterals and Chest Harnesses

Laterals and chest harnesses provide additional stability in conjunction with the back supports. Laterals come in various shapes, sizes, and contours. Identifying the positioning goals to select the appropriate size, shape, and

Table 14-3 Seat Cushions

Cushion Type	Image	Application	Benefits	Limitations
Plain rectangular foam		Low-risk patients	Inexpensive	No pressure relief regions Wears out in 6 months to a year Low maintenance
Contoured foam with skin		Provides cutaway regions to relieve pressure on bony prominences	Reduces risk of pressure ulcers Less expensive than custom-made cushion	Application limited to individuals without asymmetries Cushion has limited life expectancy
Carve and assemble foam		For patients with asymmetries needing custom cutouts	Low-cost method of custom fabrication Lightweight	Custom-fitted, hard to replicate
Contour-molded with gel-filled inserts		Higher risk patients prone to ulcers	Semiliquid gel will mold to body contours	Heavier than regular foam cushions Uncomfortable when cold
Air cushion with insert padding		For patients with asymmetries The air-filled tetrahedron "balloons" can be nested together to build shape	Lightweight, personalized fit No special tools required	Moderate cost Lower life expectancy Customization harder to replicate
Matrix of air-filled elastic capsules		High-risk patients who cannot maintain skin integrity with foam products	Improved pressure relief Bladders can be tied off to create pressure relief regions	More expensive than foam cushion Loss of trunk stability Bladders can be punctured High maintenance
Alternating air cell inflation		Very–high-risk patients with intractable ulcers	Battery-powered air compressor sequentially inflates and deflates cells	Cost >$2000 Requires charging Electronics add complexity

contour is important. Laterals can be removed or swung away from the wheelchair. This option allows the user to have minimal disruption during transfers. Furthermore, individuals may only use swing-away or removable laterals for specific activities such as driving or during transportation. Harnesses can be divided into shoulder and chest harnesses. They come in various shapes and sizes as well as materials.

Shoulder harnesses are designed to provide shoulder retraction, good head control, and to correct shoulder rotation. They typically attach to the top of the wheelchair near the clavicle and at the bottom of the back support near the inferior/posterior aspect of the rib cage. Chest harnesses provide more support than shoulder harnesses and offer increased support to the trunk. Chest harnesses can be incorporated into the shoulder harness for full support or can simply be attached horizontally across the chest for stability. Single chest harnesses cover the lateral aspect of the chest and do not interfere with the shoulders. Chest harnesses are commonly used in driving for stability, but do not replace the occupant restraint system. Most school systems require pediatric wheelchair users to use a chest harness, a positioning belt, and a headrest when being transported in a school bus.

Headrests

Headrests can also come in various shapes and sizes. They may range in function from providing minimal head control when an individual tilts a wheelchair to providing maximal head control in all situations. Proper assessment of the needs and ability of the user is necessary to assure the headrest is providing support and not completely holding the head up. Headrests can be removable or swing away. Removing a headrest is important for transfers and can also be convenient if the headrest is not used all the time. Some headrests are only used during transportation and the user may not need it during the day.

Footrests, Leg Rests, and Footplates

Footrests, leg rests, and footplates are referred to collectively as front rigging (Table 14-4). These components provide support for the legs and feet. Footrests can come

Table 14-4 Front Riggings

Description	Image	Application	Benefits	Limitations
Fixed frame integrated		Used on ultralight and sport frame wheelchairs	Lightweight, no detachable parts	Limited to no adjustability Minimal foot stabilization provided
Swing-away tubular footrests with folding footplates and heel loops		Standard hardware used on most manual wheelchairs Tube lengths can be adjusted	Easy removal for transfers Footplates typically fold Convenient for travel	Additional weight No footplate angle adjustments Fixed angle tubing
Higher adjustability footrests and calf supports		Elevating footrest provides leg and footplate angle adjustability	Better foot support for individuals with lower limb abnormalities Permits leg elevation for comfort	More expensive More weight and complexity
Power-elevating leg rests		Accessory for power chairs Provides appropriate leg support for power tilt and recline users	Allows for independent positioning through joystick or other input method Removable or swing away	Extra cost Additional complexities of motor drive and requires power supply cable
Flip-up–flip-down footplate for power wheelchairs	A B	Unimpaired lower extremity posture	Less stigmatizing Easier to operate Improved driving clearances	Transfers might be more difficult

in options that are removable, flip-up, or rigid to the chair. The footrests and footplate support the feet and the leg rests support the calves.

Removable leg rests are important for transfers and when using the feet during propulsion. Footrests can be flip-up and mounted on swing-away hangers to get them out of the way of transfers or they can be center-mounted and flip-up. Power wheelchairs may have a center-mount, flip-up footplate. Ultralight rigid chairs have a footplate mounted in the center of the rigid front end. Angle adjustable footplates accommodate lack of ankle range of motion. Ankle huggers, heel loops, footstraps, or shoe cup holders on footplates can be provided for additional positioning for the user.

The angle of the footrests can vary from a standard angle of 70 degrees to a more custom angle of 85 degrees. Elevating leg rests allow the foot to extend out independent of the hip moving.

Ultralightweight chairs commonly have rigid foot riggings and the footplate is integrated in the frame to reduce the overall weight of the wheelchair. These can be tapered (closer to the legs) or standard to allow more room near the calves/legs. The degree of taper is dependent on the preference of the individual. A tightly tapered foot rigging allows for greater maneuverability and less bulkiness of the frame.

Careful attention to hamstring length during the seating evaluation will allow the feet to rest in a comfortable position on the footplates. Tight hamstrings are a common cause of poor pelvis and foot positioning. The chair should not be used to stretch the legs, but should accommodate for any range-of-motion limitations.

Wheels and Tires

There are several factors to consider when choosing the most suitable wheel and tire configuration, including type of indoor and outdoor terrain, activity level, maintenance, weight, and cost. Many standard and lightweight wheelchairs come equipped with either mag-style or spoke wheels (Figure 14-12). Mag wheels are made from composite plastics or metal (initially they were made from magnesium, hence the term *mag*). They are usually heavier than spoke wheels, but are more durable and require less maintenance. Newer types of mag wheels are composed of high-strength lightweight materials and can even be lighter than spoke wheels, but are more costly. Spoke wheels have a tendency to get out of alignment (wheel wobbles when spun), requiring a trip to a bicycle shop or a wheelchair dealer to true the wheels.

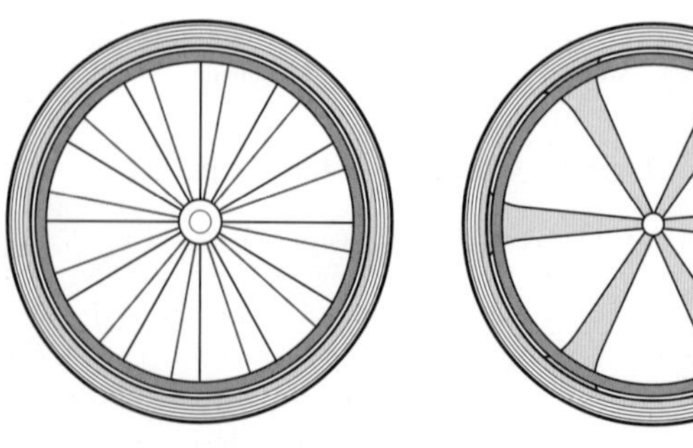

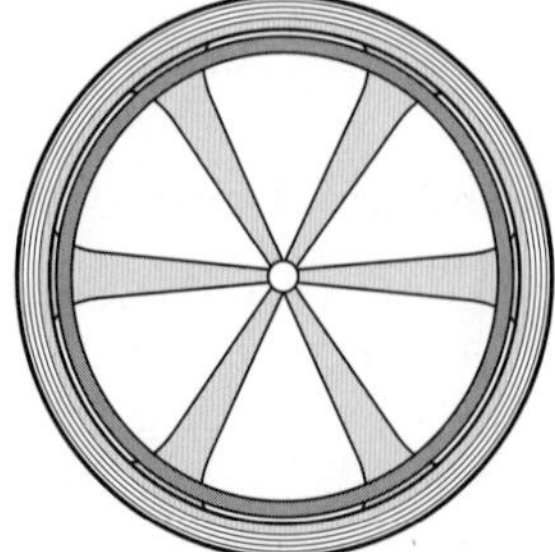

FIGURE 14-12 Mag and spoke wheels.

Wheels are available in many different sizes. The most common rear tire diameters for manual wheelchairs are 22, 24, and 26 inches. Smaller tires can be found on pediatric manual wheelchairs and wheelchairs that are foot-propelled to keep the seat-to-floor height at a minimum.

Tires are available in many different tread designs and widths to accommodate almost any type of terrain, as well as the mobility needs of the individual. Treads range from very smooth to extremely knobby, such as those typically seen on high-performance mountain bikes. Smoother tread and skinnier tires result in a lower rolling resistance. If the wheelchair is primarily used indoors, a smooth to lightly treaded skinny tire is most desirable. If the wheelchair will be used outdoors, however, a wider tire with a medium knobby tread provides increased traction on rougher surfaces. The inner part of the tire or insert can either be air-filled (pneumatic) or solid foam. A pneumatic tire has a smoother ride for indoor or outdoor propulsion and has lower rolling resistance than solid tires,[52] but requires more maintenance (e.g., need to be able to repair a flat). Many standard and lightweight wheelchairs are equipped with solid plastic or foam tires, which require less maintenance than air-filled tires, but tend to be heavier than pneumatic wheels.

Caster wheels also come in various sizes and configurations. Smaller casters provide for greater foot clearance and agility, but are more apt to get stuck in cracks and at bumps, causing forward falls. They are often found on high-performance, ultralight, and sports wheelchairs. The smallest casters available for manual wheelchairs are approximately 2 inches in diameter and are the same type used on most "in-line" skates. Casters may be as large as 8 inches in wheelchairs designed for daily use. The larger casters can provide the user with more security because they roll over changes in surface height more easily. Similar to the rear tires, casters can be either pneumatic or solid (usually made of polyurethane). The polyurethane casters are very durable, but do not offer the user as much comfort as the pneumatic tires.

Wheel Locks

Wheel locks are also commonly referred to as brakes. They come in various styles but basically consist of two levers hinged together. When one lever is pulled (or pushed), the other presses against the wheel and holds it in place. Sometimes the levers are difficult for people to reach or manipulate. Devices called wheel lock extensions can be added to lengthen the lever arm. Wheel locks are essential for safety; however, some wheelchair users opt not to have them on their wheelchair. This is usually due to the user's hands interfering with the braking levers or parts when the user propels the wheelchair. Not having wheel locks requires that users be able to stabilize themselves well enough with the upper body, either by grasping the tires or nearby surfaces, or both. This unfortunately can result in awkward postures and excessive strain on the upper body and back. A wheelchair without wheel locks also makes it more difficult to keep stable when transferring to and from the wheelchair.

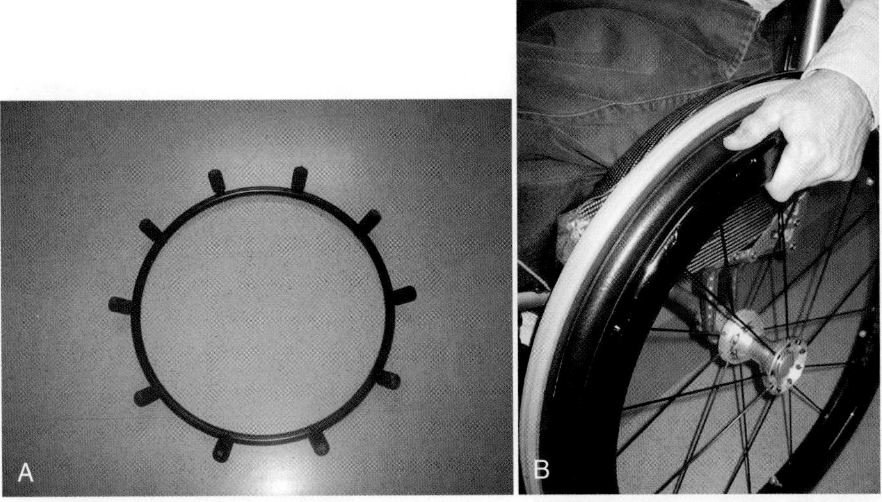

FIGURE 14-13 **A,** Pushrim with angled projections. **B,** Contoured pushrim with large surface area for gripping.

Grade Aids

Grade aids are devices that attach to the frame and are used for people who have difficulty with slopes and have a tendency to roll backward down hills. These devices prevent the wheelchair from rolling backward.

Pushrims

Pushrims are available in different sizes, shapes, and surface finishes. The pushrim most commonly found on wheelchairs is approximately 0.5 of an inch in diameter with a smooth surface finish and round cross-sectional area (Figure 14-13). People who have limited gripping ability (e.g., low-level cervical injuries) might need a larger diameter pushrim or a high-friction surface finish (e.g., vinyl or foam), or both. Sometimes these individuals need a pushrim with vertical, horizontal, or angled projections (see Figure 14-13, *A*) to be able to effectively propel their wheelchairs. New designs provide for greater surface area via an oval cross-section (see Figure 14-13, *B*) and are contoured for a more natural hand grip.

Lever Drives

Propelling the wheelchair with levers versus pushrims has proven to be more mechanically efficient. Dual-lever drive wheelchairs are more common in Europe, China, and other countries of the Far East. They are well suited for people who frequently propel long distances and over outdoor terrain (e.g., dirt roadways). The drawbacks to using a lever drive system include difficulties with maneuvering in tight places, transfers, and transportability. Single-lever drive systems are very popular in the United States and allow for the wheelchair to be propelled with one arm (Figure 14-14).

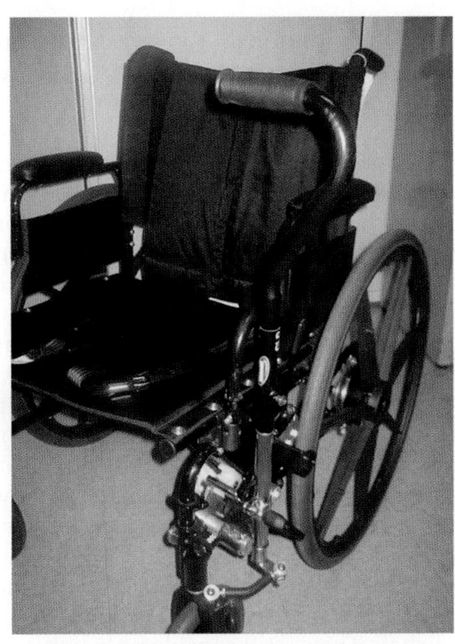

FIGURE 14-14 One-arm lever drive system.

Antitippers

Antitippers are devices that attach to the rear of the wheelchair frame and usually have adjustable length tubes with small wheels at the end (see Figure 14-9). These devices protect the user from tipping the wheelchair backward, but can make it difficult for the user to ascend a curb or pop a wheelie. The tube length can be adjusted to allow the user to traverse over small obstacles while still providing some stability. New manual wheelchairs generally come equipped with antitippers; however, high-end users often remove them after receiving the wheelchair.

Geared and Power-Assisted Wheelchairs

Geared and power-assist devices are appropriate for individuals who use or prefer their manual wheelchairs for mobility, but who need some assistance to reduce the physical effort required to self-propel. These devices are recommended for individuals with muscle paralysis or weakness, overuse, and fatigue. They are also ideal for individuals who are apprehensive about transitioning to a power wheelchair. A power wheelchair is often viewed by

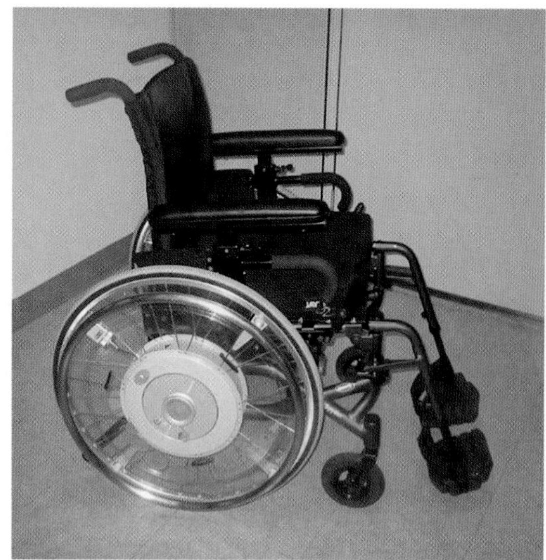

FIGURE 14-15 Pushrim-activated power-assist wheelchair.

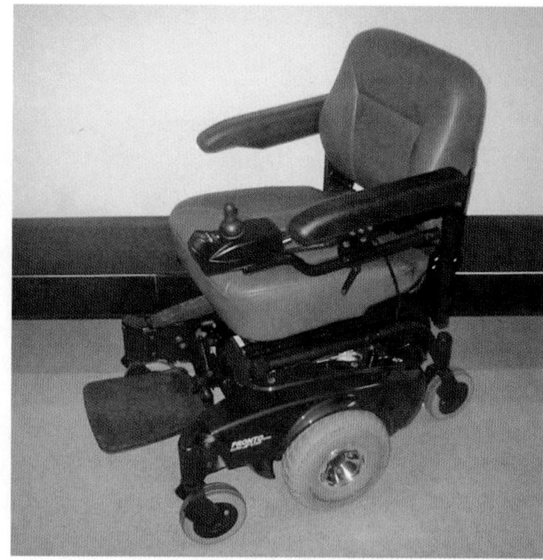

FIGURE 14-16 Basic power wheelchair.

peers as being "more disabled," too large for use in a home, too expensive, or too difficult to transport. A geared wheelchair does not require batteries and works similar to a bicycle, allowing the user to shift into a lower gear when climbing hills or rolling over uneven or rough terrain. Power-assist devices include stand-alone powered units that are partially powered by pushrim activation. Figure 14-15 shows a pushrim-activated system with motors in the wheelchair hubs. Geared and power-assist devices cost less than a fully powered wheelchair system, but require that the individual has a manual wheelchair that is compatible with the power-assist device.

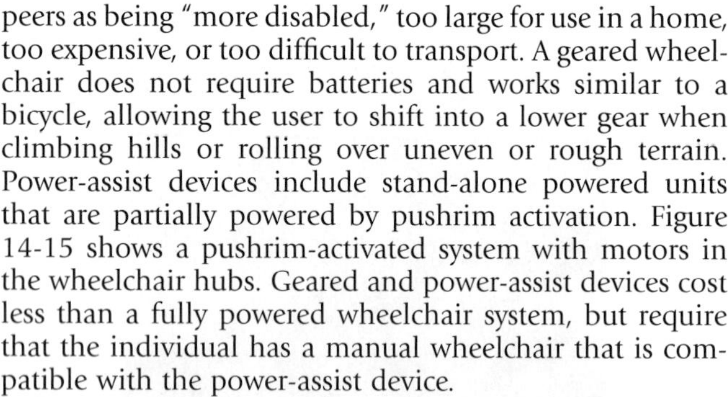

Research has shown that using a geared or pushrim-activated wheelchair results in significant reductions in the physical and physiologic demands of propulsion compared with using a manual wheelchair.[19,30] Power-assist devices can increase the width or length of the manual wheelchair base a few inches. Both geared and power-assist devices are more difficult to transport than manual wheelchairs because the equipment adds between 10 and 50 lb to the wheelchair. This is still considerably lighter, however, than a power wheelchair.

Power Wheelchairs

People who do not have the strength or stamina to propel manual wheelchairs typically need power wheelchairs for mobility independence. Power wheelchairs can be grouped into four broad categories based on wheelchair features and their intended use: (1) basic power wheelchairs, (2) folding and transport power wheelchairs, (3) combination indoor-outdoor power wheelchairs, and (4) all-terrain power wheelchairs.[42] All the power wheelchair categories include standard bases that support individuals who weigh up to 250 or 300 lb, depending on the model. Heavy-duty and extra–heavy-duty base options are available to support heavier and larger individuals. Power wheelchairs now provide a flexible platform for mobility when a manual wheelchair or power-assist wheelchair no longer meets the unique characteristics of an individual.

Basic Power Wheelchairs

Basic power wheelchairs have simple electronics, a standard proportional joystick, and limited seating options (Figure 14-16). They are low cost and low quality (see the section on Wheelchair Standards later). They are designed for light use on indoor surfaces.[23] They are appropriate for limited indoor use for individuals with a short-term disability who have good trunk control and do not need specialized seating.

Folding and Transport Power Wheelchairs

Folding and transport power wheelchairs are designed for disassembling to facilitate transport (Figure 14-17). They are usually compact for indoor use and have a small wheelchair footprint (i.e., area connecting the four wheels) for greater maneuverability in confined spaces. They might not, however, have the stability or power to negotiate obstacles outdoors. The batteries are often housed in separate boxes having easy-to-separate electrical connectors. These wheelchairs are typically used by individuals with reasonably good trunk and upper body control.

Combination Indoor-Outdoor Power Wheelchairs

Combination indoor-outdoor power wheelchairs (Figure 14-18) are intended for individuals with long-term disabilities and are designed for indoor surfaces and on finished surfaces (e.g., sidewalks, driveways, etc.) in the community. These wheelchairs, depending on the model, will support simple to advanced controllers, a wide range of input devices (e.g., proportional and nonproportional), and power seating options (e.g., tilt, recline, leg rests). Some of the power chairs in this category incorporate drive wheel suspension to reduce road vibrations. They come with either simple seating (such as that shown in Figure 14-19) or rehabilitation seating (see Figure 14-18). Rehabilitation seating allows for the attachment of modular

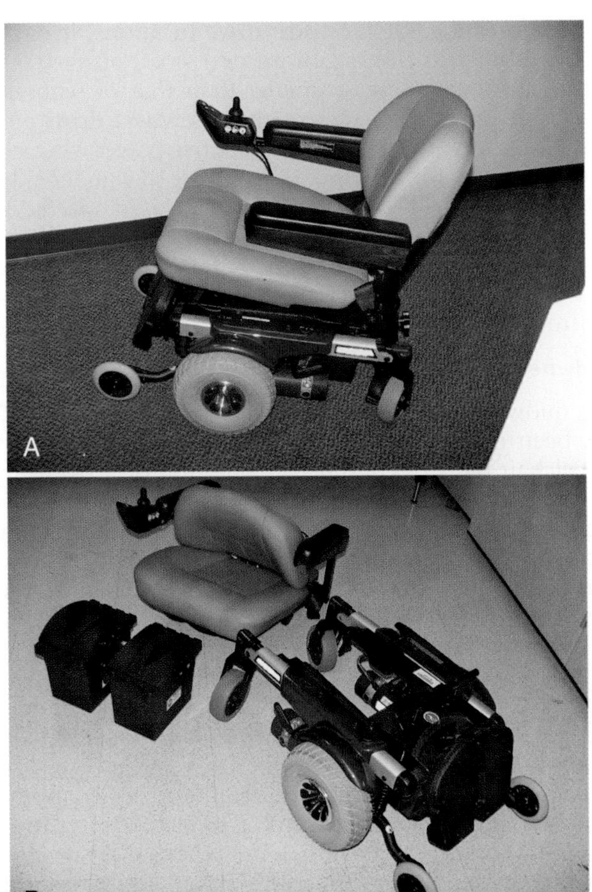

FIGURE 14-17 **A** and **B,** Transportable, lightweight power wheelchair.

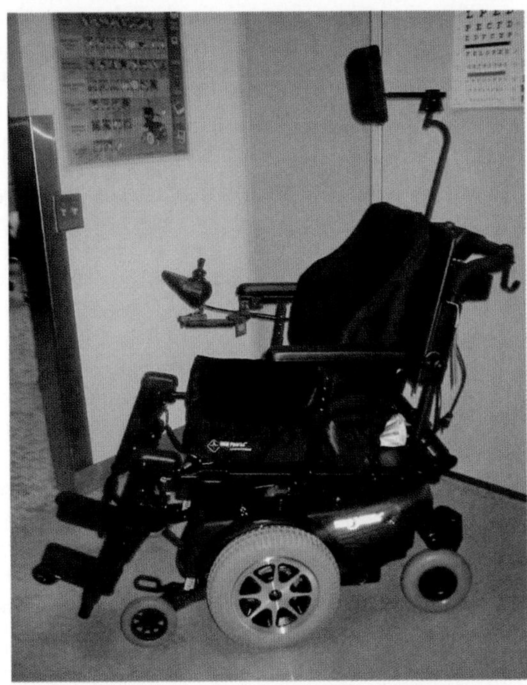

FIGURE 14-18 Indoor-outdoor power wheelchair shown with rehabilitation seating, a power tilt and recline seating system, headrest, and power-elevating leg rests.

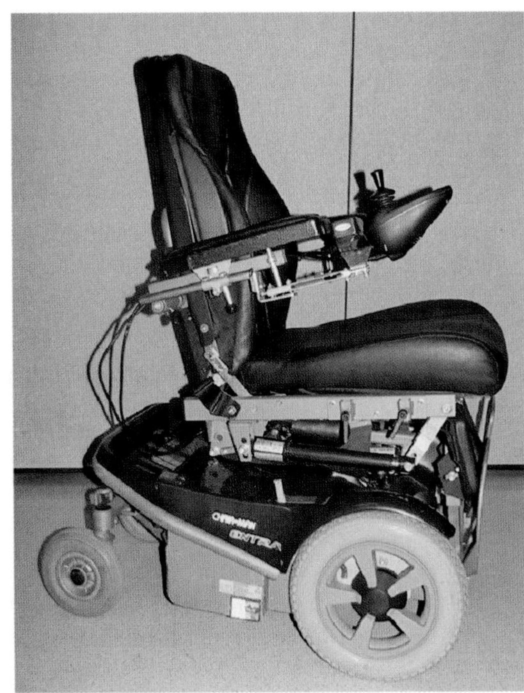

FIGURE 14-19 Front-wheel drive power wheelchair.

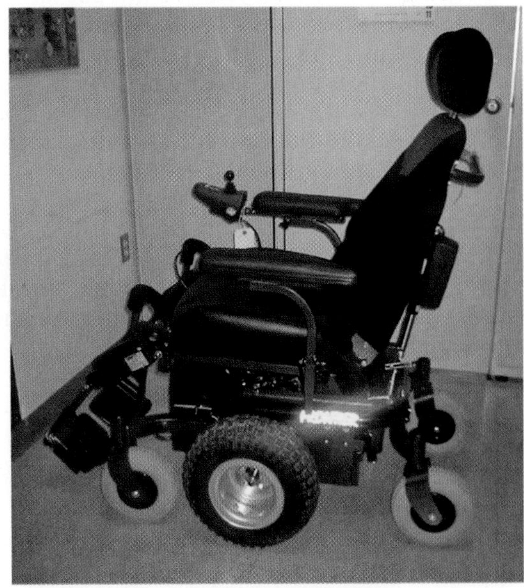

FIGURE 14-20 Heavy-duty indoor-outdoor power wheelchair.

seating hardware (e.g., backrests, cushions, laterals, hip guides, and headrests).

All-Terrain Power Wheelchairs

All-terrain indoor-outdoor power wheelchairs (Figure 14-20) are for use by people who live in communities without finished surfaces. These wheelchairs usually have more powerful motors, drive wheel suspensions, large-diameter drive wheels with heavily treaded tires, or four-drive wheels for climbing obstacles and traversing rough terrains. They are capable of faster speeds and offer greater stability on steeper inclined surfaces than the wheelchairs in the other categories.

Power wheelchairs typically use two deep-cycle lead-acid batteries in series, each producing 12 V, for a total of 24 V. The two most common types of lead-acid batteries found in power wheelchairs are the absorbent glass mat (AGM) and gelled electrolyte lead-acid (GEL) batteries. The AGM batteries are a newer technology that delivers greater power, range, and battery life over the GEL type.

Power Drive Wheel Location

There are three basic drive wheel locations for power wheelchair bases: front-wheel, midwheel, and rear-wheel drive. The drive configuration of a power wheelchair plays an important role in how well a chosen power wheelchair fits the lifestyle and environment of the user.

Rear-Wheel Drive

Rear-wheel drive is characterized by large drive wheels in the rear and small pivoting casters in the front (Figure 14-21). The rear-wheel drive power wheelchair steers and handles predictably, and naturally tracks straight, making it the most appropriate drive configuration for high-speed applications. Traditionally, rear-wheel drive was preferred by people who drive with special input devices (chin joystick, head array, etc.) or have reduced fine motor coordination because of its consistent tracking. However, this is changing because of the improved control systems on midwheel and front-wheel drive power wheelchairs. The disadvantages of rear-wheel drive include limited obstacle climbing by the small front casters. It also has the largest turning radius among the three drive locations.

Front-Wheel Drive

The front-wheel drive power wheelchair features large drive wheels in the front and small pivoting casters in the rear (see Figure 14-19). It is a very stable setup for uneven terrain and hills. Of the three drive locations, it has the best capability to climb forward over small obstacles. The overall turning radius is smaller than that of rear-wheel drive, but larger than that of the midwheel drive power base. Traditionally, the front-wheel drive power wheelchair has a tendency for the back of the chair to wander side to side ("fishtailing"), especially with increased speeds. This directional instability requires steering corrections that could make the wheelchair difficult for some users to steer. However, this is no longer an issue as a result of improved control systems.

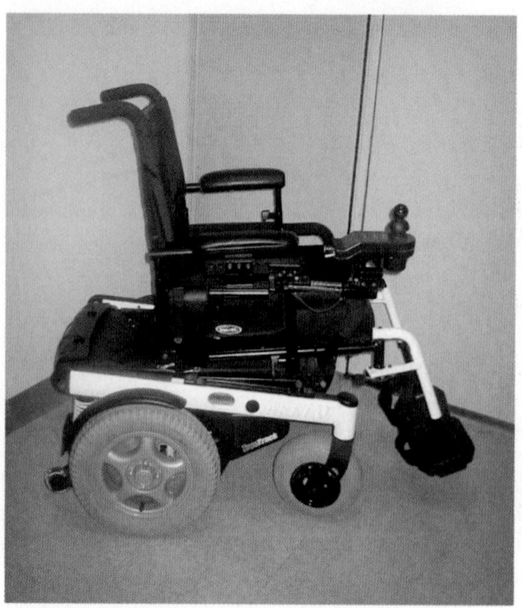

FIGURE 14-21 Rear-wheel drive power wheelchair.

Midwheel Drive

The midwheel drive power wheelchair (see Figure 14-20) has been one of the fastest growing power bases in the wheelchair industry. In this configuration the drive wheels are located near the center of the power wheelchair, allowing the user to seemingly turn in place, dramatically increasing indoor maneuverability. The midwheel drive is among the most effective at both ascending and descending obstacles for skilled, practiced users. Most midwheel drive wheelchairs have front and rear antitip casters that actively raise or lower to keep the wheelchair stable when ascending or descending curbs and to compensate for changes in the terrain while driving. A center-wheel drive location (e.g., type of midwheel drive where the drive wheels are located directly under the user) enables for a more compact footprint and a tighter turning radius. One of the concerns with a midwheel drive location, however, is that when riding on uneven terrain or up and down curb cuts with a steep transition, there is a possibility of getting "stuck" on the front or rear casters. This can suspend the drive wheel in midair with no contact with the ground.

Overall, there is no perfect drive configuration for a power wheelchair, as all have their advantages and disadvantages. The mobility of an individual is optimized by aligning his/her needs with the characteristics of each configuration, and evaluating models within the categories.

Input Methods

The interface between the wheelchair user and the wheelchair itself is often the most crucial component of a power wheelchair. A safe, consistent, and reliable method of accessing powered mobility can sometimes be the most difficult step in wheelchair assessment and evaluation.[10] Newer plug-and-play technology allows individuals to try different input devices during the evaluation. As the medical condition of the individual changes, expandable electronics allow for changes in the input device without replacing the electronics or the wheelchair.

There are many different types of input devices and control methods that can be used to operate a power wheelchair. The most common input device is a joystick that is programmed for proportional control (Figure 14-22). If an individual cannot use a joystick, then a myriad of alternative controls are available. These controls range from mechanical switches, pneumatic switches, fiber-optic sensors, and proximity sensors to joysticks placed at the head, chin, or foot.

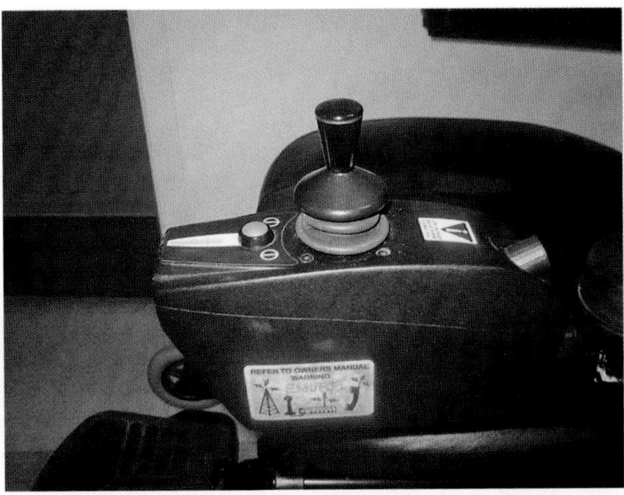

FIGURE 14-22 Conventional position-sensing joystick.

Proportional Control Versus Switched Control

Proportional control is usually the optimum solution for wheelchair control because it provides continual adjustment of speed and direction. A proportional joystick can use either a position-sensing or force-sensing method. The control output from a position-sensing joystick is proportional to the deflection of the joystick from a neutral position. A change in electrical resistance or inductance can be used to signal the position of the joystick. The control output from a force-sensing joystick is proportional to the force exerted on the stick by the user.[25] A strain gauge bridge is usually instrumented to the joystick shaft to measure forces. Force-sensing joysticks could be effective for individuals with tremors, spasms, and limited range of motion.

For users with limited hand function or fine motor control, the joystick can be mounted on a wheelchair and positioned to operate by the chin, head, shoulder, elbow, arm, knee, foot, or tongue. Although chin or head control joysticks can be effective, they are visually intrusive and could obstruct some of the daily functional activities. They are also difficult to use to steer accurately over uneven and rough surfaces because of the relative movements of the joystick and head. With the proportional head control, if users do not have refined head control their speed might be erratic. Users also tend to forcefully extend the neck and sustain pressure on the headrest to move the wheelchair forward, which could increase muscle tone and trigger other reflexive reactions. Switched head control does not require any pressure to activate and prevents further increases in muscle tone.

Joysticks can be ordered in various sizes (e.g., "mini" for small movements) and with different shaped handles (e.g., round, oblong, goalpost-shaped). Alternative joysticks are available that require a smaller range of motion and less force to deflect the lever. A touchpad, which works similar to a mouse pad on a laptop computer, is another type of proportional input device that can be used to operate a power wheelchair.

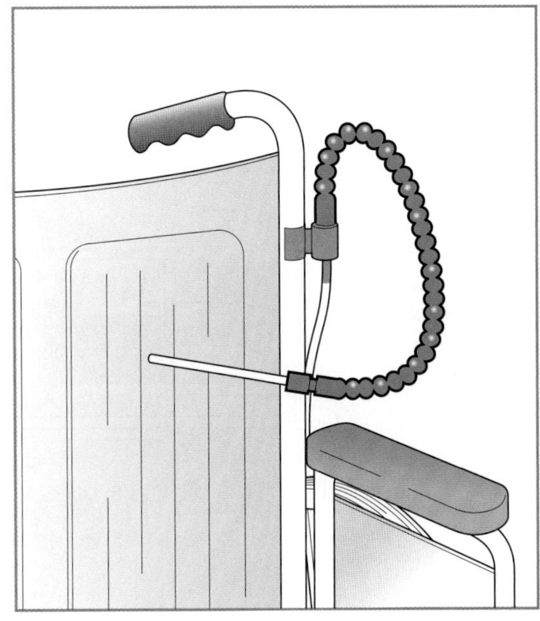

FIGURE 14-23 Sip-and-puff input device.

Nonproportional Drive Control

If the user does not have the fine motor skills necessary for reliable control of a proportional joystick, a nonproportional joystick could be chosen. A nonproportional joystick moves in a limited number of discrete directions (usually four or eight). These directions typically are forward, reverse, left and right, and the four diagonal directions. Speed is not directly controllable when the joystick is configured for nonproportional control and must be preprogrammed.

A variety of switches are available for nonproportional drive control. Switches can be either mechanical or electrical. Mechanical switches require physical contact with the switch and range in size and the amount of force required to activate them. The placement site of the switch is also crucial to achieving the accuracy and consistency needed to use the wheelchair safely. A sip-and-puff input device is a type of mechanical switch for users who cannot reliably access a switch with any other part of the body but their mouth (Figure 14-23). Sip-and-puff systems consist of a tube mounted near the mouth that the user can either puff air into or sip from. The direction of air into and out of the tube and the strength of the puff or sip (e.g., a hard puff versus a soft puff) allow for differencing between different movements of the wheelchair.

Electrical switches do not require a direct touch to operate. When motor control and coordination is impaired, a head array with proximity switches may be considered. A head array consists of a three-piece headrest (two side pads and one center) with proximity switches built into each pad. By placing the head near to the switch imbedded in the center pad, the individual moves the wheelchair forward. Activating the side pads moves the wheelchair in the corresponding direction. A separate reset switch toggles between the forward and reverse functions. Similar to the switched joystick, the head array offers control in four or

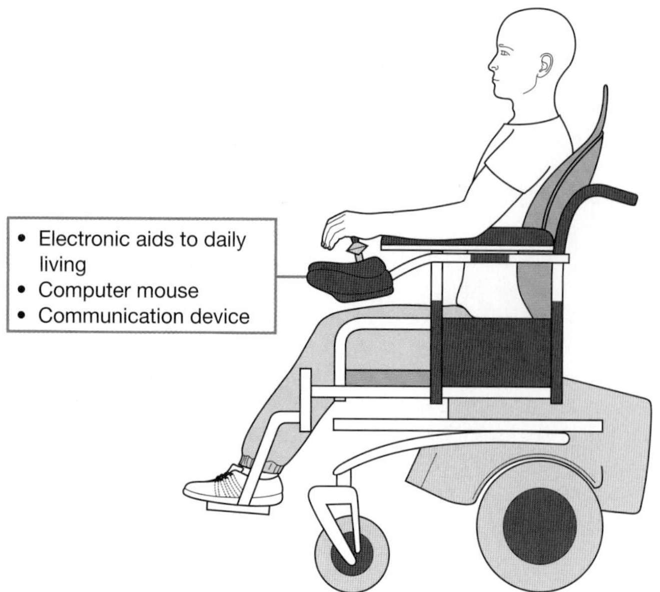

FIGURE 14-24 Diagram of integrated control system.

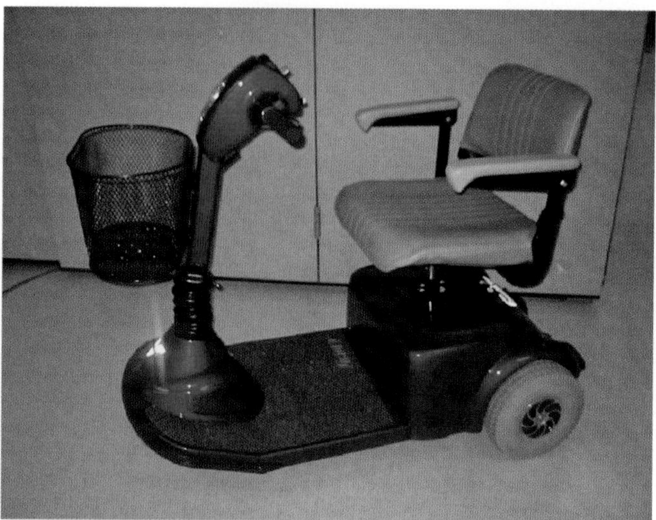

FIGURE 14-25 Three-wheeled scooter.

eight directions if an individual can simultaneously activate two switches at the same time (e.g., forward/right or forward/left). Fiber-optic switches are another type of electrical switch that activates when a body part interrupts a beam of light.

The use of alternative input devices and nonproportional drive control requires an expandable controller on the power wheelchair. If an alternative input method is thought to be required eventually as the medical condition of the user diminishes, an expandable controller should be considered at the time of initial wheelchair prescription to allow for anticipated use of an alternative control. Trying out different input devices and types of drive control during the initial assessment is essential to ensuring success with wheelchair mobility.

Integrated Controls

Wheelchair input devices are used for controlling both wheelchairs and electronic aids to daily living, speech-generating devices, or computers. When a single control interface (e.g., joystick, touchpad, or switch) is used to operate two or more assistive devices, the system is called an integrated control system (Figure 14-24).[24] Although integrated control is beneficial, users can lose access to every operation mode if the input device is broken. Therefore, it is important to consider the overall goals, the local technical support, and the training requirements when integrating the controls into a single system.

Programmability

Performance of a power wheelchair depends on the setup and configuration of the wheelchair controller. Programming or fine-tuning the wheelchair to meet the needs of the individual user can improve control, safety, and maneuverability. Fast and simple adjustments can be made for directional control (forward, reverse, and turning), speeds (acceleration and deceleration), and sensitivity of the joystick. These adjustments affect how the wheelchair responds to different commands.

The maximum speed of power wheelchairs varies significantly among different manufacturers and models. Wheelchairs are typically programmed for higher speeds when they are used outdoors. A slow mode of operation is needed for maneuvering indoors. Braking or deceleration is another crucial adjustment for maintaining a safe position for users in the wheelchair. An extremely sensitive setting can cause users to be thrown forward when they release the joystick, whereas a mildly sensitive setting can cause the wheelchair to coast and not stop in time to avoid an obstacle. The sensitivity of an input device can compensate for physical limitations or unintentional movements of users so that they have full and safe control of the power wheelchair.

Scooters

A scooter is designed to provide intermittent mobility support for individuals with good arm strength, trunk balance, and ability to transfer in and out of the device. Scooters typically have a single motor for the rear wheels and a tiller for steering (which looks and acts like the handlebar on a bicycle). The tiller can be tilted forward or back and locked at any desired position. Thumb levers are used to generate forward and reverse motion and to control speed. Scooters are usually equipped with automatic braking (similar to power wheelchairs) and are not able to coast. Three-wheeled scooters (Figure 14-25) are more common than four-wheeled scooters (Figure 14-26), which can traverse more rugged terrain but are large for most indoor settings. Scooters cost less than a typical power chair.

Scooters usually have a wide turning radius, therefore requiring more room and effort to maneuver in closed or tight environments. They lack the capacity to modify the seating system to accommodate postural deformities and have limited control options. They cannot accommodate for changes as the user's needs change, and are not recommended for people with progressive medical conditions such as multiple sclerosis and amyotrophic lateral sclerosis.

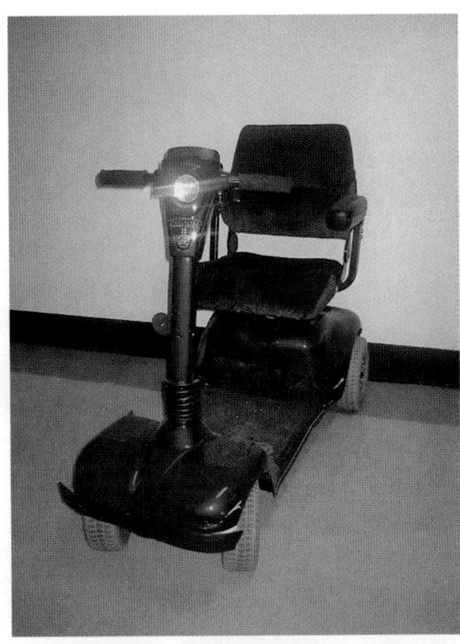

FIGURE 14-26 Four-wheeled scooter.

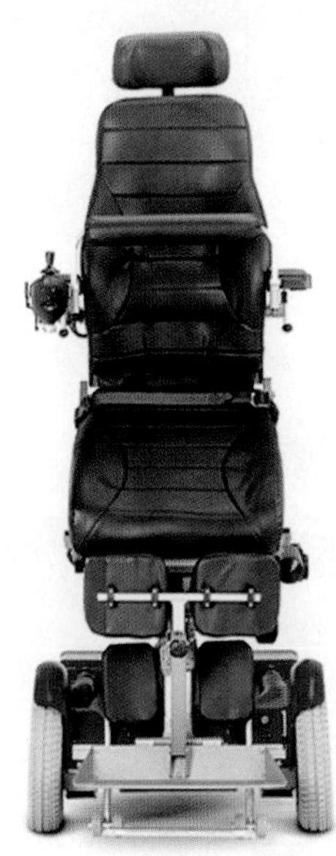

FIGURE 14-27 Standing wheelchair. (Courtesy Permobil, Lebanon, Tenn.)

Standing Wheelchairs

Standing wheelchairs offer a variety of advantages over standard wheelchairs. The ability of a person to achieve an almost vertical position has several advantages, including physiologic (i.e., pressure relief, improved circulation and digestion, and improved bone density), practical (i.e., improved reach to higher surfaces, which increases functional independence), and psychological (i.e., interacting with colleagues face to face) (Figure 14-27).[27]

Standing options are available on manual and power wheelchair bases. The standing option consists of a manual or powered lifting mechanism. Manual wheelchairs have either a manual or powered lift mechanism, whereas power wheelchairs have only powered lifting mechanisms. Powered lifts on power wheelchairs are generally activated with the same input device used for driving and require an expandable power wheelchair controller. When in the elevated position, the wheelchair has a higher center of gravity and for this reason the individual should use extreme caution when driving in a standing position outdoors or when on a cracked, rough, or broken floor indoors. Some systems incorporate an automatic wheel base adjustment that increases their stability when driving on nonlevel or uneven outdoor surfaces. Standing wheelchairs are safest when used on flat and smooth flooring and when the user is properly strapped and secured to the seat and seat back. People who have not stood for a long time might not have the hip, knee, or ankle range of motion to accommodate standing, and can experience orthostatic hypotension and injury. Although the standing mechanism adds weight to the wheelchair making it more difficult to lift and transport, advancements in design and material selection now make standing wheelchairs a good alternative to traditional manual and power wheelchairs.

Wheelchair Transportation

Wheelchair transportation primarily involves three components: (1) entering/exiting the vehicle, (2) securing the wheelchair, and (3) securing the occupant. The most common ways to get wheelchair users on/off of vehicles are ramps and lift systems. The most common methods for securing a wheelchair are the use of a stud-and-clamp–locking system or a four-point tie-down system. The most common occupant restraint system is the three-point system. The combination of these systems provides for safe travel. Wheelchair transportation has significant implications for an individual's overall mobility throughout the community.

Lifts

Lifts provide access to a vehicle through vertical translation of the wheelchair and occupant. A platform lift (Figure 14-28, *A*) folds out from the van similar to a drawbridge, and requires perpendicular access to load or unload a wheelchair. It also uses minimal storage space within the van, folding upright against the door. When a pull-in type of parking space is used, the equivalent of two parking spaces (8 to 10 feet) is needed to lower the platform lift and load or unload a wheelchair. A platform lift can also be installed on the rear door of the vehicle, but this often requires loading or unloading the wheelchair in a traffic lane. Rear door mounting also eliminates the use of space for extra passenger seats.

An overhead strap lift (Figure 14-28, *B*) uses an arm with nylon straps that attach to several points on the wheelchair and hook onto the arm of the lift. The lift has no platform and uses little storage space in the van. The wheelchair is loaded and unloaded perpendicular to the van, but less space is required because there is no platform to lower.

Several systems are available to ease transfers to the driver or passenger side seats. These systems provide a motorized option that allows for lowering and raising either the vehicle seat itself (Figure 14-28, *C*) or a platform that extends out from the vehicle (Figure 14-28, *D*) that the person can transfer to first. These systems usually do

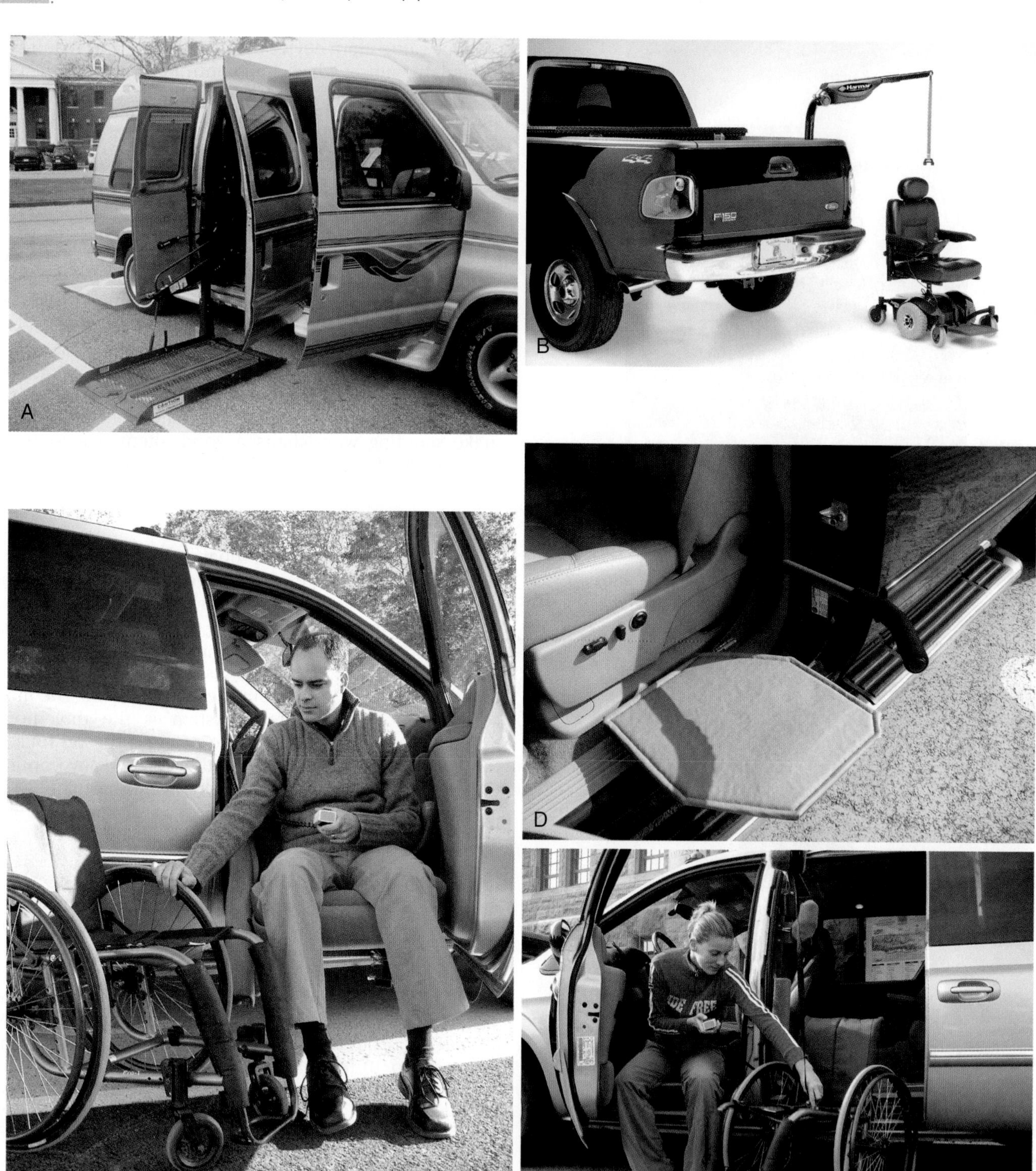

FIGURE 14-28 Vehicle lift systems. **A,** Platform lift. **B,** Overhead strap lift. (Courtesy Braun Corp., Winamac, Ind.) **C,** Automated height adjustable vehicle seat. **D,** Automated height adjustable platform. (Courtesy St. Lambert, Quebec, Canada.) **E,** Side-door overhead wheelchair lift system.

not require structural modifications to the vehicle and enable a safe and easy transfer because the surface the person is transferring to can be set at the same height as the wheelchair seat. Transferring to a higher surface is more difficult and strenuous because it requires greater force and range of motion to overcome the effects of gravity and should be avoided when possible. These systems align the seat next to the wheelchair and reduce the space separating the two surfaces, which further assists with transfers. For manual wheelchair users who are independent and drive, one potential solution would be to combine a transfer system with an overhead strap lift that attaches to the side door opening of a van. The lift stows the wheelchair behind the driver's seat (Figure 14-28, *E*).

Ramps

Ramps are the inexpensive alternatives to vehicle lifts.[56] They can be portable, mounted inside the vehicle (non-powered or powered), or integrated into the frame of the vehicle. Typically, they are installed in full-sized vans, mini-vans, and pick-up trucks. They are usually installed on the side or at the rear of the vehicle and have either a single track or double track with a nonslip surface. With powered ramps, a remote entry button opens the door and extends the ramp. Vehicles having powered ramps (Figure 14-29) can also have a "kneeling" feature that lowers the vehicle before extending the ramp to minimize the ramp slope. Selection of a ramp is based on the size and weight of the user and wheelchair. Also, the user's ability to push or drive up a ramp is a consideration when choosing a ramp or lift.

Tie-Downs and Securement

If a wheelchair user is going to remain in a wheelchair while riding, special tie-down or restraint systems for the wheelchair and the occupant must be used for safety. The wheelchair securement and occupant restraint system, when used properly, significantly increases the overall safety of the individual.[13,53] Wheelchairs are not designed to withstand crash-level forces like automobile seats are, and can be tipped over easily by even a minor collision or sudden braking of the vehicle. A tie-down system with an occupant restraint as well as wheelchair anchorage provides the best protection (Figure 14-30, *A*). A typical four-point restraint system has four webbing straps that are secured to the main frame of the chair. The preferred angles for rear wheelchair tie-down are between 30 and 45 degrees to the horizontal plane. The preferred angles for front tie-down are between 40 and 60 degrees to the horizontal plane. The wheelchair tie-down system only stops the chair from tipping or moving; it does not stop the occupant from being thrown out of the wheelchair in a collision or an emergency maneuver (e.g., sharp turn). In addition to the four-point wheelchair restraint system, a three-point lap and shoulder belt combination is required as the occupant restraint. Properly positioned lap and shoulder belts can prevent an occupant from falling out of the wheelchair or from being ejected from the vehicle. It can reduce chest and head excursions in a crash environment.[14] Although the four-point, strap-type securement system has been shown to be one of the most effective and versatile methods for securing a wide range of wheelchairs, it is also a system that is difficult and time-consuming to use.

A docking system (Figure 14-30, *B*) is another type of wheelchair restraint system. Docking systems typically include a stud or bolt that extends from the bottom of the wheelchair and is secured by a clamping mechanism mounted to the vehicle floor. The automatic clamping mechanism simply requires that the occupant guide the wheelchair over the top of the clamp until the interface on the wheelchair is fully engaged. A conveniently located push-button switch is used to release the wheelchair from the system. The advantages are that it is quick and easy to operate, and offers increased user independence. However, it is typically two to five times as expensive as standard belt restraint systems. Docking devices have been shown to work reasonably well for private (rather than public) vehicles in which the matching components can be individually configured to the specific wheelchair and vehicle.[14] A

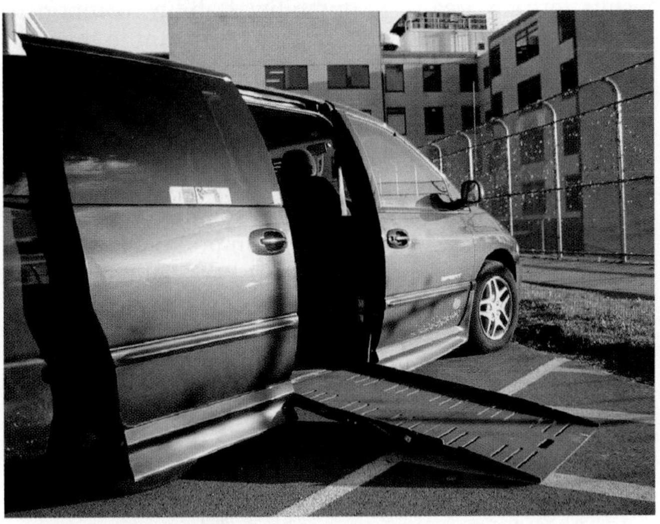

FIGURE 14-29 Modified minivan with powered ramp system.

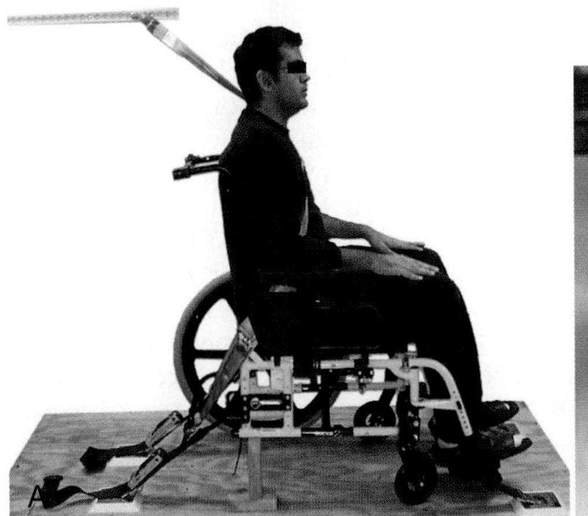

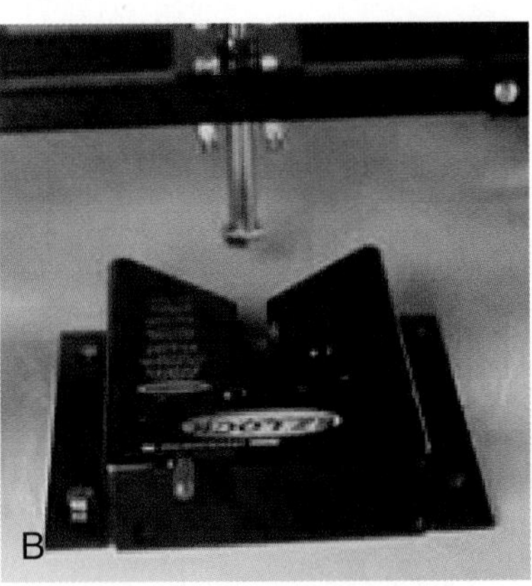

FIGURE 14-30 Wheelchair tie-downs and securement. **A,** Wheelchair and occupant restraint system. **B,** Wheelchair docking system.

universal design for docking systems does not currently exist; therefore, they are not used in public vehicles. Wheelchair tie-down and occupant restraint systems in conjunction with safe methods for entering and exiting vehicles provide increased community access for individuals using a wheelchair.

Wheelchair Standards

Wheelchair standards were developed to provide a means to objectively compare the durability, strength, stability, and cost-effectiveness of commercial products. Wheelchair standards are voluntary in the United States, but the test results are accepted by the U.S. Food and Drug Administration, which approves commercial marketability of the device. Most countries have adopted the International Organization for Standardization (ISO), which acts to continually develop and refine wheelchair standards. The ANSI and RESNA are member organizations of the ISO for the United States.

Fatigue testing is one of the procedures used to assess the strength and durability of a wheelchair and its components. This test involves subjecting the wheelchair to a large number of low-level stresses, similar to stresses experienced during daily use of the wheelchair. This is accomplished with two machines: a double-drum tester and a curb-drop tester. The double-drum tester consists of two rollers with 12-mm-high, 30-mm-wide slats attached to each drum to simulate bumps and small obstacles. The wheelchair or scooter is positioned over the rollers, which turn at 1 m/s for 200,000 cycles. The curb-drop tester lifts the wheelchair 5 cm and allows it to free-fall to a hard surface for a total of 6666 drops. The combination of double-drum and curb-drop testing simulates 3 to 5 years of wheelchair use. Some wheelchairs and scooters are tested until failure as opposed to stopping at the minimum number of cycles or drops. This information is used to calculate their cost-effectiveness.[31] Other tests include testing the durability and strength of wheelchair components (e.g., armrests, footrests, seat, backrest, wheels, casters, and pushrims), as well as static and dynamic stability (how stable the wheelchair or user is on various slopes). Wheelchair standards provide stakeholders (e.g., patients, clinicians, physicians, policymakers, and manufacturers) with information on safety and performance, thereby increasing the value of the mobility device to the patient.

Manual Wheelchair Performance

Ultralight wheelchairs have been shown to last approximately 13 times longer than standard wheelchairs and cost approximately three and a half times less to operate.[17] Ultralight wheelchairs last approximately five times longer and cost approximately two times less to operate than lightweight wheelchairs.[18] When tested to failure, ultralight wheelchairs had the longest survival rate and fewer catastrophic failures in comparison with standard and lightweight wheelchairs.[31] Ultralight models with suspension elements incorporated into the frame, the casters, or both perform similarly to lightweight wheelchairs with respect to wheelchair durability and cost-effectiveness.[39] Folding ultralight models are more durable and cost-effective than rigid ultralight models. However, folding models are not necessarily the better choice over rigid frames.[42] Although folding frames are collapsible to compress the overall size, their extra weight and bulkiness increases the stress on the upper limb joints of a user when lifting and manipulating the wheelchair into or out of a motor vehicle. Ultralight models in which the frame and parts are composed of titanium metal offer the lightest possible option in the ultralight category and have other advantages such as anticorrosive properties and a smoother ride. Wheelchairs made with titanium cost more up-front than those made with aluminum. However, they are as cost-effective as aluminum models when the initial cost is normalized by the fatigue life (e.g., number of double-drum and curb-drop cycles completed before failure).[42]

Power Wheelchair Performance

Power wheelchairs undergo all the same tests as manual wheelchairs in addition to a series of tests on the power and control systems and batteries. Power wheelchair test results indicate that combination indoor-outdoor models perform better than basic models in terms of durability (total equivalent cycles on the double-drum and curb-drop machine).[29,48] However, it is important to look at the test results in each area (e.g., durability, stability, component strength, etc.), in relation to what is important to the individual. For instance, a wheelchair might outperform others in terms of durability but have poor static and dynamic stability results. If durability is an important factor (most health insurance companies limit the patient to one wheelchair per 5 years), the user might choose to sacrifice the performance of the wheelchair for stability. Stability for certain individuals can be a more important factor than durability if the patient has a high risk for falling from the wheelchair or frequently traverses up and down steep ramps.

Power wheelchairs perform similarly to ultralight wheelchairs in terms of their durability.[29] With regard to value, power wheelchairs are more costly than ultralight and lightweight manual wheelchairs. They are, however, more economical than standard wheelchairs when considering how long they last, the number of repairs, the cost of repairs, and the initial cost of the device. Few test data have been reported on scooters and power-assist wheelchairs. Scooters and power-assist wheelchairs vary widely in performance, depending on the model.[34,54,] Scooters with bigger wheel bases and overall larger dimensions are more stable than scooters with smaller wheel bases. Overall, scooters and power wheelchairs are more durable than power-assist and manual wheelchairs.[59]

Using wheelchairs that are less prone to failure is safer for individuals.[35,57] Component failures and engineering factors are responsible for 40% to 60% of the injuries to power wheelchair users.[32,35] The number of wheelchair breakdowns and associated consequences (e.g., injuries, left stranded, missed work/school or medical appointments) have increased in recent years.[62] According to a recent survey, 60.4% of participants reported requiring one or more repairs to their power wheelchair over a 6-month period and 30.8% experienced one or more adverse consequences.[62] Additional research shows that the durability of wheelchairs has not improved significantly with the improvements in materials and technologies over time, which points to possible deficiencies in the design of the wheelchair or the quality control processes.[59] It is important that the reliability and cost-effectiveness data associated with the wheelchair make and model of interest be part of the wheelchair selection process.

Seat Functions: Tilt, Recline, and Elevation

Tilt and recline are useful for handling complex seating needs through pressure distribution management. If the individual has upper limb weakness or pain that limits independent weight relief (e.g., "push-up" or leaning to the side or forward), a wheelchair equipped with tilt or recline, or both, is needed. Seat elevators increase independence, productivity, and social interactions by extending reach capability, enabling and facilitating transfers, and providing peer height at different ages.[3,26] Table 14-5 provides an overview of the seating configurations possible.

Tilt

Tilt is also called "tilt-in-space" and refers to rotating the person's entire body, the seat base, and back and front rigging as a single unit in the sagittal plane. The traditional rocking chair provides an example of the tilt-in-space maneuver. Both manual and power wheelchairs can be ordered with a tilt feature. Tilt provides weight relief for the sitting surfaces by redistributing the effects of gravity away from the buttocks and onto the back. Tilt can also provide a position of rest and relaxation. A wheelchair with tilt is less stressful to the body than a reclining wheelchair because shear forces to the skin are almost negligible.

Recline

Recline refers to a means of increasing the angle between the seat base and back, typically between 90 and 170 degrees. The pivot point at the seat back does not match the pivot point of the hip; therefore the individual's back will slide down the back support when reclining. This is a risk factor for skin injury in some individuals. Furthermore, the contours of the back support will no longer match the contours of the back support. Many power wheelchairs have special linkages or mechanical compensation to minimize skin shear during recline. Recline is less frequently prescribed for this reason, but is often required for self-catheterization, transfers, and pressure-relieving activities.

Elevation

Seat elevators provide 6 to 9 inches of additional height and can make transfers easier by placing the wheelchair at the same height as the target surface. A seat elevator adds additional weight to the wheelchair and can increase the seat-to-floor height in some models.

Wheelchair-Mounted Accessories: Assistive Technology

In addition to mobility, wheelchairs serve as a platform for assistive technology devices for many daily activities. They are often equipped with lap trays, tote bags, mobile phones, portable entertainment devices, and even cup holders. In addition to these common accessories, wheelchairs frequently carry advanced electronic assistive technology to enhance communication or access the environment. Categories of devices include electronic ADLs (also known as environmental control systems), computer access products, and speech-generating devices. All devices must be properly mounted to the wheelchair for safety and function.

Table 14-5 Seating Configurations Possible with Tilt, Recline, and Leg Rest Elevation

Position	Image	Use
Normal driving position		Travel position
Leg elevation		Comfort and improved circulation
Recline		Rest, pressure relief, self-catheterization
Recline plus leg elevation		Rest, pressure relief, self-catheterization
Tilt		Rest, comfort, pressure relief
All combined: Tilt recline leg elevation		Rest, comfort, sleep

Electronic Aids to Daily Living

Individuals often have difficulty reaching standard doorknobs, switches, appliances, and home entertainment systems because of the postural restrictions imposed by the wheelchair. Access is limited even if they have unimpaired arm function. Seat elevators and standing wheelchairs are one solution but are not always feasible because of the cost and limited funding opportunities. One way to gain increased access to items in the environment is to use wireless electronic aids to daily living (EADL) systems. These systems operate by transmitting ultrasound, radio frequency, or infrared signals to receivers that are connected to the appliance or device. Examples of devices include door openers, lights, televisions, radios, fans, and thermostats. Some power wheelchairs are equipped with an "EADL" mode so that the individual can operate items directly from their wheelchair.

Speech-Generating Devices

Speech-generating devices (also known as augmentative and alternative communication devices) are computer-based systems that provide an electronic voice for individuals unable to speak. These can be accessed by keypads of various sizes, optical pointers, or with single-switch scanning strategies. To keep the device in reach, they are typically mounted on a swing-away arm that attaches to the wheelchair frame. The control input method must be positioned so that the user can readily reach it, which can require additional wheelchair-mounting hardware. The placement of the speech-generating device is predicated on the type of wheelchair and seating system.

Summary

Successful wheelchair outcomes require current knowledge about the equipment available, the intended application, and the seating and positioning parameters. It also requires an interdisciplinary team to execute a systematic approach to wheelchair assessment. The team should consider the patient's mobility goals; medical, physical, and functional variables; environments where the device will be used; transportation needs; past experience with wheelchair and seating technology; and reimbursement. Ideally the individual should try various technologies in the actual environments where the device will be used before making the final decision. Adequate fitting, training, and follow-up are essential in ensuring comfort, satisfaction, and a successful match between the patient and mobility device.

REFERENCES

1. Arledge S, Armstrong W, Babinec M, et al: *RESNA wheelchair service provision guide*, Arlington, 2011, Rehabilitation Engineering and Assistive Technology Society of North America.
2. Armstrong W, Borg J, Krizack M, et al: *Guidelines on the provision of manual wheelchairs in less-resourced settings*, Geneva, 2008, World Health Organization.
3. Arva J, Schmeler MR, Lange ML, et al: RESNA position on the application of seat-elevating devices for wheelchair users, *Assist Technol* 21:69–72, quiz 74–75, 2009.
4. Askari S, Kirby RL, Parker K, et al: Wheelchair propulsion test: development and measurement properties of a new test for manual wheelchair users, *Arch Phys Med Rehabil* 94:1690–1698, 2013.
5. Beekman CE, Miller-Porter L, Schoneberger M: Energy cost of propulsion in standard and ultralight wheelchairs in people with spinal cord injuries, *Phys Ther* 79:146–158, 1999.
6. Boninger ML, Baldwin M, Cooper RA, et al: Manual wheelchair pushrim biomechanics and axle position, *Arch Phys Med Rehabil* 81:608–613, 2000.
7. Boninger ML, Souza AL, Cooper RA, et al: Propulsion patterns and pushrim biomechanics in manual wheelchair propulsion, *Arch Phys Med Rehabil* 83:718–723, 2002.
8. Boninger ML, Koontz AM, Sisto SA, et al: Pushrim biomechanics and injury prevention in spinal cord injury: recommendations based on CULP-SCI investigations, *J Rehabil Res Dev* 42(Suppl 1):9–20, 2005.
9. Boninger ML, Waters RL, Chase T, et al: Preservation of upper limb function following spinal cord injury: a clinical practice guideline for health-care professionals. Paralyzed Veterans of America Consortium for Spinal Cord Medicine, *J Spinal Cord Med* 28:434–470, 2005.
10. Brienza D, Angelo J, Henry K: Consumer participation in identifying research and development priorities for power wheelchair input devices and controllers, *Assist Technol* 7:55–62, 1995.
11. Brubaker CE: Wheelchair prescription: an analysis of factors that affect mobility and performance, *J Rehabil Res Dev* 23:19–26, 1986.
12. Brubaker C: Ergonometric considerations, *J Rehabil Res Dev Clin Suppl* 2:37–48, 1990.
13. Buning ME, Bertocci G, Schneider LW, et al: RESNA's position on wheelchairs used as seats in motor vehicles, *Assist Technol* 24:132–141, 2012.
14. Chaves ES, Cooper RA, Collins DM, et al: Review of the use of physical restraints and lap belts with wheelchair users, *Assist Technol* 19:94–107, 2007.
15. Cooper RA: *Wheelchair selection and configuration*, New York, 1998, Demos Medical Publishing.
16. Cooper RA: Introduction. In Cooper RA, Ohnabe H, Hobson DA, editors: *An introduction to rehabilitation engineering*, Boca Raton, 2006, CRC Press, pp 1–18.
17. Cooper RA, Robertson RN, Lawrence B, et al: Life-cycle analysis of depot versus rehabilitation manual wheelchairs, *J Rehabil Res Dev* 33(1):45–55, 1996.
18. Cooper RA, Gonzalez J, Lawrence B, et al: Performance of selected lightweight wheelchairs on ANSI/RESNA tests. American National Standards Institute-Rehabilitation Engineering and Assistive Technology Society of North America, *Arch Phys Med Rehabil* 78:1138–1144, 1997.
19. Cooper RA, Fitzgerald SG, Boninger ML, et al: Evaluation of a pushrim-activated, power-assisted wheelchair, *Arch Phys Med Rehabil* 82:702–708, 2001.
20. Cowan RE, Boninger ML, Sawatzky BJ, et al: Preliminary outcomes of the SmartWheel users' group database: a proposed framework for clinicians to objectively evaluate manual wheelchair propulsion, *Arch Phys Med Rehabil* 898:260–268, 2007.
21. Dempsey PG, McGorry RW, Maynard WS: A survey of tools and methods used by certified professional ergonomists, *Appl Ergon* 36:489–503, 2005.
22. Dey ZR, Nair NR, Shapcott N: Evaluation of the force sensing application pressure mapping system, *J Med Eng Technol* 37:213–219, 2013.
23. Dicianno BE, Tovey E: Power mobility device provision: understanding Medicare guidelines and advocating for clients, *Arch Phys Med Rehabil* 88:807–816, 2007.
24. Ding D, Cooper RA, Kaminski BA, et al: Integrated control and related technology of assistive devices, *Assist Technol* 15:89–97, 2003.
25. Dicianno BE, Spaeth DM, Cooper RA, et al: Force control strategies while driving electric powered wheelchairs with isometric and movement-sensing joysticks, *IEEE Trans Neural Syst Rehabil Eng* 15:144–150, 2007.
26. Dicianno BE, Arva J, Lieberman JM, et al: RESNA position on the application of tilt, recline, and elevating leg rests for wheelchairs, *Assist Technol* 21:13–22, quiz 24, 2009.
27. Dicianno BE, Morgan A, Lieberman J, Rosen L: *RESNA position on the application of wheelchair standing devices: 2013 current state of the literature*, Arlington, 2013, Rehabilitation Engineering and Assistive Technology Society of North America.
28. Eggers SL, Myaskovsky L, Burkitt KH, et al: A preliminary model of wheelchair service delivery, *Arch Phys Med Rehabil* 90(6):1030–1038, 2009.
29. Fass MV, Cooper RA, Fitzgerald SG, et al: Durability, value, and reliability of selected electric powered wheelchairs, *Arch Phys Med Rehabil* 85:805–814, 2004.
30. Finley MA, Rodgers MM: Effect of 2-speed geared manual wheelchair propulsion on shoulder pain and function, *Arch Phys Med Rehabil* 88:1622–1627, 2007.
31. Fitzgerald SG, Cooper RA, Boninger ML, Rentschler AJ: Comparison of fatigue life for 3 types of manual wheelchairs, *Arch Phys Med Rehabil* 82:1484–1488, 2001.
32. Gaal RP, Rebholtz N, Hotchkiss RD, Pfaelzer PF: Wheelchair rider injuries: causes and consequences for wheelchair design and selection, *J Rehabil Res Dev* 34:58–71, 1997.

33. Inkpen P, Parker K, Kirby RL: Manual wheelchair skills capacity versus performance, *Arch Phys Med Rehabil* 93:1009–1013, 2012.
34. Karmarkar A, Cooper RA, Liu H, et al: Evaluation of pushrim-activated power-assisted wheelchairs using ANSI/RESNA standards, *Arch Phys Med Rehabil* 89:1191–1198, 2008.
35. Kirby RL, Ackroyd-Stolarz SA: Wheelchair safety—adverse reports to the United States Food and Drug Administration, *Am J Phys Med Rehabil Assoc Acad Physiatr* 74:308–312, 1995.
36. Kirby RL, Thoren FA, Ashton BD, Ackroyd-Stolarz SA: Wheelchair stability and maneuverability: effect of varying the horizontal and vertical position of a rear-antitip device, *Arch Phys Med Rehabil* 75:525–534, 1994.
37. Kirby RL, Smith C, Parker K, et al, editors: *Wheelchair Skills Test (WST) © Version 4.1 Manual*, Halifax, 2012, Dalhousie University.
38. Kumar A, Schmeler MR, Karmarkar AM, et al: Test-retest reliability of the functional mobility assessment (FMA): a pilot study, *Disabil Rehabil Assist Technol* 8:213–219, 2012.
39. Kwarciak AM, Cooper RA, Ammer WA, et al: Fatigue testing of selected suspension manual wheelchairs using ANSI/RESNA standards, *Arch Phys Med Rehabil* 86:123–129, 2005.
40. Kwarciak AM, Sisto SA, Yarossi M, et al: Redefining the manual wheelchair stroke cycle: identification and impact of nonpropulsive pushrim contact, *Arch Phys Med Rehabil* 90:20–26, 2009.
41. LaPlante MP, Kaye HS: Demographics and trends in wheeled mobility equipment use and accessibility in the community, *Assist Technol* 22:3–17, quiz 19, 2010.
42. Liu HY, Pearlman J, Cooper R, et al: Evaluation of aluminum ultralight rigid wheelchairs versus other ultralight wheelchairs using ANSI/RESNA standards, *J Rehabil Res Dev* 47:441–455, 2010.
43. Masse LC, Lamontagne M, O'Riain MD: Biomechanical analysis of wheelchair propulsion for various seating positions, *J Rehabil Res Dev* 29:12–28, 1992.
44. McClure LA, Boninger ML, Oyster ML, et al: Wheelchair repairs, breakdown, and adverse consequences for people with traumatic spinal cord injury, *Arch Phys Med Rehabil* 90:2034–2038, 2009.
45. McLaurin CA, Brubaker CE: Biomechanics and the wheelchair, *Prosthet Orthot Int* 15:24–37, 1991.
46. Mills T, Holm MB, Trefler E, et al: Development and consumer validation of the Functional Evaluation in a Wheelchair (FEW) instrument, *Disabil Rehabil* 24:38–46, 2002.
47. Mukherjee G, Samanta A: Physiological response to the ambulatory performance of hand-rim and arm-crank propulsion systems, *J Rehabil Res Dev* 38:391–399, 2001.
48. Pearlman JL, Cooper RA, Karnawat J, et al: Evaluation of the safety and durability of low-cost nonprogrammable electric powered wheelchairs, *Arch Phys Med Rehabil* 86:2361–2370, 2005.
49. Porter ME: What is value in health care?, *N Engl J Med* 363:2477–2481, 2010.
50. Rosen L, Arva J, Furumasu J, et al: RESNA position on the application of power wheelchairs for pediatric users, *Assist Technol* 21:218–225, quiz 228, 2009.
51. Rushton PW, Kirby RL, Miller WC: Manual wheelchair skills: objective testing versus subjective questionnaire, *Arch Phys Med Rehabil* 93:2313–2318, 2012.
52. Sawatzky BJ, Kim WO, Denison I: The ergonomics of different tyres and tyre pressure during wheelchair propulsion, *Ergonomics* 47:1475–1483, 2004.
53. Schneider LW, Klinich KD, Moore JL, MacWilliams JB: Using in-depth investigations to identify transportation safety issues for wheelchair-seated occupants of motor vehicles, *Med Eng Phys* 32:237–247, 2009.
54. Souza AE, Pearlman JL, Cooper R, et al: Evaluation of scooters using ANSI/RESNA standards, *J Rehabil Res Dev* 50:1017–1034, 2013.
55. Sprigle S, Dunlop W, Press L: Reliability of bench tests of interface pressure, *Assist Technol* 15:49–57, 2003.
56. Storr T, Spicer J, Frost P, et al: Design features of portable wheelchair ramps and their implications for curb and vehicle access, *J Rehabil Res Dev* 41(3B):443–452, 2004.
57. Ummat S, Kirby RL: Nonfatal wheelchair-related accidents reported to the National Electronic Injury Surveillance System, *Am J Phys Med Rehabil* 73:163–167, 1994.
58. van der Woude LH, Veeger DJ, Rozendal RH, Sargeant TJ: Seat height in handrim wheelchair propulsion, *J Rehabil Res Dev* 26:31–50, 1989.
59. Wang H, Liu HY, Pearlman J, et al: Relationship between wheelchair durability and wheelchair type and years of test, *Disabil Rehabil Assist Technol* 5:318–322, 2010.
60. Waugh K: *Glossary of wheelchair terms and definitions*, Denver, 2013, University of Colorado.
61. Worobey L, Oyster M, Nemunaitis G, et al: Increases in wheelchair breakdowns, repairs, and adverse consequences for people with traumatic spinal cord injury, *Am J Phys Med Rehabil Assoc Acad Physiatr* 91:463–469, 2012.
62. Worobey L, Oyster M, Pearlman J, et al: Differences between manufacturers in reported power wheelchair repairs and adverse consequences among people with spinal cord injury, *Arch Phys Med Rehabil* 95:597–603, 2014.

CHAPTER 15

THERAPEUTIC EXERCISE

Robert P. Wilder, Jeffrey G. Jenkins, Preeti Panchang, Siobhan Statuta

I repeat my advice to take a great deal of exercise on foot. Health is the first requisite after morality.

Thomas Jefferson

General Principles

Regular physical activity is an important component of a healthy lifestyle. Increases in physical activity and cardiorespiratory fitness have been shown to reduce the risk for death from coronary heart disease as well as from all causes. The primary focus on achieving these health-related goals in the past has been on prescribing exercise to improve cardiorespiratory fitness, body composition, and strength. Recently, the Centers for Disease Control and Prevention (CDC) and the American College of Sports Medicine (ACSM) suggested that the focus be broadened to address the needs of more sedentary individuals, especially those who cannot or will not engage in structured exercise programs. There is increasing evidence showing that regular participation in moderate-intensity physical activity is associated with health benefits, even when aerobic fitness remains unchanged. To reflect this evidence, the CDC and ACSM are now recommending that every adult in the United States accumulates 30 minutes or more of moderate-intensity physical activity on most, and preferably all, days of the week. Those who follow these recommendations can experience many of the health-related benefits of physical activity, and if they are interested are ready to achieve higher levels of fitness.[52,53,124,137]

Important in prescribing exercise is an understanding of the principles of specificity and periodization. The principle of specificity states that metabolic responses to exercise occur most specifically in those muscle groups being used. Furthermore, the types of adaptation will be reflective of the mode and intensity of exercise. The principle of periodization reflects the importance of incorporating adequate rest to accompany harder training sessions. Overall training programs (macrocycles) are divided into phases (microcycles), each with specific desired effects (i.e., enhancing a particular energy system or sport-specific goal).

This chapter provides a brief overview of the basic fundamentals of exercise physiology, including the metabolic energy systems, and the basic muscle and cardiorespiratory physiology associated with exercise. It will then provide an overview of the exercise prescription according to the current ACSM guidelines, and the fundamentals of exercise programming, including preexercise screening.

Energy Systems

A 70-kg human has an energy expenditure at rest of approximately 1.2 kcal/min, with less than 20% of the resting energy expenditure attributed to skeletal muscle. During intense exercise, however, total energy expenditure can increase 15 to 25 times above resting values, resulting in a caloric expenditure between 18 and 30 kcal/min. Most of this increase is used to provide energy to the exercising muscles that can increase energy requirements by a factor of 200.[31,119]

The energy used to fuel biological processes comes from the breakdown of adenosine triphosphate (ATP), specifically from the chemical energy stored in the bonds of the last two phosphates of the ATP molecules. When work is performed, the bond between the last two phosphates is broken, producing energy and heat:

$$\text{ATP} \xrightarrow{\text{ATPase}} \text{ADP} + \text{Pi} + \text{energy}$$

The limited stores of ATP in skeletal muscles can fuel approximately 5 to 10 seconds of high-intensity work (Figure 15-1). ATP must be continuously resynthesized from adenosine diphosphate (ADP) to allow exercise to continue.[78,130] Muscle fibers contain three metabolic pathways for producing ATP: the creatine phosphate system, rapid glycolysis, and aerobic oxidation.[31,119,124]

Creatine Phosphate System

When limited stores of ATP are nearly depleted during high-intensity exercise (5 to 10 seconds), the creatine phosphate system transfers a high-energy phosphate from creatine phosphate to rephosphorylate ATP from ADP:

$$\text{ADP} + \text{creatine phosphate} \xrightarrow{\text{creatine kinase}} \text{ATP} + \text{creatine}$$

Because it involves a single reaction, this system can provide ATP at a very rapid rate. Because there is a limited supply of creatine phosphate in the muscle, however, the amount of ATP that can be produced is also limited.

There is enough creatine phosphate stored in skeletal muscle for approximately 25 seconds of high-intensity work (see Figure 15-1). The ATP–creatine phosphate system lasts for approximately 30 seconds (5 seconds for the stored ATP and 25 seconds for creatine phosphate). This provides energy for activities such as sprinting and weightlifting. The creatine phosphate system is considered an anaerobic system because oxygen is not required.[31,119,124]

Rapid Glycolysis (Lactic Acid System)

Glycolysis uses carbohydrates primarily in the form of muscle glycogen as a fuel source. When glycolysis is rapid,

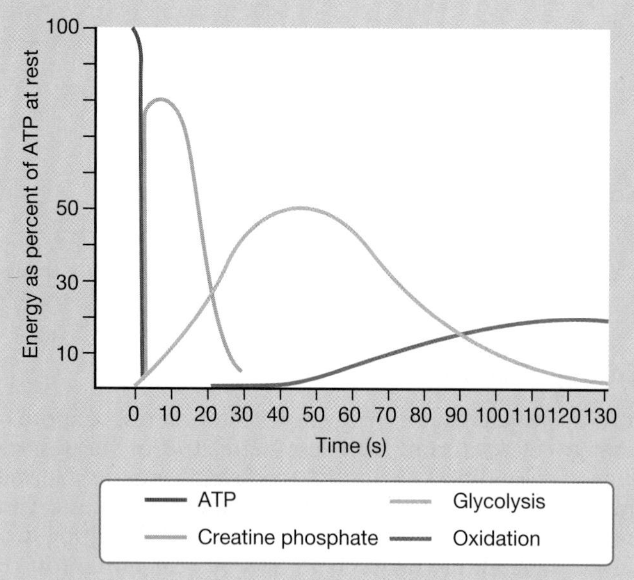

FIGURE 15-1 Energy sources in relation to duration of contraction. Muscular metabolism available from the various substrates participating in supplying energy during the first 2 minutes of an attempted maximal contraction. The relative contribution of each substrate at any moment is indicated. The intensity of metabolic activity over the 2-minute period is adjusted to the change of the isometric tension produced during a sustained voluntary maximal contraction. (Redrawn from DeLateur BJ: Therapeutic exercise to develop strength and endurance. In Kottke FJ, Stillwell GK, Lehmann JF, editors: *Krusen's handbook of physical medicine and rehabilitation*, Philadelphia, 1982, Saunders, with permission.)

the pathways that normally use oxygen to make energy are circumvented in favor of other, faster yet less efficient paths that do not require oxygen. As a result, only a small amount of ATP is produced anaerobically, and lactic acid is produced as a byproduct of the reaction.

For many years, lactic acid was considered to be the waste product caused by inadequate oxygen supply. Lactic acid limited physical activity by building up in muscles and leading to fatigue and diminished performance. Since the early 1980s, there has been a fundamental change in thought, and evidence now shows that a limited oxygen supply is not required for lactic acid production. Lactate is produced and used continuously under fully aerobic conditions. This is referred to as the cell-to-cell lactate shuttle in which lactate serves as a metabolic intermediate tying together glycolysis (as an end product) and oxidative metabolism.

Once lactic acid is formed, there are two possible venues it can take. The first involves conversion into pyruvic acid and subsequently into energy (ATP) under aerobic conditions (see section on "Aerobic Oxidation System"). The second involves hepatic gluconeogenesis using lactate to produce glucose, which is known as the Cori cycle.

Anaerobic oxidation starts as soon as high-intensity exercise begins and dominates for approximately 1.5 to 2 minutes (see Figure 15-1). It would fuel activities such as middle-distance sprints (400-, 600-, and 800-m runs) or events requiring sudden bursts of energy, such as weightlifting.

Although glycolysis is considered an anaerobic pathway, it can readily participate in the aerobic metabolism when oxygen is available and is considered the first step in the aerobic metabolism of carbohydrates.[31,119,124]

Aerobic Oxidation System

The final metabolic pathway for ATP production combines two complex metabolic processes: the Krebs cycle and the electron transport chain. The aerobic oxidation system resides in the mitochondria. It is capable of using carbohydrates, fat, and small amounts of protein to produce energy (ATP) during exercise, through a process called oxidative phosphorylation. During exercise, this pathway uses oxygen to completely metabolize the carbohydrates to produce energy (ATP), leaving only carbon dioxide and water as byproducts. The aerobic oxidation system is complex and requires 2 to 3 minutes to adjust to a change in exercise intensity (see Figure 15-1). It has an almost unlimited ability to regenerate ATP, however, limited only by the amount of fuel and oxygen that is available to the cell. Maximal oxygen consumption, also known as $\dot{V}O_{2max}$, is a measure of the power of the aerobic energy system, and is generally regarded as the best indicator of aerobic fitness.[31,119,124]

All the energy-producing pathways are active during most types of exercise, but different exercise types place greater demands on different pathways. The contribution of the anaerobic pathways (creatine phosphate system and glycolysis) to exercise energy metabolism is inversely related to the duration and intensity of the activity. The shorter and more intense the activity, the greater the contribution of anaerobic energy production, whereas the longer the activity and the lower the intensity, the greater the contribution of aerobic energy production. In general, carbohydrates are used as the primary fuel at the onset of exercise and during high-intensity work. However, during prolonged exercise of low to moderate intensity (longer than 30 minutes), a gradual shift from carbohydrate toward an increasing reliance on fat as a substrate occurs. The greatest amount of fat use occurs at approximately 60% of maximal aerobic capacity ($\dot{V}O_{2max}$).[31,119,124]

Cardiovascular Exercise

Cardiorespiratory Physiology

The cardiorespiratory system consists of the heart, lungs, and blood vessels. The purpose of this system is the delivery of oxygen and nutrients to the cells, as well as the removal of metabolic waste products to maintain the internal equilibrium.[78,119,124]

Cardiac Function

Heart Rate

Normal resting heart rate (HR) is approximately 60 to 80 beats/min. HR increases in a linear manner with the work rate and oxygen uptake during exercise. The magnitude of HR response is related to age, body position, fitness, type of activity, the presence of heart disease, medications, blood volume, and environmental factors such as temperature and humidity. HR during maximal exercise can exceed 200 beats/min, depending on the individual's age and training state. With the onset of dynamic exercise, HR increases in proportion to the relative workload. The maximal HR (HR_{max}) decreases with age, and can be estimated in healthy men and women with the following formula: $HR_{max} = 220 - age$. There is considerable variability in this estimation for any fixed age, with a standard deviation of ±10 beats/min.[78,119,124]

Stroke Volume

Stroke volume (SV) is the amount of blood ejected from the left ventricle in a single beat. SV is equal to the difference between end-diastolic volume and end-systolic volume. Greater diastolic filling (preload) will increase SV. Factors that resist ventricular outflow (afterload) will result in a reduced SV.

SV is greater in men than in women. At rest in the upright position, it generally ranges from 60 to 100 mL/beat, whereas maximal SV approximates 100 to 120 mL/beat. During exercise, SV increases in a curvilinear relationship with the work rate until it reaches near maximal at a level equivalent to approximately 50% of aerobic capacity. SV starts to plateau, and further increases in workload do not result in increased SV, primarily because of reduced filling time during diastole.

SV is also affected by body position, with SV being greater in the supine or prone position and lower in the upright position. Static exercise (weight training) can also cause a slight decrease in SV because of increased intrathoracic pressure.[78,119,124]

Cardiac Output

Cardiac output (Q) is the amount of blood pumped by the heart each minute. It is calculated by the following formula:

$$Q\ (L/min) = HR\ (beats/min) \times SV\ (mL/beat)$$

Resting cardiac output in both trained and sedentary individuals is approximately 4 to 5 L/min, but during exercise the maximal cardiac output can reach 20 L/min. Maximum cardiac output in an individual depends on many factors, including age, posture, body size, presence of cardiac disease, and physical conditioning. During dynamic exercise, cardiac output initially increases with increasing exercise intensity by increases in SV and HR. Increases in cardiac output initially beyond 40% to 50% of $\dot{V}O_{2max}$, however, are accounted for only by increases in HR.[78,119,124]

Blood Flow

At rest, 15% to 20% of the cardiac output is distributed to the skeletal muscles, with the remainder going to visceral organs, the brain, and the heart. During exercise, 85% to 90% of the cardiac output is selectively delivered to working muscles and shunted away from the skin and splanchnic vasculature. Myocardial blood flow can increase four to five times with exercise, whereas blood supply to the brain is maintained at resting levels. The difference between the oxygen content of arterial blood and the oxygen content of venous blood is termed the arteriovenous oxygen difference. It reflects the oxygen extracted from arterial blood by the tissues. The oxygen extraction at rest is approximately 25%, but at maximal exercise the oxygen extraction can reach 75%.[78,119,124]

Venous Return

Venous return is maintained or increased during exercise by the following mechanisms[78,119,124]:

- Contracting skeletal muscle acts as a "pump" against the various structures that surround it, including deep veins, forcing blood back toward the heart.
- Smooth muscle around the venules contracts, causing venoconstriction. This increases the pressure on the venous side, maintaining blood flow toward the heart.
- Diaphragmatic contraction during exercise creates lowered intrathoracic pressure, facilitating blood flow from the abdominal area and lower extremities.

Blood Pressure

Blood pressure is the driving force behind blood flow. Systolic blood pressure (SBP) is the maximal force of the blood against the walls of the arteries when cardiac muscle is contracting (systole). Normal resting SBP is less than 130 mm Hg. Diastolic blood pressure (DBP) is the force of the blood against the walls of the arteries when the heart is relaxing (diastole). Normal resting DBP is less than 85 mm Hg.[119]

SBP increases linearly with increasing work intensity, at 8 to 12 mm Hg per metabolic equivalent (MET) (where 1 MET = 3.5 mL of O_2 per kilogram per minute). Maximum values typically reach 190 to 220 mm Hg. Maximum SBP should not be greater than 260 mm Hg. DBP remains unchanged or only slightly increases with exercise.[78,119]

Because blood pressure is directly related to cardiac output and peripheral vascular resistance, it provides a noninvasive way to monitor the inotropic performance (pumping capacity) of the heart. Failure of SBP to rise, decreased SBP with increasing work rates, or a significant increase in DBP are all abnormal responses to exercise, and indicate either severe exercise intolerance or underlying cardiovascular disease.[78,119,124]

Postural Considerations

In the supine position, gravity has less effect on return of blood to the heart, thus the SBP is lower. When the body is upright, gravity works against the return of blood to the heart, thus SBP increases. DBP does not change significantly with body position in healthy individuals.[51,117,124]

Effects of Arm and Leg Exercises

At similar oxygen consumptions, HR, SBP, and DBP are higher during arm work than during leg work. This is primarily because the total muscle mass in the arms is smaller, and consequently a greater percentage of the available mass is recruited to perform the work. In addition, arm work is less mechanically efficient than leg work.[78,119,124]

Pulmonary Ventilation

Pulmonary ventilation ($\dot{V}e$) is the volume of air exchanged per minute, and generally is approximately 6 L/min at rest in an average sedentary adult man. However, at maximal exercise, $\dot{V}e$ increases 15- to 25-fold over resting values. During mild to moderate exercise, $\dot{V}e$ increases primarily by increasing tidal volume, but during vigorous activity it increases by increasing the respiratory rate.[51,117]

Increases in $\dot{V}e$ are generally directly proportional to an increase in oxygen consumption ($\dot{V}O_2$) and carbon dioxide that is produced ($\dot{V}CO_2$). At a critical exercise intensity (usually 47% to 64% of the $\dot{V}O_{2max}$ in healthy untrained individuals and 70% to 90% $\dot{V}O_{2max}$ in highly trained individuals), however, $\dot{V}e$ increases disproportionately relative to the $\dot{V}O_2$ (paralleling an abrupt increase in serum lactate and $\dot{V}CO_2$). This is called the anaerobic (ventilatory) threshold.[51,117,124]

Anaerobic Threshold

The anaerobic threshold signifies the onset of metabolic acidosis during exercise, and traditionally has been determined by serial measurements of blood lactate. It can be noninvasively determined by assessment of expired gases during exercise testing, specifically $\dot{V}e$ and carbon dioxide production ($\dot{V}CO_2$). The anaerobic threshold signifies the peak work rate or oxygen consumption at which the energy demands exceed the circulatory ability to sustain aerobic metabolism.[51,117,124]

Maximal Oxygen Consumption

The most widely recognized measure of cardiopulmonary fitness is the aerobic capacity, or $\dot{V}O_{2max}$. This variable is defined physiologically as the highest rate of oxygen transport and use that can be achieved at maximal physical exertion.

The resting oxygen consumption of an individual (250 mL/min) divided by body weight (70 kg) gives the resting energy requirement, 1 MET (approximately 3.5 mL/kg per minute). Multiples of this value are used to quantify levels of energy expenditure. For example, running a 6-mph pace requires 10 times the resting energy expenditure, giving an aerobic cost of 10 METs, or 35 mL/kg per minute. Because there is little variation in HR_{max} and maximal systemic arteriovenous oxygen difference with physical training, $\dot{V}O_{2max}$ virtually defines the pumping capacity of the heart. When expressed as milliliters of oxygen per kilogram of body weight per minute (mL/kg per minute) or in METs, it is considered the best index of physical work capacity or cardiorespiratory fitness.[51,117,124]

Oxygen Pulse

The oxygen pulse (mL/beat) is the ratio of $\dot{V}O_2$ (mL/min) to HR (beats/min), when both measures are obtained simultaneously. Oxygen pulse increases with increasing work effort. A low value during exercise indicates an excessive HR for workload and can be an indicator of heart disease.[34]

Respiratory Quotient and Respiratory Exchange Ratio

The respiratory quotient (RQ) is the ratio of CO_2 produced by cellular metabolism to O_2 used by tissues. It quantifies the relative amounts of carbohydrate and fatty acids being oxidized for energy. An RQ of 0.7 implies dependence on free fatty acids. An RQ of 1.0 indicates dependence on carbohydrate. The RQ does not exceed 1.0.

The respiratory exchange ratio (RER) reflects pulmonary exchange of CO_2 and O_2 at rest and during exercise. The RER also ranges between 0.7 and 1.0 during rest, and can also reflect substrate preference. During strenuous exercise, however, the RER can exceed 1.0 because of increasing metabolic activity not matched by $\dot{V}O_2$ and additional CO_2 derived from bicarbonate buffering of lactic acid. The terms *respiratory quotient* and *respiratory exchange ratio* are often used interchangeably, but their distinction is important.[34]

Effects of Exercise Training

Cardiovascular System

The effects of regular exercise on cardiovascular activity can be grouped into changes that occur at rest, during submaximal exercise, and during maximal work (Box 15-1).[119,124] Regular exercise can also affect a number of physiologic measurements (Box 15-2).

Detraining

The changes induced by regular exercise training generally are lost after 4 to 8 weeks of detraining. If training is reestablished, the rate at which the training effects occur does not appear to be faster.[119,124]

Overtraining

Overtraining fatigue syndrome presents as a prolonged decreased sport-specific performance, usually lasting greater than 2 weeks. It is characterized by premature fatigability, emotional and mood changes, lack of motivation, infections, and overuse injuries. Recovery is markedly longer and variable among affected athletes, sometimes taking months before the athlete returns to baseline performance (Box 15-3).[119,124]

Exercise Prescriptions

Exercise prescriptions are designed to enhance physical fitness, promote health by reducing risk factors for chronic disease, and ensure safety during exercise participation. The fundamental objective of the prescription is to bring about a change in personal health behavior to include habitual physical activity. The optimal exercise prescription for an individual is determined from an objective evaluation of that individual's response to exercise, including observations of HR, blood pressure, rating of perceived exertion (RPE) to exercise, electrocardiogram when appropriate, and $\dot{V}O_{2max}$ measured directly or estimated during a graded exercise test. The exercise prescription should be developed with careful consideration of the individual's health status, medications, risk factor profile, behavioral characteristics, personal goals, and exercise preferences.[53,124,137]

Components of an Exercise Prescription

- Mode is the particular form or type of exercise. The selection of mode should be based on the desired outcomes, focusing on exercises that are most likely to sustain participation and enjoyment.
- Intensity is the relative physiologic difficulty of the exercise. Intensity and duration of exercise interact and are inversely related.

BOX 15-1

Effects of Regular Exercise on Cardiovascular Activity

Changes at Rest

- Heart rate decreases, probably secondary to decreased sympathetic tone, increased parasympathetic tone, and a decreased intrinsic firing rate of the sinoatrial node.
- Stroke volume increases secondary to increased myocardial contractility.
- Cardiac output is unchanged at rest.
- Oxygen consumption does not change at rest.*

Changes at Submaximal Work†

- Heart rate decreases, at any given workload, because of the increased stroke volume and decreased sympathetic drive.
- Stroke volume increases because of increased myocardial contractility.
- Cardiac output does not change significantly because the oxygen requirements for a fixed workload are similar. The same cardiac output is generated, however, with a lower heart rate and higher stroke volume.
- Submaximal oxygen consumption does not change significantly because the oxygen requirement is similar for a fixed workload.
- Arteriovenous oxygen (a-vO_2) difference increases during submaximal work.
- Lactate levels are decreased because of metabolic efficiency and increased lactate clearance rates.*

Changes at Maximal Work

- Maximum heart rate does not change with exercise training.
- Stroke volume increases because of increased contractility and/or increased heart size.
- Maximal cardiac output increases because of increased stroke volume.
- Maximal oxygen consumption ($\dot{V}O_{2max}$) increases primarily because of increased stroke volume.
- Ability of the local mitochondria to use oxygen is improved.* (Because measured a-vO_2 difference represents whole-body a-vO_2 difference, there is generally little change in the measured a-vO_2 difference.)

*From Rupp JC: Exercise physiology. In Roitman JL, Bibi KW, Thompson WR, editors: *ACSM health fitness certification review,* Philadelphia, 2001, Lippincott Williams & Wilkins; Seto C: Basic principles of exercise training. In O'Connor F, Sallis R, Wilder R, et al, editors: *Sports medicine: just the facts,* New York, 2005, McGraw-Hill.

†Submaximal work is defined as a workload during which a steady state is achieved.

- Duration or time is the length of an exercise session.
- Frequency refers to the number of exercise sessions per day and per week.
- Progression (overload) is the increase in activity during exercise training, which, over time, stimulates adaptation.[53,119,124,137]

These five essential components apply when developing an exercise prescription for individuals of all ages and fitness levels. Each component of fitness (e.g., cardiorespiratory endurance, muscular strength and endurance, and flexibility) has its own specific exercise prescription associated with it. The following section reviews the ACSM guidelines for each component of fitness.

BOX 15-2

Physiologic Changes After a Regular Exercise Program

Blood Pressure

- In normotensive individuals, regular exercise does not appear to have a significant impact on resting or exercising blood pressure. In individuals with hypertension, there can be a modest reduction in resting blood pressure as a result of regular exercise.*

Blood Volume Changes

- Total blood volume increases because of an increased number of red blood cells and expansion of the plasma volume.*

Blood Lipids

- Total cholesterol can be decreased in individuals with hypercholesterolemia.
- High-density lipoprotein cholesterol increases with exercise training.
- Low-density lipoprotein cholesterol can remain the same or decrease with regular exercise.
- Triglycerides can decrease in those with elevated triglycerides initially. This change is facilitated by weight loss.*

Body Composition

- Total body weight usually decreases with regular exercise.
- Fat-free weight does not normally change.
- Percent body fat declines.*

Biochemical Changes

- Stored muscle glycogen increases.
- The percentage of fast- and slow-twitch fibers does not change, but the cross-sectional area occupied by these fibers may change because of selective hypertrophy of either fast- or slow-twitch fibers.*

Energy System Changes

- Specificity of training refers to the fact that the changes that occur are specific to the muscles and energy systems that are being used.
- Chronic anaerobic training using the ATP–creatine phosphate system results in improved capacity and power of this system because of enhancement of enzyme activity and increases in the amount of ATP and creatine phosphate in the muscle.
- Anaerobic glycolysis is improved if the training program uses this system, resulting in increased stores of muscle glycogen and improved ability of enzymes in the system.
- Regular aerobic training improves $\dot{V}O_{2max}$. It increases muscle glycogen and triglyceride stores, as well as the rate at which carbohydrates and fat are metabolized.*

*From Rupp JC: Exercise physiology. In Roitman JL, Bibi KW, Thompson WR, editors: *ACSM health fitness certification review,* Philadelphia, 2001, Lippincott Williams & Wilkins; Seto C: Basic principles of exercise training. In O'Connor F, Sallis R, Wilder R, et al, editors: *Sports medicine: just the facts,* New York, 2005, McGraw-Hill.

ATP, Adenosine triphosphate; $\dot{V}O_{2max}$, maximal oxygen consumption.

Exercise Prescription for Cardiorespiratory Endurance

Cardiorespiratory endurance is the ability to take in, deliver, and use oxygen. It is dependent on the function of the cardiorespiratory system (heart and lungs) and the cellular metabolic capacities. The degree of improvement that

BOX 15-3

Symptoms of Overtraining Syndrome

- Sudden decline in quality of work or exercise performance
- Extreme fatigue
- Elevated resting heart rate
- Early onset of blood lactate accumulation
- Altered mood states
- Unexplained weight loss
- Insomnia
- Injuries related to overuse

can be expected in cardiorespiratory fitness is directly related to the frequency, intensity, duration, and mode of exercise. $\dot{V}O_{2max}$ can increase between 5% and 30% with training. It has become apparent recently, however, that the level of physical activity necessary to achieve the majority of health benefits is less than that needed to attain a high level of cardiorespiratory fitness.[53,124,137]

ACSM Recommendations for Cardiorespiratory Endurance Training

Mode

- The best improvements in cardiorespiratory endurance occur when large muscle groups are engaged in rhythmic aerobic activity.
- Various activities can be incorporated into an exercise program to increase enjoyment and improve compliance.
- Appropriate activities include walking, jogging, cycling, rowing, stair climbing, aerobic dance ("aerobics"), water exercise, and cross-country skiing as examples.[53,124,137]

Intensity

- ACSM recommendations describe minimal exercise intensity as exercise of at least moderate intensity (i.e., 40% to 60% of $\dot{V}O_{2max}$ that noticeably increases HR and breathing).
- A combination of moderate and vigorous exercise (≥60% of $\dot{V}O_{2max}$ that results in substantial increases in HR and breathing) is ideal for the attainment of improvements in health and fitness in most adults.[53,124,137]

Calculating Intensity. Because of limitations in using $\dot{V}O_2$ calculations for prescribing intensity, the most common methods of setting the intensity of exercise to improve or maintain cardiorespiratory fitness use HR and RPE.[53,115,124]

Heart Rate Methods. Heart rate is used as a guide to set exercise intensity because of the relatively linear relationship between HR and percentage of $\dot{V}O_{2max}$. It is best to measure HR_{max} during a progressive exercise test whenever possible, because HR_{max} declines with age. HR_{max} can be estimated with the following equation: $HR_{max} = 220 - \text{age}$. This estimation has significant variance, with a standard deviation of 10 beats/min.[53,115,124,137]

MAXIMUM HEART RATE METHOD. One of the oldest methods of setting the target HR range uses a straight percentage of the HR_{max}. Using 70% to 85% of an individual's HR_{max} approximates 55% to 75% of $\dot{V}O_{2max}$ and provides the stimulus needed to improve or maintain cardiorespiratory fitness.[53,115,124,137] For example, if the HR_{max} is 180 beats/min, then the target HR (70% to 85% of HR_{max}) would range from 126 to 153 beats/min. (See also Chapter 27.)

HEART RATE RESERVE METHOD. The HR reserve (HRR) method is also known as the Karvonen method. In this method the target range is calculated as follows: subtract standing resting HR (HR_{rest}) from HR_{max} to obtain HRR. Calculate 50% and 85% of the HRR. Add each of these values to the HR_{rest} to obtain the target range. Therefore the target range is as follows:

$$\text{Low Target HR} = [(HR_{max} - HR_{rest}) \times 0.50] + HR_{rest}$$
$$\text{High Target HR} = [(HR_{max} - HR_{rest}) \times 0.85] + HR_{rest}$$

The small but systematic differences between the two HR methods occur because the percentage HR_{max} is 55% to 75% of $\dot{V}O_{2max}$, whereas the percentage HRR_{max} is 60% to 80% of $\dot{V}O_{2max}$. Either method can be used to approximate the range of exercise intensities known to increase or maintain cardiorespiratory fitness or $\dot{V}O_{2max}$.[53,124,137]

Rating of Perceived Exertion. The RPE is a subjective grading of how hard individuals feel they are exercising. Use of RPE is considered an adjunct to monitoring HR. It has been shown to be a valuable aid in prescribing exercise for individuals who have difficulty with HR palpation, and in cases where the HR response to exercise may have been altered because of a change in medication. The most commonly used scale of perceived exertion is the Borg Scale (Table 15-1). The average RPE range associated with physiologic adaptation to exercise is 13 to 16 ("somewhat hard" to "hard") on the Borg Scale category. One should suit the RPE to the individual on a specific mode of exercise and not expect an exact matching of the RPE to a percentage HR_{max} or percentage HRR. It should be used only as a guideline in setting the exercise intensity.[53,108,115,124,137]

Table 15-1 Borg Scale of Perceived Exertion

Level	Perceived Exertion
6	—
7	Very, very light
8	
9	Fairly light
10	
11	
12	
13	Somewhat hard
14	
15	Hard
16	
17	Very hard
18	
19	Very, very hard
20	

From Noble B, Borg G, Jacobs I: A category-ratio perceived exertion scale: relationship to blood and muscle lactates and heart rate, *Med Sci Sports Exerc* 15:523-528, 1983.

The appropriate exercise intensity is one that is safe and compatible with a long-term active lifestyle for that individual and achieves the desired outcome given the time constraints of the exercise session. The ACSM recommends an intensity that will elicit an RPE within a range of 12 to 16 on the original 6 to 20 Borg Scale (see Table 15-1).

Duration

- Duration can be measured by duration of physical activity or by the total caloric expenditure.
- A dose-response relationship exists between the number of calories used during activity and the health and fitness benefits.
- Physical activity may be continuous or intermittently accumulated during a day through one or more sessions of activity lasting greater than 10 minutes.
- The ACSM recommends the following quantity of physical activity for most healthy adults: 1000 kcal/wk (or approximately 150 min/wk or 30 min/day).
- For most adults, larger quantities of exercise (i.e., ≥2000 kcal/wk or ≥250 min/wk or 50 to 60 min/day) results in greater health benefits.[53,115,124,137]

Frequency

- As above, activity can be continuous or intermittent and accumulated over the course of a day through more than one session of activity lasting greater than 10 minutes.
- The ACSM recommends exercise 3 to 5 days per week.
- Less conditioned people can benefit from lower intensity, shorter duration exercise performed at higher frequencies per day and/or per week.[53,124,137]

Progression

- The rate of progression depends on health and fitness status, individual goals, and compliance rates.
- Frequency, intensity, and/or duration can be increased to provide overload.
- The ACSM notes a 5- to 10-minute increase every 1 to 2 weeks over the first 4 to 6 weeks of an exercise is reasonable for a healthy adult.[53,124,137]

Medical Clearance

Exercise training might not be appropriate for everyone. Patients whose adaptive reserves are severely limited by disease processes might not be able to adapt to or benefit from exercise. In this small subpopulation of people with severe or unstable cardiac, respiratory, metabolic, systemic, or musculoskeletal disease, exercise programming can be fatal, injurious, or simply not beneficial, depending on the clinical status and condition of the individual.[54,137]

The recommended level of screening before beginning or increasing an exercise program depends on the risk for the individual and the intensity of the planned physical activity. For individuals planning to engage in low- to moderate-intensity activities, the Physical Activities Readiness Questionnaire (PAR-Q) (Box 15-4) should be considered the minimal level of screening. The PAR-Q was designed to identify the small number of adults for whom physical activity might be inappropriate or those who should receive medical advice concerning the most suitable type of activity.[54,124,137]

BOX 15-4

Physical Activity Readiness Questionnaire*

- Has your doctor ever said that you have a heart condition and that you should only do physical activity recommended by a doctor?
- Do you feel pain in your chest when you do physical activity?
- In the past month, have you had chest pain when you were not doing physical activity?
- Do you lose your balance because of dizziness or do you ever lose consciousness?
- Do you have a bone or joint problem that could be made worse by a change in your physical activity?
- Is your doctor currently prescribing drugs (e.g., water pills) for your blood pressure or heart condition?
- Do you know of any other reason why you should not do physical activity?

*A "yes" answer to any of the questions indicates the necessity of a physician's referral for a preexercise evaluation before the individual begins or increases physical activity (Franklin B, Whaley M, Howley E, editors: General principles of exercise prescription. In *ACSM's guidelines for exercise testing and prescription*, ed 6, Philadelphia, 2000, Lippincott Williams & Wilkins; Thompson WR, editor: *ACSM's guidelines for exercise testing and prescription*, ed 8, Philadelphia, 2010, Lippincott Williams & Wilkins.)

Preexercise Evaluation

A preexercise evaluation by a physician is more comprehensive and should include a patient history and a determination of whether the patient needs an exercise stress test.

Patient History

- Current and previous exercise patterns
- Discussion of motivations and barriers to exercise
- Beliefs regarding risks and benefits of exercise
- Preferred types of exercise activity
- Review of heart disease risk factors:
  - Family history of heart disease before the age of 50 years
  - Diabetes, hypertension, smoking, and hyperlipidemia
  - Sedentary lifestyle and obesity
- Physical limitations
- Current medical problems (cardiac, pulmonary, and musculoskeletal)
- History of exercise-induced symptoms (chest pain, shortness of breath, and hives)
- Time and scheduling considerations
- Social support for exercise
- Current medications[55,137]

Identification of Those Who Need an Exercise Stress Test

Indications for an exercise stress test according to the American College of Cardiology and American Heart Association are as follows[130]:

- To evaluate patients for suspected coronary artery disease (typical and atypical angina pectoris).
- To evaluate patients with known coronary artery disease after myocardial infarction or intervention.
- To evaluate patients with suspected or confirmed pulmonary limitations.
- To evaluate healthy, asymptomatic individuals in the following categories:
  - Individuals in high-risk occupations such as pilot, firefighter, law enforcement officer, and mass transit operator;
  - Men older than 40 years and women older than 50 years who are sedentary and plan to start vigorous exercise; and
  - Individuals with multiple cardiac risk factors or concurrent chronic diseases.
- To evaluate exercise capacity in patients with valvular heart disease (except severe aortic stenosis).
- Individuals with cardiac rhythm disorders for the following reasons:
  - To evaluate response to treatment of exercise-induced arrhythmia, and
  - To evaluate response of rate-adaptive pacemaker setting.

The ACSM guidelines are summarized in Box 15-5 and Tables 15-2 and 15-3.[88,137] Contraindications to exercise testing are listed in Box 15-6.

Muscle Physiology

Each skeletal muscle is made of many muscle fibers, which range in diameter between 10 and 80 μm. Each muscle fiber, in turn, contains hundreds to thousands of myofibrils. Each myofibril comprises approximately 1500 myosin (thick) filaments and 3000 actin (thin) filaments, which are responsible for muscle contraction (Figure 15-2).[69,136]

Myosin and actin filaments partially interdigitate, causing myofibrils to have alternate light and dark bands. The light bands contain only actin filaments and are called I bands (because they are isotropic to polarized light). Dark bands contain myosin as well as the ends of the actin filaments where they overlap the myosin, and are called A bands (because they are anisotropic to polarized light). Small projections, called cross-bridges, protrude from the surface of myosin filaments along their entire length, except in the very center. The interaction between the myosin cross-bridge and the actin filaments results in contraction.[69,136]

The ends of actin filaments are attached to Z disks. From the Z disk, actin filaments extend in either direction, interdigitating with the myosin filaments. The Z disk passes from myofibril to myofibril, attaching the myofibrils across the muscle fiber. Thus the entire muscle fiber has light and dark bands, as do individual myofibrils, and thus the striated appearance of the muscle fiber.[69,136]

The portion of a myofibril or the whole muscle fiber between two Z disks is called a sarcomere. The myofibrils within the muscle fibers are suspended in a matrix called

BOX 15-5

Major Symptoms or Signs Suggestive of Cardiopulmonary Disease

- Pain and discomfort (or other anginal equivalent) in the chest, neck, jaw, arms, or other areas that may be ischemic in nature
- Shortness of breath at rest or with mild exertion
- Dizziness or syncope
- Orthopnea or paroxysmal nocturnal dyspnea
- Ankle edema
- Palpitations or tachycardia
- Intermittent claudication
- Known heart murmur
- Unusual fatigue or shortness of breath with usual activities

From Kenny W, Humphrey R, Bryant C, editors: *ACSM's guidelines for exercise testing and prescription,* ed 5, Philadelphia, 1995, Williams & Wilkins; Thompson WR, editor: *ACSM's guidelines for exercise testing and prescription,* ed 8, Philadelphia, 2010, Lippincott Williams & Wilkins.

Table 15-2 American College of Sports Medicine Recommendations for Medical Examination and Exercise Testing Before Participation and for Physician Supervision of Exercise Tests

		Apparently Healthy		*Increased Risk*[a]		
Guideline		**Younger**[b]	**Older**	**No Symptoms**	**Symptoms**	**Known Disease**[c]
Medical examination and clinical exercise test recommended before participation	Moderate exercise[d]	No[e]	No	No	Yes	Yes
	Vigorous exercise[f]	No	Yes[g]	Yes	Yes	Yes
Physician supervision recommended during exercise test	Submaximal testing	No[e]	No	No	Yes	Yes
	Maximal testing	No	Yes[g]	Yes	Yes	Yes

From Kenny W, Humphrey R, Bryant C, editors: *ACSM's guidelines for exercise testing and prescription,* ed 5, Philadelphia, 1995, Williams & Wilkins, with permission of Williams & Wilkins.

[a]Individuals with two or more risk factors (see Table 15-3) or one or more signs or symptoms (see Box 15-5).

[b]Younger implies ≤40 years for men, ≤50 years for women.

[c]Individuals with known cardiac, pulmonary, or metabolic disease.

[d]Moderate exercise as defined by an intensity of 40% to 60% of $\dot{V}O_{2max}$; if intensity is uncertain, moderate exercise may alternatively be defined as one that has an intensity well within the individual's current capacity, that can be comfortably sustained for a prolonged period of time (i.e., 60 minutes), that has a gradual initiation and progression, and that is generally noncompetitive.

[e]A "No" response means that an item is deemed not necessary and is generally noncompetitive.

[f]Vigorous exercise is defined by an exercise intensity greater than 60% of $\dot{V}O_{2max}$; if intensity is uncertain, vigorous exercise may alternatively be defined as exercise intense enough to represent a substantial cardiorespiratory challenge or if it results in fatigue within 20 minutes.

[g]A "Yes" response means that an item is recommended. For physician supervision, this suggests that a physician is in close proximity and readily available should there be an emergent need.

Table 15-3 Coronary Artery Disease Risk Factor Thresholds for Use With American College of Sports Medicine Risk Stratification

Risk Factors	Defining Criteria
Positive	
Family history	Myocardial infarction, coronary revascularization, or sudden death younger than 55 years of age in father or other male first-degree relative (i.e., brother or son) or younger than 65 years of age in mother or other female first-degree relative (i.e., sister or daughter)
Cigarette smoking	Current cigarette smoker or those who quit within the previous 6 months
Hypertension	Systolic blood pressure of ≥140 mm Hg or diastolic ≥90 mm Hg, confirmed by measurements on at least two separate occasions, or on antihypertensive medication
Hypercholesterolemia	Total serum cholesterol of >200 mg dL (5.2 mmoL/L) or high-density lipoprotein cholesterol of <35 mg/dL (0.9 mmoL/L) or on lipid-lowering medication. If low-density lipoprotein cholesterol is available, use >130 mg/dL (3.4 mmoL/L) rather than total cholesterol of >200 mg/dL
Impaired fasting glucose	Fasting blood glucose of ≥110 mg/dL (6.1 mmoL/L) confirmed by measurements on at least two separate occasions
Obesity*	Body mass index of ≥30 kg/m^2 or waist girth of >100 cm
Sedentary lifestyle	Individuals not participating in a regular exercise program or meeting the minimal physical activity recommendations in the U.S. Surgeon General's report
Negative	
High serum high-density lipoprotein cholesterol†	>60 mg/dL (1.6 mmoL/L)

Modified from Thompson PD, editor: Preparticipation health screening. In *ACSM's guidelines for exercise testing and prescription*, ed 9, Philadelphia, Williams & Wilkins, 2014, with permission.

*Professional opinions vary regarding the most appropriate markers and thresholds for obesity; therefore, exercise professionals should use clinical judgment when evaluating this risk factor.

†Accumulating 30 minutes or more of moderate physical activity on most days of the week. It is common to sum risk factors in making clinical judgments. If high-density lipoprotein (HDL) cholesterol is high, subtract one risk factor from the sum of positive risk factors because high HDL decreases coronary artery disease risk.[3]

sarcoplasm. The sarcoplasm contains potassium, magnesium, phosphate, enzymes, and mitochondria. The sarcoplasm also contains the sarcoplasmic reticulum, an extensive endoplasmic reticulum important in the control of muscle contraction.[65,136]

Physiology of Muscle Contraction

Sliding Filament Mechanism

Muscle contraction occurs by a sliding filament mechanism. In the relaxed state the ends of actin filaments, derived from two successive Z disks, barely overlap each other while at the same time completely overlapping the myosin filaments. In the contracted state the actin filaments overlap each other to a great extent, and the Z disks are pulled up to the end of the myosin filaments (Figure 15-3).

The muscle contraction is initiated by the release of acetylcholine from the motor nerve. Acetylcholine opens protein channels in the muscle fiber membrane, allowing sodium to flow into the muscle fiber membrane and initiating a muscle action potential. The action potential depolarizes the muscle fiber membrane, causing the sarcoplasmic reticulum to release calcium. Calcium, in turn, generates attraction between actin and myosin cross-bridges, causing them to slide together.[69,79,136]

Molecular Characteristics of the Contractile Filaments

Each myosin filament is composed of 200 or more myosin molecules. Each myosin molecule is composed of six polypeptide chains: two heavy chains and four light chains. The two heavy chains are wrapped around each other to form a double helix, the tail and arm of the myosin molecule.

BOX 15-6

Contraindications to Exercise Testing

Absolute

- A recent significant change in the resting electrocardiogram suggesting significant ischemia, recent myocardial infarction (within 2 days), or other acute cardiac event
- Unstable angina
- Uncontrolled cardiac dysrhythmias causing symptoms or hemodynamic compromise
- Symptomatic, severe aortic stenosis
- Uncontrolled symptomatic heart failure
- Acute pulmonary embolus or pulmonary infarction
- Acute myocarditis or pericarditis
- Suspected or known dissecting aneurysm
- Acute systemic infection accompanied by fever, body aches, or swollen lymph glands

Relative

- Left main coronary stenosis
- Moderate stenotic valvular heart disease
- Electrolyte abnormalities
- Severe arterial hypertension (i.e., systolic blood pressure >200 mm Hg and/or a diastolic blood pressure >110 mm Hg) at rest
- Tachydysrhythmia or bradydysrhythmia
- Hypertrophic cardiomyopathy and other forms of outflow tract obstruction
- Neuromuscular, musculoskeletal, or rheumatoid disorders that are exacerbated by exercise
- High-degree atrioventricular block
- Ventricular aneurysm
- Uncontrolled metabolic disease (i.e., diabetes, thyrotoxicosis, or myxedema)
- Chronic infectious disease (i.e., mononucleosis, hepatitis, acquired immunodeficiency syndrome)
- Mental or physical impairment leading to inability to exercise adequately

From Franklin B, Whaley M, Howley E, editors: Physical fitness testing and interpretation. In *ACSM's guidelines for exercise testing and prescription*, ed 6, Philadelphia, 2000, Lippincott Williams & Wilkins; Thompson WR, editor: *ACSM's guidelines for exercise testing and prescription*, ed 8, Philadelphia, 2010, Lippincott Williams & Wilkins.

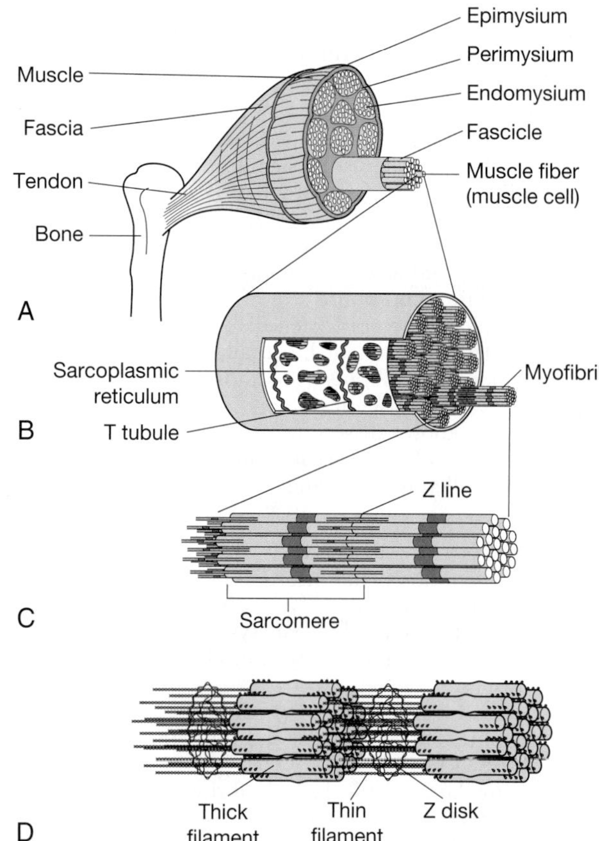

FIGURE 15-2 Structure of skeletal muscle. **A,** Skeletal muscle organ, composed of bundles of contractile muscle fibers held together by connective tissue. **B,** Greater magnification of a single fiber, showing smaller units, myofibrils, in the sarcoplasm. Note the sarcoplasmic reticulum and T tubules forming a three-part structure called a triad. **C,** A myofibril magnified further to show sarcomere between successive Z lines. Cross striae are visible. **D,** Molecular structure of a myofibril, showing thick myofilaments and thin myofilaments. (Redrawn from Thibodeau GA, Patton KT: *Anatomy and physiology,* St Louis, 1999, Mosby, with permission.)

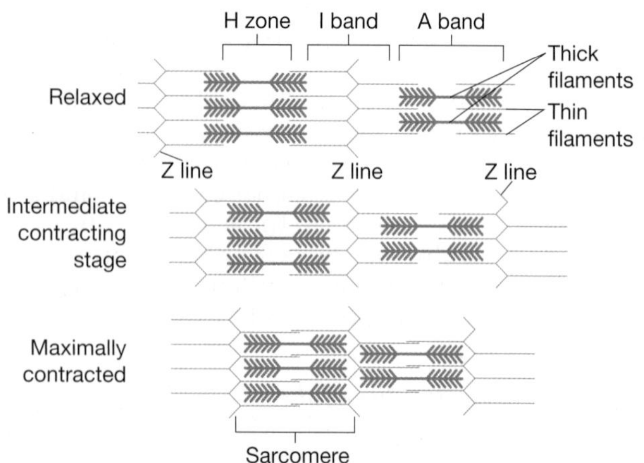

FIGURE 15-3 Sliding filament theory. During contraction, myosin cross-bridges pull the thin filaments toward the center of each sarcomere, thus shortening the myofibril and the entire muscle fiber. (Redrawn from Thibodeau GA, Patton KT: *Anatomy and physiology,* St Louis, 1999, Mosby, with permission.)

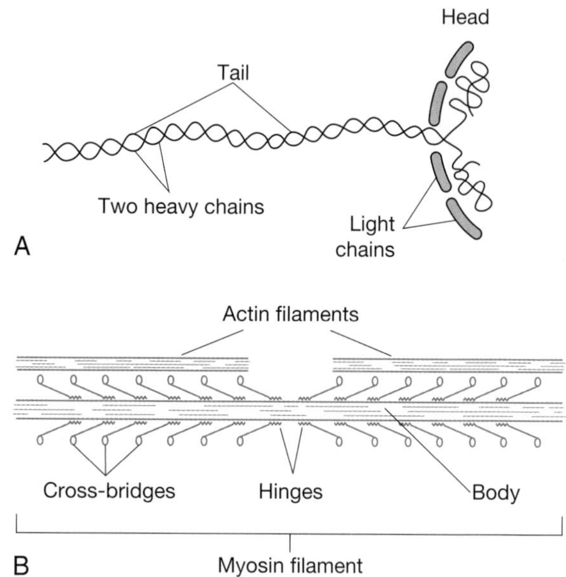

FIGURE 15-4 The myosin filament. **A,** The myosin molecule. **B,** The combination of many myosin molecules to form a myosin filament. Also shown are the cross-bridges and the interaction between the heads of the cross-bridges and adjacent actin filaments. (Redrawn from Guyton A: *Textbook of medical physiology,* Philadelphia, 1996, Saunders, with permission.)

One end of each of the chains is folded into a globular mass called the myosin head. Therefore two myosin heads are lying side by side. The four light chains are also parts of the myosin heads, two to each head (Figure 15-4).

The tails of myosin molecules are bonded together, forming the body of the myosin filament. Protruding from the body, the arm and heads of the myosin molecules are called cross-bridges, which are flexible at two points called hinges. In addition to serving as a component of the cross-bridge, the myosin head also functions as adenosine triphosphatase (ATPase), allowing the head to cleave ATP and energize contraction (Figure 15-5).

Actin filaments are composed of three protein components: actin, tropomyosin, and troponin (Figure 15-6). Several G-actin molecules form strands of F-actin. Two F-actin strands are then wound in a double helix. One molecule of ADP is attached to each G-actin molecule. These ADP molecules represent the active sites of the actin filaments with which myosin cross-bridges interact to cause muscle contraction.

Tropomyosin molecules are wrapped around the F-actin helix. In the resting state, tropomyosin covers the active sites of the actin strands, preventing contraction. Attached near one end of each tropomyosin molecule is a troponin molecule. Each troponin molecule consists of three protein subunits. Troponin I has a strong affinity for actin, troponin T for tropomyosin, and troponin C for calcium.

In the resting state the troponin-tropomyosin complex is thought to cover the active sites of actin, inhibiting contraction. In the presence of calcium, this inhibitory effect is removed, allowing contraction to proceed.[69,136]

Muscle Fiber Types

Muscle fibers can be characterized based on their speed of contraction or twitch. Type 1 fibers (slow oxidative) are

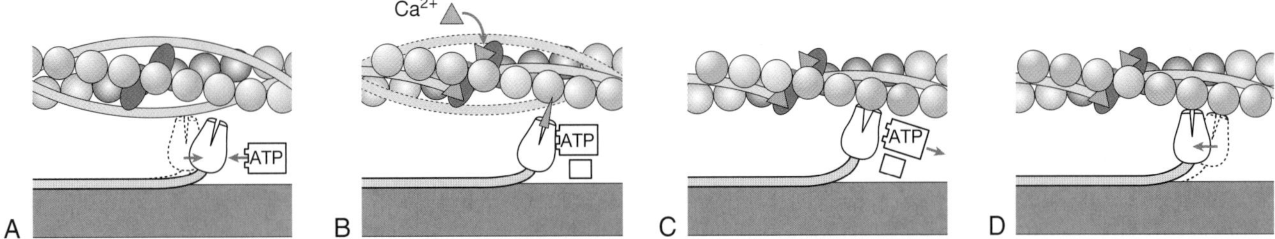

FIGURE 15-5 The molecular basis of muscle contraction. **A,** Each myosin cross-bridge in the thick filament moves into a resting position after an ATP binds and transfers its energy. **B,** Calcium (Ca^{2+}) ions released from the sarcoplasmic reticulum bind to troponin in the thin filament, allowing tropomyosin to shift from its position blocking the active sites of actin molecules. **C,** Each myosin cross-bridge then binds to an active site on a thin filament, displacing the remnants of ATP hydrolysis: ADP and inorganic phosphate. **D,** The release of stored energy from step **A** provides the force needed for each cross-bridge to move back to its original position, pulling actin along with it. Each cross-bridge will remain bound to actin until another ATP binds to it and pulls it back to its resting position (**A**). *ADP,* Adenosine diphosphate; *ATP,* adenosine triphosphate. (Redrawn from Thibodeau GA, Patton KT: *Anatomy and physiology,* St Louis, 1999, Mosby, with permission.)

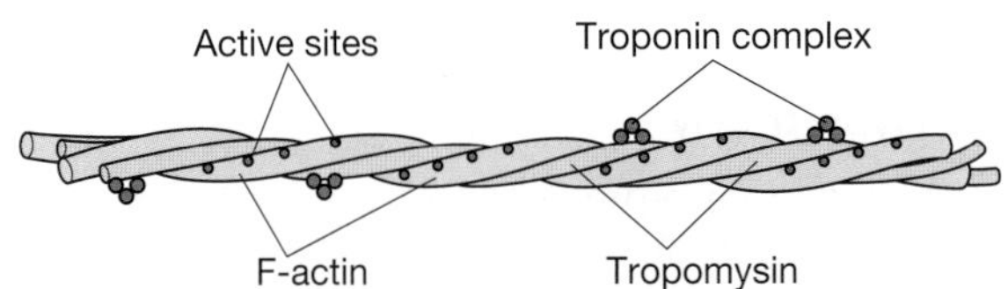

FIGURE 15-6 Tropomyosin molecules. The actin filament, composed of two helical strands of F-actin and tropomyosin molecules that fit loosely in the grooves between the actin strands. Attached to one end of each tropomyosin molecule is a troponin complex that initiates contraction. (Redrawn from Guyton A: *Textbook of medical physiology,* Philadelphia, 1996, Saunders, with permission.)

best suited for endurance activities requiring aerobic metabolism. Type 2 fibers (fast twitch) are most active during activities requiring strength and speed. Type 2 fibers are further categorized into type 2A (fast, oxidative glycolytic) and type 2B (fast glycolytic). Type 2A represents a type of hybrid that retains some oxidative capacity. Features of each muscle type are summarized in Table 15-4.

During anaerobic activity, slow oxidative fibers (type 1) are used almost exclusively at intensities below 70% of $\dot{V}O_{2max}$. Beyond this intensity, anaerobic pathways are stimulated. At $\dot{V}O_{2max}$, both type 1 and type 2 are relied on, and oxygen debt eventually occurs secondary to aerobic metabolism.

During isometric contractions, type 2 fibers are generally recruited when force exceeds 20% of the maximal voluntary contraction. If sustained for long periods, however, type 2 units can be recruited at thresholds below 20% of maximal voluntary contraction.[29,65,136]

Muscle Fiber Orientation

Parallel muscles have their fibers arranged parallel to the length of the muscle and produce a greater range of motion than similar-sized muscles with pennate arrangement. Pennate muscles have shorter fibers that are arranged obliquely to their tendons (similar to the makeup of a feather), increasing cross-sectional area and the power produced.

Types of Muscle Contraction

Isometric contractions are contractions in which there is no change in the length of the muscle. No joint or limb motion occurs. Isotonic contractions occur when the muscle changes length, producing limb motion. Concentric contractions occur when the muscle shortens. Eccentric contractions occur when the muscle lengthens. More fast-twitch fibers are recruited during eccentric contractions. Isokinetic contractions occur when muscle contraction is performed at a constant velocity. This can be done only with the assistance of a preset rate-limiting device. This type of exercise does not exist in nature.

Factors Affecting Muscle Strength and Performance

Determinants of Strength

The ability of a muscle to produce force is directly proportional to its cross-sectional area. For parallel muscles, this corresponds to the cross-section at the bulkiest part of the muscle. For pennate muscles, multiple cross-sections are taken at right angles to each of the muscle fibers. Pennate muscles are particularly adapted to force production because many more muscle fibers are contained in pennate muscles and these fibers are shorter.[88]

Length-Tension Relationship

Maximum force of contraction occurs when a muscle is at its normal resting muscle length. For the muscles, this corresponds to about midrange of joint motion or slightly longer, and is the length at which tension just begins to exceed zero. If a muscle is stretched beyond resting length before contraction, resting tension develops, and active tension (the increase in tension during contraction) decreases.

Efficiency (percentage of energy that is converted into work instead of heat) occurs at a velocity of contraction of approximately 30% of maximal.[28,29]

Torque-Velocity Relationship

The greatest amount of force is generated by a muscle during fast eccentric (lengthening) contractions.[28,29] The least amount of force is produced during fast concentric (shortening) contractions. The amount of force developed in the order of most force to least force can be summarized as follows: fast eccentric, isometric, slow concentric, and fast concentric (Figure 15-7).

Table 15-4 Skeletal Muscle Fiber Characteristics

	Type I (Slow Oxidative)	Type 2B (Fast Glycolytic)	Type 2A (Fast Oxidative Glycolytic)
Major source of ATP	Oxidative phosphorylation	Glycolysis	Oxidative phosphorylation
Mitochondria	High	Low	High
Myoglobin content	High	Low	High
Capillarity	High	Low	High
Muscle color	Red	White	Red
Glycogen content	Low	High	Intermediate
Glycolytic enzyme activity	Low	High	Intermediate
Myosin ATPase activity	Low	High	High
Speed of contraction	Slow	Fast	Fast
Rate of fatigue	Slow	Fast	Intermediate
Muscle fiber diameter	Small	Large	Intermediate

ATP, Adenosine triphosphate.

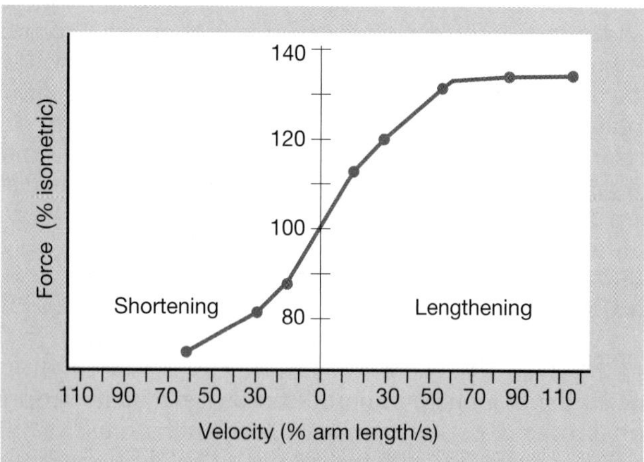

FIGURE 15-7 Relationship of maximal force of human elbow flexor muscles to velocity of contraction. Velocity on the abscissa is designated as a percentage of arm length per second. (Redrawn from Knuttgen HG: Development of muscular strength and endurance. In Knuttgen HG, editor: *Neuromuscular mechanisms for therapeutic and conditioning exercises,* Baltimore, 1976, University Park Press, with permission.)

Effects of Exercise Training

The SAID principle (*s*pecific *a*daptations to *i*mposed *d*emands) states that a muscle will adapt to a specific demand imposed on it, making it better able to handle the greater load.

Neural Adaptations

Observed strength gains within the first few weeks of a weightlifting program are mostly because of neuromuscular adaptations. The nervous system recruits larger motor units with higher frequencies of stimulation to provide the force necessary to overcome the imposed resistance. Early strength gains and increased muscle tension production from training therefore result from a more efficient neural recruitment process. This means that most of the improvement in strength-related functional activities gained on inpatient rehabilitation units is attributable to neural recruitment rather than muscle hypertrophy, as a result of the relatively short length of stays.[92]

Muscle Hypertrophy

Muscle hypertrophy represents enlargement of total muscle mass and cross-sectional area. Muscle hypertrophy is more common in fast-twitch than in slow-twitch muscles. Type 2A fibers exhibit the greatest growth, more so than type 2B and type 1 fibers. Muscle hypertrophy is typically experienced after 6 to 7 weeks of resistance training.[33,73] Conversely, muscle atrophy resulting from disuse occurs primarily in type 2 fibers.

Virtually all muscle hypertrophy occurs from hypertrophy of the individual muscle fibers. During muscle hypertrophy the rate of muscle contractile protein synthesis is greater than decay, leading to greater numbers of actin and myosin filaments in the myofibrils. The myofibrils within each muscle fiber split, resulting in more myofibrils in each muscle fiber. Only under very rare conditions of extreme muscle force generation do the numbers of muscle fibers increase (fiber hyperplasia), and even then by only a few percent.[29,69]

Another type of muscle hypertrophy occurs when muscles are stretched to a greater-than-normal length, causing new sarcomeres to be added at the ends of muscle fibers where they attach to the tendons. Conversely, when a muscle remains shortened at less than its resting length, sarcomeres at the end of the muscle fibers disappear.[27,29]

Exercise Prescription

Advancing in a training program can include increasing the amount of weight lifted (progressive resistive exercise), increasing repetitions, or increasing the velocity of training. A commonly used term to express an individual's current strength level is the one-repetition maximum (1-RM), which is the most weight that can be lifted one time. The current strength fitness level for a particular exercise can be expressed in terms of an individual's multiple RM (e.g., 10-RM is the amount of weight that an individual is capable of lifting 10 times).

Progressive Resistance Exercise

Popular protocols include the DeLorme, Oxford, and daily adjusted progressive resistance exercise (DAPRE) methods.

DeLorme. In the DeLorme method, three sets are performed for each exercise. Ten repetitions are performed in each set. The weight for the first set is 50% of the 10-RM; the second set, 75% of the 10-RM; and the third set, 100% of the 10-RM.[30] This is usually referred to clinically as progressive resistive exercise.

Oxford. In the Oxford technique, an individual starts with 10 repetitions at 100% of the 10-RM, then 10 repetitions at 75% of the 10-RM, then a third set of 10 repetitions at 50% of the 10-RM. This is usually referred to in the clinical setting as regressive resistive exercise.

Daily Adjusted Progressive Resistance Exercise. The DAPRE method of strength training guides the athlete through four sets of exercise per muscle group. The first set in DAPRE involves 10 repetitions at 50% of the athlete's predetermined 6-RM. The second set consists of six repetitions at 75% of the athlete's 6-RM. The third set consists of as many repetitions as can be performed at the athlete's 6-RM. The number of repetitions performed in the third set determines the resistance for the fourth set. If five to seven repetitions were performed in the third set, resistance stays the same. If fewer than five repetitions were performed in the third set, the weight is lowered by 5 lb. If more than seven repetitions are performed in the third set, the weight is raised by 5 lb. The fourth set consists of as many repetitions as can be performed to fatigue. The working weight for the next day is established based on the athlete's performance during the fourth set, with the same formula for determining resistance change from the third to the fourth set.[73,91]

It is important to note that none of these three types of resistive training programs have been determined to be superior to the others.

Increasing Number of Repetitions or Rate

Critical to developing muscle strength is to exercise to the point of fatigue. Both high weight–low repetition and low weight–high repetition programs can be effective in achieving strength as long as exercise proceeds to muscle fatigue. Far more repetitions must be carried out with low weights to reach this point of fatigue. In fact, the amount of mechanical work required by low weight–high repetition exercise to reach muscle fatigue might be much greater than during higher weight exercise. Although circumstances exist where low weight–high repetition exercise can be appropriate for training (such as during injury or when training for a highly repetitive task), in general the use of higher weights to fatigue is a more effective means of strength training.

Hellebrandt and Houtz[75] advocate increasing the rate of contraction (controlled by a metronome) each session while lifting the same number of repetitions (10 to 20).[29]

Effects of Aging

Although it was previously believed that strength training in older adults was attributable only to learning or neural factors,[105] reports have also demonstrated that the muscles of older individuals can demonstrate hypertrophy after strength training.[56,88]

Table 15-5 Recommended Guidelines for Strength Training

Component	Details
Mode	Perform a minimum of 8 to 10 exercises that train the major muscle groups
Intensity	One set of 8 to 12 repetitions resulting in volitional fatigue for each exercise*
Duration	The entire program should last no more than 1 hour. Programs lasting longer than 1 hour are associated with a higher dropout rate
Frequency	At least 2 days per week*

From Thompson WR, editor: *ACSM's guidelines for exercise testing and prescription*, ed 8, Philadelphia, 2010, Lippincott Williams & Wilkins.

*Although more frequent training with additional sets or repetitions might elicit additional strength gains, the additional improvement is considered relatively small (Kabat H: Proprioceptive facilitation in therapeutic exercise. In Licht S, editor: *Therapeutic exercise*, ed 2, New Haven, 1961, E Licht.)

ACSM Guidelines for Prescription of Strength-Training Exercise

Muscular strength and endurance can be developed with both dynamic and static exercise. Both forms have their indications, but for most individuals dynamic exercise is recommended. Strength exercise should be rhythmic, performed at low to moderate speed, and performed through a full range of motion. Normal breathing should be maintained. Heavy resistance training associated with breath holding can result in dramatic rises in SBP and DBP.

A specific technique for each exercise should be closely adhered to. Both the lifting (concentric) and lowering (eccentric) phases of resistance exercise should be performed in a controlled manner. When possible, training with a partner can provide feedback, assistance, motivation, and safety.

Recommended guidelines for strength training are listed in Table 15-5.

Flexibility

Flexibility generally describes the range of motion commonly present in a joint or group of joints that allows normal and unimpaired function.[17] More specifically, flexibility has been defined as "the total achievable excursion (within limits of pain) of a body part through its range of motion."[120] With regard to flexibility, the following generalizations can be made. Flexibility is an individually variable, joint-specific, inherited characteristic that decreases with age; varies by gender and ethnic group; bears little relationship with body proportion or limb length; and most important for the purposes of this chapter, can be acquired through training.[22,59,66–68,141]

From a developmental standpoint, flexibility is greatest during infancy and early childhood. Flexibility reaches minimal levels between 10 and 12 years of age. It then improves again toward early adulthood, but not sufficiently to allow ranges of motion seen in childhood.[38] The early adolescent growth spurt results in short-term tightness of the joints, probably as a result of increased tension in the connective tissue. Girls are generally more flexible than boys,[11,90,111,118] and this advantage probably persists into adulthood.

Achieving a maximal functional range of motion is an important goal of many therapeutic exercise regimens. Most typically, increased range of motion is achieved via the process of stretching. The term *stretching* defines an activity that applies a deforming force along the rotational or translational planes of motion of a joint.[120] Stretching should respect the lines of geometry of the joint as well as its planes of stability. In addition to stretching, mobilization is used to maintain flexibility. Mobilization moves a joint through its range of motion without applying a deforming force.

Importance of Flexibility

Flexibility has only recently been identified as an important component of therapeutic exercise. Cureton[26] emphasized flexibility as an important component of physical fitness after working with swimmers during the 1932 Olympic Games. Later, Kraus[94] stressed the importance of flexibility in preventing low back pain. His work inspired much of the subsequent research on flexibility. It was not until 1964 that Fleishman[49] proved flexibility to be an independent factor in physical fitness that was unrelated to other factors, including strength, power, endurance, and coordination. During the same decade and in another landmark work, DeVries and Housh[37] proved the value of passive stretching in improving flexibility and range of motion. Subsequent studies have demonstrated the value of flexibility training for patients in the industrial and athletic settings, for patients with back pain, and for patients who are status postorthopedic surgical procedures.

Subsequent to Kraus's work, biomechanical studies have shown that lower limb flexibility is needed for the prevention of lumbar spine injuries.[47] An increased frequency of spondylolysis and spondylolisthesis in individuals with severe hamstring inflexibility has been reported.[110] Cady et al.[14] demonstrated an inverse relationship between flexibility and the incidence of back injuries and workers' compensation costs in a cohort study of firefighters placed on a fitness program.

The work of Salter and associates[89,122,143] has emphasized the importance of maintaining motion and flexibility postoperatively in patients who have undergone orthopedic procedures. The benefits of the mobilization of postoperative joints to the surrounding ligamentous and musculotendinous structures have been well established.

In the realm of athletic training, flexibility has been both extensively applied and extensively studied. The proposed benefits of flexibility to athletes include injury prevention, reduced muscle soreness, skill enhancement, and muscle relaxation.* With regard to injury prevention, muscles possessing greater extensibility are less likely to be overstretched during athletic activity, lessening the possibility of injury. A 1987 review of all studies of soccer injuries suggested an important role for flexibility in the prevention of injury, and attributed up to 11% of all injuries to poor flexibility.[87] A prospective study of a flexibility program in soccer players demonstrated a correlation between improvement in range of motion and reduction in incidence of muscle tears.[45] There is some evidence that delayed muscular soreness can be prevented and treated by static stretching.[35,36]

Flexibility has generally been hypothesized to improve athletic performance through skill enhancement. For example, mastery of the serve in tennis requires sufficient shoulder flexibility. Similarly, proficient golf skills require flexibility throughout the hips, trunk, and shoulders.[21] On the biomechanical level, prestretching a muscle has been shown in several studies to enhance the force of muscle contraction.[8,9,16,17]

There is, however, considerable uncertainty regarding two of the most important proposed benefits of flexibility training for athletes: prevention of injury and improvement of performance. Although currently held teaching states that stretching is a preventive measure for athletic injury, it has been pointed out that little conclusive epidemiologic evidence supports this idea.[71,74] In fact, it has been proposed that a certain degree of tightness might protect against injury by allowing load sharing when joints are stressed.[74] Hypermobility or excessive stretching could theoretically result in increased stress on the ligaments, bone, and cartilage at the joint, resulting in injury or arthritis.[66,107] In support of this is the fact that there is general agreement that the major predictive factor for joint injury is a previous joint injury or indeed the presence of excessive joint laxity, rather than inadequate flexibility.† Presently, the role of preexercise stretching in the prevention of sports-related injury is unclear. A systematic review performed by Thacker et al.[135] for the ACSM failed to find "sufficient evidence to endorse or discontinue routine stretching before or after exercise to prevent injury among competitive or recreational athletes."

With regard to athletic performance, several laboratories have shown that among runners, less flexible individuals have a lower rate of oxygen consumption while covering the same distance at the same speed as their more flexible cohorts.[23] In addition, the aforementioned improvement in contraction strength resulting from prestretching has not been consistently observed in the world of athletics. In fact, it has been shown repeatedly that passive stretching can result in an acute loss of strength.‡ Along the same lines, a recent study of elite female soccer players demonstrated that static stretching before sprinting resulted in worsened performance.[123] Prior stretching does appear to have one reproducible benefit with regard to performance, however: maintenance of strength with the muscle in a lengthened position during and after eccentric exercise.[103] This benefit might be important in resisting injurious muscle elongation during continued sport performance.[103]

The athletic literature seems to show in general that flexibility training, when used appropriately, plays a positive role in sports injury and performance. However, excessive flexibility can actually be both a risk factor for injury and a detriment to performance. Stiff structures appear to benefit from stretching, whereas hypermobile structures require stabilization rather than additional mobilization.

*References 11, 21, 27, 39, 41, 45, 60, 82.

†References 44, 45, 62, 85, 87, 125.

‡References 24, 25, 46, 50, 93, 100.

Determinants of Flexibility

The determinants of joint mobility can be subdivided into static and dynamic factors. Static factors include the types of tissues involved, the types and state of collagen subunits in the tissue, the presence or absence of inflammation, and the temperature of the tissue. Dynamic factors include neuromuscular variables such as voluntary muscle control and the length-tension "thermostat" of the musculotendinous unit, as well as external factors such as pain associated with injury.[120]

Static Factors

The most important tissue with regard to flexibility is the muscle-tendon unit, which is the primary target of flexibility training.[120] This structure includes the full length of the muscle and its supporting tissue, the musculotendinous junction, and the full length of the tendon to the tendon-bone junction. Within the muscle-tendon unit, it is the muscle that has the largest capacity for percent lengthening[81,131,132] of the tissues involved in a stretch. A ratio of 95% to 5% for the muscle-to-tendon length change has been demonstrated.[132]

From a mechanical standpoint, muscle is composed of contractile and elastic elements arranged in parallel.[69] Muscle can respond to an applied force or stretch with permanent elongation. Animal studies have shown that this results from an increase in the number of sarcomeres, which translates to increased peak tension of a muscle at longer resting lengths. By contrast, muscle at rest has a tendency to shorten because of its contractile element. This shortening can be permanent and is associated with a reduction in sarcomeres.[64,66,142] Tendon has a much more limited capacity for lengthening than muscle, probably because of its proteoglycan content and collagen cross-links (2% to 3% of its length, compared with 20% for muscle).[131,132,145] Of the external static factors, temperature has been studied the most. Warmer tissues are generally more distensible than cold ones.[42,140,141]

Dynamic Factors

Perhaps the most clinically and physiologically significant dynamic determinant of flexibility is the muscle length–tension thermostat or feedback control system. Intrafusal fibers (muscle spindles), innervated by gamma motor neurons, lie in parallel with extrafusal contractile fibers. The intrafusal fibers serve the purpose of regulating the tension and length of the muscle as a whole. Muscle spindle length and tension are regulated by the gamma motor neuron, which in turn is subject to influences from the central nervous system. These include segmental input at the spinal cord level and suprasegmental input from the cerebellum and cortex. Consequently, muscle length and tension can be subject to multiple influences simultaneously.

An additional complicating factor is that receptors in the musculotendinous unit called the Golgi tendon organs act to inhibit muscle contraction at the point of critical stresses to the structure. The Golgi tendon organs allow lengthening and facilitate relaxation. When acting in conjunction, these dynamic mechanisms facilitate a response to a stretch in the following way. As the muscle spindle is initially stretched, it sends impulses to the spinal cord that result in reflex muscle contraction. If the stretch is maintained longer than 6 seconds, the Golgi tendon organ fires, causing relaxation.[120]

The relative contribution of static muscle factors and dynamic neural factors to flexibility remains somewhat controversial. It seems clear that the changes in flexibility noted immediately after the institution of a stretching program occur too rapidly to be attributable solely to structural alteration of the muscle and connective tissue. The consensus view is that neural factors probably play the major role in this early flexibility. After prolonged periods of training, changes in sarcomere number can play a role in the establishment of a new elongated muscle length.[120]

Assessment of Flexibility

Flexibility is generally assessed in terms of joint range of motion. Joint range of motion in turn is generally assessed with a goniometer or similar device. A goniometer consists of a 180-degree protractor designed for easy application to joints. The methods used with a goniometer, as well as the normal ranges of motion encountered with these methods, are well standardized.[44,114] Interobserver and intraobserver reliability are good.[41] Limitations of the standard goniometer include application to only single joints at a given time, static measurements only, and difficulty of application to certain joints (e.g., costoclavicular).

The Leighton Flexometer contains a rotating circular dial marked in degrees and a pointer counterbalanced to remain vertical. It can be strapped to a body segment, and range of motion is determined with respect to the perpendicular. Its reliability is good but is not fully equivalent to that of the standard goniometer.[72]

The electrogoniometer substitutes a potentiometer for a protractor. The potentiometer provides an electrical signal that is directly proportional to the angle of the joint. This device is able to give continuous recordings during a variety of activities, allowing a more realistic assessment of functional flexibility and dynamic range of motion during actual physical activity.

With regard to measuring trunk flexibility, goniometric devices are generally considered inadequate. The Schober test, originally designed to measure spinal flexion and extension in patients with ankylosing spondylitis, is commonly used, as modified by Moll and Wright.[104a] Two marks are made along the proximal and distal ends of the lumbar spine, and tape measurements are made between them with the spine in flexion, neutral, and extension. This test has been shown to be more reliable than other methods, including fingertip to floor measurements and the inclinometer technique of Loebl. "Eyeball" measurements show marked variability. These tests of trunk flexibility are all nonspecific, and each is limited to a gross measurement of compound motion of the entire thoracolumbar spine. None of these methods can assess articular mobility in the translational and rotational planes.[120] The optimal measurement of trunk flexibility is probably that obtained with plain films, but these have the obvious disadvantages of cost and radiation exposure.

Methods of Stretching

It is important to take several factors into consideration when using a stretching program. Prevention of injury and treatment of specific joint injury, as well as the presence and effects of pain or muscle spasm, require modification of the program. Stretching can be dangerous and might result in significant injury if performed incorrectly.[121,124,126] As with any form of therapeutic exercise, flexibility training must be approached within a program aimed at addressing the specific functional needs of the individual.

Numerous options now abound for improving flexibility with stretching techniques. A distinct superiority of any one method has not been demonstrated. For the purposes of this chapter, stretching techniques are divided into the following four categories: ballistic, static, passive, and neuromuscular facilitation.

Ballistic

Ballistic stretching uses the repetitive rapid application of force in a bouncing or jerking maneuver. Momentum carries the body part through the range of motion until the muscles are stretched to their limits. This method is less efficient than other methods because muscle will contract under these stresses to protect itself from overstretching. Additionally, the rapid increase in force can cause injury.[125,133] An example would be the 10-count bouncing toe touches popularized in the 1970s, but has since been abandoned because of lack of efficacy and risk for injury.

Passive

Passive stretching is done by a partner or therapist who applies a stretch to a relaxed joint or extremity. This method requires excellent communication and the slow and sensitive application of force. This method is most appropriately and most safely used in the training room or in a physical or occupational therapy context. Outside these contexts, passive stretching can be dangerous for recreational or competitive athletes because of an increased risk for injury.

Static

Static stretching applies a steady force for a period of 15 to 60 seconds. This method is the easiest and probably the safest type of stretching. Static stretching seems to be particularly helpful as a warm-up to any other form of therapeutic or recreational exercise, including athletic activity. Static stretching has the added advantage here of being associated with decreased muscle soreness after exercise.

Neuromuscular Facilitation

The efficacy of stretching afforded by neuromuscular facilitation techniques has been documented in several studies.[121,134] These methods typically require a trained therapist, aide, or trainer. The specific activities most frequently used include hold-relax and contract-relax techniques, characterized by an isometric or concentric contraction of the musculotendinous unit followed by a passive or static stretch. The prestretch contraction is thought to facilitate relaxation and flexibility via the muscle length–tension thermostat discussed previously in this chapter.

Table 15-6 Recommended Guidelines for Flexibility Training

Component	Details
Mode	Static, dynamic, and PNF stretching of major muscle groups including the low back and posterior thigh
Intensity	To a mild degree of tightness without discomfort
Duration	Static stretches are held 15 to 60 seconds. A 6-second contraction followed by 10 to 30 seconds-assisted stretch for PNF
Frequency	At least 2 to 3 days per week
Repetitions	Four or more per muscle group

From Thompson WR, editor: *ACSM's guidelines for exercise testing and prescription*, ed 8, Philadelphia, 2010, Lippincott Williams & Wilkins.
PNF, Proprioceptive neuromuscular facilitation.

ACSM Guidelines for Prescription of Exercise for Musculoskeletal Flexibility

Optimal musculoskeletal function requires that adequate range of motion be maintained in all joints. Particularly important is maintenance of flexibility in the low back and posterior thigh muscles. Poor flexibility in these regions can predispose to low back pain.[88,137]

Some common stretching exercises might not be appropriate for all people, particularly those with a previous injury, joint insufficiency, or other conditions that could place them at risk for injury. Furthermore, exercises requiring substantial flexibility or skill are not recommended for older, less flexible, or less experienced individuals.[83]

Recommended guidelines for flexibility training are listed in Table 15-6.[88,137]

Plyometrics

Plyometrics is a relatively recent addition to the panoply of therapeutic exercise. This class of exercises is used primarily in the training of athletes. Proponents of plyometrics advocate it because of its apparent muscle strengthening and injury prevention effects. Plyometric exercises are generally defined as brief, explosive maneuvers that consist of an eccentric muscle contraction followed immediately by a concentric contraction. An example is the action of planting and jumping during sport activity. Here, the process of planting the feet and flexing the hips, knees, and ankles while loading the lower extremities (eccentric contraction) is followed by a quick changeover to concentric contractions while these joints are extended to propel upward into a jump. This type of stretch-shortening cycle is analogous to a spring coiling and uncoiling.

Plyometrics allows the body to store elastic energy briefly in the muscle during the eccentric phase. This stored energy, combined with activation of the myotatic stretch reflex, results in a more powerful concentric contraction than is otherwise possible. This type of relatively complex action relies more heavily on the interplay between central nervous system and muscular system than do many other forms of exercise. Feedback from the central nervous system to the muscles influences the length of each muscle at any point during the movement, as well as the tension required for maintaining postural stability and initiating or stopping movement.[20] With training, according to proponents of plyometrics, this neuromuscular interplay can be finely tuned. The widespread use of plyometric training in the athletic community suggests general acceptance of these methods by trainers, therapists, and athletes. However, many techniques in use have not been adequately studied. Results of research so far have generally been promising.

Hewett et al.[77] have reported that plyometric jump training improved lower body strength in high school–age girls. Specifically, hamstring isokinetic strength and vertical jump height were improved after a 6-week program. A 22% decrease in peak ground reaction forces and a 50% decrease in the abduction-adduction moments at the knee during landing were also observed. In a later study using the same plyometric program, Hewett et al.[76] prospectively analyzed the effect of this neuromuscular training on the incidence of serious knee injuries in female athletes. The authors reported a statistically significant decrease in the number of knee injuries sustained by the trained group versus the matched control group.

Plyometric exercises vary in intensity, from simple, two-footed, in-place jumps, to hopping and bounding for maximum distance, to depth jumps from boxes of varying height. Plyometrics has been shown to result in ground reaction forces of four to seven times the body weight.[7,144] Clearly these exercises should be approached with caution and begun at an elementary level. Progression to more advanced exercises should be based on the individual's proficiency with the basic movements, taking into account baseline levels of strength, stability, and coordination.

Proprioception

Proprioception denotes the process by which information about the position and movement of body parts is related to the central nervous system. Proprioceptive organs, including muscle (particularly intrafusal spindle fibers), skin, ligaments, and joint capsules, generate afferent information that is crucial to the effective and safe performance of motor tasks. The process of proprioception is unfortunately subject to impairment from injury and disease. For example, knee and ankle ligament injuries have been shown to reduce proprioception. The same is true for both osteoarthritis and rheumatoid arthritis.[6,48] Neuropathies, most notably diabetic neuropathy, can also cause significant loss of proprioception.[127] Proprioception has also been shown to decrease with age.[128]

The importance of proprioception to injury prevention and rehabilitation from injury is generally accepted. Impaired proprioception has been associated with an increased risk for joint damage, athletic injury, and falls. Decreased joint proprioception is thought to influence the progressive joint deterioration associated with osteoarthritis, rheumatoid arthritis, and Charcot disease.[5,6] In a study of soccer players, a significantly greater incidence of ankle injury was observed among players with abnormal proprioceptive testing results as compared with those who tested within normal measurements.[139] Some findings also suggest that return to sport after knee injury might be more dependent on proprioception than on ligament tension.[6] It has also been demonstrated in several studies that the risk for falling in the older adult population correlates with postural sway, a variable that is determined in large part by proprioception.[95,97,98,138]

Proprioceptive exercise regimens, by definition, seek to improve joint and limb position sense. These exercises are typically used after an injury has occurred to a joint that has resulted in a deficit in proprioception. For example, the tilt or wobble board is commonly used after ankle ligamentous injuries. Classically, the unidirectional boards are used first, with a progression to multidirectional boards. This type of training has led to measurably improved position sense in athletes.[58] Other proprioceptive exercises include carioca (sideways running) and backward walking or running. It has also been shown that elastic bandaging improves position sense in individuals with previously impaired proprioception,[6] perhaps through stimulation of proprioceptors in the skin.

Neurofacilitation Techniques

Central nervous system dysfunction poses a unique set of challenges to both the patient and the treatment team. The following therapeutic exercise techniques were developed specifically for patients with central nervous system impairment, particularly impairment resulting from an acquired cortical lesion (i.e., stroke or brain injury).

Proprioceptive Neuromuscular Facilitation

This form of therapy uses resistance to indirectly facilitate movement. The therapist provides maximal resistance to the stronger motor components of specific spiral and diagonal movement patterns, thereby facilitating the weaker components of the patterns. Proprioceptive neuromuscular facilitation techniques are best applied to patients with hypotonia associated with supraspinal lesions to promote normalization of tone. In patients with spasticity, these techniques can actually further increase tone in a potentially detrimental manner.[83,84]

Brunnstrom

These techniques use resistance and primitive postural reactions to facilitate gross synergistic movement patterns and increase muscle tone during early recovery from central nervous system injury.[10] During later stages, Brunnstrom techniques emphasize development of isolated movement and control. Similar to proprioceptive neuromuscular facilitation, this approach is thought to be effective in normalizing tone in a patient with hypotonic or flaccid hemiplegia.

Bobath

The neurodevelopmental techniques developed by Berta Bobath and Karel Bobath differ significantly from proprioceptive neuromuscular facilitation and Brunnstrom methods. The Bobath techniques use reflex inhibitory movement patterns to inhibit increased tone. These inhibitory patterns, which are generally antagonistic to the primitive synergistic patterns, are performed without resistance. Neurodevelopmental techniques also incorporate advanced postural reactions to stimulate recovery. Advocates of these techniques claim reduction of hypertonicity and facilitation of motor recovery as their primary benefits.[57]

The techniques described in this section are all in common clinical use, with most therapists using an eclectic approach, borrowing some from each. There is no convincing evidence, however, that any of these methods actually alter the natural history of recovery from neurologic insult. These approaches to therapy seem to be most useful in providing compensatory techniques during the course of recovery. Using these methods, patients are able to improve performance in and gain independence with such tasks as making transfers, stretching, bed mobility, and safe ambulation.[57]

Exercise for Special Populations

Physical Inactivity and Obesity

Physical inactivity is associated with increased fat and visceral adipose tissue accumulation. Not only does physical inactivity contribute to development of heart disease but it also increases chances of breast and colon cancer, depression, diabetes, and metabolic syndrome. Sedentary jobs have significantly increased in recent years and physical activity demanding jobs constitute only 25% of the workforce. Regular activity is protective by regulating weight and improving the body's use of insulin. Being active is beneficial for blood pressure, blood lipid levels, glucose levels, clotting factors, the health of blood vessels, and inflammation, which is a powerful promoter of cardiovascular disease. A total of 48% of adults meet the 2008 ACSM Physical Activity Guidelines. Based on age-adjusted estimates, non-Hispanic black (41.1%) and Hispanic (42.2%) adults were more inclined to be inactive compared with non-Hispanic white adults. People who are insufficiently physically active have a 20% to 30% increased risk of all-cause mortality compared with those who engage in at least 30 minutes of moderate-intensity physical activity most days of the week.[61]

Although most of the comorbidities relating obesity to coronary artery disease increase as body mass index (BMI) increases, they also relate to body fat distribution. Visceral fat causes central adiposity and increases risk of insulin resistance and diabetes mellitus, heart disease, stroke, and dementia. Long-term longitudinal studies, however, indicate that obesity not only relates to but can also independently predict coronary atherosclerosis. This holds true for both men and women with minimal increases in BMI. In a 14-year prospective study, middle-aged women with a BMI greater than 23 but less than 25 had a 50% increase in risk of nonfatal or fatal coronary heart disease,[99] and men aged 40 to 65 years with a BMI greater than 25 but less than 29 had a 72% increased risk.[116] It has been shown that weight loss also shortens the QT interval, thus further reducing the risk of heart disease.[15] Treatment of obesity should be tailored according to severity and the presence of comorbidities, such as congestive heart failure, hypertension, dyslipidemia, non–insulin-dependent diabetes, and obstructive sleep apnea.[43]

Exercise for Fat Reduction

Successful weight loss requires a combination of diet and exercise. The threshold for change in body weight appears to be 30 minutes of exercise per day, with more marked losses noted with 60 min/day. Moderate-intensity land–based activity such as cycling, brisk walking, or pushing a lawn mower is safe for most adults and will reduce the risk of coronary heart disease by approximately 30%. The aim should be to reach 60% to 85% of resting HR during exercise. If exercising for an extended period is not possible, it may be broken into periods of 10 minutes at a time of continuous moderate-vigorous activity. This regimen should be performed with major muscle group activation (all extremities, chest, abdomen, back) at least 2 days per week.[18] Swimming in the absence of caloric restriction did not appear to result in weight loss. In fact, individuals gained weight, although this appeared to be all muscle weight, thus increasing lean body mass. It stands to reason, however, that swimming can be effective in weight loss if combined with caloric restriction.[29,70]

Exercise is broadly categorized into aerobic and anaerobic. Aerobic, or cardiovascular, exercise builds endurance. It uses O_2 to burn carbohydrates and fats for energy production. Protein and amino acids are used as energy substrates only in cases of starvation, severe caloric deprivation, and "overexercising." Anaerobic exercise builds muscle and strength through short bursts of strenuous activity.

Isotonic and isometric exercises are performed during strength training. Isotonic exercise causes a muscle to contract to overcome a resistance and creates movement of the attached joint. It aids in building strength and endurance without overtaxing the cardiovascular system. By contrast, isometric activity involves contraction of the muscle against a fixed resistance and is more stressful on the heart and circulatory system.

Exercise prescription for strengthening should include frequency, intensity, and volume. Strengthening regimen in older adults should focus on multiple muscle groups to avoid overuse and injury of one particular muscle. Strength training is an effective way to improve muscle strength, mass, and neuromuscular activity in older adults, which in turn translates to improved functional capacity while performing everyday activities. It should be performed at least twice weekly, on nonconsecutive days at high to moderate intensity with two to three sets per exercise (set = 8 to 12 repetitions).[13,18]

Maintaining a BMI less than 25 throughout adult life has been recently recommended. For most patients with a BMI between 25 and 30, lifestyle modifications including diet and exercise are appropriate. For individuals over 51 years of age getting 20 to 30 minutes of moderate activity each day should be combined with daily caloric intake restricted to 1600 for women and 2000 for men. The current *Dietary Guidelines for Americans* recommends limiting sodium intake to 2300 mg (approximately 1 teaspoon) per day for adults, and further reduce to 1500 mg for those over 51 years of age, as well as African-American adults and those with hypertension, diabetes, and kidney disease.[40]

Pharmaceuticals should be considered with a BMI greater than 30 or a BMI greater than 27 with an obesity-related disorder. Currently, Tenuate (diethylpropion), Adipex (phentermine), Didrex (benzphetamine), and Bontril (phendimetrazine) are approved for short-term use to provide weight loss. In 2014, the U.S. Food and Drug Administration (FDA) approved a new antiobesity medication, Contrave (combination of naltrexone and bupropion), for long-term use. Other medications approved for long-term use include Xenical (orlistat), Belviq (lorcaserin), and Qsymia (phentermine and topiramate extended-release).

Pregnancy

Special considerations exist during pregnancy because of the possible competition between exercising maternal muscle and the fetus for blood flow, oxygen delivery, glucose availability, and heat dissipation. Metabolic and cardiorespiratory adaptations to pregnancy can alter the responses from exercise training. The acute physiologic responses to exercise are generally increased during pregnancy compared with prepregnancy levels. There are no data in humans to indicate that pregnant women should or should not limit exercise intensity and lower target HRs because of potential adverse effects.[89,137] Healthy, pregnant women without exercise contraindications are encouraged to exercise throughout the pregnancy. Regular exercise during pregnancy provides health and fitness benefits to the mother and child.[32,137] Exercise might also reduce the risk for developing conditions associated with pregnancy, such as pregnancy-induced hypertension and gestational diabetes mellitus.[32,113] For women who do not have any additional risk factors for adverse maternal or perinatal outcomes, the American College of Obstetricians and Gynecologists (ACOG) has established guidelines for the safe prescription of exercise.[1,2] The Canadian Society for Exercise Physiology Physical Activity Readiness Medical Examination, termed the PARmed-X for Pregnancy, should be used for the health screening of pregnant women before their participation in exercise programs.[137] Participation in a wide range of recreational activities appears to be safe during pregnancy. The safety of each sport is determined largely by the specific movements required by that sport. Participation in recreational sports with a high potential for contact, such as ice hockey, soccer, and basketball, could result in trauma to both the woman and the fetus. Recreational activities with an increased risk for falling, such as gymnastics, horseback riding, downhill skiing, and vigorous racquet sports, have an inherently high risk for trauma in pregnant and nonpregnant women. Those activities with a high risk for falling or for abdominal trauma should be avoided during pregnancy. Scuba diving should be avoided throughout pregnancy because during this activity the fetus is at increased risk for decompression sickness secondary to the inability of the fetal pulmonary circulation to filter bubble formation. Exertion at altitudes of up to 6000 feet appears to be safe, but engaging in physical activities at higher altitudes carries various risks.

- During pregnancy, women can continue to exercise and derive health benefits even from mild to moderate exercise routines. Regular exercise (at least three times per week) is preferable to intermittent activity. Thirty minutes or more of moderate exercise per day on most, if not all, days is recommended.
- Women should avoid exercise in the supine position after the first trimester. Such a position is associated with decreased cardiac output in most pregnant women. Because the remaining cardiac output is preferentially distributed away from splanchnic beds (including the uterus) during vigorous exercise, such regimens are best avoided during pregnancy. Prolonged periods of motionless standing should also be avoided.
- Women should be aware of the decreased oxygen available for aerobic exercise during pregnancy. They should be encouraged to modify the intensity of their exercise according to maternal symptoms. Pregnant women should stop exercising when fatigued and not exercise to exhaustion. Weight-bearing exercises can under some circumstances be continued at intensities similar to those before pregnancy throughout the pregnancy. Non–weight-bearing exercises, such as stationary cycling or swimming, will minimize the risk for injury and facilitate the continuation of exercise during pregnancy.
- Exercise should be terminated should any of the following occur: vaginal bleeding, dyspnea before exertion, dizziness, headache, chest pain, muscle weakness, calf pain or swelling, preterm labor, decreased fetal movement, and amniotic fluid leakage. In the case of calf pain and swelling, thrombophlebitis should be ruled out.
- Pregnant women may participate in a strength-training program that incorporates all major muscle groups, with a resistance that permits multiple repetitions (i.e., 12 to 15 repetitions) to be performed to a point of moderate fatigue. Isometric muscle actions and the Valsalva maneuver should be avoided, as should the supine position after the first trimester.
- Morphologic changes in pregnancy should serve as a relative contraindication to types of exercise in which loss of balance could be detrimental to maternal or fetal well-being, especially in the third trimester. Any type of exercise involving the potential for even mild abdominal trauma should be avoided.
- Pregnancy requires an additional 300 kcal/day to maintain metabolic homeostasis. Women who exercise during pregnancy should be particularly careful to ensure an adequate diet.
- Pregnant women who exercise in the first trimester should augment heat dissipation by ensuring adequate hydration, appropriate clothing, and optimal environmental surroundings during exercise (exercising in cool environments whenever possible).[137]

The ACOG recommends that women who currently participate in a regular exercise program can continue their training during pregnancy, following these recommendations listed. Studies have demonstrated that women naturally decrease their exercise duration and intensity as their pregnancy advances. Those who begin an exercise program after becoming pregnant are advised to receive physician authorization and begin exercising with low-intensity, low-impact (or nonimpact) activities, such as

BOX 15-7

Contraindications to Aerobic Exercise During Pregnancy*

Absolute Contraindications
- Hemodynamically significant heart disease
- Restrictive lung disease
- Incompetent cervix or cerclage
- Multiple gestation at risk for premature labor
- Persistent second- or third-trimester bleeding
- Placenta previa after 26 weeks' gestation
- Premature labor during the current pregnancy
- Ruptured membranes
- Preeclampsia or pregnancy-induced hypertension

Relative Contraindications
- Severe anemia
- Unevaluated maternal cardiac arrhythmia
- Chronic bronchitis
- Poorly controlled type 1 diabetes
- Extreme morbid obesity
- Extreme underweight (body mass index <12 kg/m^2)
- History of extremely sedentary lifestyle
- Intrauterine growth restriction in current pregnancy
- Poorly controlled hypertension
- Orthopedic limitations
- Poorly controlled seizure disorder
- Poorly controlled hyperthyroidism
- Heavy smoker

Further Reasons to Discontinue Exercise and Seek Medical Advice During Pregnancy[†]
- Vaginal bleeding
- Dyspnea before exertion
- Dizziness
- Headache
- Chest pain
- Muscle weakness
- Calf pain or swelling (need to rule out thrombophlebitis)
- Preterm labor
- Decreased fetal movement
- Amniotic fluid leakage

*From Thompson WR, editor: *ACSM's guidelines for exercise testing and prescription*, ed 8, Philadelphia, 2010, Lippincott Williams & Wilkins.
[†]From American College of Obstetricians and Gynecologists: Exercise during pregnancy and the postpartum period, *Obstet Gynecol* 99:171-173, 2002; Kenny W, Humphrey R, Bryant C, editors: *ACSM's guidelines for exercise testing and prescription*, ed 5, Philadelphia, 1995, Williams & Wilkins; Thompson WR, editor: *ACSM's guidelines for exercise testing and prescription*, ed 8, Philadelphia, 2010, Lippincott Williams & Wilkins.

walking and swimming.[1,2] Contraindications for exercise during pregnancy have also been established by the ACOG (Box 15-7).[2,137]

Many of the physiologic and morphologic changes of pregnancy persist 4 to 6 weeks postpartum. Therefore, the ACSM recommends in general to resume exercise 4 to 6 weeks after delivery. This will vary from one individual to another, with some women able to resume an exercise routine within days of delivery. There are no published studies to indicate that, in the absence of medical complications, rapid resumption of activities will result in adverse effects. Having undergone detraining, resumption of activities should be gradual. No known maternal complications are associated with resumption of training.[137]

Activity for Older Adults

According to the American College of Sports Medicine, it is estimated that the population age 65 years and older will reach 70 million in the United States by 2030. Senior adults age 85+ years will constitute the fastest growing segment of the population.

The loss of strength and stamina attributed to aging is in part caused by reduced physical activity. Inactivity usually increases with age. By age 75 years, approximately one in three men and one in two women engage in no exercise. Among adults aged 65 years and older, walking, gardening, and yard work are the most popular physical activities. Social support from family and friends has been consistently and positively related to regular physical activity.[19]

Exercise should focus on improving balance, strength, flexibility, and endurance.

Senior adults who are physically active have lower rates of coronary artery disease, hypertension, cerebrovascular accident, type 2 diabetes mellitus, osteoporosis, and a higher level of cardiorespiratory function, muscular strength, and endurance. They demonstrate higher levels of functional health, better cognitive function, and overall have a reduced risk of moderate to severe functional limitations.

Effect of Aging on Muscle

Loss of muscle mass, sarcopenia, results from disuse of the muscle. Aging muscle is also affected by decrease in growth factors, modifications of motor units, and innervation of the fibers. Although functional motor units decline with age, the surviving axons are required to innervate a higher number of muscle fibers. By age 50 years, total muscle area has shrunk by approximately 10%. The rate of muscle loss accelerates significantly thereafter.[101]

Maximal oxygen consumption (VO_{2max}) is used to assess cardiovascular function and maximal capacity. VO_{2max} decreases approximately 5% to 15% per decade starting at 25 to 30 years of age. Similarly, HR_{max} decreases by approximately 6 to 10 beats/min per decade, which contributes to most of the age-related decrease in cardiac output. In older adults, diminishing SV during exercise also causes a drop in HR.

Age-related declines in oxidative competence of the muscle and in vascular capacity cause a drop in maximal a-vO_2 difference. These factors along with diminished oxygen delivery mechanisms and mitochondrial changes further reduce the capacity to use oxygen at the level of the active skeletal muscle. With exercise training, older adults can attain the same 10% to 30% increase in VO_{2max} as their younger counterparts. This may be attributed to improvements in maximal cardiac output and a-vO_2 difference. The magnitude of change depends on the intensity of the physical activity; low intensity exercise produces minimal changes.

Exercise is highly beneficial for those with arthritis. Some advantages include muscle strength and flexibility, bone health, and reduced joint pain and fatigue. Improving range of motion of the joint and strengthening the surrounding muscles helps decrease the discomfort associated with arthritis during activity.

Aquatic therapy (pool therapy) is particularly helpful for those with both peripheral joint and spinal facet arthropathy. Such a gravity–reduced environment relieves friction and reduces stress on the joints and the spine. Mind-body integrative approaches such as yoga, tai chi, and Pilates are safe and viable alternatives that are thought to lessen inflammation in the body, improve posture, and alleviate stress, although more scientific studies are required.

Age-specific barriers and motivators unique to this cohort are relevant and must be acknowledged. The identification of reliable predictors of exercise adherence will allow health care providers to effectively intervene and change patterns of physical activity in sedentary older adults. In particular, because older patients often respect their physician's advice and have regular contact with their physician, physicians can play a pivotal role in the initiation and maintenance of exercise behavior among the older adult population.

Specific recommendations for older adults are outlined in Table 15-7.[12,88] Individualization of resistance training prescriptions is also essential and should be based on the health and fitness status and specific goals of the participant. Some guidelines follow, with reference to the intensity, frequency, and duration of exercise (Table 15-8).[88,137]

Table 15-7 Guidelines for Aerobic Exercise Prescription for Older Adults

Component	Details
Mode	The exercise modality should be one that does not impose significant orthopedic stress.
	The activity should be accessible, convenient, and enjoyable to the participant; all factors directly related to exercise adherence.
	Consider walking, stationary cycling, water exercise, swimming, or machine-based stair climbing.
Intensity	Intensity must be sufficient to stress (overload) the cardiovascular, pulmonary, and musculoskeletal systems without overtaxing them.
	High variability exists for maximal heart rates (HR_{max}) in individuals older than 65 years. It is always better to use a measured HR_{max} rather than age-predicted HR_{max} whenever possible.
	For similar reasons, the HR reserve method is recommended for establishing a training HR in older adults, rather than a straight percentage of HR_{max}.
	The recommended intensity for older adults is 50% to 70% of HR reserve.
	Because many older adults have a variety of medical conditions, a conservative approach to prescribing aerobic exercise is warranted.
Duration	During the initial stages of an exercise program, some older adults can have difficulty sustaining aerobic exercise for 20 minutes. One viable option can be to perform the exercise in several 10-minute sessions throughout the day.
	To avoid injury and ensure safety, older adults should initially increase exercise duration rather than intensity.
Frequency	Alternate between days that involve primarily weight-bearing and non–weight-bearing exercise.

From Thompson WR, editor: *ACSM's guidelines for exercise testing and prescription*, ed 8, Philadelphia, 2010, Lippincott Williams & Wilkins.

Flexibility Training

Static stretching is considered safer than dynamic stretching for older adults (Table 15-9). The American Heart Association recommends holding each stretch for 10 to 30 seconds, with 3 to 4 repetitions.[106]

Regardless of which specific protocol is adopted, several common-sense guidelines pertaining to resistance training for older adults should be followed[88,137]:

- The major goal of the resistance training program is to develop sufficient muscular fitness to enhance an individual's ability to live a physically independent lifestyle.

Table 15-8 Guidelines for Resistance Exercise Prescription for Older Adults

Component	Details
Intensity	Perform one set of 8 to 10 exercises that train all the major muscle groups (e.g., gluteals, quadriceps, hamstrings, pectorals, latissimus dorsi, deltoids, and abdominals). Each set should involve 8 to 12 repetitions that elicit a perceived exertion rating of 12 to 13 (somewhat hard).
Frequency	Resistance training should be performed at least twice a week, with at least 48 hours of rest between sessions.
Duration	Sessions lasting longer than 60 minutes can have a detrimental effect on exercise adherence. Following the above guidelines should permit individuals to complete total body resistance training sessions within 20 to 30 minutes.

From Thompson WR, editor: *ACSM's guidelines for exercise testing and prescription*, ed 8, Philadelphia, 2010, Lippincott Williams & Wilkins.

Table 15-9 Physical Activity Counseling For Older Adults: A Quick Guide

Recommendations
Aerobic
• ≥30 min or three sessions of ≥10 min/day • ≥5 days/week • Moderate intensity = 5 to 6 on a 10-point scale (where 0 = sitting, 5 to 6 = "can talk," and • 10 = all-out effort) • In addition to routine activities of daily living
Strength
• 8 to 10 exercises (major muscle groups), 10 to 15 repetitions • ≥2 nonconsecutive days/week • Moderate to high intensity = 5 to 8 on a 10-point scale (where 5 to 6 = "can talk" and 7 to 8 = shortness of breath)
Flexibility/Balance
• ≥10 min ≥2 days/week • Flexibility to maintain/improve range of motion (i.e., stretching of major muscle/tendon groups, yoga) • Balance exercises for those at risk for falls (i.e., tai chi, individualized balanced exercises)
Prevention
• Create a single physical activity plan that integrates preventive and therapeutic treatment of chronic conditions

- The first several resistance training sessions should be closely supervised and monitored by trained personnel who are sensitive to the special needs and capabilities of older adults.
- Begin (the first 8 weeks) with minimal resistance to allow for adaptations of the connective tissue elements.
- Teach proper training techniques for all the exercises to be used in the program.
- Instruct older participants to maintain their normal breathing pattern while exercising.
- As a training effect occurs, achieve an overload initially by increasing the number of repetitions, and then by increasing the resistance.
- Never use a resistance that is so heavy that the exerciser cannot perform at least eight repetitions.
- Stress that all exercises should be performed in a manner in which the speed is controlled (no ballistic movements should be allowed).
- Perform the exercises in a range of motion that is within a "pain-free arc" (i.e., the maximal range of motion that does not elicit pain or discomfort).
- Perform multijoint exercises (as opposed to single-joint exercises).
- Given a choice, use machines to resistance train, as opposed to free weights (machines require less skill to use, protect the back by stabilizing the user's body position, and allow the user to start with lower resistances, to increase by smaller increments, and to more easily control the exercise range on motion). Heavy free weights should be used only by those who have had special training in how to lift properly, and who have a spotter with them during the exercise.
- Do not overtrain. Two strength-training sessions per week are the minimum number required to produce positive physiologic adaptations. Depending on the circumstances, more sessions might not be productive.
- Participants with arthritis should never participate in strength-training exercises during active periods of joint pain or inflammation.
- Engage in a year-round resistance-training program on a regular basis.
- When returning from a layoff, start with resistances of less than 50% of the intensity at which the participant had been previously training (as tolerated), then gradually increase the resistance.
- Flexibility exercises should be performed on major muscle groups with prolonged (not ballistic) stretching at an intensity of 50% to 60% maximal at least 2 days/wk. Balance exercises should be incorporated for frequent fallers or those with mobility problems.

Children

Children tend to be more active than adults, and accordingly tend to maintain adequate levels of physical fitness. Healthy children should be encouraged, nonetheless, to engage in physical activity on a regular basis. However, because children are anatomically, physiologically, and psychologically immature, special precautions should be applied when designing exercise programs. Children can experience a higher incidence of overuse injuries, or damage the epiphyseal growth plates if endurance exercise is excessive. The risk for injury can be significantly decreased by ensuring appropriate matching of competition in terms of size, maturation, or skill level, the use of properly fitted protective equipment, liberal adaptation of rules toward safety, proper conditioning, and appropriate skill development. Children have less efficient thermoregulation than that of adults and are more prone to hyperthermia and hypothermia.[88,137]

The current rise in childhood obesity underscores the importance of regular exercise. In the United States, 32% of children are overweight or obese.[96,109] This increase in obesity has been linked to increases in comorbidities including glucose intolerance, type 2 diabetes, hypertension, and hyperlipidemia.[96] Studies have demonstrated that monitored programs of moderate to vigorous exercise can result in a decrease in percent body fat and improvement of insulin resistance.[102] Consensus guidelines for 2005 recommend that schools provide for 30 to 34 minutes of daily vigorous activity.[129] The Endocrine Society recommends 60 minutes of daily vigorous activity.[4]

Specific considerations for children include the following[137]:

- Children and adolescents may safely participate in strength-training activities after proper instruction and supervision. Eight to 15 repetitions of an exercise should be performed to the point of moderate fatigue with good mechanical form before the resistance is increased.
- Because of immature thermoregulatory systems, youth should exercise in thermoneutral environments and be properly hydrated.
- Children and adolescents who are overweight or physically inactive may not be able to achieve 60 min/day of physical activity. Therefore, gradually increase the frequency and time of physical activity to achieve this goal.
- Efforts should be made to decrease sedentary activities (i.e., television and video games) and increase activities that promote lifelong activity and fitness (i.e., walking and cycling).

ACSM guidelines for exercise prescription in children are detailed in Table 15-10.[137]

Table 15-10 Guidelines for Strength Training in Children

Component	Details
Frequency	At least 3 to 4 days/wk and preferably daily
Intensity	Moderate (physical activity that noticeably increases breathing, sweating, and HR) to vigorous (physical activity that substantially increases breathing, sweating, and HR) intensity
Time	30 min/day of moderate and 30 min/day of vigorous intensity to total 60 min/day of accumulated physical activity
Type	A variety of activities that are enjoyable and developmentally appropriate for the child or adolescent

From Thompson WR, editor: *ACSM's guidelines for exercise testing and prescription*, ed 8, Philadelphia, 2010, Lippincott Williams & Wilkins.
HR, Heart rate.

Hypertension

The ACSM makes the following recommendations regarding exercise testing and training of individuals with hypertension[88,137]:

- Mass exercise testing is not advocated to determine those individuals at high risk for developing hypertension in the future as a result of an exaggerated exercise blood pressure response. However, if exercise test results are available and an individual has an exercise blood pressure response above the 85th percentile, this information does provide some indication of risk stratification for that patient and the necessity for appropriate lifestyle behavior counseling to ameliorate this increase.
- Endurance exercise training by individuals who are at high risk for developing hypertension can reduce the rise in blood pressure that occurs with time, justifying its use as a nonpharmacologic strategy to reduce the incidence of hypertension in susceptible individuals.
- Endurance exercise training elicits an average reduction of 10 mm Hg for both SBPs and DBPs in individuals with mild essential hypertension (blood pressures in the range of 140/90 to 180/105 mm Hg) and secondary hypertension resulting from renal dysfunction.
- The recommended mode, frequency, duration, and intensity of exercise are generally the same as those for apparently healthy individuals. Exercise training at somewhat lower intensities (e.g., 40% to 70% of $\dot{V}O_{2max}$) appears to lower blood pressure as much, or more, than exercise at higher intensities. This can be especially important in specific hypertensive populations, such as older adults.
- Based on the high number of exercise-related health benefits and low risk for morbidity and mortality, it seems reasonable to recommend exercise as part of the initial treatment strategy for individuals with mild to moderate essential hypertension.
- Individuals with marked elevations in blood pressure should add endurance exercise training to their treatment regimen only after a physician's evaluation and the initiation of pharmacologic therapy. Exercise can reduce their blood pressure further, allowing them to decrease their antihypertensive medications and attenuate their risk for premature mortality.
- Resistance training is not recommended as the primary form of exercise training for individuals with hypertension. With the exception of circuit weight training, resistance training has not consistently been shown to lower blood pressure. Resistance training is recommended as a component of a well-rounded fitness program, but it should not be the only form of exercise in the program.
- If resting SBP is greater than 200 mm Hg and/or DBP is greater than 110 mm Hg, do not exercise. When exercising, it appears prudent to maintain a SBP of 220 mm Hg or less, and/or a DBP of 105 mm Hg or less.

Specific guidelines for exercise in patients with hypertension are listed in Table 15-11.[88,137]

Table 15-11 Guidelines for Exercise Prescription in Patients with Hypertension

Component	Details
Frequency	Aerobic exercise on most, preferably all, days of the week; resistance exercise 2 to 3 days/wk
Intensity	Moderate-intensity aerobic exercise (i.e., 40% to <60% $\dot{V}O_2R$) supplemented by resistance training at 60% to 80% 1-RM
Time	30 to 60 min/day of continuous or intermittent aerobic exercise; if intermittent, use a minimum of 10-minute sessions
Type	Emphasis should be placed on aerobic activities

From Thompson WR, editor: *ACSM's guidelines for exercise testing and prescription*, ed 8, Philadelphia, 2010, Lippincott Williams & Wilkins.
RM, Repetition maximum; *$\dot{V}O_2R$*, oxygen uptake reserve.

Peripheral Vascular Disease

Patients with peripheral vascular disease experience ischemic pain (claudication) during physical activity as a result of a mismatch between active muscle oxygen supply and demand. The symptoms can be described as burning, searing, aching, tightness, or cramping. Pain is most often experienced in the calf, but can begin in the buttock region and radiate down the leg. The symptoms typically disappear on cessation of exercise, although some patients can have claudication at rest in severe cases.

Severe peripheral vascular disease is treated initially with exercise and medications that decrease blood viscosity. Treatment with angioplasty or bypass grafting might also be indicated. Weight-bearing exercise is preferred to facilitate greater functional changes, but might not be well tolerated initially. Prescription of non–weight-bearing exercise (which can permit a greater intensity or longer duration) is a suitable alternative.[88,137] Specific guidelines for exercise in patients with peripheral vascular disease are listed in Table 15-12.[88,137]

Diabetes

The response to exercise in the patient with type 1 diabetes mellitus depends on a variety of factors, including the adequacy of control by exogenous insulin. If the patient is under appropriate control or only slightly hyperglycemic without ketosis, exercise can decrease blood glucose concentration and lower the insulin dose required. Patients with type 1 diabetes mellitus must be under adequate control before beginning an exercise program. Serum glucose concentrations in the general range of 200 to 400 mg% (mg/dL) require medical supervision during exercise, and exercise is contraindicated for those with fasting serum values greater than 400 mg%. Exercised-induced hypoglycemia is the most common problem experienced by exercising patients with diabetes.

Hypoglycemia can occur not only during the exercise but for up to 4 to 6 hours after an exercise session.[88,137] The risk for hypoglycemic events can be minimized by taking the following precautions:

- Monitor blood glucose frequently when initiating an exercise program.

Table 15-12 Guidelines for Exercise Prescription in Patients with Peripheral Vascular Disease*

Component	Details
Frequency	Weight-bearing aerobic exercise 3 to 5 days/wk; resistance exercise at least 2 days/wk.
Intensity	Moderate intensity (i.e., 40% to <60% $\dot{V}O_2R$) that allows patients to walk until they reach a pain score of 3 (i.e., intense pain) on a 4-point pain scale.[†] Between sessions of activity, individuals should be given time to allow ischemic pain to subside before resuming exercise.[†‡]
Time	30 to 60 min/day, but initially some patients may need to start with 10-minute sessions.
Type	Weight-bearing aerobic exercise, such as walking, and non–weight-bearing activity, such as arm ergometry. Cycling may be used as a warm-up, but should not be the primary type of activity. Resistance training is recommended to enhance and maintain muscular strength and endurance.

*From Thompson WR, editor: *ACSM's guidelines for exercise testing and prescription*, ed 8, Philadelphia, 2010, Lippincott Williams & Wilkins.
†From Topper AK, Maki BE, Holliday PJ: Are activity-based assessments of balance and gait in the elderly predictive of risk of falling and/or type of fall? *J Am Geriatr Soc* 41:479-487, 1993.
‡From Goldspink D: The influence of immobilization and stretch on protein turnover of rat skeletal muscle, *J Physiol* 264:267-282, 1977.
$\dot{V}O_2R$, Oxygen uptake reserve.

Table 15-13 Guidelines for Exercise Prescription in Patients with Diabetes*

Component	Details
Frequency	3 to 7 days/wk.
Intensity	50% to 80% $\dot{V}O_2R$ or HRR corresponding to an RPE of 12 to 16 on a scale from 6 to 20.[†]
Time	20 to 60 min/day continuous or accumulated in sessions of at least 10 minutes to total 150 min/wk of moderate physical activity, with additional benefits of increasing to 300 minutes or more of moderate-intensity physical activity.
Type	Emphasize activities that use large muscle groups.
Resistance training should be encouraged for individuals with diabetes mellitus in the absence of contraindications, retinopathy, and recent laser treatments.	
Frequency	2 to 3 days/wk with at least 48 hours separating the exercise sessions.
Intensity	2 to 3 sets of 8 to 12 repetitions at 60% to 80% 1-RM.
Time	8 to 10 multijoint exercises of all major muscle groups in the same session (whole body) or sessions split into selected muscle groups.

*From Thompson WR, editor: *ACSM's guidelines for exercise testing and prescription*, ed 8, Philadelphia, 2010, Lippincott Williams & Wilkins.
†From DeLateur BJ: Therapeutic exercise. In Braddom RL, editor: *Physical medicine and rehabilitation*, Philadelphia, 1996, Saunders.
HRR, Heart rate reserve; *RM*, repetition maximum; *RPE*, rating of perceived exertion; *$\dot{V}O_2R$*, oxygen uptake reserve.

- Decrease insulin dose (by 1 to 2 units as prescribed by the physician) or increase carbohydrate intake (10 to 15 g carbohydrate per 30 minutes of exercise) before an exercise session.
- Inject insulin in an area such as the abdomen that is relatively inactive during exercise.
- Avoid exercise during periods of peak insulin activity.
- Eat carbohydrate snacks before and during prolonged exercise sessions.
- Be knowledgeable of the signs and symptoms of hypoglycemia and hyperglycemia.
- Exercise with a partner.

Other precautions that should be taken include the following[88,137]:

- Use proper footwear and practice good foot hygiene.
- Be aware that beta-blockers and other medications can interfere with the patient's ability to discern hypoglycemic symptoms and/or angina.
- Be aware that exercise in excessive heat can cause problems in diabetic patients with peripheral neuropathy.
- Patients with advanced retinopathy should not perform activities that cause excessive jarring or marked increases in blood pressure.
- Patients should have physician approval to resume exercise training after laser treatment.

Specific guidelines for exercise in patients with diabetes are listed in Table 15-13.[88,137]

Myofascial Pain Syndrome and Fibromyalgia

Chronic musculoskeletal pain of various etiologies affects many adults. It is characterized by fascial contraction and trigger points in the muscles, causing pain and decreased range of motion. This adversely affects quality of life. Patients may present with a knot or fibrous band in the muscle, most commonly located in the upper traps, rhomboids, and paraspinals. There are multiple interventions for myofascial pain syndrome, including nonsteroidal anti-inflammatory drugs and trigger point injections; however, massage, stretching, and activity are most effective in the management and prevention of myofascial pain.

Prevalence of fibromyalgia is approximately 2% to 4%, most commonly affecting women. It is characterized by widespread muscular pain, headache, fatigue, sleep disturbances, and memory/cognitive problems. Working women with fibromyalgia who are hospitalized for chronic musculoskeletal issues were almost 10 times less likely to return to work and 4 times less likely to retain work 1 year posthospitalization.

Low-intensity aerobic exercise combined with gentle stretching should be prescribed for patients with fibromyalgia. The goal is to maintain function in day-to-day activities. Pain is the most common limiting factor. Clinical trials have shown that aerobic exercise decreases pain levels, thereby improving function and quality of life. One particular study trained patients for 25 min/day two to three times per week with an average intensity of 50% VO_{2max}. Unlike the control group, the testing group demonstrated a decrease in the number of tender points and painful body surface area. A study published by the American College of Rheumatology suggests that there is a linear relationship between the number of steps taken daily and relief from symptoms of fibromyalgia. It is recommended that patients gradually accumulate at least 5000 additional steps daily.[86] McLoughlin et al.[104] proved that using functional magnetic resonance imaging that increased physical activity was associated with decreased perception of pain in women with fibromyalgia.

Patient education and cognitive therapy is also an important aspect in the management of fibromyalgia. Patients should be counseled on how to prioritize their time to achieve a balance among work, daily responsibilities, and leisure.

Acupuncture is increasing in popularity to alleviate the symptoms; however, data supporting this is sparse and further investigations are required. Other modalities such as yoga, tai chi, massage, deep breathing, and meditation therapy are widely employed.[12]

Organ Transplantation

Postcardiac transplantation, abnormal aerobic tolerance is caused as a result of deconditioning before transplant, chronotropic incompetence from denervation, skeletal muscle weakness, and immunosuppressive medications (steroids, cyclosporine). Long-term use of cyclosporine causes muscle atrophy and a shift toward a larger amount of fast-twitch muscle fibers at the expense of the slow-twitch fibers, whereas corticosteroids result in mitochondrial dysfunction.

A study of patients with a left ventricular assist device and cardiac transplant demonstrated improved quality of life and physical activity within the first 3 months of surgery but stayed relatively unchanged thereafter and always remained well below their healthy counterparts.[80]

The importance of cardiac rehabilitation was illustrated in a study that randomized 27 patients within 2 weeks of cardiac transplantation to a 6-month structured rehabilitation program or unstructured therapy at home. Compared with the control group, the exercise group had a greater increase in peak oxygen consumption (49% versus 18%) and workload (59% versus 18%) and a greater reduction in the ventilatory equivalent for carbon dioxide (20% versus 11%).[112]

As a result of persistent sinus node denervation, the HR cannot be used as a measure of work intensity. Most commonly, the Borg Rate of Perceived Exertion Scale is used to quantify the intensity of the activity being performed.

Patients with an organ transplant are deconditioned and weak postoperatively. Although data are limited, rehabilitation after solid organ transplantation appears highly beneficial. A study of patients with renal transplant showed that rehabilitation posttransplant is helpful in aiding psychological and physical recovery, thereby improving quality of life.[146]

Summary

The benefits of exercise for health and human performance are well known. Applying appropriate exercise prescriptions based on the physiologic response to exercises and the principle of specificity of training will ensure an appropriate training response and minimize the risk for injury. Special populations, including the young, older adults, and those with disease states, might require specific modifications in exercise programs to maximize safety.

KEY REFERENCES

2. American College of Obstetricians and Gynecologists: Exercise during pregnancy and the postpartum period, *Obstet Gynecol* 99:171–173, 2002.
4. August GP, Caprio S, Fennoy I, et al: Prevention and treatment of pediatric obesity: an endocrine society clinical practice guideline based on expert opinion, *J Clin Endocrinol Metab* 93:4576–4599, 2009.
6. Barrett DS: Proprioception and function after anterior cruciate reconstruction, *J Bone Joint Surg Br* 73:833–837, 1991.
10. Brunnstrom S: *Movement therapy in hemiplegia*, New York, 1971, Harper & Row.
12. Busch A, Webber S, Brachaniec M, et al: Exercise therapy for fibromyalgia, *Curr Pain Headache Rep* 15:358–367, 2011.
13. Cadore EL, Pinto RS, Bottaro M, Izquierdo M: Strength and endurance training prescription in healthy and frail elderly, *Aging Dis* 5:183–195, 2014.
18. Centers for Disease Control and Prevention: *How much physical activity do older adults need?*, Atlanta, 2014, Centers for Disease Control and Prevention.
19. Centers for Disease Control and Prevention: *Physical activity and health: a report of the Surgeon General*, Atlanta, 1999, Centers for Disease Control and Prevention.
20. Chu D: *Jumping into plyometrics*, Champaign, 1998, Human Kinetics.
23. Craib MW, Mitchell VA, Fields KB, et al: The association between flexibility and running economy in sub-elite male distance runners, *Med Sci Sports Exerc* 28:737–743, 1996.
25. Cramer JT, Housh TJ, Weir JP, et al: The acute effects of static stretching on peak torque, mean power output, electromyography and mechanomyography, *Eur J Appl Physiol* 93:530–539, 2005.
28. DeLateur BJ: Therapeutic exercise to develop strength and endurance. In Kottke FJ, Stillwell GK, Lehmann JF, editors: *Krusen's handbook of physical medicine and rehabilitation*, Philadelphia, 1982, Saunders, pp 457–462.
29. DeLateur BJ: Therapeutic exercise. In Braddom RL, editor: *Physical medicine and rehabilitation*, Philadelphia, 1996, Saunders.
31. Demaree SR, Powers SK, Lawler JM: Fundamentals of exercise metabolism. In Roitman JL, Haver EJ, Herridge M, et al, editors: *ACSM's resource manual for guidelines for exercise testing and prescription*, Philadelphia, 2001, Lippincott Williams & Wilkins, pp 133–140.
32. Dempsey FC, Butler FL, Williams FA: No need for a pregnant pause: physical activity may reduce the occurrence of gestational diabetes mellitus and preeclampsia, *Exerc Sport Sci Rev* 33:141–149, 2005.
34. Deuster P, Keyser D: Basics in exercise physiology. In O'Connor F, Sallis R, Wilder R, et al, editors: *Sports medicine: just the facts*, New York, 2005, McGraw Hill.
40. *Dietary guidelines for Americans, 2010, executive summary*, Washington, 2010, U.S. Department of Agriculture and the U.S. Department of Health and Human Services. Available at: http://www.cnpp.usda.gov/sites/default/files/dietary_guidelines_for_americans/ExecSumm.pdf.
51. Franklin BA: Normal cardiorespiratory response to acute aerobic exercise. In Roitman JL, Haver EJ, Herridge M, editors: *ACSM's resource manual for guidelines for exercise testing and prescription*, Philadelphia, 2001, Lippincott Williams & Wilkins.
52. Franklin B, Whaley M, Howley E, editors: Benefits and risks associated with exercise. In *ACSM's guidelines for exercise testing and prescription*, ed 6, Philadelphia, 2000, Lippincott Williams & Wilkins, pp 3–15.
53. Franklin B, Whaley M, Howley E, editors: General principles of exercise prescription. In *ACSM's guidelines for exercise testing and prescription*, ed 6, Philadelphia, 2000, Lippincott Williams & Wilkins.
54. Franklin B, Whaley M, Howley E, editors: Health screening and risk stratification. In *ACSM's guidelines for exercise testing and prescription*, ed 6, Philadelphia, 2000, Lippincott Williams & Wilkins, pp 22–33.

57. Frontera WR, Moldover JR, Borg-Stein J, et al: Exercise. In Gonzalez EG, Myers SJ, editors: *Downey and Darling's physiological basis of rehabilitation medicine*, ed 3, Boston, 2001, Butterworth-Heinemann.
59. Gleim GW, McHugh MP: Flexibility and its effects on sports injury and performance, *Sports Med* 24:289–299, 1997.
61. Go A, Mozaffarian D, Roger V, et al on behalf of the American Heart Association Statistics Committee and Stroke Statistics Subcommittee: Heart disease and stroke statistics—2013 update: a report from the American Heart Association, *Circulation* 127:e6–e245, 2013.
62. Godshall RW: The predictability of athletic injuries: an eight-year study, *J Sports Med* 3:50–54, 1975.
65. Golnick P, Karlsson J, Peihl K: Selective glycogen depletion in skeletal muscle fibers of man following sustained contractions, *J Physiol* 241:59–67, 1974.
66. Grahame R: Joint hypermobility: clinical aspects, *Proc R Soc Med* 64:692–694, 1971.
69. Guyton A, editor: *Textbook of medical physiology*, Philadelphia, 1996, Saunders.
73. Hart J, Ingersoll C: Weightlifting. In O'Connor F, Sallis R, Wilder R, et al, editors: *Sports medicine: just the facts*, New York, 2005, McGraw-Hill, pp 543–548.
75. Hellebrandt FA, Houtz SJ: Methods of muscle training: the influence of pacing, *Phys Ther Rev* 38:319–322, 1958.
78. Holly RG, Shaffrath JD: Cardiorespiratory endurance. In Roitman JL, Haver EJ, Herridge M, et al, editors: *ACSM's resource manual for guidelines for exercise testing and prescription*, Philadelphia, 2001, Lippincott Williams & Wilkins.
80. Jakovljevic D, McDiarmid A, Hallsworth K: Effect of left ventricular assist device implantation and heart transplantation on habitual physical activity and quality of life, *Am J Cardiol* 114:88–93, 2014.
88. Kenny W, Humphrey R, Bryant C, editors: *ACSM's guidelines for exercise testing and prescription*, ed 5, Philadelphia, 1995, Williams & Wilkins.
96. Lieb DC, Snow RE, DeBoer MD: Socioeconomic factors in the development of childhood obesity and diabetes, *Clin Sports Med* 28:349–378, 2009.
101. Mazzeo RS: Exercise and the older adult, Indianapolis, American College of Sports Medicine. Available at www.acsm.org/docs/current-comments/exerciseandtheolderadult.pdf.
103. McHugh MP, Neese M: Effect of stretching on strength loss and pain after eccentric exercise, *Med Sci Sports Exerc* 40:566–573, 2008.
115. Pollock M, Gaesser G, Butcher J: American College of Sports Medicine position stand. The recommended quantity and quality of exercise for developing and maintaining cardiorespiratory and muscular fitness, and flexibility in healthy adults, *Med Sci Sports Exerc* 30:975–991, 1998.
117. Roitman JL, Haver EJ, Herridge M, editors: *ACSM's resource manual for guidelines to exercise testing and prescriptions*, Philadelphia, 2010, Lippincott Williams & Wilkins.
119. Rupp JC: Exercise physiology. In Roitman JL, Bibi KW, Thompson WR, editors: *ACSM health fitness certification review*, Philadelphia, 2001, Lippincott Williams & Wilkins.
120. Saal J: Flexibility training. In Kibler W, editor: *Functional rehabilitation of sports and musculoskeletal injuries*, Gaithersburg, 1998, Aspen.
121. Sady SP, Wortman M, Blanke D: Flexibility training: ballistic, static or proprioceptive neuromuscular facilitation?, *Arch Phys Med Rehabil* 63:261–263, 1982.
124. Seto C: Basic principles of exercise training. In O'Connor F, Sallis R, Wilder R, et al, editors: *Sports medicine: just the facts*, New York, 2005, McGraw-Hill, pp 75–83.
130. Stephens MB, O'Connor F, Deuster P: Exercise and nutrition. In *American Academy of Family Physician's home study self-assessment program, monograph 283*, Leawood, 2002, American Academy of Family Physicians.
131. Stolov WC, Weilepp TG, Jr: Passive length–tension relationship of intact muscle, epimysium, and tendon in normal and denervated gastrocnemius of the rat, *Arch Phys Med Rehabil* 47:612–620, 1966.
132. Stolov WC, Weilepp TG, Jr, Riddell WM: Passive length–tension relationship and hydroxyproline content of chronically denervated skeletal muscle, *Arch Phys Med Rehabil* 51:517–525, 1970.
136. Thibodeau GA, Patton KT: *Anatomy and physiology*, St Louis, 1999, Mosby.
137. Thompson WR, editor: *ACSM's guidelines for exercise testing and prescription*, ed 8, Philadelphia, 2010, Lippincott Williams & Wilkins.
141. Wiktorsson-Moller M, Oberg B, Ekstrand J, et al: Effects of warming up, massage, and stretching on range of motion and muscle strength in the lower extremity, *Am J Sports Med* 11:249–252, 1983.
145. Zarins B: Soft tissue repair: biomechanical aspects, *Int J Sports Med* 3:9–11, 1982.
146. Zhirnova T, Achkasov E, Tsirul'nikova O, et al: Influence of physical rehabilitation on quality of life after renal transplantation, *Vestn Ross Akad Med Nauk* 3-4:65–70, 2014 [in Russian].

The full reference list for this chapter is available online.

CHAPTER 16

MANIPULATION, TRACTION, AND MASSAGE

Christopher J. Wolf, Jeffrey S. Brault

The "laying on of hands" has been a diagnostic and therapeutic modality used since antiquity and has created a special bond between practitioner and patient. Over the millennia a multitude of "hands-on" techniques have been used to treat human suffering. This therapeutic touch has had varied connotations from spiritual healing to physical healing to emotional support and beyond. Although the use of these techniques have waxed and waned in popularity, these modalities and techniques have been gaining acceptance in recent years. These methods have been used as a nonsurgical approach to the treatment of musculoskeletal disorders, particularly neck and low back pain. This approach has been used as the primary form of treatment at times, but also has been as an adjunct to aid in pain relief or gaining mobility to aid the overall treatment. Neck and low back pain have reached epidemic proportions in many industrialized nations. It has been estimated that approximately 80% of all adults will experience low back pain in their lives, and approximately 50% of individuals will experience neck pain.[60] The global prevalence of low back pain is expected to continue to rise in coming years.[84] This escalation of axial pain has created great financial ramifications for society. In recent years, there has been an attempt to reduce morbidity and improve the cost-effectiveness of therapy options.

Many physiatrists use these modalities or lead a multidisciplinary team that does. Understanding the basic principles behind manipulation, traction, and massage, their application, and their potential for complications is highly important in physiatric practice.

Manipulation

Definition and Goals

The International Federation of Manual Medicine[142a] defines *manipulation* as "the use of the hands in the patient management process using instructions and maneuvers to maintain maximal, painless movement of the musculoskeletal system in postural balance." The goal of manipulation or manual medicine is to help maintain optimal body mechanics and to improve motion in restricted areas. Enhancing maximal, pain-free movement in a balanced posture and optimizing function are major goals.[42,45,122] These goals are accomplished by treatments that attempt to restore the mechanical function of a joint and normalize altered reflex patterns,[103,122] as evidenced by optimal range of motion, body symmetry, and tissue texture. The indications for successful use of manual medicine techniques are determined by structural evaluation before and after treatment.[42,100]

Manual medicine can involve manipulation of spinal and peripheral joints as well as myofascial tissues (muscles and fascia). The most fundamental use of manual medicine is to relieve motion restriction and improve motion asymmetry. Improved motion and flexibility are helpful in restoring optimal muscle function and ease of motion. This restoration of function is often accompanied by a decrease in pain, which is often the end point most noticeable to the patient. The ultimate goal of manipulation is to improve the function and well-being of the patient. Examples of this include reduction of pain, improved ambulatory ability, and improved efficiency of biomechanical motion. There are physiologic objectives, such as decreasing nociceptive input, decreasing gamma gain, enhancing lymphatic return, and improving circulation to the tissues. Sometimes therapy is directed at reduction of afferent (nociceptive) input to the spinal cord. Endorphin release increases pain threshold and reduces pain severity.[70,85,103]

Manual medicine continues to be widely practiced and is in high demand by patients.[46] It is estimated that 12 to 17.6 million Americans[124,130] receive manipulations each year, with a high degree of patient satisfaction.[27] Providers who perform manual medicine include physicians from osteopathic medical schools (D.O.), who have this training as part of their core curriculum, and also include allopathic physicians (M.D.) who have obtained additional training in manipulation. Chiropractic providers are taught manual medicine as their primary form of treatment and typically provide this as their only or most primary service to patients. Indeed, in 2002, 7.4% of the population used chiropractic care.[151] Physical therapists can also receive training in some manual therapy techniques and provide this service to patients.

Overview of Various Types of Manual Medicine

Barrier Concept

Central to the application of manual medicine techniques is the barrier concept. This concept recognizes limitation of motion of a normal joint in which asymmetric motion is present. Motion is relatively free in one direction, with loss of some motion in the other direction. Motion loss occurs within the normal range of motion for that joint (Figure 16-1).

The barrier concept implies that something is preventing a full range of motion of a joint. The term *pathologic barrier* was initially used to describe that point where

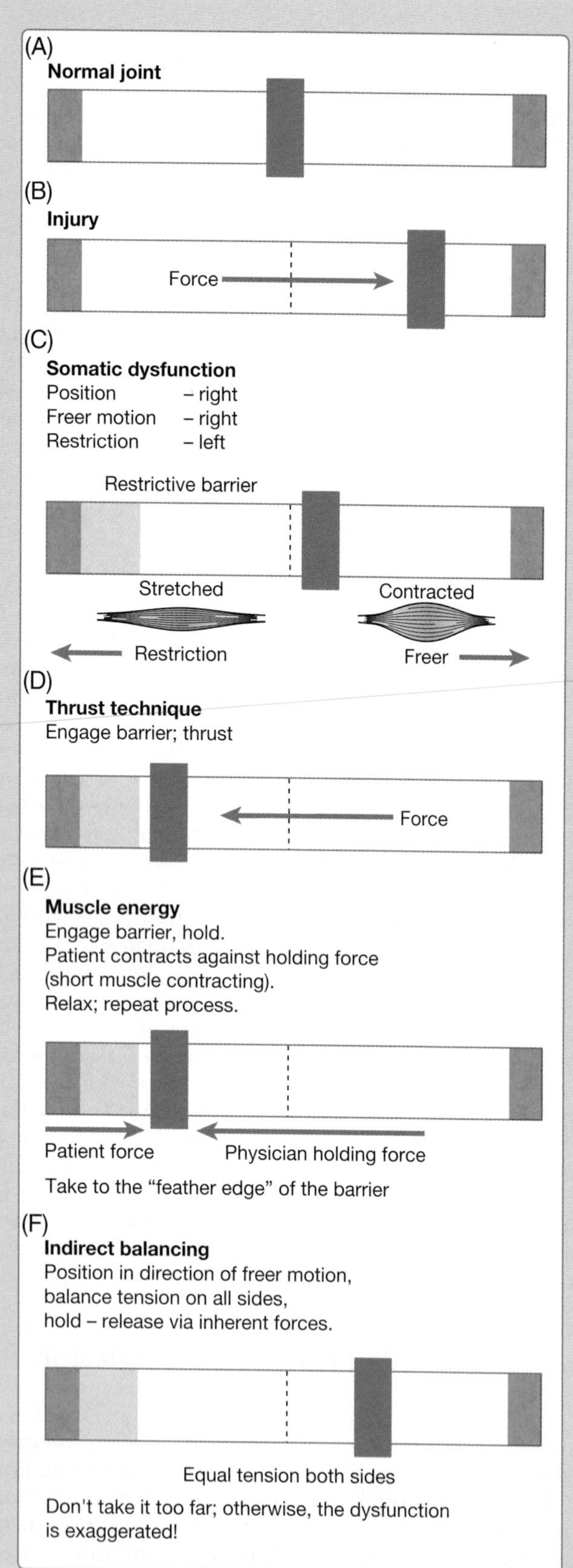

FIGURE 16-1 A model of somatic dysfunction. The first three panels depict production of somatic dysfunction from a mechanical cause. The last three panels depict treatment positions with thrust technique, isometric muscle energy technique, and indirect balancing. **A,** A *normal joint* is positioned in the center, with free motion available in either direction. The shaded area at either end depicts the end of permitted motion. The outside line is termed the *anatomic barrier.* If joint motion goes beyond this point, structural damage will occur. The *Glossary of Osteopathic Terminology* describes the anatomic barrier as the end point of passive motion and the physiologic barrier as the end point of active motion. **B,** This panel, *injury,* shows a force moving the center of the joint to the right. **C,** The third panel, *somatic dysfunction,* shows the effect of the injury. The neutral point is now positioned to the right. The muscle on the right is contracted and shortened; the muscle on the left is stretched (strained). Motion to the right is freer; motion to the left exhibits bind or restriction. This is asymmetric motion, which is typical of spinal somatic dysfunction. There is restriction of motion to the left so that the range of motion is impaired. The end point of this restriction of motion to the left is termed the *restrictive barrier.* Think of the barrier as a series of restrainers that are preventing motion to the left, as contrasted to a brick wall preventing motion. The short, tight muscle on the right prevents full motion to the left. The last three panels show treatment position. **D,** *Thrust technique* (impulse, high velocity, and low amplitude) is a direct technique. The barrier is engaged by moving the joint to the left. The final corrective force is a practitioner force. **E,** Direct isometric *muscle energy* technique looks very similar on the panel. The barrier is engaged by moving the joint to the left. The physician holds and asks the patient to contract against the holding force. The shortened, contracted muscle is the one that is contracting. **F,** *Indirect balancing* involves moving the joint to the right, away from the restrictive barrier. The tension should be balanced on both sides. Final corrective force is a release by inherent forces.

normal motion is limited. The current term used is *restrictive barrier,* which means that no organic pathology can be seen under the microscope; these are functional restrictions. The motion restriction associated with this somatic dysfunction occurs within the normal range of motion of the joint. The new neutral position has shifted in the direction of less restricted motion. This gives rise to positional asymmetry, which leads to physical diagnosis. The lay terms "out" and "out of place" are often used to describe this positional asymmetry. Manipulation is designed to restore normal motion. Manipulation does not put the joint back in place. If a joint is dislocated, this is not somatic dysfunction. Dislocation involves movement beyond the anatomic barrier and outside the normal range of motion and involves associated tissue damage.

Technique

Manual medicine techniques can be classified in different ways. Techniques may be classified as soft tissue technique, articulatory technique, or specific joint mobilization.[100] The objective of a given treatment is specific to the treatment technique applied, but this treatment then has an overall objective for the patient. For example, mobilization of a joint would be a specific goal of a technique but when combined with the overall mixture of techniques in a full treatment the goal is increased pain-free range of motion for the patient.

The terms *direct* and *indirect* are used to classify technique, with several types of technique in each category. Direct technique means that the practitioner moves the body part(s) in the direction of the restrictive barrier. Indirect technique means the practitioner moves the body part away from the restrictive barrier.

Direct techniques include the following:

- *Thrust (impulse, high velocity, low amplitude):* The final activating force is operator force.
- *Articulation:* Low velocity, high amplitude.
- *Muscle energy (direct isometric types):* The final activating force is a patient contraction.
- *Direct myofascial release:* Load (stretch) tissues, hold, and wait for release.

Indirect techniques include the following:

- Strain-counterstrain
- Indirect balancing
- Multiple names (functional, balanced ligamentous tension)
- Indirect myofascial release
- Craniosacral

Historical Perspective and Practitioners

Manual medicine has regained popularity over the past 30 to 40 years, but its practice dates back to the time of Hippocrates (460-377 BC) and Galen (131-202 AD).[74,76] Many other physicians (e.g., Sydenham, Hahnemann, Boerhaave, and Shultes) deviated from the traditional disease-oriented form of medicine during the sixteenth and seventeenth centuries,[76] but manual medicine fell out of favor until the nineteenth century. The pioneers of manual medicine at that time included the "bonesetters" of England: Richard Hutton, Wharton Hood, and Sir Herbert Baker.[23,76]

Manual medicine today is most closely linked to the pioneers of the late nineteenth century, including Andrew Taylor Still, the founder of osteopathic medicine in 1874,[69] and Daniel David Palmer, the founder of chiropractic medicine in 1895.[69,76]

Still's philosophy stressed wellness and wholeness of the body.[106] Osteopathic principles describe the body as a unit that possesses self-healing mechanisms, and that structure and function are interrelated. All of these principles are incorporated into practice.[28] Manual medicine was and is an integral part of this treatment. Today, graduates of one of the 30 colleges of osteopathic medicine, awarded a Doctor of Osteopathy, or D.O., have all had these tenets and training in manual medicine as part of their training curriculum.[5a]

Chiropractic philosophy describes a fundamental relationship between the spine and health and its mediation by the nervous system. Mechanical impairments of the spine are thought to impair health, and the correction of these subluxations can bring about improvements in health.[156] There are currently 18 chiropractic colleges in the United States graduating Doctors of Chiropractic Medicine.[5b]

"Traditional" medical professionals have also shown interest in manual medicine. Mennell and his son John M. Mennell[114] espoused the use of joint manipulation within the British medical community. Beginning in the 1940s James Cyriax,[37] a British orthopedic surgeon, published several works related to manipulation, incorporating massage, traction, and injections. The use of manual techniques for examination purposes by Janet G. Travell, M.D., has been widely accepted.[152] Today, the Fédération Internationale de Médecine Manuelle represents manual medicine practitioners throughout the world.

Normal and Abnormal Coupled Spinal Motion

Motion of the spine follows principles of spinal motion often attributed to Harrison H. Fryette.[59] Flexion (forward bending) and extension (backward bending) are sagittal plane motions and are not coupled. However, rotation and side bending are coupled. The amount of pure rotation or pure side bending of spinal joints is limited and varies depending on the site within the spine. Rotation and side bending occur together in normal spinal joints. Fryette stated that when there is an absence of marked flexion or extension (termed *neutral*) and side bending is introduced, a group of vertebrae rotate into the produced convexity, with maximum rotation at the apex. Rotation and side bending occur to opposite sides when compared with the original starting position. This is sometimes referred to as neutral mechanics or type 1 dysfunction. Nonneutral, or type 2, mechanics involve a component of flexion or extension with rotation and side bending to the same side. This is usually single-segment motion, although several segments may be involved. The cervical spine (C2 to C7) exhibits rotation and side bending to the same side whether flexed, neutral, or extended.

Some atypical joints (occiput, atlas, and sacrum) do not have an intervertebral disk. Their motion patterns are dictated by anatomy. The major motions of the occiput are flexion and extension. Rotation and side bending occur to opposite sides because of the anatomic construction of the joint. The major motion of the atlas is rotation. The atlas rotates around the dens (odontoid process). Half the rotation of the cervical spine occurs at the atlas. Flexion and extension occur but are not involved in motion restriction of the atlas. The atlas does not side bend as it rotates. Actually, both sides of the atlas translate inferiorly during rotation, but side bending does not occur. Trauma can produce atypical motion patterns.

Nomenclature

Somatic Dysfunction

Manual medicine or manipulation involves treating motion restrictions. Nomenclature to describe this motion restriction has changed. The term *manipulatable lesion* is a generic term to describe musculoskeletal dysfunction that might respond to manipulation. Previous terms included *osteopathic lesion, subluxation, joint blockage, loss of joint play,* and *joint dysfunction*.[102,103,122]

Somatic dysfunction is a diagnostic term listed in the Draft for *International Classification of Diseases, Tenth Revision* classification of diagnoses codes M99.0 to M99.09.[123a] It is defined as impaired or altered function of related components of the somatic (body framework) system: skeletal, arthrodial, and myofascial structures, and related vascular, lymphatic, and neural elements.[42] Somatic dysfunction represents a critical concept in manipulative medicine. Somatic dysfunction is diagnosed by palpation. Dysfunctions that are palpated include changes in tissue texture, increased sensitivity to touch (hyperalgesia), altered ease or range of motion, and anatomic asymmetry or positional change.[160]

The *Glossary of Osteopathic Terminology*[28] describes the following three ways of naming somatic dysfunction:

Type 1: Where is it or what position is it in (e.g., right rotated)?

Type 2: What will it do or what is the direction of freer motion (e.g., right strain)?

Type 3: What will it not do or what is the direction of restriction (e.g., restriction of left rotation)?

A dysfunction should be named in three planes of motion, with the upper segment described in relation to the lower. For type 2 dysfunctions, an example of proper nomenclature would be T3 in relation to T4, flexed, rotated, and side bent right. Abbreviations are often used. An example of naming a type 1 group curve would be "L1-L5 neutral, rotated right, side bent left." This would be a lateral curve, convex right.

The Educational Council on Osteopathic Principles has described the point for naming vertebral motion as the most anterior superior part of the vertebral body. For flexion, this point moves forward; for extension, it moves backward. For side bending right, the point moves to the right. Naming rotation is the most common problem. Right rotation involves this point moving right. With left rotation, this point moves left. With right rotation, the right transverse process moves posteriorly. Some practitioners describe rotation using movement of the spinous process. An easy way to remember rotation is to consider riding a bicycle. The handlebars represent the transverse processes. How do you turn the handlebars to turn right? Turning right is an example of right rotation.

Segmental dysfunctions are named for the anterior superior portion of the upper vertebrae in relation to the lower (e.g., T3 in relation to T4). Nomenclature can be expanded to include the three planes of motion (e.g., "T3 flexed, rotated, and side bent right").

Physiologic Rationale for Manual Therapies

Gamma System

Two types of motor neurons exit the spinal cord through the ventral rami to innervate skeletal muscle. Alpha motor neurons innervate large skeletal muscle fibers. A motor unit consists of a single alpha motor neuron and the skeletal muscle fibers it innervates. Gamma motor neurons innervate intrafusal fibers in the muscle spindle. These intrafusal fibers have annulospiral and flower spray endings that report information about muscle length or rate of change of muscle length. Increased gamma activity of the muscle spindles results in increased alpha motor neuron activity to extrafusal fibers of skeletal muscle causing contraction. However, decreasing gamma gain activity is one mechanism that results in muscle relaxation.[44] From a clinical perspective, if a muscle is too tight, the practitioner attempts to bring about muscle relaxation.

Golgi Tendon Reflex

Golgi tendon organs are encapsulated sensory mechanoreceptors located in tendons between the muscle and tendon insertions. These receptors report on tension, and at the spinal cord level they synapse with inhibitory interneurons. Increased tension in a skeletal muscle inhibits alpha motor neurons to that muscle, which causes decreased firing of motor units.

If the muscle spindle is stretched, increased activity of the gamma system stimulates muscle activity. This is just the opposite activity of the Golgi tendon reflex. The gamma system functions to prevent tearing or overstretching of the belly of a muscle. The Golgi apparatus serves to protect the tendon. If a muscle is shortened sufficiently, the stretch receptors cease firing and the alpha motor neurons are turned off.

Muscle Stretch Reflexes

Muscle stretch reflexes, such as the patellar tendon reflex, are considered to be monosynaptic. With the knee flexed to 90 degrees, the quadriceps muscle is placed in a mild stretch. A sudden strike of a hammer against the tendon results in a dynamic stretch. This stimulates the alpha motor neurons to contract the quadriceps muscle, extending the knee.

Spinal Facilitation

Spinal cord facilitation is maintenance of a pool of neurons in a state of subthreshold excitation. In this state, less afferent stimulation is required to produce a response. Consider a model of a sound system with a microphone, amplifier, and speaker. Facilitation acts as if the gain control on the amplifier is turned up. Given a normal input to the microphone, the speaker is too loud. In patients with somatic dysfunction, the muscles are hypertonic and shortened. Spinal facilitation results in hyperactivity of both the general somatic system and the sympathetic nervous system.

Early research studies on facilitation demonstrate how behavior of the spinal cord is altered. Korr[102] applied pressure to spinous processes and measured how much pressure was necessary to produce an electromyographic response in the muscle. A facilitated segment requires less pressure to produce a response. The sympathetic nervous system innervates sweat glands (although this is a cholinergic response). Spinal cord facilitation results in increased sweating at the segmental level. Other factors affect spinal cord behavior. Patterson[125] demonstrated that the spinal cord has "memory" that results in conditioned reflexes. If a stimulus is maintained for a certain period, then removal of the stimulus does not eliminate the response. At one time it was considered that the amount of afferent input produced facilitation. However, when the mix of afferent input is altered, it is as if the cord listens more carefully to the signals (sensitization) coming in. Afferent input from dysfunctional visceral structures produces viscerosomatic reflexes and facilitation.

Originally it was thought that the muscle spindle with increased gamma tone was the basic factor in maintaining facilitation. Subsequent studies have shown that nociception maintains facilitation.[154] Animal studies have been conducted in which afferent fibers from the spindle to the cord were cut, and facilitation continued. Blocking nociceptive input tends to cause facilitation to disappear.

The previous discussion of neurophysiology only scratches the surface. The spinal cord is connected to the brain. There is a vertical component to nerve conduction to and from the brain, as well as a horizontal component between dorsal and ventral roots. There is a neuroendocrine immune system at work. Neuropeptides can sensitize primary afferent fibers as well as fibers within the central nervous system. The practitioner needs to understand the physiologic mechanisms behind muscle tightness, motion restriction, nociception, and inflammation that create dysfunction. Manipulation is one of the treatments used to decrease dysfunction and help the patient. Much of the data necessary to use manipulation effectively come from palpatory assessment rather than high-tech testing. Simple soft tissue techniques are designed to relax tight muscles and fascia. Forces applied too fast or too heavy will cause the muscle to fight back. The response to the application of force is continuously monitored to make sure the muscle relaxes. The focus of the practitioner during treatment is to assess how the patient is responding to the treatment rather than whether the gamma gain has been reduced. Figure 16-1 illustrates how a shortened and contracted muscle can restrict motion.

Indications and Goals of Treatment

Somatic dysfunction is the indication for manual medicine and is diagnosed by palpatory examination. If manual medicine is being considered as a treatment option, there are several questions. Are there signs of a musculoskeletal component to the patient's complaint? Does the somatic dysfunction found in the patient rationally seem to be contributing to the patient's complaint? If the answer to these questions is "yes," then manual medicine may be considered as a potential treatment.

Somatic dysfunction can coexist with "orthopedic disease" (e.g., osteoarthritis or disk disease).[65] Manual medicine treatment helps the somatic dysfunction and helps the patient, but the underlying orthopedic disease process will remain. Other confounding factors are causes for the somatic dysfunction. The patient might have an anatomic short leg, which will continue to maintain sacroiliac and low back dysfunction. Certain activities might be too stressful for the musculoskeletal system. In a controlled study of low back pain, it is impossible to control for these confounding factors. Despite these factors, manual medicine may still be an appropriate option in conservative treatment before more aggressive measures are taken.

Examination and Diagnosis

An examination is a process of data gathering. Subjective data can be obtained by taking a history. On taking a history from a patient, Dr. Max Gutensohn stated, "I always had a feeling that if I could talk to patients long enough, they would tell me what was wrong with them."[16] Pain, discomfort, or functional loss is a frequent complaint. Additional information such as predisposing factors, patient motivation, postural issues, and stresses can all be elicited from a good history.

Physical examination includes acquiring a sufficient physical examination database to enable appropriate diagnosis and treatment. The musculoskeletal examination goes beyond the standard examination of looking for problems in a system (Video 16-1). The practitioner should look for clues about the health status and function of the patient. Is there a somatic component to the patient's problem? The musculoskeletal screening examination looks at gait, posture, and symmetry or asymmetry. This is ordinarily done with the patient standing. A standardized 12-step biomechanical screening examination may be done,[42] or the screening examination may be nonstandard, with a systematic approach used to evaluate all body regions. This examination can be integrated into a comprehensive physical examination.

A standardized examination is ordinarily used by students, whereas experienced physicians often raise questions, and the examination is tailored to finding answers to the questions. For efficiency the patient should be examined in multiple positions: standing, seated, supine, and prone. To conserve time and enhance efficiency, all tests should be completed with the patient in one position before moving the patient to the next position. The mnemonic for a musculoskeletal examination is TART: *T*, tenderness or sensitivity; *A*, asymmetry (look); *R*, restriction of motion (move); *T*, tissue texture abnormality (feel). The diagnosis of somatic dysfunction is based on a palpatory examination with TART.

Palpation for Tissue Texture Abnormality

Tissue texture abnormality is palpable evidence of physiologic dysfunction. The approach to palpation is to compare right versus left and above versus below. When evaluating a single area without comparing with adjacent areas, it is difficult to come to a meaningful conclusion. Description of dysfunctional areas is done relative to these adjacent areas. Palpation is done in layers, projecting your sense of touch to the depth required.

Acute tissue texture change can be described and remembered by thinking of acute inflammation and the four cardinal signs: red, puffy, painful or tender, and warm. With acute tissue texture changes, sweating is increased and the skin is usually moist (increased sympathetic tone). Chronic tissue texture abnormality is associated with thin, dry, atrophic skin that is cool. The palpatory quality is firm or fibrotic. Motion testing reveals motion loss.

Paraspinal viscerosomatic reflexes have palpatory qualities that are characteristic and give the experienced clinician clues that these changes may be as a result of visceral disturbances. The maximum intensity of the findings is reported to be at the costotransverse and rib angle areas. The greatest number of findings is in the skin and subcutaneous tissue.

Palpating for tissue texture abnormalities can be an accurate and efficient method of identifying problem areas, as well as their acuity, in the musculoskeletal system that require further examination.

Motion Testing

There are multiple methods for motion testing. Because manipulative treatment has as its immediate objective the improvement of motion, motion testing skills and treatment skills become intertwined with the motion testing being used for ongoing diagnosis throughout the treatment.

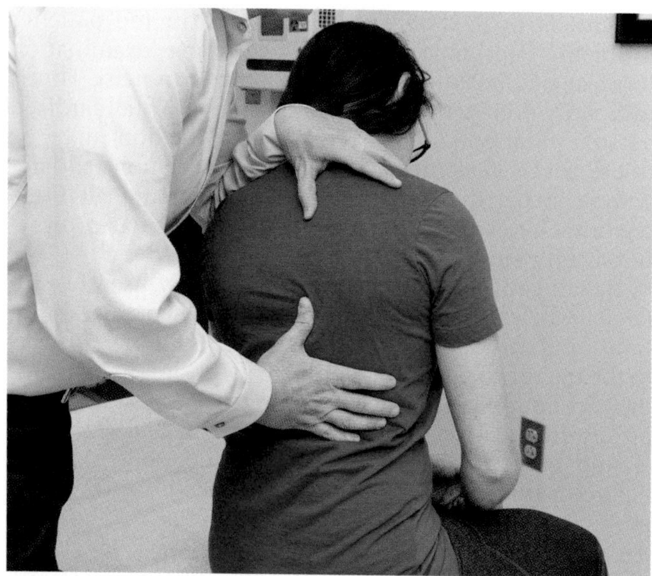

FIGURE 16-2 Motion testing or articulatory treatment of the thoracic spine. The patient is seated, and the practitioner stands behind the patient with the arm draped over the patient's shoulder girdles. This enables the practitioner to comfortably induce forces from above that can be used for diagnosis and treatment. These forces include rotation, side bending, lateral translation, and flexion-extension. The opposite hand is placed on the opposite side of the spine to monitor motion for diagnosis. Articulatory treatment can occur with the same hand position but with forces combined from both hands or arms.

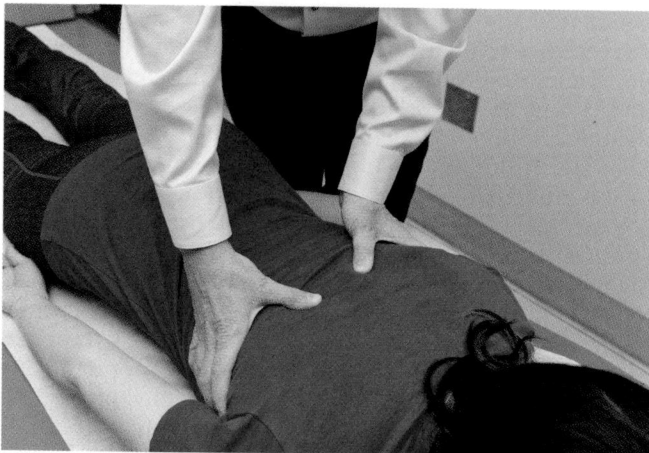

FIGURE 16-3 Segmental motion testing. The practitioner's hands are positioned with the thumbs overlying the transverse processes on either side of the segment in question. Alternating pressure on the thumbs induces rotation at the segment while side bending can be induced with medial pressure directed from the hand itself. Flexion and extension preference is tested separately.

Types of motion testing include the following:

- Observation of active motion.
- Palpation of active motion with palpating fingers over the facet area.
- Rib motion, which is often tested by palpating motion as the patient inhales and exhales.
- Active hand/passive hand, which is motion testing in which one hand does the moving and the other hand assesses motion (e.g., moving the head and neck while palpating in the upper thoracic spine).
- Direct passive motion testing in which the physician's hands provide the force and also monitor response to this force. Terms to describe the "feel" might be *ease* and *bind* or *freedom* and *resistance* (Figure 16-2).

The muscle energy type of motion testing looks for the most posterior transverse process. Place the palpating fingers on the transverse process area of both sides of the segment to be tested. Instruct the patient to flex and extend. For example, assume T3 is extended, rotated, and side bent right. When T3 is flexed (this is the barrier), the muscle on the right side "balls up" under the palpating finger, and the right transverse process becomes more posterior. When T3 is extended, the findings on either side are decreased. The concept demonstrated is that positional asymmetry is increased when the barrier is engaged.

Using the same example of T3 extended, rotated, and side bent right, flex T3 by flexing the head and neck. Attempt to rotate right and left. Left rotation will be very restricted. Extend T3 and again rotate. Left rotation will be much freer. This confirms that the barrier is flexion, and the dysfunction is extended.

Segmental motion testing can also be induced with pressure through the hands without relying on patient movement for diagnosis (Figure 16-3).

There are other approaches to diagnosis, but they share the evaluation of relative motion differences in one of the cardinal planes. The choice of technique for motion testing varies depending on the physician's preference, the body type of the practitioner and the patient, as well as the physical layout of the treatment area.

Assessment of Fascia

Fascia has unique features that include the formation of sheets with multidirectional fibers giving it tensile strength, and sheets with nonlinear motion that allow for shortening and elongating, thus accounting for its flexibility and pliability. By contrast, there is little or no motion in scar tissue. Fascia is three-dimensional and can form sleeves to compartmentalize, act as cables, or form diaphragms. All these properties must be considered when assessing fascia.

Assessment of fascia starts with placement of the hands to perceive the combined vector force in the tissue.[47] Hand placement varies depending on the area to be assessed and treated. Assessment of an extremity would start with hand placement proximal and distal to the area. An example of this would be the assessment of the forearm. One hand grasps the patient's hand and the other hand grasps the proximal forearm near the elbow.

In the assessment of a three-dimensional region, such as the chest cage, the hands will start with one anterior and the other posterior on the thorax. The hands should be placed in such a manner that they are 180 degrees to one another. Assessment of a large area, such as the thoracolumbar fascia, might begin with the hands placed in the same direction, on either side of the spine, adjacent to each other.

Once the hands are placed, the fascia must be "entered" by adding tension to the area to engage the viscoelastic property of fascia. The viscoelastic property allows fascia to deform. With tension in place, the practitioner can now "read" the tissue and simultaneously assess and treat. The practitioner can move the fascia to a tightened position by combining multiple motion vectors (clockwise-counterclockwise rotation, anterior-posterior motion, cephalad-caudad motion, pronation-supination) as in a direct release, or follow the combined vector to a point of balance as in an indirect release. Examination of the fascia and myofascial structures may include looking for special "points" or "triggers." These include counterstrain tender points, the myofascial triggers of Simon and Travell, and acupuncture points.

Types of Technique

Overview of Various Types of Manual Medicine

As mentioned earlier, manual medicine techniques can be classified in different ways, including soft tissue technique, articulatory technique, or specific joint mobilization. These are applied directly or indirectly. Combined technique starts with indirect technique, and once the release has occurred, the practitioner may switch to direct technique. Detailed descriptions of the most commonly used techniques are listed below.

Direct Techniques

Soft Tissue Technique. The purpose of soft tissue technique is to relax muscles and fascia. There are an infinite number of modifications of soft tissue technique. Usually they involve lateral force to stretch the muscle, direct longitudinal stretching, or careful kneading. Sensitive hands and experience are necessary to assess the response of the tissues to the treatment. Apply forces slowly and release slowly. Do not allow tissues to snap back quickly or spasm might occur. Do not allow your fingers to slide over the skin. Avoid excess force per unit area; instead, spread the forces out. Avoid direct pressure over bony prominences. Soft tissue technique can be the primary approach. It can be used to prepare an area for specific mobilization. It can be used to facilitate movement of fluids. It can reduce or modify pain. This is similar to massage, but there is a different end point of the treatment. The focus here is on moving tissue rather than relaxing muscles.

Articulatory Treatment. This procedure moves a joint back and forth repeatedly to increase freedom of range of motion. Articulatory treatment may be classified as a low-velocity, high-amplitude approach. Sometimes articulatory treatment is a form of soft tissue treatment in which the only way to access deep muscles is to move origin and insertion (see Figure 16-2). Articulatory treatment is very useful for stiff joints and for older patients. It might be the only form of treatment applicable for some patients. There are many modifications to articulatory technique.

Mobilization with Impulse (Thrust; High Velocity, Low Amplitude). Thrust technique is often considered synonymous with manipulation. In Europe, thrust techniques are reserved for the physician, whereas other techniques are termed *mobilization*. Thrust techniques are applicable for restriction of motion in joints. Thrust technique is often the quickest form of addressing restriction of joint motion. An audible pop can occur with application of the technique. The noise has no effect on treatment outcome. To assess the effectiveness of treatment, reevaluation is required.

A diagnosis of motion restriction is essential before application of thrust technique, and this diagnosis should incorporate the three planes of motion: flexion-extension, rotation, and side bending. The first principle of thrust technique is to engage the barrier. With an accurate diagnosis, engaging the barrier is specific. The barrier must feel solid, not rubbery. A thrust should not be applied if the barrier does not feel solid. Instead of addressing the restriction of motion of the joint, the force is dissipated by muscles and fascia. The thrust must be low amplitude, meaning a very short distance. The thrust should be high velocity (Figures 16-4 to 16-6). There is no place for high-velocity, high-amplitude technique.

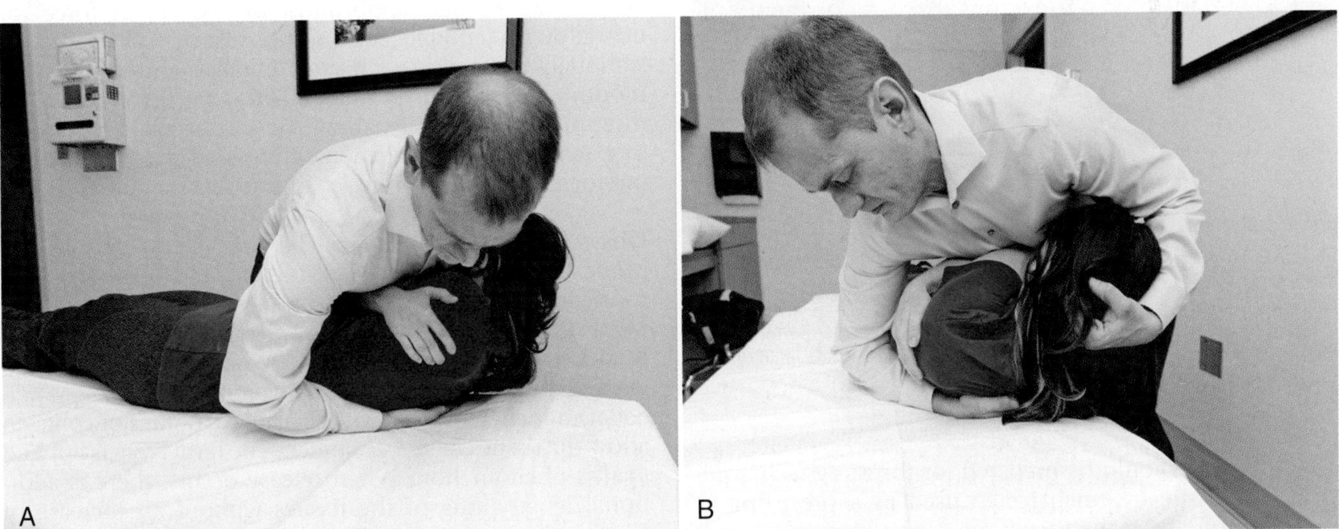

FIGURE 16-4 Supine treatment of thoracic somatic dysfunction. There are multiple variations of this technique, sometimes referred to as the "Kirksville krunch." It can be modified to treat type 1 and type 2 dysfunctions, as well as ribs. The technique pictured involves T5 flexed, rotated, and side bent to the left. The practitioner stands on the right side of the patient. The patient's arms are folded across the chest (position can vary with technique). The practitioner's fulcrum hand is placed posteriorly over the T6 left side (segment below, side opposite) (**A**). The patient's torso is rolled back and the patient's body is moved adjusting side bending and flexion-extension to localize force over fulcrum hand (**B**). The patient is flexed to the segment, and extension is created at the fulcrum as the corrective high-velocity, low-amplitude force is applied.

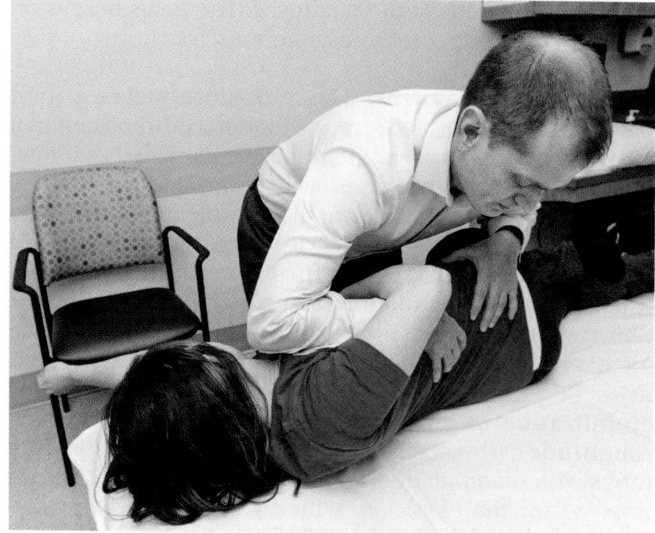

FIGURE 16-5 Treatment of lumbar somatic dysfunction. There are many variations of technique for treating the lumbar region with the patient on their side. This technique shown is for an L2 dysfunction that is flexed, rotated, and side bent to the left. The posterior transverse process from diagnosis is placed down (left side down). The patient's torso is perpendicular to the table. The patient's hips and knees are flexed with the upper leg flexed more. Extension at L2 is obtained from above by torso movement. Side bending is maintained by stretching out the right side. Rotation from below is obtained by pushing the shoulder posteriorly. The final corrective force on the iliac crest emphasizes side bending toward the patient's head; rotation is automatic with the force.

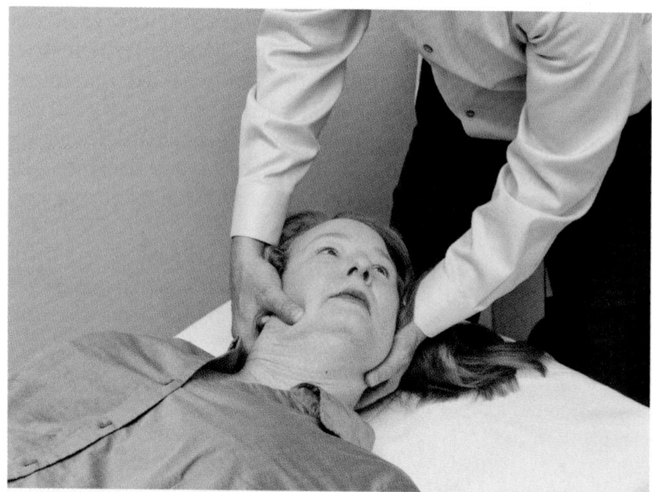

FIGURE 16-6 Treatment of cervical spine C2 to C7. In this example, the diagnosis is C4 flexed, rotated, and side bent left. The lateral mass of C4 is contacted with the index finger. An extension break at C4-C5 keeps forces localized at the segment to be treated. Rotation to the left is performed to lock out the rotation component. The corrective force is a side bending into the barrier.

The tissues should be prepared for thrusting technique with soft tissue treatment often used as a precursor to thrust technique. If the tissues are not properly prepared, it is more difficult to engage the barrier and more force must be used. The dissipation of excess force can cause iatrogenic problems. The patient must be relaxed. There is no substitute for skilled hands that allow the patient to relax. Often the thrust is given during exhalation because the tissues are more relaxed at this time. The final activating force is operator force.

Muscle Energy: Direct Isometric Types. Muscle energy technique[66,118] was introduced by Fred Mitchell, Sr.[117] Muscle energy technique involves the patient voluntarily moving the body as specifically directed by the practitioner. This directed patient action is from a precisely controlled position against a defined resistance by the practitioner. The initial classification of muscle energy techniques was based on whether the force was equal (isometric), greater (isotonic), or less (isolytic) than the patient force. Most muscle energy techniques used by physicians are direct isometric techniques. This technique has been used extensively by therapists and is often referred to as contract relax technique.

Muscle energy technique requires a specific diagnosis incorporating all three planes of motion (Video 16-2). The first step is moving the dysfunctional component into the restrictive barrier. Fred Mitchell Jr.[116] emphasizes that the practitioner moves the dysfunctional component to the "feather edge" of the barrier. The practitioner holds this position and instructs the patient to contract against the holding force. The patient controls the amount of force, so injury is not likely. Additionally, the manner in which the practitioner holds the patient position suggests the amount of force. A heavy-handed vice grip will suggest more force than a lighter touch. The muscle contraction is held for 3 to 5 seconds. Then there is a period of relaxation, sometimes termed *postisometric relaxation*. The practitioner then reengages a new barrier, and the process is repeated several times. If there is no further increase in the range of motion, it is time to stop. Three repetitions are the usual number, followed by reassessment.

Most direct isometric muscle energy techniques involve the patient actively contracting the shortened (sometimes referred to as the "sick") muscle. The usual mistakes in using muscle energy technique are failure to properly engage the barrier, application of too much force, or not allowing enough time for postisometric relaxation. Although engaging the barrier involves three planes of motion, the patient contraction may be in one, two, or three planes. Often the patient contraction will be a flexion or extension. In muscle energy technique, the final activating force is a patient muscle contraction (Figure 16-7).

Direct Myofascial Release. The goal of myofascial technique is to identify tissue restriction and to remove the restriction. This requires sensing arms and hands. Direct myofascial technique involves loading the myofascial tissues (stretch), holding the tissues in position, and waiting for release. Release is by inherent forces. When collagen is stretched, the viscoelastic properties of collagen allow the tissues to slowly stretch. The term *creep* is applied to this phenomenon. When release occurs, there is additional lengthening of the tissues without an increase of force being applied. This phenomenon takes several seconds. This release might be likened to an ice cube melting. The release is perceived by the practitioner treating the patient. Reevaluation of the patient reveals a decrease of the restriction being treated, with increased freedom of range of motion (Figure 16-8).

Indirect Techniques

Strain-Counterstrain. Counterstrain is a type of manipulative treatment that uses spontaneous release by positioning, and uses tender points serving as a monitor to achieve the proper position. Lawrence Jones, D.O.,[92] developed this method of treatment (Video 16-3). Counterstrain is classified as an indirect technique. The objective is to relieve painful dysfunction through a reduction of inappropriate afferent proprioception activity. Referring to Figure 16-1, the shortened muscle remains shortened because of inappropriate proprioceptive activity. Tender points are located in the muscle belly, tendon (usually at or near the bony attachment of the tendon), or dermatome of the shortened muscle. Treatment position further shortens the short muscle, as a "counterstrain" is applied to the originally strained muscle on the other side. The neurophysiologic mechanism is based on the fact that shortening the muscle quiets the muscle and breaks into the inappropriate strain reflex.

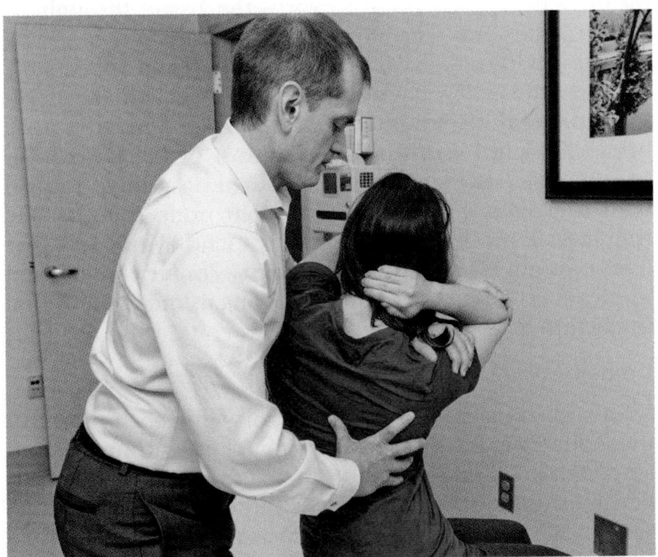

FIGURE 16-7 Treatment of thoracic spine with seated, direct muscle energy technique. In this example, the diagnosis is T5 to T8 flexed, rotated right, side bent to the left. The patient is asked to place right hand behind neck and grasp right elbow with left hand and maintain this arm position. The practitioner then reaches in front of the patient to grasp the patient's right arm to allow for movement to engage the dysfunctional barrier, and in this case it is slight extension of the trunk, rotation to the left, and side bending to the right. The practitioner's right hand then monitors motion to ensure localization to proper segments and provide some counter force. The activating force is an isometric contraction from the patient.

Tender points are related to specific dysfunctions. The practitioner must know where to look for these specific points.[93] For example, if the patient has a dysfunction at L3 that is flexed, rotated, and side bent left, an anterior lumbar tender point is located in the abdominal wall in the vicinity of the anterior inferior iliac spine. The use of counterstrain requires a structural evaluation and assessment for tender points. Tender points are tissue areas that are tender to palpation. They are sometimes described as "pealike" areas of tension. The common denominator is the tissue change and tenderness.

Treatment involves identifying the tender point, maintaining a palpating finger on the tender point, and placing the patient in a position so that tenderness in this point is eliminated or reduced significantly. This position is in a pain-free direction of ease. Also, the position places the patient in the original position of injury. Counterstrain is not a form of acupressure. The monitoring finger continues to palpate and assess the point, but pressure is not applied. The amount of time that the treatment position is held is 90 seconds, 120 seconds for ribs. It is essential that the patient be slowly returned from the treatment position to the starting point. The patient should remain passive during the entire process. After return, the tender point is reassessed. If the physician's palpating finger stays on the tender point, and tenderness is now absent, both practitioner and patient know that a change was made (Figure 16-9).

Counterstrain is a very gentle technique with an extremely low risk of injury. However, patients can become

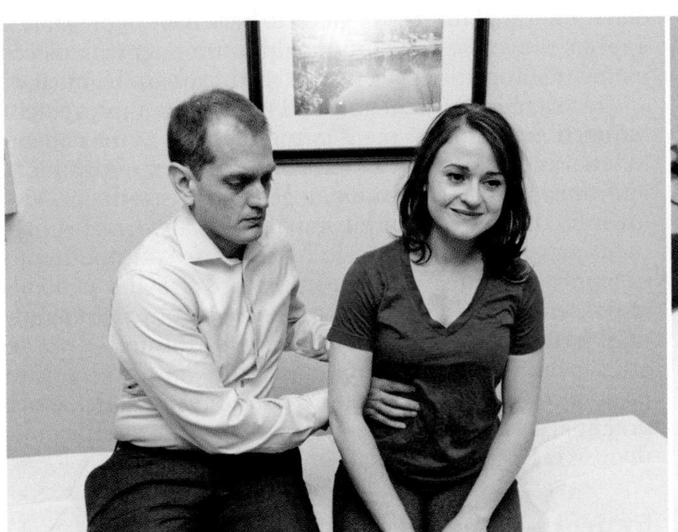

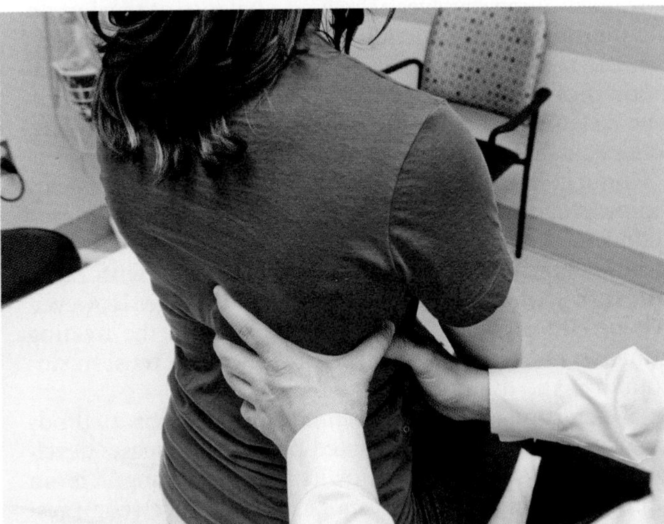

FIGURE 16-8 Direct myofascial/indirect treatment for rib. In this example, the diagnosis is right rib 8 exhalation preference. The hand position approximates the length of the rib. Slight pressure is placed anteriorly and posteriorly on the rib to free the rib. For a direct myofascial technique, the rib is taken into the restrictive barrier with slight consistent pressure until release is felt. In an indirect technique, the rib is positioned in the position of ease away from the restrictive barrier exaggerating the exhalation preference.

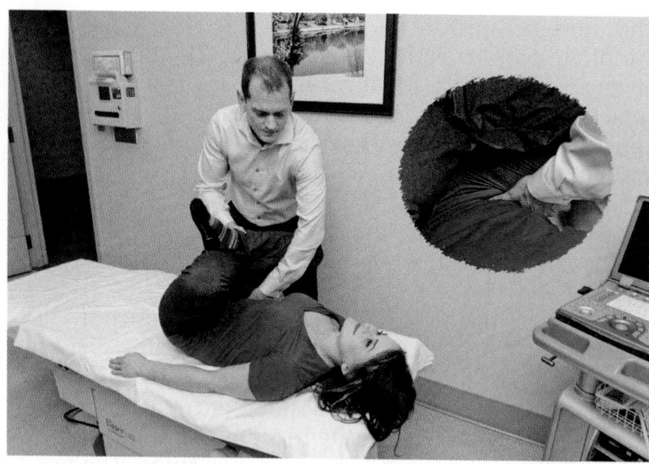

FIGURE 16-9 Counterstrain for iliacus tender point. The patient is in supine position. The tender point is palpated in the anterior pelvis deep in iliac fossa (see inset). Treatment is achieved by flexion of the legs and bilateral hip rotation until tenderness is decreased by more than 80% while tension in the tender point is continuously monitored. The position is then held for 90 seconds or until palpable release. The practitioner then slowly removes the patient from the treatment position and rechecks tenderness for resolution.

very sore after counterstrain treatment. It is appropriate to caution patients that they might become sore after treatment. Sometimes analgesics are used to treat the soreness. Patients are often advised to drink plenty of water to maintain adequate hydration. Counterstrain can be used to treat tenderness that remains after other manual treatments have addressed motion restriction. These techniques are also often a good starting point for those learning manual medicine techniques.

Indirect Balancing. There are multiple names to describe types of indirect technique. These names include functional technique and balanced ligamentous tension. The common denominator in all these technique types is that they are indirect, in that the dysfunction is positioned in a direction of freer motion away from the restrictive barrier. The positioning involves achieving a balance of tension on all sides of the dysfunction. The functional technique of Johnston[91] involves balancing tension in the three translations (front-back, side to side, up-down) and respiration. The more perfect this balance, the quicker the release. Release is by inherent forces.

Indirect balance techniques are difficult for some practitioners and much easier for others. With counterstrain, a tender point helps in finding the proper treatment position. Achieving the proper treatment position with other forms of indirect technique can be a challenge. However, when release occurs, this is very apparent to the treating clinician because there is a decrease of overall tension surrounding the dysfunction.

Some forms of indirect technique use various methods to facilitate a release. Facilitated positional release, developed by DiGiovanna, Schiowitz, and Downing,[44] is an indirect technique that uses a facilitating force (compression, distraction, or torque) to speed the release. DiGiovanna was once asked about the difference between counterstrain and facilitated positional release. She thought for a moment and replied, "About 85 seconds!"

Combined technique or a combined approach is often used with indirect technique. As release is occurring, the original barrier is softening, and the dysfunction is moved into the restrictive barrier. Combined technique means that one starts with indirect technique and finishes with direct technique. Still technique, based on the surviving evidence of how A.T. Still approached manual therapy, has been described by several sources and is a type of combined technique. It involves positioning a joint into the position of ease (indirect), then inducing a light force of compression or traction into the joint. This is followed by then using this force to carry the tissue through its range of motion and through the restrictive barrier[153] (Figure 16-10).

Craniosacral. Craniosacral technique is applied to the bony calvarium and the sacrum. Most of the techniques are indirect. For example, if the patient has a right torsion with the right sphenoid and the left occiput high, take the cranial mechanism into right torsion, which is the freer motion. Hold and wait for release. Some cranial techniques are direct; for example, disengagement of sutural impaction.

Common Clinical Uses of Manual Medicine

Manual therapy has a variety of uses within the practice of medicine. It can serve as a primary treatment modality in some cases. Acute pain with somatic dysfunction as a pain generator can often involve early treatment with manual therapy. The goals of improved function with manual therapy are truly a universal goal for all patients. Therefore, although the use of manual therapy can be used for many different patients, the groups most helped by this treatment are not well defined in the literature. One group that seems to derive benefit is the pregnant population. Pregnant patients with low back and pelvic discomfort can benefit from the conservative treatment provided by manual therapy (Figure 16-11). Osteopathic manipulative treatment of back and pelvic pain in pregnancy is found to be better than usual care overall.[127] Additionally, the deterioration of function related to back pain in pregnancy appears slowed or halted in the third trimester with osteopathic manipulation as a part of the treatment regimen.[108]

The overall treatment goal still remains as improvement in function or improvement in specific goals of the patient. Manual medicine may be just one part of the treatment and thus secondary treatment or adjunct treatment. Frequently, there are postural imbalances, abnormal movement patterns, or core instability that are contributing to not only the somatic dysfunction but also the patient's major symptomatology. Home exercises or physical therapy may be beneficial as a component of the treatment to aid resolution of the symptoms. This can also work to prolong the benefits of the manual therapy and remove potential predisposing factors for the somatic dysfunctions themselves.

Evidence-Based Use of Manual Therapies in Practice

The effectiveness as well as the risks of manual medicine continues to generate controversy. Adequate randomized

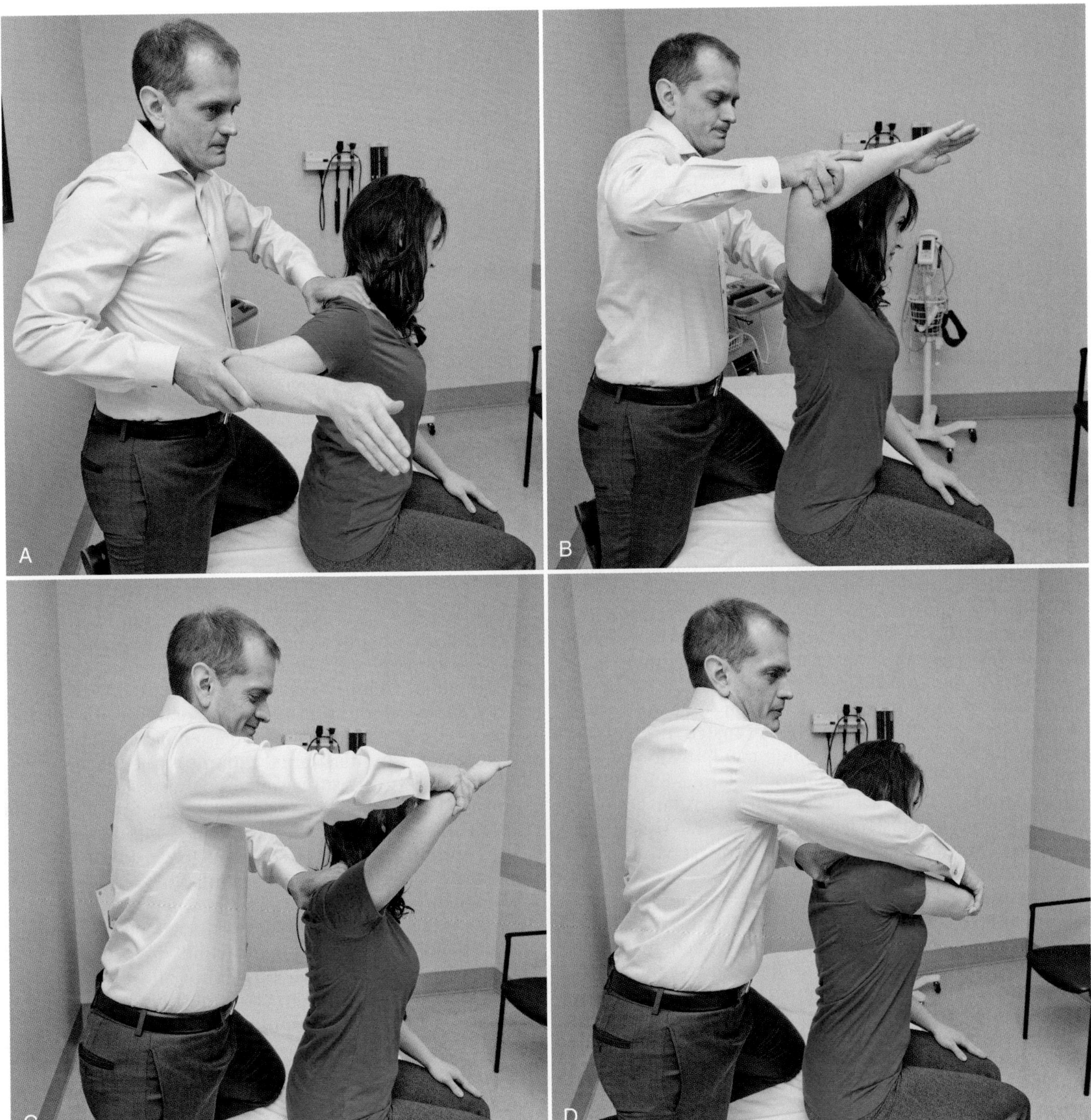

FIGURE 16-10 Still technique for acromioclavicular joint. The tissues are taken to the point of ease (**A**). Force vector loads the joint while in position of ease. Then the practitioner keeps this force while the tissue is taken through its range of motion (**B** to **D**). The correction of dysfunction occurs through this range as the restrictive barrier is breached.

controlled studies to determine long-term benefits are not available. Available studies have been limited by the heterogeneity of patients, duration of pain, variety of manual medicine techniques used, difficulty of "blinding" patients, and lack of widely accepted or validated outcome measures.[5] Recent reviews of manual medicine studies[5] indicate effectiveness in some subpopulations, especially in people with low back pain of 2 to 4 weeks' duration.[73,112] These reports contributed to the support for their use in *Guidelines for Acute Low Back Problems* by the Agency for Health Care Policy and Research.[12] There are no current guidelines for treatment regimens for the cervical and thoracic spine. However, several studies support the use of manipulation in these areas.[9,25,71,86] A recent study by Mills et al.[115] supports the effectiveness of manipulation in the treatment of acute otitis media. For chronic back pain, recent studies showed that patients report more pain improvement, more satisfaction with their treatment, and less medication use than those not receiving manual medicine.[109]

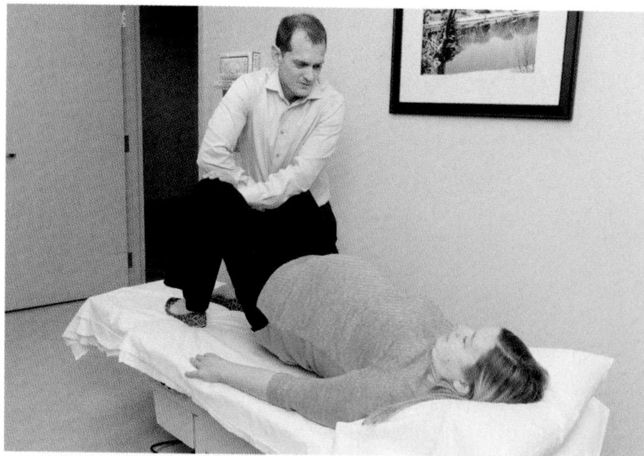

FIGURE 16-11 Pelvic treatment in a pregnant patient. In this example, pubic somatic dysfunction is safely treated with a muscle energy technique in a pregnant woman. Many techniques can be modified to be used safely in the pregnant patient by the experienced practitioner.

Contraindications and Side Effects

Perhaps the most serious complication of cervical manipulation is stroke associated with vertebrobasilar artery dissection.[49] Approximately 275 cases of adverse events with cervical spine manipulation have been reported in the literature since 1925.[7,146,155] It has been suggested there might be an underreporting of adverse events.[75] The number of cervical spine manipulations is estimated to be from a low of 33 million to a high of 193 million annually in the United States and Canada.[86] The estimated risk for an adverse outcome after cervical spine manipulation ranges from 1 in 400,000 manipulations to 1 in 3.85 million manipulations.[104] The risk for a vertebrobasilar accident occurring spontaneously is nearly twice the risk as for a vertebrobasilar accident resulting from cervical spine manipulation.[86]

In an attempt to identify patients who might be at risk for vertebral artery injury from cervical spine manipulation, some provocative tests were developed, with the DeKline test proving the most popular. This test and others like it have been found to be unreliable.[35] Complications from cervical spine manipulation most often occur in patients who have had previous cervical spine manipulation uneventfully and without obvious risk factors for vertebrobasilar artery dissection.[86] The most common risk factors for vertebrobasilar artery dissection are migraine, hypertension, use of oral contraceptives, and smoking.[75] Most vertebrobasilar dissections occur in the absence of cervical manipulation, either spontaneously or after trivial trauma or common daily movements of the neck, such as backing out of a driveway, painting the ceiling, playing tennis, sneezing, or engaging in yoga.[146]

Most complications are associated with high-velocity thrusting techniques. Box 16-1 shows a list of conditions that are contraindications to thrusting technique. Contraindications can arise from several causes. Practitioner errors involve diagnostic errors, lack of manual skill, and failure to obtain a needed consultation. There are patient pathologies that contraindicate thrusting techniques. There are other patient-related problems of a psychological or behavioral nature that are also contraindications to the technique. Side effects can occur with manipulation and are not always complications. Patients sometime experience a rebound phenomenon with a temporary increase of symptoms, which often occurs several hours after the treatment. These symptoms subside spontaneously, and the patient is usually much improved after the rebound symptoms subside. Counterstrain technique is a gentle, nontraumatic technique. Posttreatment pain can occur several hours later. Patients should be informed they might experience this posttreatment pain and that it will subside.

The practitioner must consider the risks versus the potential benefits whenever manipulation is considered. A comprehensive list of contraindications does not replace this assessment by the physician. Experience in treating patients with manipulation is helpful in making these judgments. There is also a possibility of an overdose of manipulative treatment. The dose must be limited by the ability of the patient to respond to the treatment.

BOX 16-1

Contraindications for High-Velocity Manipulation Techniques

- Unstable fractures
- Severe osteoporosis
- Multiple myeloma
- Osteomyelitis
- Primary bone tumors
- Paget disease
- Any progressive neurologic deficit
- Spinal cord tumors
- Cauda equina compression
- Central cervical intervertebral disk herniation
- Hypermobile joints
- Rheumatoid arthritis
- Inflammatory phase of ankylosing spondylitis
- Psoriatic arthritis
- Reiter syndrome
- Anticoagulant therapy
- Congenital bleeding disorder
- Acquired bleeding disorder
- Inadequate physical and spinal examination
- Poor manipulative skills

Traction

Definition

Traction is a technique used to stretch soft tissues and to separate joint surfaces or bone fragments by use of a pulling force.[79] The force applied must be of sufficient magnitude and duration in the proper direction while resisting movement of the body with an equal and opposite force.

Historical Perspective

Traction dates back to the time of Hippocrates, who recommended its use for scoliosis, kyphosis, and fractures of the femur.[79,81] Throughout history, it has most commonly been used to reduce fractures and dislocations. For many centuries after Hippocrates, it was the preferred method of treating femur fractures.

The use of traction to treat spinal disorders has become more widespread in the past 50 years, being popularized by Cyriax.[37,39] He proposed traction for the treatment of lumbar disk disorders. He hypothesized that patients should be in constant traction for at least 20 minutes to produce stretch and decompression of spinal structures. Judovich[94-96] stated that higher forces were poorly tolerated with constant traction and that the greater forces needed to overcome surface resistance were best used with intermittent traction. He discovered that 20 to 25 lb of force was required to produce distraction in the cervical spine. In the 1960s, Colachis and Strohm[30-33] studied the biomechanics of traction and attempted to define the optimal angle of pull for cervical traction, as well as the optimal duration of traction for both the lumbar and the cervical regions. They concluded that 24 degrees of flexion intermittently for 25 minutes produced optimal distraction. Further studies regarding the optimal angle of pull, duration, and force have produced varying results.[11,38,81]

Traction continues to be used in the treatment of cervical and lumbar pain disorders. More recent advances have included inversion techniques,[63] motorized systems,[134,138,143,162] and the development of stabilizing tables.[64,134,143,149]

Types of Traction

Traction can be delivered by several different methods, including manual, mechanized,[79] motorized, or hydraulic,[134,138,143,162] or with the assistance of gravity via inversion.[63] Irrespective of the method, the surface resistance must be overcome. It is approximately equal to half the weight of the body segment.[95,96] The force can be continuous, sustained, or intermittent. *Continuous* traction uses a low force over a long period, such as 30 to 40 hours.[79] Continuous traction is typically not well tolerated and is not used very commonly. *Sustained* traction uses a larger force but for a shorter period (typically 30 to 60 minutes).[79] Sustained traction is still difficult to tolerate, but is commonly used in the lumbar spine with a split traction or autotraction table. *Intermittent* traction uses greater forces over shorter periods.[79] The traction force can be increased or decreased during each treatment cycle, and the duration of pull can be adjusted. The cycle is usually repeated for 15 to 25 minutes, with the traction phase ranging from 5 to 60 seconds, and the rest phase ranging from 5 to 15 seconds.[30,32] The magnitude, duration, and direction of the pull can be varied.

Cervical traction is commonly performed manually, mechanically, or motorized with a head or chin sling, or with a supine posterior distraction unit.[79] The optimal angle of pull ranges between 20 degrees and 30 degrees of flexion,[33,38] while 25 lb of force is required to reverse the normal cervical lordosis and bring about the earliest distraction of vertebral segments.[95] Mechanical cervical traction can be applied in the supine position, which reduces the weight of the head but increases the frictional resistance. This position also allows for better control of the head by the patient and is typically more comfortable (Figure 16-12).[162] Traction in the sitting position allows

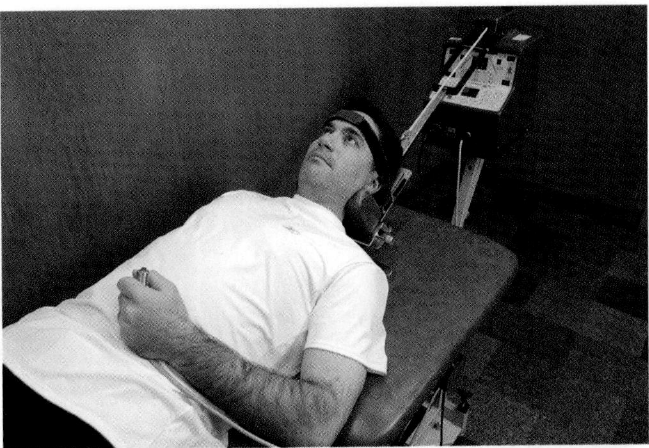

FIGURE 16-12 Mechanical cervical traction. Cervical traction can be performed with a mechanical device. The patient is placed in a comfortable supine position with the neck flexed slightly.

more accurate positioning for the correct angle of pull, but usually affords less head control and is less comfortable. Cervical traction can be used at home with a traditional over-the-door unit (Figure 16-13) or a supine posterior distraction unit (Figure 16-14).

Lumbar traction requires significantly greater force to create distraction of the vertebral segments than cervical traction. Common traction systems include a thoracic or chest belt with a pelvic belt (Figure 16-15), inversion, a split traction table, or an autotraction table.[143] Split traction tables have a mobile and a stationary half. The lower body rests on the mobile half, which separates from the stationary portion. The force necessary to overcome resistance is reduced, and the force required for distraction is significantly less.[79,81,95,134,143] The autotraction table allows both segments of the table to move and is controlled by the patient. The patient assumes the most pain-free position and performs the active traction by pulling on an overhead bar. The patient then uses his or her feet to activate a bar, which alternates compressive and distracting forces.[149] There has been no study of lumbar traction to determine the most efficacious angle of pull, magnitude, or duration of pull.

Vertebral axial decompression (VAX-D) has been more recently advocated for lumbar pain with or without leg pain. This method of traction uses a split traction table with the patient lying prone. An initial study by Ramos and Martin[134] suggested that negative intradiscal pressures of 100 mm Hg could be obtained during VAX-D treatment. However, Nachemson[121] stated that these results were probably invalid because of improper calibration, lack of accounting for temperature, and the fact that this was not a closed system. Three clinical studies suggest clinical efficacy for back or leg pain, or both, but none were blinded.[67,133,144] Only one of the studies was randomized, compared with transcutaneous electrical stimulation. One case report of an enlarged disk herniation during VAX-D treatment has been published.[83] Despite its rising popularity, the definitive benefit is still unknown.

Another decompression device, the DRX9000, has received significant attention in the lay literature. It is promoted as nonsurgical spinal decompression for treating

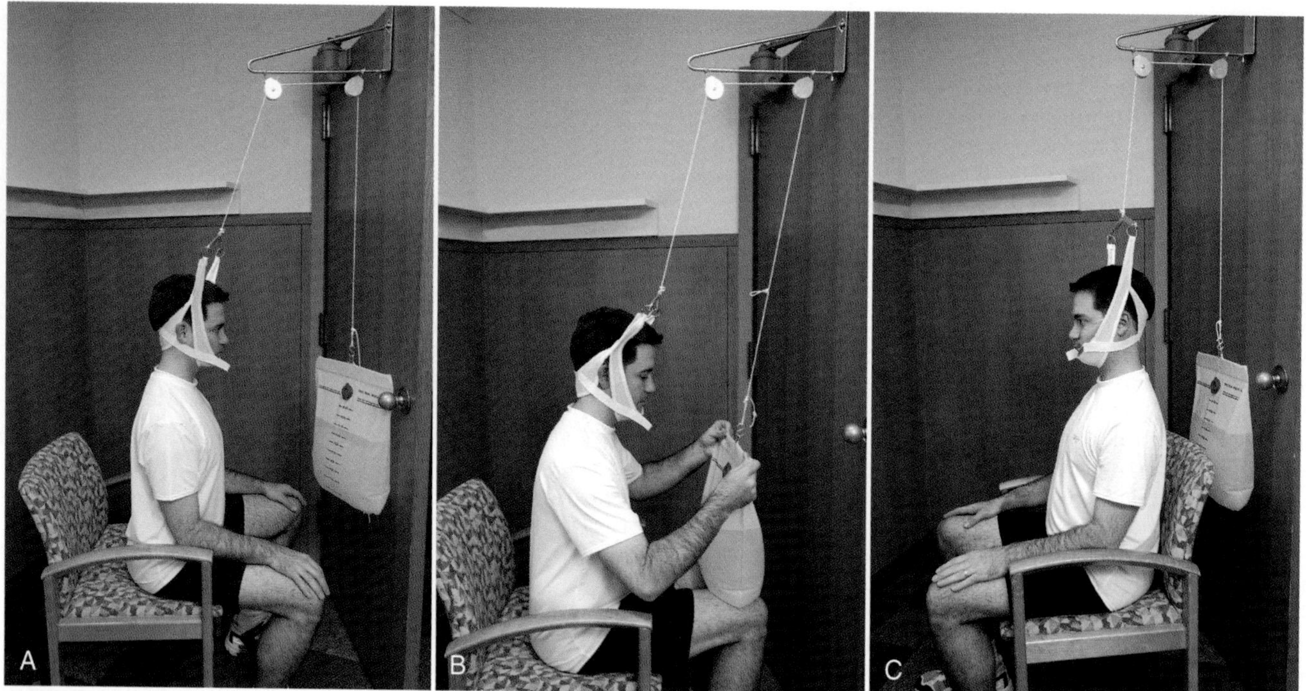

FIGURE 16-13 Home cervical traction. **A,** Cervical traction performed with an over-the-door pulley system. This type of traction is performed with the patient facing the door to allow for the cervical spine to be slightly flexed. Movement of the door should be avoided during treatment. **B,** Intermittent traction can be performed by resting the weight (water bag) on the patient's lap, producing a slack in the tension rope. The cervical posture is maintained throughout the course of traction. **C,** The patient is improperly positioned, with the back to the door. This can lead to extension and possible worsening of the cervical condition.

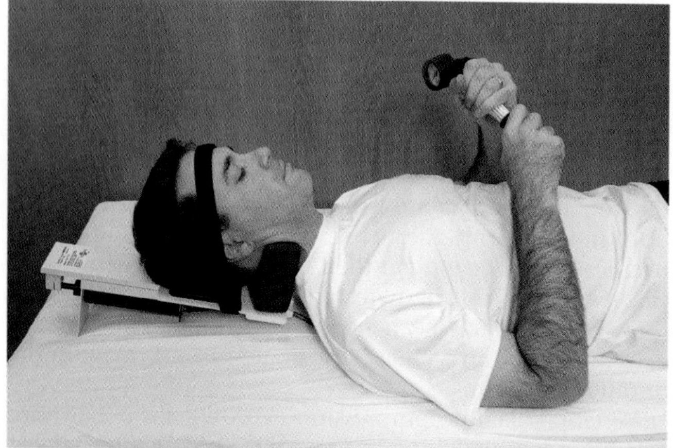

FIGURE 16-14 Alternative home traction device. The patient is placed in a supine position with gravity eliminated. The neck is positioned in slight flexion against a padded groove. The edges of the groove come in contact with the base of the skull. The amount of distraction pressure is controlled by the patient, using a hand pump.

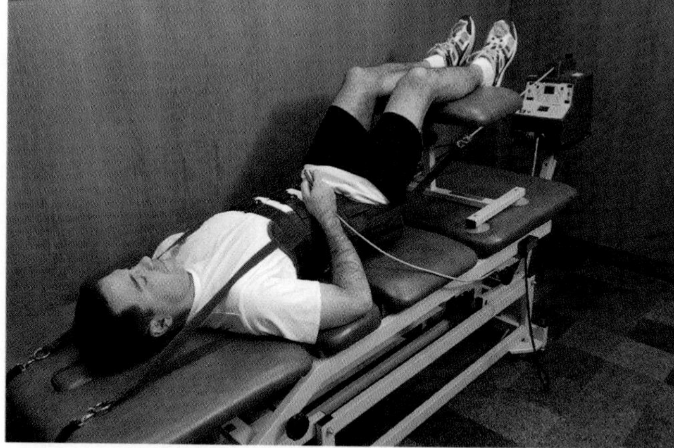

FIGURE 16-15 Motorized lumbar traction. The patient is placed in a supine position with the hips and knees flexed. The distraction force is mechanically created by pulling on a pelvic belt. The upper body is stabilized by another strap around the chest. Additional distraction force can be accomplished on a traction table that allows the upper and lower segments to separate.

lumbar pain with or without leg pain. A retrospective study by Macario et al.[111] showed that a drop in the mean numerical pain intensity rating equaled 6.05 at presentation and decreased to 0.89 at the completion of treatment. There is also a report of increased disk height after treatment.[6] There have not been any randomized, placebo-controlled trials involving the DRX9000. Its definitive efficacy is still unknown and the actual efficacy is subject to some controversy as lawsuits have been filed in three states for false claims of efficacy.[58]

Physiologic Effects

The physiologic effects of traction have been extensively evaluated and reported. Traction can stretch muscles and ligaments, tighten the posterior longitudinal ligament to exert a centripetal force on the annulus fibrosis,[79] enlarge the intervertebral space,[33] enlarge the intervertebral foramina, and separate apophyseal joints.[30-33] It naturally follows that indications for traction include conditions in which these physiologic effects would be deemed beneficial.

Indications, Goals of Treatment, and Efficacy

There is no consensus on the definitive indications for traction, but the condition having the most support for its use is cervical radiculopathy. The use of traction with lumbar radiculopathy, neck pain, and low back pain is more controversial, with contradictions existing in the literature.[79] In the absence of contraindications, traction can be used to treat any condition in which the physiologic effects of traction would theoretically be beneficial. Traction is most commonly prescribed to treat cervical radiculopathies.[140] The literature supporting this practice is scant, with two case series suggesting good resolution of symptoms.[34,119] The use of traction for axial neck pain is even less well established. Three articles extensively reviewed this topic and concluded that the efficacy of traction in treating cervical pain is unknown.[83,158]

The popularity of lumbar traction in treating low back pain, with or without radicular features, has declined over the past few decades.[43] This change came about because of the lack of efficacy and an emphasis on more active treatment programs. A case series of 49 patients with sciatica of greater than 6 weeks' duration found 79% improvement with traction, but the study was uncontrolled.[64] One study compared traction with a sham treatment,[11] whereas another compared traction plus physical therapy with physical therapy alone.[19] Both studies found no difference in outcome between the respective treatment groups. Gianakopoulos et al.[63] found improvement in 13 of 16 patients with low back pain treated with an inversion device. Side effects, however, including elevated blood pressure, headaches, and periorbital and pharyngeal petechiae, were significant. Three review articles concluded that there was not enough information to support the use of traction for lumbar spine disorders, or that there simply was no indication for its use.[95,113,158]

Contraindications

Absolute contraindications to traction include malignancy, infection, such as osteomyelitis or diskitis, osteoporosis, inflammatory arthritis, fracture, pregnancy, cord compression, uncontrolled hypertension or cardiovascular disease, and in the setting of carotid or vertebral artery disease.[79,95] Caution should also be used in the elderly, in the setting of midline disk herniations, and in the lumbar region when abdominal problems are present. Inversion traction involves more risks because increases in blood pressure and decreases in heart rate are known to occur,[63] leading to headaches and periorbital petechiae. Most practitioners are in agreement that traction should be discontinued if there is exacerbation of symptoms, discomfort from the traction device, or with production of systemic symptoms, such as dizziness.

Massage

Definition

The application of a "soothing hand" to a sick person can be considered the prototype of any therapeutic treatment.[101] *Massage* is the term used to describe certain manipulations of the soft tissue of the body. Massage has further been defined as a group of procedures, which are usually done with the hands, and include friction, kneading, rolling, and percussion of the external tissues of the body. This is done in a variety of ways, with a curative, palliative, or hygienic objective in view.[68] Massage is administered for the purpose of producing effects on the nervous and muscular systems, as well as the effects on the local and general circulation of the blood and lymph.[10]

Massage and manipulation have common historical roots. In early descriptions of these two techniques, the words are used interchangeably. More recently they have been separated into two distinct modalities, but continue to share similar terminology, philosophy, and technique.

History

Massage has waxed and waned in popularity throughout the millennia in different cultures. Even the etymology of the term massage fosters debate.[99] The postulated origins of this word include the Arabic verb *massa*, which means "to touch"; the Greek word *massein*, meaning "to knead"; or the Sanskrit term *makek*, which means "to press or condense."[68,99] All these terms were derived at different times and in different cultures, depicting the significant role that massage played in these societies. The earliest known reference to massage is in cave paintings in the Pyrenees that date back to 15,000 BC and depict the use of hands for therapeutic touch.[36] The ancient medical records depicting massage as a therapeutic intervention originate out of China, India, and Babylon.

In a Chinese text written on kung fu in 2700 BC, references are made on the use of massage for the relief of ailing muscles.[99] In 1000 BC, *Nei Ching*, also known as *The Yellow Emperor's Classic of Internal Medicine*, describes how massage of the skin and flesh and breathing exercises were used in the treatment of complete paralysis.[99,120] The *Ayur Veda* (1500-1200 BC) is considered the oldest medical text written in India, and it makes frequent reference to massage. In Babylon of Assyria, around 900 BC, massage was prescribed to expel demons and to aid in healing.[99]

The ancient Greek and Roman medical literature makes abundant references to the use of massage as a therapeutic modality. Hippocrates, who is generally considered the father of modern medicine, wrote extensively on the use of massage in his book *On Articulations*.[99] Plato (427-347 BC) and Socrates (470-399 BC) made reference to anointing with oils when performing massage. The Greek physician Asclepiades (129-40 BC), who practiced in Rome and is considered the father of physical medicine, wrote about hydrotherapy, exercise, and massage as the three most important therapeutic modalities to use in the treatment of patients.[99]

In the Middle Ages, the "Church of Rome" discouraged the use of massage as a healing practice, and it fell out of favor.[131] Massage practitioners during this time were thought to be practicing quackery by the medical profession. This dealt a crushing blow to the advancement of massage as a therapeutic modality. During the Renaissance, medical scholars resurrected massage and attempted to understand the physiology and anatomy this modality affected. The French medical community embraced "friction of the skin" and described many different techniques for providing massage. Many of the terms for these techniques, such as *effleurage, pétrissage, tapotement,* and *friction massage,* are still in use today.[99]

The roots of modern-day massage are derived from the work of Per Henking Ling (1776-1839) of Sweden.[99] He was the founder of curative gymnastics, an approach that incorporated massage and exercise. Ling used many of the previously described French techniques and nomenclature. He also used terms such as *rolling, sliding, pinching, shaking,* and *vibration* to define massage techniques. Ling was instrumental in establishing the Central Royal Institute for Gymnastics, which practiced, taught, and promoted what has become known as "Swedish" massage. Several of Ling's students immigrated to New York and established the Swedish Institute of Massage in 1916.[99]

In the past century, two physicians strongly advocated the use of massage in their orthopedic practices. James Mennell wrote the book *Physical Treatment by Movements, Manipulation, and Massage* in 1917.[99] This book greatly influenced the field of physical therapy to use massage as a therapeutic modality. James Cyriax wrote extensively on the use of manipulation and deep friction massage, which today is used for the treatment of musculoskeletal and other sports injuries.[99,129]

The popularity of massage as a therapeutic intervention has continued to fluctuate over the past several decades. In recent years, however, there has been a resurgence of interest in massage that has generated scientific inquiry into its usage as a therapeutic modality.*

Indications and Goals of Treatment

Massage has multiple effects on the body, including mechanical, reflexive, neurologic, and psychological.[23,40,163] The exact therapeutic mechanism by which massage works is not fully understood and probably represents a combination of the above. The method and application of massage correlate with the magnitude of these effects. The goals of therapeutic massage are to produce relaxation, relieve muscle tension, reduce pain, increase mobility of soft tissues, and improve circulation. These techniques can be used on patients who would benefit from mobilization of tissues and reduction of swelling and discomfort. Massage for patients with cancer has been providing these benefits and reducing the need for additional pain-relieving medications.[107,110,139,159]

Mechanical and Physiologic Effects

The mechanical effects of massage are the most apparent and are well understood. These effects are brought on by the physical forces applied to the body tissues, such as compression, shearing, or vibration. The mechanical pressure created by massage moves fluid from areas of relative stasis (low pressure) to higher pressure areas by creating a hydrostatic pressure gradient. Once fluids leave the cells or interstitial fluid, they can enter the lymphatic or vascular system. Valves within the lymphatic and venous system prevent return of the fluid to the tissue.[24,129,161]

Massage can have an immediate effect on cutaneous blood flow, with hyperemia being noticed even with superficial techniques.[65] The mechanism of action for this is not well understood, but is most likely as a result of stimulation of the mast cells and release of histamines. This local histamine release causes the triple response of Lewis, including flare, redness, and wheal formation at the site of stimulation.

Deep massage has an effect on the underlying fascia and deep connective tissues.[23,163] Injury to this deeper tissue can result in restrictions, adhesions, and scarring. These fascial constrictions can potentially cause restriction of fluid movement within the vasculature, as well as reduction in muscle activity. Deep massage can help to release these restrictions, adhesions, and microscarring.[163]

Pain, inactivity, and debilitation result in insufficient muscle to mobilize fluids.[163] This hypomobility can result in increased fluid stasis, producing a self-perpetuating feedback loop. This can result in fluid accumulation, and can also result in the accumulation of metabolic byproducts. These metabolic byproducts can create an osmotic influence on fluid shifts and result in stimulation of pain fibers. Massage increases the mobility of these metabolic byproducts and the dispersion of fluid accumulations. Once this self-perpetuating cycle of pain, stasis, and hypomobility is broken, the body can restore its normal healing mechanism.[17,72]

It has been postulated that massage results in neural reflex reactions.[14,102,103,126] It is thought that these reactions are what account for the global effects produced with massage techniques. Somatic afferent nerve fibers carry information from the somatic system to the spinal cord. Dysfunction within the somatic structure can result in increased afferent neural input. This increased input results in a change in the efferent activity at the same spinal cord level through interneurons and can result in muscle hypertonicity and contraction. This hypertonic region can localize to a specific spinal cord level and has been considered by many to be called "facilitative spinal segment." See the manipulation section for a more extensive discussion.

Types of Massage

A vast array of techniques has been used to perform a therapeutic massage. These techniques can be categorized by geographic region of origin, either classic western (European) or eastern (Asian) forms of massage. The most common western (European) techniques are those outlined by the Swedish system. These four basic massage strokes are effleurage, pétrissage, friction massage, and tapotement as originally described by the French. Several treatment schemes combine massage with other techniques, such as structural reintegration, function restoration, and movement therapies.

Western Forms of Massage

Effleurage. Effleurage involves gliding the palms, fingertips, and/or thumbs over the skin in a rhythmic circular pattern with varying degrees of pressure.[40,80,163] This stroke is performed by maintaining continuous contact with the

*References 29, 46, 48, 62, 87, 124, 131.

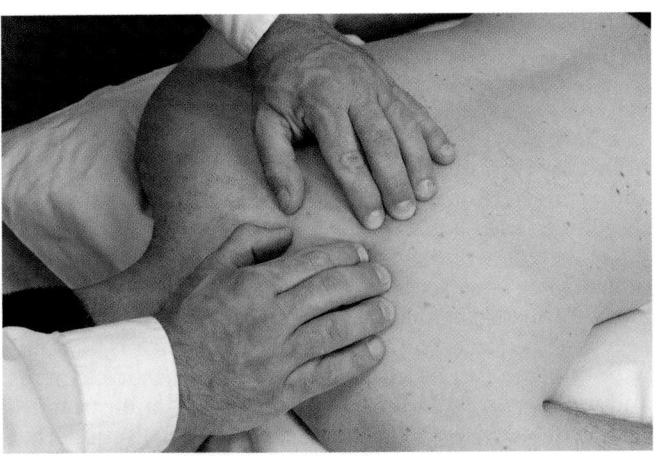

FIGURE 16-16 Effleurage massage. This type of massage being performed on the patient's posterior shoulder is a rhythmic, circular motion with the fingertips. Pressure can be varied to massage deeper structures.

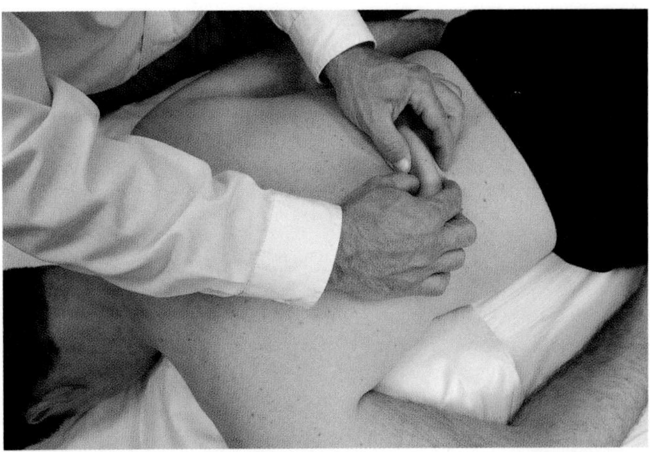

FIGURE 16-17 Pétrissage massage ("rolling"). In this form of pétrissage, the skin or muscle is gathered up between the fingers and thumb and rolled continuously; new skin and muscle are gathered.

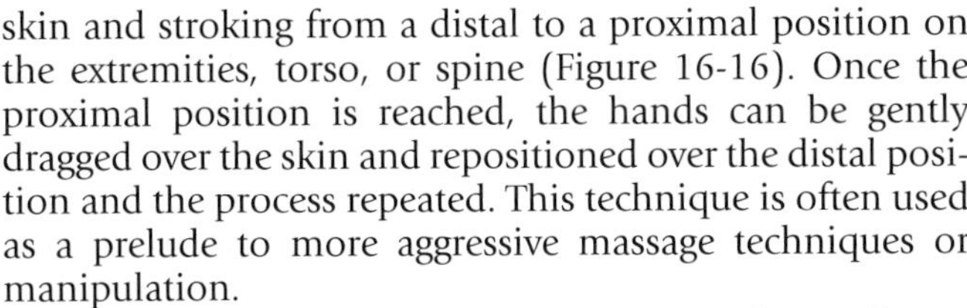

skin and stroking from a distal to a proximal position on the extremities, torso, or spine (Figure 16-16). Once the proximal position is reached, the hands can be gently dragged over the skin and repositioned over the distal position and the process repeated. This technique is often used as a prelude to more aggressive massage techniques or manipulation.

Effleurage performed superficially can result in reflexive and psychological changes. The blood flow to the area is increased, introducing relaxation when done slowly, and stimulation when done more quickly. Deeper mechanical stroking can result in mechanical effects on the circulatory and deep myofascial systems. Effleurage is used to stimulate lymphatic drainage and to relieve joint sprain–type pain, muscle strains, and bruising, as well as vascular congestion related to surgery, peripheral vascular disease, or complex regional pain syndrome.

Pétrissage. Pétrissage is also known as "kneading massage." It involves both hands compressing the skin between the thumb and fingers.[40,69,80,163] The tissue is grasped from the underlying skeletal structures, lifted, and massaged. Both hands alternate rhythmically in a rolling motion. The depth of pétrissage can determine the mechanical effect. Superficial techniques promote relaxation, whereas deeper techniques increase blood flow, mobilize fluid and tissue deposits, decrease adhesions, and increase tissue pliability.

Pétrissage is also considered compression massage, and several variations exist, including kneading or picking up, wringing, rolling, or shaking the tissue. "Kneading" involves circular movements of one hand superimposed on the other. The finger pads and thumb compress tissue and distract it from the deeper underlying structures. "Picking up" involves four basic steps: compression of the soft tissue against the underlying structures, grasping the soft tissue, and compression, release, and repositioning the hands in a more proximal position to repeat the process. "Wringing" resembles picking up, except that once tissue is grasped, one hand pushes while the other one pulls, creating a shearing-type force in the tissue planes. "Rolling" involves grabbing a small amount of tissue between the finger pads and thumb, and rolling the tissue as if moving a small object under the skin (Figure 16-17). "Shaking" is a technique in which the tissue is grabbed and vigorously shaken between the hands. The hands are then repositioned along the course of the muscle being treated.

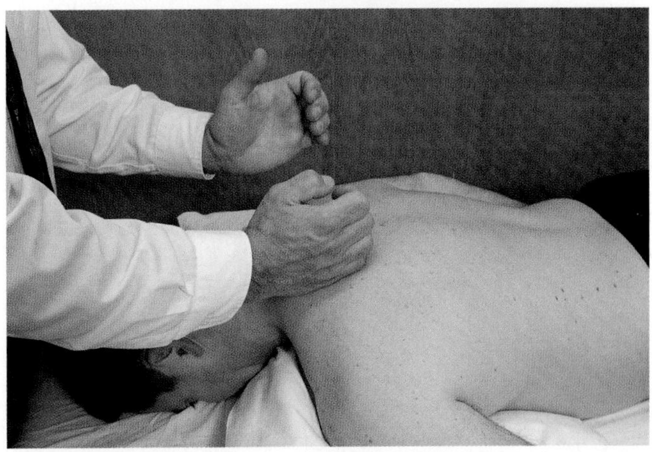

FIGURE 16-18 Tapotement massage ("hacking"). Hacking involves striking the body at right angles with the ulnar aspect of the hands.

Tapotement. Tapotement, or percussion massage, uses rhythmic alternating contact of varying pressure between the hands and the body's soft tissue.[40,80,163] Various techniques are used to produce this type of massage, including hacking, clapping, beating, pounding, and vibration. "Hacking" involves using the ulnar aspect of the hands to alternately strike the body tissues. These rapid strokes at 2 to 6 Hz are delivered in a sequential pattern along the entire region to be treated (Figure 16-18). "Cupping" involves the use of a cupped palm, which is percussed against the chest wall. This technique is frequently used to loosen secretions in disease processes, such as cystic fibrosis (Figure 16-19). "Beating" involves using a clenched fist to repetitively pummel the tissue. This is a very aggressive type of tapotement and is not frequently used. "Tapping" uses the finger pads, typically of the index and middle fingers, to percuss. The finger pads strike the underlying

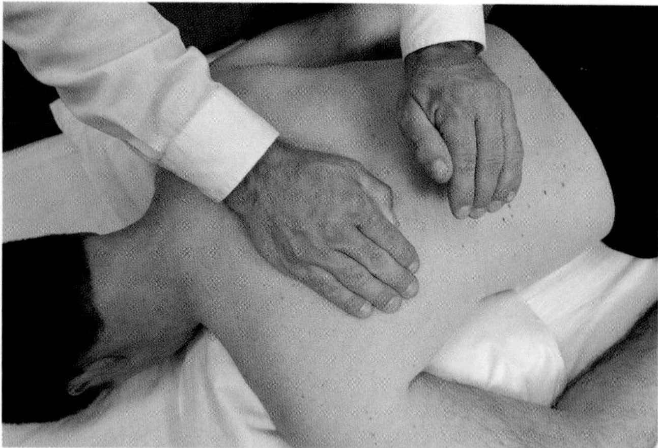

FIGURE 16-19 Tapotement massage ("cupping"). Cupping is frequently performed over the rib cage to loosen secretions in the lungs.

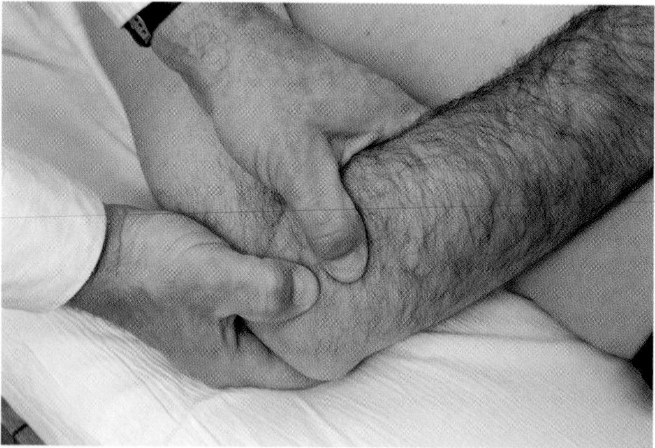

FIGURE 16-20 Friction massage being performed on the lateral epicondyle to promote tendon healing.

tissue in rapid succession. This technique is frequently used over the sinuses to loosen secretions.

Friction Massage. Friction massage is a circular, longitudinal, or transverse pressure applied by the fingers, thumb, or hypothenar region of the hand to small areas.[69,80,163] Cross-friction massage is perpendicular to the fibers and was used extensively by Cyriax.[40] Very little motion occurs at the fingertips overlying the skin. The tissues are massaged from superficial to deep by increasing the pressure applied. The goal of friction massage is to break down adhesions in scar tissue, loosen ligaments, and disable trigger points. It is often uncomfortable and can even result in some bruising. Despite this, it is an effective treatment for tendonitis or tendinopathy, subacromial bursitis, plantar fasciitis, and trigger points as described by Travell[152] (Figure 16-20).

Other Western Techniques

Other techniques that integrate massage, structure, function, and movement into a rehabilitation program include Tager psychological integration, Alexander and Feldenkrais techniques, "Rolfing," myofascial release, and manual lymphatic drainage (MLD). Although these techniques are not used as much as the common Swedish techniques, they are gaining in popularity.

Tager Psychological Integration. This treatment method was developed by Milton Tager, M.D., in the 1940s. This technique combines the use of gentle hands-on tissue work and reintegration of movement through reeducation and relaxation exercises. The technique teaches patients to move with ease and efficiency. The hands-on work consists of gently rocking, stretching, or rolling movements to relax and diminish tension. The movement component of the Tager technique is coined "mentastics," which is a combination of mental, psychological, and gymnastic elements, and focuses on making movements lighter and easier.[36]

Tager therapists use "hook-up," which involves the therapist attaining a calm and focused state of mind. They use this hook-up to connect with the patient's needs and how the patient is responding to treatment. Information is communicated from the therapist's hands to the patient's body and assists in easing movements.

Alexander Technique. F.M. Alexander (1869-1955) was a Shakespearean actor who had recurrent neck and vocal problems. After much self-reflection and postural reeducation, he noted that his vocal problems could be corrected by postural reeducation. He developed a series of techniques for the treatment of chronic neck and low back pain.[36]

His approach centers on balance between head and neck movement "primary control," and a state of dynamic postures and breathing exercises. This technique teaches patients to engage their mind to understand beneficial patterns and overcome motion patterns, which are considered automatic. It is thought that these nonbeneficial patterns can be broken through conscious training.[89,142]

Feldenkrais Pattern. Moshe Feldenkrais, D.Sc. (1880-1967), was a physicist and mechanical engineer who had a knee dysfunction and was told that he most likely would have to be a wheelchair user. Using his black belt judo techniques and physics background, he studied movement and the interrelationship between muscle contraction and motion. Through self-rehabilitation of his knee problem, he developed several techniques.[36] He began teaching his students these simple exercises that could be performed during functional tasks. The goals of these techniques are to learn efficient and pain-free motion. Feldenkrais emphasizes multiple repetitions to lay down new neuromuscular patterns, and considers the entire body, even in the simplest of movements.[89]

Rolfing Structural Integration. Ida Rolf (1896-1979), a chemist who had health problems, was inspired by such medical philosophies as osteopathy, Alexander technique, and yoga. She viewed the body as a group of units and studied their relationship to each other. Rolf saw gravity as one of the primary causes of dysfunction. The primary tenet of her structural integration system was to help clients achieve proper vertical alignment and efficient movement.[36] The typical regimen consists of a series of ten 60- to 90-minute sessions. Superficial massage is performed initially, with progression to deeper friction massage. This is in an attempt to stretch fascia and allow muscles to relax and lengthen. The sessions build on one another, and additional treatments are frequently required to accommodate for the changes promoted. The deep friction massage traditionally performed with Rolfing techniques can be painful. Newer techniques have been implemented, which are less painful and less invasive. Other techniques have been influenced by Rolfing, including Keller work and Aston patterning.

Myofascial Release. The term *myofascial release* was coined by Robert Ward, D.O., in the 1960s[157] and further developed by John Barnes, P.T.[8] This technique is founded on the premise that the body is encased in connective tissue (i.e., fascia). Fascia is the ground substance that interconnects all bones, muscles, nerves, and other internal organs and tissues. Injury or tension within one area of the fascia can result in pain and tenderness. Because of the interconnections, injury in one area of the fascia can result in pain and dysfunction at a distant point. Practitioners of myofascial release use gentle stretching and massage to release the fascial tension, and can often work on areas that seem unrelated to the primary pain or injury. Myofascial release is frequently used to treat chronic pain and restore normal range of motion.

Manual Lymphatic Drainage. MLD was developed in Europe in the 1930s by Danish physiotherapists Estrid and Emil Vodder as a technique to control postmastectomy lymphedema. MLD is a gentle and superficially focused massage in which lymph is moved from areas of lymphatic vessel damage to watershed regions.[18] The first part of the treatment involves massage of the proximal region of the extremity to be treated. This is thought to dilate the watershed lymph vessels and allows them to accept fluid from distal areas. After proximal areas have been gently massaged, a more rhythmic massage is performed from a distal to a proximal part of the extremity. The typical session lasts 45 to 60 minutes. Complex lymphedema therapy includes MLD combined with other modalities, such as sequential pumping, low-tension wraps, skin care, compressive garments, and exercise.[105] Long-term maintenance is required for sustained edema control. It has been demonstrated that the limb volume can be reduced by as much as 25% to 63% after this treatment.[18,90] MLD is quickly becoming popular in the United States, and many therapists have become trained in these techniques.

Eastern Forms of Massage

Acupressure. Acupressure has been defined as digital pressure performed in a circular motion to treat areas that are typically treated with acupuncture needles and for the same reason.[148] Acupuncture was developed more than 3000 years ago in China. The basic philosophy behind this technique is to restore energy flow or *qi*. *Qi* has two basic components that flow along 12 meridians: *yin* is associated with passivity, rest, and cold, whereas *yang* is associated with activity, stimulation, and heat. A balance of these forces is thought to be associated with health, and an imbalance with disease.

The goal of treatment is to restore energy balance or homeostasis. Acupressure is performed with the patient lying on a table. Deep pressure is applied to the acupuncture points in a circular manner without the use of lubrication. Acupressure can be used for the treatment of nausea and vomiting associated with chemotherapy, to decrease postoperative pain, for the treatment of headaches, and to decrease temporomandibular joint pain. Acupressure is a technique that can easily be converted to a self-performed treatment modality.

Shiatsu. *Shi* (meaning finger) *atsu* (meaning pressure) is the Japanese type of body work based on acupuncture.[148] This technique was initially practiced by visually impaired clinicians. Pressure is applied in particular meridians similar to acupuncture. This type of treatment has been westernized and is being increasingly used in the United States.

Reflexology. Ancient medical practitioners hypothesized that there is a homuncular representation of the body on the sole of the feet.[148] This philosophy probably dates back to ancient Egypt, but the Chinese medical literature demonstrated a homunculus of the body on the ears, feet, and hands. Palpations of specific areas on the feet were thought to be tender if their corresponding body part was dysfunctional. Reflexology is the application of deep circular pressure applied to specific dysfunctional points on the soles of the feet. This is considered a separate discipline in the United States, but is used by some Swedish massage practitioners to treat areas of extreme tenderness. It has been used to treat hypertension, stress, fatigue, and digestive complaints.

Evidence-Based Use of Massage

Massage has been used in multiple forms for the treatment of many conditions. Traditional research is difficult to perform on these techniques because of the lack of a standardized sham treatment. Although there is a paucity of quality research on these techniques, there has been a renewed interest in establishing the efficacy of massage.

At least one large randomized controlled trial supports the use of massage in the treatment of anxiety and stress*; arthralgias and various arthritides[51,52,128]; fibromyalgia[20]; lymphedema[21]; musculoskeletal disorders, such as whiplash, low back pain,[62] and sports-related injuries[26,88,98,132]; and sleep disorders.[135,136]

There are recommendations suggesting that massage therapy might be useful as an adjunct treatment or possible alternative treatment for the following conditions (research data for these are less compelling than a randomized controlled trial): burn care,[54,55,78] care of people with cancer,[13,21,50,107,159] chronic pain,[41,61,97] exercise-induced injury,† headaches,[132] and human immunodeficiency virus infection and acquired immunodeficiency syndrome.[15,141] Although massage therapy is obviously not curative in these conditions, it might enhance the effectiveness of other therapeutic interventions.

---

*References 29, 50, 53, 56, 57, 123.

†References 22, 77, 82, 137, 145, 147, 150.

Contraindications to Massage

Massage therapy is a relatively safe modality. Complications are rare and usually not serious. There are several absolute and relative contraindications to traditional Swedish massage. Potential complications for shiatsu, reflexology, and acupuncture have not been specifically delineated. Massage should not be performed over areas of malignancy, cellulitis, or lymphangitis.[101] The effect of massage on these regions can cause mobilization of tumor cells into the vascular lymphatic supply or the spread of infection.

Areas of trauma or recent bleeding should not be treated with deep tissue massage. Mobilization of these areas can increase the propensity for rebleeding. Patients who are taking anticoagulants should be treated with gentler techniques and observed for bruising and ecchymoses. Deep tissue work should be used with extreme caution in those receiving anticoagulants or who have a bleeding diathesis.

Massage should not be used over areas of known deep venous thrombosis or atherosclerotic plaques. This could result in dislodgment of these vascular thrombi, resulting in embolic infarcts affecting the pulmonary, cerebral, or peripheral systems. Special care should be observed in patients with osteoarthritis or severe osteoporosis to avoid any excess range of motion or stretching that could alter articulating surfaces. Patients with low blood pressure might experience postural hypotension after treatment and should be observed carefully. Patients who have been physically or sexually abused can reexperience elements of trauma during treatment. Special care regarding touch is especially warranted with these individuals. People with edema should not undergo deep tissue massage or any other massage technique that could result in local accumulation of interstitial fluid.

Conclusion

Manipulation, traction, and massage have been an integral part of health care since ancient times. The popularity of these techniques ebbs and flows with changes in the traditional medical paradigm of the time. They have enjoyed a resurgence in popularity in recent years. Research efforts, although in their infancy, have shown that a spectrum of beneficial physiologic and clinical changes can be associated with these modalities. Manipulation, traction, and massage are becoming increasingly recognized as a valuable adjunct to standard medical care. Many medical centers now have dedicated departments to the practice, education, and research of these modalities.

KEY REFERENCES

5. Abenhaim L, Bergeron AM: Twenty years of randomized clinical trials of manipulative therapy for back pain: a review, *Clin Invest Med* 15(6):527–535, 1992.
9. Beal MC, Vorro J, Johnston WL: Chronic cervical dysfunction: correlation of myoelectric findings with clinical progress, *J Am Osteopath Assoc* 89(7):891–900, 1989.
10. Beard G: *Massage: principles and techniques*, Philadelphia, 1964, WB Saunders.
11. Beurskens AJ, de Vet HC, Koke AJ, et al: Efficacy of traction for nonspecific low back pain: 12-week and 6-month results of a randomized clinical trial, *Spine* 22(23):2756–2762, 1997.
12. Bigos S, Bowyer O, Braen G: *Acute low back problems in adults*, Rockville, 1994, Agency for Health Care Policy and Research, U.S. Department of Health and Human Services.
18. Boris M, Weindorf S, Lasinkski S: Persistence of lymphedema reduction after noninvasive complex lymphedema therapy, *Oncology* 11(1):99–109, discussion 110, 113–114, 1997.
19. Borman P, Keskin D, Bodur H: The efficacy of lumbar traction in the management of patients with low back pain, *Rheumatol Int* 23(2):82–86, 2003.
23. Cantu RL, Grodin AJ: *Myofascial manipulation: theory and clinical application*, New York, 1992, Aspen.
27. Cherkin DC, MacCornack FA: Patient evaluations of low back pain care from family physicians and chiropractors, *West J Med* 150(3):351–355, 1989.
31. Colachis SC, Jr, Strohm BR: Effect of duration of intermittent cervical traction on vertebral separation, *Arch Phys Med Rehabil* 47(6):353–359, 1966.
33. Colachis SC, Jr, Strohm BR: A study of tractive forces and angle of pull on vertebral interspaces in the cervical spine, *Arch Phys Med Rehabil* 46(12):820–830, 1965.
39. Cyriax J: Conservative treatment of lumbar disc lesions, *Physiotherapy* 50:300–303, 1964.
40. Cyriax J, Russell G: *Textbook of orthopaedic medicine, vol 2, treatment by manipulation, massage, and injection*, London, 1980, Bailliere Tindall.
41. Day JA, Mason RR, Chesrown SE: Effect of massage on serum level of beta-endorphin and beta-lipotropin in healthy adults, *Phys Ther* 67(6):926–930, 1987.
42. DeStefano L: *Greenman's principles of manual medicine*, ed 4, Philadelphia, 2011, Lippincott Williams & Wilkins.
43. Deyo RA, Tsui-Wu YJ: Descriptive epidemiology of low-back pain and its related medical care in the United States, *Spine* 12(3):264–268, 1987.
44. DiGiovanna EL, Schiowitz S, Downing DJ: *Osteopathic approach to diagnosis and treatment*, Philadelphia, 1997, Lippincott-Raven.
45. Dvorak J, Dvorak V: *Manual medicine: diagnostics*, Stuttgart, 1990, Thieme.
49. Fernandez-Carnero J, Fernandez-de-las-Penas C, Cleland JA: Immediate hypoalgesic and motor effects after a single cervical spine manipulation in subjects with lateral epicondylalgia, *J Manipulative Physiol Ther* 31(9):675–681, 2008.
59. Fryette HH: *Principles of osteopathic technique*, Kirksville, 1980, merican Academy of Osteopathy.
60. Frymoyer JW: Back pain and sciatica, *N Engl J Med* 318(5):291–300, 1988.
62. Furlan AD, Imamura M, Dryden T, Irvin E: Massage for low back pain: an updated systematic review within the framework of the Cochrane Back Review Group, *Spine* 34(16):1669–1684, 2009.
63. Gianakopoulos G, Waylonis GW, Grant PA, et al: Inversion devices: their role in producing lumbar distraction, *Arch Phys Med Rehabil* 66(2):100–102, 1985.
65. Goats GC: Massage: the scientific basis of an ancient art. Part 1. The techniques, *Br J Sports Med* 28(3):149–152, 1994.
68. Graham D: *Practical treatise on massage*, New York, 1884, William Wood.
69. Greenman P: *Principles of manual medicine*, Baltimore, 2003, Williams & Wilkins.
70. Greenman PE: Models and mechanisms of osteopathic manipulative medicine, *Osteopath Med News* 4:1–20, 1987.
75. Haldeman S, Kohlbeck FJ, McGregor M: Risk factors and precipitating neck movements causing vertebrobasilar artery dissection after cervical trauma and spinal manipulation, *Spine* 24(8):785–794, 1999.
76. Harris JD: History and development of manipulation and mobilization. In Basmajian JV, editor: *Manipulation, traction and massage*, Baltimore, 1985, Williams & Wilkins.
79. Hinterbuchner C: Traction. In Basmajian JV, editor: *Manipulation, traction and massage*, Baltimore, 1985, Williams & Wilkins.
84. Hoy D, Bain C, Williams G, et al: A systematic review of the global prevalence of low back pain, *Arthritis Rheum* 64(6):2028–2037, 2012.
86. Hurwitz EL, Aker PD, Adams AH, et al: Manipulation and mobilization of the cervical spine. A systematic review of the literature, *Spine* 21(15):1746–1759, discussion 1759–1760, 1996.

92. Jones LH: *Strain and counterstrain*, Newark, 1992, American Academy of Osteopathy.
94. Judovich B, Nobel GR: Traction therapy, a study of resistance forces: preliminary report on a new method of lumbar traction, *Am J Surg* 93(1):108–114, 1957.
95. Judovich BD: Herniated cervical disc: a new form of traction therapy, *Am J Surg* 84(6):646–656, 1952.
96. Judovich BD: Lumbar traction therapy: elimination of physical factors that prevent lumbar stretch, *J Am Med Assoc* 159(6):549–550, 1955.
99. Kanemetz HL: History of massage. In Basmajian JV, editor: *Manipulation, traction and massage*, Baltimore, 1985, Williams & Wilkins.
100. Kimberly PE: Formulating a prescription for osteopathic manipulative treatment, *J Am Osteopath Assoc* 79(8):506–513, 1980.
102. Korr IM: Proprioceptors and somatic dysfunction, *J Am Osteopath Assoc* 74(7):638–650, 1975.
103. Korr IM: Somatic dysfunction, osteopathic manipulative treatment, and the nervous system: a few facts, some theories, many questions, *J Am Osteopath Assoc* 86(2):109–114, 1986.
108. Licciardone JC, Buchanan S, Hensel KL, et al: Osteopathic manipulative treatment of back pain and related symptoms during pregnancy: a randomized controlled trial, *Am J Obstet Gynecol* 202(1): 43.e1–8, 2010.
109. Licciardone JC, Minotti DE, Gatchel RJ, et al: Osteopathic manual treatment and ultrasound therapy for chronic low back pain: a randomized controlled trial, *Ann Fam Med* 11(2):122–129, 2013.
116. Mitchell FL: *The muscle energy manual* (vols 1–4). East Lansing, 1995, MET Press.
117. Mitchell FL: *Structural pelvic function*, Indianapolis, 1958, American Academy of Osteopathy.
121. Nachemson AL: Advances in low-back pain, *Clin Orthop Relat Res* 200:266–278, 1985.
127. Pennick V, Liddle SD: Interventions for preventing and treating pelvic and back pain in pregnancy, *Cochrane Database Syst Rev* (8):CD001139, 2013.
152. Travell J: *Myofascial pain and dysfunction: the trigger point manual*, Baltimore, 1983, Williams & Wilkins.
153. Van Buskirk R: *The still technique manual*, Indianapolis, 2006, American Academy of Osteopathy.
163. Wood EC: *Beard's massage: principles and techniques*, Philadelphia, 1974, Saunders.

The full reference list for this chapter is available online.

CHAPTER 17

PHYSICAL AGENT MODALITIES

Wen-Shiang Chen, Thiru M. Annaswamy, Weibin Yang, Tyng-Guey Wang

The use of physical agent modalities dates back to the early days in the development of the field of physical and rehabilitation medicine. The term *physiatrist* is derived from the Greek words *physis*, pertaining to physical phenomena, and *iatreia*, referring to healer or physician. Thus, a physiatrist is a physician who uses physical agents to relieve a patient's discomfort. Modalities are physical agents used to produce desired therapeutic effect. They include cold, heat, sound, electromagnetic waves, electricity, and mechanical forces. In this chapter, their physiologic effects, indications, techniques, and precautions are reviewed and discussed. Acupuncture and moxibustion, which use needling and heat to produce therapeutic effect, are also included. Physical agent modalities, although generally considered adjunctive rather than curative treatments, are widely used and important in the daily practices of most physiatrists.

Cryotherapy

Physiology

Cryotherapy refers to treatment by the lowering of local tissue temperature. The major physiologic effects of cryotherapy include changing local sensation, muscle relaxation, and vasoconstriction, which are possibly followed by vasodilation.[141] Cold decreases the excitability of free nerve endings of peripheral nerve fibers, thus decreasing the nerve conduction velocity of pain fibers and causing local analgesic effect.[63] When local temperature is decreased, patients usually report an uncomfortable sensation of cold followed by stinging or burning, then an aching sensation, and finally complete numbness, around 15 minutes after cold is applied.[110] When cold is applied directly to the skin, the skin vessels constrict progressively to a temperature of approximately 50° F (10° C), at which point the vessels reach their maximum constriction. At a temperature bel 50° F (10° C), usually after cold is applied for 15 minutes, the vessel begins to dilate. The vasodilation of applying cold may be from a spinal cord reflex to preserve local temperature or partially from the changing sensitivity of vessel to local nerve stimulation. The cold itself may also paralyze the vessel wall muscle through blockage of nerve impulse to the vessels and cause local dilation of vessels.[44] As the temperature approaches 32° F (0° C), the skin vessels reach maximum vasodilation.[76] Local application of cold decreases local neuronal activity, including small fibers located in the muscle spindle and Golgi tendon organ. By decreasing the rate of afferent muscle fiber activity of muscle fiber, cold reduces muscle spasm.[115]

Indications and Evidence Basis

Cryotherapy is commonly used in acute soft tissue injury,[25,90,110] especially in sports-related injury. It is also applied to control pain and edema after surgical procedures,[103,184] and to decrease acute inflammation of local tissues.[121] Cold is used in acute soft tissue injury on the basis of the rationale that cold causes local vasoconstriction[141] and reduces local edema and hemorrhage. Furthermore, lowering the local temperature reduces the metabolic rate with a corresponding decrease in the production of metabolites and metabolic heat of the injured tissues. This helps the injured tissue survive the relative hypoxia and limits further tissue damage.[26] Cold is also used in the acute phase of inflammation in conditions such as tenosynovitis, bursitis, acute exacerbation of osteoarthritis, and rheumatoid arthritis.[162] Cryotherapy is often used in reducing postsurgical pain and edema, such as after anterior cruciate ligament repair or reconstruction.[134,184] Research shows that cryotherapy not only reduces pain and swelling after surgery but also helps with muscle power recovery.[103]

Cryotherapy is sometimes used in chronic pain, mostly because of its effect on reducing muscle spasm. It has been demonstrated that cryotherapy is effective in the treatment of myofascial pain syndrome (MPS), especially combined with stretching exercise.[177] MPS is often characterized by active trigger points with referred pain and is associated with sensitized local nerve endings. A trigger point may be palpated as a small nodule or a strip of tense muscle tissue.[14] Cold can block the sensitized nerve endings, reduce local pain, and decrease muscle spasm.

Contraindications and Precautions

Cryotherapy is contraindicated in patients with hypersensitivity to cold, impaired local circulation, local skin infection, and impaired sensitivity. Table 17-1 lists some of the common indications and contraindications for cryotherapy.

Types of Devices and Techniques

Types of cryotherapy include ice pack, ice massage, cold whirlpool, chemical cold spray, and contrast baths. The most commonly applied methods are ice pack and chemical cool spray. Depth of cold penetration depends on the intensity and duration of cold application. The temperature reduction by cryotherapy generally occurs in the superficial layer, subcutaneous and superficially located muscles, and the therapeutic effect of cryotherapy decreases with increasing tissue depth.[43] Because at least 15 minutes is necessary to achieve analgesia effect by cryotherapy, 20 minutes is the usually recommended treatment duration. The temperature of cryotherapy for limited local tissue treatment is generally set between 32° F and 50° F (0° C to 10° C). For a larger area, cryotherapy such as cold whirlpool, 50° F to 60° F (10° C to 15° C) is commonly used. For whole body cryotherapy, 65° F to 80° F (18° C to 27° C) is recommended. Routine local cold application typically does not result in too much body heat depletion, but in patients with impaired circulation cold application must be used cautiously.

Table 17-1 Indications and Contraindications for Cryotherapy

Indications	Contraindications
Acute injury including acute swelling (controlling hemorrhage and edema)	Impaired circulation (i.e., Raynaud phenomenon)
	Peripheral vascular disease
Acute contusion	Hypersensitivity to cold
Acute muscle strain	Skin anesthesia
Acute ligament sprain	Open wounds or skin conditions (cold whirlpools and contrast baths)
Bursitis	Local infection
Tenosynovitis	
Tendinitis	
Muscle spasm	
Muscle guarding	
Chronic pain	
Myofascial trigger points	

Ice massage, which can be applied by either the therapist or the patient, can cool soft tissue more rapidly than an ice pack.[186] Ice massage can be initiated fairly easily with the use of paper cups. A cup is filled with water, and a wooden tongue depressor is placed in the cup, which is then placed in a freezer. Once frozen, the paper cup is torn off. An ice bar on a stick is now ready to be used for ice massage (Figure 17-1). Before it is used, the rough edges of the ice cup can be smoothed by gently rubbing along the edges. There are also other ways to make ice bars for ice massage.

Applying ice massage can be in a circular or a longitudinal motion, with each succeeding stroke covering half the previous stroke (Video 17-1). When ice massage is done, comfort of the patient should be considered at all times. In general, ice massage can be applied for 15 to 20 minutes. However, when the ice massage is done, the local tissues of the patient should be monitored at all times. Once the skin is numb to light touch, ice massage can be terminated. With this technique followed in patients with intact circulation, frostbite can be avoided.

Ice packs are commercially available cold packs that are filled with a chemical substance such as petroleum distillate gel (Figure 17-2, *A*; Video 17-2). It must be cooled to 60° F (15° C) in the refrigerator before use. When used, it should be covered with a towel to slow down the loss of coldness. Ice packs are commonly used in acute or subacute injury. The patient should not lie on top of the cold pack. Checking the sensation of the applied area after application is important. Treatment time required for onset of numbness is usually around 20 minutes. The other simple way to apply ice packs is to put crushed or cubed ice into a plastic bag (Figure 17-2). The bag is then covered with a towel and placed on the area to be treated. Sometimes, moist towels are used to facilitate cold transmission and reach the target temperature. An elastic bandage is sometimes used to hold the plastic ice pack in

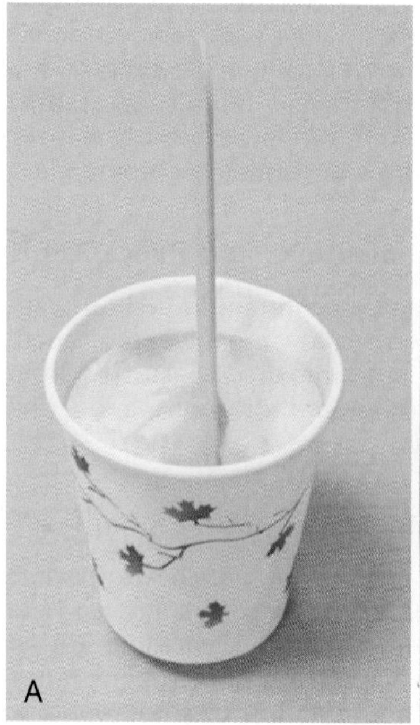

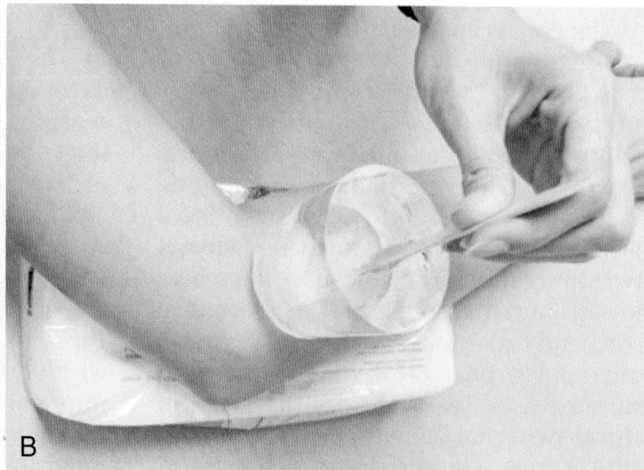

FIGURE 17-1 Making an ice bar for ice massage by **(A)** freezing water in a paper cup with a tongue depressor, and **(B)** then stroking the tissue with the ice bar either in a circular or longitudinal pattern.

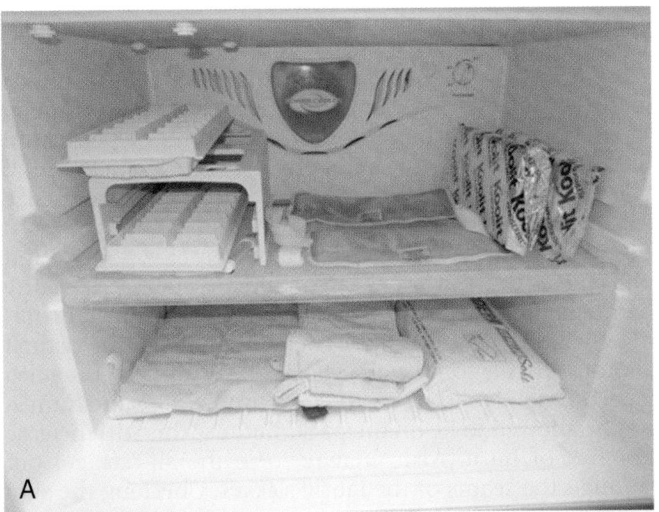

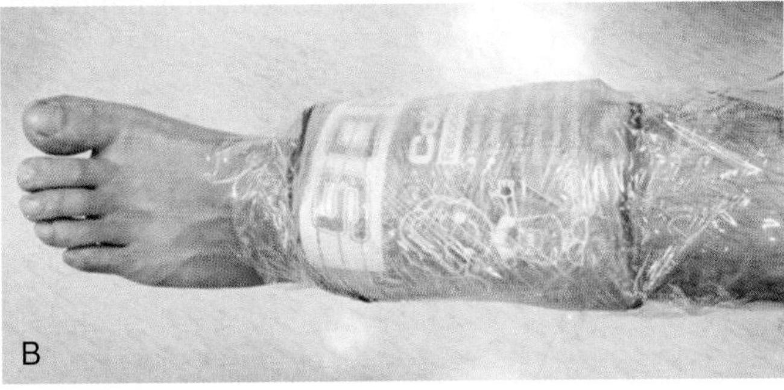

FIGURE 17-2 Commercial cold pack. **A,** Different cold packs stored in a refrigeration unit. **B,** Cold pack molded to the injured part.

place and to apply compression, which is reported to produce a significantly greater decrease in intramuscular temperature.[117,163] With chemical ice packs, the temperature decreases with time. In a plastic bag containing ice cubes or crushed ice, melting ice gives off more energy and therefore can get colder initially. The therapist may add salt to the ice to facilitate melting of the ice to create a colder slush mixture. Once again, checking the condition of the local tissue at all times when applying an ice pack or icing is important to prevent frostbite.

Of late, cold spray, such as Fluori-Methane, has been used less commonly because it does not provide adequate deep penetration of cold. The primary action of cold spray is to stimulate Aβ fiber to reduce painful arc as well as muscle spasm. It can be used in the field to reduce the pain and muscle spasm in acute sports injury. Cold spray is also commonly used to treat MPS. It is used in the technique of "spray and stretch" to relieve the muscle spasm.[177] When doing the spray, the therapist holds the spray bottle (upside down) 12 to 18 inches (30 to 45 cm) away from the treatment surface, allowing the jet stream of coolant to meet the skin at an acute angle (Figure 17-3; Video 17-3). If spraying occurs near the face, the patients' eyes, nose, and mouth should be covered. Apply the spray in one direction at a rate of 4 in/sec (10 cm/sec). Three or four sweeps of the spray in one direction are sufficient. It is possible that too many sweeps of the spray can freeze the skin and cause frostbite.

Contrast baths, a therapy technique with alternately applied hot and cold packs, are used to treat subacute swelling through vasodilation-vasoconstriction response. Two containers, one container holding cold water at 50° F to 60° F (10° C to 15° C) and the other holding hot water at 104° F to 108° F (40° C to 42° C), are needed. Hot and cold water immersions are alternated. Treatment time should be at least 20 minutes. Treatment consists of five 1-minute cold immersions and five 3-minute warm immersions. Alternate vasoconstriction and vasodilation occurs and reduces local edema.[110]

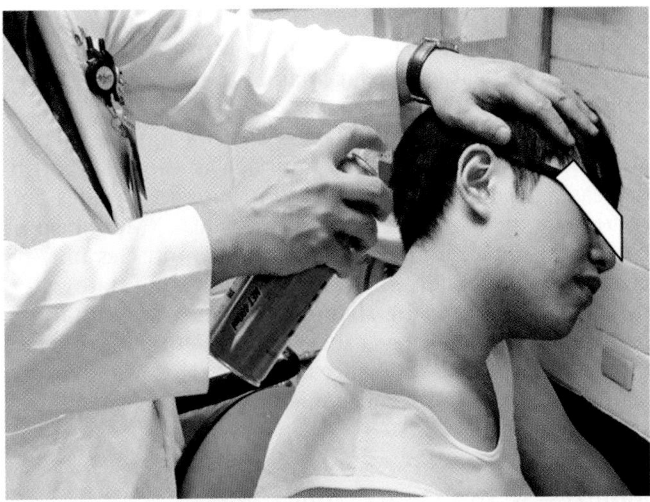

FIGURE 17-3 Spray-and-stretch technique with Fluori-Methane.

Superficial Heat

Physiology

Thermotherapy is used to increase tissue temperature. Thermotherapy can be divided into superficial and deep heat (diathermy). Superficial heat is named as such because penetration of heat is superficial and usually less than 1 cm deep, whereas diathermy can reach as deep as 3 to 5 cm without heating superficial tissues.[57,80] As a result of poor penetration, superficial heat generally only affects cutaneous blood flow and cutaneous nerve receptors. When superficial heat is applied, absorption of energy in the subcutaneous tissues causes its temperature to rise and cutaneous blood flow to increase, whereas subcutaneous blood flow in both muscles and fat layers decreases initially.[57] If energy is absorbed cutaneously over a long enough period to increase blood flow, the hypothalamus will reflexively increase blood flow to the underlying tissues such as subcutaneous fat and muscles as well.[1]

In addition to increasing local blood flow by applying heat, the higher cutaneous temperature also has an analgesic effect.[135] Three types of sensory receptors are found in the superficial tissues: cold, warm, and pain. Temperature and pain signals are transmitted to the brain via the lateral spinothalamic tract. These nerve fiber responses change with changing temperature.[2] The gate control theory suggests that more temperature signals would reduce the pain signals. Both cold and warm receptors discharge minimally at 91° F (33° C), and discharge maximally between 99° F and 104° F (37° C to 40° C). At a temperature greater than 113° F (45° C), the pain receptors are stimulated again. This explains how proper application of superficial heat will reduce pain, but high temperatures would induce pain.

Heat has the effect of relaxing skeletal muscle.[57] Local application of heat relaxes muscle by simultaneously decreasing the stimulus threshold of muscle spindles and decreasing the gamma efferent firing rate.[129a] Muscle spindles are easily excitable.[172] Consequently, muscles may be electromyographically silent while in a resting state when heat is applied, but the slightest amount of voluntary or passive movement may cause the efferent to fire, thus increasing muscular resistance to stretch. This negative biofeedback explains the mechanism by which heat relaxes skeletal muscle.

Indications and Contraindications

Superficial heat is used in subacute conditions for reducing pain, inflammation, facilitation of tissue healing, and muscle relaxation. The primary effect of superficial heat includes increased local blood flow and local circulation,[57] produces analgesia,[135] increases muscle relaxation, and reduces inflammation[153] through removal of metabolites and other products. They are often used in muscle spasm, chronic tenosynovitis, osteoarthritis, and chronic inflammation and pain (Table 17-2).

Types of Devices and Techniques

The superficial heating devices include heating pad, hydrocollator packs, paraffin bath, hot whirlpool, and infrared.[28] The most common used superficial heat at home is hot tower, hot water bath, and electrical heating pad. The temperature from these devices is unreliable and decreases rapidly.

Hydrocollator Pack

The most commonly used superficial heat in institutions is the commercial hydrocollator pack (Figure 17-4; Video 17-4). The pack comprises canvas pouches of petroleum distillate. A thermostat maintains the high temperature of 170° F (76° C) and helps prevent burns. The regular size for the low back or middle back is 24 × 24 inches (61 × 61 cm) and the cervical is 6 × 18 inches (15 × 45 cm) and is removed by tongs or scissor handles before use. The hydrocollator packs are immersed in the thermostat completely. When hydrocollator packs are applied, the patient should be in a comfortable position. Treatment duration is recommended to be 15 to 20 minutes. The patient must not be allowed to lie on the packs because this will increase the risk of burn. Also, it may force the silicate gel out through the seams of the fabric sleeves. Checking the skin condition frequently to prevent a local burn is important, especially in the older patient.

Table 17-2 Indications and Contraindications for Thermotherapy

Indications	Contraindications
Subacute and chronic inflammatory conditions	Acute musculoskeletal conditions
Subacute or chronic pain	Impaired circulation
Subacute muscle strain	Peripheral vascular disease
Subacute contusion	Skin anesthesia
Subacute ligament sprain	Open wounds
Muscle guarding	Infection
Muscle spasm	
Decreased range of motion of joint	
Myofascial trigger points	

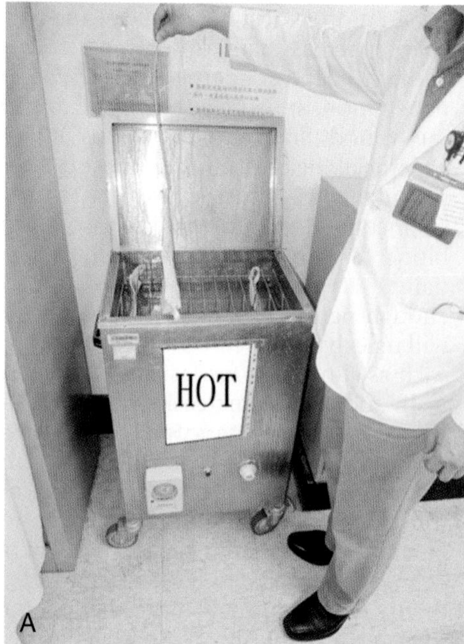

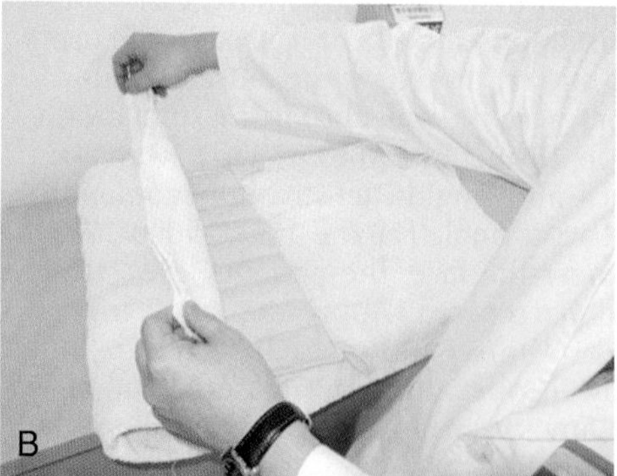

FIGURE 17-4 Commercial hot pack. **A,** Hydrocollator packs stored in a tank. **B,** Technique of wrapping hydrocollator packs; six layers of toweling should be provided to prevent the patient from burns.

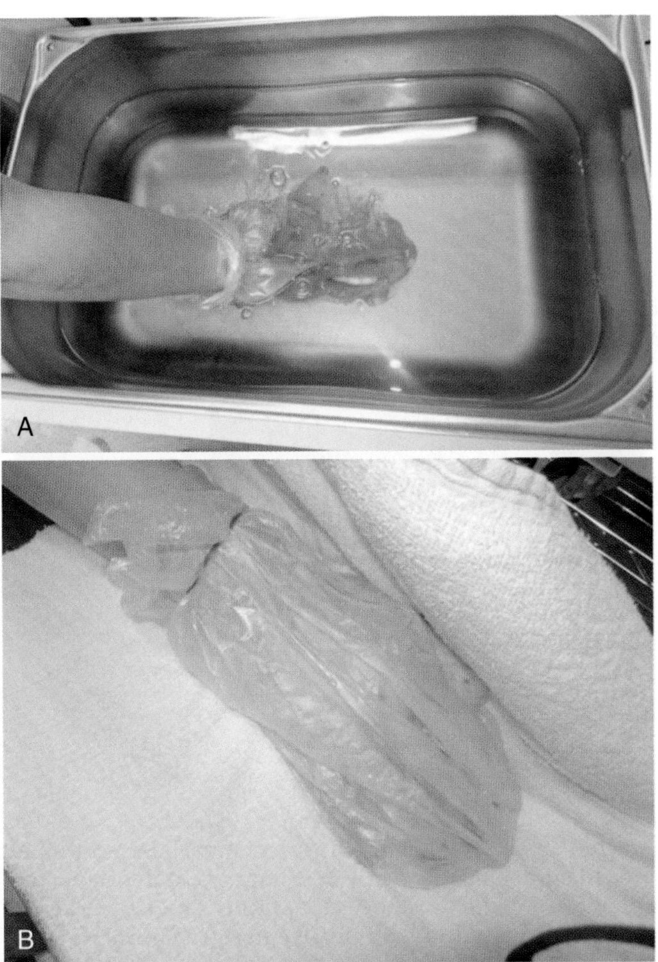

FIGURE 17-5 Paraffin bath. **A,** Hand being dipped in paraffin bath. **B,** After being dipped in paraffin, the hand should be wrapped in plastic bags and toweling.

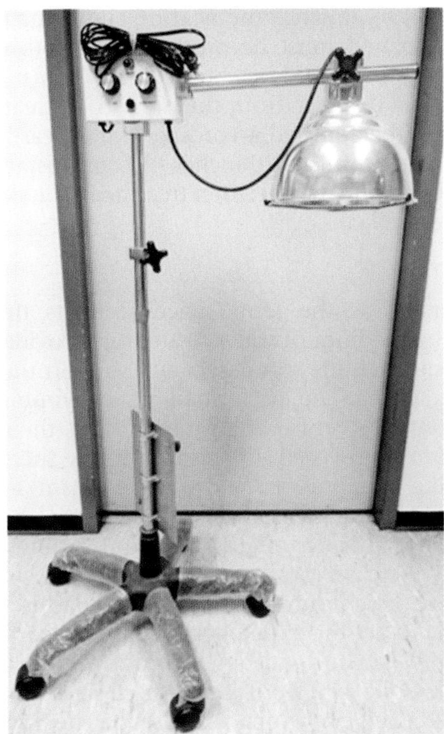

FIGURE 17-6 Infrared heating lamp.

Paraffin Bath

A paraffin bath (Figure 17-5) is a simple and efficient method to apply superficial heat, especially to the small joints of the body such as the interphalangeal joints. It is most commonly used in rheumatoid arthritis[153] and osteoarthritis (Video 17-5).[135] Paraffin treatments provide six times the amount of heat available in water because the mineral oil in the paraffin lowers the melting point of paraffin.[110,153] The combination of paraffin and mineral oil has a low specific heat, which enhances the patient's ability to tolerate heat from paraffin better than from water of the same temperature. The mixture ratio of paraffin to mineral oil is 1 gal of mineral oil to 2 lb of paraffin. The mineral oil reduces the ambient temperature of the paraffin, which is set at 126° F (52° C). The paraffin is stored in the thermostat. Some thermostats can elevate the temperature to 212° F (100° C), thus killing any bacteria that may grow in the paraffin. If the paraffin becomes soiled, it should be dumped and replaced at no longer than 6-month intervals. The treated extremity should be dipped in the paraffin for a couple of seconds and then removed to allow the paraffin to harden slightly for a few seconds. The procedure is repeated until six layers have accumulated on the part to be treated. It is important to build six layers of paraffin, in which the first layer is the highest on the body segment and each successive layer lower than the previous one. This is important because when dipping the extremity in paraffin, if the second layer is allowed to get between the skin and the first layer of the paraffin, the heat will not dissipate and the patient could be burned. The therapist should then enclose the paraffin in paper towels, plastic bags, and toweling to maintain the heat. The treatment is applied for approximately 20 to 30 minutes. Removing the paraffin calls for extra care not to contaminate the used portion so that it does not affect the entire bath when it is used again.

Infrared

Infrared is classified as superficial heat, although it is an electromagnetic energy modality rather than a conduction energy modality. It is generally agreed that no form of infrared energy can have a depth of penetration greater than 1 cm. Infrared is a dry heat modality compared with other types of superficial heat. Dry heat from an infrared lamp tends to elevate superficial temperatures more than moist heat; however, moist heat probably has a greater depth of penetration.[89] The commonly used infrared modality is the infrared lamp (Figure 17-6). The advantage of the infrared lamp over other superficial heat modalities is that it can raise the temperature without the unit touching the patient. This characteristic makes the infrared lamp the only superficial heating choice when the patient has skin defects. It is also commonly used to elevate the temperature of patients during or after surgical procedures.

Superficial skin burns occur sometimes because of intense infrared radiation and the reflector becoming extremely hot (4000° F/2004° C). Avoiding touching the reflector cannot be overemphasized. It is recommended that a warm moist towel be placed over the body segment to be treated to enhance the heating effect. Areas that are not being treated must be protected by clothing or dry towels. The skin should be checked every few minutes for mottling. The distance from the area to be treated to the lamp should be adjusted according to the treatment time. The standard formula is 20 inches (50 cm) distance equals 20 minutes treatment time. After treatment, the skin surface should be checked.

Hydrotherapy

Hydrotherapy, as the term suggests, treats the patient through the medium of water. Water can provide the temperature, moisten the soft tissue, and support the tissue.[59a] Hydrotherapy can be performed in a swimming pool, Hubbard tank, or whirlpool. Among them, the whirlpool is most commonly used. In addition to the thermal effect on reducing pain, edema, and muscle spasm, a quick jet stream or stroking motion during whirlpool has a local massage effect, which might cause further muscle relaxation and increase local circulation. When whirlpool is applied, the patient can move the treated part in the whirlpool easily to get the added benefit of exercise.[197a]

Whirlpool can be divided into cold whirlpool and warm whirlpool. Cold whirlpool is indicated in acute and subacute conditions in which exercise of the injured part during a cold treatment is needed. Cold whirlpool has been discussed earlier in the section on cryotherapy. For warm whirlpool, the temperature should be 98° F to 110° F (37° C to 45° C) for treatment of the arm, hand, or legs. For full body treatment, the temperature should be 98° F to 102° F (37° C to 39° C). Time of application should be 15 to 20 minutes. Jet flow should be 6 to 9 inches (15 to 23 cm) from the body segment. In addition to increased circulation and reduction of spasm from the heat, benefits of the warm whirlpool include the massaging and vibrating effects of the water movement (Figure 17-7). Warm whirlpool is an excellent treatment for rheumatoid arthritis and osteoarthritis to increase systemic blood flow and mobilization of the affected body part without too much pressure of the joints.[51,54]

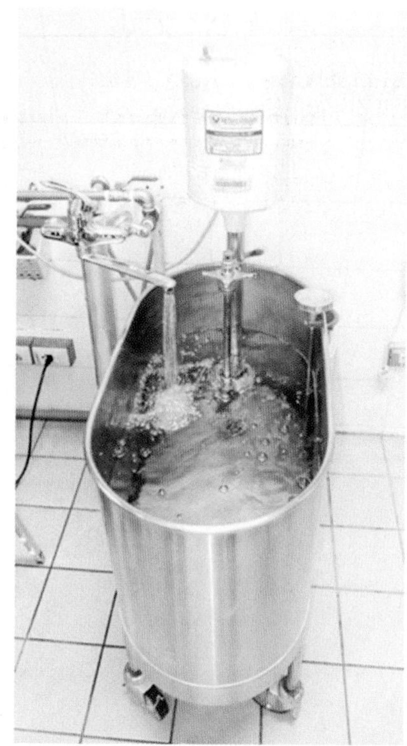

FIGURE 17-7 Whirlpool with jet flow.

The whirlpool should be cleaned frequently to prevent bacterial growth. When a patient with any open or infected lesion uses the whirlpool, it must be drained and cleaned immediately after. Cleaning should be done with both a disinfecting and antibacterial agent. Particular attention should be focused on cleaning the turbine by placing the intake valves in a bucket containing the disinfecting solution and turning the power on. Bacterial cultures should be monitored periodically from the tank, drain, and jets. Aerobic exercise in the water is to increase range of motion, flexibility, and muscle power, which is appropriate for patients with lower leg arthritis.[149]

Spinal Traction

Physiology

Traction has been used in the treatment of painful spinal conditions since ancient times. Traction is defined as applying a tension or force to a body segment. Clinically, traction can be classified as mechanical (using a traction machine to apply a traction force), manual, and positional. The manual traction involves clinical judgment and personal skill, which is too complicated to be addressed here.[56] This section will focus on mechanical traction (machine-derived force).

Spinal traction moves the spine overall and at each individual spinal segment.[29,142] The amount of movement varies according to the position of the spine, the amount of force, and the traction duration.[14,102,142] Separation of intervertebral space up to 1 to 2 mm has been reported, but it is transient and the spine returns to the previous condition quickly when applied force has stopped.[78,122,146]

The major physiologic effect of spinal traction comes from the distraction of the spine, which may stretch the ligament, muscle, and facet joint.[14] It also reduces the disk pressure and facilitates the disk to return to its origin position.[142,146] An intermittent traction with a rhythmic on-and-off cycle not only provides distraction load but also promotes movement of the facet joints. The ligamentous structures of the spinal column are stretched by traction. Loading should be applied slowly and comfortably because slow loading rates allow the spinal ligament to lengthen as it absorbs the force of load. The amount of ligament deformity accompanying a low rate of loading is higher than in the rapid loading situation. The ligament deformity from the traction allows the spinal vertebrae to move apart. In patients with ligaments shortened or contracted by an injury or a long-term poor posture, traction may be beneficial in restoring the normal length of spinal ligament. The traction force should provide the stress that encourages the ligament to make adaptive changes in length and strength but not heavy enough to damage the ligament. The mechanical force created by traction has an excellent effect on disk protrusion and disk-related pain.[146]

The intervertebral disk helps to dissipate compression forces when the spine is in the erect posture. When the disk is injured, the vertebral bodies move closer together and the annular fibers bulge out just like an underinflated car tire. Then, the disk nucleus will shift to the less pressure site. The bulging disk might compress the surrounding tissues including the nerve root and causes pain as well as nerve irritation symptoms. Traction could separate the vertebral bodies and thus decrease the central pressure in the disk space and facilitate the disk nucleus to return to the central position. Return of the nucleus pulposus relieves the pain and symptoms of nerve or vascular structure compression. Decreasing the compressive forces through spinal traction also allows for the better fluid interchange within the disk and spinal canal. However, the reduction of disk herniation or disk pressure by spinal traction is not sustained and tends to recur when the compression force returns. Minimizing compressive forces after traction, such as the use of a brace or rest, may be equally as important to the success of the treatment as the traction itself.

The articular joints of the spine (facet joint) can also be affected by traction.[78,123] Traction can separate the joint surfaces, which releases the impingement of meniscal structures, synovial fringes, and osteochondral fragments between joint space, and symptom reduction may occur. Increased joint separation lessens the compression pressure of articular cartilage, encourages synovial fluid exchange, nourishes the cartilage, increases proprioceptive discharge from the facet joint, and thus decreases pain perception. Spinal traction also stretches the specific paraspinal muscle group, allows better muscular blood flow, and also activates muscular proprioceptors, providing a gating influence on the pain.[78,94] Part of the spinal pain is originally from the spinal nerve impinged.[14,102,146] The impingement of nerve may be from bulging disk material, irritated facet joint, bony spur, or narrowed foramen. Tingling is usually the first clinical sign indicating a nerve compression, followed by numbness, motor weakness, and loss of reflexes. Spinal traction, as mentioned earlier, could relieve the possible local nerve compression and increase the blood flow to the nerve, decreasing edema, and allowing the nerve to return to normal function. The treatment plan should include the clinical criteria for judging the success and continued use of traction. Positive change should occur within five to eight treatments if traction is going to be successful.

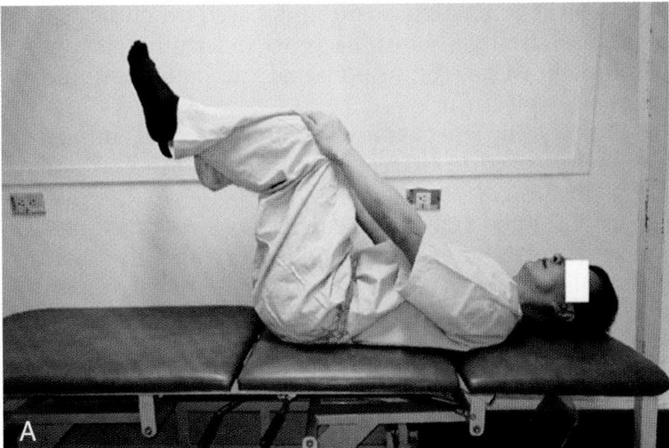

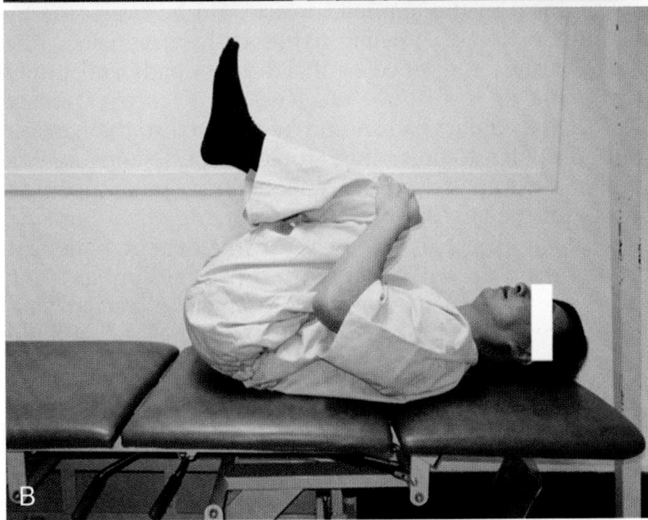

FIGURE 17-8 Positional traction: knees to chest posture can be used to increase the size of the lumbar foramen bilaterally. **A,** Beginning position. **B,** Terminal position.

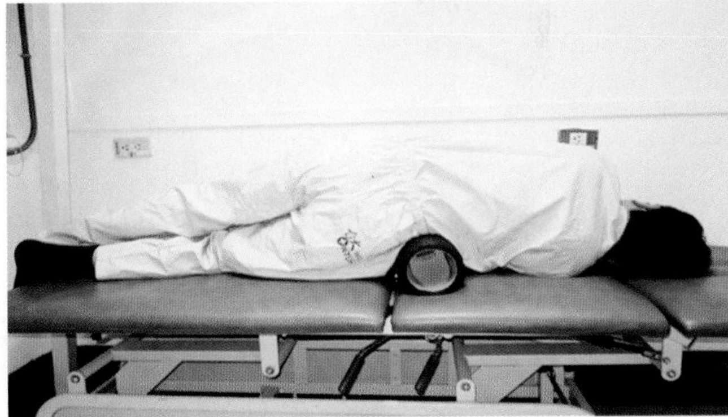

FIGURE 17-9 Positional traction: patient positioned side-lying with a blanket roll between the iliac crest and the lower border of the rib cage. This increases the intervertebral foramen size of the left side of the lumbar spine.

Types of Devices and Techniques

Positional traction is to use a proper position to stretch the specific spinal structures. It is a simple method and sometimes has good results. It is mostly used in the lumbar spine. Normal spinal mechanics allow movement to occur that narrows or enlarges the intervertebral foramina.[146,161] If the patient is placed in the supine position with the hip and knee flexed, and the lumbar spine bends forward, the spinous processes separate. This motion would open the intervertebral foramen bilaterally (Figure 17-8). The flexion postures used to treat low back pain are an example of the lumbar positional traction. Unilateral foraminal opening occurs by positioning the patient sidelying with a pillow or blanket roll between the iliac crest and lower border of the rib cage (Figure 17-9). The side on which foraminal opening is desired should be on top. The pillow or blanket roll should be close to the level of spine where the foramen is desired to be opened.[146,161] Maximum opening can be achieved with the addition of trunk rotation toward the side of the superior shoulder. Positional traction is normally used when the patient is on a very restricted activity program from low back pain and cannot tolerate active treatment. The traction position is based on clinical judgment and trial-and-error basis to determine maximum comfort; however, the response of the patient should be the main concern.

When doing mechanical traction, several important parameters need to be set, including traction equipment, body position, force used, traction pattern (intermittent versus sustained traction), and duration of traction. The research on mechanical lumbar traction with well-described protocols to decrease disk protrusion and nerve root symptoms is promising. However, outcome in other pathologies is not as well supported by research.[72,125]

A split table (Figure 17-10) or other mechanisms to eliminate friction between body segments and the table surface is a prerequisite to effective lumbar traction. Otherwise, most of the applied force would be overcome by the friction force. A pelvic harness is always used. The pelvic harness is applied so that contact pads and upper belt are at or just above the level of iliac crest (Figure 17-10). The contact pad should be adjusted so the harness loop provides a posteriorly directed pull, encouraging lumbar flexion. In general, the neutral spinal position allows for the largest intervertebral foramen opening, and it is usually the position of choice whether the patient is prone or supine. Extension beyond neutral lumbar spine causes the bony elements of the foramen to create a narrower opening. Lumbar spine flexion beyond neutral causes the ligamentum flavum and other soft tissues to constrict the opening of the foramen.[152] Saunders[160] recommended the prone position with a normal to slightly flattened lumbar lordosis as the position of choice in disk protrusion. The amount of lordosis can be controlled with the use of a pillow under the abdomen. The prone position also allows the easy application of other modalities such as heat packs and an easier assessment of the amount of spinous process separation. When lumbar traction is applied to a patient in the supine position, the degree of hip flexion affects vertebral separation. As hip flexion increases from 0 to 90 degrees, traction produces a greater posterior intervertebral space separation. Overall, the patient's positioning for lumbar traction should be varied according to the patient's need and comfort. Although clinical judgment on positioning is important to maximize the effect of traction on the patient, patient comfort is far more important. If the patient cannot relax his or her back muscles, the traction will not be successful in causing vertebral separation.

Several research articles have indicated that no lumbar vertebral separation will occur with traction forces less than a quarter of the patient's body weight. The traction force necessary to cause effective vertebral separation will usually range between 65 and 200 lb.[123,160] This effective force is not necessary to be reached in the first attempt, and progressive steps are often necessary to comfortably reach the therapeutic load. A force equal to half the patient's body weight is a good guideline to use in selecting a force high enough to cause vertebral separation. These high weight levels do not cause damage, because research on cadavers indicates that a force of 440 lb or greater is necessary to cause damage to the lumbar spine.[122,123] It is recommended that during an initial lumbar traction trial a maximum of 30 lb is used to determine whether or not

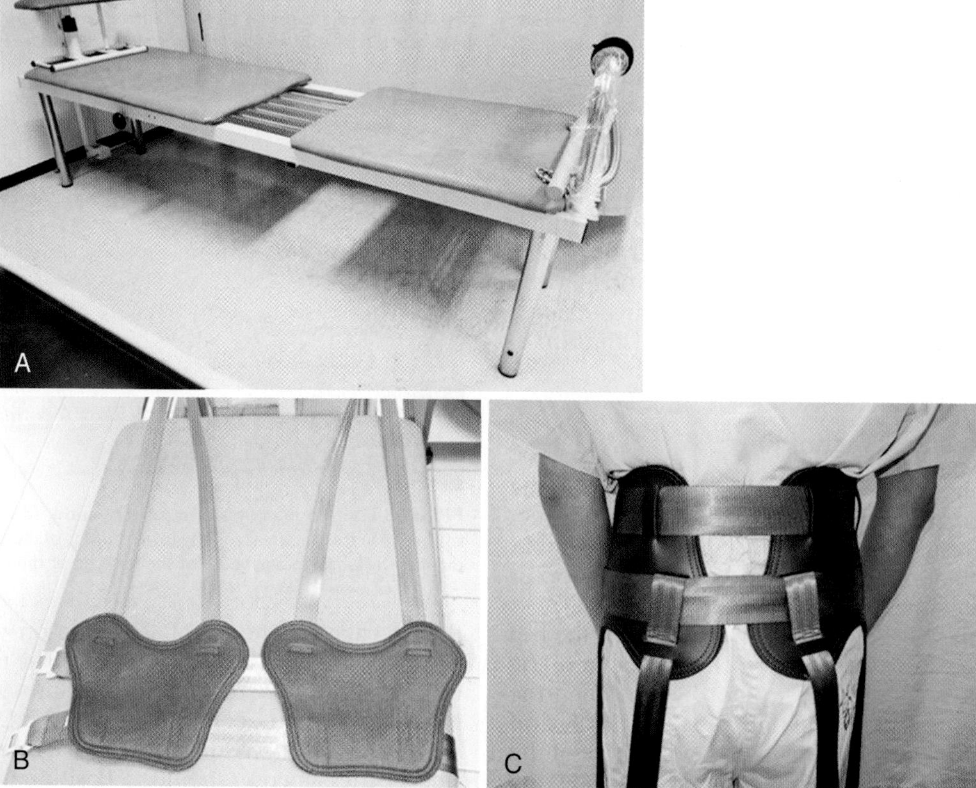

FIGURE 17-10 Lumbar spine traction. **A,** Split table with movable section to decrease frictional forces. **B,** Traction harness. **C,** Pelvic harness for mechanical lumbar traction. The contact pads are applied so that the upper belt is at or just above the level of the iliac crest.

traction will have a negative effect. As previous research has shown, traction certainly has therapeutic effects at forces that are not associated with vertebral separation, and if these effects are desired, using lower levels of force may be necessary to achieve them.

The effects of traction have been reported either from intermittent or sustained traction. Partial reduction in disk protrusion was observed in 4 minutes of sustained traction.[14,122,123,160] Separation of the posterior intervertebral space was noted with a 10-second hold intermittent traction.[86] In general, sustained traction is favored in treating intervertebral disk herniation because sustained traction allows more time with the disk uncompressed to cause the disk nuclear material to move centripetally and reduce the pressure of the disk herniation on nerve structures. Most other traction-appropriate diagnoses may be treated with intermittent traction. Intermittent traction is usually more comfortable when compared with sustained traction with the same force, especially in higher forces. There is no conclusive evidence supporting the choice of one method over the other. For intermittent traction, the timing of traction and rest phases has not been well studied. Short traction phase (less than 10 seconds) causes only minimum interspace separation but will activate joints and muscles and create facet joint movement. Longer traction phases (greater than 10 seconds) tend to stretch the ligament and muscular tissue to overcome their resistance to movement and create a longer-lasting mechanical separation.[72] The rest time should be relatively short but allow the patient to recover and feel relaxed before the next traction cycle. The therapist should monitor the patient undergoing traction frequently to adjust traction and rest time to maintain the patient in a relaxed comfortable state. The total treatment time of sustained traction and intermittent traction are not well studied. For sustained traction in a disk-related problem, traction should start at less than 10 minutes, and up to 30 minutes treatment may be eventually needed.

The literature provides a relatively clear protocol in trying to achieve cervical vertebral separation with a mechanical traction apparatus.[125] The patient should be supine or sitting with the neck flexed between 20 and 30 degrees (Figure 17-11). The traction harness must be arranged comfortably so the majority of pull is placed on the occiput rather than the chin, in which the traction force is effectively transferred to the structures of the cervical spine. The cervical traction force greater than 20 lb is applied intermittently for a minimum of 7 seconds of traction time, and adequate rest time for recovery is recommended. The traction duration is approximately 20 to 25 minutes. A higher force (up to 50 lb) has been reported to increase separation of intervertebral space. The average separation at the posterior vertebral area is 1 to 1.5 mm/space, whereas the anterior vertebral area separates approximately 0.4 mm/space.[70,72]

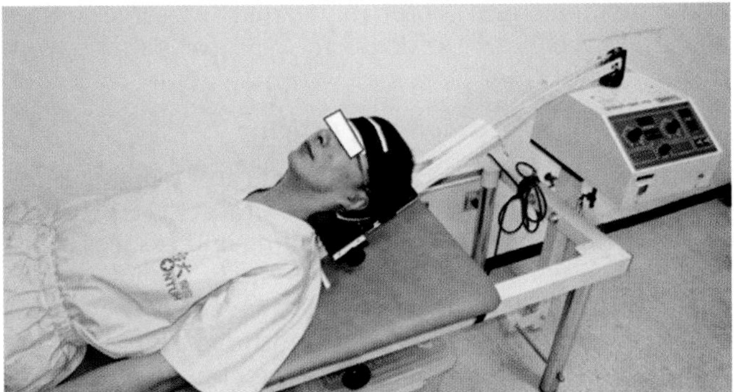

FIGURE 17-11 Mechanical cervical traction. The patient is in the supine position with the traction harness placed so that maximum pull is exerted on the occiput and the patient is in a position of approximately 20 to 30 degrees of neck flexion.

Indications and Contraindications

Spinal traction is indicated in patients with nerve impingement from disk herniation, spondylolisthesis, narrowed intervertebral foramen, spur formation, degenerative facet joints, joint hypomobility, diskogenic pain, and muscle spasm.[158,189] Spinal traction is contraindicated in acute sprain or strain, acute inflammation, or vertebral joint instability. Tumors, bone disease, severe osteoporosis, and infection in bones or joints are also contraindications (Table 17-3).

CASE 1

Hot Pack and Spinal Traction

Background: A 69-year-old woman developed lower back pain for years. She reports radiating pain to the right buttock and the posterior lateral part of her right thigh. Daily activity such as walking and housework increases her discomfort. Oral medications including nonsteroidal antiinflammatory drugs (NSAIDs) have provided limited relief. Physical examination including straight-leg raising test and piriformis muscle stretching showed negative findings. X-rays indicate degenerative changes such as spur formation and L4 to L5, L5 to S1 disk space narrowing with marginal spur formation.

Impression: Lumbar spondylosis with right sciatica.

Treatment plan: Physical therapy was prescribed, which included hydrocollator packing of low back followed by intermittent lumbar traction. A 3-day-per-week course of traction was arranged. The patient was positioned supine on the traction table and the traction unit was adjusted to have approximately 25 degrees of lumbar flexion during traction. For the first week, 15 kg of intermittent traction force (body weight 60 kg) was applied, with progressive 1 to 2 kg step up weekly. Each traction cycle consisted of 15 seconds of tension, followed by 20 seconds of rest. The total treatment time was 25 minutes. The maximum traction force was 26 kg because higher load induced discomfort after traction. Therapeutic exercises consisted of core muscle strengthening, and back stretching was also taught and monitored.

Response: The patient reported to have gradual pain reduction and the traction was completed after 2 months of treatment.

Discussion:

- Is the pain reduction related to spinal traction or just a natural course?
- Is epidural block indicated if the response to traction is limited?
- What are the added benefits of therapeutic exercises?
- What are the contraindications, such as osteoporosis, to the use of spinal traction?
- What is the adequate duration of traction before failure is determined?

Table 17-3 Indications and Contraindications for Spinal Traction

Indications	Contraindications
Impingement on a nerve root	Acute sprains or strains
Disk herniation	Acute inflammation
Narrowing within the intervertebral foramen	Fractures
Osteophyte formation	Any condition in which movement exacerbates the existing problem
Degenerative joint diseases	Tumors
Spondylolisthesis	Bone diseases
Joint hypomobility	Pregnancy
Diskogenic pain	**Relative Contraindications**
Muscle spasm or guarding	Vertebral joint instability
Spinal ligament or connective tissues contractures	Osteoporosis

Deep Heat

The forms of heat having deeper penetration into tissue, including ultrasound, shortwave, and microwave, are classified as deep heat or diathermy. The term *diathermy* is derived from the Greek words *dia* and *therma*, and literally means "heating through." Deep heat is the form of heat which can maximally deposit its energy on deep tissue such as ligament, tendon, muscle, and joint capsule, avoiding excessive heat in skin and subcutaneous fat. The mechanism of heat transfer for deep heat modalities is conversion, referring to the transformation of energy (e.g., acoustic or electromagnetic) to heat. Deep heat modalities include ultrasound, shortwave, and microwave.

Ultrasound

Physics and Devices

Ultrasound is an oscillating sound pressure wave with a frequency greater than the upper limit of the human hearing range, usually 20 kHz. Medical uses of ultrasound can be divided into diagnostic and therapeutic. Diagnostic ultrasound emits and receives ultrasonic waves and is used for the evaluation of various organs and systems, such as uterus, heat, lung, kidney, etc., and for physiatrists, the musculoskeletal system. The applications of ultrasound on disease diagnosis are outside the scope of this chapter and will not be discussed further. Therapeutic ultrasound emits high-frequency acoustic energy to produce thermal and mechanical effects in tissue. It has been widely used in the field of physical medicine for soft tissue disorders. Other applications, such as liposuction, bony nonunion, chronic wound healing, dental scaling, skin lift, and tumor ablation, are also under rapid development. However in this chapter, we will only focus our discussion on ultrasound diathermy for soft tissue disorders.

A typical therapeutic ultrasound unit consists of an applicator, a matching electrical circuit, a high-frequency electrical generator, and a power amplifier. The transformer converts the 110- or 220-voltage alternating current to a high-frequency one, and the matching circuit quarantines the efficient oscillation of the piezoelectric crystal inside the applicator in resonant frequency. Figure 17-12 shows the major components of an ultrasound diathermy unit.

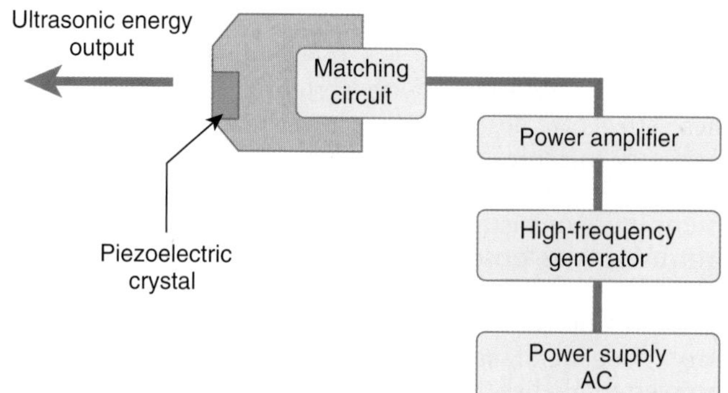

FIGURE 17-12 Schematic of the components of an ultrasound diathermy unit.

Table 17-4 Attenuation of Human Tissues at 1 MHz of Ultrasound

Material	Attenuation Coefficient (dB/cm)
Water	0.0022
Fat	0.6
Blood	0.18
Brain	0.85
Liver	0.9
Kidney	1
Muscle (along fibers)	1.2
Muscle (across fibers)	3.3
Skull	20
Lung	10

History

Medical ultrasound initially started with its applications in therapy rather than diagnosis. The destructive ability of high-intensity ultrasound was recognized in the 1920s from the time of Paul Langévin when he noted the killing of fish and pain induced in his hand when placed in a water tank insonated with high-intensity ultrasound. In the 1950s, William Fry and Russell Meyers used ultrasound to destroy parts of the basal ganglia in patients with parkinsonism. Ultrasonic energy used in physical and rehabilitation medicine was probably started by Jerome Gersten at the University of Colorado in 1953 for patients with rheumatic arthritis.[191]

Physiology and Mechanism of Action

The physiologic effects of ultrasound can be divided into thermal and nonthermal (or mechanical) effects. The loss of ultrasound energy while propagating into tissue is called attenuation, which includes the effects of both scattering and absorption. Heat is produced when acoustic energy is absorbed, especially at or near the surfaces of structures with high-attenuation coefficients (e.g., bone). Table 17-4 lists selected attenuation coefficients of typical materials encountered during daily ultrasound treatments.[81] Bony structures and lungs, which contain air, have the largest attenuation at 1 MHz of ultrasound. The localized heating

Table 17-5 Half-Value Thickness (HVT) of Different Materials at 1 MHz and 5 MHz

	HVT (cm)	
Material	**1 MHz**	**5 MHz**
Water	1360	54
Fat	5	1
Blood	17	3
Brain	3.5	1
Liver	3	0.5
Muscle	1.5	0.3
Bone	0.2	0.04
Air	0.25	0.01

by ultrasound near bony surfaces (e.g., the soft tissue–bone interfaces) preferably produces hyperemia and enhances extensibility of tissues such as ligaments, tendons, and joint capsules. The attenuation in a specific material can be quantified in terms of the ultrasonic half-value thickness (HVT) or half-value layer. HVT is defined as the distance in a specific material that reduces the intensity of the ultrasonic beam to half of its original value (Table 17-5).[81] Ultrasound of higher frequency has smaller HVT and thus can penetrate less.

Nonthermal effects include cavitation, media motion (acoustic streaming and microstreaming), and standing waves. Cavitation is the oscillation of bubbles in a sound field.[113] These bubbles expand and contract with alternating compressions and rarefactions of the ultrasound waves periodically, usually called stable cavitation. Bubbles may also grow and collapse violently, creating more bubbles in unstable or transient cavitation. High temperature and pressure are generated and induce various forms of bioeffects, such as vessel ruptures, platelet aggregation, and tissue damage.

As the ultrasound wave travels through medium, it may be absorbed and the momentum absorbed manifests itself as a bulk flow of the medium in the direction of the sound field, usually termed acoustic streaming.[113] Microstreaming refers to the flow of interstitial fluids near small obstacles or vibrating bubbles in a sound field. The shear forces set up within the medium may disrupt cell membranes around, resulting in certain bioeffects.[113] Standing waves are produced by the superimposition of incident and reflected ultrasound waves, and can result in local heating in tissue. The clinical significance or application of nonthermal effects of ultrasound is still unclear and is under intense investigation.

Techniques

Ultrasound is usually applied on a target area with a stroking technique, which allows a more even energy distribution. The ultrasound probe is moved over an area of approximately 25 cm^2 (4 square inches) slowly in a circular or longitudinal manner for 5 to 10 minutes. Keeping the probe in a stationary position should be avoided because of the potential for creating standing waves and local hot spots. Output is specified by power (watts) or intensity (watts per square centimeter) and is adjusted to just below the pain threshold. A coupling agent between the probe and the skin is essential because ultrasound is unable to penetrate even a thin layer of air. Coupling agents should not be salt-based such as those used for electromyography or electrocardiography, because the salt may damage the ultrasound probe.

Ultrasound can also be applied with an indirect or immersing method, especially when treating irregular surfaces such as the foot and ankle is necessary. The target body part is placed in a container filled with degassed water. The ultrasound probe is held a short distance away (0.5 to 3.0 cm) and moved without touching the skin. Degassed water can be produced by allowing the tap water to sit for several hours or by using commercial vacuum suction devices. Dissolved gasses in water may form bubbles during treatment and attenuate the ultrasound energy. Unwanted cavitation-related bioeffects may also be generated in gaseous water. If for some reason the treatment area cannot be immersed in water, an ultrasound gel pad or a water-filled bag can be used instead. Both sides of the gel pad or water bag should be coated with gel to ensure better contact.

Ultrasound delivery can be continuous or pulsed, depending on whether thermal or nonthermal effect is preferable. Pulsed delivery involves the emission of brief bursts or pulses of ultrasound, interspersed with pause periods. Thus, heating is minimized and ultrasound nonthermal effect is emphasized. Additional parameters are defined for pulsed ultrasound output. For most commercial machines, duty factor or cycle, commonly ranging from 10% to 50%, is the only variable the users need to select. The smaller the duty factor, the less heat will be produced. Duty factor is defined as the fraction of total time during which ultrasound is emitted. For example, a 10% duty factor means 10% of time in a certain period (e.g., 1 second) ultrasound is emitted. Other parameters—pulse duration (ultrasound on-time) and pulse repetition frequency (number of pulses per second)—are not controllable by users.

The ultrasound transducer, also referred to as an applicator, consists of a piezoelectric crystal that converts electrical energy to acoustic energy through vibrating the crystal in the thickness direction periodically. The U.S. Food and Drug Administration (FDA) requires the technique information of the applicator, which includes operating frequency, effective radiating area (ERA), beam nonuniformity ratio (BNR), and type of applicator, that is, whether focusing, collimating, or diverging. Most of the therapeutic ultrasound used in diathermy has frequencies, the vibration frequency of the piezoelectric crystal, ranging between 0.8 and 3 MHz after considering its focusing, penetration, heat generation, and standardization for clinical applications. Low-frequency ultrasound has better penetration, and high-frequency ultrasound generates more heat in the superficial area. The ERA indicates the portion of the applicator surface that actually produces sound waves and is described in square centimeters. The ERA is determined by scanning the applicator surface at a distance of 5 mm by a listening hydrophone in a water bath, and recording the area with power output of more than 5% of the maximum power output on the applicator surface. The ideal ERA is the area of the applicator but is always smaller. The BNR is the ratio of the spatial-maximum intensity to the spatial-average intensity across the applicator surface. For example, a BNR of 2:1 means that when the average output intensity is 1 W/cm^2, the peak point intensity of the beam is 2 W/cm^2. An optimal BNR is 1:1 but is not possible. Ideal BNR should fall between 2:1 and 5:1. The lower the BNR, the more uniform the output energy of the applicator is, and thus a lower chance for a focal hot spot to induce tissue overheating.

Indications and Evidence Basis

Therapeutic ultrasound is widely used in the treatment of various soft tissue disorders. Because fibroblasts are the basic cellular components of soft tissue and are responsible for the production of collagen to form connective tissue matrix, their responses to ultrasound exposure have been extensively studied.[46,79] Ultrasound has been found to significantly enhance the proliferation, collagen production, and noncollagen protein synthesis through the upregulation of interleukin-1β and vascular endothelial growth factor of cultured fibroblasts.[46] Both continuous and pulsed ultrasound promotes fibroblast proliferation in a process related to the upregulation of proliferating cell nuclear antigen.[179] Pulsed ultrasound at an intensity ranging from 0.1 to 1.0 W/cm^2 and 20% duty cycle stimulates the migration of primary tendon fibroblasts in an intensity-dependent manner associated with upregulating the expression of alpha-smooth muscle actin.[178] In addition, the upregulation of a more upstream signal mediator, transforming growth factor-β, demonstrates the pivotal role of ultrasound in regulating the proliferation, migration, and protein synthesis, including collagen, of tendon fibroblasts (Figure 17-13).[180,181] Ultrasound treatment was found to increase calcium uptake for intensities and duration at the range of diathermy, and the calcium uptake increased with increasing exposure time.[133] The physical mechanism underlying the stimulating effect was shown to be related to acoustic cavitation or shear wave stress on cell membranes, which increases cytoplasmic calcium levels.[53,182,187,188]

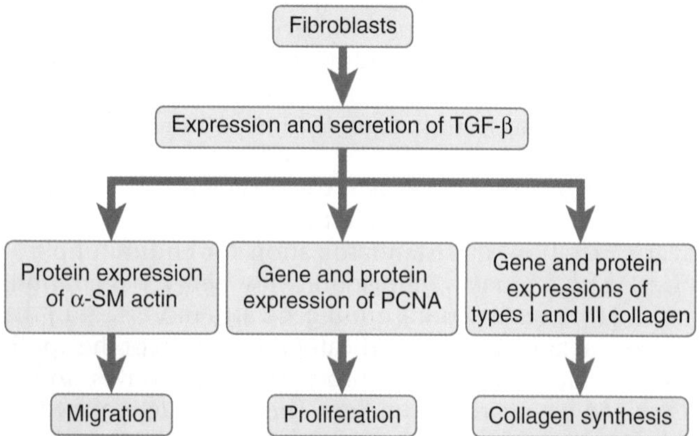

FIGURE 17-13 Proposed mechanisms for ultrasound to promote the migration, proliferation, and collagen expression of tendon cells. *α-SM actin*, alpha-smooth muscle actin; *PCNA*, proliferation cell nuclear antigen; *TGF-β*, transforming growth factor-beta. (From Tsai WC, Tang SFT, Liang FC: Effect of therapeutic ultrasound on tendons, *Am J Phys Med Rehabil* 90:1068-1073, 2011.)

Low-Intensity Pulsed Ultrasound

It is generally believed that excessive heating may have a detrimental effect on wound healing. Thus low-intensity pulsed ultrasound (LIPUS) with a duty cycle around 20% to 25% is a preferred form of ultrasound energy delivery. LIPUS treatment was shown to promote the healing process of surgically lacerated flexor tendons in animal models. Increasing range of movement, faster scar maturation, and reduced inflammatory infiltrate around the repair site was found after ultrasound treatment.[64] LIPUS was also found to promote the restoration of mechanical strength and collagen alignment in healing tendons, especially when applied at early healing stages.[60] LIPUS is able to accelerate bone–tendon junction repair by stimulating angiogenesis, chondrogenesis, and osteogenesis in a rabbit model.[119] The upregulation of biglycan, collagen I, and vascular endothelial growth factor may be responsible for enhancing the bone–tendon junction healing.[118,144]

Ultrasound diathermy is in widespread use and many physiatrists and physical therapists remain convinced that ultrasound has benefits in the treatment of musculoskeletal disorders. Figure 17-14 shows a typical ultrasound diathermy device being applied on a patient with lateral epicondylitis. However, surprisingly there is little clinical evidence documenting the efficacy of ultrasound in tendinopathy or to promote tendon healing.* Few clinical

*References 6, 9, 50, 75, 137, 183, 185.

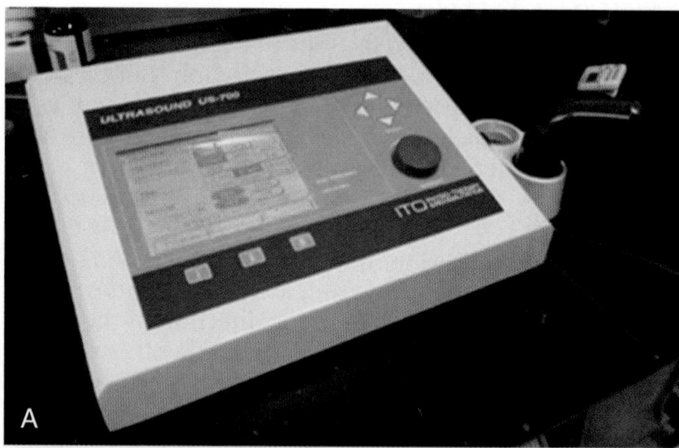

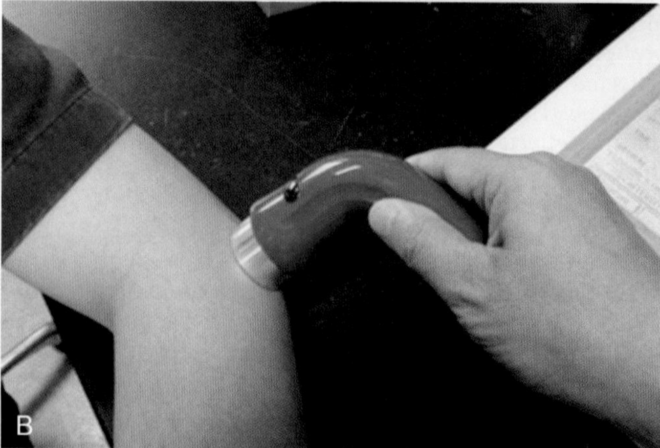

FIGURE 17-14 A, A commercial ultrasound device. **B,** Its application on a patient with lateral epicondylitis.

studies have proved its effects on soft tissue injuries. For example, a randomized controlled trial showed significant benefits of ultrasound in the treatment of calcified tendinitis at the end of an intensive 6-week treatment program. However, this difference disappeared 9 months later.[52] Another recent randomized controlled trial showed that therapeutic ultrasound provided no additional benefit in improving pain and function in addition to exercise training for patients with osteoarthritic knees.[33] That is not too surprising because penetration of ultrasound into knee joints is poor. Nonetheless, current available trials on the efficacy of ultrasound are usually poor in quality. Well-designed studies are still needed to establish the effectiveness of ultrasound treatment to support its popularity.

Sonophoresis

It has long been known that application of ultrasound to the skin increases its permeability (sonophoresis or phonophoresis) and enables the delivery of various substances into and through the skin. Transdermal drug delivery offers several important advantages over traditional oral delivery or injections, including minimizing gastric irritation, first pass effect, and pain. Ultrasound of low to medium frequencies (20 to 200 kHz and 0.2 to 1 MHz, respectively) is predominantly used for sonophoresis resulting from the relatively stronger cavitation effects. In 2004, the FDA granted the use of the SonoPrep ultrasonic skin permeation device (Sontra Medical, Franklin, Mass.) for use with topical lidocaine to achieve rapid (within 5 minutes) skin anesthesia. For musculoskeletal disorders, phonophoresis with topical steroidal or nonsteroidal anti-inflammatory cream has been shown to be effective in pain reduction for patients suffering from, for example, MPS, knee osteoarthritis, carpal tunnel syndrome, and epicondylitis.[17,30,120,159]

Contraindications and Precautions

General contraindications and precautions of the use of ultrasound diathermy are summarized in Box 17-1. Ultrasound produces focal and intense heat and in certain conditions may induce detrimental mechanical effects such as vessel ruptures or tissue damage. Heat should generally be avoided in areas of impaired sensation or in patients with cognitive impairment. Heat can exacerbate acute inflammation; thus ultrasound should be avoided in the management of acute tendinitis, arthritis, or ligament sprain. Applying ultrasound near structures vulnerable to thermal injury, such as nerve, brain, eyes, and reproductive organs, should be avoided. Similarly, applying ultrasound near the laminectomy sites may induce spinal cord heat and is contraindicated. Heat theoretically may increase the rate of tumor growth or hematogenous spread; thus ultrasound diathermy should be avoided in known areas of malignancy.[110] Controversies exist in the use of therapeutic ultrasound near implants. Applying ultrasound near a pacemaker is generally contraindicated because ultrasound may cause its malfunction.[20] Plastics such as methyl methacrylate or polyethylene have high acoustic attenuation coefficients and will be overheated during ultrasound exposure. Therefore, ultrasound should be avoided near implants containing plastic materials, such as artificial hip joints with polyethylene liner or breast implants. Metal has a lower acoustic attenuation coefficient and higher thermal conductivity than bone and soft tissues, and has been shown to have no focal temperature increase when exposed to ultrasound.[67,100,111,112] Different from shortwave or microwave diathermy, ultrasound is believed to be the only type of diathermy that can be used in areas with surgical metallic implants.

BOX 17-1

Contraindications and Precautions of Ultrasound Diathermy

General heat precautions
Acute injury/inflammation
Near nerve, brain, eyes, reproductive organs
On pregnant uterus
Near spine or laminectomy sites
Malignancy
Near pacemaker
On epiphysis
Implants containing plastic materials

Shortwave

Physics

Shortwave diathermy (SWD) is a modality that produces heat by converting electromagnetic energy to thermal energy. Shortwave generates heat by oscillating high-frequency electrical and magnetic fields to move ions, rotate polar molecules, and distort nonpolar molecules in body tissues. The U.S. Federal Communications Commission restricts industrial, scientific, and medical use of shortwave to 13.56 MHz (wavelength, 22 m), 27.12 MHz (wavelength, 11 m), and 40.68 MHz (wavelength, 7.5 m). However, in certain countries (e.g., the United Kingdom), frequency-modulated bandwidths between 88 and 108 MHz, which includes the fourth harmonic of the 27.12-MHz diathermy bandwidth, are allocated for medical use.[18,154] Most SWD machines operate at 27.12 MHz.

The temperature increase of tissue during SWD can be quantitatively described by the specific absorption rate (SAR), which represents the rate of energy absorbed per unit area of tissue mass. SAR is proportional to the square of the induced electrical current and inversely to the electrical conductivity of the tissue.[110] Therapeutic changes only occur when the temperature of the tissue rises to 40° C to 45° C. At higher temperatures, protein denaturing may occur, resulting in irreparable cell damage and acute pain.

History

The medical use of shortwave can be traced back to the early twentieth century. Although widely used in the field of physical therapy, the first medical application of SWD was in the gynecologic field. In 1910, the Spanish scientist and radiologist Celedonio Calatayud applied SWD for the first time in the treatment of gynecologic diseases.[148]

Techniques

Shortwave energy can be delivered to the target tissue via ether capacitor or inductor electrodes. Capacitor electrodes consist of two condenser plates (Figure 17-15) and in between a strong electrical field is created. The area to be treated is placed between the electrodes and becomes part of the circuit. The plates and the patient's treated area act like a capacitor; thus the term *capacitor electrodes* was given. Because there are many free ions with either positive or negative charges, the alternating electrical field will attract or repel these ions periodically and rapidly, which generate heat by friction among molecules. The highest temperature increase occurs in areas with the highest electric current density, usually those near the plate surface and closer to its center. The capacitor electrodes are thought to induce more power absorption and heat generation in areas with higher resistance to the passage of the electrical field, such as subcutaneous fat.[110]

Inductive electrodes consist of induction coils that produce, unlike capacitor electrodes, a stronger magnetic field (Figure 17-16). The alternating magnetic field also moves ions and charged molecules, and results in heat generation. The inductor electrodes produce more power absorption and higher heat generation in the deeper high-water-content tissue such as muscle than in subcutaneous fat. Commercially, there are different shapes of inductive electrodes available for different clinical settings. For example, pad electrodes are separately placed on the two sides of the back pain area to induce deep heat in the back muscles. Cable applicators consist of rubber-coated cables that are usually wrapped around an extremity such as the knee joint for the treatment of knee arthritis. Careful placement of the inductive coil to avoid crossover is important to avoid overheating. A drum-shaped applicator with coils encased in rigid housing can be positioned toward the target area. A 20- to 30-minute total treatment time for one body area is usually necessary to achieve enough heating and maximum therapeutic effects in the deep tissues.

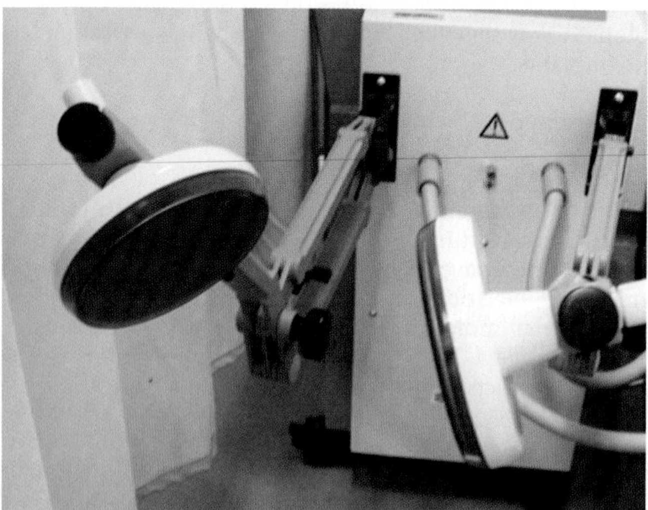

FIGURE 17-15 Capacitor electrodes of shortwave diathermy produce a strong electrical field in between the two condenser plates.

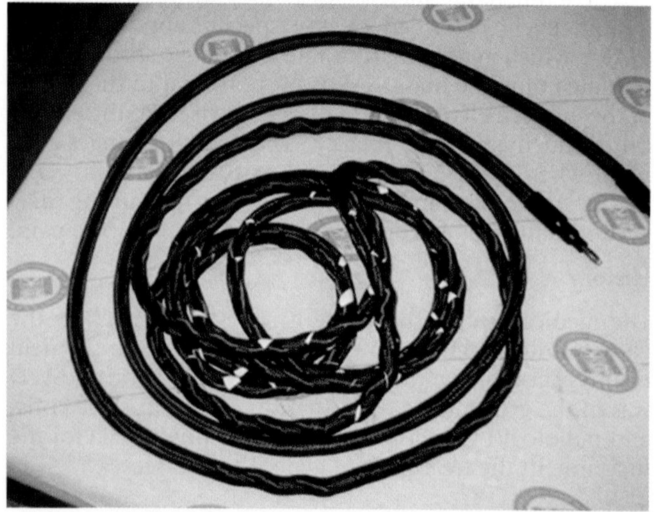

FIGURE 17-16 Inductor cable electrodes are usually wrapped around the treatment area (e.g., knee joint). They produce a strong magnetic field at the center of the coiled cable and generate heat.

Recently, pulsed SWD has also been used in the treatment of various soft tissue injuries and joint arthritis.[62] Pulsed SWD is produced by interrupting the output of conventional continuous SWD at consistent intervals. As a result of the heat dissipation during the off-time, pulsed SWD is believed to function on cellular levels by its nonthermal effects. Pulsed SWD was found to induce dose-dependent increased rates of fibroblast and chondrocyte proliferation in vitro.[85] Pulsed SWD has also been theorized to induce membrane repolarization of damaged cells, thus correcting cell dysfunction. However, a recent meta-analysis found small, significant effects of pulsed SWD on pain and muscle performance only when the power levels of SWD were high enough to induce a local thermal sensation, suggesting the role of thermal effect.[107]

Indications and Evidence Basis

Continuous SWD is the technique of choice when uniform elevation of temperature is required in the deep tissues and inside joints. As a result of the strong attenuation of ultrasound on bony structures, SWD is preferable if the target area is the interior of large joints, such as the knee, hip, or ankle. Subacute or chronic conditions respond well to continuous SWD, whereas acute lesions are better treated with pulsed SWD.[68] Heat reinforces acute inflammation, promoting further edema with exacerbation of pain. Thus, pulsed SWD is used more appropriately in the acute situation. Continuous SWD, when applied properly, is believed to have the ability to relieve pain and muscle spasm, resolve inflammation, reduce swelling, promote vasodilation, and increase soft tissue extensibility and joint range of motion.

SWD, similar to other heating modalities, may elevate pain threshold and retard nerve transmission of pain signals, resulting in the reduction of chronic pain. Muscle spasm secondary to pain from musculoskeletal disorders could be effectively reduced by deep heat provided by SWD and this in turn will contribute to the lessening of pain. Heat can also increase the elasticity of connective tissue and joint capsule if effectively delivered to the target areas, and SWD is thus ideal for the treatment of joint contracture.

Controversy exists for the effects of SWD on the treatment of osteoarthritis. Two recent control studies showed that both continuous and pulsed SWD treatments are effective short term for pain relief and improvement of function and quality of life in women with knee osteoarthritis.[16,62] However, other studies compared the additional effect of SWD on exercise training and found no further benefit.[8,151]

Contraindications and Precautions

In general, the common contraindications and precautions of SWD are similar to those for other methods of heating. For example, heating in areas with impaired sensation or patients with cognitive disability may result in burn injury. Owing to good bone penetration, heating of the epiphyseal plates in the long bones of children may affect growth, hence injudicious application of SWD to a child may lead to late side effects. SWD is contraindicated in areas with metal implants. Excessive heating and burn may be generated. SWD has also been found to have a definite adverse effect on some cardiac pacemakers. The adverse effects on pacemakers include an increase or decrease in pacemaker rate or rhythm, ventricular fibrillation, a total loss of pacing, or cessation of impulses.[95]

The FDA has issued an alert to the risk of serious injury or death if patients with implanted electrical leads are exposed to diathermy treatments, such as SWD or microwave diathermy (MWD). Deaths have been reported in patients with implanted deep brain stimulators after receiving diathermy therapy. Interaction of the diathermy energy with the implanted lead would cause excessive heating in the tissue surrounding the lead electrodes.[55]

Electromagnetic waves may selectively heat water; thus areas with excessive fluid, such as edematous tissue, moist skin, eyes, fluid-filled cavity, and pregnant or menstruating uterus, should be avoided for both SWD and microwave treatment. Towels are usually necessary to be placed between the SWD applicators and the treatment areas to absorb moisture and avoid focal hot spots on body surfaces. A rule of "no water and no metal" is generally recommended for the use of both SWD and MWD on patients (Box 17-2).

Microwave

Physics

Similar to SWD, MWD is also a modality that produces heat by converting electromagnetic energy to thermal energy. However, microwave has a shorter frequency than SWD and generates heat by oscillating the high-frequency electrical field with a lesser extent of the magnetic field to induce internal vibration of molecules that are high in polarity. The U.S. Federal Communications Commission approves industrial, scientific, and medical use of microwaves to 915 MHz (wavelength, 33 cm) and 2456 MHz (wavelength, 12 cm, more commonly used). Microwave does not penetrate tissue as deeply as shortwave or ultrasound, and its penetration decreases with the increase of microwave frequency. Focusing ability becomes more difficult for low-frequency MWD, resulting from a longer wavelength.

Techniques

A commercial MWD device usually has one or two electrodes, or applicators, operating in continuous or pulsed mode. The applicator can be round or rectangular in shape and is applied perpendicularly to the skin surface of the target site. The penetrating depth of MWD is estimated to be 3 to 5 cm. As a result of penetration limit, MWD is best for use in the area covered with low subcutaneous fat content; thus tendons, muscles, and joints can be effectively heated.

Indications and Evidence Basis

In general, the tissue response to MWD compares closely with that of SWD, and their indications and contraindications are similar. Microwave is absorbed significantly by water and thus is theoretically able to selectively heat muscle. Owing to limitation in penetration, SWD is preferable to heat superficial muscles and shallow joints.

MWD is usually used in patients with chronic neck pain, back pain, and joint arthritis. A double-blinded randomized clinical trial of MWD delivered three times a week for 4 weeks significantly improved pain and function in patients affected by moderate knee osteoarthritis, with benefits retained for at least 12 months.[150] However, recent randomized controlled studies of MWD treatment for chronic and low back pain failed to show additional benefits.[11,48]

Contraindications and Precautions

MWD treatment should be avoided in areas close to epiphysis, reproductive organs, nervous system, and fluid-filled cavity. MWD is contraindicated to be placed on, or near, a patient with a cardiac pacemaker or lead electrodes.[55,95] Epidemiologic studies on workplace safety suggest a statistically significant increase in chance of miscarriages among pregnant therapists. The risk increases with increasing level of MWD exposure.[143] Physical therapists are advised to keep at least 1 m away from MWD devices, and intermittent exposure is suggested for physical therapists who use MWD on a daily basis.[143] Currently, the use of MWD is rare because of miscarriage or health concerns of therapists (see Box 17-2).

BOX 17-2

Contraindications and Precautions of Shortwave Diathermy and Microwave Diathermy

General heat precautions
Areas with acute injury/inflammation
Reproductive organs such as ovaries or testes
Pregnant uterus
Metal implants
Near pacemaker
On epiphysis
Fluid-filled areas or organs, such as joint with effusion or inflamed synovial cavity or eyes
Menstruating uterus
On patients sitting on metal chairs or lying on metal beds

Extracorporeal Shock Wave Therapy

History

Shock wave has been used for the treatment of kidney stones for more than 30 years. The first treatment of kidney stones in patients was performed in 1980 in Munich with a prototype machine called Dornier Lithotripter HM1. The first commercial shock wave lithotripter, the Dornier HM3, was brought to the market in 1983. Currently, extracorporeal shock wave lithotripsy (ESWL) is considered the "gold standard" for the management of kidney stones. The application of shock wave in musculoskeletal disorders started from nonunion of osseous tissue (pseudarthrosis) in the late 1980s and in calcified tendinosis in the early 1990s. The first specialized shock wave device for musculoskeletal disorders, OssaTron (HMT AG), which was equipped with a free moveable therapy head, became available in 1993.[175] The term *extracorporeal shock wave therapy* (ESWT) was introduced to describe the applications of shock waves in numerous chronic disorders of the musculoskeletal system (Video 17-6).

Physics

The shock waves used in medicine are high-intensity pulsed mechanical waves with relatively low repetition frequency. Unlike therapeutic ultrasound, the temperature increase in the focal area is negligible for intensities used in therapeutic applications. Pressure amplitudes (peak positive pressure) currently used in therapeutic applications range from a few bars (atmospheric pressure) to more than 100 megapascals or MPa (1 MPa = 10 bar). Shock wave travels in a speed slightly greater than sound. At the wave front, the positive pressure rises extremely rapidly followed by a longer phase of negative pressure (Figure 17-17).

Focused shock waves can be generated in three different ways, by electrohydraulic, electromagnetic, or piezoelectric generators. The electrohydraulic generator has an electrode placed in the first focal point of a semiellipsoid reflector and high voltage is switched to the tips of the electrode to generate an electrical spark. A shock wave is released by the vaporization of the water between the electrode tips. The spherical shock waves are reflected by the metal ellipsoid reflector and focused into the second focal point, for which the therapy is adjusted to the target side of the patient's body.

The electromagnetic shock wave generator features a flat coil and an isolated conductive membrane. When a high current pulse is released through the coil, a strong magnetic field is generated and induces a secondary magnetic field with opposite polarization in the opposite membrane. The electromagnetic forces repulse and accelerate the metal membrane away from the coil to create an acoustic pulse, which is focused by an acoustic lens. Treatment target is placed at the focal point of the lens.

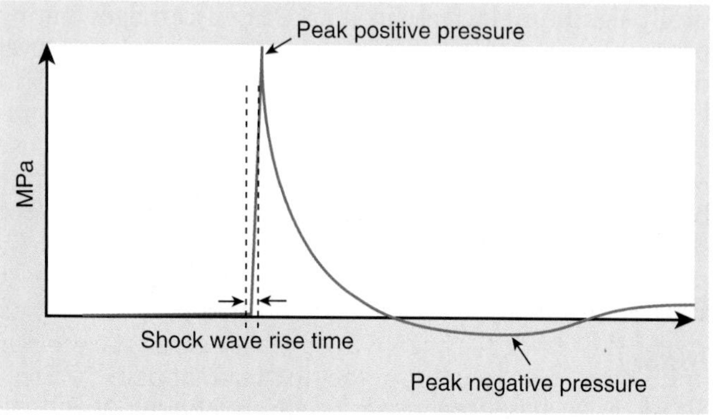

FIGURE 17-17 The pressure profile of a shock wave.

The piezoelectric shock wave generator has a few hundred to some thousand piezoelectric crystals mounted to the inner side of a spherical surface. When switching a high-voltage pulse to the crystals, they immediately contract and expand to generate pressure pulses in the surrounding medium. The pressure pulses are focused by the geometric shape of the sphere and increase in amplitudes during the propagation of the wave to the focal point where the target side of the patient is positioned.

The generated pressure pulses are concentrated into small focal areas of 2 to 8 mm in diameter, depending on the generators, to optimize therapeutic effects and minimize side effects on surrounding tissues. The term *energy flux density* (EFD, in mJ/mm^2) is used to describe the "dose" of shock wave energy in a perpendicular direction to the direction of propagation. There remains no consensus as to the definition of "high" and "low" energy ESWT, but as a guideline, low-energy ESWT has EFD from 0.08 to 0.28 mJ/mm^2, medium energy from 0.28 to 0.60 mJ/mm^2, and high energy greater than 0.60 mJ/mm^2.[155,170] Another frequently used definition has low-energy ESWT as EFD less than 0.12 mJ/mm^2 and high energy as greater than 0.12 mJ/mm^2.[170]

In recent years, a new type of shock wave, radial shock wave, emerged for the treatment of tendinopathy and has been shown to be effective.[36] Radial shock wave therapy (RSWT), compared with conventional focused shock wave, does not have a focus at the site of the effect. The waves disperse eccentrically from the applicator tip and have the advantage of wider effective regions without the requirement of precisely locating the painful points. Pressure waves of RSWT are generated by accelerating a projectile, with compressed air, through a tube at the end of which an applicator is placed. The projectile hits the applicator and the applicator transmits the generated pressure waves into the body. The pressure amplitude is usually a few bars instead of tens of megapascals in focused shock waves.

Techniques

Two to three thousand shock waves for three consecutive sessions applied at weekly intervals are usually recommended. Ultrasonography is usually used to determine the location and depth of the pathologic site as shock wave target. However, there is no consensus as to the appropriate number of sessions and impulses of shock waves, as well as treatment on either the painful site or the lesion site. Setting the highest and mostly tolerable energy output within medium intensity ranges is an ideal option when applying focused shock wave therapy on soft tissue disorders. High-intensity treatment is usually reserved for the treatment of bony nonunion, but may induce local swelling and pain, and usually requires local analgesia, which is known to reduce its effectiveness. Thus, high-energy ESWT is usually performed in a hospital or ambulatory surgery center, whereas medium-energy to low-energy ESWT or RSWT is usually performed in the office without anesthesia.

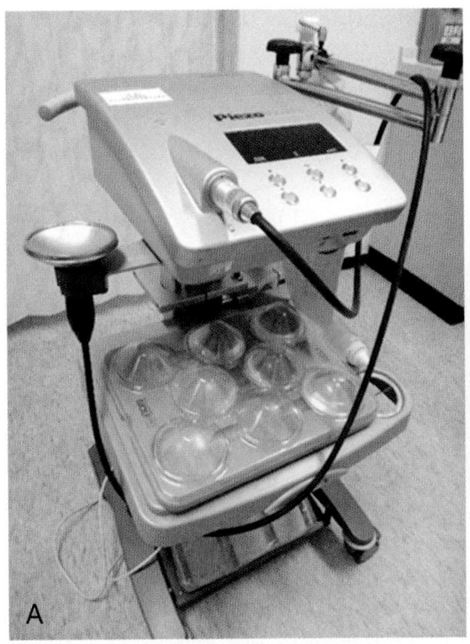

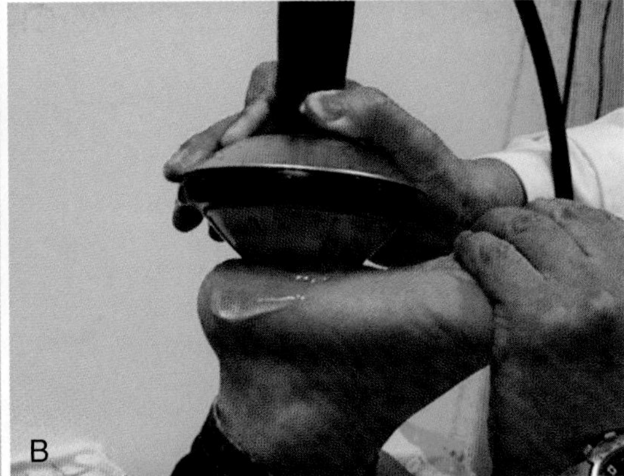

FIGURE 17-18 **A,** A commercial piezoelectric shock wave device. **B,** Shock wave treatment on a patient with plantar fasciitis.

Indications and Evidence Basis

The use of shock wave in the treatment of plantar fasciitis is well studied and approved by the FDA. The biological mechanisms are thought to include destroying sensory unmyelinated nerve fibers and eliciting neovascularization in degenerative plantar fascia[88,138] (Figure 17-18). There is level 1 evidence for the benefit of focused shock wave in the treatment of chronic plantar fasciitis, and the success rates are around 60% to 70% at 6-month follow-up.[15,170,194] High-intensity shock wave is not necessarily more effective in terms of success rate than low-intensity or radial shock wave.[194] Elevated energy efflux density tends to relieve pain more.[36,114]

ESWT has been shown to have the ability to stimulate bone remodeling. Clinical success has been reported by many authors as an alternative to surgical treatment for fractures, bony nonunion, and delayed union, and yields better short-term clinical outcomes.[31] However, controversy still exists.[196] The union rate in hypertrophic nonunions seems to be significantly higher than that in atrophic nonunions.[196]

The use of shock wave therapy in the treatment of lateral epicondylitis has been approved by the FDA. However, conflicting results exist regarding its effect. A systematic review and metaanalysis on the effectiveness for lateral epicondylitis suggests no beneficial effect.[22] There is no high-quality randomized controlled study for radial shock wave.

There is consistent level 1 evidence of at least 6 months effectiveness of focused shock wave, particular for medium-intensity regimes, in reducing pain, dissolving calcifications, and improving shoulder function for patients with rotator cuff calcified tendinopathy.[91] The treatment effects can be maintained over the following 6 months.[91] Less robust evidence is present for RSWT.[170] So far, there is no solid evidence for shock wave in noncalcified shoulder tendinopathy.

BOX 17-3

Complications of Shock Wave Treatment

Soft tissue swelling
Ecchymosis or hematoma
Redness of the skin
Increased pain
Skin erosion
Nerve lesion
Transient bone edema
Humeral head osteonecrosis

Contraindications and Precautions

Contraindications to ESWT or RSWT include bleeding disorders and pregnancy. Side effects of shock wave treatment are usually minor, especially when set at medium to low intensity for soft tissue disorders (Box 17-3). However, one should be aware that there are case reports of humeral head osteonecrosis after ESWT of rotator cuff tendinopathy, probably as a result of damage to the blood supply of the humeral head during treatment.[49,116]

Electrotherapy

History

Electrotherapy has been used for treating people since the days of ancient Egyptians and Hippocrates.[184] Electric eel and fish capable of producing electricity were used to treat headache and joint pains. The Leyden jar was invented in 1745 and was one of the first medical electrical stimulation devices used for the treatment of pain.[183a] Electrotherapy devices then underwent an evolution in technology from franklinism, through galvanism, faradism,

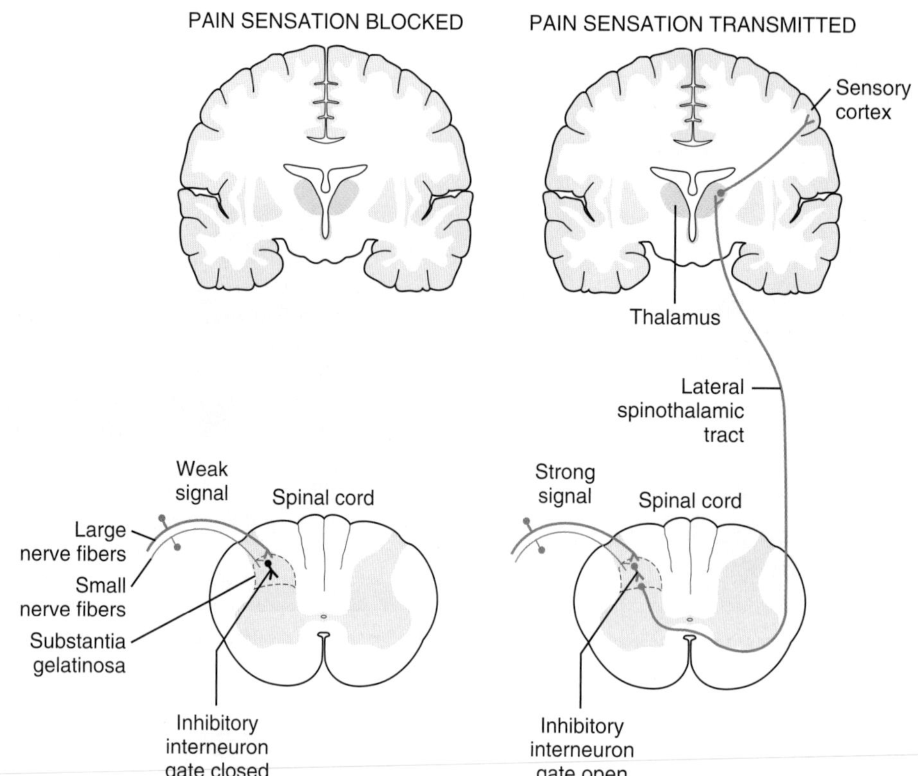

FIGURE 17-19 Several animal and human studies have supported the theories of descending inhibitory pathway stimulation and release of endogenous opioids and other neurotransmitters. (From Mathews JA: The effects of spinal traction, *Physiotherapy* 58:64-66, 1972.)

and d'arsonvalisation, reaching its golden age in the nineteenth century.[82]

Transcutaneous electrical nerve stimulation (TENS) devices have been around since the late nineteenth century,[166] with claims of use in a variety of medical indications including "reversal of apparent death." Overuse of this fancy new modality eventually led to widespread criticism by the mid-twentieth century and its use subsided.[136] However, Melzack and Wall's gate control theory of pain was published in 1965,[128] which triggered a revival of interest in the medical community for the use of electrotherapy in treating pain. TENS devices and other electrotherapy devices have been widely used since then in medicine for various indications (Video 17-7).

Physiology and Mechanism of Action

It was initially speculated that electrical stimulation dilated blood vessels and separated the clogging particles of stagnant fluid, thereby stimulating blood flow.[136] Subsequently, increased understanding of human neuromuscular and electrophysiology led to a better understanding of the mechanism of action of electrotherapy devices in the relief of pain and restoration of muscle and nerve function.

The mechanism of action of electrotherapy devices on pain can be broadly summarized as: (1) segmental inhibition of pain signals to the brain and the dorsal horn of the spinal cord (Melzack and Wall's gate control theory[128]), and (2) activation of descending inhibitory pathways and stimulation of the release of endogenous opioids and other neurotransmitters such as serotonin, gamma-aminobutyric acid, noradrenaline, and acetylcholine.[82]

The gate control theory[128] hypothesizes that small nociceptive afferents from A-delta and C fibers hold the central "gate" open, whereas stimulation of large afferents from A-beta fibers (carrying touch, pressure, and vibration sensations) can close this gate and inhibit transmission of pain signals to the brain (Figure 17-19).

Currently, electrotherapy is used in a variety of clinical indications including preventing or treating pain, neuromuscular disease, restriction of motion, wound and tissue healing, and edema management.[176] Electrotherapy is thought to help in the disorders discussed earlier based on its effect on reducing muscle spasms, slowing or preventing disuse atrophy, stimulating muscle and blood circulation, improving joint range of motion, and promoting wound and tissue healing. Electrotherapy is also used to enhance drug delivery in iontophoresis and related applications (Table 17-6).

Types of Electrotherapy

Transcutaneous Electrical Nerve Stimulation

TENS devices are small, widely used, portable (usually battery operated) units that deliver electric current to the skin through surface electrodes. After education in its use is provided (usually by a physical therapist) to the patient,

Table 17-6 Electrotherapy Modalities and Indications

Modality	Indications
Transcutaneous electrical nerve stimulation (TENS)	Nociceptive pain: Acute, subacute, or chronic pain Neuropathic pain
Percutaneous electrical nerve stimulation (PENS)	Mild to moderate pain
Electrical twitch-obtaining intramuscular stimulation (ETOIMS)	Myofascial pain syndrome (MPS)
Interferential current (IFC)	Musculoskeletal conditions Neurologic conditions Incontinence
Electrical myostimulation (EMS)	Sarcopenia MPS
High-voltage galvanic stimulation (HVGS)	Wounds Weakness Fatigue
Microcurrent	Depression Posttraumatic stress disorder Anxiety Neuropathic pain Fibromyalgia
Iontophoresis	Pain treatment: Acute, subacute, or chronic Soft tissue inflammation Pain prophylaxis Swelling

the device is self-administered by the patient as instructed. Sometimes, several instructional sessions are needed to establish optimal stimulation settings and electrode placement sites.

TENS units specifications and characteristics can vary widely among the commercially available devices used and clinician preference.[99] However, commonly used TENS units are either conventional or traditional TENS (frequency greater than 50 Hz) or low-frequency or acupuncture-like TENS (frequency of 1 to 10 Hz).[169] Within each type, the patient can usually adjust the intensity (amplitude), width (duration), rate (frequency), and mode (pattern) of flow of electric current based on their desired effect.[82] Conventional TENS provides a tingling sensation to the patient, whereas the acupuncture-like TENS provides a burning, needling sensation.[99] TENS devices may also be modified such that the stimulation parameters are cyclically changed during a single treatment application.[169]

The effectiveness of TENS devices has been studied extensively. Early on, Melzack and Wall[129] reported there was no longer any doubt that TENS was effective in chronic pain. However, effectiveness of TENS in treating pain and other clinical disorders has been researched and questioned widely since then. Poor design of clinical trials and lack of homogeneity of the patient population has severely impeded the strength and quality of evidence obtained and the generalizability of its findings.

TENS has been used extensively for treatment of chronic low back pain despite a lack of good quality studies supporting its use. An evidence-based review on treatments for chronic low back pain concluded that because of low-quality evidence there is nothing to support that TENS is any more effective than placebo or sham TENS in reducing pain or improving functional status.[37] A systematic review evaluating TENS therapy for chronic low back pain found that it was no more effective than sham TENS.[96] Based on a review of evidence, in 2012, the Centers for Medicare and Medicaid Services published a memorandum stating that "TENS is not reasonable and necessary for the treatment of CLBP (chronic low back pain)."[42]

However, in painful diabetic peripheral polyneuropathy TENS unit has been found effective in several studies.[59,82,104,105] Development of tolerance has been reported to be an issue with continued use of TENS devices limiting the long-term effectiveness of such therapy. TENS therapy has also been found useful to treat neuropathic pain in patients with spinal cord injury.[35] In MPS, one study used TENS as one of the control groups and found level 2 evidence against the use of TENS unit in the treatment of MPS[12] For myofascial trigger points, compared with placebo, TENS was found to be superior.[27] However, relief was short lived with no persistence of relief after 1 to 3 months. In comparison, relief provided by frequency-modulated neural stimulation, a variety of TENS, appeared to last longer (3 months) than the relief provided by conventional TENS.[27]

Interferential Current

Interferential current therapy (IFC) is a type of electrotherapy modality that uses alternating medium-frequency electric current (4000 Hz) signals of slightly different frequencies.

When two waves of slightly different frequencies interact, two types of "interference" take place. When the waves are in phase (the peaks or troughs of the two waves are in sync) they summate and exhibit "constructive interference." When the two waves are out of phase (the peaks or troughs of the two waves are out of sync) they subtract and exhibit "destructive interference."[69] Based on the degree of synchronization, the resultant wave may have a range of amplitudes, from double the amplitude of the two waves (when perfectly synchronized) to zero (when perfectly unsynchronized) amplitude (Figure 17-20).

This results in a new wave with cyclically modulated amplitude. The frequency of the resultant wave equals the difference in frequency between the two signals.[69] In the practical application of IFC devices, the parameters of signal frequency, beat frequency, amplitude, and cycle time can be adjusted as needed.

The purported advantage of IFC therapy over low-frequency TENS devices is the ability of IFC to decrease skin impedance, thereby penetrating tissue more easily.[61,69,164] Frequency modulation can help to limit neural adaptation.[97] Amplitude can be fixed or modulated so that the point of maximum amplitude interference changes. This provides another advantage with IFC therapy because of its ability to generate a low-frequency current deep within the treatment area resulting from its amplitude-modulated parameters.[61] IFC machines come with two, four, or six applicators that can be arranged in the same plane (planar), or in different planes (coplanar).[10] With these adjustments, IFC devices can be used effectively even when the treatment area is large or poorly defined (Figure 17-21).

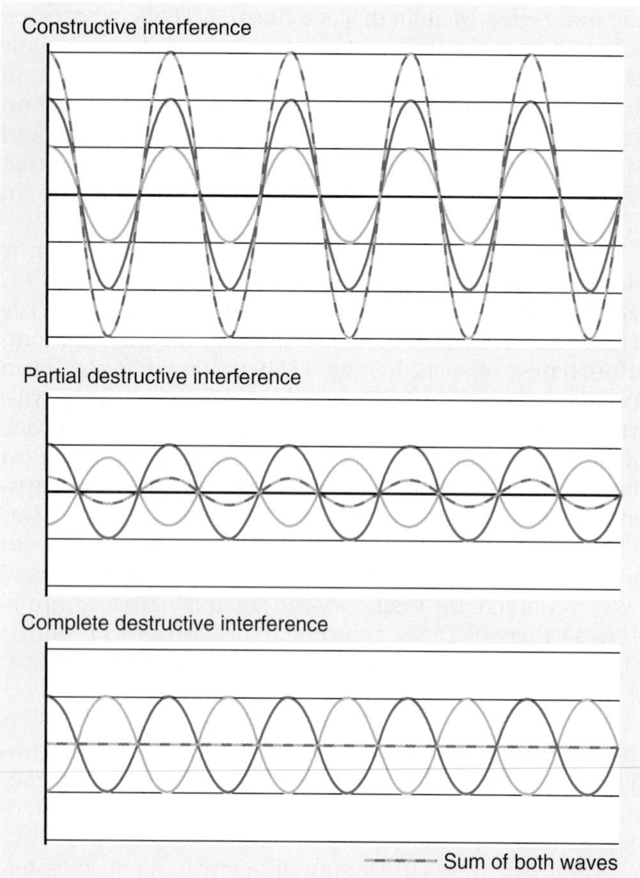

FIGURE 17-20 Constructive and destructive interference of two waves.

Some IFC devices also allow for on-off cycling. IFC treatment parameters can be manipulated to produce stimulation parameters similar to the different types of TENS devices.[97,98] However, a significant advantage that IFC has over TENS is that it can deliver higher current than a TENS device.[97]

IFC therapy has been successfully used in a variety of musculoskeletal and neurologic conditions, as well as in the management of urinary incontinence,[47,71,93,97,164] although some literature fails to demonstrate its superiority over other interventions or placebo.[61,139] Fuentes et al.[61] performed a thorough systematic review and metaanalysis on the use of IFC in musculoskeletal pain. They retrieved 2235 articles out of which only 20 met the quality threshold. Based on their review, they concluded that when applied alone, IFC does not provide any unique attributable benefit over placebo. However, in combination with a multimodal treatment plan, IFC was found to be superior to placebo. In chronic low back pain, IFC combination therapy showed effectiveness even at 3 months. They also noted that as a result of heterogeneity of the patient population and study design no conclusive statements could be made about IFC monotherapy, and further research was recommended.[61,147]

Iontophoresis

Iontophoresis is the technique of using the charges of ions and particles to drive them across tissues and membranes under the influence of an imposed electrical field. Use of iontophoresis in humans was first reported by Richardson ("father of iontophoresis") when he used it in dental anesthesia with a compound of chloroform and aconite.[84] After the 1870s, iontophoresis and the study of electricity guided transdermal transport of drugs were more prevalent.[84] Iontophoresis is also referred to as "an injection without the needle." To produce this effect, a positive and

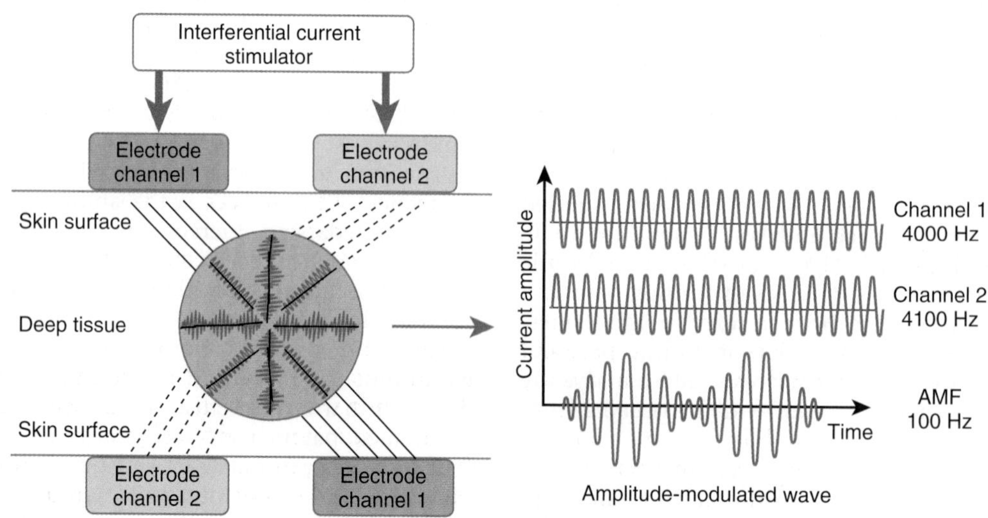

FIGURE 17-21 The principles of generating of an amplitude-modulated interference wave (amplitude modulation frequency, AMF). An interferential current that is modulated in its amplitude is thought to be produced by the delivery of two out-of-phase currents across the surface of the skin. It is claimed that AMF excites deep-seated nervous tissue, leading to analgesia, because its frequency is within the range for excitable tissue. (Reprinted from *Phys Ther* 2003;83(3):208-223, with permission of the American Physical Therapy Association. © 2003 American Physical Therapy Association.)

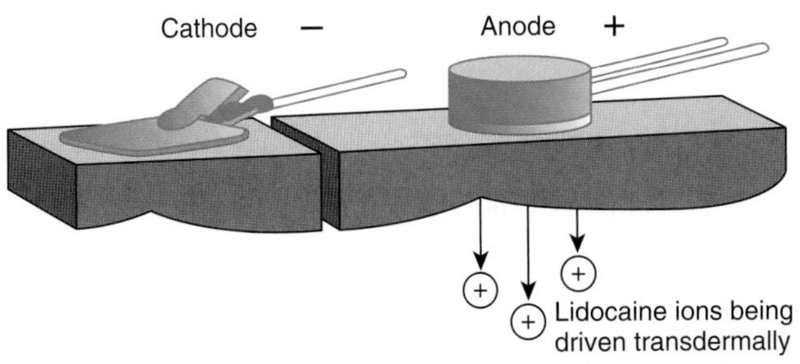

FIGURE 17-22 The dose of solution successfully transported depends on various factors including local current density, skin impedance, duration of treatment, and the solution concentration.

negative charge is applied to the skin to administer a drug transdermally (Video 17-8).

The solution to be phoresed is placed on the electrode of the same polarity, and then the negative, positive, and ground electrodes are applied to the skin. A direct current, typically between 10 and 30 mA, is applied to drive the solution away from the electrode and into the surrounding tissues.[168] For example, lidocaine is a positively charged solvent, therefore when placed under the iontophoresis anode it is repelled into the epidermal layer beneath the lead (Figure 17-22; Video 17-9).

The primary use of iontophoresis in medicine is to aid in transcutaneous systemic or local delivery of medicines and substances. It can also be used for systemic drug delivery because it avoids first-pass hepatic metabolism, and problems associated with oral or intravenous routes such as gastric irritation and variability of serum concentration; however, in physical medicine, iontophoresis is primarily used to deliver medicines directly to soft tissues such as to treat inflammatory conditions such as lateral epicondylitis[193] and shoulder tendonitis.[108] For such purposes, the drugs administered with iontophoresis include corticosteroids such as dexamethasone,[74] local anesthetics such as lidocaine,[193] and acetic acid.[108]

Lidocaine iontophoresis (1% to 4% lidocaine, with or without epinephrine, at 20 mA/min to 80 mA/min dose applied for 5 to 10 minutes) has been used effectively to mitigate pain during needle insertion procedures such as arterial or venous cannulation.[132,167] Pretreatment with iontophoresis has also been shown to significantly reduce pain associated with needle electromyography.[13]

Microcurrent

Microcurrent devices use electric current of extremely low amplitude (millionths of an ampere). Microcurrent devices can deliver the stimulation directly to the brain by means of earclip electrodes or directly to the body. Earclip electrode stimulation is typically delivered with a protocol called cranial electrotherapy stimulation (CES), and body stimulation with regular electrodes is often referred to as microcurrent electrical therapy. Alpha-Stim is a commercially available medical device that uses both microcurrent stimulation protocols. CES has been widely studied in the treatment of mental health conditions such as anxiety, depression, and insomnia.[106,157] However, CES has also been studied in painful disorders such as fibromyalgia and neuropathic pain.[173,174] A study by Taylor et al.[174] revealed some benefit in pain, fatigue, sleep, and functional improvement in patients with fibromyalgia with CES when compared with sham device or usual care. A study by Tan et al.[173] showed that CES provided small but statistically significant improvement in neuropathic pain in patients with spinal cord injury.

Other Electrical Modalities

Electrical twitch-obtaining intramuscular stimulation (ETOIMS) is an emerging type of electrotherapy device.[12] It has been used for pain relief in MPS. ETOIMS is a technique with which a clinician applies electricity through a monopolar needle electromyography electrode to potentially stimulate deep motor end plates, thereby eliciting a twitch response.[40] This technique is based on modification of the principle behind the mechanism of action of acupuncture or dry needling. Three studies by the same author reported case series studying the effect of ETOIMS in MPS.[39-41] These studies provided level 4 evidence, which is neither for nor against the use of ETOIMS, for chronic refractory pain in MPS.[12]

One study reported the effect of direct current therapy in MPS and found similar effect in both groups: direct current therapy alone or lidocaine iontophoresis with direct current therapy.[12]

High-voltage galvanic stimulation (HVGS) uses intensities of 50 to 75 V, stimulated at a frequency of 100 pulses per second and a negative electrode polarity. HVGS has been studied extensively in wound healing,[3,145] with mixed results. It has also been used to improve fatigue and weakness.[101]

Precautions and Complications

Electrotherapy devices should not be used near implanted or temporary stimulators (pacemakers, intrathecal pumps, spinal cord stimulators, etc.) because of the potential for interference with the function of these devices.[69,97] There is also the potential for abnormal vascular responses when electrotherapy is used near sympathetic ganglia or the carotid sinus.[97] IFC should not be used near open incisions or abrasions because of the potential for concentration of electric current.[97] Electrotherapy devices should not be used near the gravid uterus because of potential adverse effects on fetal development or the possibility for stimulating uterine contractions.[69,97] There is a possibility that deep venous thrombosis can be dislodged and propagated resulting in emboli if electrotherapy induces the stimulation of vascular smooth muscle, thereby dislodging a clot within.[69,97] Other precautions include insensate skin or a patient with cognitive impairment. Partial or full-thickness burns can also be a complication of incorrectly applied electrotherapy devices.[58] It is also important that the electrodes used with electrotherapy devices are recommended for that specific electrotherapy device, because not all electrodes are manufactured with the same specifications. Mismatched electrodes can result in unsafe performance, which can increase risk of burns. Iontophoresis is generally well tolerated, although some of the reported minor transient symptoms are pruritus, erythema, or a feeling of warmth.[13]

CASE 2

Electrotherapy

Background: A 49-year-old man with a 9-month history of right shoulder pain presents to the shoulder clinic. He reports pain with overhead activities such as reaching into cabinets, shelving, etc. Lifting objects or doing grooming tasks such as combing hair is also reportedly painful. Oral medications including NSAIDs have provided limited relief. Physical examination including the Neer test and the Hawkins test indicated shoulder impingement and subacromial bursitis. X-rays and other diagnostics did not indicate any structural abnormalities.

Impression: Right shoulder impingement syndrome and subacromial bursitis.

Treatment Plan: Physical therapy was prescribed. Therapeutic exercises performed in physical therapy consisted of passive and active range-of-motion exercises, and gradually progressive strengthening exercises of the scapular stabilizers and rotator cuff muscles as tolerated. However, the patient continued to report pain that limited his participation and progress. Iontophoresis with dexamethasone was initiated. The patient was treated with iontophoresis with IontoPatch to the right subacromial region with dexamethasone. He was educated regarding the use of a portable unit of IontoPatch with dexamethasone for home use. Iontophoresis was delivered at 0.12 mA/min applied for a total of 840 minutes (14 hours), delivering a total of 1.1 mg of dexamethasone for a total dose of 80 mA/min. At the end of 14 hours of treatment, the patient's pain decreased by 75%. He then proceeded further in physical therapy with therapeutic exercises as planned and was discharged home to continue his home exercises, which included range-of-motion exercises and strengthening/stabilization exercises.

Response: The patient's pain resolved and activity limitations were alleviated. He returned to his previous asymptomatic baseline.

Discussion:

- Is steroid iontophoresis a useful treatment for subacromial bursitis?
- Is steroid iontophoresis preferable to subacromial steroid injection?
- What are the added benefits of therapeutic exercises?
- What are the contraindications to use of iontophoresis?
- What are the expected outcomes of steroid iontophoresis in other inflammatory musculoskeletal disorders?
- When are modalities such as iontophoresis counterproductive to the long-term outcome of the patient?

Low-Level Laser Therapy

History

The term *laser* is an acronym for light amplification of stimulated emissions of radiation. Lasers have many important applications. They are used in common consumer electronic devices such as DVD players, laser printers, and barcode scanners in a supermarket. They are also used in industry for cutting and welding, and in the military for guiding missiles. In medicine, lasers are useful in surgical treatments for cutting and coagulation.

In 1917, Albert Einstein established the theoretical foundations for the laser in his paper "On the Quantum Theory of Radiation." Many theoretical and research works followed. The first functioning laser device was proposed in 1960 by Theodore H. Maiman at Hughes Research Laboratories. The first medical treatment with a laser on a human patient was performed in 1961 by Dr. Charles J. Campbell at Columbia-Presbyterian Hospital in Manhattan for the treatment of a retinal tumor.[156] The first report of laser applications in the musculoskeletal field was by Mester et al.[130] on wound healing in the 1960s.

Physics and Bioeffects

When an excited electron returns to its ground state, a photon is released. When having an environment with unlimited excited electrons by applying an external power source to a lasing medium, a triggering photon would cause a chain reaction to generate many photons when contained in a pumping chamber (light amplification). The chamber usually has a totally reflective mirror at one end and another semipermeable mirror at the other end. When a specific level of energy is attained, photons of a particular wavelength are released through the semipermeable mirror and produce coherent, monochromatic, and collimated laser light (stimulated emissions of radiation).

Photons of a single color move in parallel and in phase to one direction. The material capable of generating laser light is called the lasing medium, which can be gas, solid, or liquid. The red helium neon (HeNe, 632.8 nm) and infrared semiconductor diodes such as gallium arsenide (GaAs, 904 nm) or aluminum gallium arsenide (AlGaAs, 808 nm) lasers are the two principal lasers for medical applications. Currently, low-level laser therapy (LLLT) devices are commonly produced from semiconductor diodes because of the relative ease of production and the better penetration of infrared into biological tissues to treat musculoskeletal conditions. LLLT is relatively low in energy, usually from a few milliwatts (mW) to 100 to 200 mW, and is applied for short periods of time (seconds to minutes), which produces insignificant changes in tissue temperature (measured to be around 1.0° C). LLLT is thought to have a stimulating effect on target tissues and is used to decrease pain and inflammation, stimulate collagen metabolism and wound healing,[130] and promote fracture healing. The exact mechanism is still under investigation but the effect on inflammation modulation and cell proliferation has been proposed.[5,65]

Techniques

The laser probe is usually placed perpendicular to the skin surface of the target area in a short distance to maximize the energy transmission. For most commercial devices, only the treatment time and the intensity can be adjusted. However, there is lack of consensus for the dose, duration, and type of laser on therapeutic effect, leaving treatment measurements to be determined largely empirically. Combining lasers of two different wavelengths is increasing in popularity in recent devices. For example,

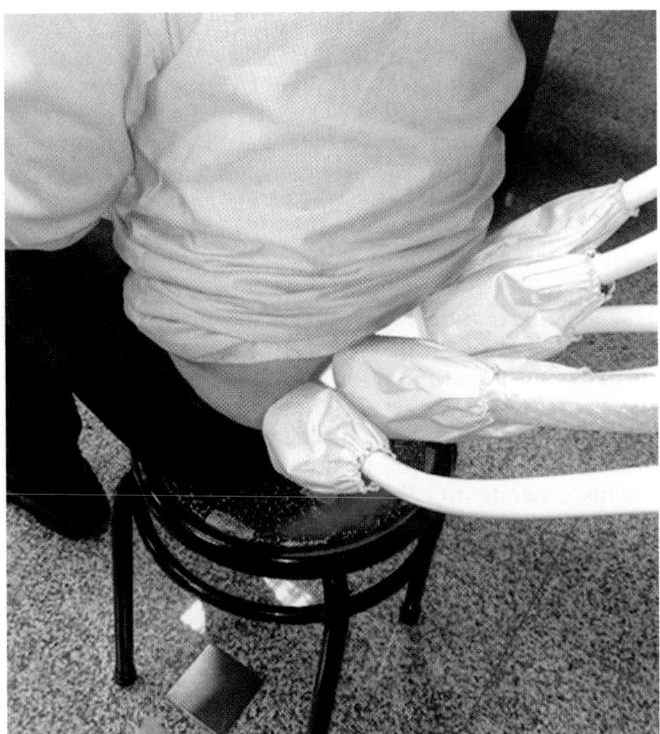

FIGURE 17-23 The application of low-level laser therapy for low back pain.

the laser device shown in Figure 17-23 has six probes, each consisting of diodes emitting lasers of two wavelengths, 660 and 780 nm. A towel is sometimes wrapped around the probe to avoid incidental reflection of laser light to eyes.

Indications and Evidence Basis

Many previous studies have shown the in vitro and in vivo effects of LLLT on wound healing,[130] but clinical trials with human models do not provide sufficient evidence to establish the usefulness of LLLT as an effective tool in wound care, especially diabetic foot ulcer, at present.[21]

Randomized controlled trials show pain reduction immediately after treatment in patients with acute neck pain, and up to 22 weeks after completion of treatment in those with chronic neck pain of various etiologies,[38,73] probably through its effect on nerves.[131] Systematic reviews and metaanalysis also show the effect of LLLT on pain reduction for different joints, including wrist, fingers, knee, temporomandibular joints, etc.[23,92] Its effect on lateral epicondylitis (tennis elbow) is debated, but a recent review suggests short-term pain relief and reduction in disability with both LLLT alone and in conjunction with an exercise regimen.[24]

Contraindications and Precautions

Laser has been well recognized as being potentially dangerous. Even the low-power lasers with only a few milliwatts of output power can be hazardous to human eyes if the beam hits the eye directly or after reflection from a shiny surface. Also, LLLT should not be used in areas with cancerous tissue.

CASE 3

Ultrasound Diathermy and Extracorporeal Shock Wave Therapy

Background: A 52-year-old woman complained of left shoulder pain of more than 3 months' duration. She felt sharp pain while lifting objects or when performing shoulder internal rotation. She visited an outpatient clinic where oral medication (including an NSAID and muscle relaxant) was given, but the effect was limited. She consulted a physiatrist in a teaching hospital, where she was found to have calcified supraspinatus tendinopathy after musculoskeletal ultrasound and physical examinations. The ultrasound report indicated a dense calcified lesion located in the medial part of a swollen and hypoechoic supraspinatus tendon. Her shoulder also showed approximately 20 degrees of limitation in internal rotation.

Impression: Supraspinatus tendinopathy, left side.

Treatment Plan: Initially, oral NSAIDs and physical therapy were prescribed. The physical therapy consisted of ultrasound diathermy for 5 minutes at the calcified spots and passive range-of-motion exercise for 10 minutes after the ultrasound treatment. She visited the physical therapy gym three times a week for 1 month, but the response was limited. She still complained of frequent sharp pain, which sometimes interrupted her sleep. Therefore, an echo-guided injection of 20 mg 0.5 mL triamcinolone mixed with 3.5 mL 1% lidocaine into the left subdeltoid bursa was performed. Her discomfort reduced 50% 2 weeks after the injection. Extracorporeal shock wave therapy was then arranged. She underwent a weekly shock wave treatment of her left shoulder with a medium intensity (0.28 to 0.45 J/mm^2) three times. The depth and frequency settings were 15 mm and 6 Hz, respectively. The patient was advised to continue her physical therapy, which included passive range-of-motion exercise and muscle strengthening.

Response: The patient's symptoms diminished (pain decreased from 7/10 to 1 to 2/10 on a visual analog pain scale) 6 months after the shock wave treatment.

Discussion:

- Is ultrasound diathermy a useful tool for calcified shoulder tendinopathy?
- Is steroid injection adequate and necessary before shock wave therapy?
- What can be done for sharp pain if an oral NSAID or a pain killer has failed?
- Is the calcified lesion responsible for the shoulder pain?
- Is the treatment effect attributable to extracorporeal shock wave therapy, physical therapy, or steroid injection?
- How to differentiate shoulder tendinopathy and the early stage of frozen shoulder?
- If steroid injection is indicated, which one, the bursa or joint space, is a better target?

Other Modalities: International Perspective

Acupuncture

History and Theory

Acupuncture is the procedure of inserting and manipulating filiform needles into various points (called acupuncture points) to relieve pain or for other therapeutic purposes. Acupuncture is an important component of traditional Chinese medicine (TCM) and medicine of some other Asian countries such as Japan and Korea. It has been used for several thousand years. Acupuncture was first systematically published in a classic Chinese book, *Huang Di Nei Jing*, meaning "Yellow Emperor's Inner Canon" in English, in the 100s BC. The principles stated in the book have guided practitioners in the past and also in modern time. Acupuncture was introduced to Europe in the eighteenth century and later to North America and other regions, and it has become steadily popular. There has been a significant increase in the use of complementary and alternative medicine (CAM) in the United States during the past 2 decades.[19] Acupuncture is the most frequently used form of CAM in the United States.

In TCM, the framework of diagnosis and point selection for treatment is based on the theoretical network of the meridian system (Figure 17-24) and the internal organ subsystem interrelated to the meridian system, where the names of the internal organs are regarded as the names for the subsystem with particular functionalities rather than the actual anatomic entities. The names of the internal organ subsystems that are used to name the meridians include Lung, Pericardium, Heart, Large Intestine, San Jiao (Triple Warmer), Small Intestine, Bladder, Gall Bladder, Stomach, Spleen, Kidney, and Liver. The twelve principal meridians consist of three pairs of Yin and Yang meridians in a limb: Hand Tai Yin—Lung, Hand Yue Yin—Pericardium, Hand Shao Yin—Heart, Hand Yang Ming—Large Intestine, Hand Shao Yang—San Jiao, Hand Tai Yang—Small Intestine, Foot Tai Yin—Spleen, Foot Yue Yin—Liver, Foot Shao Yin—Kidney, Foot Yang Ming—Stomach, Foot Shao Yang—Gallbladder, and Foot Tai Yang—Bladder. There are also eight extraordinary meridians: Conception Vessel (Ren Mai), Governing Vessel (Du Mai), Penetrating Vessel (Chong Mai), Girdle Vessel (Dai Mai), Yin-linking Vessel (Yin Wei Mai), Yang-linking Vessel (Yang Wei Mai), Yin Heel Vessel (Yin Qiao Mai), and Yang Heel Vessel (Yang Qiao Mai). Another set of points that are also commonly used are the points at each vertebra along the spine slightly lateral to the midline bilaterally, called Hua Tuo Jia Ji (HTJJ) points, named after Hua Tuo, one of the most famous ancient Chinese physicians (110-207 AD). Those points are not only important in the treatment of spine-related pain conditions but also commonly used in treating other internal organ disorders. The hypothesized mechanism is that the stimulation of the HTJJ points not only has an impact on the nerve roots but also on the paraspinal muscles and the sympathetic chain along the spine.[32]

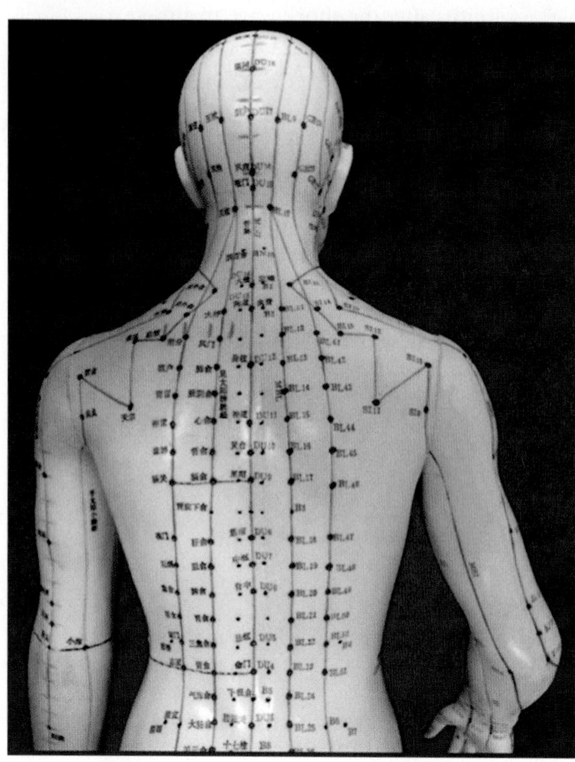

FIGURE 17-24 Acupuncture model with meridians.

According to the basic theory of TCM, the internal organs generate and the meridian system transports vital energy ("Qi" and "Blood") to every part of the body to keep the physiologic function in balance. A person is presumed to suffer from diseases when the vital energy is not flowing smoothly resulting from blockage or stagnation along the meridians. The etiology of the disease state is usually categorized as an internal pathologic condition, such as sadness, anger, or fear, and an external assault, such as "wind," cold, heat, or dampness. Acupuncture is supposed to restore the flow of vital energy and to bring the human body to a new balanced state in homeostasis.

Possible Mechanism

Even though acupuncture has been used for several thousand years and has showed clear clinical benefits, the mechanism behind it has not been fully explained by the Western medical system. In the past several decades much research has been done on the mechanism of acupuncture. Pain is the most common condition encountered in physiatric practices and acupuncture is probably the most thoroughly researched physical modality in medicine with regard to its analgesic effects. Research has indicated that the possible mechanism for the effectiveness of acupuncture includes the descending and ascending inhibition of pain (gate theory), the hormonal mechanism (endorphin regulation), the interaction with the autonomic nervous system, and local effects.[66] Melzack[127] has suggested that all pain input enters the spinal cord. Pain impulses travel along the small nerve fibers. The large myelinated nerve fibers have an inhibitory effect on pain, by closing the gate to pain at the spinal cord level. If pain is not transmitted to the brain, no pain is perceived. Acupuncture stimulates large myelinated nerve fibers, thereby closing the gate to pain.[127] It is probable that acupuncture works partially through the gate control theory, although this cannot be seen as a complete explanation of its mechanism. The effects of acupuncture on pain control involve the release of endogenous opioids and neurotransmitters in the body. Acupuncture increases the endorphin level in various parts of the central nervous system and beta-endorphin can be shown to attenuate chronic pain.[7] Analgesia produced by auricular acupuncture can be blocked by the opiate antagonist naloxone, indicating the role of endorphinergic systems in the underlying mechanisms of auriculotherapy.[140] The development of neuroimaging tools, such as positron emission tomography (PET) and functional magnetic resonance imaging (fMRI), has taken the study of the effects of acupuncture on the activity of the human brain to another level. Studies with PET have shown that thalamic asymmetry present among patients with chronic pain was reduced after acupuncture treatment. There are studies that have reported on the relationship between particular acupuncture points and visual-cortex activation on fMRI. These powerful new tools open the possibility to new scientific studies on this ancient therapy.[165]

Needles and Insertion Techniques

An acupuncture needle is divided into five parts: tip, body, root, handle, and tail. The tip and body of a needle are the parts inserted into the body on the acupuncture points. The handle and tail of a needle are the parts used by a practitioner to manipulate the needle. The root connects the body and handle of a needle. Commonly used acupuncture needles are made of stainless steel with sizes from 26 to 40 gauge and lengths from 0.5 inches to 2.5 inches. Because of its small size, very often people claim that the acupuncture needle is a "painless needle." The tip of an acupuncture needle is blunt even though it is very tiny. Compared with the tip of a regular needle with the same gauge number, the tip of an acupuncture needle has less chance of cutting the tissue (Video 17-10).

Depending on the location of acupuncture points to be used, patient's preference, and patient's tolerance to certain positions, a patient can be placed in the supine, prone, recumbent, or sitting positions. The lying position is usually preferred because of the possibility of fainting in some patients from needling, especially in a patient who has the treatment for the first time.

There are four common ways in inserting a needle: finger pressing insertion, pinching needle insertion, pinching skin insertion, and tight skin insertion.[34] The skin at the insertion site is cleaned with an alcohol pad. The needle inserting angle can be perpendicular, oblique, or horizontal to the skin surface with various depths, depending on the location of acupuncture points, treating medical conditions, as well as the patient's size and habitus.

Finger Pressing Insertion (Figure 17-25). This technique is used when a short needle is used. Before inserting, the practitioner uses one fingertip (guiding finger) of the assisting hand to gently press the acupuncture point. The needle is then inserted into the skin of the acupuncture point along the edge of the guiding finger.

Pinching Needle Insertion. This technique is used when an acupuncture point is deep and a long needle is used. Once the acupuncture point is identified, the thumb and index fingers of the assisting hand hold the distal part of the needle with a sterile gauze or sterile cotton ball, the dominant hand holds the handle of the needle. The needle is then inserted with both hands.

Pinching Skin Needle Insertion. This technique is used when the skin and muscles of the inserted site are thin or if the insertion point is close to important organs such as the lungs or eyeballs. Once the acupuncture point is identified, the skin and muscles are pinched or picked up with the thumb and index fingers of the assisting hand. The needle is then inserted through pinched skin with the dominant hand.

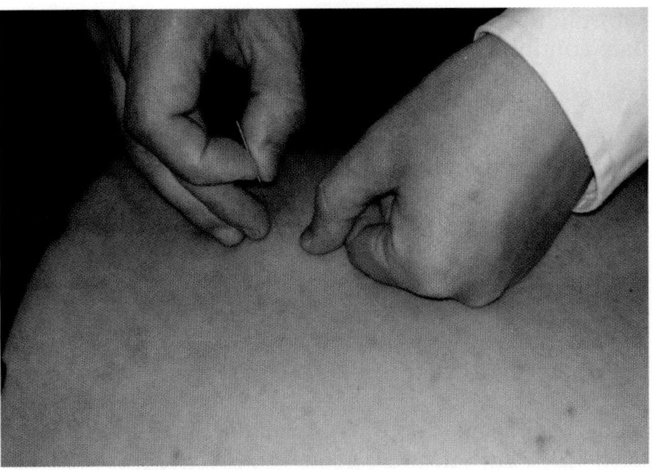

FIGURE 17-25 Finger pressing needle insertion.

Tight Skin Needle Insertion. This technique is used when the skin over the acupuncture point is loose. Once the acupuncture point is identified, the skin over the acupuncture point is stretched and tightened with the thumb and index fingers. The needle is inserted with the dominant hand.[197]

All needles are currently sold with guiding tubes. Using a guiding tube usually helps to reduce the pain and discomfort caused by the initial needle insertion through tapping the tail (top) of the needle. The guiding tubes are especially useful for those who are less experienced practitioners.

There are two basic methods of stimulating the needles after they are inserted: manual manipulation and electrical stimulation. There are various techniques in manipulating the needles manually to achieve the desired effects. The techniques are grouped by the needle effects, which are categorized in tonification (to treat deficiency), sedation (to treat excess), or in neutral. For example, tonification, a commonly used technique, is to insert the needle with an angle in the direction of energy flow on a specific meridian, and then advance the needle slowly turning it with slow, yet firm clockwise rotations as the needle is being advanced, and not penetrating too deeply. When withdrawn, the needle should be removed quickly and the skin at the inserting point should be covered by a finger and massaged in a clockwise manner. Sedation is contrary to tonification. The needle is angled against the direction of energy flow on the meridian and is inserted quickly and deeply with rapid counterclockwise rotations. The needle should be withdrawn slowly and the surface should not be touched after removal of the needle. The needles usually stay for 15 to 30 minutes. Electrical stimulation became available in modern times. The electrodes are connected to the needles. The negative lead is attached to the needle(s) where the electron flow is started, whereas the positive lead is attached to the needle(s) where the flow is directed to. The low-frequency impulse, between 2 and 8 Hz, is considered to have a tonification effect. Higher frequency impulse, between 70 and 150 Hz, is used on the points surrounding the painful area, especially in musculoskeletal pain conditions.[83]

Indications, Precautions, and Contraindications

Acupuncture has been used to treat many conditions in physiatric settings. Some conditions, such as facial pain, headache, knee pain, lower back pain, neck pain, periarthritis of the shoulder, postoperative pain, rheumatoid arthritis, sciatica, sprain, stroke, and tennis elbow, have been treated effectively by acupuncture. There are other conditions that have shown clinical improvement with acupuncture, such as Bell palsy, cancer pain, fibromyalgia and fasciitis, gout, insomnia, obesity, substance dependence, osteoarthritis, complex regional pain syndrome, acute spine pain, and stiff neck, but further research is needed.[192] Acupuncture is a safe and effective form of treatment. Complications from the clinical application of acupuncture are extremely rare, and side effects, if any, are limited. There are a number of guidelines, however, that govern the use of particular acupuncture points. A precaution or contraindication may be related to use in certain conditions, with particular techniques, or because of the location of a point. Some of the commonly accepted contraindications and precautions are no deep needling for acupuncture points close to the lungs, heart, and liver to avoid damage to those organs; the avoidance of moxibustion at certain acupuncture points such as most points on the face; the avoidance of puncturing arteries such as the radial artery at the wrist; and special precautions with the sue of certain acupuncture points to avoid miscarriage. Because needles are used in other procedures, there are possible adverse events during acupuncture treatment: fainting, hematoma, pneumothorax, and injuries to the nerve tissue including the spinal cord. There have also been other events reported, such as needle stick, bent needle, or broken needle left in the body.

Evidence-Based Research

Since the early 1970s, more and more studies on acupuncture have been published in English literature from many disciplines of basic and clinical sciences. The majority of those research studies are not well designed and cannot be used as true evidence-based research. Among well-designed studies, they can be generally divided into three categories.

The first and most common category is studies related to the effectiveness of acupuncture to treat a medical condition compared with a control measure, typically sham acupuncture, or other conventional treatment such as physical therapy or a medication. For example, Yurtkuran et al.[195] carried out a double-blind, randomized study to investigate the effectiveness of laser acupuncture in knee osteoarthritis. They compared the treating group (laser acupuncture, $n = 24$) with the control group (placebo laser to the same acupuncture point, $n = 25$). After 10 sessions (2 weeks) of treatment, the treating group showed a significant difference in knee circumference (140). The *Natural Standard Monograph* gives the highest grade (grade A) on acupuncture treatment for osteoarthritis, which means there is statistically significant evidence of benefit with supporting evidence in basic science, animal studies, or theory.[135a] Another example is that in a randomized controlled trial of 270 patients. Melchart et al.[126] concluded that acupuncture had an effect comparable with other types of Western allopathic headache treatments.

The second category of acupuncture research studies the mechanism of acupuncture. For example, Akil et al.[7] studied the possible physiologic basis of acupuncture for analgesia and found that acupuncture increases the endorphin level in various parts of the central nervous system, and beta-endorphin can be shown to attenuate chronic pain. Han[77] concluded that acupuncture or electrical stimulation in specific frequencies applied to certain body sites can facilitate the release of specific neuropeptides in the central nervous system that elicit profound physiologic effects and even activate self-healing mechanisms.

The third category of acupuncture research is related to the study of acupuncture itself. For example, Ahn et al.[4] studied the effectiveness of two different styles of acupuncture: Japanese and TCM. White et al.[190] studied whether needling sensation (De Qi) affects treatment outcome in pain. Despite the huge amount of research done, high-quality randomized studies are much needed.

Moxibustion

History and Mechanism

In addition to acupuncture, another common practice is moxibustion, which is a frequently used technique in the comprehensive acupuncture regimen (Figure 17-26). As a matter of fact, in Chinese, acupuncture is called "zheng jiu," in which "zheng" means needling and "jiu" means moxibustion. Moxibustion is a method in which moxa is burned on or above the skin at acupuncture points. The heat generated from moxa warms the Qi and the blood in the channels and is useful in the treatment of disease and maintenance of health.[87] Moxa is a bunch of dried leaves of mugwort plants that have been formed into a small cone or cigarlike stick.

Moxibustion started several thousand years ago, along with acupuncture. Moxibustion has been recorded in many classic books such as *Huang Di Nei Jing* and has been a divisible part of the comprehensive acupuncture regimen.

Current research study of the moxibustion mechanism mainly relates to thermal effects, radiation effects, and pharmacologic actions of moxa and its combustion

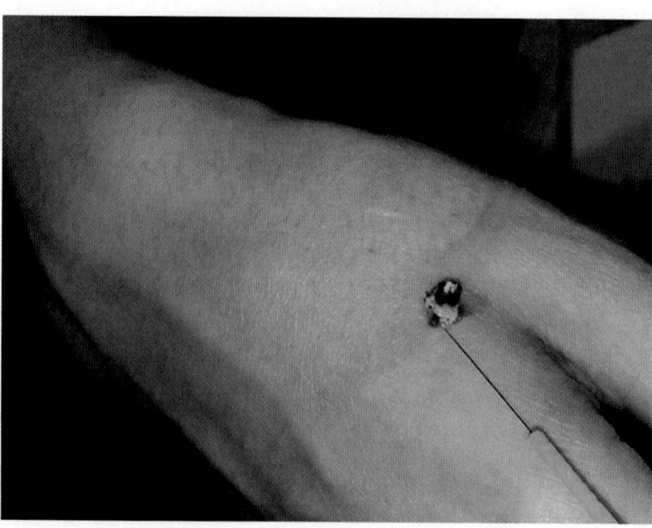

FIGURE 17-26 Moxibustion after needle insertion.

products. Experimental results showed that moxibustion thermal stimulation affects both shallow and deep tissues of the skin, and the warm heat effects of moxibustion have a close relation to the warm receptors or the polymodal receptor.[45]

Indications and Contraindications

Moxibustion is used to treat Yin syndrome, cold syndrome, and deficiency syndrome. It treats chronic conditions and Yang Qi deficiency such as chronic diarrhea, chronic dysentery, malaria, phlegm, water retention, edema, asthma cold type, impotence, enuresis, Bi syndrome, abdominal pain, stomach ache, and metrorrhagia resulting from Qi deficiency. It is also used to treat older adults with frequent urination attributable to Yang deficiency, wind stroke, profuse sweating, dying Yang syndrome, and collapse of Qi. Moxibustion can also be used for emergency treatment of collapse of Yang.

Scaring moxibustion should not be applied to the face, the pericardial region, the breast region, perineal area, the area close to large blood vessels, prominent tendons, or major creases in the skin. Moxibustion is forbidden on the abdomen region and lumbosacral region of a pregnant woman. Patients with cognitive deficit or sensory deficit should not use excessive doses of moxibustion to avoid burning injuries. Moxibustion is contraindicated for patients with febrile diseases.

Techniques and Evidence-Based Effects

There are many types of moxibustion. Three common types of techniques are moxibustion with moxa cones, moxibustion with moxa sticks, and moxibustion with warming needles.[197]

Moxibustion with moxa cones comprise two subtypes: direct moxibustion and indirect moxibustion. Direct moxibustion is a method that a moxa cone is placed directly on the skin, and is further divided into nonscarring moxibustion and scarring moxibustion. For nonscarring moxibustion, before the procedure, apply a small amount of Vaseline cream or Shiunko ointment on top of the acupuncture point. If the patient feels pain when the moxa is burnt, the moxa will be removed. This process will be repeated up to seven times or until the local skin color becomes ruddy. In contrast to nonscarring moxibustion, in scarring moxibustion moxa is placed directly on the skin and burnt. A local blister will form and eventually end with a scar. Scarring moxibustion is less favorable because of cosmetic concerns. In indirect moxibustion, by definition, the moxa does not contact directly with the skin but on some types of insulation material. Commonly used insulation material includes ginger, garlic, and salt.

Moxibustion with moxa sticks (rolls) is a method that ignited moxa is placed above or over the acupuncture points without contacting the skin. Based on how the movement of the moxa stick is controlled, this method is further divided into three subtypes: mild-warm moxibustion, "sparrow-pecking" moxibustion, and circling moxibustion.

Moxibustion with a warm needle is used when both a retaining acupuncture needle and moxibustion are needed. A needle is inserted into the acupuncture point first. Once the needle is in place, moxa wool or a short stick is wrapped or attached to the handle of the needle. The moxa is then ignited and burnt.

Compared with acupuncture, there is much less scientific research on moxibustion, especially those involved in moxibustion alone without acupuncture. Lee et al.[109] carried out a systematic review of clinical trials that used moxibustion in cancer treatment and suggested that moxibustion might help to reduce nausea and vomiting caused by chemotherapy. There were conflicting research results related to the possibility of moxibustion helping to convert fetuses in breech position to head-first position. There were other studies that examined the use of moxibustion in asthma and ulcerative colitis. Mazzoni et al.[124] carried out a small pilot study and found that moxibustion and acupuncture did not help weight control. Overall, similar to acupuncture research, there is not enough good evidence-based clinical research done on moxibustion.

CASE 4

Acupuncture

Background: A 79-year-old man who has a 40-year history of intermittent left second and third toe pain after an injury. He had surgery after the injury. He has been diagnosed with complex regional pain syndrome and peripheral neuropathy. He has tried medications and injections and none of them have worked. The pain usually starts when he lies down for 5 to 10 minutes and mainly affects him in the evening when he tries to sleep. He went to the Mayo Clinic at one point and was instructed not to take any pain medications anymore because they did not help anyway. The patient also has a history of diabetes, vitamin B_{12} deficiency, and restless leg syndrome, and all of them have been addressed. He rates his pain at 8/10 on a visual analog pain scale. He describes his pain as aching, sharp, shooting, and throbbing. Rubbing his toe, bending his knee, and icing make his pain slightly better. Physical examination was normal including light touch sensation; however, lying flat provoked pain in his left second and third toes.

Impression: Left second and third toe pain attributable to neuropathy.

Treatment: The patient initially tried to use a TENS unit to his left foot. It had helped to a certain degree initially and he only woke up once or twice each night. However, the effectiveness of a TENS unit waned several months later and his pain returned to previous levels.

The patient was started on acupuncture without electrostimulation, targeting mainly acupuncture points at left Liver, Stomach, and Gallbladder meridians on the left foot and left lower leg. He has now received the treatment on average once a week for 6 weeks.

Response: During all treatment sessions, he tolerated the procedure well and had been pain-free throughout each 30-minute treatment session. After the first treatment, pain relief lasted for 1 day; after the second treatment, it lasted 3 days; after the third treatment, it lasted 4 days; and after the fourth treatment, he was pain-free for the whole week and he no longer woke up in the evening. After he finished his sixth session, the patient has not returned to the clinic for any further acupuncture sessions.

Discussion:

- What is the possible mechanism behind acupuncture?
- What are the principles on acupuncture point selection?
- What is the efficacy of acupuncture on neuropathy based on research studies?
- What are the contraindications of the use of acupuncture?

KEY REFERENCES

1. Abramson DI, Tuck S, Jr, Chu LS, Agustin C: Effect of paraffin bath and hot fomentations on local tissue temperatures, *Arch Phys Med Rehabil* 45:87–94, 1964.
12. Annaswamy TM, De Luigi AJ, O'Neill BJ, et al: Emerging concepts in the treatment of myofascial pain: a review of medications, modalities, and needle-based interventions, *PM&R* 3:940–961, 2011.
14. Annette PNH: The effectiveness of cervical traction, *Phys Ther* 10:217–229, 2005.
33. Cakir S, Hepguler S, Ozturk C, et al: Efficacy of therapeutic ultrasound for the management of knee osteoarthritis: a randomized, controlled, and double-blind study, *Am J Phys Med Rehabil* 93:405–412, 2014.
34. Car C, Yang W, Zhou L, et al: Acupuncture in treatment of aging spine-related pain conditions. In Yue JJ, Guyer RD, Johnson JP, et al, editors: *The comprehensive treatment of the aging spine*, Philadelphia, 2011, Elsevier Saunders.
35. Celik EC, Erhan B, Gunduz B, Lakse E: The effect of low-frequency TENS in the treatment of neuropathic pain in patients with spinal cord injury, *Spinal Cord* 51:334–337, 2013.
36. Chang KV, Chen SY, Chen WS, et al: Comparative effectiveness of focused shock wave therapy of different intensity levels and radial shock wave therapy for treating plantar fasciitis: a systematic review and network meta-analysis, *Arch Phys Med Rehabil* 93:1259–1268, 2012.
37. Chou R: Low back pain (chronic), *Clin Evid* 2010:1–41, 2010.
45. Deng H, Shen X: The mechanism of moxibustion: ancient theory and modern research, *Evid Based Complement Alternat Med* 2013: 379291, 2013.
54. Escalante Y, Garcia-Hermoso A, Saavedra JM: Effects of exercise on functional aerobic capacity in lower limb osteoarthritis: a systematic review, *J Sci Med Sport* 14:190–198, 2011.
55. Feigal DW: *FDA public health notification: diathermy interactions with implanted leads and implanted systems with leads*, Silver Spring, December 19, 2002, US Food and Drug Administration. Retrieved from www.fda.gov/MedicalDevices/Safety/AlertsandNotices/PublicHealthNotifications/ucm062167.htm.
61. Fuentes JP, Armijo Olivo S, Magee DJ, Gross DP: Effectiveness of interferential current therapy in the management of musculoskeletal pain: a systematic review and meta analysis, *Phys Ther* 90:1219–1238, 2010.
62. Fukuda TY, Alves da Cunha R, Fukuda VO, et al: Pulsed shortwave treatment in women with knee osteoarthritis: a multicenter, randomized, placebo-controlled clinical trial, *Phys Ther* 91:1009–1017, 2011.
63. Galvan HG, Tritsch AJ, Tandy R, Rubley MD: Pain perception during repeated ice-bath immersion of the ankle at varied temperatures, *J Sport Rehabil* 15:105–115, 2006.
65. Gao XJ, Xing D: Molecular mechanisms of cell proliferation induced by low power laser irradiation, *J Biomed Sci* 16:4, 2009.
66. Gellman H: *Acupuncture treatment for musculoskeletal pain: a textbook for orthopedics, anesthesia, and rehabilitation*, New York, 2002, Taylor & Francis.
69. Goats GC: Interferential current therapy, *Br J Sports Med* 24:87–92, 1990.
80. Hawkes AR, Draper DO, Johnson AW, et al: Heating capacity of rebound shortwave diathermy and moist hot packs at superficial depths, *J Athl Train* 48:471–476, 2013.
81. Hedrick WR, Hykes DL, Starchman DE, editors: Basic ultrasound physics. In *Ultrasound physics and instrumentation*, ed 4, St Louis, 2005, Elsevier Mosby.
82. Heidland A, Fazeli G, Klassen A, et al: Neuromuscular electrostimulation techniques: historical aspects and current possibilities in treatment of pain and muscle wasting, *Clin Nephrol* 79(Suppl 1): S12–S23, 2013.
88. Hsu RW, Hsu WH, Tai CL, Lee KF: Effect of shock-wave therapy on patellar tendinopathy in a rabbit model, *J Orthop Res* 22:221–227, 2004.
89. Huang D, Gu YH, Liao Q, et al: Effects of linear-polarized near-infrared light irradiation on chronic pain, *Scientificworldjournal* 2012:567496, 2012.
92. Jang H, Lee H: Meta-analysis of pain relief effects by laser irradiation on joint areas, *Photomed Laser Surg* 30:405–417, 2012.
96. Khadilkar A, Milne S, Brosseau L, et al: Transcutaneous electrical nerve stimulation for the treatment of chronic low back pain: a systematic review, *Spine* 30:2657–2666, 2005.
97. Kloth L: Electrotherapeutic alternatives for the treatment of pain. In Gersh MR, editor: *Electrotherapy in rehabilitation (Contemporary perspectives in rehabilitation)*, Philadelphia, 1992, FA Davis.
99. Knight KL, Draper DO: *Therapeutic modalities: the art and science with clinical activities manual*, Baltimore, 2007, Lippincott Williams & Wilkins.
102. Krause M, Refshauge KM, Dessen M, Boland R: Lumbar spine traction: evaluation of effects and recommended application for treatment, *Man Ther* 5:72–81, 2000.
111. Lehmann JF, Brunne GD, Martinis AJ, McMillan JA: Ultrasonic effects as demonstrated in live pigs with surgical metallic implants, *Arch Phys Med Rehabil* 40:483–488, 1959.
118. Lu H, Qin L, Cheung W, et al: Low-intensity pulsed ultrasound accelerated bone-tendon junction healing through regulation of vascular endothelial growth factor expression and cartilage formation, *Ultrasound Med Biol* 34:1248–1260, 2008.
121. Macedo CS, Alonso CS, Liporaci RF, et al: Cold water immersion of the ankle decreases neuromuscular response of lower limb after inversion movement, *Braz J Phys Ther* 18:93–97, 2014.
123. Mathews JA: The effects of spinal traction, *Physiotherapy* 58:64–66, 1972.
125. McGaw SC, Fritz J, Brennan G: Factors related to success with the use of mechanical cervical traction, *J Orthop Sports Phys Ther* 36:A14, 2006.
128. Melzack R, Wall PD: Pain mechanisms: a new theory, *Science* 150:971–979, 1965.
139. Olah KS, Bridges N, Denning J, Farrar DJ: The conservative management of patients with symptoms of stress incontinence: a randomized, prospective study comparing weighted vaginal cones and interferential therapy, *Am J Obstet Gynecol* 162:87–92, 1990.
140. Oleson T: Auriculotherapy stimulation for neuro-rehabilitation, *Neurorehabilitation* 17:49–62, 2002.
141. Olson JE, Stravino VD: A review of cryotherapy, *Phys Ther* 52:840–853, 1972.
142. Onel D, Tuzlaci M, Sari H, Demir K: Computed tomographic investigation of the effect of traction on lumbar disc herniations, *Spine* 14:82–90, 1989.
149. Qubaeissy KY, Fatoye FA, Goodwin PC, Yohannes AM: The effectiveness of hydrotherapy in the management of rheumatoid arthritis: a systematic review, *Musculoskeletal Care* 11:3–18, 2013.
150. Rabini A, Piazzini DB, Tancredi G, et al: Deep heating therapy via microwave diathermy relieves pain and improves physical function in patients with knee osteoarthritis: a double-blind randomized clinical trial, *Eur J Phys Rehabil Med* 48:549–559, 2012.
154. Rogoff JB: *Therapeutic heat and cold*, Baltimore, 1972, Waverly Press.
159. Sarrafzadeh J, Ahmadi A, Yassin M: The effects of pressure release, phonophoresis of hydrocortisone, and ultrasound on upper trapezius latent myofascial trigger point, *Arch Phys Med Rehabil* 93:72–77, 2012.
169. Sluka K: *Mechanisms and management of pain for the physical therapist*, ed 1, Seattle, 2009, IASP Press.
172. Takahashi N, Nakamura T, Kanno N, et al: Local heat application to the leg reduces muscle sympathetic nerve activity in human, *Eur J Appl Physiol* 111:2203–2211, 2011.
174. Taylor AG, Anderson JG, Riedel SL, et al: Cranial electrical stimulation improves symptoms and functional status in individuals with fibromyalgia, *Pain Manag Nurs* 14:327–335, 2013.
176. Tiktinsky R, Chen L, Narayan P: Electrotherapy: yesterday, today and tomorrow, *Haemophilia* 16(Suppl 5):126–131, 2010.
181. Tsai WC, Tang ST, Liang FC: Effect of therapeutic ultrasound on tendons, *Am J Phys Med Rehabil* 90:1068–1073, 2011.
183. van der Heijden GJ, van der Windt DA, de Winter AF: Physiotherapy for patients with soft tissue shoulder disorders: a systematic review of randomised clinical trials, *BMJ* 315:25–30, 1997.
193. Yarrobino TE, Kalbfleisch JH, Ferslew KE, Panus PC: Lidocaine iontophoresis mediates analgesia in lateral epicondylalgia treatment, *Physiother Res Int* 11:152–160, 2006.
197. Zhang E: *Chinese acupuncture and moxibustion: a practical English-Chinese library of traditional Chinese medicine*, Shanghai, 1990, Publishing House of Shanghai College of Traditional Chinese Medicine.

The full reference list for this chapter is available online.

CHAPTER 18

INTEGRATIVE MEDICINE IN REHABILITATION

David F. Drake, Robert A. Schulman, Deborah Daimaru

Integrative Medicine

Complementary and integrative medicine (CIM) is a holistic, interdisciplinary approach to health, designed to treat the person, not just the disease. It is a partnership between the patient and his or her providers. The goal is to treat the mind, body, and spirit concurrently. CIM combines treatments of conventional medicine and elements of complementary and alternative medicine (CAM) when there is strong evidence of safety and effectiveness. The Osher Center for Integrative Medicine at the University of California, San Francisco, states on its website: "Integrative medicine seeks to incorporate treatment options from conventional and alternative approaches, taking into account not only physical symptoms, but also psychological, social and spiritual aspects of health and illnesses."[85] CIM encompasses Eastern and Western philosophies, mind and body, and individual and family. Most important, CIM is patient centered. It transforms the current medical model into a personalized, proactive, patient-driven approach, which enables engagement with life in accordance with how an individual wants to live. CIM focuses on empowering the consumer through comprehensive education regarding their health and wellness, thereby encouraging active participation in one's own well-being. Many practitioners in integrative medicine (IM) talk about a cultural change. The Veterans Health Administration thought this was so important that it created a central (national) office of patient-centered care and cultural transformation in 2011. The cultural change or transformation is on both the patient's and the provider's side.

The current model of health care is problem based and disease oriented. The focus is on the identification of current problems associated with the disease process and treating them. It is reactive with sporadic intervention. Care is physician-directed in which the physician makes a diagnosis and offers treatment. The Institute of Medicine (IOM) rules for the twenty-first century health care system describe the current approach to health care as focused on care-based visits, driven by professional autonomy with the control of the care left to the health care professionals. The IOM encourages a new view to include care based on continuous healing relationships and customization according to the needs and values of the patient.[23] Integrative care is wellness oriented. It focuses on the identification of and the minimization of risk and addresses the whole person. It is proactive and patient driven by engaging the patient in making pertinent decisions regarding their health. These decisions are often lifelong commitments to healthy changes.[100]

Key elements within CIM are communication and education. An open dialogue occurs between the provider and the patient to align the patient's expectations with what can realistically be achieved. Integrative health coaches (IHCs) can be an important part of the health care team. They facilitate change by helping to set realistic goals and, most important, by empowering the patients to take control of their own health and wellness, thus laying the foundation for successful, permanent change.

An IHC meets individually with participants in a supportive partnership to facilitate healthy changes in behavior. The IHC creates a dialogue that encourages discussion while offering insights and clarity that may lead to personal discovery. He or she opens the participant to changes that will include the mind, body, and spirit and assists and supports the participant in making and sustaining, often new, healthy behaviors. A wheel of health that encompasses the mind-body connection, nutrition, spirituality, movement and exercise, relationships, environment, and personal and professional development is frequently used to identify which area or areas are most important to the individual participant. This often includes discussions on complementary methods while encouraging modern medical support, blending the best of both in an individualized patient-centered approach to health. Each participant commits to changes he or she thinks are important to them. They are then held accountable for these changes, through future meetings and discussions. Through this relationship, the IHC is able to empower the participants to follow through on the course set and to identify any obstacles he or she may see while creating a path that will guide them past those obstacles.[31]

Topics, such as sleep hygiene, nutrition, and activity, may be discussed in detail and elaborated on after collecting sleep, nutrition, or activity logs from each participant. This method gives insight into the life of each person and allows for the development of one-on-one patient-centered individualized programs addressing any concerns discovered during the review of the various logs. The interventions place an emphasis on the patient's responsibility in their own health and well-being.

It is probably more appropriate to refer to patients as "participants" in the CIM approach to medical care. By recognizing the connection among the mind, body, spirit and individuals' interaction within their community, an interdisciplinary team may offer comprehensive, individualized attention facilitated through dynamic dialogue between the consumer and his or her providers. This in turn can lead to greater satisfaction with services offered, an increase in active participation in one's own health care, and, most important, lifestyle changes that lead to improved well-being.

Complementary and Alternative Medicine

The National Center for Complementary and Alternative Medicine (NCCAM) uses the term "complementary health approaches" and defines two specific subgroups: natural products and mind-body practices.[81] Natural products are herbs and supplements, such as probiotics, vitamins, and minerals. Mind-body practices include a very diverse, large group of techniques or procedures that include acupuncture, massage, meditation, mindfulness, movement therapies, relaxation techniques, spinal manipulation, traditional Chinese medicine (to include tai chi and qigong), yoga, and others not specifically listed.[41] Complementary medicine involves the use of nonmainstream techniques or treatments in conjunction with conventional medicine. Alternative medicine, by contrast, is the use of CAM in place of conventional medicine.

According to the 2007 National Health Interview Survey, approximately 38% of American adults and 12% of children used some type of CAM in the 12 months before the survey. The most commonly used therapies among adults were nonvitamin, nonmineral (i.e., herbal) natural products (18%); deep-breathing exercises (13%); meditation (9%); chiropractic or osteopathic manipulation (9%); massage (8%); and yoga (6%). Back pain (17.1%), neck pain (5.9%), and joint pain (5.2%) were the most common conditions prompting CAM use.[1]

The one area where CAM and Western medicine treatments differ dramatically is the environment in which care is delivered. Whereas Western medicine settings are almost sterile, CAM surroundings are intended to be comfortable and relaxing, thereby allowing patients to participate fully in their sessions. The atmosphere is established by providing a temperate climate, with dimmer lighting, soft music, warm room decorations, and even a mild pleasant aroma. Many hospitals are beginning to incorporate some of these concepts into their waiting rooms and grounds.

Complementary and Alternative Medicine Practices

Whole Medical Systems

Traditional Chinese medicine is probably the best known of the whole medical systems. It uses specific diagnostic evaluations, such as pulse and tongue assessment, and treatments that include herbal prescriptions and interventions, such as acupuncture.

Ayurveda[5] is a whole medical system from India that aims to provide guidance regarding food and lifestyle to either maintain wellness or improve health. It understands that there are energetic forces (Tridoshas) that influence nature and human beings and that there is a strong connection between the mind and the body.[80]

Homeopathy, developed in Germany in the late eighteenth century, focuses on two theories: "like cures like" (i.e., the disease can be treated or cured by a substance that produces similar symptoms in healthy people) and "law of minimum dose" (i.e., the effect is greater at the lowest dose of the medication). Many homeopathic remedies are so diluted that no molecules of the original substance remain.[80]

Mind-Body Medicine

Research over the past several decades has identified interactions between the brain and the immune system, suggesting that the mind-body connection is real.[95] CIM attempts to address this connection to assist and improve well-being. Many of the CAM modalities mentioned actively engage the mind and body, such as the breathing and mindfulness techniques used in qigong, tai chi, and yoga. Mindfulness-based interventions (MBIs) appear to be some of the most rapidly growing areas within CAM. Yoga, tai chi, and qigong are a few common MBIs, but much of the recent focus has been on the mindfulness-based cognitive therapy and mindfulness-based stress reduction programs, both of which are derived from ancient Buddhist and yoga philosophies. These approaches are being used in psychotherapy and can also be applied in the management of pain.[58]

Manipulative and Body-Based Practices

Osteopathy. Since its founding in the nineteenth century by Andrew Taylor Still, MD, DO, osteopathic medicine, which includes manual manipulation of the spine, has been at the forefront of IM. Dr. Still stressed the importance of the connection among mental, physical, emotional, and spiritual health and taught that each plays an important role in the patient's overall health. The evidence for manual therapy, as many refer to it, is not overwhelming. However, there does appear to be a role for osteopathic medicine in the management of pain, particularly if treated early. A 2011 Cochrane review looking at the use of manual therapy in low back pain (LBP) showed improved pain and decreased disability in the short term and decreased pain in the medium term for acute/subacute LBP.[108]

Massage. Massage is a general term for pressing, rubbing, and manipulating the skin, muscles, tendons, and ligaments to aid in relaxation and recovery from injury. Massage therapists typically use their hands and fingers but may also use their forearms, elbows, and even feet. Swedish massage is primarily used for relaxation and is most common in spa settings. Thai massage uses assisted stretching. Shiatsu is a Japanese technique in which finger pressure, often along meridians that may correspond with acupuncture points, is used. Deep tissue massage is used to target trigger points and release chronic muscle tension. Sports massage can be used before events as part of a warm-up, during the event in cases of cramping, and after the event as part of the cool down. Heat can be added to any of the above treatments via warmed stones, topical ointments, creams, or other emollients to aid in relaxation.

Movement Therapies. Transitional aquatics use aerobic exercise, stretching, and yoga poses that can be done both in and out of the water. Participants use the buoyancy and support that an aquatic environment provides to begin working out. Once muscle tone, flexibility, and balance improve, they can transition to land-based activities, including gaming systems commonly found in homes, such as the *Wii Fit*, and eventually to classes offered in the community. Other common forms of movement therapy include tai chi, qigong, and yoga.

Acupuncture. Acupuncture is a form of energy medicine and is one of the more common and more researched of the CAM modalities. It shares with the others a similar treatment setting and a conceptual framework similar to tai chi or qigong life energy called Qi (pronounced chee) and is thought to circulate through all parts of the body through energy channels called meridians. These meridians connect the exterior to the interior and the organs to each other and the exterior. The classical Chinese explanation is that channels of energy run in regular patterns through the body and over its surface. These energy channels (meridians) are like rivers flowing through the body to irrigate and nourish the tissues. An obstruction in the movement of these energy rivers is like a dam that backs up in others. Pain and illness are thought to occur when the flow of Qi becomes blocked or unbalanced. Acupuncture is one of the treatments used to reestablish the flow of Qi through the placement of needles at points along the meridians, thus allowing the body to return to a homeostasis and easing the ailment for which it was prescribed. The meridians can be influenced by needling the acupuncture points. The acupuncture needles unblock the obstructions at the dams and reestablish the regular flow through the meridians. Acupuncture treatments can therefore help the body's internal organs to correct imbalances in their digestion, absorption, and energy production activities and in the circulation of their energy through the meridians.

The modern scientific explanation is that needling the acupuncture points stimulates the nervous system to release chemicals in the muscles, spinal cord, and brain. These chemicals will either change the experience of pain or will trigger the release of other chemicals and hormones, which influence the body's own internal regulating system. The physiologic reactions of acupuncture effects are beginning to emerge. Stimulation of acupuncture points has been shown to create signal changes in the amygdala, anterior hippocampus, and subgenual cingulate cortex on functional magnetic resonance imaging (fMRI).[72] Other studies confirm these findings, defining the role of the amygdala in affect, fear, and defensive behavior, as well as the processing of pain[10,16,55] and motivation.[119] The hippocampus is thought to link affective states with memory processing. The signal decrease within the amygdala and anterior hippocampus is consistent with past acupuncture fMRI studies at acupoints LI-4 and GB-34, as well as ST-36.[51,52,115,116,120] Ahsin et al.[3] linked electroacupuncture to functional improvement by the measured rise in endorphins and fall in cortisol levels in individuals given electroacupuncture.

The improved energy and biochemical balance produced by acupuncture results in stimulating the body's natural healing abilities and in promoting physical and emotional well-being. The anatomy of acupuncture points is not clear; however, a theory proposed by Langevin and Yandow[65] suggests that the meridians are located within tissues planes. Acupuncture points occur at a convergence of these planes and meridian Qi is the biochemical and bioelectrical signaling in the connective tissue. A blockage of Qi may lead to an altered connective tissue matrix composition leading to altered signal transduction and therefore pain or other symptoms.[65]

Clinically, acupuncture does appear to be of benefit in some patients. According to the *Journal of Rheumatology*, there is sufficient evidence to warrant positive recommendations for osteoarthritis, LBP, and lateral epicondylitis in routine care of patients with rheumatic diseases.[33] Acupuncture has been shown to be effective in the treatment of LBP,[45] lateral epicondylitis,[39] shoulder pain resulting from subacromial impingement,[56] as well as headaches.[70] Nausea and vomiting have also shown to be effectively managed by acupuncture.[21,67]

Acupuncture is an ancient medical modality, with physiologic changes that appear to suggest neurologic and neurochemical effects that can lead to clinical improvement. Many people may benefit from acupuncture, although it is not a panacea.

Supplements. The National Center for Health Statistics reported that the use of dietary supplements is common among the U.S. adult population. More than 40% used supplements from 1988 to 1994, and more than 50% from 2003 to 2006.[41] Multivitamins, calcium, folate, and vitamin D were among the most commonly used. The number of adults in the United States that ever used herbs or supplements grew slightly, from 50.6 million in 2002 to 55.1 million in 2007. However, the proportion of adults who reported use of herbs or supplements in the past 12 months dropped significantly: from 18.9% in 2002 to 17.9% in 2007.[114]

Herbs and supplements are used for both health and wellness, and although research does not support many, there is a growing level of evidence for some. It is important for the medical practitioner to ask about herb and supplement use and to know where to look for information on specifics of their use. The *Natural Standard* is a good resource to provide evidence-based information about CAM, including dietary supplements and integrative therapies.[82] The NCCAM also provides evidence-based information for the health care provider.[79]

Vitamin D is a fat-soluble steroid hormone that is synthesized from 7-dehydrocholesterol through a multistep conversion process in the skin when exposed to ultraviolet light. Vitamin D is also absorbed from dietary sources of innate or fortified food. Research suggests that deficiency of vitamin D has been associated with poor health, diabetes, hyperglycemia, depression, muscle weakness, poor balance, and all-cause mortality.[50] Low vitamin D levels have also been associated with depression.[4,57] Supplementation with vitamin D may be indicated in preventing falls in the elderly with low vitamin D levels.[44] It has also been associated with decreased pain, improved functional mobility and quality of life,[96] and decreased mortality.[11,12]

N-Acetylcysteine (NAC) is a precursor to the antioxidant glutathione, which is synthesized in the body. Supplementation with NAC therefore increases the production of glutathione. Research supports NAC supplementation as a potential treatment of chronic obstructive pulmonary disease by improving function of small airways and decreasing exacerbation frequency.[106] A study of a 6-month course of treatment with NAC resulted in reduction of influenza-like episodes and severity.[26] NAC shows promise in the treatment of neuropsychiatric disorders, including the treatment of mood disorders,[75] schizophrenia,[29] addiction,[104] and autism.[46] In a study of mice, NAC was demonstrated to induce analgesia and may be useful in the treatment of inflammatory pain.[9]

S-Adenosyl methionine (SAM-E) is a methyl-donor produced and used in the liver. Studies have shown that SAM-E supplements have comparable antidepressive efficacy as imipramine in patients with major depression.[27,86] It is promising as an adjunct treatment for antidepressant nonresponders with major depressive disorder,[87] and its use resulted in lower erectile dysfunction when used with antidepressants.[30] Patients with chronic hepatitis C showed an improved response when treated with PEGylated interferon alpha and SAM-E.[38] Controlled clinical studies have also shown that SAM-E is as effective in the treatment of knee osteoarthritis as treatment with nabumetone and celecoxib.[17,60]

Glucosamine (amino sugar) and chondroitin sulfate (sulfated glycosaminoglycan) have had some controversy and mixed clinical reports regarding efficacy for the treatment of arthritis, and guidelines vary for use of these compounds in the setting of hip and knee arthritis.[19,91,97]

Methylsulfonylmethane (MSM) is frequently used in arthritis; however, there is a paucity of studies on MSM. Some trials suggest efficacy in the treatment of osteoarthritis of the knee,[18,61] decreased muscle damage after exercise,[8] and in animal models of arthritis. Other analyses suggest nonefficacy for human arthritis.[18,35]

Alpha-lipoic acid (ALA; organosulfur compound derived from octanoic acid) is used as a treatment of diabetic sensory-motor neuropathy.[20,53,122] Trial results have been mixed,[123,124] and case reports suggest a potential for precipitating insulin autoimmune syndrome.[6]

Magnesium is an alkaline earth metal. It is necessary for several hundred cellular enzymatic reactions, such as those synthesizing ATP, DNA, and RNA. Only a very small portion of the body's magnesium is stored in the extracellular compartment (1%). Sixty percent is in the skeleton, and 39% is in the intracellular compartment (20% in skeletal muscle). Therefore serum magnesium measurements are thought to be a poor reflection of total body magnesium stores. Magnesium deficiency is associated with diverse conditions, such as asthma,[37,48,98] diabetes,[25,118] metabolic syndrome, elevated C-reactive protein, hypertension, atherosclerotic vascular disease, sudden cardiac death, osteoporosis, migraine headache, asthma, and colon cancer.[93] A variety of oral forms of magnesium are available for use in supplementation. Magnesium oxide contains a high level of magnesium by weight but is insoluble in water and not bioavailable,[40,71] particularly in comparison with magnesium citrate.[107] An important note is that chronic proton pump inhibitor use is associated with hypomagnesemia.[62,64]

Calcium and strontium contain nearly the same size atomic nucleus. As a result, strontium is readily taken up by bones and tooth enamel. Strontium ranelate is approved as a prescription drug for the treatment of osteoporosis in Europe and other countries but not in the United States. Strontium ralenate is thought to be effective in both women[90] and men.[59,92] It has been found to be effective in the treatment of knee arthritis.[89] Strontium citrate is available in the United States as a nutritional supplement. Animal studies indicated that strontium citrate is taken up by bone in greater concentration than the ralenate form,[113] although no clinical trials have yet been conducted with the citrate form. The higher atomic number of strontium (38, compared with 20 for calcium) may create difficulty in the assessment of treatment efficacy based on dual-energy x-ray absorptiometry (DXA) scans.[69]

Fish oils contain the omega-3 fatty acids eicosapentaenoic acid and docosahexaenoic acid. These fatty acids are precursors of eicosanoids, signaling molecules that control myriad body functions, including those of the central nervous system, inflammation, and immune function. An uncontrolled study suggested efficacy for discogenic pain.[77] Fish oil reduces the need for rescue nonsteroidal antiinflammatory drugs (NSAIDs) in primary dysmenorrhea,[88] decreases dysmenorrhea in adolescents,[47] and increases walking distance in persons with claudication secondary to peripheral arterial disease (PAD).[74] In conjunction with a low arachidonic acid diet, fish oil has an antiinflammatory effect on persons with rheumatoid arthritis,[2] and some patients are able to discontinue taking NSAIDs[63] and concomitant antirheumatic medication.[43] Fish oil also has other important functions in the treatment of depression[101] and attention deficit hyperactivity disorder (ADHD) in children.[13] It is associated with lowered risk of breast cancer,[121] may improve function in patients with heart failure,[28,117] and may lower triglycerides.[34]

Qigong

Qigong (pronounced chee-gung) is a "moving" mindfulness practice, which uses slow graceful movements often with coordinated breathing to promote the circulation of Qi ("energy flow" or "life force") within the human body, to enhance overall health, relaxation, and mental focus. There are several forms of qigong, which allow for it to be practiced in standing, sitting, and lying positions; some with little or no movement at all. In its simplest form, the Chinese character for Qi, in qigong, can mean air, breath, or "life force." Gong means work, so qigong is therefore the practice of "working" with ones' "life force."

Qigong is often confused with the Chinese martial art of tai chi. This misunderstanding can be attributed to the fact that most Chinese martial arts practitioners will usually also practice some form of qigong. It is best to think of qigong as the roots and trunk of the tree whose branches form much of the eastern martial arts.

The great appeal of qigong is that anyone can practice it, regardless of their fitness level, age, belief system, income, or life circumstances. Qigong may benefit anyone, from the most physically challenged to the super athlete.

Most physicians in the Western world view qigong as a set of breathing and movement exercises with benefits to health through stress reduction and exercise. One of the more important long-term effects is that qigong is said to reestablish the body-mind-spirit connection. When these three aspects of our being are integrated, it is thought to encourage a positive outlook on life and help eliminate harmful attitudes and behaviors.

Research supports these thoughts in many areas. Meta-analysis and systematic reviews support the use of qigong to improve stress and anxiety,[110] as well as depression.[111] A randomized controlled trial indicated that medical qigong can improve the overall quality of life mood status of patients with cancer and reduce fatigue.[84] Evidence also supports the use of qigong in patients with fibromyalgia, showing significant improvements in pain and sleep, as well as physical and mental function, when compared with the wait list/usual care control group. The benefits extended well past the 8-week study period, with significant changes noted for 6 months.[66,73]

A review of the scientific literature published in the *American Journal of Health Promotion* suggests that there is strong evidence of beneficial health effects of both tai chi and qigong, including bone health, cardiopulmonary fitness, balance, and quality of life. Because of the apparent similarities between tai chi and qigong, the researchers reviewed the literature on both practices together. The review, conducted by the Institute of Integral Qigong and Tai Chi (Santa Barbara, California), Arizona State University, and the University of North Carolina, included 77 articles reporting on 66 randomized controlled trials that included 6410 participants of tai chi and qigong. Most of the studies used a nonexercise control group, but some included a control group that practiced other forms of exercise, whereas others included both exercise and nonexercise groups as controls. They concluded that the strongest and most consistent evidence of health benefits for tai chi or qigong is for bone health, cardiopulmonary fitness, balance, and factors associated with preventing falls, quality of life, and self-efficacy (the confidence in and perceived ability to perform a behavior). They went on to suggest that tai chi and qigong are viable forms of exercise with health benefits. Because of the similarities in philosophy and critical elements between tai chi and qigong, they thought that the outcomes could be analyzed across both types of studies.[54]

Tai Chi

Tai chi (TIE-chee) involves performing a series of postures or movements in a slow, graceful manner. It is often referred to as "meditation in motion." Each posture flows into the next without pause, ensuring that the body is in constant motion. Forms of tai chi include rhythmic patterns of movement synchronized with breathing.

Similar to qigong, most forms are gentle and suitable for everyone, regardless of age or physical ability, as technique is emphasized over speed or strength. It is inexpensive, requires no special equipment, can be done indoors or outdoors, and alone or in a group.

Beyond the study mentioned above, further evidence supports the benefits of tai chi. It has been used for years in patients with Parkinson disease. Studies have shown that tai chi training reduces balance impairments in patients with mild-to-moderate Parkinson disease.[68] Additional benefits included improved functional capacity and reduced falls.[42,105]

Practicing tai chi with defined goals as part of a rehabilitation program was found to be more effective than the rehabilitation program alone in improving the performance of activities of daily living.[76]

Tai chi practice may exert its effects by changing brain shape. A controlled study compared tai chi practitioners with controls and showed significantly thicker cortex in the precentral gyrus, insula sulcus, and middle frontal sulcus in the right hemisphere, and the superior temporal gyrus, medial occipitotemporal sulcus, and lingual sulcus in the left hemisphere. Greater intensity of tai chi practice was associated with a thicker cortex in left medial occipitotemporal sulcus and lingual sulcus. These findings suggest that committed long-term practice may induce regional structural change, suggesting that tai chi might share similar patterns of neural correlates with meditation and aerobic exercise.[112]

A National Institutes of Health (NIH) comprehensive review of health benefits of qigong and tai chi concluded that research has demonstrated consistent, significant results for a number of health benefits in randomized controlled trials, and suggested a similarity and equivalence of qigong and tai chi.[54]

Tai chi is simply a safe and effective form of physical exercise. As noted, it enhances cardiovascular fitness, muscular strength, balance, and physical function. It also appears to be associated with reduced stress, anxiety, depression, and improved quality of life. Tai chi can be safely recommended to patients with osteoarthritis, rheumatoid arthritis, and fibromyalgia as a CAM approach to affect patient health and wellness.[109]

Yoga. With many different types of yoga being practiced today, it may be difficult for patients to figure out which style fits them best, and discovering which type of yoga meets their needs. The following is a quick explanation of five of the most common yoga styles practiced.[24]

- Hatha originated in India in the fifteenth century and is slow-paced, gentle, and focuses on breathing and meditation.
- Vinyasa synchronizes breath with movement as one moves through some basic poses. It is a variety of Hatha yoga emphasizing the Sun Salutation, a series of 12 poses in which movement is matched to the breath.
- Ashtanga is a fast-paced and intense form of power yoga that incorporates lunges and push-ups.
- Iyengar covers all aspects of Ashtanga yoga and uses props, such as straps, blankets, and blocks, to assist in strengthening the body while maintaining a focus on body alignment. Standing poses are emphasized and are often held for long periods of time.
- Bikram is a series of 26 poses practiced in a room that is 95° to 100°, which allows for sweating and loosening of tight muscles.

These are only a few of the many styles of yoga.

Research has shown a benefit to yoga practice. In one study, the yoga group significantly improved standing balance, sit-to-stand test, 4-m walk, and one-legged stand with eyes closed compared with a control group.[103]

In another study, the postyoga testing showed a significant decrease in the heart rate and respiratory rate. Maximum changes were seen in autonomic variables and breath rate during the state of effortless meditation (Dhyāna). The changes were all suggestive of reduced sympathetic activity and/or increased vagal modulation.[102]

In a population with traumatic brain injury, one study revealed that the yoga group demonstrated significant longitudinal change on measures of observed respiratory functioning as well as self-reported physical and psychological well-being over a 40-week period. The control group, by contrast, showed marginal improvement on two of the six measures of respiratory health, physical and social functioning, emotional well-being, and general health. The small sample sizes precluded the analysis of between-group differences. This study suggests that breath-focused yoga may improve respiratory functioning and self-perceived physical and psychological well-being of adults with severe traumatic brain injury.[99]

One study of yoga on patients after stroke did not find significant changes in depression or anxiety in those practicing yoga. However, they did report that comparison of individual case results were clinically relevant. Participants reported no adverse events, and the study experienced high retention of participants and high compliance in the yoga program. They concluded that yoga after stroke is a feasible, safe, and acceptable intervention, but additional investigations with larger sample sizes are needed.[22]

Meditation/Mindfulness. Meditation has been practiced for thousands of years and, today, is commonly used for relaxation and stress reduction. Attention is focused to help control the stream of stressful thoughts, which may result in enhanced physical and emotional well-being. Anyone can practice meditation. It is simple, does not require special equipment, and can be practiced anywhere.

There are numerous types of meditation and ways to meditate. The following are a few examples:

- Guided imagery or visualization allows the practitioner to form mental images of relaxing places or situations, incorporating as many senses as possible.
- Mantra meditation, of which, transcendental meditation is a type, is simply the repeating of a calming word, thought or phrase, often silently, which may prevent distracting or troubling thoughts.
- Mindfulness meditation creates an increased awareness of the present moment, focusing on your experience during meditation, such as breathing, seeing, hearing, smelling, tasting, and touching. Seeing your thoughts and emotions, you let them pass without judgment.
- Prayer is the best known and most widely practiced example of meditation.

Although meditation and mindfulness have been a significant part of the human experience for millennia, modern medicine has recently shown an increased interest in meditation and mindfulness, primarily as a result of Jon Kabat-Zinn's work on stress reduction. In a 1982 article, he described a 10-week stress reduction and relaxation program to train patients with chronic pain in self-regulation. He reported on 51 patients with chronic pain who had not improved despite modern medical interventions. At the end of the 10 weeks, he noted 65% showed a reduction of 33% or more in mean total pain rating, whereas 50% showed a reduction of 50% or more. He also reported improvement in mood and psychiatric symptoms.[58]

One study used fMRI to assess the neural mechanisms by which mindfulness meditation influences pain in healthy human participants. Each participant underwent a 4-day training period in which they learned mindfulness meditation techniques. A painful stimulus was applied at rest, to establish a baseline, then applied again while they were practicing the mindfulness meditation they were taught. The study found a reduction in pain unpleasantness by 57% and pain intensity ratings by 40% when the participants were practicing mindfulness meditation. The fMRI was then reviewed, and they found that meditation reduced pain-related activation of the contralateral primary somatosensory cortex. In addition, meditation-induced reductions in pain intensity ratings were associated with increased activity in the anterior cingulate cortex and anterior insula, areas involved in the cognitive regulation of nociceptive processing. Reductions in pain unpleasantness ratings were associated with orbitofrontal cortex activation, an area implicated in reframing the contextual evaluation of sensory events. The drop in pain unpleasantness appeared to be associated with thalamic deactivation. They thought this might reflect a limbic gating mechanism involved in modifying interactions between afferent input and executive-order brain areas. This study seemed to show that meditation engages multiple brain mechanisms that may alter the pain experience from the afferent information.[36]

Mantram repetition has been shown in two randomized controlled trials to assist in managing psychological distress in patients with HIV and to reduce symptoms in self-reported and clinician-rated posttraumatic stress syndrome symptom severity.[14,15]

Economics of Complementary and Integrative Medicine

Amid soaring health spending, there is growing interest in workplace disease prevention and wellness programs to improve health and lower costs. In a critical metaanalysis of the literature on costs and savings associated with such programs, it was found that medical costs fell by approximately $3.27 for every dollar spent on wellness programs and that absenteeism costs fell by approximately $2.73 for every dollar spent. Although further exploration of the mechanisms at work and broader applicability of the findings are needed, this return on investment suggests that the wider adoption of such programs could prove beneficial for budgets and productivity as well as health outcomes.[7]

A systematic review was conducted to determine whether integrative therapies and complementary care was a cost-effective option. The review spanned the years 2001 to 2010 and used criteria based on those of the Cochrane Complementary and Alternative Medicine Group. All studies of CIM reporting economic outcomes were included. They found specific cost savings for acupuncture alone and in combination with other therapies, such as manual therapy and injections. Cost savings were also seen for manual therapy delivered by a physiotherapist, who was also a registered manual therapist for neck pain in terms of perceived recovery, pain, neck disability, and quality-adjusted life years (QALYs); for preoperative oral supplementation with arginine and omega-3 fatty acids for patients with gastrointestinal cancer undergoing surgery; for vitamin K_1 supplementation for postmenopausal women with osteopenia and osteoporosis in terms of QALYs; for supplementation with vitamins C and E and β-carotene for cataract prevention; for fish oil supplementation in men with a history of heart attack; for tai chi to prevent hip fractures in nursing home residents and for naturopathic care offered through a worksite clinic for chronic LBP in terms of both reductions in absenteeism and gains in QALYs. The comprehensive search strategy of this study identified 338 economic evaluations of CIM. The cost-utility analyses found were of similar or better quality compared with those published across all medicine. The higher-quality studies indicate potential cost-effectiveness and even cost savings across a number of CIM therapies and populations.[49]

In 2009, Abbott Northwestern Hospital in Minneapolis, Minnesota, undertook a retrospective study to examine nontoxic, nonpharmacologic integrative approaches to its inpatient population. A total of 1839 inpatients, two thirds of whom never had CIM, underwent various CIM practices that included acupuncture, massage, reflexology (foot massage), music therapy, guided imagery, relaxation response stress reduction, and aromatherapy. The researchers noted an immediate pain reduction of 55% with no side effects. When they analyzed the cost data, they found that when pain was reduced, they saved approximately $2000 per stay, or a total of approximately $2 million. They thought this was attributable to decreased medication use in those patients receiving IM.[32]

The Ford Motor Company was spending $80 million to $90 million per year on managing back pain. This accounted for approximately $400 of the price of every car they sold. Disability payments were a major factor. They recruited the University of Arizona Corporate Health Improvement Program (CHIP) to suggest a more cost-effective way to manage back pain. In 2010, workers with LBP were treated with an integrative approach that included usual care offered at Ford Motor Company clinics, onsite clinical acupuncture, mind-body stress reduction therapies, and referral to chiropractic services. Over 6 weeks, prescription drug use decreased by nearly 60% and more workers returned to their jobs, which meant a savings on disability costs. The Ford Motor Company has adopted this integrative approach in other company health clinics, with insurers covering much of the costs.[78]

A prospective observational study was designed to assess the effectiveness of an IM intervention on modifiable disease risk, patient activation, and psychosocial risk factors for stroke, diabetes, and coronary heart disease (CHD). Sixty-three adults participated in a 3-day comprehensive, multimodal health immersion program at Duke Integrative Medicine, Duke University Medical Center, Durham, North Carolina. Participants received follow-up education, physician support, and telephonic health coaching between the immersion program and the end point, 7 to 9 months later. Psychosocial functioning, readiness to change health behaviors, and risk of developing diabetes, stroke, and CHD were assessed at baseline and end point. Although cardiac risk remained unchanged during the study period, risk of diabetes and stroke decreased significantly. Perceived stress remained unchanged, but improvements were seen in mood and relationship satisfaction. Patients became more activated toward self-management of health, endorsed greater readiness to change health behaviors, and reported increased aerobic exercise and stretching following the intervention.[94]

A study was undertaken to compare health care expenditures of insured patients with back pain, fibromyalgia syndrome, or menopause symptoms who used CAM providers for some of their care with a matched group of patients who did not use any CAM care. Insurance coverage was equivalent for both conventional and CAM providers. Insurance claims data for 2000 to 2003 from Washington State, which mandates coverage of CAM providers, were analyzed. CAM-using patients were matched to CAM-nonusing patients based on age group, gender, index medical condition, overall disease burden, and prior-year expenditures. The results showed that CAM users had lower average expenditures than nonusers. (Unadjusted: $3797 compared with $4153, $P = .0001$; β from linear regression −$367 for CAM users.) CAM users had higher outpatient expenditures; however, these were offset by lower inpatient and imaging expenditures. The largest difference was seen in the patients with the heaviest disease burdens, among whom CAM users averaged $1420 less than nonusers, which more than offset slightly higher average expenditures of $158 among CAM users with lower disease burdens. This analysis indicates that among insured patients with back pain, fibromyalgia, and menopause symptoms, after minimizing selection bias by matching patients who use CAM providers to those who do not, those who used CAM had lower insurance expenditures than those who did not use CAM.[70]

To determine the return on investment (ROI) of the Highmark Inc employee wellness programs, a comparison was done between medical claims for participants of wellness programs versus risk-matched nonparticipants for years 2001 to 2005. The difference was used to define savings. It was determined that health care expenses per person per year were $176 lower for participants. Inpatient expenses were lower by $182. Four-year savings of $1,335,524 compared with program expenses of $808,403 yielded an ROI of $1.65 for every dollar spent on the program. This study suggests that a comprehensive health promotion program can lower the rate of health care cost increases and produce a positive ROI.[83]

Conclusion

IM is more accurately described as an approach to the delivery of health care, not as a separate entity in and of itself. In fact, many think that IM is the way all medical care, not just rehabilitation, will be in the future. Although it often incorporates many complementary practices, the key is a patient-centered integrative approach that includes all health and wellness practices that best serve each individual.

KEY REFERENCES

3. Ahsin S, Saleem S, Bhatti AM, et al: Clinical and endocrinological changes after electro-acupuncture treatment in patients with osteoarthritis of the knee, *Pain* 147:60–66, 2009.
4. Anglin RE, Samaan Z, Walter SD, McDonald SD: Vitamin D deficiency and depression in adults: systematic review and meta-analysis, *Br J Psychiatry* 202:100–107, 2013.
10. Bingel U, Quante M, Knab R, et al: Subcortical structures involved in pain processing: evidence from single-trail fMRI, *Pain* 99:313–321, 2002.
11. Bjelakovic G, Gluud LL, Nikolova D, et al: Vitamin D supplementation for prevention of mortality in adults, *Cochrane Database Syst Rev* (7):CD007470, 2014.
15. Bormann JE, Thorp SR, Wetherell JL, et al: Meditation-based mantram intervention for the veterans with posttraumatic stress disorder: a randomized trial, *Psychol Trauma Theory Res Pract Policy* 5(3):259–267, 2013.
16. Bornhord K, Quante M, Blauche V, et al: Painful stimuli evoke different stimulus-response functions in the amygdala, prefrontal, insula and somatosensory cortex: a single trial fMRI study, *Brain* 125:1326–1336, 2002.
17. Bradley JD, Flusser D, Katz BP, et al: A randomized, double blind, placebo controlled trial of intravenous loading with S-adenosylmethionine (SAM) followed by oral SAM therapy in patients with knee osteoarthritis, *J Rheumatol* 21(5):905–911, 1994.
21. Carlsson CP, Axemo P, Bodin A, et al: Manual acupuncture reduces hyperemesis gravidarum: a placebo-controlled, randomized, single-blind, crossover study, *J Pain Symptom Manage* 20(4):273–279, 2000.
22. Chan W, Immink MA, Hillier S: Yoga and exercise for symptoms of depression and anxiety in people with post-stroke disability: a randomized, controlled pilot trial, *Altern Ther Health Med* 18(3):34–43, 2012.
23. Committee on Quality of Health Care in America, Institute of Medicine: *Crossing the quality chasm: a new health system for the 21st century*, Washington, 2001, National Academy Press.
31. Duke University Integrative Medicine. www.dukeintegrativemedicine.org/patient-care/integrative-health-coaching.
32. Dusek JA, Finch M, Plotnikoff G, Knutson L: The impact of integrative medicine on pain management in a tertiary care hospital, *J Patient Saf* 6(1):48–51, 2010.
33. Ernst E, Lee MS: Acupuncture for rheumatic conditions: an overview of systematic reviews, *Rheumatology* 49(10):1957–1961, 2010.
34. Eslick GD, Howe PR, Smith C, et al: Benefits of fish oil supplementation in hyperlipidemia: a systematic review and meta-analysis, *Int J Cardiol* 136(1):4–16, 2009.
36. Zeidan F, Martucci KT, Kraft RA, et al: Brain mechanisms supporting the modulation of pain by mindfulness meditation, *J Neurosci* 31(14):5540–5548, 2011.
39. Fink M, Wolkenstein E, Karst M, Gehrke A: Acupuncture in chronic epicondylitis: a randomized controlled trial, *Rheumatology* 41(2):205–209, 2002.
41. Gahche J, Bailey R, Burt V, et al: *Dietary supplement use among U.S. adults has increased since NHANES III (1988-1994), National Center for Health Statistics (NCHS) Data Brief, no. 61*, Hyattsville, 2011, National Center for Health Statistics, pp 1–8.
42. Gao Q, Leung A, Yang Y, et al: Effects of tai chi on balance and fall prevention in Parkinson's disease: a randomized controlled trial, *Clin Rehabil* 28(8):748–753, 2014.
44. Gillespie LD, Robertson MC, Gillespie WJ, et al: Interventions for preventing falls in older people living in the community, *Cochrane Database Syst Rev* (9):CD007146, 2012.
45. Haake M, Muller HH, Schade-Brittinger C, et al: German acupuncture trials (GERAC) for chronic low back pain: randomized, multicenter, blinded, parallel-group trial with 3 groups, *Arch Intern Med* 167(17):1892–1898, 2007.
49. Herman PM, Poindexter BL, Witt CM, Eisenberg DM: Are complementary therapies and integrative care cost-effective? A systematic review of economic evaluations, *BMJ Open* 2:e001046, 2012.
50. Hirani V, Cumming RG, Naganathan V, et al: Associations between serum 25-hydroxyvitamin D concentrations and multiple health conditions, physical performance measures, disability, and all-cause mortality: the Concord Health and Ageing in Men Project, *J Am Geriatr Soc* 62(3):417–425, 2014.
51. Hui K, Liu J, Chen A: Effects of acupuncture on human limbic system and basal ganglia measured by fMRI, *Neuroimage* 5:226, 1997.
52. Hui KK, Liu J, Makris N, et al: Acupuncture modulates the limbic system and subcortical gray structures of the human brain: evidence from fMRI studies in normal subjects, *Hum Brain Mapp* 9:13–25, 2000.
54. Jahnke R, Larkey L, Rogers C, et al: A comprehensive review of health benefits of qigong and tai chi, *Am J Health Promot* 24(6):e1–e25, 2010.
57. Ju SY, Lee YJ, Jeong SN: Serum 25-hydroxyvitamin D levels and the risk of depression: a systematic review and meta-analysis, *J Nutr Health Aging* 17(5):447–455, 2013.
58. Kabat-Zinn J: Chronic pain patients based on the practice of mindfulness meditation: theoretical consideration and preliminary results, *Gen Hosp Psychiatry* 4:33–47, 1982.
65. Langevin HM, Yandow JA: Relationship of acupuncture points and meridians to connective tissue planes, *Anat Rec* 269:257–265, 2002.
66. Lauch R, Cramer H, Hauser W, et al: A systematic review and meta-analysis of qigong for fibromyalgia syndrome, *Evid Based Complement Alternat Med* 635182, 2013.
68. Li F, Harmer P, Fitzgerald K, et al: Tai chi and postural stability in patients with Parkinson's disease, *N Engl J Med* 366(6):511–519, 2012.
70. Lind BK, Lafferty WE, Tyree PE, Diehr PK: Comparison of health care expenditures among insured users and nonusers of complementary and alternative medicine in Washington State: a cost minimization analysis, *J Altern Complement Med* 16(4):411–417, 2010.
72. Linde K, Allais G, Brinkhaus B, et al: Acupuncture for migraine prophylaxis, *Cochrane Database Syst Rev* (1):CD001218, 2009.
73. Lynch M, Sawynok J, Kiew C, Marcon D: A randomized controlled trial of qigong for fibromyalgia, *Arthritis Res Ther* 14:R178, 2012.
76. Mańko G, Ziolkowski A, Mirski A, Klosinski M: The effectiveness of selected tai chi exercise in a program of strategic rehabilitation aimed at improving the self-care skills of patients aroused from prolonged coma after severe TBI, *Med Sci Monit* 19:767–772, 2013.
79. National Center for Complementary and Alternative Medicine (NCCAM). http://nccam.nih.Gov.
82. Natural Standard. www.naturalstandard.com.
84. Oh B, Butow P, Mullan B, et al: Impact of medical qigong on quality of life, fatigue, mood and inflammation in cancer patients: a randomized controlled trial, *Ann Oncol* 21:608–614, 2010.
85. Osher Center for Integrative Medicine. www.osher.ucsf.edu.
87. Papakostas GI, Mischoulon D, Shyu I, et al: S-Adenosyl methionine (SAMe) augmentation of serotonin reuptake inhibitors for antidepressant nonresponders with major depressive disorder: a double-blind, randomized clinical trial, *Am J Psychiatry* 167(8):942–948, 2010.
94. Wolever RQ, Webber DM, Meunier JP, et al: Modifiable disease risk, readiness to change, and psychosocial functioning improve with integrative medicine immersion model, *Altern Ther Health Med* 17(4):38–47, 2011.
96. Sakalli H, Arslan D, Yucel AE: The effect of oral and parenteral vitamin D supplementation in the elderly: a prospective, double-blinded, randomized, placebo-controlled study, *Rheumatol Int* 32(8):2279–2283, 2012.
106. Tse HN, Raiteri L, Wong KY, et al: High-dose N-acetylcysteine in stable COPD: the 1-year, double-blind, randomized, placebo-controlled HIACE study, *Chest* 144(1):106–118, 2013.
110. Wang CW, Chan CHY, Ho RTH, et al: Managing stress and anxiety thorough qigong exercise in healthy adults: a systematic review and meta-analysis of randomized controlled trials, *BMC Complement Altern Med* 14:8, 2014.
112. Wei GX, Xu T, Fan FM, et al: Can tai chi reshape the brain? A brain morphometry study, *PLoS ONE* 8(4):e61038, 2013.
114. Wu CH, Wang CC, Kennedy J: Changes in herb and dietary supplement use in the U.S. adult population: a comparison of the 2002 and 2007 National Health Interview Surveys, *Clin Ther* 33(11):1749–1758, 2011.
115. Wu MT, Hsieh JC, Xiong J, et al: Central nervous pathway for acupuncture stimulation: localization of processing with functional MR imaging of the brain—preliminary experience, *Radiology* 212:133–141, 1999.
116. Wu MT, Sheen JM, Chuang KH, et al: Neuronal specificity of acupuncture response: a fMRI study with electroacupuncture, *Neuroimage* 16:1028–1037, 2002.
120. Zhang WT, Jin Z, Cui GH, et al: Relations between brain network activation and analgesic effect induced by low vs. high frequency electrical acupoint stimulation in different subjects: a functional magnetic resonance imaging study, *Brain Res* 982:168–178, 2003.

122. Ziegler D, Ametov A, Barinov A, et al: Oral treatment with alpha-lipoic acid improves symptomatic diabetic polyneuropathy: the SYDNEY 2 trial, *Diabetes Care* 29(11):2365–2370, 2006.
123. Ziegler D, Hanefeld M, Ruhnau KJ, et al: Treatment of symptomatic diabetic polyneuropathy with the antioxidant alpha-lipoic acid: a 7-month multicenter randomized controlled trial (ALADIN III Study). ALADIN III Study Group. Alpha-Lipoic Acid in Diabetic Neuropathy, *Diabetes Care* 22(8):1296–1301, 1999.

The full reference list for this chapter is available online.

CHAPTER 19

COMPUTER ASSISTIVE DEVICES AND ENVIRONMENTAL CONTROLS

Cathy Bodine

This chapter provides an overview of assistive technology (AT) devices and services including definitions, history, and legislation. It also discusses the use of AT for people with communication disorders, impaired mobility, hearing and visual impairments, and cognitive/learning disabilities. New, in this edition, is a discussion of the use of mainstream technologies by persons with disabilities. In addition, this chapter covers the selection of appropriate technology and training in its use; suggests ways to avoid the abandonment of AT by patients and caregivers; and discusses the principles of clinical assessment and physician responsibility. Finally, it briefly discusses the future in terms of research and development and application of emerging technologies to the needs of people with disabilities.

Defining Assistive Technology

The term "assistive technology," coined in the late 1980s, describes tools used to enable people with disabilities to walk, eat and see, and otherwise conduct and participate in activities of daily living. Tools used to support persons with disabilities were recorded in use as early as the sixth or seventh century BC.[14,16] Public Law (PL) 100-407[23] defines AT as "any item, piece of equipment or product system whether acquired commercially off the shelf, modified, or customized that is used to increase or improve functional capabilities of individuals with disabilities." This definition also includes a second component, defining AT services as "any service that directly assists an individual with a disability in the selection, acquisition, or use, of an assistive technology device." PL 100-407 specified the following[23]:

- Evaluating an individual with a disability in terms of his or her goals, needs, and functional abilities in his or her customary environment
- Purchasing, leasing, or otherwise providing for the acquisition of AT by persons with disabilities
- Selecting, designing, fitting, customizing, adapting, applying, retaining, repairing, or replacing AT devices
- Coordinating and using other therapies, interventions, or services with AT devices, such as those associated with existing education and rehabilitation plans and programs
- Training or technical assistance for the person with a disability or, if appropriate, his or her family
- Training or technical assistance for professionals (including individuals providing education or rehabilitation services), employers, or other individuals who provide services to, employ, or are otherwise substantially involved in the major life functions of children with disabilities

Beginning in 1988, this definition has also been used in other federal legislation authorizing services or supports for persons with disabilities. The Individuals with Disabilities Education Act[24] (IDEA) and Reauthorization of the Rehabilitation Act[25] are both examples of legislation that further codifies PL 100-407.

History and Legislation of Assistive Technology

Education: The Individuals with Disabilities Education Act

IDEA originated in 1997 and was reauthorized most recently as PL 108-446 by the 108th Congress. Although overdue for reauthorization, the current Congress has provided continuing resolutions for multiple years. Presumably, the IDEA legislation will be evaluated for renewal in the next few years. IDEA strengthens academic expectations and accountability for the 5.8 million children with disabilities in the United States. One important impact of IDEA legislation is that it specifies that AT devices and services be provided to children from birth to age 21 years to facilitate education in a regular classroom if such devices and services are required as part of the student's special education, related services, or supplementary aids and services (Code of Federal Regulations, Title 34, Sections 300.308 [34CFR]) (Box 19-1). For students with disabilities, AT supports their acquisition of a free and appropriate public education (FAPE). All individualized education plans (IEPs) developed for children needing special education services must indicate that AT has been considered as a way "to provide meaningful access to the general curriculum" (IDEA, 1997). AT devices and services included as a component of an IEP must also be provided at no cost to the student or parents. The school, however, may use other public and private funding sources that are available (34CFR).

Part C of IDEA also includes children before they start school. It covers the needs of children as soon as their

BOX 19-1

Summary of Individuals with Disabilities Act Assistive Technology Requirements

- Assistive technology (AT) must be provided by the school district at no cost to the family.
- AT must be determined on a case-by-case basis; if needed to ensure access to free and appropriate public education, AT is required.
- If the individualized education plan team determines that AT is needed for home use to ensure free and appropriate public education, it must be provided.
- The student's individualized education plan must reflect the nature of the AT and amount of supportive AT services required.
- A parent is accorded an extensive set of procedural safeguards, including the provision of AT to the child.

From Public Law 108-446: The Individuals with Disabilities Education Act Amendments of 1997.

developmental differences are noted. It intends that infants and toddlers receive services in the home or in other places, such as preschool settings, where possible. The services provided for these children are described in individualized family service plans (IFSPs). IFSPs include parents, extended family, and early childhood interventionists and personnel of other related services in planning, identifying goals, and necessary services. IDEA also recognizes that coordination is needed to help families and children with the transition from infant and toddler programs to preschool programs. As a result, students with disabilities are being educated in preschool settings along with typically developing children in an effort to help all children reach the same developmental milestones.

Americans with Disabilities Act and the Reauthorization of the Rehabilitation Act

The American with Disabilities Act (ADA) was originally passed in 1990, and clarified the civil rights of persons with disabilities and specified equal access to public places, employment, transportation, and telecommunications. The ADA built on the foundation of the Rehabilitation Act of 1973 (updated in 2003 as the Reauthorization of the Rehabilitation Act) in recognizing the role of employment in enabling individuals with disabilities to become economically self-sufficient and integrated into communities. The ADA was amended in 2008 and these amendments became effective January 1, 2009. The amended ADA retains the Act's basic definition of "disability" as an impairment that substantially limits one or more major life activities, a record of such an impairment, or being regarded as having such an impairment.[36,37] However, in several ways it changes the way that these statutory terms should be interpreted. Most significantly, the ADA:

- Directs the Equal Employment Opportunity Committee (EEOC) to revise that portion of its regulations defining the term "substantially limits"
- Expands the definition of "major life activities" by including two nonexhaustive lists:
  - The first list includes many activities that the EEOC has recognized (e.g., walking) as well as activities that the EEOC has not specifically recognized (e.g., reading, bending, and communicating).
  - The second list includes major bodily functions (e.g., "functions of the immune system, normal cell growth, digestive, bowel, bladder, neurologic, brain, respiratory, circulatory, endocrine, and reproductive functions").
- States that mitigating measures other than "ordinary eyeglasses or contact lenses" shall not be considered in assessing whether an individual has a disability
- Clarifies that an impairment that is episodic or in remission is a disability if it would substantially limit a major life activity when active
- Changes the definition of "regarded as" so that it no longer requires a showing that the employer perceived the individual to be substantially limited in a major life activity, and instead states that an applicant or employee is "regarded as" disabled if he or she is subject to an action prohibited by the ADA (e.g., failure to hire or termination) based on an impairment that is not transitory and minor.
- Provides that individuals covered only under the "regarded as" prong are not entitled to reasonable accommodation (www.eeoc.gov/types/ada.html).

The latest reauthorization was signed on July 23, 2010, when Attorney General Eric Holder signed final regulations revising the Department of Justice's ADA regulations, including its ADA Standards for Accessible Design. The final rules took effect March 15, 2011.

Workforce Innovation and Opportunity Act (PL 113-128)

The Workforce Innovation and Opportunity Act (WIOA) was reauthorized in July 2014. It is designed to help job seekers (both those with and without disabilities) and workers access employment, education, training, and support services to succeed in the labor market and to match employees with employers. The WIOA includes authorization for vocational rehabilitation services for persons with disabilities (formerly served under the Rehabilitation Act of 1973) and is slated to take effect July 1, 2015. How does the WIOA impact working adults with disabilities?

Vocational rehabilitation services are often the key to enabling employment for adults with disabilities. This legislation mandates that AT devices and services should be considered and provided as a means to acquire vocational training, as well as to enter into and maintain employment. It also requires that AT be considered during the development and implementation of the individualized worker rehabilitation plan, the document that guides a person's vocational rehabilitation process. For example, if an individual has limited sight and needs to fill out paperwork to determine his or her eligibility for vocational rehabilitation services, assistive devices to facilitate reading must be provided at that time. In recent years, offices of vocational rehabilitation have become important sources of funding for AT devices and services to support employment for adults with disabilities.

Assistive Technology and the International Classification of Functioning

The term "disability" is not always precise and quantifiable. Further, the concept of disability is not even agreed upon by individuals who self-identify as having a disability, by professionals who study disability, or by the general public.[22,23] This lack of agreement creates an obstacle to the study of disability and to the fair and effective administration of programs and policies intended for people with disabilities.[4-8,17] With this issue in mind, the World Health Organization (WHO) developed a global common health language; one that includes physical, mental, and social well-being. The International Classification of Impairment, Disabilities, and Handicaps was first published by the WHO in 1980 as a tool for classification of the "consequences of disease." The newest version, International Classification of Functioning, Disability and Health, known as ICF, moves away from a "consequence of disease" classification (1980 version) to a more positive "components of health" classification. This latest version provides a common framework and language for the description of health and health-related domains and uses the following language[39,40]:

Body functions are the physiologic functions of body systems (including psychological functions).

Body structures are anatomic parts of the body such as organs, limbs, and their components.

Impairments are problems in body function or structure such as a significant deviation or loss.

Activity is the execution of a task or action by an individual.

Participation is involvement in a life situation.

Activity limitations are difficulties an individual may have in executing activities.

Participation restrictions are problems an individual may experience in involvement in life situations.

Environmental factors make up the physical, social, and attitudinal environments in which people live and conduct their lives.

The ICF and its language help professionals define the need for health care and related services, such as the provision of AT. It recognizes that physical, mental, social, economic, or environmental interventions can improve lives and levels of functioning for persons with diseases that affect them at the body, person, and social functioning levels.[39] It also characterizes physical, mental, social, economic, or environmental interventions that will improve lives and levels of functioning. Because AT has the potential to improve daily activities and participation in social and physical environments and thus improve the quality of life of individuals with disabilities, it clearly fits within the ICF. The common-health language of the WHO is used throughout this chapter to discuss the potential impact of appropriate AT.

Overview of Assistive Technology Devices

AT devices are designed to facilitate functional abilities and to meet the needs of humans throughout their varied life stages and roles. It is important to remember that AT device usage and requirements will change over time as individuals mature and take on different life roles. Consequently, there is no "one size fits all" technology available. It is also equally important to recognize the exponential growth and change in available technologies. The AT and mainstream technologies described in this chapter may or may not be relevant in just a few short months or years. It is crucial that practitioners keep an eye out for new developments and opportunities to choose the most timely and relevant technologies for their patients.

Human-Technology Interface

AT devices have the potential to compensate or facilitate immobility, low endurance, difficulty reaching, grasping or accurately touching keys or switches, problems with seeing or hearing, verbal communication, and the complex skills necessary for reading, writing, and learning. This section will focus on specific categories of AT devices as they are related to these areas of human function.

Considering one's own interaction with technology gives insight into the issues involved in the concept of human-technology interface (HTI). Devices await activation or input from the people who use them. This commonly occurs through dials, switches, keyboards, handlebars, joysticks, or handgrips. This interface typically requires fine motor control, hearing, and vision within normal limits. People know they have successfully interacted with devices by the physical, visual, or auditory feedback these devices provide, for example, the sight of brewing coffee, images on a computer monitor, or the sound of a telephone ringing.

Individuals with impairments that affect their interaction with items in their environment need special consideration in the design, function, or placement of the devices they want or need to use. For many individuals, it is essential that they are first seated or positioned for optimal use of their residual abilities by means of orthotic or ergonomic seating and positioning interventions. (Please refer to Chapter 14 for more on this topic.)

Direct Selection

Once optimal positioning is established, assessment of an individual's reliable, low-effort, high-accuracy hand movements, vision, communication, and hearing will help an evaluator determine whether they are able to use a typical "interface" or need one that is adapted. Using a typical interface (e.g., a computer keyboard, steering wheel, TV remote control) is called direct selection because all possible options are presented at once and can be directly selected by the individual. For those without the ability to accurately choose an intended item within the available selection set, a different selection method must be considered.

Scanning or Indirect Selection

Scanning is the most common indirect selection method used by persons with significant motor impairments. A selection set is presented on a display (e.g., a series of

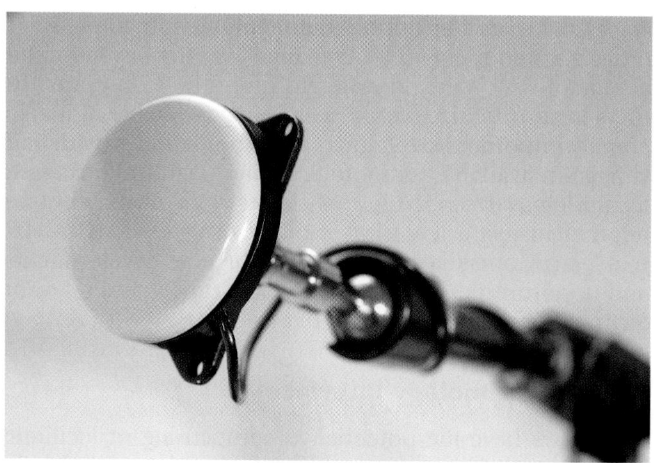

FIGURE 19-1 Head switch. (Courtesy AbleNet Technologies, Roseville, Minn.).

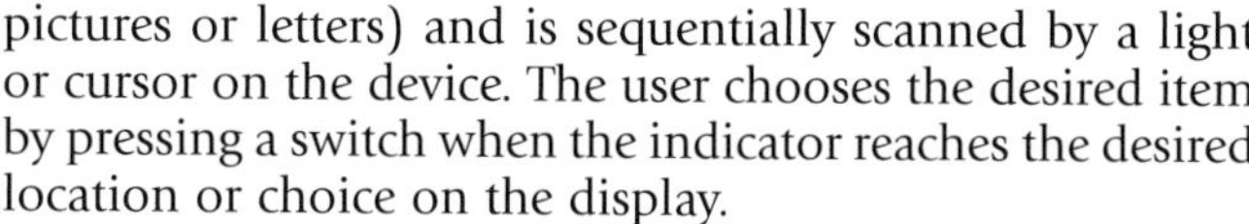

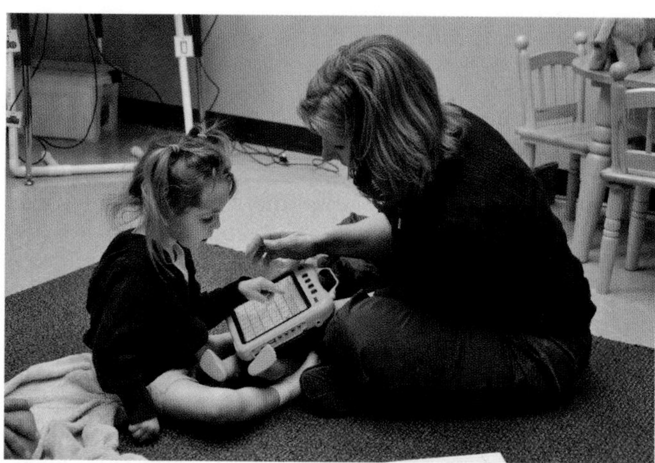

FIGURE 19-2 A child using the Accent 800 (Prentke Romich Company, Wooster, Ohio), an augmentative and alternative communication device.

pictures or letters) and is sequentially scanned by a light or cursor on the device. The user chooses the desired item by pressing a switch when the indicator reaches the desired location or choice on the display.

Switches come in many styles and are selected based on the body part that will be activating them (e.g., elbow or chin) and the task or setting for using them (e.g., watching TV in bed or using a communication device while eating). A switch can be as simple as a "wobble" switch that is activated by a gross motor movement such as hitting the switch with the head (Figure 19-1), hand, arm, leg, or knee. Other switches are activated by tongue touch, by sipping and puffing on a straw, or through very fine movements such as an eye blink or a single muscle twitch. Regardless, switch use and timing accuracy can be very difficult for new users and must be taught. One common method to teach switch activation and use is to interface a switch with battery-operated toys and games or home/work appliances to increase motivation and teach the concepts used in indirect selection.

Fairly recent developments include the eye gaze switch and head mouse. The eye gaze switch calibrates intentional eye movement patterns and selects targets such as individual keys on an onscreen keyboard. Other new developments include brainwave technology (e.g., an eye and muscle operated switch [EMOS]) that responds to excitation of alpha waves to trigger a selection.

Displays

HTI also applies to completing the feedback loop from devices back to the user. Examples include software that enlarges images on a computer display for a person with low vision, installing flashing alarms for persons without hearing, and using devices that convert printed text into synthesized speech or Braille for persons with blindness or a learning disability.

These HTI concepts apply to all forms of AT whether it is being used for seating, mobility, communication, computer activity, or control of the environment. Good assessment skills and a focus on patients and their goals and needs are essential for HTI success and prevention of assistive device abandonment.

Assistive Technology for Communication Disorders

Vocal communication allows humans to interact, form relationships, and direct the events of their lives to enable choice and participation. Human communication is based on having both receptive and expressive language abilities and the physical capacity to reliably produce intelligible speech sounds. Communication impairment can result from congenital conditions such as intellectual and developmental disability, cerebral palsy, developmental verbal apraxia, and developmental language disorders. Other impairments can be acquired through traumatic brain injury, stroke, multiple sclerosis, amyotrophic lateral sclerosis, tetraplegia, ventilator-dependence, and laryngectomy resulting from cancer.[3] AT devices that meet the needs of persons with many types of speech and language impairment are commonly called augmentative and alternative communication (AAC) devices because they can either support or substitute for expressive language impairments. More recently, the term "speech-generating device" has entered into the medical vocabulary to differentiate AAC devices from basic computer devices, especially when seeking third-party funding such as Medicaid and Medicare.[8]

Some individuals are completely unable to speak or have such severe expressive difficulties that only those very familiar with them are able to communicate effectively with them. For these individuals, many devices are available, ranging from simple, low-tech picture books to high-end, sophisticated electronic devices with digitally recorded or synthetic text-to-speech output capable of producing complex language interactions (Figure 19-2).

Although AAC devices are extremely useful to nonspeaking individuals, they do not replace natural communication. AAC device use should be encouraged along with all other available communication modalities such as gestures, vocalizations, sign language, and eye gaze.[27] There are no firm cognitive, physical, or developmental prerequisites for using an AAC device. Instead, comprehensive evaluation techniques are used to match the individual's abilities and communication needs with the appropriate

AAC technologies and intervention strategies. A qualified team of clinicians performs this evaluation with input from the individual and their family members, teachers, employers, and others. Because speaking is considered to be a crucial human function, many parents and family members wait to seek out AAC devices in the hope that natural speech will develop. However, research shows that accessing an AAC device and services can actually support verbal language development and can, in fact, increase the potential for natural speech to develop.[3] Children and adults with severe communication impairments can benefit socially, emotionally, academically, and vocationally from using a device that allows them to communicate their thoughts, learn and share ideas, and participate in life activities.[2]

In the past several years, the use of touchscreen tablets, such as the iPad, has become highly popular. Many potential users and their families express a preference for using these ubiquitous mainstream technologies. They are less expensive and have the added advantage of being perceived as "cool." There are numerous AAC applications, or apps, available for these devices. At issue, however, is a current debate (2014-2015) regarding Medicare's willingness to pay for technologies that include access to computing functions. Medicare will cover the cost of "medically necessary" technologies, including AAC devices. However, Medicare will not pay for any other functional capabilities and, in fact, has required manufacturers to lock-down any computing functions before funding computer-based AAC technologies. Although the jury is still out, it is important for practitioners to be aware of this issue.

Additionally, although tablet-based AAC devices are popular, there are some drawbacks. Namely, volume settings require additional amplification, battery life, and robustness. Many tablets have a limited (4- to 6-hour) battery life and almost all are prone to breakage or damage when dropped or thrown. In addition, the apps that are available for these tablet devices do not always incorporate robust, research-based language programs. For young consumers in particular, these devices often prove distracting as many who understand how to use the technology prefer Web browsing, games, and videos over voice output communications. Clinicians, caregivers, and end users must carefully weigh these considerations before prescribing and/or purchasing.

Nonelectronic Systems

Low-tech, nonelectronic AAC systems are often used in addition to an electronic voice output system (or as a backup system in case an electronic device fails or cannot be used during certain activities such as during a swimming lesson). Low-tech systems can be made with digital photographs, pictures from books or catalogs, or a marker to draw letters, words, phrases, or pictures. Picture library software is also available commercially. This software (e.g., BoardMaker and PCS Symbols) incorporates thousands of line drawings and pictures that can be used to quickly and easily fabricate a low-tech, nonelectronic communication system.

Adults with progressive diseases such as amyotrophic lateral sclerosis or multiple sclerosis can also choose to use low-tech picture or alphabet boards as a supplement to verbal communication as a result of fatigue during the day or as their ability to verbally communicate decreases. Many of these adults choose to use both low-tech and high-tech communication systems depending on the environment they are in, available communication partners, and their comfort level with technology.[9]

Electronic Voice Output Systems: Digital Speech

A variation in low-tech communication systems has developed as a result of the manufacture of low-cost microprocessors capable of storing digitized speech. These low-tech, digital voice output devices allow recording and storing of simple phrases into memory within the device. When the user wants to speak, he or she simply presses a button and the device speaks the prerecorded message.

Devices such as One Step, Step by Step, and BIGmack communication aids (Figure 19-3) are simple and relatively inexpensive, and are designed to communicate quick, simple messages such as "Hi," "Let's play," or "Leave me alone." These technologies are often used with very young children who are beginning communicators, or for those who have significant cognitive impairments. They are not appropriate for individuals needing or wanting to communicate complex thoughts and feelings.[12]

Complex digitized devices store several minutes of recorded voice that is usually associated with representative pictures or icons on a keyboard. These devices are often used by individuals who are not yet literate, have intellectual and developmental disabilities, or simply wish to have a simple device to use when going to the store or out to eat. Examples are the SuperTalker Progressive, the GoTalk (Figure 19-4), and the TechSpeak.

Electronic Voice Output Systems: Synthesized Speech

Synthesized speech is created by software that uses rules of phonics and pronunciation to translate alphanumeric text into spoken output through speech synthesizer hardware.

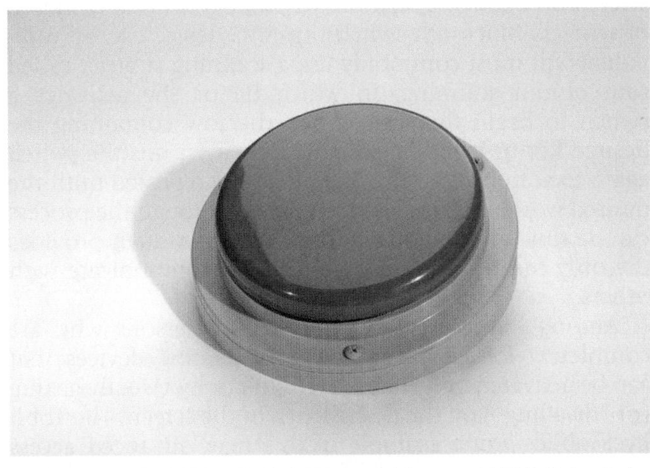

FIGURE 19-3 The BIGmack Communicator. (Courtesy AbleNet Technologies, Roseville, Minn.).

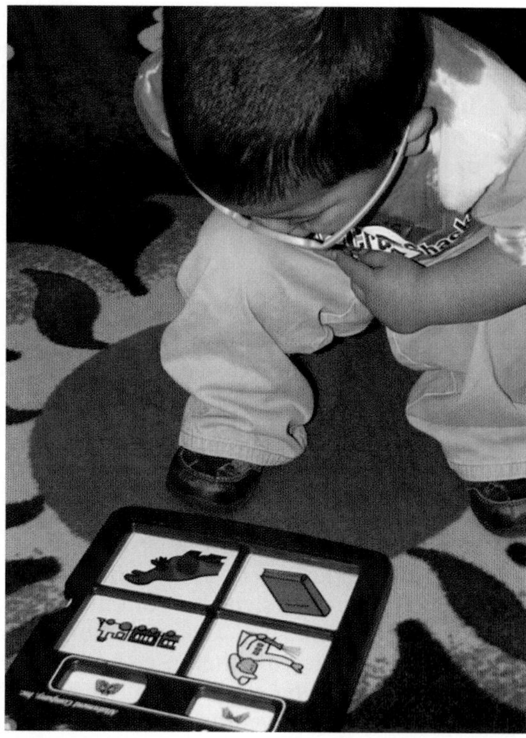

FIGURE 19-4 A child using GoTalk (Attainment Company, Verona, Wis.), an electronic voice output system.

Voice output systems such as Lightwriter, DynaVox T Series, and ECO2 are examples of high-tech text-to-speech devices with built-in speech synthesis that speak words and phrases that have been typed and/or previously stored in the device. The advantage of these systems is that they allow users to speak on any topic and use any words they wish to use. These systems, which can encode several thousand words, phrases, and sentences, are expensive (costing from $6000 to $9000). They form, however, an essential link to the world for people with severe expressive communication disabilities.

All of these voice output systems, whether digital or text-to-speech, can be activated by direct selection (e.g., using a finger or a pointing device such as a mouth stick or head pointer). They can also be activated with indirect selection (e.g., using a scanning strategy with an infrared or wireless Bluetooth switch). In AAC device use, an individual will most commonly use a scanning strategy called row-column scanning, in which he or she activates a switch to begin the scan. When the row containing the desired key or icon is highlighted, the user hits the switch again to scan by column. The process is repeated until the desired word or phrase is assembled. Although the process can be slow and tedious, indirect selection often provides the only means many people have to communicate with others.

Among the latest developments for persons who are completely locked-in are speech-generating devices that can be activated by a simple eye blink or by visually gazing (or "dwelling") on the desired area of the screen. The Tobii EyeMobile is one example of this new, advanced access method. It is composed of two parts: a Windows-based tablet and a PCEye Go accessory.

AAC devices differ in mapping and encoding strategies used to represent language, and in storing and retrieving methods used for vocabulary. However, all systems use either orthographic or pictographic symbols, which vary in ease of learning. When selecting a set of symbols for an individual as part of the user interface, it is important to consider these factors and compare them with the individual's cognitive and perceptual abilities.

Portable Amplification Systems

For people who speak quietly because of low breath support or other difficulties with phonation, portable amplification systems that function like a sound system in a large lecture hall are available. The Speech Enhancer processes speech sounds for people with dysarthria and enables improved recognition by others. The user wears a headset with a microphone attached to a portable device, and their clarified voice is projected via speakers attached to the unit.

Assistive Technology for Mobility Impairments

Motor impairments greatly affect the ability of individuals to interact with their environment. Infants are compelled to roll, then crawl, and as toddlers being able to walk in their efforts to explore their surroundings. Any motor impairment can greatly impact overall development. This is often the situation with cerebral palsy, spina bifida, arthrogryposis, and other diagnoses that impact motor skills. Early intervention and supporting caregivers and families available to create modifications and incorporate AT devices into activities can help children achieve critical developmental milestones.

The loss of acquired motor abilities through trauma or disease is experienced as a severe loss for children and adults and occurs with spinal cord injury, stroke, multiple sclerosis, amputation, and so forth. There are many forms of AT that help compensate for impaired motor skills, and they should be introduced as early as possible in rehabilitation to ensure the best outcome possible.

Upper Body Mobility Devices

Given the importance of computer use in education, training, and employment, many AT devices have been developed to give individuals with upper body mobility impairment such as poor hand control or paralysis access to computers. But what if someone is unable to use a standard mouse and keyboard?

Alternate computer keyboards come in many shapes and sizes. There are expanded keyboards such as the IntelliKeys (AbleNet Technologies, Roseville, Minn.) (Figure 19-5), which provides a larger target or key surrounded by inactive space than a standard keyboard. Options such as delayed activation response help individuals who have difficulty with pointing accuracy or removing a finger after activating a key. Individuals unfamiliar with a standard QWERTY keyboard layout have the option for alphabetical layout. This is often helpful for young children who are

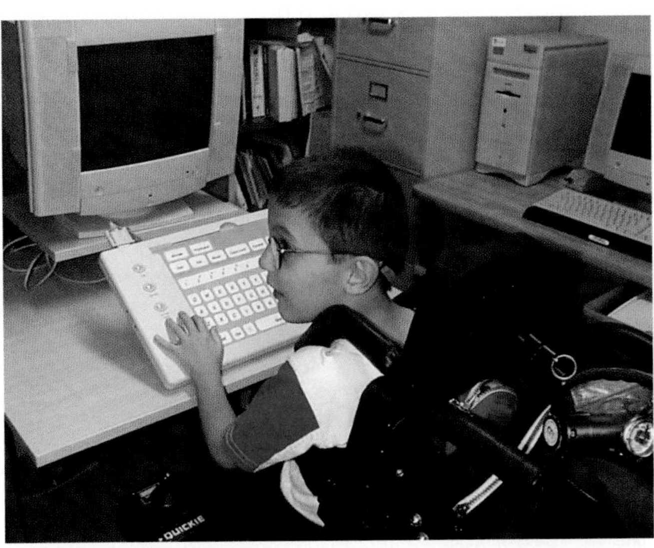

FIGURE 19-5 A child using an expanded keyboard.

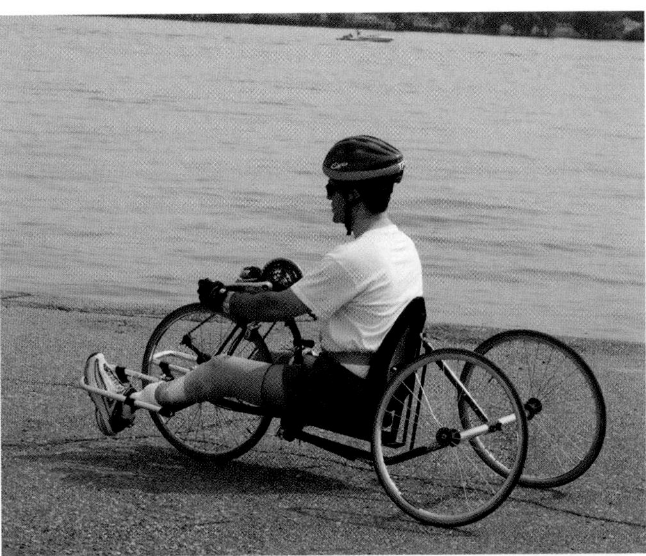

FIGURE 19-6 The hand bike, an example of a low-tech recreation aid.

developing literacy skills, as well as for adults with cognitive or visual impairments.

There are also smaller keyboards (e.g., Tash Mini Keyboard) designed for persons with limited range of motion and endurance. They are also helpful for individuals who type with one hand, or use a head pointer or mouth stick to type. These keyboards use a "frequency of occurrence" layout. The home or middle row in the center of the keyboard holds the space bar and the letters in English words that occur most frequently (e.g., "a" and "e"). All other characters, numbers, and functions (including mouse control) fan out from the center of the keyboard based on how frequently they are used in common computer tasks.

Voice recognition (VR) is a mass-market technology that has become essential for computer access for many individuals with motor impairment. Instead of writing via the keyboard, VR users write or speak words out loud. The computer processor uses information from the user's individual voice file, compares it with digital models of words and phrases, and produces computer text. If the words are accurate the user proceeds, if not, the user corrects the words to match what was said. As the process continues, the computer updates its voice file and VR accuracy improves. This software is cognitively demanding, yet can offer "hands-free" or greatly reduced keyboarding to many individuals with motor impairment.

Another group of computer input methods include devices that rely on an onscreen keyboard visible on the computer monitor such as the Head Mouse Extreme and TrackerPro. The user wears a head-mounted signaling device or a reflective dot on the forehead to select keys on the onscreen keyboard, choose commands from pull-down menus, or direct mouse movement. Onscreen keyboards are typically paired with rate enhancement options such as word prediction or abbreviation expansion to increase a user's word-per-minute rate. Because so many tasks can be accomplished through computers, individuals with disabilities—even those with the most severe motor impairments—can fully participate in life. They can perform education- and work-related tasks and monitor and control an unlimited array of devices/appliances at home, work, and school.

Lower Body Mobility Devices

Individuals with spinal cord injury, spina bifida, or cerebral palsy often have lower body mobility impairments. AT solutions can include crutches, a rolling walker, a powered scooter, or a manual or powered wheelchair (see Chapter 14). Simple environmental modifications or adaptations such as installing a ramp instead of stairs, raising the height of a desk, or widening doorways can be indispensable facilitators for these individuals and might be all that is needed. For other activities or to increase participation, adding automobile hand controls, adapted saddles for horseback riding, or sit-down forms of downhill skiing (Figure 19-6) are possible.

There are literally thousands of low-tech assistive devices available for individuals with motor impairments. Commonly referred to as aids or adaptive devices for completing activities of daily living, these devices include weighted spoons and scoop plates to facilitate eating; aids for personal hygiene such as bath chairs and long-handled hairbrushes; items for dressing such as sock aides and one-handed buttoners; adapted toys for play; built-up pencil grips for writing and drawing; and many others. Many low-tech mobility aids can be handmade for just a few dollars, whereas others, such as an adult rolling bath chair, can cost several hundred dollars. All share the common goal of reducing barriers and increasing participation in daily life.

Assistive Technology for Ergonomics and Prevention of Secondary Injuries

A rapidly growing area of concern for AT practitioners is the development of repetitive strain injuries (RSIs) among both individuals who are able-bodied and individuals who are disabled. Although specialized keyboards and mouse control have provided computer access for many individuals, the pervasiveness of computer technology has also increased the possibility of RSIs. Over the past few years, an entire industry of AT has developed to deal with repetitive motion disorders.

Computer desks, tables, and chairs used in computer laboratories, classrooms, and offices do not always match the physical needs of users. When people with and without disabilities spend hours repetitively performing the same motor movement, they can and do develop RSIs. Potential solutions include properly supporting seated posture, raising or lowering a chair or desk for optimal fit, implementing routine breaks, and using ergonomically designed keyboards and other ATs.

Many of the AT devices described in this chapter (i.e., alternate and specially designed ergonomic keyboards, VR software, and strategies to minimize keystrokes) can also provide useful solutions for individuals with RSIs. There are also internet-based resources that target ergonomic issues such as those found in Table 19-1.

Table 19-1 Internet-Based Resources for Ergonomics

Organization	Website Address
Government Sites	
NIOSH Web	www.cdc.gov/niosh/topics/ergonomics/
OSHA Web	www.osha.gov/SLTC/ergonomics/index.html
Educational Institution Sites	
Cornell University Ergonomics	http://ergo.human.cornell.edu/
Ergonomic Design Standard—University of Melbourne	http://safety.unimelb.edu.au/docs/manual-handling-and-ergonomics-procedure.pdf
Ergonomic Guidelines for Video Display Terminal	http://ehs.fiu.edu/Programs/General%20Safety/Pages/Ergonomic-Guidelines.aspx#vdt
Ergonomic Workstation Guidelines—North Carolina State University	www.ncsu.edu/ehs/www99/right/handsMan/office/ergonomic.html
Loughborough University Ergonomics	www.lboro.ac.uk/departments/lds/ergonomics/research/
Office Ergo Guidelines—University of Sydney	http://sydney.edu.au/whs/guidelines/ergonomics/index.shtml
Office Ergonomic Standard—University of Toronto	www.ehs.utoronto.ca/services/Ergonomics.htm
Ohio State University Ergonomics	http://ergonomics.osu.edu/
University of California, Berkeley, San Francisco Ergonomics	http://ergo.berkeley.edu/
University of California Los Angeles Ergonomics	http://ergonomics.ucla.edu/
University of Michigan Ergonomics	http://ioe.engin.umich.edu/degrees/grad/gradspecial.php
University of Nebraska Ergonomics	http://rsi.unl.edu/
Additional Ergonomic Resources	
ANSI BHMA Search	www.buildershardware.com/bhma-standards
Ergonomics for Notebooks	www.ergoindemand.com/laptop-workstation-ergonomics.htm
Human Factors Standards	www.12207.com/human_factors.htm
Ergonomic Edge	www.ergonomicedge.com/
Ergonomic Resources	www.ergoweb.com/
Ergonomics for Teacher and Student	www.ergonomics4schools.com/
Next Gen Ergo	www.nexgenergo.com/
Stress Ergonomics	www.spineuniverse.com/wellness/ergonomics/ergonomics-human-body-injury-prevention
Industry Sites	
3M Ergo	http://solutions.3m.com/wps/portal/3M/en_US/ergonomics/home/advice/workspacecomfortguide/
American Ergonomics Corporation	http://americanergonomics.com/
Basic Ergo Standard	https://ergoweb.com/knowledge/ergonomics-101/faq/
Hewlett Packard Ergo Guidelines—Working in Comfort	www8.hp.com/us/en/hp-information/ergo/index.html
Office Ergonomics Training	http://office-ergo.com/
Office Ergonomics	www.healthycomputing.com/office/
Repetitive Strain Injury FAQs by CTD Resource Network, Inc.	www.tifaq.org/information.html
Work-Related Musculoskeletal Disorders	www.nsc.org/learn/Safety-Training/Pages/Courses/ergonomics-managing-results.aspx

Electronic Aids to Daily Living

Electronic aids to daily living (EADLs) provide alternative control of electrical devices within the environment and increase independence in tasks of daily living. This technology is also referred to as environmental control units (ECUs). Within the home, EADLs can control audiovisual equipment (i.e., TV, video players and recorders, cable, digital satellite systems, stereo), communication equipment (i.e., telephone, intercom, and call bells), doors, electric beds, security equipment, lights, and appliances (i.e., fan, wave machine). EADLs are controlled directly by pressing a button with a finger or pointer or by voice command, or indirectly by scanning and switch activation. Some AAC devices or computer systems also provide EADL device control of devices within the environment.

Almost anyone with limited control over his or her environment can benefit from this technology. Children and adults with developmental delays often benefit from low-tech EADLs that increase independence in play through intermittent switch control of battery-operated toys or electrical devices such as a disco light. For those unable to operate a TV remote control, switches or voice commands to an EADL device allow access to devices they would otherwise be unable to control. Many EADLs also accommodate cognitive and visual deficits. For example, an AAC device can display an icon instead of text for an individual without literacy or who cannot read English. The same device can also use auditory scanning so that choices can be heard if the individual has impaired vision.

EADLs are primarily used in the home, but can also be used in a work or school setting. An individual can use EADL technology to turn on the lights at a workstation and use the telephone. A child who uses a switch can participate more fully in the classroom by advancing slides for a presentation or by activating a tape player with a story on cassette for the class.

The term EADL was chosen over ECU for two primary reasons. First, the term more accurately defined this area of AT by emphasizing the task (i.e., communication is a daily living activity) rather than the item being controlled (i.e., the telephone). Second, the term was chosen to improve reimbursement by third-party providers because the category of ECUs has been poorly funded in the past. In contrast, aids to daily living (ADL) equipment is traditionally funded very well. ADL equipment, which is designed to make the individual more independent in a specific daily living task, includes bath seats, toileting aids, built-up spoon handles, and zipper pulls. This equipment is defined by the "daily living" task it "aids."

ECU devices had the same general goal, but the name failed to reflect the goal, particularly to funding agencies. EADL expands ADL equipment to include equipment that happens to use batteries or plug into the wall, but still shares the same goal: increasing independence in tasks of daily living.

Home Automation Systems

During the past decade a number of "smart-home" technologies have become available. Initially targeted to high-end consumers, many AT practitioners and others have begun to recognize the growing utility of these devices for persons with disabilities and older adults. For example, sensors placed in the home can assist in physiologic monitoring, and alert systems are now available for medication reminders. Automated heating and cooling controls can be used for persons who have difficulty regulating internal temperature. Remote video monitoring and automated door locks and openers can be used to facilitate entry, safety, and security. New developments that will be readily available in 2015 include the ability to incorporate technologies manufactured by differing companies into a single application, enabling direct or indirect control of various technologies.

Assistive Technology for Hearing Impairments

Hearing impairment and deafness affect the feedback loop in the human-environment interaction. Because most individuals can hear, it is commonly recognized as a significant barrier in communication and can compromise safety in situations where sound is used to warn of danger.

Hearing Aids

Individuals who are deaf or hard of hearing deal with two major issues: lack of auditory input and compromised ability to monitor speech output and environmental sound. AT devices such as hearing aids and FM (frequency modulation or radio wave) systems can be used to facilitate both auditory input and speech output. Other types of AT devices provide a visual representation of the auditory signal. These include flashing lights as an alternate emergency alarm (e.g., for fire or tornado) or the ring of a telephone or doorbell.

Cochlear Implants

When the hearing system is impaired at the level of the middle ear or the cochlea, a highly specialized form of AT is used to create an alternate means of stimulating the auditory nerve. This technology is implanted surgically with an electrode array placed within or around the cochlear structure. The external portion, a microphone, relays speech and environmental sound to the implanted portion, which is programmed to process, synchronize, and stimulate electrodes appropriately. This system requires a battery pack worn on the body or behind the ear.[8] It also requires an experienced audiologist to teach the individual to use the acoustic cues produced by the cochlear implant as a substitute for natural hearing.

Other Hearing Technologies

Another recent adaptation for persons with significant hearing impairments is computer-assisted real-time translation (CART). This AT solution involves a specially trained typist or stenographer who captures what is being spoken on a computer. The text is then projected onto a display, resulting in close to "real-time" translation. The advantage of this technology is that it can be used by individuals with hearing impairment who are not fluent in sign language as well as others who might need listening help, such as those who use English as a second language. In addition to use in group environments such as conferences or meetings, a variation of this technology can be used to assist a single student or employee in a small setting.

Environmental Adaptations

For individuals who wear hearing aids, there are additional technologies that can facilitate hearing in large rooms or in noisy, crowded environments such as a restaurant. The Conference Mate and Whisper Voice are specially designed for these environments. In the case of the Conference Mate, an individual with hearing loss wears a "neckloop" that acts as an antenna and is capable of broadcasting directly to a hearing aid. A microphone placed near the speaker transmits directly to the neckloop, eliminating background sound. This is also an excellent solution for office and school environments. The Whisper Voice is similar, except it uses a smaller microphone and is more portable. It can be passed from speaker to speaker with sound transmitted to the neckloop and then onto the hearing aid for amplification.

Environmental adaptations can frequently support individuals who are deaf or hard of hearing. For example, a person speaking to someone who has difficulty hearing can take care not to stand in front of a light source (windows, lamps, etc.) and not to overexaggerate or hide lip movements. Gestures can also be helpful.

Assistive Technology for Visual Impairments

The term visual impairment technically encompasses all types of permanent vision loss, including total blindness. Low vision refers to a vision loss that is severe enough to impede performing everyday tasks, but still provides some usable visual information. Low vision cannot be corrected to normal by eyeglasses or contact lenses.

Low-Tech Visual Aids

A variety of AT devices and strategies can help individuals with visual impairments perform daily activities such as reading, writing, personal care, mobility, and recreational activities. Among low-tech solutions are simple handheld magnifiers, the use of large print, or mobility devices (e.g., a white cane, Figure 19-7) for safe and efficient travel. High-contrast tape or markers can also be used to indicate hazards, what an item is, or where it is located.

Other low-tech solutions include items such as using wind chimes to help with direction finding, using easily legible type fonts such as Verdana (16 point or larger), and using beige-colored paper rather than white to improve the visibility of text. In recreational activities, solutions include beeper balls, three-dimensional puzzles, and outdoor trails with signage called "Braille trails" designed to improve access to wilderness and other outdoor activities.

Brailed text, although less used than in the past because of the advances of computer and other technologies, is still the first choice of many individuals for reading. Many restaurants now provide large print, Braille, and picture-based menus for customers with a variety of abilities.

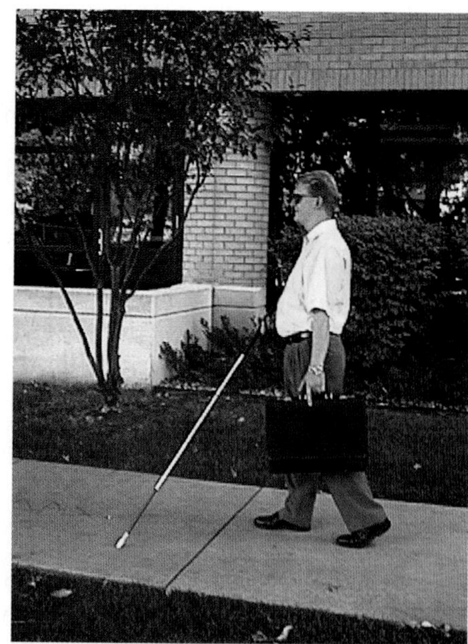

FIGURE 19-7 Use of a cane by a person with visual impairment.

Books-on-tape are another resource for individuals with severe visual impairments. In addition to commercially available tapes for sale and at public libraries, special libraries provide print materials in alternate formats for persons with visual, physical, and learning impairments. Borrowers can arrange to have textbooks and other materials translated into alternate formats. For more information, contact the American Federation for the Blind or the National Library Service for the Blind and Physically Handicapped (www.loc.gov/nls/) (Box 19-2).

High-Tech Visual Aids

Numerous high-tech solutions exist for persons with visual impairments. Computers outfitted with a speech synthesizer and specialized software such as Jaws or Window-Eyes allow navigation of the desktop, operating system, applications, and documents, as well as the entire internet. Any digital text can be heard aloud by the person using this software. For text that is printed (e.g., menus, memos, letters), using a technology called optical character recognition allows a page scanner and software to convert print into digital form. It can then be listened to through the computer's speech synthesizer, or converted to Braille or large print.

Another category of high-tech aids are portable note takers with either Braille or speech synthesizer feedback for the user. These devices are specialized personal digital assistants with calendars, contacts, memo, and document capabilities, and can be purchased with either a QWERTY or Braille keyboard.

For individuals with some degree of visual ability, screen magnification software such as Zoomtext (Figure 19-8) and MAGic enable the user to choose the amount (2 to 20

BOX 19-2

Resources for Persons with Low Vision or Blindness

- **American Academy of Ophthalmology**
  PO Box 7424
  San Francisco, CA 94120
  Tel 415 561-8500
  www.eyenet.org
- **American Council of the Blind in Colorado**
  910 16th Street, Suite 1240
  Denver, CO 80202
  Tel 303 831-0117
  www.acbco.org
- **American Council of the Blind**
  2200 Wilson Boulevard, Suite 650
  Arlington, VA 22201
  Tel 202 467-5081
  www.acb.org
- **American Foundation for the Blind**
  2 Penn Plaza, Suite 1102
  New York, NY 10121
  Tel 800 232-5463
  www.afb.org
- **American Printing House for the Blind**
  1839 Frankfort Avenue
  Louisville, KY 40206
  Tel 502 895-2405
  www.aph.org
- **Lighthouse International**
  111 E 59th Street
  New York, NY 10022-1202
  Tel 800 284-4422
  http://lighthouse.org/navh
- **National Braille Association, Inc.**
  95 Allen Creek Road, Building 1, Suite 202
  Rochester, NY 14618
  Tel 585 427-8260
  www.nationalbraille.org
- **National Braille Press, Inc.**
  88 St. Stephen Street
  Boston, MA 02115
  Tel 888 965-8965
  www.nbp.org
- **Learning Ally**
  20 Roszel Road
  Princeton, NJ 08540
  Tel 800 221-4792
  www.learningally.org
- **Rehabilitation Engineering and Assistive Technology Society of North America State Technology Projects**
  1700 N Moore Street, Suite 1540
  Arlington, VA 22209-1903
  Tel 703 524-6866
  www.resna.org
- **Assistive Technology Partners**
  601 E 18th Avenue, Suite 130
  Denver, CO 80203
  Tel 303 315-1280
  www.ucdenver.edu/academics/colleges/medicalschool/Programs/atp/Pages/AssistiveTechnologyPartners.aspx
- **Guide Dogs for the Blind, Inc.**
  PO Box 151200
  San Rafael, CA 94915-1200
  Tel 800 295-4050
  www.guidedogs.com
- **Guide Dogs for the Blind, Inc.**
  32901 SE Kelso Road
  Boring, OR 97009
  Tel 503 668-2100
  www.guidedogs.com
- **Helen Keller National Center for Deaf-Blind Youth and Adults**
  141 Middle Neck Road
  Sand Point, NY 11050
  Tel 516 944-8900
  www.helenkeller.org
- **National Federation of the Blind**
  200 East Wells Street at Jernigan Place
  Baltimore, MD 21230
  Tel 410 659-9314
  www.nfb.org
- **National Library Services for the Blind-Physically Handicapped**
  Library of Congress
  1291 Taylor Street, NW
  Washington, DC 20542
  Tel 202 707-5100
  www.loc.gov/nls

times) and type of magnification preferred for optimal computer access. Many magnification applications combine enlargement with speech synthesis or text-to-speech.

A recent addition to the list of screen magnification software is called Bigshot. This software is less expensive ($99) and provides fewer features than some other programs. However, it appears to be a highly affordable alternative for users who do not need access to the more sophisticated computer functions.

Environmental Adaptations

Persons with visual impairments usually keep the setup of their home and work environments constant, because this helps in locating items. However, they usually need specialized training for mobility in the community. They learn to use environmental cues such as traffic sounds, echoes, or texture of the sidewalk in combination with mobility aids such as a white cane or a guide dog.

To supplement these less technical aids, some individuals use electronic travel aids that have the capability of detecting obstacles missed by a cane such as overhanging branches or objects that have fallen. This technology (Talking Signs) uses ultrasound or information embedded in the environment expressly for users who have limited vision. The demands for independence in community mobility by persons with significant visual impairments are huge because of the high cognitive demand for remembering routes and because environments constantly change. Many individuals use these types of technologies to increase their independent mobility in both familiar areas and the larger community.

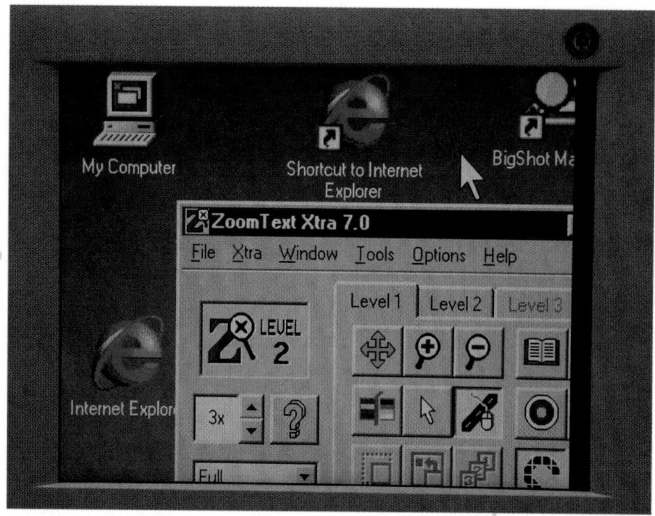

FIGURE 19-8 Screen magnification software (Zoomtext) for persons with visual impairment.

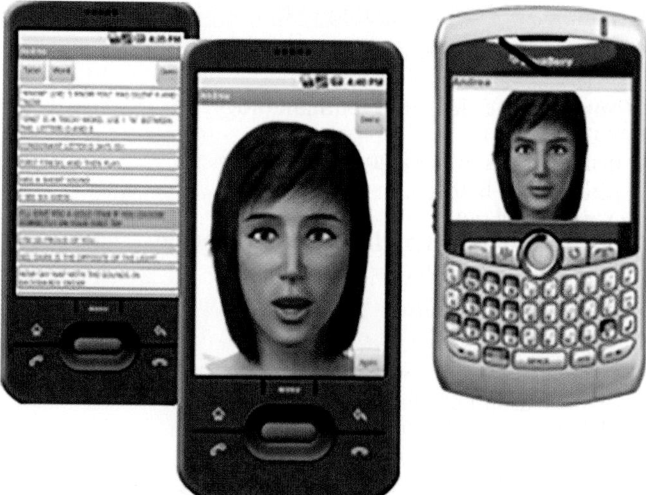

FIGURE 19-9 Animated intelligent agent.

Assistive Technology for Cognitive/Learning Disabilities

Cognitive disabilities include disorders such as traumatic brain injury, intellectual and developmental disabilities, autism, Alzheimer disease, learning disability, Fragile X syndrome, and other disorders, both developmental and acquired. Although improving, most individuals in this group have not had the benefit of using AT devices because relatively few products have been specifically developed to date for intellectual impairments. In addition, families, teachers, and others providing support services for individuals with cognitive impairments have generally not been aware of its usefulness.[38]

Most have looked to simple solutions for persons with learning and/or cognitive impairments using strategies such as colored highlighter tape, pencil grips, enlarged text, reminder lists, and calendars. Others try low-tech adaptations such as using a copyholder to hold print materials for easy viewing and making cardboard windows to help eyes follow text when reading.

In 2004, the U.S. Department of Education, National Institute on Disability Research and Rehabilitation, recognizing the need to increase AT development for persons with cognitive disabilities, funded the first Rehabilitation Engineering Research Center for the Advancement of Cognitive Disabilities (RERC-ACT; www.rerc-act.org) in the United States. This RERC-ACT, refunded from 2009 to 2014, worked to develop a wide range of ATs focused on developing vocational and literacy skills, service provision, and enhanced caregiving supports for persons with significant cognitive impairments.

One of the developments of the RERC-ACT is the use of intelligent agents to interactively help people with everyday tasks in education, health care, and workforce training. The systems were designed to assess, instruct, or assist new readers and learners, as well as people who have speech, language, reading, or cognitive difficulties. The intelligent or "animated" system is available on desktop or mobile computing devices. It is being used to assist persons with cognitive disabilities to learn new job tasks and/or to prompt persons through various steps within a task (Figure 19-9).

Other RERC-ACT work includes the development of "battery-less" micropower sensors. Access to low levels of power and the elimination of batteries in sensor technologies for persons with cognitive and physical disabilities enables additional prompts or inputs based on time, weight, location awareness, and other context-aware sensor capabilities. It enables developers to use context-aware sensors in a multitude of environments and technologies to facilitate the safety, capacity, and well-being of persons with cognitive disabilities. This new field of "cognitive technologies" promises numerous advances during the next decade.

The RERC-ACT was again refunded in 2014 for an additional 5 years and reflects the current and growing attention being paid to persons with cognitive impairments worldwide. In this iteration of the RERC-ACT, enterprise-level solutions with indoor navigation, nonlinear context-aware prompting, and easy-to-use setup systems for nontechnical implementers are under development. International standards work focused on technology design and human interface solutions are also in process across multiple workgroups in the United States and internationally.

Literacy Technologies

There are a number of both low- and high-technology solutions available to assist literacy development. Individuals who are unable to read print materials often use books-on-tape or some of the text-to-speech software solutions mentioned earlier, such as Jaws. Co: Writer is an example of a specially designed application that predicts the word or phrase an individual is trying to spell as they begin to type a word. Other applications (e.g., Write: OutLoud and Kurzweil 3000) provide multisensory feedback by both visually highlighting and speaking the text he or she is generating on the computer.

In addition to those with mobility impairment, VR can sometimes be helpful for persons with learning disabilities so significant they are unable to develop writing skills. VR software enables such an individual to speak words, phrases, or sentences into a standard computer word-processing program such as Microsoft Word. A review or playback feature in the application allows the writer to hear the text they have written repeated back to them.

Although VR software is a rapidly developing technology, the user must currently have a fifth grade reading ability to read the text used to generate a voice file, which hinders its usability by those with significant learning disabilities. Dragon Naturally Speaking has developed a VR version for children 9 years and older, but its success rate for children with learning and other cognitive disabilities has not yet been published.

Other limitations of VR include reduced accuracy in the presence of ambient noise (such as that found in a typical classroom) and fluctuating vocal abilities related to fatigue or some types of disabilities. In general, it takes more than 20 hours to train the software to an acceptable level of accuracy (greater than 90%). Although caution is currently in order when prescribing this type of software, the rapid pace of development bodes well for future use of this type of software for persons with disabilities.

Other applications for persons with cognitive impairment focus on a range of topics including academics, money management, personal skills development, behavior training, development of cognitive skills, memory improvement, problem solving, time concepts, safety awareness, speech and language therapy, telephone usage, and recreation and games.

Prompting Technologies

Recent mainstream technology developments include handheld personal digital assistants. AT software developers, such as AbleLink Technologies, Inc. (Colorado Springs, Colo.), have used this technology and developed software applications (Figure 19-10) that provide auditory prompts for individuals with cognitive disabilities. This software can be set up to prompt an individual through each step of a task as simple as mopping a floor, up to the complexity of solving a math problem. The latest version of this software combines both voice prompts with visual prompts (Visual Assistant). The individual setting up the system for a user can simply take a digital picture with the accompanying camera and combine them with digitally recorded voice prompts to further facilitate memory and cognition.

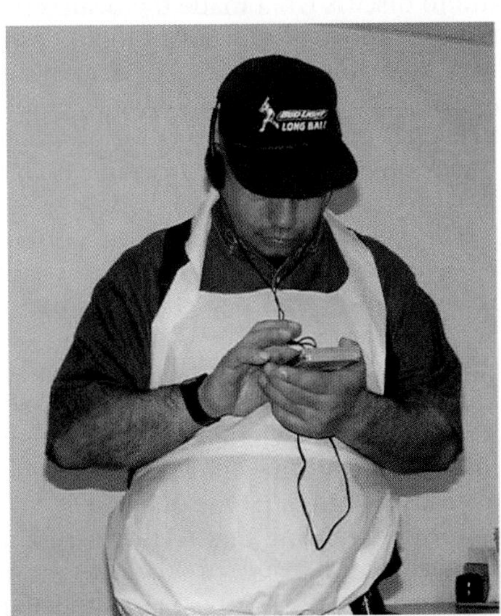

FIGURE 19-10 Use of digital prompting software in a handheld personal digital assistant device (Pocket Coach).

Selecting Appropriate Assistive Technologies

Abandonment

Practitioners are sometimes surprised to learn that not everyone with a disability enjoys using technology, however useful it might appear. Depending on the type of technology, nonuse or abandonment can be as low as 8% or as high as 75%. On average, one third of more optional ATs are abandoned, most within the first 3 months.[21]

Research has not yet been done to determine the number of individuals who are unhappy with their devices, but who must continue to use them because they cannot abandon them without severe consequences.[21,28,31,32] For example, an individual who has just received a new wheelchair that does not meet expectations simply cannot stop using the chair, but must wait until third-party funding becomes available again (typically several years). Alternatively, the individual must engage in potentially difficult and unproductive discussions with the vendor, who has more than likely provided the chair as it was prescribed by the assessment team.

Research does tell us that the main reason individuals with disabilities choose not to use assistive devices is because practitioners failed to consider their opinions and preferences during the process of selecting the device. In other words, the person with a disability was not included as an active member of the team during the evaluation process.[10,11,21,26]

Principles of Clinical Assessment

The goal of an AT evaluation is to determine if AT devices and services have the potential to help an individual meet their activity or participation goals at home, school, work, or play. Other goals include (1) providing a safe and supportive environment for the person with a disability and his or her family to learn about and review available assistive devices; (2) identifying the need for AT services such as training support staff or integrating an AT device into daily activities, (3) modification or customization needed to make the equipment effective; and (4) developing a potential list of recommended devices for trial usage before a final selection of technology is made. In addition, the individual and his or her family, as well as the AT team, should specify exactly what they hope to achieve as a result of the evaluation (i.e., equipment ideas, potential success with vocational or educational objectives, etc.).

When selecting team members to conduct an AT evaluation, professional disciplines should be chosen based on the identified needs of the person with the disability. For example, if the individual presents with both severe motor and communication impairments, team members should include an occupational or physical therapist with expertise in HTI as well as a speech-language pathologist with a background in working with persons with severe communication impairments and alternative forms of communication. If a cognitive impairment has been identified, someone versed in learning processes such as a psychologist, neurolinguist, teacher, or special educator would be an appropriate member(s) of the team. If there is an ergonomic issue (i.e., repetitive stress injury), an evaluator with training in ergonomic assessment or a background in physical or occupational therapy is a necessary component for a successful experience.

It is not appropriate for an AT vendor to be called in to perform an AT evaluation. Although vendors can and should be members of the evaluation team, it must be recognized that they have a conflict of interest, because they earn a living by selling products. When working with a manufacturer or vendor, it is important to work with a credentialed provider. When requested by the team, vendors demonstrate their products, discuss pertinent features, and assist in setting up the equipment for evaluation and trial usage. However, other team members, including the end user and their family, should perform the evaluation and make the final recommendation(s).

Phase I Assistive Technology Assessment

Knowledge within the field of AT continues to expand and change, sometimes on a daily basis. This directly impacts whether or not the AT device recommended by the assessment team will be used or abandoned by the consumer.[15,18] As a result of rapidly changing information, the evaluation process continues to be refined. Many researchers are working to develop standardized AT measurement tools,* but the fact remains that there are few available resources to guide practitioners who have not received formalized training in AT assessment.

As mentioned earlier in this chapter, the most common reason AT is abandoned is because the needs and preferences of the consumer are not taken into account during the evaluation process. Other reasons cited for abandonment of devices include the following[21]:

- Changes in consumer functional abilities or activities.
- Lack of consumer motivation to use the device or do the task.
- Lack of meaningful training on how to use the device.
- Ineffective device performance or frequent breakdown of the device.
- Environmental obstacles to use, such as narrow doorways.
- Lack of access to and information about repair and maintenance.
- Lack of sufficient need for the device functions.
- Device aesthetics, weight, size, and appearance.

Given the relationship that must develop between individuals and AT devices, it is common sense that these factors be considered during the evaluation process. The AT assessment process has evolved from a random process of trying out any number of devices with the individual, to a team process that begins with the technology out of sight.

Phase 1 of the assessment process begins when a referral is received. Standard demographic and impairment-related information is collected, usually over the telephone. In the majority of cases, cognitive, motor, vision, and other standard clinical assessments have already been performed, and a release of information is requested from the individual or his or her caregiver so that information can be forwarded to the team. If appropriate assessments have not been conducted, they are scheduled as a component of phase 2 of the assessment process.

Based on the preliminary information, an appropriate team of professionals is assembled and a date is chosen for the evaluation. The team leader takes responsibility for ensuring that the individual with the disability, his or her family, and any other significant individuals are invited to the evaluation.

At the initial meeting, team members spend some time getting to know the individual. Using methods described by Cook and Hussey[8] and Galvin and Scherer,[10] the team identifies the life roles of the consumer (e.g., student, brother, musician) and the specific activities engaged in by the individual to fulfill that life role. For example, if a young man is a "brother," that means he might play hide and seek with a sibling, squabble over toys, or otherwise engage in brotherly activities. If he is a musician, then he might want or need to have access to musical instruments, sheet music, or simply a radio.

Next, the team identifies any problems that might occur during the individual's daily activities. For example, the musician might not have enough hand control to manage recording equipment or could experience visual or cognitive difficulties with sheet music. The team asks specific questions about where and when these difficulties occur (activity limitations). Perhaps problems occur when the individual is tired or not properly positioned, or when he or she is trying to communicate with others. The individual is also asked to describe instances of success with these activities and to discuss what made them successful (previous history with and without technology). Typically the team is then able to recognize patterns of success and failure from the individual's perspective as common limitations across environments emerge.

Finally, the team prioritizes the order in which to address barriers to participation, and a specific plan of action is developed. This specific plan of action contains "must statements" such as "the device must have a visible display in sunlight" or "the technology chosen must weigh less than 2 lb."

It is at this point the team may be reconfigured. For example, if the individual is not properly seated and positioned, he or she is referred to the occupational or physical therapist for seating and positioning evaluation before proceeding further. Some members of the team may leave after determining that further assessment from their perspective is not needed. In other situations as additional needs becomes apparent, new members are invited to join the team (e.g., a vision specialist). At all times, the assessment team includes the individual and his or her caregivers as the primary members.

*References 1, 7, 10, 15, 19, 20, 21, 32, 33, 35.

Phase 2 Assistive Technology Assessment

Once the team has agreed upon the specific plan of action and those things that "must" occur, phase 2 of the assessment process begins. The person with the disability and/or his or her caregivers are asked to preview any number of AT devices that might serve to reduce activity limitations and increase participation in chosen environments. These AT devices are tried along with various adaptations, modifications, and placements to ensure an appropriate match of the technology to the individual.

It is at this point that the clinician's AT skills become crucial. If trial devices are not properly configured or if the wrong information is given to the consumer, he or she will be unable to make an appropriate selection. Because many devices require extensive training and follow-up, it is essential that realistic information about training and learning time is provided and appropriate resources within the local community identified. With very few exceptions, the wise course of action involves borrowing or renting the AT device before making a final purchase decision. For many individuals the actual use of technologies on a day-to-day basis raises new issues that must be resolved. For instance, there might not be the local supports necessary for the technology that appears to be best for an individual. In these cases, it is best to first identify local resources or local AT professionals willing to seek additional training before sending the device home with the user. Consumers and their families should always be informed so that they can make the final decision regarding when and where the equipment will be delivered.

Unexpected benefits of trial use occur as a result of improved functioning, including changes in role and status. In some cases, these unexpected benefits create an entirely new set of problems. For most individuals, these problems can be resolved with time, energy, and patience. Others decide that they either prefer the old way of doing things or that they are interested in adding or changing the technology once they have had a chance to experiment with it in different settings.

AT professionals, in consultation with the physician, should also anticipate future needs (e.g., physical and cognitive maturation), and final decisions should consider both the expected performance and durability of the device.[31]

Writing the Assistive Technology Assessment Report

The evaluation report documents the AT assessment process and must include several components. First and foremost, it is helpful to use layman's terms to help case managers, educators, and others unfamiliar with ATs understand the process.

In cases where medical insurance is being used to purchase technology, it is essential to document the medical need for the device(s) within the report. This information will be included in the "letter of medical necessity" required by medical insurers before funding approval. For example, the evaluation report might state, "Mr. Jones will use this wheelchair to enable safe and independent mobility in the home and community and to meet the functional or activities of daily living goals as listed." In instances where educational or vocational funding is being requested to purchase the technology, the report should focus on the educational or vocational benefit of the assistive devices and how relevant goals will be met with the recommended equipment.

It is also extremely important that all components of the AT device be included in the list of recommended equipment (e.g., cables, ancillary peripherals, and consumable supplies). In many instances, devices are recommended for purchase as a "system." As a result, acquisition can be delayed for months because an item was not included in the initial list. An estimate of the amount of time, cost, and source of training should also be included at this point. Purchasing AT devices without paying for the AT services needed to learn how to use the device(s) and/or integrate it into identified life activities will result in low use or abandonment.[28,31,32]

Finally, it is also important to include contact information for the vendors who sell the equipment. Many purchasers are unfamiliar with rehabilitation technology supply companies, and acquisition can be delayed if this information is not included in the report.

Physician Responsibilities

Prescribing the Technologies

The American Medical Association[35] recommends that the following items be considered when prescribing AT and certifying medical necessity:

- The physician must provide evidence of individual medical necessity for the specific AT being prescribed and be prepared to talk with insurance company representatives about the medical necessity of complex ATs (e.g., power wheelchairs, AAC devices, etc.). Reviewing a comprehensive assessment report from the AT assessment team should supply all the needed information.
- Health insurance requires an "appropriate" prescription that includes mention of the comprehensive assessment process, the individual's motivation, the availability of training, and the potential functional outcome(s) for the patient, as compared with the cost of the products. Success with reimbursement also includes using the appropriate medical necessity forms and previous authorization procedures.

Documentation in the Health Care Record

In addition to prescribing and certifying medical necessity on various forms, physicians must maintain complete patient health care records that include:

- Patient diagnosis or diagnoses.
- Duration of the patient's condition.
- Expected clinical course.
- Prognosis.
- Nature and extent of functional limitations.
- Therapeutic interventions and results.
- Past experience with related items.
- Consultations and reports from other physicians, an interdisciplinary team, home health agencies, etc.

- A complete listing of all assistive devices the patient is using, including copies of prescriptions and certification forms or letters.
- A system to track device performance, including follow-up assessment schedules and lists of professionals and vendors to contact if problems occur.

This comprehensive health care record supplies the background information needed to substantiate the need for the AT devices and services regardless of the funding source.

Funding Letters of Medical Necessity

Physicians are frequently asked to write "letters of medical necessity." Well-written letters of medical necessity help ensure that the AT needs of patients are met. These letters should include the diagnoses (International Classification of Diseases codes) and the functional limitations of the patient (e.g., balance disorder, developmental delay, etc.). In addition, there should be a statement about the patient's inability to perform specific tasks such as activities of daily living, work activities, and walk functionally.

For example, patients with severe communication disorders typically cannot communicate verbally and/or in writing and are often unable to communicate independently over the telephone. This would also mean that they are unable to adequately communicate their health care needs to medical personnel and are therefore unsafe or at risk. These details should be included in a letter of medical necessity.

The letter should also include a paragraph stating why the equipment is necessary. For example, the use of the equipment will allow the patient to do the following:

Function independently or improve the patient's functional ability.
Perform independent wheelchair mobility in the home and community.
Return home or move to a less expensive level of care.
Be required as a lifetime medical need (if shorter duration, explain need).

Next, the letter needs a rationale for choosing this specific equipment. This requires a description of the specific equipment features and listing all required components. This might include the following:

Features that provide safety or safe positioning for an activity
Cost-effectiveness of preventing secondary complications (e.g., pressure ulcers)
Mobility restrictions preventing independent activity
Access to areas in the home, such as the bathroom and kitchen
Durability of the product over its alternatives
Past experience, interventions, and results (failure of less expensive solutions)

Funding Assistive Technology

The funding sources for AT devices and services fall into several categories. The AT assessment process often helps to identify which source will be used. One source is private or government medical or health insurance. Health insurance defines AT as "medical equipment necessary for treatment of a specific illness or injury," and a physician's prescription is usually required. When writing a prescription for an AT device, it is important the physician is made aware of the costs and benefits of the devices and is prepared to justify their prescriptions to third-party payers. Funding includes not only the initial cost of the device but also the expense involved in equipment maintenance and patient education or training, as well as the potential economic benefits it provides to the patient (e.g., a return to work).

AT is usually covered under policy provisions for durable medical equipment, orthoses, and prostheses, or ADL and mobility aids. With private health insurance, with government insurance policies, such as Medicaid and Medicare, coverage is based on existing law and regulations. In 2002, AAC devices were included for reimbursement by Medicare. AT professionals and other health care providers should continually advocate for adequate coverage of AT in all health care plans.

Funding for AT is also available from other federal and state government entities, such as the Veterans Administration, State Vocational Rehabilitation Agencies, State Independent Living Rehabilitation Centers, and State Department of Education Services. Local school districts might also fund educational-related AT for children.[13]

Each agency or program sets criteria for the funding of AT devices based on their mission and the purpose of the technology. For example, vocational rehabilitation agencies pay for AT devices and services that facilitate or help maintain paid employment; and education systems fund AT that enable students to perform or participate in school.

Funding is generally available for AT, but persistence and advocacy by the AT provider are required for success.[29,30,34] The AT provider must also keep abreast of the requirements of various funding sources to direct the patient to appropriate organizations. Private funding is often available through subsidized loan programs, churches, charitable organizations, and disability-related nonprofit groups. Often funding from several sources is needed to reduce personal out-of-pocket costs. It is important that the presumed availability of funding not drive the evaluation process and limit the options that are considered for an individual. When the need and justification for a particular AT solution is clear, then it becomes much easier to locate a source of funding and make the case for purchase of the AT device or service.

Beukelman and Mirenda[3] identify five steps in developing a funding strategy:

1. Survey the funding resources available to the individual.
2. Identify various funding sources for the various steps in the AT intervention (i.e., assessment, funding, training, etc.).
3. Prepare a funding plan with the patient and family members or advocates.
4. Assign responsibility to specific individuals for the funding of each step of the AT intervention.
5. Prepare the necessary written documentation for the funding source so that there is a record in the event an appeal is needed.

Summary and Future Directions

The world of AT is moving at a very rapid pace, fed in large part by the growth in mainstream technologies, cloud-based systems, and the "Internet of things." There is a growing culture of inclusion that is changing traditional concepts about disability and impairment. Space travel, satellite-supported telecommunications, wireless networks, robotics, new materials with advanced performance properties, miniaturization of integrated circuits, and innovation in batteries and power sources are all crossing over into the field of AT. Social assistive robotics, along with rehabilitation robotics, are fueling tremendous changes in how clinicians address disability These technologies hold great promise and are beginning to provide a real opportunity to rethink how and when and where clinicians provide interventions, as well as how families can be more engaged in the rehabilitation process. Federal funding supports rehabilitation and engineering research centers for the development and testing of new AT concepts. Funds also support the transfer of technologies from the federal laboratory system to AT manufacturers. The convergence of these factors is leading to AT products that are more likely to meet the needs of persons with disabilities.

REFERENCES

1. Anonymous: The Rehabilitation Act of 1973, as amended. 1973.
2. Ball L, Beukelman D, Patee G: Augmentative and alternative communication: clinical decision making for persons with ALS, *Perspect Augment Altern Commun* 11:7–12, 2002.
3. Beukelman DR, Mirenda P: *Augmentative and alternative communication: management of severe communication disorders in children and adults*, ed 2, Baltimore, 1998, Paul H Brookes.
4. Blake DJ, Bodine C: An overview of assistive technology for persons with multiple sclerosis, *J Rehabil Res Dev* 39:299–312, 2002.
5. Bodine C, Beukelman DR: Prediction of future speech performance among potential users of AAC systems: a survey, *Augment Altern Commun* 7:100–111, 1991.
6. Bromley BE: Assistive technology assessment: a comparative analysis of five models, Los Angeles, 2001, Home Modification Resources. Available at www.homemods.org/resources/pages/ATAssess.shtml.
7. Chatman A, Hyams S, Neel J, et al: The Patient Specific Functional Scale: measurement properties in patients with knee dysfunction, *Phys Ther* 77:820–829, 1997.
8. Cook AM, Hussey SM: *Assistive technologies: principles and practice*, ed 2, St Louis, 2002, Mosby.
9. De Ruyter F, Kennedy MR, Doyle M: Augmentative communication and stroke rehabilitation: who is doing what and do the data tell the whole story? In *The Third Annual National Stroke Rehabilitation Conference*, Boston, May 10-11, 1990.
10. Galvin JC, Scherer M: Evaluating, selecting, and using appropriate assistive technology, Gaithersburg, 1996, Aspen.
11. Gray DB, Quatrano LA, Lieberman M: *Designing and using assistive technology: the human perspective*, Baltimore, 1998, Paul H Brookes.
12. Grove N: Augmentative and alternative communication: management of severe communication disorders in children and adults, *J Intellect Disabil Res* 38:219–220, 1994.
13. Hager RM: *Funding of assistive technology: State Vocational Rehabilitation Agencies and their obligation to maximize employment*, Buffalo, 1999, Neighborhood Legal Services.
14. James P, Thorpre N: *Ancient inventions*, New York, 1994, Ballantine Books.
15. Jutai J: Quality of life impact of assistive technology, *Rehabil Eng* 14:2–7, 1999.
16. Klund J: A crash course on alternative access, *Technol Spec Interest Sect Q* 1–3, 2001. Available at http://www.aota.org/-/media/Corporate/Files/Secure/Publications/SIS-Quarterly-Newsletters/T/TSIS0301.pdf.
17. La Plante MP: The demographics of disability, *Milbank Q* 69(Suppl 1–2):55–77, 1991.
18. Nagi S: Some conceptual issues in disability and rehabilitation. In Sussman M, editor: *Sociology and rehabilitation*, Washington, 1965, American Sociological Association, pp 100–113.
19. Patterson DJ, Liao Lin, Fox D, et al: Inferring high-level behavior from low-level sensors. In McCarthy AD, editor: *UBICOMP 2003: the Fifth International Conference on Ubiquitous Computing*, New York, 2003, Springer-Verlag, pp 73–89.
20. Pentland A: Machine understanding of human action. In *The Seventh International Forum on Frontier of Telecom Technology*, Tokyo, November 29-30, 1995. Available at: http://www.white.media.mit.edu/vismod/demos/ive/.
21. Phillips B, Zhao H: Predictors of assistive technology abandonment, *Assist Technol* 5:36–45, 1993.
22. Pope AM: Tarlove AR, editor: *Disability in America: toward a national agenda for prevention*, Washington, 1991, National Academy Press.
23. Public Law 100-407: Technology Related Assistance for Individuals with Disabilities Act of 1988. *Federal Register* 41272, August 19, 1991.
24. Public Law 108-446: The Individuals with Disabilities Education Act Amendments of 1997. 1997.
25. Public Law 93-113: Section 508 of the *Rehabilitation Act of 1973*, as amended 29 USC 794 (d). 1998.
26. Riermer-Reiss ML, Wacker Robbyn R: Factors associated with assistive technology discontinuance among individuals with disabilities, *J Rehabil* 66:44–49, 2000.
27. Romski MA, Sevcik RA: *Language learning through augmented means: the process and its products*, Baltimore, 1993, Paul H Brookes.
28. Scherer M: Assistive technology use, avoidance and abandonment: what we know so far. In *Proceedings of the Sixth Annual Technology and Person with Disability Conference*, Los Angeles, March 20-23, 1991.
29. Scherer MJ: *Living in a state of stuck: how technology impacts the lives of people with disabilities*, Cambridge, 1993, Brookline Books.
30. Scherer MJ: *Living in the state of stuck: how technology impacts the lives of people with disabilities*, ed 3, Cambridge, 2000, Brookline Books.
31. Scherer M: *Assistive technology: matching device and consumer for successful rehabilitation*, Washington, 2002, American Psychological Association.
32. Scherer M, Coombs FK: Ethical issues in the evaluation and selection of assistive technology. Available at http://www.gatfl.gatech.edu/documents/ethical.pdf.
33. Scherer MJ, Cushman LA: Measuring subjective quality of life following spinal cord injury: a validation study of the assistive technology device predisposition assessment, *Disabil Rehabil* 23:387–393, 2001.
34. Scherer MJ, McKee BG: Assessing predispositions to technology use in special education: music education majors score with the "Survey on Technology Use." In *RESNA '94 Annual Conference*, Arlington, 1994, Rehabilitation Engineering and Assistive Technology Society of North America.
35. Schwartzberg JG, Kakavas VK, Malkind S: *Guidelines for the use of assistive technology: evaluation, referral, prescription*, ed 2, Chicago, 1996, American Medical Association.
36. US Congress: Americans with Disabilities Act of 1990. 1990.
37. US Congress: Americans with Disabilities (ADA) accessibility guidelines for buildings and facilities, Washington, 1991, US Architectural and Transportation Barriers Compliance Board.
38. Wehmeyer ML, Kelchner K, Richards S: Individual and environmental factors related to the self-determination of adults with mental retardation, *J Vocat Rehabil* 5:291–305, 1995.
39. World Health Organization: *International classification of functioning, disability and health: literature review on environmental factors*, Geneva, 2000, World Health Organization.
40. World Health Organization Committee for the International Classification of Functioning: *International classification of functioning: ICF checklist*, Geneva, 2002, World Health Organization.

SECTION 3

Common Clinical Problems

CHAPTER 20

BLADDER DYSFUNCTION

Lance L. Goetz, Adam P. Klausner, Diana D. Cardenas

The primary functions of the urinary bladder are storage of urine and coordinated emptying. Incontinence and urinary retention are common presenting symptoms of bladder dysfunction in patients with neurologic disorders cared for by physiatrists. Optimal management of the neurogenic bladder requires an understanding of the neuroanatomy, physiology, and classification of neurogenic bladder types. Clinical evaluation and individualized management, including behavioral, pharmacologic, and surgical techniques, are outlined and common complications are reviewed.

Neuroanatomy and Physiology

Detrusor and Sphincter Muscle Characteristics

Previously, the detrusor muscle in humans was said to have no gap junctions and a one-to-one innervation ratio. Although this is not likely to be correct,[4] innervation of the bladder is nevertheless dense and complex. Contraction of the detrusor muscle is initiated by phosphorylation of the light myosin chain and terminated by dephosphorylation. Contraction is initiated by an increase in intracellular calcium released from intracellular sources and an influx of extracellular calcium. This influx is controlled by as many as four calcium channels (three voltage-sensitive and one receptor-sensitive), which probably explains why calcium channel blockers are not effective inhibitors of detrusor activity in the clinical setting. Relaxation of the detrusor is associated with an influx of potassium into the cell. In addition to smooth muscle, collagen forms nearly 50% of the bladder wall in healthy individuals. This proportion increases considerably in disease states. In the striated muscle of the distal sphincter, the majority of fibers are slow twitch, whereas those in the pelvic floor are a mixture of fast and slow twitch. Maintenance of sphincter tone facilitates continence, but not a fast contractile response, which probably explains why suddenly stopping a urine stream is difficult.

Lower Urinary Tract Pharmacology: Receptors and Neurotransmitters

The bladder contains cholinergic muscarinic and nicotinic receptors and α- and β-adrenergic receptors.

Muscarinic Receptors and Transmitters

The receptors active during bladder contraction are cholinergic muscarinic (M_2 and M_3) receptors widely distributed in the body of the bladder, trigone, bladder neck, and urethra. The M_2 receptors predominate structurally in normal bladders, but the M_3 receptors might be more important functionally. This distribution of M_3 receptors explains the widespread use of antimuscarinic agents for the treatment of overactive bladder (OAB) and the relatively recent rush by pharmaceutical companies to develop more M_3-selective compounds.[50]

Cholinergic nicotinic receptors are primarily located in the striated sphincter.

Adrenergic Receptors and Transmitters

Adrenergic receptors are concentrated in the trigone, bladder neck, and urethra and are predominantly α_1. These have recently been subdivided into α_{1a}, α_{1b}, and α_{1d}. Identification of these α_1 subgroups allows increased specificity with regard to therapeutic agents. For example, α_{1a}-selective antagonists (i.e., tamsulosin and silodosin) are widely used in the treatment of benign prostatic hyperplasia and disorders of bladder neck dysfunction. Likewise, α_{1d} receptors may be more important in the symptom of bladder urgency, and naftopidil, a combined α_{1a}/α_{1d} drug, is being studied in the treatment of benign prostatic hyperplasia and OAB, and is approved for clinical use in Japan.[69]

Norepinephrine-containing nerve cells are also found in the paravesical and intramural ganglia. Some authors describe norepinephrine terminals in the striated muscle of the distal sphincter, although most would dispute this. When these cells are active, they have excitatory effects and maintain continence by contraction of the bladder neck and urethral smooth muscle. β_2-Adrenergic and β_3-adrenergic receptors are found in the bladder neck and also in the body of the bladder. These receptors are inhibitory when activated and can produce relaxation at the bladder neck on initiation of voiding and relax the bladder body to enhance storage (Figure 20-1). In fact, a β_3-antagonist, mirabegron, the first new drug for the treatment of OAB that is not an antimuscarinic, was approved by the U.S. Food and Drug Administration (FDA) in 2012, and studies demonstrate similar efficacy to standard antimuscarinic agents.[20]

Other Receptors and Transmitters

Other lower tract transmitters have been considered, but much of the evidence for their presence and activity is from preclinical animal models. The role of these other transmitters in normal and disease states in humans is uncertain. Many lower tract transmitters have opposing effects on lower tract function, depending on their site of action. Purine receptors (P_1, stimulated by adenosine, and P_2, stimulated by adenosine triphosphate [ATP]) have their effects at the pelvic ganglia and the neuroeffector junction. They have inhibitory and facilitative effects, respectively,

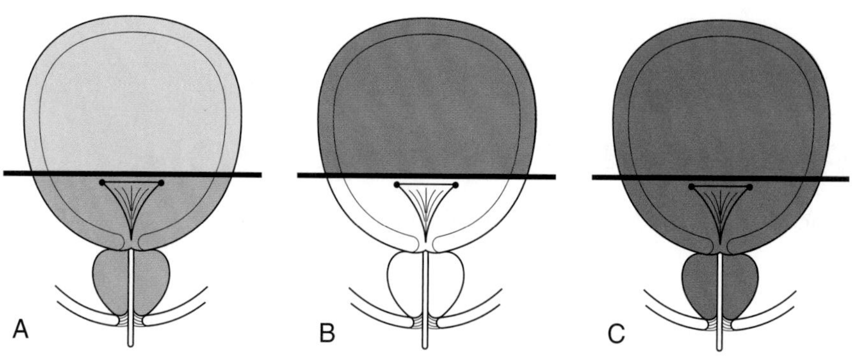

FIGURE 20-1 A, Distribution of the α-adrenergic receptors, with few in the dome of the bladder and more in the base of the bladder and prostrate. **B,** Distribution of the β-receptors, which are largely in the dome. **C,** Distribution of the cholinergic receptors, which are widely distributed throughout the dome and the base of the bladder and the urethra.

on the detrusor muscle. Vasointestinal polypeptide, by contrast, enhances transmission of acetylcholine in pelvic ganglia and inhibits acetylcholine-mediated contraction in the detrusor. Neuropeptide Y has excitatory functions on the detrusor muscle and indirect facilitative effects by inhibiting norepinephrine release. This transmitter also has inhibitory effects by blocking acetylcholine release and blocks the atropine-resistant bladder contraction. Tachykinins are found mostly in afferent nerves, where their effects are to augment the micturition reflex and also transmit pain sensation. Tachykinins augment the contractile and vascular response in inflammatory states. Prostaglandins cause the slow onset of contractions of the detrusor, whereas parathyroid hormone–related peptide causes relaxation. ATP is heavily involved in urothelial to detrusor signaling and is likely to represent the nonadrenergic noncholinergic transmitter that mediates bladder contraction.[11]

The main effector transmitter for contraction of the urethra is norepinephrine, via the α_1 receptors. Smooth muscle relaxation is mediated by the effects of acetylcholine in the pelvic ganglia. This releases nitric oxide (NO) in the urethral wall, resulting in relaxation of urethral smooth muscle. NO has been studied as a potential treatment for detrusor sphincter dyssynergia. However, systemic effects have limited its utility.[59,75]

Prostaglandins, in contrast to their effects on the detrusor, cause a relaxation of the urethral muscle. Prostaglandins have been tried in various clinical states of urinary retention but without consistent results and may be important in the generation of low-amplitude spontaneous rhythmic contractions during the filling phase of micturition.[22] Because of its stimulatory effect on the detrusor smooth muscle, prostaglandin E_2 has been used as a preclinical model of detrusor overactivity.

Serotonin appears to be an antagonist that causes urethral muscle contraction. It might be important in the production of irritative urethral symptoms and in bladder neck and sphincteric contraction. The combined norepinephrine and serotonin reuptake inhibitor, duloxetine, has been used for the treatment of stress urinary incontinence in Europe but is not approved for this indication in the United States. It may also have uses in the treatment of some forms of neurogenic voiding dysfunction.[31,32]

Estrogens

The role of estrogens on the lower urinary tract in women is confined to secondary effects on tissues and receptors because they do not appear to have direct transmitter effects.

Transmitter Function Depends on Location

In the brainstem and spinal cord the various transmitters described earlier can have a variety of inhibitory and facilitative actions, depending on their site of action. Serotonin might have inhibitory detrusor effects at the midbrain level, and uptake of serotonin might be blocked by tricyclics (used in the treatment of nocturnal enuresis). Activation of opiate receptors in the brainstem and sacral spinal cord inhibits voiding. This might partly explain the retention of urine seen with the use of these agents.[77] The pudendal motor neuron bodies are situated in the lateral border of the ventral horn of the sacral cord (Onuf nucleus). Serotonin and norepinephrine reuptake inhibitors prolong the effect of these agents in the synaptic cleft of Onuf nucleus and increase the activity of the external sphincter.

A complete discussion of the pharmacology of the lower urinary tract can be found in Steers.[77]

Lower Urinary Tract Innervation

Peripheral Innervation

The afferent and efferent peripheral pathways include autonomic fibers that are carried in the pelvic (parasympathetic) and hypogastric (sympathetic) nerves, and somatic fibers that are carried in the pudendal nerves (Figure 20-2 and Table 20-1). In healthy individuals, the micturition reflex is triggered by sensory information regarding bladder filling volume. Once a threshold filling volume is reached, afferent Aδ fibers relay information back to the central nervous system. In pathologic states, stimulation of capsaicin or vanilloid receptor subtype 1 (VR1) (receptors expressed by unmyelinated afferents in the bladder) lead to excitation of C-afferent fibers, possibly mediating bladder dysfunction as a result of inflammatory reactions. These receptors are cation channels, expressed almost exclusively by the primary sensory neurons involved in nociception and neurogenic inflammation, which can also be activated by noxious heat and changes in pH. In suprasacral neurogenic bladder disease, these capsaicin-sensitive vanilloid receptors and C-afferent fibers have a major role in the pathogenesis of detrusor overactivity. Intravesical capsaicin and resiniferatoxin, which block transmission through C-afferent fibers for several months, have been used experimentally to treat detrusor overactivity when it

Table 20-1 Bladder Afferent Pathways

Receptor	Pelvic (Parasympathetic)	Hypogastric (Sympathetic)	Pudendal (Somatic)
Bladder wall tension	+	—	—
Bladder mucosal nociception (pain, temperature, chemical irritation)	+	+	—
Urethral mucosal sensation (pain, temperature, passage of urine)	—	—	+

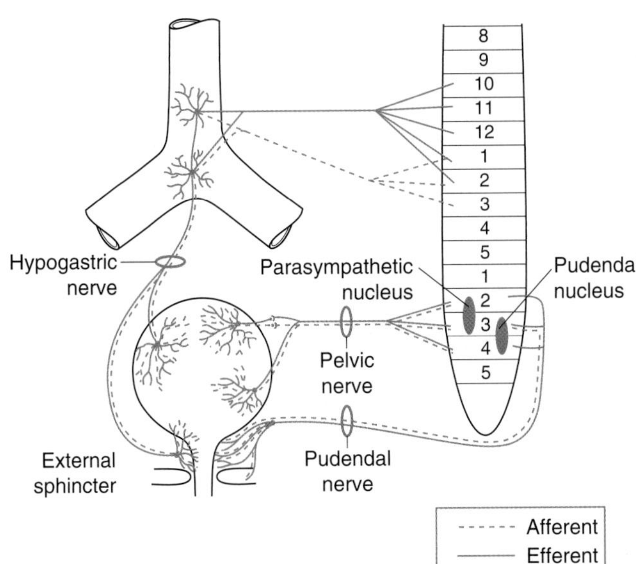

FIGURE 20-2 The parasympathetic, sympathetic, and somatic nerve supply to the bladder, urethra, and pelvic floor. (Redrawn from Blaivas JG: Management of bladder dysfunction in multiple sclerosis, *Neurology* 30:12-18, 1980.)

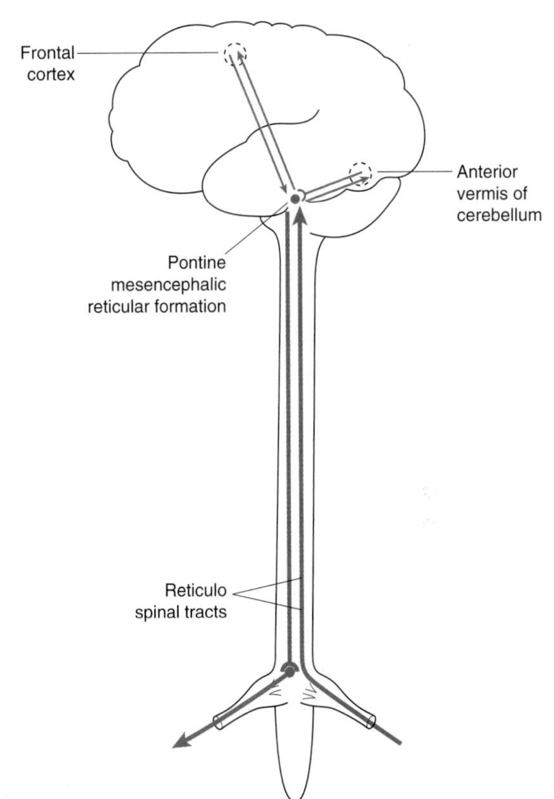

FIGURE 20-3 The central connections of the bladder reflex are shown, with the afferents ascending possibly in the reticulospinal tracts or the posterior columns to the pontine mesencephalic reticular formation and the efferents running down to the sacral outflow in the reticulospinal tracts. The pontine center is largely influenced by the cortex but also by other areas of the brain, particularly the cerebellum and basal ganglia. (Redrawn from Bradley WE: Physiology of the urinary bladder. In Walsh PC, Gittes RF, Perlmutter AD, et al, *Campbell's urology*, ed 5, Philadelphia, 1986, Saunders, pp 129–185.)

does not respond to the usual pharmacologic agents.[40,47] Larger studies are needed to clarify the clinical role of these agents.[39]

Micturition Reflex

The reflex center for the coordination and control of lower urinary tract function, referred to as the pontine micturition center (PMC), lies in the pons along with the other autonomic centers (Figure 20-3). Coordination of bladder and sphincter activity is dependent on intact connections to the PMC. For the micturition reflex to be successfully completed, timing is crucial. In this regard, the sphincter must relax just before the onset of a bladder contraction to achieve unobstructed voiding. Thus, disruptions in pathways between the PMC and the sacral outflow to the bladder can lead to detrusor sphincter dyssynergia, a leading cause of obstruction in individuals with suprasacral spinal cord injury (SCI).

Other Lower Urinary Tract Reflexes

Not shown in Figure 20-3 is a facilitatory reflex with afferent axons originating from the bladder and synapsing on the pudendal nerve nucleus at S2, S3, and S4 (Onuf nucleus). This allows inhibition of pelvic floor activity during voiding. Another important reflex uses the local segmental innervation of the external sphincter with afferents from the urethra, sphincter, and pelvic floor, and efferents in the pudendal nerve. Higher (voluntary) control over the pelvic floor is achieved through afferents that ascend to the sensory cortex. Descending fibers from the motor cortex synapse with the pudendal motor nucleus.[9]

Lower Urinary Tract Function

Urodynamic studies in both healthy individuals and those with neurologic disease have yielded clinical insights into the normal and abnormal function of the lower urinary tract that occur with development and aging (Figure 20-4).

Voiding Function in Infants and Young Children

Neonates and infants have involuntary reflex voiding that occurs at approximately 50 to 100 mL volumes. Sometime after the first year of life, the child begins to show some awareness of bladder evacuation and can begin to delay

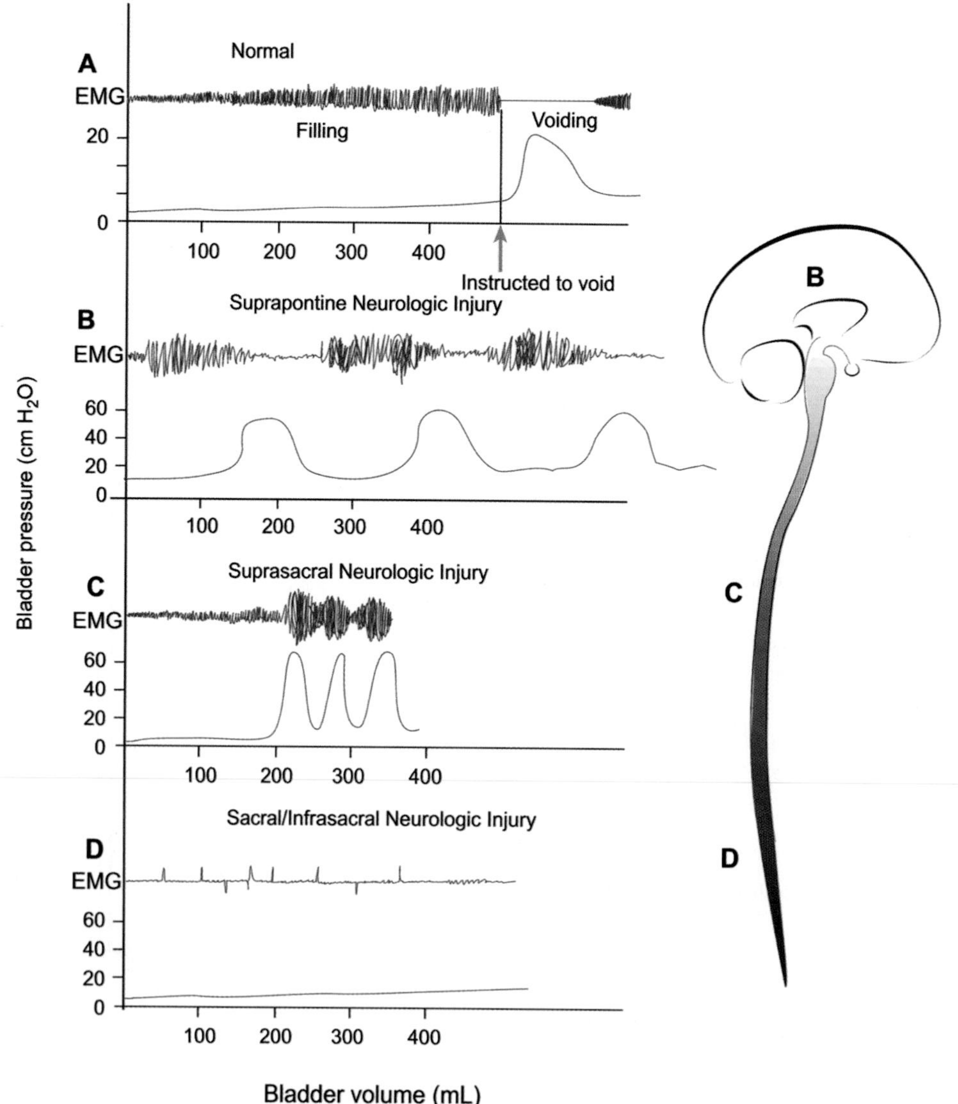

FIGURE 20-4 Diagrams of external sphincter electromyography (*EMG*) and bladder pressure during filling and voiding. **A,** Normal pattern. No contractions occur during filling. Voiding is initiated by relaxation of the sphincter before the bladder contracts. Low pressure emptying occurs. **B,** Suprapontine neurologic lesion. Contractions occur during filling, which the patient tries to suppress. Coordinated sphincteric relaxation occurs, leading to incontinence. **C,** Infrapontine/suprasacral neurologic lesion. Contractions occur during filling and sphincteric cocontraction (detrusor sphincter dyssynergia) occurs, leading to high detrusor pressure. **D,** Sacral or infrasacral neurologic lesion. Minimal or no bladder contraction or sphincteric activity is present.

urination for a brief period by contracting the voluntary sphincter. For normal control, the detrusor reflex has to be inhibited by the higher centers above the level of the PMC. By 5 years of age, approximately 90% of children have volitional control of voiding. The remaining 10% have a more infantile or immature pattern, with involuntary detrusor activity that occurs between voluntary voids producing frequency, urgency, and occasionally urge incontinence and nocturnal enuresis. Most of these children gradually have inhibition of the detrusor reflex and resolution of enuresis by the onset of puberty. Treatment is almost always with reassurance and observation.

Voiding Function in Adults

With bladder filling, there is only a minimal increase in intravesical pressure (known as accommodation) together with an increase in recruitment of activity in the pelvic floor and voluntary sphincter. Normal voiding is initiated by voluntary relaxation of the pelvic floor with subsequent release of inhibition of the detrusor reflex at the pontine level, resulting in detrusor contraction. Detrusor contraction is maintained steadily throughout voiding, and the pelvic floor remains quiescent.

Voiding Function in Older Adults

OAB is a symptom syndrome identified as elevated urinary urgency usually with increased daytime frequency and nocturia in the absence of identifiable causes.[3] The prevalence of OAB in the adult U.S. population is estimated at nearly 20% and increases with age, making it a common and bothersome geriatric condition.[70] Lower urinary tract symptoms including frequency, urgency, and incontinence with incomplete emptying are common in older adults. Urodynamic studies show that many older adults have involuntary bladder contractions during filling that may explain these symptoms. These contractions may be poorly sustained and result in incomplete emptying. This condition, now called detrusor underactivity by the International Continence Society, is poorly understood and may be neurogenic or myogenic in origin.[85]

Older adult men can have prostatic obstruction caused by benign prostatic hyperplasia, and women can have incontinence related to impaired sphincter activity or stress incontinence. However, in the absence of these well-defined mechanical factors, changes in bladder function in older adults have been ascribed to loss of cerebral inhibition resulting from minor strokes as well as changes in the bladder wall caused by collagen deposition. Changes in bladder function can also result from polyuria secondary to reduced renal concentrating ability, diuretic use, lack of normal increase in antidiuretic hormone secretion at night, and mobilization of lower extremity edema during sleep. In this regard, the American Urological Association now recommends completion of a frequency-volume chart in the workup of all men with benign prostatic hyperplasia and as a consideration in patients with OAB. Patients with more than 3 L of total urine production in 24 hours can be diagnosed with polyuria and can often be treated with behavioral modifications. Likewise, patients with more than 33% of their total 24-hour urine production occurring in the overnight period are diagnosed as having nocturnal polyuria and may have underlying medical conditions rather than primary bladder dysfunction.[64]

Classification of Neurogenic Bladder Dysfunction

The neurogenic bladder has been classified in a variety of ways, beginning with the anatomic classification of Bors and Comarr.[8] The first functional classification was based on cystometric findings, and five basic groups were described: (1) reflex, (2) uninhibited, (3) autonomous, (4) motor paralytic, and (5) sensory neurogenic bladders.[63] Later, a more anatomic classification system was proposed, in which the neurogenic bladder was subdivided into types including supraspinal, suprasacral spinal, infrasacral, peripheral autonomic, and muscular lesions (Figure 20-5). At the same time, others developed functional classifications, all of which were based on conventional urodynamic evaluations. This was an attempt to categorize the lower urinary tract according to the passive storage ability of the bladder and the activities and coordination of the detrusor and sphincter mechanisms (Table 20-2). In practice, it is common to use a combination of both anatomic and functional classifications. Clinical management is based on functional changes demonstrated by urodynamic testing.

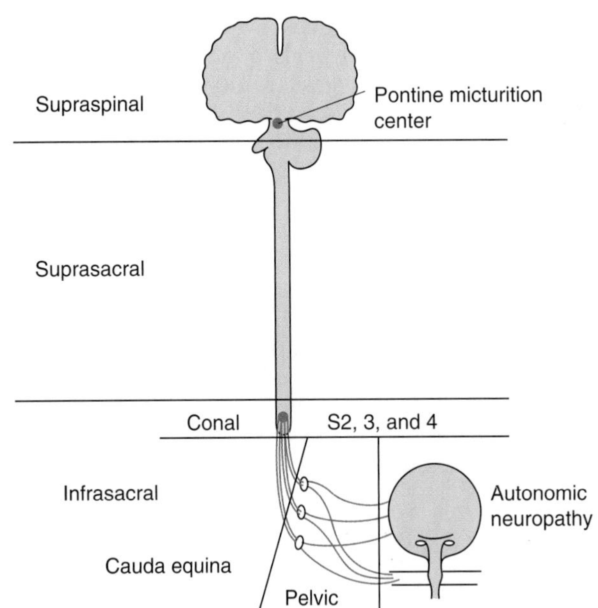

FIGURE 20-5 Anatomic classification of the neurogenic bladder.

Table 20-2 Functional Classification of the Neurogenic Bladder

Type of Failure	Bladder Factors	Outlet Factors
Failure to store	Hyperactivity Decreased compliance	Denervated pelvic floor Bladder neck descent Intrinsic bladder neck sphincter failure
Failure to empty	Areflexia Hypocontractility	Detrusor sphincter dyssynergia (striated sphincter and bladder neck) Nonrelaxing voluntary sphincter Mechanical obstruction (benign prostatic hypertrophy or stricture)

Evaluation of Neurogenic Bladder Dysfunction

History and Physical Examination

Although the symptoms associated with neurogenic bladder dysfunction are often misleading and correlate poorly with objective findings, relief of symptoms is often the patient's main concern. It is often helpful to have the patient or attendant complete a standardized "void diary" to record fluid intake, output, and incontinence episodes over several 24-hour periods. A history of recurrent urinary tract infection (UTI) can be directly associated with acute changes in voiding function. The patient's ability to sense bladder fullness and notice incontinence can also be useful. The history should help determine whether there were voiding symptoms before the causative neurologic event or any premorbid conditions such as diabetes, stroke, and previous urologic or pelvic surgery. The neurologic diagnosis, especially the level of the lesion and its completeness, is important in predicting the type of lower urinary tract dysfunction that might be expected.

The physical examination should assess mental status and confirm the level of the neurologic deficit (if present). Perineal sensation and pelvic floor muscle and rectal tone are particularly important. Reflexes are also important, but the bulbocavernosus, cremasteric, and anal reflexes are sometimes difficult to elicit. The skin of the perineum and the amount of bladder support should be assessed. In women, a pelvic examination is warranted to assess for adequate estrogenization and any evidence of vaginal wall support defects. Good estrogenization is evidenced by a pink and moist vaginal mucosa with good rugae, whereas lack of estrogenization reveals a pale, dry, and smooth vaginal mucosa. In this regard, evidence now supports the use of topical vaginal estrogen for the prevention of recurrent UTIs in postmenopausal women.[74] Physical examination findings of cystocele or pelvic organ prolapse can indicate vaginal wall support defects. The evaluation of voiding dysfunction in men should include a prostate examination.[64] Prostate size or consistency alone is not a good indicator of obstruction, which can only be established with formal pressure-flow urodynamic studies. However, prostate size has clearly been associated with the development of urinary retention in randomized trials.[61] It is also important to assess the patient's motivation, lifestyle, body habitus, and physical impairments including upper limb function, lower limb function, and spine range of motion.

Diagnostic Testing for Neurogenic Bladder Dysfunction

Indications for Diagnostic Testing

The extent of upper and lower urinary tract testing has to be individualized for each patient and each neurologic condition. The upper tract needs evaluation if there are symptoms suggestive of pyelonephritis or history of renal disease. Some neurologic conditions such as stroke, Parkinson's disease, and multiple sclerosis infrequently cause upper tract involvement. For these conditions, a simple baseline screening test such as renal ultrasonography (US) is sufficient. Persons with spinal cord lesions and myelodysplasia need more extensive and regular upper tract surveillance with both structural and functional tests. The lower urinary tract evaluation can be simple, from urinalysis to urine culture to measurement of postvoid residual (PVR). A full urodynamic evaluation might be necessary, however, especially if incomplete bladder emptying, incontinence, recurrent bacteriuria, or upper tract changes are present.

Bladder findings on urodynamic studies cannot be used alone to determine the level of neurologic lesion. For example, a suprasacral neurogenic bladder from a complete SCI can remain areflexic, and a conal or cauda equina bladder can exhibit high pressures from poor compliance (Table 20-3). Although the anatomic level of the neurologic lesion can suggest to the clinician the most likely pattern of bladder dysfunction, urodynamic testing should be performed to confirm this. Functional bladder studies in traumatic SCI are best deferred until spinal shock has resolved.

Table 20-3 Urodynamic Definitions

Term	Definition
Bladder	
Hyperactivity	Contractions of the detrusor during filling
Hypocontractility	Unsustained contractions causing failure to empty
Areflexia	Absent contractions with attempt to void
Compliance	Change in volume divided by change in baseline pressure with filling (<10 mL/cm H_2O abnormal; 10 to 20 mL/cm H_2O borderline if capacity reduced)
Outlet	
Detrusor sphincter dyssynergia	
At bladder neck	Usually in patients with tetraplegia and autonomic hyperactivity
At striated sphincter	Uncoordinated pelvic floor and striated sphincter contraction with detrusor contraction during attempts to void
Nonrelaxing sphincter	Poor voluntary relaxation of voluntary sphincter in patients with areflexia attempting to void by the Valsalva maneuver
Decreased outlet resistance	Incontinence caused by damage to the bladder neck or striated sphincter, pelvic floor descent, or denervation

Upper Tract Tests

Ultrasonography

US is a low-risk and relatively low-cost test for routine evaluation of the upper urinary tract, and is also easy for the patient. It is not sensitive enough to evaluate acute ureteral obstruction, and in this clinical setting non–contrast-enhanced computed tomography (CT) should be performed. US is adequate for imaging chronic obstruction and dilation, scarring, renal masses (both cystic and solid), and renal stones. The ureter is seen on US imaging only if dilated. The bladder, unless empty, can be evaluated for wall thickness, irregularity, and the presence of bladder stones.

Plain Radiography of the Urinary Tract: Kidneys, Ureter, and Bladder

A kidney, ureter, and bladder (KUB) study is often combined with US to identify any possible radiopaque calculi in the ureter or bladder stones not seen on US.

Computed Tomography

CT is often performed without contrast enhancement, and this study has replaced KUB, US, and excretory urography in the evaluation of the upper tracts when acute obstruction from stones is a possibility. It is also the most sensitive study for detecting small bladder stones in patients with an indwelling catheter in whom the bladder is collapsed around the catheter.

Excretory Urography or Computed Tomography/Intravenous Pyelogram

A CT without and then with intravenous contrast, with a delayed phase, has largely replaced the excretory urogram. The delayed phase can be used to reconstruct a complete urogram and, hence, the study is now called a "CT-Urogram" or CTU. If the serum creatinine concentration is greater than 1.5 mg/dL, or if the patient has insulin-dependent diabetes, intravenous contrast agent administration increases the risk of contrast-related nephropathy. In these cases, alternative studies include US, radioisotope renography, and possibly cystoscopy with retrograde pyelography. The "gold standard" for the workup of patients with asymptomatic microscopic hematuria (defined as greater than three red blood cells per high powered field in the absence of identifiable causes) is the CTU.[25] Imaging choices should be made in the context of results of a formal microscopic urine analysis.

Creatinine Clearance Time

This has been the gold standard for assessing renal function and is said to approximate the glomerular filtration rate (GFR). Its accuracy depends on meticulous urine collection, and it can be misleading in some clinical situations. For example, in patients with low muscle mass and a 24-hour creatinine excretion of less than 1000 mg, the calculated creatinine clearance time can be too inaccurate to be clinically useful. Because of such limitations, more endogenous markers of GFR are being increasingly studied.[29] Chief among these has been serum cystatin C, which is a low-molecular-weight protein filtered at the glomerulus. It is produced by all nucleated cells, and unlike creatinine, it is not secreted by the renal tubule and is not affected by muscle mass. Cystatin C is, however, increased in inflammation. Efforts are under way to improve agreement among commercially available assays.[57]

Isotope Studies

The technetium-99m dimercaptosuccinic acid (DMSA) scan is still the best study for both differential function and evaluation of the functioning areas of the renal cortex. The renogram obtained with technetium-99m mertiatide (MAG-3) also gives information on urinary tract drainage, as well as a good assessment of differential function. In patients who might have ureteral reflux, these studies should be done only after the bladder has been drained with an indwelling catheter. Iothalamate is another contrast medium used in excretory urography. It is of low molecular weight and is handled by the kidney in a manner identical to inulin. Both unlabeled and radioisotopic iothalamate have been used to measure GFR.

Lower Tract Tests

Urinalysis, Culture, and Sensitivity Testing

These tests are done routinely for all patients with neurogenic bladder disease and should be repeated as often as necessary or at the very least at routine follow-up annually. These would also be recommended before invasive procedures in cases of suspected UTI (i.e., with cloudy, foul-smelling, or bloody urine) or with new lower urinary tract symptoms such as incontinence, frequency, or dysuria. In persons with SCI who lack sensation, UTI symptoms may also include increased spasticity or autonomic dysreflexia. Bacteriuria should be treated before any invasive urologic procedure or test is performed.

Postvoid Residual

The PVR is simple to determine and clinically useful, especially when compared with previous recordings and considered in conjunction with the bladder pressure, clinical symptoms, and the appearance of the bladder wall. PVRs can vary throughout the day. A catheter insertion has been used for PVR in the past, but there are now simple US machines that noninvasively obtain the PVR.[13] A low (less than 20% of bladder capacity) PVR is not by itself indicative of a "balanced" bladder, as it was once defined, because high intravesical pressures can be present despite low PVR values.

Cystography

This study is usually performed to test for the presence or absence of ureteral reflux, and it also shows the outline and shape of the bladder. Findings suggestive of increased bladder pressure, such as diverticuli or an irregular bladder contour due to trabeculation, can be observed. However, it does not provide information about bladder pressure corresponding to reflux; for this, urodynamic testing is needed (discussed later).

Significant bacteriuria should be treated before the test is performed. Blood pressure should be monitored in persons with SCI at risk for, or with a history of, autonomic dysreflexia. In many cases urodynamic studies, which include fluoroscopy of the bladder and monitoring of the intravesical pressure, are more clinically useful.

Urodynamics

Urodynamics, a pressure-flow study of lower urinary tract function, remains the gold standard for the evaluation of lower urinary tract function and dysfunction. The study involves insertion of a catheter into the bladder and a second catheter to measure abdominal pressures into the rectum, ostomy, or vagina. The catheter in the bladder serves as a filling catheter and is also used for real-time pressure monitoring. An abdominal pressure tracing is helpful to distinguish intravesical pressure variations (resulting from intraabdominal transmission) from contractions of the detrusor itself. Reported filling rates vary, but usually range from 25 to 60 mL/min and should be reported as physiologic (≤weight [kg]/4 in mL/min) or nonphysiologic for rates above this threshold.[3]

During filling, patients are asked to suppress voiding. Normal values include a capacity of 300 to 600 mL, with an initial sensation of filling at approximately 50% of capacity. In children younger than 2 years, the formula 2 × age (years) + 2 will give the expected bladder capacity in ounces.[46] For children aged 2 years and older, the appropriate formula to calculate the bladder capacity in ounces is age (years)/2 + 6.[46] To convert to mL, multiply the ounces by 30. The sensation of normal fullness is said to be appreciated in the lower abdomen with a sense of urgency in the perineum. Bladder compliance is the change in volume divided by the increase in baseline pressure during filling (i.e., before a detrusor contraction). This value should be greater than 30 mL/cm H_2O, with 10 to 20 mL/cm H_2O usually defined as borderline and less than 10 mL/cm H_2O defined as poor compliance.[51] The patient is asked to suppress detrusor contractions during this test. Any detrusor contraction during the filling phase of the test, usually defined as a phasic pressure change of more than 15 cm H_2O, is abnormal and is labeled as an involuntary detrusor contraction. Individuals with involuntary detrusor contractions are classified as having "detrusor overactivity" in the absence of an identifiable cause or "neurogenic detrusor overactivity" when the voiding dysfunction is clearly associated with a neurogenic etiology. It is important to distinguish "detrusor overactivity," which is reserved purely for urodynamic findings, from the term OAB, which is a purely clinical term.

Although patients can be instructed to try to void at capacity, many are unable to generate a detrusor contraction. The presence of an easily obtainable involuntary detrusor contraction confirms the presence of detrusor overactivity in a patient with a suprasacral or supraspinal lesion. However, the absence of a contraction does not necessarily imply true acontractility in a patient with an infrasacral lesion.

Urethral Pressure Profiles

Urethral pressure profiles are obtained by withdrawing a measuring device (microtip transducer or perfused side-hole catheter) gradually down the urethra and measuring centrally oriented forces. It has limited value except in determining whether a sphincter-active area is still present after a sphincterotomy, which can also be evaluated by fluorourodynamics.

Sphincter Electromyography

Sphincter electromyography (EMG) can be combined with the cystometrogram (CMG) or preferably with a full multichannel videourodynamic study.[60] Recordings have been made with a variety of electrodes (monopolar, coaxial needle, and surface electrodes) from the levator, perianal, or periurethral muscles. Because some authors claim there is a functional dissociation between these muscle groups, periurethral recordings are preferred. The integrated EMG is displayed on the same trace as the bladder pressure. Normally, EMG activity gradually increases as bladder capacity is reached during bladder filling, and then becomes silent just before voiding. Low levels of EMG activity with no recruitment during filling are a common pattern in complete SCI. When a reflex detrusor contraction occurs in these patients, the EMG activity in the sphincter can increase rather than decrease. With this detrusor sphincter dyssynergia, voiding often occurs toward the end of the detrusor contraction because the striated sphincter relaxes more quickly than the smooth muscle of the bladder. This type of sphincter EMG does not display individual motor units and cannot be used for the evaluation of infrasacral denervation of the pelvic floor musculature (for which standard needle EMG is needed). Diagnostic integrated EMG recordings from the external urethral sphincter are difficult to obtain, invasive, and painful in patients who are sensate. The fluoroscopic appearance of the urethra is an alternative method of determining sphincter dysfunction and is preferred after distal sphincterotomy if recurrent distal sphincter dyssynergia is suspected (Figure 20-6).

Videourodynamics/Fluorourodynamics

This study is designed to give the maximum information about the filling and voiding phases of lower urinary tract function, and every effort is made to make it as physiologic as possible.[7] A videourodynamic study is indicated in the following patients: those with incomplete spinal cord lesions with incontinence who have some ability to void and inhibit voiding voluntarily but empty incompletely; persons with mechanical obstruction (e.g., benign prostatic hyperplasia) with neuropathy; candidates for sphincterotomy, to assess detrusor contraction and the presence or absence of bladder neck obstruction in addition to striated sphincter dyssynergia; those who fail to respond to pharmacotherapy; those who may be candidates for surgical procedures such as augmentation, continent diversion, or placement of an artificial sphincter or a suprapubic catheter; patients who have deterioration of the upper tracts; and patients who relapse frequently with symptomatic bacteriuria. The procedure requires placement of a seven-French two-channel catheter in the bladder and an eight-French balloon catheter in the rectum. EMG of the sphincter can be recorded along with bladder, rectal, and detrusor (bladder minus rectal) pressures. A contrast solution delivered at physiologic or supraphysiologic rates (i.e., ≥ weight [kg]/4 in mL/min) is used to fill the bladder, with the patient sitting or lying as appropriate. The blood pressure is recorded in patients with spinal cord lesions above T6 to monitor for autonomic dysreflexia. The bladder image is monitored intermittently with fluoroscopy, and the combined radiographic and urodynamic image is mixed on the same screen and can be recorded on videotape (see Figure 20-6). If the patient can sit and void during the study, a flow rate can also be recorded. A videourodynamic study in children with myelodysplasia or SCI might have to be modified, and adequate clinical information can often be obtained by recording bladder pressure combined with fluoroscopy. Table 20-3 lists urodynamic terms used to categorize bladder and outlet abnormalities.

Cystoscopy

The only routine indication for cystoscopy is the presence of a long-term indwelling suprapubic or urethral catheter because the presence of the catheter increases the risk for bladder tumor development.[77] Cystoscopy is recommended after 5 years in high-risk patients, such as smokers, or after 10 years in those with no risk factors. Cystoscopy should also be performed after CTU in patients who have gross or microscopic hematuria that cannot be attributed to UTI, stones, or trauma. Often a noncontrast CT is the only study that will pick up small bladder stones, especially if the bladder is collapsed around an indwelling catheter. Repeated lower tract infections can be an indication for cystoscopy and can reveal nonopaque foreign bodies, such as hairs, that have been introduced by catheterization.

Nonpharmacologic Treatment of Neurogenic Bladder Dysfunction

General Principles

Bladder management should be undertaken in the context of the whole person. Patient goals are to empty the bladder not more than every 3 to 4 hours, remain continent, sleep without interference from incontinence or a urinary drainage system, and avoid recurrent UTI or other complications. Less than optimal bladder management decreases the person's social, vocational, and avocational potential. The following discussion describes specific management approaches (Table 20-4).

Behavioral Management

Timed Voiding

For patients with detrusor overactivity producing urgency or involuntary leakage, a timed voiding program can help by having the patient urinate before the anticipated detrusor contraction. The limitation to this program is that persons with dementia need continual reminding. It is also

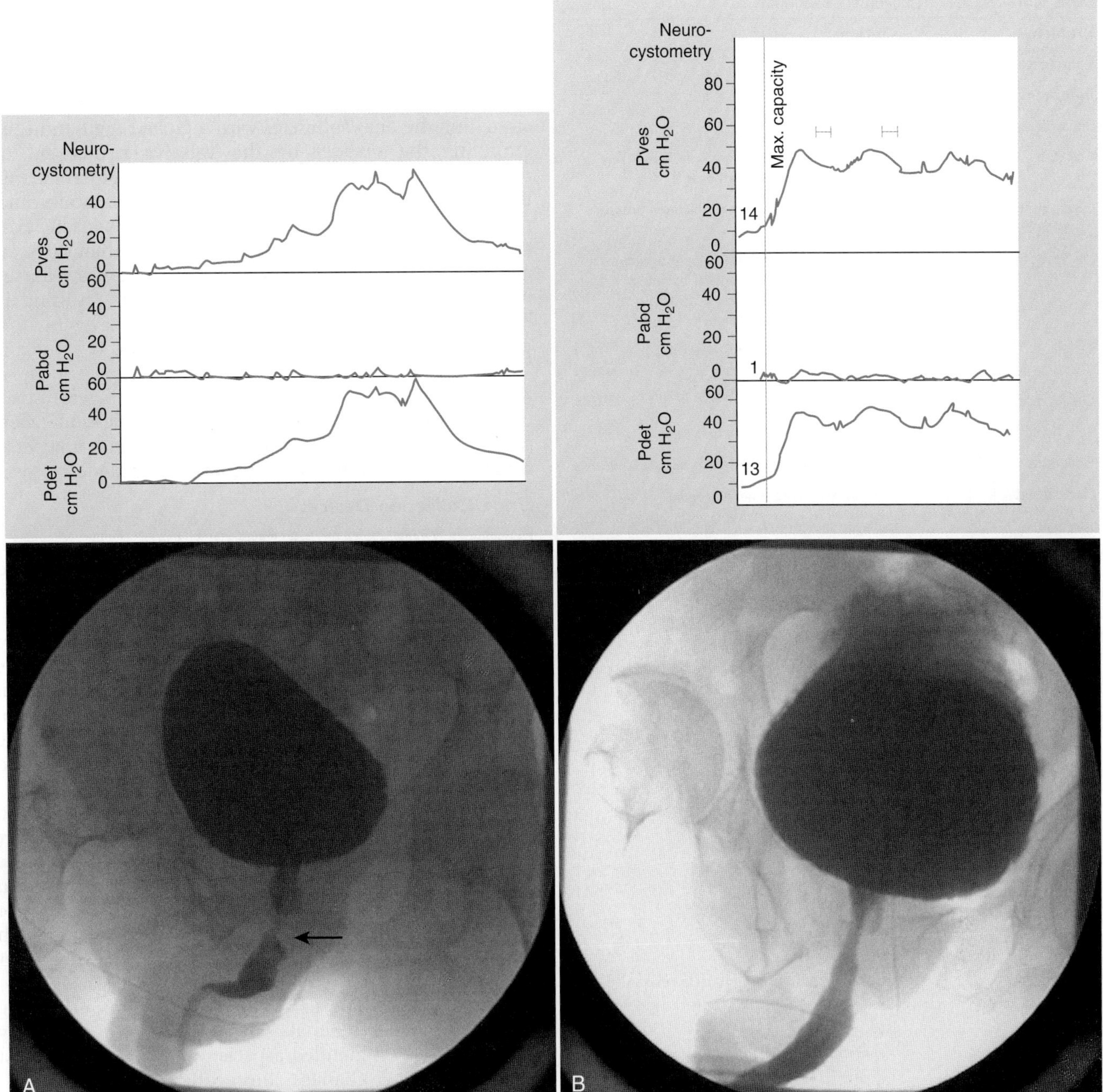

FIGURE 20-6 **A,** A videourodynamic study in a male patient with tetraplegia showing recurrent distal sphincter dyssynergia *(arrow)*. **B,** A study in a similar patient showing no evidence of dyssynergia.

useful in patients with sphincter weakness because the incontinence is worse when the bladder is full, and timed voiding reduces the amount of urine leakage. Pads may be needed to control accidents. This can be combined with monitoring fluid intake patterns and educating the patient in the relationship between fluid intake and urine output.

Bladder Stimulation

Various maneuvers have been used to stimulate bladder emptying. Stroking or pinching the perineal skin to cause reflex emptying is not consistently effective. Suprapubic tapping or jabbing over the bladder causes a mechanical stretch of the bladder wall and subsequent contraction. Controlled studies have shown that deeper indentation of the bladder with a jabbing technique is the most effective maneuver.[14] This can be used with condom catheters by patients with SCI. It is most effective in patients with paraplegia who have good upper limb function. Studies evaluating efficacy and safety of these techniques are lacking, however.

Valsalva and Credé Maneuvers

Patients with areflexia and some denervation of the pelvic floor (infrasacral lesions) may be able to void by doing a Valsalva maneuver or straining. This is most effective in women because even the partially paralyzed pelvic floor descends with straining, and the bladder neck opens, although over time the pelvic floor descent increases as the

Table 20-4 Bladder Management Options

Problem	Options
Failure to Store	
Bladder factors	
Behavioral	Timed voids
Collecting devices	Diaper, external ("condom" or "Texas") catheter, indwelling catheter
Clean intermittent catheterization	With medications to lower bladder pressure
Medications	Antimuscarinics, intravesical onabotulinum toxin injections, intrathecal baclofen,* calcium channel blockers,* intravesical vanilloids (resiniferatoxin)*
Surgery	Augmentation, continent diversion, denervation procedures*
Outlet factors	
Behavioral	Timed voids, pelvic floor exercises
Collecting devices	Diaper, condom catheter, indwelling catheter
Medications	α-Agonists, imipramine, estrogens
Surgery	Collagen injection, fascial sling, artificial sphincter, coaptite injection, Teflon*
Failure to Empty	
Bladder factors	
Behavioral	Timed voids, bladder stimulation, Valsalva and Credé maneuvers
Collecting devices	Indwelling catheter
Clean intermittent catheterization	
Medications	Bethanechol
Surgery	Neurostimulation*
Outlet factors	
Behavioral	Anal stretch void
Collecting devices	Indwelling catheters
Clean intermittent catheterization	
Medications	α-Blockers, oral striated muscle relaxant, intrathecal baclofen*
Surgery	Sphincterotomy incision, stent sphincterotomy, bladder neck incision, prostate resection, pudendal neurectomy*
Failure of storage and emptying with nonusable urethra	
Surgery	Suprapubic catheter with or without bladder neck closure, ileal conduit urostomy, ileovesicostomy, continent diversion

*Experimental or nonstandard management.

paralyzed muscles atrophy and stretch, and the patient complains of worsening stress incontinence. In men, complete flaccidity of the pelvic floor can allow emptying by straining. The Credé maneuver, usually performed by an attendant, mechanically pushes urine out of the bladder in patients with tetraplegia. The abdominal wall must be relaxed to allow the Credé maneuver to be effective, and there is a theoretical risk of producing ureteral reflux by the long-term use of this method.

Anal Stretch Voiding

In patients with paraplegia who have a spastic pelvic floor, effective voiding has been achieved by an anal stretch technique. This technique involves relaxing the pelvic floor by stretching the anal sphincter with a gloved digit and then emptying the bladder by the Valsalva maneuver.[49] It requires transfer onto a toilet, absence of anal pain sensation, and the ability to generate adequate intraabdominal pressure. For these reasons it is not widely used, even though the technique was described more than 30 years ago. In addition, anal stretch can induce reflex bowel activity that could occur concurrently or later, resulting in bowel incontinence.

Pelvic Floor Exercises

Kegel exercises are effective only in women with stress incontinence resulting from pelvic floor descent. Most patients with infrasacral neuropathy need surgery to achieve continence. Otherwise, pads are needed.

Urine Collection Devices

External ("Condom" or "Texas") Catheters. External catheters are convenient and may be an acceptable method of management for men with tetraplegia who are unable to perform self-catheterization, provided that any outflow obstruction is adequately treated. The combination of sphincterotomy and condom drainage, although attractive for men with tetraplegia, often fails over time because of inadequate detrusor contractions[88] or penile skin problems. Problems with skin breakdown and urethral damage can occur if the condom is applied too tightly. An increased risk of UTI can result from poor hygiene.

Indwelling Catheters. Indwelling catheters can be either urethral or suprapubic and are typically used either because other programs have failed or for patient convenience. In the past, indwelling catheters had a justifiably negative reputation, but studies report that some patients with indwelling catheters do no worse than those using other methods of management.[28,36]

This change is due to a number of factors, including improved catheter materials. Good catheter care is still very important. Recommended aspects of care include at least monthly catheter changes (more often if frequent infections occur), generous fluid intake (2 L or more daily), control of hyperactivity with medication,[48] changing or sterilization of urine collection devices, and avoidance of traction on the catheter. Catheter-related traction can result in severe injury, causing splitting of the urethra, referred to as traction or traumatic hypospadias. Catheter securement devices can help prevent this.[24] Suprapubic placement can also avoid some of the complications associated with urethral indwelling catheters.[36] The prevalence of squamous cell carcinoma of the bladder associated with an indwelling catheter might be lower than reported.[71,81]

Adult Diapers and Other Protective Garments. Protective garments have improved considerably over the past few years, and a high-absorbency gel-impregnated material is now used that allows the lining against the patient's perineal skin to stay dry. Protective garments are commonly used in incontinent patients with dementia who have adequate bladder emptying and in persons who leak as a result of low outlet resistance.

Clean Intermittent Catheterization. Intermittent catheterization with a sterile technique was introduced by Guttmann and Frankel in the 1950s for the management of patients with acute SCI. Lapides et al.[55] in 1972 proposed a nonsterile but "clean" technique for the management of chronic retention and infection. The technique has since been used extensively for neurogenic bladder disease. However, it is important to recognize that no catheter has ever been approved for reuse by the FDA. An intermittent catheter program requires a low-pressure bladder of adequate capacity (greater than 300 mL) and enough outflow resistance to maintain continence with normal daily activities. If the bladder is not sufficiently compliant, antimuscarinic anticholinergic medications can be used. People with SCI lesions at C6 and below can often manage self-catheterization. Although attendants and family members can perform intermittent catheterization in persons who cannot manage self-catheterization, the program often breaks down if the patient is at school or work. Patients should restrict fluid intake as needed to allow reasonable catheterization intervals. Some patients have enough sensation to be able to catheterize based on urge, but most must do so on a timed schedule. A minimum of three catheterizations per 24 hours is recommended because longer intervals between catheterizations theoretically increase the risk of symptomatic bacteriuria.[67] Many patients do wash their catheters with soap and tap water and reuse them. In those patients with recurrent UTIs, other types of catheters (touchless, enclosed systems, or hydrophilic catheters) or sterilization of catheters can be helpful in reducing infections.[16,26] A completely sterile technique can also be used but is rarely done in clinical practice.

The most common problems with self-catheterization are symptomatic bacteriuria, urethral trauma, and incontinence. Occasionally a bladder stone formed on a nidus of hair or lint is found. Patients should be warned to avoid introducing foreign material into the bladder with the catheter. Urethral trauma and catheterization difficulties can be caused by sphincter spasm. This can be managed with extra lubrication and local anesthetic urethral gel (lidocaine 2%). Sometimes a curved-tip (coudé) catheter is helpful. Hydrophilic catheters may also be useful for persons with urethral strictures, bleeding, or discomfort with catheterization.[79]

Repeated urethral bleeding suggests the presence of a break in the urethral mucosa or a false passage, and using an indwelling urethral catheter for a period of time might be necessary for this to resolve. Urethroscopy and unroofing of a false passage is occasionally necessary.

Pharmacologic Treatment of Neurogenic Bladder Dysfunction

General Principles

Many drugs for lower urinary tract management have been tried, with the rationale for their use often based on animal and in vitro experiments. Bladder management drugs in humans have generally been disappointing. The most effective groups are those that inhibit detrusor activity.

Antimuscarinic Agents

Antimuscarinic agents have been used for many years for the suppression of detrusor activity. Atropine, from belladonna, is the original compound from which numerous agents have followed. Propantheline bromide (15 to 30 mg three times a day) and hyoscyamine (0.125 to 0.25 mg three or four times a day) are agents that have been in use for many years. Oxybutynin is currently the most commonly used agent. Oxybutynin hydrochloride is given at doses up to 5 mg four times daily, or sustained release 15 mg once or twice daily in patients with no renal impairment. Lower doses are needed in patients with severe hepatic impairment. Oxybutynin in solution can be administered as an intravesical instillation in patients requiring intermittent catheterization and appears to be effective. The somewhat delayed serum levels are almost as high as when given orally. Side effects include primarily dry mouth and constipation that appear to be less severe than when the drug is given orally.[58] However, this requires a tablet to be crushed and dissolved in sterile water. A transdermal oxybutynin preparation is available, which minimizes hepatic metabolism and reduces side effects that are related to the hepatic metabolite. Skin irritation can limit its use in some persons.

Tolterodine is a long-acting muscarinic receptor antagonist used at a dose of 4 mg daily with lower dosing available for individuals with severe renal or hepatic impairment or with concomitant ketoconazole administration. Fesoterodine is a similar but newer agent. It has been demonstrated to be effective for OAB in a dose-dependent manner[87] and is one of the few agents supported by level I evidence for use in vulnerable older adult patients.[34]

Several new muscarinic receptor antagonists are now available for clinical use. Darifenacin is available as an extended release tablet (7.5 to 15 mg daily), which binds M_3 receptors to a much greater extent and might, therefore, be more bladder-selective. No renal adjustment is needed with limitation to the 7.5-mg dose in hepatic impairment and with concomitant ketoconazole use. Solifenacin is available at 5 to 10 mg daily. It should not be used in cases of severe hepatic impairment; only 5 mg should be used in cases of severe renal impairment and when used concurrently with ketoconazole. Solifenacin has been shown to improve urodynamic parameters in persons with SCI.[53] Trospium is used at a dose of 20 mg twice daily or sustained release at 60 mg daily, but it cannot be used in cases of severe hepatic impairment and must be limited to 20 mg every other day in cases of severe renal impairment. It has a quaternary amine structure, does not cross the blood-brain barrier, and has been suggested as a preferred agent in older adults or persons who are cognitively impaired.[17] Major side effects include dry mouth, blurry vision, constipation, and trospium should be used with caution in patients with narrow-angle glaucoma. A recent study found persistent detrusor overactivity, involuntary detrusor contractions, and incontinence in a significant percentage of persons with SCI despite therapy with trospium, oxybutynin, or combination therapy.[44]

Imipramine is recommended by several authors for its presumed anticholinergic actions. It is said to be additive in its effectiveness when combined with other anticholinergic agents. It does not seem to increase side effects.

Cholinergic Agonists

Bethanechol. The detrusor is innervated by cholinergic muscarinic (M_2 and M_3) receptors. In theory, bethanechol, a cholinergic agonist, might be helpful in detrusor hypocontractility by increasing detrusor activity. Although a pharmacologic effect can be seen with a parenteral dose when the bladder is partially innervated, oral doses are not effective at levels that can be tolerated by patients. Controlled clinical trials are lacking and the use of this drug has greatly declined.[38]

Adrenergic Antagonists

The α-adrenergic receptor antagonist phenoxybenzamine (10 to 30 mg daily) has α_1- and α_2-blocking actions and has been used for inhibiting smooth muscle activity at the bladder neck and in the prostate. Newer agents with more specific α_1-blocking actions are available, such as prazosin, terazosin, and doxazosin.[82] These are typically given in doses of 1 to 20 mg daily as tolerated. These agents have a number of effects. They appear to reduce the irritative symptoms in men with obstruction resulting from benign prostatic hyperplasia and to increase emptying in patients with neurogenic voiding dysfunction. Even more selective α_{1a}-selective agents, including tamsulosin (0.4 to 0.8 mg daily) and silodosin (4 to 8 mg daily), have been used for the treatment of benign prostatic hyperplasia. These agents have fewer vascular effects and rarely cause hypotension. However, increased α_{1a} selectivity may lead to high rates of retrograde ejaculation and may be unacceptable in sexually active individuals who may be interested in fertility. Data for tamsulosin in neurogenic bladder dysfunction suggest that this agent improves bladder storage and emptying and decreases the symptoms of autonomic dysreflexia in suprasacral SCI.[2] All of these agents are effective in control of the vascular manifestations of autonomic dysreflexia. Phenoxybenzamine, with its α_1- and α_2-blocking action, might be a better choice in this regard than the pure α_1-blocking agents.

Adrenergic Agonists

Adrenergic agonists have been used to increase urethral resistance in patients with mild stress incontinence. Anecdotally, ephedrine (25 to 75 mg/day) has been effective in controlling mild stress incontinence in children with myelodysplasia, but controlled studies are lacking. This is also a consideration when treating congestion from upper respiratory infections in patients with SCI, depending on their bladder emptying system. Adrenergic agonists are rarely used in adults with bladder neuropathy. Prolongation of the α-adrenergic effects on the external urethral sphincter could be possible in the future with duloxetine, a serotonin and norepinephrine reuptake inhibitor, which acts on the pudendal (Onuf) nucleus in the sacral cord. This drug may be effective for the treatment of neurogenic stress urinary incontinence but is not FDA-approved for this indication. The drug mirabegron, which acts on β_3-adrenergic receptors in the detrusor muscle, is now approved for treatment of OAB. Mirabegron has demonstrated efficacy for OAB symptoms, including incontinent episodes, urgency, and frequency, in three large-scale, randomized, placebo-controlled studies. Its effect was shown to increase with increasing severity of incontinence.[20]

Estrogens

Postmenopausal women often have atrophy of the urethral submucosa, which can lead to stress incontinence. Estrogen administration by local application often restores or maintains this tissue and can be helpful in women with a partially denervated pelvic floor and stress incontinence.

Muscle Relaxants

Baclofen, tizanidine, diazepam, and dantrolene sodium are frequently used for skeletal muscle spasticity (see Chapter 23) but have never been shown to be effective in controlled studies in patients with detrusor-striated sphincter dyssynergia. Anecdotally, some patients report better emptying with diazepam. Baclofen given intrathecally by infusion pump for severe lower extremity spasticity depresses pelvic floor reflexes but also depresses the detrusor reflex.[78] The net result is a lower-pressure bladder that might empty less effectively. Insofar as intrathecal baclofen is indicated in some patients with tetraplegia, this overall decrease in bladder emptying might not be desirable. A theoretical advantage exists of reduction in outlet resistance for those using reflex voiding, but its clinical significance is unknown.

Intravesical Therapy

Botulinum toxin type A, or onabotulinumtoxinA, given via cystoscopic injection as 200 units distributed in 30 sites in the bladder wall reduces or abolishes detrusor overactivity for 6 to 9 months. This is the only FDA-approved therapy for neurogenic detrusor overactivity that is refractory to medications. Repeated injections have been given with success for refractory cases of OAB.[33] Level I evidence now clearly supports the use of onabotulinumtoxinA for the treatment of both idiopathic and neurogenic detrusor overactivity. A large randomized, placebo-controlled trial in women confirmed the efficacy and safety of botulinum toxin type A for treatment of detrusor overactivity.[84] Another large randomized, placebo-controlled trial demonstrated the efficacy of onabotulinumtoxinA for symptom reduction in persons with idiopathic OAB.[68] In addition, Ginsberg et al.[41] demonstrated the efficacy and safety of onabotulinumtoxinA for the treatment of neurogenic detrusor overactivity.

Resiniferatoxin instillations are also under trial. These are not as effective as botulinum toxin type A but may be simpler to administer.[40,47]

Surgical Treatment of Neurogenic Bladder Dysfunction: To Increase Capacity

Bladder Augmentation

Bladder augmentation is sometimes recommended for patients who have detrusor overactivity, reduced compliance, and decreased functional storage capacity that fails to respond to medical therapy.[76] The advent of intravesical onabotulinum toxin is reducing its role. The patient must be motivated to reliably perform clean intermittent catheterization indefinitely, have adequate outlet resistance, and be informed of immediate surgical risks and possible long-term sequelae of the procedure. Immediate surgical risks include prolonged intestinal ileus or obstruction, anastomotic leak with peritonitis, wound infection, and pulmonary complications such as pneumonia and deep venous thrombosis with pulmonary emboli. Bladder augmentation has been performed since the 1950s, especially in children with myelodysplasia and developmentally small bladders. Long-term complications reported so far have included chronic bacteriuria, a theoretical risk of neoplastic change, possible diarrhea or malabsorption from a shortened gut or decreased intestinal transit time, and hyperchloremic acidosis caused by absorption of urine with secondary mobilization of skeletal calcium (acting as a buffer).[30]

The bladder is opened widely in this procedure, and a detubularized and reconfigured segment of bowel is sewn in. A 20- to 30-cm segment of distal ileum is usually used, but an ileocecal segment, sigmoid, or even a wedge of stomach can also be used (Figure 20-7). The procedure is intended to result in a 600-mL, low-pressure reservoir without the use of any drugs. Mucus production is the main day-to-day problem initially. Mucus production can increase with an active urinary infection. Mucus production is rarely a problem after the first 3 months if a good intermittent catheterization technique is used. Bladder irrigation may be used as needed. Because the risk of neoplastic change is unknown with this procedure, yearly cystoscopy should probably begin 10 to 15 years after the augmentation.

Bladder Augmentation with Continent Catheterizable Stoma

In this procedure, a section of bowel is used not just to increase effective bladder capacity but also to form a continent catheterizable channel that opens onto the abdominal wall. It is particularly useful in women for whom intermittent self-catheterization via the urethra is difficult or impossible because of leg spasticity, body habitus, severe urethral incontinence, or the need to transfer from a wheelchair. Men who are unable to perform intermittent catheterization because of partial hand function, strictures, false passages, or fistulas are also potential candidates. Severe urethral disease in men is frequently the result of poor personal care, and it is inappropriate to perform these procedures on patients who cannot or will not follow through with appropriate techniques. If the patient fails to catheterize after augmentation and continent diversion, the bowel segment can rupture internally before overflow incontinence occurs through the urethra or catheterizable channel.

The procedure involves enlarging the bladder and constructing some form of continent catheterizable channel. The terminal ileum and the ileocecal valve work well, but the intussuscepted small bowel, the appendix, and the defunctioned segments of the ureter have all been used. The bladder neck might require closure if there is sphincter-related incontinence.

Urinary Diversion

If the bladder cannot be preserved because of malignant disease, contracture, or ureteral reflux, a standard ileal conduit is recommended with removal of the bladder in most cases. Usually a 10- to 15-cm segment of the small bowel is used. In theory, a nonrefluxing ureterointestinal anastomosis should reduce risk of infections; however, evidence has not supported this and refluxing anastomoses are expected to have similar long-term outcomes with decreased rates of anatomic strictures.

Denervation Procedures

Denervation techniques for bladder hyperactivity are theoretically attractive but not widely used. Operative approaches include sectioning of the sacral nerve roots or interrupting the peripheral nerve supply near the bladder. Selective sacral rhizotomies have been attempted. The

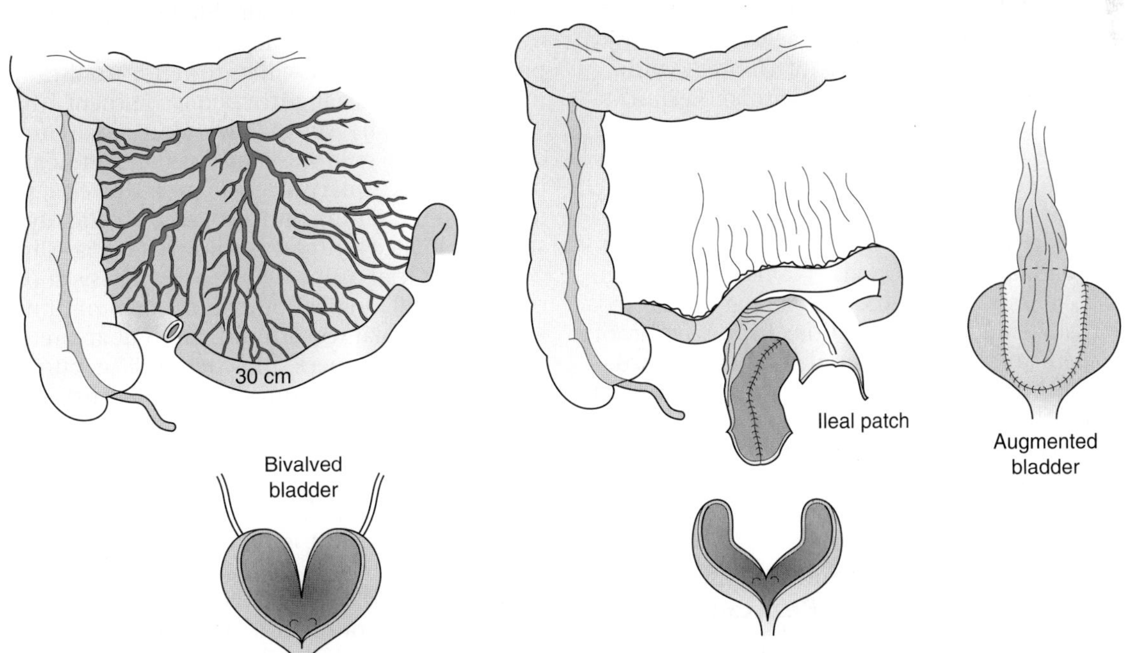

FIGURE 20-7 Augmentation cystoplasty. A 30-cm segment of the small bowel is opened and reconstructed as a U-shaped patch and then sewn into the bivalved bladder.

technique involves identifying the nerve root (usually S3 on one side) that carries the detrusor reflex by doing differential sacral local anesthetic blocks while monitoring the detrusor reflex with CMG. Surgical or chemical destruction of S3 usually results in only temporary acontractility. Over time the detrusor reflex typically reroutes through the intact sacral nerves. Bilateral S2, S3, and S4 rhizotomies permanently abolish the reflex but at the expense of loss of reflex erections and loss of reflex colon emptying. Improvements in cystometric capacity have been demonstrated in small numbers of patients with percutaneous radiofrequency sacral rhizotomy techniques.[21,37]

Peripheral denervation of the detrusor has been attempted by transecting the detrusor above the trigone and resuturing it, by removing the paravesical ganglia via a vaginal approach, or by overdistending the bladder with the intent of damaging the intramural nerves and muscle fibers. In one clinical study of patients with complete paraplegia, the bladder was intentionally distended in the spinal shock phase with the intent of preventing the return of the bladder reflex. The prevalence of areflexia in the short term following distention was 63%.[45] None of these peripheral denervation procedures have become commonly accepted, and long-term results of intentional overdistention of the bladder in spinal shock have not yet been reported. Chemical denervation procedures have been discussed under intravesical therapy.

Surgical Treatments for Neurogenic Bladder Dysfunction: To Increase Contractility

Electrical Stimulation

Detrusor contraction can be elicited electrically with electrodes implanted on the bladder wall, pelvic nerves, sacral roots, and conus.[10] The electrodes are placed on the anterior roots either intradurally or extradurally. To prevent spontaneous hyperactive contractions and antidromic reflex contractions, bilateral S2, S3, and S4 dorsal rhizotomies are usually performed. Pelvic floor contraction with anterior root stimulation can obstruct voiding, and thus intermittent stimulation is used. This leads to intermittent voiding because the striated pelvic floor muscle relaxes more quickly than the smooth muscle detrusor. In a center developing this device in the United States, pudendal neurectomies were performed to decrease outflow resistance.[83] Adequate bladder emptying at acceptable intravesical pressures with preservation of the bladder wall and upper tract morphology and function has been reported.[10,53] One disadvantage of bilateral S2, S3, and S4 rhizotomies is that reflex erections are abolished, and usable erections from sacral root stimulation occur infrequently. Stimulated bowel evacuation, however, is improved in many patients. Refinements being studied include supraselective rhizotomies, modification of stimulus parameters, and electrode designs. Sacral anterior root stimulation is approved for clinical use in the United States but is not widely available.[52]

Surgical Treatment of Neurogenic Bladder Dysfunction: To increase Outlet Resistance

Incontinence resulting from decreased outlet resistance is relatively uncommon in bladder dysfunction secondary to neurologic disease. It is seen in children with myelodysplasia and in women with infrasacral lesions and a denervated pelvic floor. It can occur in active men with complete pelvic floor denervation, but this is rare. Although α-adrenergic agonists might help minor incontinence, more severe leakage typically requires some form of urethral compressive procedure. The options include injection therapy into the bladder neck and urethra to increase the bulk of tissue under and around the bladder neck muscle, a fascial sling, or an artificial sphincter. Electrical stimulation of pelvic floor muscles or nerves via rectal, vaginal, or implanted electrodes has been tried but has not been effective enough to achieve widespread popularity.

Urethral Bulking Agents

Injection of periurethral bulking agents has been a widely used technique for certain types of stress incontinence. Teflon (DuPont, Wilmington, Del.) has been used with some success for many years but has never been made available in the United States because of the potential danger of particle migration. Likewise, hyaluronic acid was voluntarily removed from the market because of injection site complications. Other agents including autologous fat, bovine collagen, and hydroxyapatite have been tried, and may be beneficial in some patients with more mild degrees of incontinence. The injection procedure has few potential side effects and is especially suitable for older adults and poor-risk patients. Recently, injection of autologous stem cells is being investigated and has the potential to offer a longer term and more effective treatment for stress urinary incontinence.[80]

External Compressive Procedures

In the autologous fascial sling procedure, a 2-cm strip of fascia is taken from the anterior rectus abdominis fascia or tensor fascia latae, positioned beneath the bladder neck, and fixed anteriorly to the abdominal fascia or pubic tubercle. Patients who are candidates for this procedure must have compliant low-pressure bladders. They will be unable to void by the Valsalva maneuver after a successful sling procedure and must be willing to perform self-catheterization indefinitely in exchange for being continent. More recently, synthetic (mesh) slings have been used and are now considered the gold standard for the treatment of uncomplicated stress urinary incontinence. However, stress incontinence in the setting of neurogenic bladder dysfunction is still best treated with an autologous fascial sling.

The artificial urinary sphincter consists of a cuff, a pressure-regulating balloon, and a control pump. The cuff is usually implanted around the bulbar urethra in men and the bladder neck in women. The pump is placed in the labia or scrotum allowing the patient to voluntarily open the cuff for voiding. The cuff reinflates automatically over 2 minutes. Mechanical failure, cuff erosion, and infection can occur with this device, especially if sensation is impaired. The device can be used in the neurogenic bladder[54] but is not in widespread use in the SCI population.

Some persons may be able to empty using the Valsalva maneuver and not require intermittent catheterization. In patients with myelodysplasia, uncontrolled hyperactivity occurs in 10% in the first year after implantation of an artificial sphincter. This is despite the fact that preoperatively the detrusor was naturally areflexic or was rendered so by drugs. This probably results from activation of dormant urethrovesical reflexes. Careful follow-up evaluation is essential and, if hyperactivity occurs, intravesical botulinum toxin (BTX) or bladder augmentation can be performed.

Surgical Treatment of Neurogenic Bladder Dysfunction: To Decrease Outlet Resistance

Sphincterotomy

In male patients with SCI who are unable or unwilling to do self-catheterization, the use of an external catheter is one alternative. Because it is unusual to find a lower urinary tract that has adequate detrusor contraction and a coordinated pelvic floor in these patients, some procedure to decrease outflow resistance is usually indicated. The results are poor in patients without adequate detrusor contractions. Ablation of the striated sphincter, usually by incision, is the standard procedure. It is now performed anteriorly to avoid the cavernous artery and nerve, which both lie lateral to the membranous urethra because damage to these structures can result in erectile dysfunction. Some patients also have bladder neck obstruction resulting from primary hyperactivity (in persons with high SCI) or bladder wall hypertrophy as a result of chronic striated sphincter dyssynergia. These patients need bladder neck ablation either by resection or by incision. In older men, prostatic obstruction from hypertrophy can also contribute to increased outflow resistance and might require prostatic resection. The immediate morbidity from sphincterotomy, bleeding, clot retention, and infection, is relatively high. The long-term results can be compromised because of recurrent obstruction from stricture or recurrent dyssynergia. Residual urine with pyuria, worsening urinary retention, and hydronephrosis resulting from elevated pressure and poor emptying are all potential long-term problems.[88] However, a laser sphincterotomy technique may have similar results with reduced side effects.[73]

Urethral Stents

Implantable stainless steel stents, previously used for the treatment of urethral strictures[5] have been utilized in the sphincteric position instead of sphincterotomy[18,19] or after failed sphincterotomy.[72] Urothelial ingrowth incorporates the stent.[62] A small 20-year follow-up SCI cohort has been reported.[1] Although the procedure is described as reversible, removal can be difficult, requiring wire-by-wire extraction. The stent is not well tolerated in men with sensory incomplete SCI and complications such as migration, encrustation, and epithelial overgrowth have occurred.

Other Methods of Decreasing Outflow Resistance

Intrathecal baclofen given for severe spasticity decreases pudendal reflexes and pelvic floor muscle tone, but the detrusor reflex and contractions are also reduced. Consequently, it cannot be used as a chemical sphincterotomy. Botulinum toxin type A injected into the striated sphincter has also been used experimentally, but (as in the bladder) its effects last only a few months.[35]

Differential Diagnosis of Neurogenic Bladder Dysfunction

Diseases of the Brain

Stroke. After an initial period of areflexia, patients with stroke typically have hyperactivity with frequency and urge incontinence but coordinated voiding and complete emptying (see Chapter 44). Antimuscarinics frequently help ameliorate symptoms without adversely affecting emptying. Persistent areflexia and retention can occur with bilateral lesions. Prostatic obstruction can cause retention in older adult men after a stroke. Videourodynamic studies are helpful in differentiating these conditions.

Parkinson Disease. The prevalence of bladder symptoms in patients with Parkinson disease is high (see Chapter 45). Most have frequency, urgency, and urge incontinence, and 50% complain of difficulty voiding. Evaluation typically shows bladder hyperactivity, but the contractions are poorly sustained and result in incomplete emptying. Failure to empty can also be caused by bradykinesia, secondary to failure of pelvic floor relaxation, adrenergic effects of levodopa, or even the anticholinergic effects of other antiparkinsonian drugs.[6] Treatment is difficult because there is frequently a combination of incontinence and retention. Detrusor inhibition with drugs worsens emptying, and α-adrenergic blockers have a marginal effect in decreasing outflow resistance.[82] Intermittent catheterization and detrusor inhibition are often the best choice, but many patients do not have sufficient upper extremity dexterity to catheterize independently.

Dementia, Brain Tumors, and Trauma. Dementia, brain tumors, and trauma can all cause hyperactivity with reflex or urge incontinence with complete emptying. If cognitive impairment is severe, incontinence often persists despite detrusor inhibition. Some type of collecting device is appropriate for many of these patients (see Chapter 43).

Diseases of the Brain and Spinal Cord. Multiple sclerosis is the most common disease in this category with 90% of patients developing urinary manifestations in the course of the disease (see Chapter 46). The bladder symptoms usually present because of an incomplete spinal cord lesion with hyperactivity and hypocontractility. Detrusor inhibition with drugs worsens emptying in this case. In the rare, predominantly encephalopathic variety of multiple sclerosis, these agents might be useful. Patients with multiple sclerosis and a predominantly conal lesion have bladder areflexia. Intermittent catheterization is eventually indicated in most patients with multiple sclerosis, but few are able to undertake it because of poor upper extremity strength and coordination. High-pressure bladders resulting from hyperactivity and detrusor sphincter dyssynergia are uncommon in multiple sclerosis.[56]

Diseases of the Spinal Cord. Injury, tumors, and vascular lesions of the spinal cord cause the majority of suprasacral neurogenic bladder problems (see Chapter 49). The detrusor reflex typically returns after a varying period of spinal shock. The center for the detrusor reflex develops in the sacral cord in patients with complete injury. Inhibitory control by the higher center is impaired, and because the long-routed detrusor reflex is interrupted, the detrusor contraction might not be completely sustained. Coordination and control of the pelvic floor are also impaired, leading to lack of voluntary contraction and relaxation. In complete lesions there is often dyscoordinated activity during voiding. This dyscoordination or detrusor sphincter dyssynergia affects the striated voluntary sphincter, but in patients with high complete tetraplegia, excessive sympathetic activity can also lead to detrusor bladder neck dyssynergia. Incomplete spinal cord lesions can produce the supraspinal pattern with urgency and adequate emptying, whereas patients with complete lesions have reflex incontinence and incomplete emptying because of detrusor sphincter dyssynergia (in most cases). Some patients have hypocontractility or areflexia and retention. A truly balanced bladder with sustained detrusor contraction and coordinated pelvic floor is uncommon.

The onset and severity of the symptoms vary with the cause of spinal cord dysfunction, but the management discussed here is in relation to traumatic SCI. An indwelling catheter is typically maintained until the patient's medical state is stable and fluid intake can be regulated to achieve a urine output of 1500 to 2000 mL per day. Intermittent sterile catheterization is then started, preferably by a dedicated catheterization team. The patient should learn self-catheterization when able to do so. A sterile technique is ideal in the hospital, but a clean technique can be used when the patient is discharged home. In some patients, however, daytime fluid retention in the lower limbs while the patient is upright, with subsequent mobilization and dumping at night, is frequently a problem. The use of compressive stockings such as TED hose, recumbency early in the evening, and an extra catheterization in the middle of the night can be tried to manage this.

In the majority of patients with SCI, the detrusor reflex returns within the first 6 months. Its return is often indicated by episodes of incontinence, but the presence of the detrusor reflex should be confirmed by urodynamics. Antimuscarinics can be given to suppress the reflex and allow intermittent catheterization to continue. Patients with lesions at the level of C7 and below who can do self-catheterization can continue this in the long term. If the detrusor reflex cannot be suppressed, BTX injections should be considered. BTX has replaced bladder augmentation as the second-line option for achieving low-pressure urine storage.

In male patients unable or unwilling to do self-catheterization, as well as for those who refuse augmentation, sphincterotomy followed by use of an external catheter is probably the best alternative. Other options include intermittent catheterization by an attendant, although this has a greater risk of febrile UTIs.[15] An external collector alone can be considered, but few men with SCI have a suitable, "balanced" bladder with coordinated voiding at low pressure. Some external catheter users end up with an indwelling catheter because of sphincterotomy failure, inadequate detrusor contractions, or skin breakdown on the penile shaft. Women using intermittent catheterization who are unable to control urinary incontinence with medications might also choose to use an indwelling catheter, but chronic use of urethral indwelling catheters should be avoided in women, as their short urethra can become dilated, resulting in severe leakage. A regular long-term urinary tract surveillance program (Box 20-1) should be set up for patients with SCI who might, with good care, have a near-normal life expectancy.

BOX 20-1

Routine Urinary Tract Surveillance After Spinal Cord Injury

Initial Rehabilitation Admission

- Urinalysis, initial and as needed
- Urine culture and sensitivity, initial and as needed
- Renal and bladder ultrasound; add KUB in patients with a Foley catheter
- CT-IVP only if US is abnormal or noncontrast CT renal protocol
- PVR if voiding
- CMG or urodynamics if clinically indicated
- CrCl, 24-hour urine

Routine Evaluations (Yearly for the First 5 Years and, if Stable, Every Other Year Thereafter)

- Renal US and KUB for all annual evaluations
- CT-IVP only if indicated by clinical status or US findings
- Urodynamics determined on individual basis (often needed annually for the first few years)
- CrCl, 24-hour urine, annually
- PVR if voiding
- Other tests of renal function as needed

Cystoscopy

Generally performed in patients after 10 years of chronic, continuous indwelling catheterization (urethral or suprapubic), or earlier (at 5 years) if at high risk (heavy smoker, age >40 years, or history of complicated UTIs) or in any patient with symptoms that warrant such a procedure.

CMG, Cystometrography; *CrCl*, creatinine clearance; *CT-IVP*, computerized tomography-intravenous pyelography; *IC*, intermittent catheterization; *KUB*, kidneys, ureters, and bladder, plain film study; *PVR*, postvoid residual; *US*, ultrasound; *UTI*, urinary tract infection.

Diseases of the Conus, Cauda Equina, and Peripheral Nerves. Trauma, disk disease, lumbar stenosis, arachnoiditis, and tumors are some of the mechanical lesions that can affect this region of the spinal canal. The resulting bladder is typically areflexic or noncontractile and insensate. Pelvic floor innervation is frequently affected in conal lesions, which can lead to incontinence, especially in women. In cauda equina lesions, the nonmyelinated pelvic nerve roots are more easily damaged and pelvic floor innervation is usually relatively more intact than the detrusor nerve supply. In autonomic neuropathy secondary to diabetes and multiple system atrophy, the detrusor afferents and efferents are affected, and because of lack of sensation, overstretching contributes to the result, which is a noncontractile and insensate bladder.

Intermittent catheterization is the initial treatment if retention is present. If the pelvic floor is severely paralyzed, patients might be able to void by straining. α-Adrenergic blocking agents can help decrease outflow resistance in men. Women can often empty by straining but tend to develop severe stress incontinence. Some patients can be candidates for a fascial urethral sling or artificial sphincter.

Reduced bladder compliance, usually found in patients after radical pelvic surgery, does not respond well to medications. An augmentation might be indicated in these cases, particularly if the outflow resistance is high and the upper tracts begin to dilate. In the early stages of diabetes, patients can often maintain bladder function and contractility and avoid overdistention by timed voidings.

Diseases of the Spinal Cord and Conus. Myelodysplasia is the most common disease producing a mixed pattern of lower urinary tract dysfunction. Any combination of detrusor and sphincter activity can be found, but it is most common to have a hyperactive or noncompliant bladder with dyssynergia or a nonrelaxing sphincter. Intermittent catheterization is used initially along with medication in infancy and childhood. In many cases, reconstructive surgery is necessary early if more conservative measures fail.

Complications of Neurogenic Voiding Dysfunction

Bacteriuria

Approximately half of all hospital-acquired infections originate in the urinary tract in association with urinary catheters and other drainage devices. These are referred to as catheter-associated UTIs. UTIs are a common source of morbidity in patients with neurogenic bladders. UTI is the most common infection after SCI; occurring an average of 2.5 times per year.[24] Frequent exposure to antibiotics increases the risk of infection with antibiotic-resistant organisms, further complicating the treatment of UTI. The diagnosis of UTI can be delayed or missed in patients with neurologic disorders affecting bladder sensation. In patients with spinal cord disorders, signs and symptoms suggestive of UTI include fever, onset of urinary incontinence, increased spasticity, autonomic dysreflexia, increased sweating, cloudy and malodorous urine, malaise, lethargy, and sense of unease.[43,65] Unexplained signs and symptoms suggestive of UTI in the presence of pyuria warrant empirical therapy for UTI. The absence of pyuria makes the diagnosis of UTI unlikely, but does not exclude it.

Asymptomatic bacteriuria is very common in patients with neurogenic bladder, especially those using intermittent or indwelling catheterization. Most authorities recommend against routine treatment of asymptomatic bacteriuria, although the presence of significant bacteriuria with urease-producing organisms that are associated with stone formation might warrant treatment.[66]

The spectrum of uropathogens that cause catheter-associated UTI is much broader than that causing uncomplicated UTI. *Escherichia coli* causes the majority of uncomplicated UTIs. *E. coli* and organisms such as species of *Proteus, Klebsiella, Pseudomonas, Serratia, Providencia,* enterococci, and staphylococci are relatively more common in patients with catheter-associated UTI.[65] Polymicrobic bacteriuria is frequent in patients with indwelling catheters.

Patients with mild to moderate illness can be treated with an oral fluoroquinolone such as ciprofloxacin, levofloxacin, or gatifloxacin. Fluoroquinolones are associated with an increased risk of tendonitis and tendon rupture in patients of all ages. The risk is further increased in those older than 60 years, with concomitant steroid use, or organ transplant. This group of antibiotics provides coverage for most expected pathogens, including most strains of *Pseudomonas aeruginosa.* Trimethoprim-sulfamethoxazole is another commonly used antibiotic for patients who are less ill, but it does not provide coverage against *P. aeruginosa*. It is less expensive than the fluoroquinolones and can be used empirically and continued according to the results of susceptibility testing. Ampicillin and nitrofurantoin are poor choices for empirical therapy because of the high prevalence of resistance to these agents among uropathogens typically involved in complicated UTIs.

In patients who are more seriously ill and hospitalized, piperacillin plus tazobactam, ampicillin plus gentamicin, or imipenem plus cilastatin provide coverage against most expected pathogens, including *P. aeruginosa* and most enterococci.[12] A number of other parenteral antimicrobial agents can also be used. Patients can be switched to oral treatment after clinical improvement. At least 7 to 14 days of therapy is generally recommended, depending on the severity of the infection.[66] No convincing evidence shows that regimens longer than this are beneficial. Patients undergoing effective treatment for UTI with an antibiotic to which the infecting pathogen is susceptible should have definite improvement within 24 to 48 hours. If not, a repeat urine culture and imaging studies (US or CT) are indicated.

In a patient who has had UTI with high fever or hemodynamic changes suggestive of sepsis, or who is having recurrent symptomatic UTIs, a CT-KUB, cystogram, or urodynamic evaluation might be indicated after successful treatment to look for correctable anatomic or functional abnormalities.

Autonomic Dysreflexia

Afferent stimulation into the spinal cord from nociceptive sources, such as a distended bladder, can trigger this phenomenon. Because of the lack of supraspinal inhibition resulting from an SCI, exaggerated reflex sympathetic outflow occurs, resulting in autonomic dysreflexia symptoms, which can include sudden hypertension, sweating, piloerection, headache, and reflex bradycardia. Autonomic dysreflexia occurs more commonly in persons with more complete lesions. Spinal cord injuries below T6 are rarely associated with this problem. Afferent stimuli from the bladder from high pressure or other irritation are the most common cause of autonomic dysreflexia. The best treatment is prevention of such stimuli. If symptoms persist when the bladder has been emptied or if the blood pressure is at a dangerously high level, apply 0.5 to 1 inch of nitroglycerin ointment on the skin because this can be wiped off when hypertension resolves or if hypotension occurs. Sublingual nifedipine 10 mg was used more commonly in the past, but has fallen out of favor because of the risk of hypotension. If a patient has recently ingested sildenafil, then prazosin or captopril can be used instead.[23] Long-term management with phenoxybenzamine (10 to 30 mg daily) has been used to prevent autonomic dysreflexia when all detectable causes have been eliminated (see Chapter 49 for further explanation of the treatment of autonomic dysreflexia). Further research is needed to evaluate the efficacy of agents used for the treatment of this condition.

Hypercalciuria and Stones

Loss of calcium from the bones occurs in all patients with SCI and is worse in young males. Increased urinary calcium (greater than 200 mg/24 hours) begins approximately 4 weeks after injury, reaches a maximum at 16 weeks, and can persist for 12 to 18 months. Renal stone incidence in the first 9 months is approximately 1.0% to 1.5% and is mainly attributable to hypercalciuria. Over the next 10 years upper tract stones are found in 7% of cases, with many of these secondary to infection. The incidence of bladder stones in the first 9 months in patients on intermittent catheterization is 2.3%. In the presence of an indwelling catheter, and despite greater urine output, the prevalence is higher (8.8%).[27]

Bladder stones are effectively treated with cystoscopy and laser lithotripsy. Small stones and particles can be dissolved by daily bladder irrigations with 30 mL of 10% hemiacidrin (Renacidin) solution, which is left in the bladder for 30 minutes. Some patients with recurrent stones use this once or twice a week for prophylaxis. In patients who have ureteral reflux, it should be used with caution because of potential nephrotoxicity and absorption of magnesium. Calyceal calculi that are small (less than 1 cm) and asymptomatic can be followed expectantly, but 50% of these patients become symptomatic over 5 years, and half of these will need some sort of invasive procedure.[42] Calculi that are growing or that are located in the renal pelvis should probably be treated before they pass into the ureter and cause obstruction (Figure 20-8). Extracorporeal shock wave lithotripsy (ESWL) is the standard treatment. For large stones (greater than 3 cm

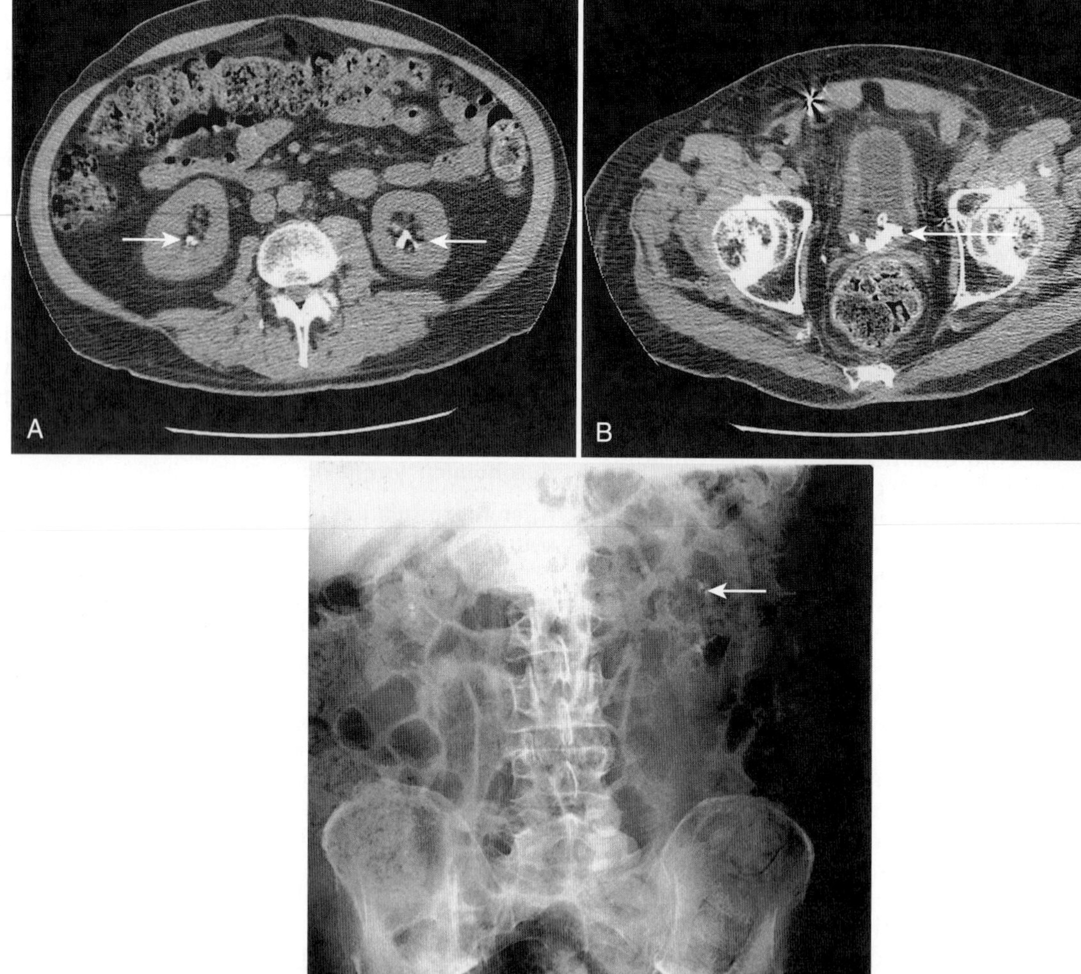

FIGURE 20-8 A computed tomography of the kidney, ureter, and bladder (CT-KUB) **(A** and **B)** and a standard KUB **(C)** showing renal *(short arrows)* and bladder *(long arrows)* stones in a patient with tetraplegia. The stones can be seen on the standard KUB in this patient, but in many patients visualization is difficult because of the size and density of the stones, the size of the patient, and the state of the overlying bowel. CT-KUB is more sensitive.

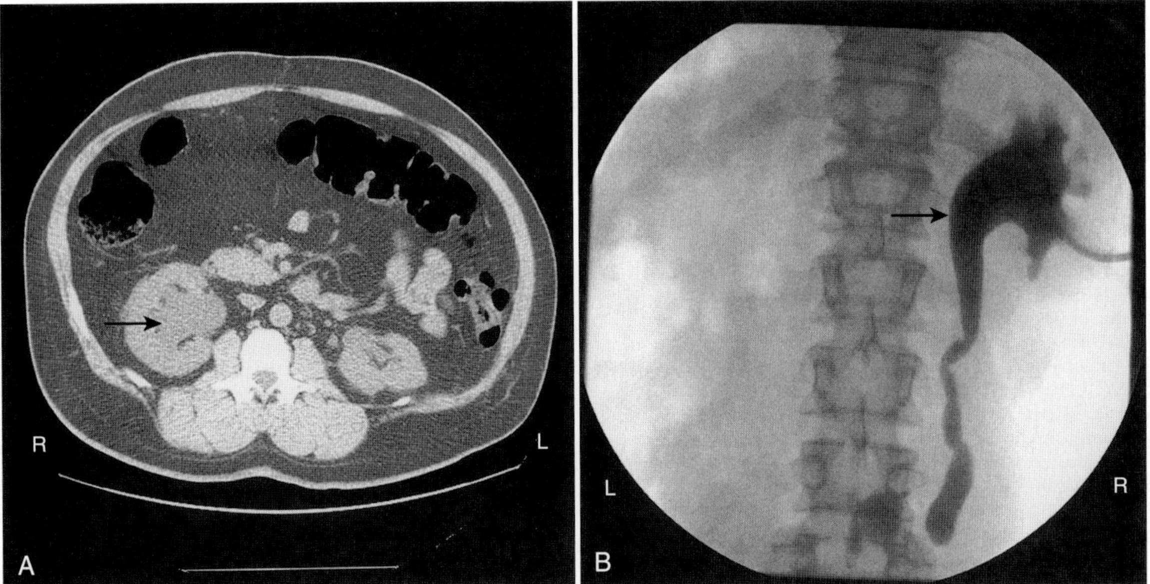

FIGURE 20-9 A computed tomography of the kidney, ureter, and bladder (CT-KUB) **(A)** and a prone antegrade nephrostogram **(B)** demonstrating right hydronephrosis with a dilated ureter *(arrows)* down to the ureteroileal junction. The patient is a male with spina bifida whose bladder was augmented and the ureters reimplanted 10 years before. The cause of the obstruction was an inflammatory stricture.

diameter), a percutaneous approach is preferred because clearance of fragments is poor if patients are inactive.

Ureteral stones are potentially dangerous in patients with no renal sensation. These can be managed expectantly if they pass down within 2 to 3 weeks. Patients with reduced sensation might not perceive continuous pain, which would normally suggest severe continuing obstruction. This results in an increased risk of renal damage. When obstruction and infection occur together, they require an emergent drainage procedure with a percutaneous nephrostomy or a retrograde stent. This is typically followed by an endoscopic lithotripsy, stone removal, or ESWL.

Lower Urinary Tract Changes

Trabeculation occurs in the majority of patients after SCI. In many cases, trabeculation happens despite appropriate management strategies. Sacculation and diverticula can occur when obstruction and high pressure are severe. If a diverticulum occurs at the ureteral hiatus, ureteral reflux is almost inevitable. Chronic infection of dilated prostatic ducts can be an important source for relapsing UTIs in men.

Ureteral Reflux and Upper Tract Dilation

Ureteral reflux or high bladder pressure in the absence of reflux can cause upper tract dilation (Figure 20-9). Dilation without reflux is said to be caused by decreased compliance, but data from long-term monitoring suggest that baseline pressure elevations are minimal with natural rates of filling and that increased phasic activity might be more important.[86] With reflux, or ureteral dilation without reflux, the bladder pressure should be lowered with intermittent catheterization, antimuscarinic medication, or botulinum toxin injections. If bladder pressure responds but reflux fails to improve, surgery to repair the reflux can be considered. If bladder pressures do not improve, surgical urinary diversion is indicated.

Summary

The ultimate goal of bladder management is to establish a program for the patient that optimizes quality of life while preventing renal deterioration and reducing morbidity such as UTIs. A history and physical examination followed by appropriate testing will allow classification of the patient's bladder dysfunction. This will allow, with careful consideration of other medical problems and social issues, choice of the best method of bladder management to meet these stated goals.

KEY REFERENCES

1. Abdul-Rahman A, Ismail S, Hamid R, Shah J: A 20-year follow-up of the mesh wallstent in the treatment of detrusor external sphincter dyssynergia in patients with spinal cord injury, *BJU Int* 106:1510–1513, 2010.
2. Abrams P, Amarenco G, Bakke A, et al; European Tamsulosin Neurogenic Lower Urinary Tract Dysfunction Study Group: Tamsulosin: efficacy and safety in patients with neurogenic lower urinary tract dysfunction due to suprasacral spinal cord injury, *J Urol* 170:1242–1251, 2003.
3. Abrams P, Cardozo L, Fall M, et al; Standardisation Sub-committee of the International Continence Society: The standardisation of terminology of lower urinary tract function: report from the Standardisation Sub-committee of the International Continence Society, *Neurourol Urodyn* 21:167–178, 2002.
8. Bors E, Comarr AE: *Neurological urology*, Baltimore, 1971, University Park Press.
10. Brindley GS, Rushton DN: Long-term follow-up of patients with sacral anterior root stimulator implants, *Paraplegia* 28:469–475, 1990.
11. Burnstock G: Purinergic signalling in the lower urinary tract, *Acta Physiol* 207:40–52, 2013.
15. Cardenas DD, Mayo ME: Bacteriuria with fever after spinal cord injury, *Arch Phys Med Rehabil* 68:291–293, 1987.
16. Cardenas DD, Moore KN, Dannels-McClure A, et al: Intermittent catheterization with a hydrophilic-coated catheter delays urinary tract infections in acute spinal cord injury: a prospective, randomized, multicenter trial, *PM R* 3:408–417, 2011.
19. Chancellor MB, Gajewski J, Ackman CF, et al: Long-term follow-up of the North American multicenter UroLume trial for the treatment

of external detrusor-sphincter dyssynergia, *J Urol* 161:1545–1550, 1999.
20. Chapple C, Khullar V, Nitti VW, et al: Efficacy of the β_3-adrenoceptor agonist mirabegron for the treatment of overactive bladder by severity of incontinence at baseline: a post hoc analysis of pooled data from three randomised phase 3 trials, *Eur Urol* 67:11–14, 2015.
21. Cho KH, Lee SS: Radiofrequency sacral rhizotomy for the management of intolerable neurogenic bladder in spinal cord injured patients, *Ann Rehabil Med* 36:213–219, 2012.
22. Collins C, Klausner AP, Herrick B, et al: Potential for control of detrusor smooth muscle spontaneous rhythmic contraction by cyclooxygenase products released by interstitial cells of Cajal, *J Cell Mol Med* 13:3236–3250, 2009.
23. Consortium for Spinal Cord Medicine: Acute management of autonomic dysreflexia: individuals with spinal cord injury presenting to health-care facilities, *J Spinal Cord Med* 25(Suppl 1):S67–S88, 2002.
24. Darouiche RO, Goetz L, Kaldis T, et al: Impact of StatLock securing device on symptomatic catheter-related urinary tract infection: a prospective, randomized, multicenter clinical trial, *Am J Infect Control* 34(9):555–560, 2006.
25. Davis R, Jones JS, Barocas DA, et al: *Diagnosis, evaluation and follow-up of asymptomatic microhematuria (AMH) in adults: AUA guideline*, 2010, American Urological Association. Available at: www.auanet.org/education/guidelines/asymptomatic-microhematuria.cfm.
26. De Ridder DJ, Everaert K, Fernández LG, et al: Intermittent catheterisation with hydrophilic-coated catheters (SpeediCath) reduces the risk of clinical urinary tract infection in spinal cord injured patients: a prospective randomised parallel comparative trial, *Eur Urol* 48:991–995, 2005.
28. Dewire DM, Owens RS, Anderson GA, et al: A comparison of the urological complications associated with long-term management of quadriplegics with and without chronic indwelling urinary catheters, *J Urol* 147:1069–1071, discussion 1071–1072, 1992.
29. Dharnidharka VR, Kwon C, Stevens G: Serum cystatin C is superior to serum creatinine as a marker of kidney function: a meta-analysis, *Am J Kidney Dis* 40:221–226, 2002.
30. Dahl DM, McDougal WS, Wein AJ, et al: Use of intestinal segments in urinary diversion. In Wein AJ, Kavoussi LR, Novick AC, et al, editors: *Campbell-Walsh urology*, ed 10, Philadelphia, 2012, Elsevier.
32. Dmochowski RR, Miklos JR, Norton PA, et al; Duloxetine Urinary Incontinence Study Group: Duloxetine versus placebo for the treatment of North American women with stress urinary incontinence, *J Urol* 170:1259–1263, 2003.
33. Dowson C, Watkins J, Khan MS, et al: Repeated botulinum toxin type A injections for refractory overactive bladder: medium-term outcomes, safety profile, and discontinuation rates, *Eur Urol* 61(4):834–839, 2012.
34. Dubeau CE, Kraus SR, Griebling TL, et al: Effect of fesoterodine in vulnerable elderly subjects with urgency incontinence: a double-blind, placebo controlled trial, *J Urol* 191:395–404, 2014.
36. Feifer A, Corcos J: Contemporary role of suprapubic cystostomy in treatment of neuropathic bladder dysfunction in spinal cord injured patients, *Neurourol Urodyn* 27:475–479, 2008.
38. Finkbeiner AE: Is bethanechol chloride clinically effective in promoting bladder emptying? A literature review, *J Urol* 134:443–449, 1985.
39. Foster HE, Lake AG: Use of vanilloids in urologic disorders, *Prog Drug Res* 68:307–317, 2014.
40. Giannantoni A, Di Stasi SM, Stephen RL, et al: Intravesical resiniferatoxin versus botulinum-A toxin injections for neurogenic detrusor overactivity: a prospective randomized study, *J Urol* 172:240–243, 2004.
41. Ginsberg D, Gousse A, Keppenne V, et al: Phase 3 efficacy and tolerability study of onabotulinumtoxinA for urinary incontinence from neurogenic detrusor overactivity, *J Urol* 187:2131–2139, 2012.
43. Goetz LL, Cardenas DD, Kennelly M, et al: International Spinal Cord Injury Urinary Tract Infection Basic Data Set, *Spinal Cord* 51:700–704, 2013.
45. Iwatsubo E, Komine S, Yamashita H, et al: Over-distension therapy of the bladder in paraplegic patients using self-catheterisation: a preliminary study, *Paraplegia* 22:210–215, 1984.
47. Kim JH, Rivas DA, Shenot PJ, et al: Intravesical resiniferatoxin for refractory detrusor hyperreflexia: a multicenter, blinded, randomized, placebo-controlled trial, *J Spinal Cord Med* 26:358–363, 2003.
48. Kim YH, Bird ET, Priebe M, Boone TB: The role of oxybutynin in spinal cord injured patients with indwelling catheters, *J Urol* 158:2083–2086, 1997.
50. Klausner AP, Steers WD: Antimuscarinics for the treatment of overactive bladder: a review of central nervous system effects, *Curr Urol Rep* 8:441–447, 2007.
51. Klausner AP, Steers WD: The neurogenic bladder: an update with management strategies for primary care physicians, *Med Clin North Am* 95:111–120, 2011.
52. Krasmik D, Krebs J, van Ophoven A, Pannek J: Urodynamic results, clinical efficacy, and complication rates of sacral intradural deafferentation and sacral anterior root stimulation in patients with neurogenic lower urinary tract dysfunction resulting from complete spinal cord injury, *Neurourol Urodyn* 33:1202–1206, 2014.
53. Krebs J, Pannek J: Effects of solifenacin in patients with neurogenic detrusor overactivity as a result of spinal cord lesion, *Spinal Cord* 51:306–309, 2013.
54. Lai HH, Hsu EI, Teh BS, et al: 13 years of experience with artificial urinary sphincter implantation at Baylor College of Medicine, *J Urol* 177(3):1021–1025, 2007.
55. Lapides J, Diokno AC, Silber SJ, Lowe BS: Clean, intermittent self-catheterization in the treatment of urinary tract disease, *J Urol* 107:458–461, 1972.
57. Levey AS, Fan L, Eckfeldt JH, Inker LA: Cystatin C for glomerular filtration rate estimation: coming of age, *Clin Chem* 60:916–919, 2014.
58. Madersbacher H, Jilg G: Control of detrusor hyperreflexia by the intravesical instillation of oxybutynine hydrochloride, *Paraplegia* 29:84–90, 1991.
59. Mamas MA, Reynard JM, Brading AF: Nitric oxide and the lower urinary tract: current concepts, future prospects, *Urology* 61:1079–1085, 2003.
61. McConnell JD, Roehrborn CG, Bautista OM, et al; Medical Therapy of Prostatic Symptoms (MTOPS) Research Group: The long-term effect of doxazosin, finasteride, and combination therapy on the clinical progression of benign prostatic hyperplasia, *N Engl J Med* 349:2387–2398, 2003.
64. McVary KT, Roehrborn CG, Avins AL, et al: *American Urological Association guideline: management of benign prostatic hyperplasia (BPH)*, Linthicum, 2014, American Urological Association. Available at: www.auanet.org/education/guidelines/benign-prostatic-hyperplasia.cfm.
66. National Institute on Disability and Rehabilitation Research Consensus Statement: The prevention and management of urinary tract infection among people with spinal cord injuries, *J Am Paraplegia Soc* 15:194–204, 1992.
67. Newman DK, Willson MM: Review of intermittent catheterization and current best practices, *Urol Nurs* 31:12–28, 48; quiz 29, 2011.
68. Nitti VW, Dmochowski R, Herschorn S, et al; EMBARK Study Group: Onabotulinumtoxin A for the treatment of patients with overactive bladder and urinary incontinence: results of a phase 3, randomized, placebo controlled trial, *J Urol* 189:2186–2193, 2013.
69. Oh-oka H: Usefulness of naftopidil for dysuria in benign prostatic hyperplasia and its optimal dose—comparison between 75 and 50 mg, *Urol Int* 82:136–142, 2009.
71. Pannek J: Transitional cell carcinoma in patients with spinal cord injury: a high risk malignancy? *Urology* 59(2):240–244, 2002.
72. Pannek J, Göcking K, Bersch U: Clinical usefulness of the Memokath stent as a second-line procedure after sphincterotomy failure, *J Endourol* 25(2):335–339, 2011.
74. Perrotta C, Aznar M, Mejia R, et al: Oestrogens for preventing recurrent urinary tract infection in postmenopausal women, *Cochrane Database Syst Rev* (2):CD005131, 2008.
75. Reynard JM, Vass J, Sullivan ME, Mamas M: Sphincterotomy and the treatment of detrusor-sphincter dyssynergia: current status, future prospects, *Spinal Cord* 41:1–11, 2003.
76. Sidi AA, Becher EF, Reddy PK, Dykstra DD: Augmentation enterocystoplasty for the management of voiding dysfunction in spinal cord injury patients, *J Urol* 143:83–85, 1990.
77. Steers WD: Physiology and pharmacology of the bladder and urethra. In Walsh PC, Retch AB, Vaughan ED, Jr, et al, editors: *Campbell's urology*, ed 7, Philadelphia, 1998, WB Saunders.
78. Steers WD, Meythaler JM, Haworth C, et al: Effects of acute bolus and chronic continuous intrathecal baclofen on genitourinary dysfunction due to spinal cord pathology, *J Urol* 148:1849–1855, 1992.

79. Stensballe J, Looms D, Nielsen PN, Tvede M: Hydrophilic-coated catheters for intermittent catheterisation reduce urethral micro trauma: a prospective, randomised, participant-blinded, crossover study of three different types of catheters, *Eur Urol* 48:978–983, 2005.
80. Strasser H, Marksteiner R, Margreiter E, et al: Transurethral ultrasonography-guided injection of adult autologous stem cells versus transurethral endoscopic injection of collagen in treatment of urinary incontinence, *World J Urol* 25:385–392, 2007.
81. Subramonian K, Cartwright RA, Harnden P, Harrison SCW: Bladder cancer in patients with spinal cord injuries, *BJU Int* 93:739–743, 2004.
84. Tincello DG, Kenyon S, Abrams KR, et al: Botulinum toxin A versus placebo for refractory detrusor overactivity in women: a randomised blinded placebo-controlled trial of 240 women (the RELAX study), *Eur Urol* 62:507–514, 2012.
85. Van Koeveringe GA, Vahabi B, Andersson KE, et al: Detrusor underactivity: a plea for new approaches to a common bladder dysfunction, *Neurourol Urodyn* 30:723–728, 2011.
86. Webb RJ, Griffiths CJ, Ramsden PD, Neal DE: Ambulatory monitoring of bladder pressure in low compliance neurogenic bladder dysfunction, *J Urol* 148:1477–1481, 1992.
87. Wyndaele JJ, Schneider T, MacDiarmid S, et al: Flexible dosing with fesoterodine 4 and 8 mg: a systematic review of data from clinical trials, *Int J Clin Pract* 68:830–840, 2014.
88. Yang CC, Mayo ME: External urethral sphincterotomy: long-term follow-up, *Neurourol Urodyn* 14:25–31, 1995.

The full reference list for this chapter is available online.

CHAPTER 21

NEUROGENIC BOWEL: DYSFUNCTION AND REHABILITATION

Gianna Rodriguez, Steven A. Stiens

Gastrointestinal dysfunction is most often characterized by a conglomeration of symptoms that indicate lower gastrointestinal impairment, including constipation, diarrhea, and fecal incontinence. It can also present as upper gastrointestinal impairment heralded by bloating, nausea, early satiety, burning, and gaseousness. Neurogenic bowel dysfunction can be a clinically elusive condition. It is often eclipsed by other, more noticeable associated motor deficits. Neurogenic bowel dysfunction itself can be particularly life-limiting, if it is not thoroughly assessed and treated with rehabilitation principles. Interdisciplinary rehabilitative interventions focus on establishing a total management plan for bowel function, termed a bowel program, and for assisted defecation, known as bowel care.[114] Sensation and mobility might be limited, affecting a person's ability to anticipate the need for and to physically perform independent bowel care and hygiene.

In spite of many abilities regained during the rehabilitation process, bowel care capabilities at the time of discharge are not always comparable to other skills that would be expected for a given level of function. Bowel continence is one of the greatest predictors of return to home for survivors of stroke.[36] In fact, bowel management has been found to be one of the areas of least competence among rehabilitated persons with spinal cord injury (SCI).[54] More than one third of surveyed persons with SCI rated bowel and bladder dysfunction as having the most significant effect on their lives after SCI. In a recent Swedish review of medical problems after SCI, 41% of patients rated bowel dysfunction as a moderately to severely life-limiting problem.[79]

Epidemiology

Gastrointestinal dysfunction is frequently seen in people with neurologic diseases who require rehabilitation. Besides the direct effects of neurologic disease on gut function, debility, insufficient fluid intake, and use of anticholinergics and other medications can play a huge role in the development of enteric problems. Digestive tract problems and neurogenic bowel problems in stroke, brain injury, multiple sclerosis, Parkinson disease, neuromuscular diseases, muscular dystrophy, dysautonomias, peripheral nerve injuries, SCI, myelomeningocele, and other neurologic disorders have been shown to be difficult and challenging to manage and can be a primary disabling and handicapping feature for patients.*

Neurogenic bowel dysfunction results from autonomic and somatic denervation, and produces fecal incontinence, constipation, and difficulty with evacuation (DWE). These symptoms are common. The prevalence of fecal incontinence and fecal impaction ranges from 0.3% to 5.0% in the general population. The prevalence of DWE ranges from 10% to 50% among the hospitalized or institutionalized older adult population.[121] Although many gastrointestinal disorders can contribute to fecal incontinence or DWE, disorders that impair the extrinsic (sympathetic, parasympathetic, or somatic) nervous control of the bowel and anorectal mechanisms are more common among the patient populations seen by physiatrists.

Impact

Living with nausea, vomiting, bloating, abdominal pain, constipation, diarrhea, or fecal incontinence profoundly affects the quality of life. It significantly affects nutrition, overall health, and sense of well-being. Loss of voluntary control over bowel function alters every facet of a person's life at home, at work, and in the community. The ability to spontaneously regulate and direct bowel function is essential for participation in everyday activities at home, work, or school. It plays a major role in one's ability to create and maintain relationships. It has a significant impact on activities such as recreation or travel. Problems with constipation and fecal incontinence can create considerable psychological, social, and emotional trauma.

Fecal incontinence decreases the return-to-home rates for patients with stroke. Almost one third of persons with SCI report or exhibit worsening of bowel function 5 years beyond their injury, with 33% developing megacolon, suggesting inadequate long-term management.[55,117] Recent evidence has shown some improvement outcomes for SCI bowel management.[70] Nursing home costs are higher for patients with fecal incontinence.[121] When restoring normal defecation is not possible, social continence becomes the goal. Social continence is defined as predictable, scheduled, adequate defecations without incontinence at other times. It is often achievable by persons with neurogenic

*References 2, 21, 36, 67, 114, 127.

bowel dysfunction. Embarrassment and humiliation from fecal incontinence frequently result in vocational and social disability, and adds substantial costs to the care related to neurogenic bowel dysfunction.

Neuroanatomy and Physiology of the Gastrointestinal Tract

In the past two decades, there has been significant advancement in the science of neurogastroenterology. This includes new discoveries in the basic physiology of the gastrointestinal tract and interactions with the brain and spinal cord, autonomic and enteric nervous systems, and somatomotor system (pharyngeal muscles and swallowing, pelvic floor muscles and defecation, continence. and pelvic pain).

Normal functioning of the stomach and intestines entails coordination of muscle contraction, digestion and absorption of nutrients, and regulation of blood flow. The neural schema of the gastrointestinal tract is much more complex than previously thought. Neural control of the gastrointestinal tract is an extremely organized and integrated hierarchy of mechanisms that involve the central nervous system (CNS; brain and spinal cord), autonomic nervous system (sympathetic and parasympathetic), and the enteric nervous system (ENS) (Figures 21-1 and 21-2).[131,134]

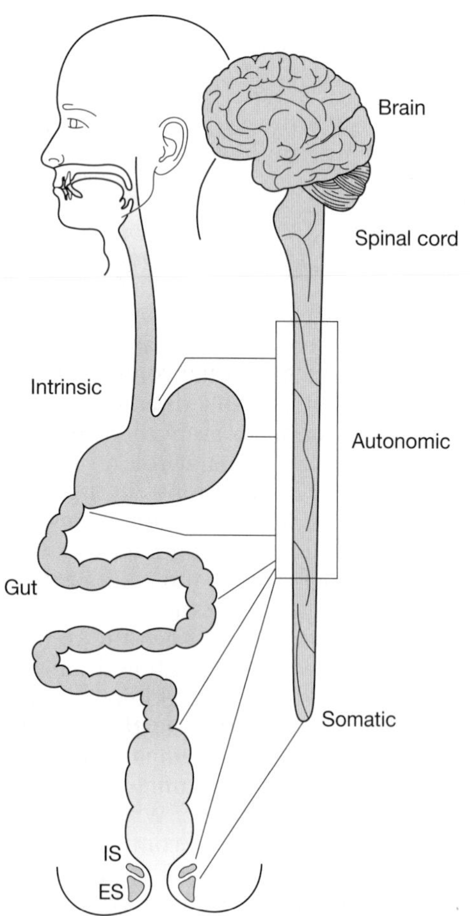

FIGURE 21-1 Gastrointestinal function is coordinated by three nervous systems: somatic, autonomic, and the enteric nervous system intrinsic to the gut wall. *ES*, External sphincter; *IS*, internal sphincter.

Enteric Nervous System

The ENS is a distinct system that has its own set of neurons that coordinate sensory and motor functions. In the ENS, the ganglia are interconnected, which allows for integration and processing of data (as opposed to autonomic ganglia, which only serve as relay centers for stimuli transmitted from the CNS). There are three different types of neurons in the ENS based on function: sensory neurons, interneurons, and motor neurons.[131,134] Sensory neurons perceive thermal, chemical, or mechanical stimuli and transform these sensations into action potentials that are conducted to the nervous system. Interneurons serve as conduits between the sensory and motor neurons. The numerous synapses between interneurons create a highly organized circuitry that processes sensory input from the gut and other parts of the nervous system and integrates and generates reflex responses to these stimuli. Motor neurons are the final common pathway. They receive and translate signals to the gut (mucosa, muscle, vasculature) that affect digestive, interdigestive, and emetic functions based on the transmitters released.[131,134]

Automatic feedback control is present in the ENS, with the neurons being in close proximity to the stomach and intestines. This can be manifested as reflex circuits that systematize reflex responses to sensory signals, integrative circuits that coordinate motor patterns (migrating motor complex, digestive activity, giant migratory contractions [GMCs]),[131,134] or as a pattern-generating activity that is generated when a "command neuron" is actuated and a rhythmic, repetitive behavior occurs.[134]

The ENS is the key to proper functioning of the entire gastrointestinal tract. This collection of highly organized neurons is situated in two primary layers: the submucosal (Meissner) plexus and the intramuscular myenteric (Auerbach) plexus. These plexuses have an estimated 10 to 100 million neurons, plus two to three glial cells per neuron. The ENS glial cells resemble CNS astrocytes, and are much less abundant than the 20 to 50 glial cells per neuron in the CNS.[50] The coordination of segment-to-segment function is largely regulated by the ENS.[129] The ENS also has its own blood-nerve barrier, similar to the blood-brain barrier of the CNS.[25]

Enteric Nervous System Relationship to the Spinal Cord and Brain

Sensory information from vagal afferents in the ENS is relayed to the nodose ganglia (caudal ganglion of the vagus) and consequently to the nucleus tractus solitarius (NTS) and area postrema in the medullary area of the brainstem. The NTS and the area postrema send signals to the rostral centers in the brain.[131,134] The brain processes the data and projects descending connections to the dorsal vagal complex. The brain also participates in vagovagal reflex circuits that continuously monitor and promptly modify responses to changes in the chemical, thermal, and mechanical environment in the whole gut (mostly in the

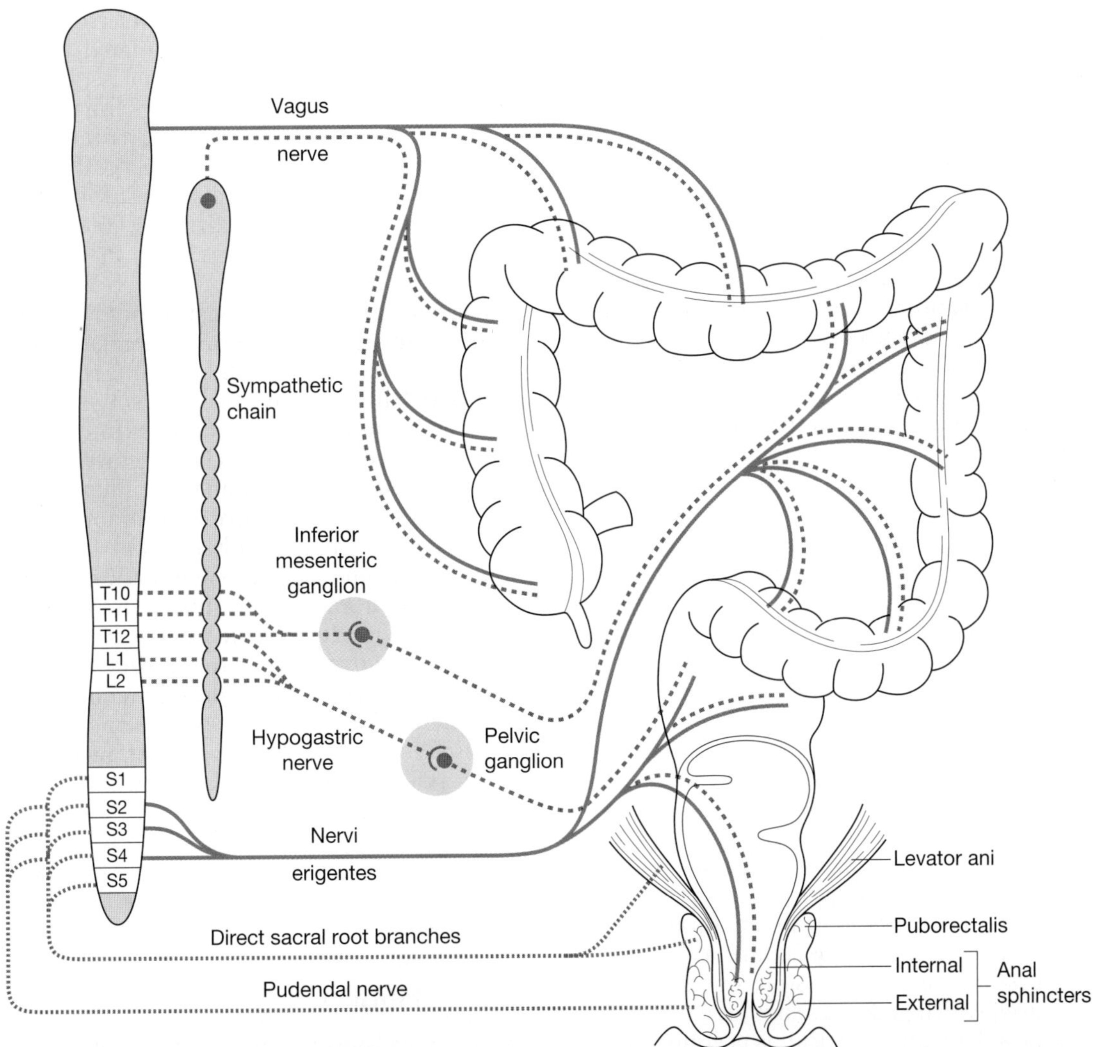

FIGURE 21-2 Neurologic levels and pathways for the sympathetic, parasympathetic, and somatic nervous system innervation of the colon and anorectum. Not shown is the enteric nervous system, which travels along the bowel wall from the esophagus to the internal anal sphincter and forms the final common pathway to control the bowel wall smooth muscle.

esophagus, stomach, duodenum, gall bladder, and pancreas). Sensory stimulation through this vagal circuit does not appear to reach the level of consciousness.[131,134]

Besides making connections with the NTS and the area postrema in the brainstem, vagal afferents synapse with the dorsal motor nucleus of the vagus (DVN) and the nucleus ambiguus, creating the dorsal vagal complex. The incoming sensory information is integrated and shared with the forebrain and brainstem by the dorsal vagal complex. Brain coordination and influences (conscious and nonconscious) are translated to the dorsal vagal complex, where the DVN and nucleus ambiguus represent the efferent arm of the reflex pathway. It is the final common pathway from the brain responsible for precise control of muscle, glandular, and circulatory responses of the gastrointestinal tract.[131,132,134] Multiple neurotransmitters are involved in the intricate conduction of impulses between the neuronal circuits in the dorsal vagal complex. Approximately 30 are identified and consist of acetylcholine, biogenic amines, amino acids, nitric oxide, and peptides.[131,134]

Spinal afferents (splanchnic and pelvic) send sensory impulses to the dorsal root ganglia (or prevertebral sympathetic ganglia), which are then conducted to the dorsal horn (laminae I, II, V, and X) of the spinal cord and the dorsal column nuclei.[51,93] The dorsal column is thought to play a greater role in nociceptive transmission of messages from the gut than the spinothalamic or spinoreticular tracts. The conscious perception of pain in the digestive tract is largely mediated through spinal afferents. The spinal cord modulates the conduction of neural messages (both nociceptive and nonnociceptive) to the higher brain.[51] Other somatic and visceral sensory stimuli from the vagina, uterus, bladder, colon, and rectum are also conveyed through the dorsal horn and dorsal column in the spinal cord. Likewise, somatic afferents supply sensory input from the muscles of the pelvic floor through the pudendal nerve to the sacral region of the spinal cord.[11,51,93,94]

Brain centers modulate the nociceptive impulses from the bowel that are relayed to the dorsal horn of the spinal cord. These descending pathways are facilitative or inhibitory or both, based on the visceral stimulus, and can alter the perception of pain in the digestive tract.[51,105] The neurotransmitters serotonin, noradrenalin, and dopamine are released by these descending pathways as they synapse with the spinal cord.[134]

The secondary somatosensory cortex and, to a lesser extent, the paralimbic and limbic areas (anterior insular, anterior and posterior cingulate, prefrontal and orbitofrontal cortices) mediate emotional, volitional, and psychological responses to sensory input from the gut. These are manifested by abdominal pain, anorexia, nausea, vomiting, hyperphagia, constipation, or diarrhea.[51,78,111] The somatosensory cortex regulates the awareness and recognition of pain, and the paralimbic and limbic areas contribute to the cognitive and affective aspects of pain.[51,111,134]

Data from the brain and descending vagal pathways are conducted to the spinal cord, and then with the preganglionic neurons in the thoracolumbar area (modulates the sympathetic response) and the sacral area (modulates the parasympathetic response). Sympathetic or parasympathetic output is translated to the neurons in the ENS circuitry, which can be excitatory or inhibitory to motor neurons, gastric or digestive glands, and secretory mechanisms.[51,134]

Gastrointestinal Neuromotor System

The muscles of the gastrointestinal tract carry out essential functions throughout the gut, including propulsion, grinding, mixing, absorption, storage, and disposal. The gut wall is composed of "self-excitable" smooth muscles that contract in an all-in-one manner. It spontaneously responds to stretch and can be independent of neural or endocrine control. The interstitial cells of Cajal act like a pacemaker and allow propagation of electrical slow waves into the circular muscle layer, which generates spontaneous muscle contraction. It acts like an electrical syncytium where action potentials are conducted in three dimensions from one smooth muscle fiber to another through gap junctions.[51,134]

The gastrointestinal tract muscles respond to influences of the vagal efferents and the ENS microcircuitry based on excitatory or inhibitory innervation of motor neurons. Contraction is mediated by the release of excitatory neurotransmitters by vagal afferents at the neuromuscular junctions, acetylcholine (at the muscarinic receptor), and substance P (at the neurokinin-1 receptor).[32,51,87,134] Conversely, the release of nitric oxide, adenosine triphosphate, and vasoactive intestinal peptide from the inhibitory motor neurons (which express the serotonergic 5-HT_1 receptor) impedes contractile activity and facilitates relaxation. The aboral direction of propulsive activity throughout the digestive tract is achieved by segmental inactivation of inhibitory motor neurons distally.[16,17,51,62,134] Contraction can only occur in the segments where the inhibitory motor neurons are inactivated. With passing of the food bolus or stool, the esophageal and internal anal sphincters (IASs) (smooth muscle sphincters), and inhibitory motor neurons are usually shut off and are inactivated. During vomiting, however, the inhibitory motor neurons are deactivated and propulsive forces work in the opposite direction.[51,134]

The sympathetic and parasympathetic nervous systems seem to modulate the ENS, rather than directly controlling the smooth muscles of the bowel.[129] The smooth muscles of the bowel also have their own electromechanical automaticity, which is directly modulated by the inhibitory control of the ENS.[25,50] Sympathetic nervous system stimulation tends to promote the storage function by enhancing anal tone and inhibiting colonic contractions, although little clinical deficit occurs from bilateral sympathectomy.[39] Parasympathetic activity enhances colonic motility, and its loss is often associated with DWE, including impactions and functional obstructions, such as Ogilvie pseudoobstructive syndrome.[39]

The ENS and sympathetic postganglionic neurons transmit excitatory or inhibitory messages to secretomotor neurons. These secretomotor neurons release acetylcholine and vasoactive intestinal polypeptide when there is excitatory activation from paracrine stimulation by mucosal and submucosal cells such as enterochromaffin cells, mast cells, and other immune and inflammatory cells. Acetylcholine and vasoactive intestinal polypeptide are released at the neuroepithelial and neurovascular junctions. This promotes secretion into the gut of water, sodium chloride, bicarbonate, and mucus drawn from the intestinal glands. In addition, dilatation and increase in blood flow occurs with release of nitric oxide from vascular endothelium.[7,13,51] Inhibitory influence reduces neuronal firing from secretomotor neurons by hyperpolarization of membranes. Sympathetic release of norepinephrine from nerve endings of the alpha$_2$-noradrenergic receptors inhibits secretomotor actuation, preventing the release of excitatory neurotransmitters. As a result, there is a decrease in secretion of water and electrolytes into the lumen and a congruent shunting of blood from the splanchnic to systemic circulation.[51,82,96]

Gastric Motility

Based on its motility pattern the stomach is divided into an upper and lower portion. The upper portion (fundus) has sustained, low-frequency contractions and has a tonic pattern. The lower portion (antrum) has intermittent, powerful contractions and has a phasic pattern. The fundus acts as a reservoir and accommodates incoming food, which inhibits contraction and allows the stomach to stretch without significant increase in pressure. The antrum is a mixer that generates propulsive waves that accelerate as food is propagated towards the pylorus. The amount and consistency of food in the fundus regulates excitatory and inhibitory influence and adjustments to volume and pressure.[51,71]

Intestinal Motility

The ENS is designed to control the various patterns of motility in the intestinal tract. The interdigestive migrating motor complex pattern occurs during fasting in the stomach and the small intestine.[51,128] It seems to be influenced by the hormone motilin, and is responsible for removal of waste from the intestinal lumen throughout the fasting period.[51,83] When a meal is ingested, the postprandial segmentation ("mixing") pattern of motility commences as digestion transpires. The brainstem sends signals that are transmitted to vagal efferents, which convert migrating motor complex motility to segmentation motility with the increase in bulk and nutrients, especially lipids (medium-chain triglycerides). This subsequently becomes peristaltic motility, which is propagated through brief segments of the intestine at a time.[37,51] Peristaltic activity gradually develops into powerful contractions sustained through long portions of circular muscle along the small and large bowel. These "GMCs" propel waste through the lumen, particularly in the large intestine.[51,65,107]

Motility of the Anus, Rectum, and Pelvic Floor

Normal defecation and maintenance of fecal continence entail a highly coordinated mechanism that involves the levator ani, puborectalis, and the external anal sphincter (EAS) and IAS muscles. The pelvic floor is composed of the levator ani, the underlying sheets of which form a sling. The levator ani, puborectalis, and EAS are skeletal muscles that constantly maintain tone and sustain pelvic organs in place against the forces of gravity.[40,51] Simultaneous contraction of these muscles prevent the involuntary loss of stool and help maintain the regular pattern of defecation.[46,51]

Physiology of Normal Defecation

The colon is a reservoir for food waste until it is convenient for elimination. It also acts as a storage device as long as the colonic pressure is less than that of the anal sphincter mechanism. Fecal elimination occurs when colonic pressure exceeds that of the anal sphincter mechanism. Another function of the colon is to reabsorb fluids (up to 30 L/day can be reabsorbed from the large and small bowel walls with typically only 100 mL of water loss in feces). The colon also reabsorbs gases (90% of the 7 to 10 mL of gases produced by intracolonic fermentation is absorbed rather than expelled). The colon also provides an environment for the growth of bacteria needed to assist in digestion, and also serves to absorb certain bacterial breakdown products.[53] The layers of the colon wall are depicted in Figure 21-3.

The rectum is usually empty until just before defecation. Perception of rectal contents and pressures[112] is essential for signaling voluntary contraction of the anal sphincter. Normal defecation begins with reflexes triggered by rectosigmoid distention produced by approximately 200 mL of feces (Figure 21-4).[99] A rectorectal reflex occurs in which the bowel proximal to the distending bolus contracts and the bowel wall distally relaxes, serving to propel the bolus further caudad. Reflex relaxation of the internal sphincter and stretching of the puborectalis muscle also occurs, which is enhanced by, but does not require, an extrinsic nerve supply. This relaxation, called the rectoanal inhibitory reflex, correlates with the urge labeled "the call to stool."[129] One can then volitionally contract the levator ani to open the proximal anal canal and relax the external sphincter and puborectalis muscles. This allows a straighter, shorter, and more open anorectal passage (see Figure 21-4), which permits the bolus to pass. Increasing the intraabdominal pressure by squatting and by the Valsalva maneuver assists bolus elimination. For 90% of normal individuals only the contents of the rectum are expulsed, whereas 10% will clear the entire contents of the left colon from the splenic flexure distally.[39]

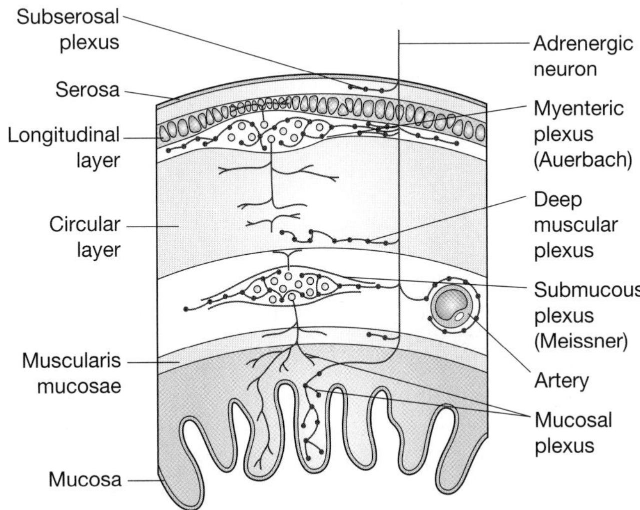

FIGURE 21-3 A transverse section of the gut, showing the enteric plexus and the distribution of adrenergic neurons. Note the ganglionic plexuses of Auerbach and Meissner. The deep muscular plexus contains a few ganglia, the subserosal contains an occasional ganglion, and the mucosal plexus shows none. The adrenergic fibers are all extrinsic and arise from the prevertebral sympathetic ganglia. The adrenergic fibers are distributed largely to the mesenteric, submucous, and mucosal plexuses and to blood vessels. (From Goyal RK, Crist JR: Neurology of the gut. In Sleisenger MH, Fordtram JS, editors: *Gastrointestinal disease*, Philadelphia, 1989, WB Saunders, pp 21-52, with permission.)

One can elect to defer defecation, however, by volitionally contracting the puborectalis muscle and EAS. The reflexive IAS relaxation subsequently fades, usually within 15 seconds, and the urge resolves until the IAS relaxation is triggered again. The rectal wall accommodates to the bolus by decreasing its wall tension with time, resulting in less sensory input and less reflex triggering from that particular accommodated bolus. This continence and reflex process is somewhat analogous to the function of the striated external urethral sphincter in volitional control of urinary voiding (see Chapter 20).

The external sphincter generally tenses in response to small rectal distentions via a spinal reflex, although reflexive relaxation of the external sphincter occurs in the presence of greater distentions.[112] These spinal cord reflexes are centered in the conus medullaris and are augmented and modulated by higher cortical influences. When cortical control is disrupted, as by SCI, the external sphincter reflexes usually persist and allow spontaneous defection. During sleep the colonic activity, anal tone, and protective responses to abdominal pressure elevations are all decreased, whereas rectal tone is increased.[25,129]

The "gastrocolonic response" or "gastrocolic reflex" refers to the increased colonic activity (GMCs and mass movements) in the first 30 to 60 minutes after a meal. This increased colonic activity appears to be modulated both by hormonal effects, from release of peptides from the upper gastrointestinal tract (gastrin, motilin, cholecystokinin) that increase contractility of colonic smooth musculature, and by a reduction in the threshold for spinal cord–mediated vesicovesical reflexes.[25] Upper gastrointestinal receptor stimulation also results in increased activity in the colon, possibly because of reflexively increased parasympathetic efferent activity to the colon. The possibility of a purely ENS-mediated activation exists, although the small bowel and colon motor activities do not seem to be

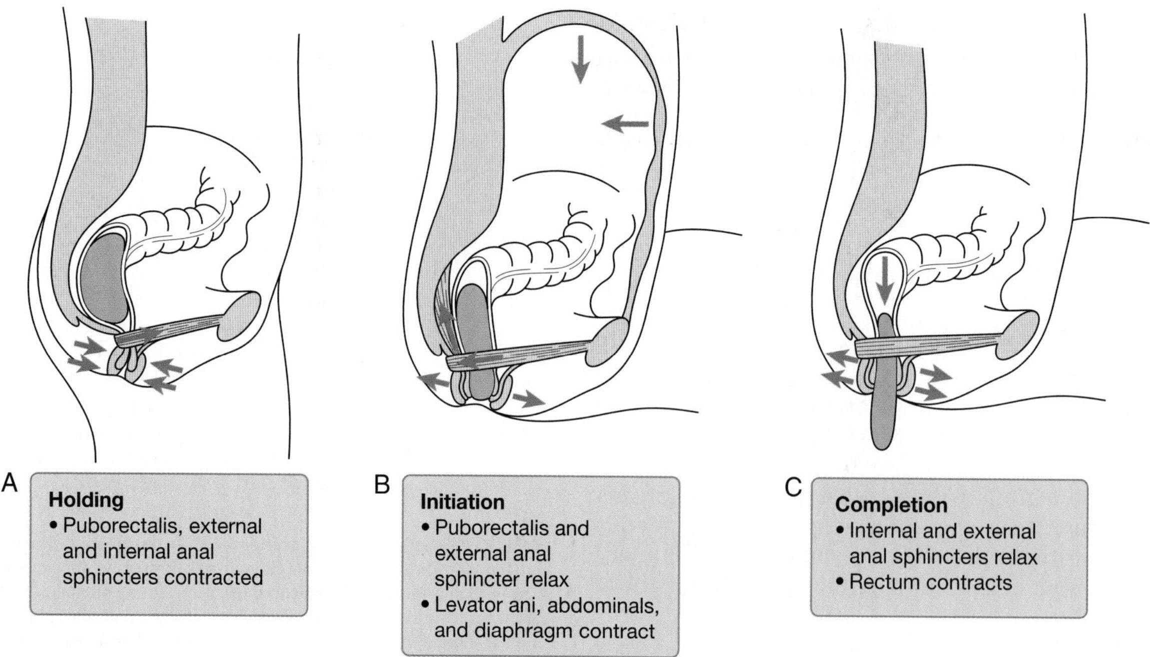

FIGURE 21-4 **A,** Defecation is prevented by a statically increased tone of the internal anal sphincter (IAS) and puborectalis, as well as by the mechanical effects of the acute anorectal angle. Dynamic responses of the external anal sphincter (EAS) and puborectalis to rectal distention reflexes or increased intraabdominal pressures further impede defecation. **B,** To initiate defecation, the puborectalis muscle and EAS relax while intraabdominal pressure is increased by the Valsalva maneuver, which is facilitated by squatting. The levator ani helps reduce the acute anorectal angle to open the distal anal canal to receive the stool bolus. **C,** Intrarectal reflexes result in continued IAS relaxation and rectal propulsive contractions, which help expel the bolus through the open canal. (From Schiller LR: Fecal incontinence. In Sleisenger MH, Fordtran JS, editors: *Gastrointestinal disease*, Philadelphia, 1993, WB Saunders, pp 934-953.)

synchronized. In persons with SCI, the measured increase in colonic activity after a meal is blunted as compared with that in normal individuals.[25] The gastrocolonic response is often used therapeutically, even in patients with SCI, to enhance bowel evacuation during this 30- to 60-minute postprandial time frame.[1] Occasionally certain foods can serve as trigger foods that are especially likely to induce bowel evacuation shortly after consumption.

The resting anal canal pressure is largely determined by the angulation and pressure at the anorectal junction by the puborectalis sling and smooth muscle internal sphincter tone. Continence is maintained by the anal sphincter mechanism,[86,114] which consists of the IAS, EAS, and the puborectalis muscle.[86] Only approximately 20% of the anal canal pressure is attributable to the static contraction of the somatically innervated striated EAS.[10] The EAS and puborectalis muscle are the only striated skeletal muscles whose normal resting state is tonic contraction. These muscles consist mainly of slow-twitch fatigue-resistant type I fibers (unlike the situation in nonupright animals such as the cat or dog, in which it consists of predominately type II fibers).[10] Anal pressure can be increased volitionally by contracting the EAS and puborectalis muscles. Maximum volitional squeeze pressures, however, are not as high as can be generated reflexively against Valsalva pressure. The EAS is physically larger than the internal sphincter, and its contraction is under both reflex and volitional control. The volitional control is learned during the course of normal maturation. Normal baseline reflex action of the anorectal mechanism allows spontaneous stool elimination.[109] The EAS is innervated by the S2 to S4 nerve roots via the pudendal nerve. The puborectalis muscle is innervated by direct branches from the S1 to S5 roots (see Figure 21-1).[97] The remarkable degree of learned EAS coordination allows the selective discrete passage of gas while juggling a variable mixture of solids, liquids, and gases.

Pathophysiology of Gastrointestinal Dysfunction

A whole range of neurologic diseases affecting central, peripheral, and intrinsic enteric nervous innervation have been demonstrated to result in disorders in various segments of the bowel. These are predominantly characterized by disturbances in gastroesophageal, small or large intestinal motility, and sensation. Symptoms of dysphagia, vomiting, bloating, abdominal discomfort and pain, constipation, and incontinence have been described in individuals with neurologic ailments.[5,19,20,98]

Exact and detailed pathophysiologic mechanisms of gastrointestinal dysfunction in the various neurologic diseases are not very well understood. Recent studies, however, have been able to identify various mechanisms of symptom production that might facilitate therapeutic strategies.

Nausea, Vomiting, Bloating, and Early Satiety

The syndrome of nausea, vomiting, bloating, and early satiety in the setting of neurologic conditions without mechanical obstruction can herald motility problems in the gastrointestinal tract. Neurologic dysfunction that affects the inhibitory motor neurons in the ENS at any level of the neural axis from the brain, spinal cord, and afferent and efferent nerves can lead to spasticity of the gastric or intestinal/colonic musculature. When inhibitory motor neurons are inactivated or destroyed by disease there is a continuous, nonsystematic contraction of the circular muscles incapable of forward propulsion, causing functional obstruction.[131,133] This can be manifested as dysphagia, gastroparesis, or chronic intestinal/colonic pseudoobstruction, which might be associated with anorexia, abdominal pain, diarrhea, and constipation. Inhibitory motor neurons can be affected by autonomic neuropathy, dysfunction of neurons in the myenteric plexus, or from degeneration of smooth muscle.*

Abdominal Pain and Discomfort

Abdominal pain and discomfort arise from gastrointestinal tract distention and powerful contractions. High threshold and silent mechanoreceptors sense severe distention and intense contractions when there is ischemia, injury, inflammation, or obstruction. Mechanical and chemical irritants stimulate mechanoreceptors in the ENS and translate signals to the brain and spinal cord from muscle stretching and contractions.[94,133]

- The presence and persistence of ischemia, injury, and inflammation can elicit abdominal pain from the following mechanisms:
- The spinal afferent nerves express receptors for inflammatory mediators. Release of bradykinin, adenosine triphosphate, adenosine, prostaglandins, leukotrienes, histamine, and mast cell proteases heighten sensitivity of the spinal sensory endings.[133]
- Amplified levels of 5-HT_3 released from hyperactive 5-HT_3 receptors at the vagal and spinal nerve endings facilitate production of pain. By contrast, there can be excessive induction of serotonergic receptors by 5-HT_3 resulting from a defective serotonin transporter.[60,74,133]
- Central sensitization occurs in the spinal cord from constant stimulation of the C fibers in the dorsal horn and dorsal column nuclei. Neurons become hypersensitive and are persistently activated. The "wind-up" phenomenon develops with the actuation of *N*-methyl-D-aspartate receptors from the release of glutamate from C fibers. The reactive state of dorsal horn and dorsal column neurons becomes a memory imprint in the spinal cord.[3,4,133]
- Mechanoreceptors in the gut wall can receive a deluge of signals from mechanical irritation. This barrage of impulses conducted to the brain can be inferred as nociceptive because of the overwhelming stimulation.[133,134]
- The descending facilitative modulation of the brain through the dorsal horn can promote recognition of ordinary sensory input as innocuous. The brain misreads normal nonconscious signals relayed from mechanoreptors as noxious.[105,133]

Diarrhea

Neurologic dysfunction can present with frequent passage of watery stools. Diarrhea occurs when there is overstimulation of secretomotor neurons by histamine from inflammatory and immune-mediated cells in the mucosa and submucosa, and/or vasoactive intestinal peptide and serotonin from mucosal enterochromaffin cells. Moreover, these substances influence presynaptic inhibitory receptors to block the release of norepinephrine from the postganglionic sympathetic fibers that inhibit secretomotor neurons.[132,133]

Defecation Dysfunction

Constipation

Constipation can be an enigma in neurologic states. Infrequent, incomplete, emptying of hard stools is a result of a decrease in secretion of water and electrolytes into the lumen attributable to reduced excitation of the secretomotor neurons in the ENS. Norepinephrine released by sympathetic stimulation inhibits the firing of secretomotor neurons by hyperpolarization. Release of excitatory neurotransmitters is reduced in the secretory epithelium, decreasing the secretion of water and electrolytes.[133,134] Lack of rectal sensation and decreased urge to defecate can be strongly associated with constipation in various conditions that present with lesions in the brain, spinal cord, sacral nerves, and hypogastric and pudendal nerves. Outlet obstruction can ensue because of delayed colonic transit times and lack of perineal and rectoanal sensation.[133]

Fecal Incontinence

True fecal incontinence described as unconscious loss of stool often occurs in neurologic conditions with lesions affecting the lumbar spinal cord, cauda equina, S2 to S4 nerves, pudendal nerve, and pelvic floor nerves. Denervation leads to impaired perineal and rectoanal sensation, aberrant contraction, loss of tone, and weakening of the pelvic floor muscles and the EAS. This underlies unexpected loss of stool and abnormal defecation, and diminished support for pelvic structures.[29,51] Parasympathetic augmentation can occur and might further complicate matters, because it contributes to weakness in the internal sphincter and increases the risk for incontinence. It is always important to rule out overflow incontinence resulting from constipation.

Upper Motor Neurogenic Bowel

Any destructive CNS process above the conus, from SCI to dementia, can lead to the upper motor neurogenic bowel (UMNB) pattern of dysfunction. Spinal cortical sensory pathway deficits lead to a decreased ability to sense the urge to defecate. Most persons with SCI, however, sense a vague discomfort when excessive rectal or colonic distention occurs. It has been reported that 43% have chronic complaints of vague abdominal distention discomfort that eases with bowel evacuation.[84,117] These sensations might be mediated by autonomic nervous system afferent fibers bypassing the zone of SCI via the paraspinal sympathetic chain, or by means of vagal parasympathetic afferents.

Colonic compliance and sphincter tone[109] have been experimentally evaluated in patients with SCI. Studies of

*References 8, 33, 58, 59, 113, 124, 133.

colonic compliance in response to a continuous infusion of saline initially suggested rapid pressure rises and a hyperreflexic response.[92,125] More recent studies have demonstrated normal colonic compliance in patients with SCI who have UMNB.[85,95] Passive filling of the rectum leads to increases in the resting sphincter tone.[120] These increases are associated with increased external sphincter pressure development resulting from sacral reflexes that can be abolished by pudendal block.[10] This form of rectal sphincter dyssynergia has unfortunately been labeled decreased colonic compliance, even though intermittent or slow filling in the rectum appears to be associated with normal bolus accommodation and pressure relaxation.[85] This contrasts with the true decreased compliance found in ischemic or postinflammatory rectal bowel wall resulting from fibrosis, which cannot accommodate and relax regardless of flow rates.

Colonic motility and stool propulsion are known to be affected by SCI. De Looze, et al.[36] used a questionnaire method to study patients with SCI levels above L2 and found that 58% of patients with chronic SCI had constipation (defined as two or less bowel movements per week or the requirement for digital evacuation). Only 30% (P = 0.002) of patients with paraplegia below T10 and above L2, however, were prone to constipation. Actual stool propulsion was studied later by Krogh et al.[76] using swallowed markers and serial radiographs. In patients with chronic SCI with supraconal lesions, transit times were significantly prolonged in the ascending, transverse, and descending colon and rectosigmoid. Total gastrointestinal transit time averaged 3.93 days (control group, 1.76 days) for chronic complete SCI above the conus. In an attempt to demonstrate a difference that may have been conferred by sympathetic innervation, mean total gastrointestinal transit times were compared for patients with lesions above T9 (2.92 ± 2.41 days), and from T10 down to L2 (2.84 ± 1.93 days). No statistically significant differences could be found even with comparison of transit times for individual colonic segments.

Patients with SCI who had complete upper motor neuron bowel lesions were studied during the acute phase (5 to 21 days) after SCI. These same patients were reevaluated 6 to 14 months later. Total gastrointestinal transit time was longer during the acute rather than the chronic phase. The upper motor neuron neurogenic colon tended to have slower transit throughout the colon with less severe rectosigmoid dysfunction.[76] Patients with UMNB have spared reflex arc control of the rectosigmoid and pelvic floor. Internal sphincter relaxation upon rectal distention occurs in persons with SCI as well as in neurologically intact persons. Sufficient rectal distention might cause the external sphincter to completely relax, resulting in expulsion of the fecal bolus. Rectal sphincter dyssynergia does not necessarily correlate with bladder sphincter dyssynergia, but it often results in DWE.[97] The protective vesicorectal reflex, in which the external sphincter pressure increases in response to increased intraabdominal pressure, is usually intact (Table 21-1).[10] Patients with UMNB also have normal or increased anal sphincter tone, intact anocutaneous (or anal wink) and bulbocavernosus reflexes,[114] a palpable puborectalis muscle sling, and normal anal verge appearance (Figure 21-5).

Lower Motor Neurogenic Bowel

Polyneuropathy, conus medullaris or cauda equina lesions, pelvic surgery, vaginal delivery, or even chronic straining during defecation can impair the somatic innervation of the anal sphincter mechanism. Persons with benign joint hypermobility syndrome might be more predisposed to these lesions.[88] These conditions can also produce sympathetic and parasympathetic innervation deficits. If an isolated pudendal insult has occurred, colonic transit times are normal and fecal incontinence predominates. Distal colonic sluggishness can occur as a result of loss of parasympathetic supply. Segmental stool transit studies demonstrate prolonged transit through the rectosigmoid segments resulting from the lack of direct innervation from the conus.[76] The addition of constipation and DWE to fecal incontinence compounds difficulties. This is an especially problematic combination because the accumulation of a large amount of hard stool that can result from such colonic inertia can overstretch the weakened anal mechanism. This can result in a gaping, patulous, incompetent anal orifice, often with associated rectal prolapse. The denervation, atrophy, and overstretching of the EAS and IAS lead to loss of the protective IAS tone, which can result in stool soilage from the increased abdominal pressures associated with everyday activities. Rectal distention leads to the expected internal sphincter relaxation, but attenuated or absent external sphincter protective contractions can result in fecal incontinence or fecal smearing whenever boluses are present at the rectum. The presence of a large bolus in the rectal vault can further compromise the rectoanal angulation at the pelvic floor and contribute to paradoxical liquid incontinence around a low impaction, called the ball-valve effect.[10,118,135]

Patients with lower motor neurogenic bowel (LMNB) dysfunction have decreased anal tone because of the smooth muscle that makes up the internal sphincter. If no tone is found initially upon inserting the examining finger, the examiner should wait up to 15 seconds to allow IAS reflex relaxation to recover and restore tone. Chronic overstretching has probably occurred if tone does not return. The anal-to-buttock contour typically appears flattened and "scalloped" (see Figure 21-5) because of atrophy of the pudendal-innervated pelvic floor muscles and EAS.[10] The anocutaneous reflex is absent or decreased (depending on the completeness of the lesion). The bulbocavernosus reflex is also weak if present (see Table 21-1). The anal canal is shortened (as compared with the normal 2.5- to 4.5-cm length) and the puborectalis muscle ridge might not be palpable. Excessive perineal descent and even rectal prolapse can occur with the Valsalva maneuver.

Gastrointestinal Dysfunction in Common Neurologic Disorders

Brain Disorders

Strokes (ischemic or hemorrhagic), cerebral trauma, mass, infection, or other lesions cause a whole range of neurologic damage and complications to many areas of the brain. They commonly present with dysphagia, delays in

Table 21-1 Features of Colorectal Function in Normal Individuals and in Those With Upper Motor Neurogenic Bowel, Upper Motor Neurogenic Bowel With Posterior Rhizotomy, and Lower Motor Neurogenic Bowel

	Normal	Upper Motor Neurogenic Bowel	Upper Motor Neurogenic Bowel With Posterior Rhizotomy	Lower Motor Neurogenic Bowel
Bowel dysfunction	Normal colon activity and defecation	Chronic intractable constipation, fecal impaction, reflex defecation with or without incontinence	Chronic constipation, no reflex defecation	Chronic constipation, fecal impaction maximal in the rectum
Transit time (cecum to anus)	12 to 48 hours	Prolonged >72 hours	Very prolonged unless sacral nerve stimulator used	Prolonged >6 days, especially left side of colon
Colonic motility at rest	GMCs approximately 4 per 24 hours	GMCs may be reduced in frequency	Reduced GMCs	Reduced GMCs
Colonic motility in facilitation response to stimuli	GMCs facilitated by defecation, exercise, and food ingestion	Less GMC facilitation by defecation, exercise, or food ingestion	Less GMC facilitation by defecation, exercise, or food ingestion	Less GMC facilitation by defecation, exercise, or food ingestion
Anal Sphincter Pressure (mm Hg)				
Resting tone	>30	>30	Normal	Reduced
Volitional squeeze	>30 (up to 1800)	Absent	Absent	Absent
Rectal compliance	Normal	Normal but sigmoid compliance decreased	Normal or increased	Rectum dilated, increased distention volume, increased compliance
Rectal Balloon Distension				
Effect on IAS	Normal rectoanal inhibitory reflex	Normal rectoanal inhibitory reflex	Normal rectoanal inhibitory reflex	Normal rectoanal inhibitory reflex
Effect on EAS	Causes contraction	Causes contraction	No contraction	No contraction
Sensory perception threshold	<20 mL volume	None	None	None
Stimulation of rectal contraction	Induced by balloon distention	Giant rectal contractions stimulated readily	Rectal contraction stimulation	Rectal contraction stimulation
Vesicoanal reflex	Present (>50 mm Hg)	Present	Absent	Absent
Valsalva Protective Reflex				
Reflex defecation	Yes	Yes	Impaired	Impaired
Perianal sensation (cutaneous sensation of touch, pinprick)	Normal	No sensory perception	No sensory perception	Loss of perianal buttock sensation resulting from injury to sacral nerves
Anocutaneous reflex ("anal wink")	Present	Present, may be increased	Absent	Absent as a result of injury to afferent or efferent sacral pathways
Bulbocavernosus reflex	Present	Present, may be increased	Absent	Absent
Anal appearance	Normal	Normal	Normal	Flattened, scalloped, attributable to loss of EAS bulk

From Banwell JG, Creasey GH, Aggarwal AM, Mortimer JT: Management of the neurogenic bowel in patients with spinal cord injury, *Urol Clin North Am* 20:517-526, 1993; Schiller LR: Fecal incontinence. In Sleisenger MH, Fordtran JS, editors: *Gastrointestinal disease*, Philadelphia, 1993, WB Saunders, pp 934-953.)

EAS, External anal sphincter; *GMCs*, giant migratory contractions; *IAS*, internal anal sphincter.

gastric emptying and ileus (intestinal pseudoobstruction), constipation, and fecal incontinence. Brainstem or cranial nerve involvement often causes dysphagia. Studies report that dysphagia occurs in approximately 45% of patients with stroke during the acute phase. Cerebral edema and high intracranial pressure play a role in gastrointestinal ulceration, gastroparesis, or ileus through unknown mechanisms. Depending on the severity of the cerebral or brainstem involvement, dysphagia and ileus progressively improve. Approximately 23% of patients with stroke were shown to have fecal incontinence in stroke research, and constipation has been observed to be very common in clinical practice.[5,20,56,98]

Parkinson Disease and Parkinson Plus Diseases

Parkinson disease and Parkinson plus diseases (multiple system atrophy, progressive supranuclear palsy, corticobasal degeneration) are neurodegenerative diseases that affect various parts of the nervous system including the cerebral cortex, basal ganglia, brainstem, cerebral cortex, cerebellum, and spinal cord. They are characterized by dementia, muscle rigidity, bradykinesia, resting tremor, dystonia, shuffling gait, and dysphagia. They also have dysautonomia, which is manifested as orthostatic hypotension, sexual incompetence, gastric dysmotility, and

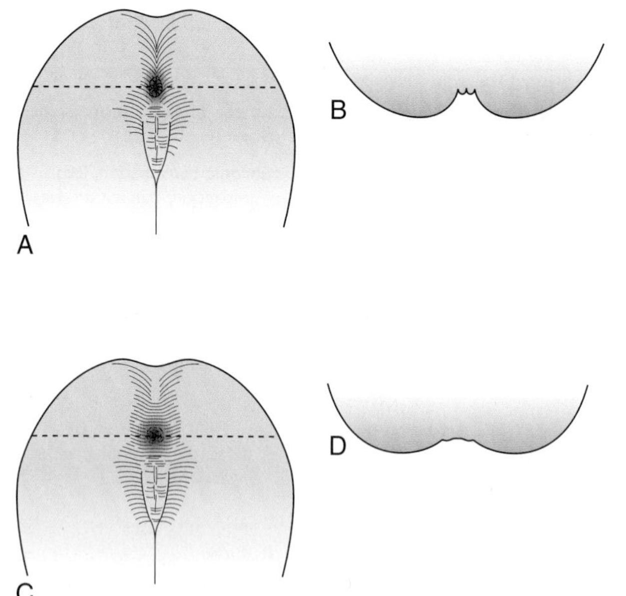

FIGURE 21-5 Upper motor neurogenic bowel presents an appearance similar to normal (**A,** rear view; **B,** profile from above). Anal contour of the lower motor neurogenic bowel (**C,** rear view; **D,** profile from above), with its atrophic external anal sphincter, shows a flattened, scalloped-appearing anal area.

constipation. Up to 50% of persons with Parkinson disease have been found to have dysphagia and problems with defecation in a study done on 98 persons. In this group, 52.1% had dysphagia, 28.7% had constipation, and 65% had problems with defecation. These gastrointestinal problems can be severe enough to compromise nutrition and cause severe morbidity.[29,42,42a,43,77,102]

Multiple Sclerosis

Multiple sclerosis is a demyelinating disease caused by an autoimmune process that involves different regions of the brain and spinal cord (see Chapter 46). Presentation can be any neurologic sign or symptom, which can consist of paresis, spasticity, ataxia, paresthesias, visual problems, cognitive deficits, mood disorders, dysphagia, gut dysmotility, urinary incontinence or retention, fecal incontinence, diarrhea, or constipation. In a study done on patients with multiple sclerosis, 68% were reported to have gastrointestinal problems, with 43% having constipation and 53% having fecal incontinence. The bowel and bladder problems in these diseases are believed to be caused by supraspinal or spinal lesions associated with autonomic sympathetic and parasympathetic system impairment.[20,29,47,126]

Spinal Cord Disorders

Trauma, masses, infection, hemorrhage, or ischemia to the spinal cord causing tetraplegia or paraplegia primarily affects colonic motility, perineal and anorectal sensation, and function in the acute and chronic phases (see Chapter 49). Upper gastrointestinal tract problems resulting from disorders of the spinal cord, however, are increasingly being recognized. Depending on the level of the injury, brain and autonomic modulation of the ENS is impaired. The bowel dysfunction is principally one of motility rather than secretion or absorption. It has been demonstrated that the upper digestive tract is more involved in people with tetraplegia rather than with paraplegia, and is characterized by gastroparesis, impaired gastric emptying, and delayed gastrointestinal times. Dysphagia is common in people with cervical cord lesions during the acute phase and often eventually resolves. Gastric and duodenal ulcerations have also been prevalent in persons with myelopathy. Across all levels of injury, there is a loss of voluntary control over bowel movements resulting in constipation or fecal incontinence. For lesions occurring above the conus medullaris (above T12), rectoanal reflexes are preserved with the sphincters being spastic. This is usually called the upper motor neuron bowel. Lesions below the conus medullaris (below T12) display flaccidity of the sphincters with loss of reflexes. This is referred to as the lower motor neuron bowel.*

Peripheral Neuropathy

There are multiple causes of peripheral neuropathy, including metabolic, viral, traumatic, toxic, metastatic, and genetic (see Chapter 41). Sensory and motor deficits are associated with autonomic involvement. Disturbances in gastrointestinal transit are most often caused by peripheral neuropathies. Motility problems might result in diarrhea (from bacterial overgrowth) or in constipation. Well-known complications of diabetes include gastroparesis and decreased intestinal motility primarily from autonomic dysfunction. In paraneoplastic syndromes in small cell carcinoma of the lung or pulmonary carcinoid, immunoglobulin G antibody against enteric neurons has been found to be responsible for esophageal dysmotility, gastroparesis, and constipation. Injury to the pudendal nerve (from childbirth or persistent and protracted straining), S2 to S4 nerve root lesions, or cauda equina underlies fecal incontinence and abnormal defecation.

Comprehensive Evaluation

History

A comprehensive investigation for nausea, vomiting, bloating, early satiety, abdominal pain, diarrhea, constipation, and fecal incontinence must be completed. The gastrointestinal history should not only review for cardinal symptoms but should also address the patient's general neuromuscular and gastrointestinal function. A detailed review of the patient's bowel program includes an assessment of fluids, diet, activity, medications, and aspects of bowel care. Careful consideration must be given to drugs that seriously decrease gastrointestinal motility such as opiates, anticholinergics, tricyclics, antihistamines, calcium channel blockers, and phenothiazines. A review of the technique and outcome of bowel care should include a description of schedule, initiation method (chemical or mechanical stimulation), facilitative techniques, time requirements, and characteristics of stool results. The

*References 5, 12, 20, 23, 68, 130.

history should include premorbid bowel pattern information, such as defecation frequency, typical time(s) of the day, associated predefecatory activities, bowel medications and techniques or trigger foods, and stool consistency. It is important to elicit any history of premorbid gastrointestinal disease or dysfunction. The presence of gastrointestinal pain, warning sensations for defecation, sense of urgency, and ability to prevent stool loss during Valsalva activities such as laughing, sneezing, coughing, or transfers should be noted. Excessively large-caliber hard stool can be ascertained by a history of toilet plugging. The patient's goals and willingness to alter previous bowel patterns or management need to be established. All aspects of impairment and disability that limit a person's ability to maintain continence and volitionally defecate must be assessed within the perspective of the entire person. All aspects of personal performance should be addressed in person-centered rehabilitation, with the overall goal of maximizing independence in bowel management or direction of a bowel program.

Physical Examination

The physical examination should include the gastrointestinal system and the associated parts of the musculoskeletal and nervous systems required for adequate management of the bowel program. The examination should be completed at the onset and then annually for SCI.[114] The purpose of the examination is to detect functional changes, screen for complications, and identify any new masses or lesions.

The abdomen should be inspected for distention, hernias, and other abnormalities. Careful assessment for the presence or absence of bowel sounds should be done. Percussion and auscultation should precede palpation for masses and tenderness. With the abdomen relaxed, the examiner transabdominally palpates the colon for hard stool. Palpable hard stool should not be present on the right side of the abdomen (ascending colon). Gastroparesis, intestinal, and colonic pseudoobstruction present with an abdomen that is distended, tympanitic with hypoactive bowel sounds, and tender. This can be accompanied by autonomic dysreflexia in persons with SCI. The patient can show signs of malnutrition and dehydration, including loss of weight, pale skin, dry mucous membranes, poor skin turgor, orthostatic hypotension, and tachycardia.

The rehabilitation evaluation should be interdisciplinary in approach and include assessment not only for colon and pelvic floor dysfunction but also for impairments of other organs or systems that could affect rehabilitative strategies to make bowel care independent or prevent unplanned bowel movements.

Physical examination continues with inspection of the anus. A patulous, gaping orifice suggests a history of overdistention and trauma by a previous regimen. A normal anal-buttock contour (see Figure 21-5) suggests an intact EAS muscle mass, whereas its loss results in a flattened, fanned-out, scalloped-appearing anal region. The patient should perform a Valsalva maneuver while the examiner observes the anus and perineum for excessive descent. Perianal cutaneous sharp stimulation normally results in an externally visible anal sphincter reflexive contraction. This is the anocutaneous reflex, mediated by the inferior hemorrhoidal branch of the pudendal nerve (S2 to S5). Sensation to light touch is tested at the same time. The tone and voluntary squeeze strength of the EAS and tone of the IAS should be assessed. Integrity of the pelvic floor muscles can be examined by the ability to contract and relax. The length of the anus, where pressure is sensed, is normally 2.5 to 4.5 cm. The point where the pressure decreases marks the anorectal junction. Along the posterior wall, 1.5 to 2.5 cm from the anal verge, the puborectalis muscular sling can be palpated as a ridge that will push the finger forward as the patient resists defecation. No palpable ridge or push suggests puborectalis atrophy or dysfunction. A shortened length of anal pressure zone suggests EAS muscle atrophy. With the examiner's finger in place, the bulbocavernosus reflex can be elicited by rapidly tapping or squeezing the clitoris or glans penis. The response can be delayed up to a few seconds in pathologic conditions. Insertion of the finger in the anal canal occasionally triggers IAS relaxation, but more often triggers a tightening squeeze that is efferently equivalent to the bulbocavernosus reflex. The patient is asked to volitionally squeeze the anus before removing the finger ("resist defecation") to check for volitional EAS and puborectalis tone and control. In addition, the patient is asked to bear down and relax alternately to evaluate contraction, relaxation, and coordination of the pelvic muscles.

Diagnostic Testing

The history and physical examination provide most of the necessary information. The clinical cause of neurogenic bowel dysfunction in most patients who are referred to physiatrists is readily apparent. Additional objective laboratory testing can be helpful when the cause of fecal incontinence or DWE is obscure, the history appears doubtful, conservative interventions fail, or surgical interventions are contemplated. Table 21-2 lists some of the many tests available.

Basic laboratory tests complement the physical examination. A flat plate radiograph of the abdomen can be helpful to rule out impaction, megacolon, obstruction, and a perforated viscus.

Management

Management of Nausea, Vomiting, Bloating, and Early Satiety

Nausea, vomiting, bloating, and early satiety may indicate gastroparesis, a small intestinal, or colonic pseudoobstruction in persons with neurologic disease. Acute or chronic episodes of subocclusion can occur. During episodes of acuity, there are findings of distended bowel loops and air-fluid levels requiring gastrointestinal decompression with nasogastric and rectal tubes. The patient must be placed on bowel rest and take nothing by mouth. Nutrition, fluid, and electrolyte support must be provided with intravenous infusion. Drugs such as opiates, anticholinergics, tricyclics, antihistamines, calcium channel blockers, and phenothiazines (all of which profoundly diminish motility) must be minimized or discontinued. Once decompression is achieved, feeding is slowly advanced to

Table 21-2 Diagnostic Tests for Gastrointestinal Dysfunction

Test	Purpose
Colonoscopy, rectosigmoidoscopy, anoscopy	Visualize anatomy to identify lesions Limited benefit to assess function
Anal endosonography	Evaluate structure and continuity of pelvic muscles
Radiography	
Defecography	Visualize kinesiology of defecation
Barium enema	Identify structural defects, fluoroscopy time too limited to assess function in any detail
Serial radiographs of tiny radiopaque plastic beads ingested with food	Evaluate colonic transit time, useful to confirm constipation history and to identify dysfunctional segments that help plan colostomy level
Manometry	Assess giant migratory contractions and anal pressures; with intrarectal balloon inflation, to evaluate rectoanal inhibitory reflex
Kymography	Measure pressure and volume change by intraluminal balloons
Catheter	Measure pressures by catheter in various compartments of the bowel
Solid sphere retention test	Measure maximal anal resistance force to extraction of spheres of standard sizes
Rectally infused saline continence test	Quantitative reproducible assessment of liquid continence ability
Electromyography	
Traditional	Assess motor nerve supply to puborectalis, anococcygeus, levator ani, and external anal sphincter; assess sensory pelvic afferents by nerve conduction studies, bulbocavernosus reflex testing, or somatosensory-evoked potentials
Mucosal electrosensitivity	Assess degree of mucosal wall sensibility
Intraluminal catheter	Research tool to assess colonic smooth muscle electrical potential activity

From Christensen J, editor: *The motor function of the colon,* Philadelphia, 1991, JB Lippincott; Schiller LR, editor: *Fecal incontinence,* Philadelphia, 1993, WB Saunders; Stone JM, Nino-Murcia M, Wolfe VA, Perkash I: Chronic gastrointestinal problems in spinal cord injury patients: a prospective analysis, *Am J Gastroenterol* 85:1114-1119, 1990.

a general diet. Prokinetic agents such as metoclopramide and domperidone (dopamine antagonists), erythromycin (macrolide antibiotic, motilin receptor agonist) have been found to be beneficial in facilitating gastric emptying and intestinal motility and improving symptoms. A review of studies with high-quality randomized clinical controlled trials showed good results for prucalopride (Resolor; not available in the United States), neostigmine (Prostigmin, Vagostigmin; administered both with and without glycopyrrolate), and fampridine (Fampyra, Ampyra in the United States; Dalfampridine).[75] Effects of tegaserod (Zelnorm) and cisapride (Propulsid), 5-HT_4 receptor agonists, were more favorable but these drugs were pulled from the US market as a result of serious cardiovascular adverse events including myocardial ischemia, acute angina, arrhythmias, and stroke. For chronic subocclusive states, enteral nutrition is preferred in patients with satisfactory digestive function. Meals should be small; frequent; liquid; contain polypeptide and hydrolyzed protein; be low in fat, fiber, and lactose; and contain multivitamins (iron, folate, calcium, and vitamins D, K, and B_{12}). If oral intake is not tolerated, enterostomies can be helpful to optimize nutrition. Total parenteral nutrition to satisfy nutrition requirements should be reserved for very severe cases. It generates various complications such as pancreatitis, glomerulonephritis, liver abnormalities, and septicemia or thrombosis from chronic catheter use.

Bacterial overgrowth syndrome may also present with nausea, vomiting, bloating, and early satiety. It can also present with diarrhea in chronic inflammatory conditions. This occurs when there is an overwhelming increase in bacteria or other pathogens in the upper gastrointestinal tract (stomach, duodenum, jejunum, and proximal ileum) where there are normally low amounts of bacteria.[103] There are many causes of bacterial overgrowth syndrome, but in persons with neurologic disease, it is most likely caused by upper gastrointestinal tract dysmotility, which leads to decreased clearance of unwanted bacteria and undigested substances.[15] To diagnose this condition, the glucose hydrogen breath test is the simplest to perform. Levels of exhaled hydrogen to 20 ppm indicate a positive test. This test is 82% sensitive and 62.5% specific.[49] Treatment with 1200 or 1600 mg/day of rifaximin (Rifagut) is recommended.[48] Alternatively, a combination of ciprofloxacin (Cipro) and metronidazole (Flagyl) were also shown to be very effective.[22]

Management of Diarrhea

Occurrence of diarrhea in neurologic disease is commonly a result of severe constipation. When solid stools are not passed regularly, they become very hard and are difficult to pass causing a blockage of more watery stool behind it. Eventually, there is overflow of the watery stool around the hard stool causing diarrhea. Therefore, it is necessary to determine if diarrhea is actually a result of constipation through history, physical examination, and abdominal x-ray to evaluate for fecal loading or impaction.

As a result of repeated use of antibiotics for treatment of urinary tract infections, pneumonia, and other infections, diarrhea is frequently caused by *Clostridium difficile* colitis. In can be associated with abdominal pain and cramps, anorexia, malaise, lower abdominal tenderness, and in more severe cases fever and dehydration. A stool test confirms the presence of the toxin or the cytotoxin.[6] Treatment with metronidazole is used to treat mild to moderate colitis. Oral vancomycin (Vancocin) is used to treat severe or complicated disease producing faster symptom resolution and fewer treatment failures. In fulminant cases, combined therapy with intravenous metronidazole and oral (or per rectum) vancomycin is recommended.[31] Fecal transplantation is considered investigational in the treatment of recurrent colitis.[123]

More recently, there has been the increasing use of probiotics that are live nonpathogenic bacteria (*Lactobacillus*, *Bifidobacterium*) or yeast (*Saccharomyces boulardii*) to treat illnesses that result in diarrhea. Probiotics are thought to block the production of microbial toxins, inhibit pathogen adhesion, modulate the immune system, and improve the gut barrier function. In a Cochrane review of 63 randomized control trials (RCTs), probiotics were shown to reduce duration of illness with diarrhea lasting less than 4 days and decrease stool frequency.[91]

Management of Defecation Dysfunction: Constipation and Fecal Incontinence

A bowel program is a comprehensive individualized patient-centered treatment plan focused on preventing incontinence, achieving effective and efficient colonic evacuation, and preventing the complications of neurogenic bowel dysfunction. The subcomponents of a bowel program address diet, fluids, exercise, medications, and scheduled bowel care. Bowel care is the individually developed and prescribed procedure for defecation that is carried out by the patient or attendant.[69,114]

Neurogenic bowel dysfunction results in problems with fecal storage and elimination. Inability to volitionally inhibit spontaneous defecations leads to incontinence, whereas the inability to adequately empty leads to constipation and impactions. Paradoxically, impactions can result in diarrhea and incontinence. Providing adequate timely emptying must be combined with the inhibition of spontaneous defecations except at desired times to achieve social continence.[115] The role of the individual that occurs after the acute rehabilitation process is complete determines the timing and content of the bowel care schedule. The demands of life activities, the duration of bowel care, and the needs of other members of the household should all be considered in scheduling the bowel program.[70,114]

Goals of the Bowel Program

It is essential to outline the goals of the bowel program as a person-centered plan for each patient. Each person responds differently to various techniques and medications used to treat constipation and fecal incontinence. Regular bowel emptying is recommended as the primary means for enhancing both elimination and decreasing incontinence between stooling. The goals of the bowel program should include the following[70,115]:

- Regular passage of stool on a daily or every-other-day basis.
- Bowel evacuation at a consistent time of day (AM or PM).
- Complete emptying of the rectal vault with every bowel care session.
- Stools that are soft, formed, and bulky.
- Completing the bowel care within half an hour (at most within 1 hour).

Fully appreciating an individual's premorbid "normal" bowel function is important in the planning and goal setting for a new neurogenic bowel program. A wide range of "normal" bowel patterns exist. Ninety-five percent of individuals have a frequency of between three times per day and three times per week. Stool consistencies vary from liquid to pudding, pasty, semisolid, soft-formed, medium-formed, and hard-formed.[69,70]

The choice of the frequency and specific timing of bowel care to induce adequate colonic emptying can be based on previous elimination patterns. It is best, however, to plan for everyday or every-other-day bowel movements to avoid episodes of fecal impaction. Waiting more than 2 days to have a bowel movement increases episodes of constipation and incomplete emptying of the rectum. Establishing a consistent schedule for bowel care facilitates predictability and planning. Ensuring complete emptying of the rectum decreases incontinence or multiple stooling during the course of the day. Incontinence is reduced by less stool accumulation, because stool is not presented to the rectum between desired defecation times. Adequate emptying is accomplished by making stools easier to move by means of softening, adding bowel stimulant medication if needed, and triggering the defecatory reflex at consistent desired times to promote habituation and if unable to use the defecatory reflex, using mechanical means of cleaning out stools.[69,70,115]

Bowel programs and techniques for bowel care training can begin during inpatient rehabilitation and are then monitored and maintained or modified at outpatient visits. Some patients need attendants who are well trained to help with bowel care.[114] The burden of care for persons with neurogenic bowel is much higher if continence is not achieved or if bowel care evacuation times are excessive. It is crucial that the patient takes a decisive leadership role in designing a bowel program that includes a convenient bowel care schedule. Educating patients about their altered neurogenic bowel physiology empowers them with options and techniques to construct a bowel care regimen compatible with their daily routine. Making them independent with their bowel care is an important aspect of the overall rehabilitation process.[69,70,114]

Dietary Considerations

Food and fluid choices are important when colonic transit time is prolonged, such as in SCI where the transit time is often 96 hours versus the 30 hours typically found in normal individuals. The main goal of dietary choices is to achieve soft but well-formed, bulky stools. Excessive fluid resorption can result in stool hardening and subsequent constipation. Gases and liquids are propelled by the colon 30 to 100 times faster than solids. Stools that have lost their plasticity might not be kneaded and folded properly by the haustra, impeding the transit time. Food fiber has been used to maintain a more fluid content. Fiber increases stool bulk and plasticity, especially in the more physically coarse forms of fiber, which also tends to decrease colonic pressures.[135] Control of excessive stool hardness requires higher-fiber foods in preference to lower-residual foods. It is important to remember, however, that sufficient intake of fluids (preferably water) is imperative when taking a high-fiber diet. The Institute of Medicine recommends daily fluid intake of 3 L for men and 2.2 L for women.[100] Otherwise, a high-fiber diet with insufficient intake of fluids can promote constipation. It should also be remembered that highly caffeinated fluids such as coffee, tea, and energy drinks can lead to dehydration from diuresis.

A diet that contains at least 38 g for men and 25 g for women of fiber daily is recommended (15 g initially and gradually increase as tolerated).[63,115] Aside from fiber from vegetables, fruits, and grains, artificial fiber products can be used such as psyllium (Metamucil, Fiberall), calcium polycarbophil (FiberCon), and methylcellulose (Citrucel). One study showed that taking psyllium for 8 weeks increased the number of stools per week and stool weight in patients with Parkinson disease without affecting colonic transit time. A recent case series study proposes that an increase in fiber in individuals with SCI may not improve but impair bowel function compared with people with normal bowels.[18,75] The effects of fiber intake on stool consistency, frequency, and efficacy of evacuation should be evaluated in each individual patient and fiber intake should be titrated accordingly. High pressures involved in moving solid feces probably contribute to the 90% incidence of hemorrhoids in Americans and to premature diverticula formation and hemorrhoidal complications in greater than 70% of patients with SCI.[114] Constant straining at stool can contribute to peripheral neuropathic deficits in the anal sphincter musculature.[114] Acceptance of softer stools, from a higher-fiber diet, might help reduce these complications and is often recommended for their treatment.

Treatment Approaches and Rationale

To select the best approach, the UMNB must be delineated from the LMNB. Brain disease and spinal cord disorders above T12 present with UMNB, and peripheral neuropathy and spinal cord disorders below T12 present with LMNB. Colonic transit time and fecal elimination are enhanced by softer stool. If the stool becomes too liquid, however, the protective angle provided by the puborectalis becomes less effective, and greater EAS pressures are required to maintain continence. Neurogenic bowel resting anal pressures are usually normal to slightly decreased but are unable to develop the protective increases in EAS tone needed to control more liquid stool.[40] Some degree of stool firmness must be tolerated to prevent incontinence. To avoid incontinence upon straining, more firmness (medium-formed) is required for the weaker anal sphincter mechanism of LMNB than for UMNB (semi-formed to soft-formed).

Fiber more consistently softens stool, but also adds bulk. Bulkier stools can help stimulate the defecatory response more easily in LMNB, although less stimulus is needed in UMNB.

The presentation of stool to the rectum, triggering defecation, can be associated with GMCs and mass movements more than with the slow accumulation of sufficient rectal stool to trigger reflex defecation. The GMC might be what is actually habituated.[116]

Choosing long intervals between elimination allows more fluid reabsorption, resulting in harder stools, which can worsen DWE. Because 95% of unimpaired persons defecate three or more times per week, choosing a frequency of at least as often as every other day would seem more physiologic and less likely to contribute to constipation. One study of well-managed patients with SCI found frequencies of bowel care to be chosen as daily by 24%, every other day by 46%, and more often than three times per week by 85%. The desire to avoid the unpleasant task of stool elimination leads some to elect longer time intervals between bowel care sessions, but this carries the attendant risk for impaction or sphincter damage caused by rectal distention by larger-caliber, harder stools.

Management of Upper Motor Neuron Defecatory Dysfunction

In the UMNB the defecatory reflex is intact, so that triggering of defecation can be accomplished by digital stimulation, rectal stimulant medications, enemas, or electrical stimulation. All of these cause reflex relaxation of the IAS, and if strong enough can also reflexively relax the EAS. This activates preserved anorectal colonic reflexes that increase motility of the left colon and help eliminate any stool that is present.[73,75] The GMC and mass movement associated with the "call to stool" for many intact persons often occurs at consistent times, which can be trainable.

Digital rectal stimulation is done by inserting a gloved, lubricated finger into the rectum and stimulating the rectal wall with gentle circular movements. This should be done for 20 seconds and repeated every 5 to 10 minutes until the bowel care is completed and the rectal vault is emptied.

There are a variety of rectally administered medications that are used to trigger and sustain reflex defecation. These are usually inserted into the rectum approximately 30 minutes before the intended bowel care, followed by digital rectal stimulation. The rationale for this prescription is to use the least irritating and most easily inserted and retained medication. Suppositories that are typically used include glycerine, vegetable oil–based bisacodyl (Dulcolax), and polyethylene glycol bisect bisacodyl (Magic Bullet). Options for minienema-triggered bowel care include small-volume phosphor-soda enema, bisacodyl enema, and Enemeez. Clinical efficacy studies have been conducted in attempts to measure efficiency and effectiveness of bowel care with various rectally administered medications. In a randomized blinded study, hydrogenated vegetable oil–based bisacodyl suppositories were compared with polyethylene glycol–based suppositories and the Therevac minienema. Individuals with UMNB dysfunction were studied with the events and intervals of bowel care.[61] Bowel care trials with polyethylene glycol–based suppositories showed an average time to defection of approximately 22 minutes, and a total bowel care time of 50 minutes. This was much shorter than the average time to defection of 40 minutes and total bowel care time of 85 minutes observed with hydrogenated vegetable oil–based bisacodyl suppository trials. The use of minienemas had similar efficiency as polyethylene glycol–based suppositories and have since been replaced by Enemeez. Results vary in individual patients and the use of digital stimulation alone is efficient for many persons with SCI who have UMNB.

In the UMNB, digital stimulation to induce defecatory reflexes should be favored over manual disimpaction, because the latter can easily result in inadvertent overstretching of the insensate and more delicate anal mechanisms of the neurogenic bowel. Local rectal stimulant suppositories and minienemas with bisacodyl or glycerin do not carry the same risk as oral stimulant medications and do not appear to lead to chronic inflammatory changes of the rectal mucosa.

When digital rectal stimulation and rectal medications are not sufficient to achieve the goals of the bowel program, oral colon stimulants such as senna (Senokot), bisacodyl (Dulcolax), osmotic agents such as polyethylene glycol (Miralax), lactulose (Cephulac), magnesium derivatives (Milk of Magnesia, magnesium citrate), and/ or stool softeners such as docusate (Colace) are commonly used. Determining the most appropriate oral medication is usually done by trial and error based on type, dosage, quantity, and duration of efficacy. Constantly being aware of the goals of the bowel program assists with titration, revision, and timing of intake of oral medications. Approaches that appear effective initially need longer-term studies to verify their continued benefits, especially because there is a high incidence of late gastrointestinal problems reported in an initially successfully managed population with SCI.[69]

New Medications to Treat Constipation

New medications to treat constipation have emerged in recent years, including:

Lubiprostone. Lubiprostone (Amitiza) increases intestinal fluid secretion by activating type 2 chloride channels, which promotes gastrointestinal motility. This enhances intestinal and colonic transit and helps with passage of stool. It affects prostaglandin E receptors, which facilitate gastric and colonic muscle contraction and motility.[44,91]

Linaclotide. Linaclotide (Linzess, Constella) is a 14-amino peptide agonist of guanylate cyclase-C (GC-C) receptor located on the luminal surface of intestinal epithelial cells. It increases cyclic guanosine monophosphate (cGMP), which triggers a signal transduction cascade activating the cystic fibrosis transmembrane conductance regulator that results in secretion of fluid into the lumen and promotes intestinal transit. It is further shown to relieve abdominal pain by activating GC-C expressed on mucosal epithelial cells, resulting in the production and release of cGMP, inhibiting nociceptors.[44,91]

Prucalopride. Prucalopride (Resolor; not available in the United States) is a selective 5-hydroxytryptamine receptor agonist that stimulates colonic transit and improves constipation by causing high-amplitude propagated contractions, hence enhancing segmental contractions.[119]

Methylnaltrexone and Alvimopan. For patients who have significant problems with constipation related to long-term opiate use caused by its effects on mu-receptors, there are two drugs, methylnaltrexone (Relistor) and alvimopan (Entereg), which have been shown to improve constipation without reversing analgesia and/or prompting opioid withdrawal. These drugs are peripherally acting mu-opioid receptor antagonists that selectively block mu-receptors outside of the CNS (Table 21-3).[110]

Management of Lower Motor Neuron Defecatory Dysfunction

In the LMNB the bowel is areflexic, and the most effective way of completely emptying the rectum is through manual disimpaction or the use of cleansing enemas (water, soapsuds, mineral oil, milk of molasses) that are done daily or twice a day. Sphincter and pelvic floor muscle tone is lost, increasing the likelihood of fecal incontinence. Consequently it is imperative to keep the stools well-formed and bulky, and to empty the rectal vault more regularly. Use of oral medications as outlined for the UMNB might likewise be warranted if stool is not efficiently reaching the rectum in a timely manner.

One approach to initiating neurogenic bowel training is outlined in Box 21-1. Each step is added only after a 10- to 14-day consistent trial of the previous step has been ineffective. In this stepwise approach, obtaining elimination at the desired time is emphasized as the first step and usually precedes development of complete continence by several weeks. This regimen is designed to enhance responsiveness and emptying at the habituated time with less stool presentation between bowel care sessions.

Intrinsic loss of the ENS in any segment, or surgical reanastomosis, can result in loss of the rectoanal inhibitory reflex, causing DWE. Oral laxative abuse can cause dysfunction of the ENS. If bowel training is not accomplishing defecation at the desired times or if repeated involuntary incontinence occurs, further diagnostic evaluation might be indicated (see Table 21-2).

When neurogenic bowel deficits are incomplete and some degree of control and sensation is present, biofeedback might offer a means of enhancing the patient's residual sensory and motor abilities. Improved sensory awareness after biofeedback training is an indicator of success. This typically requires only a few sessions, and most patients improve after just one session.[18] Among more severely impaired nonselected children with myelomeningocele, biofeedback and behavioral training are equally effective in restoring continence.[40] For selected individuals with some degree of volitional EAS activation and some degree of anorectal sensation, biofeedback can be a tool to help restore not just social continence but also normal defecatory control.

Physical Interventions

Bowel Irrigation

Transanal irrigation with a unique enema system that includes a pump and a rectal balloon catheter (Peristeen, Coloplast) was found to be helpful in one large multisite randomized controlled study in improving constipation, incontinence, bowel function, total time for bowel care, gastrointestinal symptoms, and quality of life in individuals with SCI compared with the regular bowel program.[27,28,75,101] Subsequent studies further demonstrated lower costs of care,[26,28] reduced or discontinued use of medications,[38,75] and prolonged successful outcomes (continued use of the device, resolution of symptoms).[45,75]

Pulse water irrigation of the bowel has been shown to be a safe and effective method for relieving fecal loading and impactions by delivering intermittent, rapid pulses of

Table 21-3 Luminally Acting Agents for Constipation

Agent Category	Mechanism of Action	Clinical Considerations
Currently Available Agents		
Bulk laxatives; for example, soluble fiber (psyllium, methylcellulose, calcium polycarbophil, partially hydrolyzed guar gum, wheat dextrin) and insoluble fiber (bran, flaxseed, rye)	Increases stool water content to soften stool; increased stool mass might stimulate peristalsis	Use in mild constipation; soluble fiber is more effective than insoluble fiber; psyllium and ispaghula husk most studied; avoid when dyssynergia present
Surfactant laxatives; for example, docusate sodium, docusate calcium	Anionic detergents lower the surface tension of stool; allows water to penetrate stool	Use in mild constipation; psyllium is more effective than docusate
Osmotic laxatives; for example, PEG, lactulose, sorbitol, magnesium salts	Generation of an osmotic gradient in gut lumen; promotes movement of water into lumen; luminal water softens stool and stimulates secondary peristalsis	PEG and lactulose effective for intermittent and chronic constipation; PEG is more effective than lactulose; might not benefit pain in IBS-C; avoid use of magnesium in patients with renal dysfunction
Stimulant laxatives; for example, diphenylmethanes (bisacodyl, sodium picosulfate), anthraquinones (senna, cascara), misoprostol, castor oil	Direct colonic wall irritant; stimulation of sensory nerves on colonic mucosa; possible inhibition of water absorption; prostaglandin-induced effects on motility and secretion with misoprostol	Efficacy for intermittent constipation; diphenylmethanes effective for chronic constipation; long-term safety not established
Chloride channel activation; for example, lubiprostone	Secretion of chloride ions into intestinal lumen through direct activation of C1 to C2 chloride channels on enterocytes; results in passive movement of sodium and water into intestine	Short-term and long-term efficacy and safety data in chronic constipation and women with IBS-C; main adverse event is dose-dependent nausea
Probiotics; for example, *Bifidobacterium lactis, Lactobacillus paracasei*	Hypothesized effects on gut transit and secretion through alteration of gut microbiota	Possible role in chronic constipation and IBS-C; no long-term efficacy or safety data; quality control issues (regulated as food additives not drugs)
Emerging Agents		
Chloride channel activation; for example, linaclotide, plecanatide	Activation of guanylate cyclase C receptor generating cGMP; secretion of chloride ions into intestinal lumen through cGMP-mediated activation of CFTR; results in passive movement of sodium and water into intestine; inhibition of visceral pain fiber firing by cGMP in animals	Effective in chronic constipation and IBS-C in phase II (linaclotide and plecanatide) and phase III clinical trials (linaclotide); main adverse event is diarrhea
Bile acid analogues; for example, chenodeoxycholic acid	Increases colonic motor activity; increases luminal secretory activity	Effective in IBS-C, as shown in phase II trial; risk of abdominal pain and/or cramps
Inhibitors of bile acid resorption; for example, elobixibat	Partial inhibition of ileal bile acid transporter; increases colonic bile acid concentrations promoting colonic motility and secretion	Effective for chronic constipation shown in phase II trial; dose-dependent abdominal pain reported
Peripherally acting mu-opioid receptor antagonists; for example, methylnaltrexone, alvimopan	Improve constipation without reversing analgesia and or prompting opioid withdrawal by peripherally acting mu-opioid receptor antagonists, which selectively block mu-receptors outside of the CNS	Effective in controlling constipation in chronic opioid users; methylnaltrexone (six RCTs) and alvimopan (four RCTs) were shown to be superior to placebo: adverse effects of abdominal pain and diarrhea

Modified from Menees S, Saad R, Chey WD: Agents that act luminally to treat diarrhoea and constipation, *Nat Rev Gastroenterol Hepatol* 9:661-674, 2012.

CFTR, Cystic fibrosis transmembrane conductance regulator; *cGMP*, cyclic guanosine monophosphate; *IBS-C*, constipation-predominant irritable bowel syndrome; *PEG*, polyethylene glycol; *RCT*, randomized control trial.

warm water into the rectum for bowel cleansing and to stimulate rectal motility.[75,101]

Abdominal Massage

Abdominal massage has been shown to promote better bowel movements, relieve abdominal distention, and improve colonic transit time in persons with SCI. This was demonstrated in 24 individuals who received 15 minutes of abdominal massage, from the cecum, throughout the colon, to the rectum, for 15 days.[9,75] Constipation score was significantly improved in patients with multiple sclerosis who received abdominal massage for 4 weeks, although the neurogenic bowel dysfunction score was not, and there was no difference in quality-of-life scores. Long-term improvement was not demonstrated when treatment was stopped after 4 weeks.[28,90]

Functional Electrical Stimulation/Functional Magnetic Stimulation

Use of an abdominal belt with electrodes for electrical stimulation of the abdominal muscles in persons with tetraplegia was shown to improve colonic transit time with overnight use in a good RCT.[28,72,75] Another study showed similar results in reducing colonic transit time with electrical stimulation of the abdominal muscles for 25 minutes, 5 days per week for 8 weeks compared with placebo.[57,75] Comparatively, individuals with SCI were shown to have shorter colonic times with functional magnetic stimulation

BOX 21-1

Protocol for Progressive Steps in Bowel Habituation Program*

1. Perform bowel cleanout if stool is present in the rectal vault or palpable proximal to the descending colon, by multiple enemas or oral cathartic.
2. Titrate to soft stool consistency with diet and bulking agents (fiber) and stool softeners (docusate).
3. Trigger defecation with a glycerin suppository or by digital stimulation 20 to 30 minutes after a meal; 10 minutes later, have the patient attempt defecation on the toilet, limited to less than 40 minutes, and relieving skin pressure every 10 minutes.
4. If defecation is not initiated, a trial of a bisacodyl suppository per rectum is initiated.
5. Digital stimulation. Start 20 minutes after suppository placement and repeat every 5 minutes.
6. Timed oral medications. Administer casanthranol–docusate sodium (Peri-Colace), senna (Senokot), or bisacodyl (Dulcolax) tablets timed so that bowel movement would otherwise result 30 minutes to 1 hour after anticipated triggered bowel timing.
7. If defecation occurs in less than 10 minutes after suppository insertion, transition to digital stimulation technique only. Once the patient is well habituated, straining alone may rarely trigger defecations at a desired time.

*Note that steps 1 to 3 are initial interventions and are always followed, with steps 4 to 6 incorporated only as needed. At least 2 weeks trial with proper technique is pursued before advancing to the next step.

of the abdominal muscles, but better quality studies are necessary.[75,80,81]

Surgical Options

Gastric Electrical Stimulation

Treatment of gastroparesis with electrical pacemakers has been studied. The most promising device was surgically implanted in nine patients with gastroparesis in whom conservative pharmacologic treatment was unsuccessful. Of the nine patients, gastroparesis in five was attributable to diabetes, in three as a result of idiopathic causes, and in one because of postoperative complications. This device delivered high-energy electrical pulses at a frequency higher than normal slow-wave impulses. Results showed improvement in gastric emptying and discontinuation of enterostomal feedings. Unfortunately, the device was too large to be implanted and was impractical for use on a long-term basis. Research is ongoing for a more feasible device.

Gastrostomies and Enterostomies

Optimization of nutrition via gastrostomies and enterostomies has been found to be beneficial in patients with gastroparesis, intestinal, or colonic pseudoobstruction. It not only helps prevent malnutrition, but it also alleviates discomfort from nausea, vomiting, and abdominal distention. For individuals on parenteral nutrition, a venting enterostomy provides symptomatic relief from gaseous distention and bloating.

Surgeries for Chronic Intestinal or Colonic Pseudoobstruction

During acute subocclusive episodes, colonoscopic decompression is successful in 75% to 90% of cases where nasogastric or rectal tubes were ineffective. A colonic decompression tube with suctioning can be used for those requiring repeated decompression. Decompression of the gastrointestinal tract also improves forward motility and coordinated propulsion. For cases in which conservative treatment has failed, subtotal colectomy with ileorectostomy has been found to be the most effective for chronic colonic pseudoobstruction. Intestinal transplantation is another option for patients with complete small intestinal failure and who cannot receive total parenteral nutrition. Intestinal transplantation is often accompanied by liver transplantation for patients who have developed liver failure from total parenteral nutrition. These patients must receive lifelong immunosuppressive therapy. Survival rates have improved with the use of tacrolimus (FK506; Prograf, Advagraf, Protopic) rather than cyclosporine (Neoral, Sandimmune, Gengraf) for immunosuppressive therapy.

Pelvic Floor Sling

Sacral nerve deficits interfere with the action of the puborectalis, levator ani, and EAS (see Figure 21-3). The resulting pelvic floor descent impairs the protective puborectalis sling angle and decreases the efficacy of protective EAS contractions. Some patients have benefited from transposition of innervated gracilis, adductor longus, gluteus maximus, or free muscle graft palmaris longus to replace puborectalis function and restore the acute anorectal junction angle that this sling provides. Chronic electrical stimulation to enhance development of fatigue resistance is used with these transplants. Sensory deficits are not improved, but continence is somewhat restored with the ability to inhibit defecation if some degree of sensation remains.

Electroprosthesis

Stimulation of anterior sacral roots S2, S3, and S4 by transrectal electrical stimulation or via a stimulator surgically placed for micturition has been performed. Stimulation of S2 tends to promote nonperistaltic, low-level electrical impulses to the sacral plexus, influencing the anal canal, colon, and pelvic floor musculature. Stimulation of S3 causes occasional high-pressure peristaltic waves, especially with repetitive stimulation; stimulation of S4 increases both rectal and anal tone; however, consistent changes in anal resting pressure and other manometric outcome measures have not been reported in the literature.

The sacral anterior root stimulator has been used in individuals with SCI to manage the neurogenic bladder with electrodes surgically placed in the S2, S3, and S4 anterior nerve roots, which is controlled with an external device that delivers short, high-voltage electrical stimulation to the bladder for emptying. Consequently, the sacral anterior root stimulator has produced good results for the neurogenic bowel in case series studies,[35,64] by facilitating colonic motility and spontaneous bowel evacuation,[24,28,75,122] reducing constipation and duration of bowel program,[24,28,64,75,122] preventing autonomic dysreflexia during bowel care, enhancing quality of life,[28,64,75] and reducing the need for caregiver assistance.[75,84] Fecal incontinence and quality of life were also shown to improve with sacral nerve root stimulation in patients with cauda equina syndrome.[52,75]

Antegrade Continence Enema

The options of the antegrade continence enema should be considered in clinical scenarios of prolonged bowel care time, recurrent fecal impactions, or poor or intermittent response to rectal medications to initiate bowel care. This is an alternative method of antegrade enema delivery that requires the surgical construction of a catheterizable appendicocecostomy stoma. The appendix and right colon are mobilized through a horizontal right lower quadrant incision and brought against the abdominal wall. The tip of the appendix is then amputated and the opening into the appendix lumen is modified into a catheterizable stoma on the abdominal wall. This procedure can now also be performed laparoscopically.[108] This stoma can be catheterized and infused with 200 to 600 mL of tap water to trigger a propulsive colonic peristalsis and defecation within 10 to 20 minutes. Bowel care can then be additionally facilitated with digital stimulation in the usual manner.

Colostomy

Colostomies are indicated in four general scenarios: (1) when conservative medical measures and training have failed; (2) when repetitive bowel impactions occur; (3) when pressure ulcers or other skin lesions occur that cannot be effectively healed because of frequent soiling; or (4) when intrinsic bowel deficits exist such as in Hirschsprung disease, Chagas disease, and colonic atresia. Colostomies have been demonstrated to be beneficial in various ways in multiple studies and systematic reviews in persons with SCI.* It has been shown that colostomies promote ease in bowel care by simplifying and decreasing time spent on bowel management,[14,66,75,104] reduce bowel symptoms,[75,104] mitigate episodes of incontinence, lower rate of hospital admissions from gastrointestinal problems,[75,104] encourage independence, and raise quality of life.[66,75,104] Patients do report a desire to have done the colostomy sooner[14,75]; therefore, a colostomy should be considered sooner. A sigmoid colostomy (left-sided, more distal) is typically recommended to allow absorption of fluid, preserve hydration, and have better-formed stools.[75,106]

Complications

For persons with gastroparesis or intestinal pseudoobstruction, the primary complication is chronic malnutrition, dehydration, and electrolyte imbalance. It is important to optimize nutrition and hydration, and monitor weight, vitamin, and electrolyte levels regularly. Oral and enteral feedings must provide adequate calories, protein, electrolytes, and vitamins despite being liquid in consistency; low in fat, fiber, and lactose; high in polypeptides and hydrolyzed protein; and received in small, frequent amounts.

In acute subocclusive episodes of colonic pseudoobstruction, it is important to achieve decompression as soon as possible. Failure to do so can result in progressive distention and cecal ischemia, causing perforation. The risk for perforation is increased when cecal diameters are 12 cm or greater. Colonic perforation requires emergent exploratory laparotomy and intestinal resection. The mortality rate is approximately 36% to 44% and is determined by age, diameter of the cecum, delay of decompression, and comorbidities.

Significant bowel complications requiring medical treatment or lifestyle alterations are reported by 27% of persons with SCI by 5 years or greater beyond their injury, even if bowel management was satisfactory during the first 5 years. More than 80% of persons with SCI reported bowel impactions and 20% had chronic bowel impaction and DWE problems.[61] Impactions have been reported to be complicated by perforation or even death. Impactions have a morbidity rate ranging up to 6% in the "normal" population, being higher in the cognitively impaired older adult population.[117] Other late gastrointestinal complications reported by patients with SCI include gastroesophageal reflux, premature diverticulosis, and autonomic dysreflexia. Morbidity from colonic perforation by enema use has also been reported.[108]

Hemorrhoids are more symptomatic when patients have intact sensation, but in one study rectal bleeding caused by hemorrhoids was reported by 74% of patients with SCI.[108] Hemorrhoids develop as a result of frequent high pressures in the anorectal marginal veins and are associated with constipated hard stool passage. Stool softening is the best preventative and chronic treatment measure, but it should be balanced with the requirement to modulate stool consistency to maintain continence.

An overstretched patulous noncompetent sphincter associated with rectal prolapse is often the end result of chronic passage of very large hard stools through a weakened anorectal mechanism in LMNB. Overdistention of the weakened neurogenic anal mechanism should be avoided by the use of stool softening and gentle care to dilate the sphincter whenever manual disimpaction is required to minimize trauma to these denervated structures. Although the anus can be significantly dilated to accommodate two fingers for breaking up low impactions, anorectal overdistention has been hypothesized to lead to atonic segments similar to bladder overdistention. The bowel, however, cannot be as easily decompressed and rested to allow recovery as can the bladder. The IAS is smooth muscle that will shorten and remodel to eventually regain competent closure if the overstretching can be eliminated. Unfortunately, this might require months of incontinent, liquid to soft pasty stools, which is seldom tolerated. Should the patient require a temporary colostomy for some other disease process, it might be possible after many months to then train toward social continence with the decompressed and restored IAS. Such patients have usually had long courses of constant soiling, however, and often prefer to keep their colostomy and continence rather than pursue surgical reversal and training.

Autonomic dysreflexia occurs in patients with SCI who have lesions at or above the midthoracic region. Fecal impaction is a common and potentially dangerous cause

*References 14, 28, 30, 66, 75, 104.

of autonomic dysreflexia because of the substantial time that can be required for its clearance (see Chapter 49). If manual disimpaction is required, lubrication with lidocaine gel is recommended to decrease additional nociceptive sensory input from the richly innervated anal region.

Bloating and abdominal distention are common complaints of patients with neurogenic bowel dysfunction. These complaints can be reduced in patients with SCI by increasing the frequency of bowel care. This complaint can be especially severe in those with hyperactive EAS protective responses to rectal distention, which can preclude the passing of flatus. Digital release of flatus might be required, in addition to diet modification to eliminate foods that produce excessive gases. The workup should also include assessment for any contributing aerophagia (air swallowing).

Treatment Outcomes

Bowel habituation training in children with myelomeningocele by means of suppositories, digital stimulation, or both resulted in 83% of compliant patients having less than one incontinent stool per month.[39] The continence catheter enema, which has a distal rectal balloon to avoid immediate enema expulsion, when used daily or every other day, reduced fecal incontinence to fewer than three episodes per month in children with myelomeningocele.[89]

Nursing home residents with fecal incontinence and dementia evaluated to have UMNB were treated by medically constipating them (with codeine) and giving biweekly enemas. Those diagnosed to have LMNB had their stools softened with lactulose and received weekly enemas. Fecal continence was restored in 80% of those who were consistently treated with these protocols.

Although all patients with complete SCI have episodic fecal incontinence, this is a chronic problem for only 2%. DWE appears to be a progressive problem that develops 5 years or more after SCI. This is rarely reported after training in the first 4 years but occurs in 20% by a mean of 17 years after injury. Gastrointestinal problems in SCI are not merely nuisances, because they also account for 10% of SCI late mortality.[34]

Patients with multiple sclerosis, Parkinson disease, or muscular dystrophy have also been helped by methods to enhance bowel storage or elimination in the setting of deteriorating neuromuscular and anorectal function.[86] Colostomy can also provide a means of achieving social continence in these patients. As noted earlier, colostomy complications include embarrassing gas problems, appliance loosening and leakage, and cosmetic difficulties.

Patients who develop social bowel continence are able to venture into public without fear of malodorous embarrassment and unpredictable social disasters that humiliate as well as require substantial clean-up time. When fear of such adverse events persists, full social and vocational reintegration is impeded. A major hurdle that many patients with neuromuscular compromise can overcome is control of the seemingly automatic neurogenic functions of defecation and bowel elimination. Such patients should not needlessly suffer because inadequate attention has been paid by care providers to this potentially functionally impairing and socially disabling deficit.

Many solutions are yet to come for the large number of persons who cope with neurogenic bowel dysfunction. The colon will continue to be a fertile area for research.

KEY REFERENCES

1. Aaronson MJ, Freed MM, Burakoff R: Colonic myoelectric activity in persons with spinal cord injury, *Dig Dis Sci* 30:295–300, 1985.
10. Bartolo DC, Read NW, Jarratt JA, et al: Differences in anal sphincter function and clinical presentation in patients with pelvic floor descent, *Gastroenterology* 85:68–75, 1983.
12. Bittinger M, Barnert J, Wienbeck M: Autonomic dysfunction and the gastrointestinal tract, *Clin Auton Res* 9:75–81, 1999.
13. Bornstein JC, Furness JB: Correlated electrophysiological and histochemical studies of submucous neurons and their contribution to understanding enteric neural circuits, *J Auton Nerv Syst* 25:1–13, 1988.
18. Cameron KJ, Nyulasi IB, Collier GR, Brown DJ: Assessment of the effect of increased dietary fibre intake on bowel function in patients with spinal cord injury, *Spinal Cord* 34:277–283, 1996.
19. Camilleri M: Disorders of gastrointestinal motility in neurologic diseases, *Mayo Clin Proc* 65:825–846, 1990.
25. Christensen J, editor: *The motor function of the colon*, Philadelphia, 1991, JB Lippincott.
27. Christensen P, Bazzocchi G, Coggrave M, et al: A randomized, controlled trial of transanal irrigation versus conservative bowel management in spinal cord-injured patients, *Gastroenterology* 131: 738–747, 2006.
28. Coggrave M, Norton C, Cody JD: Management of faecal incontinence and constipation in adults with central neurological diseases, *Cochrane Database Syst Rev* (1):CD002115, 2014.
30. Coggrave MJ, Ingram RM, Gardner BP, Norton CS: The impact of stoma for bowel management after spinal cord injury, *Spinal Cord* 50:848–852, 2012.
35. Creasey GH, Grill JH, Korsten M, et al: An implantable neuroprosthesis for restoring bladder and bowel control to patients with spinal cord injuries: a multicenter trial, *Arch Phys Med Rehabil* 82:1512–1519, 2001.
39. Devroede G, Lamarche J: Functional importance of extrinsic parasympathetic innervation to the distal colon and rectum in man, *Gastroenterology* 66:273–280, 1974.
41. Dubrovsky B, Filipini D: Neurobiological aspects of the pelvic floor muscles involved in defecation, *Neurosci Biobehav Rev* 14:157–168, 1990.
44. Eswaran S, Guentner A, Chey WD: Emerging pharmacologic therapies for constipation-predominant irritable bowel syndrome and chronic constipation, *J Neurogastroenterol Motil* 20:141–151, 2014.
46. Filipini DL, Dubrovsky B: Pelvic floor muscles response to graded rectal distension and cutaneous stimulation, *Dig Dis Sci* 36:1761–1767, 1991.
51. Grundy D, Al-Chaer ED, Aziz Q, et al: Fundamentals of neurogastroenterology: basic science, *Gastroenterology* 130:1391–1411, 2006.
55. Harari D, Minaker KL: Megacolon in patients with chronic spinal cord injury, *Spinal Cord* 38:331–339, 2000.
56. Harari D, Norton C, Lockwood L, Swift C: Treatment of constipation and fecal incontinence in stroke patients: randomized controlled trial, *Stroke* 35:2549–2555, 2004.
58. Hasler WL: Gastroparesis: symptoms, evaluation, and treatment, *Gastroenterol Clin North Am* 36:619–647, 2007.
61. House JG, Stiens SA: Pharmacologically initiated defecation for persons with spinal cord injury: effectiveness of three agents, *Arch Phys Med Rehabil* 78:1062–1065, 1997.
65. Kamath PS, Phillips SF, O'Connor MK, et al: Colonic capacitance and transit in man: modulation by luminal contents and drugs, *Gut* 31:443–449, 1990.
68. Kiba T: Relationships between the autonomic nervous system, humoral factors and immune functions in the intestine, *Digestion* 74:215–227, 2006.
69. King R, Biddle A, Braunschweig C, et al: Neurogenic bowel management in adults with spinal cord injury, *J Spinal Cord Med* 21:248–293, 1998.

70. Kirshblum SC, Gulati M, O'Connor KC, Voorman SJ: Bowel care practices in chronic spinal cord injury patients, *Arch Phys Med Rehabil* 79:20–23, 1998.
73. Korsten MA, Singal AK, Monga A, et al: Anorectal stimulation causes increased colonic motor activity in subjects with spinal cord injury, *J Spinal Cord Med* 30:31–35, 2007.
75. Krassioukov A, Eng JJ, Claxton G, et al: Neurogenic bowel management after spinal cord injury: a systematic review of the evidence, *Spinal Cord* 48:718–733, 2010.
76. Krogh K, Mosdal C, Laurberg S: Gastrointestinal and segmental colonic transit times in patients with acute and chronic spinal cord lesions, *Spinal Cord* 38:615–621, 2000.
78. Ladabaum U, Minoshima S, Hasler WL, et al: Gastric distention correlates with activation of multiple cortical and subcortical regions, *Gastroenterology* 120:369–376, 2001.
85. MacDonagh R, Sun WM, Thomas DG: Anorectal function in patients with complete supraconal spinal cord lesions, *Gut* 33:1532–1538, 1992.
91. Menees S, Saad R, Chey WD: Agents that act luminally to treat diarrhoea and constipation, *Nat Rev Gastroenterol Hepatol* 9:661–674, 2012.
92. Meshkinpour H, Nowroozi F, Glick ME: Colonic compliance in patients with spinal cord injury, *Arch Phys Med Rehabil* 64:111–112, 1983.
95. Nino-Murcia M, Stone JM, Chang PJ, Perkash I: Colonic transit in spinal cord-injured patients, *Invest Radiol* 25:109–112, 1990.
103. Quigley EM, Abu-Shanab A: Small intestinal bacterial overgrowth, *Infect Dis Clin North Am* 24:943–959, 2010.
104. Rosito O, Nino-Murcia M, Wolfe VA, et al: The effects of colostomy on the quality of life in patients with spinal cord injury: a retrospective analysis, *J Spinal Cord Med* 25:174–183, 2002.
105. Saab CY, Park YC, Al-Chaer ED: Thalamic modulation of visceral nociceptive processing in adult rats with neonatal colon irritation, *Brain Res* 1008:186–192, 2004.
106. Safadi BY, Rosito O, Nino-Murcia M: Which stoma works better for colonic dysmotility in the spinal cord injured patient?, *Am J Surg* 186:437–442, 2003.
107. Sarna SK: Giant migrating contractions and their myoelectric correlates in the small intestine, *Am J Physiol* 253:G697–G705, 1987.
109. Shafik A, Shafik AA, Ahmed I: Role of positive anorectal feedback in rectal evacuation: the concept of a second defecation reflex: the anorectal reflex, *J Spinal Cord Med* 26:380–383, 2003.
110. Sharma A, Jamal MM: Opioid induced bowel disease: a twenty-first century physicians' dilemma. Considering pathophysiology and treatment strategies, *Curr Gastroenterol Rep* 15:334, 2013.
111. Silverman DH, Munakata JA, Ennes H, et al: Regional cerebral activity in normal and pathological perception of visceral pain, *Gastroenterology* 112:64–72, 1997.
113. Stanghellini V, Cogliandro RF, de Giorgio R, et al: Chronic intestinal pseudo-obstruction: manifestations, natural history and management, *Neurogastroenterol Motil* 19:440–452, 2007.
114. Stiens SA, Bergman SB, Goetz LL: Neurogenic bowel dysfunction after spinal cord injury: clinical evaluation and rehabilitative management, *Arch Phys Med Rehabil* 78(3 Suppl):S86–S102, 1997.
115. Stiens SA, Braunschweig C, Cowel F, et al: *Neurogenic bowel: what you should know. A guide for people with spinal cord injury*, vol 53, Washington, 1999, Consortium for Spinal Cord Medicine.
117. Stone JM, Nino-Murcia M, Wolfe VA, Perkash I: Chronic gastrointestinal problems in spinal cord injury patients: a prospective analysis, *Am J Gastroenterol* 85:1114–1119, 1990.
120. Tjandra JJ, Ooi BS, Han WR: Anorectal physiologic testing for bowel dysfunction in patients with spinal cord lesions, *Dis Colon Rectum* 43:927–931, 2000.
126. Wiesel PH, Norton C, Glickman S, Kamm MA: Pathophysiology and management of bowel dysfunction in multiple sclerosis, *Eur J Gastroenterol Hepatol* 13:441–448, 2001.
128. Wingate DL, Ewart WR: The brain–gut axis. In Yamada T, editor: *Textbook of gastroenterology*, Philadelphia, 1991, JB Lippincott.
131. Wood JD: Neuropathy in the brain-in-the-gut, *Eur J Gastroenterol Hepatol* 12:597–600, 2000.
132. Wood JD: Enteric neuroimmunophysiology and pathophysiology, *Gastroenterology* 127:635–657, 2004.
133. Wood JD: Neuropathophysiology of functional gastrointestinal disorders, *World J Gastroenterol* 13:1313–1332, 2007.

The full reference list for this chapter is available online.

CHAPTER 22

SEXUAL DYSFUNCTION AND DISABILITY

Kelly M. Scott, Kate E. Temme

Sexuality is one of the most complex aspects of human life, with myriad physiologic and psychosocial influences. It is a topic that may be challenging to comfortably discuss in a physician's office. It may promote feelings of embarrassment and discomfort on the part of the patient and the physician, and yet it is one of the most important determinants of quality of life. Disability often has a dramatic negative impact on sexual functioning, but it does not change the inherent human yearning for intimacy, companionship, and physical satisfaction that sexuality affords. The physiatrist who has the willingness and knowledge to openly address issues of sexual dysfunction with patients will enrich their lives immeasurably.

The goal of this chapter is to provide an overview of sexual function and dysfunction, with an emphasis on the sexual challenges faced by people with disabilities. Great care has been taken to give equal treatment to the sexual dysfunctions of both men and women, as female sexuality is often overlooked both in society and in the medical literature.

Sexual Response and Behavior

Human Sexual Response

The classic model of human sexual response was formulated by Masters and Johnson[130] in the 1960s, based on a study of 600 able-bodied men and women. The model depicts women and men as having similar sexual responses throughout four phases: excitement, plateau, orgasm, and resolution (Box 22-1).[131] In the Masters and Johnson model, men tend to pass through each phase faster than women and achieve only one orgasm per cycle, often with a very short plateau phase. Women can achieve multiple orgasms in the same sexual response cycle. Masters and Johnson[130] also noted that women could become "stalled" at the plateau phase and then pass straight to resolution without achieving orgasm.

There have been many critics of the Masters and Johnson sexual response model, primarily because it places too much emphasis on genital responses and does not acknowledge the role of central neurophysiologic control.[16,165,205] In the late 1970s, Kaplan[107] devised a new model of sexual response with three phases: desire, excitement, and orgasm. In the Kaplan model, desire always precedes arousal, and is described as "the specific sensations that motivate the individual to initiate or become responsive to sexual stimulation."[107,113,165] The Kaplan model, like that of Masters and Johnson, proposes that human sexual response is linear and basically invariant between men and women.[113]

More recent research has furthered our understanding of human sexual response, particularly the ways in which the sexual response cycle is different in women and men. The Masters and Johnson and Kaplan models ignore major components of women's sexual satisfaction, such as the importance of trust, intimacy, affection, respect, and communication.[16] Basson[16-18] proposed a new model for the female sexual response to address these gender differences (Figure 22-1).[113]

Basson's circular model emphasizes that sexual response in women is much more complex than that in men. In women a sexual encounter does not necessarily start from a place of spontaneous sexual drive or desire. Women often approach becoming intimate from a point of sexual neutrality, and the decision to become sexually engaged can result from numerous and varied factors, including a wish to emotionally connect with their partner.[16,113] Sexual arousal and sexual satisfaction often do not occur solely through physical means, such as clitoral stimulation and orgasm, but may also be dependent on intangible factors, such as the ability to focus the mind on the present moment and a feeling of security or psychological well-being.[20] The circular sexual response cycle may be repeated many times within the same sexual encounter.[20] Janssen et al.[102] have also proposed a circular model of human sexual response, which is similar to that of Basson, which might be more applicable to both genders.[102]

Sexual Behavior and Aging

The frequency of sexual activity has been well documented to decline with age.[64,104] Recent research has shown that the degree of decline is much less than was previously thought and that sexuality remains an important contributor to quality of life throughout the entire life span.[64,104] An important reason for the discrepancy is that older studies tended to quantify sexual activity only as intercourse, but more modern research looks at all aspects of sexuality.[64,104] The 2009 National Survey of Sexual Health and Behavior found that although sexual activity declined with age, in participants aged 70 years or older, 43% of men and 22% of women reported vaginal intercourse in the year before the study.[94] Solo masturbation was reported in 46% of men and 33% of women in this age group.[94]

Many medical factors influence sexual activity in the elderly, including sexual dysfunction caused by medical illness, increasing frailty, and the side effects of medications. Postmenopausal women tend to experience

BOX 22-1

Masters and Johnson Model of Sexual Response

Excitement

- Associated with the senses, memory, and fantasy
- Increases in heart rate, blood pressure, and respiratory rate
- Myotonia develops late in the arousal phase
- *Men:* Engorgement of the corpus cavernosa of the penis, testicular elevation, scrotal skin flattening, possible nipple erection
- *Women:* Clitoral enlargement, vaginal lubrication, constriction of the lower third of the vagina with dilation of the upper two thirds, uterine elevation out of the deep pelvis, nipple erection, areolar enlargement

Plateau

- Further increases in heart rate, respiratory rate, and muscle tone
- Sex flush may develop (rash over the chest, neck, and face)
- *Men:* Increase in diameter and color of the glans penis, increase in testicular elevation and size of 50% to 100% over baseline
- *Women:* Breast engorgement by up to 50% and clitoral shaft and glans retraction
- Lasts seconds to minutes, and described as a "general sense of well-being"

Orgasm

- Further increases in heart rate, respiratory rate, and blood pressure
- Involuntary rhythmic contractions of the pelvic floor muscles
- *Men:* Only one orgasm per cycle
- *Women:* Can have multiple orgasms per cycle or can skip this phase altogether and go straight from plateau to resolution

Resolution

- Generalized perspiration in conjunction with gradual reversal of the above changes in heart rate, blood pressure, and respiratory rate
- Lasts 5 to 15 minutes, but the penis does not return to its normal size for 30 to 60 minutes after orgasm

From Masters WH, Johnson VE: *Human sexual response,* Boston, 1980, Bantam Books.

vulvovaginal atrophy and vaginal dryness, which cause pain with vaginal penetration.[105] Men have decreased testosterone with advancing age, which contributes to diminished sexual drive and also has physical effects that contribute to increased frailty.[104] Psychosocial barriers to sexual activity in the elderly are numerous, including decreased partner availability, alterations in body image and change in self-perception, cognitive decline, and environmental issues, such as the loss of privacy experienced in many residential settings.[75,104]

Types of Sexual Dysfunction

Classification

Sexual dysfunction is most frequently classified according to the *Diagnostic and Statistical Manual, fifth edition* (DSM-5), which was published in 2013.[10] To qualify as a sexual dysfunction, a person's sexual problem must cause "significant distress."[10] This distinction is important to remember for patients with disabilities, because they might experience altered sexual response but not have a sexual dysfunction in need of further workup or treatment.[191] In the same way that spasticity after stroke or phantom sensations after amputation are not always problems that need to be addressed by the physician, a patient's sexual difficulties only need to be treated when the patient's quality of life is adversely affected.

The DSM-5 stipulates that sexual dysfunction diagnoses require a minimum of 6 months' duration and that symptoms must be present 75% to 100% of the time (with the exception of medication-induced sexual dysfunction disorders). The DSM-5 also allows for two subtypes to be applied to all primary diagnoses to further clarify the nature of the dysfunction. The first subtype describes the onset of the disorder, lifelong or acquired (which means it developed after a period of normal functioning). The second subtype is used to designate the context in which the dysfunction occurs, generalized or situational (meaning limited to certain types of stimulation, situations, or partners). The

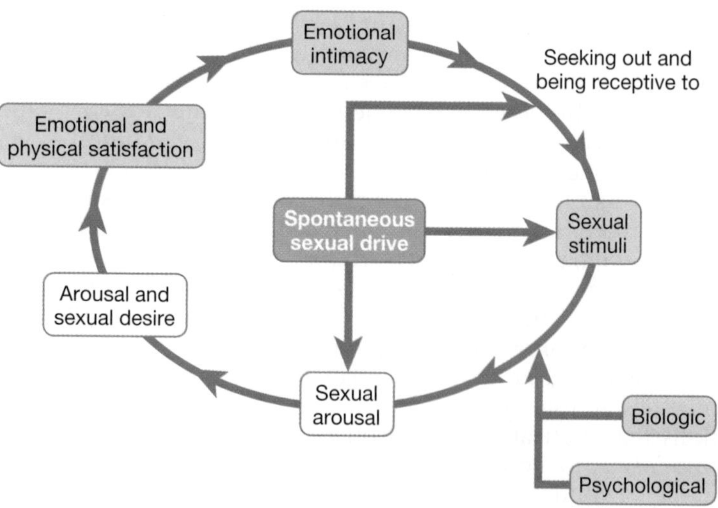

FIGURE 22-1 Female sexual response cycle. (Redrawn from Kingsberg SA, Janata JW: Female sexual disorders: assessment, diagnosis, and treatment, *Urol Clin North Am* 34:497-506, 2007.)

Table 22-1 Sexual Dysfunctions in the DSM-5

Male Dysfunctions	Female Dysfunctions	Other Dysfunctions
Male Hypoactive Sexual Desire Disorder	Female Sexual Interest/Arousal Disorder*	Substance/Medication-Induced Sexual Dysfunction
Premature (Early) Ejaculation	Female Orgasmic Disorder	Other Specified Sexual Dysfunction
Delayed Ejaculation (formerly known as Male Orgasmic Disorder)	Genito-Pelvic Pain/Penetration Disorder	Unspecified Sexual Dysfunction
Erectile Disorder		

From American Psychiatric Association: *Diagnostic and statistical manual of mental disorders, fifth edition* (DSM-5), Arlington, 2013, American Psychiatric Publishing.
*Desire and arousal classifications merged in DSM-5,[10] as compared with DSM-IV-TR.[9]

patient's sexual dysfunction should not be able to be better explained by a "nonsexual mental disorder, a consequence of severe relationship distress (e.g., partner violence), or other significant stressors." The DSM-5 criteria highlight the importance of separate classification systems for men and women, and abandons the Masters and Johnson linear sexual response model for both sexes.[202] The DSM-5 sexual dysfunctions are summarized in Table 22-1.[10] In addition to the DSM-5, there have been a number of international consensus conferences which have helped to further define and classify sexual dysfunctions.[21,22,25,124,143]

Male Sexual Dysfunction

The main focus of both clinical care and research for men with sexual dysfunction has traditionally been centered on performance problems, particularly erectile dysfunction and premature ejaculation. There has been a major paradigm shift in the past 2 decades away from the psychiatric understanding of most sexual disorders in men and toward a medicalization of male sexuality (particularly with the advent of proerection medications).[133,168] Purely psychogenic male sexual disorders are much more underrepresented in the medical literature and are often misdiagnosed as erectile dysfunction by health physicians.[138] Types of male sexual dysfunction include the following:

- *Male Hypoactive Sexual Desire Disorder:* Persistent or recurrent absence or deficit of sexual fantasies and desire for sexual activity, accounting for factors that affect sexual function, such as age and life context.[10] Hypoactive sexual desire disorder has been reported in 0% to 15% of men, with a metaanalysis by Simons and Carey[188] indicating a prevalence of 0% to 3% from community samples.[138,164,188]
- *Erectile Disorder/Dysfunction (ED):* Persistent or recurrent inability to attain, or to maintain until completion of the sexual activity, an adequate erection.[10] The diagnosis is primarily based on the patient's self-report, and ED must occur on a recurrent basis to establish the diagnosis (unless there is a history of trauma or surgically induced ED).[10,143] Prevalence estimates for ED vary greatly, from 0% to 5%, to 52%.[70,180,188] Results of the Massachusetts Male Aging Study in 1994 showed that 35% of men aged 40 to 70 years demonstrated moderate to severe ED, with another 25% exhibiting mild symptoms.[74] The 2006 National Health and Nutrition Examination Study was tailored to create a racially diverse sample population, and found ED in one out of every five respondents over the age of 20 years.[175] ED is known to be associated with advanced age, cardiovascular disease, diabetes, dyslipidemia, smoking, obesity, and depression, so the prevalence of this disorder is predicted to grow in keeping with the prevalence of these conditions.[156,180] ED was previously known as impotence, but the term has been phased out because of its pejorative implications and lack of precision.[147,180]
- *Premature (Early) Ejaculation Disorder:* Persistent or recurrent ejaculation before or within approximately 1 minute of intravaginal penetration and before the person wishes it.[10] This contrasts the average intravaginal ejaculation latency time (IELT) of 5.4 minutes in multinational populations.[208] Factors that affect duration of the excitement phase must be taken into account, such as age, novelty of the sexual partner or situation, and recent frequency of sexual activity. Consensus opinions also recognize that psychological distress in the patient and/or in the patient's partner is a critical diagnostic component.[6,143,169] Prevalence data for premature ejaculation are often limited to self-report, with estimates of up to 30% across all age cohorts.[122,166,169] However, when the IELT time parameter is applied to diagnostic criteria, prevalence drops to 1% to 3%.[6] Approximately 30% of men with premature ejaculation have concomitant ED, which typically results in early ejaculation without full erection.[89] Premature ejaculation is often caused by a combination of organic, psychogenic, and relationship-based causes.[6,169] More recently, neurobiologic and genetic variations have been proposed as contributing factors in premature ejaculation.[6]
- *Delayed Ejaculation:* Persistent or recurrent unwanted delay in, or absence of, ejaculation following a normal sexual excitement phase during sexual activity, which is adequate in focus, intensity, and duration.[10,136,143] This condition was formerly termed male orgasmic disorder.[9] Delayed ejaculation can originate through a variety of anatomic, neurogenic, and endocrine-related causes, as well as medication-related side effects and psychogenic etiologies.[136] As the least common sexual complaint among men, the prevalence of delayed ejaculation in the general population is thought to be in the range of 0% to 9%, and is more likely to affect partnered versus masturbatory ejaculatory responses.[136,188]
- *Dyspareunia:* Recurrent or persistent genital pain associated with sexual intercourse. Male dyspareunia was eliminated as a separate entity in the DSM-5 (compared with previous editions of the DSM).[9,10,202] This change was apparently made because dyspareunia in

men is much less prevalent than in women; however, estimates do range from 0.2% to 8%.[188,202] In gay men, the prevalence has been estimated at 3% (insertive) and 16% (receptive).[167]

Female Sexual Dysfunction

Female sexual dysfunction is very common, with a reported prevalence of 40% to 50% in multiple population-based studies.[11,122] Sexual dysfunction in women has become a focus of renewed research interest in the past 10 to 15 years, in part based upon the new understanding of the female sexual response cycle proposed by Basson[16] and the implications of that understanding toward diagnosis and treatment.[16,113] In contrast to sexual dysfunction in men, the psychological aspect of women's sexual functioning typically receives far more attention than organic etiologies of dysfunction. This discrepancy is partially because of institutional bias, but it is also based on a growing body of data suggesting that psychological factors correlate more strongly with sexual dysfunction in women than do medical problems.[25,113] It is especially important to remember that personal distress is necessary to make a diagnosis of sexual dysfunction when dealing with female patients. Up to 50% of women who report a problem with sexual functioning do not have any associated personal distress, and thus they cannot be classified as having a sexual dysfunction.[181] Types of female sexual dysfunction include the following:

- *Female Sexual Interest/Arousal Disorder:* With updated DSM-5 criteria, female sexual interest/arousal disorder is a convergence of the female desire and arousal disorders formerly termed female hypoactive sexual desire disorder and female sexual arousal disorder in DSM-IV-TR.[9,10] For diagnosis, at least three of the following six criteria must be absent or reduced: (1) interest in sexual activity, (2) sexual/erotic thoughts or fantasies, (3) initiation of sexual activity or receptiveness to a partner's initiation attempts, (4) sexual excitement/pleasure during sexual encounters, (5) sexual interest/arousal response to internal/external sexual/erotic cues, and (6) genital/nongenital sexual activity sensations during almost all or all sexual encounters.[10] Owing to the recent classification of female sexual interest/arousal disorder as a unique disorder, the prevalence is currently unknown. Prevalence data for the previous DSM-IV-TR disorders of female hypoactive sexual desire disorder and female sexual arousal disorder have been well established:
  - Female hypoactive sexual desire disorder was previously defined as absent or diminished feelings of sexual interest or desire, absent sexual thoughts or fantasies, and a *lack of responsive desire*.[9] Lack of interest was described as being beyond what would be considered normal for the woman's age and relationship duration, and must have been a frequent and persistent problem not related to changes in life situation or relationship dynamics.[21,181] The lack of responsive desire was the key to diagnosis, because many normal women do not have spontaneous sexual thinking, fantasizing, or desire ahead of sexual activity.[19] Despite traditional notions, female hypoactive sexual desire disorder has not been clearly linked to menopause or advancing age.[92,113,181] Prevalence estimates in population-based studies have been typically quoted at 24% to 43%, but may be much lower when strict diagnostic criteria are applied (closer to 5.4% to 13.6%).[181]
  - Female sexual arousal disorder was previously defined as persistent or recurrent inability to attain, or to maintain until completion of the sexual activity, sufficient sexual excitement, which may be expressed as a lack of subjective excitement, or as a lack of adequate genital (lubrication-swelling) or other somatic response.[9,22] The prevalence has been estimated to be 6% to 21%.[188]
- *Female Orgasmic Disorder:* Persistent or recurrent lack of orgasm, markedly diminished intensity of orgasmic sensations, or marked delay of orgasm from any type of stimulation despite the self-report of high sexual arousal/excitement.[10,25] Orgasmic disorder in women is often difficult to distinguish from an inadequate arousal response without a careful history, because women with decreased arousal will also not be able to achieve orgasm.[113] Many women are situationally orgasmic, in that they can reliably achieve orgasm with some forms of stimulation but not others. Vaginal intercourse alone is not a reliable way for many women to achieve orgasm, and the need for clitoral stimulation to achieve orgasm is not considered abnormal.[113] The prevalence of female orgasmic disorder was estimated at 24% in the National Health and Social Life Survey.[122] Other estimates range from 4% to 42%, based on research setting and methodology.[160,188]
- *Genito-Pelvic Pain/Penetration Disorder:* defined by persistent or recurrent difficulties with vaginal penetration, genito-pelvic pain during vaginal intercourse or other penetration attempts, fear or anxiety of genito-pelvic pain or vaginal penetration, and/or increased pelvic floor tension during attempted vaginal penetration.[10] This disorder encompasses the former DSM-IV-TR disorders of dyspareunia (persistent or recurrent pain with attempted or complete vaginal entry and/or penile vaginal intercourse) and vaginismus (the persistent or recurrent difficulties of the woman to allow vaginal entry of a penis, a finger, and/or any object, despite the woman's expressed wish to do so).[9,21] Vaginismus was originally defined as persistent spasm of the outer third of the vaginal musculature, which interferes with vaginal penetration. More recent research and consensus opinion dispute the classic definition because muscle spasm and even pain are not always present.[21,113,159] Prevalence rates for vaginismus have been reported at 1% to 6%.[124] Vaginismus is one of many potential causes of dyspareunia. Dyspareunia was previously thought to be primarily of psychogenic origin, but it is now known that biologic factors often contribute to the presentation.[113] Some even characterize dyspareunia as a pain disorder that interferes with sexuality instead of a sexual disorder characterized by pain.[31,113] The differential diagnosis of dyspareunia in women includes vulvovaginal atrophy, postmenopausal vaginal dryness, pelvic floor myofascial pain or dysfunction, vulvodynia (vulvar pain without visible signs of pathology and with no known etiologic diagnosis), and vestibulodynia/vulvar vestibulitis

syndrome (a type of vulvodynia localized only to the vulvar vestibule, which may or may not have associated inflammatory changes visible on physical examination).[24,85,113] Urethral disorders, cystitis, bladder pain syndrome (formerly known as chronic interstitial cystitis), anatomic variations, pelvic adhesions, infections, endometriosis, inflammatory bowel disease, abdominal wall pain, cancer, late effects of pelvic radiation, vulvovaginal dermatologic diseases (such as lichen sclerosis or lichen planus), and pelvic congestion syndrome can also cause chronic dyspareunia.[24,113,210] Dyspareunia prevalence estimates range from 3% to 18% in the general population, 3% to 46% in a primary care setting, and 9% to 21% in postmenopausal women.[188]

Sexual Dysfunction in Disability and Chronic Disease

The development of sexual dysfunction after the onset of disability is usually related to myriad diverse etiologic factors that can be grouped into five different categories: primary physical changes, secondary physical limitations, psychosocial contributions, the effect of comorbid conditions, and medication-related factors.

Primary physical changes derive from the disease pathophysiology and directly affect sexual response. These primary physical changes could include altered genital sensation, decreased vaginal lubrication, ED, or anorgasmia. Secondary physical limitations also play a significant role in the development of sexual difficulties after disability. These are indirect effects of the disease process that do not affect genital function or sexual response, but which make sexual activity unpleasant or challenging. Examples of secondary physical limitations include fatigue, pain, weakness, spasticity, contractures, ataxia, bowel and bladder dysfunction, and cognitive impairment. The psychosocial contribution to the development of sexual dysfunction includes psychological, emotional, relational, situational, social, and cultural factors. People with disabilities often have difficulty adjusting to their new life circumstances. They can have poor self-esteem and body image, fear of isolation and abandonment, anger, shame, guilt, strained relationships with loved ones, anxiety, and depression. All of these issues can affect sexual functioning. The fourth category to consider is the effect of comorbid conditions, particularly diabetes, cardiovascular disease, and depression, which can cause sexual dysfunction independent of the pathology of the primary disability. Finally, many medications commonly prescribed for people with disabilities can lead to the development of sexual dysfunction. It is important for the physician to consider factors from all five categories when diagnosing and treating a disabled patient with sexual dysfunction. Disability-specific sexual dysfunctions are discussed later.

Spinal Cord Injury

In contrast to many of the other disabilities discussed in this chapter, sexual dysfunction in patients with spinal cord injury (SCI) has been well studied in both genders. The type of sexual dysfunction the patient will ultimately experience depends in large part upon the spinal cord level and the degree of completeness of the injury.[142] Multiple studies have shown that the frequency of sexual activity and the level of sexual satisfaction decreases in both men and women after sustaining an SCI.[4,49,56,117,193]

Upper motor neuron (UMN) SCI allows for reflexogenic erection to occur in men, because the parasympathetic sacral reflex arc is intact. Psychogenic erection, however, is usually not possible unless the injury is incomplete. Ejaculation is difficult for these patients because it is sympathetically mediated from T11-L2. Lower motor neuron (LMN) SCI has preserved integrity of the thoracolumbar sympathetic outflow tract, and thus psychogenic erections and ejaculation are theoretically more likely to be intact but reflexogenic erections are not.

Bors and Comarr[36] conducted a pivotal study in 1960 detailing the prevalence of erectile and orgasmic dysfunction in 529 men with SCI. They found that in men with complete UMN lesions, 93% of patients were able to achieve reflexogenic erections, and none were able to attain psychogenic erections. Anterograde ejaculation in complete UMN SCI was seen in 4% of patients. Men with incomplete UMN SCI achieved erection 99% of the time, with 80% of men having only reflexogenic erections and 19% having combined reflex and psychogenic erections. Ejaculation was possible in 32% of patients with incomplete UMN SCI, with 72% of those occurring after reflexogenic erection and 26% occurring after psychogenic erection. Complete LMN lesions showed a very different picture, with 26% of patients able to achieve psychogenic erections and none attaining reflexogenic ones. Ejaculation was possible in 18% of these men. Incomplete LMN lesions fared far better, with 90% retaining the ability to achieve erection and 70% the ability to ejaculate. The results of the Bors and Comarr study are summarized in Figures 22-2 and 22-3.

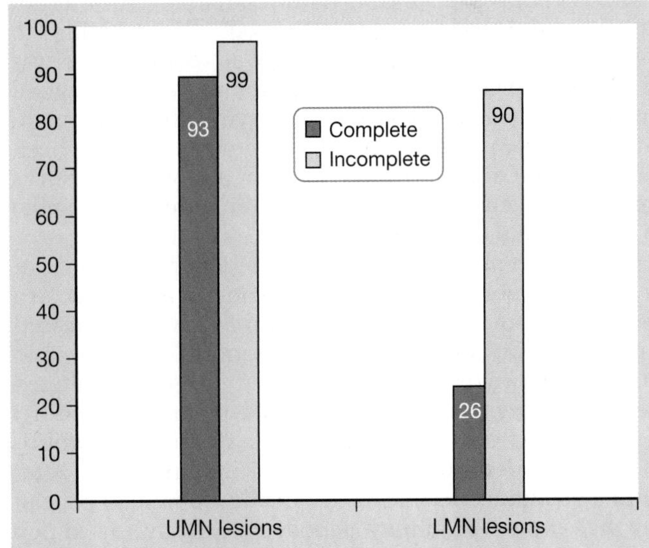

FIGURE 22-2 Percentage of men with spinal cord injury able to achieve erection. *LMN*, Lower motor neuron; *UMN*, upper motor neuron. (Data from Bors E, Comarr AE: Neurological disturbances of sexual function with special reference to 529 patients with spinal cord injury, *Urol Surv* 110:191-221, 1960.)

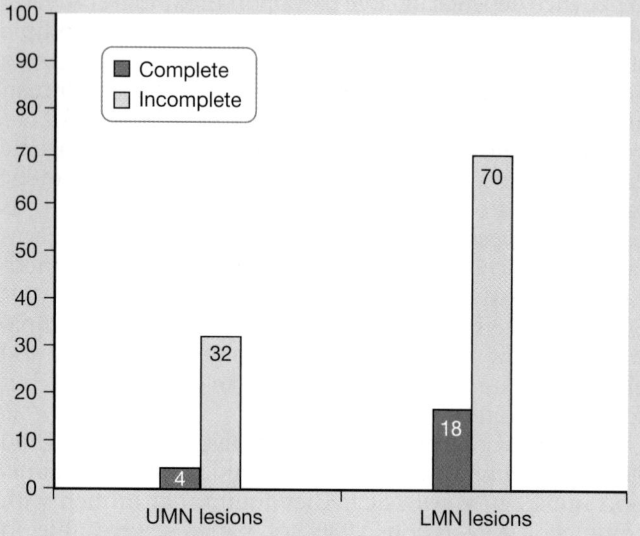

FIGURE 22-3 Percentage of men with spinal cord injury able to achieve anterograde ejaculation. *LMN*, Lower motor neuron; *UMN*, upper motor neuron. (Data from Bors E, Comarr AE: Neurological disturbances of sexual function with special reference to 529 patients with spinal cord injury, *Urol Surv* 110:191-221, 1960.)

Orgasmic ability has been shown to be preserved in 38% to 50% of men with complete UMN SCI, 78% to 84% of men with incomplete UMN injury, and 0% of men with complete LMN injury.[4,5,154,190] It should be noted, however, that a majority of studies on men have focused on ability to ejaculate instead of ability to have an orgasm, which have more recently been noted to be separate occurrences.[5] Some men are also occasionally able to achieve orgasm without anterograde ejaculation, possibly indicating either anejaculation or retrograde ejaculation into the bladder.[190]

Women with SCI have been shown to have similar sexual responses to men, with arousal and vaginal lubrication as the female correlate to penile erection.[56,194,195] In women with complete UMN injuries, reflexogenic but not psychogenic lubrication is preserved.[56,195] Sensation to light touch and pinprick in the T11-L2 dermatomes was found to be predictive of the ability for psychogenic vaginal lubrication, which is thought to be sympathetically mediated.[56,194] From 44% to 54% of women with SCI have been shown to be able to achieve orgasm, although orgasm is much less likely in women with LMN injuries affecting the S3-S5 segments.[49,56,101,193,194]

Fertility in men with SCI is impaired, in part because of a decreased ability to ejaculate.[158] Semen quality has also been found to be poor in men with SCI, with decreased sperm motility, decreased mitochondrial activity, and increased sperm DNA fragmentation.[161] Reasons for altered semen quality have been postulated to include seminal fluid stasis, testicular hyperthermia, recurrent genitourinary tract infections, and hormonal dysfunction.[161] After initial postinjury decline, semen quality appears to plateau in the chronic postinjury period.[37,99] Fertility in women with SCI is preserved once menstruation resumes, on average about 5 months postinjury.[12] Family planning counseling should include these post-SCI fertility considerations.

Stroke

Stroke is the world's second leading cause of death and the leading cause of adult disability.[51] Sexual dysfunction is a common finding after stroke in both men and women. The most common findings for men are erectile and ejaculatory dysfunction (in 40% to 50%) and decreased sexual drive.[47,103,115,128,203] Women tend to experience decreased sexual drive, decreased vaginal lubrication (in approximately 50%), decreased orgasm (in approximately 20% to 30%), and decreased overall sexual satisfaction.[47,111,115,128,203] Prevalence of decreased sexual drive has been reported to be between approximately 25% to 50% in both genders after stroke, with similar effects in spouses.[111,115] Stroke also leads to significantly decreased frequency of sexual activity in both genders, and in one study, approximately 50% of stroke survivors reported no sexual activity whatsoever by 1 year poststroke.[82,115,203]

The physical effects of stroke that contribute to sexual dysfunction include hemiparesis with its effect on body positioning and movement, hemineglect, hemianopsia, neurogenic bowel and bladder, and spasticity.[144,158] Not much is known about the functional neuroanatomy of sexual behavior and control, but some studies have indicated that the right cerebral hemisphere may play a more important role in sexual functioning than the left side.[54,80,103] Many studies have suggested that sexual dysfunction following stroke is related to the presence of medical comorbidities (cardiac disease, diabetes, hypercholesterolemia, depression), medications, and psychosocial factors (inability to discuss sexuality with the partner, unwillingness for sexual activity, fear of another stroke, sexuality being unimportant) rather than the direct effect of stroke.*

Traumatic Brain Injury

The prevalence of sexual dysfunction after traumatic brain injury (TBI) has been reported at 4% to 71%, a wide range that is likely to represent the limited number of quality studies and the varied types and severities of injury that are possible.[177] In a recent TBI model systems multicenter study of post-TBI community-dwelling individuals, 20% met criteria for sexual dysfunction.[178] Greater impairments were correlated with female gender, older age, higher TBI severity, and decreased social participation.[178] Although sexual dysfunction prevalence and type may be associated with both global and focal brain tissue injury, previous studies have not shown a consistent relationship to injury severity and sexual dysfunction.[35,158,177] Types of sexual dysfunction reported have been similar to those seen in stroke patients, including reduced sexual desire and frequency of sexual activity in both genders, ED and ejaculatory dysfunction in men, and dyspareunia, anorgasmia, and reduced lubrication in women.[95,116,158,177,178] In addition, brain injury can cause hypersexual behavior, such as excessive masturbation. This can occur in particular with injury to the limbic system or prefrontal regions, which can cause disinhibition; or to bilateral temporal poles, which produces the Klüver-Bucy syndrome of hypersexuality and hyperorality.[40,123,189] This can be treated with

*References 47, 50, 82, 103, 111, 115, 158.

anticonvulsants, such as Depakote, but it is important to remember that such medications can also greatly contribute to the sexual dysfunction witnessed after brain injury.[84] Psychosocial factors seems to play a major role in sexual functioning after brain injury, with the presence of depression being the most sensitive indicator for sexual dysfunction.[95] Other important psychological factors include perceived health status and quality of life, low self-esteem, anxiety, and perceived decline in personal sex appeal.[95,118]

Multiple Sclerosis

Multiple sclerosis (MS)-induced sexual dysfunction is present in 40% to 80% of women and 50% to 90% of men.[65] Historically, the sexual disorders have been attributed directly to the location and duration of the spinal cord or brain lesion, but more recent research tends to describe a multitude of other factors that also contribute to the development of sexual dysfunction in MS.[41,121,198]

In MS, sexual dysfunction is now conceptualized into three levels of dysfunction.[41] Primary sexual dysfunction relates to neurologic impairments in libido, lubrication, and orgasm. Secondary sexual dysfunction includes the effects of fatigue and physical limitations on sexual expression. Physical limitations may include bowel and bladder dysfunction, weakness, incoordination, positioning and body control during sexual encounters, numbness, paresthesias, pain, and cognitive impairment.[121,198] Tertiary sexual dysfunction reflects the psychological, emotional, social, and cultural implications of MS on sexual function. Psychosocial factors contributing to tertiary sexual dysfunction include poor self-image, poor self-esteem, fear of isolation and abandonment, shame, dependency on one's partner to provide for one's basic needs, and depression.[179,198] Additionally, side effects of medication management may contribute to sexual dysfunction.

Women with MS tend to have decreased sexual desire, anorgasmia, decreased vaginal lubrication, and increased spasticity with sexual activity.[58,97,158] Many of these symptoms are thought to be related to the decreased genital sensitivity experienced by 62% of women with advanced MS.[97] Men with MS have ED, ejaculatory dysfunction (premature, delayed, or absent), orgasmic dysfunction, decreased genital sensation, and decreased sexual drive.[58,158] In one study, sexual dysfunction in men with MS was found to be correlated with lower-limb disability and bladder dysfunction, whereas in women, sexual disorders were most strongly correlated with fatigue.[77] Women report more symptoms of sexual dysfunction, whereas men report more dissatisfaction with sexual function.[41,148]

Other Neurologic Disorders

Parkinson disease (PD) is often associated with low testosterone levels and therefore decreased sexual drive.[144] In one study of young men with PD (ages 36 to 56 years), up to 40% had low sexual desire.[211] Men with PD also can experience ED and premature or delayed ejaculation.[42,158] In women, decreased lubrication and involuntary urination can occur during intercourse.[42] Treatment with dopamine and dopamine agonist medications, by contrast, have been documented to cause hypersexual behavior, which often accompanies mania.[206] Hypersexuality has also been described with deep brain stimulation of the subthalamic nucleus.[162]

Peripheral neuropathy can cause sexual dysfunction, particularly when the etiology is diabetes, amyloid, and some of the inherited neuropathies with urogenital symptoms as prominent early features.[158] Guillain-Barré syndrome has been linked to ED when there is residual neurologic deficit or disability after recovery.[46]

Chronic Pain

The reasons for sexual dysfunction in patients with chronic pain are multifactorial, often related to physiologic, pharmacologic, and psychological factors.[151] In one study, 73% of patients with chronic pain had pain-related difficulty with sexual activity. The reasons for this included decreased arousal, positioning issues, exacerbations of pain, low confidence, performance worries, and relationship issues.[8] In another study, sexual problems were reported in 46% of patients with low back pain.[69] Women with low back pain have been shown to have decreased frequency of sexual activity, more pain during sexual intercourse, and decreased sexual desire compared with men with low back pain or patients of either gender with neck pain.[126] Sexual dysfunction in patients with chronic pain has been correlated most strongly with the presence of depression, poor coping skills, and shorter pain duration.[119] Many of the medications used to treat chronic pain (including opioids, antidepressants, and anticonvulsants) can independently contribute to sexual dysfunction.[204]

Rheumatologic Disease

Osteoarthritis (OA) impacts sexual function primarily through associated joint pain, stiffness, and fatigue, and the hip joint is the most often implicated in leading to sexual difficulties.[32,57,144] Total hip replacement often significantly improves sexual functioning; in one study, 65% of patients found relief from sexual difficulties after the surgery.[201] It is important to instruct patients in proper positioning after joint replacement to reduce the risk of dislocation, and many surgeons instruct patients to refrain from sexual intercourse for 1 to 2 months after hip replacement for this reason.[192]

Rheumatoid arthritis (RA), similar to OA, can cause problems in sexual functioning through joint pain, stiffness, and fatigue.[146] RA in men has also been shown to be associated with decreased sexual desire and ED during periods of active inflammation.[87] One study of women with RA identified 62% with difficulties in sexual performance caused by joint pain and stiffness and 92% with diminished sexual desire or satisfaction.[2] Difficulties in sexual performance were related to overall level of disability and hip involvement, whereas decreased sexual desire and satisfaction were correlated more with perceived pain, age, and depression.

Amputation

Patients with limb amputation usually have preserved sexual genital functioning (unless a comorbid condition, such as diabetes or cardiac disease, or the side effects of their medications play a significant detrimental role).[98] But their sexual life can be significantly affected by a variety of factors associated with their amputation, including depression, poor self-esteem and body image, phantom sensations and pain, problems with balance and movement, and difficulties with body positioning during sexual activity.[184] Preservation of the knee joint can be helpful for maintaining balance during sexual intercourse, although transfemoral amputees can use a pillow to aid in positioning.[44] Upper limb amputees would benefit from side-lying or supine positioning to allow for free movement of both the intact arm and the residual limb.[192] Sexual dissatisfaction ranges from 13% to 75% among amputees, with increased levels of sexual dysfunction despite preserved sexual desire, and therefore deserves increased focus during postamputation reintegration counseling.[34,79,98]

Diabetes Mellitus

Diabetes mellitus (DM) is one of the major comorbidities affecting people with disabilities, as its presence is a significant risk factor for subsequent stroke and amputation. DM plays a clear role in the development of sexual dysfunction in men. ED is three times more common in men with DM than in the general population, with prevalence estimates ranging from 35% to 75%.[26,127,198] Premature ejaculation and hypoactive sexual desire disorder have also been documented in 40% and 25%, respectively, of men with diabetes.[127] Diabetes-related sexual dysfunction in men is strongly correlated with glycemic control, duration of disease, and burden of diabetic complications.[26] The pathogenesis of sexual dysfunction in DM is likely to be multifactorial, including vasculopathy, autonomic neuropathy, and diminished nitric oxide production, which leads to decreased neurogenic vasodilation.[11,198]

Diabetes in women has a much less clear effect on sexual functioning, as research is limited and at times contradictory.[144] The most commonly reported condition is sexual arousal disorder, with its accompanying decreased vaginal lubrication.[11] Low sexual desire, decreased clitoral sensation, orgasmic dysfunction, and dyspareunia have also been infrequently reported.[48] Factors for the development of sexual dysfunction in women with diabetes have been analyzed, and a far different picture has emerged than for men with diabetes. In women, there has been no documented correlation with diabetic complications, length of disability, or level of glycemic control.[11,71,72] A recent meta-analysis demonstrated a relationship between sexual function and elevated body mass index.[155] Associations have been previously shown for cardiovascular comorbidity, depression, and age.[209]

Cardiac Disease

Cardiovascular disease is another common comorbidity in patients with disabilities. Hypertension, coronary artery disease, and congestive heart failure have all been associated with increased prevalence of sexual dysfunction.[28,33,198] Hypertension is the most prevalent comorbidity among men with ED.[45,198] ED has been noted in 40% to 95% of men with hypertension and is correlated with duration of hypertensive disease.[74,140] Control of blood pressure often leads to restoration of erectile function.[144] ED is also common in cardiac disease, with a prevalence of 42% to 75%.[157] ED is often one of the earliest indicators of cardiovascular disease, and men (with or without disabilities) who present with ED with no obvious cause should be worked up for this potentially deadly comorbidity.[198] It has been reported that 25% to 63% of women with cardiac disease experience sexual dysfunction, including decreased sexual desire, vaginal dryness, dyspareunia, decreased genital sensation, and decreased orgasmic ability.[3,28,198]

Cardiac disease, especially after myocardial infarction has been sustained, is often associated with depression and anxiety, which contribute to sexual dysfunction.[78,86,163] Other psychological factors that are likely to play a role include fear of recurrence of cardiac symptoms or fear of death with resumption of sexual activity.[93] Cardiovascular deaths during sexual intercourse are actually very rare, with the rate in men estimated to be 0.2 per 100,000 and the risk in women 12 times lower than in men.[153]

Many cardiovascular medications (including antihypertensives and digoxin) have been known to contribute to the sexual dysfunction seen in cardiac disease.[204]

Depression

Depression is one of the most common comorbidities in patients with all types of disabilities, and it has been shown to contribute to sexual dysfunction in a variety of ways, including medical, pharmacologic, and psychosocial.[52] There has been intense research and publicity about the sexual side effects of antidepressant medications, but untreated depression has also been strongly correlated with sexual dysfunction.[182] Clinically, it can be difficult to distinguish whether a patient's sexual dysfunction is secondary to the depression itself or to the antidepressant medication.[14] In one study of 134 patients with major depressive disorder who were not taking any medication to treat their illness, hypoactive sexual desire was seen in 40% to 50% of men and women, decreased arousal was observed in 40% of women, ED was seen in 50% of men, and ejaculatory or orgasmic dysfunction was seen in 15% to 20% of men and women.[109] Psychosocial factors in patients with depression that are likely to play a role in the development of sexual dysfunction include interpersonal relationship difficulties and poor body image and self-esteem.[52]

Sexual Dysfunction Related to Medication Use in Individuals with Disability

Sexual dysfunction is a common side effect of many medications used routinely in patients with disabilities. It is important for the physician to maintain open communication with patients, understand these sexual side effects, and explain the risks to patients before prescribing these drugs. If sexual dysfunction occurs secondary to the use of a medication, it is often necessary to switch to a

Table 22-2 Medications and Sexual Dysfunction*

Drug Category	Drug Class†	Impact on Sexual Function (most common listed first)
Cardiac	Diuretics (**thiazides, spironolactone,** loop diuretics, chlorthalidone)	ED, decreased sexual desire, impaired ejaculation, retrograde ejaculation
	Centrally acting sympatholytics (clonidine, α-methyldopa)	ED, decreased sexual desire
	β-Blockers	ED, decreased sexual desire (men and women)
	α-Blockers (prazosin, terazosin)	ED, priapism (rare), retrograde ejaculation
	Vasodilators (hydralazine)	Priapism (rare)
	Antiarrhythmics (**digoxin,** disopyramide)	ED, decreased sexual desire
	Anticholesterolemics (statins, fibrates, niacin)	ED, decreased sexual desire
Psychiatric	**Selective serotonin reuptake inhibitors (SSRIs)**	Ejaculatory dysfunction, anorgasmia (men and women), decreased sexual desire (men and women), ED
	Serotonin-norepinephrine reuptake inhibitors (SNRIs)	ED, decreased sexual desire
	Tricyclic antidepressants (TCAs)	decreased sexual desire, ED
	Trazodone	Priapism
	Antipsychotics	Decreased sexual drive (men and women), ejaculatory/orgasmic dysfunction, ED, priapism
	Benzodiazepines	Orgasmic dysfunction (women), delayed ejaculation, decreased sexual desire
	Neurostimulants (methylphenidate, amantadine)	Hypersexual behavior
Gastrointestinal	**H_2-blockers** (especially **cimetidine**)	ED, decreased sexual desire, painful erections, gynecomastia
	Proton pump inhibitors	ED, gynecomastia
	Metoclopramide	Decreased sexual drive, ED
Other	Baclofen (especially **intrathecal baclofen**)	Ejaculatory dysfunction, ED, decreased orgasmic function (men and women)
	Gabapentin, pregabalin and other anticonvulsants **(phenytoin)**	Ejaculatory dysfunction, anorgasmia (men and women), and decreased sexual desire (men and women)
	Opioids	Decreased sexual desire, anorgasmia, ED, hypogonadism
	Tramadol	Delayed ejaculation
	NSAIDs	ED
	Corticosteroids	Decreased sexual desire
	Methotrexate	ED, decreased sexual desire, gynecomastia

*From references 24, 29, 53, 59, 88, 134, 139, 176, 187, 200, 204, 207, 212.
†The medications that cause sexual side effects most commonly are listed in boldface.
ED, Erectile disorder/dysfunction; *NSAIDs,* nonsteroidal antiinflammatory drugs.

different class of medications to regain the function that has been lost or altered. Another alternative, especially in men, is to use a medication, such as a phosphodiesterase-5 (PDE-5) inhibitor, to counteract the sexual side effects of the initial medication. Table 22-2 presents an overview of the sexual dysfunctions associated with various classes of medications commonly encountered in a physiatry practice.[24,139,204] The medications that cause sexual side effects most commonly are listed in boldface in Table 22-2. It should be noted that a majority of the research in this area has been focused on male sexual dysfunction; therefore, less is known about the effects of these medications on sexuality in women.

Evaluation of Sexual Dysfunction

Sexual History Taking

The idea of obtaining a sexual history can be daunting to some physicians. Remember that patients' quality of life can be significantly improved if their physicians are unafraid to discuss this topic with them. Because sexuality is a sensitive topic, it is best to maintain an attitude of openness and flexibility throughout the interview. There are multiple validated tools for assessing sexual dysfunction.[114] "ALLOW," "PLISSIT," and "BETTER" models are three different approaches for facilitating such a conversation (Box 22-2).[76,90,96]

When asking a patient about sexual dysfunction, it is important to assess the nature of the problem and the time course of the complaint (including whether it started in relation to a certain disability, medical comorbidity, or medication administration). It is equally vital to ascertain whether the patient is experiencing dissatisfaction or disruption of quality of life as a result of the sexual dysfunction. The Brief Sexual Symptom Checklist is a self-report tool that can be a useful adjunct to the physician's comprehensive sexual history (Figure 22-4).[90]

A thorough inquiry into the patient's sexual dysfunction also includes obtaining information about the medical, sexual, and psychosocial history of the patient.[90,106] The basic medical history includes both medical and surgical history, medication use (including over-the-counter and herbal medications), substance use (including smoking, alcohol abuse, and recreational drug use), and family medical history.[76] Important medical conditions to inquire about include cardiovascular disease, diabetes, hypertension, hyperlipidemia, cancer, benign prostatic hypertrophy or the presence of lower urinary tract symptoms, neurologic diseases (e.g., SCI, MS, TBI, stroke), thyroid conditions, and endocrine deficiencies (e.g., hypogonadism, androgen insufficiency, or estrogen deficiency).[27,90,112,180] In women, it is also necessary to ask about reproductive

BOX 22-2

ALLOW, PLISSIT, and BETTER Models for Facilitating Communication About Sexuality

A—**Ask** the patient about sexual function and activity.
L—**Legitimize** the patient's problem and acknowledge that sexual dysfunction is a relevant clinical issue.
L—**Limitations** in the evaluation of the sexual dysfunction should be identified.
O—**Open up** the discussion: Potentially refer the patient to a subspecialist.
W—**Work together** to develop goals and a treatment plan.

P—**Permission** should be obtained from the patient to discuss sexuality.
LI—**Limited Information** should be given (e.g., about normal sexual functioning and effects of disability).
SS—**Specific Suggestions** should be given about the patient's particular complaint.
IT—**Intensive Therapy** may be required, including referral to a subspecialist or therapist.

B—**Bring up** the topic of sexuality.
E—**Explain** that sexuality is important and that you are open to discussion of it with your patient.
T—**Tell** your patient about resources that you will use to assist them.
T—**Time** the discussion to the patient's preference.
E—**Educate** the patient about the side effects of treatment medications and the disability itself.
R—**Record** that you had a conversation about sexuality in the patient's medical record.

Data from Frank JE, Mistretta P, Will J: Diagnosis and treatment of female sexual dysfunction, *Am Fam Physician* 77:635-645, 2008; Hatzichristou D, Rosen RC, Broderick G, et al: Clinical evaluation and management strategy for sexual dysfunction in men and women, *J Sex Med* 2004; 1:49-57,2004; Hordern A: Intimacy and sexuality after cancer: a critical review of the literature, *Cancer Nurs* 31:E9-E17, 2008.

history, history of gynecologic disease (e.g., fibroids or endometriosis), and current menstrual status.[112]

The basic sexual history includes age of first sexual experience, types of sexual practices, gender of partners, history of sexually transmitted diseases, inquiry into safe sex practices, and type of birth control used.[15] It should never be assumed that the patient is heterosexual, and gender-neutral terms (such as "partner" or "spouse" instead of "boyfriend" or "wife") are preferable until the issue has been clarified by the patient.[15,106]

The psychosocial history relevant to sexual dysfunction includes a history of depression, anxiety, disordered sleep, or other psychiatric illness.[27] Major life stressors and relationship dynamics should be discussed.[90,112] Any history of abuse (physical, sexual, verbal, or emotional), sexual trauma, or domestic violence should also be sensitively explored.[106]

Physical Examination

Although physical examination findings can be normal in patients with sexual dysfunction, it is important to do a thorough evaluation to identify pathology as well as provide patient education about what is normal for their disability or disease state.[76] A comprehensive examination includes height, weight, and vital signs; auscultation of the heart and lungs; examination of the thyroid, lymph nodes, breasts, and abdomen; a check of peripheral pulses; evaluation for lower extremity edema; a neurologic examination; and a thorough genital examination.[180,215] In particular, it is important to look for signs of cardiovascular disease (obesity, hypertension, diminished peripheral pulses, lower extremity edema) and endocrinopathies (thyromegaly, gynecomastia).[27]

The neurologic examination should include mental status, motor and sensory testing; measurement of the range of motion of joints; and evaluation of muscle tone, coordination, and reflexes.[215] Range-of-motion measurements of the hips, knees, shoulders, and hands are particularly important. It is necessary to note whether the patient has UMN or LMN findings. Sensory testing should include light touch, pinprick, and proprioception in the lower limbs.[215] Paying particular attention to the sensory evaluation of T11-L2 and S2-S5 is especially important because they represent the sympathetic and parasympathetic outflow tracts.[194,215] Reflexes should be checked in the upper and lower limbs. The anal wink and bulbocavernosus reflexes both evaluate the integrity of the pudendal nerve and should be performed in both men and women.[180,215]

In men, the genital examination consists of examining the penis for lesions and urethral position.[180] The penis should also be palpated in the stretched position to detect fibrous plaques consistent with Peyronie disease (an acquired disorder of the tunica albuginea characterized by the formation of fibrous tissue and often accompanied by penile pain and deformity on erection).[27] The testes should be checked for size, masses, and position, and the rectum evaluated for sphincter tone, pelvic floor muscle tenderness and strength, prostate size, masses, and lesions.[180,215]

In the genital examination of women, it is important to check the appearance of external genitalia, looking for inflammation or atrophy of the vulva, episiotomy or childbirth laceration scarring or strictures, and external dermatologic lesions.[106,112] A vaginal examination with one or two fingers inserted into the vagina is a good way to assess many of the common problems associated with female sexual dysfunction.[215] Vaginismus can be appreciated by resistance or inability to insert a finger into the vagina.[106] Tenderness of the levator ani and obturator internus muscles can be assessed, as well as pelvic floor muscle strength, coordination, and hypotonicity or hypertonicity.[76,215] The presence of pelvic organ prolapse should be noted.[106] Bimanual examination can be performed to assess for uterine and adnexal abnormalities, including tenderness and masses.[106,112] Rectal examination should also be performed to assess for anal sphincter muscle tone, pelvic floor muscle tenderness, and voluntary and involuntary pelvic floor muscle contraction and relaxation ability.[215]

In both genders, the physician should check for signs of infection or sexually transmitted diseases, including discharge, rashes, or ulcerations.[106]

Diagnostic Evaluation

A large number of laboratory tests, as well as specialized diagnostic procedures, can be used to determine the

Brief sexual symptom checklist: men's version

Please answer the following questions about your overall sexual function in the past **3 months** or more.

1. Are you satisfied with your sexual function?
   ☐ Yes ☐ No
   If no, please continue.
2. How long have you been dissatisfied with your sexual function?
   ____
3a. The problem(s) with your sexual function is: (mark one or more)
   ☐ 1 Problems with little or no interest in sex
   ☐ 2 Problems with erection
   ☐ 3 Problems with ejaculating too early during sexual activity
   ☐ 4 Problems taking too long, or not being able to ejaculate or have orgasm
   ☐ 5 Problems with pain during sex
   ☐ 6 Problems with penile curvature during erection
   ☐ 7 Other:
3b. Which problem is most bothersome (circle) 1 2 3 4 5 6 7
4. Would you like to talk about it with your doctor?
   ☐ Yes ☐ No

Brief sexual symptom checklist: women's version

Please answer the following questions about your overall sexual function in the past **3 months** or more.

1. Are you satisfied with your sexual function?
   ☐ Yes ☐ No
   If no, please continue.
2. How long have you been dissatisfied with your sexual function?
   ____
3a. The problem(s) with your sexual function is: (mark one or more)
   ☐ 1 Problems with little or no interest in sex
   ☐ 2 Problems with decreased genital sensation (feeling)
   ☐ 3 Problems with decreased vaginal lubrication (dryness)
   ☐ 4 Problems reaching orgasm
   ☐ 5 Problems with pain during sex
   ☐ 6 Other:
3b. Which problem is most bothersome (circle) 1 2 3 4 5 6
4. Would you like to talk about it with your doctor?
   ☐ Yes ☐ No

FIGURE 22-4 The Brief Sexual Symptom Checklist for men and women. (Redrawn from Hatzichristou D, Rosen RC, Broderick G, et al: Clinical evaluation and management strategy for sexual dysfunction in men and women, *J Sex Med* 1:49-57, 2004.)

pathologic origin of a patient's sexual dysfunction. In general, however, the selection of treatment options is based on the presenting complaint and not the etiology behind the sexual dysfunction. Consequently, complicated diagnostic testing is usually unnecessary. Recommended laboratory testing for all men and women with sexual dysfunction includes complete blood cell count, chemistry panel, fasting glucose, and fasting lipid profile.[90,106,143] Other laboratory testing can be warranted based on history and physical examination findings, including thyroid studies and serum free testosterone, prolactin, and prostate-specific antigen levels.[7,27,90,145,180] Measurement of other sex hormones, such as estrogen, follicle-stimulating hormone, luteinizing hormone, or total testosterone, has been shown to have far less utility in a majority of cases.[7,145] In women, androgen levels do not correlate with sexual dysfunction and are not currently recommended for diagnosis.[62,114] Vaginal wet mount testing or screens for gonorrhea, chlamydia, or human immunodeficiency virus can be done if infection is clinically suspected.[106]

For men with ED, a variety of specialized diagnostic procedures are used to determine the specific etiology of disease, usually in preparation for surgical treatment.[90] The use of these tests has declined since the advent of oral PDE-5 inhibitor medications, with their ease of use, high level of effectiveness, and low side effect profile. The procedures include penile color duplex ultrasound, nocturnal penile tumescence monitoring, pharmacoarteriography, pharmacocavernosometry or pharmacocavernosography (PHCAS or PHCAG), and electrodiagnostic testing.[81] Penile color duplex ultrasound is the most practical and commonly used diagnostic modality. It is a good tool to diagnose vasculogenic ED and is minimally invasive.[81] Nocturnal penile tumescence monitoring measures sleep-related erections and has traditionally been used to distinguish psychogenic and organic ED.[81,90] Penile pharmacoarteriography, PHCAS or PHCAG, and electrodiagnostic testing, such as dorsal nerve stimulation or somatosensory evoked potentials, are more invasive and time-consuming and are rarely used.[81,197]

In women, pelvic ultrasound can be indicated if uterine or adnexal pathologic disorders are suspected. The use of objective measures of genital blood flow, as measured by vaginal photoplethysmography, and advanced imaging techniques, such as functional magnetic resonance imaging, are currently primarily limited to the research setting.[7,120]

Treatment of Sexual Dysfunction

Male Hypoactive Sexual Desire Disorder

Limited research has been done on hypoactive sexual desire disorder in men, and thus little is known about treatment options. Secondary hypoactive sexual desire in men is thought to develop most frequently in response to another type of sexual dysfunction, usually ED or premature ejaculation.[133] It follows that treatment of the primary sexual dysfunction would improve desire. Secondary hypoactive sexual desire disorder is also often related to medication side effects, and thus changing the drug dose or category will often improve the patient's sexual drive. Primary hypoactive sexual desire is thought to typically relate to a "sexual secret," such as a variant arousal pattern (e.g., a man who is aroused by Internet pornography but not by his partner), a preference for masturbatory sex over partner sex, a history of poorly processed sexual trauma, or conflict about sexual orientation.[133] Treating these psychosocial factors and getting the patient to be honest with himself and his partner about his true motivations will be helpful.

Hypogonadism and low testosterone levels certainly contribute to hypoactive sexual desire in men, and treatment with testosterone supplementation is beneficial.[138] It is less clear whether treatment with testosterone in eugonadal men with hypoactive sexual desire disorder can improve their sexual drive, but at least two studies have shown this to be the case.[13,150]

Erectile Dysfunction

The treatment of ED was revolutionized in 1998 with the Food and Drug Administration (FDA) approval of sildenafil, the first of the now ubiquitous PDE-5 inhibitors, which have low side effect profiles and excellent efficacy across the spectrum of disease states that cause ED.[125] There are four PDE-5 inhibitors currently approved for use in the United States: sildenafil (Viagra), vardenafil (Levitra), tadalafil (Cialis), and avanafil (Stendra). Avanafil received FDA approval in 2012 and may prove to have the earliest onset of action of available PDE-5 inhibitors.[156] Other new PDE-5 inhibitors, such as lodenafil, udenafil, and mirodenafil, have shown promise in metaanalyses of recent clinical trials and are currently available for use in a few countries.[67,68,91,156]

Sildenafil and vardenafil have similar pharmacokinetics, with onset of action within 30 to 120 minutes and duration of efficacy of 4 to 5 hours.[70] Tadalafil has an onset of action of 30 to 60 minutes and duration of efficacy of 12 to 36 hours.[70] High-fat intake is known to significantly affect the action of sildenafil and vardenafil.[156] Tadalafil has been approved for on-demand or daily dosing and is effective for the concomitant treatment of symptoms related to ED and benign prostatic hyperplasia.[156] PDE-5 inhibitors have been studied and proven effective in patients with cardiovascular disease, hypertension, diabetes, SCI, MS, and depression.[70,156] These medications have been reported to significantly improve erectile function as evidenced by successful vaginal penetration in as many as 79% to 87% of patients.[156] Men with SCI achieve 80% success rates.[63,83]

Side effects reported with PDE-5 inhibitors include headache, flushing, rhinitis, back pain, and hearing loss.[70] Nonarteritic anterior ischemic optic neuropathy (NAION) has been reported but to date no causal link has been confirmed to PDE-5 inhibitor use.[156] These medications are strictly contraindicated in patients taking nitrates for chest pain.[125] In the setting of documented underlying hypogonadism, concurrent treatment with testosterone replacement therapy increases the effectiveness of PDE-5 inhibitors.[143,156]

PDE-5 inhibitors are known to be less effective in patients with very severe ED, uncontrolled diabetes with neuropathy, severe vascular disease, and in those who have undergone radical prostatectomy. Currently, few other oral agents show treatment benefit. Those available include sublingual apomorphine and yohimbine.[125] Bremelanotide, a melanocortin receptor agonist, was efficacious in multiple clinical trials, including those in patients who had been unsuccessfully treated with sildenafil.[174,183] Development was halted, however, as a result of blood pressure side effects. Future oral therapies potentially include other melanocortin receptor agonists, dopamine receptor agonists, L-arginine, and Rho-kinase inhibitors.[91,156]

Second-line treatments after PDE-5 inhibitor treatment failure include intracavernosal injection therapy, intraurethral alprostadil (medicated urethral system for erection [MUSE]) therapy, topical alprostadil, and vacuum constriction devices.

Intracavernosal penile injections have been used for decades with treatment satisfaction rates of 87% to 93.5%, relatively low adverse effects, and rapid onset of action (Figure 22-5).[70,125] However, considerable training is required for effective use. High discontinuation rates have been noted secondary to penile pain and complications that can occur include priapism and Peyronie disease.[70] The most commonly injected medications include various combinations of FDA-approved alprostadil and the "off-label" use of papaverine and phentolamine.[125]

Intraurethral treatment of alprostadil with the MUSE system can be an alternative in patients who cannot take PDE-5 inhibitors and who do not want to try more intracavernosal injection therapy (Figure 22-6). Its efficacy ranges from 37% to 53% and penile pain is a common complaint.[156] It is rarely associated with hypotension and syncope.[70,125] Topical alprostadil formulations are currently undergoing clinical trials with modest efficacy results, but this treatment is not currently recommended as

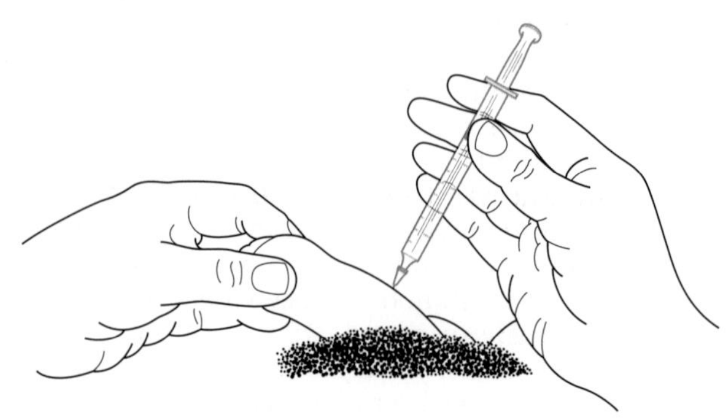

FIGURE 22-5 Penile injection.

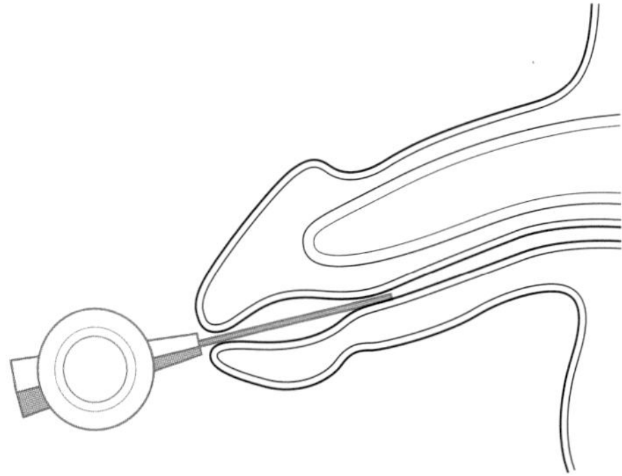

FIGURE 22-6 Intraurethral therapy.

monotherapy for ED.[156] Side effects include penile burning and partner vaginal pain.[91]

Vacuum constriction devices apply a negative pressure to draw blood into the corpora cavernosa, which is then retained by the application of a constriction band at the base of the penis (Figure 22-7).[125] Efficacy rates are as high as 90%, but satisfaction rates tend to be lower because of the unnatural appearance of the erection, penile pain, and trapped ejaculate.[70,156] Constriction devices are contraindicated in patients with a history of severe bleeding disorder, priapism, or severe penile curvature.[156] Anticoagulant therapy is a relative contraindication.[125] These devices are often preferred in men who do not want to take medications. The constriction band cannot be left in place longer than 30 minutes because of the risk of ischemia, especially in patients who are insensate, such as those with SCI.[70,156]

Third-line treatments for ED include surgical options, such as penile prostheses (Figure 22-8). Penile prostheses come in two types: semirigid (malleable) and inflatable. Semirigid prostheses have malleable silicone elastomer rods with central metal cables that can be bent or straightened to produce erection.[70] Inflatable prostheses have cylinders that are implanted into the corpora cavernosa, a reservoir with fluid, and a pump that is placed in the scrotum.[70] Erection is achieved by compressing the scrotal pump to transfer fluid from the reservoir to the cylinders.[70] Infection rates have been reduced to approximately 1% because of antibiotic and hydrophilic coatings that are now available on the prostheses.[70] Mechanical failure rates are 5% at 1 year, 20% by 5 years, and 50% at 10 years.[125]

Premature Ejaculation

The mainstay of treatment until recently for premature ejaculation was cognitive-behavioral therapy (CBT) and psychological counseling. Various CBT approaches include the start-pause and frenulum squeeze techniques, as well as experimentation with positioning, rhythm, speed, breathing, and depth of penile penetration.[6,152,169] These strategies have success rates of up to 70% in the short-term, but long-term treatment satisfaction has only been reported at 25% to 60%.[169] Cognitive-behavioral approaches to treatment are often very time-consuming, expensive, and perceived as intrusive and mechanistic, affecting intimacy and spontaneity during a sexual encounter.[152,169]

Although no medications are FDA-approved for the treatment of premature ejaculation, many pharmacologic approaches have been well studied and show significant benefit. (It should be noted that the following medications are "off-label" for the treatment of premature ejaculation.) Selective serotonin reuptake inhibitors (SSRIs) are the most commonly used medications for premature ejaculation, with paroxetine being the most effective, followed by fluoxetine and sertraline.[6,171] The tricyclic antidepressant (TCA) clomipramine has also been used successfully, but anticholinergic side effects limit its tolerance.[6,152] Both SSRIs and clomipramine are usually given daily because of their slow onset of action (5 hours), long half-lives, and

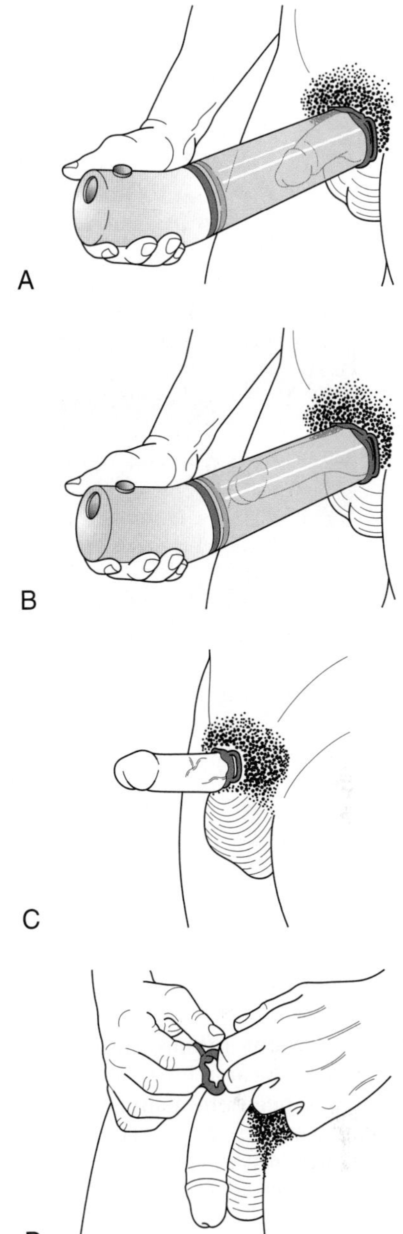

FIGURE 22-7 Use of a vacuum-assisted device. Patient instructions are as follows: **A,** Place your penis inside the cylinder and use the ErecAid system's specially designed pump to produce the vacuum that pulls blood into the penis. **B,** The vacuum allows you to create a near-natural erection within a few minutes. **C,** After you slip the tension ring off the cylinder and onto the base of your penis and remove the cylinder, you can safely and easily keep the erection for up to 30 minutes, using only the tension ring. **D,** Once you remove the tension ring, your penis returns to its soft state.

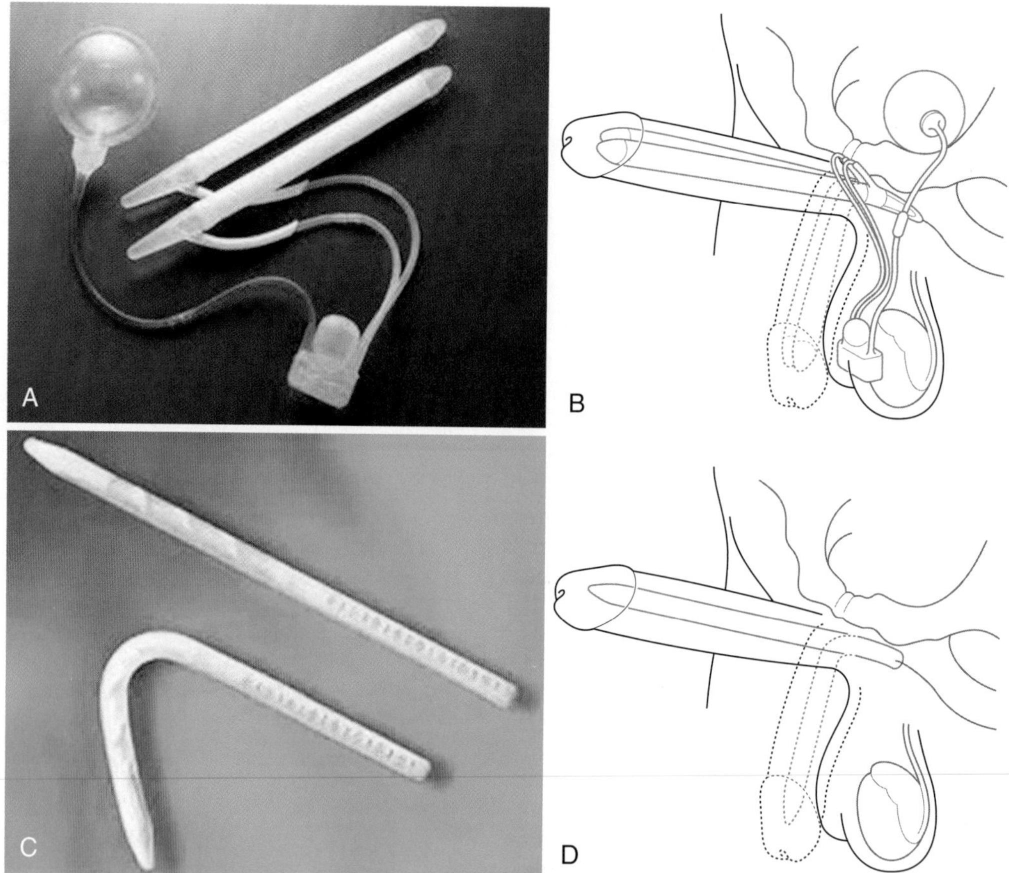

FIGURE 22-8 Penile prostheses. **A, B,** Inflatable. **C, D,** Malleable.

long treatment time (up to 4 weeks) to achieve a steady state.[6,152,171]

On-demand treatment for premature ejaculation has been the holy grail of research into this disorder, and some recent advances have been promising. Conventional SSRIs have been studied for "as needed" use, with less profound effects on IELT versus daily dosing.[6,171] Dapoxetine is a new, short-acting SSRI developed specifically for on-demand use for premature ejaculation. It achieves peak plasma concentration within 1 hour and has a half-life of 1.5 hours.[152] It has been shown to significantly increase IELT and improve patient satisfaction.[108,152] Dapoxetine has been approved for use in several countries but is not yet available in the United States.[6] Tramadol has also been shown to be an excellent on-demand treatment for premature ejaculation, with one study showing a 13-fold increase in mean time to ejaculation.[6,171,173,214] Longer-term safety studies and comparison to SSRIs are needed. Topical agents, such as lidocaine or EMLA cream, can be helpful by decreasing sensory perception in the penis, thereby prolonging ejaculation.[6,171] In the absence of concurrent ED, PDE-5 inhibitors are contraindicated in premature ejaculation treatment.[6]

Delayed Ejaculation, Anejaculation, and Anorgasmia in Men

Assisted ejaculation methods that have proved effective for fertility treatment in men with SCI, MS, and other disabilities include penile vibratory stimulation (PVS) and rectal probe electroejaculation (EEJ) (Figures 22-9 and 22-10).[199] PVS is the most commonly used technique because it is able to produce superior sperm quality, is more comfortable and preferable to patients, and can be used in a home setting.[38,55,161] PVS only produces ejaculation in 60% to 80% of cases, whereas EEJ is 80% to 100% successful.[161] EEJ is usually only used in patients in whom PVS has been unsuccessful, because it produces lower quality semen, must be conducted in a physician's office setting, and often requires the use of anesthesia to perform the procedure and retrieve ejaculate.[38,55,161] Chemically

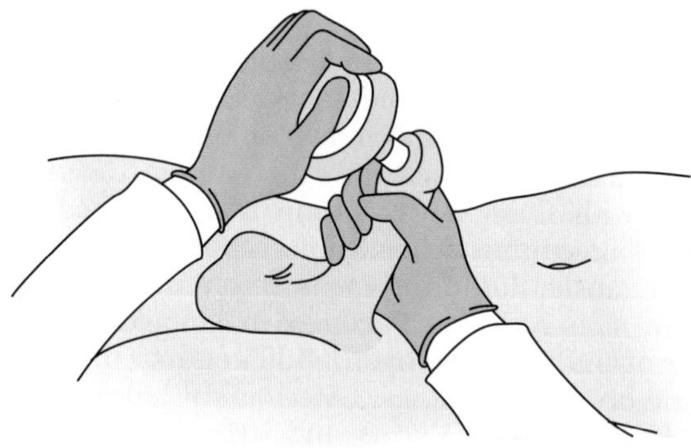

FIGURE 22-9 Vibrator disc position during penile vibratory stimulation. (Redrawn from Sonksen J, Ohl DA: Penile vibratory stimulation and electroejaculation in the treatment of ejaculatory dysfunction, *Int J Androl* 25:324, 2002.)

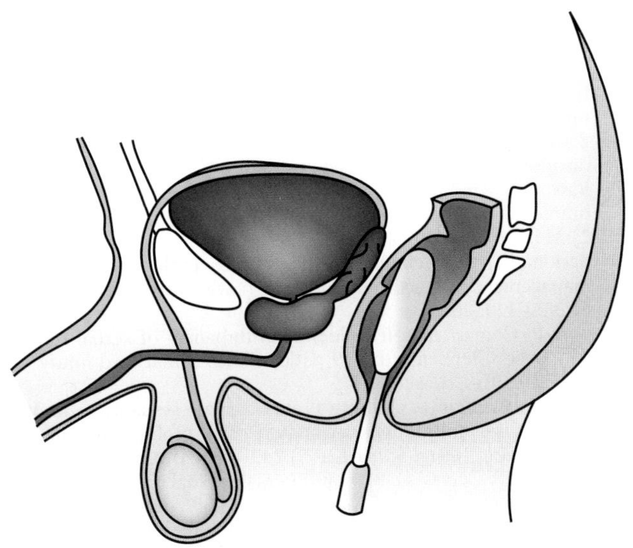

FIGURE 22-10 **Rectal probe position during an electroejaculation procedure.** (Redrawn from Sonksen J, Ohl DA: Penile vibratory stimulation and electroejaculation in the treatment of ejaculatory dysfunction, *Int J Androl* 25:324, 2002.)

assisted ejaculation is also a possibility, particularly with the use of midodrine to improve ejaculation success rates in combination with PVS.[55] Vardenafil has been shown to improve ejaculation rates in men with SCI.[83] Care must be taken to monitor blood pressure and look for signs of autonomic dysreflexia in men with SCI undergoing assisted ejaculation.[199]

Delayed ejaculation in men is much harder to treat when the goal is enhanced sexual function as opposed to fertility. Pharmacologic treatment for ejaculatory and orgasmic dysfunction in men is still largely unproved, although there have been some case series and small controlled trials with sildenafil, bupropion, amantadine, buspirone, cyproheptadine, and yohimbine that showed modest benefits.[135,136,141] Cognitive-behavioral modification and psychotherapy are indicated in men with psychogenic (situational or relational) orgasmic dysfunction.[125]

Female Sexual Interest/Arousal Disorder

When considering treatment for women with low sexual desire or arousal, it is important to remember that the sexual response cycle of women is very different from that of men. Many women experience only responsive, as opposed to spontaneous, sexual desire.[18] The first step in treating a woman with a complaint of low sexual desire is educating her as to what is normal for women, because there are many misconceptions fueled by popular culture about what a woman should feel.[76] Referring the patient to the work of Dr. Rosemary Basson may facilitate reassurance and improved understanding.[16-18]

Despite limited research, psychotherapy remains a mainstay for the treatment of female sexual interest/arousal disorder. In one of the few empirically tested outcome studies, mindfulness-based CBT improved sexual desire and arousal in gynecologic cancer survivors.[43] Sexual behavioral techniques, sex therapy, and couples counseling (originally conceived by Masters and Johnson[129]) have been shown to be beneficial by helping to reduce anxiety and exaggerated sexual expectations.[129,132]

The major pharmacologic treatment for female hypoactive sexual desire is testosterone therapy. Many treatment preparations are available, but a transdermal patch is the most commonly studied and prescribed method.[1] Many studies have confirmed the effectiveness of transdermal testosterone for increasing sexual desire and satisfaction in postmenopausal women or "surgically menopausal" women who have had bilateral oophorectomies.[39,73,186] Less robust data exist in premenopausal women, and potential fetal exposure remains a concern.[60,114] Side effects are usually related to masculinization, such as hirsutism and acne. The FDA has not approved the use of testosterone to treat female sexual interest/arousal disorder in women despite its effectiveness and relatively low side effect profile, largely because long-term safety data have not been established.[73] Theoretical concerns include effects on breast and endometrial cancer risks, as well as cardiovascular health. In a large phase 3 trial of transdermal testosterone gel, interim data demonstrated no increased adverse cardiovascular outcomes in postmenopausal women with preexisting cardiovascular risks.[61,213] Current available safety data, although not conclusive, are reassuring with regard to breast, endometrial, and cardiovascular outcomes.[61,114] Further research is necessary.

Other medications that show promise for treating female hypoactive sexual desire include tibolone (a synthetic steroid), melanocortins, flibanserin (a proposed serotonin receptor 5-HT_{1A} agonist/5-HT_{2A} antagonist), and combinations of testosterone with PDE-5 inhibitors or buspirone.[66,114,132,183]

Pharmacologic interventions for female arousal and lubrication disorders have been increasingly studied in recent years, with mixed results. Given that the physiology of female arousal should theoretically parallel that of male erectile function, there was much anticipation that sildenafil would prove to be a promising treatment option. Research trials have been largely disappointing, however, especially compared with the effectiveness of PDE-5 inhibitors in men with ED. The medication has been well tolerated, but the overall summation of research conducted to date does not show a benefit for sildenafil in most women with generalized arousal disorder without a known organic cause.[23,132,185] In women with disabilities, however, PDE-5 inhibitors remain a viable treatment option, because trials have been positive in limited, small populations of women with an acquired genital arousal disorder of an organic nature (premenopausal type 1 diabetics, women with SCI, patients with MS, and women taking SSRIs).[48,132,149,196] More research is needed on PDE-5 inhibitors in women, both with and without acquired disabilities.

Other medications have shown more promise than sildenafil for treating female arousal disorders in the general population, particularly in postmenopausal women. These include melanocortins, phentolamine, L-arginine, and alprostodil.* Acquired arousal disorder in postmenopausal women is often treated with systemic or local estrogen therapy to improve vaginal lubrication and

*References 66, 100, 110, 170, 172, 183.

blood flow.[113] Mechanical devices can also aid in increasing arousal, including vibratory stimulators and the Eros Clitoral Therapy Device, a clitoral vacuum that has been approved by the FDA to augment female arousal and orgasm.[30]

Female Orgasmic Dysfunction

Female orgasmic dysfunction in the absence of a concomitant arousal disorder is usually considered to be a psychogenic problem. Beneficial treatments include CBT (to focus on decreasing anxiety and promoting changes in attitudes and sexual thoughts), sensate focus therapy (which guides a woman and her partner through a series of exercises with increasing level of sexual intimacy), and directed masturbation (educating a woman that masturbation is healthy and normal and having her use self-stimulation to discover what is effective for her).[76,113] These behavioral treatments have been shown to be effective in 60% of women.[137] Bupropion has been shown in at least one study to help orgasmic dysfunction in women.[141] As with decreased arousal, mechanical devices can help with attainment of orgasm.[30]

Genito-Pelvic Pain/Penetration Disorder

Dyspareunia and vaginismus have a variety of organic and psychogenic causes, and proper treatment depends on etiology. Certainly, the diagnosis and treatment of any underlying pelvic pathology is of paramount importance. The treatment of pelvic floor dysfunction and vulvodynia, which are two of the major underlying pathologies contributing to genito-pelvic pain/penetration disorder, are expanded on in Chapter 38.

Conclusion

Disability does not diminish the importance of sexuality to the overall quality of an individual's life. A thorough understanding of the diagnosis and treatment of sexual dysfunction within the context of disability, and the willingness to be open to discussions about sexuality with patients will enable the physician to have a significant impact on quality of life and bring a measure of comfort and hope to those who need it most.

KEY REFERENCES

5. Alexander M, Rosen RC: Spinal cord injuries and orgasm: a review, *J Sex Marital Ther* 34(4):308–324, 2008.
6. Althof SE, Abdo CH, Dean J, et al: International Society for Sexual Medicine's guidelines for the diagnosis and treatment of premature ejaculation, *J Sex Med* 7(9):2947–2969, 2010.
7. Amato P: Categories of female sexual dysfunction, *Obstet Gynecol Clin N Am* 33(4):527–534, 2006.
10. American Psychiatric Association: *Diagnostic and statistical manual of mental disorders*, ed 5 (DSM-5), Arlington, 2013, American Psychiatric Publishing.
11. Aslan E, Fynes M: Female sexual dysfunction, *Int Urogynecol J Pelvic Floor Dysfunct* 19(2):293–305, 2008.
16. Basson R: The female sexual response: a different model, *J Sex Marital Ther* 26:51–65, 2000.
17. Basson R: Human sex-response cycles, *J Sex Marital Ther* 27:33–43, 2001.
18. Basson R: Using a different model for female sexual response to address women's problematic low sexual desire, *J Sex Marital Ther* 27(5):395–403, 2001.
21. Basson R, Althof S, Davis S, et al: Summary of the recommendations on sexual dysfunctions in women, *J Sex Med* 1(1):24–34, 2004.
24. Basson R, Weijmar Schultz W: Sexual sequelae of general medical disorders, *Lancet* 369(9559):409–424, 2007.
25. Basson R, Wierman ME, van Lankveld J, et al: Summary of the recommendations on sexual dysfunctions in women, *J Sex Med* 7(1 Pt 2):314–326, 2010.
27. Beckman TJ, Abu-Lebdeh HS, Mynderse LA: Evaluation and medical management of erectile dysfunction (cover story), *Mayo Clin Proc* 81:385–390, 2006.
36. Bors E, Comarr AE: Neurological disturbances of sexual function with special reference to 529 patients with spinal cord injury, *Urol Surv* 110:191–221, 1960.
41. Bronner G, Elran E, Golomb J, et al: Female sexuality in multiple sclerosis: the multidimensional nature of the problem and the intervention, *Acta Neurol Scand* 121(5):289–301, 2010.
47. Calabro RS, Gervasi G, Bramanti P: Male sexual disorders following stroke: an overview, *Int J Neurosci* 121(11):598–604, 2011.
56. Cramp JD, Courtois FJ, Ditor DS: Sexuality for women with spinal cord injury, *J Sex Marital Ther* 41:238–253, 2013.
61. Davis SR, Braunstein GD: Efficacy and safety of testosterone in the management of hypoactive sexual desire disorder in postmenopausal women, *J Sex Med* 9(4):1134–1148, 2012.
64. DeLamater J: Sexual expression in later life: a review and synthesis, *J Sex Res* 49(2–3):125–141, 2012.
70. Ellsworth P, Kirshenbaum EM: Current concepts in the evaluation and management of erectile dysfunction, *Urol Nurs* 28(5):357–369, 2008.
76. Frank JE, Mistretta P, Will J: Diagnosis and treatment of female sexual dysfunction, *Am Fam Physician* 77:635–645, 2008.
90. Hatzichristou D, Rosen RC, Broderick G, et al: Clinical evaluation and management strategy for sexual dysfunction in men and women, *J Sex Med* 1:49–57, 2004.
91. Hatzimouratidis K, Hatzichristou DG: Looking to the future for erectile dysfunction therapies, *Drugs* 68(2):231–250, 2008.
96. Hordern A: Intimacy and sexuality after cancer: a critical review of the literature, *Cancer Nurs* 31(2):E9–E17, 2008.
104. Kaiser FE: Sexuality in the elderly, *Urol Clin North Am* 23(1):99–109, 1996.
106. Kaplan C: Assessing and managing female sexual dysfunction, *Nurse Pract* 34(1):42–48, quiz 49–50, 2009.
112. Kingsberg SA: Taking a sexual history, *Obstet Gynecol Clin North Am* 33(4):535–547, 2006.
113. Kingsberg SA, Janata JW: Female sexual disorders: assessment, diagnosis, and treatment, *Urol Clin North Am* 34(4):497–506, 2007.
114. Kingsberg SA, Rezaee RL: Hypoactive sexual desire in women, *Menopause* 20(12):1284–1300, 2013.
125. Lue TF, Giuliano F, Montorsi F, et al: Summary of the recommendations on sexual dysfunctions in men, *J Sex Med* 1(1):6–23, 2004.
131. Masters WH, Johnson VE: *Human sexual response*, Boston, 1980, Bantam Books.
133. McCarthy B, McDonald D: Assessment, treatment, and relapse prevention: male hypoactive sexual desire disorder, *J Sex Marital Ther* 35(1):58–67, 2009.
136. McMahon CG, Jannini E, Waldinger M, et al: Standard operating procedures in the disorders of orgasm and ejaculation, *J Sex Med* 10(1):204–229, 2013.
139. Miller TA: Diagnostic evaluation of erectile dysfunction, *Am Fam Physician* 61(1):95–104, 2000.
143. Montorsi F, Adaikan G, Becher E, et al: Summary of the recommendations on sexual dysfunctions in men, *J Sex Med* 7(11):3572–3588, 2010.
144. Morley JE, Tariq SH: Sexuality and disease, *Clin Geriatr Med* 19(3):563–573, 2003.
152. Palmer NR, Stuckey BG: Premature ejaculation: a clinical update, *Med J Aust* 188(11):662–666, 2008.
156. Porst H, Burnett A, Brock G, et al: SOP conservative (medical and mechanical) treatment of erectile dysfunction, *J Sex Med* 10(1):130–171, 2013.
158. Rees PM, Fowler CJ, Maas CP: Sexual function in men and women with neurological disorders, *Lancet* 369(9560):512–525, 2007.
169. Rowland DL, Rose P: Understanding and treating premature ejaculation, *Nurse Pract* 33(10):21–27, 2008.

178. Sander AM, Maestas KL, Nick TG, et al: Predictors of sexual functioning and satisfaction 1 year following traumatic brain injury: a TBI model systems multicenter study, *J Head Trauma Rehabil* 28(3):186–194, 2013.
180. Seftel AD, Miner MM, Kloner RA, et al: Office evaluation of male sexual dysfunction, *Urol Clin North Am* 34(4):463–482, 2007.
181. Segraves R, Woodard T: Female hypoactive sexual desire disorder: history and current status, *J Sex Med* 3:408–418, 2006.
188. Simons JS, Carey MP: Prevalence of sexual dysfunctions: results from a decade of research, *Arch Sex Behav* 30:177–219, 2001.
194. Sipski ML, Alexander CJ, Rosen R: Sexual arousal and orgasm in women: effects of spinal cord injury, *Ann Neurol* 49(1):35–44, 2001.
198. Somers KJ, Philbrick KL: Sexual dysfunction in the medically ill, *Curr Psychiatry Rep* 9(3):247–254, 2007.
199. Sonksen J, Ohl DA: Penile vibratory stimulation and electroejaculation in the treatment of ejaculatory dysfunction, *Int J Androl* 25:324, 2002.
202. Sungur MZ, Gunduz A: A comparison of DSM-IV-TR and DSM-5 definitions for sexual dysfunctions: critiques and challenges, *J Sex Med* 11(2):364–373, 2014.
203. Tamam Y, Tamam L, Akil E, et al: Post-stroke sexual functioning in first stroke patients, *Eur J Neurol* 15(7):660–666, 2008.
204. Thomas DR: Medications and sexual function, *Clin Geriatr Med* 19(3):553–562, 2003.
215. Yang CC: The neurourological examination in women, *J Sex Med* 5(11):2498–2501, 2008.

The full reference list for this chapter is available online.

CHAPTER 23

SPASTICITY

Gerard E. Francisco, Sheng Li

Spasticity is a significant complication of many neurologic conditions. In itself it predisposes to other complications, such as joint contractures and joint deformities, but, as a comorbidity, spasticity amplifies the effects of weakness and other motor disorders and contributes to limitations in activity and participation. Although it has become common practice to label any condition presenting as muscle tightness "spasticity," it is important to point out that it is only one of myriad consequences of the upper motor neuron (UMN) syndrome. Other important UMN syndrome features include weakness, exaggerated stretch reflexes, clonus, impaired coordination, and motor control/planning.[149] These numerous abnormalities evolve over time and interact with each other, and produce a dynamic picture of varying clinical presentations after a UMN lesion.[83,84] For example, weakness tends to result in immobilization in a shortened muscle length and predisposes to contracture. This in turn exacerbates the development of spasticity in the same muscles. Further, spasticity exacerbates contracture and triggers a vicious cycle that worsens the condition.[83,84,174]

Owing to the lack of a strict definition and clinical measurement of spasticity, estimates of spasticity incidence and prevalence vary. It is estimated to occur in around 85% of people with multiple sclerosis,[190,215] and 65% to 78% in those with spinal cord injuries (SCIs).[151,196] There is little known about the occurrence in persons with traumatic brain injuries (TBIs), but in those with severe brain stem involvement, spasticity can exist in up to 40%.[224] Prevalence in stroke has a wide range, anywhere from 19%[211] to 92%.[146] Within the first year of stroke, spasticity was found in 38% of survivors.[223] In persons with stroke, involvement of the basal ganglia, thalamus, insula, and white matter tracts (internal capsule, corona radiata, external capsule, and superior longitudinal fasciculus) were significantly associated with severe upper limb spasticity,[181] whereas those with multiple sclerosis will typically develop spasticity if plaques affect the corticospinal tract (CST), brain stem, and callosal radiations.[15]

Pathophysiology

Stretch Reflex and Its Regulation

To understand the physiology of stretch reflex and its regulations is fundamental to understand abnormal muscle tone and spasticity in various pathologic conditions. Muscle tone has been viewed as a manifestation of stretch reflex neuromotor control ever since Sherrington conducted his landmark experiments demonstrating that reflexes were not isolated phenomena within a single reflex arc, but the product of integrated activation as a result of reciprocal innervation of muscles.[147,148] The following brief review provides a theoretical basis to understand abnormalities of stretch reflex after UMN injury or disease.

Stretch reflex is a monosynaptic reflex that provides automatic regulation of skeletal muscle length. When a muscle is lengthened by passive stretch, both the change in muscle length and its rate are detected by muscle spindles (primarily group Ia afferent fibers, and secondarily group II afferent fibers). Golgi tendon organs also send information on muscle tension through group Ib afferent fibers. The increase in neuronal activity in these fibers in turn increases alpha motor neuron activity in the stretched muscles, causing the muscle fibers to contract and thus resist muscle lengthening or stretching. Meanwhile, Ia afferent fibers also synapse with Ia inhibitory interneurons, producing relaxation of the antagonist muscles ("reciprocal inhibition"). Gamma motor neurons regulate muscle spindle (fusimotor system) and reflex sensitivity. Excitability of spinal motor neurons is influenced by a host of factors: local intraspinal mechanisms, such as recurrent inhibition from Renshaw cells; reciprocal Ia inhibition; inhibition from group II afferents; nonreciprocal Ib inhibition; and presynaptic inhibition. In addition to these intraspinal mechanisms, excitability of the stretch reflex pathway (afferent fiber, spinal motor neuron, and efferent fiber) is further regulated by excitatory and inhibitory descending supraspinal signals.

In the human motor system, there are five important descending pathways: corticospinal, reticulospinal, vestibulospinal, rubrospinal, and tectospinal. The CST originates from the cerebral cortex and is primarily involved in voluntary movement. Isolated lesions in the corticospinal pathway produce weakness, loss of dexterity, hypotonia, and hyporeflexia, instead of spasticity.[31,167,203] The other four descending pathways originate from the brain stem. The tectospinal tract originates from the tectum (superior colliculus) in the midbrain and contributes to visual orientation. The reticulospinal tract (RST) and the vestibulospinal tract (VST) provide balanced excitatory and inhibitory descending regulation of spinal stretch reflex. The rubrospinal pathway emanates from the lateral brain stem and is almost absent in humans.[169] Imbalance of these descending inhibitory pathways, along with facilitatory influences on stretch reflex, are thought to be the cause of spasticity.[26,167,203]

There are two principal excitatory and inhibitory systems from the brain stem that modulate excitability of spinal reflexes. They are anatomically distinct and differ in cortical control. The dorsal RST,[136] which originates from the ventromedial reticular formation[211] in the medulla, provides a powerful inhibitory effect on the spinal stretch reflex. The medullary reticular formation receives cortical facilitation from the motor cortex via corticoreticular fibers, which act as the suprabulbar inhibitory system. Corticospinal and corticoreticular tracts run adjacent to each other in the corona radiata and internal capsule. Below the medulla, the dorsal RST and the lateral CST descend adjacent to each other in the dorsolateral funiculus.

The medial RST and VST exert excitatory effects on spinal stretch reflexes. The medial RST has a diffuse origin, mainly in the pontine tegmentum, and has efferent connections passing through and receiving contributions from the central gray and tegmentum areas of the midbrain, and the medullar reticular formation (distinctly different from the inhibitory area). In contrast to the dorsal RST, the medial RST is not affected by stimulation of the motor cortex or internal capsule. The VST originates from the lateral vestibular nucleus and is virtually uncrossed. Both the RST and VST descend onto the ventromedial cord, anatomically distant from the lateral CST and dorsal RST in the dorsolateral cord.

It is worth mentioning that although the reticular formation is diffusely distributed throughout the brain stem, it is highly organized.[4,105] It has four longitudinal columns with ill-defined boundaries: paramedian zone, paramedian-medial zone, intermediate zone, and lateral zone. The reticular formation has connections with the spinal cord and various centers in the brain stem, thalamus, cerebellum, basal ganglia, and cortices. In addition to the above-mentioned role in regulating spinal reflexes, the reticular formation is also involved in the coordination of fine movement, autonomic regulation of respiration, heart rate, and blood pressure, as well as in arousal, consciousness, and modulation of pain.

Abnormal Regulation of the Stretch Reflex

Excitability of the spinal stretch reflex arc is maintained both by descending regulation from the inhibitory dorsal RST and facilitatory medial RST and VST, and intraspinal processing of the stretch reflex. Recent reports suggest that abnormalities in the supraspinal pathways predominate, whereas intraspinal mechanisms represent secondary plastic rearrangements responsible for the development of spasticity. For more details, the reader is referred to some excellent reviews of the contribution of intraspinal processing in the evolution of spasticity.[31,84,167,172] In summary, abnormal intraspinal processing could result from (1) increased afferent inputs to spinal motoneurons, where sensitivity of spindles is enhanced through activation of the gamma fusimotor system and/or adaptive changes after immobilization, resulting in increased gain of stretch reflex; (2) altered interneuronal reflex circuits resulting in enhanced motoneuronal excitability, including reduction in presynaptic inhibition on Ia afferents, group Ib facilitation (instead of inhibition), group II facilitation, and reduced reciprocal inhibition (these changes result in less inhibition from intraspinal reflex circuits on spinal motor neurons, such that motoneurons are at subthreshold or at spontaneous firing); and (3) changes in intrinsic properties of the spinal motor neurons. Disruption of descending inputs could cause spinal motoneurons to activate voltage-dependent persistent inward currents.[96] Persistent inward currents can lead to the development of plateau potentials in motoneurons and self-sustained firing in response to a transient input. These changes in reflex circuits and intrinsic properties of spinal motoneurons can lead to decreased reflex threshold, which has been considered as the primary change in patients with spasticity (Figure 23-1).[118,142]

Abnormal intraspinal processing is likely to represent a plastic rearrangement secondary to an imbalance in excitatory and inhibitory descending inputs to the intraspinal network. Plastic rearrangement at segmental levels has been demonstrated after complete (e.g., complete SCI) or incomplete disruption (e.g., stroke, TBI, multiple sclerosis, and incomplete SCI) of descending supraspinal inputs to spinal reflexes. Recently, Sist et al.[210] demonstrated in an animal model that following a cortical sensorimotor stroke, there is a time-limited period of heightened structural plasticity in the brain and spinal cord. The plastic change correlates with severity of cortical injury and promotes behavioral recovery. Elevated structural spinal plasticity is highest during the first 2 weeks and returns to baseline levels by 28 days poststroke. By contrast, alpha motor neuron hyperexcitability, including spontaneous discharges from these neurons, has been consistently reported in patients with spasticity.* For example, spontaneous motor unit discharges were observed at rest in the spastic biceps brachii muscle. The firing frequency of the firing unit was increased with increases in voluntary elbow flexion force. The spontaneous unit continued to fire after activation despite verbal cueing to relax the muscle and the patient perceived having the muscle in a relaxed state.[164] The firing frequency of spontaneous units was found be greater in the postcontraction resting period than in the precontraction resting period.[39] The specific mechanisms of spontaneous motor unit discharges are not known. However, these observations suggest that spontaneous discharges in spastic muscles are likely to be caused by supraspinal mechanisms, but not under voluntary control.[39,164,165]

Abnormal descending regulation of spinal stretch reflex results from an imbalance between the descending inhibitory dorsal RST and facilitatory medial RST and VST. The VST is important in maintaining decerebrate rigidity but has a limited role in human spasticity, whereas abnormalities in RST outflow are considered to be the main abnormality in the latter. These views are based on findings from invasive lesion studies in animals in the past century (see reviews by Brown,[26] Mukherjee and Chakravarty,[167] and Sheean[203]). For example, a section of the unilateral or bilateral VST in the anterior cord only caused a transient reduction in the extensor tone in the lower limbs. After more extensive cordotomies, including the medial RST, spasticity was drastically reduced, but tendon hyperreflexia, clonus, and adductor spasms persisted.

The CST and the corticoreticular tract travel adjacent to each other from their origins in the motor cortex, via the corona radiata and internal capsule, to the medullary bulge and medullary reticular inhibitory center. The CST and dorsal RST continue to run adjacent to each other in the dorsolateral spinal cord. Isolated lesions of the CST rarely occur and only result in weakness, hypotonicity, and

*References 32, 39, 112, 113, 142, 164, 165.

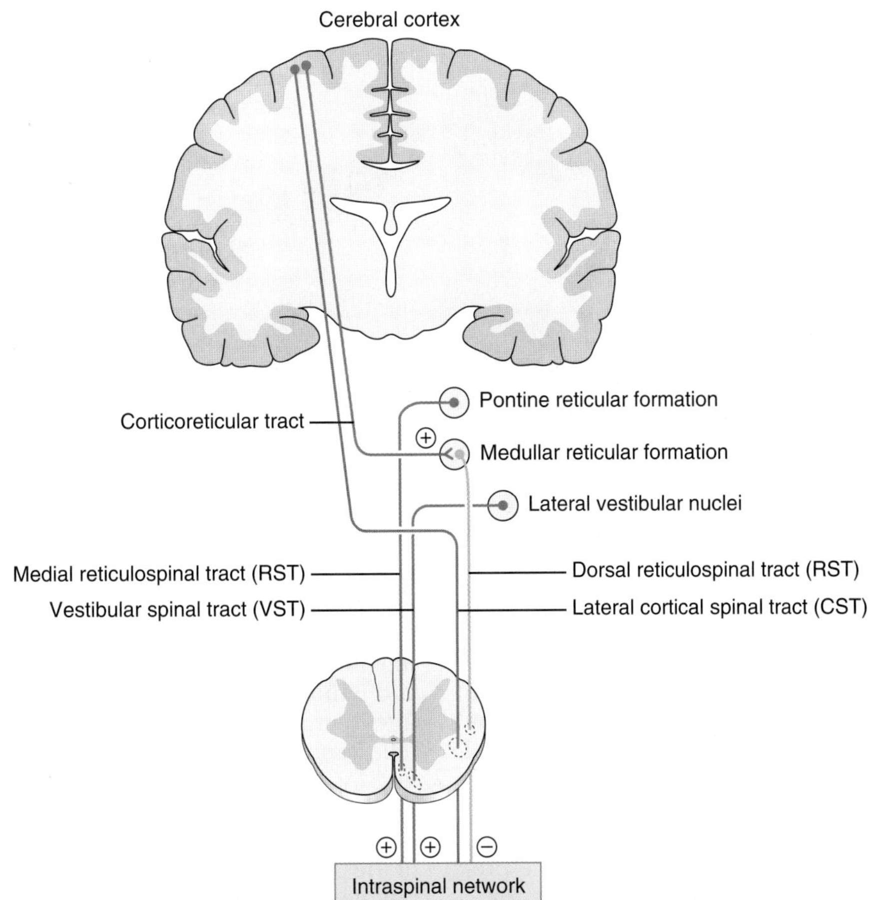

FIGURE 23-1 Illustration of supraspinal control of spinal stretch reflex. *CST,* Corticospinal tract; *RST,* reticulospinal tract; *VST,* vestibulospinal tract; *(+),* facilitation; *(–),* inhibition. For simplicity, the other descending pathways, such as rubrospinal, tectospinal, and medial CST are not shown.

hyporeflexia, but not spasticity. In cortical and internal capsular lesions, however, damage often involves both the CST and the corticoreticular tract, resulting in loss of cortical facilitatory input to the medullary inhibitory center. This leaves the facilitatory medial RST unopposed, because it is not under cortical control. As a result, spastic hemiplegia with antigravity posturing is often seen. However, flexor spasms are unusual in this type of suprabulbar lesion, because flexor spasms are a release phenomenon of flexor reflexes as a result of damage to the dorsal RST.

In humans, RST excitability could be examined indirectly through the acoustic startle reflex (ASR), a brain stem–mediated reflex via reticulospinal pathways.[27,51] The ASR has been used to examine reticulospinal excitability after stroke.[45,102,109,141,221] ASR responses were elicited in flaccid muscles of some patients in the acute phase after cerebral infarcts, but no muscle response to magnetic cortical stimulation was elicited in any of these patients.[221] The presence of ASR responses was considered to be a result of corticoreticular disinhibition after stroke.[221] In patients with chronic stroke, exaggerated ASR responses have been reported in spastic muscles.[109] However, for those who have a full motor recovery from stroke or no motor recovery at all (flaccid) at the chronic stage when further recovery is arrested (Figure 23-2), ASR responses are within normal limits.[141] These results suggest hyperexcitability of reticulospinal pathways at rest in the spastic stages, but not in recovered nonspastic stages. Reticulospinal pathways usually have bilateral projections.[50] During voluntary contraction, biceps electromyographic (EMG) activity of the resting nonimpaired limb increased proportionally in the spastic group, but no such correlation was found in the recovered nonspastic group. Such results of contralateral motor overflow from the impaired limb extend the findings of the previous study and further support reticulospinal hyperexcitability in the spastic stages, but not in the nonspastic stages. Collectively, these findings also support the concept that spasticity is a phenomenon of abnormal plasticity.

The reticulospinal mechanism for spasticity could account for commonly observed clinical features associated with spasticity. For example, reticulospinal activation involves divergent projections to multiple muscles and flexor bias in the upper extremity.[50] This could account for commonly observed flexor synergies in the upper extremity[56] and interlimb coupling[126] in patients with stroke and spasticity. The regulation of basic survival functions, such as breathing, posture, pain, temperature, and muscle tone, could be related to the divergent but well-organized function of reticular formation and reticulospinal projections.[171] Reticulospinal hyperexcitability could enhance interactions among these functions. For example, in the spastic condition recruitment of both the plantar flexor and dorsiflexor muscles was observed during normal

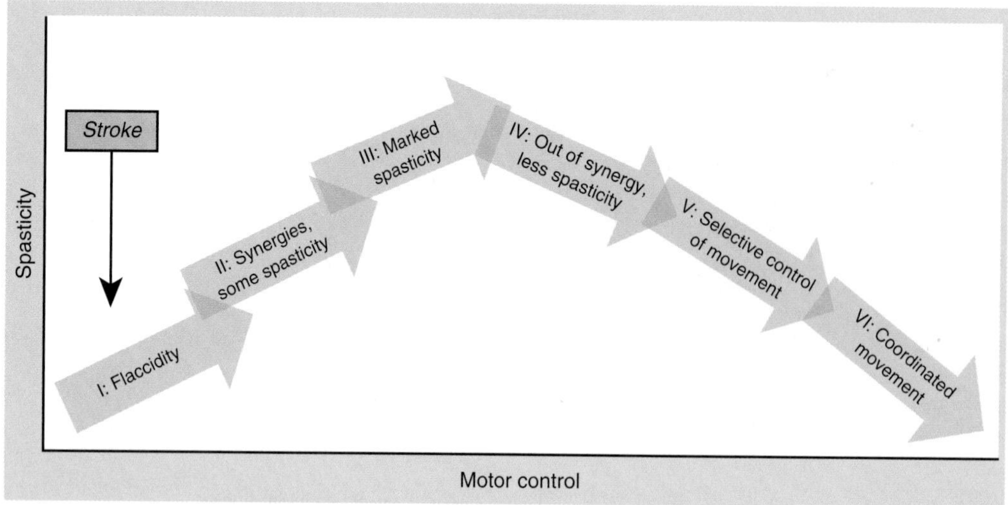

FIGURE 23-2 Brunnstrom stages of motor recovery after stroke.

breathing at rest, but with a predominance of plantar flexion during coughing.[84] Similarly, this mechanism could also account for other common clinical observations that, as mentioned previously, spasticity changes with posture (dynamic tone), ambient temperature, pain, emotional states, time of day (temporal fluctuation), and breathing.

The clinical presentation of spasticity varies among supraspinal lesions and spinal lesions. Spasticity can be classified as either *tonic* or *phasic*, depending on the predominant involvement of phasic (dynamic) or tonic (static) components of muscle stretch reflex. Spasticity can also be classified as either *extrinsic* or *intrinsic*. The former refers to involuntary muscle spasms that occur in response to a perceived noxious stimulus originating from sources extrinsic to the muscle. For example, flexion withdrawal spasms commonly seen in people with SCI are triggered by afferent input from the skin, muscle, subcutaneous tissues, and joints, collectively referred to as "flexor reflex afferents." As a result of the disruption of descending inhibition after SCI, flexor withdrawal reflexes occur in response even to normal stimuli. Intrinsic phasic spasticity, by contrast, describes symptoms, such as tendon hyperreflexia and clonus. Tendon hyperreflexia is caused by exaggeration of the phasic component of the stretch reflex secondary to reduced presynaptic Ia inhibition. Clonus is defined as "involuntary rhythmic muscle contraction that can result in distal joint oscillation" and most often occurs at the ankle. The dominant view of the underlying mechanism is that clonus is caused by recurrent activation of stretch reflexes; for example, ankle clonus is the outcome of mutual and alternating activation of plantar flexor and dorsiflexor stretch reflexes. Intrinsic tonic spasticity results from an exaggeration of the tonic component of the stretch reflex. When a sustained passive stretch is imposed to the muscle, both primary and secondary muscle afferents are activated and facilitate contraction of stretched muscles.[54]

The pathophysiology of incomplete and complete SCIs is also mediated by different mechanisms. In incomplete spinal cord lesions, both the CST and dorsal RST are often damaged in the dorsolateral cord. Damage to the dorsal RST could also lead to a release phenomenon, producing flexor spasms and hyperreflexia, in addition to spasticity. In complete SCI, the situation is different. Both excitatory and inhibitory supraspinal descending inputs to spinal interneuronal network are absent, and thus both stretch reflex and flexor reflex afferents are completely disinhibited. As such, a strong flexor pattern follows, resulting in paraplegia with predominant flexion features.[167,203]

More recent investigations offer a deeper understanding of the pathophysiology of spasticity. In rodents with experimentally induced SCI, downregulation of the potassium chloride cotransporter, KCC2, in motor neuron membranes appears to be involved. This downregulation depolarizes the chloride equilibrium potential and reduces the strength of postsynaptic inhibition. This downregulation appears to be countered by brain-derived neurotropic factor after SCI.[20]

Does Spasticity Result from Maladaptive Plasticity?

Motor recovery commences almost immediately after the onset of a central nervous lesion, when reversible changes resolve. For instance, following a stroke regardless of type (hemorrhagic or not) or location (cortical or subcortical), a relatively predictable pattern of recovery sets in.[219] Brunnstrom[28,29] empirically describes the stereotypical stages of motor recovery from flaccidity to full recovery of motor function, which are summarized in Figure 23-2. As a stroke survivor improves, progression from one recovery stage to the next toward recovery of normal movement occurs in an orderly manner, but evolution may be arrested at any stage.[29,219]

Interestingly, as motor recovery progresses, spasticity decreases. However, the same pattern of motor recovery and emergence and disappearance of spasticity may not be seen in other etiologies of the UMN syndrome. What is common is the observation that there is a period of "shock" after the initial injury (traumatic or acquired), which is followed by a gradual return of reflexes, but not a sudden progression to hyperreflexia. This implies that there must be some sort of neuronal plastic change after the initial injury. This process occurs at any time, but is usually seen between 1 and 6 weeks after the initial injury.[8] Plastic rearrangement occurs within the brain and spinal cord (see reviews*), and is regarded as an attempt at restoration of function through emergence of novel neuronal circuitry. This process of plastic rearrangement often results in muscle overactivity and hyperreflexia, and thus spasticity.[66] In a recent longitudinal study that examined the time course of development of spasticity and contractures at the wrist after 6 weeks of stroke, the authors reported that patients who recovered arm function showed signs of spasticity at all assessment points but did not develop contractures. In contrast to this, patients who did not recover useful arm function had signs of spasticity and changes associated with contracture formation tested over a follow-up course of 36 weeks,[146] suggesting that spasticity, a harbinger of contractures, persisted. Collectively, emergence and disappearance of spasticity in the course of complete motor recovery implies that presence of spasticity reflects a phenomenon of abnormal plasticity. Spasticity may be maintained after its emergence if further plastic rearrangement and recovery are arrested. That spasticity is a manifestation of maladaptive plasticity is further supported by recent studies demonstrating that abnormal cortical reorganization can be modulated by interventions directed at decreasing spasticity.[106]

Peripheral Contribution

Spasticity can be differentiated from hypertonia arising from other mechanisms by its dependence on the speed of the muscle stretch.[204] However, spasticity may also be explained by changes in mechanical properties of muscles and not only by hyperreflexia.[58,215] The increased mechanical resistance may be caused by alterations in tendon compliance and physiologic changes in muscle fibers. These muscle property changes may be adaptive and secondary to paresis. When a paralyzed muscle is held in a shortened position, it loses sarcomeres to "adjust" its length so that it can produce optimal force at the shortened muscle length. As a result, muscle fibers are almost twice as stiff as in nonspastic muscles.[78] These changes in mechanical properties of muscles occur gradually and may also lead to contracture and increased muscle stiffness[160] and are not easily detected during usual clinical examination.[220] The effect of blood flow restriction on Ia afferent activity has also been implicated. Animal studies have shown that a decrease in blood flow can increase Ia afferent firing through the activation of group III and group IV afferent fusimotor activity that responds to accumulation of metabolites within the muscle.[57]

Clinical Presentation, Goal Setting, and Assessment

Problem Identification

What is the problem?
What is the main cause of the problem?
What other factors contribute to the problem?

Patients rarely express their complaint as spasticity. Rather, they typically use words that describe the manifestations of spasticity, such as muscle tightness or that a limb could not be moved, or more often the resultant functional limitations, such as the inability to release a grasped object or difficulty with walking as a result of an in-turned foot. Also, patients usually complain of symptoms resulting from other UMN abnormalities, such as spasms or clonus triggered by walking, weakness, and difficulty manipulating objects due to decreased hand dexterity. Thus the importance of obtaining a thorough, yet focused, history is of paramount importance in guiding the examination and formulation of mutually agreed upon treatment goals and plans.

When a patient presents with tight muscles and limb deformities, and complains of inability to perform certain tasks, it is often tempting to attribute all problems to spasticity. The clinician should keep in mind that spasticity is but one of the multitude of problems resulting from UMN disease. Often weakness, rather than spasticity, is the primary cause of limitations. Thus, although spasticity is present, it may not be the immediate cause of a particular problem, which is a consequence of different, but related, UMN pathologies.

Postural Abnormalities

Although the clinical presentation varies widely across individuals within and across patient populations, there are postural patterns that are commonly observed. They are manifestations of imbalance of agonist and antagonist strength and hypertonia. Thus, a flexed elbow posture is not necessarily as a result of flexor muscle group hypertonia solely, but may be a combination of hypertonic flexors and weak extensors; or it could also be that both flexor and extensor muscle groups are both hypertonic, but the former predominates. It has been suggested that knowledge of the abnormal postural patterns help inform treatment, goal setting, and outcome of interventions, such as chemodenervation.[97] Table 23-1 lists muscles that, when they are hypertonic, are potentially involved in commonly observed abnormal postures.

Impaired Movement

Similar to abnormal postures, impaired movements usually result from the interaction among spasticity, weakness, and other features of the UMN syndrome, such as loss of coordination and dexterity, and dystonia, or sustained contraction of muscles.

Functional Limitation

Activity limitation is even more complex because the causes of impaired movement not only are further aggravated by abnormalities other than the UMN disorder, but are also a direct result of the underlying disease. Tactile and proprioceptive sensory loss, visual field cut and hemineglect, and cognitive difficulties, such as learning a novel task and procedural sequencing, can magnify the motor challenges imposed upon by spasticity and weakness. Thus, a rehabilitation effort that will be effective in enhancing activity participation should address not just spasticity and deficits in strength and coordination but also concurrently tackle the related impairments.

*References 8, 31, 83, 84, 167, 172, 173.

CASE 1

Problem Identification

O.A. is a 50-year-old male who sustained a nonpenetrating brain injury caused by a motorcycle crash 16 years ago. He complains of the difficulty in reaching for objects because "it feels like something is holding my elbow back," and of foot drop that causes him to trip occasionally, especially after walking a long distance. He used to take oral baclofen 10 mg three times daily, which helped relax his arm and allowed easier reaching. However, he also thought that he has been tripping more often since starting baclofen, and elected to discontinue the drug 3 months earlier. At rest, he held the right elbow in 30 degrees of flexion and the wrist and hand in normal anatomic position. An attempt to extend the right elbow with the shoulder abducted to around 70 degrees was characterized by coarse jerking (alternating elbow flexion and extension) and clenched fist. It took him approximately 30 seconds to extend the elbow to about −20 degrees from the resting position. He had difficulty dorsiflexing the right ankle, being able to move it only through about a 20-degree range. On passive ranging, the right ankle lacked 35 degrees of dorsiflexion while the knee was in either extended or flexed position. Ashworth Scale scores were 1 in the right shoulder adductor, elbow extensor, knee extensor, and ankle dorsiflexor; 2 in the right elbow flexor; and 0 elsewhere. Based on these clinical findings alone, the clinician thought that the inability to reach was most likely as a result of abnormal cocontraction of the elbow extensors (agonist) and flexors (antagonist) and the inability to grasp as a result of synkinesis, or associated reaction, of the finger and thumb flexors triggered by elbow extension movement. The clinician also linked the history of increased tripping when the patient was receiving baclofen with the observation that the patient had right ankle dorsiflexor weakness and plantar flexor contracture. Thus in this patient, the two presenting problems, inability to reach and gripping, were most likely not attributable to spasticity, but to other UMN disease features, such as weakness, abnormal agonist-antagonist cocontraction or loss of reciprocal inhibition, and synkinesis.

Table 23-1 Common Postural Abnormalities Due to Spasticity and Potential Muscle Involvement

Postural Abnormality		Muscles Potentially Involved
Shoulder adduction	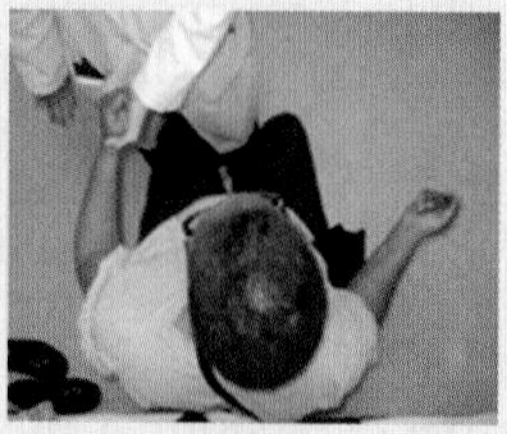	Pectoralis major and minor Latissimus dorsi Coracobrachialis (especially when shoulder is forward flexed)
Shoulder internal rotation		Subscapularis Teres major Pectoralis major and minor
Elbow flexion	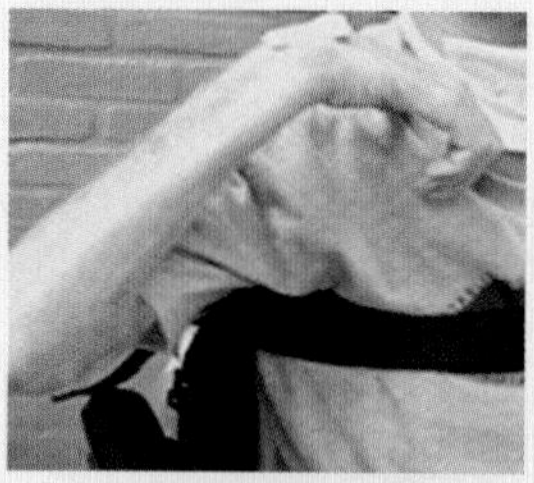	Brachialis Biceps Brachioradialis Pronator teres
Elbow extension	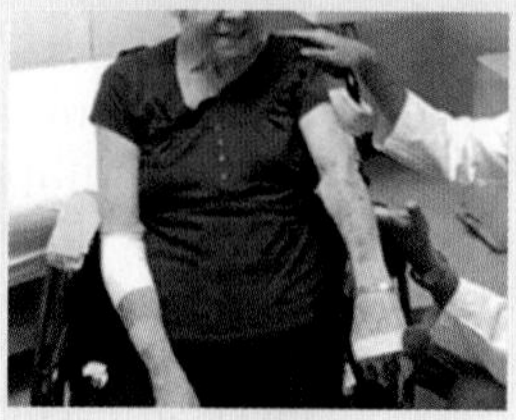	Triceps Anconeus

Table 23-1 Common Postural Abnormalities Due to Spasticity and Potential Muscle Involvement—cont'd

Postural Abnormality	Muscles Potentially Involved
Forearm pronation	Pronator teres Pronator quadratus
Wrist extension	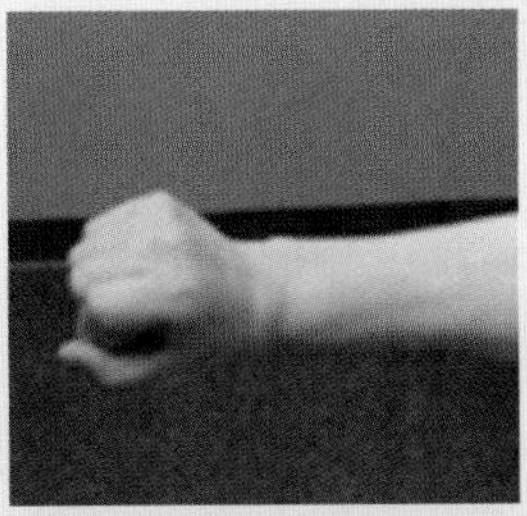 Extensor carpi radialis Extensor carpi ulnaris
Wrist flexion	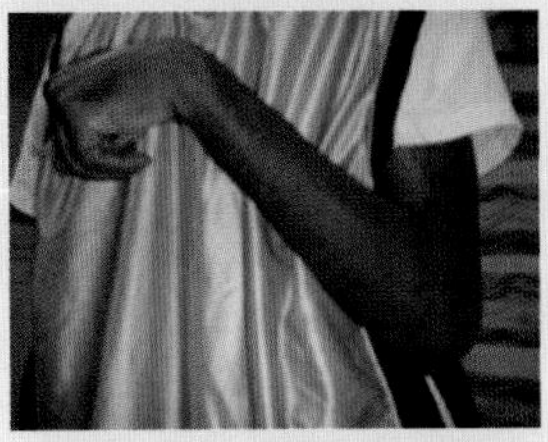 Flexor carpi radialis Flexor carpi ulnaris
Metacarpophalangeal (knuckle) flexion	Lumbricals
Finger flexion	Flexor digitorum superficialis (proximal phalanx) Flexor digitorum profundus (distal phalanx)
Thumb flexion	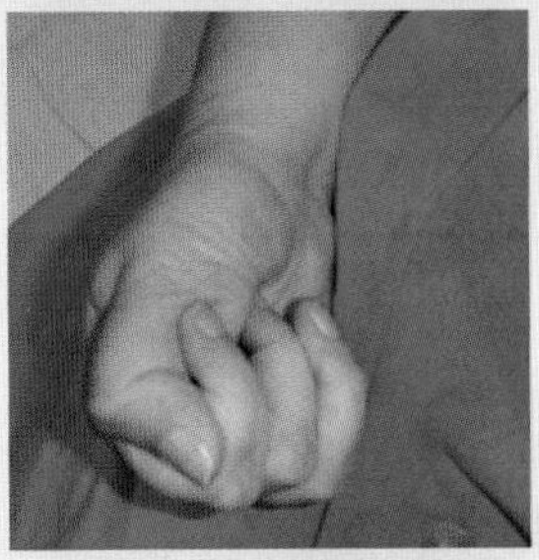 Flexor pollicis brevis (proximal) Flexor pollicis longus (distal phalanx)
Trunk flexion, lateral	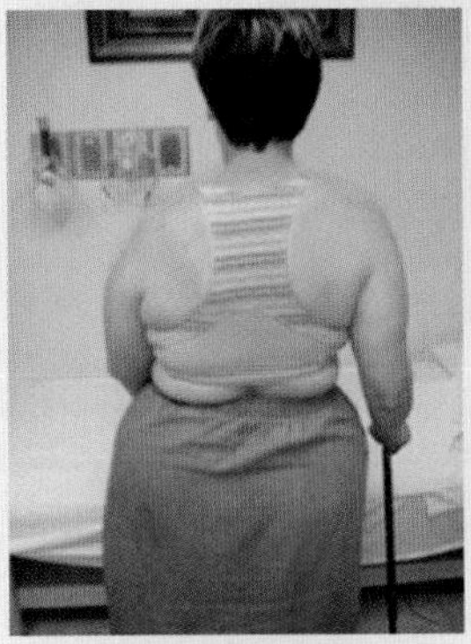 Quadratus lumborum Latissimus dorsi
Hip Flexion	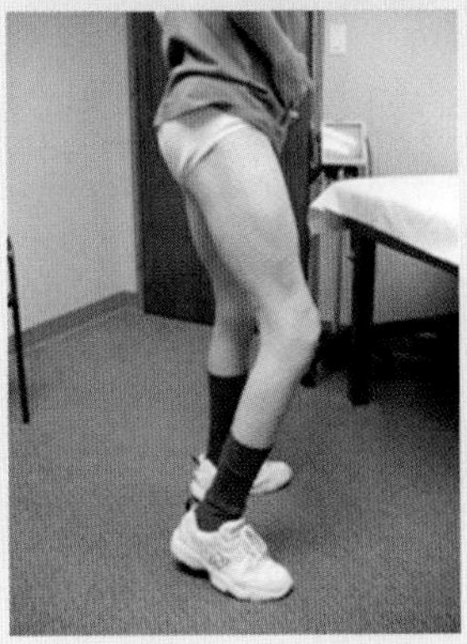 Psoas Iliacus Rectus femoris

Continued on following page

Table 23-1 Common Postural Abnormalities Due to Spasticity and Potential Muscle Involvement—cont'd

Postural Abnormality	Muscles Potentially Involved
Hip extension	Gluteus maximus
Hip adduction	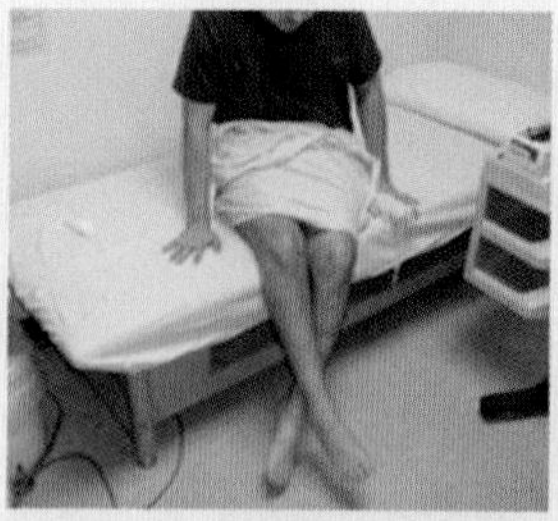 Adductor complex
Knee extension	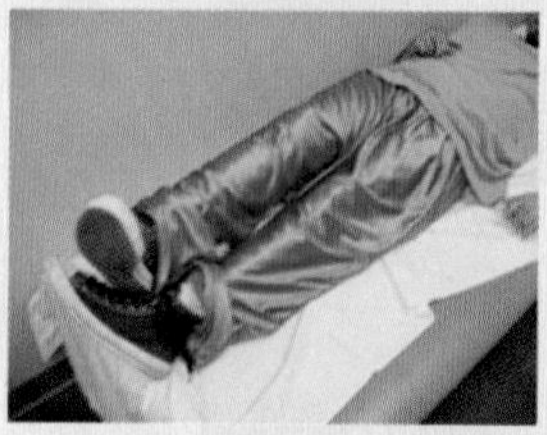 Quadriceps complex
Knee flexion	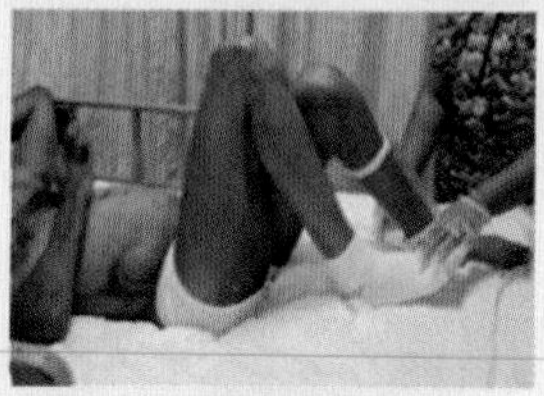 Hamstrings Gastrocnemius
Ankle plantar flexion	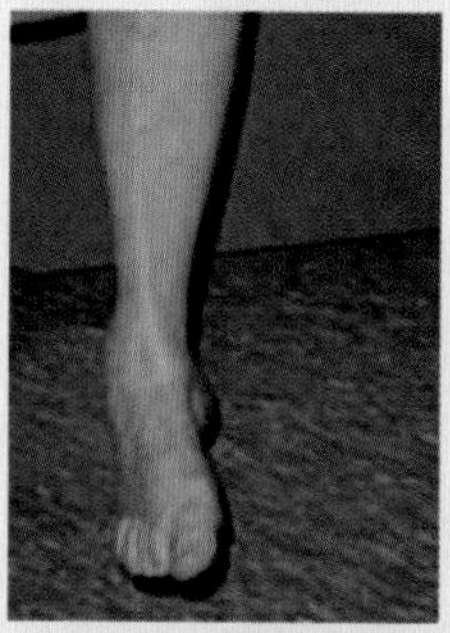 Gastrocnemius Soleus Tibialis posterior Tibialis anterior Flexor digitorum longus
Ankle inversion	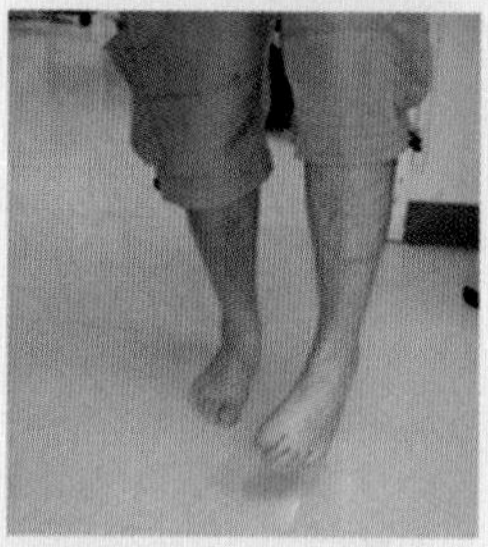 Tibialis posterior Tibialis anterior Extensor hallucis longus
Small toe flexion	Flexor digitorum brevis (proximal) Flexor digitorum longus (distal)
Great toe hyperextension	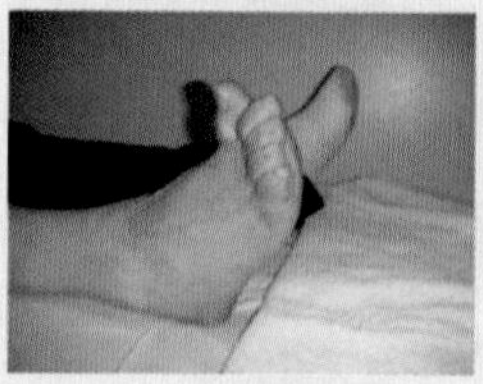 Extensor hallucis longus

Goal Setting

What will help the patient and caregivers?
Are the goals "SMART"?
How will one know whether the treatment goal has been achieved?

An important component of assessment and management decision making is arriving at treatment goals that are mutually agreed upon by the patient (or caregiver) and clinician. Identifying goals a priori provides a context for identifying pertinent problems and their solutions, and in the process manage the use of resources. It is not uncommon for patients to desire goals of regaining normal form and function, but because this is not always achievable, a discussion regarding goal setting before initiating treatment can help manage expectations of treatment outcomes. Goal setting can also help identify the best treatment strategy at a particular time in the course of a person's rehabilitation and recovery. A useful method uses the SMART acronym, originally used in the business sector.[59] Each of the letters in the acronym stands for a criterion that characterizes goals and objectives and that has appeared in various iterations to fit different purposes. For the purpose of goal setting in spasticity management, SMART, or SMARTER, can stand for:

- S—Specific (well defined and targets a specific problem to be addressed)
- M—Measurable (either quantitatively, as for technical goals, or qualitatively as for symptom-directed goals); Meaningful (achievement of goal should be beneficial to the patient or caregiver)
- A—Agreed upon (the patient or caregiver and clinician work toward a common end)
- R—Realistic (will the patient's potential for improvement and available resources support achievement of treatment goal?)
- T—Time bound (achievement of goal should be within a reasonable amount of time)
- E—Evaluated (at predetermined points in time, goal achievement and progress in doing so should be performed to determine effectiveness of intervention)
- R—Revised (based on evaluation of goal achievement, new treatment goals may be identified or previous ones revised)

Clinical Assessment

Spasticity assessment typically consists of a combination of quantitative and qualitative measures. Although it is true that quantitative measures are desirable because of their inherent objectivity and reliability, they may not be practical and discourage clinicians from assessing and managing spasticity. Ideal measures include biomechanical and electrophysiologic tests, but many of the devices needed to carry these out are not available to a typical clinician, and time needed to perform them properly may impose excessive demands in a busy practice. Thus, a combination of clinical measures, some of which appear to correlate with biomechanical and electrophysiologic assessment, is a practical approach. Table 23-2 summarizes many of these evaluation tools and techniques.

Table 23-2 Measures of Spasticity Categorized According to the World Health Organization International Classification of Function

Domain	Measure	Examples
Body function and structure	Clinical	Visual Analog Scale Goniometric Ashworth Scale (and its modified version)* Tardieu Method Tone Assessment Scale Spasm Severity Scale Spasm Frequency Scale
	Physiologic	H_{max}/M_{max} ratio Vibratory Inhibitory Index Tendon reflex gain Angular joint velocity Reflex threshold angle Torque measurement Pendulum test Myotonometer
Activity	Impairment†	Fugl-Meyer Jebsen-Taylor Hand Test Wolf Motor Test Action Research Arm Test Berg Balance Scale
	Function†	Functional Independence Measure Barthel Index Disability Assessment Scale* Frenchay Arm Test Timed Walking Test Motion Analysis Individualized functional tasks
Participation	Quality of life†	SF-36 Health Survey Satisfaction with Life Scale EuroQol (EQ-5D)

*Measure was developed specifically for spasticity.
†Measure is not specific for spasticity.

Platz et al.[185] proposed a rating scale coined REsistance to PASsive movement, or REPAS. Test items for various passive limb motions based on the Ashworth Scale were analyzed and compared with other scales that measure spasticity and related phenomena, motor impairment, and activity limitation. This summary rating scale was found to be highly internally consistent and reliable for the clinical assessment of resistance to passive movement in patients with UMN disorders. Further, the REPAS scores were associated with a patient's functional abilities and a caregiver's difficulty in assisting with hygiene. The REPAS Scale offers an alternative that may be able to more accurately assess spasticity and effects of therapeutic interventions clinically. In Box 23-1 and Table 23-3, a systematic approach to history taking and clinical assessment of spasticity is proposed, which can be modified to suit different clinical scenarios. REPAS, or more popularly used scales, such as the Ashworth Scale can be made part of this proposed examination sequence.

Biomechanical and Electrophysiologic Assessment

Biomechanical Assessment: Spasticity or Contracture?

Resistance to passive stretch is composed of three components: passive muscle stiffness, active muscle stiffness, and

CASE 2

Goal Setting and Clinical Assessment

W.T. is a 49-year-old right-handed female administrative assistant who had a left basal ganglia hemorrhage attributable to hypertension a year earlier. She presented with tightness of her right index finger flexors. Going deeper into the nature of her presenting concern, the clinician learned that although the patient is able to actively flex her fingers, when she attempts to type she is unable to extend the right index finger to lift the digit off the keyboard. The clinician also inquired about how else the tightness of her finger has affected her ability to do things. To this, the patient expressed her concern that her limited typing ability may be grounds for dismissal from work, as preparing written communication is an essential function of her current job. Upon further question the clinician also found out that the patient has difficulty extending her right elbow each time she attempts to reach, and that she has no other problems related to muscle tightness. The clinician's examination consisted of observing the patient actively flex and extend the right elbow. He noticed that the patient slowly, but smoothly flexed her right elbow, but that she struggled as she attempted to extend the same elbow, often jerking the arm. The patient was not able to actively extend the right elbow against minimal resistance. The patient demonstrated her ability to actively flex the right digits, but difficulty of extending the index and middle fingers. Ashworth Scale testing of the right upper limb yielded the following results: shoulder adductors and internal rotators—1, elbow flexors—1, elbow extensors—0, wrist flexors and extensors—0, finger and thumb flexors—0.

The patient asked the clinician about his treatment recommendation based on the examination, to which the clinician replied that he suggests botulinum toxin injections to the right elbow flexors and the right index and middle finger flexors. The patient asked the clinician why the shoulder adductors will not be treated because she heard that the "score was a 1, whereas the fingers had a score of 0." The clinician confirmed with the patient that she has trouble neither cleaning her underarm nor donning shirtsleeves, and thus felt that muscle tightness alone is reason enough for treatment. Intervention should be considered only if spasticity causes or predisposes to the development of problems and complications. Further, the clinician pointed out that although the Ashworth score, which is done passively, is not as important as the patient's report of functional problems with the two finger flexors that tend to tighten up in relation to a particular task. The patient also asked about other treatment options. The clinician replied that he did not think that the systemic side effects of oral drugs justify its use treating a problem that is limited to two muscle groups in a single limb. He also pointed out that another injection technique with phenol carries more risks for adverse events than botulinum toxin. The clinician and patient mutually agreed on the following goals, treatment plan, and measure of success:

Problem	Goal	Treatment Approaches	Outcome Measure	Target Date
Difficulty reaching caused by spastic elbow flexors and, possibly, weak elbow extensors	Increase active elbow extension to at least −30 degrees to allow positioning of forearm close to keyboard	Botulinum toxin chemodenervation of brachialis, biceps, and brachioradialis, immediately followed by strengthening of the elbow extensors and functional reaching exercises	Technical: Elbow flexor Ashworth score—0; increased smoothness of elbow extension-flexion Functional: Ability to actively extend elbow far enough to reach the keyboard	Two months postinjection with botulinum toxin
Unable to type with index finger due to tight flexor	Type with right index finger	Botulinum toxin chemodenervation of flexor digitorum superficialis and profundus, immediately followed by task-specific home program consisting of practicing typing with index finger	Technical: Finger flexor Ashworth score—0; recovery of isolated active index finger flexion and extension Functional: Ability to type using index finger (short term) with 100% accuracy in hitting desired keyboard tiles (long term)	Two months postchemodenervation (short term); may need to have a reinjection and further therapeutic exercises to achieve long-term outcome (4 to 5 months after first chemodenervation)
Minimally tight shoulder adductors and internal rotators	Not applicable	No intervention, as the tightness of the shoulder is not causing any difficulty currently	Not applicable	Not applicable

Table 23-3 Practical Clinical Examination Sequence

Examination Phase	What to Look for	What Can Be Gleaned
Observation	Observe limb posture at rest and how it changes with position	Posture at rest—Sustained muscle contraction (dystonia) or contractures Position-dependent postural changes—Synkinesis or associated reactions
Active (patient performs actions)	How limbs move and how much active range is available Pain and discomfort as the patient moves	Functional strength, coordination, spastic cocontraction, contractures, presence of other movement disorders
Passive (examiner performs maneuvers)	Passive range of motion, strength, muscle tone, velocity-dependent "angle of catch," clonus Pain and discomfort as a maneuver is performed	Spasticity Rigidity Contracture
Functional	Gait characteristics and associated upper limb and trunk postural abnormalities Performance of specific tests and tasks (both formal tests, such as Frenchay Arm Test, and improvised tasks, such as demonstrating ability to pick up a bottle of water and pour its contents into a cup)	Impact of multiple impairments (e.g., spasticity, weakness) on performance

BOX 23-1

Some Important Historical Points in Spasticity Assessment

- Is the limb tight all the time or only at certain times?
- Does a particular position or movement trigger tightness?
- Is the tightness related to spasms?
- Does the tightness cause pain?
- Have there been episodes of skin compromise resulting from tightness or spasm?
- Does the tightness result in difficulty with cleaning?
- Does the tightness result in difficulty donning splints?
- Does the tightness limit ability to move limbs, reach for objects, and use the hands?
- Does the tightness of the lower limbs result in problems with transferring from one surface to another or with walking?
- What treatments for muscle tightness have been tried previously and what are their outcomes?
- What are the current medications?
- Was there a recent increase in tightness (that may warrant further diagnostic testing to rule out a new neurologic problem)?
- Any recent medical problems?

neutrally mediated reflex stiffness. Experimentally, total joint stiffness is first measured in response to a controlled angular perturbation. The measured total stiffness is then decomposed into reflex and nonreflex components. Changes in nonreflex muscle stiffness could presumably be as result of changes in peripheral muscle tissue, such as fibrosis, fat infiltration, and muscle atrophy. Change in reflex stiffness could be caused by a change in the descending influences on the monosynaptic reflex between the muscle spindle afferents and the alpha motor neurons. Therefore the mechanical changes may provide insights into the underlying neural pathway or muscle tissue changes, or both. When applied to spastic muscles, the common findings are velocity-dependent increase in reflex component during controlled passive stretch.* The findings are consistent with the commonly used definition of "velocity-dependent increase in tonic stretch reflex."[132] It has also been reported that there is increased nonreflex intrinsic muscle stiffness.[209] This finding suggests that there was a change in the muscle itself rather than just a change in the nervous system that accounted for the clinical presentation of the spastic limb.

Although useful, these quantification devices are cumbersome and the analysis is time-consuming, making it difficult to be directly used in the clinical settings. Findings from these biomechanical approaches, however, can be translated into clinical practice and help better assess spasticity clinically. It has been demonstrated from animal studies that primary muscle spindles (Ia) are velocity-sensitive and secondary spindle afferents are length-dependent, and there are interactions between the two in animal models.[104,136] In patients with spastic finger flexors after stroke, Li et al.[142] confirmed that velocity dependence was greater at longer lengths and length was greater with faster stretches. Overall, stretch responses are both velocity-dependent and length-dependent. Essentially, this study provides evidence that spasticity is also position-dependent in addition to velocity-dependent. Therefore pay attention to joint position (equivalent to muscle length) when examining spastic muscles at bedside. Clinically, the Tardieu method, rather than the Ashworth Scale, estimates the velocity-dependent nature of spasticity much better.[94] The Myotonometer, a portable device, measures muscle stiffness at rest and during voluntary contraction by recording displacement of the probe perpendicular on the target muscle and the amount of force applied to the probe by the examiner. The Myotonometer measurement is found to have good intrarater and interrater reliability, and is correlated well with clinical measurement of spasticity by the Modified Ashworth Scale.[137,138] This measurement, however, does not provide the reflex component of the stretch response.

Electrophysiologic Measurement

Reflex stiffness from torque angle relations can be obtained quantitatively as described earlier. However, certain precautions should be taken when interpreting this reflex

*References 43, 114, 115, 142, 209, 232, 233.

stiffness. Mechanical property of the muscle, such as viscosity, changes and is influenced by stretching velocities.[36] An analysis of neuromuscular response (EMG) could provide electrophysiologic insight into measurement of spasticity. In spastic muscles, a normal passive stretch could elicit an exaggerated stretch reflex response. The angle at which an EMG response is first detected when the limb is displaced at one or more velocities is defined as the threshold of stretch reflex.[140] The threshold indicates the onset of motoneuronal recruitment in response to external stretch. Based on this concept, Calota et al.[35] developed a portable device and demonstrated velocity-dependent dynamic stretch reflex threshold for spasticity measurement. This method provides electrophysiologic measures of spasticity. It is able to distinguish hypertonia between spasticity and rigidity.[168] However, it is not able to measure mechanical properties of spastic muscles that are associated with contracture. Furthermore, clinical application is somewhat limited to muscles of major joints. So far, it has been limited to the elbow flexors.[35,168]

Management

How can the problem be solved?
What are the safety-risk ratios and benefit-risk ratios of the chosen treatment?
Is the chosen management cost-effective?

Nonpharmacologic

Although spasticity is a neurologically based condition, its obvious manifestation is physical, and thus physical modalities are considered to be a mainstay in the first line of treatment, because they are widely available and innocuous relative to drugs. Passive stretching has been shown to be effective in reducing tone and increasing range of motion (ROM) in patients with brain injury.[212] Splinting and casting are often used in the acute setting for sustained stretching.[18,21,163,186,189] Casting alone seems sufficient to prevent contracture and to reduce spasticity if the intervention is initiated early after severe brain injury. A systematic review on the use of upper extremity casting found high variability in casting protocols, which indicates no consensus in technique.[133] Individualized stretching has been shown to be clinically promising to reduce wrist and finger spasticity and passive ROM.[46]

Electrical stimulation may be used to reduce spasticity temporarily.[200] A novel technique demonstrated a long-lasting effect on spasticity reduction if electrical stimulation was triggered by voluntary breathing.[143] The efficacy of electrical stimulation on spasticity reduction was not observed in more recent studies.[139,147]

Pharmacologic

There is more than one way to approach the pharmacologic management of spasticity. Historically there was a step ladder paradigm, beginning with the least invasive treatment and culminating with surgical procedures should nonoperative options fail. More recently, this sequential approach has been abandoned in favor of concurrent use of both "noninvasive" and "invasive" procedures (e.g., injection therapy concurrent with therapeutic exercises or the use of injection therapy for residual focal spasticity in persons' whole generalized spasticity is simultaneously managed with intrathecal drugs). This reflects better appreciation of the magnitude of the problem, that is, spasticity alone does not account for the presenting problem, and that other features of the UMN syndrome contribute significantly, and that different treatments may be required to increase the chances of successful outcome. There are also different methods when deciding on pharmacologic intervention for spasticity. One approach is to base drug choice on the clinical presentation and the number of limbs involved. The algorithm in Figure 23-3 illustrates this.

Another method is to determine the choice of drug on the underlying pathophysiology of spasticity, which in turn is influenced by neuroanatomic involvement in the disease process[26,54] (Figure 23-4). This can be particularly challenging, as it is not always easy to determine the exact pathophysiologic process responsible for spasticity.

Oral Spasmolytics

Various medications with different mechanisms of action have been used to treat spasticity, of which the most commonly used are baclofen, a gamma amino butyric acid B agonist,[49] tizanidine, an alpha-2 adrenergic receptor agonist, and dantrolene, a hydantoin derivative (Table 23-4). Others include benzodiazepines, which are $GABA_A$ agonists and gabapentin, a likely selective inhibitor of voltage-gated calcium channels, both antiepileptic drugs (AEDs). On the basis of a suggestion made by a few case reports and a series of studies, AEDs, including levetiracetam, pregabalin, phenytoin, and carbamazepine, also appear to exert a spasmolytic effect,[22,95] although their mechanisms of action vary. In general, oral spasmolytics are associated with similar and related adverse events, such as sedation, drowsiness, and weakness. These side effects limit the effective use of oral spasmolytics. A retrospective analysis that used medical and pharmacy claims data from a large, national U.S. health plan speculated that poor adherence could be a function of the adverse effects associated with oral baclofen, tizanidine, or dantrolene, or of the perception of the limited efficacy of these drugs. Oral drug adherence did not vary across patient populations, including stroke, SCI, TBI, cerebral palsy, and multiple sclerosis.[92]

Broadly, the evidence for therapeutic efficacy for all spasmolytic agents is supported by only a few placebo-controlled trials. Consequently, there is no evidence-based treatment algorithm for drug choice and dose. Instead, medication choice is based on practical reasons, such as favoring certain medications to avoid, or in some situations capitalize on, certain known adverse effects. For instance, a person with SCI and painful nocturnal spasms may be best managed by tizanidine, which has an analgesic effect independent of its spasmolytic effect. Because one of its common side effects is sedation, tizanidine may also help promote sleep that is disturbed by the spasms. However, if the same patient has orthostatic hypotension, or is taking clonidine, another alpha agonist, tizanidine may not be the best choice because of its potential hypotensive effect.

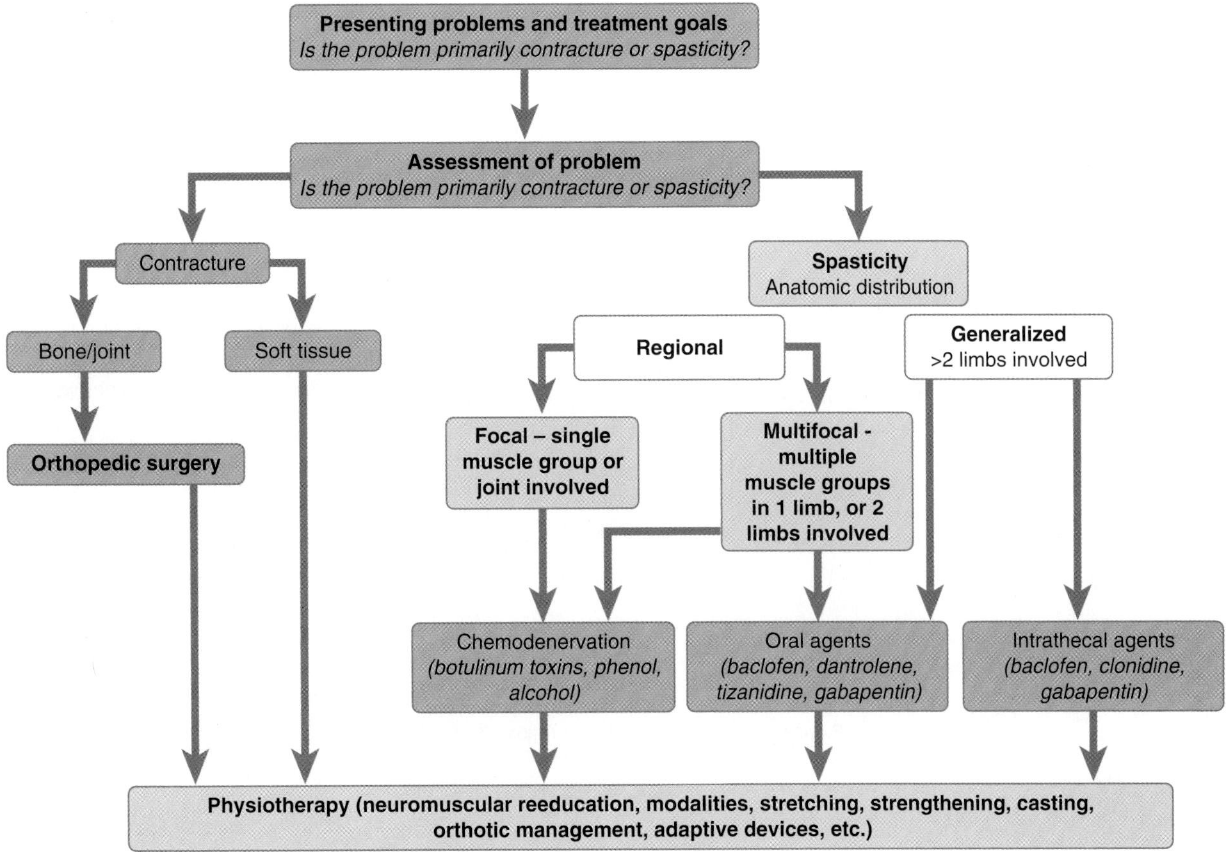

FIGURE 23-3 Clinical treatment decision making.

Medication dosages vary from person to person, largely resulting from the tolerability of side effects. Deficits in alertness and attention in people with cerebral disease are magnified by the sedating effects of oral spasmolytics. It is not uncommon to bypass oral drugs in this patient population and instead use focal injection therapy as first-line treatment. As a result of the therapeutic effect of spasmolytics, a reduction in muscle hypertonia may unmask latent weakness[213] in people with incomplete SCI or multiple sclerosis, who may lose the ability to ambulate should the weakness become pronounced. In this situation, a lower dose of the spasmolytic drug is preferred even though spasticity will not be adequately controlled. Another option is to use a combination of different medications, although at lower doses, to circumvent a particular side effect typical of a drug.

As presented earlier in this chapter, there are various independent or interacting pathophysiologic processes that are postulated to cause spasticity. Yet, in the absence of solid scientific evidence medication choices are typically empirical or to a certain extent based on the side effect profile of a drug. This common practice may explain why a particular medication is not consistently effective both within and across patient populations. Corollary to this, the fact that different pathomechanisms are involved resulting from varying disease types and severity or anatomic involvement may explain why a single medication cannot be always effective for a specific disease condition. This also imposes an important challenge in designing comparative efficacy and safety because of the heterogeneity of the likely pathomechanisms underlying the spastic condition and the mechanisms of action of various spasmolytic drugs.

Baclofen is an analog of GABA, the most potent inhibitory neurotransmitter. It binds to $GABA_B$ receptors that are widespread in Ia sensory afferent neurons and alpha motor neurons. It is the most widely studied oral spasmolytic in various patient populations, including SCI, multiple sclerosis, cerebral palsy, and acquired brain injuries (TBI, stroke, anoxia, or encephalopathy).* As with many spasticity medication trials, the studies involving baclofen demonstrated reduction in hypertonia and spasms, but did not investigate functional impact. Adverse effects of baclofen include drowsiness and weakness, which are shared by other oral spasmolytics. Abrupt discontinuation of baclofen may result in a withdrawal syndrome, characterized by rebound spasticity, hallucinations, and seizures.

Tizanidine is believed to exert its effects by inhibiting the facilitatory ceruleospinal tracts and the release of excitatory amino acid from spinal interneurons. As a result, presynaptic interneuronal excitation is suppressed manifesting as a reduction in tonic and phasic stretch reflexes and agonist-antagonist cocontraction.[213] Similar to baclofen, its efficacy in reducing muscle hypertonia and clonus, but not in improving function, has been demonstrated by various investigations.[153] However, in patients with stroke or TBI, tizanidine was deemed inferior to botulinum toxin in efficacy and safety in treating upper limb

*References 12, 62, 152, 157, 159, 184.

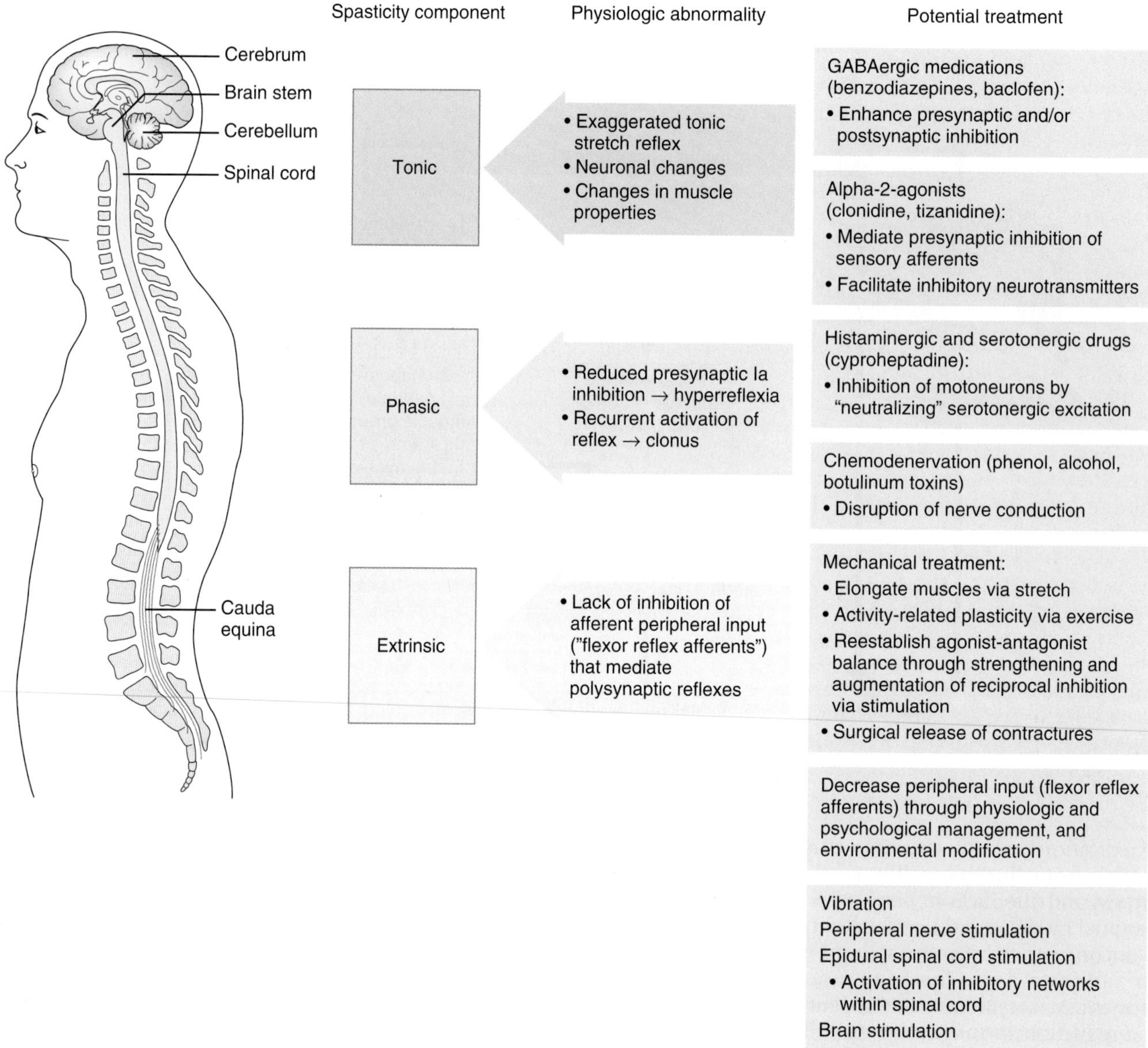

FIGURE 23-4 Spasticity treatment based on pathophysiology. (Adapted from references 26 and 54.)

Table 23-4 Classification of Drugs with Spasmolytic Activity According to Mechanism of Action

General Mechanism of Action	Drugs with Spasmolytic Activity
GABAergic	$GABA_A$: Benzodiazepines, Carisoprodol $GABA_B$: Baclofen
Monoaminergic	Tizanidine Clonidine Cyproheptadine Cyclobenzaprine
Ion flux blockade	Dantrolene (blocks calcium) 4-Aminopyridine (blocks potassium) Antiepileptic drugs, e.g., lamotrigine, phenytoin (blocks sodium); pregabalin (blocks calcium)
Excitatory amino acid suppression	Orphenadrine
Others	Cannabinoids

spasticity.[208] In addition to the typical side effects of oral spasmolytics, hepatotoxicity may also occur. Thus, monitoring liver function testing is important, especially in those patients who concomitantly take hepatically cleared drugs. Being a central alpha-2 adrenergic receptor agonist, tizanidine should be used carefully in patients with hypotension or are concomitantly taking other alpha agonists, such as clonidine. Likewise, caution should be used when coadministering tizanidine with fluoroquinolone antibiotics, which may increase the serum concentration of the former. Tizanidine is a peculiar spasmolytic in that it has a dose-dependent antinociceptive effect, presumably resulting from a reduction in the release of substance P and activity of excitatory amino acids at the spinal level.[194] This makes tizanidine a suitable choice for those with concurrent spasticity and pain. Concerns for its side effects, mainly drowsiness, sedation, reduced attention and memory impairment, and the potential for physiologic dependence have limited the use of benzodiazepines as first-line treatment for spasticity. They appear to be used more often when spasticity is accompanied by other conditions that are also amenable to benzodiazepine therapy, such as seizures, anxiety, insomnia, spasms, and other movement disorders. Similar to baclofen, benzodiazepines exert their effects through modulation of GABAergic transmission, but, unlike baclofen, which bind $GABA_B$ receptors, benzodiazepines bind $GABA_A$ receptors. Also similar to baclofen, abrupt discontinuation of benzodiazepines may result in a withdrawal syndrome.

Another GABAergic agent, gabapentin, is commonly used for the treatment of seizures and neuropathic pain, but through its selective inhibitory effect on voltage-gated calcium channels containing the $\alpha_2\delta$-1 subunit decreases muscle hypertonia. A few studies have demonstrated the beneficial effect of gabapentin on spasticity, although it seems that a dose as high as 2400 mg/day are needed.[49,63,72,89,166] Similar to other oral spasmolytics, the main adverse effects of gabapentin include drowsiness, sedation, and dizziness.

Dantrolene is used to manage a myriad of conditions, such as neuroleptic malignant syndrome and 3,4-methylenedioxymethamphetamine (MDMA; "ecstasy") overdose, but its first reported therapeutic use was for spasticity.[121] Unlike baclofen and tizanidine, which act on the central nervous system, dantrolene works directly on skeletal muscle. Although it is widely regarded to exert its muscle relaxant effect by inhibiting the release of calcium from the sarcoplasmic reticulum during excitation-contraction coupling, its exact mechanism of action has not been elucidated until recently. It appears that a direct or indirect inhibition of the ryanodine receptor, the major calcium release channel of the skeletal muscle sarcoplasmic reticulum, is fundamental in the molecular action of dantrolene in decreasing intracellular calcium concentration.[127] Several investigations have supported the beneficial effect of dantrolene on spasticity.[12,117,121,225] Although it is peripherally acting, dantrolene has also been associated with side effects that appear to be centrally mediated, such as drowsiness, dizziness, fatigue, and weakness, perhaps through alteration of neuronal calcium homeostasis.[69,117] Owing to its potential for hepatotoxicity, regular monitoring of liver function is recommended.

A systematic review of 101 randomized trials[41] found that baclofen, tizanidine, and dantrolene are effective in reducing spasticity relative to placebo, particularly in the multiple sclerosis population. It also found evidence that baclofen and tizanidine are equivalent in effectiveness, but that there was insufficient evidence to compare with dantrolene. The review also found fair evidence that the overall side effect rate between baclofen and tizanidine is similar, and that the former is more associated with weakness and the latter with dry mouth.

Other agents that have been observed to exert a spasmolytic effect in various patient populations with UMN disease include the alpha-adrenergic agonist clonidine, which has more affinity to alpha-2 rather than alpha-1 receptors.[145] 4-Aminopyridine, a potassium-channel blocker that is thought to enhance neural transmission by improving axonal conduction and synaptic neurotransmitter release has also been shown to reduce spasticity in patients with SCIs.[188] Cyproheptadine, a serotonergic antagonist, has been demonstrated to decrease spasticity in persons with SCI.[222] Cannabis and its active ingredient, delta-9-tetrahydrocannabinol, are believed to decrease spasticity,[47,179] especially in those with pain. Its use is limited owing to concerns about potential cognitive impairment and possible increased risk of psychosis associated with cannabis.

Focal Treatment: Botulinum Toxin Chemodenervation

Chemodenervation with botulinum toxins has become a widely used spasticity treatment. It is preferred for the management of focal spasticity, or when the treatment plan targets a particular muscle. Botulinum toxin exerts its effect through inhibition of acetylcholine release at the neuromuscular junction. The clinical effects of the toxin do not manifest until several days following an injection, largely caused by a complex process involved, which include: (1) internalization of the toxin; (2) reduction and translocation of disulfide bonds holding the light and heavy polypeptide chains of the toxin; and (3) inhibition of acetylcholine release. The last effect occurs because the internalized toxin cleaves so-called SNARE (soluble *n*-ethylmaleimide sensitive fusion attachment receptor) proteins that facilitate neuronal membrane adherence of synaptic vesicles, a necessary step before extrusion into the neuromuscular junction. The clinical effects last approximately 3 months, and was previously thought to be attributable to neuronal resprouting. However, it has been shown that functional repair of the previously affected neuromuscular junctions is the likely mechanism for the duration of action.[53] Up until recently, there had been only seven serotypes (A, B, C1, D, E, F, G) of *Clostridium botulinum* identified. The discovery of a new serotype, H, was the first for a neurotoxin in approximately 4 decades.[9] Currently, only serotypes A and B are used clinically: *abobotulinumtoxinA, incobotulinumtoxinA, onabotulinumtoxinA, rimabotulinumtoxinB*. All serotypes share common properties in that they are all clostridial neurotoxins with a bichain structure. They all inhibit acetylcholine release and the muscle paralysis they produce is reversible. However, they are antigenically distinct, and they have varying neuronal binding site and enzymatic actions on different SNARE proteins. They may also have different species specificity. Table 23-5 summarizes these differences and other properties of pharmaceutical preparations of these toxins.

Consensus and review papers support the use of botulinum toxins for the management of spastic conditions in pediatric and adult populations.[52,192,205,207,228] Although overwhelming evidence demonstrates that botulinum toxin chemodenervation results in significant improvement at the body function and structure level,* it has not been shown unequivocally to be significantly efficacious in improving the activity and participation domains of the International Classification of Functioning.[24,37,70,75] Perhaps, published studies failed to show the impact on function as a result of methodological limitations, such as in subject selection and sensitivity of outcome measures.

---

*References 7, 14, 33, 101, 131, 192, 193, 202, 205, 207, 214, 228.

Table 23-5 Comparison of Some Commercially Available Botulinum Toxin Preparations

	AbobotulinumtoxinA	IncobotulinumtoxinA	OnabotulinumtoxinA	RimabotulinumtoxinB
Clostridium botulinum strain	Ipsen strain	Hall A	Hall A	Bean B
SNARE target	SNAP-25	SNAP-25	SNAP-25	VAMP
Preparation	Powder for reconstitution	Powder for reconstitution	Powder for reconstitution	Ready-to-use-solution
Storage	Below 8 degrees	Below 25 degrees	Below 8 degrees	Below 8 degrees
Shelf life	15 months	36 months	24 to 36 months	24 months
pH of solution	7.4	7.4	7.4	5.6
Stabilization	Freeze dried	Vacuum dried	Vacuum dried	pH reduced
Excipients	Human serum albumin 125 µg/vial; Lactose 2500 µg/vial	Human serum albumin 1 mg/vial; sucrose 5 mg/vial	Human serum albumin 500 µg/vial; NaCl 900 µg/vial	Not reported
Biological activity	500 MU-I/vial	100 MU-M/vial	100 MU-A/vial	1/2.5/10 kMU-E/vial

Adapted from Dressler D, Benecke R: Pharmacology of therapeutic botulinum toxin preparations, *Disabil Rehabil* 29:1761-1768, 2007.

Clinical Issues Related to Botulinum Toxin Chemodenervation

Dosing. Clinical experience, regulatory and insurance coverage restrictions, and manufacturers' recommendations based on a few studies largely dictate the choice of doses of the various botulinum toxins. There are a handful of dose-ranging studies that define dose-related therapeutic and adverse effects in spasticity.* Doses that are used in current practice, recommended by consensus statements[228] and described in retrospective studies,[60,81] appear to be higher than doses used in published randomized controlled studies. The use of escalating doses of botulinum toxins was becoming a common practice until safety concerns were raised and fueled by mandates from the U.S. Food and Drug Administration (FDA). Responding to reports suggestive of systemic botulinum toxins, in 2009 the FDA required new label warnings and a risk mitigation strategy that requires clinicians to discuss the risks and provide written material that details the warnings. The current experience of many clinicians is that using dosages of incobotulinumtoxinA and onabotulinumtoxinA as high as 600 to 800 units is effective and safe.[197,227]

Dilution. It is believed that increasing the volume of botulinum toxin solution injected magnifies its therapeutic effects by facilitating the ability of the toxin to reach more motor end plates. This has been demonstrated in animal studies,[124,201] where muscle paralysis and atrophy were greater when a more dilute preparation, that is, higher volume relative to dose, or lower concentration, of botulinum toxin is injected. Humans studies are equivocal in demonstrating superiority of higher volumes of botulinum toxin injections,[76,135] largely as a result of methodological limitations of studies, although some investigations have found that high-volume or end plate–targeted botulinum toxin injections result in more profound neuromuscular blockade and spasticity and cocontraction reduction, as compared with low-volume, non–end plate–targeted injections.[87] As much as high-volume injections appear attractive, it may be a double-edged sword in that it may facilitate distant spread of the toxin. Cases have been reported wherein patients with poststroke spasticity who receive large dilution volumes in proximal upper limb muscles developed transient weakness in the noninjected contralateral upper limb. Based on electrophysiologic abnormalities documented following the injection, weakness was attributed to neuromuscular blockade.

Techniques to Enhance Toxin Effectiveness. There is a lot of interest in techniques to enhance the clinical effects of botulinum toxin, without concomitantly increasing the risk for adverse events. Prohibited by recommended total toxin dose and cost, clinicians continuously seek ways to extend the clinical effects of toxin through modification of injection technique and use of adjunctive modalities. Although no standard currently exists, spreading the toxin within a muscle by using a higher volume/more dilute toxin solution (already discussed earlier) and injecting at multiple sites within a muscle are regarded as ways to increase effectiveness by spreading the toxin to reach more muscle end plates, where neuromuscular junctions lie. It has also been suggested that targeting the muscle innervation zone, not just the motor points, can optimize the effects of botulinum toxin administration.[91] In some muscles, these areas where intramuscular nerve endings are distributed may also result in better outcomes.[108] Other techniques used to attempt enhancement of toxin effectiveness include guided injection by listening to EMG activity, identifying motor points through electrical stimulation, or visualizing target sites by sonography. The superiority of one guidance technique over another is yet to be established, but consistently studies have demonstrated that either electrical stimulation or sonography is better than anatomic localization through muscle palpation.[180-182,199]

The beneficial role of adjunctive therapy modalities in enhancing clinical outcomes of botulinum toxin chemodenervation has not been well studied. The few investigations described the potentially beneficial effects of casting[176] and adhesive taping,[196] but in the case of the latter, subsequent studies did not yield consistent results.[116] Casting may also enhance the effect of onabotulinumtoxinA,[65] because prolonged stretching of spastic muscles after botulinum toxin chemodenervation affords long-lasting therapeutic benefit.

*References 6, 16, 40, 86, 107, 206.

Table 23-6 Potential Reasons for Poor Outcome of Botulinum Toxin Chemodenervation

Patient-Related	Injector-Related	Drug-Related
• Age and size • Disease condition • Concurrent medications that interact with spasmolytic drugs or alter muscle tone • Unrealistic goals • Immunoresistance • Genetics (?)	• Incorrect diagnosis • Incorrect muscle selection • Improper injection technique	• Incorrect dose • Incorrect preparation • Inactive medication

Another promising technique to magnify the clinical effect of botulinum toxin chemodenervation is pairing it with superficial electrical stimulation, which influences activity of synaptobrevin-2[211] receptors that facilitate neuronal binding and subsequent uptake of botulinum toxins.[11,99,150,226] More recently, extracorporeal shockwave therapy has been shown to have a greater magnitude of enhancement of botulinum toxin enhancement than electrical stimulation, most likely through modulation of muscle rheology and neurotransmission.[197,226]

Reasons for Poor Response to Botulinum Toxin Chemodenervation. Botulinum toxin is widely regarded as an effective treatment of spasticity, but the response to treatment varies from person to person. In most cases, spasticity relief is not sufficient, whereas in others even relatively small doses may result in weakness and other adverse events. Table 23-6 summarizes some potential reasons for poor outcomes of botulinum toxin chemodenervation.

Immunoresistance. In addition to unintended toxin diffusion to neighboring nerve endings and to distant areas owing to still yet to be defined mechanisms,[191,216] other undesirable effects of botulinum toxin therapy include sustained blockade of neural transmission that results in prolonged effects similar to anatomic denervation, such as muscle atrophy and immunoresistance. The latter accounts for loss of responsiveness to the spasmolytic effects of botulinum toxins. Thus, there is growing interest in incobotulinumtoxinA, which is free of excipient proteins and, as such, may have a lower propensity to induce an immunogenic response relative to the other botulinum toxin preparations with complexing proteins[13,111] Based on early reports in the cervical dystonia population, high doses and frequent injections of botulinum toxin were identified as risk factors for immunoresistance.[88,234] This also provided support for the practice of allowing no less than 90 days in between exposures to botulinum toxins. A much higher incidence of antibody formation has been associated with cervical dystonia than in spasticity.[170] A metaanalysis of 16 clinical trials involving a total of 3006 participants with various diagnoses found that neutralizing antibodies determined by mouse protection assay appeared in 1.28% of cervical dystonia, as opposed to only 0.32% poststroke patients. In another pooled analysis involving three 12- to 42-week clinical poststroke spasticity studies, the formation of neutralizing antibodies was found to be 0.5% (1 out of 191 patients).[231]

Bioassay of neutralizing antibodies to botulinum toxin is considered the gold standard in confirming immunoresistance, but more practical clinical tests, such as the FTAT (frontalis antibody test) or UBI (unilateral brow injection), can be easily performed by injecting a small dose of botulinum toxin in either the frontalis (FTAT) or corrugator (UBI) muscle.[25] Another method to assess nonresponse is the EDB (extensor digitorum brevis) test that involves measurement of compound muscle action potential amplitude elicited by electrical nerve stimulation of the peroneal nerve before and after injection of a small dose of botulinum toxin into the EDB.[120]

Repeated Injections: When Is "Enough" Enough? Most studies involving the use of botulinum toxin for spasticity involve only a few cycles of injection. A rare few have reported safety and sustained efficacy up to five injection cycles over a few years.[64,82,130] In clinical practice, many patients receive multiple injections over a period of many years, sometimes decades, and the long-term effects are not systematically documented. The fact that patients continue to receive botulinum toxin over a long period of time implies that the patients continue to enjoy the benefits of the treatment without experiencing adverse events. However, some studies have claimed that safety concerns remain about the long-term effect of botulinum toxins on muscles following repeated injections. An animal study concluded that the contractile properties of target and nontarget muscles did not fully recover within 6 months of a botulinum toxin injection treatment protocol.[73] The same investigators also found that following repeated botulinum toxin injections, muscle atrophy sets in and contractile material is replaced by fat.[74] Recognition of the effects of botulinum toxin on muscle length and force[217] is also emerging, although how this translates clinically is still unclear. These concerning findings need to be studied further in clinical studies emphasizing muscle changes in recovery after botulinum toxin chemodenervation.

Another area that warrants further investigation is the determination of when other treatment interventions should be considered after repeated botulinum toxin injections. For example, how many botulinum toxin injections need to be done to address a spastic-dystonic "clenched fist" before surgical release of the finger and thumb flexor tendons should be considered? How many times should a person with spastic paraplegia receive botulinum toxins before intrathecal baclofen therapy is considered? The economic impact of these clinical decisions will also need to be weighed to better appreciate the cost-effectiveness of spasticity interventions.

Early Treatment. There is no standard in how early botulinum toxins can be safely and effectively administered. A few studies reported that treatment as early as 3 to 6 months of disease onset effectively manages muscle hypertonia and decreases risk of later complications, such as contracture development.[67,98]

Recovery of Function. The effect of botulinum toxins is primarily in decreasing muscle hypertonia resulting from spasticity and other related conditions, such as rigidity. However, there are unusual, but not rare, cases when the

CASE 3

Delayed Recovery of Function

P.J. is a 69-year-old right-handed male who presented with a 3-year history of multiple cerebral insults. He was involved in a motor vehicle crash that resulted in a moderate traumatic brain injury. During the difficult extrication from the vehicle, he lost blood that resulted in hypotension on the scene. While recovering from these at the intensive care unit he had a brain stem stroke and a suspected hypoxic event. Upon recovery, he had proximal muscle weakness and profound difficulty with walking. He subsequently developed spasticity in the right upper limb, characterized by a "clenched fist," involving severe flexion of the fingers and thumb, which prevented his caregivers from cleaning his hand and trimming his fingernails (Figure 23-5, A). He was on oral baclofen 10 mg three times daily at the time of presentation. On examination, he had limb weakness (at best 4 out of 5 in most limbs) and an Ashworth score of 4 in the right finger, metacarpal (MCP) and thumb flexors, 1 in the wrist and elbow flexors. The third distal interphalangeal joint was hyperextended. Given the focality of the spasticity, the clinician suggested weaning the oral baclofen with intent to discontinue after approximately 4 weeks and botulinum toxin injection of the flexor digitorum superficialis (onabotulinumtoxinA, 100 units) and profundus (75 units), and flexor pollicis longus (25 units). Around 1 month after the injection, the Ashworth score of the finger and thumb flexors decreased to 2. The patient received another injection of onabotulinumtoxinA 3 months after the first injection to the same muscles with the same doses. An additional 20 units were injected into the lumbricals to address the MCP flexion spasticity. Approximately 1 month later, the patient reported not only a significant decrease in tightness but also a new ability to actively extend his fingers and open his hand (Figure 23-5, B, C, and D). He also received occupational therapy that focused on "forced-use" activities and functional retraining. Subsequently, he recovered full active movement of the right hand and the ability to perform functional tasks, such as picking up objects including utensils and a drinking glass during meals, combing his hair, and buttoning his shirt.

CASE 4

Therapeutic Weakness

T.P. is a 53-year-old right-handed female who sustained a hemorrhagic right middle cerebral artery stroke 3 years earlier. She had finger flexor spasticity and residual weak finger/wrist extension. She received 50 units of botulinum toxin type A injection, each of the left flexor digitorum superficialis and flexor digitorum profundus, respectively. As expected, botulinum toxin injection led to tone reduction and weakness of the spastic finger flexors. However, she was able to open her hand more quickly probably as a result of improved ability to more quickly release handgrip. She also reported increased ability to engage the impaired hand when performing various activities of daily living. This correlated with reduced finger extensor muscle electromyography activity, as shown in Figure 23-6. The improvement in voluntary control of hand opening and grip release was probably realized by a decrease in the abnormal cocontraction of finger flexors during voluntary finger extension. This case suggested that a reduction in finger flexor spasticity following botulinum toxin injection is associated with improvement in voluntary control of residual finger extension.

outcome of botulinum toxin injection surpasses this expectation and results in an increase in functional abilities, particularly when appropriate therapeutic exercise is included in the treatment regimen. Although an obvious explanation for the outcome in this particular case is the uncovering of latent finger and thumb extensors strength once flexor spasticity is controlled, alternative mechanisms should be considered. Could it be that botulinum toxin merely controlled spasticity of the finger flexors and it was the ensuing "forced use" and task-specific exercises that accounted for the increased function? Natural recovery may be dismissed because the improvement occurred almost 4 years after the onset of neurologic disease, but it may be postulated that controlling spasticity may have allowed the progression of natural recovery that was stalled when spasticity set in? Did altering muscle hypertonia and stretch properties also modify afferent input into the spinal cord, and subsequently influence motor output?[161] Or could it be that botulinum toxins have yet-to-be defined direct central nervous system effects, as suggested by some reports?[5,48,79]

"Therapeutic Weakness." Botulinum toxin injection to the spastic muscles concurrently results in both spasticity reduction and muscle weakness, the latter either as a latent phenomenon uncovered by spasticity reduction or a direct consequence of the toxin. It has been observed that in some patients, this weakness could lead to less resistance to voluntary activation of the antagonist muscles, resulting in improvement of voluntary control of the weakened spastic muscles and their antagonist muscles. For this reason, it is coined "therapeutic weakness." This phenomenon is revealed in a recent case of improved voluntary grip and release control after botulinum toxin type A injection to spastic finger flexors.[38]

This concept is further supported by another study,[14] where 15 patients with spastic hemiparesis from stroke or TBI were instructed to perform reaching movements within the available ROM before and 1 month after botulinum toxin injections. All patients performed reaching movements better, including reaching velocity and smoothness after injections. However, clinical outcomes, such as the Action Research Arm Test and the Box and Block Test, remained unchanged. These findings cannot be explained by spasticity reduction alone. Although EMG activity of flexors and extensor muscles was not recorded, the authors postulated that improved reaching performance after injections to the flexors was likely to be related to better control of antagonist extensor muscles. In other words, voluntary control of extensor muscles during reaching movements is achieved from decreased flexors spasticity and weakening of flexors after injections. Collectively, these findings showed better voluntary control of extensor muscles and subsequent functional improvement after reduction in spasticity of (elbow, wrist, and finger) flexors in a selected group of spastic hemiparesis after stroke and TBI. It is also important to point out that these patients had preserved voluntary, although weak, control of extensor muscles before injection. Improvement in voluntary

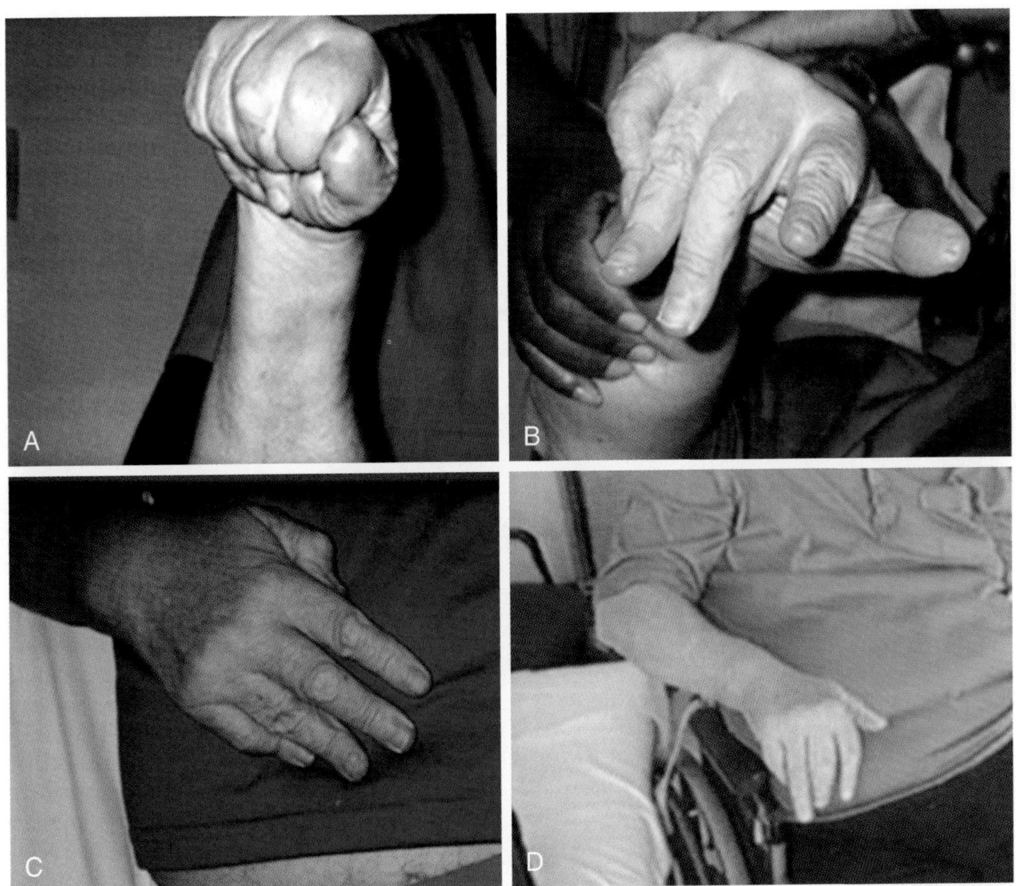

FIGURE 23-5 **A,** Severe flexion of the fingers and thumb. **B, C, D,** After injection of onabotulinumtoxinA, a significant decrease in tightness is seen, but also a new ability to actively extend the fingers and open the hand.

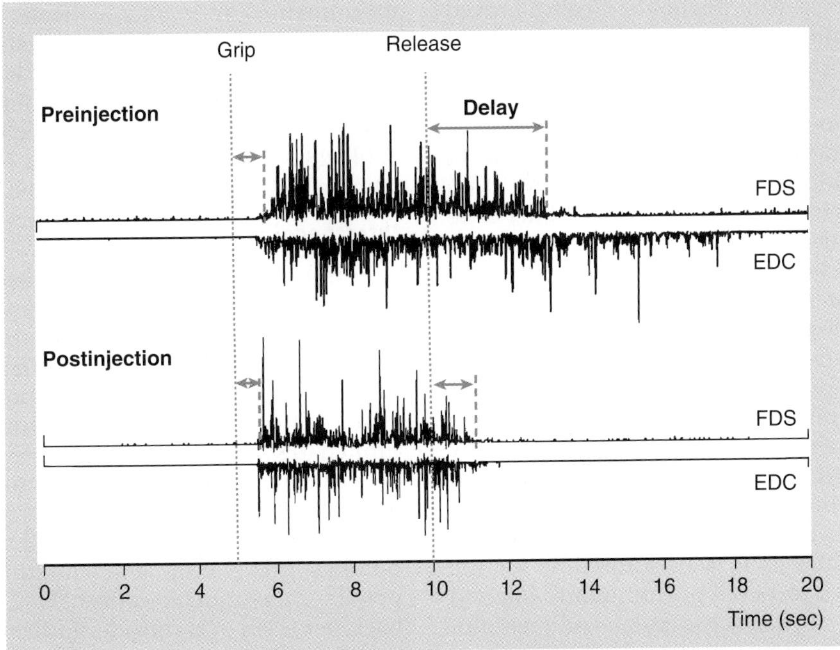

FIGURE 23-6 A representative electromyography (EMG) of flexor digitorum superficialis (FDS) and extensor digitorum communis (EDC) before and 10 days after botulinum toxin injection. The patient was asked to grip as soon and as hard as possible after the "grip" signal and relax after the "release" signal (dashed lines). The release delay time decreases after injection, along with shortened EDC activities. (From Chang SH, Francisco GE, Li S: Botulinum toxin (BT) injection improves voluntary motor control in selected patients with post-stroke spasticity, *Neural Regen Res* 7:1436-1439, 2012.)

Table 23-7 Comparison of Clinical Characteristics of Botulinum Toxins and Phenol

	Phenol	Botulinum Toxin
Mechanism of action	Neurolysis	Blockade of acetylcholine release into neuromuscular junction
Onset	Immediate (anesthetic effect); within 24 to 48 hours (neurolytic effect)	5 to 10 days
Duration	Variable: dose-dependent	3 months
Dose titration to desired effect	Yes	Yes
Target injection site	Muscle (motor end plates)	Nerves, typically motor branches
Injection technique	Percutaneous with electrical stimulation or sonographic guidance	Intramuscular with electromyography, electrical stimulation, or sonographic guidance
Ease of administration	Requires more training and expertise	Relatively easy
Evidence of efficacy	Randomized controlled trials published	Randomized controlled trials published
Pain during injection	More	Some
Pain days after injection	Higher risk	Rare
Adverse events	Higher incidence of dysesthetic pain and swelling, among others	Less common dysesthetic pain; also refer to U.S. Food and Drug Administration "Black Box Warning"

control of extensor muscles is likely to be a result of reduced reciprocal inhibition from the spastic flexors after injection. Previous results have shown that injections can paralyze afferent fibers,[68] in addition to blocking acetylcholine release presynaptically at neuromuscular junctions.

Focal Pharmacologic Treatment: Nerve Block (Neurolysis)

Before the introduction of botulinum toxins, nerve block with either alcohol or phenol was the only option for focal spasticity management. It was used in the 1950s to chemically ablate nerves to manage cancer-related pain, and subsequently applied to relieve spasticity. Over time, percutaneous nerve blocks with phenol or alcohol proved to be effective in controlling focal spasticity across different populations, including cerebral palsy, TBIs, and stroke.[42,122] Phenol (5% to 7%) and alcohol (35% to 60%) denature proteins in neural tissues, leading to blockade of nerve transmission. In addition, phenol appears to result in degeneration of muscle spindles[229] and damage to both afferent and efferent nerve fibers.[17] This chemical denervation is thought to be irreversible and to lead to permanent control of spasticity; however, this is not commonly observed clinically, because spasticity tends to return several months after the percutaneous block. This may be explained by partial nerve regrowth and sprouting.

Percutaneous injections can either be at the nerve or motor branch level, guided by electrical stimulation or ultrasound. Because phenol is also an anesthetic, especially at concentrations less than 3%, muscle relaxation commonly observed immediately after injection is as a result of the anesthetic effect. The neurolytic effect may not set in until a few hours later as it takes some time for the effects on neural tissues to develop. Commonly injected upper limb nerves are pectoral, subscapular, and musculocutaneous. In the lower limb, the obturator and tibial nerves and their branches are commonly treated. Care must be exercised in injecting nerves with a significant sensory component to mitigate risk of developing postinjection dysesthesia. Other side effects include localized swelling and excessive weakness. Inadvertent intravascular injection or systemic absorption may result in cardiovascular or central nervous system effects, including hypotension and tremor or convulsions, respectively.

Nerve blocks with phenol and alcohol have taken a backseat to chemodenervation with botulinum toxins, which appear to have a better safety profile and are easier to administer. Although both treatments are effective when applied to the appropriate clinical indication and perform well, there is no evidence demonstrating superiority of one over the other in managing spasticity. To date, there is only one peer-reviewed publication comparing onabotulinumtoxinA and phenol 5%.[125] In this study, both onabotulinumtoxinA and phenol were effective in reducing spasticity as measured by the Ashworth scores of ankle plantar flexors and invertors, but that the former was better in decreasing muscle tone and ankle clonus at 2 and 4 weeks, but not at 8 and 12 weeks, following injection. Table 23-7 presents a comparison of the clinical characteristics of botulinum toxins and phenol.

Intrathecal Therapies

As early as the 1950s, intrathecal phenol was used to reduce pain and spasticity. Its popularity has waned owing to its many potential complications, such as sensory, respiratory, bladder, bowel, and sexual dysfunction, and the introduction of baclofen, which appears to have a better adverse effect profile. The use of intrathecal phenol is now limited to specific situations, where severe spasticity cannot be managed through any of the other currently available techniques.[110] Other drugs that have been administered intrathecally primarily manage pain, among which are opioids, gabapentin, and clonidine, the last one with possible spasmolytic effect.[158] Continuous intrathecal baclofen (ITB) was introduced in the 1980s to treat spasticity in SCI. Since then, several trials demonstrated similar beneficial effects in other patient populations, such as cerebral palsy,[1] brain injuries,[155] stroke,[154] and multiple sclerosis.[178]

The physiologic effect of ITB involves a decrease in monosynaptic and polysynaptic reflex responses,[134] and reduction in resistance to passive stretch.[198] At the cellular level, the mechanism of action of ITB is similar to that of the oral form; however, it has the advantage of more direct access to $GABA_B$ receptors in the spinal cord because the blood-brain barrier will not have to be traversed. Thus, intrathecal administration allows greater hypertonia reduction and reflex inhibition at doses lower than the oral form, and hence decreases the risk of adverse events.

ITB is usually considered only when less invasive management options are ineffective in controlling spasticity, although use within the first few months of disease onset may be warranted in situations where spasticity of the lower limbs is so severe such that waiting for other less invasive options to take effect may predispose to more complications. An investigation on the use of ITB within 3 months of acquired brain injuries showed significant reduction of spasticity and spasm frequency at 1-year follow-up, and their global outcome measures did not differ from those who received ITB therapy later (between 3 and 6 months of disease onset).[187] Another situation where very early use has been shown to be beneficial is in people with severe dysautonomia following a brain injury.[77] Concern exists that early use of ITB may retard recovery as a result of the inhibitory effects of GABA,[23] but a more recent study suggests otherwise. In an animal model, ITB treatment was initiated at 1 week postclosed TBI and maintained for 1 month. It appeared to block the early onset of spasticity and significantly diminish late-onset spasticity and anxiety-like behavior, without causing any significant adverse effect on cognitive and balance performance of rats. Concurrently, it was observed that there was a marked upregulation of GABA, norepinephrine, and brain-derived neurotropic factor expression in spinal cord tissue.[19]

The intrathecal system consists of a programmable pump that has an accessible drug reservoir that is implanted subcutaneously in the abdominal area. A catheter that is connected to the side port of the implanted pump is tunneled under the skin and enters the spine at the lumbar level. The catheter tip is advanced cephalad and usually left at the thoracic level, although it is not uncommon for it to be placed at the cervical area,[2] or sometimes intraventricularly.[218] Before surgical implantation of the catheter and pump, a "trial" is performed to confirm the effectiveness of ITB in decreasing spasticity, spasms, or pain. The trial typically involves bolus administration of baclofen into the intrathecal space through a spinal needle. An alternative method is to continuously infuse baclofen intrathecally through an external catheter.[93] Given risks associated with this technique, performance of the trial usually requires hospital admission, as compared with the former method, which is carried out in the ambulatory setting. Superiority of one over the other has not been established, although the former appears to be more commonly employed because it is not as labor or resource intensive. A successful screening trial is generally defined as a 1- to 2-point drop on the Ashworth scale. However, in certain situations the Ashworth Scale is not always applicable. For instance, the indication for considering ITB may be painful, intermittent, spasms, where the use of the Ashworth Scale as an assessment tool and outcome measure is not valid. Sometimes, the indication is to decrease tone (regardless of Ashworth scores) just enough to facilitate positioning for care and transfers, or to allow participation in a therapeutic exercise program. In addition to the usual assessment with the Ashworth Scale and ROM testing, videotaping while performing tasks actively or passively may help clinicians and patients and caregivers to decide on whether or not intrathecal infusion of baclofen may help with spasticity or spasms. The recommended intrathecal bolus dose of baclofen during a screening trial is 50 µg. If ineffective, the option is to try higher doses sequentially: 75 and 100 µg. Some patients, such as those with multiple sclerosis and incomplete SCI, demonstrate profound weakness confounding spasticity and may experience exaggeration of the underlying weakness immediately after a screening trial. First, the patient must be assured that weakness during the trial is reversible and that it does not mean the same degree of weakness will occur after ITB pump implantation. The finding of increased postscreening trial weakness merely demonstrates that ITB has the potential to abolish spasticity and suggests that the patient will most likely require a low dose of ITB following pump implantation. Thus, instead of starting with the "usual" starting dose after pump implantation (determined by doubling the dose used during the screening trial that resulted in significant decrease in spasticity), the starting daily dose may be the same bolus dose used during the trial. To illustrate, if a patient experienced good control of spasticity or spasms with a 50-µg *bolus* of baclofen but also experienced an increase in weakness, the initial dose postpump implantation may be 50 µg infused continuously over a 24-hour period. Another strategy to assuage concerns about excessive weakness during the screening trial is to use a lower dose (e.g., a 25-µg bolus). Although 97% of patients with spasticity resulting from SCI[177] and 94% with cerebral origin spasticity[80] respond positively to bolus screening trials, it is still advantageous to perform the screening trial to allow the patients and caregivers an opportunity to experience a state of low or no spasticity. The trial results can also guide the physician regarding future dose targets and a patient's peculiar response to intrathecal baclofen.

When planning ITB therapy, nonmedical conditions need to be considered, such as the patient's ability to comply with dose titration and pump management, which will require regular visits with the clinician. Management does not end with implantation of the pump; frequent dose adjustments will be needed subsequently to reach appropriate ITB dose. We define *optimal dose* as one that adequately controls (not completely abolishes) spasticity without causing any unwanted effect. Thus optimal dose can be determined only by titrating the dose upward until a side effect occurs (e.g., excessive weakness, bladder retention, constipation), and then decreased to a level that does not cause the adverse event. The frequency of regular refills of the pump reservoir depends on the dose and concentration of the drug. The importance of patient and caregiver education regarding the need for pump maintenance, including refills, and recognition of potential ITB system-related problems cannot be overemphasized.

This case demonstrates the importance of recognizing the signs and symptoms of ITB withdrawal, especially when they appear concurrently with other abnormalities.

CASE 5

Intrathecal Baclofen Withdrawal

L.Y. is a 27-year-old female in a minimally conscious state secondary to anoxic brain damage 10 years earlier who presented to the emergency room with generalized seizures. Before this, her seizures had been well controlled with carbamazepine. Her mother reported that a few days earlier the patient "just did not seem like herself" and that since the day before she was "a lot more tight in the legs than usual." The mother reported that the patient's urine seemed to be cloudier, but did not pay much attention to this. The mother had difficulty pointing out the exact day she noticed these changes in the patient owing to the patient's inability to meaningfully communicate. Past medical history is significant for seizure disorder that developed after the anoxic event, but has been well controlled by carbamazepine. An intrathecal baclofen (ITB) pump was implanted 7 years earlier to better control seizures and extensor posturing. Current (ITB) dosage is 974.8 μg/day, which controls lower limb spasticity well enough to facilitate care and transfers, and the most recent intrathecal pump refill was 6 weeks earlier. Aside from ITB and baclofen, the patient was not on any other medication. At the emergency room, she also had a temperature of 102.1° F. Blood pressure was 120/70, and heart rate 110/min. The mother added that the patient seemed more restless and uncomfortable. The patient was subsequently admitted to the critical care unit, where her temperature increased to 104.0° F. Efforts to decrease hyperthermia with a cooling blanket and acetaminophen failed to resolve fever. While awaiting the blood and urine test results, including culture, she was empirically started on broad-spectrum intravenous antibiotics because the clinician was suspecting that sepsis may have triggered the seizure. Chest radiograph was normal, and a noncontrast computed tomography scan of the brain did not show any acute lesion. Six hours after admission to the unit, she had status epilepticus in spite of intravenous lorazepam and phenytoin. Her temperature increased to 106.8° F. Urinalysis, complete blood count, and electrolytes were normal. Later that evening the patient went into cardiac arrest.

A suspicion of sepsis-triggered seizure in this case was justified owing to the report of changes in urine color and fever. However, there were other earlier signs that should have indicated ITB withdrawal, such as recurrence of spasticity ("a lot more tight in the legs than usual"). This, in addition to the nonspecific change in her overall condition ("just did not seem like herself"), sudden recurrence of seizures, and fever, should have raised the suspicion of ITB withdrawal in its advanced stage. The ITB pump should have been interrogated to assess function, a plain radiograph of the pump and catheter should have been done to assess gross catheter integrity, and intrathecal or enteral bolus of baclofen should have been considered. ITB withdrawal evolves over 1 to 3 days[44] and usually results from an abrupt decrease in GABA activity. Supportive measures and drugs, such as benzodiazepines, intravenous dantrolene,[123] and cyproheptadine,[156] may help mitigate withdrawal symptoms, but a definitive treatment is restitution of intrathecal baclofen delivery. Figure 23-7 presents an algorithm for troubleshooting suspected ITB problems.

The most common drug-related side effect is hypotonia, followed by somnolence, headache, convulsion, dizziness, and urinary retention. Pump-related adverse events include pump stall, but catheter-related problems, including dislodgement, fracture, and kinking, are more common. Finally, clinician-related complications, such as dosage and programming error that can lead to either underdose or overdose, can occur.

Surgical Intervention

Surgical management of spasticity is a well-accepted treatment option for contractures, as it primarily addresses joint deformities rather than spasticity itself. Surgical interventions include neuroablative procedures, such as peripheral neurotomies and dorsal rhizotomies, and orthopedic reconstructive procedures, such as tendon lengthening and tendon transfer. Surgical intervention is a permanent treatment. Optimal management of spasticity by nonsurgical means should be attempted before surgical treatment is employed. Therefore it is often viewed as a treatment of "last resort." However, surgical intervention could be pursued earlier in cases where other options are unavailable owing to lack of availability or resources. When excessive spasticity and contracture are not sufficiently controlled by therapy and pharmacologic treatment, tendon lengthening is often considered. This involves correction of abnormal joint posture alignment, allowing for improved ability to move joints and in many cases facilitate activity and exercise.[119] Common tendon procedures include split anterior tibial tendon transfer (SPLATT) and Achilles tendon lengthening to manage spastic equinovarus.[55] Tendon lengthening and release can also help with upper limb management.[3] Surgical interventions primarily manage joint deformities rather than spasticity itself. Tendon lengthening elongates the tendon, and subsequently corrects the abnormal joint position. But it does not change the contractile and mechanical properties of muscle and its innervation. In other words, the unchanged spastic muscle has a new resting position at a corrected joint position via the elongated tendon. The reflex responses are both velocity and muscle (not tendon) length-dependent[142] and related to muscle fiber length and sarcomere numbers.[71,78,144] The exaggerated reflex responses are still expected to remain unchanged, if the same stretch is applied with reference to the new resting position. Therefore tendon lengthening can improve posture, but is not likely to correct altered stretch reflex in spastic muscles. Other procedures, such as neurotomy, have also been shown to benefit spastic conditions.[30,61]

Emerging Therapies

In addition to the various treatment options described earlier, other modalities are emerging as potential primary or adjunctive spasticity management options. These include acupuncture[103] vibration,[34,195] and noninvasive brain,[10,90,129,230] spinal,[183] and transcutaneous[100,175] nerve stimulation. The effect of peripheral nerve stimulation appears inconsistent.[128] Extracorporeal shockwave therapy is also being investigated.[162,197] Currently, there is very little research evidence or clinical experience to support the use of these interventions and, as such, they are not widely used in clinical practice.

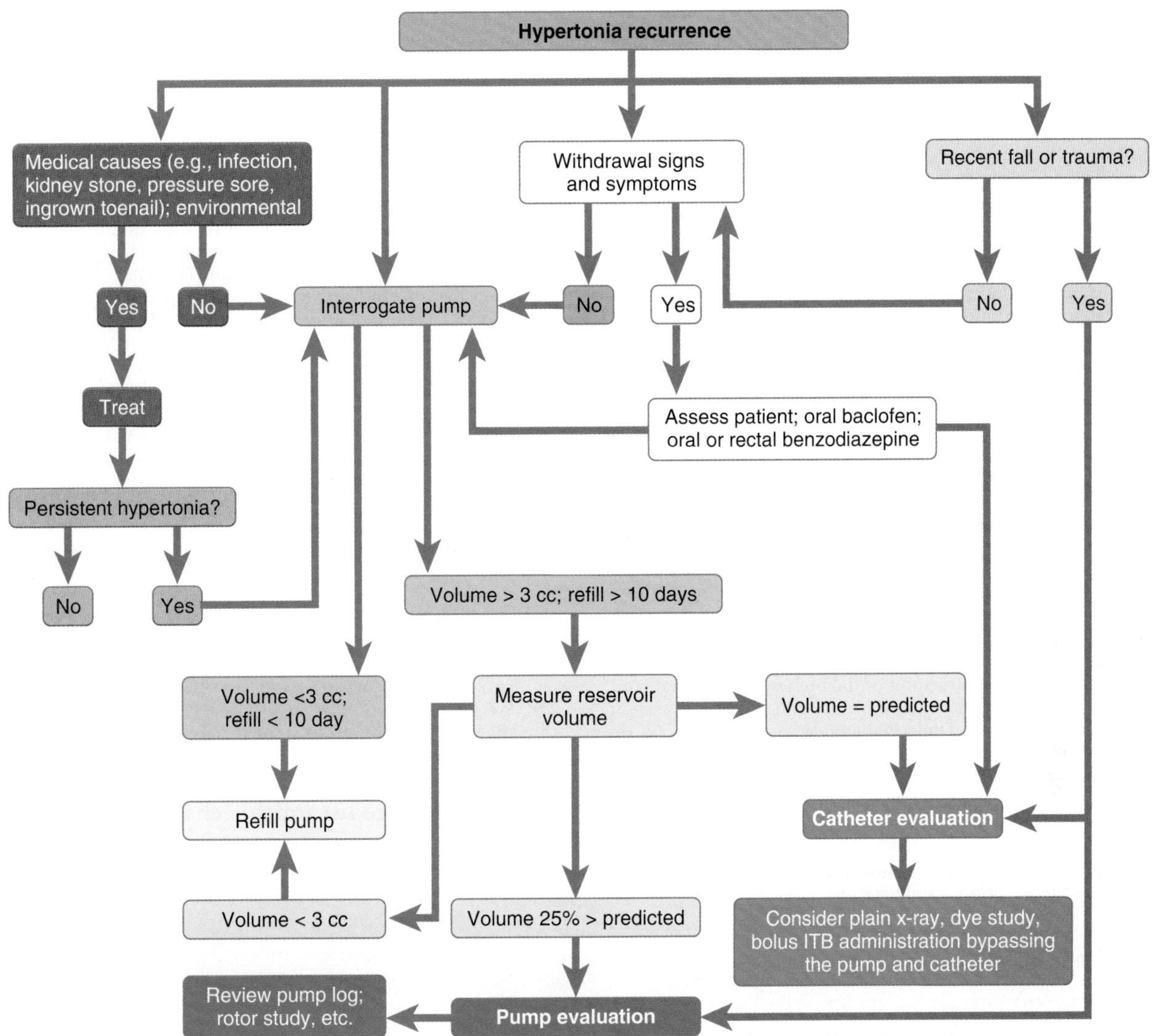

FIGURE 23-7 **Algorithm for assessing suspected intrathecal baclofen (ITB) withdrawal syndrome.** (From Francisco GE, Saulino M: Intrathecal baclofen management of spasticity. In Brashear A, Elovic E, eds: *Spasticity: diagnosis and management*, New York, 2015, Demos Medical Publishing.)

KEY REFERENCES

7. Bakheit AMO, Thilmann AF, Ward AB, et al: A randomized, double-blind, placebo-controlled, dose-ranging study to compare the efficacy and safety of three doses of botulinum toxin type A (Dysport) with placebo in upper limb spasticity after stroke, *Stroke* 31:2402–2406, 2000.
17. Bodine-Fowler SC, Allsing S, Botte MJ: Time course of muscle atrophy and recovery following a phenol-induced nerve block, *Muscle Nerve* 19:497–504, 1996.
21. Bovend'Eerdt TJ, Newman M, Barker K, et al: The effects of stretching in spasticity: a systematic review, *Arch Phys Med Rehabil* 89:1395–1406, 2008.
24. Brashear A, Gordon MF, Elovic E, et al: Intramuscular injection of botulinum toxin for the treatment of wrist and finger spasticity after a stroke, *N Engl J Med* 347:395–400, 2002.
26. Brown P: Pathophysiology of spasticity, *J Neurol Neurosurg Psychiatry* 57:773–777, 1994.
32. Burne JA, Carleton VL, O'Dwyer NJ: The spasticity paradox: movement disorder or disorder of resting limbs? *J Neurol Neurosurg Psychiatry* 76:47–54, 2005.
33. Burridge JH, Wood DE, Hermens HJ, et al: Theoretical and methodological considerations in the measurement of spasticity, *Disabil Rehabil* 27:69–80, 2005.
35. Calota A, Feldman AG, Levin MF: Spasticity measurement based on tonic stretch reflex threshold in stroke using a portable device, *Clin Neurophysiol* 119:2329–2337, 2008.
44. Coffey RJ, Edgar TS, Francisco GE, et al: Abrupt withdrawal from intrathecal baclofen: recognition and management of a potentially life-threatening syndrome, *Arch Phys Med Rehabil* 83:735–741, 2002.
53. de Paiva A, Meunier FA, Molgó J, et al: Functional repair of motor endplates after botulinum neurotoxin type A poisoning: biphasic switch of synaptic activity between nerve sprouts and their parent terminals, *Proc Natl Acad Sci U S A* 96:3200–3205, 1999.
54. Decq P: [Pathophysiology of spasticity], *Neurochirurgie* 49:163–184, 2003 [in French].
56. Dewald JP, Pope PS, Given JD, et al: Abnormal muscle coactivation patterns during isometric torque generation at the elbow and shoulder in hemiparetic subjects, *Brain* 118:495–510, 1995.
60. Dressler D, Benecke R: Pharmacology of therapeutic botulinum toxin preparations, *Disabil Rehabil* 29:1761–1768, 2007.
74. Fortuna R, Aurélio Vaz M, Rehan Youssef A, et al: Changes in contractile properties of muscles receiving repeat injections of botulinum toxin (Botox), *J Biomech* 44:39–44, 2011.
75. Francis HP, Wade DT, Turner-Stokes L, et al: Does reducing spasticity translate into functional benefit? An exploratory meta-analysis, *J Neurol Neurosurg Psychiatry* 75:1547–1551, 2004.
79. Gilio F, Curra A, Lorenzano C, et al: Effects of botulinum toxin type A on intracortical inhibition in patients with dystonia, *Ann Neurol* 48:20–26, 2000.
83. Gracies JM: Pathophysiology of spastic paresis. I: paresis and soft tissue changes, *Muscle Nerve* 31:535–551, 2005.
84. Gracies JM: Pathophysiology of spastic paresis. II: emergence of muscle overactivity, *Muscle Nerve* 31:552–571, 2005.

99. Hesse S, Reiter F, Konrad M, Jahnke MT: Botulinum toxin type A and short-term electrical stimulation in the treatment of upper limb flexor spasticity after stroke: a randomized, double-blind, placebo-controlled trial, *Clin Rehabil* 12:381–388, 1998.
106. Huynh W, Krishnan AV, Lin CSY, et al: Botulinum toxin modulates cortical maladaptation in post-stroke spasticity, *Muscle Nerve* 48:93–99, 2013.
109. Jankelowitz SK, Colebatch JG: The acoustic startle reflex in ischemic stroke, *Neurology* 62:114–116, 2004.
132. Lance JW: Symposium synopsis. In Feldman RG, Young RR, Koella WP, editors: *Spasticity: disordered motor control*, Chicago, 1980, Year Book Medical Publishers, pp 485–494.
149. Mayer NH, Esquenazi A: Muscle overactivity and movement dysfunction in the upper motoneuron syndrome, *Phys Med Rehabil Clin N Am* 14:855–883, 2003.
154. Meythaler JM, Guin-Renfroe S, Brunner RC, Hadley MN: Intrathecal baclofen for spastic hypertonia from stroke, *Stroke* 32:2099–2109, 2001.
164. Mottram CJ, Suresh NL, Heckman CJ, et al: Origins of abnormal excitability in biceps brachii motoneurons of spastic-paretic stroke survivors, *J Neurophysiol* 102:2026–2038, 2009.
170. Naumann M, Carruthers A, Carruthers J, et al: Meta-analysis of neutralizing antibody conversion with onabotulinumtoxinA (BOTOX®) across multiple indications, *Mov Disord* 25:2211–2218, 2010.
174. O'Dwyer N, Ada L, Neilson P: Spasticity and muscle contracture following stroke, *Brain* 119:1737–1749, 1996.
177. Penn RD, Savoy SM, Corcos D, et al: Intrathecal baclofen for severe spinal spasticity, *N Engl J Med* 320:1517–1521, 1989.
183. Pinter MM, Gerstenbrand F, Dimitrijevic MR: Epidural electrical stimulation of posterior structures of the human lumbosacral cord: 3. Control of spasticity, *Spinal Cord* 38:524–531, 2000.
192. Rosales RL, Chua-Yap AS: Evidence-based systematic review on the efficacy and safety of botulinum toxin-A therapy in post-stroke spasticity, *J Neural Transm* 115:617–623, 2008.
201. Shaari CM, Sanders I: Quantifying how location and dose of botulinum toxin injections affect muscle paralysis, *Muscle Nerve* 16:964–969, 1993.
203. Sheean G: Neurophysiology of spasticity. In Barnes MP, Johnson GR, editors: *Upper motor neurone syndrome and spasticity: clinical management and neurophysiology*, ed 2, Cambridge, 2008, Cambridge University Press, pp 9–63.
204. Sheean G: The pathophysiology of spasticity, *Eur J Neurol* 9(Suppl): 3–9, 2002.
205. Sheean G, Lannin NA, Turner-Stokes L, et al: Botulinum toxin assessment, intervention and after-care for upper limb hypertonicity in adults: International Consensus Statement, *Eur J Neurol* 17(S2): 74–93, 2010.
206. Simpson DM, Alexander DN, O'Brien CF, et al: Botulinum toxin type A in the treatment of upper extremity spasticity. A randomized, double-blind, placebo-controlled trial, *Neurology* 46:1306, 1996.
207. Simpson DM, Gracies JM, Graham HK, et al: Assessment: botulinum neurotoxin for the treatment of spasticity (an evidence-based review). Report of the Therapeutics and Technology Assessment Subcommittee of the American Academy of Neurology, *Neurology* 70:1691–1698, 2008.
208. Simpson DM, Gracies JM, Yablon SA, et al: Botulinum neurotoxin versus tizanidine in upper limb spasticity: a placebo-controlled study, *J Neurol Neurosurg Psychiatry* 80:380–385, 2009.
210. Sist B, Fouad K, Winship IR: Plasticity beyond peri-infarct cortex: spinal up regulation of structural plasticity, neurotrophins, and inflammatory cytokines during recovery from cortical stroke, *Exp Neurol* 252:47–56, 2014.
211. Sommerfeld DK, Eek EU, Svensson AK, et al: Spasticity after stroke: its occurrence and association with motor impairments and activity limitations, *Stroke* 35:134–139, 2004.
219. Twitchell TE: The restoration of motor function following hemiplegia in man, *Brain* 74:443–448, 1951.
227. Wissel J, Manack A, Brainin M: Toward an epidemiology of post-stroke spasticity, *Neurology* 80:S13–S19, 2013.
228. Wissel J, Ward AB, Erztgaard P, et al: European consensus table on the use of botulinum toxin type A in adult spasticity, *J Rehabil Med* 41:13–25, 2009.

The full reference list for this chapter is available online.

CHAPTER 24

CHRONIC WOUNDS

Robert J. Goldman, Jean M. de Leon, Adrian Popescu, Richard (Sal) Salcido

The economic and quality-of-life burden of chronic wound care is immense and is expected to increase with the aging population demographics, particularly in industrialized countries. The global market for wound care is estimated to reach approximately $18.5 billion by 2020.[141] Separately, the cost of wound care in the United States is estimated to be $11 billion annually. The average cost to treat an individual with an "unstageable" ulcer or a "deep tissue injury" (DTI) is estimated to be $43,180. The mean hospital cost for management of pressure ulcers in the United States is $14,426 per patient.[141] The average length of stay in hospital is almost three times longer in patients with chronic wounds. Additionally, other common wound types significantly contribute to the economic burden of chronic wound care. For example, the cost treating diabetic foot ulcers (DFUs) is estimated to range between $9 billion and $13 billion in addition to the cost associated of treating diabetes itself.[115] Similarly, the expenditures for venous stasis disease resulting in venous leg ulcers are an economic burden for the Centers for Medicare and Medicaid Services (CMS) and also private insurers, with an annual U.S. payer burden of $14.9 billion.[116]

With a new emphasis on ambulatory care models, there is a proliferation of outpatient wound care centers, including treatment centers offering hyperbaric oxygen therapy (HBOT).[40] Spending on outpatient "wound services" in the United States is estimated at $50 billion per annum.[40]

Recent advances in wound care treatment strategies derives from the current revolution in molecular biology, gene therapy, biomaterials, bioengineering, tissue engineering, and stem cell research.[66] Stem cells are now being applied to chronic wounds in animal model research and also in human trials.

Chronic wound products derived from recombinant DNA technology have been in place since the late 1990s.[52] Dramatic changes in wound care will continue as gene therapy involving growth factors undergoes human trials. A diversity of synthetic and natural skin grafts are now commercially available for various wound types.[123] The use of biologic extracellular matrices for "scaffolding," or the provision of a living framework to initiate wound repair, is on the horizon.[76]

In the clinical setting, the practice of using autologous platelet-rich plasma (PRP) in the treatment of chronic wounds is trending, albeit with the need for more evidence to support its use.[90] The CMS issued a Medicare National Coverage Determination on August 2, 2012, which allows coverage of autologous PRP under Coverage with Evidence Development with certain conditions.[7]

Physiatrists should maintain chronic wound care as a clinical competency because of the focus of the specialty on optimizing the musculoskeletal function of patients, prescribing orthoses, modalities, understanding gait biomechanics, protected weight-bearing, and the management of interprofessional rehabilitation teams. This chapter emphasizes the role of the physiatrist as a wound care consultant, promoting limb salvage and functional preservation of the largest organ of the body, the skin, and the underlying musculoskeletal system. In the update of this chapter, the use of HBOT and autologous PRP and the quality of wound care is emphasized.

Scope of the Problem

Definitions

The National Pressure Ulcer Advisory Panel (NPUAP) defines a pressure ulcer as localized injury to the skin and/or underlying tissue, usually over a bony prominence, as a result of pressure or pressure combined with shear and/or friction[104] (Figure 24-1). Pressure ulcers are associated with immobility, impaired mental status or sensation, poor hygiene or nutrition, dark skin color (associated with difficulty in detecting early-stage ulcers), and multiple comorbid factors. High standards of nursing and medical management are the key to prevention of ulcers in patients who are immobilized.

Chronic venous or edematous ulcers of the leg typically arise on the lower third of the leg ("gator area"). They are associated with impaired venous return, incompetence of venous perforators, or loss of integrity of the leg fascia (e.g., from trauma) in patients with normal arterial inflow. The cornerstone for this treatment is compression.

Neuropathic ulcers result from repetitive trauma to hyposensate distal extremities (e.g., feet and, not uncommonly, tips of the fingers), usually on weight-bearing bony prominences such as metatarsal heads. In the case of uncomplicated neuropathic ulcers, the circulation is usually functionally intact.[34]

The presence of neuropathic ulcers requires immediate relief of abnormal repetitive pressure and shear stress, and addressing the etiologic and treatment strategies associated with the underlying neuropathy.

Ischemic ulcers occur on extremities with impaired arterial inflow caused by arteriosclerotic disease and, in the setting of diabetes, microvascular disease. Often initiated by minor trauma or shoe pressure on the medial or lateral foot margins, they are typically painful and blanched. Ischemic ulcers are frequently associated with neuropathy or edema. Healing of these ulcers depends on reestablishing arterial circulation.

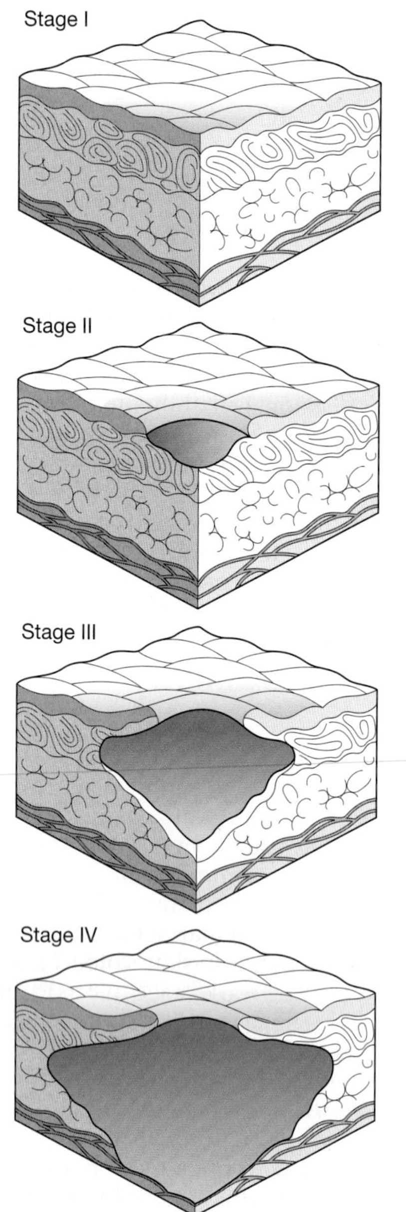

FIGURE 24-1 Pressure ulcer staging system. Although there is no consensus on generalizing the Shea Index to leg ulcer types, for reimbursement purposes, practitioners are frequently asked to describe stasis or neuropathic wounds according to the Shea Index. (Modified with permission of the National Pressure Ulcer Advisory Panel, Washington, DC.)

Epidemiology of Chronic Wounds

Pressure Ulcers

Despite more attention to prevention and patient safety in acute care hospitals; individuals who develop hospital-acquired pressure ulcers are more are more likely to die, incur longer hospital lengths of stay, and be readmitted within 30 days after discharge. Considerable variability exists in the reported pressure ulcer rates depending on the diagnosis, methodology used, and clinical setting. A working knowledge of the incidence and prevalence of chronic wounds provides medical/disease intelligence about this pervasive problem and enhances patient safety. Ultimately, a high level of clinical vigilance is needed irrespective of the setting or diagnosis.[111]

A national survey of 51,842 randomly selected hospitalized fee-for-service Medicare beneficiaries discharged from hospital between January 1, 2006, and December 31, 2007, was conducted with a retrospective secondary analysis of the Medicare Patient Safety Monitoring System. The hospital-acquired pressure ulcer incidence rate was 4.5%, and the pressure ulcer prevalence on admission was 5.8%. Of the 2999 individuals who entered the hospital with a pressure ulcer, 16.7% developed at least one new pressure ulcer at a different anatomic site during their hospitalization. The majority of participants who developed at least one pressure ulcer were nonwhite and aged 75 to 84 years. They had significantly higher rates of congestive heart failure, chronic obstructive pulmonary disease, cerebrovascular disease, diabetes mellitus, and use of corticosteroids during hospitalization. Obesity was significantly associated with hospital-acquired pressure ulcers.[85]

Pressure ulcers are particularly high in critical care settings with estimated prevalence rates in the range of 15% to 20% and at least one third at stage III pressure ulcers.[78] In the nursing home setting, incidence studies are confounded by methodological variabilities. However, most studies demonstrate an 8% to 12% prevalence range.[16]

Another group at risk for pressure ulcers are older adult patients with hip fractures and the inherent complications associated with immobility and major surgery. In a large multisite study (n = 685, including 9 hospitals and 105 postacute facilities) of patients 65 years of age or older who underwent surgical repair of hip fracture, the cumulative incidence of hospital-acquired pressure ulcers after 32 days posthospital admission was 36.1%.[13]

The incidence and prevalence of pressure ulcers in the pediatric population are lower than that in adults. However, children with severe illnesses, including neurologic impairments consequent to cerebral palsy, spina bifida, and traumatic and acquired spinal cord injury (SCI), are at significant risk.[141,142]

Pressure ulcers related to medical devices in hospitalized infants are increasingly problematic. The most prevalent devices associated with mechanical skin friction include oxygen saturation probes, noninvasive ventilation masks, orthotics, vascular access tubing, tracheostomies, and other mechanical-catheter–related devices.[102]

Individuals with SCI and associated comorbidity are at increased risk for the formation of pressure ulcers. These individuals are paralyzed below a certain level of the body, limiting their ability to relieve the pressure impinging on the immobile portions of the body. The sensory loss resulting from SCI also renders the patients unaware of the impending or existing injury caused by prolonged pressure. Another factor is that the neural and metabolic regulatory mechanisms for the maintenance of adequate tissue blood flow are impaired in patients with SCI.[82]

In patients (n =185) with SCI,[120] the prevalence rate of at least one pressure ulcer was 49.2% inclusive of the following anatomic sites: the foot (36.1%) and the coccyx/sacrum (15.1%). The risk for occurrence of a pressure ulcer was lower for patients with the American Spinal Injury Association (ASIA) Impairment Scale (AIS) of C or D compared with patients with an AIS of A.[120] Patients with SCI who are at least 50 years of age compared with those who are aged 15 to 29 years are at a 30% higher risk for the development of a pressure ulcer.[32]

Diabetic, Ischemic, and Neuropathic Ulcers

Neuropathy, arteriosclerosis, and microvascular disease are part of the natural history of diabetes. These comorbidities create a high risk for development of ischemic or neuropathic ulcers in individuals with diabetes, as evidenced by a 12% to 25% lifetime risk for developing a foot ulcer.[91] Diabetic foot ulcers (DFUs) in turn increase the likelihood of lower limb amputations. Cumulative rates of reamputation per person have been estimated at 26.7% at 1 year, 48.3% at 3 years, and 60.7% at 5 years.[43,70] Historically, hospitalization rates for lower limb amputation are much higher for individuals with diabetes than for the general Medicare population. Health inequities persist; for example, amputation rates in the African-American population are estimated to be five times larger than in non–African-American population in the United States.[101] The first major limb amputation for those with diabetes is often followed by a second major amputation.

The first statewide amputee database of a population was carried out in Minnesota during a 4-year period (2005 to 2008). The age-adjusted incidence was 20.0 years per 100,000 cases. Amputations increased significantly with age, were more common in men and in individuals with diabetes, and were slightly more common in rural residents. The number of amputation-related hospitalizations was steady over 4 years. The median total charge for each amputation was $32,129 and hospitalization charges were $56.5 million in 2008.[107] In 2005, 1.6 million individuals in the United States were living with the loss of a limb; 42% were nonwhite and 38% had an amputation secondary to dysvascular disease and diabetes mellitus. It is projected that the number of people living with the loss of a limb will more than double by the year 2050 to 3.6 million, which challenges the health system to provide preventative measures, such as education and prevention and treatment of diabetes.[145]

There are some positive trends in recent years. From 1988 to 2008, the age-adjusted nontraumatic lower extremity amputation rate for diabetics older than 40 years old decreased significantly from 8.5 to 3 per 1000.[81] However, the rate of amputation is still eight times the rate for individuals who are nondiabetic. Over the same time, the rate for "lower extremity ulcer" hospital discharges decreased from 8.3 to 5.6 per 1000, and peripheral arterial disease from 6.2 to 2.8 per 1000.[5] Unfortunately, the prevalence of diabetes has increased substantially. After remaining at 6 million cases from 1980 to 1990, the prevalence increased sharply to 22 million by 2010.[6] Therefore, the total number of amputation hospital discharges for lower extremity amputation may reciprocally increase, indicating the need for intense preventative services, including new strategies for patient teaching by interprofessional wound care teams.

Chronic Venous Leg Ulcers

Chronic venous leg ulcers begin as aberrancies in the peripheral venous system manifesting as varicose veins, and they end as discrete chronic ulcers.[14] Of venous ulcers, 20% to 30% are intractable, are present for more than 1 year, and have a surface area exceeding 10 cm^2. Epidemiologic estimates indicate that greater than 11 million men and 22 million women between the ages of 40 and 80 years in the United States have varicose veins, greater than 2 million adults have advanced chronic venous disease, and chronic venous leg ulcers are the most common leg ulcers.[80]

Chronic venous leg ulcers affect between 500,000 and 2 million individuals annually in the United States and account for over 50% of leg ulcers. Chronic venous leg ulcers are an underrecognized and undertreated disease.[50] At an average cost of $3000 per ulcer, the total direct cost is estimated at $2 billion, which does not include the hidden costs of untreated ulcers.[116] Venous ulcers also cause an estimated 2 million lost workdays.[109] A recent evaluation of Venous Ulcer (VU) Clinical Practice Guidelines conducted by Morton et al.[99] reviewed strength of evidence ratings for treatments and found that "good clinical science informs more than two thirds of the decisions recommended for VU management." For the remaining recommendations better strength is needed to improve outcomes and resource use.

Wound Physiology and Pathophysiology

Definitions

The Wound Healing Society defines healing as complete closing of the integument. Surgically induced skin wounds heal by primary intention and heal rapidly without complication in 3 to 14 days. Wounds that heal by secondary intention are usually large tissue defects that fill by granulation followed by epithelialization and ultimate contraction of the wound.

Process of Normal Healing

The major phases of wound healing are inflammation, proliferation/provisional matrix formation, repair, and remodeling.[52] After tissue injury, protective mechanisms promote hemostasis in the form of platelet plugs and platelet-derived growth factors (PDGFs). Subsequently, procoagulant molecule activation converts fibrinogen to fibrin. Fibrin-mesh scaffolding is created by platelet adhesion, stimulating growth factors.

The inflammatory phase of wound healing is characterized by remodeling of the preexisting tissue scaffolding and cleanup of extracellular and pathogen debris. Matrix breakdown stimulates chemotactic migration of neutrophils, macrophages, epidermal cells, and fibroblasts into the site of injury, for repair. The proliferation of extracellular matrix (ECM) components (a provisional matrix of glycosaminoglycans, which are protein-sugar complexes and fibronectin) attached to "integrins" (transmembrane receptors or linkages for cell-cell and cell-ECM interactions). This evolving framework is reinforced by type I collagen, which is secreted in sections (fibrils) and self-assemble extracellularly. Over this framework, a "ceiling" of epidermal cells advance over the defect to provide a durable cover, with a collateral neovascularization that supplies oxygen and nutrients. Remodeling of the dermal matrix occurs after closure, during which collagen fibers are preferentially retained along lines of stress forming a functional cicatrix.

Each stage of wound healing is orchestrated by signaling between cells and matrix components (dynamic reciprocity). These signaling components include cytokines, growth factors, proteases, and protease inhibitors.[52] "Gasotransmitters" also interact with nitric oxide to enhance neovascularization of the healing wound.[103]

Biochemistry of Normal Healing

Wound healing and remodeling of tissues[25] are activated by chemical stimuli such as PDGF, vascular endothelial growth factor (VEGF), and transforming growth factor-beta (TGF-β). In a parallel process, a complex cascade of procoagulant molecule activation culminates in the conversion of fibrinogen to fibrin, creating a fibrin mesh that forms the scaffolding of a blood clot.[25]

Growth factors such as TGF-β, PDGF, fibroblast growth factor (FGF), and cytokines (including interleukin-1 [IL-1] and tumor necrosis factor-α [TNF-α]) stimulate the fibroblasts to migrate to the injury site, proliferate, and secrete matrix metalloproteinases (MMPs). The released MMPs aid in the breakdown of ECM. Degradation of ECM results in the release and activation of growth factors such as TGF-β1, PDGF, basic fibroblast growth factor (bFGF), and interferon-γ (IFN-γ).[25]

Various immune cells including neutrophils, monocytes, macrophages, mast cells, and lymphocytes are recruited to the wound site by growth factors derived from platelets and ECM. These cells clear tissue debris, bacteria, and foreign materials from the wound site by phagocytosis and synthesize various growth factors and cytokines. Neovascularization is also promoted by VEGF.[25]

Activated fibroblasts further synthesize and deposit major ECM components such as collagen and fibronectin that impart strength to the healing wound. Collagen is secreted into the ECM in the form of tropocollagen. Three strands of tropocollagen then polymerize to form collagen.[25] A portion of fibroblasts are converted to myofibroblasts under the combined influence of mechanical tension, TGF-β, and cellular fibronectin extra domain type A (ED-A).[44] Myofibroblasts aid in shrinking and closing the wound with the use of an actin-myosin contractile system that involves alpha-smooth muscle actin. These cells also synthesize collagen types I and III. Myofibroblasts disappear after epithelialization via apoptosis (preprogrammed cell death).[67]

In parallel with the changes in the wound stroma, the epithelial cells around the wound margin migrate over the defect to provide a durable cover of the wound. The epithelial cells undergo a series of phenotypic changes termed epithelial-mesenchymal transition. In this transition, epithelial cells assume a fibroblast-like appearance and gain motility and invasiveness. E-cadherin molecules facilitate epithelial adhesion to the basement membrane and to adjacent epithelial cells, whereas adhesion is suppressed by N-cadherin molecules found in the mesenchymal cells.[138]

The stimuli that trigger the migration of epithelial cells include gradients of chemoattractants, pressure from adjacent cells, and endogenous microelectric fields.[144] Basement membrane components are deposited as the cells move. After the migrating fibroblast-like cells have covered the wound site, they revert to epithelial cells through a process known as mesenchymal-epithelial transition.[138]

Pathophysiology of Chronic Wounds

Chronic wounds appear to be in a chronic inflammatory state synonymous with healing arrest. Six commonly identified factors dynamically interact to arrest healing and perpetuate wound stasis: (1) pathomechanics, (2) chronic hypoxia, (3) reperfusion injury, (4) edema and impaired oxygen and nutrient exchange, (5) growth factor abnormalities, and (6) chronic inflammation.

Pathomechanics

Pathomechanics implies noxious application of pressure on and shear stress tangential to the skin surface. Unrelieved pressure is the critical factor in the development of pressure ulcers. Prolonged pressure leads to ulcers if it exceeds the tissue capillary pressure of 32 mm Hg. Known as the critical tissue interface pressure, it serves as a basis for the design of clinical pressure-relieving surfaces.[119]

The critical interface pressure is the pressure above which a tissue cannot be loaded for an indefinite period without resulting ulceration. An inverse, hyperbolic relationship exists between pressure and the duration of pressure application necessary to cause ulcers. Unrelieved pressure four to six times the systolic blood pressure causes necrosis in less than 1 hour. Pressure below systolic blood pressure, however, might require 12 hours to produce a similar lesion. This hyperbolic relationship has been confirmed for several animal models.[77,119]

The surface pressure, however, might not be a good measure of the true pressure in deep tissues. Deep muscle layers that cover bony prominences are often exposed to higher stresses than overlying skin surfaces. Prolonged compression increases muscle stiffness around the bone-muscle interface, which further stresses the muscles. This makes the muscle even more prone to ischemia and infarction. The injury progresses from deep to superficial tissues in an inverted cone shape. As a result, when we see the injury on the skin, it is literally "the tip of the iceberg."[117,118]

Shear stresses exacerbate the tendency for ulceration caused by pressure by lowering the ulceration threshold. The classic example of shear stress generation is when a patient reclines in a hospital bed with the head of the bed elevated; the human-machine interface. This position places the sacrum at increased risk for tissue breakdown. Once ulcers form, they are empirically more sensitive to pressure and shear stress than intact skin.

Recent evidence from cell and tissue culture studies suggest that sustained cellular deformation can cause tissue death primarily as a result of apoptosis even under normal supply of nutrients and oxygen. These results indicate that pure compression without any metabolic derangements associated with hypoxia/ischemia might be an etiologic factor leading to tissue damage. In particular, this mechanism of injury is implicated in the formation of DTIs.[47,48]

Chronic Hypoxia

Chronic hypoxia results from poor inflow of blood typically caused by arteriosclerotic narrowing proximal to hypoxic skin. Chronic ischemia blunts granulation tissue deposition, proliferation of fibroblasts, mononuclear cell infiltration, delayed epithelialization, and probability of wound closure. On the subcellular level, α1(I) procollagen is downregulated, and TGF-β signaling in fibroblasts is altered (e.g., lower TGF-β1 mRNA levels and downregulated TGF-β type II receptors) under the condition of chronic hypoxia.[74] These changes associated with chronic hypoxia contrast with the stimulatory effect of acute hypoxia on wound healing.[130]

Reperfusion Injury

The current practice for managing pressure ulcers is turning the patient every 2 hours. The question still remains about the appropriate turning frequency for patients at risk because of an inadequate evidence base for turning schedules.[15] Ischemia-reperfusion injury involves reactive oxygen species that overwhelm endogenous antioxidants, resulting in a cascade of events including mast cell degranulation, recruitment of neutrophils to the endothelial wall, arteriolar constriction that limits tissue perfusion, and increased vascular permeability leading to inflammation and edema.

Animal studies have shown that in young animals, chemotaxis, oxidant release, and phagocytosis by neutrophils play key roles in tissue damage after reperfusion. In older animals, increases in oxidative stress and mast cell density and action appear to have a more significant perturbation on the antioxidant defense.[119]

Patients with diabetes mellitus are at increased risk of reperfusion injury because there are decreased levels of microvessel nitric oxide (which is a potent vasodilator that protects the vascular endothelium from reperfusion injury).

Edema, Impaired Oxygen, and Nutrient Exchange

Edema is one of the major factors associated with the pathogenesis and maintenance of chronic wounds. Venous ulcers extravasate fibrinogen and fluid across the microvasculature endothelium resulting from venous congestion and back pressure, leading to excess protein-rich interstitial fluid. The excess osmotic pressure of interstitial fluid is thought to sequester growth factors, which are then unavailable to heal the edematous skin. Venous congestion can also lead to endothelial damage, causing neutrophils to marginate and release free radicals and collagenases. This process further increases membrane permeability to macromolecules, osmotic pressure and fluid shifts, and worsening edema.

Growth Factor Abnormalities

Growth factor abnormalities can occur in one of four categories: (1) reduced synthesis, (2) increased protein or matrix sequestration, (3) increased breakdown, or (4) insensitivity of target cells (i.e., reduced growth factor receptor concentration). As wounds heal with optimum conservative treatment, these abnormalities tend to resolve.

Chronic wounds contain elevated levels of a variety of proteases such as interstitial collagenases (MMP-1 and MMP-8), gelatinases (MMP-2 and MMP-9), and stromelysins (MMP-3, MMP-10, and MMP-11). Chronic wounds also have various levels of serine proteases and elastases, all of which collectively degrade the ECM of the wound bed. Tissue inhibitor of metalloproteinase, plasminogen activator inhibitor, alpha$_1$-protease inhibitor, alpha$_1$-antichymotrypsin, and alpha$_2$-macroglobin usually balance the activity of the MMPs but are overwhelmed in a chronic wound mainly by the influx of large numbers of neutrophils.[31]

Chronic Inflammation

Although colonization with bacteria is normal and can even be helpful during the initial healing phase, critical colonization and local infection impede healing. Wounds that have greater than 10^5 organisms per gram of tissue tend not to heal,[64] and are "stuck" in the inflammatory stage. The process of decreasing bacterial bioburden through "wound bed preparation" is discussed later.

Comorbidities

The factors that contribute to chronic wound persistence are diverse, interactive, and cumulative, and they affect the whole person. Predisposing conditions include aging, SCI, and diabetes, among many others (Table 24-1). These comorbidities interact and are cumulative at many levels to contribute to pathomechanics, hypoxia, reperfusion injury, and local inflammation. Pressure ulcers in individuals with SCI are slow to heal. This slow healing process is thought to be caused by neural and metabolic derangements in the denervated skin such as a limited inflammatory response as a result of vascular impairments, decreased availability of oxygen, reduced synthesis of collagen molecules, and decreased fibronectin resulting in impaired fibroblast activity. Aging is also associated with slower wound healing and subsequent functional wound closure. Reduced proliferation of fibroblasts, keratinocytes, and vascular endothelial cells, decreased collagen synthesis, and diminished fibroblast response to growth factors are associated with advanced age.[113]

Clinical Wound Assessment

Wound Area and Volume Assessment

Assessments are performed weekly or biweekly to document the effectiveness of therapy, make changes in treatment if necessary, and support the overall treatment plan.

Wound Area

The most straightforward technique is to document the perpendicular linear dimensions of the wound (typically in centimeters): the maximum distance is length and perpendicular distance is width.[2] Although linear dimensions can be performed rapidly, they have limited sensitivity to change in wound size, limited information about shape, and overestimate the wound area by up to 25%.[57] Because of these concerns, serial wound outlines are often performed. Manual tracing, a useful and inexpensive technique, involves drawing the wound outline on clear plastic

Table 24-1 Comorbidities Associated With Chronic Wounds

Condition	Pathophysiologic Effect Related to Wound Healing
Spinal cord injury	Vasomotor instability (>T6 level), insensitivity, denervation atrophy, spasticity, contractures, bowel/bladder alterations[45]
Older adult	Reduced skin elasticity and altered skin microcirculation,[136] comorbidities, reduced healing rate noted clinically and in animal models[58]
Diabetes	Insensitivity, microangiopathy, and altered inflammatory response,[97] foot deformities (intrinsic minus, Charcot), blunted reactive hyperemia, reduced incision breaking strength,[108] and contraction[59] in diabetic models
Malnutrition	Negative nitrogen balance, cachexia, immunosuppression
Anemia	Local hypoxia
Arteriosclerosis	Local hypoxia
End-stage renal disease	Transient dialysis–related hypoperfusion, arteriosclerosis, microangiopathy
Steroid medications	Reduced healing rate in animal models, immunosuppression
Transplant recipients	Immunosuppression
Smoking	Hypoxia, vasoconstriction, increased blood viscosity
Parkinson disease	Immobility
Osteoporosis	Bony prominences
Upper motor neuron disease	Immobility, contractures, bowel/bladder alterations
Dementia	Immobility, malnutrition, contractures, bowel/bladder alterations
Acutely ill (intensive care unit–related)	Hypotension, immobility, bowel/bladder alteration, malnutrition, increased metabolic demands
Noncompliance, abuse, and neglect	Multifactorial

(e.g., acetate sheet for transparencies) with an indelible marker. Counting the number of squares inside the wound periphery on the acetate sheet gives an estimate of wound area. These drawings then become part of the patient's permanent record. Inspection allows immediate appraisal of progress and modification of the treatment without delay.

Wound Volume

For a first approximation of volume, area is multiplied by depth to find volume. The volume of a rectangular solid calculated in this manner overestimates the volume of pressure ulcers. Computing volume of a spheroid is more accurate.[57] By either calculation, using depth is most accurate for deep cavities and least accurate for shallow, irregularly shaped wounds.

Wound Appearance

To describe wound appearance, the red-yellow-black system is often used (wounds classically transform from black, to yellow, to red as they heal (Figure 24-2). One method is to classify a wound as the least advantageous of the three colors that it displays. This method has been criticized as simplistic. The color of the wound surface can be alternatively described as a relative percentage of the three colors. Digital photography, with patient consent, makes it convenient to serially classify with wound color.

Computerized Assessment of Wound Geometry

Video technology[46] and computerized systems have been developed for more accurate and automated assessment of wound geometries. Digital planimetry enables automatic calculation of the wound area once the wound edge is traced manually or digitally. Excellent interrater and intrarater reliabilities and concurrent validity have been reported for computerized planimetry compared with other methods of wound area determination.[63,79] Regions of fast and slow healing (e.g., via granulation tissue induction) can also be tracked by following the geometry of the wound surface (Figure 24-3).

In summary, wound measurement techniques need to be accurate, reliable, and reproducible. When used for clinical and research purposes, any measurement technique must possess a high level of sensitivity and specificity. Measurement techniques must also be easy to use. Volumetric wound assessment is paramount for the refinement and advancement of modern wound measurement techniques. No definitive conclusions can be reached about the best method of studying diameter and depth of chronic wounds.

Efforts to obtain combined sensitivity and specificity are hampered by methodological and statistical differences in analyzing products and components and heterogeneous wound types.[105]

Perfusion Assessment

It is exceedingly rare that large vessel disease contributes to the formation of pressure ulcers of the trunk, occiput, hips, or buttocks. As a result, perfusion is more commonly assessed on distal wounds of the leg and foot. It is very important to have a regional assessment of perfusion because (1) in the setting of poor perfusion, therapeutic compression might cause pressure necrosis; and (2) the degree of perfusion is predictive of wound closure.

Macrocirculation

Macrocirculation refers to blood flow through named anatomic arteries, such as the iliac, femoral, posterior tibial, and plantar arteries.

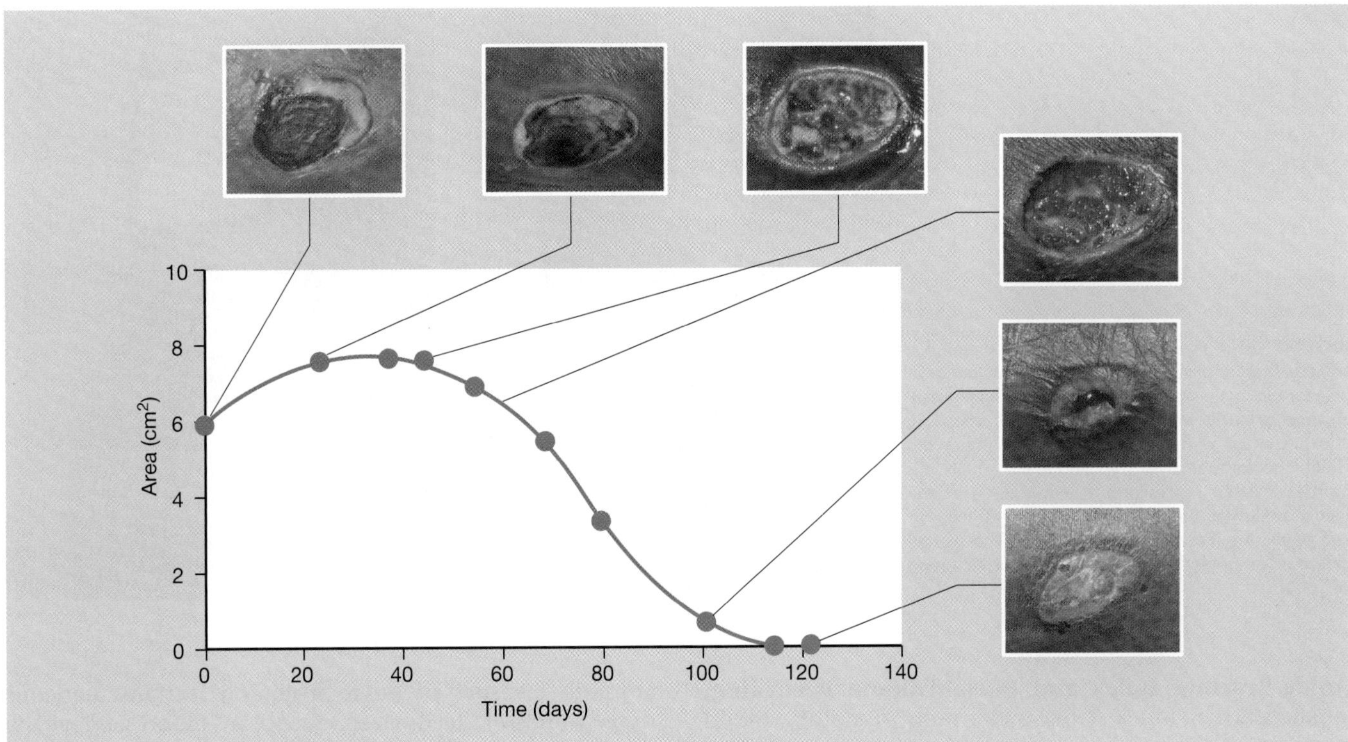

FIGURE 24-2 Illustrated is the transformation of wound bed from black eschar, to yellow slough, to beefy red granulating base. As the wound bed granulates, area (determined by serial outlines) first increases, then stabilizes, then decreases as epithelialization commences over a granulating wound base. Of the 16 weeks spent in healing this wound, almost half was devoted to wound bed preparation and half to epithelialization. The patient is a 38-year-old man with type I diabetes and "small vessel disease," which is often associated with black eschar. Lines connect the wound photographs to corresponding time points. (From Goldman R, Salcido R: More than one way to measure a wound: an overview of tools and techniques, *Adv Skin Wound Care* 15:236-243, 2002.)

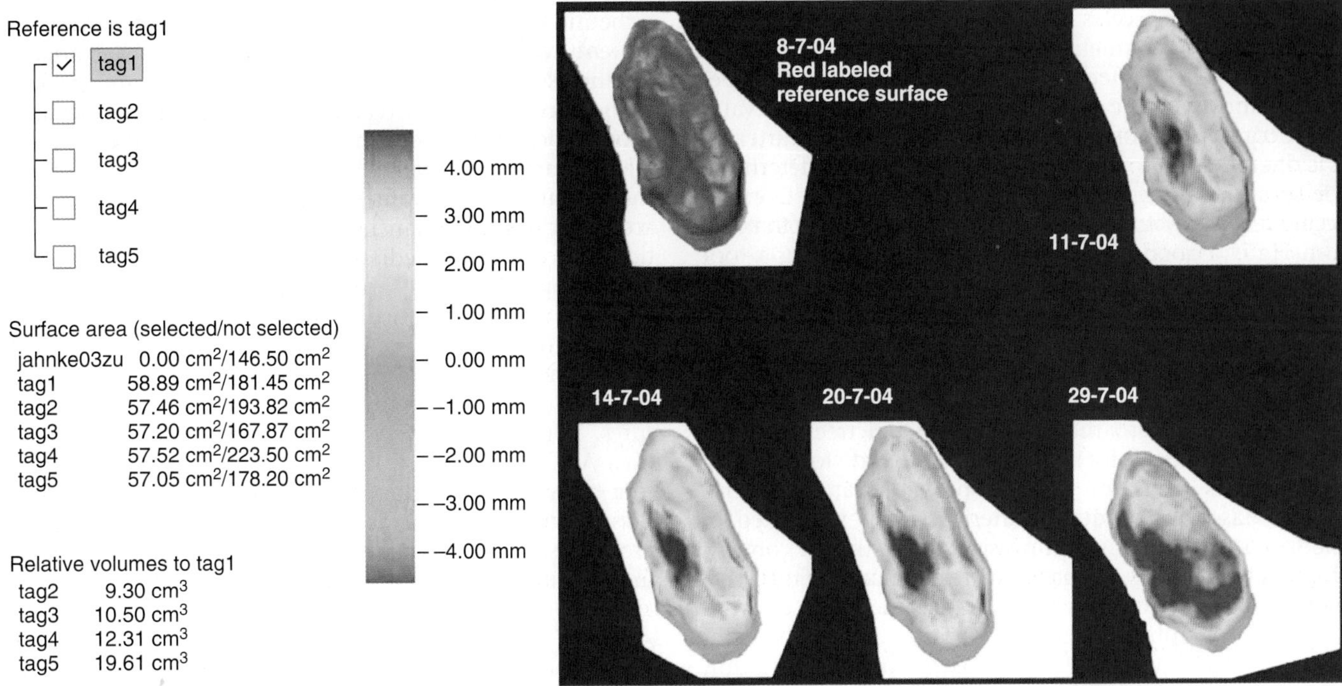

FIGURE 24-3 Monitoring the change in the elevation/depression of the wound geometry (from baseline) with a stereo photographic wound measurement system (DigiSkin). (Modified with permission from Körber A, Reitkötter J, Grabbe S, et al: Three-dimensional documentation of wound healing: first results of a new objective method for measurement, *J Dtsch Dermatol Ges* 4:848-854, 2006.)

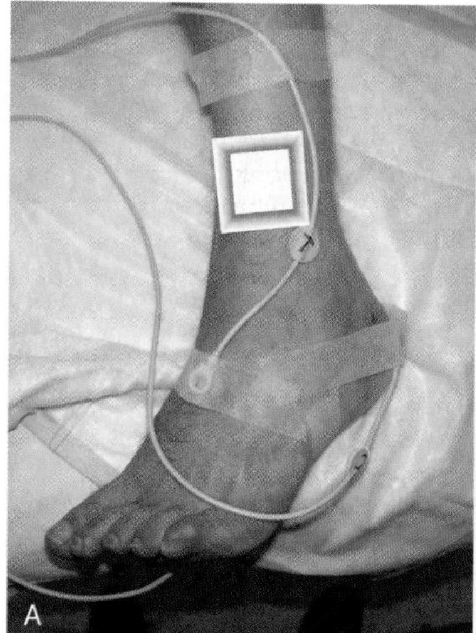

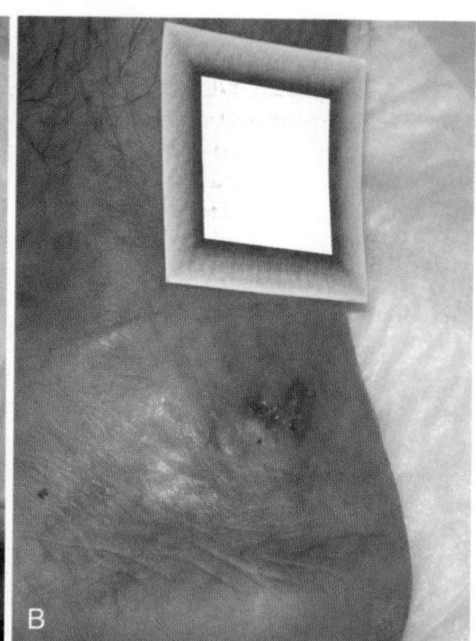

FIGURE 24-4 **A** and **B,** Electrode placement for transcutaneous oxygen ($TcPO_2$) determination on a 39-year-old man status postiliac artery angioplasty and medial ankle wound of 8 months' duration. He also presented with "blue toe syndrome" (note the violet discoloration over toes and medial ankle in a mottled pattern representing livedo). $TcPO_2$ at the medial ankle was 0 mm Hg, foot dorsum 40 mm Hg, and upper leg (not shown) 50 mm Hg. The wound closed after 4 months, coincident with normalization of $TcPO_2$.

Ankle-Brachial Index and Pulse Volume Recording. Ankle-brachial index (ABI) is the ratio of systolic blood pressure of the ankle to that of the arm (brachium).[57] Normal ABI is 0.8 to 1.3 and can be determined by a portable Doppler instrument and a blood pressure cuff. A series of cuffs can be used to obtain a pulse volume recording, which is continuous monitoring of pressure within cuffs applied to the thigh, calf, and ankle. These segmental pressure traces are checked for bilateral symmetry and waveform shape. Pulse pressure curves of normal arteries resemble steep isosceles triangles. Flattened pulse pressure waveforms or asymmetric indices suggest proximal flow compromise from arteriosclerosis. For patients with diabetes, calcinosis of the tunica media often falsely elevates ABI. Because calcinosis is less likely to involve foot arteries, it is often helpful to determine toe pressures. To determine toe pressure, a tiny cuff fits over the hallux and a Doppler probe records systolic pressure. A pressure greater than 40 mm Hg is a good prognostic indicator of healing a foot ulcer. Toe pressure and ABI determination use a portable Doppler instrument and do not require a dedicated vascular laboratory.

Angiography. Angiography typically involves injecting radiopaque dye into the proximal arterial tree. Conventional dye angiography is the "gold standard" for imaging macrovessels. It is an accurate prognosticator of limb salvage based on burden of arteriosclerosis visualized in the lower extremity. A noninvasive alternative to conventional angiography is magnetic resonance angiography, which requires no contrast dye and is superior to conventional angiography in visualizing arteries of the ankle and foot. However, use is limited for glomerular filtration rate less than 30 resulting from the well-known risk of gadolinium-induced nephrogenic systemic sclerosis.

Microcirculation

In the skin, blood flows through arterioles, capillaries, and venules in the papillary and reticular dermis. A direct and absolute measure of microcirculation is transcutaneous oxygen ($TcPO_2$). $TcPO_2$ is in essence a "blood gas" of the skin. The normal $TcPO_2$ is greater than 50 to 60 mm Hg. Wound healing is considered impaired at pressures less than 40 mm Hg. $TcPO_2$ levels at 20 mm Hg are associated with rest, pain, ischemic ulcers, and pressure levels less than 20 mm Hg are at risk for amputation.[106] A typical pattern of electrode placement is the upper leg, foot dorsum, and periwound (Figure 24-4).

$TcPO_2$ prognosticates the healing rate of neuropathic and ischemic ulcers. Its predictive value is uniquely strong for patients with diabetes who typically have distal arterial calcinosis.[106] For this population, $TcPO_2$ is more accurate than toe pressures to prognosticate healing. $TcPO_2$ may also prognosticate success of incisional healing at the transtibial level and foot level.[110] A disadvantage of $TcPO_2$ is that the technique gives values that are inaccurately low over areas of callus and transiently low in the setting of infection and in the immediate postoperative situation. $TcPO_2$ measuring instruments are expensive ($2500 to $5000 per channel) and time-consuming (20 minutes to 1 hour to obtain a reading).

The most complete picture of lower extremity perfusion comes from combining $TcPO_2$ and segmental pressures. For example, very low distal segmental pressures (i.e., ABI less than 0.4) but normal foot $TcPO_2$ can indicate collateralization around an arterial blockage. Under these conditions, normal $TcPO_2$ suggests good healing prognosis and a favorable chance of limb salvage despite the low ABI.[57]

Pressure and Shear Stress Assessment

Sensor arrays and point sensors are commercially available that can help to ensure that insoles and seating cushions distribute pressure over a maximum surface area.[57] Two-dimensional sensor arrays (e.g., resistive, capacitive, and piezoresistive types) provide accuracy and good resolution of pressure distribution. Although pressure is well quantified, transducers for shear stress have yet to be perfected for routine clinical use.

Skin Biopsy

Although there are many biopsy types (e.g., excisional, incisional, and shave), the 3-mm punch technique is amenable for physiatric practice (low risk of bleeding and small skin defect). The method for biopsy involves selecting a site over soft tissue that is distant from subcutaneous arteries, fascia, or bone. The site selected should include periwound skin and a small sample of the wound base. Lidocaine without epinephrine (1 to 2 mL) is infused through intact periwound skin toward the wound center. The punch is inserted with a pressing, twisting motion, and a sample is harvested for histologic analysis.[130,134]

General Principles of Treatment

Wound Bed Preparation

Chronic wounds (unlike acute wounds) tend to be heavily colonized by bacteria. Colonization, however, does not equal infection.[124] Wounds exist on a continuum between frank bacterial invasion, critical colonization, colonization, and healing. As wounds heal (and bacterial virulence decreases), wound appearance transforms from black, to yellow, to dull red, to bright red (see Figure 24-2). With beefy granulation tissue formation, there is a substantial decrease of drainage and pain, with management implications. The therapeutic processes for "coaxing" a chronic wound to granulate have been referred to as "wound bed preparation."[124] Once the wound bed is prepared, the goal is to maintain a moist environment. In a moist environment the epithelium advances and adjoins without having to digest eschar (i.e., "scab"), which optimizes the rate of healing. Wound fluid is also rich in growth factors that help promote closure.

Débridement

Surgical Débridement

Surgical débridement is well established as an approach to the care of pressure ulcers and other chronic wounds. Surgical débridement is performed under general or regional anesthesia as needed. It is indicated for abscesses or wounds that traverse tissue planes and has a moderate to high risk for significant bleeding.

Sharps Débridement

Less aggressive outpatient or bedside sharps débridement is performed by professionals from many disciplines, including physiatrists, and has been recognized as a distinct débridement method as a time honored practice. A series of sharps débridements is typically required to have the same effect as one surgical débridement. Sharps débridement is commonly performed in the outpatient setting as part of routine wound care with minimum blood loss. Any pain concerns are managed with topical analgesia. A local anesthetic, lidocaine 5%, or EMLA cream (lidocaine 2.5% and prilocaine 2.5%) can be applied 5 to 15 minutes before débridement. Premedication with a fast-acting oral nonopiate and/or oral opiate analgesic can also be helpful. Débridements should be performed at regular intervals to ward off infection because devitalized tissue supports the proliferation and growth of pathogens.

Pain is usually not a problem for patients with neuropathic ulcers. These ulcers develop callus or a pseudocapsule that is débrided in an inverted-cone pattern with a scalpel and forceps, which is referred to as "saucerization." Débridements should be done periodically because neuropathic ulcers readily form calluses even with very little weight bearing, and a callus increases the mechanical tension in the wound. Venous ulcers do not develop calluses but frequently produce a yellow fibrinous slough over the wound bed (which can be removed with curettage). If a stasislike leg ulcer expands after débridement, the diagnosis of pyoderma gangrenosum should be considered.

Note that slough and necrosis can be similarly removed from pressure ulcers. Because pressure ulcers tend to be deeper than they are wide, knowledge of pelvic anatomy is essential, such as the location of the inferior gluteal artery. Particular concern is raised if the pressure ulcer is "unstageable" (e.g., when it has a 100% yellow surface). A completely nonviable surface raises concern that the pressure ulcer extends well into deep tissue planes. Such wounds should be sharp débrided with great care (because of the risk of bleeding), with a very low threshold for surgical referral.

Ischemic wounds must also be sharp débrided with great care because the blood supply might not be adequate to support a repair response (which can lead to further necrosis). If eschar appears to be contiguous with bone (e.g., black eschar over the calcaneus), that bone will likely not heal if exposed. In this circumstance, the eschar should be left dry unless infection supervenes. Where black eschar overlies soft tissue and reperfusion is possible, the authors advocate topical use of silver sulfadiazine, which has a broad antibacterial spectrum and softens eschar. This forms "pseudoeschar," which can self-dislodge or is readily removed by careful periodic sharps débridement.[55]

Mechanical Débridement

Mechanical débridement is accomplished by whirlpool treatments, forceful irrigation, or use of wet-to-dry dressings. Wet-to-dry dressings involve placing an unraveled, moist gauze into the lesion so that all sections of it are touching the dressing, then allowing the dressing to dry. When the dry dressing is subsequently removed, necrotic tissue is removed with it and this can be painful.

Enzymatic Débridement

Several major types of enzymatic débridement agents are currently on the market. These include collagenase (e.g., Santyl). In the United States, papain-urea (e.g., Accuzyme and Gladase) is currently off the market. Urea denatures protein, which increases the effectiveness of the nonspecific protease papain. Collagenase may be better for preparing the wound bed because it does not digest growth factors or matrix proteins.[37]

The use of enzymatic débriding agents can be the most cost-effective method for treating well-perfused partially necrotic pressure ulcers where sharps débridement is not readily available, such as in the skilled care setting.[94] They are applied with daily change of dressings, until wounds are free of slough or eschar. It should be noted that enzymatic débridement might increase pain and drainage, requiring adjustments to dressing change schedules. The efficiency of enzymatic débriding agents is increased by "cross-hatching" the eschar with a scalpel.

Autolytic Débridement

Autolytic débridement involves the use of natural proteases and collagenases in wound fluid to digest nonviable material. This method can be very effective when used under semiocclusive or occlusive dressings. Autolytic débridement is contraindicated, however, when wounds are infected or critically colonized. It should also be kept in mind that if slough or necrotic material is excessive, drainage can accelerate the maceration of periwound skin and increase wound size. As a rule of thumb, in a healing wound, the area of viable granulating base should be greater than 50% of the entire wound surface.[94]

Dressings

Dressings are typically applied in layers. The primary dressing is contiguous with the wound surface. A secondary dressing is applied external to the primary for absorption, protection, or fixation. For primary or secondary application, the dressing categories in Table 24-2 roughly correspond to the order in which they would be used in the process of wound bed preparation. The dressing categories in Table 24-2 are organized from most to least absorptive. Note the following caveats: (1) it is unusual to use more than a few categories for a given wound; (2) composites, specialty absorptives, and foams are more likely to be used for a longer period, or until healing; and (3) in small, clean stage II and stage III wounds, use of hydrocolloids, hydrogels, and films is the norm.

Hyperbaric Oxygen Therapy

HBOT is the delivery of O_2 at 10-fold or higher partial pressure than ambient O_2 for therapeutic effect. In the field of critical care, HBOT treats decompression sickness and carbon monoxide poisoning among other indications. In the area of wound care for the past 3 decades, HBOT has been used: (1) for complex DFUs with "hospital level" infection and/or gangrene (i.e., Wagner III or IV lesions); (2) acute arterial obstruction post revascularization; (3) refractory osteomyelitis; (4) flap failure (e.g., transtibial amputation dehiscence); (5) crush injury; and (6) radiation therapy–induced ulcers or mucosal injury.[131]

For those with diabetes at high risk of major lower extremity amputation, HBOT is associated with improved odds of limb preservation.[53,73] The usual "dose" for wound healing is 2.0 to 2.5 atmospheres pure oxygen daily and 30 to 50 daily treatments spanning 6 to 10 weeks. Each

Table 24-2 Advantages, Disadvantages, and Examples of Dressing Types*[66]

Product Type	Structure	Advantages	Disadvantages	Examples
Composites	Combine physically distinct components into one dressing, include an adhesive border	Well reimbursed Absorbent May be used on infected wounds Are easy to apply and remove Used also in children	Requires a border of intact skin for anchoring the dressing	Alldress (Molnlycke Health Care) Telfa Island (Tyco Healthcare/Kendall) 3M Tegaderm + Pad Transparent Dressing with Absorbent Pad (3M Health Care) CovRSite Plus (Smith & Nephew Wound Management) Stratasorb (Medline Industries, Inc.)
Antimicrobials	Release ionic silver or polyhexamethylene biguanide to reduce bacterial virulence	Provides a broad range of antibacterial activity Reduces infection Used also in children	May cause staining, stinging, or sensitization Expensive, not covered by all payers	Acticoat Antimicrobial Dressing (Smith & Nephew Wound Management) Contreet Foam Cavity Dressing with Silver (Coloplast Corporation) TELFA AMD (Tyco Healthcare/Kendall) SilvaSorb hydrogel (Medline Industries, Inc.) Maxorb (Medline Industries, Inc.)
Specialty absorptives	Unitized, multilayered fibers of absorbent cellulose, cotton, or rayon; gauze dressings of this type	Very absorbent Can be used as secondary dressings Are semiadherent or nonadherent Easy to apply and remove May have an adhesive border Used also in children	May not be appropriate as a primary dressing for deep or undermining wounds	Tendersorb Wet-Pruf Abdominal Pads (Tyco Healthcare/Kendall) Primapore Specialty Absorptive Dressing (Smith & Nephew Wound Management) BreakAway Wound Dressing (Winfield Laboratories, Inc.)
Alginates	Packaged dry, derived from brown seaweed, absorbs up to 20 times its own weight	Very absorbent Fills in dead space Are easy to apply and remove Used also in children	Can dehydrate the wound bed Requires a secondary dressing	Aquacel Hydrofiber Wound Dressing (ConvaTec) Sorbsan (Mylan Bertek Pharmaceuticals) 3M Tegagen HI Alginate Dressing (3M Health Care) Algisite M (Smith & Nephew Wound Management) Maxorb (Medline Industries, Inc.) SeaSorb (Coloplast Corporation)

Table 24-2 Advantages, Disadvantages, and Examples of Dressing Types—cont'd

Product Type	Structure	Advantages	Disadvantages	Examples
Foams	Foam of polyurethane, silicone, etc.	Very absorbent May repel contaminants May be used under compression Used also in children	Not effective for dry wounds May macerate periwound skin if saturated No adhesive, requires secondary dressing for fixation	Allevyn Adhesive Hydrocellular Polyurethane Dressings (Smith & Nephew Wound Management) Mepilex Border Self-adherent Soft Silicone Foam Dressing (Molnlycke Health Care) PolyMem (Ferris Mfg. Corp.) 3M Foam dressing (3M Health Care) Lyofoam (ConvaTec) Optifoam (Medline Industries, Inc.)
Wound fillers	Beads, pasts, powders, gels, and pads; they absorb several time their weight in exudates	Very absorbent, reduces odor Promotes autolytic débridement Easy to apply and remove Fills dead space	Not recommended for use in dry wounds Requires secondary dressing	FlexiGel Strands Absorbent Wound Dressing (Smith & Nephew Wound Management) Iodoflex Pad/Iodoflex Gel (Healthpoint) Multidex Maltodextrin Wound Dressing Gel or Powder (DeRoyal)
Collagens	Sheets, pads, particles, and gels	Promote granulation Are absorbent Maintain a moist environment May combine with topical agents	Not recommended for black wounds Requires a secondary dressing	BCG Matrix Wound Dressing (Brennen Medical, Inc.) FIBRACOL PLUS Collagen Wound Dressing with Alginate (Johnson & Johnson Wound Management) Kollagen-Medifil Pads (Biocore Medical Technologies, Inc.) PROMOGRAN Matrix (Johnson & Johnson Wound Management)
Contact layers	Thin, porous interface between wound and dressing	Can protect the fragile wound base May be applied beneath topical medications, wound fillers, or gauze dressings for easy removal	Not recommended for stage I pressure ulcers or dry wounds Requires a secondary dressing	Mepitel Soft Silicone Wound Contact Layer (Molnlycke Health Care) Profore Wound Contact Layer (Smith & Nephew Wound Management) Silon-TSR Temporary Skin Replacement (Bio-Med Sciences, Inc.)
Hydrocolloids	Occlusive hydroactive wafers, beads, pastes, or granules; forms gel on contact with wound	Provides minimum to moderate absorption Promote autolytic débridement Are self-adhesive and protective May be used under compression products Used also in children	Not for infection, heavy exudates, or high percentage eschar Not for exposed tendon or bone May injure fragile skin upon removal Not for most stage III or stage IV wounds	Comfeel Plus Hydrocolloid Ulcer Dressing (Coloplast Corporation) DuoDERM SignaDress (ConvaTec) Exuderm (Medline Industries, Inc.) Replicare Hydrocolloid Dressing (Smith & Nephew Wound Management)
Hydrogels	Glycerin and water-based products for wound hydration	Provides minimum to moderate absorption Facilitates autolytic débridement Fills in dead space (Hydrogel gauzes) Easy to apply and remove Used also in children	Some require secondary dressing Dehydrates easily if not covered Some might be difficult to secure Some might cause maceration	CarraSmart Gel Wound Dressing with Acemannan Hydrogel (Carrington Laboratories, Inc.) ClearSite Hydrogel Wound Dressing (CONMED Corporation) Curagel (Tyco Healthcare/Kendall) Dermagran Hydrophilic Wound Dressing (Derma Sciences, Inc.) Vigilon Primary Wound Dressing (Bard Medical Division, C.R. Bard, Inc.) Intrasite (Smith & Nephew Wound Management) Skintegrity Hydrogel (Medline Industries, Inc.) Tegagel (3M Healthcare)
Transparent films	Semipermeable polyurethane membrane dressings; transparent and waterproof	For wounds with minimum drainage Retain moisture Facilitates autolytic débridement Allows wound observation Does not require secondary dressings Used also in children	Not indicated for infected wounds, nor on fragile skin Requires a border of intact skin May be difficult to apply and handle May dislodge in high-friction areas	Bioclusive Transparent Dressing (Johnson & Johnson Wound Management) Mefilm (Molnlycke Health Care) Opsite (Smith & Nephew Wound Management) 3M Tegaderm Transparent Dressing (3M Healthcare) SureSite (Medline Industries, Inc.)

Note: no single product provides optimum coverage for all wounds. Therefore, practitioners are urged to understand dressing characteristics and functions. This table is not intended as an exhaustive list nor does it imply endorsement of any product.

session begins with a "descent" from 1.0 atmosphere to higher target pressure over 5 to 25 minutes, and after 90 to 120 minutes, a similar "ascent." There are many mechanisms that support effectiveness of HBOT for wound healing inflammation, repair, and remodeling. HBOT enhances the natural mechanism of phagocytosis, which requires large quantities of oxygen. This response is blunted in hypoxic environments such as infected bone. HBOT also reduces inflammation and reperfusion injury by reducing activity of intracellular adhesion molecule-1 (ICAM-1) by a nitric oxide–related mechanism. ICAM-1 makes damaged endothelium "sticky" to leukocytes. By decreasing "stickiness," HBOT reduces leukocyte margination and extravasation into formerly ischemic tissue. During repair, HBOT increases VEGF and neovascularization. It is also associated with release of endothelial progenitor stem cells from bone marrow. Also, during repair, HBOT enhances cross-linking of collagen in the ECM.[131] HBOT is most effective if hyperoxia reaches tissue at risk, as would be expected for any therapeutic dose-response relationship. A retrospective cohort study of 6100 hyperbaric patients found that a robust increase in periwound oxygenation during a HBOT session (greater than 200 mm Hg) lead to better granulation tissue formation and healing than a marginal increase (less than 100 mm Hg).[39]

There are two types of risk from HBOT: barotrauma and oxygen toxicity. The most common is otic barotrauma, commonly referred to as "ear squeeze." This can be mild to severe, from mild inflammation to (rarely) rupture of the tympanic membrane. To prevent the latter, training on "clearing the ears" for the patient is usually all that is required. Pulmonary barotrauma may occur in the setting of chronic obstructive pulmonary disease. Lung barotrauma may rarely lead to pneumothorax on "ascent."[53]

Oxygen is a vasoconstrictor and can increase both afterload and may (speculatively) increase coronary artery tone. For high-risk patients such as diabetic patients, there is likely preexisting atherosclerosis. Coronary artery disease and increased tone can potentiate ischemic symptoms or even acute coronary syndrome. Therefore, a chemical stress test on diabetic patients is often performed as part of the HBOT workup. Oxygen seizures rarely occur and are unrelated to seizure disorder. Risk is mitigated by use of "air breaks," breathing air at-pressure for 5 to 10 minutes during each 90-minute session. Air breaks are often used where there are medications (such as opiates) that lower the seizure threshold.[53]

In 2014, the American College of Hyperbaric Medicine published a consensus paper providing guidelines for hospital credentialing recommendations for physicians wanting to practice hyperbaric medicine. These recommendations represent the consensus opinion of leaders in the field of hyperbaric medicine and are subject to local determinations.[121]

Gene Therapy and Exogenous Application of Growth Factors

Exogenous application of growth factors has been proposed as a means of promoting wound healing because these factors are often deficient in chronic wound environments. Despite the obvious rationale, clinical application of recombinant growth factors has been limited, partly because the growth factors tend to be digested by the proteolytic enzymes in the wound bed, and only a small fraction of these factors survive and diffuse into the wound tissue. Recombinant human platelet-derived growth factor BB (PDGF-BB) was approved by the U.S. Food and Drug Administration (FDA) for use in diabetic ulcers. For the recombinant PDGF to reach therapeutic levels in the wound site, however, a dose 50 times the minimum effective dose is required. Clinical trials testing the efficacy of recombinant human keratinocyte growth factor-2 and recombinant human granulocyte colony-stimulating factor continue.[87]

Gene therapy refers to the insertion of a desired gene into recipient cells. The large surface area and superficial location of wounds renders the skin a good candidate for gene therapy. Gene therapy has been introduced to wound care practice for more efficient delivery of growth factors. Permanent insertion of DNA to the genome of recipient cells and transient transformation for short-term expression of a gene are two approaches to reach this goal.[18] A variety of techniques, such as viral transfection, naked DNA application, liposomal delivery, and high-pressure injection, have been applied to facilitate the transfer of growth factor genes to the target wounds. High-pressure injection applied to cationic cholesterol-containing liposomal constructs, in particular, has shown great promise.[18]

Stem Cell Therapy

Stem cells are classified as autologous (patient-derived) and therefore not subject to immunologic rejection. Adult stem cells can undergo "differentiation" in that they are adipogenic, osteogenic, and neurogenic. Stem cells possessing the most potential to develop into skin are bone marrow–derived stem cells or mesenchymal cells.[92] Adipose-derived stem cells can differentiate into chondrogenic, myogenic, and osteogenic cells and are readily harvested from liposuction or solid fat tissue.[4] Randomized controlled trials to test the efficacy of these approaches and in the wound care space are needed.

Platelet-Rich Plasma

Autologous PRP is a treatment that contains fibrin and high concentrations of growth factors and has the potential to aid wound healing.

In the clinical setting, the practice of using autologous PRP in the treatment of chronic wounds is trending downward. Although not widely used in wound care currently, clinical research continues, and PRP may reemerge as an important modality in the future.[29,33,42,127]

PRP is an autologous concentration of platelets suspended in plasma. It is derived from whole blood with a centrifuge to separate the PRP from the red blood cells. Typically 20 to 30 mL of blood is drawn from the patient to be centrifuged. The plasma level is drawn off and combined with calcium chloride and thrombin (Figure 24-5).

The fibrin from the fibrinogen is polymerized with exposure to calcium chloride and thrombin creating a gel consistency. Once platelets are activated, they degranulate and release a variety of growth factors, including PDGF, VEGF, and TGF involved in wound healing.[10] The gel, rich

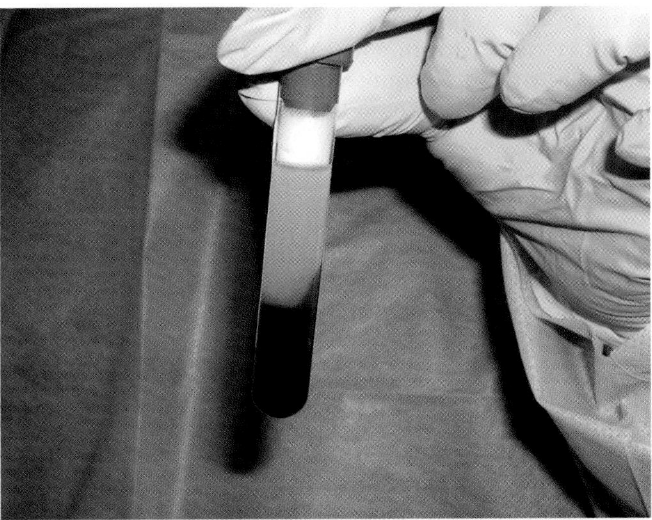

FIGURE 24-5 Platelet-rich plasma is derived from whole blood with a centrifuge to separate the platelet-rich plasma from the red blood cells. Typically, 20 to 30 mL of blood is drawn from the patient to be centrifuged. The plasma level is drawn off and combined with calcium chloride and thrombin.

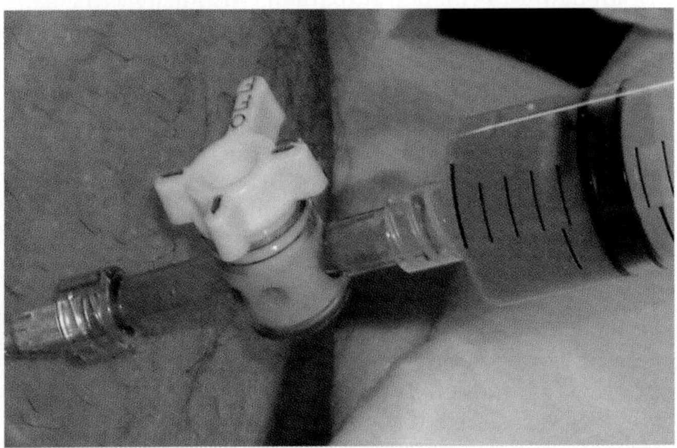

FIGURE 24-6 Injection of Aurix into the left trochanteric region with a three-way stopcock attached to a barrel syringe.

in platelets and growth factors, can then be applied to wounds to promote hemostasis and/or accelerate healing.

The first retrospective study based on 49 patients treated with PDGF is considered an index study, and Knighton et al.[75] patented this treatment mixture. The plasma was initially separated from the white blood cells and red blood cells with a centrifuge, and then the platelets were separated from the plasma and resuspended in a buffer solution. This platelet solution was then added to a collagen preparation to create a topical salve. The mixture was named Procuren and it was available in 150 wound care centers from 1986 to 2001. It is no longer produced.

Current PRP preparations include the Aurix system (Nuo Therapeutics, Gaithersburg, Md.) (Figure 24-6). This product is different from previous products in that they contain whole cells including white cells, red cells, plasma, platelets, fibrinogen, stem cells, macrophages, and fibroblasts. The high concentration of leukocytes also has an added antimicrobial effect. These preparations are specifically marketed for wound care, but there are other PRP preparations proposed for the treatment of musculoskeletal conditions such as epicondylitis, plantar fasciitis, degenerative disorders of the joint, Achilles tendinopathy, and Dupuytren contracture. PRP is different from fibrin glues or sealants. The glues and sealants are created from pooled homologous human donors. They consist of mainly fibrinogen and can be created from platelet-poor plasma.[22]

In 2012, a Cochrane database review for "Autologous PRP for treating chronic wounds" was conducted,[90] including the data on the small number of trials eligible ($n = 9$) for evidence-based review to support the clinical use for PRP. The authors concluded there was insufficient evidence to recommend the use of PRP in the adjunctive treatment of wounds. However, this conclusion is based on a small number of randomized controlled trials (RCTs), most of which were either at high or unclear risk of bias.[90] Similarly, a clinical research study in which platelet lysate was used for the healing of chronic venous ulcers on 86 patients (36 men and 50 women, median age 70 years) found no difference in healing between platelet lysate and placebo application. The methods used in this study had no influence on the healing of chronic venous ulceration.[126]

Margolis et al.[88] evaluated the effectiveness of platelet releasate administered by a proprietary group of wound care centers for the treatment of diabetic neuropathic foot ulceration using a database of 26,599 patients (1988 to 1997) with diabetic plantar ulcers. The methodology included the use of a retrospective cohort study, which incorporated the use logistic regression–derived propensity scores (controlling for treatment selection bias). The research group concluded that in large surface areas and anatomically deep wounds, platelet releasate was more effective than standard care.[88] As in most novel therapies, well-designed and adequately powered clinical trials are needed to substantiate that their use are warranted.

Currently, the CMS and most private carriers do not believe there is enough evidence to support PRP treatments for wounds. However, the CMS did issue a Medicare National Coverage Determination on August 2, 2012, which allows coverage of autologous PRP only under coverage with evidence development, with certain conditions. Therefore, patients would only be able to receive PRP treatments in the outpatient setting if they are part of an approved study that is collecting outcome data that is submitted to the CMS.[7]

Therapeutic Ultrasound

Ultrasound usage on wounds results in two types of therapeutic effect: thermal and nonthermal. Thermal effects are generated by high-intensity ultrasound and are manifested as increased tissue temperature. Thermal effects include increased blood flow and collagen extensibility.[12] Nonthermal effects are largely attributable to acoustic streaming and cavitation. Streaming refers to the bulk fluid flow that can displace biomolecules and is caused by the sound forces. Cavitation involves the formation and oscillation of microbubbles. Both streaming and cavitation appear to alter cell membrane activity, cell signaling, and cellular metabolism. Nonthermal effects of ultrasound include stimulation of protein synthesis, proliferation of fibroblasts and inflammatory cells, increased angiogenesis, collagen deposition and fibrinolysis, and release of cytokines and growth factors.[122]

High-frequency ultrasound (1 to 3 MHz) at intensities of 0.5 to 1 W/cm^2 has been used in wound care, particularly on periwound tissues. A metaanalysis pooling four trials compared ultrasonic therapy with standard/sham therapies in the care of venous leg ulcers. The number of ulcers healed was greater (relative risk = 1.51, 95% confidence interval = 1.09 to 2.09) and the percentage of remaining ulcer area was smaller (weighted mean differences = −5.34%, 95% confidence interval = −8.38 to −2.30) in the ultrasound treatment group than in the control group. Therapeutic ultrasound for the treatment of pressure ulcers was compared with sham therapy in a metaanalysis pooling two studies involving 128 patients with pressure ulcers. No significant benefit of ultrasound on pressure ulcer healing rates was found (relative risk = 0.97, 95% confidence interval = 0.65 to 1.45).[27]

The use of low-frequency (40 kHz), noncontact ultrasound was recently approved by the FDA for use in the treatment of wounds. Ultrasound is delivered to the wound bed via a saline mist without direct contact of the ultrasound transducer with the body. Mechanical energy at this frequency range is believed to exert débriding and cleansing action, as well as bactericidal activity through enhanced cavitation and streaming.[122] RCTs have shown that this therapy accelerates healing and alleviates pain in chronic wounds of diverse causes.[72]

Electrical Stimulation and Electromagnetic Therapy

The rationale behind the use of electrical stimulation in the management of wounds is based on the observation that the endogenous microelectric field created in the wound serves as a sentinel cue to guide the migration of epithelial cells in the process of wound healing.[144] In a wound with disrupted epithelium, the normal transepithelial potential is short-circuited. This results in a decrease in electric potential in the exposed stroma and results in an endogenous electric field that points to the center of the wound. Application of an externally generated electric potential that amplifies this endogenous electric field toward the wound center is expected to facilitate the migration of epithelial cells and promote wound healing. Electrotherapy was approved in the United States for the treatment of pressure, arterial, diabetic, and venous stasis ulcers. A variety of modes for delivering electric fields to the wound bed have been developed (e.g., continuous or pulsed currents, high or low voltage, and direct or alternating currents).

Electromagnetic therapy provides a low-frequency field effect rather than direct current of electrical stimulation or high-frequency radiation of laser therapy. Low-frequency electromagnetic field is known to influence the biologic tissue in a variety of ways: change in the permeability of cell membrane ion channels and signal transduction, altered expression of genes controlling cellular proliferation such as *fos*, *myc*, *jun*, and *p53*, increased cellular proliferation and epithelialization, and enhanced angiogenesis via upregulation of FGF-2.[20]

RCTs in the 1990s failed to provide evidence of significant benefit of electromagnetic therapy for healing of venous and pressure ulcers. More recently, however, a number of studies consisting of stringent instrumental parameters and treatment regimens have been tried and have shown some promise in the use of electromagnetic therapy for wound care in animal models.[20]

Negative Pressure Wound Therapy

Topical negative pressure (TNP) treatment involves negative pressure on the wound surface to promote wound healing. TNP is indicated for acute, chronic, traumatic, and dehisced wounds, partial-thickness burns, flaps, and grafts. The following have been proposed as mechanisms of action of TNP: increase in local blood flow, reduction of edema and wound exudates, decrease in bacterial colonization, stimulation of cell proliferation, induction of granulation tissue, and provision of moist wound environment. A pressure of −125 mm Hg is commonly used because this level of pressure has been demonstrated to promote maximum increase in tissue blood flow and maximum granulation tissue formation. A metaanalysis involving 7 RCTs and 10 non-RCTs concluded that "negative pressure wound therapy (NPWT) may improve wound healing, but the strength of evidence available is insufficient to clearly prove an additional benefit of NPWT."[60] Clinically, the use of various modes of NPWT devices has gained acceptance and is in common use in various settings, including the military. However, the literature suggests that the strength of evidence claims that "edema reduction and bacterial clearance mechanisms have not been proven with basic research" and more evidence is needed.[100]

Skin Substitutes

Skin substitutes afford rapid temporary or permanent coverage of various types of wounds by providing epidermal or dermal components to the wound base. They are viable in a less vascularized wound bed and can enhance the tempo of healing, improve survival rate, and improve the function and appearance of the wound. Living keratinocytes and fibroblasts embedded in cellular substitutes can secrete collagen and other ECM components, supply cytokines and growth factors for angiogenesis and induction of host fibroblast proliferation, and produce antimicrobial host defense peptides.[11] Some skin substitutes further improve the healing environment by absorbing inhibitory factors from the wound bed.[123] New products are in the pipeline, and currently a variety of xenografts, autografts (split-thickness, full-thickness, and cultured autologous), allografts (epithelial/epidermal, acellular dermal, cellular dermal, and composite), and synthetic monolayer/bilayer substitutes are available on the market (Table 24-3).[123]

Diagnosis and Treatment of Specific Ulcer Types

Pressure Ulcers

Presentation

According to the NPUAP Pressure Ulcer Staging System, pressure ulcers are staged based on the extent of the lesion

Table 24-3 Examples of Commercially Available Skin Substitutes

Categories of Skin Substitutes		Product	Uses in Wound Management
Xenograft		Permacol	Temporary coverage of burn and clean partial-thickness wounds
		OASIS	Temporary coverage of burns and chronic wounds
Autograft	Cultured autologous skin	Epicel	Deep partial-thickness and full-thickness burns >30% TBSA
		Laserskin	Chronic wounds, deep partial-thickness and full-thickness burns >30% TBSA
Allograft	Acellular dermal allograft	AlloDerm	Deep partial-thickness and full-thickness burns
	Cellular dermal allograft	TransCyte	Superficial partial-thickness wounds not requiring skin grafts, deep wounds requiring subsequent skin grafts
	Composite allograft	Apligraf	Chronic wounds, excision sites, epidermolysis bullosa
		OrCel	Skin graft donor sites, chronic wounds, epidermolysis bullosa
Synthetic monolayer substitute		Suprathel	Split-thickness skin graft donor sites, partial-thickness burns
Synthetic bilayer substitute		Biobrane	Superficial partial thickness burns, temporary coverage of excised wounds, split-thickness skin graft donor sites
		Integra	Coverage after excision of deep burns, chronic wounds, traumatic wounds, draining wounds

TBSA, Total body surface area.

as revealed by clinical observation. Stage I pressure ulcers are characterized by intact skin with nonblanchable redness of a localized area, usually over a bony prominence. Stage II or above requires that the integrity of dermis is compromised. Lesions with partial-thickness and full-thickness loss of dermis are classified as stage II and stage III pressure ulcers, respectively. In stage IV pressure ulcers, bone, tendon, or muscle is exposed. Full-thickness lesions with wound bed covered with slough or eschar are called "unstageable." Recently added to the staging system is suspected DTI, where the skin is intact but discolored. DTI can also be present when a blood-filled blister is present as a result of damage of underlying soft tissue. DTIs are lesions confined to the deep tissues but with intact skin. They arise in deep muscle layers covering bony prominences as a result of high tissue stresses adjacent to the prominences and are aggravated by muscle stiffening caused by prolonged compression.[47,48]

The vulnerability of skeletal muscles to ischemia/hypoxia,[62] as described previously, is an etiologic factor of DTI.

Deep Tissue Injury

Deep tissue injury (DTI) is an elusive diagnosis and defies accurate measurement in time and space. Many hypotheses exist. The working paradigm is that the "DTI" clinically manifests as a "bruise, purple hue or bogy tissue," and that there is damage to the underlying "tissues."[104]

Advancing DTIs from clinical discussions to scientific debate and then to clinical practice keeps the DTI agenda in the forefront.[17] Salcido et al.[117-119] have established an oxygen-free radical pathophysiologic basis for DTI. They demonstrated that, in response to sustained pressure, the oxygen-free radical destruction of the muscle is primary. They confirmed that the muscle tissue (deep tissues) is more sensitive to ischemia and reperfusion injury than the skin. Additionally, they analyzed sequential histopathologic changes that occurred in the development of pressure ulcers experimentally induced in the fuzzy rat model. Computer-controlled pressure was applied for 6 hours at a maximum of five sessions to skin over the greater trochanter of anesthetized rats. Lesions were similar, but more pronounced after the third, fourth, and fifth sessions as compared with the first or second sessions. Lesions developed first in the muscle rather than the dermis or epidermis. The lesion most often associated with pressure was necrosis of the panniculus carnosus muscle, often accompanied by damage to underlying adipose tissue. They concluded that recurrent pressure results in increasingly severe damage to the vascular system and parenchyma, consistent with an ischemia/reperfusion insult, initiated through a free-radical mechanism.[119] More recently, Salcido has described the phenomena as a "myosubcutaneous-dermal infarct."[117]

The understanding of DTI and moving beyond the standard clinical model of pressure ulcer staging is appropriate. In the model of DTI, there exists a deep zone of infarction or inverted cone of injury that has yet to manifest visually as a "stage I." This DTI is certainly beneath or subserosally under the skin; this DTI is a serious ulcer emanating from DTI or what is now called stage III or stage IV. The DTI-focused model puts importance on the early detection and prevention of DTI, not the prevention of stage I and stage II pressure ulcers, although counterintuitive; stage I and stage II pressure ulcers are most likely not the precursors of most stage III and stage IV pressure ulcers. Early intervention systems should be focused not on superficial insults to the skin but to insults that can cause harm to the more susceptible deeper tissues. This should be the first line of defense.[128] The prevention and treatment of pressure ulcers by pressure relief should not necessarily match the particular stage. Variable pressure relief and distribution for a DTI should be the same as for all other stages, including a stage IV. The pressure ulcer staging system is illustrated in Figure 24-1. *Decubitus ulcer* and *bed sore* are terms used interchangeably with *pressure ulcer*. These terms, however, have a connotation of describing pressure ulcers arising in bedridden patients only and consequently are not recommended.

Patients with intact sensorimotor function can use periodic movements to relieve noxious mechanical stimuli prone to cause pressure ulcers. However, patients who are comatose, severely demented, or who are insensate (e.g., patients with SCI) are at increased risk. Spasticity, contractures, immobility, incontinence, cachexia, diabetes, and advanced age also increase risk. It has been suggested that

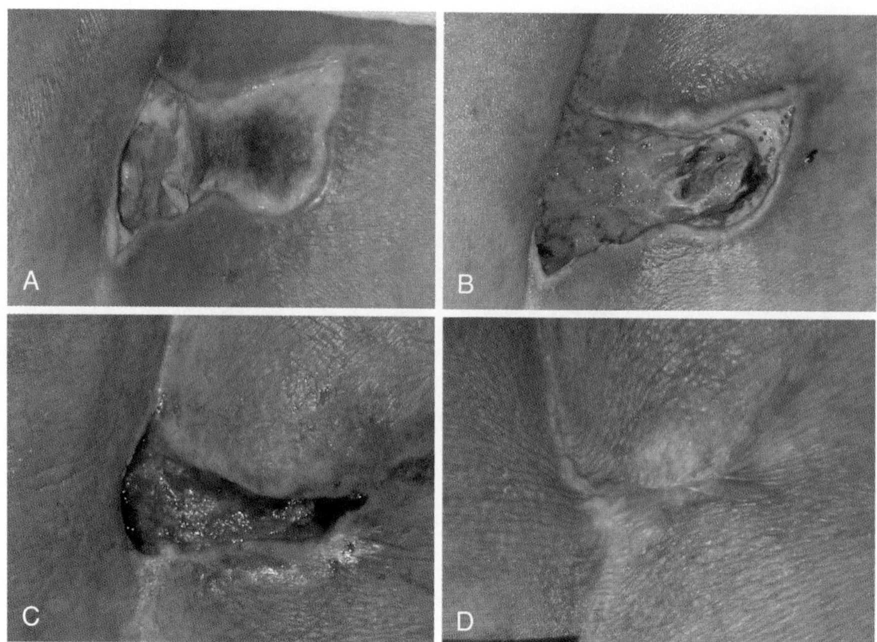

FIGURE 24-7 The course toward healing for a 66-year-old woman with type 2 diabetes mellitus who had a stage III sacral pressure ulcer during prolonged acute hospitalization for bilateral iliofemoral bypass complicated by congestive heart failure. On initial evaluation, 2 months postoperatively, the wound had a foul odor and was covered with yellow-green eschar laterally. Wound size was 4 × 8 cm and 2.5 cm deep (**A**). The patient received a pressure-relieving surface, nutritional interventions, two sharps débridements, and saline/dilute Betadine (1:100) wet to dry. **B,** Wound 3 weeks after initial evaluation, after the second sharps débridement. After this, topical treatment included papain-urea-chlorophyllin copper complex (Panafil) with a specialty adsorptive (ABD) and overlying composite (Alldress), changed daily at first. Nine weeks later the wound is actively contracting (**C**). With contraction, the wound reached 95% closure 28 weeks after initial evaluation but took an additional 12 weeks to achieve full closure (**D**).

patients with darkly pigmented skin are at higher risk because nonblanching erythema of stage I pressure ulcers might not be readily visible on casual inspection.[125]

The most common sites of pressure ulcer formation are ischium (28%), sacrum (17% to 27%), trochanter (12% to 19%), and heel (9% to 18%). A case history of a sacral pressure ulcer on an older adult patient is provided in Figure 24-7. Sacral and trochanteric pressure ulcers are also common in patients with SCI, as noted above.

Treatment

The mainstay of pressure ulcer treatment is evidence-based medical and nursing care, including continence care. In the long-term care setting or at home, the debilitated or partially dependent patient with a pressure ulcer should be turned at a minimum every 2 hours.[114] The sidelying position should be avoided as much as possible, however, because of high pressures against the trochanteric region. Much lower pressures are recorded for the 30-degree sidelying positions[28] between which patients should be transferred during position changes. Wound area, depth, undermining, and appearance should be assessed at least weekly, and treatment should be modified as necessary to maintain healing rate. Nutrition management is a crucial issue for patients with pressure ulcers (see discussion on nutrition in this chapter). Total enteral nutrition should be considered if oral intake is inadequate and likely to remain so.

Pressure ulcers with necrosis or fibrin must be periodically débrided (e.g., sharp, mechanical, or enzymatic). Deep wounds should be irrigated. Irrigation can also be done at the bedside with normal saline with the use of a 50-mL syringe with a 19-gauge flexible catheter. After irrigation, all "dead space" should be loosely packed. Significant drainage is managed with foams, alginates, or specialty absorptives at an adequate change schedule, so that the dressing can be moist (but not soaked). Hydrogels are appropriate once drainage has diminished and is minimum to moderate, and the wound is completely granulating. Without an underlying absorptive layer, hydrocolloids (e.g., DuoDERM) are appropriate by themselves for stage II ulcers or small, clean stage III wounds.

Pressure relief in bed includes placing pillows or other cushioning between trochanteric prominences and bed surface for sidelying, keeping the bed as horizontal as possible, and using heel protectors. The efficiency of pressure and shear stress relief correlates positively with cost (Table 24-4). The most expensive systems are called "pressure relieving" because they theoretically maintain tissue interface pressure below capillary closing pressure of 32 mm Hg. Those systems with peak pressures greater than 32 mm Hg but that are better than hospital mattresses are called "pressure reducing." Pressure-reducing surfaces work with the use of air, gel, water, or foam to passively redistribute pressure and are referred to as "static" types of devices. Pressure-relieving devices can also be "dynamic" (i.e., they require an energy source to redistribute pressure). An example of a dynamic system is a low air loss (e.g., the SAR Low Air Loss Mattress System). Pressure-relieving, dynamic systems are required for high-risk patients (e.g., those with complete SCI) who cannot turn themselves off the ulcerated surface (i.e., they need assistance for bed mobility).

Table 24-4 Advantages and Disadvantages of Support Surfaces

Surface	Advantages	Disadvantages
Static Overlays		
Air	Low maintenance Inexpensive Multipatient use Durable	Can be punctured Requires proper inflation
Gel	Low maintenance Easy to clean Multipatient use Resists puncture	Heavy Expensive Little research
Foam	Lightweight Resists puncture No maintenance	Retains heat Retains moisture Limited life
Water	Readily available in the community Easy to clean	Requires heater Transfers are difficult Can leak Heavy Difficult maintenance Procedures difficult
Dynamic Overlays	Easy to clean Moisture control Deflates for transfers Reusable pump	Can be damaged by sharp objects Noisy Assembly required Requires power
Replacement mattresses	Reduced staff time Multipatient use Easy to clean Low maintenance	High initial cost May not control moisture Loses effectiveness
Low air loss	Head and foot of bed can be raised Less frequent turning required Expensive Pressure relieving Reduces shear and friction Moisture control	Noisy Difficulty with transfers Requires energy source Restricts mobility Skilled setup required Rental charge
Air-fluidized	Reduces shear and friction Lowest interface pressure Low moisture Less frequent turning required	Expensive Noisy Heavy Dehydration can occur Electrolyte imbalances can occur May cause disorientation Difficulty with transfers Hot

From Bryant R: *Acute and chronic wounds: nursing management*, St Louis, 1992, Mosby Yearbook.

Seating systems for wheelchairs are prescribed to many patients who lack protective sensation. Examples include air-filled villous cushions (e.g., ROHO), contoured foam with a gel insert (e.g., Jay), or contoured foam on a solid-seat wheelchair (e.g., polyurethane). For patients who cannot perform weight shifts, mechanical weight shift devices (i.e., tilt-in-space) are appropriate. "Doughnut-type" devices should be avoided because they might be more likely to cause pressure ulcers than prevent them.

Studies on adjunctive treatments have the goal of improving these outcomes. Those therapies that are commercially available and are supported by prospective RCTs include electrical stimulation and normal temperature therapy. The use of growth factor therapy PDGF-BB for pressure ulcers, although supported by several RCTs, remains controversial. The increased use of NPWT and the strength of evidence for its clinical use is evolving.

Prevention

A good argument can be made that some pressure ulcers cannot be avoided, especially on moribund patients, particularly at the end of life. Formation of multiple stage III and stage IV pressure ulcers near the end of life has been termed skin failure.

For patients with advanced age and with a reasonable chance of long-term survival, education, inspection, and continued pressure and shear stress optimization are the key to prevent the first or recurrent ulcerations. In the long-term care setting, assessments by the Norton or Braden Scales are reliable and valid. The Braden Scale might be more cost-effective and is widely used in the United States. It comprises six subscales that reflect sensory perception, skin moisture, activity, mobility, shear force, and nutritional status. A score of 12 or less indicates high risk necessitating aggressive inspection, nutritional, and support surface interventions. For the assessment of pressure ulcer risk in the pediatric population, the Braden Q Scale, the Neonatal Skin Risk Assessment Scale, and the Glamorgan Scale have been clinically validated in terms of efficacy and reliability.

Surgery of greater than 4 hours' duration is associated with the development of pressure ulcers that involve the heels and sacrum.

Screening of Pressure Ulcers

Detection of early-stage pressure ulcers is an important goal because in stage I pressure ulcers the skin is still intact and recovery is typically easier than in later stages. The early detection of pressure ulcers has recently become even more crucial in light of the Inpatient Prospective Payment System of the CMS. The Hospital-Acquired Conditions provision in the regulation requires hospitals to identify whether certain specified diagnoses, such as pressure ulcer, are present when the patient is admitted. For discharges occurring on or after October 1, 2008, full reimbursement might not be available to hospitals to cover the extra cost incurred in the treatment of stage III or stage IV pressure ulcers that had not been documented on admission.

The clinical procedure for identifying a stage I pressure ulcer is the manual blanch test. A stage I pressure ulcer is diagnosed when redness persists after the release of pressure exerted by the finger on that area suspected of having a pressure ulcer. The disadvantage of this test is its limited use in patients with dark skin color in whom redness is often difficult to observe. This might be a contributing cause of the high proportion of patients developing stage III and stage IV pressure ulcers in African-American and Hispanic populations.

A multitude of screening tools drawing on various technologies are being developed to detect stage I pressure ulcers irrespective of the patient's skin tone, although none are yet ready to be used in the clinical setting. These technologies purport to detect substantive biophysical changes in skin tissue that accompany ulcerations.

Uncomplicated Chronic Venous Ulcers

Presentation

Patients with chronic venous ulcers usually have a history of previous venous ulcer, dependent edema, previous deep venous thrombosis, pelvic surgery, vein stripping, or vein harvest for coronary artery bypass graft. Peripheral pulses are typically intact (although it is sometimes difficult to palpate pulses through edematous skin). A well-granulating ulcer with irregular borders positioned about the medial malleolus is typical of saphenous vein dysfunction. Although the "gator area" (i.e., lower third of the leg) is typical, venous ulcers can be located anywhere on the lower leg, ankle, or edematous foot dorsum. Frequently associated with venous ulcer are lower leg hyperpigmentation and a "knobby" induration of subcutaneous tissue "lipodermatosclerosis." Edema of the leg is a hallmark of venous stasis disease, and stasis ulceration is the end result of long-standing venous congestion (Figure 24-8).

Normally the contraction of skeletal muscles in the lower limb results in the compression of deep veins and cephalad propulsion of blood in the deep venous system. This muscle pump is powered by the contraction mainly of calf muscles within an unyielding leg fascial envelope, creating cyclic pressure peaks, which can reach 100 mm Hg. During muscle relaxation, blood in the superficial venous system drains into deep veins through perforator veins, which are aided by valves in the perforator veins that resist blood flow from deep to superficial veins. This siphoning effect lowers the superficial venous pressure in the lower limb during standing.

The valves in the deep venous system and perforator veins can become incompetent, however, because of the presence of an old clot or proximal vein occlusion (e.g., from organized clot, pelvic mass, or fibrosis). The ensuing superficial venous hypertension during standing in turn is transmitted to dermal exchange vessels. The venoarteriolar reflex (which is arteriolar constriction in response to an increase in precapillary pressure) is also often abnormal in cases of severe chronic venous insufficiency. This results in failure to prevent the increased arterial pressure during standing from being transmitted to dermal capillaries. The increased hydrostatic pressure in the superficial microvasculature results in fluid filtration and extravasation of plasma proteins into the ECM, which can overwhelm the lymphatic drainage system and cause protein-rich edema that limits nutrient delivery. Extravasated fibrinogen molecules aided by suboptimal fibrinolytic activity form fibrin cuffs around dermal capillaries. The microenvironment in the edematous region can also induce fibroblast dysfunction and can impede wound healing. Furthermore, capillary plugging by white blood cells reduces the number of perfused capillaries and can cause epithelial injury and inflammation. This further decreases tissue nutritional support and aggravates edema.

The differential diagnosis of venous stasis ulcers includes ulcers related to congestive heart failure, lymphedema, or sickle cell anemia. Other diagnoses requiring alternative

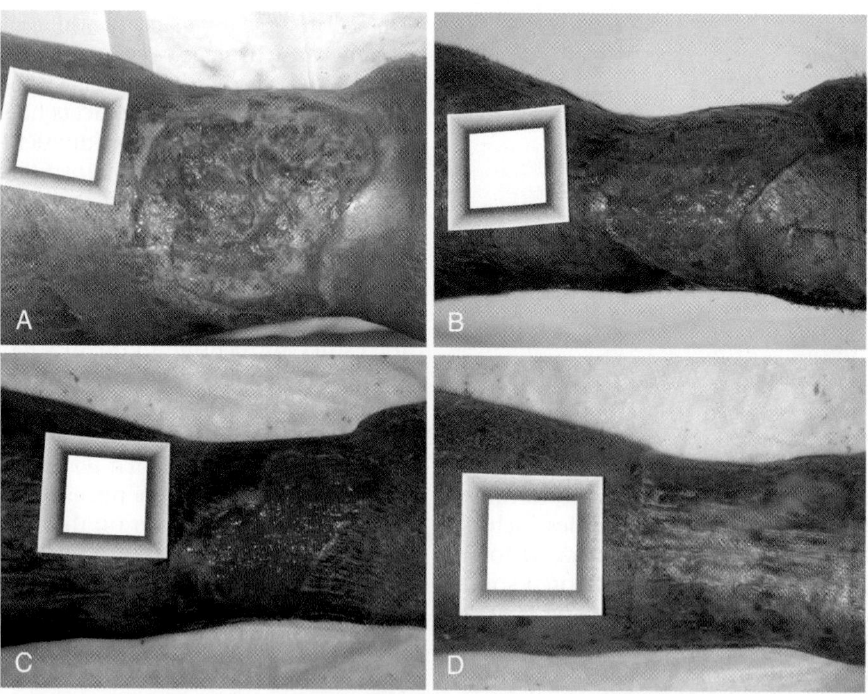

FIGURE 24-8 The course of healing a venous stasis ulcer of 1 year's duration and area greater than 100 cm^2 on an 81-year-old woman with good blood flow (ankle-brachial index = 1.2). On initial presentation, pain was significant (20 mg hydrocodone/day) as was edema (+4 pitting). Dramatic edema is also evident in the initial appearance (**A**). Initial care included a course of systemic antibiotics for wound infection without systemic signs (amoxicillin/clavulanate). Topical care included silver sulfadiazine to the wound with rolled gauze (Kerlix) and loose long-stretch compression bandaging toe to knee (Coban), with substantial reduction of edema by week 4 of treatment (**B**). Over the first 4 weeks, to decrease eschar burden there were twice per week curettage débridements, with daily dressing changes because of significant drainage. Also at 4 weeks and with a moderately red base, silver sulfadiazine was changed to a hydrocolloid with an overlying specialty absorptive dressing. Compression was tapered up to 1.5 rolls of Coban/leg at 4 weeks and 2 rolls at 8 weeks of treatment. The wound at week 12 is illustrated (**C**). Opiate intake continued to decrease: at 12 weeks she consumed hydrocodone 5 to 10 mg/day, and 5 mg/week at 16 weeks. With pain decrease, drainage also decreased, resulting in the need for dressing changes twice per week by week 20 and once per week by week 23. The wound closed by week 26 (**D**).

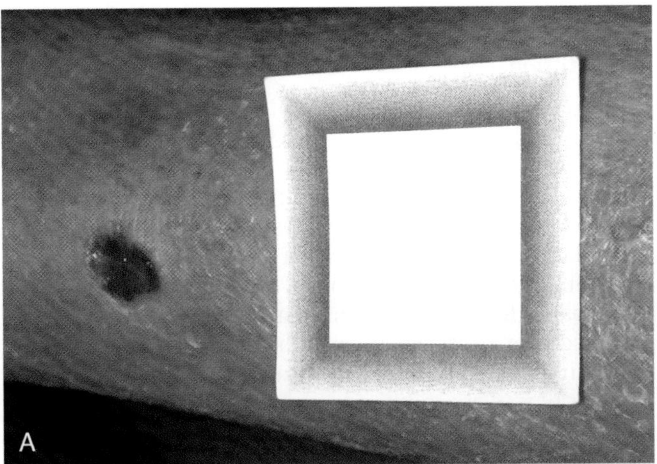

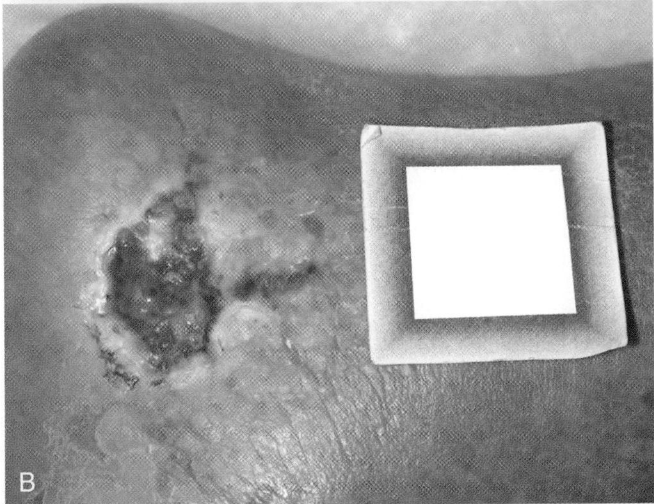

FIGURE 24-9 Differential diagnosis of venous stasis ulceration: Basal cell carcinoma established by 3-mm punch biopsy for stasislike ulcer on posterior leg of an elderly man with chronic obstructive pulmonary disease (**A**); Kaposi sarcoma (by wedge biopsy) on a 45-year-old man with epidemic AIDS on medial ankle (**B**). Both lesions were unresponsive to compression therapy.

treatment approaches include squamous or basal cell carcinoma, cutaneous T-cell lymphoma, Kaposi sarcoma,[135] cutaneous tuberculosis, vasculitis (such as in the setting of rheumatoid arthritis), and pyoderma gangrenosum. A wound that does not respond within 4 to 6 weeks or one that occurs on an unusual location (i.e., popliteal fossa, foot dorsum) might be an indication for a biopsy (Figure 24-9).[110]

Diagnostic Tests

Best practice indicates the need for a pretreatment ABI evaluation. For a normal ABI, standard care including compression (see discussion later) works well for most stasis ulcers. If arterial disease is suspected, segmental studies (e.g., pulse volume recordings or arterial Doppler studies) are useful to ensure that therapeutic compression is safe. Measurement of $TcPO_2$ is considered when the ABI is less than 0.8 or where microcirculation might be impaired (e.g., diabetes mellitus or end-stage renal disease). If the presentation warrants, venous studies including Doppler and venogram are useful to rule out acute venous thrombosis on an urgent basis. A venous duplex study might confirm venous insufficiency or postphlebitic syndrome.

Treatment

Compression therapy has emerged over time as the standard of care for venous stasis ulcers. Edema reduction typically results in pain reduction and wound healing. A common denominator for applying compression is application from toe to knee (distal to proximal). Two major types of compression are used: elastic and nonelastic (with long-stretch and nonstretch bandaging, respectively). Nonelastic nonstretch compression, classically the Unna paste boot, is effective. Edema is reduced by the inelastic dressing, which serves as a "fascial envelope" against which calf muscles can increase pressure during ambulation and reestablish a venous ankle pump. Ambulators obtain the best edema reduction.

Elastic compression provides compression of 30 to 40 mm Hg continuously, depending on the elastic compression brand. Because of the "high" static pressure, elastic dressings typically have three layers to increase tolerability: (1) a primary dressing over the wound; (2) a secondary layer of padding from toe to knee, applied distal to proximal (e.g., bulky 4-inch Kerlix); and (3) an overlying long-stretch compression layer (e.g., Coban). The entire three-layer system can be purchased as a unit (e.g., Profore). Over-the-counter elastic wraps (e.g., ACE) tend not to supply an adequate and uniform compression needed to heal venous ulcers, unless the patient can adhere to a most-of-the-day schedule of waist-level leg elevation.

A common error in the treatment of venous ulcers is inadequate attention to drainage management, such as in the presence of infection. If infection is suspected and is being treated, compression therapy can be used with frequent dressing changes and débridements, or with primary dressings that are more efficient at collecting or "wicking away" drainage. Frequent dressing changes are also required for draining wounds to prevent maceration of surrounding tissues and shear stress.

Inadequate drainage management is a likely common reason for failure of the weekly applied Unna boot. Although the Unna boot is durable, a disadvantage is that it requires training to apply. The Unna boot increases interstitial leg pressure during the toe-off phase of the gait cycle as a substitute for the natural ankle pump of the leg, which facilitates the flow of venous blood back to the central circulation. Because of the cyclic rather than constant pressure, the Unna boot could be the most appropriate method for mixed venous-arterial ulcers. Elastic compression is, in contrast, relatively easy to apply by caregivers in the home setting (with training). Elastic compression is best for those who are nonambulators.

McGuckin et al.[95] have incorporated the above set of treatments into a guideline that demonstrates efficacy; if the guideline is not used, the healing time is four times longer and costs six times more. With treatment consistent with this guideline, approximately 50% of ulcers heal after 12 weeks of treatment, and another 35% heal after 24 weeks. Wounds that do not close typically have these characteristics in common: ulcer size greater than 10 cm^2, wound present more than 12 months, and ABI less than 0.8.

For intractable wounds for which the wound bed is optimally prepared, bioengineered skin substitutes can be applied beneath compressive dressings with a bolster and without suturing. Because of their high cost, prudence dictates that skin substitutes should be reserved for venous ulcers that remain open for an extended period despite the best conservative treatment outlined earlier.

Prevention: Compression Stockings

Once venous ulcers heal, the patient remains at risk for recurrence because the underlying venous or fascial anatomic defect remains. Compression must be a lifelong practice. Compression garments (e.g., Jobst and Juzo) look and feel like stiff stockings and come in many sizes, colors, and pressures. Most patients do well with 20-to 30-mm Hg pressure. If an adherent patient ulcerates at the 20- to 30-mm Hg level, they are then prescribed the 30-to 40-mm Hg level. With this stepwise approach, only a few patients will require 40-to 50-mm Hg compression. Most garments are off the shelf, and only very obese patients or those with unusual-shaped legs (e.g., posttrauma) require custom-fitted stockings. Several pairs of stockings should be purchased to allow washing and rotation, and stockings should be replaced at 6-month intervals. Patient education and "buy-in" are the key to long-term ulcer prevention, and follow-up evaluation at 6-month intervals can maximize adherence.

Uncomplicated Neuropathic Ulcers

Presentation

Neuropathic or "insensate" foot ulcers can occur as a result of neuropathy of any cause (e.g., diabetes, leprosy) or congenital sensory neuropathy (e.g., heredity sensory motor neuropathy type 2, lumbar meningomyelocele). The most common type in the United States, however, is neuropathy secondary to diabetes mellitus (Figure 24-10). The sensorimotor neuropathy of diabetes is a "dying back" distal neuropathy leading to preferential denervation atrophy of intrinsic foot muscles (intrinsic minus foot). This results in an unbalanced pull of long flexors and extensors leading to pes cavus, claw toes, and subluxation of the metatarsal heads. This "intrinsic minus" deformity increases the pressure on bony prominences of already insensate feet. Insensitivity most often affects the plantar forefoot first, thus neuropathic ulcers commonly affect plantar toes, hallux, or metatarsal heads. Neurotrophic osteoarthropathy, or Charcot foot, frequently causes midfoot collapse and plantar-grade subluxation of the navicular or cuboid, leading to especially problematic neuropathic midfoot ulcers.

The physical examination of an uncomplicated foot ulcer typically shows peripheral pulses to be intact, but

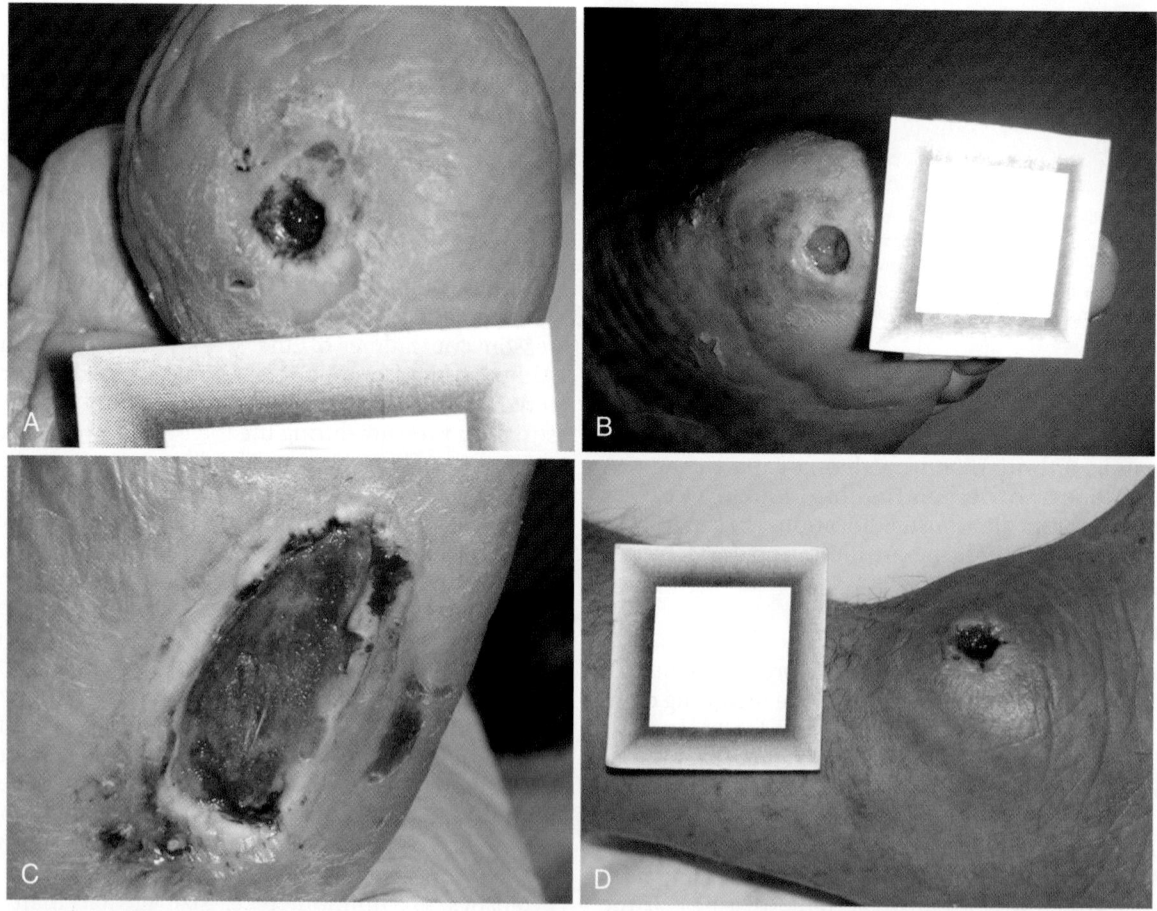

FIGURE 24-10 Presentations of neuropathic ulceration as circular or ovoid granular wounds surrounded by callus on weight-bearing bony prominences. For each example, weight bearing is excessive because of foot deformity such as claw toe (**A**), subluxation of first metatarsal head (**B**), and Charcot foot with calcaneal bony prominence (**C**). These patients have diabetes mellitus with peripheral neuropathy and local insensitivity to the 5.07 Semmes-Weinstein monofilament. **D,** A 31-year-old man with lumbar meningomyelocele with a left medial malleolar "fat pad" as an adaptation to ambulation on pronated feet as a child. As an adult he no longer ambulates, but a neuropathic ulcer has occurred on this prominence as a result of repetitive trauma.

sensation is diminished or absent in the vicinity of the ulcer, as measured by the 5.07 Semmes-Weinstein monofilament. Ulcers are most frequently located on bony prominences of the plantar metatarsals, midfoot, or heel. Ulcers can also be associated with digital abnormalities such as claw toes or hallux rigidus. Ulcers usually have regular borders and exuberant surrounding callus formation (see Figure 24-10 for examples of neuropathic ulcers).

Diagnostic Tests

Segmental arterial pressures, including toe pressures, are often used to assess perfusion. If these are equivocal, $TcPO_2$ can prognosticate healing as long as hyperkeratotic skin is avoided (e.g., the plantar foot). If there is clinical suspicion of osteomyelitis, magnetic resonance imaging (MRI) or combined indium-leukocyte bone scan is useful before initiating conservative treatment.

Treatment

Treatment strategies involve "off weighting" the ulcer, which promotes healing by reducing mechanical irritation, inflammation, and edema. Neuropathic patients might not feel pain on ambulation, making it challenging to adhere to weight-bearing restrictions. Limited weight bearing must be implemented after a complete physiatric assessment. This assessment should result in prescriptions for orthoses, assistive devices, weight-relief shoes, physical therapy, and limited weight bearing.

Local care of neuropathic ulcers follows general "good wound care" principles. The moist wound environment can be maintained by antibiotic ointments, such as mupirocin (Bactroban), or a hydrogel. Débridement (i.e., "saucerization") is also used on a weekly or biweekly basis (see the section on débridement in this chapter).

With the use of standard methods, approximately 24% of neuropathic wounds are healed at 12 weeks and 31% to 47% at 20 weeks. Factors positively associated with healing are wound areas less than 2 cm^2 and duration at time of presentation of less than 2 months.[86] The disappointing results with standard care have prompted many clinicians to seek adjunctive and complementary treatment strategies for their patients with neuropathic wounds.

A very popular and effective treatment for recalcitrant neuropathic ulcers with good circulation is total contact casting (TCC), which many consider to be the "gold standard" of care. TCC uses very little padding, usually only around the toes, the malleoli, and the tibial crest. In contrast to a conventional orthopedic cast for fractures, TCC is lightweight and is mainly designed for protection, immobility, and uniform pressure application. Pressure concentration is avoided by virtue of the custom contour of the set plaster, and there is minimum shear stress because of negligible amount of space inside the cast to allow movement. TCC is contraindicated where $TcPO_2$ is less than 35 mm Hg or ABI is less than 0.45 in the affected leg.[65]

The effectiveness of TCC has been accepted in clinical applications and practice; however, the cast application is a time-consuming, labor-intensive, expensive, and technically challenging process. Even in specialized centers, the technique might be best reserved until other, simpler methods fail to be effective.

Because of the difficulties associated with casting, simpler off-loading techniques are commonly used. These include the healing shoe, the forefoot relief shoe (i.e., "half shoe"), the removable cast walker, and the DH walker. The DH walker is a well-padded knee-high "boot" with a unique insole. The insole comprises hundreds of removable hexagonal pieces, each of which moves freely in multiple directions to reduce shear stress. For wounds at the toes or metatarsal heads, the DH walker might be as effective as TCC.

Healing shoe insoles have prominences proximal to or surrounding plantar ulcers to relieve high pressure. If prepared by trained professionals, healing shoes can be effective in healing digital plantar ulcers. The IPOS forefoot relief shoe (half shoe) reduces pressure to forefoot ulcers because the forefoot is "hanging in space." The half shoe can be effective if used as directed, but not as effective as TCC. One problem with healing shoes, half shoes, and walker boots is that they are removable: patients tend to "cheat," and only a few steps taken without them can defeat the healing process.

An alternative and very novel strategy is recombinant growth factor technology. Regranex, a formulation of recombinant PDGF-BB isoform (rh-PDGF-BB), has been approved by the FDA for healing of foot ulcers of neuropathic and diabetic etiology. In a randomized, prospective, double-blind, placebo-controlled trial and after 20 weeks of treatment, 45% of wounds closed in the rh-PDGF-BB group compared with 25% closure for the standard care group.[127] Application of Regranex is straightforward (topical, once per day, alternated with standard topical care). Disadvantages include the expense and the fact that it requires refrigerated storage. Because of the requirement for daily application, it cannot be used with casting, which is arguably a much more effective technique based on the evidence. If a patient with a well-perfused neuropathic ulcer cannot be casted, however, topical PDGF-BB might be a good choice.

Another method of treatment is application of bioengineered skin substitutes. Skin substitutes can be used with TCC. Where casting is to be done on an immunosuppressed patient with an expected slow healing rate, a skin substitute might be considered.

Prevention

The most cost-effective predictor of risk of neuropathic ulceration is testing with the 5.07 Semmes-Weinstein monofilament. If positive, the individual is at risk of the development of a wound or a recurrence. Neuropathic ulcers often recur without periodic follow-up evaluation and by not prescribing orthopedic oxford shoes. Even if the shoe prescription is filled correctly so that pressure and shear stress are minimized, there is a recurrence rate of up to 30% per year, even with good compliance. Recurrence rates are high for patients who refuse to wear prescription shoes. Every effort should be made to optimize the shoe prescription and to educate the patient about the benefits to his or her health by adhering to the treatment strategies that have been proven to minimize or eliminate the risk.

During the period of skin maturation, a shoe prescription can be filled by a certified pedorthist. A pedorthist has been specifically trained and certified in making specialty shoes and is well versed in insole and outsole modifications. A typical accommodative shoe prescription is for orthopedic oxford shoes with high toe box, removable PPT-Plastazote insoles, and modified rocker bottom. Each element is important. Rocker bottoms reduce pressure at the metatarsal heads. Insoles should be replaced at 3-month intervals because of a tendency to "bottom out", and shoes should be replaced at 1-year intervals. Patient education involves daily inspection of the feet and legs to make sure there are no ecchymoses or excessive callus, which are harbingers of reulceration. Emollients, such as lanolin or Lac-Hydrin, help prevent the drying and cracking of skin, especially between toes, that can be portals for entry of pathogens. A professional (e.g., podiatrist) should perform nail and callus débridements every 2 to 3 months on routine follow-up evaluation.

Ischemic Ulcers

Presentation

Patients with ischemic ulcers typically have peripheral arterial disease, that is, calcification, stenosis, or blockage of named arteries anywhere from the aortic bifurcation to the plantar and digital arteries. The term *arterial ulcer* is equally acceptable. Peripheral arterial disease and cardiovascular disease have similar risk factors, including hypertension, diabetes, smoking, hypercholesterolemia, and family history. In addition to arteriosclerosis, patients with ischemic wounds (including those with diabetes and end-stage renal disease) have microvascular disease or microcirculation abnormality, which contributes to chronic local hypoxia. Classic ischemic symptoms such as intermittent claudication are uncommon, partly because patients with ischemic ulcers have limited mobility or they have peripheral neuropathy and sometimes can be insensate to pain.

Ischemic leg and foot ulcers are of multiple subtypes: pure, postsurgical, venous, pressure, or neuroischemic. Neuroischemic ulcers (i.e., neuropathy is present) typically occur at areas of trauma or repeated pressure. Neuroischemic ulcers do not occur on the plantar surface but on the foot margins (e.g., lateral heel, lateral fifth metatarsal head, and medial hallux). Also occurring at the foot margins are pressure-related ischemic wounds. A particularly common scenario seen in the rehabilitation setting is pressure necrosis of the lateral heel margins as a result of prolonged immobility during anesthesia or on the operating table.

A postsurgical ischemic wound can occur as a result of dehiscence of a residual limb incision within an ischemic region. Venous ischemic wounds can occur anywhere on the leg and foot and are associated with edema or venous insufficiency (see Figure 24-11 for examples of ischemic ulcers). Pure ischemic ulcers occur in the setting of acute proximal arterial blockage, distal emboli, or macroangiopathy or microangiopathy not otherwise classified (see Figure 24-4).

Ischemic ulcers tend to be exceedingly painful for sensate patients and are exacerbated by leg elevation and relieved by placing the leg in a dependent position. Some patients with painful ischemic ulcers are able to sleep only in the sitting position. In addition to wound pain, the skin over the affected area is hairless and appears fragile and friable. The ischemic ulcer frequently has a blanched base, has a "punched out" appearance, and is painful to probe, and the area surrounding the ulcer might have a bright or dusky red hue that has been termed ischemic livedo. The color can be purple or black, signaling the onset of

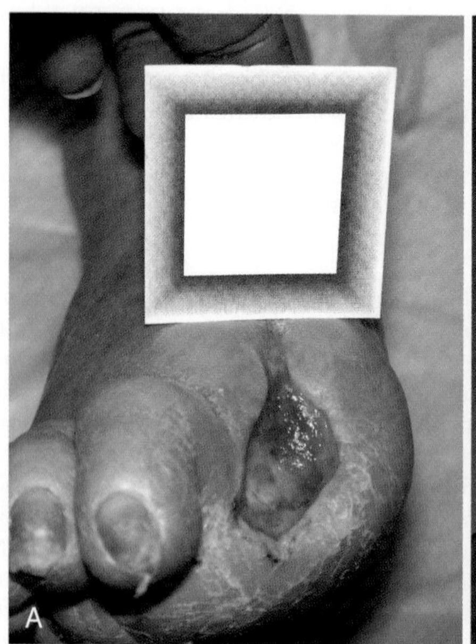

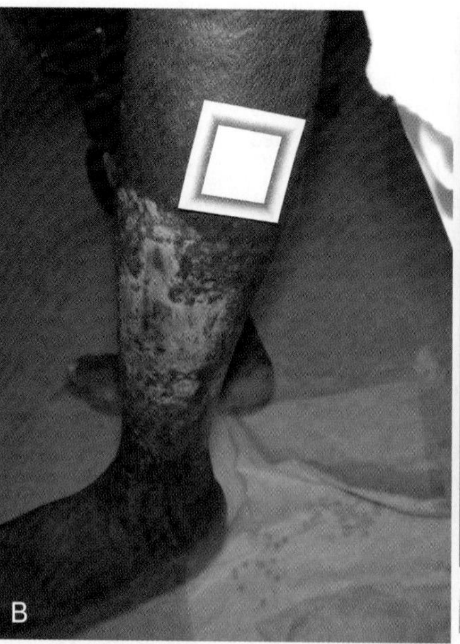

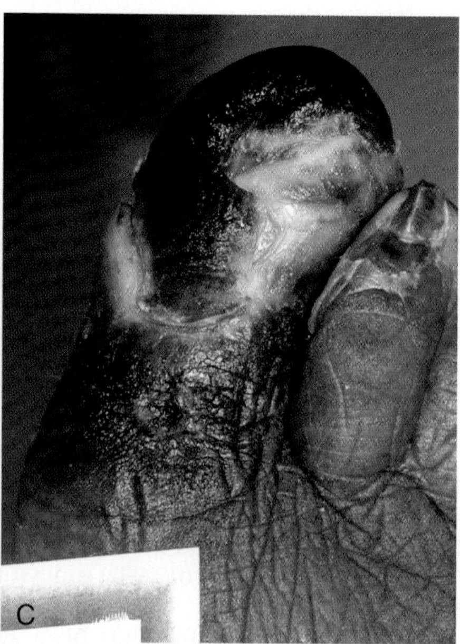

FIGURE 24-11 Examples of ischemic ulcers. **A,** An ischemic postsurgical wound on a 70-year-old man with adult-onset diabetes and peripheral neuropathy who presented with hallux gangrene and an occluded femoral-popliteal bypass. **B,** A stasis-ischemic wound on an older adult nursing home resident, which responded to leg elevation rather than compression. **C,** An ischemic hallux on an elderly woman with end-stage renal disease. For each case, initial periwound transcutaneous oxygen ($TcPO_2$) was less than 10 mm Hg; each patient had documented peripheral arterial disease, and each ultimately healed coincident with increase of $TcPO_2$ out of ischemic range. In addition to standard care, case C received a 24-week course of daily high-volt pulsed current (HVPC) electrotherapy; case A received 4 weeks of hyperbaric oxygen and then 28 weeks of HVPC.

gangrene. Any suspicion of gangrene or cellulitis requires an urgent surgical referral.

The natural history and the healing course of ischemic wounds are highly variable, much more than might be expected for other wound types. They might heal slowly, be quasi-stable for an indefinite period, or aggressively increase in size. Ischemic wounds that expand can lead to deep soft tissue infection, osteomyelitis, and limb loss. An ischemic wound typically has a periwound $TcPO_2$ less than 20 mm Hg,[106] with the most hypoxic wounds (i.e., $TcPO_2$ less than 10 mm Hg) typically demonstrating the most ominous course. A particularly aggressive form of cutaneous gangrene is calciphylaxis, an unusual and grave condition noted in the setting of renal osteodystrophy in dialysis patients.[93]

Diagnostic Tests

Vascular studies are crucial to establish a prognosis for conservative healing. Pulse volume recordings might show an asymmetrically low value, although an ABI of less than 0.4 is not uncommon and tends to carry a poor prognosis. A useful definition of ischemia is periwound $TcPO_2$ less than 20 mm Hg.[55] Healing requires oxygenating the wound by increasing the blood supply.

Treatment

If the wound is truly ischemic, a revascularization vascular surgical referral is needed to determine whether proximal flow can be reestablished by angioplasty or a bypass procedure. The outcome in terms of healing and limb preservation is much more favorable with successful revascularization.[133] Whether or not the surgical consultant concludes that bypass or angioplasty is indicated, noninvasive methods contribute immeasurably to reversal of wound area expansion and even to healing. Conservative, nonsurgical, standard wound care must be optimized, including liberal use of padding and weight-relief strategies. The usual guidelines concerning the "moist wound environment," however, do not hold for ischemic wounds. Many have advocated keeping ischemic wounds dry in an effort to avoid "wet gangrene." Others use dilute Betadine, which is a strong antimicrobial and desiccating agent. A good argument exists to use silver sulfadiazine sparingly (an eschar-softening agent, broad-spectrum antimicrobial that is usually well tolerated) on ischemic wounds for which the goal is healing but around which ischemia has not yet resolved.

Techniques that address pathomechanics are crucial and involve optimizing gait mechanics, with limited weight-bearing to or near the ischemic wound (i.e., limited weight bearing with an assist device). Overly aggressive rehabilitation of a patient with an ischemic wound can be detrimental. For example, consider the common scenario of a patient with a "black/purple heel" undergoing preprosthetic inpatient rehabilitation. A "black/purple heel" should be considered ischemic until proven otherwise.[118] Progressive ambulation that involves "hopping" and repetitive trauma on the ischemic heel wound could worsen inflammation, pain, and ischemia and cause wound expansion and loss of the functional remaining limb. In this case, the short-term goal might best be downgraded to transfer activity.

The evidence base is expanding for noninvasive techniques to promote oxygenation and blood flow to ischemic wounds. These treatments are intended for patients for whom revascularization does not lead to healing, who experience graft failure, or who are not revascularization candidates because of multiple high-risk comorbidities. Currently available treatments include hyperbaric oxygen, the circulator boot, and high-volt pulsed current (HVPC) electrotherapy. HVPC has been shown in case series,[54,55] a controlled retrospective trial, and a small prospective randomized study[56] to prevent area expansion and promote healing of nonsurgical ischemic wounds. Positive outcomes are associated with long-lasting resolution of hypoxia according to serial $TcPO_2$ determination (Figure 24-12).

$TcPO_2$ can be helpful in assessing which patients will respond to systemic HBOT. A sea-level air $TcPO_2$ less than 15 mm Hg combined with an in-chamber $TcPO_2$ less than 400 mm Hg predicts failure of HBOT with reliability and a positive predictive value of 75%.[38]

Prevention

Prevention of ischemic wounds requires a high index of suspicion. For ischemic wounds with a neuropathic, pressure, or venous component, similar guidelines apply as for uncomplicated wounds of these respective types. For prevention of ischemic pressure wounds, the Braden Scale is helpful but might not predict formation of ischemic heel wounds. Frequent skin checks and vigilance are required. In the posthealing phase of venous ischemic wounds, careful attention should be paid to compression pressure to avoid necrosis (i.e., use 5 to 10 mm Hg antiembolism stockings or 10 to 20 mm Hg compression hose, rather than 20 to 30 mm Hg stockings). Cigarette smoking lowers $TcPO_2$, which complicates healing of chronic wounds (especially ischemic wounds) and makes recurrence more likely.

Infection, Surgical Repair, and the Transition from Outpatient to Acute Inpatient Management

Presentation

It is crucial to make the distinction between wounds that are static (i.e., healing "arrest") because they are critically colonized or locally infected, and those with frank tissue invasion with systemic signs and symptoms of infection. Patients with systemic infection benefit from hospitalization, close monitoring, and intravenous antibiotics. Oral antibiotics, débridement, and topical therapies best manage locally infected wounds. The signs and symptoms of local infection are increased pain, friable granulation tissue, wound breakdown (i.e., small openings in newly formed epithelial tissue not caused by reinjury or trauma), and foul odor. These "secondary" signs and symptoms have better sensitivity, specificity, and a positive predictive value than the classic signs of infection (i.e., heat, pain, redness, and swelling).

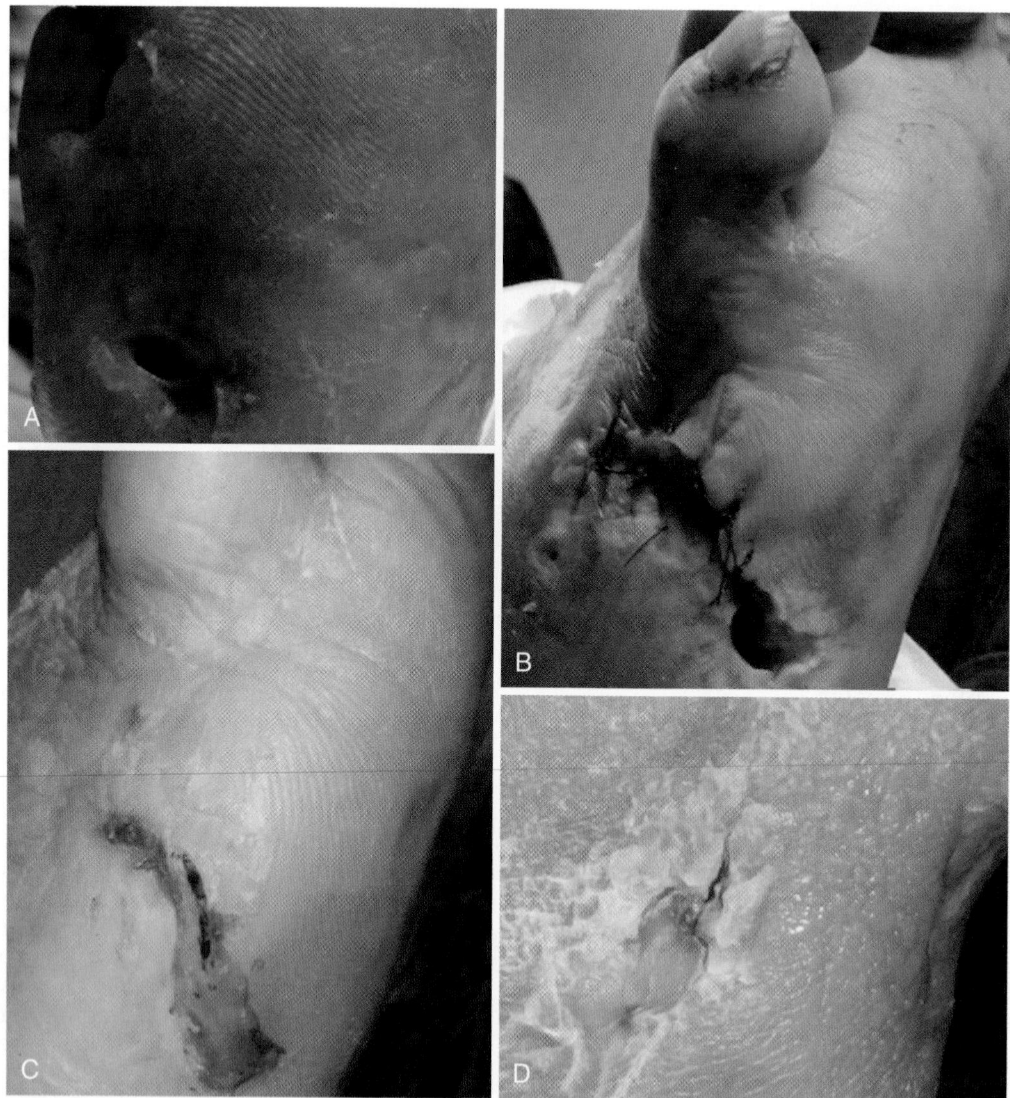

FIGURE 24-12 Case study of complex Wagner III diabetic foot ulcer that resolved after minor amputation and hyperbaric oxygen therapy (HBOT) with preservation of function. EP is a 76-year-old man with adult-onset diabetes, aortic stenosis, systolic dysfunction, and coronary artery disease. He was admitted on November 1, 2013, to a regional hospital with cellulitis from a right fifth metatarsal plantar ulcer (**A**). Magnetic resonance imaging (MRI) revealed osteomyelitis of the right fifth proximal phalanx and metatarsal head. Wound culture revealed coagulase negative staph and alpha-hemolytic strep. He was placed on intravenous Ertapenem (which ended 67 days later). He was discharged after 2 weeks to a local nursing facility and 3 weeks later evaluated at the Fort Healthcare Wound and Edema Center, Johnson Creek, Wis. On examination, there was an ulcer on the right plantar fifth metatarsal head 1.5 × 0.9 × 0.7 cm deep. There was tunneling 4 cm to the dorsal surface. He was an independent ambulator with assist device. Peripheral arterial disease was mild. An arterial Doppler including the past 9 months revealed an ankle-brachial index of 1.1 bilaterally with incompressible vessels but no evident occlusive disease. Toe indices were 0.99 on the right, and 0.53 on the left. A transcutaneous oxygen measurement on the right leg/foot revealed very distal small vessel disease, but ankle and leg electrodes yielded normal response at baseline, leg elevation, and 100% oxygen challenge. Because this was Wagner III disease, podiatric surgery was consulted. The surgeon noted bone destruction on plain film. The surgeon concluded that conservative healing was not possible, and on December 20, 2013, resected the fifth toe and the distal half of the fifth metatarsal head. **B,** The wound pictured 3 days postoperatively of lateral fifth metatarsal head. Cardiac clearance for HBOT was received and treatment was started on December 31, 2013, at the wound center. This continued until March 3, 2014, on weekdays at 2.0 atm with two 5-minute air breaks for 90 minutes per session Sutures remained in place for a few weeks but the wound never closed and sutures were removed (**C**). The remaining wound tracked as deep as 1.5 cm, but as treatment progressed it "filled in" to zero depth. Area was typically less than 0.1 cm. By April 22, 2014, the wound healed (**D**). After healing, a repeat MRI was negative for osteomyelitis.

Systemic signs of inflammation or infection indicate the need for acute care or hospitalization. These include fever, chills, sweats, nausea, vomiting, or loss of appetite; elevated or depressed temperature; elevated white count; change in mental status; and/or increased glucose intolerance in patients with diabetes. For patients with diabetes or immunosuppressed status (e.g., patients with HIV, organ transplant recipients, and those with end-stage renal disease), there is a lower threshold for hospitalization. For venous leg ulcers, cellulitis is an indication for hospitalization when erythema extends more than 2 cm from the ulcer margin with systemic signs. Frank purulence or abscess necessitates an urgent surgical referral.

Soft Tissue Infections: Wound Culture, Microbiology, and Antibiotic Therapy

Because the surfaces of all ulcers are colonized by bacteria, ulcer cultures should not be routinely performed. Routine cultures do not have meaning in the absence of suspected "critical colonization" or infection. For identifying the causative organisms, there are five major culturing techniques: semiquantitative swab, quantitative swab, needle aspiration, curettage, and quantitative culture. Quantitative cultures are obtained by performing a punch biopsy. Results are described in terms of colony-forming units per gram of tissue. Many consider quantitative culture to be the "gold standard." A high false-positive rate is observed, however, for quantitative culture of burn wounds.[94] Additionally, not all microbiology laboratories are able to perform the technique. In contrast, nearly all microbiology laboratories can analyze swabs. Semiquantitative swabs are readily available, and their use is straightforward, but they have a sensitivity, specificity, and predictive value of less than 50%. Quantitative swabs are more accurate, in that they correlate with quantitative culture if wounds are prewashed before swabbing.[94]

Mixed bacterial infections can also occur in patients who are not diabetic or immunosuppressed. Infection involving deep tissue invasion and hospitalization is almost always polymicrobial, including strict anaerobes and facultative aerobes. Aerobic organisms are usually found in surface swabs, whereas anaerobes are more often isolated from deep tissue or in larger pressure ulcers. Deep tissue isolates can reveal *Proteus mirabilis,* group B or D streptococci, *Escherichia coli, Staphylococcus aureus, Pseudomonas aeruginosa, Peptostreptococcus* species, *Clostridia,* and *Bacteroides fragilis. B. fragilis* is often found in blood cultures associated with clinical sepsis. Surgical diabetic foot infections often reveal similar organisms. In recent years, methicillin-resistant *S. aureus* (MRSA) and vancomycin-resistant *Enterococcus* have emerged as important virulent organisms within wounds.[94]

Débridement, antimicrobial dressings, or topical antibiotic agents are required for clinically infected wounds. Outpatient management of infections requires treatment with broad-spectrum oral antibiotics that cover gram-positive and gram-negative bacteria and anaerobes.[35] Choices for aerobes include cephalexin, sulfamethoxazole-trimethoprim, and quinolone (e.g., ciprofloxacin or levofloxacin). For anaerobes, choices include metronidazole and clindamycin. Clindamycin also covers some gram-positive bacteria and can be used in simple infections as a single agent. Another choice as a single agent is amoxicillin trihydrate-clavulanate potassium. Linezolid is a member of the oxazolidinone antibiotic class, can be used for MRSA, and is broadly active against gram-positive bacteria, with the advantage of being an oral agent. Intravenous antibiotics for inpatient infections are typically best determined in conjunction with infectious disease or internal medicine consultants.

Osteomyelitis

Subclinical untreated osteomyelitis often leads to nonhealing ulcers. Approximately 25% of all nonhealing ulcers contain bone infection[51] and osteomyelitis should be considered and ruled out on the initial presentation if there is a reasonable suspicion. Although bone biopsy is 96% sensitive,[30] surgeons are often reluctant to perform one unless there is some other compelling indication to operate.[134] In the outpatient setting, osteomyelitis is most easily diagnosed by imaging studies.

Imaging Studies

Plain films are positive for osteomyelitis if they show reactive bone formation and periosteal elevation. Plain films are the least expensive imaging study but have a sensitivity of 78% and specificity of only 50%. Because of the deficiencies of plain films, test combinations have been suggested. A combination of the leukocyte count, erythrocyte sedimentation rate, and plain films provided a combined sensitivity of 89% and specificity of 88%. If all three test results are positive, the positive predictive value of this combination is 69%. If all are negative, the negative predictive value is 96%.[30] The combination is less helpful if only one or two tests are positive.

Conventional three-phase bone scan is more sensitive for osteomyelitis than plain films, but specificity is still only 50%. Specificity is low because bone scans are poor at differentiating osteomyelitis from soft tissue infection contiguous to bone.[98] Indium leukocyte scanning has been reported to overcome this deficiency, with a sensitivity of 89%. When combined with a three-phase bone scan, the sensitivity of indium white blood cell scanning is 100% and the specificity is 81%.[19] Radionuclide tests either singly or in combination have the drawback of not revealing anatomic detail.

MRI reveals anatomic detail and is extremely sensitive to the presence of marrow edema on the T2-weighted image. A recent study confirmed that the high sensitivity and specificity of MRI in the evaluation of osteomyelitis of the diabetic foot, using a probe-to-bone test (PTBT) method and a standard MRI. The PTBT method had a sensitivity of 82.5% and a specificity of 76.9%. The standard MRI had a sensitivity of 97% and a specificity 88.5% with a positive predictive value of 96.3%. Although the PTBT method is less accurate than the MRI, it remains an alternative.[143] Other entities that cause marrow edema, such as resolving fracture or recent surgery, have to be considered. The combined sensitivity and specificity of biopsy and MRI is cumulative in diagnostic power.

Adjunctive Treatment for Osteomyelitis

After a surgical evaluation, with or without surgical débridement and biopsy, management of osteomyelitis requires 6 weeks of antibiotics. Such treatment for up to 12 weeks has been suggested for more aggressive treatment of osteomyelitis for individuals with diabetes. For recurrent osteomyelitis or an initial presentation of osteomyelitis in an immunosuppressed patient (e.g., transplant recipient), HBOT is considered in parallel with intravenous antibiotics. An oxygen-rich environment in bone enhances leukocytic killing and is synergistic with antibiotics.

Surgical Management

The physiatrist on the "front line" of wound care understands that many, if not most, chronic wounds heal with conservative care. While the physiatrist focuses on the functional aspects of medical management, the physical medicine and rehabilitation services must have access to consultants to effectively manage infections. Although conservative care has its place, it might not be prudent for scenarios illustrated in the following sections, and others as professional judgment dictates.

Surgical Management of Infection

At no time is the surgeon more critical than on presentation of a wound with frank tissue invasion, abscess, frank purulence, fistulae, or acute osteomyelitis, any of which might lead to sepsis (Figure 24-13). These infections require operating room débridement and culture (see discussion on débridement in this chapter) because the infection will not resolve with antibiotics alone.

Soft Tissue Reconstruction

Musculocutaneous flaps are usually the best choice for stage IV pressure ulcers of the buttocks[8] in patients with SCI, or when the concomitant loss of muscle function does not contribute to comorbidity or deficits in functional status. Tissue expanders serve to optimize wound coverage and are now commonly used. Musculocutaneous flaps are also occasionally used for well-vascularized pressure ulcers of the heel. Musculocutaneous flaps can help heal osteomyelitis and limit further damage caused by shearing, friction, and pressure. Split-thickness skin grafts can also be used to repair recalcitrant venous ulcers and neuropathic ulcers.

In individuals with advanced age or patients who are chronically ill, the benefits of reconstructive surgery might be outweighed by the risks. In addition to the risk of surgery, musculocutaneous flaps have a significant recurrence rate in ulceration, with a short-term failure rate (most commonly the result of suture line dehiscence) with a high likelihood of recurrence. The recurrence rate can be minimized by carefully attending to mechanical factors. If the biomechanical defect that led to the ulcer in the first place is not corrected (by means of specialty shoes, orthoses, stockings, seating systems, or beds), the ulcer is likely to recur postoperatively.

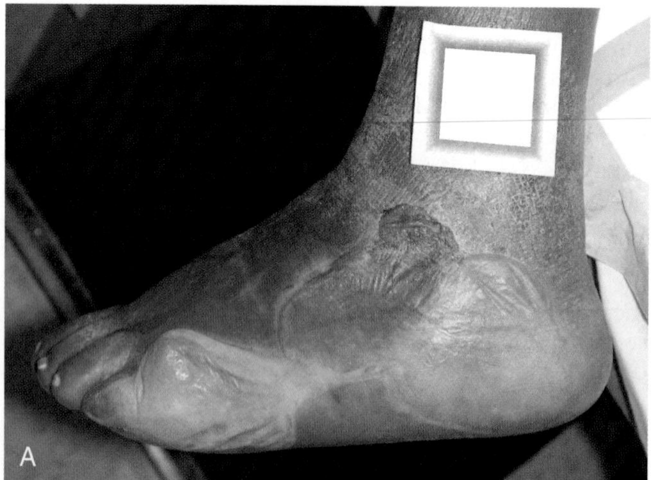

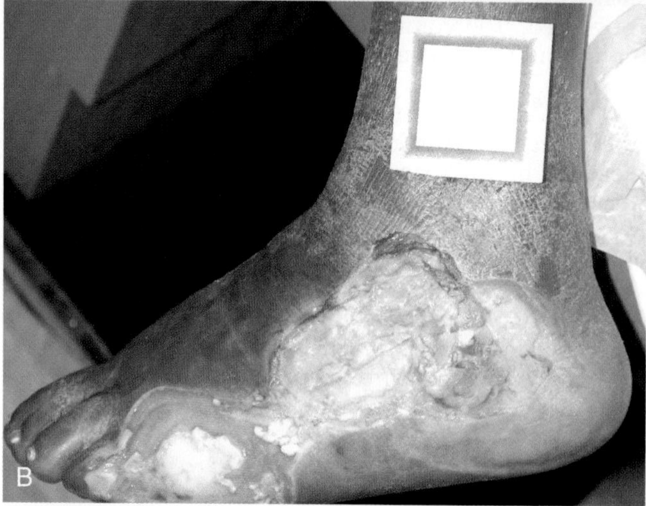

FIGURE 24-13 An example of a case requiring surgical referral. A 51-year-old man with L3 meningomyelocele complained of a 2-week history of chills and poor appetite. On presentation to the wound clinic he was afebrile with a warm, blistered erythematous foot (**A**). A podiatric surgeon was immediately called, who performed a sharps débridement (**B**) and admitted the patient for treatment of abscess/cellulitis with intravenous antibiotics, surgical débridement, and split-thickness skin grafting, which ultimately achieved closure.

Bone Repair and Reconstruction

The diabetic foot has deformities that predispose to ulceration. If the ulcer heals and then recurs several times, the orthopedic or podiatric surgeon should evaluate the patient for foot reconstruction, osteotomies, or tendon recessions to relieve the source of pathomechanical risk factors.

Revascularization

Revascularization has become the standard of care for the limb at risk. A review of the Cochrane database for peripheral arterial disease does not identify a RCT for revascularization versus no revascularization.[41] However, in clinical practice, it is known that revascularization is associated with limb preservation.[36]

Bypass procedures became much more commonplace after 1979.[49] Three decades later, the paradigm has shifted again, in favor of angioplasty. Angioplasty and bypass produce similar results, although angioplasty enjoys lower periprocedural morbidity for high-risk wound patients.[129]

Indeed, a blinded RCT (the BASIL trial) of 500 enrollees with critically ischemic arterial ulcers (40% diabetes, 50% smokers) were randomized into bypass-first and angioplasty-first cohorts.[1] At 1 year, there were higher costs, length of stay, and slightly higher mortality in the bypass group. At 2 years, there was 60% amputation-free survival and 70% overall survival for both groups. The BASIL trial did not report on healing of arterial ulcers, which 80% of enrollees had. At 3 years, there seemed to be better overall survival and graft patency in the bypass group. At 5 years, for both groups survival was approximately 50%. The 5-year survival for patients after dysvascular amputation is also approximately 40%, suggesting it is an underlying disease rather than amputation itself that leads to high mortality. A study of quality of life 7 years after revascularization found end-point survival of 37%. For the one third that survived, two thirds retained functional limbs (i.e., independent in-house ambulatory status).[68]

Amputation

Major amputation secondary to significant dysvascular disease can be done at the digital, transmetatarsal, Symes, transtibial, or transfemoral level for rapidly expanding gangrene or overwhelming infection. The following statement summarizes clear decision-making surrounding major amputation: "Amputation should be performed if tissue loss has progressed beyond the point of salvage, if surgery is too risky, if life expectancy is very low, or if functional limitations obviate the benefit of limb salvage."[9]

The physiatrist should be involved in "staging" the amputation. The team approach should take into account the patient's function, ambulation, the cardiopulmonary burden arising from increased energy expenditure, and oxygen consumption associated with preprosthetic and postprosthetic gait training.

Nutrition

A major sign of poor nutrition is body weight less than 90% of ideal body weight. Laboratory markers include albumin less than 3.5 g/mL and prealbumin less than 15 mg/mL.[24] An established link exists between poor nutrition and pressure ulcer formation.

Nutritional therapy for patients with stage III or stage IV pressure ulcers includes (1) 30 to 35 kcal/kg/day; (2) 1.2 to 1.5 g/kg/day protein by means of oral, enteral, or parenteral routes; and (3) fluid intake at 1 mL/kcal.[96] Patients with SCI or AIDS wasting syndrome and pressure ulcers might additionally benefit from oxandrolone to build lean muscle mass. Oxandrolone is an anabolic steroid that is approved by the FDA to promote weight gain after severe physiologic stress (recommended dose of 10 to 15 mg/day). Oxandrolone is not, however, specifically FDA-approved for treatment of pressure ulcers and should probably be considered as an off-label use.

The evidence base for vitamin and mineral supplementation is not established for patients without specific vitamin deficits. The relative safety of these compounds, however, suggests that it is reasonable to include them in a complete wound-healing nutritional program. Arginine might enhance collagen concentration and wound-breaking strength.[140]

Vitamin C is an essential nutrient in wound healing because of its role as a cosubstrate in the hydroxylation of proline and lysine, which form collagen cross-links. When specific deficiencies are diagnosed, it is reasonable to recommend up to 750 mg/day for women and 900 mg/day for men. Vitamin A deficiency results in delayed wound healing and increased susceptibility to infection, especially in patients treated with corticosteroids. Zinc is a zymogen for DNA syntheses and metalloproteinases. Oral zinc might have a beneficial effect on healing of venous ulcers in individuals with lower serum zinc level at baseline.[139] A reasonable dose of zinc sulfate is 220 mg/day.

Management of Wound Pain

Wound pain bears similarities to both acute and chronic pain: chronic, because the pain is considered long-lasting; acute, because the pain (with few exceptions) resolves when the wound heals. Any wound pain concerns associated with débridement, as mentioned previously, are managed with topical analgesia. A local anesthetic, lidocaine 5%, or EMLA cream (lidocaine 2.5% and prilocaine 2.5%) can be applied up to 15 minutes before débridement. Premedication with a fast-acting oral nonopiate and/or oral opiate analgesic can also be helpful. Because the acute pain is of moderate to severe intensity, most patients receive opiate analgesics. They make the patient comfortable, foster sleep, and improve adherence to treatment. In the absence of substance abuse history, nearly all patients easily wean off opiates after the wound heals. (For older adults or those at fall risk, it is reasonable to prescribe nonopiate analgesics.) Of note, of foremost importance, is the adequate pain management for other health ailments that can influence the patient's position while sitting or lying in bed. In the particular case of pressure ulcers, the patient may maintain an antalgic position secondary to another issue such as knee pain or hip pain. This position maintained for a prolonged time can lead to pressure over a bony prominence that makes him or her susceptible to pressure ulcers in that specific area. A comprehensive approach to managing any other sources of pain, to prevent prolonged antalgic positions that can contribute to the development of pressure ulcers, should be undertaken.[112]

The patient can be dispensed "as needed" codeine (e.g., 30 mg), oxycodone (e.g., 5 mg), morphine sulfate (e.g., 15 mg), or hydromorphone (e.g., 2 mg), depending on the patient's history of allergies, adverse reactions, opiate tolerance, and physician experience. If the oral morphine-equivalent intake per day exceeds 30 mg, the physician should consider using long-acting opiates based on opiate equivalence. Choices include oxycodone slow release (10 mg every 12 hours) or morphine sulfate slow release (15 mg every 12 hours), or fentanyl transdermal patches (a 25-μg patch applied to the skin every 3 days). Long-acting opioids avoid the high peak/low trough effect associated with on-demand doses. "Breakthrough" doses should follow predictable patterns, but total equivalent dose per week should gradually decrease as inflammation subsides and the wound heals. Wound pain requires an assessment scale to judge the effectiveness of treatment. The most basic assessment is a numerical rating scale, which is an 11-point scale where 0 is no pain and 10 is the worst possible pain. Patients are asked to quantify their pain levels by choosing a single number from the 11-point scale.[71] The number of "pain pills" per day consumed by the patient is a concrete and readily understood measure of patient discomfort. The American Pain Society coined the phrase "pain: the fifth vital sign" to elevate awareness of pain treatment among health care professionals. The Joint Commission has declared that pain should be treated as a vital sign. The traditional vital signs—pulse, blood pressure, respiration, and temperature—are called signs for a reason. They follow the medical axiom that signs must be objective, measurable, and quantifiable. Pain is not a sign, it is a symptom. Symptoms are what patients describe subjectively as a feeling, and feelings are not easy to quantify. One should, however, measure and treat a patient's pain with the same degree of urgency as is done with other vital signs.[112]

Wound Care Centers

Wound care lends itself to guideline-driven care. This is because there are major categories of chronic wounds, each with an evidence-based guideline. This chapter outlines four categories: arterial, venous, pressure, neuropathic. Postsurgical wounds constitute a fifth category. Once an ulcer is diagnosed within one or more categories, a guideline is straightforward to implement and track. Wound progress is monitored week by week. If progress stalls, practitioners make collaborative course corrections.

Wound care is an interprofessional endeavor: close collaboration of medical, surgical, podiatric, nursing, and rehabilitation specialists. Successful wound care is also time and material intensive, and education is crucial to build cooperation and buy-in. Once the wound heals, all staff participates in education and secondary prevention.[61]

In the United States, this model has propagated in the private sector. There are approximately 5700 hospitals in the United States in 2014 (www.aha.org/research/rc/stat-studies/fast-facts.shtml). In 2012, approximately 3100 hospitals offered "wound management services." Since 2008, this number has grown by 3% per year (American Hospital Association, personal communication). Wound care centers follow a continuum from a single practitioner to a full-scale hospital-based outpatient center. A Wound Management Organization often administers the center under contract and installs a dedicated wound electronic medical record (EMR). Dedicated wound care EMRs complement guideline-driven care and are an industry standard in this age of "meaningful use." All told, a quarter of U.S. hospitals have fully organized outpatient wound centers.

BOX 24-1

Wagner Classification System for Complex Diabetic Foot Ulcers

Wagner grade	(1) A Wagner designation is retained as long as a wound persists. For instance, if toe gangrene occurs and the toe is amputated and the incision does not "durably" heal, the Wagner IV designation continues. When durable healing occurs, the foot reverts to Wagner 0. (2) Wagner II is to some degree an archaic designation. This is because of improved imaging methods. When the scale was first published in 1980, magnetic resonance imaging was not available for clinical use.
Wagner I	Is an uncomplicated neuropathic ulcer through skin and subcutaneous tissue (discussed earlier).
Wagner II	Through fascial plane but no infection by clinical appearance.
Wagner III	In general, diabetic foot ulcer with "hospital level infection": cellulitis beneath fascial plane, osteomyelitis, septic arthritis, or tendonitis.
Wagner IV	Localized gangrene (likely to involve deep soft tissue or bone).
Wagner V	Extensive gangrene.

From Wagner F: The dysvascular foot: a system for diagnosis and treatment, *Foot Ankle* 2:64-122, 1981.

Team Form and Function

For challenges such as Wagner III or IV DFU, the interdisciplinary team includes the diabetes management specialist, surgeon, vascular, and HBOT specialists. In fact, comprehensive care of a dedicated, multidisciplinary guideline-driven diabetic foot clinic in the United Kingdom correlates with lower amputation rate. Over 5 years of implementation, there was a reduction over the entire region in major amputation rates from 5.8 to 1.7 per 1000.[21] There was a far greater decrease in major lower extremity amputation (LEA) than minor LEAs. Although correlation is not causality, at the same time there was a rise for nondiabetic LEA, suggesting the multidisciplinary diabetic foot program itself was limb preserving. It is an open question as to whether major amputation rates in the United States are decreasing in part as a result of the diffusion of the comprehensive wound center model across the country.

Limb Preservation and the Diabetic Foot Ulcer

DFUs are characterized according to the Wagner scale (I through V).[137] Wagner III and IV lesions are the focus and template of limb preservation protocols (Box 24-1). Complex DFUs represent a hybrid of ischemic and neuropathic types, often presenting with limb-threatening infection. For DFU prevalence in general, 35% are neuropathic, 15% are arterial or "ischemic," and 50% are mixed (arterial plus neuropathic, or "neuroischemic").[8] For mixed DFU disease, apply treatment protocols of both types: for a neuropathic ulcer the standard of care is off-loading, and for an arterial ulcer it is revascularization. A misconception in treatment of the complex Wagner III to IV DFU is that the goal is healing. Although primary healing is preferred, presence of (for instance) toe gangrene or metatarsal osteomyelitis may make primary healing unrealistic. In this case, the question is if there is enough blood flow and oxygenation to heal a distal minor amputation level or bone resection. The goal is actually to preserve a functional heel and avoid major amputation.

Limb-threatening Wagner III and IV diabetic foot disease is best addressed as part of a comprehensive wound care plan, including planning for revascularization, surgical strategy, infectious disease consultation, orthotics, and comprehensive diabetic management. The interdisciplinary treatment paradigm lends itself to comprehensive management at a wound center.

Hyperbaric Oxygen and Limb at Risk

Many wound centers have hyperbaric oxygen. Goldman[53] has addressed the question of whether HBOT improves odds of limb preservation in the setting of Wagner III or IV DFUs. He conducted a metaanalysis of articles from 1978 to 2008. There were seven articles identified with high or moderate level of evidence. For patients with DFUs complicated by surgical infection, HBOT reduced chance of amputation (odds ratio = 0.242, 95% confidence interval = 0.137 to 0.428). Typically for these studies, the major amputation rate was approximately 10% versus 30% for the HBOT and non-HBOT cohorts, respectively. An earlier Cochrane database review yielded similar results.[131]

The most rigorous study included in this metaanalysis was the unblinded RCT by Faglia et al.[35] For HBOT/

non-HBOT groups, respectively, ABI was 0.64/0.65, foot transcutaneous oxygen measurement of 23/21, and there were 13/13 revascularization procedures, respectively. The amputation surgeon was blinded to HBOT treatment. In HBOT/non-HBOT cohorts there were 3/11 major amputations, which occurred with 4.5 months of presentation. The greatest difference for Wagner IV (gangrene) was 2 out of 22 major amputations in the HBOT group, and 11 out of 20 in the non-HBOT group. Therefore HBOT appears especially useful in limb preservation where there is gangrene, where "tissue at risk" is accompanied by severe peripheral arterial disease. HBOT can also improve primary healing of Wagner III and IV lesions. A double-blind RCT performed on HBOT or sham HBOT for treatment of Wagner III and IV DFUs demonstrated this improvement.[84] Patients had stable nonreconstructable peripheral arterial disease with maximum blood flow and were not candidates for revascularization at the time of entry into the study. Many had previous amputation. Average toe pressure was 50 mm Hg. After enrollment, there was no significant difference in amputation rate. By intent to treat analysis, 1 year after enrollment, there were 52% (25/49) healed in the HBOT group and 29% (12/42) in the control group ($P < 0.05$). For individuals that fully participated in the HBOT/sham HBOT treatment, more ulcers healed in both groups 9 and 12 months after enrollment: 58%/19% ($P < 0.01$) and 61% versus 27% ($P < 0.01$), respectively.

HBOT and limb preservation is not without controversy: a retrospective effectiveness study of 6259 patients treated by a wound management organization (National Healing Corporation) found that HBOT is less effective in healing Wagner II to IV DFUs than standard care.[89]

However, this study by Margolis et al.[89] has raised multiple concerns: (1) for this large retrospective cohort study, DFUs with any arterial component were excluded. However, 65% of complex DFUs and those most likely to lead to amputation are arterial;[8] (2) Included were Wagner II lesions, which is not standard practice; (3) The observation period was limited to 20 weeks after hyperbarics, whereas HBOT benefits occur at least 1 year after hyperbarics;[84] and (4) the end point was primary healing. Minor amputation, although often limb preserving, was considered a treatment failure. (Note the case study in Figure 24-12 would have been a treatment failure.) The controversy surrounding this article underscores the importance of mutually acceptable inclusion, exclusion, and effectiveness criteria for HBOT DFU clinical trials.

Quality in Wound Care

Background

The Institute of Medicine has defined quality as "the degree to which health services for individuals and populations increase the likelihood of desired health outcomes and are consistent with current professional knowledge."[83] To accomplish this, six aims for improvement were defined: safety, effectiveness, patient-centeredness, timeliness, efficiency, and equity.[26]

In 2001, The Joint Commission announced that the four initial core measures for acute care hospitals were acute myocardial infarction, heart failure, pneumonia, and pregnancy and related conditions. These measures were formally adopted by Congress in 2003 for a reimbursement incentive for voluntary reporting among hospitals "The Quality Initiative" by the U.S. Department of Health and Human Services involved a consensus-derived set of hospital quality measures from the National Quality Forum (NQF) that were appropriate for public reporting and a standardized Hospital Patient Perspectives on Care Survey (HCAHPS) by the Agency for Healthcare Research and Quality (AHRQ). The NQF is a nonprofit public service organization created in 1999 that reviews, endorses, and recommends use of standardized health care performance or quality measures. The AHRQ was originally created as the Agency for Health Care Policy and Research (AHCPR) and later was changed to AHRQ in 1999 under the Healthcare Research and Quality Act of 1999.

In November of 2004, the CMS introduced a guideline for the prevention and treatment of pressure ulcers in long-term care facilities. The regulation published in the Federal Register is called "F-tag 314." State surveyors use F-tag 314 as a guide in assessing the quality of pressure ulcer prevention and treatment in nursing homes. Based on the comprehensive assessment of a resident, the facility must ensure that (1) a resident who enters the facility without pressure sores does not develop pressure ulcers unless the individual's clinical condition demonstrates that they were unavoidable; and (2) a resident having pressure ulcers receives necessary treatment and services to promote healing, prevent infection, and prevent new sores from developing.[132] This guideline splits pressure ulcers off from other chronic wounds such as diabetic neuropathic ulcers, venous insufficiency ulcers, and arterial ulcers. The remaining chronic wounds are grouped under F-tag 309, Quality of Care, thus it is important for clinicians to accurately diagnose and distinguish ulcers caused by pressure from other etiologies.

By October of 2007, hospitals were required to submit data on their claims for payment indicating whether diagnoses were present on admission (POA). Ten hospital-acquired conditions (HACs) were identified that would no longer be assigned a higher paying diagnosis-related group if acquired during hospitalization (October 2008). The specific diagnosis of concern for the practice of wound care is the failure to document, prevent, and treat a pressure ulcer and/or hospital-acquired stage III and stage IV pressure ulcers. For a complete list of these conditions, see Hospital-Acquired Conditions in Acute Inpatient Prospective Payment System Hospitals Fact Sheet.[69]

POA status for pressure ulcers is determined by physician documentation. For example, if the admission evaluation by the physician noted "sacral pressure ulcer" and a few days later the wound team documented a stage IV sacral wound, then the stage IV sacral wound would be considered POA and not a HAC. Ideally the documentation would read "necrotic sacral pressure ulcer unable to stage or full thickness sacral pressure ulcer," but simply documenting sacral pressure ulcer allows reviewers to trace the initial presentation. Documenting "no rash" on the admission evaluation does not adequately document POA and could cause the health care system to lose reimbursement for the care of that wound.

In October 2012, the quality measure of "no new or worsened pressure ulcers" described in the F-tag 314 in long-term care facilities was extended to inpatient rehabilitation facilities and long-term care hospitals as measure NQF#0678.

Quality Measures

Ideally there would be one set of nationally accepted and implemented measures that harmonize across all the health care settings of short-term acute care, long-term acute care, long-term care, inpatient rehabilitation, home health, hospice, and outpatient care. Unfortunately, it is not that unified. A quality measure is exactly that. It is a measure of something whether it is a process, a rate of prevalence or incidence, or an outcome. Measures can be bundled into composite measures, which combine multiple separate measures. For instance, a measure requiring performance of a risk assessment can be combined with measures for plan of care and implementation. A measure is first created by an organization or society, tested with data collection, validated, and then sent for endorsement. Not all measures are endorsed by the NQF, but many of the measures accepted by the CMS have received endorsement.

The AHRQ developed Patient Safety Indicators (PSIs) that illustrate the quality of care inside acute care hospitals. They include patient mortality for selected medical conditions and procedures, as well as measures of procedure volume and appropriate use. They are both process and outcome measures that allow hospitals to be compared to peer facilities and for consumers to be aware of the level of quality at a particular hospital. For example, PSI #3 Pressure Ulcer looks at the number of stage III and stage IV pressure ulcers acquired during hospitalization (HAC) per 1000 discharges among patients ages 18 years and older. PSI #3 is one component of the AHRQ Composite Measure PSI#90. In 2009, the CMS adopted eight PSIs developed for the Reporting of Hospital Quality Data for Annual Payment Update Program. PSI #90 was included in the adopted PSIs and thus hospital systems are required to report all patients with hospital-acquired stage III and stage IV pressure ulcers to the CMS.[3] Additionally, the NQF also has several endorsed measures that involve pressure ulcers. These are listed in Table 24-5.

Not all measures are applicable to each health care setting but there is a movement toward harmonizing the measures between health care settings.

In addition to these quality organizational acronyms, HAC, PSI, AHRQ, and NQF, there is another organization called the National Data Base of Nursing Quality Indicators (NDNQI). The membership is formed by acute care inpatient hospitals and it is a national database of the American Nurses Association. It provides hospitals with nursing unit-level comparison data on several nursing sensitive measures, including pressure ulcer prevalence of all stages (stages I to IV, unable to stage). This measure is based on overall documentation and not just physician documentation.

In 2006, the CMS created the Physician Quality Reporting Initiative (PQRI), also known as "pay for performance." The reporting has been voluntary. It was developed as a

Table 24-5 National Quality Forum-Endorsed Measures for Pressure Ulcers

NQF No.	Title	Description	Source
0678	Percentage of residents or patients with pressure ulcers that are new or worsened (short stay)	Percentage of short-stay (LOS <100 days) nursing home residents, or LTCH or IRF patients, with one or more pressure ulcers stage II to IV that are new or worsened since the previous MDS, LTCH CARE data set, or IRF-PAI assessment	MDS 3.0, LTCH CARE data set, IRF-PAI
0201	Pressure ulcer prevalence (hospital acquired)	Number of patients who have hospital-acquired stage II or greater pressure ulcers on the day of the prevalence measurement	
0679	Percentage of high-risk residents with pressure ulcers (long stay)	Percentage of residents who were identified as high risk living in a nursing facility for 100 days or longer who have one or more stage II to IV pressure ulcer(s). High-risk populations are those who are comatose, or impaired in bed mobility or transfer, or suffering from malnutrition	MDS 3.0
0181	Increase in number of pressure ulcers (home health care)	Percentage of patients who had an increase in the number of pressure ulcers at the end of care	
0538-0540	Pressure ulcer prevention and care	Pressure ulcer risk assessment conducted: percentage of home health episodes of care in which the patient was assessed for risk of developing pressure ulcers at the start and resumption of care (#540) Pressure ulcer prevention included in plan of care: percentage of home health episodes of care in which the physician-ordered plan of care included interventions to prevent pressure ulcers (#0538) Pressure ulcer prevention implemented during short-term episodes of care: percentage of short-term home health interventions of care during which interventions to prevent pressure ulcers were included in the physician-ordered plan of care and implemented (#0539)	OASIS-C
0337	Pressure ulcer rate (PD12) (AHRQ)	Percentage of discharges among cases meeting the inclusion and exclusion rules for the denominator with ICD-9-CM code of pressure ulcer in any secondary diagnosis field and ICD-9-CM code of pressure ulcer stage III or IV (or unstageable) in any secondary diagnosis field	

AHRQ, Agency for Healthcare Research and Quality; *CARE*, Continuity Assessment Record and Evaluation; *ICD-9-CM*, International Classification of Disease, Ninth Revision, Clinical Modification; *IRF*, inpatient rehabilitation facilities; *LOS*, length of stay; *LTCH*, long-term care hospital; *MDS*, minimum data set; *OASIS-C*, Outcome and Assessment Information Set-C; *NQF*, National Quality Forum; *PAI*, patient assessment instrument.

way of having medical practices report more detail on patient progress and outcomes. In 2008, the Medicare Improvements for Patients and Providers Act authorized a 2% bonus for those who successfully reported quality measures and an additional 2% bonus for electronic prescribing. The final program year for participating and reporting in the Medicare Electronic Prescribing (eRx) Incentive Program was 2013.

PQRI is transitioning to PQRS, the Physician Quality Reporting System. PQRS is a reporting program that uses a combination of incentive payments and payment adjustments to promote quality reporting by individual clinicians. It is limited in wound care specific measures, but clinicians can combine these with other measures such as tobacco cessation counseling, nutrition counseling, screening for falls, diabetic control, etc. Medical societies such as the American Society of Plastic Surgeons and the National Committee for Quality Assurance and Improvement have also been active in setting quality measures within the domain of their specialty interest.

Physicians are key participants in caring for patients with wounds. With the growing number of quality measures and incentive programs focused on documentation and implementation of care,[22,23] physicians need to be aware of their important role. The climate has evolved from understanding the terms *avoidable* and *unavoidable* to realizing the importance of physicians actively evaluating the skin on initial assessments to document POA and accurately describing the level of injury as partial (stage I, stage II) or full thickness (stage III, stage IV, unable to stage, suspected DTI). PQRS is driving best practice in proper evaluation of patients with wounds as well as the most appropriate treatment strategy based on evidence. The goal is still to provide the right care for every individual every time.

Summary

Prevention and early aggressive intervention are the cornerstones of chronic wound management. The "medical" wound care outlined in this chapter can be used by physiatrists to heal difficult wounds in the outpatient setting while minimizing complications to proactively save limbs. Chronic wound care offers new practice opportunities and competency attainment for physiatrists in the twenty-first century.

ACKNOWLEDGMENTS: We thank the following: Barbara Brewley, RN-C, CRC, Joachim Dissemond, M.D., and Peter Plassmann for photographs; Vista Medical Ltd. (Winnipeg, Manitoba, Canada) and Chattanooga Group (Hixson, Tenn.) for equipment; and the National Institutes of Health [NIH 1R41HL61983-01, NIH K08HD01065-01, and NIH 5T32HD007425-15] and University of Pennsylvania Research Foundation for grant funding.

KEY REFERENCES

2. Ahn C, Salcido RS: Advances in wound photography and assessment methods, *Adv Skin Wound Care* 21:85–93, quiz 94–95, 2008.
4. Akita S, Yoshimoto H, Akino K, et al: Early experiences with stem cells in treating chronic wounds, *Clin Plast Surg* 39:281–292, 2012.
8. Armstrong DG, Cohen K, Courric S, et al: Diabetic foot ulcers and vascular insufficiency: our population has changed, but our methods have not, *J Diabetes Sci Technol* 5:1591–1595, 2011.
9. Aronow WS: Management of peripheral arterial disease of the lower extremities in elderly patients, *J Gerontol A Biol Sci Med Sci* 59:172–177, 2004.
10. Atri SC, Misra J, Bisht D, Misra K: Use of homologous platelet factors in achieving total healing of recalcitrant skin ulcers, *Surgery* 108:508–512, 1990.
15. Bergstrom N, Horn SD, Rapp MP, et al: Turning for ulcer reduction: a multisite randomized clinical trial in nursing homes, *J Am Geriatr Soc* 61:1705–1713, 2013.
16. Berlowitz D: Incidence and prevalence of pressure ulcers. In Thomas DR, Compton G, editors: *Pressure ulcers in the aging population: a guide for clinicians*, New York, 2014, Humana Press, pp 19–26.
17. Bouten CV, Oomens CW, Baaijens FP, et al: The etiology of pressure ulcers: skin deep or muscle bound? *Arch Phys Med Rehabil* 84:616–619, 2003.
22. Carter MJ, Fylling CP, Parnell LK: Use of platelet rich plasma gel on wound healing: a systematic review and meta-analysis, *Eplasty* 11:e38, 2011.
23. Carter MJ, Warriner RA: Evidence-based medicine in wound care: time for a new paradigm, *Adv Skin Wound Care* 22:12–16, 2009.
24. Collins N: The difference between albumin and prealbumin, *Adv Skin Wound Care* 14:235–236, 2001.
29. de Leon JM, Driver VR, Fylling CP, et al: The clinical relevance of treating chronic wounds with an enhanced near-physiological concentration of platelet-rich plasma gel, *Adv Skin Wound Care* 24:357–368, 2011.
33. Driver VR, Hanft J, Fylling CP, Beriou JM: Autologel Diabetic Foot Ulcer Study Group. A prospective, randomized, controlled trial of autologous platelet-rich plasma gel for the treatment of diabetic foot ulcers, *Ostomy Wound Manage* 52:68–70, 72, 74, 2006.
34. Edmonds M: Classification and staging of diabetic foot. In Pendsey SK, editor: *Contemporary management of the diabetic foot*, New Delhi, 2014, Jaypee Medical, pp 55–62.
38. Fife CE, Buyukcakir C, Otto GH, et al: The predictive value of transcutaneous oxygen tension measurement in diabetic lower extremity ulcers treated with hyperbaric oxygen therapy: a retrospective analysis of 1,144 patients, *Wound Repair Regen* 10:198–207, 2002.
39. Fife CE, Buyukcakir C, Otto G, et al: Factors influencing the outcome of lower-extremity diabetic ulcers treated with hyperbaric oxygen therapy, *Wound Repair Regen* 15:322–331, 2007.
40. Fife CE, Wall V, Carter MJ, et al: Revenue in US hospital based outpatient wound centers: implications for creating accountable care organizations, *J Hospital Admin* 2:38, 2013.
42. Frykberg RG, Driver VR, Carman D, et al: Chronic wounds treated with a physiologically relevant concentration of platelet-rich plasma gel: a prospective case series, *Ostomy Wound Manage* 56:36–44, 2010.
43. Frykberg RG, Zgonis T, Armstrong DG, et al: Diabetic foot disorders. A clinical practice guideline (2006 revision), *J Foot Ankle Surg* 45(Suppl 5):S1–S66, 2006.
45. Garber S, Biddle A, Click C, et al: *Pressure ulcer prevention and treatment following spinal cord injury: a clinical practice guideline for health care professionals*, Washington, DC, 2000, Paralyzed Veterans of America.
47. Gefen A: Bioengineering models of deep tissue injury, *Adv Skin Wound Care* 21:30–36, 2008.
49. Gillum RF: Peripheral arterial occlusive disease of the extremities in the United States: hospitalization and mortality, *Am Heart J* 120:1414–1418, 1990.
50. Gloviczki P, Comerota AJ, Dalsing MC, et al: The care of patients with varicose veins and associated chronic venous diseases: clinical practice guidelines of the Society for Vascular Surgery and the American Venous Forum, *J Vasc Surg* 53:2S–48S, 2011.
52. Goldman R: Update on growth factors and wound healing: past, present and future, *Adv Skin Wound Care* 17:24–35, 2004.
53. Goldman RJ: Hyperbaric oxygen therapy for wound healing and limb salvage: a systematic review, *PM&R* 1:471–489, 2009.
56. Goldman R, Brewley B, Zhou L, et al: Electrotherapy reverses inframalleolar ischemia: a retrospective, observational study, *Adv Skin Wound Care* 16:79–89, 2003.
57. Goldman R, Salcido R: More than one-way to measure a wound: an overview of tools and techniques, *Adv Skin Wound Care* 15:236–243, 2002.
60. Gregor S, Maegele M, Sauerland S, et al: Negative pressure wound therapy: a vacuum of evidence? *Arch Surg* 143(2):189–196, 2008.
61. Gottrup F: A specialized wound-healing center concept: importance of a multidisciplinary department structure and surgical treatment

facilities in the treatment of chronic wounds, *Am J Surg* 187(5A):38S–43S, 2004.

73. Kessler L, Bilbault P, Ortega F, et al: Hyperbaric oxygenation accelerates the healing rate of nonischemic chronic diabetic foot ulcers: a prospective randomized study, *Diabetes Care* 26:2378–2382, 2003.
76. Kollar EW, Dearth CL, Badylak SF: Biologic scaffolds composed of extracellular matrix as a natural material for wound healing. In Brennan AB, Kirschner CM, editors: *Bio-inspired materials for biomedical engineering*, Hoboken, 2014, Wiley, pp 111–124.
78. Lahmann NA, Kottner J, Dassen T, Tannen A: Higher pressure ulcer risk on intensive care? Comparison between general wards and intensive care units, *J Clin Nurs* 21:354–361, 2012.
80. Lazarus G, Valle MF, Malas M, et al: Chronic venous leg ulcer treatment: future research needs, *Wound Repair Regen* 22:34–42, 2014.
81. Li Y, Burrows NR, Gregg EW, et al: Declining rates of hospitalization for nontraumatic lower-extremity amputation in the diabetic population aged 40 years or older: U.S., 1988-2008, *Diabetes Care* 35: 273–277, 2012.
84. Londahl M, Katzman P, Nilsson A, Hammarlund C: Hyperbaric oxygen therapy facilitates healing of chronic foot ulcers in patients with diabetes, *Diabetes Care* 33(5):998–1003, 2010.
85. Lyder CH, Wang Y, Metersky M, et al: Hospital-acquired pressure ulcers: results from the National Medicare Patient Safety Monitoring System Study, *J Am Geriatr Soc* 60:1603–1608, 2012.
88. Margolis DJ, Kantor J, Santanna J, et al: Effectiveness of platelet releasate for the treatment of diabetic neuropathic foot ulcers, *Diabetes Care* 24:483–488, 2001.
89. Margolis DJ, Gupta J, Hoffstad O, et al: Lack of effectiveness of hyperbaric oxygen therapy for the treatment of diabetic foot ulcer and the prevention of amputation: a cohort study, *Diabetes Care* 36:1961–1966, 2013.
90. Martinez-Zapata MJ, Martí-Carvajal AJ, Solà I, et al: Autologous platelet-rich plasma for treating chronic wounds, *Cochrane Database Syst Rev* (10):CD006899, 2012.
91. Martins-Mendes D, Monteiro-Soares M, Boyko EJ, et al: The independent contribution of diabetic foot ulcer on lower extremity amputation and mortality risk, *J Diabetes Complications* 28:632–638, 2014.
92. Maxson S, Lopez EA, Yoo D, et al: Concise review: role of mesenchymal stem cells in wound repair, *Stem Cells Transl Med* 1:142–149, 2012.
99. Morton LM, Bolton LL, Corbett LQ, et al: An evaluation of the association for the advancement of wound care venous ulcer guideline and recommendations for further research, *Adv Skin Wound Care* 26:553–561, 2013.
100. Mouës CM, Heule F, Hovius SE: A review of topical negative pressure therapy in wound healing: sufficient evidence? *Am J Surg* 201:544–556, 2011.
101. Moxey PW, Gogalniceanu P, Hinchliffe RJ, et al: Lower extremity amputations – a review of global variability in incidence, *Diabetic Med* 28:1144–1153, 2011.
103. Nowak WN, Borys S, Kusińska K, et al: Number of circulating pro-angiogenic cells, growth factor and anti-oxidative gene profiles might be altered in type 2 diabetes with and without diabetic foot syndrome, *J Diabetes Investig* 5:99, 2014.
107. Peacock JM, Keo HH, Duval S, et al: The incidence and health economic burden of ischemic amputation in Minnesota, 2005-2008, *Prev Chronic Dis* 8:A141, 2011.
111. Pieper B, editor: *Pressure ulcers: prevalence, incidence, and implications for the future*, Washington, DC, 2012, National Pressure Ulcer Advisory Panel.
112. Popescu A, Salcido R: Wound pain: a challenge for the patient and the wound care specialist, *Adv Skin Wound Care* 17:14–20, quiz 21–22, 2004.
116. Rice JB, Desai U, Cummings AK, et al: Burden of venous leg ulcers in the United States, *J Med Econ* 17:347–356, 2014.
117. Salcido R: Myosubcutaneous infarct: deep tissue injury, *Adv Skin Wound Care* 20(5):248–250, 2007.
118. Salcido R, Augustine L, Chulhyun A: Heel pressure ulcers: purple heel and deep tissue injury, *Adv Skin Wound Care* 24:374–380, 2011.
123. Shores JT, Gabriel A, Gupta S: Skin substitutes and alternatives: a review, *Adv Skin Wound Care* 20:493–508, quiz 509–510, 2007.
124. Sibbald RG, Goodman L, Woo KY, et al: Special considerations in wound bed preparation 2011: an update, *Wound Heal South Africa* 4:55–72, 2011.
129. Suding PN, McMaster W, Hansen E, et al: Increased endovascular interventions decrease the rate of lower limb artery bypass operations without an increase in major amputation rate, *Ann Vasc Surg* 22:195–199, 2008.
131. Thom SR: Hyperbaric oxygen: its mechanisms and efficacy, *Plast Reconstr Surg* 127(Suppl 1):131S–141S, 2011.
134. Trent JT, Federman D, Kirsner RS: Skin and wound biopsy: when, why, and how, *Adv Skin Wound Care* 16:372–375, 2003.
145. Ziegler-Graham K, MacKenzie EJ, Ephraim PL, et al: Estimating the prevalence of limb loss in the United States: 2005 to 2050, *Arch Phys Med Rehabil* 89:422–429, 2008.

The full reference list for this chapter is available online.

CHAPTER 25

VASCULAR DISEASES

Karen L. Andrews, Laurie L. Wolf

The rehabilitation professional is often asked to evaluate the patient with a painful, swollen, or ulcerated limb. A thorough understanding of the pathophysiology, available diagnostic testing, and clinical evaluation help the practitioners choose the appropriate vascular diagnosis and treatment program.

Arterial Diseases

Arterial diseases include those acute and chronic disorders that result in partial or complete, functional or anatomic occlusion, or aneurysmal dilatation of the arteries. An example of functional occlusion is abnormal vascular reactivity of the arteries supplying a given tissue, such as vasospasm. Recognition of the broad differential diagnosis of lower extremity arterial disease is important to optimize management.

Peripheral arterial disease (PAD) affects more than 8 million adults in the United States alone.[50] PAD is a disease of aging with an increase in disease prevalence from 10% in individuals age 65 years to more than 30% in octogenarians.[43] Patients with PAD commonly present with symptoms of intermittent claudication or critical limb ischemia. In general, symptoms occur distal to the level of stenosis. If the patient is active, intermittent claudication is the typical presenting complaint. If the patient is inactive, rest pain, ulceration, dependent rubor, or gangrene may be the presenting finding (Figure 25-1).

Patients with intermittent claudication have a significantly higher mortality than age-matched controls, approximately 12% per year.[39] Of these deaths, 66% are caused by heart disease, and 10% are caused by strokes. Only one in four patients with intermittent claudication will develop critical limb ischemia. Longitudinal studies have shown that the amputation rate in this group of patients is only 1% to 7% at 5 to 10 years.[15]

Arteriosclerosis Obliterans

The clinical presentation of acute arterial occlusion is described as "6 Ps," pain, pallor, paresthesias, paralysis, pulselessness, and polar (cold).[68] Some or all of these findings may be present. The limb with acute arterial occlusion is at risk if blood flow is not restored quickly.

Historically, it has been thought that 4 to 6 hours (following the onset of symptoms) is the maximal length of tolerable ischemia. However, patients with previous chronic limb ischemia tend to tolerate longer periods of acute ischemia. The physiologic state of the limb, determined mainly by a balance between metabolic supply and demand, rather than the elapsed time from the onset of occlusion, is actually the best predictor of limb salvage.

Intermittent claudication indicates an inadequate supply of arterial blood to contracting muscles. It occurs primarily in chronic arterial occlusive disease or severe arteriospastic disease. Intermittent claudication is brought on by walking and is relieved promptly by rest without change of position of the affected limb. Patients describe claudication as leg numbness, weakness, buckling, aching, cramping, or pain. It may change in character as the underlying lesions progress. Claudication occurs at a predictable distance or time. When the workload is increased (rapid pace, walking up hills, or walking over rough terrain), the time to claudication decreases.[68] Claudication may worsen over a period of inactivity (when the patient is hospitalized) but usually returns to baseline with reconditioning.[68] When claudication abruptly increases, one must consider thrombosis in situ or an embolic event. Claudication at the arch of the foot suggests occlusion at or above the ankle; claudication at the calf suggests occlusion at or above this region. Claudication is less frequent above the knee (probably because of the rich collateral circulation in the thigh); however, occlusion of the iliac arteries or aorta may cause thigh, lumbar region, and buttock claudication.

Although many other disorders can cause symptoms of lower extremity arterial insufficiency (thromboangiitis obliterans, arterial thromboemboli), these conditions account for only a small percentage of lower extremity arterial disease.

Vasculitic Syndrome

Vasculitis or angiitis is an inflammatory disease of blood vessels. It often causes damage to the vessel wall, stenosis, or occlusion of the vessel lumen by thrombosis, and progressive intimal proliferation. Vasculitic symptoms reflect systemic inflammation and the ischemic consequences of vascular occlusion. The distribution of the vascular lesions and the size of the blood vessels involved vary considerably in different vasculitic syndromes and in different patients with the same syndrome. Vasculitis can be transient, chronic, self-limited, or progressive. It can be the primary abnormality or secondary to another systemic process. Histopathologic classification does not distinguish local from systemic illness or secondary from primary insult.

Rheumatoid Vasculitis

Rheumatoid vasculitis manifests almost exclusively in patients with rheumatoid autoantibodies and often occurs in the context of other extraarticular manifestations.[66] The vasculitis is mediated by the deposition of circulating

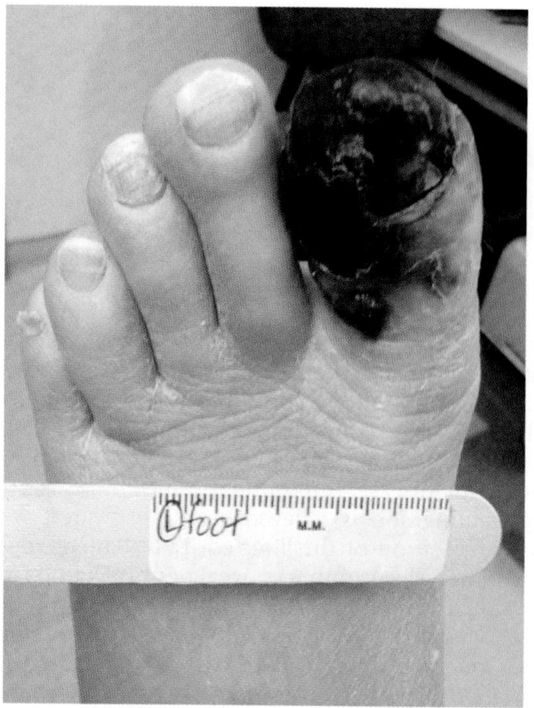

FIGURE 25-1 Left great toe gangrene in a 76-year-old man with diabetes, peripheral arterial disease, and previous right partial foot amputation.

immune complexes on the blood vessel wall with activation of complement. Proliferation of the vascular intima and media causes an obliterative enteropathy. Leukocytoclastic or small vessel vasculitis produces palpable purpura or cutaneous ulceration. The presence of HLA-C3 (human leukocyte antigen-C3) and smoking are independent predictors of vasculitis in patients with rheumatoid arthritis. Smoking, rheumatoid factor, and antinuclear antibodies are all associated with severe extraarticular disease manifestations.[66]

Cryoglobulinemia

Cryoglobulins are immunoglobulins that reversibly precipitate at reduced temperatures. Type I consists of monoclonal immunoglobulin, generally IgM or IgG. Type II cryoglobulins are a mixture of monoclonal IgM and polyclonal IgG. Type III cryoglobulins are a mixture of polyclonal IgM and IgG. Cryoglobulinemia is associated with many illnesses, which can be broadly grouped into infections (hepatitis C), autoimmune disorders, and malignancy. More than 90% of cases of cryoglobulinemia have a known underlying cause; treatment is focused on the cause of the disorder rather than merely symptomatic relief.[46]

Polyarteritis

Polyarteritis occurs by itself (polyarteritis nodosa [PAN]) or in association with another disease (secondary polyarteritis). PAN is an acute necrotizing vasculitis that affects primarily medium-sized and small arteries. It is a systemic disorder that may involve the kidneys, joints, skin, nerves, and various other tissues. The prognosis of PAN is heavily dependent on the severity and organ distribution at the time of diagnosis. PAN has a tendency to involve medium-sized muscular arteries. It spares the aorta and its major branches as well as capillaries and small arterioles that lack muscular coats. PAN also spares the venous system. Vasculitis of medium-sized arteries usually produces one of the following: livedo reticularis, nodules, ulcerations, and digital ischemia.[62] For cases of idiopathic PAN, corticosteroids and cytotoxic agents remain the cornerstone of treatment.[22]

Other Vasculitides

A wide variety of other vasculitides may affect small and medium-sized vessels. These include allergic angiitis (Churg-Strauss syndrome), Henoch-Schönlein purpura, various forms of hypersensitivity vasculitis, and numerous nonspecific necrotizing and nonnecrotizing vasculitides.

Thromboangiitis Obliterans (Buerger Disease)

Thromboangiitis obliterans (TAO) or Buerger disease is a nonatherosclerotic segmental vasculitis that affects small and medium-sized arteries and veins of the extremities and is strongly associated with tobacco exposure. The immunopathogenesis of TAO remains largely unknown.[29] The first manifestation of Buerger's disease may be superficial phlebitis. TAO occurs predominantly in young adult male smokers. Few, if any, cases occur in the absence of tobacco use. If smoking is discontinued, the process is frequently arrested.

Raynaud Syndrome

Raynaud syndrome is characterized by episodic attacks of vasospasm in response to cold or emotional stress. The fingers and hands are most often affected. In certain patients, the toes and feet may be involved. Classic episodes of vasospasm cause an intense pallor of the distal extremity followed in sequence by cyanosis and rubor on rewarming. Most patients do not experience the complete triple color response. Typically, only pallor or cyanosis is noted during attacks. Generally, the attacks are over within 30 to 60 minutes and these episodes are usually bilateral. Attacks may occur infrequently, for example, some may only have symptoms during the winter, whereas other patients may have a significant impairment/disability with multiple daily episodes. Digital ulcerations are rare but may occur. Females are affected more commonly than males.

Raynaud disease refers to a primary vasospastic disorder where there is no identifiable underlying cause. Raynaud phenomenon refers to vasospasm, secondary to another underlying condition or disease. Predisposing factors include atherosclerosis, arteritis, cancer, collagen vascular disease, thoracic outlet syndrome, embolic occlusion, occupational disease, and certain medications.[59] Secondary Raynaud phenomenon is occasionally unilateral and may produce skin breakdown.

Vibration Syndrome

Vibratory tools, such as chainsaws, grinders, and jack hammers, can induce hand dysesthesias and Raynaud phenomenon when used for several years. Symptoms initially occur during use of the instrument. Subsequently, dysesthesias and cold sensitivity persist when the vibratory tool is not being used. During exposure to vibration, there is a reduction in finger blood flow in both vibrated and nonvibrated fingers. The acute vascular responses during and after exposure to vibration may not be separate independent effects of vibration frequency, magnitude, and duration; there may be complex interactions between the effects of these variables.[7]

Hypothenar Hammer Syndrome

Occlusive disease in the hands can result from trauma to the hypothenar area caused by using the palm of the hand as a hammer in an activity that involves pushing, pounding, or twisting. This results in intimal injury to the ulnar artery as it crosses the hamate bone. Such injuries of the ulnar artery may lead to severe vascular insufficiency in the hand with thrombosis and distal embolization of the digital arteries.[69]

External Iliac Syndrome in Cyclists

Exercise-induced external iliac artery endofibrosis is rare and has been described primarily in endurance male cyclists. Clinically, it presents as claudication during maximal exercise with quick resolution after exercise. Most patients have fibrotic changes within the external iliac artery. Vasospasm may be more important than wall thickening for the reduction of blood flow during extreme exercise in affected athletes.[57]

Arterial Evaluation

Vascular diagnostic testing is typically performed to confirm a clinical diagnosis and document the severity of disease.

Noninvasive Arterial Studies

Vascular diagnostic laboratories can use segmental pressures, Doppler waveform analysis, pulse volume recordings, or Ankle-Brachial Index (ABI) with duplex ultrasonography (or some combination of these methods) to document the presence and location of PAD.[51]

Ankle-Brachial Index

The ABI provides objective data about arterial perfusion of the lower limbs. Pressures are obtained with a blood pressure cuff placed around the patient's lower calves or ankles. A handheld Doppler detects systolic blood pressure in the dorsalis pedis and the posterior tibial arteries. The brachial (arm) pressure is also obtained. In a healthy individual, because of peripheral amplification of the pulse pressure, the ankle pressure should be higher than the brachial arterial systolic pressure. A normal ankle to arm systolic blood pressure ratio is 1.0 to 1.4. Values greater than 1.4 indicate noncompressible arteries. ABI values of 0.91 to 0.99 are considered "borderline". ABI values are considered mildly diminished when they are less than or equal to 0.90 and more than or equal to 0.80, moderately diminished between 0.50 and 0.80, and severely decreased when less than 0.50.[51] An ABI identifies individuals who are at risk for developing rest pain, ischemic ulcerations, or gangrene, and it is a marker of generalized atherosclerosis. The risk of death, usually from a cardiovascular event, increases dramatically as the ABI decreases. The 5-year mortality rate in patients with an ABI less than 0.85 is 10%. When the ABI is less than 0.40, the 5-year mortality rate approaches 50%.[36]

The ABI is known to be unreliable in patients with vascular stiffness and fails to detect the early phase of atherosclerotic development. The toe vessels are less susceptible to vessel stiffness, which makes the toe-brachial index (TBI) useful.[26] The incidence of noncompressible (artifactually high), calcified conduit arteries is highest in patients with diabetes, patients with chronic renal failure, and elderly patients. Despite high recorded systolic pressure, these patients may have severe disease. The TBI should be used to establish the lower extremity PAD diagnosis in patients in whom lower extremity PAD is clinically suspected but in whom the ABI test is not reliable as a result of noncompressible vessels (usually patients with longstanding diabetes or advanced age).[9] Other diagnostic tests (arterial duplex studies, segmental pressure measurement, Doppler waveform analysis, pulse volume recording, transcutaneous oximetry [$TcPO_2$], or photoplethysmography) may also be performed to rule out significant arterial occlusive disease.

Segmental Pressure Measurements

Segmental pressure is the arterial closing and opening pressure at a specific anatomic location.[68] Systolic blood pressure obtained in this manner can be indexed relative to the brachial artery pressure in a manner analogous to the ABI. Segmental pressure analysis is often used to determine the location of arterial stenosis. Arterial pressure can be measured with blood pressure cuffs placed at various levels (upper thigh, lower thigh, upper calf, and lower calf above the ankle) sequentially along the limb. The presence of a significant systolic pressure gradient (greater than 10 to 15 mm Hg) between the brachial artery pressure and the upper thigh systolic pressure usually signifies the presence of aortoiliac obstruction. A pressure gradient located between the upper and lower thigh cuffs signifies obstruction in the superficial femoral artery. A gradient between the lower thigh and upper calf cuffs indicates distal superficial femoral or popliteal artery obstruction. A gradient between the upper and lower calf cuffs identifies infrapopliteal disease. Gradients of 10 to 15 mm Hg between adjacent sites may represent physiologically important obstruction.[68]

Continuous Wave Doppler (See Videos 25-1 to 25-3)

A normal continuous wave Doppler is triphasic, with a rapid upstroke or forward flow, a downstroke to below baseline as flow reverses, and finally a short period of forward flow is seen again. When stenosis is present, and as it increases, the reversal of flow is lost and the upstroke may be delayed. With greater stenosis, the upstroke becomes smaller, further delayed, sinusoidal, and eventually absent. A change from triphasic to monophasic waveforms provides reasonable, accurate information about the location and extent of specific lower extremity lesions. Doppler waveform analyses are reliable even in highly

Table 25-1 Doppler Signals of the Patient in Figure 25-1 Showing Right Multilevel Popliteal and Infrapopliteal and Left Infrapopliteal Arterial Occlusive Disease

	Right	Left
Common femoral	Biphasic	Biphasic
Superficial femoral	Biphasic	Biphasic
Popliteal	Reduced biphasic	Biphasic
Posterior tibial	Monophasic	Monophasic
Dorsalis pedis	Monophasic	Monophasic

Table 25-2 Transcutaneous Oximetry ($TcPO_2$) Values of the Patient in Figure 25-1 Showing Severely Reduced Perfusion by $TcPO_2$ Criteria at the Left Foot

Electrode Site	Supine	Elevated	Dependent
Chest (reference)	58	66	65
R foot	58	58	64
L above knee	60	59	64
L below knee	38	35	44
L foot proximal	2	1	7
L foot distal	3	1	3

L, Left; *R*, right.

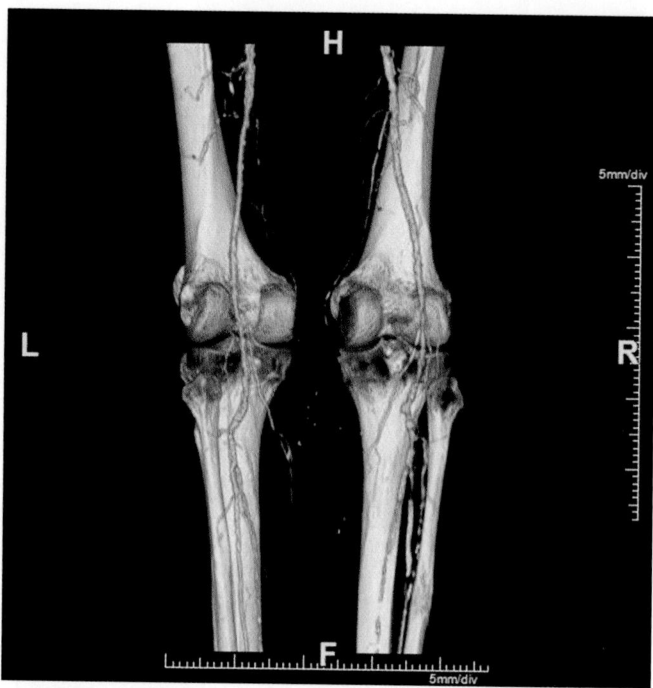

FIGURE 25-2 Computed tomography angiography of the patient in Figure 25-1 showing heavily calcified atheromatous disease, including occlusion of the bilateral anterior tibial and posterior tibial arteries. Dominant runoff via diseased peroneal arteries with probable occlusion of the proximal right peroneal artery.

calcified vessels that are not amenable to pressure determinations (Table 25-1).

Transcutaneous Oximetry

$TcPO_2$ determinations provide a very sensitive means to assess skin perfusion and the potential for cutaneous healing at a specific site.[1] $TcPO_2$ values less than 20 to 30 mm Hg suggest inadequate perfusion for healing.[1] A decrease in the $TcPO_2$ value of 10 mm Hg with leg elevation also suggests tenuous perfusion[1] (Table 25-2).

Photoplethysmography

Photoplethysmography is a noninvasive optical technique used to measure changes in the cutaneous microcirculation by detecting the reflection of infrared light. The amount of blood under the source beam affects the absorption of light.

Duplex Scanning

Duplex scanning with B-mode imaging combined with directional Doppler can visualize and assess arterial aneurysms and detect flow velocity changes at sites of localized stenosis or occlusion. Duplex scanning is particularly helpful in assessing proximal iliofemoral stenosis that may be amenable to angioplasty, providing follow-up data to assess continued patency of both venous and prosthetic arterial grafts, and evaluating the patency of previous angioplasty sites or intravascular stents.

Imaging Techniques

Advances in technology are enabling computed tomography angiography (CTA) and magnetic resonance angiography (MRA) to replace conventional angiography as a means of identifying arterial stenoses and occlusions.

Computed Tomography Angiography

CTA has become a standard noninvasive imaging modality for vascular anatomy and pathology (Figure 25-2). With continued improvement in spatial resolution, CTA is now a mainstay for preoperative imaging of abdominal aortic aneurysms. It provides accurate information not only of the size of an aneurysm but also the exact location and critical measurements needed for repair.

Magnetic Resonance Angiography

MRA can be used to determine the morphology of blood vessels, assess blood flow velocity, evaluate the lumen for the presence of thrombosis, and evaluate for the presence of hemorrhage, infection, or the status of the end organ. Unlike ultrasound, MRA is not compromised by overlying bone, bowel gas, or calcification. MRA is relatively expensive and its use is limited in situations in which metallic instrumentation may be required. MRA is the optimum imaging alternative in patients who are pregnant and patients with severe iodinated contrast allergy. Reports that gadolinium may play a role in inducing nephrogenic systemic fibrosis (NSF) are a concern. Although rare, NSF, can be catastrophic. Caution is recommended in patients with reduced glomerular filtration rate (GFR) (definitely a GFR less than 30, possibly less than 60).[16]

Contrast Arteriography

Contrast angiography has been the traditional "gold standard" for lower extremity arterial evaluation.[68]

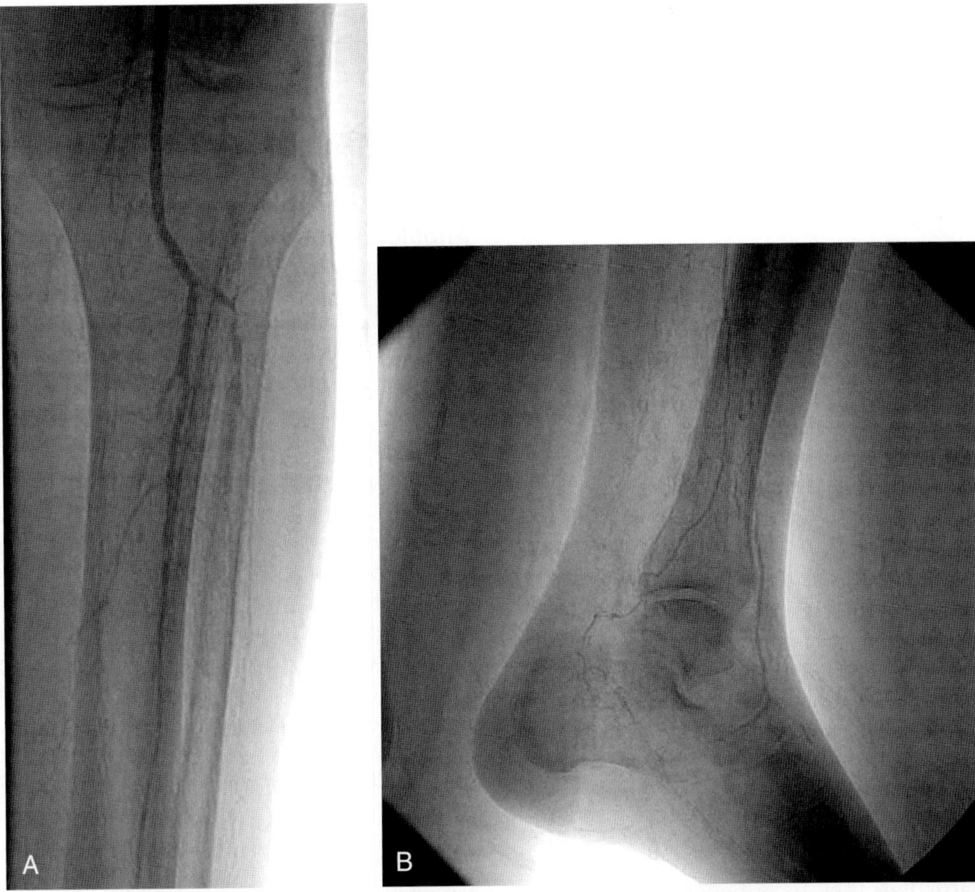

FIGURE 25-3 **A** and **B,** Angiogram of the patient in Figure 25-1.

Angiography remains the definitive approach for perioperative evaluation in patients requiring revascularization. Preprocedure arteriography is an essential part of endovascular procedures (Figure 25-3).

Management

The goals of management in patients with PAD should be to reduce cardiovascular risk and alleviate symptoms. Medical therapies can effectively modify both the natural history of atherosclerotic lower extremity arterial occlusive disease and significantly reduce the morbidity of this disorder.

On average, an age-matched control group has an all-cause mortality rate of 1.6% per year. This rate increases to 4.8% per year for patients with PAD. Cardiovascular mortality rates are similarly affected with an overall event rate of 0.5% per year in controls and 2.5% per year in patients with PAD. The presence of PAD is an independent risk factor for mortality even when other known risk factors are controlled.[47] Treatment needs to focus on both the effects of atherosclerosis in the peripheral circulation and the systemic nature of the disease. Appropriate therapy should be instituted to decrease the risk for both peripheral progression and cardiovascular mortality. The increased cardiac event rate in patients with PAD underscores the importance of intensive medical management to reduce the risk for cardiovascular morbidity and mortality.

Risk Factor Management

A transition in the pattern of atherosclerotic risk factors in the United States and worldwide is being witnessed.[20] Certain traditional atherosclerotic risk factors are on the wane (as a result of decreased rates of smoking, antihypertensive medications, statins). The astounding increase in obesity in the U.S. population has led to a significant increase in the prevalence of the components of the clustered risk factors often referred to as the metabolic syndrome. The metabolic syndrome is characterized by a constellation of interrelated pathologic conditions of a metabolic or hemodynamic nature (abdominal obesity, atherosclerosis, impaired glucose control, or hypertension) that appear to directly promote the development of cardiovascular disease.[5]

All patients presenting for treatment of PAD should have their risk factors rigorously assessed. Patients with known PAD should be treated aggressively with a combination of an HMG-CoA (3-hydroxy-3-methylglutaryl-coenzyme A) reductase inhibitor (statin), an angiotensin-converting enzyme (ACE) inhibitor, an antiplatelet agent, and a beta-blocker (if there is a history of coronary disease). Blood pressure and glucose control is imperative and aggressive smoking cessation counseling is recommended for every medical interaction.[55]

Diabetes is a strong independent predictor for stroke, myocardial infarction (MI), and PAD.[40] The need for amputation in patients with diabetes for lower extremity arterial occlusive disease is 10 times that for patients who do not have diabetes. In patients with diabetes, for every 1% increase in hemoglobin A1c, there is a corresponding 26% risk of PAD.[55]

Cigarette smoking has been identified as an independent predictor of vascular disease and the reason why vascular procedures and interventions fail. More than 80% of patients with PAD are current or former smokers.[54]

Patients with PAD consistently have higher levels of homocysteine when compared with controls. The data suggest that hyperhomocysteinemia may either be a marker of PAD or etiologically implicated in the development of PAD.[30] Elevated homocysteine levels can be lowered by folic acid and other vitamin supplementation. Randomized trials that have used vitamin treatments to lower homocysteine levels have not documented improvement in cardiovascular outcomes.[3]

Lipid Management

Effective lipid management should be considered a mandatory component of the medical therapy of patients with objective evidence of atherosclerotic peripheral arterial occlusive disease. Statins have favorable effects on multiple interrelated aspects of vascular biology important in atherosclerosis. In particular, they have beneficial effects on inflammation, plaque stabilization, endothelial function, and thrombosis.

Lipid-lowering therapy is effective in reducing the cardiovascular mortality and morbidity associated with PAD and likely improves the most common symptoms of PAD, intermittent claudication.[42] The goal for hyperlipidemia management is to maintain a low-density lipoprotein level of less than 100 mg/dL in the general population and less than 70 mg/dL in patients with atherosclerotic disease.[51]

Health care providers should increase statin therapy in a graduated manner to adequately determine the patient's response and tolerance. Because statins are cleared hepatically, it is recommended that liver enzymes be tested before initiating the medication, 12 weeks following initiation of therapy, upon any elevation of the medication dose, and every 6 months. Other side effects of HGM-CoA reductase inhibitors include myopathy and rhabdomyolysis with acute renal failure secondary to myoglobinuria. Statins should be prescribed with caution in patients with predisposing factors for myopathy and they should be discontinued if markedly elevated creatine kinase levels or myopathy is diagnosed or suspected.

Angiotensin-Converting Enzyme Inhibitors

The Heart Outcomes Prevention Evaluation (HOPE) study showed that ACE inhibitors reduce cardiovascular events by 25% in patients with symptomatic PAD.[70] In addition, treatment with ACE inhibitors improves walking ability in patients with intermittent claudication. This was not associated with significant improvement in the ABI. Patients with intermittent claudication may benefit from treatment with a high tissue affinity ACE inhibitor for a period of 6 months.[56] The overall treatment effect achieved by ACE inhibitors is more than that of other therapeutic agents for intermittent claudication, such as cilostazol and pentoxifylline, but less than that of a supervised exercise program.[56]

Antiplatelet Therapy

Antiplatelet therapy may decrease the rate of atherosclerotic disease progression, decrease the incidence of thrombotic events in the limbs, and decrease the rate of adverse coronary and cerebrovascular ischemic events. Aspirin in doses of 75 to 325 mg is recommended as safe and effective platelet therapy to reduce the risk of MI, stroke, or vascular death in individuals with atherosclerotic lower extremity PAD.[35]

Antiplatelet therapy is indicated to reduce the risk of MI, stroke, and vascular death in individuals with symptomatic atherosclerotic lower extremity PAD including those with intermittent claudication or critical limb ischemia, previous lower extremity revascularization (endovascular or surgical), previous amputation or lower extremity ischemia.[10,11] Long-term administration of clopidogrel in patients with atherosclerotic vascular disease has been reported to be more efficient than aspirin in reducing the combined risk for ischemic stroke, MI, or vascular death.[10]

Agents for Intermittent Claudication

Cilostazol and pentoxifylline have been shown to modestly improve walking distances in patients with intermittent claudication. Cilostazol has significant antiplatelet, vasodilatory, and vascular antiproliferative properties.[37] It is contraindicated in patients with either systolic or diastolic heart failure. Cilostazol (100 mg orally two times per day) is indicated as an effective therapy to improve symptoms and increase walking distances in patients with lower extremity PAD and intermittent claudication (in the absence of heart failure).[35] Pentoxifylline has diminished estimated efficacy when compared with cilostazol.[37] Minimal efficacy and caffeine-like side effects limit use of this medication.

Rehabilitation

Patients with PAD should be instructed to wear protective footwear at all times (never walk barefoot or in socks) and monitor their extremities carefully for redness or skin breakdown. Extremes of temperature should be avoided. The feet should be washed carefully with mild soap and warm water. Drying is best performed by blotting or patting with a soft clean towel (rubbing should be avoided because it may injure the skin). The skin between the toes should be carefully dried to avoid maceration. Emollients without preservatives or perfume should be used (avoid between the toes) to prevent cracking of the skin. Proper footwear, which does not produce areas of point pressure, should be used. Whenever new shoes are purchased, the patient should gradually (over a period of a week) wear-in shoes to make sure that there are no areas of point pressure with the new footwear. Warm outer footwear should be used in the winter to protect against thermal injury. Decreased activity secondary to symptomatic lower extremity arterial occlusive disease can result in deconditioning, which further contributes to disease impairment. Deconditioning may also be "iatrogenic" as a result of a prolonged period of limited mobility to avoid trauma to ischemic wounds.

Regular lower extremity exercise in the form of a structured or a supervised walking program is critical for patients with PAD. Ambulation can help to develop collateral blood flow and in time may lead to resolution or improvement of intermittent claudication. A minimum of 30 minutes of moderate activity at least three times per week is beneficial.[61] Regular training has been shown to improve oxygen extraction from blood, muscle enzyme activity, and hemorheology.[61] Regular exercise training produces a reduction in the inflammatory markers associated with endothelial damage.[25] Evidence suggests that patients following an exercise regimen improve both their claudication distance and cardiovascular risk profile. Exercise improves maximal walking ability by an average of 150%.[33] Remarkably, increased walking capacity increased further 6 months after supervised exercise training cessation, suggesting an ongoing benefit of the intervention.[52]

In summary, current recommendations are that all patients with PAD should receive antiplatelet therapy, stop smoking, exercise, and be screened and treated for hyperlipidemia, hypertension, diabetes, and hypercoagulability in accordance with national guidelines and community standards.[13]

Gene Therapy

Molecular therapies to induce angiogenesis are appealing in the claudicant population because ischemia is subacute, time is available for angiogenesis to occur, and collateral development is associated with increased walking distance.

Revascularization

Ischemic rest pain and tissue necrosis, including ischemic ulcerations or gangrene, are well-accepted indicators of advanced ischemia and threatened limb loss. Without treatment, most limbs with these symptoms experience disease progression and require major amputation. Previously, surgical revascularization was considered for patients with rest pain, impending tissue loss, or significant limitations of lifestyle who failed medical treatment. Endovascular intervention coupled with aggressive proactive medical management is replacing this conventional paradigm. The multicenter BASIL (Bypass Versus Angioplasty in Severe Ischaemia of the Leg) trial found no significant difference between surgical and endovascular revascularization in amputation-free survival or overall survival. A bypass surgery first approach, was associated with a significant increase in overall survival of 7.3 months and a trend toward improved amputation-free survival of 5.9 months for those patients who survived for at least 2 years after randomization.[8] If early and long-term patency is to be achieved, it is important that the site for vascular reconstruction has a relatively unobstructed inflow and a patent distal runoff.

Attempts at revascularization should be avoided in the presence of life-threatening sepsis, chronic flexion contracture, paralysis, and in patients with markedly reduced life expectancy. Revascularization should be delayed in most individuals with a significant acute comorbidity (recent MI), unless the limb is imminently threatened and high perioperative morbidity is acceptable.[49]

Intermittent Pneumatic Compression

Intermittent pneumatic foot and calf compression has been shown to improve walking distance comparable with supervised exercise.[27] External compression briefly raises the tissue pressure, emptying the underlying veins and transiently reducing the venous pressure without occluding arterial blood flow. The proposed mechanism to explain the increased flow is analogous to the pumping action of the calf muscle during walking. The transient inflation (quick impulse) imitates the effects of normal gait by generating a vigorous hemodynamic impulse throughout the veins each time the lower extremity is compressed. An increase in the hydrostatic pressure gradient is thought to be a major mechanism for the enhancement of arterial leg inflow. In addition, the altered flow and shear forces generated by the inflation of the pneumatic cuff may mediate the release of endothelial and humeral factors having local and systemic effects. A direct reduction in the peripheral resistance is also postulated via release of nitrous oxide secondary to shear stress across the vessel wall.[14]

Venous Disease

Venous disease includes acute or chronic occlusion of the systemic venous or pulmonary arterial system, usually as a result of thromboembolism. Chronic venous disease is a spectrum of diseases and disorders of the limbs with spider veins and varicosities on one end of the spectrum and edema, skin changes (stasis, hyperpigmentation), and ulceration on the other end (Figure 25-4). The cause is

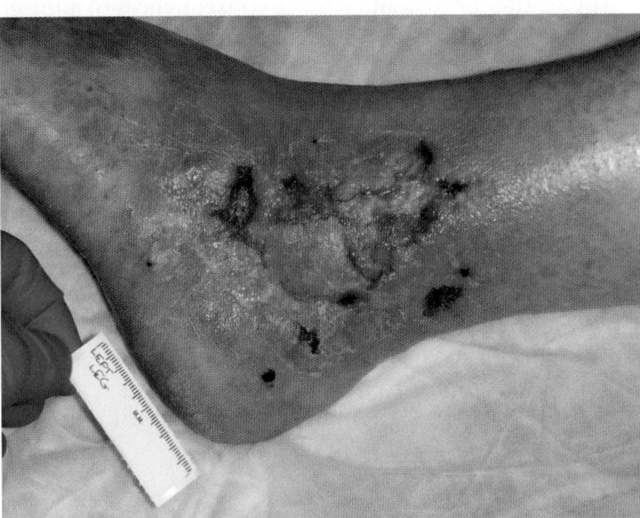

FIGURE 25-4 Photo of recurrent perimalleolar wound in a 67-year-old woman with chronic venous insufficiency with varicose veins and stasis dermatitis.

either primary valvular incompetence or postphlebitic/postthrombotic syndrome secondary to previous deep vein thrombosis (DVT).

Venous Thromboembolism

The disease burden from venous thromboembolism (VTE) is major. Each year there are an estimated 900,000 patients with clinical evidence of VTE in the United States resulting in an estimated 300,000 deaths from pulmonary embolism.[23] When a patient presents with the possibility of a DVT, predisposing risk factors, such as prolonged immobilization during car or plane trips, use of estrogen, previous DVT, or family history of thrombosis, should be elicited. Hypercoagulable states, such as those associated with cancer or inherited coagulopathies and those caused by vessel wall injury from surgery or local trauma, are major predisposing factors for thrombosis. Approximately 30% of surviving cases develop recurrent VTE within 10 years.[23] Independent predictors for recurrence include increasing age, obesity, malignant neoplasm, and extremity paresis.[23] Approximately 28% of patients develop venous stasis syndrome within 20 years.[23] To reduce VTE incidence, improve survival, and prevent recurrence and complications, patients with these characteristics should receive appropriate prophylaxis.[24] Thrombosis may occur anywhere but most commonly involves the deep veins of the leg. Once a thrombosis forms, several events may occur: (1) the thrombosis may propagate; (2) it may embolize; (3) it may be removed by fibrinolytic activity; and (4) it may undergo organization (including recanalization and retraction).

An initial inflammatory response leads to fibroblast and capillary ingrowth, which helps to stabilize the thrombus. Organization occurs over weeks to months as the thrombus becomes incorporated into the vessel wall. Once luminal flow is disturbed, prograde and retrograde propagation of the thrombus may also be promoted by hemodynamic factors. The competing process of recanalization and recurrent thrombus determine the extent of acute DVT and its sequelae. Venous thrombi rarely lyse completely unless they are subjected to pharmacologic lysis.

The natural history and clinical consequences of a lower extremity venous thrombosis depends on the site of thrombus. If the thrombotic process is close to the saphenofemoral junction, vascular surgery consultation is warranted for possible high ligation of the saphenofemoral junction.

Small calf vein thrombi frequently occur, especially in postoperative patients. Of those that are asymptomatic, 50% lyse spontaneously and are unlikely to proceed to deep vein incompetence. A calf thrombosis may remain asymptomatic; the thrombosis often dissolves without sequelae by natural fibrinolysis. However, 5% to 20% of calf vein thrombi propagate proximally. If extension occurs into the popliteal or more proximal veins, the chance of pulmonary embolism increases from less than 5% to approximately 50%.[58] Laboratory surveillance of lesions is required if anticoagulants are not used.

Phlegmasia Cerulea Dolens

Phlegmasia cerulea dolens is a rare complication of DVT, characterized by rapid and massive edema, severe pain, and cyanosis.[58] Distal cyanosis may indicate extensive blockage to venous return. Phlegmasia cerulea dolens most commonly occurs with proximal, iliofemoral obstruction with extensive distal thrombus of deep and superficial veins. In phlegmasia, the arterial pulses may not be palpable, although anatomically the arteries are patent. In severe cases, gangrene, which may necessitate amputation, occurs.[58] Urgent treatment, including placing a caval filter, heparinization, and surgical thrombectomy or thrombolysis if possible, is essential to minimize loss of life or limb. Thrombolytic therapy is often given from both the venous and arterial sides.

May-Thurner Syndrome

May-Thurner syndrome is defined as isolated left lower extremity swelling caused by compression of the left iliac vein by the right common iliac artery. Treatment of May-Thurner syndrome has historically involved anticoagulation therapy. Advances in interventional management have allowed relief of the associated mechanical compression by open surgical or endovascular repair. Endovascular stents are the most common treatment.

Chronic Venous Insufficiency

Chronic venous disease is an important cause of discomfort and disability, and is present in a significant percentage of the population worldwide. A clinical score of Clinical-Etiologic-Anatomic-Pathophysiologic (CEAP) has been developed as a standard for reporting venous disease.[4] Many factors can result in the development of venous insufficiency, including heredity, local trauma, thrombosis, and intrinsic defects in the veins or valves themselves. Venous flow is based on a force that pushes the blood proximally, an adequate outflow, and the presence of competent valves limiting reflux. Any disruption of these components results in chronic venous hypertension. Normally, the pressure in the leg veins is equal to the hydrostatic pressure from a vertical column of blood extending to the right atrium of the heart. At the ankle level, the hydrostatic pressure is approximately 90 mm Hg.[34] The pumping action of the calf muscles during exercise reduces this venous pressure by two thirds. Even slight muscular movements during normal standing will lower the pressure.[34] Patients with venous insufficiency might fail to reduce ankle pressure or show a rapid return of venous pressure to resting levels at the end of the exercise. The time required for the ankle vein pressure to return to resting levels after exercise is an indicator of the degree of reflux in the limb. Elevated ambulatory venous pressure is associated with an increased incidence of ulceration.[41] When ambulatory, venous ankle pressure is below 30 mm Hg, and the incidence of ulceration is close to 0%. The incidence of ulceration increases linearly when ankle pressure is above 30 mm Hg, reaching 100% when the ambulatory venous pressure is greater than 90 mm Hg.[41] The superficial leg veins normally carry 10% to 15% of the venous return. Incompetent valves in the superficial veins alone rarely cause serious venous hypertension, although 10% of patients with venous ulcers have superficial venous incompetence alone.

Primary deep venous reflux is more often observed in patients who are obese and is more persistent following eradication of the superficial reflux than observed for patients who are of normal weight.[67]

A quarter of patients with a first, unprovoked, unilateral, proximal DVT who were free of clinically significant primary venous insufficiency showed postthrombotic syndrome 5 to 7 months after the index event. Obesity, mild contralateral venous ectasia, poor international normalized ratio (INR) control, and the presence of ultrasonographic residual venous obstruction significantly increased the risk of postthrombotic syndrome in this population.[19] Venous insufficiency may present up to 5 to 10 years after resolution of the acute episode of thrombosis. Postphlebitic damage in the deep veins is an important cause of chronic venous insufficiency. Advanced venous insufficiency develops when the valves in the perforator or deep veins are also incompetent. Ultimately, venous hypertension is the result of valve damage and retrograde venous blood flow to the superficial veins.

Venous Evaluation

Continuous Wave Doppler

Continuous wave Doppler (described earlier) is portable, inexpensive, and used clinically as a screening tool to test the integrity of the venous system. This method can identify the presence of venous obstruction or incompetence, quantify the severity of the venous disease, and localize these abnormalities to a particular segment of the limb. The venous flow signal is obtained at several sites in the limb. The patency, spontaneous flow, phasicity, augmentation, competency, and pulsatility of the venous flow are determined and graded. Normal venous flow is spontaneous and phasic with respiration. Obstruction of a vein is characterized by the absence of normal spontaneous venous flow or by the loss of phasic variation with respiration. If the Doppler probe is placed directly over an obstruction, there is absence of spontaneous flow. If the probe is placed below the site of obstruction, there is a loss of phasic change in the venous flow with respiration (a monophasic low-frequency signal). Several maneuvers (deep breathing, Valsalva, and distal compression of the calf or forearm) can produce augmentation of venous flow. Continuous wave Doppler provides subjective information. If positive for obstruction, findings should be followed by an objective test. Because of this and other limitations, continuous wave Doppler ultrasound has largely been replaced by venous duplex scanning for the diagnosis of DVT (combines Doppler principles with real-time B-mode and color-flow ultrasound imaging).

Duplex Ultrasound

Duplex scanning has become the method of choice for testing veins of the superficial, deep, and perforating systems. Duplex ultrasound directly visualizes and locates intraluminal obstruction; assesses the characteristics of venous flow distal to the inguinal ligament; identifies the presence of collateral veins around an obstructed venous segment; permits direct detection of valvular reflux; allows visualization of specific venous valves and valve leaflet motion; quantifies the degree of incompetence; locates and assesses veins before harvest for bypass procedures; evaluates venous perforator incompetence; and evaluates conditions that may mimic venous disease.

Computed Tomography and Magnetic Resonance Venography

Early venous disease rarely requires advanced imaging studies other than duplex ultrasonography. Computed tomography (CT) and magnetic resonance imaging (MRI) have progressed tremendously in the past decade. Both modalities are suitable to identify pelvic or iliac venous obstruction in patients with lower limb varicosities when proximal obstruction or iliac vein compression (May-Thurner syndrome) is suspected. Gadolinium-enhanced MRI is especially useful in evaluating patients with vascular malformations including those with congenital varicose veins.[32]

Contrast Venography

Lower extremity contrast venography remains a powerful, but decreasingly used, tool in the evaluation of both acute and chronic DVT. With advances in duplex ultrasonography, venography has been largely replaced by duplex scanning to evaluate patients with suspected deep venous obstruction or incompetence. In chronic venous disease, ascending venography demonstrates the location and extent of postthrombotic disease (Figure 25-5), as manifested by occlusion, venous recanalization, collateral channels, and superficial varicosities. Ascending venography may also help with planning of endovascular and open surgical procedures, such as iliac and inferior vena cava recanalizations and venous bypass grafts. Ascending contrast venography is performed primarily in patients with significant chronic deep venous occlusive disease who are candidates for endovascular treatment with stents, surgical venous bypass, venous valve repair, or valve transplantation. Descending venography is used in concert with ascending venography to distinguish primary valvular incompetence from thrombotic disease. Descending venography identifies the level of deep vein reflux and evaluates the morphology of the venous valve.

D-Dimer

Fibrin D-dimer is the final product of the plasmin-mediated degradation of cross-linked fibrin. The plasma concentration of D-dimer depends on fibrin generation and subsequent degradation by the fibrinolytic system.[45] D-dimer levels have a high sensitivity for patients with acute venous thrombosis.[48] However, the specificity for acute thrombosis is rather poor.[48] D-dimer levels can be elevated in other clinical conditions that are associated with enhanced fibrin (malignancy, trauma, increased age, disseminated intravascular coagulation, inflammation, infection, sepsis, postoperative states, and preeclampsia).

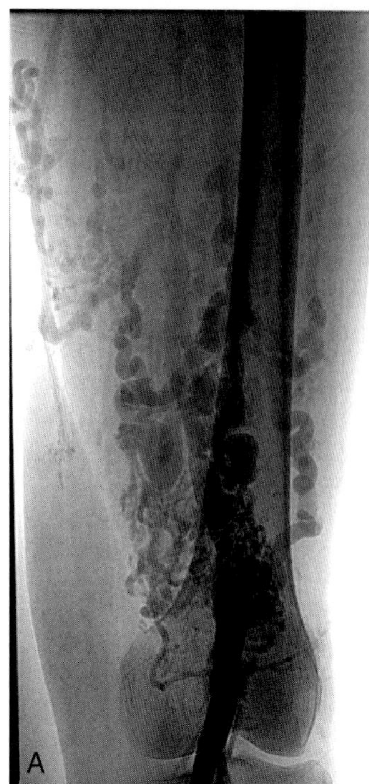

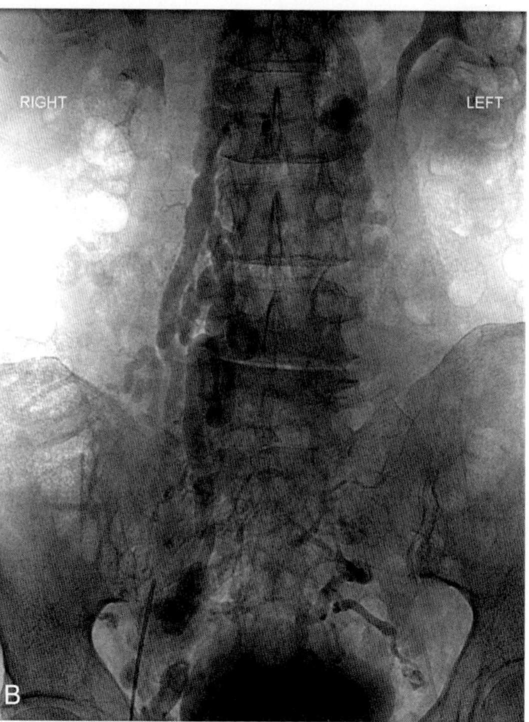

FIGURE 25-5 Venogram of the patient in Figure 25-4. **A,** The femoral vein is severely narrowed at the upper thigh level and drains preferentially via a large incompetent perforator to the great saphenous vein at the midthigh level. **B,** The external iliac veins are occluded bilaterally with extensive pelvic collaterals draining via the paraspinal venous plexus.

Management

Compression

Compression therapy is the mainstay of treatment for chronic venous insufficiency. Because venous hypertension in the upright position and during ambulation is the physiologic cause of the damage in chronic venous insufficiency, the first step of treatment should be to reduce the ambulatory venous pressure.

Compressive dressings aid venous return by compressing the leg and increasing the interstitial tension. Compression of dilated, engorged, superficial, and intramuscular veins indirectly increases the efficiency of the calf pump mechanism.[34] After the volume stabilizes, the patient can be measured for stockings. Typically, knee-length graduated compression stockings with a pressure of 30 to 40 mm Hg (at the ankles) are prescribed. Graduated compression providing decreasing pressure from distal to proximal has been the standard of care for both thromboprophylaxis and management of venous and lymphatic disorders. A recent study showed that a negative graduated compression bandage applied with higher pressures over the calf showed significant hemodynamic superiority in patients with severe venous incompetence. Bandages exerting a higher pressure over the calf compared with the ankle were more effective in increasing the venous pump function in patients with venous insufficiency compared with graduated compression.[38] The superior effect of stronger compression over the calf could be explained by more intense squeezing on the venous blood pooled in the calf or a more complete hindrance to venous reflux during walking.[38] To prevent postthrombotic syndrome, compression stockings should be used routinely following diagnosis of a proximal DVT and continued for a minimum of 1 year.[60]

Elevation

When elevation is used for edema control, the extremity is typically elevated above the level of the heart. The patient should lie on a sofa or sit in a recliner to elevate the legs appropriately. The correct duration and frequency of leg elevation should be tailored to the severity of disease. The leg should be elevated whenever possible and long periods of standing or sitting with the legs dependent should be avoided. In patients with concomitant arterial disease, lower compression and modified elevation is used to avoid further compromise of arterial inflow.

Intermittent Pneumatic Compression

With no history of congestive heart failure and no evidence of venous obstruction (on noninvasive studies), lower extremity volume can be stabilized with an intermittent pneumatic compression pump (40 to 50 mm Hg). Compression wraps should be used between pumping sessions.

Exercise

The value of exercise in the management of chronic venous insufficiency has not been conclusively demonstrated. Exercises involving the leg musculature, such as walking, bicycling, or swimming, promote muscle tone in the calf and enhance venous return. Exercise, however, produces variable reductions in venous hypertension. Patients with chronic venous stasis as a result of incompetent deep vein valves generally do not obtain as much reduction in venous pressure as do those in which the primary defect is caused by incompetent perforator valves.[18]

Lymphatic Disease

Lymphatic diseases result from congenital or acquired disorders that cause obstruction, incompetence, or destruction of lymphatic vessels or the lymph-conducting elements of lymph nodes. The most frequent form of obstructive lymphatic disease is lymphedema.

Lymphatic System

The lymphatic system is a vascular system composed of endothelial-lined channels that parallel the arterial and venous systems. The lymphatics originate in the tissue interstitium as specialized capillaries. These capillaries are porous and readily permit the entry of even large macromolecules, such as albumin.[63] The distribution of fluid between the peripheral vascular system and the tissues depends on the transcapillary balance between hydrostatic and protein osmotic pressure gradients. Interstitial osmotic pressure results from small amounts of proteins in the interstitial fluid, which draws fluid out of the capillaries. This filtrate or lymph is collected by the lymphatics and returned to the venous circulation. A primary function of the lymphatic system is to return not only fluid but also high-molecular-weight substances, such as protein and particulate matter, which are unable to reenter the venules or capillaries. The lymphatic system serves as a buffer system to decrease edema during fluid overload. As interstitial fluid volume increases, interstitial fluid pressure increases. This results in a marked increase in local lymph flow.[63]

The volume of lymph formed depends largely on the balance between intravascular and extravascular hydrostatic forces, osmotic forces, and the permeability of the filtering capillaries.[65] When lymphatic blockage occurs (lymphadenectomy or radiation-induced lymph node fibrosis), intralymphatic pressure distal to the site of blockage increases. As lymphatic vessels dilate, their valves become incompetent. Increased intralymphatic pressure also decreases lymph formation and increases tissue fluid volume.[65]

Lymphedema

Lymphedema is the result of protein-rich interstitial volume overload, secondary to lymph drainage failure in the face of normal capillary filtration. This occurs whenever there is an imbalance between capillary filtration and lymph drainage no matter the etiology. Lymphedema may be characterized as either high-lymph-output failure or low-lymph-output failure. High-lymph-output failure results from an overproduction of capillary filtrate (congestive heart failure, ascites, nephrotic syndrome) and leads to a greatly expanded extracellular fluid space. Low-lymph-output failure (decreased lymph absorption) occurs with deficient or obliterated lymphatics.

Edema that resolves after elevating the affected area overnight is likely secondary to increased capillary filtration (e.g., chronic venous insufficiency/high-lymph-output failure). Edema that does not improve much with overnight elevation often indicates lymphedema with failure of the lymph-conducting pathways (low-lymph-output failure).[28] Fibrosis may result from the inability of local macrophages to digest the excessive protein load. The accumulation of protein promotes chronic inflammation and scar formation. Although the exact mechanism of this scarring is unknown, interstitial fibrosis results in the brawny, nonpitting soft tissue swelling seen in chronic lymphedema.

Classification of Lymphedema

Clinical lymphedema is classified as either primary or secondary. Primary lymphedema occurs with aplasia, hypoplasia, or abnormal development of the lymphatic system. In addition, primary fibrosis of the lymphatics during puberty or at a later age also results in primary lymphedema. Several forms of heritable primary lymphedema are presently recognized.[17] Congenital lymphedema is usually observed at birth with asymmetric presentation in a lower extremity. Lymphedema praecox, which typically appears in the peripubertal period, can occur anytime from after birth into the third decade. Lymphedema tarda is primary lymphedema occurring after the age of 35 years.[64]

Secondary lymphedema occurs much more commonly. Disrupted lymphatic flow may occur because of infection, trauma, tumor, obstruction, surgery, or radiation. Secondary lymphedema from filariasis, usually affecting the lower extremities, is the most common cause of lymphedema worldwide. Breast cancer–associated lymphedema is the most common form of lymphedema in the United States.[2] High body mass index, axillary surgery, radiation therapy (particularly the breast and axilla), and the number of positive lymph nodes are risk factors for developing upper limb lymphedema.[31] Secondary lymphedema commonly presents within the first year after surgery, but can also present many years later.[44]

Lymphedema may also be classified into clinical stages. Grade I edema easily pits in response to pressure and is reduced in response to elevation. There is no evidence of thickened spongy fibrosis on examination. Grade II edema does not easily pit with pressure and does not reduce with elevation. Some degree of fibrosis may be present. Grade III edema is irreversible with fibrosis and sclerosis of the skin and subcutaneous tissues. This severe, organized tissue stage is often not responsive to mechanical treatment measures.

Evaluation

The differential diagnosis for new onset unilateral limb lymphedema is important. Acute DVT must be ruled out whether the edema is presenting in the upper or lower extremity. Other possibilities for diagnosis include postphlebitic syndrome, chronic venous insufficiency, tumor obstruction, chronic infection, and lipidemia. Edema secondary to deep vein thrombophlebitis usually develops suddenly. Chronic venous insufficiency is generally associated with slowly progressing edema. Lymphedema may develop with either of these presentations. Unlike venous edema, there is often involvement of the foot and toes with loss of dorsal vascular and joint markings. Systemic reasons for edema accumulation, such as congestive heart failure, liver or renal disease, and fluid-retaining medications (antiinflammatory drugs and some antihypertensive drugs), should be considered.

Imaging Techniques

Lymphoscintigraphy

Lymphoscintigraphy performed by injecting a radioactive colloid and observing uptake into the lymphatic system has become the standard evaluation tool to establish lymphatic flow patterns.[21] This test can be performed in both upper and lower extremities by injecting the colloid between the digits of the hands or toes, respectively. Lymphoscintigraphy assesses the most basic function of the lymphatic system, mainly the clearance of interstitial macromolecules that are too large to reenter the blood capillaries. When lymphedema is present, the images often show a highly characteristic dermal backflow pattern or rerouting of tracer away from the main lymphatic trunks and into fine collateral lymphatic vessels of the skin. Images may also suggest distal or proximal lymphatic obliteration, hyperplasia, or aplasia/hypoplasia of the lymphatic vessels. Because lymphatic disease occurs so rarely, the skills for administration and accurate interpretation of this test are often available only in larger medical centers where higher volumes of testing occur.

Lymphangiography

Lymphangiography should not be considered unless specific surgical intervention is being contemplated. It is invasive and may damage the (remaining) lymphatic vessels.

Treatment of Lymphedema

Lymphedema treatment is directed at minimizing the swelling, restoring normal function, and avoiding infection of the affected region. Often a patient is offered a diuretic for lymphatic edema. Short-term diuretic use, during hospitalization for acute edema reduction, accompanied by elevation and compression bandaging may be useful. Diuretics are usually not helpful for chronic management of lymphedema because the effect is temporary and the diuresis leaves behind large protein molecules that create a concentrated state in the interstitium.

Antibiotic therapy is indicated in the management of infection associated with lymphedema (focal cellulitis). Inflammatory destruction of remaining lymphatics secondary to repeated infections can worsen the clinical problem. As a result, a program of 1-week per month prophylaxis of Pen VK 250 mg or 500 mg four times daily has been advocated for patients with several episodes of cellulitis per year. For those with a penicillin allergy, a first-generation cephalosporin, clindamycin, or erythromycin can be considered.

Comprehensive treatment regimens for lymphedema (complex decongestive therapy) have become the standard of care. This includes the following:

1. Skin care management and treatment of infection
2. Specialized massage techniques to promote the movement of lymph
3. Compression of the lymphedematous regions
4. Elevation and exercises to reduce swelling and supplement the massage

After an active reduction phase (phase I), an ongoing maintenance phase (phase II) includes daily use of compression garments (and often nocturnal compression) to maintain reduction. A recent study compared the effects of applying manual lymph drainage (MLD) and postural drainage techniques to lower extremity edema of patients after bariatric surgery. Although both interventions were efficient in reducing the edema resulting from the surgery, MLD achieved the best results.[6]

General contraindications to aggressive lymphedema management include acute infection, cardiopulmonary edema, and ongoing malignant disease. Conditions such as pregnancy, recent abdominal surgery, radiation fibrosis, DVT, and aortic aneurysm may preclude some portions of the treatment. Palliative lymphedema management is appropriate.

Compression

Compression of a lymphedematous region causes increased total tissue pressure, decreases the hydrostatic pressure gradient from the blood to the tissues, and increases the hydrostatic pressure gradient from the tissues to the initial lymphatics. The pressure gradient along the lymphatic trunk is also increased. Compression of the affected region is necessary to maintain reductions in edema during and after the treatment. Lymphedematous regions may be compressed with bandages (elastic or low stretch) or graduated compression garments.

There are two basic types of compression bandages. Elastic high-stretch compression bandages have a high resting pressure (from elastic recoil) and low working pressure because they stretch in response to muscle contraction. Low-elastic or low-stretch compression bandages have low resting pressure and a high working pressure, which increases the total tissue pressure when muscles contract. Lymphatic vessels are compressed between the muscles and the bandages enhancing transport. Bandages can be used with various types of padding beneath to reshape the limb.

In patients with moderate to severe lymphedema of the legs, adjustable compression wraps (Velcro closure) achieved more pronounced reduction in volume after 24 hours than inelastic multicomponent compression bandages.[12] Patients were able to apply and adjust the device after being instructed in its use after an initial 2-hour period of wear. Autonomous handling of adjustable compression wraps seems to improve the clinical outcome and is a promising step toward effective self-managed compression.

Once reduced, stable, limb volume is achieved, graduated compression garments are necessary to prevent fluid reaccumulation. Similar to compression bandages, compression garments enhance the pumping action of lymphatics and veins and decrease the hydrostatic pressure gradient from the blood to the tissues. Compression garments are available in various levels of compression. For lymphedema, pressures of 30 to 40 mm Hg often suffice. Recalcitrant edema may require 40 to 50 mm Hg of support. Appropriate compression and fit of the garment along with instruction in donning and doffing are critical to a successful management program.

Elevation

Elevation of a lymphedematous limb can decrease the hydrostatic pressure gradient from the vasculature to the tissues and reduce the amount of fluid and protein moving out of the capillaries. Elevation can also increase the lymphatic flow by increasing the hydrostatic pressure gradient along lymphatic trunks. Patients are encouraged to elevate the involved limb periodically through the day.

Exercise

Exercises improve mobility and muscular activity and lead to the internal compression of lymph vessels. Lymph drainage is stimulated by intermittent pressure changes between muscles and external compression (bandages or compressive garments). Resistance exercises seem to increase strength and decrease the exacerbation of lymphedema, as well as decrease symptoms associated with lymphedema.[53]

Vasopneumatic Compression Therapy

Vasopneumatic compression pumps increase the total tissue pressure in edematous limbs and push tissue fluid back into blood capillaries. Because excess protein is not removed from the tissues, the concentration of tissue protein may increase and theoretically lead to the reoccurrence of edema. Other limitations of compression pumps in the management of lymphedema are that they cannot apply pressure to the areas of the trunk adjacent to draining lymph nodes, and may exacerbate genital edema or produce a collection of high protein fluid proximal to the site of pumping, which can exacerbate inflammation and fibrosis. When compression pumps are used for lymphedema management, pressures of 40 to 50 mm Hg are sufficient for fluid removal and to lessen the risk for tissue damage. Compression pumps are more helpful in the management of chronic venous insufficiency than in the management of chronic stage II or III lymphedema.

Conclusion

The patient with vascular disease poses a significant challenge to the rehabilitation professional. Arterial, venous, or lymphatic dysfunction may be the primary issue or a critical comorbidity in many patients who present to rehabilitation. A detailed vascular history, examination, and selected diagnostic tests should be inherent in the rehabilitation evaluation. When identified early, interventions including exercise, appropriate compression, positioning, protection, and proper footwear may ameliorate the need for more aggressive medical and surgical treatments in patients with vascular disease.

REFERENCES

1. Andrews KL, Dib MY, Shives TC, et al: Noninvasive arterial studies including transcutaneous oxygen pressure measurements with the limbs elevated or dependent to predict healing after partial foot amputation, *Am J Phys Med Rehabil* 92:385–392, 2013.
2. Armer JM: The problem of post-breast cancer lymphedema: impact and measurement issues, *Cancer Invest* 23:76–83, 2005.
3. Armitage JM, Bowman L, Clarke RJ, et al: Effects of homocysteine-lowering with folic acid plus vitamin B_{12} versus placebo on mortality and major morbidity in myocardial infarction survivors: a randomized trial, *JAMA* 303:2486–2494, 2010.
4. Beebe HG, Bergan JJ, Bergqvist D, et al: Classification and grading of chronic venous disease in the lower limbs. A consensus statement, *Eur J Vasc Endovasc Surg* 12:487–492, 1996.
5. Bellis A, Trimarco B: Pharmacological approach to cardiovascular risk in metabolic syndrome, *J Cardiovasc Med* 14:403–409, 2013.
6. Bertelli DF, de Oliveira P, Gimenes AS, et al: Postural drainage and manual lymphatic drainage for lower limb edema in women with morbid obesity after bariatric surgery: a randomized controlled trial, *Am J Phys Med Rehabil* 92:697–703, 2013.
7. Bovenzi M, Lindsell CJ, Griffin MJ: Acute vascular responses to the frequency of vibration transmitted to the hand, *Occup Environ Med* 57:422–430, 2000.
8. Bradbury AW, Adam DJ, Bell J, et al: Bypass Versus Angioplasty in Severe Ischaemia of the Leg (BASIL) trial: an intention to treat analysis of amputation free and overall survival in patients randomized to a bypass surgery-first or a balloon angioplasty-first revascularization strategy, *J Vasc Surg* 51:5S–17S, 2010.
9. Brooks B, Dean R, Patel S, et al: TBI or not TBI: that is the question. Is it better to measure toe pressure than ankle pressure in diabetic patients? *Diabet Med* 18:528–532, 2001.
10. CAPRIE Steering Committee: A randomized, blinded trial of Clopidogrel versus Aspirin in Patients at Risk of Ischemic Events (CAPRIE), *Lancet* 348:1329–1339, 1996.
11. Critical Leg Ischaemia Prevention Study (CLIPS) Group, Catalano M, Born G, Peto R: Prevention of serious vascular events by aspirin amongst patients with peripheral arterial disease: a randomized double blind trial, *J Intern Med* 261:276–284, 2007.
12. Damstra RJ, Partsch H: Prospective, randomized, controlled trial comparing the effectiveness of adjustable compression Velcro wraps versus inelastic multicomponent compression bandages in the initial treatment of leg lymphedema, *J Vasc Surg Venous Lym Dis* 1:13–19, 2013.
13. Davies MG, Waldman DL, Pearson TA: Comprehensive endovascular therapy for femoral popliteal arterial atherosclerotic occlusive disease, *J Am Coll Surg* 201:275–296, 2005.
14. Delis KT, Nicolaides AN: Effect of intermittent pneumatic compression of foot and calf on walking distance hemodynamics and quality of life in patients with arterial claudication: a prospective randomized controlled study with one-year follow up, *Ann Surg* 214:431–441, 2005.
15. Dormandy JA, Murray GD: The fate of the claudicant—a prospective study of 1969 claudicants, *Eur J Vasc Surg* 1191:131–133, 1991.
16. Ersoy H, Rybicki FJ: Biochemical safety profile of gadolinium-based extracellular contrast agents in nephrogenic systemic fibrosis, *J Magn Reson Imaging* 26:1190–1197, 2007.
17. Ferrell RE, Levinson KL, Esman JH, et al: Hereditary lymphedema: evidence for linkage and genetic heterogeneity, *Hum Mol Genet* 7:2073–2078, 1998.
18. Fitzpatrick JE: Stasis ulcers: update on a common geriatric problem, *Geriatrics* 44:19–31, 1989.
19. Galanud JP, Holcroft CA, Rodger MA, et al: Predictors of post-thrombotic syndrome in a population with a first deep vein thrombosis and no primary venous insufficiency, *J Thromb Haemost* 11:474–480, 2013.
20. Gaziano JM: Fifth phase of epidemiologic transition: the age of obesity and inactivity, *JAMA* 303:275–276, 2010.
21. Gloviczki P, Calcagon D, Schierger A, et al: Non-invasive evaluation of the swollen extremity: experiences with 190 lymphoscintigraphic examinations, *J Vasc Surg* 9:683–689, 1989.

22. Guillevin L, Lhote F: Treatment of polyarteritis nodosa and microscopic polyangiitis, *Arthritis Rheum* 41:2100–2105, 1998.
23. Heit J: The epidemiology of venous thromboembolism in the community, *Arterioscler Thromb Vasc Biol* 28:370, 2008.
24. Heit JA, Silverstein MD, Mohr DN, et al: The epidemiology of venous thromboembolism in the community, *Thromb Haemost* 86:452–463, 2011.
25. Hirsh AT, Haskal ZJ, Hertzer NR, et al: ACC-AHA guidelines for the management of patients with peripheral arterial disease (lower extremity, renal, mesenteric, and abdominal aortic): a collaborative report from the American Associations for Vascular Surgery/Society for Vascular Surgery, Society for Cardiovascular Angiography and Interventions, Society for Vascular Medicine and Biology, Society of Interventional Radiology, and the ACC-AHA Taskforce on Practice Guidelines, *J Vasc Interv Radiol* 17:1383–1397, 2006.
26. Hoyer C, Sandermann J, Petersen LJ: The toe-brachial index in the diagnosis of peripheral arterial disease, *J Vasc Surg* 58:231–238, 2013.
27. Kakkos SK, Geroulakos G, Nicolaides AN: Improvement of the walking ability in intermittent claudication due to superficial femoral artery occlusion with supervised exercise and pneumatic foot and calf compression: a randomized controlled trial, *Eur J Vasc Endovasc Surg* 30:164–175, 2005.
28. Kerchner K, Fleischer A, Yosipovitch G: Lower extremity lymphedema update: pathophysiology, diagnosis, and treatment guidelines, *J Am Acad Dermatol* 59:324–331, 2008.
29. Ketha SS, Cooper LT: The role of autoimmunity in thromboangiitis obliterans (Buerger's disease), *Ann N Y Acad Sci* 1285:15–25, 2013.
30. Khandanpour N, Locke YK, Meyer FJ, et al: Homocysteine and peripheral arterial disease: systematic review and meta-analysis, *Eur J Vasc Endovasc Surg* 38:316–322, 2009.
31. Kwan ML, Darbinian J, Schmitz KH, et al: Risk factors for lymphedema in a prospective breast cancer survivorship study: the pathway study, *Arch Surg* 145:1055–1063, 2010.
32. Lee BB, Bergan JJ, Gloviczki P, et al: Diagnosis and treatment of venous malformations. Consensus document of the International Union of Phlebology (IUP)—2009, *Int Angiol* 28:434–451, 2009.
33. Leng GC, Fowler B, Ernst E, Leng GC: Exercise for intermittent claudication, *Cochrane Database Syst Rev* (7):CD00990, 2000.
34. Lofgren KA: Surgical management of chronic venous insufficiency, *Acta Chir Scand Suppl* 544:62–68, 1988.
35. Marso SP, Hiatt RW: Peripheral arterial disease in patients with diabetes, *J Am Coll Cardiol* 47:921–929, 2006.
36. McKenna M, Olfson S, Kuller L: A ratio of ankle and arm arterial pressure as an independent predictor of mortality, *Atherosclerosis* 87:119–128, 1991.
37. Momsen AH, Jensen MB, Norager CB: Drug therapy for improving walking distance in intermittent claudication: a systematic review and meta-analysis of robust randomised controlled studies, *Eur J Vasc Endovasc Surg* 38:463–474, 2009.
38. Mosti G, Partsch H: High compression pressure over the calf is more effective than graduated compression in enhancing venous pump function, *Eur J Vasc Endovasc Surg* 44:332–336, 2012.
39. Muluk SC, Muluk VS, Kelley ME, et al: Outcome events in patients with claudication: a 15-year study in 2,777 patients, *J Vasc Surg* 33:251–257, 2001.
40. Muntner P, DeSalvo KB, Wildman RP, et al: Relationship between HBA1c level and peripheral arterial disease, *Diabetes Care* 28:1981–1987, 2005.
41. Nicolaides AN, Hussein MK, Szendro G, et al: The relation of venous ulceration with ambulatory venous pressure measurements, *J Vasc Surg* 17:414–419, 1993.
42. Norgren L, Hiatt WR, Dormandy JA, et al: on behalf of the TASC II Working Group: Inter-Society Consensus for the Management of Peripheral Arterial Disease (TASC II), *J Vasc Surg* 45:S5–S67, 2007.
43. Ostchega Y, Paulose-Ram R, Dillon CF, et al: Prevalence of peripheral arterial disease and risk factors in persons age 60 and older: data from the National Health and Nutrition Examination Survey 1999-2004, *J Am Geriatr Soc* 55:583–589, 2007.
44. Petrek JA, Senie RT, Peters M, et al: Lymphedema in a cohort of breast carcinoma survivors 20 years after diagnosis, *Cancer* 92:1368–1377, 2001.
45. Prisco D, Grifoni E: The role of D-dimer testing in patients with suspected venous thromboembolism, *Semin Thromb Hemost* 35:50–59, 2009.
46. Ramos-Casals M, Stone JH, Cid MC, Bosch X: The cryoglobulinaemias, *Lancet* 379:348–360, 2012.
47. Rice TW, Lumsden AB: Optimal medical management of peripheral arterial disease, *Vasc Endovascular Surg* 40:321–327, 2006.
48. Righini M, Perrier A, De Moerloose P, et al: D-Dimer for venous thromboembolism diagnosis: 20 years later, *J Thromb Haemost* 6:1059–1071, 2008.
49. Rivers SP, Scher LA, Gupta SK, et al: Safety of peripheral vascular surgery after recent acute myocardial infarction, *J Vasc Surg* 11:70–75, 1990.
50. Roger VL, Go AS, Lloyd-Jones DM, et al: Heart disease and stroke statistics—2012 update. A report from the American Heart Association, *Circulation* 125:e2–e220, 2012.
51. Rooke TW, Hirsch AT, Misra S, et al: 2011 ACCF/AHA focused update of the guideline for the management of patients with peripheral artery disease (updating the 2005 guideline): a report of the American College of Cardiology Foundation/American Heart Association Task-force on Practice Guidelines, *Circulation* 124:2020–2045, 2011.
52. Schlager O, Giurgea A, Schuhfried O, et al: Exercise training increases endothelial progenitor cells and decreases asymmetric dimethylarginine in peripheral arterial disease: a randomized controlled trial, *Atherosclerosis* 217:240–248, 2011.
53. Schmitz K, Ahmed R, Troxel A, et al: Weightlifting in women with breast cancer-related lymphedema, *N Engl J Med* 361:664–711, 2009.
54. Selvin E, Erlinger TB: Prevalence of and risk factors for peripheral arterial disease in the United States: results from the National Health and Nutrition Examination Survey 1999-2000, *Circulation* 110:738–743, 2004.
55. Selvin E, Marinopoulos S, Berkenbilt G, et al: Meta-analysis: glycosylated hemoglobin in cardiovascular disease in diabetes mellitus, *Ann Intern Med* 141:421–431, 2004.
56. Shahin Y, Barnes R, Barakat H, et al: Meta-analysis of angiotensin converting enzyme inhibitors effect on walking ability and ankle brachial pressure index in patients with intermittent claudication, *Atherosclerosis* 231:283–290, 2013.
57. Shalhub S, Zierler RE, Smith W, et al: Vasospasm as a cause for claudication in athletes with external iliac artery endofibrosis, *J Vasc Surg* 58:105–111, 2013.
58. Shephard RF: Acute deep vein thrombosis, *Cardiovasc Clin* 22:47–66, 1992.
59. Shephard RF, Shephard JT: Raynaud's phenomenon, *Int Angiol* 11:41–45, 1992.
60. Snow D, Qaseem A, Barry P, et al: Management of venous thromboembolism: a clinical practice guideline from the American College of Physicians and the American Academy of Family Physicians, *Ann Fam Med* 5:74–80, 2007.
61. Stewart KJ, Hiatt WR, Regensteiner JG, et al: Exercise training for claudication, *N Engl J Med* 347:1941–1951, 2002.
62. Stone JH, Nousari HC: "Essential" cutaneous vasculitis: what every rheumatologist should know about vasculitis of the skin, *Curr Opin Rheumatol* 13:23–34, 2001.
63. Thibodeau GA, Patton KT: *Structure and function of the body*, ed 14, Saint Louis, 2011, Mosby.
64. Tiwari A, Cheng K, Button M, et al: Differential diagnosis, investigation, and current treatment of lower limb lymphedema, *Arch Surg* 138:152–161, 2003.
65. Toratora GJ, Derrickson BH: *Principles of anatomy and physiology: organizational support and movement and control systems of the human body* (vol 2), ed 12, Hoboken, 2009, John Wiley and Sons.
66. Turesson C, Schaid DJ, Weyand CM, et al: Association of HLA-C3 and smoking with vasculitis in patients with rheumatoid arthritis, *Arthritis Rheum* 54:2776–2783, 2006.
67. Vines L, Gemayel G, Christenson JT: The relationship between increased body mass index and primary venous disease severity and concomitant deep primary venous reflux, *J Vasc Surg Venous Lym Dis* 1:239–244, 2013.
68. Wennberg PW: Approach to the patient with peripheral arterial disease, *Circulation* 128:2241–2250, 2013.
69. Yuen JC, Wright E, Johnson LA, Culp WC: Hypothenar hammer syndrome: an update with algorithms for diagnosis and treatment, *Ann Plast Surg* 67:429–438, 2011.
70. Yusuf S, Sleight P, Pogue J, et al: Effects of an angiotensin converting enzyme inhibitor, ramipril, on cardiovascular events in high-risk patients. The Heart Outcomes Prevention Evaluation Study Investigators, *N Engl J Med* 342:145–153, 2000.

BURNS

Vincent Gabriel, Radha Holavanahalli

Significant advances in management have resulted in an increase in survival after burn injury. As a consequence, burn survivors, who tend to be young adults, have long-term sequelae that impact return to work and community reintegration. Up to 1 million burns require treatment annually in North America and over 10 times as many burns occur worldwide. In low- and middle-income countries, mortality is significantly greater than in high-income countries.[106] The future of burn care will be challenged by the expense and complexity of treatment, a predicted shortage of qualified burn surgeons, and an aging population.[63]

Epidemiology of Burn Injury

The American Burn Association has led a long-term initiative to collect information from burn centers in the United States and Canada. Most individuals with burn are male, with a mean age of 33 years, and with burns affecting less than 10% of the total body surface area (TBSA). The most common etiologies of burn injuries are flames and scalds. Over 95% of burned individuals survived their hospitalization, with predictors for burn mortality including increasing age, higher TBSA, and the presence of inhalation injury. Increasing mortality in elderly individuals with burns is predicted by the inhalation injury, burn size, and increasing age, with 60 and 70 years being significant age thresholds (Figures 26-1 and 26-2).[88] With the large majority of burned individuals surviving their hospital stay, mortality may not be an outcome measure of choice for burn research in North America. The National Institute on Disability and Rehabilitation Research (NIDRR) has funded the Burn Model Systems project to research the long-term outcomes of burn survivors in the United States.[74] Burn centers also admit individuals with other acute skin-related disorders and injuries, such as Stevens-Johnson syndrome, toxic epidermal necrolysis (TEN), and necrotizing fasciitis, which adds to the complexity of care provided in these burn centers.[10,39]

Burn epidemiology differs in the rest of the world, with approximately 90% of all burn deaths worldwide occurring in low- and middle-income countries. Intentional burn injuries, rare in the United States but seen most commonly in young men, are more common in young women in India and middle-aged men in Europe.[105,106] Unintentional burn injuries are also more common in girls than boys, in low- to middle-income countries.[5] Changing burn mortality in the future may be focused on improved treatments for inhalation injury and preventing burns in the elderly and in low- to middle-income countries.

Acute Physiatric Assessment of the Burned Individual

Because the majority of burns in the United States are less than 10% TBSA, many do not require surgical intervention.[10] In the inpatient setting, the burn physiatrist may manage many different medical aspects of burn care as part of the larger burn team. There is a long-term shift of burn care to outpatient settings.[93] In an outpatient setting, the modern burn physiatrist should be competent in managing small nonoperative burns independent of a surgical team, yet also recognize those individuals who may benefit from hospital admission, acute excision, and reconstruction of their wounds, and who may also benefit from scar reconstruction.

Size, location, and depth of burn injury are important predictors for complications and mortality, and should be assessed acutely.[11,60] Assessment of TBSA may be calculated by using a clinical tool, such as a Lund and Browder chart (Figure 26-3), by following the "rule of nines," or by estimating for small focal burns (e.g., the palmar surface of the adult hand is approximately 1% TBSA).[61]

High temperature thermal burns are divided into superficial, partial-thickness, and full-thickness injuries. Superficial wounds are red, painful, and have little exudate. A typical example of a superficial burn is sunburn. These burns injure the epidermis only, and healing typically occurs within 7 days. They do not require dressings or surgical interventions, and the risk of scarring is very low. These injuries are not usually managed in a specialized burn center.

Partial-thickness burn injuries are divided into superficial partial thickness and deep partial thickness. Superficial partial-thickness burns injure the superficial layers of the dermis and have mild to moderate wound exudate. Serous-filled blisters are typically present. These wounds are painful but typically heal within 7 to 14 days. The risk of scarring from this injury is low, but there might be pigmentation changes in the skin in the long term.

Deep partial-thickness burns injure the deeper layers of the dermis, have fewer blisters than superficial partial-thickness injuries, but have moderate to extensive exudates present. These wounds are painful but might heal within 14 to 28 days. Some deep partial-thickness injuries, however, do not heal in this time frame. The prolonged inflammatory wound healing seen in deep partial-thickness burn injuries significantly increases the risk of scarring and may be an indication for acute surgical intervention. This depth of burn may result in particularly painful recovery because of a combination of exposed

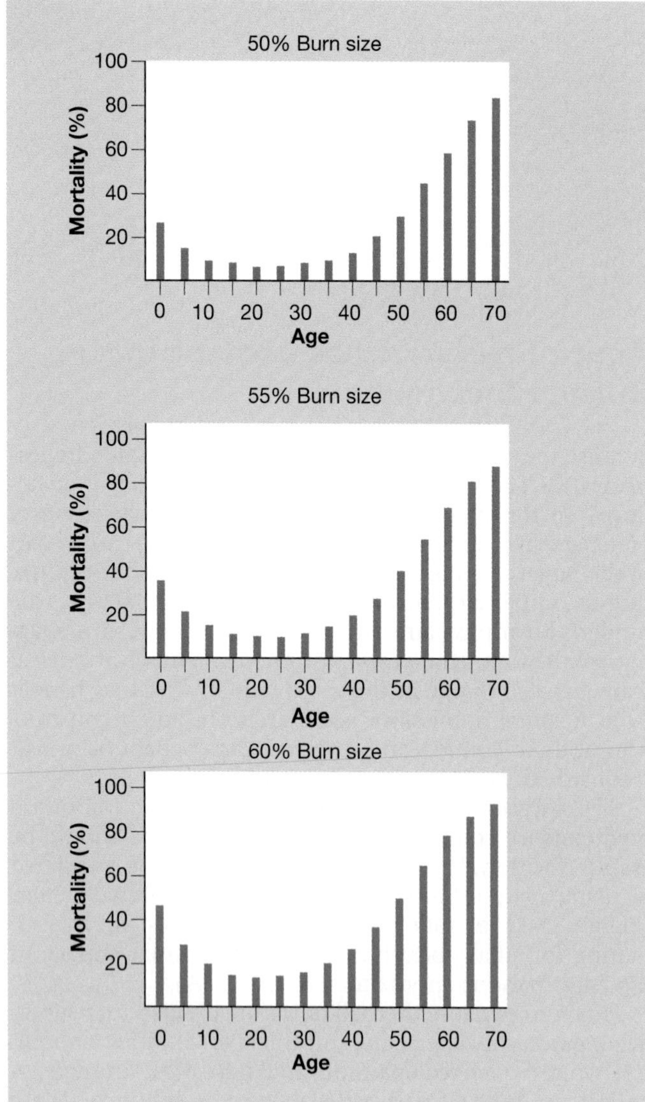

FIGURE 26-1 Effect of age on percent mortality at three discrete burn sizes. (From Pruitt BA Jr, Goodwin CW, Mason AD: Epidemiological, demographic, and outcome characteristics of burn injury. In Herndon DN, ed: *Total burn care*, ed 2, New York, 2002, Saunders, with permission.)

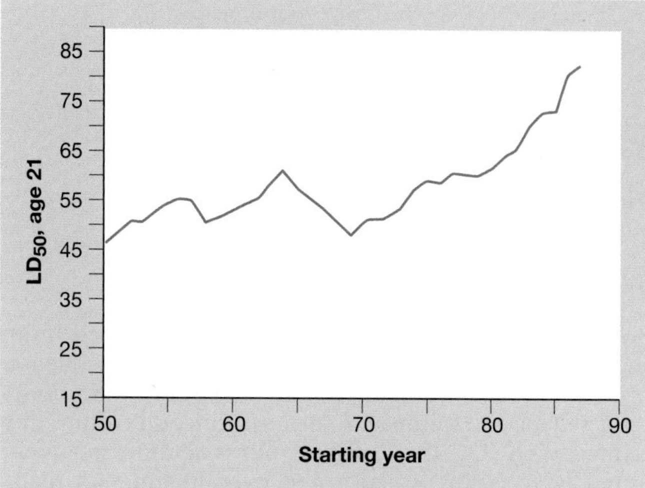

FIGURE 26-2 Changes in the LD_{50} in individuals 21 years of age over time, illustrating the increased survival of individuals with large burns. (From Pruitt BA Jr, Goodwin CW, Mason AD: Epidemiological, demographic, and outcome characteristics of burn injury. In Herndon DN, editor: *Total burn care*, ed 2, New York, 2002, Saunders, with permission.)

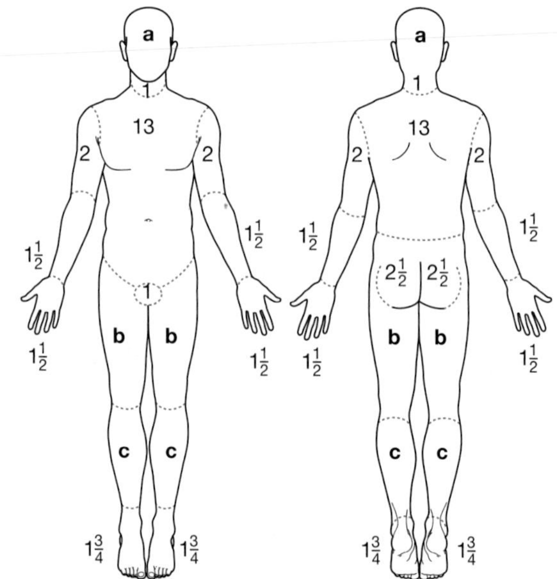

Age in years						
	0	1	5	10	15	Adult
a - $\frac{1}{2}$ of head	$9\frac{1}{2}$	$8\frac{1}{2}$	$6\frac{1}{2}$	$5\frac{1}{2}$	$4\frac{1}{2}$	$3\frac{1}{2}$
b - $\frac{1}{2}$ of one thigh	$2\frac{3}{4}$	$3\frac{1}{4}$	4	$4\frac{1}{4}$	$4\frac{1}{2}$	$4\frac{3}{4}$
c - $\frac{1}{2}$ of one leg	$2\frac{1}{2}$	$2\frac{1}{2}$	$2\frac{3}{4}$	3	$3\frac{1}{4}$	$3\frac{1}{2}$

FIGURE 26-3 The Lund and Browder method for calculation of burn size is reliable for different body proportions in children. (From Artz CP, Moncrief JA, Pruitt BA: *Burns: a team approach*, Philadelphia, 1979, Saunders, with permission.)

cutaneous peripheral nerve endings and a different regenerative capacity from deeper dermal cell types that may result in more fibrosis in healing than more superficial dermal cells.[143,145]

Full-thickness burn injuries damage all of the epidermis and the dermis, and can extend into deeper structures. The area of the burned skin may have reduced somatic sensation, but there can be pain from underlying necrotic tissue, surrounding burns, or damage to nearby structures. These wounds typically appear pale with minimal exudate. Significant scarring is almost certain from ungrafted, full-thickness burn injuries, and acute surgical intervention to excise necrotic tissue and reconstruct the wound is indicated. A summary of burn depth and skin sections is shown in Figures 26-4 and 26-5.

Electrical injuries also have special characteristics compared with thermal injuries. They are arbitrarily divided into high voltage (>1000 V) and low voltage (<1000 V). High-voltage injuries are usually work-related, whereas most low-voltage injuries occur at home.[8,56] The total extent of soft tissue damage may be greater than expected based on the cutaneous injury observed, as electrical

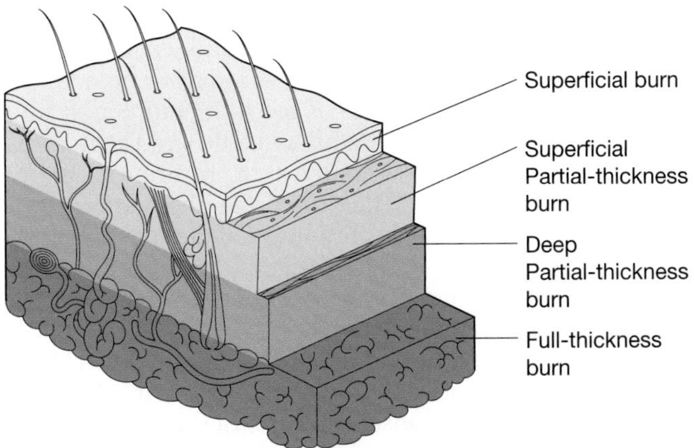

FIGURE 26-4 A superficial (first-degree) burn involves only the epidermis. A partial-thickness (second-degree) burn involves the superficial or deep dermis, and a full-thickness (third-degree) burn extends to subdermal tissues. (From Achauer BM, Eriksson E: *Plastic surgery indications, operations and outcomes*, St Louis, 2000, Mosby, with permission.)

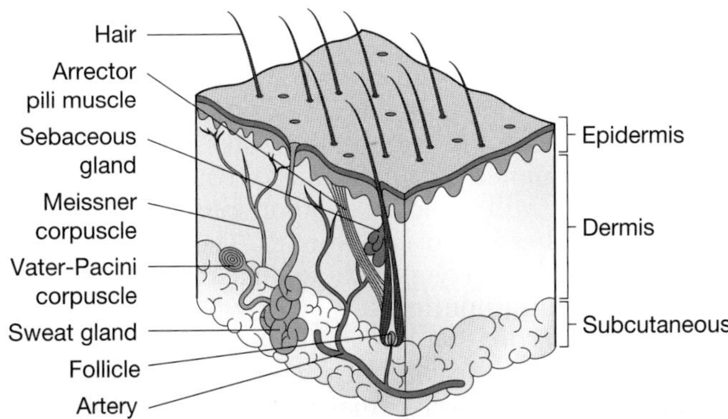

FIGURE 26-5 Cross-section of normal skin, illustrating the epidermis, the dermis, and the epidermal appendages (hair follicles, sweat, and sebaceous glands). (From Achauer BM, Eriksson E: *Plastic surgery indications, operations and outcomes*, St Louis, 2000, Mosby, with permission.)

current will affect the tissues of the least electrical resistance, resulting specifically in significant peripheral and central nervous system damage. Although risks for myocardial necrosis and arrhythmias are present following an electrical injury, individuals who do not have an arrhythmia in the first 24 hours after injury do not appear at elevated risk for later arrhythmias.[8] Survivors of high-voltage electrical injuries account for a large number of burn-related amputations and neuropathies, and have longer lengths of stay than individuals with thermal injuries. Both high-voltage and low-voltage injuries may be associated with impairments in function and complications with returning to work.[91,136] Ocular complications of electrical injury, such as the development of cataracts or macular holes, may present late after injury.[19]

Other acute wounds may be seen in the burn center. Frostbite may occur from environmental or industrial exposures to cold and the resultant wounds are more difficult to classify by depth than flame or hot contact burns. Other than rewarming, pain management, and a longer, nonoperative observation period, there is no convincing medical treatment that changes the outcome of frostbite injury. There is some early evidence that thrombolytic therapies have some benefit in the first 24 hours after injury.[154] Challenging burns may occur after medical use of ionizing radiation as these wounds tend to arise at unpredictable times. The healing potential following a radiation burn is difficult to predict.[142] Because there may be multiple wounds of varying depths within a single burn or areas of indeterminate depth, there may be a role for complementing physical examination of the injury with additional imaging, such as laser Doppler.[115,126]

Acute Wound Care

Removal of necrotic material and the establishment of a clean, moist wound bed are the primary goals of acute wound management. There are a large number of commercially available products that are acceptable to use for management of acute burns. Unfortunately, few high-quality comparative studies have been performed on these products. Silver sulfadiazine remains a mainstay in burn care because of its low cost and the fact that many wounds heal quickly regardless of the wound treatment.[147] Meta-analyses of the literature suggest superior healing outcomes from the use of biosynthetic, silver-based or hydrogel dressings compared with silver sulfadiazine. Although adequate wound healing for nonoperative burns is the ultimate goal, other considerations, such as cost and minimization of pain during dressing changes, should be taken into account when choosing a product.[71]

Management of blisters remains controversial in burn care.[120] However, in general, tense blisters associated with pain or limitation in function can be drained, allowing the separated epithelium to act as a temporary biological dressing that may reduce pain and functional limitation in the affected area.

The use of immersion hydrotherapy is no longer commonly practiced in modern burn centers. Immersion wound care in hydrotherapy tanks may result in lowering of core temperature or sodium, may be a source of gram-negative bacteria, such as *Pseudomonas*, and may cause cross-contamination of wounds. Also, the expense of draining and cleaning the tanks may be cost-prohibitive. The minimization of immersion hydrotherapy has been associated with a reduction in serious skin infections.[125] Acute wound care is superior with local wound cleaning rather than with immersion hydrotherapy. The environment must be kept warm to avoid a significant drop in core temperature for individuals with large (>20% TBSA) burns.

Acute Pain Management

Acute burn pain is typically significant and is magnified by procedural pain associated with dressing changes, mobility, stretching, and surgery. Opioids remain the mainstay of acute pain management. Treatment requires frequent reassessment because an individual's pain may change drastically around events, such as wound closure or participation in therapies.[132] Adjuncts to opioids, such as distraction, hypnosis, or anxiolytics, may be used, particularly for the pediatric burned individual.[72]

Acute Surgical Procedures in Burn Injuries

In full-thickness burn injuries, the damaged tissues are adherent to underlying structures. Wound edema and the fluids required for resuscitation after burn injury increase the risk for development of compartment syndrome, which must be monitored. Thick eschar on the trunk region can inhibit respiration and the surgical team can perform escharotomy (surgical incision through the eschar) to relieve this pressure. Escharotomies in the limbs and trunk typically are left open in the acute phase and will usually require skin grafting once the edema has resolved.[61] Limbs requiring escharotomies should be elevated and splinted in a neutral position for 24 hours before initiating passive range of motion.

Early excision of necrotic tissue and eschar, combined with autologous, split-thickness skin grafting, has greatly improved survival after burn injury. This surgical approach reduces the inflammatory stimulation from the burn eschar and the risk of infection. Donor skin is removed from an unburned area of skin through the use of a powered dermatome (Figure 26-6). The donor skin is then prepared and placed on the surgically prepared wound bed. The donor skin is held in place by staples, sutures, or, in some cases, dermal glues.[99] A compressive postoperative dressing is then applied to the skin graft area, and an appropriate dressing is applied to the skin graft donor site. As only the epidermis and superficial dermis are harvested, the donor site is normally expected to heal spontaneously in 2 weeks. Much like other acute wounds, there are a large number of products available to dress the skin graft donor site.[70] Individuals should be aware that the donor site area may be very painful postoperatively. The benefits of donor site products vary, with some more comfortable for individuals but slow healing, and others cheaper but more uncomfortable. Individual decisions are based on regional preferences.

The donor skin can be prepared by meshing, to broaden the area of wound covered. Meshing also allows for any blood or wound exudates to escape from underneath the skin graft. The donor skin can be applied as a sheet over areas of special function, such as the hands and face. Sheet grafts generally do not scar as much as meshed grafts, resulting in improved motion and aesthetic function.[69] As there is no route of escape for wound exudates from beneath the unmeshed sheet graft, seromas or hematomas can form and even cause loss of the skin graft. Small fluid collections may be drained with a needle and the material rolled out to preserve the grafted skin. To improve adherence of the skin graft to the donor site, the grafted site is typically immobilized in the immediate postoperative phase. Early (1 to 4 days after surgery) initiation of therapies and mobilization improve individual function and reduce length of hospital stay.[23]

Although lifesaving for individuals with severe burn injuries, split-thickness skin grafting results in abnormal skin as a result of the absence of the dermal appendages. Thus, the grafted skin is chronically dry, itchy, and mechanically inferior to normal skin. The grafted skin does not regenerate the dermal appendages, resulting in chronic impairments in skin function.[29]

Other Acute Conditions Treated in the Burn Center

The expertise in managing large wounds and skin grafts present in burn centers results in referrals to provide care for other acute wound conditions. After excision of the affected tissue in necrotizing fasciitis or Fournier gangrene, the individual will typically require split-thickness skin grafting to address his or her wounds. The acute management afterward is very similar to that required in skin grafting after burn injuries.[15]

Stevens-Johnson syndrome (<30% TBSA) or TEN (>30%), acute hypersensitivity reactions that result in wounds analogous to a partial-thickness burn injury, is associated with some drug exposures, such as carbamazepine, particularly in individuals with Asian ancestry.[135] Ocular involvement requires consultation with an ophthalmologist. SCORTEN (*SCORe* of *T*oxic *E*pidermal *N*ecrosis) is a good prognostic tool to predict survival following Stevens-Johnson syndrome (Table 26-1).[153] The use of intravenous immunoglobulin or intravenous steroids remains controversial in this population.[84] The main rehabilitation issues in this population are debility and neuropathy. Encouraging individuals to be up out of bed early will decrease the rate of complications.

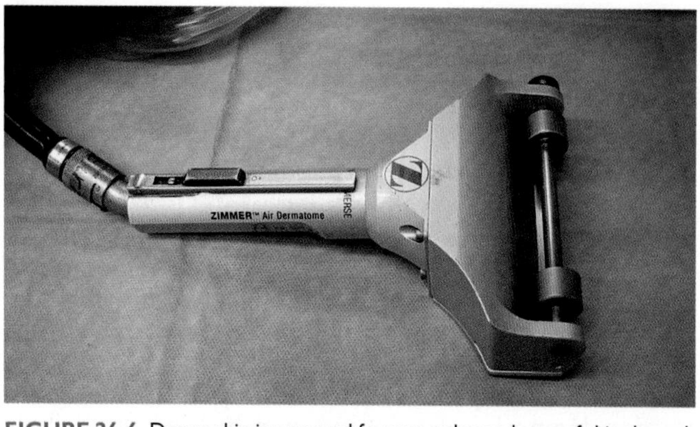

FIGURE 26-6 Donor skin is removed from an unburned area of skin through the use of a powered dermatome.

Table 26-1 SCORTEN (*SCORe* of *T*oxic *E*pidermal *N*ecrosis) Prognostic Tool to Predict Survival Following Stevens-Johnson Syndrome

Age (years)	<40	>40	0 to 1	3.2%
Associated malignancy	No	Yes	2	12.1%
Heart rate (beats/min)	<120	>120	3	35.3%
Serum blood urea nitrogen (mg/dL)	<27	>27	4	8.3%
Total body surface area involved	<10%	>10%	5 or more	>90%
Serum bicarbonate (mEq/L)	>20	<20		
Serum glucose (mg/dL)	<250	>250		

Presence of Inhalation Injury

Inhalation injury associated with burns is a significant risk factor for morbidity, especially in children and older adults.[56,88] Little has been documented regarding the incidence of hypoxic brain injury in burned individuals with inhalation injury, but the reduction of available oxygen, combined with toxic smoke components, such as carbon monoxide and cyanide, puts the burned individual with inhalation injury at risk for hypoxic brain injury.[3] Burned individuals with inhalation injuries are at risk for developing pneumonia, adult respiratory distress syndrome, and multisystem organ failure, during the acute periods of recovery.[62] Early tracheostomy in individuals likely to require prolonged intubation has not been shown to change pulmonary outcomes, but it does offer advantages for oral hygiene and management of facial burns.[112] It is not known whether inhalation injury predisposes burned individuals to pneumonia in the rehabilitation setting and, as a result, routine oxygen monitoring during therapies varies among practitioners.

Polytrauma and Burns

It is estimated that approximately 5% of traumatically injured individuals will have a concomitant burn injury.[117] Fractures outside of the burned area can be treated with standard fracture care. An individualized approach is necessary when the fractures occur in regions that also have burn injury.[73] Individuals with a history of major trauma can have delayed diagnoses, including fractures or other neurologic and musculoskeletal injuries, which the physiatrist should consider during the ongoing assessment of the burned individual.[21]

Catabolism and Metabolic Abnormalities

In all individuals with burn injuries greater than 30% TBSA, the physiatrist should anticipate a significant metabolic abnormality that results in loss of bone mineral density, lean body mass, and increased insulin resistance.[60] These metabolic abnormalities indicate that individuals with large burn injuries have increased caloric and nutritional needs that should be addressed with early enteral feeding and supplementation.[25] Progressive loss of lean body mass is associated with increasing loss of function and an increased incidence of medical complications, such as pneumonia and poor wound healing.[33]

The management of the hypermetabolic state in individuals with a large TBSA burn has been improved with the use of anabolic agents, beta-blockers, and exercise. Oxandrolone is a synthetic testosterone analog that has been shown to reduce mortality and length of hospital stay.[151] Lean body mass and bone mineral density might be improved by maintaining individuals on oxandrolone beyond their hospital discharge because the hypermetabolic state can persist beyond the time of wound closure. The typical dosage of oxandrolone for adult burned individuals is 10 mg twice a day and 0.1 mg/kg for children. Although human growth hormone (HGH) has shown some promise as an additional anabolic agent in burn injury, reports of increased mortality with the use of HGH in critically ill adults have limited research.[134]

The stress response after burn injury is thought to be mediated by circulating catecholamines. An association of increased cortisol and catecholamine levels with infections and poor wound healing has been demonstrated in children.[97] Beta-blockade is helpful in managing the increased catecholamines and the stress response to burn injury. The administration of propranolol, in doses high enough to reduce resting heart rate by 20%, has been shown in children to reduce the metabolic rate and help preserve protein and lean body mass. Beta-blockade might also have benefits for improving wound healing and preventing post-traumatic stress disorder (PTSD) in both adults and children.[59,130]

Dysfunction in insulin action is also observed as part of the metabolic response to large burn injury. The mechanism for this is not entirely clear, but it can be related to insulin antagonists emanating from inflammatory cells in the burn region. Individuals with burn injuries greater than 40% TBSA and those over age 60 years should have close monitoring of blood glucose, with a goal of euglycemia in the acute phase. They might also need glucose monitoring for months to years after injury. Besides maintaining appropriate blood glucose levels, insulin has an added benefit to improving the metabolic state of the burned individual, thus minimizing lean body mass losses.[66]

Mobilization and exercise should be initiated early in the burned individual. The frequency of active and passive therapeutic interventions by the rehabilitation team caring for acute care of burned individuals has increased over time.[148] In the acute stages after a large burn, passive therapies, including splinting and positioning, should be initiated to minimize the risk of burn scar contracture, improve respiration, and reduce the risk of ventilator-associated pneumonias.[54] As soon as the individual is able, active exercise should be started to help maintain function and to address the hypermetabolic state. Exercise is also an essential component for maximizing the benefits of anabolic hormones.[131]

Nutrition and Swallowing in Burns

Enteral feeding should be instituted early for individuals unable to feed normally. This helps maintain gut immunity and motility, while providing the necessary calories and nutrients to counter the hypermetabolic response to burn injury.[79,85] The total caloric requirements for adults with burn injuries can be estimated at 25 kcal/kg plus 40 kcal/1% TBSA burn/day.[30] In addition to the changes in lipid and carbohydrate metabolism seen in individuals with a large burn injury, important changes in protein and amino acid metabolism are also of special importance. The administration of glutamine appears to have benefits in individuals with large burn injuries.[107] Using body weight measurement to assess nutritional status can be difficult because of surgical procedures, dressings, and fluid changes.

The serum prealbumin level can be very helpful as a marker of protein synthesis.[25]

Dysphagia (see Chapter 3) can be a barrier to achieving adequate nutrition. Dysphagia can develop from inhaled irritants, mechanical complications of tube placement, or neurologic injury. Larger TBSA burns, higher number of days with a tracheostomy, and higher number of days on a ventilator are all associated with dysphagia after burn injury.[36] An abnormal bedside swallowing assessment is predictive of abnormal barium swallowing studies, but there is still uncertainty regarding the best protocols for assessing swallowing in burned individuals.[35] Although some very complex cases might have prolonged dysphagia, studies have described between 42% and 90% of individuals having normal swallowing function by the time of hospital discharge.[118,146]

Peripheral Neuropathies

Approximately 10% of burned individuals will develop peripheral neuropathies from a variety of etiologies, such as direct thermal injury, electrical current, compression, and metabolic derangements.[77] Several patterns of neuropathy are seen, including mononeuropathies, peripheral polyneuropathies, and patterns that resemble mononeuritis multiplex. Deeper and larger TBSA burns are more associated with axonal rather than demyelinating neuropathies.[87] Mononeuropathies are seen with electrical injuries and flame burns. The pattern of peripheral polyneuropathy seen in those who have prolonged stays in intensive care units is similar to critical illness polyneuropathy.

The physiatrist performing electrodiagnostic testing on burned individuals should be mindful that the changes after burn injury can alter the results of both nerve conduction testing and electromyography. The increased skin thickness seen with hypertrophic burn scars can have an inverse relationship with the amplitude of the responses seen in nerve conduction testing.[57] After large burn injuries there can be upregulation of nicotinic acetylcholine receptors in the muscle cell membrane that results in electrodiagnostic features suggestive of membrane instability or acute denervation.[66] As a result, electromyographic studies must be interpreted with caution in the burned individual because these neuromuscular changes can be indistinguishable from true neuropathic changes.

Median sensory neuropathies are the most common peripheral nerve abnormality after burn injury. Conservative electrodiagnostic studies can help to define the extent of nerve injuries in burned individuals. Over the course of approximately 1 year, repeated nerve conduction tests typically show improvement in burn-related neuropathy, without requiring intervening surgical treatments. For burn-associated neuropathies not explained by compression or direct electrical injury, the mechanism leading to development and recovery is not well known.[51]

Heterotopic Ossification

In individuals with burn injuries greater than 30% TBSA, there is a risk of development of heterotopic ossification (HO). The most common site of HO in burned individuals is the posterior elbow (Figure 26-7). HO can develop in an unburned limb, but is more common in an affected limb, and can be associated with delayed wound closure over the elbow.[75]

The best treatment and prevention for HO in burns is still controversial. This is particularly the case regarding the use of bisphosphonates, with some evidence suggesting etidronate is not helpful.[64] It is possible that etidronate is ineffective because of the significant postinjury inflammatory state seen in burn injury, and higher potency bisphosphonates might be more effective.[119] Some physicians

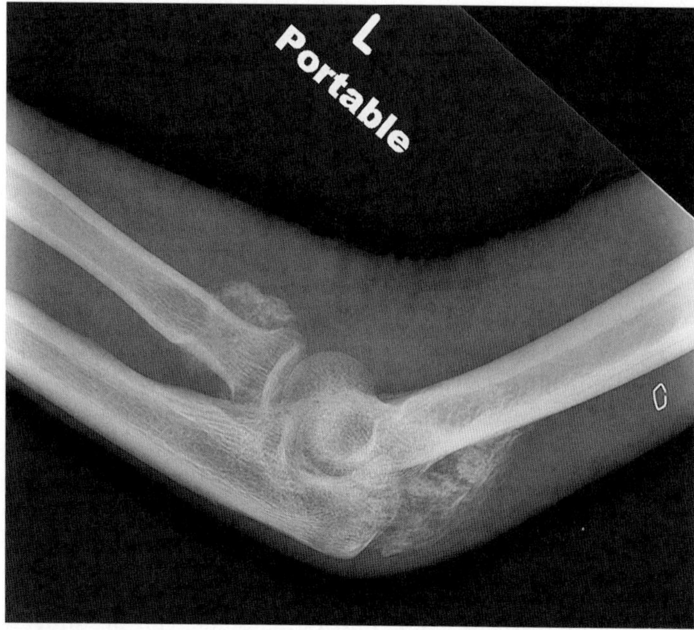

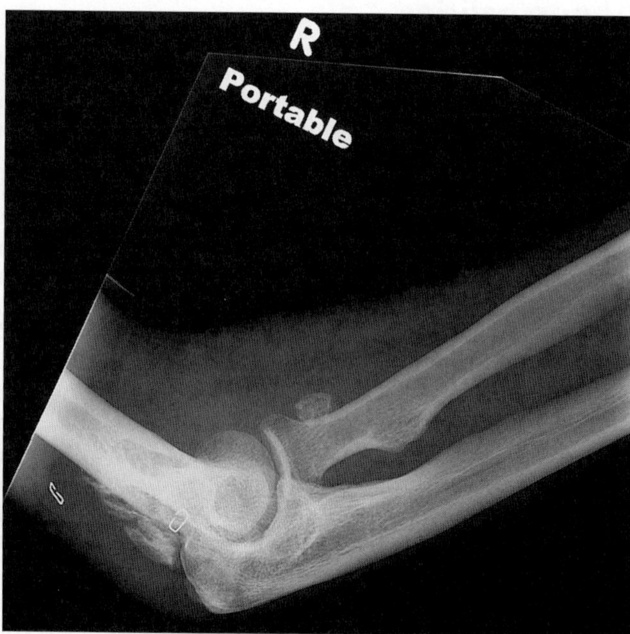

FIGURE 26-7 Heterotopic ossification of the posterior elbow.

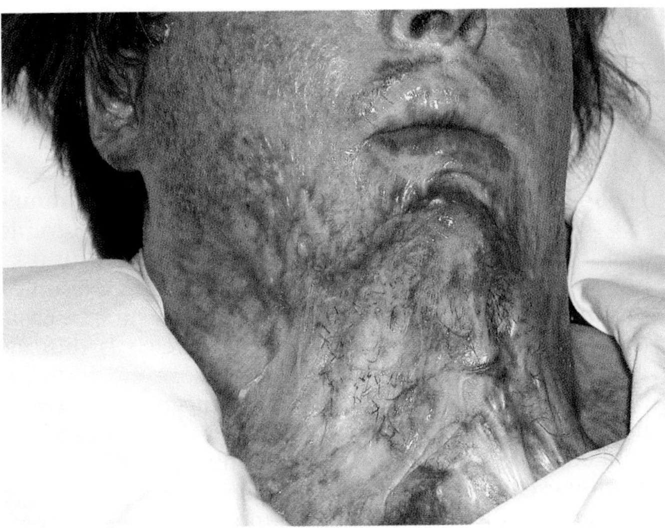

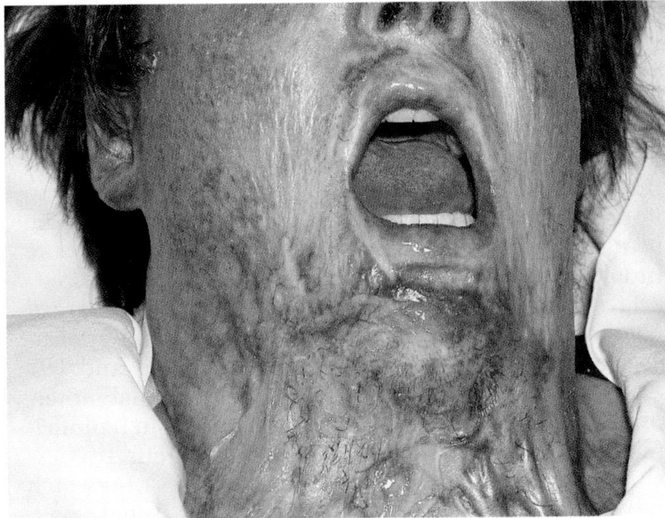

FIGURE 26-8 Hypertrophic scarring.

might be concerned regarding the potential development of osteonecrosis of the jaw with bisphosphonate administration, but this complication has been described primarily in individuals receiving zoledronate or pamidronate, and in the setting of cancer treatment. No osteonecrosis has been reported in osteoporosis trials using risedronate or alendronate.[113] If used, therapies should be maintained in limbs affected by HO, and surgical resection should be considered when the bone is mature. HO can restrict the performance of activities of daily living or result in neurovascular compromise. Particularly of concern is loss of ulnar nerve function at the elbow.

Recurrence is common, even after resection and the use of postoperative continuous passive motion. Surgical resection, however, might have to be delayed in burns compared with other diagnoses to allow for adequate soft tissue coverage in the proposed surgical site.[64] The timing of surgical resection is made based on the severity of functional deficit.

Hypertrophic Scarring

Hypertrophic scarring is the most common complication after burn injury, with a prevalence of 67%.[18] Hypertrophic scarring, such as keloids, is a dermatoproliferative disorder. Hypertrophic scars are raised, red, painful, pruritic, and contractile and stay within the margins of the original injury.[38,39] Keloid scars have some of the same characteristics as hypertrophic scars, but they also extend beyond the original injury and invade into local soft tissues.[124] Hypertrophic burn scars tend to develop in the first few months of injury, while increasing in volume and erythema. After several months, they can regress, becoming less erythematous and flatter, but the skin never returns to its original state. Although there have been some advances in the prediction of wound healing, there is no accurate predictor of who will develop hypertrophic burn scars.[115] Younger individuals, particularly adolescents, and those with darker skin pigmentation tend to have a higher incidence of hypertrophic scarring. Wounds with a prolonged inflammatory wound healing phase and those that are open longer than 3 weeks are more likely to develop hypertrophic scars (Figure 26-8).[7]

One of the limitations of studying hypertrophic burn scarring is the lack of a widely accepted animal model for burn scarring. Although some progress has been made in creating thick scars in an excisional porcine wound model, there are no well-validated scar models in other species.[40] Despite this, some progress has been made in the understanding of the development of hypertrophic burn scars. A key signal in scar development appears to be transforming growth factor-β (TGF-β).[143] TGF-β is a ubiquitous protein and part of a larger family of proteins known as bone morphogenic proteins. It exists in a latent form that can be activated through a variety of inflammatory signals. TGF-β acts through a dimerized cell membrane receptor that activates the Smad signaling proteins to increase the expression of proteins related to increased extracellular matrix production.[152] Beyond local inflammatory signals, there are also likely to be systemic effects on the development of hypertrophic burn scars, from bone marrow–derived fibrocytes that become present in burn wounds and scars. Over time, fibroblasts can develop an autocrine feedback loop between TGF-β and the Smad proteins that might perpetuate the excessive production of extracellular matrix.[145,152] The overexpression of extracellular matrix alone does not entirely account for the development of hypertrophic scars. A balance of both extracellular matrix formation and remodeling of the matrix and new skin is necessary for normal wound healing. In dermatoproliferative disorders, an imbalance in both production and breakdown is present. Important components in the balance of burn scarring are likely to be also derived from keratinocyte signals.[52] As an example, keratinocyte-derived stratifin has been demonstrated to activate matrix metalloproteinases, which can be an important component of extracellular matrix breakdown and reorganization.[52]

Many treatment options are available for addressing the symptoms associated with hypertrophic burn scars, but none completely remove the scar. The best treatment is to prevent the scar through adequate wound care. When scars are present, early and aggressive treatment is indicated. The first-line treatment for any burn scar is regular moisturizer cream, applied several (four to six) times per day, avoidance of mechanical insults, and the minimization of direct heat and sun exposure.[13] Deficiencies in skin, such as sweat and sebaceous glands, can cause scars to be dry and pruritic, and a moisturizer cream is helpful in managing these problems. Individuals with burn scars should also be instructed to minimize direct sunlight and heat exposure through the use of clothing and sunscreen.[156]

Pressure garments have been used in burn scar treatment for decades. They are thought to improve the appearance of burn scars by making the scar flatter and less erythematous and by offering some environmental protection.[139] Some evidence exists that pressure aids in remodeling hypertrophic burn scars. The overall clinical effectiveness is controversial, however; and in metaanalyses of research into pressure garment use, the overall effect seems small, with minor benefits on scar height but not necessarily on secondary measures of scar.[6] If they are used, pressure garments should be prescribed with monitoring by the rehabilitation physician or therapist, for adequate fit and wear tolerance, because friction in the garment can create or perpetuate superficial wounds in the burn scar.

Silicone gel sheeting can also be used alone or in combination with pressure garments. If worn for 12 to 24 hours per day, silicone is thought to change hypertrophic burn scars through a combination of temperature and perfusion changes.[94] Some evidence exists that silicone sheeting might be helpful in improving the volume in hypertrophic burn scars.[92] Reviews note, however, that the evidence is weak for the use of silicone sheeting in the treatment or prevention of hypertrophic burn scars.[99]

Intralesional corticosteroid injection can also be of some benefit in the treatment of hypertrophic burn scars.[76] The injections are done with an injection tangential to the skin. The injection is usually painful, particularly when used on the face, and force is necessary to infiltrate the injectate into the fibrotic scar tissue. A combination of triamcinolone with other agents, such as 5-fluorouracil, or the addition of a second modality, such as pulsed dye laser treatment, may be considered to potentiate the effects of the intralesional steroid.[9]

The use of pulsed dye laser in the treatment of hypertrophic scars is controversial. In some studies the use of laser resulted in the formation of new wounds and little clinically relevant benefit in the scar,[4,20] whereas other studies have shown benefit with this type of laser for the treatment of burn-related hyperpigmentation. Pulsed dye laser appears to have some benefits compared with carbon dioxide or argon lasers, which have also been used to attempt to obliterate hypertrophic scars and keloids. Significant scar recurrence with carbon dioxide laser has been described.[9] The use of pulsed dye laser in burn scar treatment is not yet routine in most North American burn centers. Some preclinical evidence supports the effect of interferon-α as a promising treatment for hypertrophic burn scars, but larger human studies have yet to be done.[144]

Massage is routinely applied to hypertrophic burn scars, although the evidence for its effectiveness is lacking.[28] Massage of hypertrophic burn scars can be applied by the therapist or individual, but the skin must be monitored for potential development of pain and superficial wounds in the scar.[103]

Contractures

Contracture after burn injury is common, with the shoulder, elbow, and knee being the most common joints affected in individuals discharged from the burn unit.[122] The contractures seen in burn scars might be as a result of the effect of myofibroblasts and free actin in the scar. Basic research on the mechanical effects of stretch is difficult to translate into clinical practice because small forces observed in the in vitro setting would suggest that stretching can increase the risk of contracture.[68,78] The large forces applied through splinting, positioning, and range-of-motion exercise, however, can likely overcome the changes seen at the cellular level to give a more acceptable clinical outcome.

The appropriate positioning for burned individuals has been described in an attempt to minimize burn scar contracture development (Figure 26-9). More burn centers are making use of appropriate positioning and splinting in the acute care setting.[148] Because any anatomic site can be affected by burn injury, however, there is a need for a number of different devices. The specific features of any particular burn splint can vary significantly between centers and individual therapists.[114]

There might be concerns regarding the application of splints in areas of an acute burn wound because of the unknown effect on the wound. In the acute setting, however, an affected area can be splinted while the individual is either sedated or asleep in an effort to minimize edema. A wrist and hand splint can be used to minimize

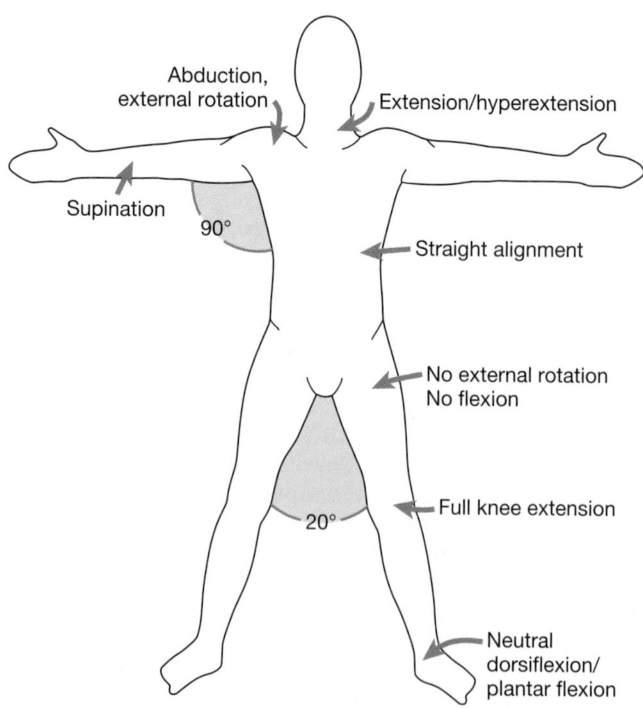

FIGURE 26-9 Suggested positioning guidelines to prevent contracture.

the "intrinsic minus" position. When the individual's mental status improves, the burned regions can be maintained in splints in positions of function during periods of sleep or sedation, and removed for wound checks and active motion. Splints for the "position of function" can be safely applied even over fresh skin grafts. A variety of splinting materials and techniques are available, none of which has been shown to be superior to others.[67,114]

Because of the frequency of axillary contractures, special consideration for the positioning and splinting of the axilla is warranted. Evidence supports early splinting and therapy for deep burns of the axilla to prevent contracture formation.[141] Concern exists that positioning the axilla in greater than 90 degrees of abduction can result in brachial plexopathy; however, this complication has infrequently been described. The shoulder can likely be safely positioned in 90 degrees of flexion with 10 degrees or less of horizontal adduction to take any potential stress off of the brachial plexus.

Burn Scar Pruritus

Another clinical feature of burn scars is the onset of pruritus in the subacute (>3 months postburn) period. The exact mechanism of burn scar pruritus is not clear, but it might be related to increased mast cell and histamine presence in the burn scar.[32] Increased nerve endings and substance P can also add to both the inflammatory state of the immature hypertrophic burn scar and the pruritic nature of scarring.[123] A variety of local and systemic treatments for pruritic burn scars are available. A topical moisturizer should be applied to all burned areas several times per day. For small regions of pruritic burn scar, topical treatments, such as colloidal oatmeal, and topical creams, such as diphenhydramine, doxepin, and gabapentin, can be helpful. Oral diphenhydramine, selective antihistamines, doxepin, hydroxyzine, and gabapentin have all shown some efficacy for large regions of burn scar.[13] Some studies show some evidence for the use of naltrexone as an antihistamine antipruritic agent.[80] Nonpharmacologic treatments with some evidence for efficacy include laser, massage, and transcutaneous nerve stimulation; however, the evidence for efficacy is not as strong as for the pharmacologic approaches.[13]

Scar Measurement

A problem for clinicians and researchers is an adequate tool for the measurement of hypertrophic burn scars. A commonly applied tool for scar measurement is the modified Vancouver Scar Scale, a subjective measurement made by a clinician that scores a scar in four domains: pliability, height, vascularity, and pigmentation.[12] Although the modified Vancouver Scar Scale can be applied quickly to measure scars, the subjective nature of the scale results in questionable validity compared with measures such as volume.[95,96] A variety of other measures can be used in assessing the characteristics of a hypertrophic scar. Ideally, a measurement tool for a hypertrophic scar would assess the volume, pliability, and color of the scar. No single instrument can provide quantitative measurements of each of these characteristics.

Scar pliability can be measured with a Cutometer, which is a device that measures deformity in the scar by applying a negative pressure to the scar through an aperture in a wand attachment. Scar pliability is then measured by an optical system that quantifies the amount of skin or scar brought up by the vacuum device. A Mexameter can be used to measure the pigmentation and vascularity of a scar. This device measures reflected light at specified wavelengths to quantify the amount of erythema as determined by the presence of hemoglobin and pigmentation as measured by the light absorbed by melanin.[95,96] Transcutaneous ultrasound can provide measurements of scar thickness. A maximum thickness can be generated by measuring the distance from the echogenic components of skin and scar and the hypoechogenic subcutaneous fat.[95,96] Each of these measurement tools has been shown to have superior interrater reliability than the modified Vancouver Scar Scale, but there are limitations to the use of these instruments. An upper limit exists on measurement with the Cutometer in very hard tissues that can be seen in a hypertrophic scar.[95,96] The erythema index used in the Mexameter might not discriminate well between normal skin and a hypertrophic scar.[96] More objective measures of scars will be important for future scar research.

Inpatient Rehabilitation Admission for Burned Individuals

Some individuals require admission to an inpatient rehabilitation facility (IRF) to maximize function. Individuals who are admitted to IRFs tend to be older individuals and have larger burn injuries (>40% TBSA burned).[127] A majority of burn centers have reported facilities available for both inpatient and outpatient burn rehabilitation services. Specialized rehabilitation units in the acute care setting have been shown to reduce length of hospital stay and improve function.[34] Centers that have a medium to high volume of annual admissions (20+ or 100+) have a significantly higher proportion of uncomplicated discharges to home than small-volume centers.[100] Although burn injury is a qualifying diagnosis for inpatient rehabilitation, it is unknown whether burned individuals are sometimes discharged to nursing homes, even though inpatient rehabilitation might be more appropriate. This may be explained by limited local resources or a shortage of physiatrists with experience in managing burn survivors.

The Functional Independence Measure (FIM) has been used to decide who to admit to inpatient rehabilitation and to describe changes during burn rehabilitation. An FIM score in the acute care setting of less than 110 has been associated with admission to an IRF.[26] In other studies using FIM as an outcome measure, however, admission FIM scores have ranged from means of 64.6 to 93.0, discharge FIM scores have ranged from means of 90.8 to 113.0, and mean days length of stay in rehabilitation has varied between 23.0 and 78.6.[129] Although FIM is used in most IRFs, it has not been shown to correlate with the size of burn injury, and the cognitive subdomain of the instrument might not be sensitive to change in burn injury.[127]

BOX 26-1

Risk Factors for Development of Depression in Burn Survivors

- Preburn affective disorders (mood disorders)
- Coping styles (adult individuals who engage in both avoidance and approach strategies of coping report greater symptoms of depression compared with those who use only one of these or other alternative strategies)
- Demographic characteristics, such as female sex
- Burn injury characteristics, such as individuals with head or neck burns
- Disposition variables, such as longer hospital stays

BOX 26-2

Risk Factors for Posttraumatic Stress Disorder Following Burn Injury

- Preburn characteristics
  - Personality
  - History of alcohol and substance abuse disorders
  - History of depression and other affective disorders
- Acute stress symptoms
- Anxiety related to pain
- Type and severity of baseline symptoms of posttraumatic stress disorder
- Injury characteristics
- Female sex
- Visibility of burn injury
- Social support
- Coping strategies

Other outcome measures have been developed and refined specific to burn injury, such as the Burn-Specific Health Scale, but there is ongoing development in creating outcome measures for burned individual rehabilitation.[49]

Psychosocial Adjustment

Comprehensive interdisciplinary rehabilitation treatment of burn injuries should focus on both physical and psychological complications.[41] Burn injury survivors are at risk of developing psychopathologies, such as depression and anxiety disorders.[140] Depression and anxiety disorders are reported to be the most prevalent (25% to 65%) in burn survivors during the first year after injury.[90,104] The largest prospective cohort study of individuals with burn injury[48] found that clinically significant psychological distress is common and tends to persist for at least 2 years postburn injury in this population.

No psychological treatment studies for depression in adult burn survivors have been published.[44] A wide discrepancy exists in the prevalence rates of depression reported across studies. Ptacek et al.[111] found a 53% prevalence rate of moderate to severe symptoms of depression within 3 days of inpatient admission, which decreased to 35% by day 5 and to 15% by day 10. Mild to moderate symptoms of depression among burn injury survivors was found to vary between 23% and 26% during hospitalization, at 1 week postdischarge and at 2 months postdischarge.[137] Although most symptoms were reported to subside after the first year postinjury,[104,140] a follow-up study[150] found a 53% prevalence rate of moderate to severe symptoms of depression at 1 month postinjury, 34% at 1 year, and 45% at 2 years postinjury. Inhospital depression was found to predict change in physical health after burn injury.[137] It is important to screen individuals for depression and acute stress disorder, both inhospital and during rehabilitation after discharge, as depression can have a negative impact on recovery.[137] A list of risk factors for development of depression in burn survivors is presented in Box 26-1.[44,47,48,150]

PTSD is now classified under the trauma-related and stressor-related disorders in which exposure to a traumatic or stressful event is listed explicitly as a diagnostic criterion.[1] The prevalence rates for PTSD among burn injury survivors, excluding the duration criterion, were found to be 11% to 25% when validated assessment methods were used, and the rates ranged from 20% to 45% in studies using validated structured clinical interviews.[44] A summary of identified risk factors for developing PTSD following a burn injury[44,47,48,140] is presented in Box 26-2.

No criteria exist for determining clinically significant levels of body image distress in burned individuals.[44] Predictors of poorer body image include burn characteristics, social and emotional variables,[82] and coping style.[46] Lawrence et al.[83] found that issues related to appearance and attractiveness are more important among female burn survivors, and body image esteem is lower among female burn survivors. Another study by Thombs et al.[138] found that female sex, TBSA burn, and importance of appearance predicted body image dissatisfaction. Body image dissatisfaction increased for women and individuals with larger burns from hospitalization up to a year, and body image dissatisfaction predicted psychosocial function at 1 year. Lawrence et al.[82] found that psychological variables, such as depression, self-acceptance, and social comfort, to be more important than burn severity and scar location in predicting body esteem. Young burn survivors appear to cope well in comparison with their normal peers, and in some areas can be coping better and reporting better body esteem.[83,110] Routine psychological screening for body image distress during hospitalization and after discharge is important.[138]

The inevitable alteration in body image and subsequent challenge to one's self-esteem is one of the most devastating consequences of a burn injury.[150] An individual's expression of sexuality remains inseparable from body image and self-esteem.[149] It is a complex human phenomenon that encompasses a broad range of feelings and behaviors and is more than just physical sexual behavior.[87] Disfiguring scars affect sexuality, as hypertrophic burn scars cause alterations in skin sensitivity.[59] Sexual dysfunction in burned individuals can be related to many factors, including adverse effects of medication, psychopathological and psychodynamic factors, and surgical and pain factors.[31] Assessment of alterations in sexual health is as important as assessments of all other areas of human function,[87] but sexuality concerns of individuals with burns rarely receive attention. Following physiologic stabilization, completing a sexual health history serves to initiate a discussion of this delicate issue.[150] Sexual health promotion and peer counseling are two types of interventions described in the literature.[140] The treatment of individuals with burns should provide the possibility of a therapeutic dialogue regarding sexuality. If that is not possible for any reason, however, the individual should be referred to a specialized counselor, sexologist, or psychiatrist as appropriate.[17] It is important for the burn team to be aware that pediatric survivors of burns, even when appearing to be adjusting well, can harbor grave self-deprecating feelings.[2] Other helpful avenues valuable for exchanging information and experience[17] include self-help groups, face-to-face peer counseling, or professionally facilitated self-help by mail.[24]

Community Reintegration

The long-term psychosocial adaptation of burn survivors depends largely on their successful reintegration into community life.[15] Community reintegration is an important aspect of every burn rehabilitation program[44] because the ultimate goal is to return the individual as close as possible to preinjury life (work, school, home, recreational, and community activities). Burn survivors have difficulty in the area of home integration, social integration, and productivity.[43] Because a large number of burn injuries happen either at work or to individuals of working age, return to work is of particular concern for the individual and the burn rehabilitation team. People with burn injuries who were employed at the time of injury are more likely to sustain hand burns and have hand surgery than the unemployed.[43] The size of the burn is inversely related to the probability of returning to work and most burn survivors are able to return to work at an average of 17 weeks postinjury.[22] A study identifying barriers to return to work after burn injuries found that although approximately 80% of individuals had returned to work by 1 year, over 30% of them had long-term disabilities.[41] Risk factors[22,121] for longer time off from work (or no return to work) and barriers[41,121] to return to work following a major burn injury are listed in Box 26-3.

BOX 26-3

Risk Factors and Barriers to Return to Work Following Major Burn Injury

Risk Factors

- Preburn psychiatric history
- Extremity burns
- Electrical etiology
- Longer stay at hospital
- Burn injury occurred at work

Barriers

- Wound issues
- Neurologic problems
- Physical abilities, impaired mobility
- Working conditions (temperature, humidity, and safety)
- Psychosocial factors
  - Drug and alcohol dependence
  - Insomnia
  - Depression
  - Posttraumatic stress (nightmares, flashbacks)
  - Anxiety
  - Appearance issues and concerns over body image

Early identification of those at risk for prolonged unemployment, referral to comprehensive rehabilitative services that include work hardening and vocational training programs, assessment of the workplace, and identification of appropriate workplace accommodations are important steps to facilitate a quicker and successful return to work.[41,121]

In school-aged individuals surviving burn injuries, returning to school is an important indicator of functional aptitude and emotional adjustment.[27] Male gender, age, and length of hospitalization were found to be significantly associated with longer time to return to school. The average time to school reentry was 10.5 days.[27]

Every person who has been touched by the experience of facial disfigurement (survivors, family members, or professionals caring for these individuals) is well aware of the challenges encountered in the course of daily life.[110] Burn injury survivors report that the single most important issue is the social anxiety and social strain accompanying community integration.[15] A study[101] investigating psychosocial adjustment of individuals 5 years after their burn injury found social reintegration of burn survivors with poor physical function unsuccessful, with feelings of social isolation, increased depression, and loss in circle of friends. Individuals with clearly apparent burn scars appeared less frequently in public, and also reported significant impairments in sexuality.[101] Social introversion is significantly associated with the development of burn-related pathologic feelings of shame.[133] Problems with social interaction include difficulties in meeting new people, making friends, and developing intimate relationships.[102,116] Commonly reported reactions in public include stares, startle reactions, remarks, and personal questions.[89,129] In the area of social adjustment, social skills training should be considered as a promising intervention to prevent social anxiety among those who suffer from interpersonal difficulties.[16,104] There are two well-known programs developed in the area of social skills training that include life skills for children, young people, adults, and families to develop self-confidence and self-esteem. (1) A program developed by *Changing Faces*[102] includes practicing skills such as the "3-2-1 Go" and includes strategies such as *3* things to do if someone stares at them, *2* things to say if someone asks what happened, and *1* thing to think if someone turns away. In addition to several informational booklets, there is a video entitled *REACH OUT* (acronym for *R*eassurance, *E*ffort, *A*ssertiveness, *C*ourage, *H*umor, *O*ver There [Distraction], *U*nderstanding, and *T*ry Again) that shows a variety of communication skills to help people cope with self-consciousness and other people's reactions to their appearance. (2) The second program, called *Beyond Surviving: Tools for Thriving After Burn Injury*, developed by The Phoenix Society for Burn Survivors, offers behavioral and enhancement skills training; life strategies to be comfortable, confident, and competent in any social, work, or school situation. Programs, such as social skills training, are now increasingly offered in major burn centers and are perceived to be of great value in facilitating successful community reentry. Another intervention is *Survivors Offering Assistance in Recovery* (SOAR), a volunteer peer support program (also developed and standardized by the Phoenix Society for Burn Survivors) that provides training to burn survivors or their family members who want to volunteer to help others whose lives have been touched by a burn injury.

The recommendations from the Psychological Outcomes Consensus Committee of the American Burn Association published in 2013[53] include the following: all inpatients should be screened for depressive and acute stress disorder (ASD) symptoms within 48 hours of accessibility (e.g., delirium cleared) at least once before discharge; all outpatients should be screened for depressive and ASD/PTSD symptoms at their first clinic visit after discharge and as indicated further; and verified burn centers should demonstrate that they have a referral process in place for an appropriate intervention by a licensed mental health physician should the individual screen positive for depressive, ASD, or PTSD symptoms. Establishment of such quality metrics for psychological outcomes after burn injuries will help establish an evidence base for raising the standard of psychosocial care for burn survivors and is clearly a movement in the right direction.

KEY REFERENCES

6. Anzarut A, Olson J, Singh P, et al: The effectiveness of pressure garment therapy for the prevention of abnormal scarring after burn injury: a meta-analysis, *J Plast Reconstr Aesthet Surg* 62:77–84, Elsevier Sci Ltd, 2009.
7. Armour A, Scott PG, Tredget EE: Cellular and molecular pathology of HTS: basis for treatment, *Wound Repair Regen* 15:S6–S17, 2007.
8. Arnoldo BD, Purdue GF, Kowalske K, et al: Electrical injuries: a 20-year review, *J Burn Care Rehabil* 25:479–484, 2004.
11. Atiyeh BS, Gunn SWA, Dibo SA: Metabolic implications of severe burn injuries and their management: a systematic review of the literature, *World J Surg* 32:1857–1869, 2008.
12. Baryza MJ, Baryza GA: The Vancouver Scar Scale: an administration tool and its interrater reliability, *J Burn Care Rehabil* 16:535–538, 1995.
13. Bell PL, Gabriel V: Evidence based review for the treatment of post-burn pruritus, *J Burn Care Res* 30:55–61, 2009.
22. Brych SB, Engrav LH, Rivara FP, et al: Time off work and return to work rates after burns: systematic review of the literature and a large two-center series, *J Burn Care Rehabil* 22:401–405, 2001.
25. Chan MM, Chan GM: Nutritional therapy for burns in children and adults, *Nutrition* 25:261–269, 2009.
29. Crandall CG, Davis SL: Cutaneous vascular and sudomotor responses in human skin grafts, *J Appl Physiol* 109:1524–1530, 2010.
33. Demling RH, Seigne P: Metabolic management of individuals with severe burns, *World J Surg* 24:673–680, 2000.
34. DeSanti L, Lincoln L, Egan F, Demling R: Development of a burn rehabilitation unit: impact on burn center length of stay and functional outcome, *J Burn Care Rehabil* 19:414–419, 1998.
38. Engrav LH, Garner WL, Tredget EE: Hypertrophic scar, wound contraction and hyper-hypopiginentation, *J Burn Care Res* 28:593–597, 2007.
39. Esselman PC: Burn rehabilitation: an overview, *Arch Phys Med Rehabil* 88:S3–S6, 2007.
40. Esselman PC, Askay SW, Carrougher GJ, et al: Barriers to return to work after burn injuries, *Arch Phys Med Rehabil* 88:S50–S56, 2007.
41. Esselman PC, Ptacek JT, Kowalske K, et al: Community integration after burn injuries, *J Burn Care Rehabil* 22:221–227, 2001.
43. Fauerbach JA, Engrav L, Kowalske K, et al: Barriers to employment among working-aged individuals with major burn injury, *J Burn Care Rehabil* 22:26–34, 2001.
48. Fauerbach JA, McKibben J, Bienvenu OJ, et al: Psychological distress after major burn injury, *Psychosom Med* 69:473–482, 2007.
51. Gabriel V, Kowalske KJ, Holavanahalli RK: Assessment of recovery from burn-related neuropathy by electrodiagnostic testing, *J Burn Care Res* 30:668–693, 2009.
53. Gibran NS, Wiechman S, Meyer W, et al: American Burn Association consensus statements, *J Burn Care Res* 34:361–385, 2013.
59. Herndon DN, Hart DW, Wolf SE, et al: Reversal of catabolism by beta-blockade after severe burns, *N Engl J Med* 345:1223–1229, 2001.
64. Hunt JL, Arnoldo BD, Kowalske K, et al: Heterotopic ossification revisited: a 21-year surgical experience, *J Burn Care Res* 27:535–540, 2006.
70. Karlsson M, Lindgren M, Jarnhed-Andersson I, Tarpila E: Dressing the split-thickness skin graft donor site: a randomized clinical trial, *Adv Skin Wound Care* 27:20–25, 2014.
71. Kessides MC, Skelsey MK: Management of acute partial-thickness bums, *Cutis* 86:249–257, 2010.
75. Klein MB, Logsetty S, Costa B, et al: Extended time to wound closure is associated with increased risk of heterotopic ossification of the elbow, *J Burn Care Res* 28:447–450, 2007.
77. Kowalske K, Holavanahalli R, Helm P: Neuropathy after burn injury, *J Burn Care Rehabil* 22:353–357, 2001.
81. Lawrence JW, Fauerbach JA, Heinberg L, Doctor M: Visible vs hidden scars and their relation to body esteem, *J Burn Care Rehabil* 25:25–32, 2004.
82. Lawrence JW, Fauerbach JA, Thombs BD: A test of the moderating role of importance of appearance in the relationship between perceived scar severity and body-esteem among adult burn survivors, *Body Image* 3:101–111, 2006.
83. Lawrence JW, Rosenberg LE, Fauerbach JA: Comparing the body esteem of pediatric survivors of burn injury with the body esteem of an age-matched comparison group without burns, *Rehabil Psychol* 52:370–379, 2007.
85. Lee JO, Benjamin D, Herndon DN: Nutrition support strategies for severely burned individuals, *Nutr Clin Pract* 20:325–330, 2005.
86. Lee MY, Liu G, Kowlowitz V, et al: Causative factors affecting peripheral neuropathy in burn individuals, *Burns* 35:412–416, 2009.
89. Macgregor FC: Facial disfigurement: problems and management of social interaction and implications for mental health, *Aesthetic Plast Surg* 14:249–257, 1990.
90. Malt U: Long-term psychosocial follow-up studies of burned adults—review of the literature, *Burns* 6:190–197, 1980.
95. Nedelec B, Correa JA, Rachelska G, et al: Quantitative measurement of hypertrophic scar: interrater reliability and concurrent validity, *J Burn Care Res* 29:501–511, 2008.
96. Nedelec B, Correa JA, Rachelska G, et al: Quantitative measurement of hypertrophic scar: intrarater reliability, sensitivity, and specificity, *J Burn Care Res* 29:489–500, 2008.
99. Orgill DP: Excision and skin grafting of thermal burns, *N Engl J Med* 360:893–901, 2009.
101. Pallua N, Kunsebeck HW, Noah EM: Psychosocial adjustments 5 years after burn injury, *Burns* 29:143–152, 2003.
105. Peck MD: Epidemiology of burns throughout the world. Part I: distribution and risk factors, *Burns* 37:1087–1100, 2011.
106. Peck MD: Epidemiology of burns throughout the World. Part II: intentional burns in adults, *Burns* 38:630–637, 2012.
108. Pereira C, Murphy K, Herndon D: Outcome measures in burn care: is mortality dead?, *Burns* 30:761–771, 2004.
114. Richard R, Ward RS: Splinting strategies and controversies, *J Burn Care Rehabil* 26:392–396, 2005.
116. Robinson E, Rumsey N, Partridge J: An evaluation of the impact of social interaction skills training for facially disfigured people, *Br J Plast Surg* 49:281–289, 1996.
121. Schneider JC, Bassi S, Ryan CM: Barriers impacting employment after burn injury, *J Burn Care Res* 30:294–300, 2009.
122. Schneider JC, Holavanahalli R, Heim P, et al: Contractures in burn injury: defining the problem, *J Burn Care Res* 27:508–514, 2006.
125. Shankowsky HA, Callioux LS, Tredget EE: North American survey of hydrotherapy in modern burn care, *J Burn Care Rehabil* 15:143–146, 1994.
129. Spires MC, Bowden ML, Ahrns KS, Wahl WL: Impact of an inpatient rehabilitation facility on functional outcome and length of stay of burn survivors, *J Burn Care Rehabil* 26:532–538, 2005.
140. Van Loey NE, Van Song MJ: Psychopathology and psychological problems in individuals with burn scars: epidemiology and management, *Am J Clin Dermatol* 4:245–272, 2003.

147. Wasiak J, Cleland H, Campbell F, Spinks A: Dressings for superficial and partial thickness burns, *Cochrane Database Syst Rev* (3):CD002106, 2008.
150. Wiechman SA, Ptacek JT, Patterson DR, et al: Rates, trends, and severity of depression after burn injuries, *J Burn Care Rehabil* 22:417–424, 2001.
151. Wolf SE, Edelman LS, Kemalyan N, et al: Effects of oxandrolone on outcome measures in the severely burned: a multicenter prospective randomized double-blind trial, *J Burn Care Res* 27:131–139, 2006.
154. Zafren K: Frostbite: prevention and initial management, *High Alt Med Biol* 14:9–12, 2013.

The full reference list for this chapter is available online.

CHAPTER 27

ACUTE MEDICAL CONDITIONS

Matthew Bartels, David Z. Prince

Medical rehabilitation medicine needs to encompass the needs of patients with cardiopulmonary disorders as well as patients with debility and renal dysfunction. There are ever greater numbers of patients who are now presenting with these issues, especially as the population ages. Cardiac disease is still the number one cause of mortality and disability in the United States, with chronic obstructive pulmonary disease now being the third leading cause of mortality.[87] Even if it is not primary rehabilitation for patients with these diseases, many patients with other disabilities will have cardiac, pulmonary, and renal disabilities, and a common theme among all of these conditions is a degree of frailty.

This issue of frailty underlies a great number of the common features of disability in these underlying conditions and will be discussed in the section on frailty. Key areas that will be addressed include sarcopenia, acute and chronic deconditioning, and the role of exercise as medicine to improve patients with all of these conditions.

Important contributors to the prevalence of all of these conditions are the aging of the population as well as the effects of combinations of these conditions on the ability to rehabilitate patients. The overall approaches to exercise treatment in these patients will be discussed and also how to approach these conditions in the acute, rehabilitation, and outpatient settings.

Cardiopulmonary Rehabilitation

It must be remembered that there are two types of cardiopulmonary patients, those with primary cardiac and pulmonary disease who need cardiac/pulmonary rehabilitation and those patients with other disabilities who have a cardiac or pulmonary secondary disability. Patients with respiratory failure and patients who have need for ventilatory support are also in this group but are beyond the scope of this chapter. Dual disability patients are more prevalent than ever in rehabilitation because more patients are now older and have multiple comorbidities. Many patients with stroke, vascular disease, or other conditions can be included in active cardiac and pulmonary rehabilitation programs or benefit from the application of cardiopulmonary rehabilitation principles to their rehabilitation. Remember also that cardiopulmonary rehabilitation is one of the most underused yet most effective treatments for patients with cardiopulmonary disease. Because we work with frail older adults and other compromised populations, it is important for rehabilitation specialists to know how to provide cardiopulmonary rehabilitation in patients with either primary or secondary cardiopulmonary disability.

To use cardiac and pulmonary rehabilitation principles for patients with cardiopulmonary disease, whether it is a primary or secondary disability, it is necessary to review some of the basic principles of cardiac and pulmonary physiology and learn how to apply these principles to improve the exercise capacity of these patients. It is also essential to have an understanding of normal exercise physiology to appreciate the issues of patients with abnormal cardiopulmonary physiology.

Assessment of Cardiopulmonary Function

History and Physical Examination

A complete cardiopulmonary history and physical examination is an essential part of the evaluation of patients with cardiopulmonary disease who participate in rehabilitation. Key parts of the history include both verbal and nonverbal cues and will allow the establishment of goals and improve patient compliance with the treatment program.

History

The history should include emotional state, concurrent illnesses, other disabilities, functional history, occupational history, social history, personal habits, family dynamics, and the effect of disability and cardiopulmonary illness on the patient in the community. Both rest and activity symptoms are reviewed with particular emphasis on the following.[13]

Dyspnea. Shortness of breath is usually the prime complaint for patients with cardiopulmonary disease. The history of dyspnea helps to differentiate the role of cardiac or pulmonary disease in the patient's symptoms. Cardiac dyspnea can be from ischemic heart disease, congestive heart failure, valvular heart disease, and arrhythmias. Pulmonary dyspnea can come from pulmonary vascular disease, restrictive lung disease, and obstructive lung disease. In some patients both cardiac and pulmonary issues may be present, and in all cases physical conditioning needs to be assessed. Because psychological factors are also important, patients should also be screened for anxiety and depression. Finally, an assessment for hypoxemia should be done. See Table 27-1 for a list of common causes of dyspnea.

Chest Pain. Chest pain and tightness is not only a mark of coronary insufficiency but can also be seen with valvular heart disease or arrhythmia. Assessing the duration, quality, provocation, location of the pain, and any ameliorating factors can help assess functional limitations and help design the appropriate therapy program. In addition, Lung conditions can cause chest pressure in both obstructive and

Table 27-1 Causes of Dyspnea

	Site of Pathology	Pathophysiology
Pulmonary Causes		
Airflow limitation	Airways	Limitation to ventilation through flow through airways
Restriction (intrinsic)	Lung parenchyma	Poor lung compliance
Restriction (extrinsic)	Chest wall	Poor chest wall compliance with or without poor chest wall strength
Acute pulmonary disease	Lungs	Increased ventilation/perfusion (V/Q) mismatch
Cardiac Causes		
Valvular disease	Heart valve stenosis or incompetence	Limited cardiac output
Coronary disease	Heart muscle ischemia	Coronary insufficiency leads to myocardial ischemia
Heart failure	Ventricular failure	Limited cardiac output from decreased stroke volume
Circulatory		
Anemia	Low hemoglobin can be from blood loss or from hemoglobinopathies	Limited oxygen-carrying capacity
Peripheral circulation	Peripheral arterial disease	Inadequate oxygen supply to metabolically active tissues, leading to early anaerobic threshold
Whole Body		
Obesity	Excess adipose tissue with associated physiologic changes	Increased work of movement, decreased efficiency May have respiratory restriction if severe—both extrinsic chest wall restriction and upper airway obstruction
Psychogenic	Emotional	Hyperventilation, anxiety
Deconditioning	Multiple organ systems, muscle weakness, cardiac deconditioning	Loss of ability to effectively distribute systemic blood flow, inefficient aerobic metabolism
Malingering	Emotional	Inconsistent results

restrictive lung disease, and is very common in pulmonary vascular disease.

Palpitations. Symptoms of palpitations can be indicative of serious arrhythmias.

Syncope. Cardiac syncope is usually abrupt with no warning or only a brief warning (with the patient feeling as if he or she were about to pass out) and can be caused by aortic stenosis, idiopathic hypertrophic subaortic stenosis, primary pulmonary hypertension, hypercarbia, hypoxemia, ventricular arrhythmias, reentrant arrhythmias, high-degree atrioventricular block, or sick sinus syndrome. Pulmonary syncope is often gradual in onset and can be caused by hypercarbia, hypoxemia, or pulmonary vascular disease. Orthostatic syncope can be caused by autonomic dysfunction, neurologic disease, vagal stimuli, or psychological stimuli.

Edema. Peripheral edema may be an indication of heart failure and may indicate the onset of right ventricular failure in pulmonary vascular disease.

Fatigue. Fatigue is likely to be the most common complaint in cardiopulmonary disease and may be worsened by the presence of depression, physical exhaustion, medication side effects, and deconditioning.

Cough. Cough can be from both cardiac and pulmonary diseases. "Cardiac" cough is often nocturnal and postural, with little to no sputum production, relieved by assuming an upright position. Cough is common in both restrictive and interstitial lung disease, with or without sputum production.

Physical Examination

A description of the complete and detailed physical examination of the patient with cardiopulmonary disease is beyond the scope of this chapter. Still, some important elements of the examination include a general survey of the patient for exophthalmos (possible thyrotoxicosis), xanthelasma (hypercholesterolemia), acrocyanosis (chronic hypoxemia), clubbing (chronic hypoxemia), ankylosis (aortic valve disease and conduction defects), Down syndrome (cardiac abnormalities), myasthenia gravis, or neuromuscular disease (cardiomyopathy, conduction disease, and ventilatory failure). A good cardiopulmonary examination and history can help to prevent complications in a cardiopulmonary rehabilitation program and should be done as a part of the physiatrist's initial history and physical examination.

A few key cardiopulmonary examination findings are highlighted here.

Cardiac auscultation can indicate an atrial septal defect, a midsystolic click may indicate mitral valve prolapse, and a murmur may indicate valvular heart disease. Pulmonary hypertension typically produces a heightened second heart sound, a noncompliant ventricle can be detected via an atrial gallop at the cardiac apex, and a left ventricular gallop may reveal heart failure. The pulse contour, split heart sounds, and the quality of the murmur can help differentiate aortic sclerosis from aortic stenosis. In younger patients, pulmonary stenosis or valvular heart disease needs to be differentiated from idiopathic hypertrophic subaortic stenosis. Diastolic murmurs may be mitral stenosis or pulmonary hypertension with pulmonary valve regurgitation, and continuous murmurs may be from ventricular septal or atrial septal defects. New findings or changes in findings are important as they may indicate the need for further evaluation or alterations in the program of cardiopulmonary rehabilitation.

Lung physical examination may have decreased breath sounds and/or barrel chest in obstructive disease, whereas interstitial lung disease may have diffuse or basilar crackles. Inspiratory stridor may indicate upper airway obstruction, whereas expiratory wheezing and rhonchi can be seen with obstruction or secretions. It is also important to assess symmetry of breathing, accessory muscle use, and possible compromise to diaphragmatic function.

Cardiac Anatomy and Physiology

Cardiac Anatomy

To supervise cardiac rehabilitation, it is essential to be familiar with the normal distribution of the major arteries of the heart, the anatomy of the heart valves, and the distribution of ischemia or infarction from the coronary arteries.

The heart has paired atria and ventricles, with deoxygenated venous blood entering the right atrium, traversing the right ventricle through the tricuspid valve, and entering the pulmonary artery through the pulmonic valve. Oxygenated blood enters the left atrium, goes to the left ventricle through the mitral valve, and is ejected into the aorta through the aortic valve. The cardiac valves ensure unidirectional unobstructed flow of blood, with atrial contraction adding up to 15% to 20% to the total cardiac output (CO). Atrial contribution to blood flow is greater with increased heart rate and in conditions with decreased ventricular compliance.[109] Atrial fibrillation can cause a loss of this atrial "kick" and may contribute to cardiac dysfunction.

The cardiac conduction system allows coordinated contraction of the atria and ventricles at a controlled rate. The normal heartbeat is initiated at the *sinoatrial* node and then travels through three atrial internodal pathways to the atrioventricular node where conduction is delayed to cause sequential atrial and ventricular contraction. Below the atrioventricular node, the signal passes into the bundle of His and divides into left and right bundles. All cardiac fibers then end in terminal branches, which excite the myocytes and cause contraction. The conduction system can be injured by myocardial infarction (MI), aging, and other conditions, and can cause heart block or sick sinus syndrome. Accessory pathways that bypass the atrioventricular node can be seen in Wolff-Parkinson-White syndrome.

Variation of Arteries

There are three main distributions of coronary circulation. Normally the left main coronary artery divides into the left anterior descending and the circumflex arteries, whereas the right coronary artery continues on as a single vessel. Right dominant circulation is seen in 60% of individuals, whereas left dominant circulation with the posterior descending artery arising from the left circumflex is seen in 10% to 15% of individuals. The remaining 30% of individuals have balanced circulation with the posterior descending artery coming from the left circumflex and right coronary arteries.[3a]

Cardiac Physiology

Cardiac myocytes extract nearly 65% of oxygen from the blood at all levels of activity (compared with 36% for brain and 26% for the rest of the body). Cardiac myocytes prefer carbohydrates as an energy source (40%), with fatty acids making up most of the remaining 60%. With high oxygen extraction and coronary blood flow only during diastole, the heart is at high risk of ischemic injury, especially in the endocardium. Coronary vasodilation with exercise is normally done via nitric oxide–mediated pathways and increases blood flow with exertion. The goal of most medical and surgical therapies for ischemia is to restore or preserve myocardial perfusion, through vasodilation, bypass, or endovascular procedures. Exercise can increase cardiac collateral circulation and also improve arteriolar vasodilation, and has long been known to be a primary therapy for cardiac ischemia.[73,94,96,121]

Another important issue to manage with patients with cardiac disease is fluid volume. Appropriate venous return can maintain appropriate cardiac "preload," whereas fluid overload can lead to too much venous return and exacerbate heart failure. In cases of mechanical cardiac constriction surgery can restore CO, and in dilated heart failure medical treatment aims to decrease the size of the ventricles to increase CO. In refractory or end-stage disease, left ventricular assist devices (LVADs) and cardiac transplantation are options.

Pulmonary Anatomy and Physiology

Pulmonary Anatomy

Important pulmonary anatomy includes the upper and lower airways (the oropharynx, larynx, trachea, main stem bronchi, and smaller bronchi), the lung parenchyma, the chest wall, and musculature (diaphragm, accessory muscles of breathing, rib cage, and pleura). Pulmonary limitations can come from abnormalities in any of these structures. The lungs also have a dual circulation with pulmonary arteries and veins, which deliver deoxygenated blood to the lungs and deliver oxygenated blood to the left atrium and intrinsic pulmonary artery circulation delivering oxygenated blood to the respiratory tree.

Stridor can result from upper airway obstruction from vocal cord paralysis or tumor, whereas asthma, bronchitis, or reactive airway disease may cause dyspnea from lower airway obstruction. Emphysema is a result of parenchymal lung disease with a loss of alveoli leading to decreased intrinsic recoil of the lung and subsequent hyperinflation and dyspnea. In interstitial lung disease and pulmonary fibrosis, there is interstitial scarring with increased recoil and decreased ability to diffuse oxygen through the lung tissues. In some patients, both restrictive and obstructive diseases can be present with one predominant over another (cystic fibrosis and sarcoidosis). In these cases, it is important to evaluate the lung parenchyma with imaging or physiologic testing (pulmonary function tests) to assess which condition may predominate.[12]

Pulmonary Physiology

Normal breathing is regulated in the medulla oblongata by the respiratory center. Respiratory signals are carried by the phrenic and other somatic nerves to the diaphragm and secondary inspiratory muscles (intercostals, sternocleidomastoids, and pectorals) and cause rhythmic breathing by generating negative pressure in the chest wall. Normal exhalation is passive, resulting from the elastic recoil of the chest wall and the lung parenchyma. Chronic obstructive lung disease (COPD) and emphysema can create the need for active exhalation, markedly increasing the work of breathing. Interstitial lung disease with scarring decreases compliance of lung tissue so severely that lung volumes decrease and hypoventilation can result. Any disease affecting the brain, spine, phrenic nerves, respiratory muscles, or changing the mechanical properties of the chest wall or diaphragm can affect normal respiration.[81,82]

Pulmonary vascular disease can result in either primary or secondary pulmonary hypertension. Primary pulmonary hypertension can be idiopathic or can result from vasculitis, thromboembolic disease, or from intrinsic parenchymal disease. Secondary pulmonary hypertension is from vascular congestion, often a result of left heart failure. Secondary pulmonary hypertension can lead to intrinsic vascular compromise if the condition is chronic. Chronic hypoxemia may also create pulmonary hypertension in individuals with obesity, obstructive sleep apnea, or high-altitude exposure through a mechanism of pulmonary vascular constriction. Chronic hypoxemia can lead to vascular intimal hypertrophy with resultant fixed pulmonary vascular resistance and pulmonary hypertension.

Basic Terminology for Exercise

Aerobic Capacity

Aerobic capacity ($\dot{V}O_2$ max) is the measure of the work capacity of an individual and is expressed as the oxygen consumed by the individual (liters of oxygen per minute or milliliters of oxygen per kilogram per minute). Oxygen consumption ($\dot{V}O_2$) increases linearly with workload, up to the $\dot{V}O_2$ max where it reaches a plateau. Maximal exercise capacity assessment can assist in rating disability and planning exercise and recovery programs.[12]

Heart Rate

Heart rate is a useful guide for exercise as a result of having a linear relationship to $\dot{V}O_2$. Maximum heart rate is best determined by testing and decreases with age. It can be estimated either by the Karvonen equation or by the equation heart rate = 220 − age.[61] Physical conditioning can alter the slope of the relationship of heart rate and $\dot{V}O_2$ with improved conditioning lowering the slope (less heart rate increase for a given $\dot{V}O_2$). A limitation to using heart rate can be the alteration of heart rate response in the setting of medications that alter vagal and sympathetic tone.[12]

Stroke Volume

Stroke volume (SV) is the volume of blood ejected with a left ventricular contraction. Maximal SV can be increased with exercise, is sensitive to postural changes (least increases in supine), with the greatest increase during early exercise. Normally SV increases in a curvilinear manner, achieving maximum at approximately 40% of $\dot{V}O_2$ max. SV declines with advancing age, with decreased cardiac compliance, after MI, and in heart failure.[36]

Cardiac Output

CO is the product of the heart rate and SV. It has a linear relationship with work and is the primary determinant of $\dot{V}O_2$ max. CO is greater in the upright position compared with the supine position.[12]

Myocardial Oxygen Consumption

Myocardial oxygen consumption ($M\dot{V}O_2$) is the oxygen consumption of the heart muscle increasing in proportion to workload. When the $M\dot{V}O_2$ exceeds the maximum coronary artery oxygen delivery, an individual will have myocardial ischemia and angina. The rate pressure product (RPP) = [heart rate × systolic blood pressure (SBP)]/100, and has a direct relationship to the $M\dot{V}O_2$. Another consideration is that arm exercise, isometric exercise, and exertion in the cold, extreme heat, after eating, and after smoking all have a higher $M\dot{V}O_2$ for a given $M\dot{V}O_2$. Supine exercises have a higher $M\dot{V}O_2$ at low intensity and a lower $M\dot{V}O_2$ at high intensity compared with erect exercises.[12]

Basic static lung volumes and dynamic responses to exercise are helpful in the assessment of exercise capacity in individuals with lung disease. Although complete pulmonary function evaluation is beyond the scope of this chapter, some important values include:

- Total lung capacity (TLC): Volume of air in the lungs at full inspiration.
- Vital capacity (VC): Volume of air between full inspiration and full expiration.
- Forced expired vital capacity (FVC): Maximum volume expired after a maximal forced expiration.
- Forced expiratory volume in 1 second (FEV_1): The maximum volume exhaled in 1 second.
- Maximal voluntary ventilation (MVV): Measurement of the maximal ventilation over 15 seconds.
- Residual volume (RV): Volume of the chest wall after a full expiration.
- Tidal volume (TV): The volume of regular resting breath.
- Diffusion of the lung for carbon monoxide (DLCO): Diffusion of carbon monoxide (oxygen analog) across the alveolar membrane.

The best evaluation of the capacity to exercise in cardiac and pulmonary conditions is with a cardiopulmonary exercise test (CPET). The CPET yields diagnostic, prognostic, and exercise prescription guidance in patients with cardiopulmonary disease. The interpretation of pulmonary exercise testing in a number of conditions is shown in Table 27-2.

Table 27-2 Effects of Physiological Conditions on Cardiopulmonary Exercise Capacity

Abnormality	Physiologic Abnormality	Gas Exchange
Obesity	• Increased work with activity • Inefficient exercise	• Rapid alveolar-arterial $p(A\text{-}a)O_2$ fall with exercise • Low VO_2 max • Rapid fatigue
Peripheral vascular disease	• Claudication can limit exercise	• Low VO_2 max • Increased lactic acidosis • Associated deconditioning often present • Low anaerobic threshold
Pulmonary vascular disease	• Impaired pulmonary blood flow • Right ventricular failure or overload • Possible right to left shunt	• Low VO_2 max • Low anaerobic threshold • Rapid pulse at low exercise • Hypoxemia • Excessive dyspnea
Anemia	• Low oxygen-carrying capacity	• Low VO_2 max • Early anaerobic threshold • Rapid pulse at low exercise • Fatigue and dyspnea
Chronic obstructive pulmonary disease	• Impairment to expiratory phase of breathing • Decreased alveolar ventilation	• Low VO_2 max • Low anaerobic threshold • Rapid pulse at low exercise • Submaximum heart rate achieved • Retention of CO_2 that increases with exercise
Restrictive lung disease (intrinsic)	• Poor diffusion capacity • Poor pulmonary compliance • Pulmonary hypertension in later disease	• Low VO_2 max • Early anaerobic threshold • Tachypnea at all levels of exertion • Low pulmonary reserve • High alveolar-arterial $p(A\text{-}a)O_2$ difference yielding marked hypoxemia • Marked dyspnea • Presence of pulmonary hypertension can cause severe hypoxemia and loss of hemodynamic response to exercise • Can trigger cough with exercise
Restrictive lung disease (extrinsic)	• Poor chest wall compliance • Chest wall muscle weakness • Loss of neural control of breathing musculature	• Low VO_2 max • Early anaerobic threshold • Tachypnea with low tidal volumes • Low pulmonary reserve • Submaximum heart rate achieved • Oxygenation and CO_2 usually preserved until severe end-stage disease
Asthma	• Restricted expiratory phase of breathing from airway obstruction • Decreased alveolar ventilation • In exercise-induced asthma, peak flows drop 5 to 10 minutes into exercise	• Most findings are normal when not symptomatic, and resemble obstructive disease with acute attack
Ventricular failure	• Compromised pulmonary blood flow • In left ventricular failure, can have pulmonary vascular congestion	• Low VO_2 max • Early anaerobic threshold • Tachypnea, dyspnea • Exaggerated heart rate response to exercise • May have hypoxemia with pulmonary congestion and loss of normal hemodynamic response to exercise
Ischemic heart disease	• Chest pain/cardiac ischemia • Can precipitate ventricular failure	• Often normal at rest or until ischemia • With onset of ischemia and ventricular stiffening/systolic dysfunction can appear like mild ventricular failure • Can have loss of normal hemodynamic response to exercise with onset of ischemia
Metabolic acidosis	• Metabolic acidosis, low HCO_3^-	• Normal diffusion • Exaggerated response of ventilation to exercise • Low VO_2 max

Interventions for Cardiopulmonary Disease

Aerobic Training

Physical exercise that increases the cardiopulmonary capacity (VO_2 max) allows for aerobic training. All aerobic training prescriptions must include four components: intensity, duration, frequency, and specificity.

Intensity. How hard an exercise is. Can be prescribed by a target heart rate, metabolic level (MET level), or intensity (wattage). Usual intensity target for cardiac primary prevention is a heart rate of 80% to 85% of the predicted maximum heart rate/peak heart rate from the exercise tolerance test (ETT). For secondary prevention in patients with known cardiopulmonary disease, exercise should be at a safe level at 60% or more of the maximum heart rate to achieve a training effect.

Duration. How long a given bout of exercise is. Usual cardiopulmonary conditioning requires 20- to 30-minute sessions, and should have a 5- to 10-minute warm-up and cool-down period. The lower the intensity of an exercise, the longer the duration will need to be to achieve a similar training effect.

Frequency. How often exercise is performed over a fixed time period (usually a week). Moderate-intensity training programs should be done at least three times per week, and low-intensity programs should be five times per week.

Specificity. The activity to be done in exercise. Training benefits specifically related to the activities performed. Thus, elliptical exercise is not as beneficial for walking as treadmill training. Specificity in prescription should be altered to adapt to the needs of each patient. For a patient with spinal cord injury, upper arm ergometry would be more functional, and cycle ergometry would be better for a patient with severe leg arthritis than a treadmill. The law of specificity of conditioning should be remembered when designing a cardiopulmonary conditioning program.[2]

The benefits of aerobic training include the following:

Aerobic capacity: Maximum capacity increases with training. Resting VO_2 is stable as is the VO_2 at a given workload. The changes are specific to the trained muscles.

Cardiac output: Maximum CO increases, whereas resting CO is stable. Resting SV increases with a corresponding decrease in resting heart rate.

Heart rate: Heart rate is lower at rest and at any given workload, whereas maximum heart rate is unchanged. The lower heart rate at rest and submaximal exercise causes a lower MVO_2 with normal activity.

Stroke volume: SV increases at rest and at all levels of exercise. CO is thus maintained at a lower heart rate and causes a lower RPP for a given level of exertion.

Myocardial oxygen capacity: After training, maximum MVO_2 does not usually change, but is less at a given workload. This reduces episodes of angina and increases safety for moderate activity. MVO_2 can also increase after pharmacologic treatments or revascularization procedures.

Peripheral resistance: Exercise training decreases peripheral vascular resistance (PVR) by reducing "afterload" through lowering arterial and arteriolar tone. The reduction in PVR results in a lower RPP and a lower MVO_2 at a given workload and at rest.

Minute ventilation: With improved conditioning, individuals will require a lower VO_2 and thus a lower minute ventilation for a given activity. For patients with pulmonary and cardiac disease, this can lead to a large reduction in dyspnea.

Tidal volume: Exercise can lead to a higher tidal volume on exertion, with a subsequent decrease in respiratory rate and decreased dyspnea.

Respiratory rate: As tidal volume is improved, respiratory rate will be lower for a given minute ventilation, decreasing dyspnea.

The application of basic physiologic principles to the design of cardiopulmonary rehabilitation programs can improve function, decrease symptoms, and improve outcomes for patients with cardiopulmonary disease. The prime effect of cardiac conditioning is in reduction of cardiac risk and improved cardiac conditioning. Reduction of cardiac risk has been well established since 1989, when pooled data from 22 randomized studies of exercise in 4554 patients following acute MI demonstrated a 20% to 25% reduction in all-cause mortality, fatal MI, and cardiac mortality in a 3-year follow-up study.[6] These benefits of cardiac rehabilitation apply across populations, including older adults, women, and patients after bypass.[6] Similar benefits have also been shown for pulmonary rehabilitation in COPD with decreased hospitalizations, improved function, and improved quality of life,[65,91,92,104] and new studies are showing that interstitial disease and pulmonary vascular disease can also benefit from exercise.[28a,38a,52a,55a,109a]

Pulmonary Rehabilitation

Abnormal Physiology: Lung

Patients with pulmonary disease demonstrate three main impairments: (1) obstructive lung disease, (2) restrictive lung disease, and (3) pulmonary vascular disease. Often more than one type of limitation may be present in a given patient and will increase the complexity of their condition. Understanding the underlying physiology can assist in the design of a specific exercise program for an individual patient.

For primary pulmonary disease, it is essential to know if the patient has primarily an obstructive or restrictive condition. Obstructive lung disease is marked by an inability to exhale resulting from either upper airway or large airway disease (sleep apnea, tracheomalacia, vocal cord disease, asthma, and bronchitis) or as a result of lower airway disease from either secretions or lung parenchymal disease (emphysema and bronchiectasis). Obstruction can also be exacerbated by a component of acute obstruction (asthma) combined with a chronic condition (COPD). The hallmark of severe COPD is carbon dioxide retention and active exhalation. Medical treatments are limited for COPD, with steroids and bronchodilators offering incomplete relief. Lung reduction surgery is only appropriate in selected individuals and transplant is only for end-stage disease. For all levels of obstructive disease, pulmonary rehabilitation is appropriate and in the "GOLD" recommendations for treatment of COPD, pulmonary rehabilitation is recommended for all patients with moderate to severe disease.[41,42]

In restrictive lung disease, the primary limitations are low tidal volumes from an inability to expand the chest wall (extrinsic restriction) or from very noncompliant lung tissue (intrinsic restriction). In extrinsic restrictive disease (neuromuscular disease, paralysis, and kyphoscoliosis), the parenchyma of the lung is normal and gas exchange is preserved, meaning that treatment is usually respiratory muscle training and mechanical ventilatory support as needed. With intrinsic restrictive lung diseases (pulmonary fibrosis, sarcoidosis, etc.), there may be a profound associated hypoxemia from severely decreased diffusion capacity of scarred lung tissue. Patients with parenchymal restrictive disease classically have severe hypoxemia and may need high-flow supplemental oxygen. Patients with end-stage intrinsic restrictive disease can have ventilatory failure with hypercarbia and hypoxemia and may be refractory to ventilatory support, and lung transplantation is then often the only remaining treatment option. Table 27-3 shows some of the lung pathologies and effects on inspiratory reserve and residual volume (obstructive diseases), and the effects of various conditions on lung compliance (restrictive diseases).[14]

Finally, patients with pulmonary vascular disease have a similar presentation in many ways to patients with heart failure. And in the end stages of the disease, right ventricular heart failure is a major part of the condition and leads to excess mortality and morbidity.[71] Rehabilitation is focused on a program that resembles exercise for patients with heart failure, with the addition of close monitoring of oxygen saturation and the use of appropriate levels of supplemental oxygen to prevent hypoxemia.

For patients with either intrinsic restrictive or obstructive disease, pulmonary rehabilitation is an important treatment to consider and should be offered for patients whether or not they have their pulmonary condition as a primary or a secondary disability. A brief overview of pulmonary rehabilitation programs for primary pulmonary disease is shown in Table 27-4.

Table 27-3 Causes of Altered Lung Physiology

Restrictive Diseases	Obstructive Diseases
Loss of inspiratory reserve Intrinsic loss of inspiratory reserve • Lung fibrosis • Pulmonary hypertension • Pulmonary edema Extrinsic loss of inspiratory reserve • Chest wall rigidity • Neurologic (central) weakness • Neurologic (peripheral) weakness • Chest wall restriction from bracing	Increase in residual volume Intrinsic increase in residual volume • Bronchial obstruction (acute asthma) • Airways collapse (chronic obstructive lung disease/ emphysema) • Bronchial obstruction (bronchiectasis, cystic fibrosis) Extrinsic increase in the residual volume • Neck obesity • Tracheomalacia

Cardiac Rehabilitation

Abnormal Physiology: Heart

An understanding of abnormal cardiac physiology in disease is necessary for appropriate cardiac rehabilitation. In general, cardiac limitation is caused by either decreased CO, or ischemic disease, or a combination of these. Ischemia causes the myocardium to have lower contractility and lower compliance reducing SV. Valvular heart disease lowers maximum CO through stenotic valves (e.g., aortic or mitral stenosis) or valvular regurgitation (e.g., aortic or mitral insufficiency). Finally, heart failure is a state of low CO, often as a result of low SV, and is associated with a reduction of Vo_2 max, increased resting heart rate, and often a greater MVo_2 for a given Vo_2.

Arrhythmias decrease CO by lowering SV and increase heart rates. For atrial arrhythmias, the mechanism can be by a loss of atrial ventricular filling (atrial "kick") during atrial fibrillation or supraventricular tachycardias, or from high heart rates without atrial coordination as in ventricular tachycardias and ventricular bigeminy.

Surgical treatments for heart disease either restore coronary circulation (e.g., bypass and intravascular procedures) or restore normal anatomy (e.g., valve replacement). Surgical treatment for heart failure can include LVADs or transplantation.[108,124] Medical treatment for heart disease either aims to improve coronary circulation for ischemia or works to improve blood flow and restore CO for heart failure by lowering afterload, reducing fluid overload, and increasing inotropy. Although medical treatment of ventricular arrhythmias has been limited, implantable defibrillators and pacemakers have been very successful. Severe end-stage heart disease of all types may require cardiac transplantation or an LVAD. In all of these conditions and

Table 27-4 Summary of Goals and Methods of Pulmonary Rehabilitation

Goals	Methods
Primary and Secondary Prevention	
Smoking cessation	Smoking cessation programs, emotional support, monitor and encourage abstinence
Immunization	Assure proper immunizations (flu and pneumonia), communicate with primary physician
Prevent exacerbations	Disease education Self-assessment skills taught Self-intervention taught Instruct on accessing private physician
Appropriate medication use	Review medication Focus on inhaler technique Review dosing schedules Review interactions and side effects Focus on appropriate use of inhalers and nebulizers
Pulmonary toilet	Review bronchial hygiene Teach cough techniques/huffing Teach appropriate use of chest physiotherapy techniques to the patient and family

Continued

Table 27-4 Summary of Goals and Methods of Pulmonary Rehabilitation—cont'd

Goals	Methods
Appropriate use of oxygen therapy	Encourage acceptance of the need for O_2 Appropriate use of oxygen at rest and with exertion Review self-monitoring with pulse oximetry Review oxygen equipment and appropriate systems for a given patient Emphasize the importance of supplemental oxygen use and the consequences of failure to use oxygen
Nutritional counseling	Aim to achieve ideal body weight For CO_2-retaining individuals, avoid high carbohydrate diet Maintenance of low sodium diets Encourage balanced nutrition, avoidance of fad diets
Family training	Disease-specific training Pulmonary toilet and chest physiotherapy Medication and oxygen use Family support group Counseling as needed
Dyspnea Relief: Exercise Training	
Exercise	Multifaceted program individualized to each patient's needs
• Strengthening	Emphasis on gradual increase in strength with a focus on proximal muscle groups Avoid injury to weakened musculotendinous structures that may have been weakened by disuse and medications Focus on high-repetition, low-intensity training
• Conditioning	Aim to increase exercise tolerance with aerobic exercises Cross-training program to avoid injury Create an independent training program Increase ambulation endurance with gait training Appropriate oxygen titration during exercise
• Respiratory muscle training for selected conditions	Isocapnic hyperpnea Inspiratory resistance training Inspiratory threshold training
• Upper extremity training	Increase strength, focus on proximal muscles Increase endurance for sustained activity, aim to decrease fatigue with ADL
• Activity of daily living (ADL) training	Energy conservation and adaptive techniques Teach anxiety and stress relief Teach pacing in activities
Dyspnea Relief: Lifestyle Modifications	
Breathing retraining	Technique of pursed lip breathing, especially in obstructive conditions Diaphragmatic breathing
Anxiety reduction	Stress relaxation techniques Paced breathing Autohypnosis Visualization Use of anxiolytics as needed Evaluate and treat any underlying depression
Improve confidence	Build compensatory techniques Build confidence in ability to exercise Provide ability to self-assess and learn disease management techniques
Disease Management	
Disease acceptance	Family and patient education regarding disease process
Coping skills	Patient and family support group Psychology and social work intervention as needed Treatment of depression as needed
Quality of life improvement	Simplify ADL management, improved coping skills Improve disease management strategies
Advance directives review	Counseling regarding end-of-life planning Establishment of health care proxy Clarification of intention for resuscitation Assistance in preparing paperwork
Encouragement	Patient support group Use of social work and psychological support
Continuing exercise and disease management compliance	Multidisciplinary team encouragement Physician (specialty and primary care) consensus Family education and involvement

treatments, cardiac rehabilitation has an important role to play. Some basic concepts to remember include that patients before transplantation are similar to patients with heart failure, whereas patients after transplantation have several physiologic changes that are unique, including high resting heart rate, limited increase in SV, and peak heart rate with exercise. The basic principles of cardiac rehabilitation are discussed as follows.[12]

Cardiac rehabilitation is either primary prevention, which includes risk factor modification and education before a cardiac event, or secondary prevention, which is cardiac rehabilitation after the onset of cardiac disease including both exercise and risk factor modification.

Primary prevention is usually performed in primary care settings rather than a rehabilitation setting. The focus is on the reduction of cardiac risk factors with a combination of education and exercise for patients in the community. Primary prevention can have a profound effect on the rate of cardiac disease with a decrease in obesity, blood pressure, and lipid profiles.[47,48,120] Ideally, behavior modification should begin in childhood with the establishment of healthy behavior and then maintained throughout life. Because populations who are disabled are generally sedentary and may have other risk factors, primary prevention should be an important component of the care of the disabled, and should include management of hypertension and lipids, along with encouraging exercise and consideration of antiplatelet agents. These are all cost-effective approaches and can decrease mortality and morbidity on a population-based scale, in addition to the individual benefits.[47,48,120]

After an episode of cardiac disease, it is essential to have secondary risk factor modification, which includes all of the features of primary prevention programs discussed earlier. In addition, disease-specific education and formal exercise is a part of the secondary prevention program. In both cardiac and pulmonary disease, smoking cessation is crucial as part of both primary and secondary prevention programs.[5,74,128]

Pulmonary Rehabilitation Programs

Rehabilitation programs for patients with pulmonary disease are similar to cardiac rehabilitation programs. After severe acute exacerbations, some patients can benefit from a short acute inpatient rehabilitation, but the majority of pulmonary rehabilitation is done in an outpatient setting. For patients who are in an intensive care setting, early mobilization programs are now being used to limit debility in these vulnerable patients.[4,17,89] Outpatient pulmonary rehabilitation programs also have primary prevention for pulmonary disease with smoking prevention and cessation, occupational safety, and prevention of exposure to environmental and infectious agents. Secondary pulmonary prevention involves medication adherence and education, smoking cessation, supplemental oxygen use and education, and environmental modification for known environmental triggers.[65,92]

For patients with ventilatory failure that cannot be supported with noninvasive ventilation, lung transplant may become necessary. Rehabilitation before transplantation is focused on both the underlying condition and transplant-specific education, whereas rehabilitation after transplantation includes education and restoration of muscle strength, which is impaired from the medical regimen for patients after transplantation.[16]

Table 27-5 Acute Phase I in Hospital Cardiac Mobilization Program

Day	Activity
Day 1	Passive range of motion (ROM), ankle pumps, introduction to the program, self-feeding Progress to dangle at side of bed, initiate patient education Progress to active assisted ROM, sitting upright in a chair, light recreation and use of bedside commode Increased sitting time by the end of the day, light activities with minimum resistance, continue patient education Progress to light activities with moderate resistance, unlimited sitting, seated activities of daily living (ADLs) by end of first day
Day 2	Increased resistance, walking to bathroom, standing ADL, up to 1 hour long group meetings Progress walking up to 100 feet, standing warm-up exercises Begin walking down stairs (not up), continued education Progress exercise program with a review of energy conservation and pacing techniques
Day 3	Advance exercise to include light weights and progressive ambulation Increase the duration of activities Progress stair activity to climbing two flights of stairs, continue to increase resistance in exercises Consolidate home exercise program teaching Aim to safely walk up and down two flights of stairs (assures safety for normal activities), complete instruction in home exercise program and in energy conservation and pacing techniques Discharge planning and education

Cardiac Rehabilitation of the Patient After Myocardial Infarction

The standard model for cardiac rehabilitation after MI was first described by Wenger and Skoropa[126] in 1971. Because revascularization is now common and infarcts are smaller than in the past, there have been modifications to the classical program with a reduction to three phases, eliminating the classical stage 2 recovery phase. A modern acute phase mobilization program is illustrated in Table 27-5.

The exception to bypassing the recovery phase for cardiac rehabilitation comes for surgical patients with sternotomy who may require recovery from their surgery before starting the training phase of rehabilitation. In summary, phase 1 rehabilitation is the acute phase in hospital immediately following a cardiac event and ends at discharge. Phase 2 is an outpatient training phase, with secondary prevention, intense education, and aerobic conditioning. Phase 3 is the most difficult, the maintenance phase where patients seek to achieve continued aerobic exercise and maintenance of lifestyle modifications. Risk factor modification is performed at all phases. This model is similar for patients with pulmonary disease. For patients with cardiopulmonary disease who are not hospitalized, the goal is essentially phase 2 and phase 3 for all patients at the time of diagnosis. A more detailed description of each of the phases follows.

Acute Phase (Phase 1)

The basics of the phase 1 program are illustrated in Table 27-5. Education about cardiopulmonary risk factor modification is introduced at the time of acute hospitalization. For patients with cardiac disease, all acute mobilizations should be done with cardiac monitoring with appropriate supervision of trained therapists or nurses. Post-MI heart rate increase with activity should be kept to within 20 beats per minute of baseline, and SBP kept within 20 mm Hg of baseline. A decrease of 10 mm Hg or more is indicative of further medical issues and exercise should be halted. The target intensity at the end of the phase I program exercise is to a level of four METs, covering most of the daily activities patients may perform at home after discharge.

For patients with pulmonary disease, similar phase 1 goals exist and there is new emphasis on early mobilization in the intensive care unit (ICU) to prevent frailty and deconditioning. Patients are aggressively mobilized, some while still on the ventilator. Innovations, including extracorporeal membrane oxygenation, are also now allowing more aggressive mobilization of patients because sedation is less, and patients may maintain better nutritional status. These patients with pulmonary disease should be enrolled in outpatient pulmonary programs to maintain their early gains and complete a full program of education and exercise.

Inpatient Rehabilitation Phase (Phase 1B)

To distinguish between patients who have a rapid recovery after their cardiopulmonary event (pure phase 1) and those patients who require either acute or subacute rehabilitation treatment before discharge home, the designation of phase 1B rehabilitation has been established. With advanced age or substantial comorbidities or other disabilities that make mobilization more difficult, many rehabilitation specialists will care for these patients in phase 1B. The guidelines for exercise are the same as they are for patients in phase 1, but with a longer recovery period extending their hospitalized care to an acute or subacute rehabilitation setting before discharge.

Training Phase (Phase 2)

Classically, phase 2 cardiopulmonary rehabilitation starts after a symptom limited full level ETT for patients with cardiac disease or a CPET for patients with complex pulmonary disease. This allows for setting target heart rates and target exercise intensity from the exercise. A target heart rate of 85% of the maximum heart rate on an ETT or a CPET is generally regarded as safe for patients at low risk. Exercise intensity targets are lower for patients at higher risk or those with underlying conditions. In patients with life-threatening arrhythmias or chest pain, target heart rates are chosen that are below notable end points. Because hypoxemia can add risk and limits participation with exercise, it is important to provide supplemental oxygen as needed (up to a rate of 15 L/min as needed) to maintain saturation above 90% for safe exercise. A target heart rate of 65% to 75% of maximum is safe and effective in a regular exercise program for patients at higher risk,[48] and with target rates as low as 60% still providing a training benefit. Monitoring also needs to be customized to accommodate the underlying risk profile.

Classically, a cardiopulmonary training program is three sessions per week for 8 to 12 weeks. Cardiac rehabilitation is covered by most insurance plans, but the major limitation is a lack of referral and/or a lack of facilities in many areas. Creative and innovative care delivery programs have been developed to increase access and include home programs (patients at low risk), telemedicine programs, and community-based programs in nonmedical facilities. Because training continues after the 8- to 12-week period, it is important for patient self-efficacy that they learn to perform self-monitoring following the guidelines presented in standard references.[49,72] Patients need to learn to begin exercise with a stretching session, then a warm-up session, a period of training exercise at designated intensity, followed by a cool-down period. The principles of specificity of training need to be remembered because training benefits generally are seen in the specific muscles exercised.

Maintenance Phase (Phase 3)

Although the maintenance phase of a cardiopulmonary rehabilitation is the most important part of the program, it often receives the least attention. The benefits of a phase 2 program can be lost in as little time as a few weeks if a patients ceases to exercise. Because of this, patient education of the importance of making exercise a part of their new health habits has to be emphasized and the patient needs to integrate exercise as a part of a healthy lifestyle. To maintain capacity, patients should perform moderate exercise at the target intensity learned in their rehabilitation program for at least 30 minutes three times a week. With low-level exercise, the frequency has to be increased to five times a week for maintenance of gains. Although telemetry monitoring is usually not used with patients with cardiac disease, patients with pulmonary disease can benefit from the use of home pulse oximetry and should be taught to adjust their supplemental oxygen as needed with exercise to maintain adequate oxygenation.[15]

Cardiac Rehabilitation Programs in Specific Conditions

Angina Pectoris

Cardiac rehabilitation for angina aims to lower heart rate at rest and with given levels of activity to decrease angina by improving fitness. Exercise benefits for patients with angina include improved peripheral efficiency and improved coronary artery collateralization.

Cardiac Rehabilitation After Revascularization Procedures

Postcoronary Artery Bypass Grafting

Cardiac rehabilitation after coronary artery bypass grafting (CABG) emphasizes secondary prevention aims to improve conditioning and fitness. For patients with low ejection fractions and heart failure, closer telemetry monitoring should be done. If a patient had a sternotomy, arm exercises will have to be limited until sternal healing occurs, usually at approximately 6 weeks after surgery. Patients who have had percutaneous interventions usually pursue the program immediately and it is similar to the program after CABG.

Cardiac Rehabilitation for Patients After Cardiac Transplantation

Because most patients after cardiac transplantation have severe heart failure and debility before transplantation, involvement in a heart failure pretransplant program can help to limit deconditioning and help to treat depression and anxiety. Heart transplantation usually improves cardiac function, therefore a posttransplant program can focus on conditioning, education, and secondary prevention. An added feature is that many patients after transplantation may have vascular and neurologic complications, which may mean a phase 1B program is needed before starting the phase 2 outpatient program. This is often done in either acute or subacute rehabilitation settings.

Remembering the alterations of cardiac physiology in the patients after transplantation is important. Transplanted hearts are denervated and have no direct sympathetic or vagal central regulation. In many patients, the loss of vagal inhibition creates a resting tachycardia of 100 to 110 beats per minute. By contrast, because there is a loss sympathetic innervation, the chronotopic response to exercise is in response to circulating catecholamines, leading to a delayed and blunted heart rate response to exercise. Posttransplant, peak heart rates are usually 20% to 25% lower than in matched controls. Other cardiovascular effects that are seen include resting hypertension from the renal effects of calcineurin inhibitors (e.g., cyclosporine and tacrolimus) and prednisone, along with diastolic dysfunction in some patients.[16] Combined, these effects usually reduce maximum work output and maximum oxygen by approximately one third compared with age-matched individuals. Of interest, despite no denervation of the heart, similar decreases in exercise capacity are also seen in patients after lung transplantation.[16] With exercise, patients after transplantation have a lower work capacity, reduced CO, lower peak heart rate, and lower oxygen uptake, with higher resting heart rate and SBP than normal individuals. Additionally, resting and exertional diastolic blood pressures are usually higher for patients after heart transplantation.[23,116] The net effect of these alterations in exercise response is higher than normal perceived exertion, minute ventilation, and ventilatory equivalent for oxygen at submaximal exercise levels.

The focus of a cardiopulmonary rehabilitation program after transplantation is on conditioning and education. Target intensity for aerobic exercise is usually approximately 60% to 70% of peak effort for 30 to 60 minutes three to five times weekly. Intensity can be regulated with rating of perceived exertion target at 13 to 14 on the Borg Scale, approximately 5 to 6 on the modified Borg Scale, with the goal being to consistently increase the level of activity. Education focuses on learning the complicated medical regimen and vocational and psychological needs. For patients after cardiac transplantation, a program of rehabilitation can help to assist them to improve work output and exercise tolerance, with some patients able to participate in competitive athletics.[62-64]

Cardiomyopathy

Fortunately, cardiac rehabilitation for heart failure is now covered by insurance plans, since Medicare regulations started to cover rehabilitation for heart failure in March of 2014 (42 C.F.R. § 410.49(b)(1)(vii)). An important consideration for heart failure rehabilitation is the increased risk of complications such as sudden death, depression, and chronic cardiac disability. Closer monitoring of telemetry and vital signs is also needed because some patients with heart failure have inconsistent responses to exercise with increased fatigue, possible exertional hypotension, and syncope. Most patients also exhibit low endurance and chronic fatigue as a result of their low-exercise capacity. However, a positive effect can be realized in their fatigue and function with even a small improvement in V_{O_2}. These changes in capacity can lead to a marked improvement in quality of life and may help patients with heart failure to continue to live independently.[6]

Because of the increased risk for complications in patients with heart failure, a graded exercise tolerance test is helpful before starting a cardiac rehabilitation program. Long warm-up and cool-down periods with gentle exercise at a limited workload helps to compensate for an impaired ability to generate a dynamic exercise response, and dynamic exercise is preferred to isometric exercise because isometric exercise can lead to an increase in diastolic pressure and cardiac afterload.[29] Heart rate targets are usually set 10 beats per minute below any notable end point found with cardiopulmonary exercise testing. Cardiac rehabilitation begins with cardiac monitoring especially when severe left ventricular dysfunction is present. Once the patient has demonstrated stability with an exercise program and has learned how to self-monitor, the patient should be taught a self-monitored program. Education of patients with heart failure also includes doing a daily body weight (to observe for fluid accumulation) and monitoring their blood pressure and heart rate responses to exercise.[6]

Patients who are on pharmacologic inotropic support or left ventricular mechanical support for end-stage heart failure can also exercise in a cardiac rehabilitation program with similar precautions to other patients with congestive heart failure.[6] Rehabilitation after an LVAD usually follows a classical postsurgical course, and may include phase 1 and phase 1B rehabilitation followed by phase 2 and phase 3 programs. Patients with an LVAD seen in acute and subacute units require staff training, close cooperation with the LVAD team, and familiarity with the devices that are used locally. Because an LVAD often restores a reasonable CO, exercise tolerance is often only limited by the peak flow of the device. In addition to normal secondary prevention education, LVAD-specific family and patient education are also essential parts of post-LVAD rehabilitation.[11]

Valvular Heart Disease

Cardiac rehabilitation for valvular heart disease resembles the program for cardiac heart failure. Postsurgical considerations are the same as for CABG, with the added consideration of anticoagulation for patients with mechanical valves. Because anticoagulation increases the risk of hemarthrosis and bruising, patients need to avoid impact exercises and need education regarding injury avoidance.[6] The overall training program is similar to that discussed for the patient post-CABG.[6]

Cardiac Arrhythmias

An essential consideration for patients with cardiac arrhythmias is the need for telemetry monitoring with increases in intensity of exercise and new exercises. Patients at high risk can benefit from an automatic implantable cardiac defibrillator (AICD), which may offer protection form ventricular arrhythmias. Cardiac rehabilitation for patients with AICD needs to be done at intensities that avoid the heart rates at which the device is set to respond to ventricular tachyarrhythmias. An exercise stress test can help to set appropriate target heart rates for an exercise program. In addition to secondary prevention and education, AICD-specific education and emotional support are important to include in the rehabilitation program.[11]

Pulmonary Rehabilitation Programs in Specific Conditions

Emphysema

Rehabilitation for patients with COPD is the standard for pulmonary rehabilitation. Goals of a pulmonary rehabilitation program include improving disease management and exercise capacity. Because pulmonary rehabilitation does not improve lung function, the goal of the rehabilitation program is to improve peripheral efficiency and decrease dyspnea. Energy conservation education (how to do a given activity at a lower level of exertion), anxiety reduction, and improved endurance all contribute to improved function and decreased dyspnea. Longer duration exercise of moderate intensity is often used, rather than high-intensity exercise. Recent investigations have started to evaluate a possible role for high-intensity interval training for patients with COPD, but this has not yet been proven to be more effective than the standard training program. Because isometric exercises increase intrathoracic pressures, they should be avoided in patients with COPD.[15] Appropriate supplemental oxygen should be given to maintain saturation above 90%, with education to lower supplemental oxygen after exercise back to baseline levels to prevent resting hypercarbia. Patients with COPD generally have relatively modest oxygen needs and can often maintain their oxygen saturation levels with 1 to 6 L of oxygen via a nasal cannula. Bilevel ventilation may have a role for patients with sleep apnea or ventilatory failure, and education for these patients should include the proper use of this modality. For patients being considered for lung volume reduction surgery, pulmonary rehabilitation is considered essential both to qualify for the surgery and after surgery to assure adequate outcomes.[15]

Airway clearance and chest physical therapy has a role in the pulmonary rehabilitation of patients with substantial secretions. A combination of external percussion devices, vibration devices, and inhaled saline in combination with cough training and huffing may help to mobilize secretions. It is also important to include family training and education about inhaled medications, supplemental oxygen use, and management of equipment.[99]

Interstitial Lung Disease

The basics of a program of pulmonary rehabilitation for interstitial lung disease are the same as for COPD. An essential issue for patients with interstitial lung disease is often profound hypoxemia that requires high-flow oxygen with exercise to maintain adequate saturation for activity. It is essential in this group of patients to avoid chronic hypoxemia to prevent secondary pulmonary hypertension because the coexistence of interstitial lung disease and pulmonary hypertension can lead to a markedly decreased life expectancy. Exercise intensity is often limited in patients with interstitial lung disease by oxygenation rather than dyspnea, and airway secretions are usually not an important issue. For some individuals with severe end-stage disease, there may be ventilatory failure with hypercarbia, but in those patients rehabilitation may no longer be possible.[118]

Because interstitial lung disease is often progressive, transplant evaluation and education or end-of-life planning may be needed to permit as many patient goals as possible to be achieved.

Pulmonary Hypertension

Patients with pulmonary hypertension have similar limitations as patients with heart failure and share many similar precautions. Effective medical treatment for pulmonary hypertension has made a once-fatal condition into a chronic disease for many patients. Patients with pulmonary hypertension now have a much longer life expectancy and improved functional status is essential for maintaining an active life. Major concerns for pulmonary rehabilitation are preventing debility and improving dyspnea. Because hypoxemia can worsen pulmonary hypertension, it is important to maintain oxygen saturation with exercise, and cardiac monitoring may be needed for patients with a history of arrhythmias and right ventricular failure. Education for this group of patients should include a review of their vasodilating medications and supplemental oxygen use. Intravenous and continuous subcutaneous vasodilator infusion is appropriate for a pulmonary rehabilitation program, but similar to patients with heart failure there may need to be long warm-up and cool-down periods. For patients with severe pulmonary vascular disease, the program should start with moderate- to low-level exercise. Definitive research of the efficacy and safety of pulmonary rehabilitation for patients with pulmonary hypertension is still ongoing.

Ventilatory Failure

For alert patients on either invasive or noninvasive ventilation for ventilatory failure, a program of pulmonary rehabilitation can help to increase mobility and prevent complications. Exercise programs for patients on nocturnal or intermittent ventilatory support aim to improve efficiency and decrease fatigue while off the ventilator. The details of ventilatory support for patients requiring noninvasive ventilation is beyond the scope of this chapter. Table 27-6 provides an overview of the types of patients who may present with ventilatory failure. A summary of the indications for ventilatory support is listed in Table 27-7.[25a]

Table 27-6 Causes of Ventilatory Failure

Central Hypoventilation	Respiratory Muscle Failure	Chronic Respiratory Disorders	Other
Intracranial hemorrhage Arnold-Chiari malformation Central nervous system trauma Congenital and central failure of control of breathing Myelomeningocele High spinal cord injury Stroke Central alveolar hypoventilation	*Amyotrophic lateral sclerosis* Congenital myopathies Botulism Muscular dystrophies Myasthenia gravis Phrenic nerve paralysis Polio/postpolio *Spinal muscular atrophy* Myotonic dystrophy	Chronic obstructive lung disease Bronchopulmonary dysplasia *Cystic fibrosis* Interstitial *lung disease* Kyphoscoliosis Thoracic wall deformities Thoracoplasty	Congestive heart failure Congenital heart disease Tracheomalacia Vocal cord paralysis Pierre Robin syndrome

Table 27-7 Indications for Ventilatory Support

Noninvasive Ventilation (NIV) Decision Tree	Mild	Moderate	Severe
Clinical syndrome	Substantial daytime CO_2 retention (>50 mm Hg with normalized pH)	Mild daytime or nocturnal CO_2 retention (45 to 50 mm Hg) with symptoms of hypoventilation	Substantial nocturnal hypoventilation or hypoxemia
Clinical diagnoses	Chronic obstructive lung disease (COPD) Neuromuscular disease	Moderate neuromuscular disease Paralysis Chest wall deformity	Central hypoventilation Marked obesity Severe neuromuscular disease End-stage lung disease
Maximum medical management options	Optimal medication Pulmonary toilet Airway management Avoidance of pulmonary exacerbations	Add management of secretions Airway protection Consider nocturnal NIV rest with daytime off NIV	Treat reversible pulmonary conditions Maximize posture and other supports Considerations for augmentative communication and assuring adequate nutrition
Indications for tracheostomy over NIV	Uncontrollable secretions	Uncontrollable secretions Chronic aspiration and chronic pneumonias *Obstructive sleep apnea* with failure to improve with continuous positive airway pressure COPD with severe hypoventilation	Uncontrollable secretions Chronic aspiration and chronic pneumonias Failure of NIV Inability to manage NIV Patient/caregiver preference

Cardiopulmonary Rehabilitation in the Physically Disabled

As the population ages and more patients survive a disabling condition, there is an increase in patients with both physical disability and cardiopulmonary disease. An issue for cardiac rehabilitation for patients with dual disability is the impaired mobility that can impair both evaluation and participation in a rehabilitation program. Individuals who are disabled tend to have lower activity levels, which puts them at increased risk of cardiac and pulmonary disease, and may present obstacles for a standard rehabilitation program for a person who is newly disabled and who has preexisting cardiopulmonary limitations. For new onset cardiac or pulmonary disease, cardiopulmonary rehabilitation is just as important and needs to be considered. Cardiopulmonary primary and secondary prevention also overlaps with the education needed for stroke and peripheral vascular disease and is especially important for patients with physical disabilities, because they are often more sedentary with a higher prevalence of obesity and deconditioning. Finally, because mobility in individuals who are disabled requires greater energy expenditure, compromised work capacity from cardiopulmonary disease may impose an even greater degree of disability on an individual who is disabled than an individual who is able-bodied.

Cardiopulmonary exercise prescription for individuals who are disabled has to be adapted for the individual disabilities that the patient has. Individuals who have a lower extremity impairment resulting from neurologic or orthopedic conditions can perform upper extremity ergometry or use modified lower extremity exercise equipment, whereas an adapted bicycle ergometer or Airdyne may be helpful for a patient with hemiplegia. The higher $M\dot{V}O_2$ requirements for upper extremity exercise compared with lower limb exercise should be considered to adapt the cardiac rehabilitation program for patients who are disabled. Patients who are disabled also need to focus on task-specific activities while increasing their aerobic conditioning and endurance, with a goal of lowering the $M\dot{V}O_2$ for any given task. Because of the expertise in dealing with physical disabilities and understanding the mechanics of motion, physiatrists are particularly well positioned to lead cardiopulmonary rehabilitation programs for the disabled. It is especially important when many traditional cardiac rehabilitation program teams are hesitant to work with patients who are physically disabled because of their lack of experience with physical disability.[102,120]

Conclusion

Cardiopulmonary rehabilitation is an area where physiatry is uniquely positioned to help manage the patient who is multidisabled, and the multidisciplinary approach is well suited to address the education and team management needed for successful cardiopulmonary rehabilitation. A goal for cardiopulmonary rehabilitation is to increase the access to cardiopulmonary rehabilitation to a greater number of patients, including populations who are underserved in rural and urban areas, women and minority groups, and patients with dual disabilities as they become a larger proportion of the patients seen with cardiopulmonary disease.

Frailty

Movement and Function

Movement is an essential part of human life and is important for the preservation of function throughout the entire life cycle. Since the beginning of human history, a high degree of physical activity has been required to maintain a livable environment and to secure adequate nutrition to ensure survival. It is only following industrialization, a relatively recent event from an evolutionary point of view, that the diseases and conditions associated with inactivity and immobility began to manifest themselves throughout human societies. Obesity and the resultant conditions of diabetes, hyperlipidemia, and decreased cardiopulmonary reserve have increased steadily throughout the past century. Much attention is focused on the "westernization" of diet, although less attention is focused on the "westernization of physical activity levels."

As physicians concerned with function, physiatrists intuitively understand the dangers of activity reduction in all settings from all causes; both medical and environmental. In fact, often physiatrists are the only physicians who have familiarity with the maintenance of function via physical activity using therapists, nurses, and family members. The knowledge of how to modify physical and social environments to maximize functional movement and overall function for their patients allows physiatrists to improve and maintain function in their patients. The physiatric focus on activities of daily living (ADLs) is an effort to return functional movements to an individual who is disabled allowing them to maintain their baseline degree of physical activity required for autonomy and independent movement.

Physiology and Consequences of Inactivity

The link between physical activity and cardiovascular disease has been well described since the 1950s,[84,85] when the relationship between workplace activity levels were directly related to higher rates of cardiovascular events. It is no surprise that less physically active daytime behavior, for example, mail sorters versus mail deliverers affected the development of cardiovascular disease. A more interesting finding is the strength of this association; primarily seated workers developed almost twice the rate of cardiovascular disease. More research investigating and elucidating the cellular biology of inactivity needs to be done until this area of physiology is as well understood as exercise physiology.

Currently, the global workforce is becoming more sedentary in numerous sectors as desk-based work responsibilities dominate the work day and after hours couch-based recreational activities including home theaters, media centers, and ubiquitous social media create prolonged voluntary immobilization after work. In the United States, the amount of daytime sedentary hours is high as revealed by data from the *National Health and Nutrition Examination Survey* (NHANES) database, which showed that 54.9% of waking hours in the population studied was spent during sedentary activities,[78] with late adolescents and older individuals being the most sedentary.

Rising "sedentarism" is not only an American phenomenon. In Australia, a large population-based study found that sedentary behavior (television viewing time) was positively associated with abnormal glucose metabolism and metabolic syndrome.[30,31] More concerning is that these associations were preserved even when controlling for what would be considered active individuals who participated in sustained and moderate-intensity recreational activities. Prolonged physical inactivity appears to be a unique risk factor for maladaptive energy metabolism. In the future it is possible that number of hours spent sitting will be recognized as a risk factor for the development of cardiovascular disease. In the context of this discussion, these observational data support the hypothesis that the physiology of inactivity is a risk factor for poor health outcomes in numerous settings. This supports the idea that there should be a paradigm shift in how all physicians view physical inactivity in their patients, especially in the hospital setting where the physiatrist is in a key position to increase patient mobility.

In addition to increased cardiovascular risk, there are numerous associations between inactivity and poor health outcomes including the metabolic syndrome, deep vein thrombosis, obesity, and serum insulin levels.

Metabolic Syndrome

Although there have not been studies to elucidate the molecular biology linking prolonged sitting to metabolic syndrome, epidemiologic data are compelling. The metabolic syndrome is the presence of three out of five of the following findings: central obesity, elevated blood pressure, low serum high-density lipoprotein cholesterol, high triglycerides, and elevated fasting glucose. Patients with this constellation of findings are at increased risk for the development of cardiovascular disease and diabetes.[1] In recent years, the recognition of the metabolic syndrome and its prevention has produced a rich literature specific to this syndrome. Prolonged inactivity (sitting) more than doubles the risk for development of metabolic syndrome.[37] Development of the metabolic syndrome has been shown to increase with each additional hour of sedentary television viewing; as opposed to having television in the background during other household activities.[30]

Deep Vein Thrombosis

The correlation with prolonged sitting and development of deep vein thrombosis has been well described.[54] This can occur even in active individuals who are immobile for prolonged periods of time. Case reports from varied settings have reported seated individuals who developed deep vein thrombosis since the 1950s. These have included observations from air raid shelters, sitting in theater, sitting on extended airplane flights, and even prolonged sitting during video game playing.[86,90] Presumed causes include rheologic changes and hemoconcentration.[52,57]

Obesity

The relationship between physical activity and body mass index is supported by the medical and epidemiologic literature. In varied populations, pediatric, adult, or older adult individuals who have a lower level of baseline physical activity generally have a higher rate of obesity. Sedentary behavior is a reversible cause of obesity in all populations,[8,34,111] and improvement of physical activity levels should begin with school-aged children.[44,125] This is especially true because there is evidence that an obese child has a significantly greater likelihood of continuing life as an obese adult.[51,127] Even high levels of physical activity in athletic adults may not be able to compensate for the deleterious effects of sedentary behavior.[59]

Insulin

Insulin resistance is a component of the metabolic syndrome, and thus it is reasonable to assume that an association would exist between amount of insulin present and sedentary behavior. Reduced leisure time physical activity levels are associated with higher levels of insulin at baseline.[38]

Numerous studies have demonstrated the relationship between prolonged sitting, obesity, and the development of type 2 diabetes, an insulin resistance state. More interestingly, however, is the suggestion that insulin levels are elevated in individuals who have prolonged sitting, even in the presence of regular exercise.[50]

Frailty Syndrome

The frailty syndrome is a recognized syndrome of decreased ability to adapt to stressors accompanied by reduced physiologic reserves and reduced energy metabolism. The frailty syndrome has been reported to vary widely depending on the population studied ranging from 4% to 60%.[39] The frailty syndrome is clearly associated with advanced age and becomes more prevalent in older groups studied; however, it is considered to be a separate syndrome and not a variant of normal aging. If it were considered the end result of normal aging it would be reasonable to expect all individuals to acquire the frailty syndrome if they lived long enough, which they do not. The potential for confusion exists when the descriptor "frail" is confused with the frailty syndrome. A universally accepted definition or set of variables to diagnose the frailty syndrome has not yet been agreed upon; however, the conversation in the medical literature is ongoing and evolving. Substantial opportunities exist for physiatric contribution to this discussion because the frailty syndrome is defined in most tools as having a strong functional component.

A true consensus on the definition of the frailty syndrome has yet to be agreed upon internationally; however, the following findings are discussed in the medical literature as possible variables in evaluating individuals thought to be at risk for the frailty syndrome:

- Increased inflammatory response
- Decreased cardiopulmonary and renal reserve
- Sarcopenia
- Weight loss
- Exhaustion
- Weak grip strength
- Slow walking speed
- Low level of physical activity

There are numerous frailty screening tools being used in a variety of settings. Two of the most commonly cited tools in the medical literature include the Fried Frailty Phenotype and the "Rockwood Indices" from the Canadian Study of Health. These measurement tools can be of use to physiatrists depending on the practice setting in which they are used.

Fried Frailty Phenotype

Fried and colleagues[39] at Johns Hopkins University developed a screening tool that identifies frailty based on a positive score in three out of five possible domains: weight loss, exhaustion, low physical activity, slow walking speed, and reduced grip strength. A positive response was assigned a score of 1 or 0 for each category.

Weight Loss

A positive value of 1 was assigned when participants responded "yes" to the following question, "In the last year, have you lost more than 10 pounds unintentionally?" Because there is considerable room for self-reported bias, follow-up measurements to confirm weight loss are recommended to confirm the initial findings.

Exhaustion

Two questions extracted from the Center for Epidemiologic Studies Short Depression Scale CES-D 10 were used as indicators of exhaustion: "I felt that everything I did was an effort" and "I could not get going." Scoring was based on the strength of participants' agreement with these statements. A positive score is assigned a value of 1.

Low Physical Activity

Kilocalories per week expended were calculated with a self-reported description of voluntary activities adapted from the Minnesota Leisure Time Activity Questionnaire. This included questions about walking, chores, outdoor gardening, and numerous types of exercise. Interpretation of the answers should be clarified to ensure that negative answers are not based on different settings (urban versus suburban) or culture. A positive value of 1 was assigned for participants with the lowest 20% of activity.

Slow Walking Speed

Measurement was the time required to walk 15 feet in seconds. Stratification by gender and height took place.

The slowest 20% of the population studied was defined as receiving a positive score and a value of 1.

Reduced Grip Strength

Results were stratified based on gender and body mass index with values recorded in kilograms with a standard dynamometer. Participants who scored in the lowest 20% after adjustment for gender and body mass index were assigned a positive value of 1.

After scores are totaled individuals who score 0 are considered "robust." The presence of one to two of the criteria listed earlier are considered to be "prefrail" and three or more positive criteria are considered "frail." This phenotypic description has been correlated with notable clinical outcomes that are recognized as important in the geriatric population including falls, hospitalizations, and mortality. This clinical applicability and relevance to important measurable outcomes has made the Fried Frailty measure a popular tool in clinical research. There are no laboratory tests or psychosocial components taken into account when determining a score with this scale. Using these criteria, Fried identified individuals who met the criteria for the frailty syndrome in 7% of the 4317 participants included in the Cardiovascular Health Study, 30% of the participants over 80 years of age, and 28% of the Women's Health and Aging Studies.[39]

Canadian Study of Health and Aging Measurement Tools

The "Rockwood Index" also known as the CSHA Frailty Index and The Clinical Frailty Scale were both derived from the Canadian Study of Health and Aging (CSHA) dataset; a prospective cohort of over 10,000 participants. Both of these scales have been widely used in medical studies. The 70-item CSHA Frailty Index is driven by clinical judgment. This is a detailed tool where clinical deficits are scored based on a 70-item index. The items include self-reported functional activities, mood, and motor symptoms, as well as signs and symptoms derived from medical history and physical examination. Each deficit is assigned a value between 0 and 1.0 to give a total score, which is then divided by 70. Some examples of variables collected are listed in Table 27-8, with division into categories provided as a conceptual framework.

This index determines clinical deficits and allows scoring based on evaluating participants for accumulation of impairments. The Clinical Frailty Index was developed as an attempt to integrate clinician judgment into a formal and universally applicable model to evaluate frailty. The authors recognized that simply evaluating frailty based on a limited number of phenotypic variables may correlate with mortality, but does not give considerably more information across all populations. Although it is of benefit to identify participants at risk for increased overall mortality, it does not guide the physician to develop interventions that can address specific and more importantly correctable impairments. The Frailty Index gives structure to an intensive review of deficit accumulation that can serve as a starting point for interventions.

These same authors recognized the utility for a shorter more clinically oriented scale that could be used by clinicians across numerous specialties. In 2005, they developed and validated the CSHA Clinical Frailty Scale.[58] This is a descriptive scale with seven categories from "very fit" to "severely frail." It has been demonstrated to be an effective measure of frailty and offers predictive information about probability of survival and likelihood of institutionalization. This is a judgment-based scale that would be more applicable in the physiatric setting, whereas the more time intensive Frailty Index would give more specific information to a primary care provider or geriatrician. Both tools are validated instruments of benefit in the research setting (Table 27-9).

Frailty: A Complex Syndrome

In addition to the functional, psychological, and musculoskeletal changes, there are also altered organ system and homeostatic responses in the frailty syndrome. These include a reduced capacity to maintain homeostasis and an increased vulnerability to stressors caused by lower energy metabolism, sarcopenia, altered hormonal activity, and decreased immune function.

Changes in the endocrine axis, specifically the growth hormone/insulin-like growth factor 1 (GH/IGF-1) axis, affect numerous metabolic systems. Hepatic IGF-1 production is controlled by pituitary growth hormone secretion and is essential for normal metabolic processes in adults. As growth hormone secretion declines with normal aging IGF-1 levels also decline, this is often referred to as the "somatopause,"[60] which accounts for the normal age-related decline in endocrine function. Decreasing circulating levels of endocrine hormones contribute in part to osteoporosis, alteration in muscle/fat ratio, and cognitive decline in addition to sarcopenia. There is an association between the frailty syndrome and abnormally low IGF-1 levels.[76] Routine testing of IGF-1 levels is not recommended because it is neither diagnostic nor cost effective.[66] However, appreciating the metabolic setting in which the frailty syndrome is more likely to occur provides a framework for understanding this complex syndrome. In the Women's

Table 27-8 Example Variables from the Canadian Study on Health and Aging Frailty Index

Medical	Functional	Psychological	Neurologic	Musculoskeletal
Lung problems	Problems cooking	Depression	Tremor at rest	Impaired mobility
Congestive heart failure	Urinary incontinence	Delirium	History of Parkinson disease	Poor muscle tone in limbs
History of stroke	Toileting problems	Restlessness	Seizures	Poor standing posture
Skin problems	Falls	Mood problems	Cognitive symptoms	Poor coordination of trunk

Adapted from Jones D, Song X, Mitnitski A, Rockwood K: Evaluation of a frailty index based on a comprehensive geriatric assessment in a population based study of elderly Canadians, *Aging Clin Exp Res* 17:465-471, 2005.

Table 27-9 Comparison of Tools Used to Measure Frailty

Measurement Tool	Variables	Scoring	Utility
Fried Frailty Phenotype[39]	Domains of physical function	Each of five domains is scored between 0 and 1. Higher scores represent greater disability. 0: "Robust" 1 to 2: "Prefrail" 3+: "Frail"	Correlated with falls, hospitalizations, and mortality Popular tool in clinical research
Canadian Study on Health and Aging (CSHA) rules-based definition of frailty[107]	Rules-based ranking from fitness to frailty.	0: Independent and continent 1: Bladder incontinent only 2: Needs assistance with one or more activities of daily living (ADLs), bowel or bladder incontinence, cognitive impairment with dementia 3: Totally dependent for transfers or at least one ADL, completely incontinent, dementia	Predictive of death or admission to an institution
CSHA Frailty Index[58]	Deficits-based ranking	70 deficits scored in varying increments from 0 to 1.0. Total divided by 70 to give an index score	Predictive of frailty and death
CSHA Clinical Frailty Scale[58]	Disabilities, comorbidities, and cognitive deficit–based scoring	1: Very fit 2: Well 3: Well, with treated comorbid disease 4: Apparently vulnerable 5: Mildly frail 6: Moderately frail 7: Severely frail	Predictive of death or admission to an institution
CSHA Function Scale[22]	ADL-based scoring	12 ADLs scored as follows: 0: Independent 1: Needs assistance 2: Incapable	

Health and Aging Study, participants who had disabilities in mobility and disabilities in ADLs were more likely to have an increase in the proinflammatory cytokine interleukin 6 (IL-6).[24] The combination of decreased IGF-1 and increased IL-6 could contribute to a theoretical shift from the normal slowly decreasing anabolic state of aging to a rapidly increasing catabolic state seen in the frailty syndrome. As the population ages the incidence of the frailty syndrome will also increase. This complex syndrome will continue to be elucidated as advances in the molecular biology of normal aging progress. For the physiatrist, early recognition of the frailty syndrome may allow multidisciplinary intervention with the intended goal of preserving function as long as possible for these patients.

Zero Physical Activity: Hospital Immobility

Traditional Hospital Practices (Bed Rest, Sedation, and Immobilization). There has been a long-standing culture of bed rest in hospital culture. The concept of "convalescence" is that an ill person's strength returns gradually and is enhanced through greater than normal rest. This word is believed to have entered regular use in the late fifteenth century[27] at a time when patients who were ill had few medical options other than rest. The deeply held belief that hospitals are places to "rest" influences sedation practices and encourages the overuse of bed rest despite there being a clear understanding of the dangers of immobility.

This is especially true in the traditional critical care setting.[100] Long-standing provider beliefs include the idea that undersedation during mechanical ventilation is painful, traumatic, and panic-inducing despite ample data to the contrary.[70,106] In a recently published study that explored nurse sedation practices in the ICU, 80% of nurses surveyed believed that sedation is necessary for patient comfort and 87% of the nurses surveyed would want sedation if they were ventilated themselves.[46] Although some degree of sedation is usually required, 56% of the nurses surveyed believed that patients who are "spontaneously moving hands and feet" are undersedated. Although overuse of sedation is associated with an increase in posttraumatic stress disorder (PTSD)[106] and prolonged mechanical ventilation[70] with the accompanying complications of total immobility, it is still a widely held belief in many institutions that "rest is best." These practices lead to accelerated and iatrogenic deconditioning resulting from immobilization.

Iatrogenic Immobilization and Deconditioning. The dangers of immobilization have been understood for a long time (Table 27-10). The often cited 4% to 5% loss of muscle strength for each week of bed rest was derived from studies that involved young healthy test individuals without underlying disease or musculoskeletal conditions.[18] It is likely that the rate of deconditioning is even faster in older adult patients with multiple comorbidities, because ambulatory function and ability to perform basic ADLs have been shown to decline in one third of hospitalized patients over the age of 70 years.[110] Some of the complications of immobility include orthostatic intolerance, skeletal muscle changes, joint contractures, pulmonary atelectasis, urinary stasis, glucose intolerance, and pressure ulcers.[68] Traditionally, physiatrists have served as advocates for increased patient activity in the hospital setting because they evaluate and identify patients who can benefit from physical and occupational therapy.

Table 27-10 Effects of Immobility

System	Impact of Immobility	Potential Functional Impact
Musculoskeletal	Atrophy of skeletal muscles Decreased core strength Joint contractures	Reduced muscle power Reduced standing balance Shift in center of gravity
Cardiovascular	Deep vein thrombosis Reduced peripheral vascular resistance Orthostatic hypotension Reduced venous return	Potential lower extremity edema Pooling of blood in lower extremities Syncope/presyncope Venous stasis
Pulmonary	Atelectasis Pneumonia	Decreased vital capacity Decreased endurance
Psychological	Delirium Depression Posttraumatic stress disorder	Extended length of stay Decreased activities of daily living Chronic depression/anxiety
Dermatologic	Pressure ulcers	Prolonged hospital admission

Adapted from Kortebein P: Rehabilitation for hospital-associated deconditioning, *Am J Phys Med Rehabil* 88:66-77, 2009.

Early Mobilization

Rationale. The importance of early mobilization is well accepted as a "best clinical practice" in every hospital setting, not just the ICU. As the complications of immobilization became more widely understood, the importance of early mobilization throughout hospital organizations becomes a logical institutional goal, ideally approached through the quality improvement methodology.[17] Less universally agreed is how to design and implement a multidisciplinary early mobilization program and how to effect the accompanying culture change that is required for success. The physiatrist, working closely with colleagues in nursing, critical care, physical therapy, and occupational therapy is ideally suited to take a major role in the effort to bring mobilization to all patients who are hospitalized. The ICU is an ideal setting in which to initiate such a program because of the increased staffing to patient ratios, extended length of stay, and awareness within the critical care community as to the important role of physical medicine and rehabilitation in these programs.

Culture of Immobility. To successfully mobilize patients who are hospitalized, one must understand the many reasons that patients are ordered to bed rest and immobilization. Only then can the root causes of reduced patient activity be addressed. The concept of therapeutic bed rest can be a difficult idea to challenge. Therapeutic bed rest has been recommended for almost every medical problem at some point in medical history, including a variety of cardiac and pulmonary conditions in both the pediatric and adult populations.[20,40,53] In the intensive care setting, long-held beliefs that the experience of mechanical ventilation was traumatic and frightening for patients gave rise to a culture of complete sedation and resultant immobility. The idea that patients who were unconscious would recover faster, "fight the vent" less, and be spared psychological suffering was essentially unchallenged. Similar to the experience of patients with cardiac disease before unit-based cardiac rehabilitation efforts began in the 1970s, survivors of critical illness were profoundly weak with substantial disabilities resulting from their prolonged immobilization. This was often interpreted as proof of how tenuous their conditions were at the time of presentation, rather than the side effects of immobilization and oversedation.

Culture of Mobility. The first step to increase patient activity is gaining the trust and "buy-in" of colleagues in medicine and nursing. The importance of having evidence-based discussions with colleagues cannot be overstated. The common ground of all health care providers is commitment to patient care and improved functional outcomes. There is now a developing medical literature on the benefits of early mobilization.[79,89,98] Journal clubs, consultative rounds, and a strong inpatient presence contributes to an understanding of the physiatric approach and will provide an appropriate venue for discussions about early mobilization.

Physiatric Involvement. As a physician who understands the important role of physical, occupational, and speech therapy, the physiatrist is ideally suited to emphasize the vital role that these services play in the hospital setting. Because of hospital-bundled payments, physical therapy expenditures have traditionally been seen as cost centers and not profit centers by hospital administrators. To address this perception, the physiatrist should be well aware of the importance and robust discussion taking place in the medical literature about the cost-effectiveness as well as clinical use of early mobilization programs in a variety of medical settings.[7,55,75,119] Familiarity with the current literature demonstrating the multiple savings to an institution is key in acquiring the resources needed to implement an early mobilization program. Having a physiatrist as part of the implementation team is optimal to represent the interests and contributions of the entire spectrum of physical medicine and rehabilitation providers.

Ambulatory Devices. Hospitalized patients who use assistive devices normally are generally unsafe to ambulate without their usual devices while in the hospital. Because of staffing ratios and constant surveillance, ambulation in the ICU would not take place unassisted; however, in a noncritical unit a mobilization program would need accommodation for patients who can ambulate independently as well as with assistance. A recently developed Fall Prevention Took Kit includes bedside signs identifying risks and required assistive devices if they are determined to be necessary for safe ambulation.[32] In one study, 45% of falls were related to attempts by patients to reach the bathroom.[123] It is logical that removing assistive devices from ambulatory patients entering the hospital will result in increased falls when patients attempt to ambulate independently.

Training. Coordinated interdisciplinary training before implementation is essential for any mobilization program. Although early mobilization is often focused on physiatric oversight and physical therapy services, without appropriate coordination by all disciplines involved successful early mobilization cannot take place. Multidisciplinary simulation training with case-based scenarios should take place in the unit where mobilization is planned. All members of the health care team should have clearly defined roles before simulation training to experience the difference between standard multidisciplinary care and interdisciplinary coordination of care, which is at the heart of early mobilization. Unit-based simulation training, ideally with an actor as the patient, is optimal when possible. Cases provided should address medical emergencies as well as the challenges of physical coordination of care. Allocating time following simulation training for team members to discuss their experiences further facilitates the team-building experience.

Treatment Considerations in the Critical Care Setting

Hemodynamic Instability/Orthostatic Hypotension

Patients hospitalized in critical care units almost universally have hemodynamic instability. The systemic inflammatory response syndrome causes peripheral vasodilation, cardiac dysfunction, capillary leak, and circulatory shunting leading to hypovolemia. A constantly changing cardiovascular environment makes daily evaluation essential. As a result of vasodilation, patients who are critically ill may be unable to tolerate bed elevation, let alone seated positioning. Observing hemodynamic response to simple turning is a bedside test of hemodynamic tone that is easily carried out by a single provider. Patients who cannot tolerate trunk elevation can be treated in a supine position with range of motion and progressive resistance. It is important for treating therapists to continually observe blood pressure response to intervention. It is strongly recommended that treating therapists consult with nursing providers to discuss any changes since last treatment resulting from rapid changes in physiologic state. With constant surveillance and gradual progression, mobilization of the patient who is critically ill is unlikely to produce any unexpected events.[17]

Ventilatory Dependence

Hypoxemic failure causes numerous pathophysiologic effects culminating in requirement for ventilator support. These include hypoxemic failure caused by ventilation/perfusion (V/Q) mismatch, shunting, and altered oxygen exchange properties. Hypercapnic failure causes decreased minute ventilation relative to physiologic demand, especially in the setting of critical illness complicated by increased dead space ventilation. Coordination of therapy in conjunction with ventilator management should take place between physical medicine and rehabilitation and respiratory therapy. In some cases, therapists may be given parameters by the primary team as to titration of oxygen during treatment sessions. Oxygen titration should always take place in coordination with respiratory therapy or nursing. Similar to hemodynamic monitoring, ventilator status and oxygen saturation can vary quickly in response to activity and should be monitored at all times. During active ambulation, a respiratory therapist is essential to monitor oxygenation as well as position of endotracheal tube.

Postparalytic/Intensive Care Unit–Acquired Weakness

ICU–acquired weakness is common following hospitalization in the intensive care setting. Approximately 50% of patients with prolonged mechanical ventilation, sepsis, or organ failure have some degree of neuromuscular dysfunction.[117] The presence of ICU–acquired weakness can cause abnormalities at any point in the gait cycle. Endurance is reduced in all patients following prolonged bed rest with or without paralytics. Ambulation trials should begin with standing at bedside and only progress out of the patient room once the entire team is assembled. This will ensure patient safety and continuous monitoring in the face of global weakness. Early and aggressive physical therapy intervention has been shown to improve recovery of muscle strength in patients in the ICU.[17,115a]

Psychology of the Patient in the Intensive Care Unit

Posttraumatic Stress Disorder

Survivors of critical illness often have symptoms of PTSD. In a recently published study, 35% of ICU survivors following admission for acute lung injury reported PTSD symptoms during the 2-year period following critical care admission.[19] Symptoms of PTSD can be persistent, given that 62% of patients who reported symptoms confirmed their persistence at 24 months. Of these, 50% had taken psychiatric medications and 40% had seen a psychiatrist since hospital discharge.[19] Clearly, the complications following an episode of critical illness are multifactorial. Although it is too early to definitively state that early mobilization programs reduce symptoms of PTSD, it is likely that the benefits of such a program include reduced psychiatric complications.

Delirium

Delirium in the intensive care setting frequently complicates patients' hospital courses with resulting negative health outcomes. It is important that all providers in the intensive care setting recognize delirium and understand how it can impact on early mobilization programs. By definition, delirium is a change in cognitive function hallmarked by a fluctuating course over a short period of time (hours to days).[3] In the critical care setting, delirium is not just a descriptive term; it is a measurable medical syndrome associated with poor outcomes. The Confusion Assessment Method, or CAM and CAM-S (short form), are measurement tools that have been validated for use in this setting.[56]

It is important for therapists to understand that the interventions the provider has been shown reduce delirium as well as improve functional outcomes.[114] Recent critical care practice guidelines state "We recommend performing early mobilization of adult ICU patients whenever feasible to reduce the incidence and duration of delirium."[10] For the rehabilitation provider, even though the fluctuating nature of delirium has the potential to interfere with physical and occupational therapy, it is essential that therapy intervention be provided whenever possible. This often necessitates frequent reevaluations throughout the day until an appropriate window of intervention can be found.

Transition of Care

The importance of care transitions is receiving greater attention in both the medical literature and the administrative realm of hospital management. An appreciation for the impact of poorly structured systems to transition care from one medical setting to another has become an area of intense focus across the health care spectrum. Transitional care programs have been studied using different combinations of licensed providers including social workers, pharmacists, nurses, and physicians with most of these programs showing some degree of benefit.[25,67,93] The use and feasibility of transitional care programs has been studied in varied environments where the transition begins including ICU, hospital, nursing home, emergency department, and rural care centers.[9,21,25,43,93] The effect of early mobilization programs on care transition has not been studied, but the current interest in ensuring continuity of communication emphasizes the importance in developing and studying systems to ensure transition of physical and occupational therapy. Without attention to appropriate transition of care of rehabilitation services, the benefits gained during early mobilization are rapidly lost following transfer. This is an area of emerging interest that justifies research efforts on the part of all disciplines involved in early mobilization programs.

Application to Patients Not in the Intensive Care Unit

Although the importance of early mobilization in the critical care setting has received substantial attention, the principles of early mobilization are applicable throughout the health care continuum. Evaluating patients at risk for immobility or reduced mobility followed by appropriate referral to trained providers can increase patient activity levels throughout a medical system. The type of provider selected is determined by the degree of assistance required for a patient to safely increase their activity level. In the hospital setting, "bed rest" orders should be replaced by systemized evaluations regarding safe patient activity levels. Allowing patients who are hospitalized to use bedside commodes and assistive devices where appropriate is an economical way to increase patient activity without skilled intervention. Providing assistive devices to appropriate and carefully selected patients who are hospitalized can increase mobility and reduce incidence of falls in the context of a structured fall-prevention program.[32]

Community Mobilization

Healthy People 2020. The U.S. Department of Health and Human Services has initiated five "Healthy People" initiatives since 1979. These are comprehensive public health programs designed to provide structure and guidance to achieve more than 1200 objectives to improve the health of all Americans. Each health objective has a reliable data source, baseline measurement, and target for specific improvements to be achieved by the year 2020 (Table 27-11).[95]

The Healthy People 2020 website is a rich resource that includes leading health indicators, tips and tools for implementation of programs, and a consortium of organizations and agencies committed to achieving the Healthy People 2020 goals.[95] Community mobilization programs can play a role in achieving targets for some of the most important leading health indicators listed as follows.

Table 27-11 Healthy People 2020 Leading Health Indicator Target Goals

Physical Activity	Adult Obesity	Obesity in Children/ Adolescents
20% of adults 18+ meet the current federal physical activity guidelines	Reduce incidence of obese adults by 14% from 36% to 30% by 2020	Reduce incidence of obese children between ages 2 and 19 years from 17% to 15%
Goal met	Goal not met	Goal not met

Wellness Centers. Chronic diseases and their cost are responsible for approximately 75% of U.S. health care costs.[103] The Prevention and Public Health Fund was established by the Patient Protection and Affordable Care Act of 2010 to administer the Community Transformation Grant program. Over 60 grantees have been funded to support Americans in adopting healthier lifestyles including healthy eating, active living, and tobacco-free living. Funding opportunities exist within this new structure to explore evidence-based community wellness initiatives.

Although the causes of preventable chronic diseases in the United States are clear (cigarette use, lack of physical activity, calorie-dense/nutrient-poor dietary patterns), the solutions are as varied as the communities throughout the country. There are many unique and innovative programs that intervene at different stages of the disease process. Preventative programs are some of the most appealing as long as the cost-benefit ratio strongly supports ongoing investment. Some programs may involve disease-specific secondary prevention, such as a traditional cardiac rehabilitation program. Others may be more broadly based and focus on increasing fitness in the context of a community.[45] Although wellness programs with general physical activity goals may be common in senior centers, some of the most innovative approaches to the overarching problem of obesity in the United States are taking place in community centers with a focus on modifying heath behavior in the context of community-based family education and counseling. The Growing Right Onto Wellness (GROW) program in Nashville, Tenn., represents an innovative program with a population of 600 parent-child pairs who will receive educational interventions from 2013 to 2016 with a goal of preventing childhood obesity from developing in children.

Wellness centers can be freestanding but with community resources (community centers, houses of worship, schools, and employers) because locations for population-specific wellness programs are an efficient way to improve health outcomes.

Regardless of the population being targeted, all wellness programs can be developed based on a standard approach, listed as follows:

Step 1: Organize Advocates and Advisors

Wellness programs are multidisciplinary in nature. Identifying a group of committed and interested leaders and creating a working group is a logical first step.

Having the input and involvement of advocate community members at an early stage can improve awareness and uptake in later stages.

Step 2: Determine the Target Population

The most common wellness programs are either community or workplace based in scope. A work-based program will by definition be multidisciplinary. A physiatrist would be ideally suited to spearhead this type of intervention within a medical center based on their understanding of function, occupational health concerns, and expertise in multidisciplinary work.

Step 3: Needs Assessment via Health Risk Appraisal

Surveying the target population by questionnaire will yield the most accurate and direct information regarding what types of conditions a population is at risk for. This in turn will guide the development of appropriate interventions. In the community setting, an open forum or informal sampling of health concerns and interests can serve the same purpose. A needs assessment survey is also an opportunity to determine the preferences and interests of the target community. For example, there are numerous ways to increase physical activity levels. Early identification of prevailing interests will guide the working group to direct its efforts where they will yield the greatest participation.

Step 4: Identify Health Goals for Intervention

Information from Health Risk Appraisals will direct the priorities for each organization or community. Some examples include: Exercise/Physical Fitness, Tobacco Reduction, Stress Management, Back Care, Nutrition, Weight Control, and Mental Health. There is no way to predict what topics will be of importance to a population without sampling opinion. In a 1994 study that queried medical students regarding priorities for a health promotion program, 49% were interested in financial planning initiatives and only 12% were interested in alcohol and drug abuse programming.[115] Targeted polling will inform where resources should be directed for maximum impact.

Step 5: Community Outreach and Resource Identification

All communities have resources; human, physical, and financial. Identifying available space, facilities, and activity leaders will clarify what types of programs are possible to develop. Publicizing the need for a service, provider, or programming space may identify participants who are willing to create programs of interest at little to no cost. Community leaders including those of faith-based organizations, political organizations, unions, and neighborhood organizations are often well aware of what resources are available for use. If community leaders have been involved from inception they are more likely to be a committed stakeholder.

Step 6: Program Development

After analyzing community data, preferences, and resources, the project leadership should be able to draft an initial plan with staged interventions and a time line for deployment. Having a written document of program components, expected outcomes, and desired metrics before beginning will not ensure success but it will create a structure where leadership can learn from experience what is working and what needs to be adjusted. There are ample resources available at the Wellness Council of America website: www.Welcoa.org.

Step 7: Evaluation Plan

Every intervention must have an evaluation plan before deployment. Specific data sampling methods should be agreed upon before implementation as should meetings to review and interpret collected data. There should be object measures collected on a regular basis that are reviewed by leadership to determine if goals are being met, and if not what action is necessary.

Step 8: Incentive Plan

Human behavior is driven by reinforcement. Creating sustainable incentives, for example, t-shirts versus weekend getaways will contribute to success over time. Newsletters, parties, recognition meals, snacks, and gift cards are all popular workplace incentives that have the added value of increasing visibility of a new program for nonparticipants. Workplace competition can be a healthy way to promote a program, especially if a substantial incentive is being offered as reward to the winning team. Geographic competitions, departmental teams, and intradisciplinary teams can all contribute to employee "buy-in" as well as team building.

Step 9: Implementation

Before implementation, additional community members, division heads, or other leaders should be included as part of the implementation team. It is just as challenging to develop programs with too many members as it is to implement a program launch with too few members on the launch team. Leaving some choices to be decided by the entire implementation team will improve participation and sense of involvement for all team members leading to better enthusiasm and community participation following deployment.

Spearheading or participating in implementation of an employee wellness program can be a gratifying and worthwhile way to improve function on a population level rather than at the individual level. Highlighting the importance of the unique physiatric approach in the health care setting as well as educating communities as to the important role physiatrists can play in keeping their community members healthy and active are additional benefits to involvement in these types of programs.

Renal Failure

Physiology of Renal Failure

Recent scientific advances have expanded our understanding of what constitutes renal failure. Once thought to be solely attributable to volume overload, urea buildup, and hypocalcemia, it is now known that uremia is a complex syndrome caused by the accumulation of organic waste products some of which have yet to be identified. Hemodialysis cannot fully duplicate the complex actions of the nephron, which filters blood, reabsorbs water and solutes, secretes toxic substances, and excretes essential hormones.

Chronic kidney damage leading to kidney failure has numerous causes; however, the most common causes are uncontrolled hypertension, poorly controlled diabetes, and glomerulonephritis.[113] Uncontrolled hypertension leads to nephrosclerosis, or localized damage to the glomeruli. There are two proposed mechanisms of hypertensive nephrosclerosis, the first glomerular ischemia and the second hypertension-induced damage and resultant hyperfiltration. Diabetic glomerulopathy has excessive extracellular matrix as the most important pathologic feature. Glomerulonephritis can be primary or secondary, each of which has many causes, a full discussion of which is beyond the scope of this chapter. Infections, immune diseases, and vasculitides can all cause primary glomerulonephritis with resulting scarring of the nephrons. Secondary causes include diabetes, hypertension, and lupus, among others.

Alternatively, chronic kidney disease can be classified based on the anatomic part of the nephron that is affected. Glomerular, interstitial, tubulointerstitial, vascular, and obstructive are all anatomic classification examples, which are listed in Table 27-12. Fluid overload with hypertension can occur when the glomerular filtration rate falls below 60 mL per minute.

Hyperkalemia

The ability to maintain normal potassium levels is preserved until the glomerular filtration rate reaches approximately 10% of normal. Although patients with chronic kidney failure can secrete potassium until an advanced stage of renal failure, the rate of excretion is reduced, causing prolonged elevations in potassium following ingestion. Caution must be used when a patient is noted to be receiving spironolactone. Spironolactone is an aldosterone agonist, which can result in dangerous hyperkalemia if not monitored closely.

Table 27-12 Anatomic Classification of Renal Disease

Type	Example
Glomerular	Postinfectious Viral Rapidly progressive Immune-mediated Membranous
Interstitial	Autoimmune (systemic *lupus* erythematosus, Sjögren syndrome, Wegener granulomatosis, Kawasaki syndrome) Medication-induced
Tubulointerstitial	Numerous conditions, including but not exclusively: Autoimmune Infection Drugs Vascular Obstruction Heavy metals Granulomatous diseases
Vascular	Renal artery thrombosis Thromboembolism Aneurysm
Obstructive	Neurogenic bladder Blood clot Tumor

Hyponatremia

Sodium metabolism is maintained until renal failure becomes advanced. As renal failure progresses the ability to conserve sodium is compromised, resulting in hyponatremia.

Uremia

Uremia literally means "urine in the blood." It is a general term that began to be used before the understanding that end-stage kidney disease was more complex than just the inability to filter urea from the blood. As nephrons die the remaining units increase their capacity in a process known as compensatory hyperfiltration.[112] Increased glomerular permeability is another adaptation to the reduced number of functioning nephrons.

Metabolic Issues

Metabolic acidosis is caused by the reduced ability of the failing kidney to excrete acid.[101] This is exacerbated by decreased ability to resorb bicarbonate. Bicarbonate serves as the main pH buffer in the body and is derived from bone stores.

Bone Issues

Hypocalcemia. Hypocalcemia is loss of calcitriol and leads to decreased calcium absorption and stimulation of parathyroid hormone release.

Hypophosphatemia. Hypophosphatemia is caused by impaired excretion. In the face of abnormal bone metabolism, soft tissues became the phosphate reservoir causing increased vascular calcification. This leads to increasing pulse pressure in advanced disease.

Weakness

Anemia of chronic disease resulting from decreased erythropoietin and iron deficiency contributes to fatigue and weakness. Supplementation with erythropoietin is recommended and overseen by the primary nephrologist.

Debility

Studies have shown that a glomerular filtration rate of less than 60 mL per minute is associated with reduced well-being and overall function.[88,105] Patients who are dependent on dialysis have multiple possible sources of debility depending on the type of dialysis they receive. Peritoneal dialysis using the peritoneum as a membranous filter typically takes place in the patient's home, causing less functional impact than hemodialysis, a facility-based intervention. Both methods of dialysis have potential for infection resulting from indwelling catheters, but peritoneal dialysis is more likely to be complicated by subacute bacterial peritonitis as opposed to bacteremia in hemodialysis. SBP is more likely to result in hospitalization, whereas hemodynamically stable bacteremia will be treated on an outpatient basis with antibiotics, and with less likelihood of iatrogenic complications during hospitalization. Patients who are hemodialysis-dependent often report substantial fatigue following dialysis sessions; this impacts on their ability to participate not only with ADLs but also rehabilitation efforts.

Issues of Dialysis: "Residual Syndrome"

The term "residual syndrome" has been applied to the syndrome of partially treated uremia, because dialysis cannot fully replace all renal functions. Electrolyte imbalances and the resultant acid-base abnormalities are responsible in part for the uremic symptoms that are seen in patients who are dialysis-dependent.

Sarcopenia/Uremia

Uremic sarcopenia has been described in chronic kidney disease.[69,77] The presence of uremia causes changes in skeletal muscle fibers including mitochondrial depletion and atrophy of both slow- and fast-twitch muscle fibers.[35,83,122] This in turn contributes to the overall sense of fatigue and weakness reported by these patients. The role of exercise in maintaining health-related quality of life and exercise capacity has been described, and patients should be enrolled in an exercise program whenever possible to preserve skeletal muscle function as soon as possible following the diagnosis of renal insufficiency.[26,129]

Rehabilitation for Patients Before Transplantation

Patients with chronic renal insufficiency are often candidates for rehabilitation in both the hospital as well as outpatient settings. Chronic deconditioning resulting from uremic sarcopenia, a predisposition to chronic pain and gait abnormalities, represent areas for substantial rehabilitative intervention.[28,80,97] Patients on dialysis should be instructed in a regular stretching program because of the potential for hip and knee contractures from prolonged sitting. Patients on hemodialysis are at risk for a substantial degree of sedentary behavior as a result of extended immobility during hemodialysis sessions and postdialysis fatigue following dialysis sessions. Three hours of dialysis followed by 2 hours of resting while watching television constitutes up to 15 hours of additional sedentary time a week. Early referral to a rehabilitation professional for institution of a home exercise program before dialysis is warranted for all patients with uremia. It has been shown to be beneficial for patients on hemodialysis to exercise during dialysis sessions, although this is rarely standard practice.

Early Mobilization After Renal Transplantation

Similar to cardiac transplantation, patients following renal transplantation are substantially disabled as a result of a long-standing chronic medical condition: uremia instead of congestive heart failure. Although a patient on hemodialysis is typically more functional than a patient with end-stage heart failure, the principles of preprocedure rehabilitation or "prehab," posttransplant evaluation, and coordination of rehabilitative care are the same.

Following transplantation, reduced mobility, prescribed corticosteroids, and a sedentary lifestyle during recovery can greatly accelerate debility even in the face of a normally functioning kidney. Unlike cardiac transplantation, there is no expected increase in CO to boost energy metabolism. It is essential that all patients be evaluated following renal transplantation for potential rehabilitation intervention whether it be for aggressive mobilization and extended monitoring or for discharge to acute or subacute facilities.

Patients following renal transplantation have complex rehabilitative needs similar to patients who are critically ill in the medical intensive care setting. Both populations have multisystem organ damage, distributive shock, hemodynamic instability, severe deconditioning, and are at risk for functional decline. Unlike the medical ICU where a comprehensive early mobilization program may be implemented previously, the patient following renal transplantation may be more reliant on physiatric consultation and coordination of care to receive required services. Applying the early mobilization model to this population would necessitate evaluation for participation with physical medicine and rehabilitation on postoperative day 1. Patients requiring ventilator support can receive physical and occupational therapy if sedation is interrupted long enough to participate with the treating therapist. Physical therapy is often automatically ordered for all appropriate patients postoperatively and coordination with the primary team should take place in the morning with an agreed upon time for treatment should an interruption in sedation be needed. Daily physiatric consultation and review of treatment session notes can guide expectations for the following treatment session. It is crucial to ensure uninterrupted therapy at least three times a week because posttransplant physical reserve is reduced and potential for accelerated deconditioning in the presence of an immunosuppressive regimen that includes corticosteroids is substantial.

Outpatient rehabilitation programs following renal transplantation should focus on controlled conditioning and education regarding the importance of exercise in maintaining exercise capacity and lifelong function. The same target heart ranges can be used for patients following both cardiac and renal transplantation: 60% to 70% of peak effort for 30 to 60 minutes three to five times weekly. Rate of perceived exertion as described in the Borg Scale is a validated method to regulate intensity. It is important to provide consistent encouragement because patients following transplantation can be extremely debilitated and depressed. Advising transplant survivors that functional improvement may not be seen for 2 weeks or more following initiation of conditioning will help maintain participation. A comprehensive rehabilitative program will offer numerous benefits following renal transplant. Physical therapy can be focused on achieving a baseline improvement to facilitate participation in activities that the patient following transplantation may have forgone in the face of declining function. Perhaps more than any other solid organ transplant, successful candidates for renal transplantation can hope to achieve maximum function with optimal rehabilitation.

KEY REFERENCES

1. Alberti KG, Eckel RH, Grundy SM, et al: Harmonizing the metabolic syndrome: a joint interim statement of the International Diabetes Federation Task Force on Epidemiology and Prevention; National Heart, Lung, and Blood Institute; American Heart Association; World Heart Federation; International Atherosclerosis Society; and International Association for the Study of Obesity, *Circulation* 120:1640–1645, 2009.

2. American Association of Cardiovascular and Pulmonary Rehabilitation: *Guidelines for cardiac rehabilitation and secondary prevention programs,* ed 4, Champaign, 2004, Human Kinetics, Inc.
5. Balady GJ, Ades PA, Comoss P, et al: Core components of cardiac rehabilitation/secondary prevention programs: a statement for healthcare professionals from the American Heart Association and the American Association of Cardiovascular and Pulmonary Rehabilitation Writing Group, *Circulation* 102:1069–1073, 2000.
6. Balady GJ, Williams MA, Ades PA, et al: Core components of cardiac rehabilitation/secondary prevention programs: 2007 update: a scientific statement from the American Heart Association Exercise, Cardiac Rehabilitation, and Prevention Committee, the Council on Clinical Cardiology; the Councils on Cardiovascular Nursing, Epidemiology and Prevention, and Nutrition, Physical Activity, and Metabolism; and the American Association of Cardiovascular and Pulmonary Rehabilitation, *J Cardiopulm Rehabil Prev* 27:121–129, 2007.
10. Barr J, Fraser GL, Puntillo K, et al: Clinical practice guidelines for the management of pain, agitation, and delirium in adult patients in the intensive care unit, *Crit Care Med* 41:263–306, 2013.
11. Bartels MN: Cardiac rehabilitation. In Stam HJ, Buyruk HM, Melvin JL, Stucki G, editors: *Acute medical rehabilitation,* Bodrum, 2012, VitalMed Medical Book Publishing, pp 251–268.
13. Bartels MN: Cardiopulmonary rehabilitation. In Cristian A, Batmangelich S, editors: *Physical medicine and rehabilitation patient centered care,* New York, 2014, Demos Publishing, pp 112–129.
14. Bartels MN: Pulmonary rehabilitation. In Cooper G, editor: *Essential physical medicine and rehabilitation,* Totwa, 2006, Humana Press, pp 119–146.
16. Bartels MN, Armstrong HF, Gerardo RE, et al: Evaluation of pulmonary function and exercise performance by cardiopulmonary exercise testing before and after lung transplantation, *Chest* 140:1604–1611, 2011.
17. Berenholtz SM, Needham DM, Lubomski LH, et al: Improving the quality of quality improvement projects, *Jt Comm J Qual Patient Saf* 36:468–473, 2010.
22. Canadian Study of Health and Aging Working Group: Disability and frailty among elderly Canadians: a comparison of six surveys, *Int Psychogeriatr* 13(Suppl 1):159–167, 2001.
24. Cappola AR, Xue QL, Ferrucci L, et al: Insulin-like growth factor I and interleukin-6 contribute synergistically to disability and mortality in older women, *J Clin Endocrinol Metab* 88:2019–2025, 2003.
47. Hamm LF, Sanderson BK, Ades PA, et al: Core competencies for cardiac rehabilitation/secondary prevention professionals: 2010 update: position statement of the American Association of Cardiovascular and Pulmonary Rehabilitation, *J Cardiopulm Rehabil Prev* 31:2–10, 2011.
48. Haskell WL, Lee IM, Pate RR, et al: Physical activity and public health: updated recommendation for adults from the American College of Sports Medicine and the American Heart Association, *Circulation* 116:1081–1093, 2007.
50. Helmerhorst HJ, Wijndaele K, Brage S, et al: Objectively measured sedentary time may predict insulin resistance independent of moderate- and vigorous-intensity physical activity, *Diabetes* 58:1776–1779, 2009.
56. Inouye SK, Kosar CM, Tommet D, et al: The CAM-S: development and validation of a new scoring system for delirium severity in 2 cohorts, *Ann Intern Med* 160:526–533, 2014.
58. Jones D, Song X, Mitnitski A, Rockwood K: Evaluation of a frailty index based on a comprehensive geriatric assessment in a population based study of elderly Canadians, *Aging Clin Exp Res* 17:465–471, 2005.
61. Karvonen MJ, Kentala E, Mustala O: The effects of training on heart rate; a longitudinal study, *Ann Med Exp Biol Fenn* 35:307–315, 1957.
65. King M, Bittner V, Josephson R, et al: Medical director responsibilities for outpatient cardiac rehabilitation/secondary prevention programs: 2012 update: a statement for health care professionals from the American Association for Cardiovascular and Pulmonary Rehabilitation and the American Heart Association, *J Cardiopulm Rehabil Prev* 32:410–419, 2012.
67. Kortebein P: Rehabilitation for hospital-associated deconditioning, *Am J Phys Med Rehabil* 88:66–77, 2009.
70. Kress JP, Gehlbach B, Lacy M, et al: The long-term psychological effects of daily sedative interruption on critically ill patients, *Am J Respir Crit Care Med* 168:1457–1461, 2003.
72. Lauer M, Froelicher ES, Williams M, Kligfield P: Exercise testing in asymptomatic adults: a statement for professionals from the American Heart Association Council on Clinical Cardiology, Subcommittee on Exercise, Cardiac Rehabilitation, and Prevention, *Circulation* 112:771–776, 2005.
74. Leon AS, Franklin BA, Costa F, et al: Cardiac rehabilitation and secondary prevention of coronary heart disease: an American Heart Association scientific statement from the Council on Clinical Cardiology (Subcommittee on Exercise, Cardiac Rehabilitation, and Prevention) and the Council on Nutrition, Physical Activity, and Metabolism (Subcommittee on Physical Activity), in collaboration with the American Association of Cardiovascular and Pulmonary Rehabilitation, *Circulation* 111:369–376, 2005.
76. Maggio M, De Vita F, Lauretani F, et al: IGF-1, the cross road of the nutritional, inflammatory and hormonal pathways to frailty, *Nutrients* 5:4184–4205, 2013.
83. Moore GE, Parsons DB, Stray-Gundersen J, et al: Uremic myopathy limits aerobic capacity in hemodialysis patients, *Am J Kidney Dis* 22:277–287, 1993.
84. Morris JN, Heady JA, Raffle PA, et al: Coronary heart-disease and physical activity of work, *Lancet* 265:1053–1057, 1953.
85. Morris JN, Heady JA, Raffle PA, et al: Coronary heart-disease and physical activity of work, *Lancet* 265:1111–1120, 1953.
89. Needham DM, Davidson J, Cohen H, et al: Improving long-term outcomes after discharge from intensive care unit: report from a stakeholders' conference, *Crit Care Med* 40:502–509, 2012.
91. Nici L, Donner C, Wouters E, et al: American Thoracic Society/European Respiratory Society statement on pulmonary rehabilitation, *Am J Respir Crit Care Med* 173:1390–1413, 2006.
92. Nici L, Limberg T, Hilling L, et al: Clinical competency guidelines for pulmonary rehabilitation professionals: American Association of Cardiovascular and Pulmonary Rehabilitation Position Statement, *J Cardiopulm Rehabil Prev* 27:355–358, 2007.
96. Oldridge NB, Guyatt GH, Fischer ME, Rimm AA: Cardiac rehabilitation after myocardial infarction. Combined experience of randomized clinical trials, *JAMA* 260:945–950, 1988.
99. Parshall MB, Schwartzstein RM, Adams L, et al: An official American Thoracic Society statement: update on the mechanisms, assessment, and management of dyspnea, *Am J Respir Crit Care Med* 185:435–452, 2012.
102. Peno-Green L, Verrill D, Vitcenda M, et al: Patient and program outcome assessment in pulmonary rehabilitation: an AACVPR statement, *J Cardiopulm Rehabil Prev* 29:402–410, 2009.
104. Qaseem A, Wilt TJ, Weinberger SE, et al: Diagnosis and management of stable chronic obstructive pulmonary disease: a clinical practice guideline update from the American College of Physicians, American College of Chest Physicians, American Thoracic Society, and European Respiratory Society, *Ann Intern Med* 155:179–191, 2011.
105. Rocco MV, Gassman JJ, Wang SR, Kaplan RM: Cross-sectional study of quality of life and symptoms in chronic renal disease patients: the Modification of Diet in Renal Disease Study, *Am J Kidney Dis* 29:888–896, 1997.
106. Rock LF: Sedation and its association with posttraumatic stress disorder after intensive care, *Crit Care Nurse* 34:30–37, quiz 39, 2014.
107. Rockwood K, Stadnyk K, MacKnight C, et al: A brief clinical instrument to classify frailty in elderly people, *Lancet* 353:205–206, 1999.
108. Rogers JG, Butler J, Lansman SL, et al: Chronic mechanical circulatory support for inotrope-dependent heart failure patients who are not transplant candidates: results of the INTREPID Trial, *J Am Coll Cardiol* 50:741–747, 2007.
110. Sager MA, Franke T, Inouye SK, et al: Functional outcomes of acute medical illness and hospitalization in older persons, *Arch Intern Med* 156:645–652, 1996.
118. Swigris JJ, Brown KK, Make BJ, Wamboldt FS: Pulmonary rehabilitation in idiopathic pulmonary fibrosis: a call for continued investigation, *Respir Med* 102:1675–1680, 2008.
120. Thomas RJ, King M, Lui K, et al: AACVPR/ACCF/AHA 2010 update: performance measures on cardiac rehabilitation for referral to cardiac rehabilitation/secondary prevention services endorsed by the American College of Chest Physicians, the American College of Sports Medicine, the American Physical Therapy Association, the Canadian Association of Cardiac Rehabilitation, the Clinical Exercise Physiology Association, the European Association for Cardiovascular Prevention and Rehabilitation, the Inter-American Heart

Foundation, the National Association of Clinical Nurse Specialists, the Preventive Cardiovascular Nurses Association, and the Society of Thoracic Surgeons, *J Am Coll Cardiol* 56:1159–1167, 2010.

126. Wenger N, Gilbert C, Skoropa M: Cardiac conditioning after myocardial infarction. An early intervention program, *J Cardiac Rehabil* 2:17–22, 1971.
128. Williams MA, Fleg JL, Ades PA, et al: Secondary prevention of coronary heart disease in the elderly (with emphasis on patients > or = 75 years of age): an American Heart Association scientific statement from the Council on Clinical Cardiology Subcommittee on Exercise, Cardiac Rehabilitation, and Prevention, *Circulation* 105:1735–1743, 2002.

The full reference list for this chapter is available online.

CHAPTER 28

CHRONIC MEDICAL CONDITIONS: PULMONARY DISEASE, ORGAN TRANSPLANTATION, AND DIABETES

J. Dennis Alfonso, Derrick B. Allred, Blessen C. Eapen

As the American and global population ages, there is an ever-increasing number of people living with chronic medical conditions, along with the multitude of complications and sequelae that may arise resulting from the primary condition. The physiatrist, trained in the tradition of optimization of function in the setting of impairments and disabilities, is in a principal position to take the lead in the management of such patients. Inevitably, individuals with chronic pulmonary disease, cardiovascular, renal and hepatic pathology undergoing solid organ transplantation, or diabetes mellitus (DM) and accompanying diabetic complications will receive the care of a physiatrist. Thus, it is mandatory for the rehabilitation medicine specialist to become knowledgeable in the diagnosis and treatment of such conditions and be well versed in the recognition and management of potential complications.

Pulmonary Rehabilitation

Definition

Pulmonary rehabilitation is defined as an evidence-based, multidisciplinary, comprehensive intervention that can be integrated into the management of individuals with chronic lung disease.[102] Pulmonary rehabilitation is a multifaceted program, which involves optimization of medical management, physical conditioning, education, nutritional counseling, coping skills, and psychosocial support with the goal of reducing symptoms, improving functional status, increasing exercise tolerance, psychological well-being, quality of life, and reducing health care resource use.[146]

Classification of Pulmonary Disease

Pulmonary disease can be classified into three major categories, which include obstructive lung disease, restrictive lung disease, and pulmonary vasculature changes. Obstructive diseases are characterized by a reduction in airflow and airflow limitation, including asthma, chronic bronchitis, chronic obstructive pulmonary disease (COPD), and emphysema. Restrictive lung diseases are characterized by a reduction in lung size or an increase in lung stiffness resulting in a decrease in the maximum volume of air that can be moved in and out of the lung such as with interstitial lung disease, neuromuscular disorders (e.g., amyotrophic lateral sclerosis or myopathic disorders), sarcoidosis, pleural disorders, or abnormalities of the chest wall. Disorders of the pulmonary vasculature include pulmonary embolism, pulmonary hypertension, and pulmonary venoocclusive disease. Many respiratory diseases fit into one of these three categories, but individuals may present with a combination or mixed pattern of disease.

Epidemiology

COPD is the most common form of lung disease and the third leading cause of chronic morbidity and mortality in the United States and worldwide, which is primarily attributable to its link with smoking.[32,86] The U.S. Centers for Disease Control and Prevention estimates that 18.1% of all adults in the United States smoke cigarettes and approximately 80% of COPD deaths are caused by smoking. In 2011, 12.7 million U.S. adults (aged 18 years and older) were estimated to have COPD.[5] Statistics regarding COPD are shown in Box 28-1.[5,145] Restrictive pulmonary disease is most commonly caused by neuromuscular disorders, thoracic injuries, such as spinal cord injury (SCI), scoliosis, or obesity. Injury to the cervical and upper thoracic spinal cord disrupts the function of inspiratory and expiratory muscles, as reflected by the reduction in spirometry and lung volume variables. According to statistics available from the National Spinal Cord Injury Statistical Center, as of March 2014 there are an estimated 240,000 to 337,000 persons with SCI or spinal cord dysfunction in the United States. Of these patients, 79% are male, 14% have complete tetraplegia, and 45% have incomplete tetraplegia. Duchenne muscular dystrophy is one of the more common neuromuscular diseases that cause restrictive pulmonary dysfunction, with an incidence of 1 per 3500 male infants in the United States.[89]

Treatment Options in Pulmonary Rehabilitation

Treatment of pulmonary disease involves a multipronged approach to achieve maximum benefit, which includes

BOX 28-1

Facts Regarding Chronic Obstructive Pulmonary Disease

- The majority of patients with chronic obstructive pulmonary disease (COPD) have asthma.
- Asthma is the most common childhood chronic disease.
- Causes of COPD: asthma, chronic bronchitis, emphysema; singly or in combination.
- Smoking is the primary risk factor for COPD. Approximately 80% of COPD deaths are caused by smoking.
- alpha$_1$-Antitrypsin deficiency is underrecognized by physicians.
- COPD is the third leading cause of death worldwide.
- Annual worldwide adult deaths from COPD: 3.1 million.
- In 2010, greater than 70,000 females died compared with greater than 64,000 males.
- In 2010, the cost to the nation for COPD was projected to be approximately $49.9 billion, including $29.5 billion in direct health care expenditures, $8.0 billion in indirect morbidity costs, and $12.4 billion in indirect mortality costs.

optimization of medical management, oxygen therapy, chest physical therapy, exercise training, and nutritional and psychosocial support. When advanced pulmonary impairment occurs, other treatment options, including mechanical ventilation, can be used. If the impairment is caused by intrinsic lung disease, partial lung resection (lung volume reduction surgery [LVRS]) and lung transplant may be helpful.

General Medical Management

Pharmacologic therapy for COPD includes inhaled quaternary anticholinergic and/or beta$_2$-adrenergic agonist bronchodilators, inhaled corticosteroids, and phosphodiesterase type-4 inhibitors.[97] Oral theophylline can improve respiratory muscle endurance and provide ventilatory stimulation. Vaccination against influenza and pneumococcal pneumonia should be initiated. For those with emphysema resulting from alpha$_1$-antitrypsin deficiency, alpha$_1$-antitrypsin augmentation therapy can be efficacious.[142] In addition, several treatments prolong life or reduce progression in this disease,[29] and these include smoking cessation, noninvasive mechanical ventilation, LVRS, combined long-acting beta-agonists with inhaled corticosteroids,[31] and oxygen therapy.

Oxygen Therapy

Long-term oxygen therapy, provided greater than 15 hours per day, improves survival and quality of life in COPD if hypoxemia is present with arterial oxygen saturation (SaO_2) less than 88% or arterial blood gas of less than 55 mm Hg. It can also improve exercise tolerance, sleep, and cognitive outcomes.[28] Long-term oxygen therapy is also needed if the patient's SaO_2 is less than 89% and there is evidence of pulmonary hypertension or peripheral edema, suggesting congestive cardiac failure, or polycythemia.[120]

Table 28-1 Characteristic Physiologic Changes Associated With Pulmonary Disorders

Measure	Obstructive Disorders	Restrictive Disorders	Mixed Disorders
FEV_1/FVC	Decreased	Normal or increased	Decreased
FEV_1	Decreased	Decreased, normal, or increased	Decreased
FVC	Decreased or normal	Decreased	Decreased or normal
TLC	Normal or increased	Decreased	Decreased, normal, or increased
RV	Normal or increased	Decreased	Decreased, normal, or increased

From *The Merck manual professional version*, edited by Robert Porter. Copyright (2015) by Merck Sharp & Dohyme Corp., a subsidiary of Merck & Co, Inc. Kenilworth, NJ. Available at http://www.merckmanuals.com/professional/. Accessed March 31, 2015.

FEV_1, Forced expiratory volume in 1 second; *FVC*, forced vital capacity; *RV*, residual volume; *TLC*, total lung capacity.

Oxygen concentrators have become the most popular method of providing oxygen in the home. Portable models are readily available and can be used with an AC or a DC inverter. Some models are as light as 6 lb, with the average weight ranging between 6 and 20 lb. Most models have batteries that can be recharged in as little as 2 hours and have battery running times as long as 6 hours. Portable concentrators can easily be carried on a pull cart or on the body with a shoulder strap or waist harness. Most units are able to deliver 1 to 6 L/min. Some companies have produced models that provide up to 8 L/min of oxygen and have two flow meters so that two individuals can use oxygen from the same concentrator if the total use is no more than 8 L/min. Other systems incorporate a refill station as part of the concentrator, so that portable oxygen cylinders can be filled over a couple of hours. An oxygen-conserving regulator allows the oxygen to last four times as long. An oxygen cylinder can now be safely mounted on a motorized wheelchair if the motors and batteries are sealed and both are covered by a rigid housing.

Chest Physical Therapy

A good understanding of pulmonary function tests (Table 28-1 and Figure 28-1), as well as the mechanics and work of breathing in normal and diseased states, is essential in planning an effective pulmonary rehabilitation program.[61] Breathing exercises begin with relaxation techniques, which then become the foundation for breathing retraining. Retraining techniques for persons with COPD include pursed lip breathing, head-down and bending-forward postures, slow deep breathing, and localized expansion exercises or segmental breathing. These techniques maintain positive airway pressure during exhalation and help reduce overinflation. Although diaphragmatic breathing is widely taught, it has been shown to increase the work of breathing and dyspnea compared with the natural pattern of breathing in the patient with COPD.[29] The other component occasionally used to reduce fatigue is respiratory muscle endurance training, which usually concentrates on inspiratory resistance training. Training of the expiratory

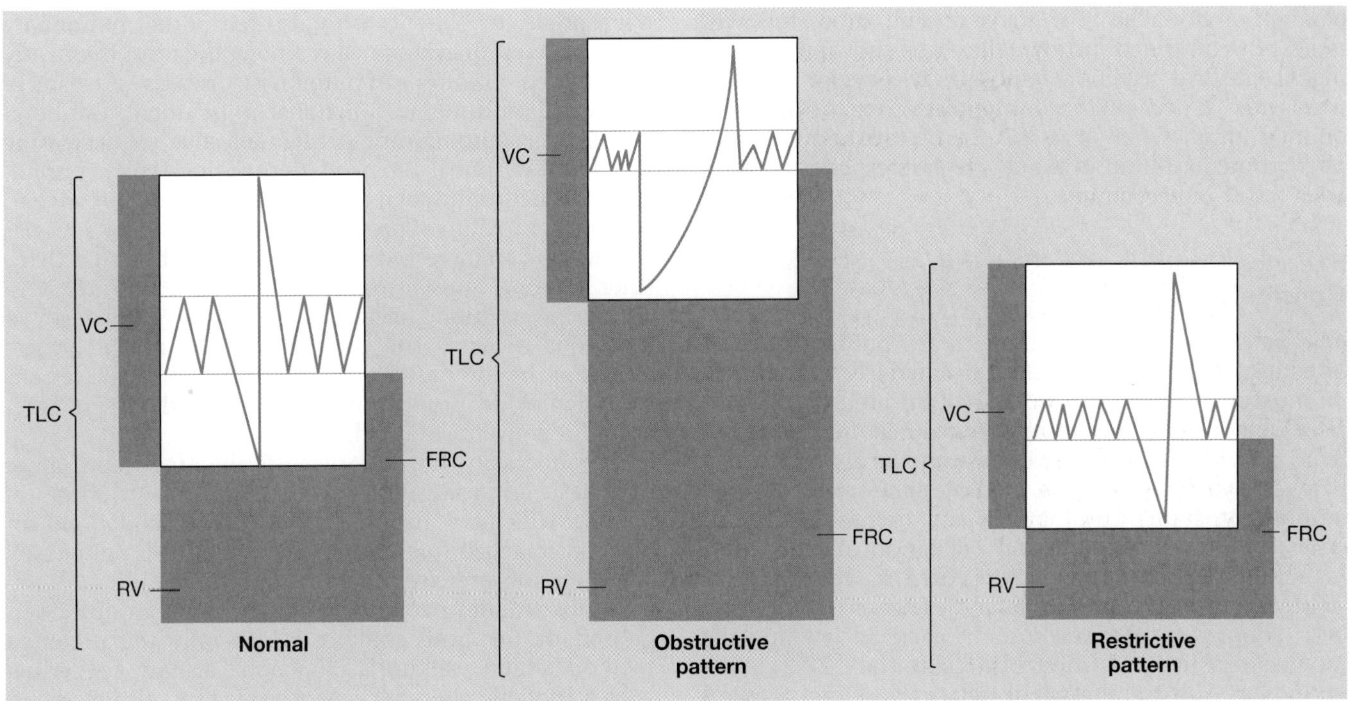

FIGURE 28-1 Lung volumes in health and disease. The breathing pattern is read from right to left. The obstructive pattern demonstrates prolonged expiration. *FRC*, Functional residual capacity; *RV*, residual volume; *TLC*, total lung capacity; *VC*, vital capacity.

muscles, however, has also been found to be of some value.[98]

Airway clearance strategies are indicated for persons with (1) abnormal cough mechanics (e.g., muscle weakness), (2) altered mucus rheology (e.g., cystic fibrosis), (3) structural airway defects (e.g., bronchiectasis), and (4) altered mucociliary clearance (e.g., primary ciliary dyskinesia).[95] Clearance of secretions is mandatory to reduce the work of breathing, improve gas exchange, and limit infection and atelectasis. For chest physical therapy to be effective, mucoactive medications must be given.[133] These include expectorants, mucolytics, bronchodilators, surfactants, and mucoregulatory agents that reduce the volume of mucus secretion. Antitussives must be used for uncontrolled coughing, which can precipitate dynamic airway collapse, bronchospasm, or syncope.

Techniques for clearing secretions include postural drainage, manual or device-induced chest percussion and vibration, device-induced airway oscillation, incentive spirometry, and other devices and measures that improve the ability to cough. Head-down tilt positions for postural drainage should be used with caution in persons with severe heart disease.[101] In a manually assisted cough, the patient's abdomen is compressed while the patient controls the depth of inspiration and the timing of opening and closing the upper airway. Noninvasive intermittent positive-pressure ventilation (NIPPV) with air stacking or glossopharyngeal breathing (GPB) is used to increase the depth of inspiration when inspiratory muscles are too weak to produce a deep breath. Air stacking is holding a portion of two or more breaths to fully inflate the lungs before exhalation. In GPB, the person uses the tongue to breathe. The technique is described more fully later in this chapter. When an upper motor neuron lesion above the midthoracic level has paralyzed the abdominal muscles, functional electrical stimulation of these muscles can produce a cough.[73]

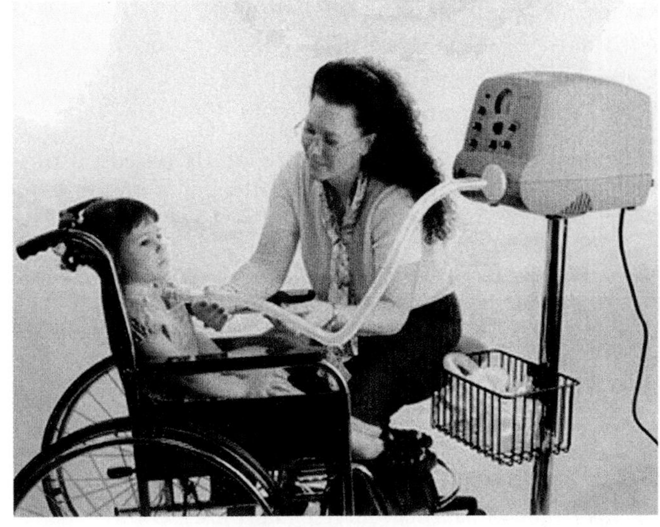

FIGURE 28-2 CoughAssist Mechanical In-Exsufflator cough machine with mother and child. The mother is using the machine at the child's tracheostomy.

Positive expiratory pressure mask therapy followed by "huff coughing" is a useful technique when other methods of mobilizing secretions are not tolerated.[90] Autogenic drainage is a secretion clearance technique that combines variable tidal breathing at three distinct lung volume levels, controlled expiratory airflow, and huff coughing. The CoughAssist Mechanical In-Exsufflator cough machine (Figure 28-2), manufactured by Philips HealthCare Respironics (Murrysville, Pa.), provides deep inspiration through a face mask or mouthpiece, or with an adapter, to the patient's endotracheal or tracheostomy tube, followed rapidly by controlled suction. It has been shown to provide highly effective secretion removal.[9] The device must be used with caution and is contraindicated in patients with bullous emphysema or a history of pneumothorax or pneumomediastinum in the recent past, especially if they are a result of barotrauma.

Exercise Conditioning: General Considerations

Aerobic exercise is the backbone of any pulmonary rehabilitation program. The inclusion criteria for exercise in pulmonary rehabilitation are straightforward.[2] A candidate must demonstrate a decrease in functional exercise capacity as a result of pulmonary disease and be able to participate safely in a rigorous cardiorespiratory endurance training program. Cardiopulmonary exercise testing is necessary for the selection and evaluation of individuals in several circumstances before exercise conditioning. Indications for cardiopulmonary exercise testing have been adopted by the American Thoracic Society and the American College of Chest Physicians (Box 28-2).[6] The pulmonary disease should be relatively stable. Medical comorbidities that contraindicate exercise should be absent. Patients should not have orthopedic or cognitive disabilities that prevent exercise. Patients must be motivated to exercise on a consistent basis. Finally, patients should abstain from tobacco products.

Exercise Prescription for Pulmonary Rehabilitation

Exercise prescription guidelines are largely based on programs in which the majority of participants are patients with COPD. These guidelines, however, appear to be

BOX 28-2

America Thoracic Society/American College of Chest Physicians Indications for Cardiopulmonary Exercise Testing

- Evaluation of exercise intolerance
- Unexplained dyspnea
- Evaluation of patients with cardiovascular disease
- Evaluation of patients with respiratory disease
- COPD
- Interstitial lung disease
- Chronic pulmonary vascular disease
- Cystic fibrosis
- Exercise-induced bronchospasm
- Preoperative evaluation
- Preoperative evaluation for lung cancer resectional surgery
- LVRS
- Evaluation for lung or heart-lung transplantation; preoperative evaluation of other procedures
- Exercise prescription for pulmonary rehabilitation
- Evaluation of impairment or disability

From American Thoracic Society, American College of Chest Physicians: ATS/ACCP statement on cardiopulmonary exercise testing, *Am J Respir Crit Care Med* 167(2):211-277, 2003.[6]

COPD, Chronic obstructive pulmonary disease, *LVRS*, lung volume reduction surgery.

appropriate for patients who also have other pulmonary diseases. Exertional dyspnea is among the most frequently experienced symptoms of pulmonary diseases and leads to physical disability and functional impairment. Cardiorespiratory exercise training is often effective for decreasing exertional dyspnea. Provided the cardiovascular, respiratory, and neuromuscular systems have adequate reserve to undergo a program of progressive exercise, skeletal muscles can develop an increased ability to sustain physical activity. After training, muscle oxygenation might be improved, which lowers blood lactate levels at any given level of strenuous exercise. The confluence of increased oxygen extraction by the muscles and lower blood lactate lessens carbon dioxide production and the ventilatory requirement for a given workload.

The American Thoracic Society,[102] the American College of Chest Physicians,[129] and the American College of Sports Medicine[121] have provided recommendations for pulmonary rehabilitation exercise. In general, pulmonary rehabilitation exercise programs should include cardiorespiratory endurance training of larger muscle groups. Overground or treadmill walking is generally the preferred method because walking is a functional activity. Leg cycling is an acceptable alternative. Arm cycling can also be incorporated. Many patients, however, might have difficulty tolerating arm cycling because of an increased ventilatory drive that could worsen the patient's dyspnea during the activity. Resistance and flexibility exercises might also improve functional capacity in patients with pulmonary diseases. The most specific exercise prescription guidelines have been provided by the American College of Sports Medicine (Table 28-2).

It is imperative that the personnel supervising the exercise program are appropriately trained in the implementation of exercise prescriptions in people with chronic illnesses and special needs. The American College of Sports Medicine offers certification programs to those with appropriate backgrounds, such as exercise science or kinesiology, nursing, occupational therapy, physical therapy, and respiratory therapy. In the initial exercise sessions, the individuals supervising the exercise program should monitor patients closely and adjust the intensity or duration of the session according to the appearance of exertional symptoms. After the patient is established at an appropriate intensity and duration, the progression of the patient must be monitored and evaluated to adjust the prescription for optimal effectiveness. The goal of the program should be a safe, effective, and enjoyable exercise regimen. Although beneficial results have been observed with exercise programs of 8 to 12 weeks in healthy individuals, those with pulmonary diseases might require longer periods of participation to show substantial results.

Exercise in Chronic Obstructive Pulmonary Disease

All studies of exercise in COPD take into account the severity of the respiratory disability (Table 28-3).[91] Numerous studies have been carried out on the effects of exercise on patients with COPD (Box 28-3).* In patients with COPD,

*References 22, 27, 42, 49, 56, 119, 172.

Table 28-2 Summary of the American College of Sports Medicine's Guidelines for Exercise Prescription

Component	Cardiorespiratory Endurance Training
Activity	Dynamic exercise of large muscle groups
Mode	Overground or treadmill walking Stationary leg cycling or outdoor bicycling Stair climbing
Frequency	3 to 5 days per week
Duration	20 to 60 minutes per session
Intensity	50% to 85% heart rate reserve 65% to 90% maximum heart rate RPE = 12 to 16 (category scale) RPE = 4 to 8 (category-ratio scale)*
Component	**Strength and Muscle Endurance Training**
Activity	Resistance training: low resistance with high repetition
Mode	Variable resistance or hydraulic weight machines Isotonic weight machines Free weights
Frequency	2 to 3 days per week
Duration	One set of 3 to 20 repetitions on 8 to 10 exercises that include all of the major muscle groups
Intensity	Volitional exhaustion on each set, *or* Stop 2 to 3 repetitions before volitional exhaustion
Component	**Flexibility**
Activity	Static stretching of all major muscle groups
Frequency	Minimum of 2 to 3 days per week Ideally 5 to 7 days per week
Duration	15 to 30 seconds per exercise, 2 to 4 stretching exercise sets
Intensity	Stretch to tightness at the end of the range of motion but not to pain

Modified from Whaley MH, Brubaker PH, Otto RM, editors: *ACSM's guidelines for exercise testing and prescription*, ed 7, Philadelphia, 2006, Lippincott Williams & Wilkins.[167]
*Warburton DE, Nicol CW, Bredin SS: Prescribing exercise as preventive therapy, *CMAJ* 174(7):961-974, 2006.[165]
RPE, Rate of perceived exertion.

Table 28-3 Classification Scheme for Chronic Obstructive Pulmonary Disease Severity: National Heart, Lung, and Blood Institute–World Health Organization Global Initiative for Chronic Obstructive Lung Disease Criteria

Stage	Criterion*
0	Normal lung function
1 (Mild)	FEV_1 ≥80% of predicted
2 (Moderate)	50% to 79% of predicted
3 (Severe)	30% to 49% of predicted
4 (Very severe)	FEV_1 <30% of predicted or presence of respiratory failure or clinical signs of right-sided heart failure

*In the presence of FEV_1/FVC ratio less than 70%.

cardiorespiratory endurance exercise therapy has been shown to improve maximum or symptom-limited aerobic capacity, timed walk distance, and health-related quality of life. Adding resistance training to the rehabilitative regimen can provide additional benefits such as increased fat-free mass and muscle strength.

BOX 28-3

Improvements Seen in Exercise Reconditioning in Moderate Chronic Obstructive Pulmonary Disease

Inspiratory Muscle Training

- Increased maximal inspiratory mouth pressure
- Increased strength of the diaphragm

Pulmonary Rehabilitation With or Without Inspiratory Muscle Training

- Increased maximal workload
- Improved activities of daily living scores
- Improved anxiety and depression scores
- Increased 6- or 12-minute walking distance

Pulmonary Rehabilitation (Cycle Ergometry, 70 W)

- Minute volume decrease of 2.5 L/min per blood lactate decrease of 1 mEq/L (normal: minute volume decrease of 7.2 L/min per blood lactate decrease of 1 mEq/L)

Several adjunct modalities might reduce the extreme breathlessness and peripheral muscle fatigue that prevent patients with severe COPD from exercising at higher intensities.[4] Continuous positive airway pressure and NIPPV during exercise might reduce the perception of dyspnea. Taking part of the work of breathing away from the respiratory muscles and reducing intrinsic positive end-expiratory pressure are considered two mechanisms by which these techniques relieve dyspnea. Nocturnal NIPPV in selected patients can improve their ability to exercise during the day. Adding electrical stimulation to strength exercises for peripheral muscles has been shown to further improve muscle strength in patients with COPD. Interval training with rest periods is capable of producing training effects in those who cannot tolerate a sustained period of exercise. Oxygen supplementation, even in patients who do not desaturate during exercise, allows for higher exercise intensities and produces a superior training effect. High-intensity physical group training in water can also produce significant benefits.[164]

After an initial exercise rehabilitation program, patients must continue to participate in routine exercise to prevent the positive effects of exercise from being lost. Continuous outpatient exercise training, home-based or community-based exercise programs, or exercise training in groups of persons with COPD is necessary to sustain the benefits acquired during the initial rehabilitation program.[147]

Exercise in Asthma

Asthma severity guidelines published in 1997 and updated in 2002 by the National Heart, Lung, and Blood Institute are based on clinical symptoms during the day and at night, and on the results of pulmonary function testing.[35] The two major categories of patients with asthma are those who have it intermittently and those who have persistent asthma. Bronchial biopsies in patients with intermittent asthma show evidence of ongoing airway inflammation. Studies have shown that aerobic exercise improves overall fitness and health of patients with asthma.

A mouse model of asthma has been developed in which the effects of exercise have been studied.[117] Exercise decreased the activation of the transcription factor nuclear factor-kappaB in the lungs of the mice. This factor regulates the expression of a variety of genes that encode inflammatory mediators. Moderate-intensity aerobic exercise training of the mice decreased leukocyte infiltration, cytokine production, adhesion molecule expression, and structural remodeling within the lungs. It is suggested that aerobic exercise in patients with asthma might reduce airway inflammation in a similar manner. By contrast, exercise itself can induce bronchoconstriction in some patients with asthma.

A study in patients with asthma found that airway vascular hyperpermeability, eosinophilic inflammation, and bronchial hyperactivity are independent factors predicting the severity of exercise-induced bronchoconstriction.[112] Rundell et al.[134] have described a laboratory method, eucapnic voluntary hyperpnea, that identifies 90% of athletes who have exercise-induced bronchoconstriction. The test is done by having athletes breathe 5% carbon dioxide and attempt to breathe for 6 minutes at a target ventilation equivalent to 30 times the baseline forced expiratory volume in 1 second (FEV_1). If eucapnic voluntary hyperpnea is positive, there is a decrease in FEV_1 of 10% to 19%.

Because exercising in cold air is known to increase bronchial responsiveness compared with exercising in warm air, a study was done to determine whether facial cooling plays a role in children with asthma.[171] It was found that facial cooling, combined with either cold or warm air inhalation, caused greater exercise-induced bronchoconstriction than with cold air inhalation. This could indicate that vagal mechanisms play a role in exercise-induced asthma.

Barreiro et al.[11] have studied the perception of dyspnea in patients with near-fatal asthma at both rest and the end point of various forms of exercise compared with other patients with asthma. Exercise tolerance was similarly reduced in both groups, but perception of dyspnea both at rest and at peak exercise was significantly lower in the group with near-fatal asthma.

Exercise in Cystic Fibrosis

An estimated 30,000 persons in the United States and 70,000 worldwide suffer from cystic fibrosis, which is an autosomal recessive disorder. The basic defect is one of chloride transport, which produces viscous mucus that inhibits the capability of the lungs to clear infection. The patient ultimately suffers from severe combined obstructive–restrictive pulmonary disease. The abnormal viscosity of the cystic fibrosis secretions is caused to a great extent by degenerating neutrophils that produce extracellular DNA. Dornase alfa (Pulmozyme), or recombinant human deoxyribonuclease, is an enzyme capable of digesting extracellular DNA. It is used daily by long-term nebulization for patients older than 5 years and whose forced vital capacity (FVC) is greater than 40%. Chest physical therapy of all pulmonary segments from one to four times daily is indicated, with increased frequency during exacerbations.

The Vest Airway Clearance System (Hill-Rom, St. Paul, Minn.) has become a popular method of providing the percussion and vibration necessary to loosen secretions. An air pulse generator rapidly inflates and deflates an inflatable vest, compressing and releasing the chest wall. This process is called high-frequency chest wall oscillation. It eliminates the need for intensive physical involvement by a caregiver. It also increases airflow velocities, which create repetitive coughlike shear forces and decrease the viscosity of secretions.

Children with cystic fibrosis have reduced anaerobic performance and do not participate in activities requiring short bouts of high-energy expenditure to the same extent as healthy children. Klijn et al.[78] carried out a study of anaerobic training on children with cystic fibrosis older than 12 years. No child had an FEV_1 less than 55% of the predicted level. Children were trained 2 days per week for 12 weeks, with sessions lasting 30 to 45 minutes. Each anaerobic activity lasted 20 to 30 seconds. Three months after the end of training, anaerobic performance and quality of life were significantly higher in the trained group. A measurable improvement in aerobic performance, however, was not sustained.

Children with cystic fibrosis are now surviving into adulthood, with the median survival in 2004 being approximately 32 years.[170] For children born and diagnosed with cystic fibrosis in year 2010, the median survival is predicted to be 37 years of age.[87] The cornerstones of treatment that have produced this increase in survival are airway clearance, nutritional support, and antibiotic therapy.[47,103]

The lung function of adults with cystic fibrosis has been studied with FEV_1. Thirty-six percent were found to have normal or mild lung dysfunction (FEV_1, 70% predicted), 39% had moderate dysfunction (FEV_1, 40% to 69% predicted), and 25% had severe dysfunction (FEV_1, less than 40% predicted). One third of adults with cystic fibrosis have multiple-resistance gram-negative organisms. A 3-year study of regular aerobic exercise in adults with cystic fibrosis has found that it reduced the expected decline in pulmonary function throughout that period. Appropriate vigorous aerobic exercise enhances cardiovascular fitness, increases functional capacity, and improves quality of life. Patients with cystic fibrosis should rarely be exercised in close proximity to one another, however, because of the possibility of transmission of *Burkholderia cepacia*, a highly transmissible bacterium that frequently infects patients with cystic fibrosis.

Survival in cystic fibrosis is correlated with maximal oxygen uptake. Blau et al.[15] have found that an intensive 4-week summer camp program for both children and young adults improved exercise tolerance and nutrition in patients with cystic fibrosis.

Exercise in Disorders of Chest Wall Function

Numerous causes of chest wall dysfunction exist with both mechanical and neuromuscular components. The chest wall can be viewed as encompassing the rib cage, spine, diaphragm, abdomen, shoulder girdles, and neck. Distortions of the trunk are also reflected in distortions of the heart, lungs, airway, and abdominal contents. Many conditions negatively affect the chest wall, including ankylosing spondylitis, pectus excavatum, obesity, the sequelae of thoracoplasty or phrenic nerve crush for the treatment of pulmonary tuberculosis, neuromuscular diseases with weakness of the respiratory bellows mechanism and superimposed spinal curvatures, and Parkinson disease. Ventilatory muscle training in these disorders can reduce respiratory muscle fatigue. Persons with Parkinson disease have shown overall improvement with pulmonary rehabilitation.[26] Patients with developmental disorders are a heterogeneous group in which severe scoliosis is commonly seen. Exercise and other ongoing rehabilitation techniques, such as positioning, and management of spasticity and dysphagia, are of value in their treatment.[159]

Exercise in Paradoxical Vocal Fold Dysfunction

Paradoxical vocal fold dysfunction is caused by the vocal folds coming together during inspiration, instead of opening normally. The diagnosis of paradoxical vocal fold dysfunction is based on patient history and laryngoscopy. The disorder can occur from adolescence to old age. In one study by Patel et al.,[118] 90% of the patients were female, 56% of them had asthma, 12% had laryngeal findings suggestive of gastroesophageal reflux disease, 12% had findings of chronic laryngitis, and 33% had additional findings of laryngomalacia, vocal fold motion impairment, sulcus vocalis, nodules, and subglottic stenosis. These additional findings were mostly seen in the exercise-induced group. If the patient is symptomatic during the examination, a flow-volume loop of the FVC shows a flattening of the inspiratory loop, indicative of the low flow associated with partial obstruction in this area during inspiration. Neurologically based dystonias are also a common cause. Throat tightness, dysphonia, and inspiratory difficulty can occur. Speech therapy can provide respiratory retraining. Acute exacerbations can be relieved by administration of helium-oxygen (70%:30%) with or without NIPPV. Direct vocal cord injection of botulinum toxin A is also used.[163]

Nutritional Issues

In moderate to severe COPD, weight loss is common and is related to decreased exercise capacity and health status and increased morbidity and mortality. To determine the exact cause of weight loss it is important to look at the underlying mechanism of weight loss and specific tissue loss. Weight loss could be a result of high insulin resistance, high catecholamine levels, and dyslipidemia.[7] More specifically, loss of fat mass is generally caused by energy imbalance, whereas fat-free mass loss could be a result of substrate and protein metabolism.[46,135]

Creutzberg et al.[36] studied nutritional treatment of the severely underweight patient in an inpatient program. Nutritional supplementation therapy with two or three 200-mL oral liquid nutritional supplements daily in these nutritionally depleted patients with COPD produced increases in body weight, fat-free mass, maximal inspiratory mouth pressure, handgrip strength, and peak workload. Symptoms and impact scores on the St. George's Respiratory Questionnaire also improved. Maintenance oral glucocorticosteroid treatment blunted the response with regard to maximal inspiratory mouth pressure and peak workload, as well as the symptom score.

Later studies found that total daily energy expenditure in patients with COPD, whether they were underweight or not, has been shown to be no different than in healthy persons.[153] Insufficient food intake was found to be the cause of the malnutrition. Patients had greater success gaining weight when their total energy intake was 1.3 times higher than their resting energy expenditure.[122] It was also found that smaller doses (125 mL) of a dietary supplement led to greater improvements. The smaller doses caused less bloating and satiety, which was found to be less compromising to diaphragmatic movement, and patients were less likely to cut out meals.[20]

The energy cost of the exercise associated with a pulmonary rehabilitation program was estimated to be 191 kcal/day. Protein supplements with a high proportion of carbohydrates over fat are necessary when vigorous exercise training results in negative energy balance and weight loss.[149] In selected well-nourished patients, it might actually increase the shuttle walking performance.

Diet counseling and self-management with changes in dietary behavior should start early in the course, when the patient with COPD is still under the care of a primary physician.[21] Practical suggestions for shopping, food preparation, and eating smaller, more frequent meals should be offered. When fatigue, dyspnea, swallowing, or poor appetite interferes with eating, a dietitian can be helpful. Involuntary weight loss is best addressed preventively.

Psychosocial Support

Biopsychosocial considerations for persons with pulmonary dysfunction include the ongoing education of the patient and family, vocational counseling, and disability evaluation. Occupational therapy can also provide patients with severe respiratory disease counseling on energy conservation and techniques for performing the basic activities of daily living.[85] Depression and anxiety are very common comorbidities associated with COPD[115] because of the often drastic limitations in functional activities and the panic associated with severe dyspnea. Antidepressant and anxiolytic medications are often useful adjuncts to counseling.

Table 28-4 presents a summary of recommendations, statements, and grades in the Evidence-Based Guidelines on Pulmonary Rehabilitation with Strength of Evidence/Balance of Benefits Grading System.

Management Options for Individuals with Severe Lung Disease and Long-Term Outcomes

Mechanical Ventilation

Within the past 25 years, there has been a dramatic reduction in the use of body ventilators (iron lungs). Their main function is to simulate the function of the inspiratory muscles. The intermittent abdominal pressure ventilator simulates the function of the expiratory muscles. Intermittent positive-pressure ventilation (IPPV) via noninvasive nasal-mouth interfaces or via tracheostomy is now the method of choice because the equipment is lightweight and portable, and powered by either AC or DC current. No contact is made with the individual other than the

Table 28-4 Summary of Recommendations, Statements, and Grades in the Evidence-Based Guidelines on Pulmonary Rehabilitation with Strength of Evidence/Balance of Benefits Grading System

Recommendation or Statement	Strength of Evidence/ Recommendation Grade
1. A program of exercise training of the ambulation muscles is a mandatory component of pulmonary rehabilitation for patients with chronic obstructive pulmonary disease (COPD).	1A
2. Pulmonary rehabilitation improves dyspnea in patients with COPD.	1A
3. Pulmonary rehabilitation improves health-related quality of life in patients with COPD.	1A
4. Pulmonary rehabilitation reduces the number of hospital days and other measures of health care use in patients with COPD.	2B
5. Pulmonary rehabilitation is cost-effective in patients with COPD.	2C
6. Insufficient evidence exists to determine whether pulmonary rehabilitation improves survival in patients with COPD.	No recommendation
7. Psychosocial benefits result from comprehensive pulmonary rehabilitation programs in patients with COPD.	2B
8A. Six to 12 weeks of pulmonary rehabilitation produces benefits in several outcomes, but these benefits decline gradually over 12 to 18 months.	1A
8B. Some benefits, such as health-related quality of life, remain above control at 12 to 18 months.	1C
9. Longer (>12 weeks) pulmonary rehabilitation programs produce greater sustained benefits than do shorter programs.	2C
10. Maintenance strategies after pulmonary rehabilitation have a modest effect on long-term outcomes.	2C
11. Lower-extremity exercise training at a higher-exercise intensity produces greater physiologic benefits than lower-intensity training in patients with COPD.	1B
12. Both low-intensity and high-intensity exercise training produce clinical benefits for patients with COPD.	1A
13. Addition of a strength-training component to pulmonary rehabilitation increases muscle strength and muscle mass.	1A
14. Current evidence does not support the routine use of anabolic agents in pulmonary rehabilitation for patients with COPD.	2C
15. Unsupported endurance training of the upper extremities benefits patients with COPD and should be included.	1A
16. The evidence does not support the routine use of inspiratory muscle training as an essential component.	1B
17. Education is an integral component of pulmonary rehabilitation and should include information on collaborative self-management and prevention and treatment of exacerbations.	1B
18. Minimal evidence supports the benefits of psychosocial interventions as a single therapeutic modality.	2C
19. Although evidence is lacking, current practice and expert opinion support the inclusion of psychosocial interventions for patients with COPD.	No recommendation
20. Use supplemental oxygen rehabilitation exercise training in patients with severe exercise-induced hypoxemia.	1C
21. In patients without exercise-induced hypoxemia, supplemental oxygen during a high-intensity exercise program can improve gains in exercise endurance.	2C
22. In selected patients with severe COPD, noninvasive ventilatory support from a mechanical ventilator might modestly improve exercise performance.	2B
23. Insufficient evidence exists to support the routine use of nutritional supplementation in pulmonary rehabilitation of patients with COPD.	No recommendation
24. Pulmonary rehabilitation benefits some patients with chronic respiratory diseases other than COPD.	1B
25. Although evidence is lacking, current practice and expert opinion suggest that pulmonary rehabilitation for patients with chronic respiratory diseases other than COPD should be modified to include treatment strategies specific to individual diseases and patients, in addition to the treatments used for patients with COPD.	No recommendation

Grading System:
Balance of Benefits to Risks and Burdens

Strength of Evidence	Benefits Outweigh Risks/ Burdens*	Risks/Burdens Outweigh Benefits†	Risks/Burdens and Benefits Balanced‡	Uncertain§
High	1A: Strong recommendation	1A: Strong recommendation	2A: Weak recommendation	
Moderate	1B: Strong recommendation	1B: Strong recommendation	2B: Weak recommendation	
Low	1C: Strong recommendation	1C: Strong recommendation	2C: Weak recommendation	2C: Weak recommendation

Modified from Ries AL: Pulmonary rehabilitation: summary of an evidence-based guideline, *Respir Care* 53:1203-1207, 2008, used with permission from RESPIRATORY CARE and the American Association for Respiratory Care. Originally modified from Guyatt et al., 2006,[60] and Ries et al., 2007.[129]
*Benefits clearly outweigh the risks and burdens (certainty of imbalance).
†Risks and burdens clearly outweigh the benefits (certainty of imbalance).
‡Risks/burdens and benefits are closely balanced (less certainty).
§Balance of benefits to risks and burdens is uncertain.

nasal-mouth interface or the attachment to the tracheostomy tube (Figures 28-3 to 28-6).

Portable ventilators are volume ventilators designed 25 years ago, high-span bilevel positive airway pressure units, and laptop volume ventilators (Figure 28-7). For further information on the wide range of noninvasive ventilator choices, the reader is referred to a publication by Benditt.[14]

Air stacking (adding consecutive quantities of air into the lungs), maximal insufflations (passively inflating the patient's lungs to maximal capacity), assisted coughing, and noninvasive ventilation are described as respiratory muscle aids by Bach.[8] Bach has also developed an oximetry feedback respiratory aid protocol. In this protocol, the oximeter is used to provide patients and their families with feedback to maintain oxyhemoglobin saturation by pulse oximeter (Spo_2) greater than 94%, which is accomplished by maintaining effective alveolar ventilation and eliminating airway secretion. If the Spo_2 decreases to less than 95% in the patient with neuromuscular disease, it is attributable to one or more of three causes: (1) hypoventilation during

Airway ventilators
IPPV
Volume ventilator — console
Volume ventilator — portable
High-span bilevel PAP
Manual ventilator (resuscitator)
Mouth to mouth, to mouth — nose, to tracheostomy
CoughAssist machine (positive phase)
High-frequency ventilator

GPB
Suctioning
Suction machine
GPB reversed
CoughAssist machine (negative phase)

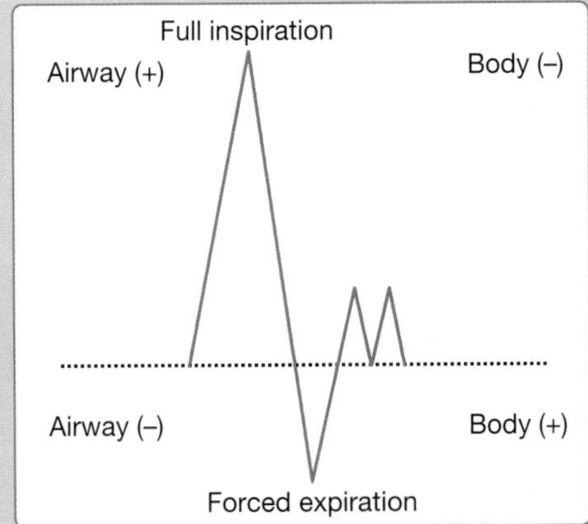

Body ventilators
NPBV
Inspiratory muscles
Iron lung or "portable" iron lung
Poncho or wrap
Cuirass or chest shell
Rocking bed — head up
Phrenic nerve stimulation

PPBV
Expiratory muscles
Intermittent abdominal pressure
Ventilator (IAPV)
Rocking bed — head down
Manual body resuscitation

FIGURE 28-3 Respiratory assistive devices superimposed on a graphic representation of the vital capacity and tidal volume. *Airway (–),* Ventilation by negative pressure on airway, producing suctioning; *airway (+),* ventilation by positive pressure on airway, producing inspiration; *body (–),* ventilation by negative pressure on body, producing inspiration; *body (+),* ventilation by positive pressure on body, producing expiration. *GPB,* Glossopharyngeal breathing; *IPPV,* intermittent positive-pressure ventilation; *NPBV,* negative-pressure body ventilator; *PAP,* positive airway pressure; *PPBV,* positive-pressure body ventilator.

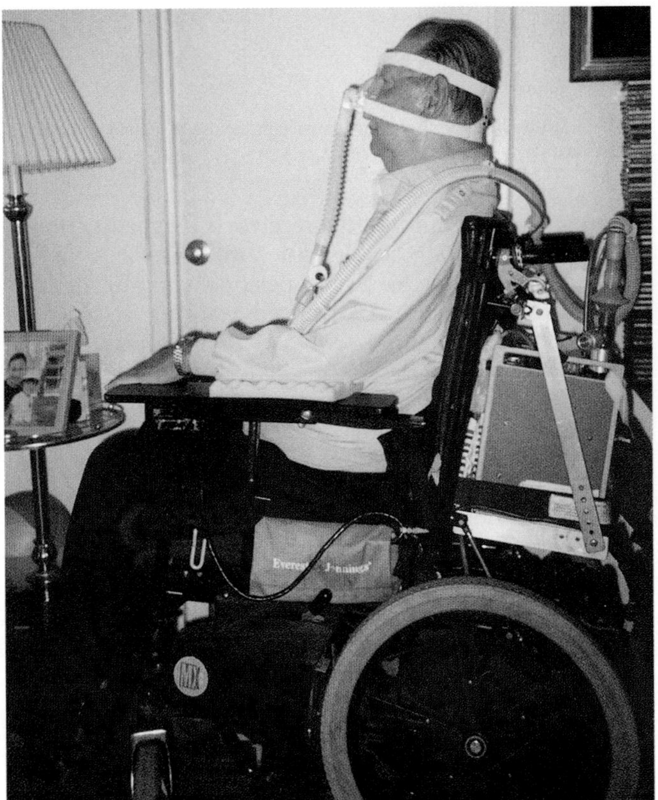

FIGURE 28-4 Nasal intermittent positive-pressure ventilation in a tetraplegic ventilator user with postpolio syndrome. The ventilator is a typical portable volume ventilator.

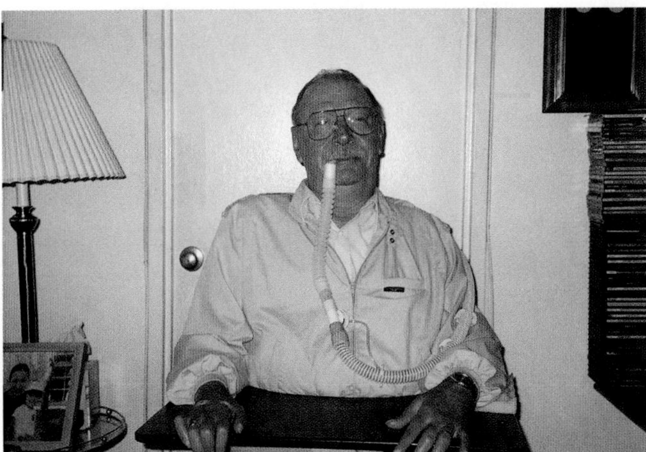

FIGURE 28-5 Mouth intermittent positive-pressure ventilation with angulated mouthpiece in a tetraplegic ventilator user with postpolio syndrome. The mouthpiece is held with teeth and lips.

which there will also be hypercapnia, (2) secretions, or (3) the development of intrinsic lung disease (usually gross atelectasis or pneumonia). Patients and families are taught to pursue airway clearance techniques conscientiously and to use NIPPV continuously. If these measures fail to bring the SpO_2 back to normal or to baseline levels, patients must be evaluated by their clinician or in the emergency room. They should be admitted if necessary. Family members or primary care providers need to remain with the patient in the hospital to perform the ongoing routine of secretion removal. The routine itself is typically too time-consuming for hospital personnel to be able to remove secretions with the frequency that is necessary during an acute respiratory infection. When there is inadequate social support, hospital personnel usually find it necessary to intubate the patient for secretion removal and ventilation.

Diaphragmatic pacing (Figure 28-8) is an alternative method of ventilation that has been available for more than 35 years. The system attained a higher level of reliability and broader application in the early 1990s. Infection and component failure are now rare complications. The need for the patient to retain a tracheostomy because of

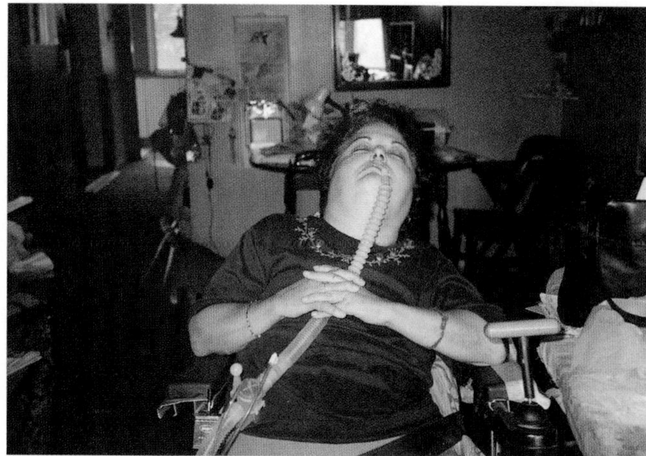

FIGURE 28-6 Mouth intermittent positive-pressure ventilation (IPPV) with angulated mouthpiece and without lip seal in a ventilator user with postpolio syndrome. She is taking a nap in her wheelchair. She can hold the IPPV hose with her hands on her chest. She has some ability to breathe on her own and is a good frog breather when she is awake.

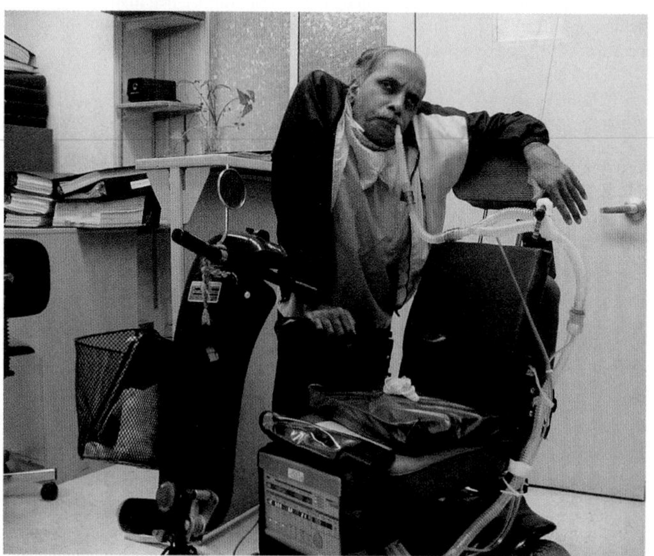

FIGURE 28-7 Mouth intermittent positive-pressure ventilation (IPPV) in a laptop ventilator user with "upside-down polio" (upper trunk weaker than lower trunk and legs) and severe kyphoscoliosis. He is breathing continuously, with abdominal muscles when erect. The ventilator allows the muscles to rest. It is mounted in front of the scooter seat. He uses console volume ventilator and tracheostomy IPPV at night. Supine, he has no "free time" off the ventilator.

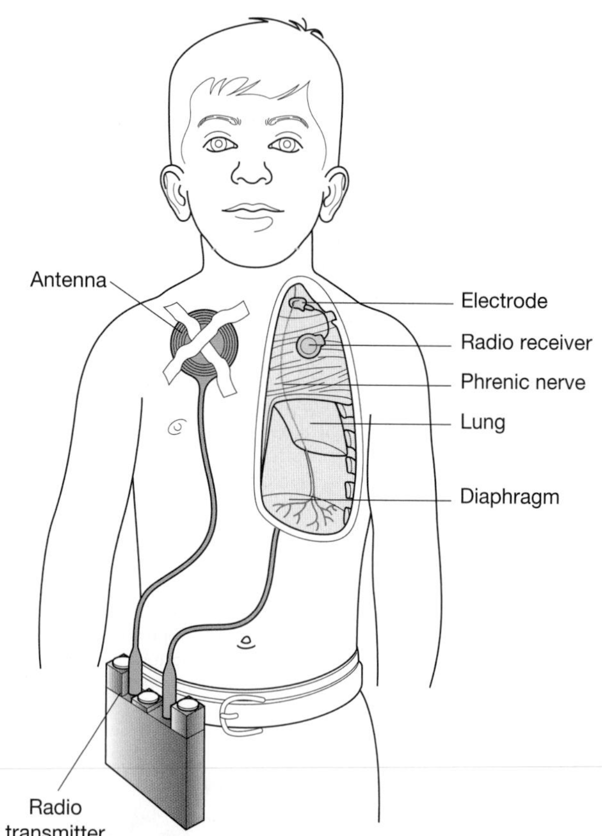

FIGURE 28-8 Bilateral diaphragmatic pacemaker use in a child with central hypoventilation syndrome.

obstructive sleep apnea remains common. Approximately 1500 phrenic nerve pacers have been implanted worldwide in persons of all ages. Many users have been successfully paced for more than 20 years.[48] Diaphragmatic pacing is indicated in patients with congenital central hypoventilation syndrome (or Ondine curse), acquired central hypoventilation syndrome, and high SCI injury.[44] Patients with inadequate social or financial support, poor motivation, or associated medical problems might not be good candidates. Although it is not common, the patient with a diaphragmatic pacer can require a mechanical ventilator as a backup during severe respiratory tract infections.

The pacing system consists of an external transmitter and antenna, and implanted electrodes and receiver. The working life expectancy of the receiver is for the lifetime of the patient, and batteries last for 2 to 3 weeks. A bipolar electrode is available for use in persons who already have demand cardiac pacers. Advanced warning is given of transmitter battery failure, with a gradual decrease in tidal volume over several days. The cervical implant is recommended in the older child and adult, with "customized" stimulation variables that enable pacing with small numbers of residual fibers. Surgery in the supraclavicular region of the neck is relatively simple, and hospitalization is typical, although the procedure can be performed in an outpatient setting. Although thoracic phrenic nerve implants for infants and younger children have required thoracotomy in the past, thoracoscopic placement of the electrodes has now been reported in children as young as 5 years.[141] Remote monitoring can be used to assess effectiveness and to diagnosis problems.

Krieger and Krieger[79] reported performing 10 nerve transfers in six patients with SCI at the C3 to C5 level, with axonal loss in the phrenic nerves to the extent that pacing was not possible. In their technique, the fourth intercostal nerve was attached to the distal segment of the phrenic nerve 5 cm above the diaphragm. The pacemaker was implanted on the phrenic nerve distal to the anastomosis. The average interval from surgery to diaphragmatic response to electrical stimulation was 9 months. All patients were able to tolerate diaphragmatic pacing as an alternative to IPPV.

Intramuscular diaphragm electrodes implanted via laparoscopic surgery were reported to successfully stimulate the phrenic nerves in one ventilator-dependent patient with tetraplegia.[45] In patients having only a single phrenic nerve that can be paced, combined intercostal muscle and unilateral phrenic nerve stimulation has also been shown to maintain ventilatory support.[141]

Long-Term Outcomes of Mechanical Ventilation

Many patients are now surviving significant illness only to become chronically ventilator-dependent. The number of long-term care hospitals in the United States has increased to greater than 250 in the past 15 years to care for these patients. Acute lung injury survivors weaned from the ventilator have been studied 1 year after hospital discharge.[38] Thirty percent still have generalized cognitive dysfunction, and 78% have decrements in attention, memory, concentration, and/or mental-processing speed. Many also have musculoskeletal complications such as weakness and numbness resulting from critical illness neuropathy and steroid-induced myopathy. Acute respiratory distress syndrome survivors weaned from the ventilator have been studied 1 year after hospital discharge.[38] Emotional dysfunction included the presence of depression, anxiety, and posttraumatic stress disorder.

Long-term outcomes of diaphragm paralysis after acute SCI have been reported.[110] Over a 16-year period, 107 patients required assisted ventilation in the acute phase of injury. Of this group, 31% (33 patients) with a level of injury between C1 and C4 (scale A in the American Spinal Injury Association Impairment Scale) had diaphragmatic paralysis at the time of respiratory failure. Twenty-one percent of the 33 patients were able to breathe independently after 4 to 14 months, with a vital capacity greater than 15 mL/kg. Another 15% (five patients) had some recovery that took more time and for whom the vital capacity remained less than 10 mL/kg.

Bach[8] has described in detail the long-term outcomes of NIPPV in neuromuscular disease. No patient with Duchenne muscular dystrophy has been tracheostomized since 1983 at the Center for Ventilator Management Alternatives and Pulmonary Rehabilitation of the University Hospital in Newark, New Jersey. Some have been using 24-hour mechanical ventilation for up to 15 to 25 years. Cardiomyopathy has become the limiting factor for survival in this population because respiratory deaths are being avoided. Wijkstra et al.[169] reported the long-term outcomes of inpatients with chronic-assisted ventilatory care over 15 years. Thirty-six percent of their 50 patients left the hospital to enter a more independent community-based environment. Better outcomes were seen among patients with SCI and neuromuscular disease than in patients with COPD and thoracic restriction. Gonzalez et al.[59] studied long-term NIPPV in kyphoscoliotic ventilatory insufficiency (thoracic restriction) over 3 years. Patients showed improved blood gas levels and respiratory muscle performance and reduced hypoventilation-based symptoms and number of hospital days.

Lung Volume Reduction Surgery

LVRS is used in patients with advanced emphysema. In LVRS, 20% to 30% of one or both lungs (usually at the apices) is removed. Decramer[41] has reported the short-term results of six randomized studies, including the National Emphysema Treatment Trial. These studies have shown reduced hyperinflation (residual volume and total lung capacity decreased) and improved FEV_1 and FVC. The 6-minute walk increased significantly and quality of life improved. In general, inspiratory muscle function (maximal inspiratory pressure and maximal transdiaphragmatic pressure) also improved. Combining LVRS with exercise produces greater benefits than exercise alone.[68]

Not all patients will benefit from LVRS. Patients with an FEV_1 less than 20% predicted and homogeneous disease, or a diffusion capacity less than 20% predicted, experience an increased mortality rate after LVRS. Additional studies suggest that patients getting the most benefit from LVRS are those with emphysema predominately in upper lobes who also have low postrehabilitation exercise capacity.[100] Conversely, patients with non–upper lobe involvement and high postrehabilitation measures of maximal work received little benefit from LVRS.[100] The results of the National Emphysema Treatment Trial suggest that all LVRS candidates should first enroll in a pulmonary rehabilitation program because some patients can improve to the point that they might not qualify for the surgery.[52] Furthermore, participation in a pulmonary rehabilitation program before LVRS helps to both identify appropriate surgical candidates[130] and helps to ensure that candidates have appropriate levels of compliance and an understanding of their condition.[152]

Bronchoscopic LVRS is an alternative treatment option, which is a less invasive and potentially beneficial intervention for patients who may not be candidates for traditional LVRS.[70] There are many different interventions, ranging from various stents, occluders, polymers, coils, and thermal vapor ablation. Stapling and plication of the most emphysematous tissue are carried out. Atelectasis can also be induced in these areas with the use of endobronchial sealants or valves. Extraanatomic tracts between the major airways and the emphysematous tissue are created and prevented from collapsing with stents to facilitate expiratory airflow.

Long-Term Results for Lung Volume Reduction Surgery

Naunheim et al.[100] provided evidence that the distribution of emphysematic changes in lung parenchyma (measured by high-resolution computed tomography) and measures of exercise capacity after rehabilitation are important factors in predicting the long-term effects of LVRS. Patients who received LVRS and had emphysema predominantly in the upper lobes with lower levels of exercise capacity continued to have improved survival rates after 4 years, improved function after 3 years, and improved dyspnea after 5 years. Patients with upper lobe involvement and high levels of exercise capacity after rehabilitation continued to have symptomatic improvements when assessed after 4 years. Patients with non–upper lobe emphysema and low exercise capacity primarily experienced improvements in health-related quality of life that became insignificant after 3 years. Patients with non–upper lobe emphysema and high exercise capacity did not experience significant benefits from LVRS, and actually experienced a higher mortality rate during the first 3 years. Improvements in all groups were no longer significant after 5 years.

Lung Transplant

Lung transplants are now performed worldwide. Living donor, lobar, and split-lung procedures are more common in children than in adults. Cystic fibrosis and primary pulmonary hypertension are the two main diseases of children for which lung transplant is performed. COPD is the main reason for lung transplant in adults, although pulmonary hypertension and pulmonary fibrosis are also common presenting diagnoses. Ongoing smoking is an absolute contraindication to lung transplant. Relative contraindications in most programs include previous cancer, psychiatric diagnosis, obesity, and correctable coronary artery disease.[83] Fifty-eight percent of programs in North America that have been queried have a minimum requirement for exercise capacity to be considered for lung transplant. Covering a minimum of 600 feet on a 6-minute walk test is the most common requirement, although some programs require only 250 feet. If an individual can only transfer from bed to chair, 46% of lung transplant centers consider this an absolute contraindication to lung transplant, and 52% consider it a relative contraindication.

Long-Term Results in Lung Transplant

Survival rates for all lung transplants from 1994 to mid-2005 were 78% at 1 year, 50% at 5 years, and 26% at 10 years, with the highest mortality rate occurring during the first year.[161] Although perioperative mortality rates are not significantly different for all age groups, patients older than 50 years tend to experience a lower survival rate beyond the first year.[161] Sepsis and bronchiolitis obliterans remain the two most common causes of death. These results, however, should be tempered with the knowledge that the mortality rate for those on the transplant waiting list is also high. For example, the 3-year survival rate for those in the sickest category of the COPD BODE Index (Body mass index, degree of airflow Obstruction, functional Dyspnea, Exercise capacity) is only 50%.[30]

Special Considerations

Obesity-Related Pulmonary Dysfunction

Data from the 2009 to 2010 National Health and Nutrition Examination Survey indicate an estimated 35.5% of adults in the United States were overweight or obese (body mass index [BMI] > 25).[53] Seventeen percent of U.S. children and adolescents are estimated to be overweight.[107] All racial and ethnic groups and both genders are affected. Primary respiratory complications associated with obesity include obstructive sleep apnea, obesity-hypoventilation syndrome, and asthma.[99] Chronic hypoxemia related to obesity-hypoventilation syndrome can lead to polycythemia, pulmonary hypertension, cardiac dysrhythmias, and right ventricular failure. One study reported that three of four adults who presented to the emergency department with acute asthma were either overweight (BMI = 25 to 29.9; 30%) or obese (BMI > 30; 44%).[158] Other conditions that can be associated with obesity include atelectasis, pneumonia, venous thrombosis, and pulmonary embolism.[99] Daily physical activity is important in preventing and treating overweight and obesity because many of the aforementioned conditions are improved with weight loss.

Obesity increases the metabolic requirements of breathing and physical activity, resulting in decreased exercise tolerance. The weight relative maximal volume of oxygen consumption ($\dot{V}O_{2\,max}$) in obese persons can be significantly decreased compared with controls. Norman et al.[104] studied severely obese adolescents (BMI > 40) and found that although absolute $\dot{V}O_{2max}$ (mL O_2/min) was similar to controls, walk/run distance was approximately 60% of the control average. Although obese adults with COPD might have greater fatigue, functional impairment, and significantly lower 6-minute walk distance compared with normal-weight individuals with COPD, similar relative improvements in walk distance are seen after pulmonary rehabilitation.[126]

Spinal Cord Injury and Pulmonary Dysfunction

In SCI, there is diminished cardiopulmonary and circulatory function, as well as lower limb muscle atrophy and bone mass reduction. Patients with high cervical cord injuries, including children as young as 3 years, can learn neck breathing[57] or GPB as forms of voluntary respiration. This allows some time off the ventilator. In GPB (or frog breathing), air is pumped into the lungs by the patient using the tongue as a piston (Figure 28-9). This technique is known as glottic press to speech pathologists. They teach it to patients who have had a laryngectomy, to pump air into the esophagus for esophageal speech. GPB can be used for a number of purposes in addition to being an alternative form of breathing. GPB can improve vocal volume and flow of speech to allow the patient to call for help, and to provide the deep breath needed for an assisted cough.

Summary

Pulmonary rehabilitation requires a team approach to management of chronic lung disease led by physiatrists who need a basic knowledge of the anatomy and pathophysiology of the cardiovascular and respiratory systems, as well as exercise physiology. Patient assessment skills include proficiency in the electromyography of the respiratory muscles and an understanding of the rapidly expanding field of cardiopulmonary imaging. The practice of pulmonary rehabilitation can be in a setting limited to this subspecialty but more commonly is practiced as a component of general rehabilitation, where patients have pulmonary dysfunction as a complication of their neurologic or musculoskeletal disabilities or as a medical comorbidity. General rehabilitative therapeutic approaches apply in either setting. Health policy, legislation, and regulations, including current health care delivery systems, must take into account the need for pulmonary rehabilitation at all ages in society. An informed public can facilitate change in this regard. The public is more informed now because of the development of online interest groups, Internet

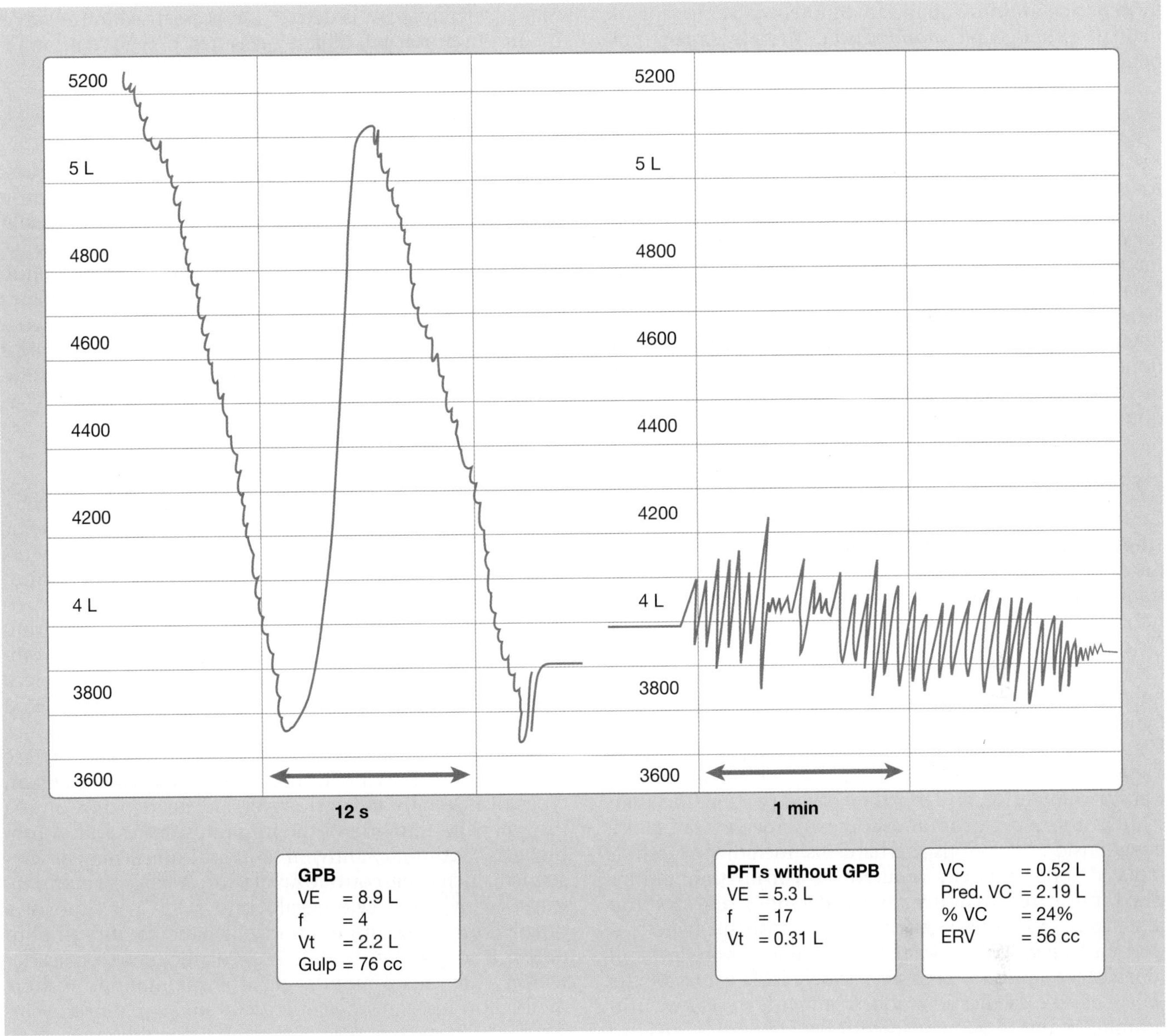

FIGURE 28-9 Glossopharyngeal breathing (GPB) tracing and results compared with pulmonary function tests without GPB in a tetraplegic ventilator user with postpolio syndrome. *ERV,* Expiratory reserve volume; *f,* frequency; *gulp,* volume or single GPB stroke; *VE,* minute ventilation; *Vt,* tidal volume.

bulletin boards, and almost 350,000 articles pertaining to pulmonary rehabilitation on the Internet.

Rehabilitation in Solid Organ Transplant Recipients

The field of transplant rehabilitation has slowly evolved over the past several years with new research assessing outcomes and the effects of exercise in transplant recipients, but there remains a paucity of literature outlining optimal transplantation rehabilitation processes. This section provides a general overview of the subject of solid organ transplantation rehabilitation with a primary focus on the kidney, heart, lungs, and liver, which are the four most common seen in physiatric practice.

Physiatric Interventions in Enhancing Outcomes

The goal of transplant rehabilitation is to improve functional outcomes and facilitate reintegration into a fulfilling life and lifestyle using a comprehensive, interdisciplinary, structured, and integrated approach between the physiatrist and primary transplant team. Long-term success of organ transplantation is largely dependent on a high-quality aftercare program that integrates essential medical management with a customized rehabilitation regimen.[138]

For all solid organ transplantation patients, a preoperative functional, psychosocial, and medical baseline must be established including a comprehensive medical history and characterization of all functional deficits associated with the patient's end-stage organ disease. This is vital to formulating an individualized comprehensive therapeutic plan of exercise and mobilization. The physiatrist must perform a detailed musculoskeletal, neurologic, and functional assessment with emphasis placed on the specific body systems adversely affected by immobilization.

During the early postoperative phase, vigilant medical surveillance and monitoring must be employed to treat transplant-associated medical complications, ensure adequate immunosuppression, minimize the risk of donor organ rejection, prevent opportunistic infections, and maintain rehabilitation goals with the implementation of measures aimed at the prevention of contractures, deep vein thrombosis and pulmonary embolism, skin breakdown, and bowel or bladder dysfunction.[24] The rehabilitation team must also be cognizant of the clinical features of acute and chronic rejection in all types of transplantation surgeries as well as other medical complications.

Hypertension

Corticosteroids and calcineurin inhibitors can have pressor effects, resulting in elevated blood pressure. In addition to the cardiovascular risk, arterial hypertension can have a significant long-term effect on morbidity and mortality in transplant patients and is one of the long-term prognostic factors for survival.[138] This is particularly problematic in renal transplant patients in whom blood pressure is frequently found to be elevated postoperatively. Arterial hypertension is prevalent in renal transplant recipients and is associated with reduced allograft and patient survival. In a single-center study, only 5% of kidney transplant patients were normotensive, as defined by blood pressure less than 130/80 mm Hg.[116] Immunosuppressive agents can cause hypertension by various mechanisms, including catechol-induced and endothelin-induced vasoconstriction, diminished nitric oxide-induced vasodilatation, and sodium retention.[93] Additional causes of posttransplant hypertension include sequelae of antibody-mediated rejection and renal artery stenosis. Calcium channel blockers may be the most useful medication for treatment of calcineurin inhibitor-induced vasoconstriction.[93] The cardioprotective and nephroprotective effects of angiotensin-converting enzyme inhibitors and angiotensin II receptor blockers are also usually preferred in transplant patients.

Hyperlipidemia

Nearly all immunosuppressive agents can lead to hyperlipidemia that is often refractory to dietary management alone. Pravastatin (Pravachol) and fluvastatin (Lescol, Canef, Vastin) are the most thoroughly studied agents in combination with immunosuppressive agents. Patients receiving treatment with statins and calcineurin inhibitors should undergo creatine kinase level monitoring because the combination may adversely lead to rhabdomyolysis.[138]

Steroid-Induced Hyperglycemia and Posttransplant Diabetes

Immunosuppression with steroids or calcineurin inhibitors has been associated with an increased incidence of insulin-dependent posttransplant diabetes. If posttransplant hyperglycemia is detected, it is essential to intervene medically either with dietary measures, oral glycemic medications, and/or insulin.[125,138]

Renal Insufficiency

Given the nephrotoxicity associated with immunosuppressants, particularly calcineurin inhibitors, renal function variables should be monitored routinely, to include serum creatinine, urea values, and glomerular filtration rate. Ensuring adequate daily fluid intake and avoiding additional nephrotoxic agents, such as nonsteroidal antiinflammatory drugs, are simple measures employed to avoid renal compromise. If the posttransplant patient exhibits renal insufficiency, changes to the immunosuppression regimen may be considered by the transplant team.[138]

Infections

Posttransplantation infections pose a significant challenge in an immunosuppressed patient. The etiologic differential of the source of infection in these patients includes nosocomial, community-acquired, or donor organ–derived and may include opportunistic pathogens that become clinically significant in the immunosuppressed.[51] The treatment team must have a very low threshold for initiating diagnostic testing, because posttransplant patients can initially present with subclinical signs and symptoms caused by an impaired inflammatory response and leukopenia. Graft rejection or graft-versus-host disease can also be confused with infection.[51] The risk for certain types of infection and inciting organisms depends on the intensity and duration of the immunosuppression. A prophylactic antibiotic, antiviral, and antifungal may be prescribed, including cotrimoxazole for *Pneumocystis carinii*, valganciclovir for cytomegalovirus (CMV) IgG-positive organ donors and nonimmunized patients and amphotericin B to prevent candidiasis.[138] Pathogens to consider within the first month posttransplantation include methicillin-resistant *Staphylococcus aureus*, vancomycin-resistant *Enterococcus*, *Clostridium difficile* colitis, as well as pulmonary infections (aspiration pneumonia, ventilator-associated or postsurgical), line-associated or catheter-associated infections, or infections of devitalized tissues and fluid collections. Other pathogens to consider in the first 6 months after transplantation are *Mycobacterium tuberculosis*, *Nocardia*, *Leishmania*, Epstein-Barr virus, herpes simplex virus, human herpes virus 6, hepatitis B virus, hepatitis C virus, and BK virus. Opportunistic infections can include *Aspergillus* and *Listeria monocytogenes*.[51] Given the diversity of these organisms and complexity of drug interactions with many of the transplant-related medications, any antimicrobial management should be under the direction of the medical-surgical transplant team.

Immunosuppression

The physiatrist must be aware of the potential adverse effects associated with the numerous immunosuppressant medications administered following transplantation. A summary of the side effects of some of the most frequently used agents is provided in Table 28-5.[62,84,132,136,162]

Table 28-5 Adverse Drug Effects of Transplant Antirejection Drugs

Drug	Adverse Effects
Azathioprine (Antiproliferative agent)	Leukopenia, anemia, thrombocytopenia Hepatotoxicity and cholestasis Hepatic venoocclusive disease Pancreatitis Increased risk of malignancy when associated with high doses of multiple agents
Mycophenolate (Antiproliferative agent)	Diarrhea, nausea, vomiting Leukopenia, thrombocytopenia Wound dehiscence Hepatotoxicity (less than azathioprine) Higher risk of opportunistic infections compared with azathioprine
Orthoclone (OKT3)	Pyrexia, malaise Respiratory distress associated with initial doses and fluid overload Increased risk of malignancy when associated with high doses of multiple agents
Antithymocyte preparations (alemtuzumab, rituximab)	Anaphylactic reactions Serum sickness associated with antibody formation to foreign protein Bone marrow depression associated with prolonged use in conjunction with azathioprine Local inflammatory reactions associated with intramuscular administration Increased risk of malignancy when associated with high doses of multiple agents
Tacrolimus (calcineurin inhibitor)	Nephrotoxicity associated with high doses Hyperkalemia Insomnia Malaise Neurotoxicity more common than in cyclosporine Drug-induced diabetes Bone marrow suppression Gum hyperplasia Less hypertension and hyperlipidemia than cyclosporine
Cyclosporine (calcineurin inhibitor)	Nephrotoxicity Malignancy Pancytopenia Neurotoxicity (posterior reversible encephalopathic syndrome, seizures, headache, tremor) Pancytopenia Gastrointestinal complaints Hypertension Hepatotoxicity Hypertrichosis Myopathy Increased risk of malignancy when associated with high doses of multiple agents Gingival hyperplasia Hyperkalemia Hypomagnesemia Impaired vision Insomnia
Sirolimus (mTOR inhibitor)	Hyperlipidemia Vasculitis Thrombocytopenia Impaired wound healing Nephrotoxic in combination of calcineurin inhibitors
Corticosteroids	Aseptic necrosis of bone, osteoporosis Hyperglycemia, steroid-induced diabetes mellitus Salt and water retention Hypertension Easy bruising Skin fragility Acne Sun sensitivity Hirsutism Growth retardation in children Gastritis/gastrointestinal ulcerations Cataracts Sleep alterations Impaired wound healing Emotional lability Weight gain and truncal obesity
Basiliximab (interleukin-2 antagonist)	Bone marrow suppression
Belatacept (costimulation blocker)	Hypertension Hyperlipidemia Diabetes mellitus Bone marrow suppression
Bortezomib	Neurotoxicity Bone marrow suppression Nausea, vomiting, diarrhea Hypotension QT prolongation

See Table 28-6 for the monitoring variables for a few immunosuppressive medications.

Renal Transplantation Rehabilitation

Impairments with activities of daily living and fatigue can present significant limitations to patients with end-stage renal disease (ESRD).[66] According to the National Kidney Foundation, as of September 2014, there were 123,175 people waiting for lifesaving organ transplants in the United States. Of those, 101,170 were awaiting kidney transplants. In 2013, 16,896 kidney transplants occurred in the United States. Of these, 11,163 came from deceased donors and 5733 came from living donors. On average, approximately 3000 new patients are added to the kidney waiting list each month and 12 people die each day while waiting for a kidney transplant.[156] Between 1980 and 2009, the prevalence of ESRD increased approximately 600%, from 290 to 1738 cases per million. The percentage of kidneys transplanted in 1980 that survived to 1990 was 25.7%. That percentage has improved with the survival rate from 1999 to 2009 rising to 44.9%. The 5-year survival rate for transplant patients is 85.5%, more than twice the 35.8% survival rate for dialysis patients.[156]

In addition to aforementioned complications associated with organ transplantation, the physiatrist must be able to recognize signs and symptoms of kidney rejection, fever, leukocytosis, anorexia, malaise, hypertension, elevated serum renal markers such as blood urea nitrogen and creatinine, kidney enlargement with focal retroperitoneal tenderness, edema, weight gain, and reduced urinary output.[123] One must be mindful of the multiple side effects of immunosuppressant medications, including prednisone, azathioprine, and cyclosporine. (See Box 28-4 for a list of clinical signs associated with renal graft rejection.)

Table 28-6 Immunosuppressive Medication Monitoring for Physiatrists

Drug	Side Effects	Monitor
Prednisone	Gastrointestinal irritability Water, fluid retention Diabetes mellitus	Stool occult blood Hematocrit Daily weight Fasting and preprandial glucose levels
Cyclosporine	Nephrotoxicity Hepatotoxicity Drug toxicity	Blood urea nitrogen, creatinine Liver function tests Cyclosporine level
Azathioprine	Pancytopenia Hepatotoxicity	Complete blood count Liver function tests

BOX 28-4

Clinical Signs of Renal Graft Rejection

- Tenderness at graft site
- Decrease in urine output
- Sudden increase in weight: 3 to 5 lb in a 24-hour period
- Edema—usually begins in hands and feet
- Elevated temperature
- Elevated serum creatinine above the individual baseline

Exercise After Kidney Transplantation

Several important physiologic elements affect the renal transplant recipient's ability to exercise. Patients with chronic kidney disease (CKD) are at risk for protein-energy wasting, abnormal body composition, and impaired physical capacity. In many circumstances, patients with CKD have an inadequate diet that also impairs physical performance promoting a sedentary lifestyle, which further contributes to loss of muscle strength and quality of life.[37] CKD is well known to induce stress on the cardiovascular system.[113] Cardiovascular disease is the most common cause of death in patients with ESRD as well as in renal transplant recipients. A recent retrospective study of 500 patients evaluated the prevalence and the types of cardiovascular disease in patients with ESRD undergoing renal transplantation and found hypertension in 62.2%, DM in 3.4%, smoking in 26.4%, dyslipidemia in 13.2%, and mean ejection fraction on echocardiogram of $51.9 \pm 7.1\%$.[17] Metabolic abnormalities, such as imbalance of electrolytes, including sodium and water retention, can cause increases in right and left ventricular preload. As circulatory volume expands, hypertension is exacerbated and increased afterload ensues, which predisposes the individual to cardiac hypertrophy and diminished compliance.

There is substantial evidence documenting the benefits of regular exercise for patients with CKD, with documented improvements in maximal exercise capacity (walking speed and distance, stair climbing, and rising from a chair) and self-reported functioning. Multiple studies have demonstrated that patients with CKD with poor levels of physical activity, regardless of age, can function at levels similar to older individuals in the general population.[114] ESRD limits exercise potential, and renal-impaired patients who engage in aerobic exercise can further diminish renal perfusion, leading to a compromised ability to conserve water. Exercise tolerance may be further reduced by comorbid anemia of chronic renal disease. Fortunately, a successful kidney transplant can greatly increase exercise capacity to near-normal values for sedentary healthy individuals,[55] although participation in exercise following renal transplant remains limited, likely resulting from skeletal muscle atrophy and cardiovascular deconditioning. Renal transplant patients have reduced peak aerobic capacity, muscle strength, arterial function, and an unfavorable cardiovascular disease risk profile. Fatigue is a major factor in up to 59% of kidney transplant recipients. Posttransplant clinical, psychosocial, and behavioral predictors of fatigue can include elevated C-reactive protein (CRP), decreased estimated glomerular filtration rate pointing to possible graft dysfunction, and reduced lean tissue index, poor sleep quality, anxiety, and depression.[33] Weight gain after transplantation is common and can be influenced by immunosuppressants, particularly corticosteroids, or delayed graft function. It is common to observe an increase in BMI in the first year after transplantation and patients must optimize diet and strive to engage in adequate physical exercise.[50]

Recent studies suggest that supervised endurance and strengthening exercise programs after kidney transplant can improve peak aerobic capacity, cardiac output, muscle strength, and quality of life. It can also result in higher levels of measured and self-reported physical functioning, although exercise alone does not necessarily yield significant improvements in body composition, lean body mass, and blood pressure.[131] However, exercise training after transplant can counteract some of the negative side effects of glucocorticoid therapy, such as muscle wasting and excessive weight gain. Rehabilitation after kidney transplant is an essential therapeutic method for improving outcomes in ESRD and transplant recipients.

Rehabilitation in Cardiac Transplantation

Heart Transplant Epidemiology

Congestive heart failure (CHF) affects 7.5 million in North America. Cardiac transplantation is considered the "gold standard" in management and is the treatment of choice for many patients with end-stage heart failure with symptoms refractory to medical therapy.[160] According to the International Society for Heart and Lung Transplantation, approximately 89,000 heart transplants have been performed worldwide since 1983 and 3500 to 4000 are performed annually, with 2400 in the United States.[3] Owing to advances in medical therapy for patients with CHF as well as the increased use of implantable cardiac devices, the annual mortality rate while on the transplant waiting list has progressively declined to 13.7% in 2009. In addition, long-term outcomes after cardiac transplantation have improved with advances in candidate selection criteria, surgical techniques, infection prophylaxis, immunosuppressive agents, postoperative care, and rehabilitation.[3,160] The median age of transplant recipients has been stable at 54 years since 2002, but the proportion of recipients at extremes of age has increased. Between the years 1982 to 1985 and 2006 to 2012, the proportion of recipients aged 60 to 69 years increased from 14% to 24%.[39] Other important changes in the demographics of heart transplant recipients over the past 2 decades include increased recipient BMI, increased proportion of females, and increasing proportion of transplant patients with diabetes, previous dialysis, hypertension, previous cardiac surgery, and previous malignancy.[39] The 1-year survival rate is 90% and 70% at 5 years, but only 20% or less survive 20 years or longer.[148] The 30-day operative mortality for cardiac transplantation spans from 5% to 10% because of graft failure, multisystem organ failure, and infection. Graft failure, acute rejection, and infection are the leading causes of death during the first year. Cardiac allograft vasculopathy and malignancy are the most significant causes of death after 1 year.[160] The joint guidelines for cardiac transplantation candidacy from the American College of Cardiology and the American Heart Association are shown in Box 28-5.[74] The absolute and relative contraindications are listed in Box 28-6.[3,74,92]

Rehabilitation Before Heart Transplantation

The inciting etiology that leads to CHF includes a broad differential, including ischemic heart disease, valve dysfunction, idiopathic cardiomyopathy, or viral myocarditis. Evaluations by both a cardiologist and physiatrist should

BOX 28-5

Indications for Cardiac Transplantation

- Refractory cardiogenic shock requiring intraaortic balloon pump counterpulsation or left ventricular assist device
- Cardiogenic shock requiring continuous intravenous inotropic therapy
- Peak VO_2 ($VO_{2\,max}$) less than 10 mL/kg per minute
- NYHA class of III or IV despite maximized medical and resynchronization therapy
- Recurrent life-threatening left ventricular arrhythmias despite an implantable cardiac defibrillator, antiarrhythmic therapy, or catheter-based ablation
- End-stage congenital heart failure with no evidence of pulmonary hypertension
- Refractory angina without potential medical or surgical therapeutic options

NYHA, New York Heart Association.

BOX 28-6

Absolute and Relative Contraindications to Heart Transplantation

Absolute Contraindications to Heart Transplantation

- Advanced irreversible renal failure with Cr >2 or creatinine clearance <30 to 50 mL/min without plans for concurrent renal transplant
- Advanced irreversible liver disease
- Advanced irreversible pulmonary parenchymal disease or FEV_1 <1 L/min
- Advanced irreversible pulmonary artery hypertension (pulmonary artery systolic pressure >60 mm Hg, pulmonary vascular resistance >4 to 5 wood units despite vasodilators) attributable to risk of acute right ventricular failure soon after transplant from insufficient accommodation of the donor heart to high pulmonary vascular resistance pressures
- History of solid organ or hematologic malignancy within the past 5 years as a result of probability of recurrence.

Relative Contraindications to Heart Transplantation Resulting from the Reversibility of the Disease Process or Lack of Direct Impact on the Transplanted Organ

- Severe peripheral vascular disease
- Severe cerebrovascular disease
- Severe osteoporosis
- Severe obesity (BMI >35 kg/m^2) or cachexia
- Acute pulmonary embolism
- Active infection (excluding LVAD-related infections)
- Advanced age (>70 years old)
- Psychological instability (e.g., PTSD)
- Active or recent (within 6 months) substance abuse (alcohol, cocaine, opioids, tobacco products, etc.)
- Diabetes mellitus with end-stage organ damage
- Lack of social support or sufficient resources to permit ongoing access to immunosuppressive medication and frequent medical follow-up

BMI, Body mass index; *Cr,* creatinine; *FEV_1,* forced expiratory volume in 1 second; *LVAD,* left ventricular assist device; *PTSD,* posttraumatic stress disorder.

be integrated to better understand the disease process and its probable impact on the patient's quality of life pretransplantation and posttransplantation. The prioritization of appropriate candidates for transplantation is based on medical comorbidities as well as the expected gains in quality of life compared against the optimization of medical and surgical resources available. Geographic distance between donor and potential recipient is also a consideration. Patients awaiting transplantation may be reassessed every 3 months for quantification of circulatory impairments, exercise performance, comorbid diagnoses, and the overall health of the patient. The most successful outcomes depend on the identification of candidates who have the physical capacity to maximally benefit from a new heart and the rehabilitation process.[144] During the period of heart procurement, a myriad of implantable devices can improve tolerance for activity and perhaps allow preliminary rehabilitation.[160]

Complications After Cardiac Transplantation

Coordination of care between the cardiac surgeon, cardiologist, and the physiatrist is essential for success. The cardiac rehabilitation team must be familiar with the complications of heart transplantation to address issues that might affect the recipient's functional performance. The main complication posttransplant is allograft failure from rejection. Signs of acute rejection include fulminant CHF, abrupt onset of new peripheral edema, new arrhythmias, such as premature atrial contractions, and sudden reduction in exercise capacity. Secondary complications include problems related to immunosuppression, such as infection, neurotoxicity, renal toxicity, hypertension, and various metabolic abnormalities. Early cardiac failure still accounts for up to 20% of perioperative deaths of heart transplant patients, with the most important causes resulting from dysfunction of the donor myocardium from acute rejection, pulmonary hypertension, and ischemic injury.[160] Right-sided heart failure is a significant cause of morbidity and mortality in the setting of increased afterload resulting in ventricular failure from pulmonary vascular resistance. The heart often requires inotropic support during the period immediately after transplant. Owing to autonomic denervation, the transplant recipient may be subject to multiple types of arrhythmias, including atrial fibrillation, flutter, supraventricular tachycardia, or bradyarrhythmias.[160]

Cyclosporine-induced renal vasoconstriction superimposed on chronic renal hypoperfusion may result in hypertension through glomerular arteriolar vasoconstriction. Tacrolimus (Prograf, Advagraf, Protopic) is associated with a lower incidence of hypertension compared with cyclosporine, which may be used under the direction of the transplant team. Blood pressures should be closely monitored, intervening with antihypertensive agents as needed. In most circumstances, this can be achieved without interruption of the exercise therapy regimen. Moderate to severe hypertension can affect up to 90% of cardiac transplant patients. Diuretics and beta-blockers should be used cautiously because of volume depletion/hypotension and blunting of the heart rate response to exercise.[160]

Careful assessment of neurologic and mental status as well as motor function is an essential part of the physiatric consultation in the postoperative phase. Neurologic complications that can occur acute posttransplantation include metabolic encephalopathy, central nervous system infection, seizures, and psychosis. Strokes can occur from particulate or air embolism, and cerebral hypoperfusion during the surgery.

One of the leading causes of death in postcardiac transplant patients is infection, including mediastinitis, pneumonia, urinary tract infections, or intravenous catheter-induced sepsis. *Escherichia coli*, *Pseudomonas aeruginosa*, and *Staphylococcus* have been shown to be the cause of the majority of bacterial infections in this patient population. However, CMV is the most significant cause of morbidity and mortality related to infection. CMV is associated with acute rejection, acceleration of coronary artery disease, and lymphoproliferative disease. CMV prophylaxis and active treatment include agents such as ganciclovir (Cytovene, Cymevene). *Aspergillus* is an opportunistic pathogen with the highest mortality and can cause serious pneumonia in 5% to 10% of recipients during the first 3 months posttransplant.[160] The incidence of *Pneumocystis carinii* pneumonia can range from approximately 1% to 10%. *Toxoplasmosis gondii* infection is a result of reactivation of latent disease in the seropositive donor heart and can cause significant infections of the central nervous system, which require treatment with pyrimethamine (Daraprim), sulfadiazine (Lantrisul, Neotrizine), or clindamycin (Cleocin).[160]

Physiology of the Transplanted Heart

An understanding of the physiology of the transplanted heart is essential to the physiatrist prescribing therapy regimen. In a normal heart, chronotropic and ionotropic regulation is dictated by the autonomic nervous system, with its sympathetic division responsible for increasing venous return, stroke volume, and cardiac output. Orthotopic heart transplantation involves extracting the native heart at the level of atrioventricular junction transecting the aorta and pulmonary artery above the semilunar valves. Immediately after the surgery, right-sided and left-sided filing pressures within the heart are elevated, which results in myocardial anoxia and pulmonary hypertension that will eventually normalize over a few weeks.[76] Postoperatively, left ventricular ejection fraction and myocardial contractility are within normal limits or slightly depressed. With the loss of vagal tone, the denervated heart has a higher than normal resting heart rate; usually 15 to 25 beats per minute above average consistent with the intrinsic rate of the sinoatrial node of the transplanted heart. This resting tachycardia is associated with a reduced stroke volume to maintain a near-normal resting cardiac output. Vagal maneuvers such as carotid massage or Valsalva does not affect the heart rate. Owing to its denervation, a transplanted heart increases to a maximum heart rate as well as return to baseline more slowly than a normal heart by a process that is principally mediated by the rise and fall of circulating catecholamines, although a minority of patients demonstrate signs of partial cardiac reinnervation several months after surgery.[148] Despite this, cardiac output in the transplanted heart does increase with total body activity mainly by the Frank-Starling mechanism, which stimulates venous return increasing cardiac preload, resulting in greater stroke volume.[76] Thus, the response of the transplanted heart to exercise is preload-dependent at the onset of increased exertion, but switches to a catecholamine-driven process through prolonged exercise that is unable to make sharp fluctuations in heart rate response. When the cardiac transplant recipient begins exercise, the Bainbridge reflex mediates a small rise in heart rate as a response to increased pressure in the right ventricular veins that can continue for up to 5 minutes, which can also contribute to a slow return to preexercise heart rate. The peak heart rate and systolic blood pressure attained during maximal exercise is lower in cardiac transplant recipients, only reaching up to 80% of normal.[25,76] Because of this chronotropic incompetence, it has historically been presumed that heart transplant recipients would not be able to fully adapt to high-intensity interval training and would be best served by enrollment in a steady-state intensity exercise regimen.[105] The patient must therefore be educated to begin any workout with a slow warm-up period and a graded progression of activity intensity.

The transplanted heart compensates for output demand mainly by increasing stroke volume. At the onset of exercise, stroke volume in the transplanted heart can rapidly increase up to 20%.[82] Successive increases in stroke volume and cardiac output during sustained submaximal exercise result from inotropic responses to circulating catecholamines.[82] See Table 28-7 for a summary of the effects of cardiac transplant on various cardiovascular variables. Owing to this catecholamine-induced tachycardic response to increased exertion, exercise prescriptions based on target heart rates are not suggested. More useful determinants of exercise intensity include blood pressure reserve (the difference between systolic and diastolic pressure), the Borg Scale of Perceived Exertion (a categorical scale from 1 to 10, with 10 representing the maximal exertion),[81] and the Dyspnea Index (a scale from 0 to 4, with 4 being the maximum shortness of breath, which prevents counting or speaking).

Resting hypertension is a common finding that may be associated with premorbid elevations in vascular resistance secondary to hypersensitivity to circulating catecholamines in the setting of chronic heart failure.[76] Diastolic blood pressure can decrease early in submaximal exercise because of reduced peripheral resistance. The peak systolic blood pressure is less than that of individuals without cardiac transplants, but diastolic blood pressure remains essentially unchanged. Cyclosporine can induce hypertension through its effect on renal function, endothelial vasodilation, or sympathetic activity to a greater extent in cardiac transplant patients than either liver or lung transplant patients.[76]

After heart transplant, patients consume less oxygen during submaximal exercise than normal controls. Oxygen consumption at the anaerobic threshold is also considerably lower than that of age-matched normal individuals. According to Braith and Edwards,[18] the decrement in peak oxygen consumption seen in transplant recipients is partly caused by changes in skeletal muscle. Skeletal myopathy associated with the heart failure syndrome produces atrophy, decreased mitochondrial counts, and decreased oxidative enzymes. Corticosteroids also promote muscle atrophy affecting primarily type II fibers, and cyclosporine further decreases oxidative enzymes.[18]

Therapeutic Exercise After Cardiac Transplantation

Aerobic cardiovascular conditioning programs and endurance training improve the ability of the heart transplant recipient to accomplish sustained involvement in higher levels of activities of daily living.[65] Regular exercise training can be effective in improving exercise capacity, particularly a regimen of at least 12 weeks in duration, involving supervision, and commencing within 1 year after the transplant surgery. Enrollment into a supervised moderate-intensity exercise training program early after cardiac transplantation has shown to improve $\dot{V}O_{2\,max}$ (by an average of 24% after 2 to 3 months), maximum power output, and body composition when compared with those recipients who did not enroll, but overall exercise capacity is still reduced

Table 28-7 Effect of Cardiac Transplantation on Selected Cardiovascular Variables

Condition	Heart Rate	Stroke Volume	Systolic	Diastolic	Pulmonary Arterial Pressure	O_2 (Oxygen Consumption)	Serum Lactate
Rest	Greater than normal	Less than normal; little (Bainbridge reflex) or no positional change	Greater than normal	Greater than normal	Slightly greater than normal (although usually lower than pretransplantation)	—	Greater than normal
Submaximal exercise	Little or no immediate increase; delayed slow increase	Increase initially resulting from the Frank-Starling mechanism; late increases as a result of circulating	Greater than normal	Fall initially as a result of reduced peripheral resistance	Greater than normal (rate of change is greater than normal)	Less than normal (absolute value)	Greater than normal
Maximal exercise	Blunted peak (less than predicted for age); peak cardiac output about 25% less than normal	Peak only 40% to 50% greater than most	Peak is less than normal	About the same	—	Less than normal (absolute value); relative anaerobic threshold is slightly higher than normal	Not markedly different

compared with normal age-controlled patients.[43,71,106] Both cardiac hemodynamic and peripheral physiologic factors most likely contribute to this reduction in exercise capacity following heart transplantation. The cardiac factors include chronotropic incompetence, possible impaired left ventricular function, or greater arteriovenous oxygen difference. Peripheral factors include decreased muscle mass, anabolic resistance as a result of reduced strength and oxidative capacity, or impaired vasodilatory capacity. Other issues to consider as possible etiology for decreased exercise capacity include advanced age of the patient, donor heart age, operative ischemic time, or premorbid deconditioning and comorbidities.[105]

Only a few randomized control trials have investigated the effect of exercise in heart transplant recipients. Most of these studies compared some form of rehabilitation or exercise program at moderate intensity with a control group without a specific form of an exercise strategy. Resistance training has been shown to increase skeletal muscle mass and strength,[81,148,154] and should not begin until 6 to 8 weeks after transplantation, permitting time for sternal healing and corticosteroid tapering.[154] Recent studies are beginning to demonstrate that heart transplant patients may be able to tolerate high-intensity interval training with benefits of overall improved exercise capacity, coronary endothelial function, and blood pressure management, but future large-scale studies are needed to confirm these effects and determine the mechanisms by which they occur.[67,81,105,106]

Early in the history of cardiac transplantation, it was considered inadvisable to start an exercise protocol immediately after the surgery. More recent research suggests, however, that early mobilization and low-level exercise should begin in the hospital after extubation barring no medical contraindications.[77,148]

Although almost every cardiac transplant patient faces episodes of acute cellular rejection (ACR), it is only rarely necessary to limit the exercise workout during episodes of moderate rejection. The risk of ACR is greatest within the first 3 months following transplantation. Greater than 60% of transplant recipients will have one or more episodes of rejection in the first 6 months. Risk factors for ACR include younger age at transplantation, female sex, black race, and greater HLA mismatch.[39] When patients show signs of new arrhythmias, hypotension, or fever, the exercise regimen can be adjusted to allow for proper medical management. Clinical and physiologic monitoring of the patient and regular review of personal life and family goals are essential to maximize the patient's prognosis, life plans, and family functioning. Patient and family education are crucial in transplantation rehabilitation (Box 28-7).[72]

BOX 28-7

Transplantation Rehabilitation: Patient-Family Education

- Basic immune system
- Purpose of immunosuppression
- Activities related to immunosuppression:
  - Avoiding crowds during high immunosuppression
  - Wearing mask in hospital and clinic
  - Care of cuts and wounds
  - Mouth care/dental visits
  - Notifying transplant team of exposure to diseases (e.g., influenza, chicken pox, measles)
- Other activities
  - Exercise (walking, bicycling, swimming if no T-tube or open wounds)
  - Restrictions on lifting and driving after major abdominal surgery (3 to 6 months)
  - Sexual activity/birth control
  - Care of T-tube (usually removed after 3 months)
- Medications—proper administration, side effects, and purpose
  - Immunosuppressants
  - Prophylactics (antivirals, antibiotics, antifungals, antacids)
  - Others (e.g., antihypertensives, multivitamins)
- Home monitoring responsibilities (how, why, and what to do if abnormal):
  - Blood pressure readings
  - Temperature
  - Stool for occult blood
  - Urine for glucose or blood
  - Daily weight
  - Quality of urine (cloudy, dark, normal)
  - Quality of stools (tan/clay color, black, maroon, normal)
- Dietary:
  - Restrictions (fat, sugar, salt)
  - Balanced diet, low-calorie snacks
  - Expected increase in appetite and fat deposition attributable to steroids
- Signs and symptoms of infection and rejection—what to do and whom to call:
  - Symptoms are so similar for these two that notifying the transplant team is paramount
- Medical follow-up:
  - Biopsies (usually 3 and 6 months, then yearly; and with dysfunction)
  - Frequent transplant clinic visits (blood tests, radiographic tests)
  - Routine checkups with referring and transplant physicians
  - Cancer monitoring (annual Pap smear, self-breast examination, testicular examination, mammogram, stool for occult blood)
  - Routine dental visits (prophylactic antibiotics before visit)

Rehabilitation in Lung Transplantation

Lung Transplants and Patient Outcomes

In 2010, 1770 lung transplant procedures were performed in the United States, and 2469 new candidates were also added to the waiting list that same year. Survival of lung transplant patients is inferior to that of recipients of other solid organ transplants owing to the great number of complications in the first postoperative year. Twenty percent of lung transplant recipients die within the first year of transplantation, suggesting an overall failing of identifying those at high risk for severe early complications.[69] The most common indications for single-lung transplants are COPD and idiopathic pulmonary fibrosis (Box 28-8).

BOX 28-8

Common Primary Diagnoses in Lung Transplant Rehabilitation Patients

- Pulmonary vascular disease
  - Primary pulmonary hypertension
  - Eisenmenger syndrome
  - Cardiomyopathy with pulmonary hypertension
- Obstructive lung disease
  - Emphysema—idiopathic
  - Emphysema—alpha-antitrypsin deficiency
  - Cystic fibrosis
  - Bronchiectasis
  - Posttransplant obliterative bronchiolitis
- Rejection
  - Acute, chronic
- Side effects of immunosuppressive therapy
- Psychosocial issues

Bilateral lung transplants are often done for cystic fibrosis and pulmonary hypertension. The most recent international guidelines for outlining candidacy for lung transplantation were issued in 2006 by the Pulmonary Scientific Council of the International Society for Heart and Lung Transplantation. The indications and absolute and relative contraindications determined by this consensus report are summarized in Box 28-9.[111]

Pretransplant Rehabilitation: Assessment, Education, and Conditioning

Pulmonary rehabilitation can be provided to a diverse group of patients with varied pulmonary conditions that limit a patient's functional capacity. Those not fully responsive to rehabilitation may be identified as transplant candidates. This requires an institution that harbors close cooperation between the rehabilitation team and pulmonary medicine.

Rehabilitation programs preceding and following transplantation have been traditionally recognized as the optimal management model for lung transplant patients. However, there remains a paucity of randomized controlled studies looking at functional outcomes.[80] Initial pretransplant workup includes pulmonary function tests, chest radiographs, computed tomography scans, ventilation perfusion scans, as well as cardiac stress testing. Well-established pulmonary rehabilitation programs are designed not only to determine baseline pulmonary function but also resultant functional deficits through physical examination and measurement of oxygen saturation at rest and with activity. Nutritional deficiencies must be evaluated by reviewing the patient's BMI, diet, and serum prealbumin and albumin levels. One of the goals of the rehabilitation team is to optimize the patient's overall nutritional status, as indicated by these clinical values, preoperatively.

A recent study by Florian et al.[54] showed that a dedicated pulmonary rehabilitation program can have positive effects on exercise capacity, specifically in functional domains of physical functioning, vitality, social functioning, and mental health. Pulmonary functional capacity, including vital capacity and FEV_1, should be monitored. A standard test used for exercise tolerance in patients with pulmonary disease is the 6-minute walk test, in which the patient is directed to ambulate as fast as possible over a flat measured course for exactly 6 minutes at submaximal exertion. Performance may be optimized by titrating oxygen supplementation to maintain blood saturations greater than 90% and using energy-efficient gait patterns.

BOX 28-9

Indications and Contraindications for Lung Transplantation

Indications for Lung Transplantation

- BODE Index* of 7 to 10 or one the following:
  - Previous hospitalization for an acute hypercapnic exacerbation (PCO_2 >50 mm Hg).
  - Pulmonary hypertension or cor pulmonale despite oxygen therapy.
  - FEV_1 <20% and either DLCO <20% or homogeneous distribution of emphysema.

Absolute Contraindications for Lung Transplantation

- Malignancy in the past 2 years, with the exception of cutaneous squamous and basal cell tumors.
- Advanced disease deemed untreatable of another major organ system.
- Coronary artery disease not amenable to percutaneous intervention or bypass grafting, or associated with significant impairment of left ventricular function, is an absolute contraindication to lung transplantation, but heart-lung transplantation could possibly be considered.
- Noncurable chronic extrapulmonary infection including chronic active viral hepatitis B, hepatitis C, and human immunodeficiency virus.
- Pronounced chest wall/spinal deformity.
- Noncompliance or inability to fully participate in medical therapy and clinic visits.
- Untreatable psychiatric or psychological condition associated with the inability to cooperate with medical therapy.
- Absence of a reliable social support system.
- Substance addiction (e.g., alcohol, tobacco, or narcotics) within the previous 6 months.

Relative Contraindications for Lung Transplantation

- Age older than 65 years.
- Critical or unstable medical condition (e.g., shock, mechanical ventilation, or extracorporeal membrane oxygenation).
- Severely limited functional status with poor rehabilitation potential.
- Colonization with highly resistant or highly virulent bacteria, fungi, or mycobacteria.
- Body mass index exceeding 30 kg/m^2.
- Severe or symptomatic osteoporosis.
- Mechanical ventilation.
- Medical conditions that have not resulted in end-stage organ damage should be optimized before transplantation. Patients with coronary artery disease may undergo percutaneous intervention before transplantation or coronary artery bypass graft concurrent with the procedure.

*BODE Index consists of measures of health quality of life that includes Body mass index, the degree of airflow Obstruction, and Dyspnea and Exercise capacity.

Quantifiable endurance testing can also be employed with the use of a treadmill or cycle ergometer. This information can be used to formulate an individualized rehabilitation regimen including exercise routines of short duration to avoid prolonged breathlessness. Patients with end-stage pulmonary disease often perform better with exercise that has a reduced ventilatory requirement, such as interval exercise training with an added focus on the conditioning of inspiratory muscles. The goal of therapy is to lengthen exercise duration and decrease the number of rest periods while minimizing adverse symptomology. Energy conservation exercises can aid in adjusting to the low functional capacity caused by end-stage pulmonary disease. The patient will need adequate education regarding effective ventilation, expectoration, strengthening, and low-level aerobic endurance. An exercise program that gradually approaches and maintains 60% of peak heart rate can effectively condition patients.[94] Exercise cessation and hospitalization may need to be considered if pulmonary function worsens. Some lung transplant programs require that the patient move closer to the transplant center to facilitate close monitoring.

Medical Complications

As with other patients having received a solid organ transplant, lung transplant recipients are medically complex and require numerous medications with potential side effects and need for routine monitoring by the rehabilitation, transplant, and cardiothoracic surgery teams. Physiatrists must be keenly aware of potential medical complications in these patients.

Lung transplant patients require a standard immunosuppressive regimen consisting of calcineurin inhibitors and systemic steroid therapy to prevent acute and chronic rejection. There is a high susceptibility to infection attributable to specific factors, including donor lung microbial flora, immunosuppression, complicated nature of the surgery, prolonged hospitalization, presence of multiple lines and tubes such as chest tubes, urinary catheters, and peripheral and central venous lines. Infection is the most common complication in lung transplantation and can lead to premature death if not promptly treated. The decreased mucociliary clearance associated with denervated lungs can contribute to increased risk for infection in the early postoperative phase. During the first month, the patient is at a particularly high risk for acquiring bacterial pneumonia, which may require the use of broad-spectrum antibiotics guided by microbial drug sensitivity. *Pneumocystis jiroveci* pneumonia prophylaxis is started immediately after transplantation, typically with drugs such as trimethoprim/sulfamethoxazole. Typical fungal pathogens can include *Candida*, *Aspergillus*, and *Pneumocystis* and prophylaxis or treatment may consist of itraconazole or amphotericin B. Prophylaxis against CMV, Epstein-Barr virus, herpes simplex virus, and varicella-zoster virus are treated with ganciclovir or valganciclovir with surveillance for adverse side effects such as leukopenia and renal injury. If pulmonary infection is suspected, the diagnosis should be made with bronchoscopic lavage and biopsy.[140] In addition, impairments in cough reflex, mucus clearance, gas exchange, and circulatory autoregulation are all postoperative risks because the transplanted lung is denervated. Inadequate clearance of airway secretions may require chest physical therapy. Diaphragmatic dysfunction may also be present prompting electrodiagnostic evaluation.

Intestinal dysmotility and constipation are common following lung transplantation secondary to medication side effects or immobilization. Measures should be taken to ensure daily bowel movements with the administration of stool softeners and laxatives as needed. Postoperative pain can limit the patient's ability to mobilize, cough, and expectorate secretions, and breathe deeply thereby diminishing aeration of all lung lobes and increasing the risk of pulmonary complications. Therefore, the implementation of adequate analgesia must be employed often with the use of opioid medications. Splinted coughing, with placement of a pillow over the postsurgical incision during coughing episodes, may help reduce postoperative pain.[140]

Antireflux measures such as reverse Trendelenburg positioning and the use of proton pump inhibitors versus histamine-2 receptor antagonists should be employed to prevent gastroesophageal reflux, which may lead to aspiration, pneumonia, or bronchiolitis obliterans.[140]

Renal and hepatic function, as well as serum electrolytes, inflammatory markers, and cell counts should all be regularly monitored. Lung transplant patients frequently have hypoalbuminemia and are commonly fluid overloaded postoperatively with a substantial increase in body weight. Intrathoracic lymphatic disruption can cause fluid retention and pulmonary edema that hinders gas exchange and reduces lung compliance. During the immediate postoperative period, maintaining a clear airway and preventing atelectasis as well as normalizing ventilatory gas exchange are primary objectives. Modified cough techniques such as breath stacking and huff coughing can increase cough effectiveness for secretion expectoration and increased airflow. Keeping the patient's head of bed upright can increase drainage from chest tubes and improve pulmonary secretions. The patient should be assisted with airway clearance, and those who are mechanically ventilated can benefit from chest percussive therapy and hyperinflation. A protein-rich diet is very important as well as the discretionary use of diuretics in the setting of fluid overload. However, both diuretics and calcineurin inhibitors increase urinary magnesium excretion necessitating serum monitoring and supplementation, because magnesium is an important cofactor in muscle function and gastrointestinal motility.[140]

Fluid management may also be complicated by heart failure, which can be attributable to new-onset atrial fibrillation commonly seen in the early postoperative phase. Therefore, any new evidence of heart failure, or unexplained hypotension or tachycardia, warrants an electrocardiogram. The cardiothoracic and transplant teams may elect to continue to perform chest radiography routinely to monitor for any concerning signs. Daily spirometry with monitoring of FEV_1 and FVC are measurements that can be used to screen for any subclinical decrement in pulmonary function that could potentially escalate to serious medical complications such as graft rejection. Graft dysfunction or rejection is life threatening with worsening of gas exchange, decreased lung compliance, and development of interstitial infiltrates on imaging. This must be considered with otherwise unexplained signs of pulmonary edema or acute respiratory distress syndrome. Critical illness polyneuropathy or myopathy may result in pronounced difficulty with ventilator weaning and profound limb muscle weakness.[140]

Postoperative Exercise Considerations

Progressive activity should be initiated on the first postoperative day, progressing from range-of-motion exercises and chest and upper limb mobilization to transfers and eventually gait and endurance training with use of a treadmill or cycle ergometer. Before discharge from the hospital, the patient should engage in stair climbing, which is one of the major milestones of recovery. Pulmonary conditioning should emphasize alveolar ventilation, mucociliary transport, and ventilation-perfusion matching to optimize the efficiency of oxygen delivery. To reduce infection risk, the lung transplant recipient may be privately roomed while on the rehabilitation unit.

Following lung transplantation, studies have shown substantial improvements in pulmonary function and exercise capacity, but peak exercise and quality of life related to physical functioning remain impaired. In other words, lung transplant recipients have an increase in exercise capacity that does not correspond to the improvement in lung function, indicating that poor strength, deconditioning, and other peripheral factors may play an important role in the noted limitation of exercise posttransplantation.[12] In the long term, approximately 30% to 50% of patients will develop comorbid conditions such as diabetes, hyperlipidemia, hypertension, and osteoporosis, which are all known to be prevented or at least controlled with exercise.[80] Peak exercise in the postlung transplant period may be reduced by up to 40% to 60% of predicted values. This exercise limitation in lung transplant patients appears to be multifactorial. Evidence suggests that although the transplanted lungs are denervated, the ventilatory response to exercise seems to be unaffected. Heart rate increases during incremental exercise to approximately 60% to 70% of age-predicted maximum, which would typically meet the patient's workload demands. However, in patients with dual heart and lung transplants, resultant impairment in ionotropic and chronotropic responses secondary to cardiac denervation can partially account for reduced exercise capacity.

A major element of reduced exercise capacity after lung transplantation is limb muscle dysfunction, such as atrophy, weakness, and alterations in muscle composition, with a reduction in type I muscle fibers likely stemming from premorbid sedentary lifestyle compounded by multiple hospitalizations. In lung transplant recipients, studies demonstrate a diminished capacity for oxidative metabolism manifested by activity-related early-onset lactic acidosis, decreased calcium uptake and release, early drop in muscle pH, and reduced peak oxygen consumption ($VO_{2\,peak}$) in the peripheral muscles. This phenomenon may play a central role in limiting posttransplant peak exercise capability. Reduced oxidative capacity may also occur secondary to the effects immunosuppressants, such as cyclosporine, which can impair mitochondrial functioning.[80,94,168]

Participation in supervised rehabilitation programs aims to improve limb muscle dysfunction and daily physical activity, which in turn improves overall quality of life and aids in reducing the risk of comorbid conditions after transplantation. There is literature to support the implementation of structured exercise training programs to optimize functional exercise capacity, skeletal muscle strength, and lumbar bone mineral density in lung transplant patients.[168] A recent small randomized controlled trial of 40 patients compared lung transplant recipients assigned after hosptial discharge to either a structured 3-month exercise training program or a control intervention and showed that after 1 year, the group that participated in the structured exercise training program had significant improvements in 6-minute walking distance, quadriceps force, self-reported physical functioning, and 24-hour ambulatory blood pressures.[80] Further studies are needed to develop standardized guidelines for exercise prescription in the lung transplant population.[168]

Rehabilitation in Liver Transplantation

Each year more than 27,000 Americans die of liver disease.[155] Liver transplantation provides a definitive cure for patients with end-stage liver disease (ESLD) secondary to cirrhosis, portal hypertension, primary sclerosing cholangitis, biliary atresia, hepatitis, and liver cancer. Individuals with chronic liver failure resulting from chronic hepatitis, alcoholic cirrhosis, or autoimmune disorders are frequently much more functionally impaired in terms of cardiovascular endurance and day-to-day functioning. Studies have shown that pretransplant health-related quality of life scores are affected by the etiology of ESLD, with hepatocellular and cholestatic causes having higher scores than alcohol or viral hepatitis.[16]

Liver transplantation has become increasingly common in the United States. As of June 2012, more than 17,000 patients in the United States were awaiting a liver transplant. Advancements in surgical techniques, improved patient selection, development of immunosuppressive medications, and improvements in postoperative management have contributed to the widespread success of liver transplantation. In the United States, the expected 1-year survival rate after liver transplantation approached 90%. However, more than 1700 people died in the United States in 2011 while awaiting a liver with the number of deceased donors remaining virtually unchanged over the past several years.[109]

Liver transplant recipients are at risk for a myriad of complications. Owing to the complex nature of liver transplant surgery with surgical disruption of areas of elevated microbial loads, such as the gastrointestinal tract, the heightened exposure to infectious pathogens during prolonged hospitalization, the use of indwelling catheters, the potential of prolonged ventilatory dependence, and the need for immunosuppressants, liver transplant patients are predisposed to nosocomial bacterial and fungal infections, especially during the first month. Opportunistic infections as a result of the patient's depressed immune system are at the greatest risk 1 month following transplantation. This elevated risk of serious infection is mitigated by the use of perioperative and prophylactic antibiotics.[127]

Acute kidney injury can also be observed in these patients. Care must be taken in interpreting traditional biomarkers, such as serum creatinine to assess renal function. Serum creatinine levels can lead to an overestimation of renal function because patients with cirrhosis have diminished creatinine resulting from malnutrition and muscle wasting. Large volumes of fluids intraoperatively can artificially lower creatinine levels through hemodilution. The use of serum creatinine as an indicator for renal function may further be misinterpreted by increasing hepatic creatinine generation with improved liver function and administration of systemic steroid therapy.[127]

Additional potential complications include prolonged intubation as a result of generalized muscle, pneumonia, pulmonary edema, or pleural effusions.[127] Hyperbilirubinemia can provoke anorexia, nausea, or vomiting, leading to profound malnutrition. Neurologic dysfunction, such as cognitive deficits, weakness, or fatigue, can be secondary to metabolic abnormalities, chronic sequelae of the liver disease, or side effects incurred from multiple transplant medications. Liver graft failure or thrombosis must be high on the differential if the patient exhibits signs of progressive sepsis, fever, altered mental status, hypotension, coagulopathy, transaminitis, leukocytosis, gastrointestinal bleeding, severe abdominal pain, worsening jaundice, hepatomegaly, or ascites.[127]

Rehabilitation Following Liver Transplant

Owing to significant sarcopenia with its associated functional decline that is typically seen in chronic ESLD, a customized rehabilitation program is essential to achieve a desirable recovery. There are several potential mechanisms for ESLD-associated physical impairments, which may be further compounded by complicated transplant surgery. Liver transplant recipients may have concomitant cardiac and pulmonary issues such as hepatopulmonary syndrome and generalized edema that can affect pulmonary function and the ability to exercise. Ascites seems to be associated with more severe impairments of fitness. These patients may also have a component of cirrhotic cardiomyopathy with a blunted ability to elevate their heart rate or left ventricular ejection fraction with exercise or posture change attributable to a postulated diminished sensitivity to a sympathetic response.[75]

Resistance training, an isometric exercise regimen, and aerobic endurance are potential approaches to reverse muscle wasting and deconditioning in these patients. When possible, a pretransplant evaluation by the rehabilitation team is desirable. There is some evidence that suggests that pretransplant exercise capacity may predict the posttransplant course and survival.[75] Physical and occupational therapies should be initiated immediately posttransplant as long as the patient is medically stable because early mobilization postoperatively is essential. Nutritional optimization must be aggressively sought after to aid in maximizing functional gains. The liver transplant patient receiving rehabilitative services should be monitored carefully for signs of rejection and liver failure, and should receive close medical surveillance from both the rehabilitation and transplant teams.

Beyond allograft-associated complications, metabolic syndrome, cardiovascular disease, renal dysfunction, and malignancies are leading causes of long-term morbidity and mortality in the liver transplant patient population.[143] Postliver transplant health-related quality of life scores are not affected by the etiology of the original liver disease, but the scores of these recipients persist significantly lower than those of healthy patient controls. During the first 6 months postliver transplantation, the majority of physical and mental components of health-related quality of life scores improve, but these increases are not sustained long term, and at 1 year following liver transplantation, these scores begin to decrease.[16] Physiatrists are in an optimal position to elucidate the cause of this phenomenon and provide long-term functional interventions to reverse this trend.

Return to Work Posttransplantation

As part of the evaluation of success of any organ transplant, return to work and social integration are essential. A recent cross-sectional analysis evaluated self-reports of 281 kidney, heart, liver, and lung transplant patients for return to competitive employment. They found that kidney transplant patients had the highest posttransplant employment rate (58.6%), followed by heart (43.6%), liver (37.5%), and lung transplant patients (28.1%). Positive predictive factors for return to work were young age at time of transplant, male sex, being married, maintaining a positive perception of one's capability to engage in work, having been employed at least 1 year before transplant, and receipt of an organ other than the lung.[40] Return to employment and even enrollment in additional vocational training after organ transplantation should be integrated into the long-term plan of any rehabilitation program.

Summary

Society has been markedly advanced by organ transplantation. Transplant patients are enjoying more active and meaningful lives as a result of comprehensive posttransplant care, which includes early rehabilitation intervention. A customized, comprehensive rehabilitation program results in transplant patients returning to a more active lifestyle. As transplant medicine continues to progress, transplant rehabilitation services will continue to develop.

Rehabilitation Management of Diabetes Mellitus

Epidemiology

In 2007, DM became the seventh leading cause of mortality in the United States, and it is estimated that 5.4% of the global population will be afflicted with this condition by year 2025.[137,157] Approximately 8% of Americans age 20 years or older suffer from DM, with two thirds remaining undiagnosed. Furthermore, DM affects nearly a quarter of the older adult population (60 years or older).[166] DM has increasingly been shown to be a destructive condition that carries profoundly devastating complications and sequelae. DM is not only the leading cause of nontraumatic lower limb amputations, blindness, and renal failure but is also a major risk factor for stroke, coronary syndromes, and low-trauma hip fractures.[157,166] Given the prevalence of DM in the United States and globally, coupled with the significant impairments with which the condition is associated, it is not surprising that there is an increasing demand for the physiatrist to become well versed in the diagnosis, management, and rehabilitation of patients with DM.

Pathophysiology and Diagnosis

DM is characterized by two hallmarks: peripheral tissue insulin resistance and dysfunction of pancreatic beta cells. In the normal fasting state, beta cells secrete basal levels of insulin. With ingestion of a meal, insulin secretion increases to match the demand within 10 minutes. In nondiabetic patients, this release of insulin should normalize blood glucose levels to basal levels within 2 hours. However, if hyperglycemia persists, beta cell function may be impaired, marking possible prediabetes or overt DM, depending on the level of blood glucose elevation. In other words, pancreatic beta cells must be highly functioning to meet metabolic demands or DM ensues. Autoimmune destruction of beta cells leads to type 1 DM (T1DM), whereas oxidative damage as a result of caloric or nutrient overburden may result in type 2 DM (T2DM). Although the exact mechanisms are yet to be fully elucidated, it appears that T2DM results in increased beta cell apoptosis, outweighing the capacity of cell replication. There seems to be a preceding "compensatory" state, during which beta cell mass increases by hypertrophy and hyperplasia in an attempt to balance body adiposity and insulin resistance. Some individuals may live in this state of compensation for years without developing overt DM, but people with poor capacity for adaptation succumb to premature beta cell death and impaired blood glucose clearance.[13] Despite its more chronic pathophysiology, T2DM is nevertheless responsible for the vast majority of DM, accounting for 90% to 95% of cases.[124]

The American Diabetes Association guidelines[34] for diagnosis of DM include:

- Glycated hemoglobin (HbA1c) of 6.5% or higher.
- Fasting plasma glucose (FPG) of at least 126 mg/dL (7.0 mmol/L).
- Two-hour plasma glucose of at least 200 mg/dL (11.1 mmol/L) during an oral glucose tolerance test with 75 g of glucose.
- Classic symptoms of hyperglycemia (polyuria, polydipsia, unexpected weight loss) or hyperglycemic crisis with a random plasma glucose of 200 mg/dL (11.1 mmol/L) or higher.
- Prediabetes: HbA1c of 5.7% to 6.4% or FPG of 100 to 125 mg/dL or 2-hour plasma glucose of 140 to 199 mg/dL following an oral glucose tolerance test.

Prevention Guidelines

Lifestyle Modifications

Current recommendations for the prevention of T2DM include lifestyle modifications, which include maintenance of healthy weight, proper and healthy nutrition intake, and participation in aerobic and resistance exercise programs.[1] Some suggest there are additional benefits to a more comprehensive lifestyle modification program that incorporates behavioral components, such as tobacco cessation, cooking lessons, use of food diaries, and attendance at annual diabetic education classes.[137] Such programs should include an interdisciplinary team with physicians, case managers, nurses, exercise advisors and trainers, behavioral therapists and counselors, psychologists, dietitians, and physiotherapists.[137] Participation in such a comprehensive program has been shown to effectively reduce body weight and BMI in high-risk individuals and prevent T2DM, although advantages are less clear for people already diagnosed with the condition.[137] In fact, participation in combined programs of dietary modification, aerobic exercise, and resistance training by at-risk individuals has been shown to reduce the incidence of T2DM by up to 58%.[1]

Preventative guidelines include participation in 2.5 hours per week of moderate-intensity physical activity, which typically consists of 30 minutes per day for 5 days per week for adults at high risk of developing DM. Although data are limited for youth and adolescent T2DM prevention, it is generally accepted that goals include limiting screen time (time watching television, playing video games, or using a personal computer) to less than 60 minutes daily and inclusion of at least 60 minutes per day of physical activity.[34]

Treatment Guidelines

Exercise and Diabetes Mellitus

Given current recommendations for lifestyle modifications as the first line of DM prevention and treatment, the physiatrist is in a prime position to take leadership of management of patients with DM. Rehabilitation physicians are uniquely trained in musculoskeletal anatomy and function, exercise physiology, and the use of physical activity as a treatment for disease. Further, the physiatrist is versed in the team approach to patient care, working closely with physiotherapists, exercise trainers, case managers, and nurses, as well as the individualization of patient care, taking into consideration the patient's unique medical needs, impairments, goals, and social background.

Assessment of Physical Activity

The American Heart Association recommends that physical activity (bodily movement produced by skeletal muscles that result in energy expenditure) and other cardiovascular risk factors be regularly assessed by clinicians. It is important to take into account an individual's overall physical activity profile, including all structured (e.g., exercise, planned activities) and incidental (e.g., activities of daily living, vocational, transport, unplanned activities) physical activity. Further, the dimensions (mode or type, frequency, duration, intensity) and domains (occupational, domestic, transportation, leisure) should be documented with each assessment.[151]

Both subjective and objective methods of evaluation exist for clinical use. Physical activity questionnaires (PAQs) such as the Global PAQ, Short Recall PAQ, and quantitative history PAQs may be completed via personal or telephone interviews or self-reported. Additionally, physical activity diaries or logs such as the Bouchard Physical Activity Record are frequently used. Objective methods of quantifying physical activity, such as indirect calorimetry, the doubly labeled water method, direct observation, heart rate monitoring, or use of motion sensors (accelerometers and pedometers), may also be used by the clinician depending on availability.[151]

Physiologic Effects of Exercise in Type 2 Diabetes Mellitus

Individuals with DM typically present limitations in physical fitness and activity, which contributes to the high cardiovascular mortality seen in this population. T2DM is associated with impaired glucose and fat metabolism as a result of impaired insulin sensitivity and lipid oxidation, as well as impaired myocardial and skeletal muscle perfusion likely resulting from vascular endothelial dysfunction.[128] T2DM risk increases with physical inactivity and occurs with more frequency in individuals with obesity, hypertension, and dyslipidemia. The objectives of physical activity in the treatment of T2DM include improvement of DM-associated abnormalities in glucose, lipid, and blood pressure control and facilitation of weight loss and maintenance.[34]

During exercise, glucose uptake into actively contracting skeletal muscles is increased, which is balanced by hepatic gluconeogenesis. This process preferentially uses carbohydrates to fuel muscular activity as intensity increases, leading to a normalization of blood glucose levels not only during physical activity but also at rest. Additionally, muscle contraction appears to circumvent DM-associated insulin resistance by inducing GLUT-4 translocation via a separate mechanism, which facilitates uptake of circulating glucose into the muscle.[150] Thus, acutely following mild-intensity to moderate-intensity physical activity, there is improved insulin activity with reduced blood glucose levels and reduction of daily time spent in hyperglycemia, an effect that may last between 2 and 72 hours postexercise.[34,88] The degree of glycemic reduction is related to the duration and intensity of the exercise, preexercise glucose levels, and the individual's state of physical training.[34]

Over the long term, exercise results in increased skeletal muscle sensitivity to insulin by increasing the expression and/or the activity of proteins involved in the glucose metabolism and insulin signaling, such as glycogen synthase and GLUT-4. Moreover, both aerobic and resistance training result in increased muscle lipid storage, oxidation, and use. T2DM has been associated with a decrease in lipid oxidation and preferential use of carbohydrate for energy. Chronic benefits of exercise also include reduction of total and low-density lipoprotein cholesterol, elevation of high-density lipoprotein levels, reduction in systolic blood pressure, and reduction of depressive symptoms in men and women of all age groups. Further, physical activity has been shown to improve vascular endothelial function, which may reduce incidence of complicating atherosclerotic cardiovascular or peripheral artery disease, prevent the onset of diabetic peripheral neuropathy, and improve autonomic function in patients with diabetic autonomic neuropathy. Overall, physical activity and physical fitness are associated with lower all-cause and cardiovascular mortality.[34]

The exact mechanisms by which physical activity improves cardiovascular function in patients with T2DM remains unclear, but recent evidence shows that exercise is associated with reductions in inflammatory markers CRP and interleukin-6 levels in individuals with T2DM. CRP is a strong independent predictor of cardiovascular disease and the outcome of acute coronary syndrome. CRP has long been identified to be generated in the liver in response to elevation in inflammatory cytokines, such as interleukin-6, but recent studies have shown production of CRP in both adipose tissue and atherosclerotic plaque.[64]

Preexercise Assessment

Participation in physical activities may undoubtedly be complicated by the presence of DM-associated complications, such as cardiovascular disease, hypertension, diabetic peripheral neuropathy, peripheral vascular disease, or retinopathy. However, current guidelines do not advise routine exercise stress testing before initiation of low-intensity physical activity, such as walking, as long as the clinician deems the individual to be of medical stability. However, patients desiring to participate in more vigorous activities should undergo more detailed medical evaluation for cardiovascular risk because coronary artery disease is greater in individuals with T2DM.

Electrocardiogram stress testing may be indicated for patients: (1) age over 40 years with or without cardiovascular disease risk factors other than DM; (2) age over 30 years and T1DM or T2DM greater than 10 years duration, hypertension, cigarette smoking, dyslipidemia, proliferative and preproliferative retinopathy, and nephropathy; and (3) with diagnosed or suspected coronary artery disease, cerebrovascular disease, peripheral artery disease, autonomic neuropathy, or advanced nephropathy with renal failure.[34]

Exercise Prescription in Type 2 Diabetes Mellitus

The beneficial effects of physical exercise in the management of T2DM may result from aerobic or resistance activities. The American Diabetes Association and the American College of Sports Medicine recommendations are outlined in Table 28-8. Although individuals with T2DM may profit from either aerobic or resistance training alone, the combination of both into an exercise regimen at least three times per week may be of greater benefit than either alone.[34] There appears to be a synergistic advantage to aerobic exercise-induced improvements in insulin sensitivity and enhanced blood glucose uptake as a result of increased muscle mass and GLUT-4 expression following resistance training.[108] Recent studies have shown statistically or clinically significant HbA1c reduction with combined exercise programs than from either exercise regimen alone.[108]

Table 28-8 Exercise Prescription Guidelines for Individuals with Type 2 Diabetes Mellitus

	Frequency	Intensity	Duration	Mode	Progression
Aerobic	At least 3 days per week with no more than 2 consecutive days per session	At least moderate intensity, i.e., 40% to 60% of $VO_{2\,max}$ (e.g., brisk walking)	At least 150 minutes per week; 30 minutes per day for 5 days per week of moderate-intensity activity OR 20 minutes per day for 3 days per week of vigorous-intensity activity	Any form of aerobic exercise that uses large muscle groups and results in sustained heart rate elevation	Gradual to reduce injury risk and increase compliance
Resistance	At least twice weekly on nonconsecutive days; ideally 3 times per week, along with aerobic activities	Moderate (50% of 1-repetition maximum) or vigorous (75% to 80% of 1-repetition maximum)	Five to 10 exercises involving major muscle groups (upper body, lower body, core), 10 to 15 repetitions per set, minimum of 1 set but as many as 4 sets	Resistance machines and free weights yield equivalent gains in strength and muscle mass	Slowly to prevent injury and increase compliance

From Colberg SR, Sigal RJ, Fernhall B, et al: Exercise and type 2 diabetes: the American College of Sports Medicine and the American Diabetes Association: joint position statement executive summary, *Diabetes Care* 33(12):2692-2696, 2010.[34]

Table 28-9 Diabetic Complications Requiring Exercise Modification

Complication	Exercise Alteration
Hyperglycemia (blood glucose >300 mg/dL without ketosis)	Patient may participate but ensure clinical stability and maintenance of hydration
Hypoglycemia	Glucose monitoring before and after physical activity (PA); Patients taking insulin or insulin secretagogues are advised to ingest carbohydrates before any PA if blood glucose is <100 mg/dL before PA; Insulin users should consume up to 15 g of carbohydrates before exercise
Vascular disease (cardiovascular disease and peripheral artery disease)	Patients with angina and type 2 diabetes mellitus should start PA in a supervised cardiac rehab setting; Patients with peripheral artery disease and intermittent claudication may participate in low to moderate walking, arm crank, and cycling
Peripheral neuropathy	Patients may participate in moderate weight-bearing exercise because moderate walking does not increase risk of diabetic foot ulceration; Patients with foot injury or diabetic foot ulcer should be restricted to non–weight-bearing activities; Closely examine feet daily
Autonomic neuropathy	Patients may proceed only with physician approval, possibly following stress testing given elevated risk for silent myocardial infarction
Retinopathy	Avoid high-intensity aerobic or resistance PA and head-down activities because these may elevate intraocular pressures; Avoid jumping and jarring activities that may increase risk of hemorrhage
Nephropathy	Patients may proceed following physician evaluation and possibly stress testing to detect associated coronary artery disease; Start at low intensity and volume because aerobic and muscle capacity are likely to be reduced

From Colberg SR, Sigal RJ, Fernhall B, et al: Exercise and type 2 diabetes: the American College of Sports Medicine and the American Diabetes Association: joint position statement executive summary, *Diabetes Care* 33(12):2692-2696, 2010.[34]

Although the guidelines provide a solid foundation upon which to build an exercise prescription for patients with T2DM, it is important to individualize exercise programs to enhance benefits, promote compliance, and reduce risk of injury. Exercise prescription should be personalized based on an individual's habits, preferences, motivation, and tolerance, rather than a general prescription with duration, intensity, and frequency.[10] A clinician developing an exercise regimen should not only consider which dose (type, intensity, duration, volume) provides the greatest health benefits but also review the risk profile relative to that dose. In other words, the clinician must balance the benefits with the risks.[10]

Additionally, it is imperative to assess for the presence of any DM-associated complications (Table 28-9), which may limit the patient's ability to participate in a desired exercise program. Of particular concern is the potential for delayed hypoglycemia (nocturnal hypoglycemia), a possibly fatal complication of the exercising individual with DM. Vigorous exercise severely depletes skeletal muscle glycogen stores, which the liver and muscles attempt to replenish postexercise by extracting circulating blood glucose, resulting in profound hypoglycemia. This condition may occur 6 to 12 hours after exercise, but may develop as late as 28 hours following physical activity. Signs and symptoms may include seizures, cardiac arrhythmias, altered mental status, altered consciousness, and death. The condition is especially threatening because it commonly develops nocturnally, during the sleeping hours.[63] Patients taking insulin or insulin secretagogues, athletes with DM, and individuals participating in repeated bouts of high-intensity exercise are at risk and are advised to consume 5 to 30 g of carbohydrates during and within 30 minutes following exercise to allow restoration of depleted glycogen.[34]

Oral Pharmacologic Treatment

The American College of Physicians recommends the addition of an oral pharmacologic agent in the treatment of patients with T2DM when lifestyle modifications, including diet, exercise, and weight loss, have failed to adequately improve hyperglycemia. According to the American College of Physicians, although treatment goals should be individualized, HbA1c level of less than 7% may be a reasonable goal for most individuals. The American College of Physicians recommends initiating therapy with metformin for most patients.[124] Metformin, however, is contraindicated in patients with CHF, renal insufficiency, COPD, age older than 80 years, and should not be used in patients receiving renal transplantation, given the possible risk of renal insufficiency.[58]

Should the combination of lifestyle therapies and treatment with metformin continue to fail to bring euglycemia, the clinician may add a second agent, such as thiazolidinediones or sulfonylurea, to the regimen.[124] Patients administered sulfonylureas should be monitored closely for evidence of hypoglycemia as a potential adverse reaction because the duration of action is typically prolonged and does not allow for rapid dose modification.[58] Thiazolidinediones have been associated with exacerbation of CHF and are contraindicated in patients with hepatic disease.[58] The clinician must remember, however, that the addition of pharmacotherapy in the management of T2DM should augment, and not replace, a comprehensive lifestyle modification program.[34]

Diabetes Mellitus Treatment with Insulin

The American Diabetes Association guidelines advise the administration of insulin for the hospitalized patient with DM to adequately control blood glucose levels because hyperglycemia, defined as blood glucose levels of 130 mg/dL or higher, contributes to poorer functional outcomes following stroke as well as longer length of stay. Three classes of insulin exist at present, depending on the onset and duration of action, and include rapid-acting (Lispro, Aspart, Regular), intermediate-acting (Neutral Protamine Hagedorn, NPH), and long-acting (Ultralente, Glargine). In determining the patient's insulin regimen, start with the calculation of the total daily dose (TDD) of required insulin by multiplying the patient's body weight in kilograms by 0.5 to 0.7 units for patients with T1DM or 0.4 to 1.0 units for T2DM. Then, 40% to 50% of the calculated TDD is administered once daily with a long-acting insulin (e.g., Glargine) or twice daily with intermediate-acting insulin (NPH), constituting the basal insulin dose. The remaining TDD minus basal insulin is then divided as nutritional insulin requirement and split into three premeal injections (if using Lispro or Aspart) or into two premeal injections before breakfast and supper (if using regular insulin). Target blood glucose levels for the hospitalized patient is less than 110 mg/dL preprandially or no greater than 180 mg/dL following meals.[58]

The Inpatient Rehabilitation Diabetes Consult Team

For many physiatrists, management of patients with T2DM is likely to start in the inpatient setting, following a DM-associated complication, such as stroke, coronary syndrome, lower limb amputation, or from a prolonged hospitalization complicated by the comorbidity of DM. A review by Weeks et al.[166] of admissions into their inpatient rehabilitation unit between 2001 and 2007, for instance, revealed that 21% of patients were admitted for stroke, 14.2% of those were undergoing orthopedic procedures, and 25% of medically complex admissions carried DM as a co-diagnosis. Therefore, it is likely that the patient is admitted to the rehabilitation unit carrying DM as a secondary diagnosis, which increases the potential for oversight. It is because of this possibility, combined with the fact that DM increases the risk for cognitive impairment, dementia, executive dysfunction, and depression, that some have advocated for the establishment of an inpatient rehabilitation diabetes consult service.[140] Such a service would follow the 2009 American Diabetes Association's guidelines for identification and management of hospitalized patients with DM by (1) identifying patients diagnosed with DM; (2) establishing standing orders and targets for blood glucose monitoring; (3) using insulin to achieve glycemic control; (4) closely monitoring and treating hypoglycemic episodes; (5) checking HbA1c levels; and (6) planning for follow-up testing and care for newly diagnosed patients upon discharge.

Advocates cite the possibility for shorter lengths of stay, improved glycemic control following acute hospitalization, and reduced readmission rates with the employment of this approach.[139]

Treatment of Diabetic Peripheral Neuropathy

Diabetic peripheral neuropathy is a diffuse, symmetrical, sensorimotor length-dependent peripheral nerve injury that afflicts up to 40% of individuals with DM.[34] The condition results in limb pain, impaired sleep and overall quality of life, and may predispose to foot injuries, diabetic foot ulcers, and lower limb amputations. Management options include anticonvulsants, antidepressants, opiates, topical medications, and physical modalities. Current evidence supports treatment of diabetic peripheral neuropathy with pregabalin, which has been shown to reduce pain and reduce sleep disturbances. Gabapentin and valproate may also be effective in the treatment of diabetic peripheral neuropathy and should be considered. However, lacosamide, lamotrigine, and oxcarbazepine are not currently recommended for use in patients with diabetic peripheral neuropathy. In the antidepressant class, amitriptyline, venlafaxine, and duloxetine have all shown efficacy in the treatment of diabetic neuropathy. Venlafaxine may be combined with gabapentin for greater response. Of the opiates, morphine sulfate, tramadol, oxycodone, and dextromethorphan have also shown efficacy, although side effect profiles and potential for dependence when used in chronic management may limit their use. Topical application of capsaicin, isosorbide dinitrate spray, and lidoderm patch may also be considered. Percutaneous electrical stimulation has also shown effectiveness in the treatment of diabetic peripheral neuropathy.[19]

Treatment of Diabetic Gastroparesis

The physiatrist should ensure that individuals with DM participating in rehabilitation or exercise programs are receiving adequate nutrition to meet metabolic demands of the prescribed physical activity. One potential complication may prove to be a serious threat to the nutritional status of the patient with DM. Diabetic gastroparesis affects 5.2% of patients with T1DM and 1% with T2DM and is characterized by delayed gastric emptying leading to nausea, vomiting, early satiety, and early postprandial fullness. Patients with diabetic gastroparesis using insulin or insulin secretagogues who are unable to consume adequate carbohydrates are therefore placed at risk for profound hypoglycemia. Thus, it is important to be vigilant about the diagnosis and management of this uncommon yet potentially deadly complication. Any patient with suspected gastroparesis should immediately undergo gastric emptying scintigraphy, which remains the standard of diagnosis. Medications that further impair gastric emptying, such as opiates and anticholinergics, should be discontinued. Should gastroparesis persist, pharmacologic agents may be used. Metoclopramide, a D2 dopamine receptor antagonist, remains the only U.S. Food and Drug Administration–approved medication for treatment of gastroparesis. Domperidone (Motilium), also a D2 dopamine antagonist, has shown equal efficacy to metoclopramide and may be considered for treatment. Erythromycin, a motilin-stimulating antibiotic, has been proven effective in the management of diabetic gastroparesis when administered intravenously. Symptomatic management of nausea and vomiting with phenothiazines, promethazine or ondansetron, may provide additional relief. At present, intrapyloric botulinum toxin injection has shown no symptomatic improvement and is therefore not recommended. Gastric electrical stimulation, by contrast, is associated with symptomatic benefits. For patients failing conservative treatment, surgical management such as venting gastrostomy, gastrojejunostomy, pyloroplasty, and gastrectomy may be considered.[23]

Conclusion

With an aging population, there is an increasing proportion of individuals living with chronic medical conditions, including pulmonary pathology, organ failure requiring transplantation, and DM with multiple diabetic complications. Given the complexity of these conditions, management cannot be compartmentalized and handled by only one medical specialist. Additionally, chronic medical diseases often directly or indirectly lead to impairments in patient function. Therefore, it is imperative for the physiatrist to become knowledgeable and involved in the management of the patient with chronic medical conditions.

KEY REFERENCES

1. Aguiar EJ, Morgan PJ, Collins CE, et al: Efficacy of interventions that include diet, aerobic and resistance training components for type 2 diabetes prevention: a systematic review with meta-analysis, *Int J Behav Nutr Phys Act* 11:2, 2014.
3. Alraies MC, Eckman P: Adult heart transplant: indications and outcomes, *J Thorac Dis* 6:1120–1128, 2014.
6. American Thoracic Society, American College of Chest Physicians: ATS/ACCP statement on cardiopulmonary exercise testing, *Am J Respir Crit Care Med* 167:211–277, 2003.
10. Balducci S, Sacchetti M, Haxhi J, et al: Physical exercise as therapy for type 2 diabetes mellitus, *Diabetes Metab Res Rev* 30(Suppl 1):13–23, 2014.
12. Bartels MN, Armstrong HF, Gerardo RE, et al: Evaluation of pulmonary function and exercise performance by cardiopulmonary exercise testing before and after lung transplantation, *Chest* 140: 1604–1611, 2011.
13. Beaudry JL, Riddell MC: Effects of glucocorticoids and exercise on pancreatic β-cell function and diabetes development, *Diabetes Metab Res Rev* 28:560–573, 2012.
16. Bownik H, Saab S: Health-related quality of life after liver transplantation for adult recipients, *Liver Transpl* 15(Suppl 2):S42–S49, 2009.
19. Bril V, England J, Franklin GM, et al: Evidence-based guideline: treatment of painful diabetic neuropathy: report of the American Academy of Neurology, the American Association of Neuromuscular and Electrodiagnostic Medicine, and the American Academy of Physical Medicine and Rehabilitation, *PM&R* 3:345–352, 352.e1–e21, 2011.
22. California Pulmonary Rehabilitation Collaborative Group: Effects of pulmonary rehabilitation on dyspnea, quality of life, and healthcare costs in California, *J Cardiopulm Rehabil* 24:52–62, 2004.
23. Camilleri M, Parkman HP, Shafi MA, et al: American College of Gastroenterology. Clinical guideline: management of gastroparesis, *Am J Gastroenterol* 108:18–37, quiz 38, 2013.
26. Casaburi R: Principles of exercise training, *Chest* 101(Suppl 5):263S–267S, 1992.
34. Colberg SR, Sigal RJ, Fernhall B, et al: Exercise and type 2 diabetes: the American College of Sports Medicine and the American Diabetes Association: joint position statement executive summary, *Diabetes Care* 33:2692–2696, 2010.
36. Creutzberg EC, Wouters EF, Mostert R, et al: Efficacy of nutritional supplementation therapy in depleted patients with chronic obstructive pulmonary disease, *Nutrition* 19:120–127, 2003.
40. De Baere C, Delva D, Kloeck A, et al: Return to work and social participation: does type of organ transplantation matter?, *Transplantation* 89:1009–1015, 2010.
43. Didsbury M, McGee RG, Tong A, et al: Exercise training in solid organ transplant recipients: a systematic review and meta-analysis, *Transplantation* 95:679–687, 2013.
53. Flegal KM, Carroll MD, Kit BK, Ogden CL: Prevalence of obesity and trends in the distribution of body mass index among US adults, 1999-2010, *JAMA* 307:491–497, 2012.
54. Florian J, Rubin A, Mattiello R, et al: Impact of pulmonary rehabilitation on quality of life and functional capacity in patients on waiting lists for lung transplantation, *J Bras Pneumol* 39(3):349–356, 2013.
58. Golden SH, Hill-Briggs F, Williams K, et al: Management of diabetes during acute stroke and inpatient stroke rehabilitation, *Arch Phys Med Rehabil* 86:2377–2384, 2005.
63. Harris GD, White RD: Diabetes in the competitive athlete, *Curr Sports Med Rep* 11:309–315, 2012.
64. Hayashino Y, Jackson JL, Hirata T, et al: Effects of exercise on C-reactive protein, inflammatory cytokine and adipokine in patients with type 2 diabetes: a meta-analysis of randomized controlled trials, *Metab Clin Exp* 63:431–440, 2014.
65. Haykowsky M, Taylor D, Kim D, Tymchak W: Exercise training improves aerobic capacity and skeletal muscle function in heart transplant recipients, *Am J Transplant* 9:734–739, 2009.
74. Jessup M, Abraham WT, Casey DE, et al: 2009 focused update: ACCF/AHA guidelines for the diagnosis and management of heart failure in adults: a report of the American College of Cardiology Foundation/American Heart Association Task Force on practice guidelines: developed in collaboration with the International Society for Heart and Lung Transplantation, *Circulation* 119:1977–2016, 2009.
75. Jones JC, Coombes JS, Macdonald GA: Exercise capacity and muscle strength in patients with cirrhosis, *Liver Transpl* 18:146–151, 2012.
76. Kavanagh T: Exercise rehabilitation in cardiac transplantation patients: a comprehensive review, *Eura Medicophys* 41:67–74, 2005.
80. Langer D, Burtin C, Schepers L, et al: Exercise training after lung transplantation improves participation in daily activity: a randomized controlled trial, *Am J Transplant* 12:1584–1592, 2012.
81. Lavie CJ, Arena R, Earnest CP: High-intensity interval training in patients with cardiovascular diseases and heart transplantation, *J Heart Lung Transplant* 32:1056–1058, 2013.

88. MacLeod SF, Terada T, Chahal BS, Boulé NG: Exercise lowers postprandial glucose but not fasting glucose in type 2 diabetes: a meta-analysis of studies using continuous glucose monitoring, *Diabetes Metab Res Rev* 29:593–603, 2013.
97. Miravitlles M, Soler-Cataluña JJ, Calle M, Soriano JB: Treatment of COPD by clinical phenotypes: putting old evidence into clinical practice, *Eur Respir J* 41:1252–1256, 2013.
105. Nytrøen K, Gullestad L: Exercise after heart transplantation: an overview, *World J Transplant* 3:78–90, 2013.
108. Oliveira C, Simões M, Carvalho J, Ribeiro J: Combined exercise for people with type 2 diabetes mellitus: a systematic review, *Diabetes Res Clin Pract* 98:187–198, 2012.
111. Orens JB, Estenne M, Arcasoy S, et al: International guidelines for the selection of lung transplant candidates: 2006 Update—a consensus report from the Pulmonary Scientific Council of the International Society for Heart and Lung Transplantation, *J Heart Lung Transplant* 25:745–755, 2006.
124. Qaseem A, Humphrey LL, Sweet DE, et al: Clinical Guidelines Committee of the American College of Physicians. Oral pharmacologic treatment of type 2 diabetes mellitus: a clinical practice guideline from the American College of Physicians, *Ann Intern Med* 156:218–231, 2012.
127. Razonable RR, Findlay JY, O'Riordan A, et al: Critical care issues in patients after liver transplantation, *Liver Transpl* 17:511–527, 2011.
128. Reusch JE, Bridenstine M, Regensteiner JG: Type 2 diabetes mellitus and exercise impairment, *Rev Endocr Metab Disord* 14:77–86, 2013.
129. Ries AL, Bauldoff GS, Carlin BW, et al: Pulmonary rehabilitation: joint ACCP/AACVPR evidence-based clinical practice guidelines, *Chest* 131(Suppl 5):4S–42S, 2007.
137. Schellenberg ES, Dryden DM, Vandermeer B, et al: Lifestyle interventions for patients with and at risk for type 2 diabetes: a systematic review and meta-analysis, *Ann Intern Med* 159:543–551, 2013.
138. Schrem H, Barg-Hock H, Strassburg CP, et al: Aftercare for patients with transplanted organs, *Dtsch Arztebl Int* 106:148–156, 2009.
139. Schumann KP, Touradji P, Hill-Briggs F: Inpatient rehabilitation diabetes consult service: a rehabilitation psychology approach to assessment and intervention, *Rehabil Psychol* 55:331, 2010.
140. Schuurmans MM, Benden C, Inci I: Practical approach to early postoperative management of lung transplant recipients, *Swiss Med Wkly* 143:w13773, 2013.
146. Spruit MA, Singh SJ, Garvey C, et al: An official American Thoracic Society/European Respiratory Society statement: key concepts and advances in pulmonary rehabilitation, *Am J Respir Crit Care Med* 188:e13–e64, 2013.
148. Squires RW: Exercise therapy for cardiac transplant recipients, *Prog Cardiovasc Dis* 53:429–436, 2011.
150. Strasser B, Pesta D: Resistance training for diabetes prevention and therapy: experimental findings and molecular mechanisms, *Biomed Res Int* 2013:805217, 2013.
151. Strath SJ, Kaminsky LA, Ainsworth BE, et al: Guide to the assessment of physical activity: clinical and research applications: a scientific statement from the American Heart Association, *Circulation* 128:2259–2279, 2013.
157. Thent ZC, Das S, Henry LJ: Role of exercise in the management of diabetes mellitus: the global scenario, *PLoS ONE* 8:e80436, 2013.
160. Toyoda Y, Guy TS, Kashem A: Present status and future perspectives of heart transplantation, *Circ J* 77:1097–1110, 2013.
162. Van Sandwijk MS, Bemelman FJ, Ten Berge IJ: Immunosuppressive drugs after solid organ transplantation, *Neth J Med* 71:281–289, 2013.
166. Weeks DL, Daratha KB, Towle LA: Diabetes prevalence and influence on resource use in Washington state inpatient rehabilitation facilities, 2001 to 2007, *Arch Phys Med Rehabil* 90:1937–1943, 2009.
168. Wickerson L, Mathur S, Brooks D: Exercise training after lung transplantation: a systematic review, *J Heart Lung Transplant* 29:497–503, 2010.

The full reference list for this chapter is available online.

CHAPTER 29

CANCER REHABILITATION

Andrea L. Cheville

Cancer rehabilitation addresses physical impairments and progressive disablement experienced by patients with cancer. A majority of impairments are directly related to cancer or its treatment; however, many arise from coexistent disease processes (e.g., ischemia and arthritis), which are increasingly prevalent among the aging cancer population. Whether impairments can or cannot be directly attributed to cancer may alter their management little. Yet, their successful rehabilitation requires consideration of cancer-specific concerns (limited prognoses, dynamic lesions, heavy symptom burden, and treatment-related toxicities) in the formulation of humane and realistic treatment plans.

Cancer is a pathologic process characterized by dysregulated cell growth and systemic spread. All tissue types have neoplastic potential and may become cancerous. Tissues distinguished by rapid cell turnover (e.g., gastrointestinal mucosa), hormone sensitivity (e.g., breast and prostate), and regular exposure to environmental mutagens (e.g., lung and skin) have higher rates of malignant transformation. The fact that any tissue can develop cancer means that cancer rehabilitation must consider all body parts and systems. Despite this broad scope, the field condenses into a manageable body of expertise predominantly focused on the effects of cancer on bones and neural tissue, maladaptive host responses (e.g., paraneoplastic syndromes), and long-term sequelae among cancer survivors.

Cancer survivorship is an important public health issue. The National Cancer Institute considers any living person who has received a cancer diagnosis, excluding skin cancers, to be a "survivor." According to the American Cancer Society, nearly 14.5 million children and adults with a history of cancer were alive on January 1, 2014, in the United States.[7] Cancer prevalence is projected to increase as a result of an aging population and an expanding arsenal of effective therapies. By January 1, 2024, it is estimated that the population of cancer survivors will increase to almost 19 million: 9.3 million males and 9.6 million females.[7] Survivors are eager to lead highly functional and productive lives despite the functional sequelae of their cancer.

This chapter is intended to provide physiatrists and other readers with an overview of the issues relevant to the rehabilitation of patients with cancer. Emphasis is placed on problems that affect the nervous and musculoskeletal systems.

Epidemiology

Cancer is a prevalent condition that becomes increasingly common with advanced age. In 2015, just less than 1.7 million new cancer cases are expected to be diagnosed, an estimate that does not include carcinoma in situ basal cell or squamous cell skin cancers, and approximately 600,000 Americans are expected to die of cancer.[6] Cancer causes one in four deaths, and is second only to heart disease as the leading cause of mortality in the United States. Approximately 76% of all cancers occur in patients 55 years of age and older. Men are more commonly affected by cancer, with a lifetime risk in the United States of one in two. The lifetime risk in women is one in three. In 2015, approximately one third of cancer deaths in the United States will be caused by tobacco smoking. Many cancers could be prevented through behavioral modification to address physical inactivity and obesity.

Demographic Disparities in Cancer

Racial, economic, and gender disparities influence cancer incidence, stage at diagnosis, and mortality. African Americans have the highest mortality associated with cancers of the lung, breast, prostate, and cervix among all racial groups in the United States. When African Americans are compared with whites, cancer death rates are 40% higher in males and 20% higher in females.[219]

The adverse impact of low economic status on cancer outcomes is being increasingly recognized. The 5-year survival rate is more than 10% higher for individuals living in affluent census tracts. The effects of economic disparity can significantly undermine cancer rehabilitation efforts through marginally covered or uncovered items, such as compression garments, high physical and occupational therapy copayments, and reduced home therapy benefits.

Disease Considerations

Staging

The specifics of cancer staging vary by disease site, but all conform to a general format geared toward describing the spread of disease from its site of origin. The T, N, and M system is the most widely used. *T* depends on the characteristics of the primary tumor, *N* on the extent of regional lymph node spread, and *M* on the presence of distant metastases. Once TNM status has been determined, a disease stage I to IV is assigned. Stage I is early, locally contained disease, whereas stage IV is advanced, characterized by distant metastases.

Cancer can also be described as in situ, local, regional, and distant. This approach distinguishes whether cancer has remained in the layer of cells where it developed (in situ) or spread beyond the tissue layer (local). Cancer staging dictates the type, duration, and aggressiveness of anticancer therapy. Staging also provides crucial information for the appropriate design of rehabilitation interventions, and for gauging each patient's risk of recurrence or progression. A safe rule of thumb during cancer rehabilitation is to attribute new or progressive signs and symptoms to malignancy until proven otherwise.

Prognosis and Metastatic Spread

Cancer presents patients and clinicians with a staggering array of prognoses, differential treatment approaches, and patterns of metastatic spread. This reflects the fact that cancer is, in truth, many diseases. In planning a long-term rehabilitation approach, it is important to anticipate where cancer is likely to spread, how it will respond to treatment, what cumulative toxicities may be associated with ongoing therapies, and how long patients are likely to live. This is not trivial, given the number of different cancer types and the varied natural histories of cancer subtypes arising from the same tissue. Treatment approaches are also continuously evolving. Nonetheless, the effort to anticipate the course of disease is crucial for the optimal delivery of cancer rehabilitation services. What follows is a synopsis of the characteristics of prevalent cancers and those that commonly lead patients to seek rehabilitative services.

Table 29-1 presents 5-year survival statistics collected between 2004 and 2010 for different cancers.[6] The implications of regional and distant spread at the time of diagnosis vary considerably by cancer type. For example, patients with prostate cancer benefit from excellent prognoses when their cancer is detected at the local or regional level, with virtually 100% 5-year survival. In contrast, among patients with lung cancer, 27% of those with regional spread and 4% of those with systemic spread are alive at 5 years. In general, cancers of the upper gastrointestinal tract (liver, pancreas, esophagus, and stomach) and of the lungs have the most limited prognoses. Prostate, breast, endometrial, and colorectal cancers have good to excellent prognoses when detected regionally. However, once systemic, all solid tumors, except thyroid and testicular, have median prognoses of 3 to 4 years. This information may inform rehabilitation goal setting, determine the emphasis placed on symptom-oriented versus disease-modifying treatments, and allow rehabilitation clinicians to gauge the appropriateness of patients' expectations.

Understanding patterns of metastatic spread can help clinicians to focus the search for metastases. Table 29-1 lists common sites of metastases for prevalent malignancies. Lung, breast, colon, and melanoma commonly spread to the brain. Regular neurologic screening examinations are therefore an important element of surveillance care. Prostate, breast, lung, renal, and thyroid cancers commonly produce bone metastases. Musculoskeletal pain in these cancer populations can be attributable to the primary or secondary consequences of bony disease and should trigger an appropriate evaluation.

Phases of Cancer

For rehabilitation purposes, cancer can be divided into several distinct stages. This approach calls clinical attention to points along the disease trajectory that may indicate a need to reevaluate functional deficits and to redefine goals. Five distinct phases of malignant disease, initial diagnosis and treatment, surveillance, recurrence, temporization, and palliation, were initially outlined in a model proposed by Gerber et al.[68a] Attention to cancer phases ensures that significant shifts in prognosis and treatment requirements inform rehabilitative efforts.

At the time of initial cancer diagnosis, patients deemed curable are treated aggressively to eradicate their disease. Box 29-1 lists rehabilitation emphases by phase of disease. A primary rehabilitation goal during initial cancer treatment is limiting the functional impact of cancer treatments: surgery, radiation, and chemotherapy. Once primary

Table 29-1 Five-Year Survival Statistics for Different Cancers, 2004 to 2010

	Five-Year Survival (%)			
Cancer	**Local**	**Regional**	**Distant**	**Common Sites of Metastatic Spread**
Lung and bronchus	54	27	4	Brain, bone, liver, mediastinal lymph nodes
Breast	99	85	25	Brain, lung, bone, liver
Prostate	>99	>99	28	Bone, pelvic lymph nodes
Colon and rectum	90	71	13	Liver, lung
Ovary	92	72	27	Peritoneum, pleura
Uterine cervix	91	57	16	Peritoneum, lung, retroperitoneal lymph nodes
Uterine corpus	95	68	18	Retroperitoneal lymph nodes, lung
Pharynx and oral cavity	83	61	37	Lung, regional lymph nodes
Melanoma	98	63	16	Brain
Stomach	64	29	4	Liver, lung, peritoneum
Esophagus	40	21	4	Liver, lung
Pancreas	26	10	2	Liver
Urinary bladder	69	34	6	Bone, intraperitoneal

From American Cancer Society: *Cancer facts and figures 2015*, Atlanta, 2015, American Cancer Society.

BOX 29-1

Rehabilitation Priorities During Cancer Phases

Initial Diagnosis

Detect and manage acute morbidity from cancer treatments
Address worsening of premorbid physical impairments

Surveillance

Physically recondition
Detect and address delayed cancer treatment toxicities
Promote reentry into vocational, social, and family roles

Recurrence

Screen for cancer treatment toxicities, given the increased risk
Proactively manage early-stage impairments

Temporization

Control symptoms
Prevent and proactively address disablement

Palliation

Preserve community integration
Support and educate caregivers
Maintain functional autonomy as feasible

cancer treatments are complete, patients enter a period of surveillance. For most patients, this is an uneasy and indefinite interval characterized by persistent vigilance for emerging treatment toxicities and recurrent cancer. For some patients, the surveillance phase ends with cancer recurrence.

If cure is possible following recurrence, patients are aggressively retreated with multimodal therapy to eliminate disease. If not, they enter the temporization phase discussed later. Patients treated for recurrent cancer are rendered extremely vulnerable to lasting functional impairments, because cancer treatments are often delivered to pretreated tissues and cumulative toxicities can be severe.

Patients who are initially diagnosed with metastatic cancer, or whose cancers are not deemed curable following recurrence, enter the temporization phase characterized by efforts to control cancer and to optimize quality of life. Anticancer therapies during this phase are geared toward reducing symptom burden, cancer spread, and the development of medical comorbidities. Patients generally undergo serial chemotherapy trials, which can contribute to progressive deconditioning and disablement. As patients enter the final, palliative phase of cancer treatment, the focus is on maximizing patients' comfort, psychological well-being, and independence in mobility and the performance of activities of daily living (ADL).

Constitutional Symptoms

Many symptoms are common in cancer, particularly among patients with stage IV disease. Inadequate treatment of symptoms such as fatigue, nausea, pain, anxiety, insomnia, and dyspnea will undermine rehabilitative efforts. The burgeoning of palliative care as a medical discipline has produced an extensive literature and several excellent textbooks detailing current strategies for managing cancer-related symptoms. Interested readers are referred to the *Oxford Textbook of Palliative Medicine* (edited by Hanks et al.) and *Principles and Practice of Palliative Care and Supportive Oncology* (edited by Berger et al.). The following is a brief discussion on strategies for managing cancer-related fatigue and pain, as these are common, function-degrading impediments to successful rehabilitation.

BOX 29-2

Reversible Sources of Cancer Fatigue

- Anemia
- Insomnia or lack of restorative sleep
- Cytokine release (e.g., tumor necrosis factor)
- Hypothyroidism
- Hypogonadism
- Depression
- Deconditioning
- Steroid myopathy
- Centrally acting medications
- Altered oxidative capacity
- Pain
- Adrenal insufficiency
- Cachexia

Fatigue

Fatigue is the most common symptom experienced by patients with cancer.[149] The prevalence of fatigue ranges from 70% to 100%, contingent on the type and stage of cancer and whether patients are receiving anticancer treatments.[151,179] A majority of patients in active treatment rate their fatigue as "severe," or 7 or higher on an 11-point numerical rating scale.[83] Because fatigue is inherently subjective, definitions of fatigue understandably differ. The National Comprehensive Cancer Network defines cancer-related fatigue as "an unusual, persistent, subjective sense of tiredness related to cancer or cancer treatment that interferes with usual functioning."[152] Experts concur that fatigue reduces the energy, mental capacity, functional status, and psychological resilience of patients with cancer.[152]

A discrete source of fatigue can be identified in some patients, leading to effective treatment and symptom reversal. More often, the responsible mechanisms are multifactorial. Box 29-2 lists possible contributing factors. In the past, anemia received the greatest attention as a source of fatigue; however, the time course of fatigue differs from fluctuations in blood counts, and normalization of hemoglobin levels often fails to reduce fatigue.

Often, cancer-related fatigue occurs in the absence of anemia or ongoing cancer therapy. In such cases, the differential diagnosis is based on patients' previous cancer treatment, medical comorbidities, and current medications. Compromise of the adrenal axis, thyroid gland, testes, and ovaries by chemical ablation, surgical resection, or irradiation can cause fatigue. Appropriate laboratory tests may identify remediable disorders in patients with suggestive treatment histories. Patients reporting poor sleep might require a sleep study if the elimination of daytime napping and use of soporifics provide no benefit. Menopausal symptoms can degrade sleep quality and warrant close scrutiny.

Deconditioning and mood-related factors (e.g., anxiety and depression)[61] are prevalent and potentially remediable contributing factors in cancer-related fatigue. Centrally acting medications can also play an important role and should be carefully reviewed in patients complaining of fatigue. A reduction or withdrawal trial of nonessential drugs can identify those producing fatigue.[152] Medications that commonly produce fatigue include opioids, benzodiazepines, antiemetics, antihistamines, tricyclic antidepressants, anticonvulsants (e.g., carbamazepine, gabapentin, and oxcarbazepine), thalidomide, and alpha$_2$-adrenergic agonists (e.g., tizanidine).

When potentially reversible sources of fatigue (see Box 29-2) have been ruled out or definitively addressed, symptom-oriented fatigue management is indicated. The National Comprehensive Cancer Network endorses a multimodal approach that includes exercise/activity enhancement[209]; psychosocial interventions; and treatments supported by category 1 evidence.[44,152] The use of aerobic exercise to reduce cancer-related fatigue is discussed at length later in this chapter under "Aerobic Conditioning and Resistive Exercise."

There are currently no validated pharmaceutical treatments for cancer-related fatigue. Both methylphenidate and modafinil have been used in the past, but evidence has accrued that indicates they are not effective.[178] Wisconsin ginseng was recently found to reduce cancer-related fatigue in a randomized controlled trial, but this result has not yet been replicated.[11]

Pain

The prevalence of cancer-related pain is 28% among patients with newly diagnosed cancer, 50% to 70% among patients receiving antineoplastic therapy, and 64% to 80% among patients with advanced disease.[214] Adequate pain control is an absolute requisite for successful rehabilitation. Patients with cancer generally experience multiple concurrent pain syndromes. Thorough evaluation therefore requires assessment of all relevant pain etiologies and pathophysiologic processes. Pain control might require the integrated use of anticancer treatments, agents from multiple analgesic classes, interventional techniques, topical agents, manual approaches, and modalities.

Important considerations in cancer pain management are listed in Box 29-3 and are explained later. One salient distinction of cancer pain management is the reliance on high-dose opioid therapy. The doses required by many patients with cancer extend far beyond the conventional levels used by physiatrists. An extensive international literature and multiple guidelines endorse the approach of opioid dosing "effect or side effect."[14,57,90,136,139] An example of the high doses that may result from this approach is the daily requirement of 15% of patients with late-stage pancreatic cancer for 5 g of oral morphine equivalent.[64]

Most cancer pain is caused by tumor effects. For this reason, disease-modifying, anticancer therapy plays a crucial role in pain management. A single radiation fraction of 8 Gy offers a definitive and effective means of controlling pain associated with symptomatic and uncomplicated bone metastases.[38,123] Cancer progression frequently causes pain to worsen and escalating analgesic requirements should be anticipated.[64] Cancer-related depression, anxiety, and existential distress can exacerbate patients' pain experience.[106,174] For this reason, contributing psychiatric factors should be sought and addressed.

Often, the enteral administration of analgesics is not feasible in patients with cancer, particularly those with advanced cancers with bowel obstruction. Analgesics with transdermal, parenteral, rectal, and transmucosal routes of administration should be preferentially used when the enteral route may be lost. Because of the limited life expectancy and intense pain associated with far-advanced cancer, the cost-benefit ratio of permanent neuroablative procedures may be acceptable. Excellent success rates have been reported with anterolateral cordotomy (84% to 95%) and myelotomy (59% to 92%).[13,215]

BOX 29-3

Considerations in Cancer Pain Management

- Therapeutic reliance on high-dose opioid analgesia
- Importance of disease-modifying analgesic approaches
- Potential loss of enteral administration
- Dynamic and rapidly progressive pain complaints
- Multiple concurrent pain syndromes
- Affective and organic psychopathology
- Feasibility of permanent ablative procedures
- Concurrent nociceptive and neuropathic pain

Acute Pain

Acute pain after surgery or radiation therapy can be successfully treated with conventional algorithms for acute postoperative pain.[3] Nerves are frequently severed, compressed, or stretched during tumor resections, making it possible for neuropathic pain to be a major factor during the postoperative period. Adjuvant analgesics should be initiated when a neurogenic contribution is suspected. As with all postoperative pain that impedes function, aggressive opioid-based and antiinflammatory analgesics should be considered. Acute pain control allows movement, minimized needless deconditioning, and enhances participation in the rehabilitation process.

Acute pain can also complicate the administration of chemotherapy, hormonal therapy, or irradiation. Most of the associated pain syndromes are transient but may produce intense discomfort warranting aggressive analgesia. Acute pain syndromes associated with cancer therapy include paclitaxel-related arthralgias and myalgias, bisphosphonate-related bone pain, radiation mucositis, steroid pseudorheumatism (following withdrawal of corticosteroids), intravesicular BCG–induced cystitis, hepatic artery infusion pain, bone pain associated with colony-stimulating factor (CSF) and granulocyte macrophage CSF administration, and radiopharmaceutical-induced pain.

Chronic Pain

Chronic cancer-related pain can arise from visceral or neural structures but is most commonly associated with bone metastases.[48] Bone metastases occur in 60% to 84% of patients with solid tumors. Pain intensity does not correlate with the number, size, or location of bone metastases, nor with tumor type and 25% of patients with bone metastases report no pain.[173] Bone pain is particularly relevant to physiatrists because moving or loading affected structures can precipitate severe pain. As mentioned earlier, bone pain responds well to local irradiation.[224]

Nonsteroidal Antiinflammatory Drugs for Bone Pain

Nonsteroidal antiinflammatory drugs (NSAIDs) are considered first-line therapy for bone pain, and a trial is warranted unless contraindicated. Cyclooxygenase (COX) nonselective inhibitors offer comparable or greater pain relief than COX-2 inhibitors but a less desirable toxicity profile.[181] Choline magnesium trisalicylate causes less inhibition of platelet aggregation than other COX nonselective inhibitors but did not statistically outperform placebo when trialed in cancer-related bone pain.[93] COX nonselective inhibitors with less desirable toxicity profiles have proven more effective. Several placebo-controlled, randomized trials found that ketoprofen reduced cancer pain to a greater extent than either codeine or morphine.[138] NSAID doses for bone pain are no different from NSAIDs at antiinflammatory doses for pain of alternative etiologies.

Adjuvant for Bone Pain

Adjuvant analgesics can augment NSAID-related control of bone pain. Corticosteroids effectively relieve bone pain.[23] Their toxicity profile (edema, bone demineralization, immunosuppression, and myopathies) is problematic and must be considered in assessing the risk-to-benefit ratio of steroid therapy, particularly with chronic administration. Parenteral bisphosphonates are also effective. Denosumab, a recently introduced monoclonal antibody therapy, was found in a metaanalysis to be as or more effective than bisphosphonates in controlling pain from bone metastases.[218] Use of calcitonin for bone pain is discouraged because of weak supportive evidence and rapid tachyphylaxis.[129,137]

Opioids for General Cancer Pain

As mentioned previously, opioid-based pharmacotherapy is the current standard of care for the management of moderate to severe cancer pain, irrespective of its origin. Opioid use should be restricted to pure mu-receptor agonists. Those most commonly used in cancer pain management include morphine, hydromorphone, oxycodone, oxymorphone, fentanyl, and methadone.

The dominant paradigm for opioid administration has a well-established track record and has been reiterated by many experts in the field with few changes over the past decades.[64,90,117] Recognizing that most patients experience constant, baseline pain punctuated by transient or incident pain, the combined use of normal and sustained-release or continuous-release opioid preparations is recommended. To rapidly estimate initial dose requirements, patients should be provided liberal access to a normal-release opioid formulation. Once their use has stabilized (this may take a day with patient-controlled analgesia pumps, or up to a week with oral dosing), mean daily or hourly consumption can be calculated and an oral or transdermal sustained-release preparation initiated. The ongoing dose titration should be driven by patients' use of supplemental normal-release, "rescue doses." Typically, rescue doses are 10% to 15% of the total daily dose.

Several practices will increase the likelihood of a successful opioid trial. First, anticipate side effects, particularly constipation and nausea, and address them proactively. Second, in the absence of dose-limiting side effects, resist the urge to switch or add additional opioids when a single mu-receptor agonist initially fails to control pain. Current recommendations urge a single agent dosing to "effect or side effect" and each agent should be adequately trialed. Third, remain vigilant for opioid-induced hyperalgesia and alterations in patients' capacity to absorb, metabolize, or eliminate opioids in the face of progressive cancer.

Opioid Conversion

Significant intraindividual variations in response to different opioids have long been recognized. An alternative opioid should be considered when an "adequate" trial of a particular agent has failed to control pain, or has caused refractory side effects. Opioid dose conversion requires calculation of the equianalgesic dose of the novel agent (Table 29-2) and reduction by 50% for incomplete cross-tolerance. Incomplete cross-tolerance describes the property of opioids to induce analgesic tolerance with sustained high-dose exposure. Tolerance is usually considerably lower to a novel agent. For this reason, patients often experience greater sedation and needless side effects when exposed to 100% of the equianalgesic dose. Opioid conversions are based on estimated dose equivalencies. Providing patients with liberal access to rescue doses is crucial during the conversion period to avoid pain crises.

Invasive and Intraspinal Analgesic Approaches

As mentioned previously, permanent ablation of central afferent tracts becomes tenable in the context of advanced

Table 29-2 Opioid Dose Conversion

Opioid (Generic)	Branded Product	Route	Dose
Morphine	MS Contin, Avinza	Oral: Tablet	30 mg
	Kadian, Oramorph SR	Oral: Elixir	30 mg
	Roxanol	Intravenous or intramuscular	10 mg
Fentanyl	Actiq	Transmucosal	500 μg
		Intravenous or intramuscular	250 μg
	Duragesic	Transdermal	250 μg
Hydromorphone	Dilaudid	Oral: Tablet	7.5 mg
		Intravenous or intramuscular	1.5 mg
Oxycodone	OxyContin	Oral: Tablet	20 mg
		Oral: Elixir	20 mg
Methadone	Dolophine	Oral	20 mg
		Intravenous or intramuscular	10 mg
Oxymorphone		Intravenous or intramuscular	1 mg

cancer, and has been used with considerable success.[31,200,205] More discrete neural blockade effectively reduces pain transmitted by one or several adjacent peripheral nerves. Intercostal, paravertebral, genitofemoral, ilioinguinal, and trigeminal nerve blocks can afford dramatic relief and reduce analgesic requirements. Nociceptive impulses of visceral origin can be blocked by ablation of sympathetic ganglia. Celiac plexus blockade affords excellent relief of visceral cancer pain.[59] Intraspinal opioid administration can reduce dose requirements and associated side effects.[195] For patients experiencing dose-limiting side effects, implantable intrathecal opioid delivery systems may achieve a superior analgesia to side effect profile.

Impairments in Cancer

Cancer can invade all tissue types, producing a wide array of functional impairments. Tumor-related deficits generally arise as a result of pain, neural compromise, loss of osseous or articular integrity, and invasion of cardiopulmonary structures. Cancer-related impairments are often dynamic, characterized by improvement or progression, depending on treatment responsiveness. Altering or initiating cancer treatment should always be considered as first-line therapy in the face of new or progressive impairments. Disability in patients with metastatic cancer is generally caused by the cumulative burden of multiple impairments and adverse symptoms.[36] In a large cohort of patients with advanced stage lung cancer, brain and bone metastases, as well as pain and fatigue, were most strongly associated with near-term functional decline.[37]

Impairments Caused by Tumor Effects

Bone Metastases

Bone metastases are highly prevalent because bone is the most common site of metastatic spread, and osseous lesions complicate the most frequently occurring cancers: lung, breast, and prostate. Thyroid cancer, lymphoma, renal cell carcinoma, myeloma, and melanoma also commonly spread to bone. Between 60% and 84% of patients with solid tumors will develop bone metastases.[118,173]

Of greatest physiatric concern are lesions involving the spine and long bones. These structures are crucial for weight-bearing and mobility, and are most prone to fracture. Bone metastases are managed with medications, radiopharmaceuticals, orthotics, radiation therapy, or surgical stabilization. The choice of intervention(s) will depend on lesion location, degree of associated pain, presence or risk of fracture, radiation responsiveness, and related neurologic compromise. The overall clinical context (e.g., prognosis, severity of medical comorbidities, and operative risk) must also be taken into consideration. Most patients with nonfractured bony lesions can be treated nonoperatively through the use of systemic therapy and radiation.

Bisphosphonates are the primary medications used to manage bone metastases. Use of these agents reduces the spread and progression of bone metastases, in addition to relieving associated pain. Use of bisphosphonates reduces the risk of vertebral fracture (odds ratio 0.69), nonvertebral fracture (odds ratio 0.65), and hypercalcemia (odds ratio 0.54).[177] Current evidence supports the empirical initiation of bisphosphonates in patients with bone metastases. Radiopharmaceuticals such as strontium-99 are predominantly used to manage severe, refractory pain associated with widely disseminated bone metastases. Drawbacks to radiopharmaceuticals include prolonged marrow suppression and potentially severe pain flares following administration.

Radiation delivered to bone metastasis offers an effective means of rapidly achieving local control of pain and tumor growth. Palliative radiation was formerly delivered in 10 fractions of 300 cGy. However, single fractions of 8 Gy also effectively alleviate pain.[38,123] At present, protocols in use range between these extremes with the choice of dose and schedule being heavily influenced by individual patient factors and institutional culture. Radiation may be delayed following surgical stabilization. However, it is an important adjunctive treatment because it suppresses tumor growth in areas where surgical management may have distributed microscopic emboli.

Painful osteolytic lesions are predominantly responsible for pathologic fractures. The incidence of pathologic fracture among all cancer types is 8%.[180] Breast carcinoma is responsible for approximately 53% of these. Other solid tumors associated with pathologic fractures are kidney, lung, thyroid cancer, and lymphoma. Sixty percent of all long bone fractures involve the femur, with 80% of these located in the proximal portion.[173]

Management bone metastases that may fracture remains a source of clinical uncertainty. Precise quantification of fracture risk has been a persistent challenge in orthopedic oncology. Table 29-3 outlines Mirel's proposed rating system for calculating fracture risk, whereby specific attributes are ascribed points.[141] Neither this, nor any other approach based on retrospective review, has been adequately validated in clinical practice.

Pathologic fractures are generally managed through well-established surgical algorithms. Four main goals direct surgical management of pathologic fractures: pain relief, preservation or restoration of function, skeletal stabilization, and local tumor control.[223] The general indications for surgery are life expectancy of more than 1 month with a fracture of a weight-bearing bone, and more than 3 months for fracture of a non–weight-bearing bone. Internal fixation or prosthetic replacements with polymethylmethacrylate are the most effective ways of relieving pain and restoring function in patients with pathologic fractures.[223] Healing rates may be low following pathologic fractures.

Table 29-3 Proposed Rating System for Calculating Fracture Risk

	Point Assigned		
Character	**1**	**2**	**3**
Anatomic location	Upper limb	Lower limb	Trochanter
Lesion type	Blastic	Blastic or lytic	Lytic
Lesion size	≤⅓ diameter	>⅓, <⅔	≥⅔
Intensity of pain	Mild	Moderate	Severe

Fractures of the pelvis are generally treated conservatively, unless pain persists after radiation or they involve the acetabulum. In the latter case, patients are generally surgically reconstructed with screws or pins, and with an acetabular component. Vertebral fractures that are not associated with neurologic compromise are generally treated conservatively with radiation and bracing. Operative decompression and stabilization may be indicated for persistent pain refractory to aggressive analgesic therapy. Vertebroplasty continues to be performed for patients who are not at risk of tumor displacement into the spinal canal. However, two large randomized controlled trials[24,94] failed to demonstrate benefit in compression fractures related to osteoporosis, and these results have raised skepticism regarding the benefit of vertebroplasty in cancer.[10]

Brain Tumors: Primary and Metastases

Brain metastases occur in 15% to 40% of patients with cancer, accounting for 200,000 new cases per year in the United States.[68] They are the most common intracranial tumors.[161] The incidence has increased in recent years, presumably as a result of prolonged patient survival and better early detection of small tumors through superior imaging modalities.[58] Lung cancer is the most common primary source of brain metastases. Up to 64% of patients with stage IV lung cancer develop brain metastases.[184] Breast cancer is the second most common source, followed by melanoma, with 2% to 25% and 4% to 20% of patients developing brain metastases, respectively.[184] Brain metastases from colorectal cancers, genitourinary cancers, and sarcomas occur with considerably less frequency (1%). The distribution of metastases reflects cerebral blood flow, with 90% situated in the supratentorial region and 10% in the posterior fossa. Brain metastases are multiple in approximately 50% to 75% of cases.

Presentation. Lung cancer and melanoma often produce multiple metastases, whereas breast, colon, and renal cancer more commonly generate single lesions.[17] Presenting symptoms at the time of diagnosis with brain metastasis, in order of decreasing frequency, are as follows (patients can have more than one): headache, 49%; mental disturbance, 32%; focal weakness, 30%; gait ataxia, 21%; seizures, 18%; speech difficulty, 12%; visual disturbance, 6%; sensory disturbance, 6%; and limb ataxia, 6%.[163] Neurologic examination reveals the following clinical signs at presentation: hemiparesis, 59%; impaired cognitive function, 58%; hemisensory loss, 21%; papilledema, 20%; gait ataxia, 19%; aphasia, 18%; visual field cut, 7%; and limb ataxia, 4%.[42]

Treatment. Corticosteroids are first-line treatment, with dexamethasone being the drug of choice. By virtue of their ability to reduce peritumoral edema, corticosteroids reverse local brain compression and associated deficits. Treatment generally involves whole brain radiation therapy with stereotactic radiosurgery or surgical resection via craniotomy.[96] Adjunctive chemotherapy can be used, contingent on patient performance status, type of cancer, and previous exposure to antineoplastics. Although seizures occur in 25% of patients with brain metastasis, studies and a metaanalysis have failed to show that antiepileptic drugs reduce their incidence.[140]

Prognosis. Untreated patients with brain metastases have a median survival of 1 to 2 months.[126] The survival of treated patients is highly variable. A number of prognostic indices have been developed for patients with brain metastases. At this point, no one index is considered definitive because their predictive capacities vary by tumor type.[71] Clinician characteristics that feature prominently in most include performance status, age, presence of extracranial metastases, and tumor type. The survival distribution is skewed, with some patients surviving more than 2 years with good functional preservation and quality of life.

The rehabilitation needs of patients with brain metastases are best determined by understanding the baseline functional status, prognoses, location and number of metastases, and antineoplastic treatment plan. Patients admitted for acute inpatient rehabilitation for primary brain tumors and brain metastases have functional independence measure (FIM) efficiencies and home discharge rates equal to or higher than patients with traumatic or ischemic brain injuries. Concurrent radiation therapy does not impact these outcomes. Brain metastasis characteristics associated with significant near-term loss of mobility are the following: (1) cerebellar or brain stem location, (2) imaging that reveals new and expanding metastases, and (3) treatment with whole brain radiation therapy.

Epidural Spinal Cord Compression

Malignant spinal cord compression (SCC) occurs in up to 5% of patients.[41] In contrast to brain metastases, which involve the brain parenchyma, most symptomatic tumors compress the spinal cord or cauda equina from the epidural space.[164] Epidural lesions generally arise from vertebral metastases and rarely breach the dura.[77] Invasion of the dural space accounts for only 5% of neoplastic SCC and is caused by either growth of tumor along the spinal roots or hematogenous spread to the cord.[42,167] The cancers that most commonly cause SCC are those that produce vertebral metastases (e.g., breast, lung, myeloma, and prostate).[20,222]

Presentation. Pain is by far the most common initial (94%) and presenting (97% to 99%) symptom of malignant SCC.[16,164] Radicular pain is present in 58% of patients at diagnosis.[16] Pain associated with SCC is generally exacerbated when supine or by coughing, sneezing, or the Valsalva maneuver. If malignant SCC is detected when pain is the only symptom, efforts to preserve function through surgical decompression or radiation therapy have high success rates.[164] Unfortunately, this is rarely the case. Reports of symptom prevalence when the diagnosis of malignant SCC is eventually made are remarkably consistent. Weakness is present in 74% to 76% of patients, autonomic dysfunction in 52% to 57%, and sensory loss in 51% to 53%.[70,164] The thoracic spine is the most common site of epidural SCC, followed by the lumbosacral and cervical spine in a ratio of 4 : 2 : 1.[164]

Diagnosis and Treatment. Magnetic resonance imaging (MRI) is the procedure of choice to evaluate the epidural space and spinal cord.[202] MRI allows rapid evaluation of the entire spine with sagittal views. Computed tomography (CT) scans are helpful if there is an absolute contraindication to MRI, or if SCC is related to tumor encroachment through the foramina. High-dose steroids and surgical decompression are the treatment of choice for operable patients.[120] Radiation is the treatment of choice for nonoperable patients.

Prognosis. Tumors that cause rapid progression of neurologic deficits are associated with poorer functional outcomes following decompression. In general, patients remain ambulatory if able to walk at the time of definitive treatment. Motor and coordination deficits rarely resolve when present at diagnosis. The recurrence rate for metastatic epidural SCC after successful treatment of the initial compression is 7% to 14%.[41]

Cancer Involving Cranial and Peripheral Nerves

Compromise of cranial and peripheral nerves is a common source of cancer-related pain and impairment. Cancer can affect nerves through local extension of primary tumors (e.g., brachial plexopathy associated with Pancoast tumors) or through metastatic spread.

Cranial Nerves

Cranial nerve palsies are caused by tumors that originate near the base of the skull or metastasize there.[32,110] Cancer can directly invade cranial nerves or exogenously compress them. Often, tumors invade the neural foramina. Bone metastases from lung, breast, and prostate cancers involving the base of the skull are also common sources of cranial nerve compromise.[172] The incidence with which different cranial nerves are affected by cancer remains poorly quantified. One series of patients with breast cancer reported a 13% incidence of cranial nerve dysfunction.[75] The trigeminal and facial nerves were most frequently involved.

Clinical presentations vary depending on the cranial nerve being compressed. Evaluation should include MRI, which is the diagnostic test of choice.[169] If patients have a bone-avid tumor (e.g., lung, breast, or prostate), a CT scan should be considered, because bone destruction is more easily observed on CT scan.[157] Positron emission tomography (PET) scanning particularly in conjunction with CT scanning can help to discretely localize the tumor if extensive postradiation change or surgical alteration of the bony architecture has occurred. Acute management should include oral steroids, unless contraindicated, to preserve neurologic function until definitive treatment is delivered. Treatment generally involves chemotherapy and radiation.

Spinal Roots

Malignant radiculopathies arise through direct hematogenous spread to the nerve roots or dorsal root ganglia, or, more commonly, by invasion from the paravertebral space. When the latter occurs, the tumor can grow longitudinally in the paravertebral space and concurrently invade multiple foramina to produce a polyradiculopathy.[165] Most cancer-related radiculopathies initially produce dysesthetic, aching, or burning pain in the affected dermatome, which can be associated with lancinations. Sympathetic hyperactivity or hypoactivity can be present.[46] Involvement of the lower cervical or upper thoracic roots can produce a Horner syndrome. In patients with a history of cancer, a new Horner syndrome should be attributed to malignancy until proven otherwise. Patients may complain of muscle cramps in affected myotomes.[196]

Diagnosis and Treatment. Evaluation of spinal roots for cancerous involvement is best achieved with MRI. MRI will permit assessment of the paravertebral space, foramina, and epidural space. Electromyography allows pathophysiologic characterization of the nerves involved and may complement the anatomic information provided by imaging studies. Steroids should be considered to minimize peritumoral edema until disease-modifying therapy can be delivered. Radiation is effective at alleviating symptoms, but its capacity to spare neurologic function has not been adequately characterized. The role of surgical decompression is generally determined on a contextual basis.

Nerve Plexuses

The brachial and lumbosacral plexuses are commonly compressed or invaded by tumor.[198] The frequency of malignant brachial plexopathy is 0.43%, and lumbosacral plexopathy 0.71%, based on retrospective case series.[92,104] The most common sources of brachial plexopathy are tumors at the lung apex and regional spread of breast cancer.[104] Because cancer generally grows superiorly to invade the lower brachial plexus, the inferior trunk and medial cord are most commonly involved. Occasionally, head and neck neoplasms grow inferiorly to invade the upper trunk.[91]

Pain in the shoulder region and proximal arm occurs in 89% of patients with malignant brachial plexopathy and is the most common presenting symptom.[65] The presence of pain helps to distinguish malignant from radiation-induced plexopathy. Only 18% of patients with radiation-induced plexopathy develop pain.[65] Radiation plexopathies also differ in their propensity to cause progressive weakness in the C5 to C6 myotomes as opposed to the lower cervical levels.[65] Horner's syndrome occurs in 23% of patients with cancer who have malignant brachial plexopathies.[91] The presence of Horner's syndrome suggests potential neuroforaminal encroachment and SCC. Numbness and paresthesias associated with malignant plexopathies typically are perceived in the C8 dermatome, especially digits 4 and 5.[165] Loss of hand dexterity and power can be the initial motor complaint. Weakness subsequently extends proximally to involve the finger flexors, wrist extensors and flexors, and elbow extensors.[165]

Malignancies responsible for lumbosacral plexopathies include colorectal carcinomas; retroperitoneal sarcomas; or metastatic tumors from breast, lymphoma, uterus, cervix, bladder, melanoma, or prostate.[92] If primary intrapelvic neoplasms are not responsible, then the lumbosacral plexus is generally invaded from lymphatic and osseous metastases.[91] Sacral plexopathies are more common than those in the lumbar region. Lumbar and sacral plexopathies can also occur concurrently.[165] Lumbosacral plexopathies are bilateral in 25% of patients, particularly when the sacral plexus is more extensively involved.[91,165] Incontinence and impotence strongly suggest bilateral involvement.[92] Back, buttock, or leg pain is present in 98% of patients with malignant lumbosacral plexopathies. Among the 60% of patients who eventually develop neurologic deficits, 86% have leg weakness and 73% have sensory loss.[91] Positive straight leg raise is present in over 50% of patients.[92] As many as 33% of patients complain of a "hot dry foot" resulting from involvement of sympathetic components of the plexus.[46]

Diagnosis and Treatment. The evaluations of a suspected brachial plexopathy should include chest radiography to assess the lung apex. MRI with gadolinium is the diagnostic test of choice for evaluating the brachial and lumbosacral plexuses.[201] Cancerous invasion of plexuses can extend along adjacent connective tissue or the epineurium of nerve trunks, without producing a discrete mass. For this reason, MRI findings can be erroneously interpreted as postradiation change. Electromyography can distinguish plexopathies from radiculopathies by defining the distribution of denervation. The presence of myokymia on needle examination is believed to be pathognomonic for radiation plexopathy.[91,198]

Acute treatment should include steroids for preservation of neurologic function. Radiation can effectively relieve pain from malignant plexopathies but is less helpful in restoring lost function.[91] Chemotherapy is commonly initiated or altered when plexus involvement heralds cancer progression; however, the success of this approach remains poorly characterized. Refractory pain requires aggressive coadministration of opioid and adjuvant analgesics, and potentially high cervical cordotomy or rhizotomy. Stellate ganglion blockade may relieve pain that is sympathetically maintained.

Peripheral Nerves

Peripheral nerves are affected most often by cancer when extension of a bone metastasis produces a mononeuropathy.[175] Rare polyneuropathy or mononeuritis multiplex resulting from myeloma, lymphoma, or leukemia has been reported.[72] More commonly, nerves are compressed where they pass directly over an involved bone or through a bony canal. Common sites of nerve compression include the radial nerve at the humerus, obturator nerve at the obturator canal, ulnar nerve at the elbow and axilla, sciatic nerve in the pelvis, intercostal nerves, and peroneal nerve at the fibular head. Pain generally precedes motor and sensory loss.

Diagnosis and Treatment. Evaluation includes plain radiographs, MRI, or electromyography. Treatment depends on the clinical context in which the mononeuropathy occurs. Radiation, surgical decompression, and chemotherapy, individually or in combination, are common treatment approaches. Significant sensorimotor recovery should not be expected, irrespective of the antineoplastic intervention.

Paraneoplastic Syndromes

Paraneoplastic syndromes are pertinent to rehabilitation because they produce refractory neurologic deficits and severe disability.[53] The incidence of paraneoplastic neurologic disorders (PNDs) is low, occurring in less than 1% of all patients with cancer.[84] PNDs may affect any level of the nervous system. Classic PNDs are listed in Table 29-4. These syndromes are produced when antibodies are made against tumors that express nervous system proteins. Most PNDs are triggered during the early stages of cancer, when primary tumors and metastases may be undetectable by conventional imaging techniques. The emergence of a PND in a patient with known cancer should trigger workup for recurrent or progressive disease. PNDs are characterized by symptoms that develop and progress rapidly in days to weeks, and then stabilize. Spontaneous improvement is rare. Diagnostic workup may include serum and cerebrospinal fluid tests, brain MRI, and PET. Screening patients' serum or cerebrospinal fluid for antineuronal antibodies known to be associated with particular cancers can direct the search for an occult malignancy. Timely diagnosis and treatment of the tumor offer the greatest chance of success in managing PNDs.[12] PNDs do not generally respond solely to immunotherapies (e.g., intravenous immunoglobulin, corticosteroids, and immunosuppressants) or to plasmapheresis. However, these may be useful adjuvant treatments.[95]

Rehabilitation of PNDs is determined by the type, distribution, and severity of the associated neurologic deficits. Potential improvement with planned antineoplastic therapy should be taken into consideration. Supportive

Table 29-4 Classic Paraneoplastic Disorders

Classic Paraneoplastic Neurologic Disorder	Associated Malignancy	Presenting Signs and Symptoms
Cerebellar degeneration	Small cell lung cancer, Hodgkin lymphoma, gynecologic, breast	Pancerebellar dysfunction with truncal and limb ataxia
Limbic encephalitis	Germ cell tumors of the testes	Anxiety, depression, confusion, delirium, hallucinations, seizures, short-term memory loss, dementia
Opsoclonus-myoclonus	Breast, gynecologic, small cell lung cancer, neuroblastoma	Chaotic, conjugate, arrhythmic, and multidirectional ocular saccades, myoclonus, truncal ataxia
Sensory neuronopathy	Small cell lung cancer	Pain, numbness, sensory deficits of cranial and spinal nerves
Lambert-Eaton myasthenic syndrome	Small cell lung cancer	Proximal muscle weakness, autonomic symptoms, strength augmentation during initial voluntary contraction
Encephalomyelitis	Small cell lung cancer, thymoma, breast	Symptoms similar to limbic encephalitis and cerebellar degeneration, sensory deficits, ataxia, bulbar deficits, weakness

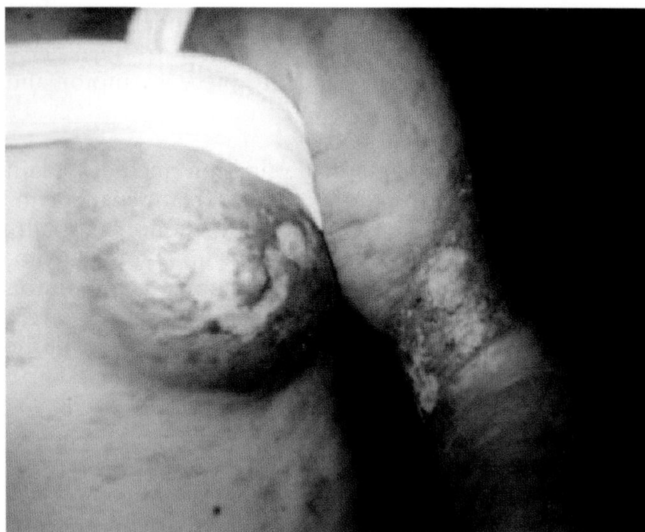

FIGURE 29-1 Skin metastases producing nonhealing wounds in a patient with breast cancer.

and preventive measures to protect the integrity of the skin, affected joints, and genitourinary symptoms are crucial while awaiting stabilization of neurologic deficits. Communication, respiratory, and nutritional issues should be addressed in patients with bulbar involvement.

Skin Metastases

Dermal metastases occur in 5.3% of patients and are most common in breast cancer.[105] Skin metastases can be a source of pain and an entry point for infectious pathogens. Because the associated wounds seldom heal, chronic wound care is necessary and becomes an integral part of patients' rehabilitation needs. Figure 29-1 shows a patient with breast cancer who has dermal metastases involving the breast and proximal arm. Dermal metastases may engender or aggravate lymphedema. Use of compression is limited only by patient tolerance. Malignant wounds should be managed with nonadherent, bacteriostatic, hyperabsorbent dressings (e.g., SilvaSorb or Aquacel Ag). Associated pain must be managed aggressively to minimize adverse functional consequences. Proactive range of motion (ROM) will prevent the formation of contractures in joints adjacent to malignant wounds, facilitating hygiene and autonomous self-care.

Cardiopulmonary Metastases

Lung, pleural, and pericardial metastases involving the heart and lungs can produce dramatic and abrupt reductions in patients' stamina and functional status. Virtually all cancers have the potential to spread to the lungs and pleura. At autopsy, 25% to 30% of all patients with cancer have lung metastases.[47] Pleural metastases occur in 12% of breast and 7% to 15% of lung cancers.[19] Metastases to the heart and pericardium are less common, although their functional impact can be similarly devastating. A series of 4769 autopsies revealed the presence of cardiac metastases in 8.4% of patients with cancer.[191] Melanoma, mesothelioma, lung tumors, and renal neoplasms had the highest prevalence of cardiac spread. The clinical diagnosis of heart or lung metastases can be generally made by CT scans. PET scans and plain x-rays may also be helpful, depending on the clinical context.

Treatment of lung, pleural, pericardial, or cardiac metastases varies considerably. The type and efficacy of anticancer treatment will depend on the primary tumor, number and location of metastases, previous antineoplastic therapies, overall medical condition of the patient, and degree of associated symptomatic distress. Surgical metastasectomy has the potential to definitively eliminate disease in certain patients.[208] Discrete metastases that are not resectable may be amenable to radiation therapy.[162]

Malignant pleural effusions should be evacuated when patients become symptomatic. However, the associated dyspnea often arises from other causes also, and reducing the effusion may fail to alleviate patients' shortness of breath if the lung is trapped because of parenchymal or pleural disease. Reaccumulation of malignant effusions can be managed through intermittent thoracentesis or pleurodesis, or placement of an indwelling pleural catheter.[35] Chemical pleurodesis has an overall complete response rate of 64% when all sclerotic agents are considered.[109] Talc appears the most effective, with a complete response rate of 91%.

The functional relevance of heart and lung metastases stems from their deleterious effect on patients' aerobic capacity. Small reductions in cardiopulmonary reserve can devastate patients who are deconditioned or have other impairments. For this reason, all potentially treatable causes should be definitively addressed. Supplemental oxygen should be initiated as soon as dyspnea becomes function-limiting. In this way, patients can engage in rehabilitation and potentially remain independent and ambulatory. If tolerated, gradual, progressive aerobic conditioning will optimize peripheral conditioning, reducing the percentage of VO_{2max} required for activities. Referral for outpatient aerobic training should be considered when patients with cancer who have cardiopulmonary disease are hospitalized for other problems (e.g., neutropenic fever). These patients are prone to rapid functional decline that usually proves permanent in the absence of structured therapy.

Impairments Caused by Cancer Treatment

Combined Modality Therapy

The push toward organ preservation in primary cancer care has led to widespread use of combined modality therapy. Clinical trials have consistently shown that concurrent or sequential administration of radiation and chemotherapy reduces the extent of tissue resection required to achieve local cancer control without compromising 5-year survival rates. The trend toward use of combined modality therapy is relevant to rehabilitation because most patients with cancer receive some combination of chemotherapy, radiation therapy, or surgery contingent on the type and stage of cancer. This renders patients vulnerable to cumulative normal tissue toxicities associated with each modality.

Surgery-Related Impairments

Primary impairments resulting from surgery depend on the extent, location, and type of tumor. Normal tissue is inevitably affected by surgical efforts to achieve local control of cancer. The principal reasons for resecting normal tissue, with the associated risk of adverse long-term consequences, include accurate staging (e.g., sampling of lymph nodes, and visceral and parietal peritoneum), definitive eradication of tumor, assurance of local disease control (e.g., removal of lymph nodes that might harbor cancer cells), and harvest for reconstructive purposes.

Cancer surgery has the greatest physiatric relevance when certain tissue types are affected. These tissues include bone, nerve, muscle, lung parenchyma, and lymphatics. Normal postoperative healing is often compromised by the previous or coadministration of additional anticancer treatment(s) (e.g., radiation and chemotherapy).

The list of established surgical approaches to eradicate tumors is vast, and readers are referred to *Surgical Oncology: Contemporary Principles and Practice* (edited by Bland) for more precise and extensive procedure-specific discussions. Operations that commonly warrant the attention of a physical medicine specialist include neck dissection for oropharyngeal carcinomas (spinal accessory nerve palsy), limb salvage or amputation for osteosarcoma (impairments vary by site), resection of truncal or limb myosarcoma (weakness, gait dysfunction, biomechanical imbalance), axillary lymph node dissection (shoulder contracture, lymphedema), and pneumonectomy or lobectomy for lung neoplasms (aerobic insufficiency). Procedures such as nephrectomy, colectomy, mastectomy, and oophorectomy may involve the resection of muscles, nerves, or vessels to achieve clean margins resulting in acute functional losses. Review of patients' surgical reports is essential to accurately identify all potential neuromuscular and lymphatic compromise.

Neurosurgical resection of central and peripheral nervous system cancers warrants physiatric evaluation, irrespective of the presence of gross deficits, given the potentially devastating effects of subtle impairments and the high likelihood of future recurrence and progression.

Secondary Impairments

Secondary surgery-associated impairments often emerge well after, presenting as familiar musculoskeletal problems (e.g., tendinopathies and arthropathies). Patients' compensatory attempts to negotiate impairments during mobility and ADL performance may produce maladaptive movement patterns, which may, in turn, engender secondary pain sources and impairments. A common example is myofascial dysfunction of the scapular retractors, middle trapezius, and rhomboid muscles as a result of pectoralis major and minor tightness following mastectomy or chest wall radiation and breast implant insertion. Secondary impairments are fortunately readily reversible through timely physiatric evaluation and treatment.

Donor Site Morbidity

Donor site morbidity associated with surgical tissue harvest for reconstructive purposes produces significant impairments less often than might be anticipated. Muscle, skin, bone, and fat are used to achieve adequate coverage of surgical defects and to optimize cosmesis. Radial forearm and fibular flaps are commonly harvested to eliminate defects produced by mandibular resection. Both are typically well tolerated and seldom produce functional deficits.

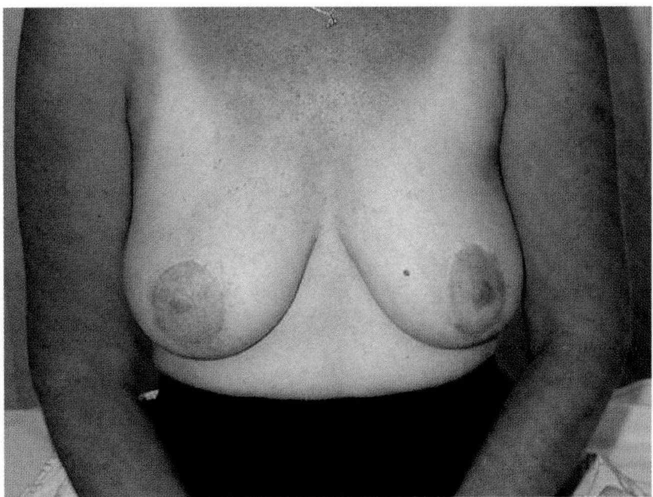

FIGURE 29-2 Excellent cosmesis achieved with bilateral transverse rectus abdominis flap breast reconstructions.

Impairments associated with the harvest of myocutaneous flaps vary by extent and site, and are no different in cancer than in other rehabilitation cohorts. Partial transposition of the pectoralis major muscle from its insertion on the humerus has been used to repair soft tissue defects involving the anterolateral neck. This procedure can destabilize the shoulder in the absence of therapeutic intervention.

By virtue of the high incidence of breast cancer, significant donor site morbidity is most prevalent with autogenous tissue transposition for breast reconstruction. Among women undergoing breast reconstruction in 2008, implants were the most common procedure (60.5%), followed by pedicled flaps (34%) and microsurgical flaps (5.5%).[5] Transverse rectus abdominis muscle (TRAM), gluteus maximus, deep inferior epigastric perforator (DIEP), and latissimus myocutaneous flaps are used, with the former being more common. With a relatively low complication rate (25.3%) and potentially excellent cosmesis (Figure 29-2), the TRAM flap procedure is a common choice, given the potential to create a natural-looking breast with normal ptosis and an inframammary fold. Comparison of functional morbidity following the TRAM and DIEP procedures suggests that they are not markedly different.[40] More patients are electing to undergo immediate breast reconstruction to reduce the risk associated with repeat operations and the psychological distress engendered by mastectomy.

The TRAM procedure involves the transposition of muscle and adipose tissue to match preoperative breast appearance (Figure 29-3). Other advantages of the TRAM procedure include relatively hidden scars and a satisfactory donor site resulting in a flat abdomen. The TRAM flap can be divided into the pedicled or free flap procedures.

These procedures differ in that the pedicled, or conventional, procedure uses the epigastric vessels supplying the rectus muscle to perfuse the subumbilical fat. Subumbilical adipose tissue is tunneled under the abdominal skin to repair the defect created by mastectomy. The inferior end of the contralateral rectus abdominis muscle is tunneled with the fat (see Figure 29-3). In contrast, the free flap procedure involves the creation of anastomoses with

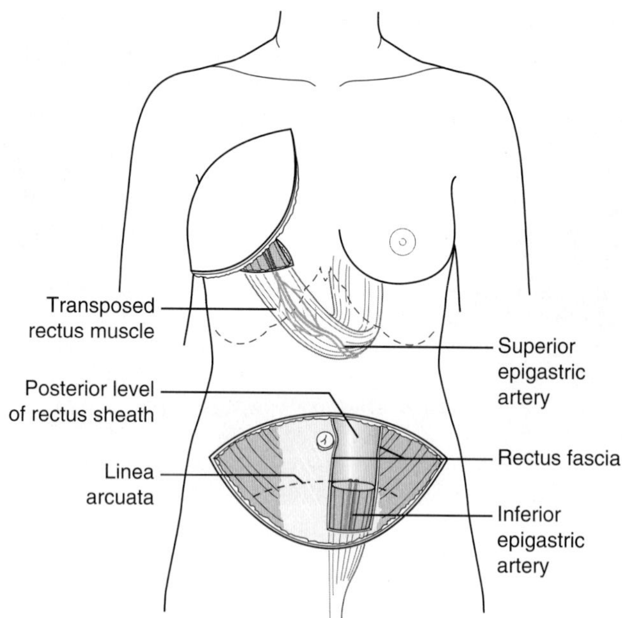

FIGURE 29-3 The transverse rectus abdominis flap procedure uses the superior epigastric artery to supply blood to the subumbilical fat, which is used to reconstruct the mastectomized breast. The fat and inferior ends of the rectus muscle are tunneled under the abdominal wall into the defect caused by mastectomy.

vessels in the chest such as the thoracodorsal or internal mammary arteries. Although the free flap procedure requires increased operative time, it is associated with decreased incidence of partial flap loss resulting from fat necrosis.[9]

Despite declining perioperative complication rates, the adverse musculoskeletal sequelae of TRAM flap breast reconstruction can be significant.[147] Donor site complications include abdominal wall bulge (2.9% to 3.8%), abdominal hernia (2.6% to 2.9%), and dehiscence (3.8%).[39,107] Patients experience abdominal weakness and reduced exertional tolerance, particularly those undergoing bilateral procedures.[143] Because the TRAM procedure produces a defect in the abdominal wall, patients have difficulty stabilizing the trunk while transferring from supine and seated positions. Partial denervation of the abdominal wall also leads to deficits in proprioception and truncal balance. Weakness of the abdominal wall can lead to exaggerated lumbar lordosis and an increased incidence of back pain. An algorithm for treatment of patients post–TRAM flap is presented later in this chapter under "Rehabilitation of Specific Cancer Populations."

Radiation Therapy–Related Impairments

Radiation therapy has become an integral part of combined modality and organ preservation therapy for many cancers. Approximately 50% of patients with cancer undergo radiation therapy during the course of their disease. Although highly effective in eliminating radiosensitive tumors, controlling regional disease, and palliating symptomatic metastases, radiation therapy also injures normal tissue. The tolerance of normal tissues surrounding tumors is the most important radiation dose-limiting consideration.[78] Radiation injury is multiphasic, characterized by discrete acute and late phases mediated by distinct pathophysiologic processes. Acute injury is predominantly caused by inflammation and the death of rapidly proliferating cell types. Cell death occurs through the induction of apoptosis and free radical–mediated DNA damage. Patients may develop desquamation of the dermis and mucous membranes, visceral inflammation (e.g., colitis, cystitis, and enteritis), and muscle hypertonicity, among other symptoms. Biological response modifiers released from injured tumor cells are thought to mediate systemic radiation effects such as fatigue and malaise.[115] The time course of acute radiation effects on normal tissue varies significantly by tissue type and radiation dose. Most patients return to their preradiation baseline by the second month after treatment. However, the distribution is highly skewed and some patients remain symptomatic as many as 12 months after treatment.

The deleterious effects of late radiation injury are attributable to tissue necrosis and fibrosis. The mechanisms underlying these end processes continue to be actively investigated. Microvascular injury predisposes to thrombus formation and produces a hypoxic interstitial environment.[60] Hypoxia is believed to favor the generation of free radical species that produce further damage and, ultimately, a self-perpetuating cycle of tissue injury and fibrosis.[216] In addition to compression from fibrosis, neural and microvascular injury may occur from occlusion of the vasa nervorum, vasorum, and lymphorum with resultant infarction.

The adverse late effects of radiation therapy depend on the extent and location of the radiation field. Identifying the tattoos placed during radiation therapy simulation can help delineate the irradiated tissue. Table 29-5 lists conditions caused by delayed radiation toxicity by system. Figure 29-4 illustrates the progressive stages and presumed pathophysiologic features of radiation-induced fibrosis. Late radiation effects most relevant to rehabilitation medicine include those involving connective tissue, muscles, and nerves. Fibrosis occurs to some degree in all muscles and connective tissue within a radiation portal. In the absence of ongoing ROM, patients may develop contractures. Because late radiation injury is an ongoing and potentially self-perpetuating process, ranging of affected muscles and fascia should continue indefinitely.

The most devastating neural effects of radiation therapy include myelopathy, plexopathy, and encephalopathy. Delayed radiation myelopathy produces symptoms 12 to 50 months after radiation therapy, and progresses over weeks or months to paraparesis or quadriparesis. The delivery of radiation in a greater number of small fractions, or "hyperfractionation," has significantly reduced the incidence of myelopathy. With conventional fractionation of 1.8 to 2 Gy per fraction to the full-thickness cord, the estimated risk of myelopathy is less than 1% and less than 10% at 54 Gy and 61 Gy, respectively, with a calculated strong dependence on dose/fraction.[98] The presenting symptom is usually a Brown-Séquard syndrome, which begins distally and ascends to reach the irradiated level of the cord.[166] MRI is useful in distinguishing radiation from malignant myelopathy. Hyperbaric oxygen may offer benefit if initiated soon after the onset of weakness; however, this remains controversial.

Radiation-induced brachial plexopathies is best characterized with incidences, in accordance with the irradiation technique, ranging from 66% for radiation-induced brachial plexopathies with 60 Gy in 5 Gy fractions in the 1960s to less than 1% with 50 Gy in 2 Gy fractions today.[52,170] Risk is dose-related and seems to increase with radiation therapy exposure greater than 5000 cGy.[97] Radiation therapy–induced brachial plexopathies develop between 3 months and 14 years (median 1.5 years) after therapy.[104] Lumbosacral plexopathies generally develop 1 to 5 years following radiation therapy. A recent cohort study reported an 8% incidence of radiation-induced plexopathy among patients treated with contoured radiation fields for cervical cancer.[212] Mean total radiation dose was significantly associated with the development of plexopathy. Characteristics of radiation therapy plexopathies that distinguish them from malignant plexopathies include lower incidence of pain, pain that develops after weakness, upper trunk involvement, and the presence of myokymia on electromyography.

Table 29-5 Conditions Caused by Delayed Radiation Toxicity

System	Adverse Late Effects
Endocrine	Hypothyroidism, hypogonadism, adrenal insufficiency, glucose intolerance caused by pancreatic insufficiency
Exocrine	Xerostomia, pancreatic enzyme deficiency
Neural	Myelopathy, plexopathy, cerebrovascular ischemia, dementia, leukoencephalopathy, cranial neuropathy
Lymphatic	Lymph node necrosis, lymphedema
Gastrointestinal	Dysmotility, malabsorption, neuroconstipation, obstruction, perforation, dysgeusia
Dermis	Atrophy, ulceration, delayed healing, hyperpigmentation
Auditory	Progressive loss of acuity, tinnitus
Vascular	Premature atherosclerosis, venous sclerosis
Pulmonary or upper respiratory	Parenchymal fibrosis tracheal stenosis, dysphonia secondary to laryngeal fibrosis
Musculoskeletal	Fibrosis, osteonecrosis, osteoporosis, soft tissue necrosis joint contracture, epimysial fibrosis
Ocular	Corneal ulceration, retinopathy, scleral necrosis
Genitourinary	Neurogenic bladder, renal failure, obstruction, perforation

Delayed radiation therapy encephalopathy resulting from necrosis of brain parenchyma occurs in 3% to 5% of patients receiving greater than 5000 cGy, and in 5% to 15% of patients receiving 6000 cGy.[128] Symptoms generally develop 2 years after completion of radiation therapy. The clinical presentation often resembles that of the primary malignancy, raising the question of local recurrence. PET scanning is of greater use in distinguishing tumor from radiation necrosis than either MRI or CT because radiation necrosis is hypometabolic.

Cerebral atrophy occurs more commonly than radiation therapy necrosis, being present invariably after whole brain radiation therapy of 3000 cGy in 10 fractions.[166] Patients manifest slowness of executive functions and profound alterations of frontal functions, such as attention focusing, mentation control, analogical judgment and insight, similar to those obtained by patients suffering from subcortical vascular dementia.[148] Virtually all patients complain of memory loss, which can be sufficiently severe to

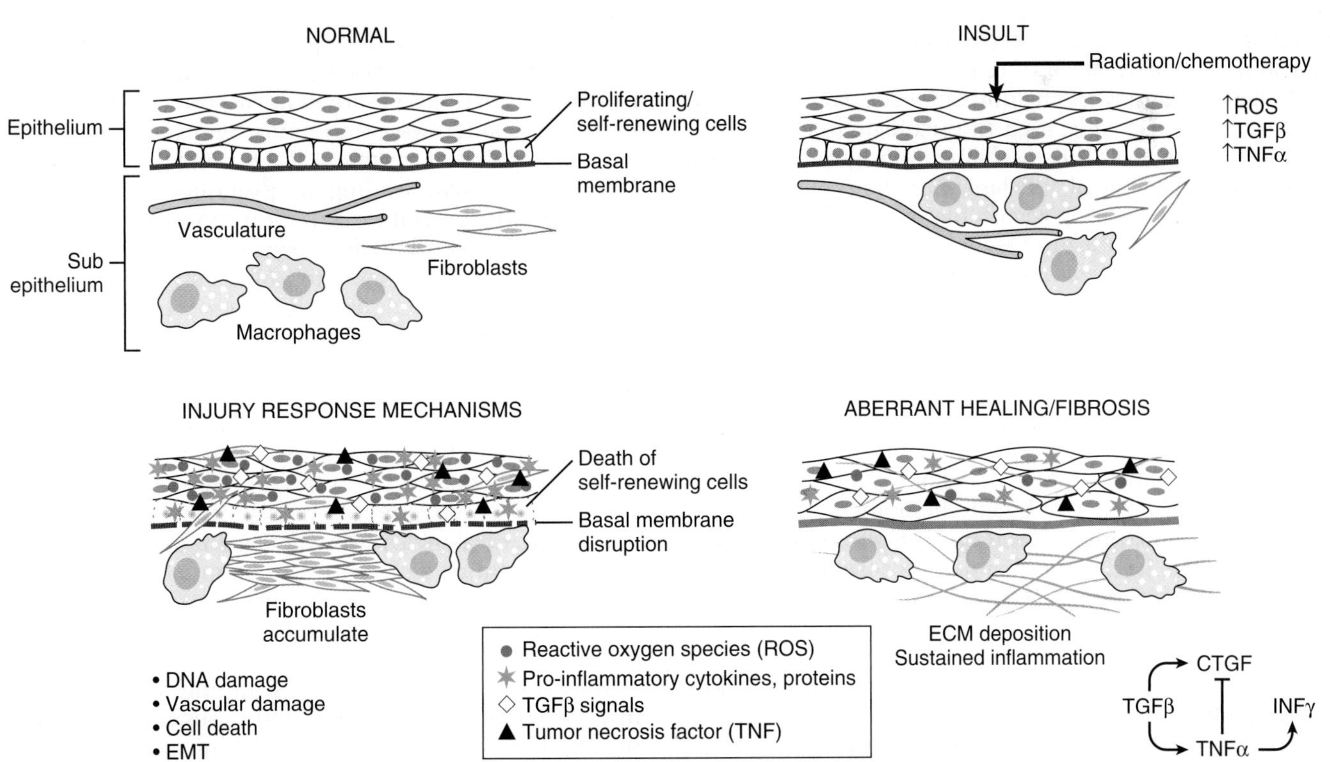

FIGURE 29-4 Sequential pathogenesis of radiation fibrosis. *CTGF*, Connective tissue growth factor; *ECM*, extracellular matrix; *EMT*, epithelial to mesenchymal transition; *INFγ*, interferon gamma; *ROS*, reactive oxygen species; *TGFα*, transforming growth factor alpha; *TGFβ*, transforming growth factor beta; *TNF*, tumor necrosis factor.

compromise vocational viability.[33] Memory loss progresses in 10% to 20% of patients to involve other cognitive domains, potentially leading to dementia.[49] Patients can also develop gait abnormalities and urinary urgency.[49]

Medical treatment of radiation therapy–associated neural compromise can include short-term steroids, anticoagulation, or hyperbaric oxygen therapy.[171] Focal radiation necrosis of brain parenchyma can require surgical resection. Increasing use of bevacizumab to reverse radiation fibrosis is based on anecdotal successes and a tenuous but growing evidence base.[119,210] Pentoxifylline, coadministered with tocopherol, attenuates radiation fibrosis.[125] The benefits of pentoxifylline have yet to be assessed in radiation therapy–related neural compromise.

Chemotherapy

Chemotherapy represents a mainstay of anticancer therapy. Chemotherapy drugs are used for different purposes and with varying efficacy in the management of cancer. Chemotherapy is used for the following four general purposes:

1. As induction therapy for advanced disease
2. As an adjunct to the treatment of localized tumor
3. As the primary treatment of localized cancer (often to reduce tumor size in preparation for surgery)
4. By direct installation into sanctuaries or site-directed perfusion of specific body regions affected by the cancer

Induction chemotherapy is administered to patients with advanced disease for which no other treatment exists. Adjuvant chemotherapy is administered after local control is achieved through surgery or radiation when no obvious tumor is present to eliminate undetectable micrometastases and reduce the risk of recurrence. Neoadjuvant therapy can be used before surgery to reduce tumor size and thereby minimize the degree of anatomic disruption. Chemotherapy is increasingly being used serially to temporize the spread of incurable, stage IV cancer.

A staggering array of chemotherapeutic agents, or antineoplastics, is currently used in oncologic practice. Antineoplastic drugs can be mechanistically grouped into a manageable number of subclasses for the nononcologist, which include alkylating agents, platins and their analogs, antimetabolites, topoisomerase interactive agents, antimicrotubule agents, differentiation agents, and miscellaneous agents. Table 29-6 lists antineoplastic drugs by class.

The type, dose, and duration of chemotherapy vary across different cancer types and stages. However, common overarching strategies apply. To exploit complementary mechanisms of action, achieve synergy, and reduce normal tissue toxicity, chemotherapeutic agents from different classes are generally coadministered or sequentially administered. Standardized combined chemotherapy regimens have given rise to a host of acronyms. Common examples include CHOP (cyclophosphamide, doxorubicin, vincristine, and prednisone), ICE (ifosfamide, carboplatin, and etoposide), and MOPP (mechlorethamine, vincristine, procarbazine, and prednisone); there are many others. It is currently rare for a single chemotherapeutic to be administered as monotherapy.

Antineoplastics are distinguished by their capacity to preferentially injure rapidly dividing cancer cells while sparing normal cells. However, all are associated with significant potential for normal tissue toxicity. The chemotherapeutic toxicities that most commonly produce functional impairments are peripheral neuropathy, cognitive dysfunction, cardiomyopathy, and pulmonary fibrosis. Fortunately, with proactive screening, the incidence of significant cardiopulmonary toxicity has been substantially reduced. Bleomycin induces acute pneumonitis. Risk factors include the cumulative dose of bleomycin, the patient's age, smoking, renal dysfunction, mediastinal radiation therapy, and administration of oxygen.[27] The incidence of bleomycin-induced pneumonitis ranges from 0% to 46%, depending on the patient population being studied and the criteria used to diagnose this entity. The risk of doxorubicin-associated cardiac toxicity directly parallels increases in cumulative dose. With cumulative doses of 550, 600, and 700 mg/m^2, the incidence is 7%, 15%, and 30%, respectively.[82] Cardiomyopathy becomes a real concern for many patients with stage IV breast cancer who resume doxorubicin treatment after having received it in the context of primary adjuvant therapy. Trastuzumab produces cardiac toxicity in 3% to 5% of patients receiving monotherapy and in 28% of patients who concurrently receive anthracyclines.[100]

Chemotherapeutic neuropathy is a prevalent and functionally morbid complication of cancer treatment. The vinca alkaloids, cisplatin, ixabepilone, the taxanes, and thalidomide are among the most important drugs inducing peripheral neurotoxicity.[192] These drugs are widely used for various malignancies, such as ovarian and breast cancer, and hematologic cancers. Chemotherapeutic neuropathy is related to cumulative dose or dose intensity.[26] Patients who already have neuropathic symptoms resulting from diabetes mellitus, hereditary neuropathies, or earlier treatment with neurotoxic chemotherapy are believed to be at higher risk.

All platin compounds (e.g., cisplatin, carboplatin, and oxaliplatin) have the potential to produce sensory neuropathy. Cisplatin is a more frequent source of neurotoxicity than the latter two compounds. Symptoms often occur after completion of treatment. Large sensory fibers are preferentially affected, leading to proprioceptive deficits.[192] Pinprick and temperature sensation, as well as motor function, are relatively spared.[26] Lower extremity deep tendon reflexes often disappear. Autonomic nerves remain unaffected. Nerve conduction studies show decreased sensory nerve action potentials and prolonged sensory distal latencies, whereas nerve conduction velocities are minimally impaired.[192]

Peripheral neuropathy related to vinca alkaloid treatment is observed most commonly with vincristine. Paresthesias in the distal extremities are the initial symptoms, and loss of lower extremity muscle stretch reflexes is the initial sign. Weakness of the wrist and digital extensors can occur. Autonomic neuropathy is common and might lead to paralytic ileus, orthostatic hypotension, and impotence.[192] Vibration sense generally remains intact.[26] Nerve conduction studies show decreased distal motor and sensory nerve action potentials, with only slight reduction in nerve conduction velocities, indicating an axonal rather than a demyelinating mechanism of injury.

Taxanes have become first-line therapy in the treatment of primary breast, ovarian, and lung cancers. Docetaxel

Table 29-6 Classes of Antineoplastic Drugs

Class	Mechanism(s)	Commonly Used Agents*	Toxicities
Antitumor	Formation of covalent bonds of alkyl groups to DNA to form reactive intermediates that attack nucleophilic sites; the DNA can no longer function as a template	Mustards: chlorambucil, cyclophosphamide, ifosfamide, alkylating agents Nitrosoureas: carmustine Tetrazines: dacarbazine Aziridines: mitomycin C, thiotepa Nonclassic alkylating agents: procarbazine	Myelosuppression (all), mucositis (busulfan), hepatotoxicity (busulfan, busulfan carmustine, dacarbazine), pulmonary fibrosis (busulfan, carmustine), cystitis (ifosfamide, cyclophosphamide), alopecia (cyclophosphamide), venoocclusive liver disease (busulfan, carmustine, mitomycin C)
Platins and their analogs	Platination of DNA with induction of apoptosis or arrest of cells in the G2 phase of the cell cycle; disruption of intracellular signaling pathways	Cisplatin, carboplatin, oxaliplatin	Nephrotoxicity, ototoxicity, neuropathy, myelosuppression
Antimetabolites	Interference with synthesis of DNA and RNA precursor molecules or DNA polymerase, thereby preventing DNA and RNA replication	Antifolates: methotrexate Fluoropyrimidines: 5-fluorouracil Pyrimidine analogs: azacitidine Gemcitabine 6-thiopurines: 6-mercaptopurine, 6-thioguanine *Streptomyces parvulus* derivatives: actinomycin D	Myelosuppression (all), gastrointestinal mucositis (all), hepatotoxicity Arabinose nucleosides: cytarabine (methotrexate, arabinose nucleosides, azacitidine, gemcitabine 6-thiopurines) Nephrotoxicity (methotrexate) Neurotoxicity (methotrexate, arabinose nucleosides, azacitidine, 6-s)
Topoisomerase-gastrointestinal interactive agents cardiotoxicity	Interaction with DNA topoisomerases (enzymes regulating DNA packing, i.e., twisting and untwisting), leading to G2 phase arrest or apoptosis in S phase	Epipodophyllotoxins: etoposide Anthracyclines: doxorubicin, daunorubicin, epirubicin, idarubicin Camptothecin analogs: topotecan, irinotecan	Myelosuppression (all), mucositis (all), anthracyclines: doxorubicin (anthracyclines), soft tissue ulceration postextravasation (anthracyclines)
Antimicrotubule agents	Disruption of microtubules that compose the mitotic spindle	Vinca alkaloids: vincristine, vinblastine, vinorelbine Taxanes: paclitaxel, docetaxel Miscellaneous antimicrotubule agents: estramustine	Peripheral neurotoxicity (vinca alkaloids, taxanes), gastrointestinal autonomic dysfunction (vinca alkaloids), neutropenia (vinca alkaloids), myelosuppression (taxanes), myalgias (taxanes), bradydysrhythmias (paclitaxel), fluid retention (docetaxel), skin toxicity (docetaxel), emesis (estramustine), congestive heart failure (estramustine)
Miscellaneous chemotherapeutic agents	Fludarabine: inhibits enzymes l-Asparaginase: exploits the inability of tumor cells to synthesize asparagine, limiting protein synthesis Bleomycin: free radical production of DNA breaks	Fludarabine, l-asparaginase, essential for DNA synthesis and repair	Myelosuppression (fludarabine), bleomycin immunosuppression (fludarabine), neurotoxicity (fludarabine), hypersensitivity reactions (l-asparaginase), pulmonary fibrosis (bleomycin), mucocutaneous toxicities (bleomycin)

*Lists are not exhaustive.

is a more frequent and severe source of neuropathy. Signs and symptoms that characterize taxane neuropathy include paresthesias, loss of muscle stretch reflexes, and diminished vibration sense.[168] Patients can develop mild proximal muscle weakness that resolves spontaneously.[66] Autonomic neuropathy occurs uncommonly. Nerve conduction studies show reduction of sensory nerve action potentials in patients treated with taxanes. Reduced motor nerve action potentials and diminished sensory and motor nerve conduction velocity have been reported.

Increasingly, targeted biopharmaceuticals displace established treatment standards. These include monoclonal antibodies to epidermal growth factor receptors (pertuzumab), small molecule tyrosine kinase inhibitors that target the various epidermal growth factor receptors (gefitinib, erlotinib), monoclonal antibodies directed at the vascular endothelial growth factor (bevacizumab), and the small tyrosine kinase inhibitors that target the vascular endothelial growth factor receptor.[25] The risk profiles of many of these agents remain inadequately characterized, particularly when administered to elderly and infirm patients who differ considerably from the cohorts studied in trials. Thromboembolic events are a concerning risk for patients receiving therapies targeting the vascular endothelial growth factor receptor.[73]

Rehabilitation Approaches

General Strategies

Rehabilitation of Bone Metastases

Strategies to rehabilitate patients with bone metastases and pathologic fractures remain largely theoretical because of a lack of empirical data. An overarching mandate is the need to coordinate therapeutic efforts with orthopedist oncologists, radiation oncologists, and medical oncologists. Bone metastases occur in complex, highly individual, and dynamic settings. Developing an integrated cross-disciplinary, long-term management plan offers patients the best chance of preserved comfort and function. Physiatric approaches can be grouped into the use of orthoses, assistive devices, therapeutic exercise, and environmental modification. All essentially deweight or immobilize compromised bones. Orthoses can be fabricated to stabilize bones in positions that limit potentially damaging forces. A common example is the use of thoracolumbosacral or spinal extension orthoses, such as cruciform anterior spinal hyperextension or Jewett braces. These orthoses limit spinal flexion, thereby reducing loads on the anterior vertebrae to protect against compression fractures. Orthoses can also be used to protect and deweight sites of fracture or impending fracture. Thermoplast arm troughs allow patients with humeral metastases to immobilize the affected extremity and reduce damaging forces. Extreme caution must be used in patients with diffuse bone metastases while redistributing weight and loading patterns. Careful radiologic evaluation of the bones to be loaded reduces the likelihood of complications. Bone metastases are rarely discrete. It can be challenging in widespread osseous disease to find sufficiently intact bone to unload weight-bearing structures.

Assistive devices and instruction in compensatory strategies may similarly unload compromised bones. Canes, crutches, and walkers are frequently used to minimize fracture risk. Identical caveats regarding the need to evaluate skeletal structures that will receive additional load via the assistive devices apply. Patients should be instructed to minimize forces by performing activities close to the body, thereby limiting torque on long bones.

Although theoretically appealing, evidence is lacking for the use of therapeutic exercise in the prevention of pathologic fractures. Nonetheless, patients at risk for vertebral fractures routinely tolerate exercise programs designed to strengthen the abdominal and spinal extensor muscles and to enhance their awareness of body positioning. A comprehensive exercise program should include postural and balance training as well as truncal strengthening. Simple environmental modifications may significantly reduce patients' fracture risk. Throw rugs and other hazards that increase fall risk should be removed. Railings can be added to stairwells and bathrooms as appropriate. Patients' prognoses should inform the decision to implement such modifications.

Exercise

Aerobic Conditioning and Resistive Exercise. Trials of aerobic conditioning in cancer populations have been conducted to determine whether exercise attenuates treatment-associated fatigue and enhances quality of life. Patients with breast cancer receiving adjuvant chemotherapy have comprised the majority of study cohorts, although Dimeo et al.[54-56] have contributed significantly to the literature with studies of aerobic conditioning immediately following bone marrow transplantation. Recently, exercise trials have been conducted in increasingly diverse cancer cohorts, including patients with advanced stage cancer.

Studies in breast and other cancer populations receiving treatment or after cancer treatment have consistently noted improved symptom burden: fatigue,[144,145,185-187] insomnia,[144] nausea,[221] and emotional distress.[144,145] Trials have varied considerably in the intensity, frequency, and duration of aerobic training, the targeted interval in cancer treatment (active, posttreatment, etc.), as well as in the level of investigator supervision.[183,193] Self-paced exercise regimens have reliably achieved modest improvements in 12-minute walk time.[144,185-187] Use of more rigorous, structured programs (more than three exercise sessions per week at 60% to 90% of maximum heart rate) increase relative lean body mass[221] and VO_{2max}.[79,88,124,155] Protocols involving less intense exercise (e.g., five times per week at 50% to 60% of VO_{2max}) have not consistently achieved statistically significant improvements in oxidative capacity (VO_{2max}),[188] suggesting a potential exertional threshold below which physiologic benefits are limited, but this remains speculative. The literature suggests that at virtually all points along the cancer trajectory, patients benefit from incremental aerobic exercise and that exercise intensities as high as 90% of maximum heart rate three times weekly may be safely tolerated. Increasingly, metaanalyses and systematic reviews replicate trial results, finding that varied types of exercise (e.g., aerobic conditioning and strengthening) positively affect diverse outcomes (e.g., fatigue,[135,158,209] quality of life,[142] and limb impairment[51]).

Aerobic conditioning alone reduces symptom burden and mitigates the physiologic impact of high-dose chemotherapy delivered in the context of bone marrow transplantation as well. Performance of cardiovascular cycling at 50% of heart rate reserve reduced participants' decline in physical performance (e.g., walking distance and speed), physiologic variables, neutropenia and thrombocytopenia, and psychological distress relative to those of controls.[54,56]

Initially, programs combining resistance training with aerobic conditioning yielded inconsistent improvement in overall quality of life, with some studies failing to note change[1,43,188] and others noting improvement.[103,189] However, recent, randomized, and adequately powered trials have consistently demonstrated marked improvements in fatigue, physical functioning, and mental health.[2,67,80,81] No study has reported compromised quality of life associated with participation in exercise programs, irrespective of their intensity. Of note, integrated physical training approaches appear to be superior to psychocognitive approaches in enhancing physical well-being and quality of life.[130]

Limited trials have evaluated the impact of resistance training in cancer populations.[45] Definitive improvement was reported with resistance training among patients with prostate cancer receiving androgen deprivation therapy,[157] as well as survivors of breast cancer[4,182] and head and neck cancer.[133] A single trial that compared resistance and aerobic training found both to be effective, but the former afforded longer-term improvements.[190] Several studies suggest that resistance training may be an effective means to reduce bone loss in postmenopausal survivors of breast cancer.[213,217] The exercise interventions were well tolerated without adverse effects in both resistance trials.

The number of trials evaluating exercise interventions in cancer populations has burgeoned in recent years. Trials have consistently demonstrated that exercise is safe, but not always effective, contingent on study end points. A comprehensive summary is well beyond the scope of this chapter. Interested readers are referred to multiple excellent and recently published systematic reviews.*

Rehabilitation of Cardiopulmonary Dysfunction. Exertional intolerance resulting from cardiopulmonary factors occurs commonly among patients with cancer. Surgical pneumonectomy or lobectomy, the current standard of care for management of local and regional lung cancer, abruptly reduces patients' aerobic capacity. Fibrosis of lung parenchyma, visceral pleura, and pericardium develops following radiation to the thorax. Review of patients' radiation treatment records can be invaluable in gauging their risk of cardiopulmonary fibrosis. Many patients requiring treatment for intrathoracic tumor have smoking histories and some degree of premorbid subclinical chronic obstructive pulmonary or reactive airway disease.[204] As a consequence, resection or irradiation of lung tissue can result in far greater dyspnea and functional compromise than anticipated. Chemotherapy and intrathoracic metastases can also produce cardiopulmonary dysfunction.

Rehabilitation of cardiopulmonary dysfunction in patients with cancer uses protocols well established in cardiac and pulmonary rehabilitation. Incremental aerobic conditioning with supplemental oxygen, as needed, usually produces a reduction in exertional intolerance. Similar to both cardiac and pulmonary rehabilitation, aerobic conditioning has limited beneficial impact on heart or lung physiology. Improvements in stamina and perceived exertion are attributable to muscle-training effects.

Flexibility Exercises. Activities to enhance ROM are crucial for rehabilitation of postsurgical and postradiation soft tissue contractures. The rationale for active and passive stretching is empirical. There is anecdotal evidence that stretching may prevent, reduce, and reverse radiation-induced contractures. Interventions to enhance flexibility are integral to the rehabilitation of other conditions associated with progressive fibrosis such as burns. Flexibility activities should be optimally tailored to the radiation port and irradiated muscles. For example, tangent beams for conventional breast irradiation encompass the pectoralis major and minor muscles (Figure 29-5). Contingent on the orientation of the posterior tangent, the serratus anterior and latissimus muscle can also be affected. Patients should be examined for secondary myofascial dysfunction, tightness in muscles outside the radiation field, and biomechanical imbalance. A single report describes the successful treatment of refractory radiation-induced contractures with botulinum toxin injections.[199]

Patients who receive radiation for intrapelvic cancers (e.g., bladder, prostate, colorectal, cervical, or uterine malignancies) often develop restricted flexibility of the muscles acting on the hip joint. Because they gradually adapt their gait and movement patterns to accommodate decreased muscle excursion, problems can arise latently as

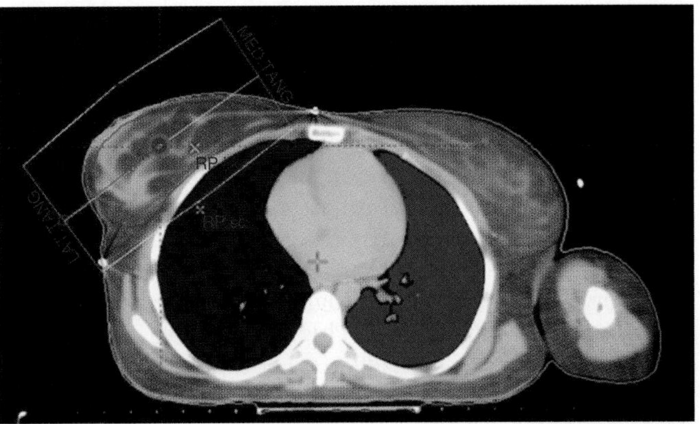

FIGURE 29-5 Conventional beams for breast irradiation that encompass the pectoral muscles.

sacroiliac or lumbar pain. Full reversal and prevention of recurrence requires that all flexibility deficits be identified and addressed.

Comprehensive Inpatient Rehabilitation

The appropriateness and potential benefits of comprehensive inpatient rehabilitation must be assessed on a case-by-case basis. The candidacy of patients with cancer is generally deemed appropriate when their deficits conform to a neurologic or musculoskeletal syndrome familiar in the inpatient rehabilitation setting—that is, hemiparesis, paraplegia, or amputation. Several studies have reported equal FIM efficacies when patients with malignant SCC are compared with patients with similar but traumatically and ischemically induced impairments. Patients with malignant SCC achieve less functional improvement but, owing to shorter lengths of stay, have comparable FIM efficiencies relative to patients with traumatic spinal cord injury.[132] Home discharge rates are equal, 84% in a retrospective case series,[131] or higher among patients with malignant SCC.

Retrospective case series of patients transferred to rehabilitation following treatment for primary brain tumors and intracranial metastases describe substantial gains in cognitive ADL and mobility domains.[87,127] The functional gains achieved by patients with brain tumors are similar to those of patients with acute stroke[85] and traumatic brain injury.[86,154] Patients with brain tumors are consistently discharged to the community more than 80% of the time,[86] and have significantly shorter lengths of stay.[85,154] Studies have differed on the impact of concurrent radiation therapy. Some describe greater FIM mobility efficiencies with radiation, whereas others report the opposite.[154]

A recent comparison of patients admitted for inpatient rehabilitation with wide-ranging cancer-related impairments noted no significant differences in FIM efficiencies or length of stay relative to noncancer patients, suggesting that inpatient admissions should be considered for patients with cancer whose debilities arise from impairments other that intracranial or epidural metastases.[206] That said, approximately 31% of patients with cancer admitted for acute inpatient rehabilitation undergo unplanned transfer back to acute care units, with predictors for transfer being low albumin, elevated creatinine, and a requirement for tube feeding or a Foley catheter.[74]

*References 19, 34, 44, 50, 89, 99, 101, 108, 122, 133, 146, 183, 194, 207.

Lymphedema Management

Lymphedema is a chronic and currently incurable condition that frequently complicates cancer therapy. Following resection or irradiation of lymph nodes and vessels, lymphatic congestion can develop in any region of the body drained by the affected lymphatics. If congestion becomes sufficiently severe, swelling can result from accumulation of protein-rich fluid.[220] Far from being a treatment-refractory and inexorably progressive condition, lymphedema is now amenable to highly effective and widely available therapy. Complete (or complex) decongestive therapy (CDT) represents the current international standard of care for lymphedema management.[15] This was formalized in a white paper published by the International Society of Lymphology in 2001.[15] CDT, an intensive integration of manual approaches, is able to achieve and maintain substantial volume reduction for the majority of patients with lymphedema. Surgical, dietary, and pharmacologic approaches offer equivocal benefit at best, but can be considered when appropriate manual and compression therapy fail to adequately reduce lymphedema.[203]

CDT is a two-phase, multimodal system that incorporates manual lymphatic drainage (MLD), short-stretch compressive bandaging, skin care, therapeutic exercise, and elastic compression garments. The initial phase, sometimes designated with a Roman numeral I or described by the term reductive, has as its primary goal decreasing lymphedema volume.[63] During daily phase I CDT sessions, patients receive approximately 45 minutes of MLD, followed by the application of compression bandages and performance of remedial exercises. Compressive bandages are left in place 21 to 24 hr/day. The efficacy of treatment delivered at this intensity has been demonstrated in numerous case series.[62,102,149] Figure 29-6 shows pre-CDT and post-CDT images in a patient with bilateral stage 3 lymphedema. Following maximum volume reduction, patients are gradually transitioned to a long-term maintenance program (phase II). In this phase, compressive garments are used during the day, with application of compressive bandages overnight. Patients perform remedial exercises on a daily basis while bandaged and receive MLD as needed.

Compression forms the basis of virtually all successful lymphedema therapy. During both CDT phases I (day and night) and II (nighttime only), compression is achieved through the use of short-stretch bandages. Short-stretch bandages have a high working pressure by virtue of contractions in the underlying muscles.[159,160,197] The bandages exert low pressure while the muscles are resting. A distal to proximal compression gradient is achieved by applying more layers of bandages distally, rather than varying the amount of tension used to apply the bandages. Compression garments are added to patients' phase II regimens for daytime compression. Compression garments achieve the following:

- Improve lymphatic flow and reduce accumulated protein
- Improve venous return
- Properly shape and reduce the size of the limb
- Maintain skin integrity
- Protect the limb from potential trauma[30]

MLD or "lymphatic massage" is a highly specialized technique designed to enhance the sequestration and transport of lymph. Specific stroke duration, orientation, pressure, and sequence characterize MLD. MLD stimulates the intrinsic contractility of the lymph vessels, leading to increased sequestration and transform of macromolecules in the interstitium.[29] Through gentle and rhythmic skin distention, congested lymph is directed through residual lymph vessels into intact lymph node beds. MLD permits shifting of congested lymph to lymphotomes (anatomic regions drained by a specific lymph node bed with preserved drainage, as illustrated in Figure 29-7). The massage is very light and superficial, limited to finger or hand pressures of approximately 30 to 45 mm Hg. MLD treatments are initiated proximally in lymphostatic regions adjacent to functioning lymphotomes. Lymph is constantly directed

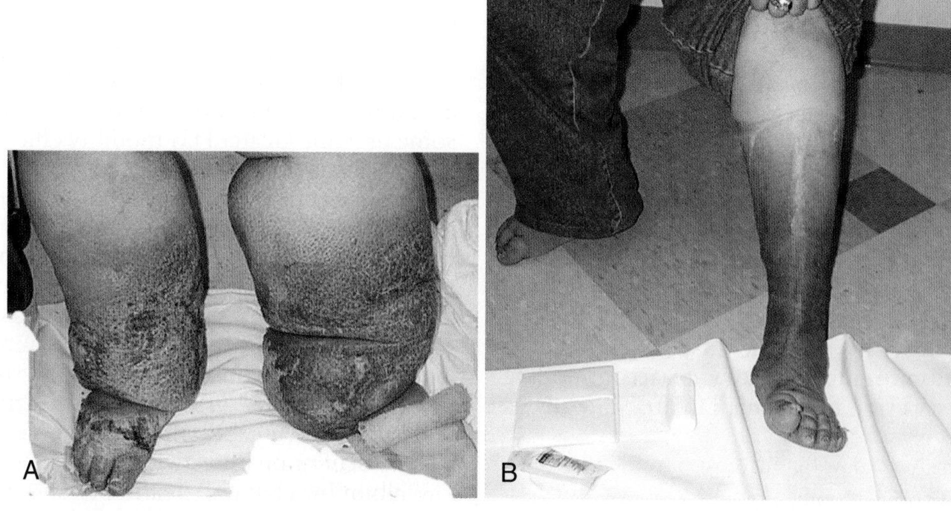

FIGURE 29-6 Lower extremity lymphedema **(A)** before and **(B)** after complete decongestive therapy, which afforded dramatic volume reduction.

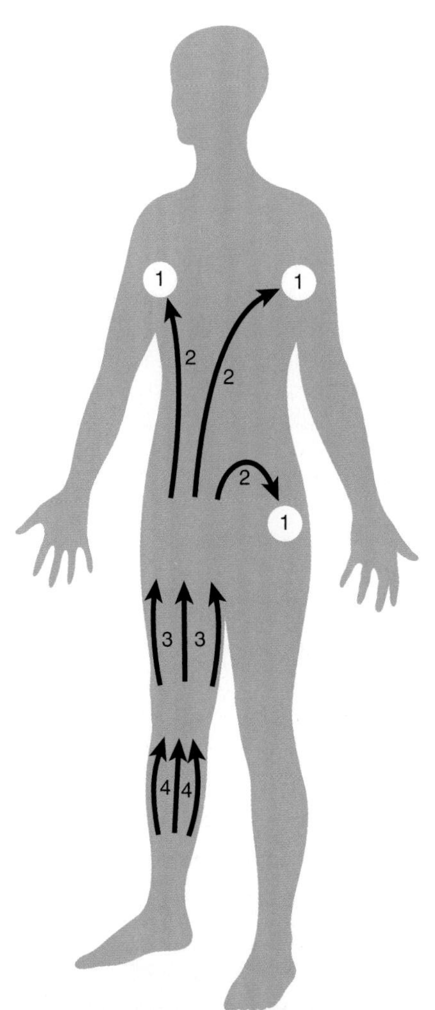

FIGURE 29-7 Manual lymphatic drainage sequence in the treatment of right lower limb lymphedema resulting from inguinal lymph node dissection: *1*, stimulate intact lymph node beds where the stagnant lymph will be directed; *2*, clear the pathways that will be used to redirect stagnant lymph into functioning lymphotomes; *3*, direct stagnant lymph proximally along the cleared pathways, working backward into the congested territory; *4*, complete treatment with proximal redirection of lymph from the most distal portions of the lymphedematous territory.

toward functional lymphotomes and lymph node beds with strategic hand movement. Treatments gradually progress distally to terminate in the regions farthest removed from intact lymphatics.

Remedial lymphedema exercises refer to repetitive movements designed to encourage rhythmic, serial muscle contractions in lymphedematous territories. Remedial exercises are always performed with external compression, most commonly compressive garments or bandages. Remedial exercises repeatedly compress the lymph vessels through sequential muscle contraction and relaxation, thereby triggering smooth muscle contraction in lymph vessel walls.[156] An internal pumping mechanism is established that encourages congested lymph to flow along the compression gradient created with bandages or garments.[113,114] Progressive strength training when supervised and gradually progressed reduced lymphedema flares in a large, randomized controlled trial. Based on this finding, strength training should be integrated into the routine management of breast cancer–related lymphedema.[182]

Skin care is stressed in manual approaches to lymphedema. The goals of skin care include controlling skin colonization with bacteria and fungi, eliminating overgrowth in skin crevices, and hydrating the skin to eliminate microfissuring. Daily cleansing with mineral oil–based soap will remove debris and bacteria while moisturizing the skin.[28]

Augmentative and Compensatory Strategies

Cancer-related impairments often render necessary daily activities challenging or impossible. The application of conventional rehabilitation paradigms for the development of alternative and compensatory strategies allows patients to remain functionally independent. Use of assistive devices for mobility and ADL performance may be necessary. Environmental modification and augmentative communication devices should be explored in appropriate cases. Pacing strategies become essential for fatigued patients receiving intensive anticancer therapy, or with advanced disease. The appropriateness and cost-benefit ratio of interventions must be determined on a case-by-case basis.

Rehabilitation of Specific Cancer Populations

Breast Cancer

Functional impairments unique to patients with breast cancer develop after surgical procedures for tumor removal and breast reconstruction. These procedures include modified radical mastectomy (MRM), lumpectomy, sentinel lymph node biopsy (SLNB), axillary lymph node dissection (ALND), and autogenous tissue transposition for reconstruction. Multifactorial physical therapy (i.e., stretching and exercises) and active exercises were effective to treat postoperative pain and impaired ROM following treatment for breast cancer.[51]

Persistent deficits in shoulder ROM occur in as many as 35% of patients following ALND[112] (Table 29-7). Even after SLNB, 16% of patients self-reported limitations.[116] Lotze et al.[121] reported that vigorous shoulder mobilization in the immediate postoperative period led to an increase in seroma formation. The time line for shoulder mobilization presented in Table 29-8 adequately restores shoulder mobility without increasing the incidence of postsurgical complications; however, it has not been empirically evaluated. MRM and ALND are performed as same-day procedures at some institutions. In such cases, a gradual, supervised, and progressive ROM program is not possible. In such cases patients are often provided with illustrated exercise sheets covering "wall walking," forward flexion assisted by the unaffected arm, shoulder rolls, etc. A growing literature suggests that physical therapy following surgery for breast cancer offers a number of compelling benefits, including reduced pain, shoulder limitations, lymphedema, as well as enhanced psychological well-being.[18,21,111,211] This evidence is arguably strong enough to mandate the inclusion of physical therapy as standard care in postsurgical breast cancer management.

For patients who have undergone immediate breast reconstruction, particularly the TRAM flap procedure,

Table 29-7 Deficits in Shoulder Range of Motion After Axillary Surgery for Breast Cancer

		Elapsed Time After Breast Cancer Surgery					
		6 week		*3 mo*		*6 mo*	
Outcome Measure	**Author**	**ALND**	**SLNB**	**ALND**	**SLNB**	**ALND**	**SLNB**
Mean decrease from ipsilateral baseline AB	Rietman et al.	26.4 degrees	24.7 degrees				
	Mansel et al.			4.2 degrees	1.9 degrees	2.3 degrees	1.5 degrees
Mean difference in AB relative to untreated shoulder	Hack et al.						
ROM <160 degrees AB	Ernst et al.						
ROM <20 degrees normal value ≥1 plane	Langer et al.						
Self-reported limit ROM	Leidenius et al.						
	Warmuth et al.						
	Veronesi et al.					27.0%	0.0%
ROM < normative values any plane	Lauridsen et al.						
Mean ROM (normal = 180 degrees)	Rietman et al.						
	Gosselink et al.			FF 126 degrees MRM 150 degrees BCT			
	Peintinger et al.						

From Ernst MF, Voogd AC, Balder W, et al: Early and late morbidity associated with axillary levels I-III dissection in breast cancer, *J Surg Oncol* 79:151-155; discussion 156, 2002; Gosselink R, Rouffaer L, Vanhelden P, et al: Recovery of upper limb function after axillary dissection, *J Surg Oncol* 83:204-211, 2003; Hack TF, Cohen L, Katz J, et al: Physical and psychological morbidity after axillary lymph node dissection for breast cancer, *J Clin Oncol* 17:143-149, 1999; Langer I, Guller U, Berclaz G, et al: Morbidity of sentinel lymph node biopsy (SLN) alone versus SLN and completion axillary lymph node dissection after breast cancer surgery: a prospective Swiss multicenter study on 659 patients, *Ann Surg* 245:452-461, 2007; Lauridsen MC, Overgaard M, Overgaard J, et al: Shoulder disability and late symptoms following surgery for early breast cancer, *Acta Oncol* 47:569-575, 2008; Leidenius M, Leivonen M, Vironen J, et al: The consequences of long-time arm morbidity in node-negative breast cancer patients with sentinel node biopsy or axillary clearance, *J Surg Oncol* 92:23-31, 2005; Mansel RE, Fallowfield L, Kissin M, et al: Randomized multicenter trial of sentinel node biopsy versus standard axillary treatment in operable breast cancer: the ALMANAC Trial, *J Natl Cancer Inst* 98:599-609, 2006; Peintinger F, Reitsamer R, Stranzl H, et al: Comparison of quality of life and arm complaints after axillary lymph node dissection vs sentinel lymph node biopsy in breast cancer patients, *Br J Cancer* 89:648-652, 2003; Rietman JS, Dijkstra PU, Geertzen JH, et al: Short-term morbidity of the upper limb after sentinel lymph node biopsy or axillary lymph node dissection for stage I or II breast carcinoma, *Cancer* 98:690-696, 2003; Rietman JS, Dijkstra PU, Geertzen JH, et al: Treatment-related upper limb morbidity 1 year after sentinel lymph node biopsy or axillary lymph node dissection for stage I or II breast cancer, *Ann Surg Oncol* 11:1018-1024, 2004; Rietman JS, Geertzen JH, Hoekstra HJ, et al: Long term treatment related upper limb morbidity and quality of life after sentinel lymph node biopsy for stage I or II breast cancer, *Eur J Surg Oncol* 32:148-152, 2006; Veronesi U, Paganelli G, Viale G, et al: A randomized comparison of sentinel-node biopsy with routine axillary dissection in breast cancer, *N Engl J Med* 349:546-553, 2003; Warmuth MA, Bowen G, Prosnitz LR, et al: Complications of axillary lymph node dissection for carcinoma of the breast: a report based on a patient survey, *Cancer* 83:1362-1368, 1998.

AB, Abduction; *ALND*, axillary lymph node dissection; *BCT*, breast conserving therapy; *FF*, forward flexion; *MRM*, modified radical mastectomy; *ROM*, range of motion: *SLNB*, sentinel lymph node biopsy.

Table 29-8 Time Line of Shoulder Mobilization

Postoperative Day	Flexion	Abduction	Internal or External Rotation
1 to 3	40 to 45 degrees	40 to 45 degrees	To tolerance
4 to 6	45 to 90 degrees	45 degrees	To tolerance
7 onward	To tolerance	To tolerance	To tolerance

shoulder mobilization should be reviewed with the plastic surgeon unless an institutional algorithm has been formulated.

Axillary web syndrome (Figure 29-8) refers to the presence of taut, palpable cords originating in the axilla and extending distally along the anterior surface of the arm, often below the elbow.[150,198] What precise tissues compromise the cords remains a source of speculation. In a limited case series resected cords were pathologically evaluated. Specimens contained either lymphatic vessels or veins and surrounding connective tissue.[150] The clinical relevance of axillary web syndrome arises from the potential for painful

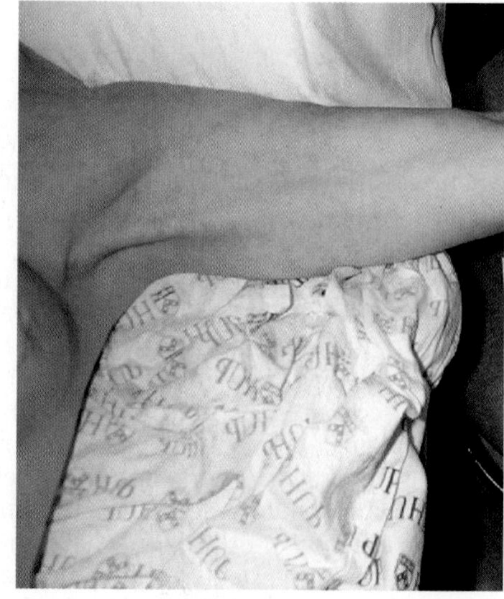

FIGURE 29-8 Axillary web syndrome manifest by thick, fibrous cords tethering the arm.

Elapsed Time After Breast Cancer Surgery					
9 to 12 mo		*24 mo*		*>2 yr*	
ALND	**SLNB**	**ALND**	**SLNB**	**ALND**	**SLNB**
		21.0 degrees	5.5 degrees		
6.3 degrees	3.1 degrees				
1.9 degrees	2.5 degrees				
14.0%				6.4 degrees	
				8.0%	
				11.3%	3.5%
				34%	16.0%
				8.0%	
		21.0%	0.0%		
				35%	
				156.6 degrees AB	
143.8 degrees AB	158.9 degrees AB				

restrictions in shoulder ROM. In severe cases, the cords tether the humerus, preventing full shoulder flexion or abduction. Pain generally responds to NSAIDs. Opioid analgesics might be necessary during passive and active-assisted ROM if the pain is severe. Therapy involves incremental ROM activities, topical heat, manipulation to soften and potentially "pop" the cords, as well as provision with a home exercise program. Heat should be used briefly if at all, given the risk of lymphedema and the almost universal presence of intercostal brachial neuropathy in the axilla and upper arm.

The surgical community has increasingly recognized the need for rehabilitation following TRAM flap breast reconstruction. The procedure denervates and disrupts the integrity of the abdominal wall, producing significant deficits in truncal stability, particularly during functional transfers. The goals of post-TRAM rehabilitation are to prevent subdermal fibrosis and adhesions, restore truncal alignment, minimize stress on the lumbar spine, optimize proprioceptive acuity in residual abdominal muscles, and encourage normal muscle recruitment patterns. The algorithm for post-TRAM flap rehabilitation (Table 29-9) was well tolerated and eliminated lasting impairment in a cohort of 52 patients. No patients developed donor site herniation or wound dehiscence.

Head and Neck Cancer

Combined modality therapy for head and neck cancer has afforded improved cure rates and reduced normal tissue compromise. The type and sequence of therapies used to treat head and neck cancer vary by the location of the primary tumor, the extent of cervical lymph node involvement, and the pathologic characteristics of the tumor. Increasingly, treatment approaches reflect a trend toward organ preservation. For example, the emphasis on "normal" tissue preservation has led to the substitution of supracricoid partial laryngectomy for total laryngectomy, and of functional neck dissection for radical neck dissection.

Treatment of head and neck cancer continues to produce some of the most challenging impairments within the scope of cancer rehabilitation. Many of the impairments directly undermine patients' ability to socialize, because of facial dysmorphism, loss of spontaneous or intelligible speech, and the inability to eat normally. Common rehabilitation problems include spinal accessory nerve palsy, radiation-induced xerostomia, soft tissue contracture of the neck and anterior chest wall soft tissues, dysphagia, dysphonia, and myofascial dysfunction. Impairments evolve over the course of head and neck cancer treatment and recovery. Rehabilitative interventions must be adjusted accordingly.

Table 29-9 Post-TRAM Procedure Rehabilitation Program

Weeks	Activities
0 to 3	Patient education: Lymphedema precautions Body mechanics Back safety (Driving permitted 3 to 4 weeks)
3 to 5	Active upper extremity range of motion (to tolerance): Supine forward flexion with wand Supine external rotation with wand Standing abduction, wall walking Postural body mechanics: Shoulder retraction—active with mirror cues Upright standing Head up or chin tucks Manual techniques as needed: Manual lymphatic drainage Scar mobilization (if healed) Gentle myofascial release if restrictions are notable Walking program if needed
6 to 7	Postural body mechanics Shoulder retraction—active with mirror cues Pectoral stretch (corner stretch) If good alignment with retraction, may initiate resistive TheraBand at yellow level for shoulder retraction Upright standing posture—posterior pelvic tilt in supine
8 to 12	Stabilization or strengthening exercises Prone lying Isometric pelvic or lumbar stabilization (in supine) Lumbar extensor strengthening or stabilization Abdominal or oblique stabilization or strengthening Physioball activities Aerobic exercise Biking Treadmill Manual techniques Manual scar mobilization Myofascial release

TRAM, Transverse rectus abdominis muscle.

Spinal Accessory Nerve Palsy

The recognition that comparable cure rates can be achieved with more conservative surgical resection has spurred the shift from radical to functional neck dissections. The former procedure removes the sternocleidomastoid muscle, the spinal accessory nerve, and the external jugular vein. The nerve to the levator scapulae muscle was also frequently resected, producing severe ipsilateral shoulder dysfunction. Functional neck dissections preserve all structures that can be safely left intact, producing dramatically lower rates of postoperative shoulder morbidity. Many patients with head and neck cancer now emerge from surgery with largely spared spinal accessory nerve function. The integrity of the spinal accessory nerve can be easily assessed with side-by-side comparison of resisted end-range forward flexion of the shoulder. Some degree of weakness can be elicited in most patients on the side of the neck dissection.

The severity and distribution of trapezius weakness secondary to spinal accessory nerve palsy (Figure 29-9) is subject to great interindividual variability. The upper, middle, and lower trapezius muscles can be innervated solely by the spinal accessory nerve or receive partial or total innervation from the cervical plexus.[22] When the spinal accessory nerve was routinely sacrificed during radical neck dissections, some patients developed little to no shoulder compromise, suggesting that innervation was predominantly derived from the cervical plexus. Baseline anatomic variability is compounded by inconsistency in the type and degree of intraoperative nerve injury. The spinal accessory nerve may be entirely spared or subject to neurapraxic, axonotmetic, or neurotmetic insult, all with different rates and degrees of recovery. Additionally, electrocautery of blood vessels can undermine blood supply to the vasa nervorum, producing ischemic injury.

The timing and intensity of rehabilitation should be guided by patients' prognosis for recovery. Spinal accessory nerve reinnervation can continue over 12 months following surgery. Two small trials have established the safety and efficacy of resistive exercise among patients with head and

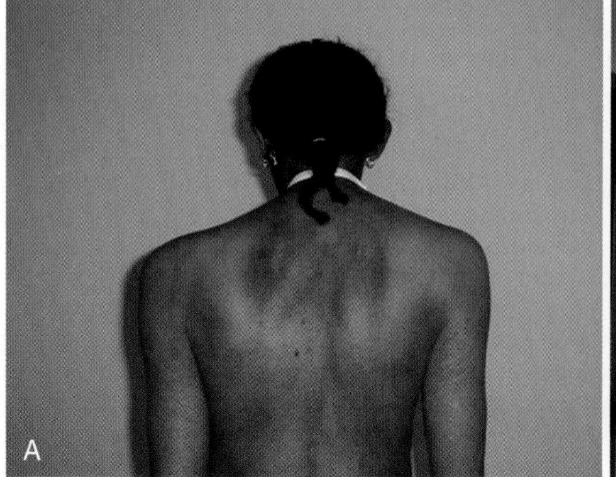

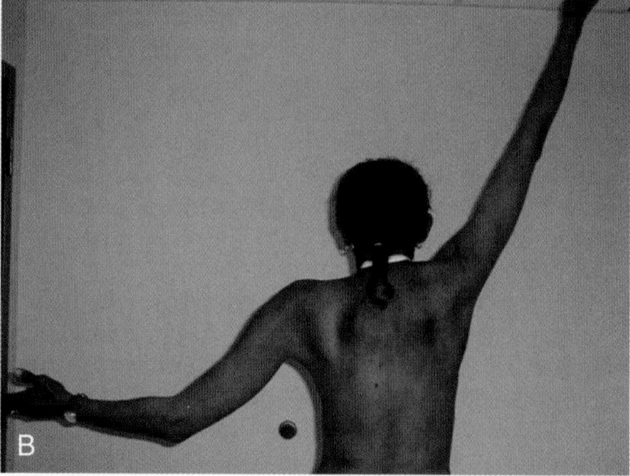

FIGURE 29-9 **A,** Resting posture of a patient with head and neck cancer and complete spinal accessory nerve palsy. **B,** Active shoulder abduction is limited to 90 degrees on the affected side resulting from middle trapezius muscle weakness.

neck cancer; one trial was conducted while patients were undergoing radiation.[133,176] Important elements of spinal accessory nerve rehabilitation include the following:

- Prevention of frozen shoulder through active ROM and active-assisted ROM
- Prevention of anterior chest wall flexibility deficits
- Strengthening of alternate scapular elevators and retractors
- Instruction in compensatory techniques for activities requiring sustained shoulder abduction and forward flexion
- Neuromuscular retraining
- Preservation of trapezius muscle tone through electrical stimulation if reinnervation is anticipated
- Postural modification
- Instruction in shoulder support to allow recovery of the levator scapulae

Patients with a complete persistent spinal accessory nerve palsy can be fitted with an orthosis. To date, none of the braces designed to substitute for absent or weak trapezius muscles have experienced widespread uptake. For patients plagued by levator scapulae fatigue and spasms, a "shelf" orthosis (Figure 29-10) designed to encircle the waist, and to provide a ledge on which patients can rest their affected arms when not in use, reduces symptoms.

Cervical Contracture

Progressive fibrosis of the anterior and lateral cervical soft tissue may be highly problematic for patients with head and neck cancer. A general approach to radiation-induced fibrosis was outlined earlier in this chapter. Because of the high radiation doses delivered to some patients with head and neck cancer, proactive ROM in all planes of neck motion should be initiated as soon as safely possible. Cervical ROM can continue throughout radiation therapy in the absence of significant skin breakdown. Ideally, ranging activities should begin immediately after surgery before radiation. The delicate balance between flexibility and postsurgical wound healing must be respected. Surgeons should be consulted regarding the length of the postoperative interval before ROM can begin. For an uncomplicated radical or functional neck dissection, 3 days is generally considered safe. Reconstruction with tissue transposition requires a longer recovery period. ROM activities should be delayed until all drains are removed to avoid seroma formation.

Irradiated patients should perform ROM activities twice daily during the first 2 years following cancer treatment and daily thereafter. As mentioned previously, radiation-induced fibrosis can be indefinitely progressive. Figure 29-11 demonstrates the head-forward posture and thoracic kyphosis characteristic of head and neck cancer patients with severe anterior cervical soft tissue fibrosis. For optimal results, patients should be taught to provide additional stretch during end-range lateral bending or rotation by exerting gentle pressure with the contralateral hand. Stretches should be held for five deep breaths and repeated between 5 and 10 times per session. Isometric strengthening of the cervical extensors, and postural modification with visual cuing, is beneficial.

Manual fibrous release techniques are indicated when ROM is restricted by robust soft tissue fibrosis or tethering of the skin to subdermal tissues. Patients can be taught self-massage to augment the efficacy of ROM activities. Compression of severely fibrotic areas breaks down established scar tissue and inhibits its reformation. Compression garments, either off the shelf or customized, are a convenient means of applying compression. Custom-cut foam pieces strategically inserted can achieve greater focal pressure on stubborn areas. Constant vigilance must be maintained to ensure that friable, irradiated skin is not compromised. Botulinum toxin injection may be tried in refractory cases.[199]

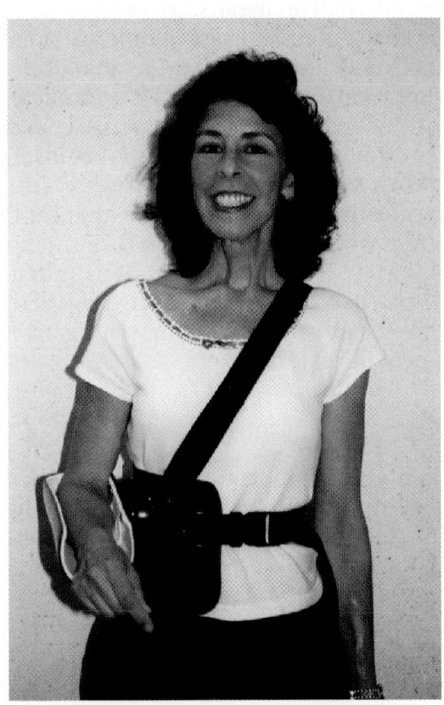

FIGURE 29-10 "Shelf" orthosis fabricated to encircle the torso of patients with complete spinal accessory nerve palsies and to provide a ledge on which they can rest their affected extremities when not in use.

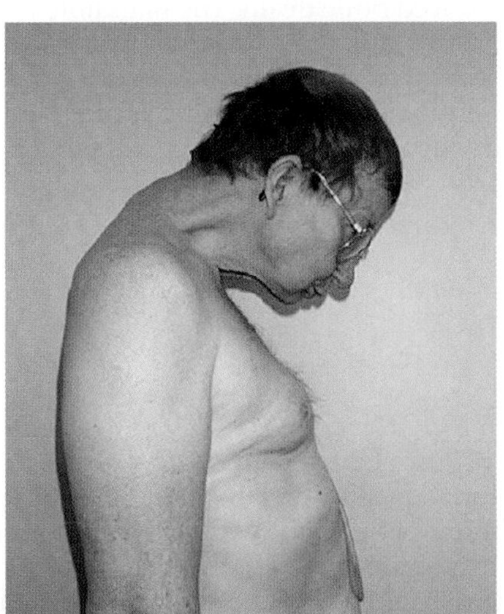

FIGURE 29-11 Head-forward posture and exaggerated thoracic kyphosis, associated with radiation-induced soft tissue contracture, in a patient with head and neck cancer.

Aphonia and Dysphonia

Impaired vocal communication occurs in the majority of patients with head and neck cancer at some point during treatment. However, this is usually transient and largely reversible because total laryngectomies have become uncommon. Radiation-induced laryngeal or pharyngeal swelling and fibrosis, tracheostomy, partial or total glossectomy, reduced oral excursion secondary to trismus, copious secretions, and neurogenic pharyngeal or laryngeal paralysis all contribute to impaired phonation. Some patients are rendered acutely voiceless after surgery. Such acute loss occurs most dramatically after total laryngectomy but is also frequent after tracheostomy and glossectomy. Gradual compromise of vocal precision, endurance, and volume is more common with organ preservation therapies. Irrespective of the acuity of onset, loss of spontaneous, intelligible speech can be profoundly isolating. It renders patients dependent in communication and can be vocationally devastating.

Various approaches to restore communication are used depending on the anticipated duration, severity, and nature of the deficit. The most common compensatory strategies used by acutely voiceless adults include mouthing words, gestures, writing, and head nods.[8,76] Patients rendered chronically aphonic by total laryngectomy can communicate through esophageal speech, tracheoesophageal speech, or use of an electrolarynx. The frequency with which these options are offered to and accepted by patients varies considerably across physician practices, institutions, and geographic regions.[134]

Additional Concerns

Patients with head and neck cancer, by virtue of their treatment and premorbid risk profile, are prone to the development of osteoradionecrosis, dental caries, and recurrent substance abuse. Comprehensive rehabilitation involves proactive screening for these conditions. Because of the high radiation doses delivered in head and neck cancer treatment, 5% to 15% of these patients develop osteoradionecrosis, an extremely painful condition caused by radiation-induced bone death. The mandible is most often affected. Patients complain of relentless jaw pain aggravated by chewing and vocalization. Associated pain should be aggressively treated with combined opioids and NSAIDs. Referral for hyperbaric oxygen treatments should be considered.

Precautions in Cancer Rehabilitation

Modalities

A climate of exaggerated caution too often limits cancer rehabilitation. Specific therapeutic precautions reflect a fear of injuring patients, or worse, spreading their cancer. Although it is important to appreciate that patients with cancer are predisposed to a host of adverse complications (e.g., hemorrhage and disease recurrence), it is equally important to recognize that a causal relationship has not been established between such complications and physiatric interventions. Inactivity causes far greater long-term morbidity for the majority of patients with cancer. Most precautions are not empirically supported and they frequently reinforce ambivalence toward structured, incremental physical activity.

Warnings against treating cancer patients with deep heat and massage are ubiquitous in the rehabilitation literature. Precautions regarding heating modalities are largely based on the concern that heat will dilate local blood vessels and increase metabolic activity in tumor cells, thereby hastening local or systemic spread. Similarly, massage is presumed to potentiate metastasis by encouraging blood and lymph flow, or by dislodging tumor cells. This line of reasoning is simplistic and at odds with several facts. First, exercise does more to promote blood and lymph flow than localized heating modalities, yet evidence suggests that exercise has a protective effect against the recurrence of breast and colon cancer. Second, thousands of patients with cancer have received MLD to deliberately stimulate lymph flow to decongest their lymphedema. Many of these patients have had known cancer at the treatment site. So far, no association has been established between lymphedema or its treatment and cancer progression. Lastly, complex genetic and biochemical alterations are required for a cell to develop metastatic potential. Tumor cells must acquire the ability to penetrate basement membranes, adhere to endothelial cells, elude the body's internal defenses, and stimulate local angiogenesis, among many other genetically determined attributes. Relative to these complex changes, being manually dislodged from a tumor mass or transiently exposed to increased blood flow probably has no impact on tumor cells.

Questioning the current rigid precautions against the use of heating modalities in cancer may be moot. Deep heat is rarely of clinical use, or therapeutic goals can be realized by alternative means. However, if the clinical context warrants a trial of ultrasound or related modalities, the option should not be reflexively abandoned because of unsubstantiated warnings. In the author's experience, patients with widespread tumors have benefited from the discrete use of ultrasound in areas of dense radiation-induced fibrosis and postsurgical scarring. Massage has the potential to greatly benefit patients with cancer through its antispasmodic, fibrolytic, and counter-stimulatory effects. Additionally, MLD is an integral part of lymphedema management. Aside from vigorous massage in the immediate vicinity of the established tumor, massage is likely to be of far greater benefit than harm.

Cytopenias

Leukopenia and thrombocytopenia commonly occur following the administration of chemotherapy. The duration and severity of cytopenias have been considerably reduced through the introduction of CSFs that accelerate bone marrow recovery. In patients with cancer who are receiving initial chemotherapy but who are not pretreated with CSFs, leukopenia and thrombocytopenia can be detected on the ninth or tenth day after chemotherapy administration. Nadir blood counts generally occur between days 14 and 18, with recovery beginning by day 21. The time course of bone marrow recovery dictates the widely used 3- to 4-week chemotherapy cycle, with new cycles being initiated 21 to 28 days after administration of the previous chemotherapy dose.

There are inconsistent guidelines limiting physical activity in the face of chemotherapy-induced cytopenias. Existing precautions are arbitrary and lack empirical testing. None has been shown to limit adverse events. Leukopenia is of less concern than thrombocytopenia, given the associated risk of intracranial hemorrhage or bleeding after a fall. Among National Cancer Institute–designated comprehensive cancer centers, cutoff platelet counts below which physical therapy is contraindicated range from 25,000 to no lower limit. No differences between institutions in the incidence of spontaneous hemorrhage have been reported. Patients undergoing allogenic and autogeneic bone marrow transplants typically spend 7 to 21 days with platelet counts of 5000 to 12,000. During this interval, most patients perform ADL independently, ambulate, transfer, and lift greater than 10 lb repeatedly without hemorrhage. When spontaneous bleeding does occur, it is typically not associated with physical activity. Given the routinely well-tolerated levels of physical activity in patients with severe thrombocytopenia, reconsideration of current precautions is warranted. Inappropriate restriction of physical therapy and exercise in this population can contribute to rapid deconditioning, bone demineralization, and contractures.

Summary

Cancer rehabilitation is a varied and challenging field of increasing public health importance. A growing evidence base suggests that conventional rehabilitative interventions succeed in preserving and restoring the functional status of patients with cancer. A marked lack of hypothesis-driven research continues to limit the field, as does a lack of experienced and interested clinicians. It is hoped that these deficits will be remedied, given the projections for steadily increasing cancer survivorship.

KEY REFERENCES

2. Adamsen L, Quist M, Andersen C, et al: Effect of a multimodal high intensity exercise intervention in cancer patients undergoing chemotherapy: randomised controlled trial, *BMJ* 339:b3410, 2009.
17. Bertolini F, Spallanzani A, Fontana A, et al: Brain metastases: an overview, *CNS Oncol* 4:37–46, 2015.
21. Box RC, Reul-Hirche HM, Bullock-Saxton JE, Furnival CM: Shoulder movement after breast cancer surgery: results of a randomised controlled study of postoperative physiotherapy, *Breast Cancer Res Treat* 75:35–50, 2002.
26. Carla C, Verstappen J, Heimans K, et al: Neurotoxin complications of chemotherapy in patients with cancer, *Drugs* 63:1549–1563, 2003.
27. Carver JR, Shapiro CL, Ng A, et al: American Society of Clinical Oncology clinical evidence review on the ongoing care of adult cancer survivors: cardiac and pulmonary late effects, *J Clin Oncol* 25:3991–4008, 2007.
33. Chang EL, Wefel JS, Hess KR, et al: Neurocognition in patients with brain metastases treated with radiosurgery or radiosurgery plus whole-brain irradiation: a randomised controlled trial, *Lancet Oncol* 10:1037–1044, 2009.
36. Cheville AL, Kornblith AB, Basford JR: An examination of the causes for the underutilization of rehabilitation services among people with advanced cancer, *Am J Phys Med Rehabil* 90:S27–S37, 2011.
38. Chow E, Zeng L, Salvo N, et al: Update on the systematic review of palliative radiotherapy trials for bone metastases, *Clin Oncol (R Coll Radiol)* 24:112–124, 2012.
41. Cole JS, Patchell RA: Metastatic epidural spinal cord compression, *Lancet Neurol* 7:459–466, 2008.
44. Cramp F, Byron-Daniel J: Exercise for the management of cancer-related fatigue in adults, *Cochrane Database Syst Rev* (11):CD006145, 2012.
50. De Backer IC, Schep G, Backx FJ, et al: Resistance training in cancer survivors: a systematic review, *Int J Sports Med* 30:703–712, 2009.
51. De Groef A, Van Kampen M, Dieltjens E, et al: Effectiveness of postoperative physical therapy for upper limb impairments following breast cancer treatment: a systematic review, *Arch Phys Med Rehabil* Published online January 13, 2015. http://dx.doi.org/10.1016/j.apmr.2015.01.006.
52. Delanian S, Lefaix JL, Pradat PF: Radiation-induced neuropathy in cancer survivors, *Radiother Oncol* 105:273–282, 2012.
53. Didelot A, Honnorat J: Update on paraneoplastic neurological syndromes, *Curr Opin Oncol* 21:566–572, 2009.
57. Dy SM, Asch SM, Naeim A, et al: Evidence-based standards for cancer pain management, *J Clin Oncol* 26:3879–3885, 2008.
58. Eichler AF, Loeffler JS: Multidisciplinary management of brain metastases, *Oncologist* 12:884–898, 2007.
67. Galvao DA, Taaffe DR, Spry N, et al: Combined resistance and aerobic exercise program reverses muscle loss in men undergoing androgen suppression therapy for prostate cancer without bone metastases: a randomized controlled trial, *J Clin Oncol* 28:340–347, 2010.
74. Guo Y, Persyn L, Palmer JL, Bruera E: Incidence of and risk factors for transferring cancer patients from rehabilitation to acute care units, *Am J Phys Med Rehabil* 87:647–653, 2008.
85. Huang ME, Cifu DX, Keyser-Marcus L: Functional outcome after brain tumor and acute stroke: a comparative analysis, *Arch Phys Med Rehabil* 79:1386–1390, 1998.
86. Huang ME, Cifu DX, Keyser-Marcus L: Functional outcomes in patients with brain tumor after inpatient rehabilitation: comparison with traumatic brain injury, *Am J Phys Med Rehab* 79:327–335, 2000.
89. Jacobsen PB, Donovan KA, Vadaparampil ST, Small BJ: Systematic review and meta-analysis of psychological and activity-based interventions for cancer-related fatigue, *Health Psychol* 26:660–667, 2007.
99. Kirshbaum MN: A review of the benefits of whole body exercise during and after treatment for breast cancer, *J Clin Nurs* 16:104–121, 2007.
102. Ko DS, Lerner R, Klose G, Cosimi AB: Effective treatment of lymphedema of the extremities, *Arch Surg* 133:452–458, 1998.
104. Kori SH, Foley KM, Posner JB: Brachial plexus lesions in patients with cancer: 100 cases, *Neurology* 31:45–50, 1981.
106. Krebber AM, Buffart LM, Kleijn G, et al: Prevalence of depression in cancer patients: a meta-analysis of diagnostic interviews and self-report instruments, *Psychooncology* 23:121–130, 2014.
112. Lauridsen MC, Overgaard M, Overgaard J, et al: Shoulder disability and late symptoms following surgery for early breast cancer, *Acta Oncol* 47:569–575, 2008.
120. Loblaw DA, Mitera G, Ford M, Laperriere NJ: A 2011 updated systematic review and clinical practice guideline for the management of malignant extradural spinal cord compression, *Int J Radiat Oncol Biol Phys* 84:312–317, 2012.
123. Lutz S, Berk L, Chang E, et al: Palliative radiotherapy for bone metastases: an ASTRO evidence-based guideline, *Int J Radiat Oncol Biol Phys* 79:965–976, 2011.
127. Marciniak CM, Sliwa JA, Heinemann AW, Semik PE: Functional outcomes of persons with brain tumors after inpatient rehabilitation, *Arch Phys Med Rehabil* 82:457–463, 2001.
131. McKinley WO, Conti-Wyneken A, Vokac CW, Cifu DX: Rehabilitative functional outcome of patients with neoplastic spinal cord compressions, *Arch Phys Med Rehabil* 77:892–895, 1996.
132. McKinley WO, Huang ME, Tewksbury MA: Neoplastic vs. traumatic spinal cord injury: an inpatient rehabilitation comparison, *Am J Phys Med Rehabil* 79:138–144, 2000.
133. McNeely ML, Parliament MB, Seikaly H, et al: Effect of exercise on upper extremity pain and dysfunction in head and neck cancer survivors: a randomized controlled trial, *Cancer* 113:214–222, 2008.
135. Meneses-Echavez JF, Gonzalez-Jimenez E, Ramirez-Velez R: Supervised exercise reduces cancer-related fatigue: a systematic review, *J Physiother* 61:3–9, 2015.

137. Mercadante S, Fulfaro F: Management of painful bone metastases, *Curr Opin Oncol* 19:308–314, 2007.
139. Miaskowski C, Cleary J, Burney R, et al: *Guideline for the management of cancer pain in adults and children,* Glenview, 2005, American Pain Society.
141. Mirels H: Metastatic disease in long bones. A proposed scoring system for diagnosing impending pathologic fractures, *Clin Orthop Relat Res* 249:256–264, 1989.
142. Mishra SI, Scherer RW, Snyder C, et al: The effectiveness of exercise interventions for improving health-related quality of life from diagnosis through active cancer treatment, *Oncol Nurs Forum* 42:E33–E53, 2015.
148. Moretti R, Torre P, Antonello RM, et al: Neuropsychological evaluation of late-onset post-radiotherapy encephalopathy: a comparison with vascular dementia, *J Neurol Sci* 229-230:195–200, 2005.
152. National Comprehensive Cancer Network (NCCN): *NCCN Clinical practice guidelines in oncology: cancer-related fatigue, 2015,* Fort Washington, 2015, National Comprehensive Cancer Network. Available at: www.nccn.org.
154. O'Dell MW, Barr K, Spanier D, Warnick RE: Functional outcome of inpatient rehabilitation in persons with brain tumors, *Arch Phys Med Rehabil* 79:1530–1534, 1998.
170. Pradat PF, Delanian S: Late radiation injury to peripheral nerves, *Handb Clin Neurol* 115:743–758, 2013.
182. Schmitz KH, Ahmed RL, Troxel A, et al: Weight lifting in women with breast-cancer-related lymphedema, *N Engl J Med* 361:664–673, 2009.
183. Schmitz KH, Holtzman J, Courneya KS, et al: Controlled physical activity trials in cancer survivors: a systematic review and meta-analysis, *Cancer Epidemiol Biomarkers Prev* 14:1588–1595, 2005.
193. Speck RM, Courneya KS, Masse LC, et al: An update of controlled physical activity trials in cancer survivors: a systematic review and meta-analysis, *J Cancer Surviv* 4:87–100, 2010.
198. Stubblefield MD, Keole N: Upper body pain and functional disorders in patients with breast cancer, *PM&R* 6:170–183, 2014.
202. Sutcliffe P, Connock M, Shyangdan D, et al: A systematic review of evidence on malignant spinal metastases: natural history and technologies for identifying patients at high risk of vertebral fracture and spinal cord compression, *Health Technol Assess* 17:1–274, 2013.
209. Tomlinson D, Diorio C, Beyene J, Sung L: Effect of exercise on cancer-related fatigue: a meta-analysis, *Am J Phys Med Rehabil* 93:675–686, 2014.
211. Torres Lacomba M, Yuste Sanchez MJ, Zapico Goni A, et al: Effectiveness of early physiotherapy to prevent lymphoedema after surgery for breast cancer: randomised, single blinded, clinical trial, *BMJ* 340:b5396, 2010.
214. van den Beuken-van Everdingen MH, de Rijke JM, Kessels AG, et al: Prevalence of pain in patients with cancer: a systematic review of the past 40 years, *Ann Oncol* 18:1437–1449, 2007.
223. Wood TJ, Racano A, Yeung H, et al: Surgical management of bone metastases: quality of evidence and systematic review, *Ann Surg Oncol* 21:4081–4089, 2014.

The full reference list for this chapter is available online.

CHAPTER 30

THE GERIATRIC PATIENT

Carlos Anthony Jaramillo

Caring for elderly patients requires an understanding of the biology and neuropsychology of aging, the diseases and conditions more common in elderly patients, and how these processes affect function, impede patient goals, and result in disability. The physical medicine and rehabilitation specialist fits well within the geriatric care paradigm because the physiatrist has experience working with multidisciplinary teams, has experience treating patients with complex conditions, and is trained to focus on patient goals and function.

Geriatric rehabilitation can be approached from a purely functional perspective, looking not so much at the pathophysiology but at function and disability. For example, tight hip extensors can impede gait efficiency, such that the person cannot walk rapidly enough to cross the street while the traffic light signals display "walk." However, aging with a disability is a separate and more challenging process. Although a physiologic insult and impairment may have been sustained earlier in life, a person's capacity to cope and compensate can change with age. Changes that occur over the course of time in health, or in psychosocial support systems, can have a negative impact on mobility, self-care, and pain.

Geriatric rehabilitation addresses problems that affect not only the individual patient but also society at large. There are major economic ramifications when individuals can no longer care for themselves. Increased longevity and global population aging will have a significant impact on society during the twenty-first century. The average life expectancy at the age of 60 years is 20 years for the global population and 23 years in the more developed countries.[87] The elderly are not a homogenous group. There are differences in health risk factors, life expectancy, and patient goals among the different elderly subgroups: 65- to 75-year-olds, who may still be working (old); persons over the age of 85 years (oldest old); and those over the age of 90 years (nonagenarian).

Changes in the Body with Aging

Changes in multiple body systems are part of the normal aging process. However, it is often difficult to determine which of these changes are as a result of the natural process of aging and which result from disease and secondary factors. The scientific study of aging (gerontology) has greatly improved our understanding of the molecular, cellular, and genetic mechanisms that underlie aging. Here, we will outline some of the physiologic changes that occur with age in organs and organ systems which are relevant to the physiatrist.

Musculoskeletal

Ability to perform daily tasks independently decreases with age even in healthy elderly adults and is greatly affected by changes in the musculoskeletal system. Such changes can lead to further disuse and injuries resulting in significant pain and disability. The musculoskeletal system is responsible for limb movement, and it provides structural support for the body and protection for soft tissue. Muscle and bone physiology is a metabolically and functionally integrated system affected by other systems (e.g., the endocrine system). The use of a systems biology approach can be valuable in that it permits the consideration of how these components interact.

Muscle

Changes in body composition that occurs in older adults result in a loss of strength and function. It is important to differentiate presumed normal loss of muscle with aging from changes attributable to an underlying disease. Cachexia is weight loss attributable to an underlying disease process resulting in the loss of both muscle and fat mass, and occurs in patients of all ages. Sarcopenia is the loss of muscle mass and strength with age and is usually accompanied by an increase in fat mass and abdominal girth. Therefore, total body weight decrease might not be observed with sarcopenia. Age-related changes in muscle may also be affected by chronic disease.[46] The mechanisms that drive sarcopenia have become a focus for basic and clinical research because of its impact on the patient and society.

Cross-sectional and longitudinal clinical studies of older adults have shown heterogeneous changes in muscle strength that vary between age subgroups and gender. Furthermore, decline in muscle strength with aging is not the same across all muscle groups. In general, however, loss in the number of muscle fibers, a decrease in fiber size and quality, and loss in whole muscle have been documented.[14,31-33] Muscle strength decreases with aging at the level of single muscle fibers resulting in a loss of force per unit area. In aging muscle, there is a disproportionate loss of type 2 muscle fibers (fast-twitch) with the muscle overall having more slow-twitch characteristics than in young adults. There is also an increased proportion of muscle fibers with multiple myosin isoforms, which suggests that characterizing muscle changes by fiber type may have limitations.[14,64]

Sarcopenia is thought to be driven by a combination of catabolic action and reduced anabolic influences. Catabolic cytokines, such as tumor necrosis factor-α, interleukin (IL)-6, and IL-1β, contribute to muscle fiber loss, but it is not clear whether these inflammatory pathways are activated during aging, by chronic disease, or because of a combination of causes.

In addition to loss of fibers, there is a loss of motor units during aging.[26] Older adults can experience limitations in maximally activating muscle as a result of several principal causes: neural changes, such as increased agonist-antagonist coactivation; decreased motor neuron excitability at the spinal cord level caused by decreased afferent input; and inefficient transmission at the neuromuscular junction.[5] With training, young adults often show adaptations in spinal cord relay components, whereas older adults might rely more on supraspinal influences.[5] Older adults typically use a higher percentage of minimal knee strength than young adults, which can lead to more fatigue because they are working near full capacity. The elderly can also experience reduced power because of a lack of rapid force development,[5] possibly resulting from a decline in voluntary neuromuscular activation.[21]

Bone

Bone mass is affected by body weight–loading and the tensile forces that the muscles exert on the skeletal structure. Insufficient load-bearing activity will result in bone demineralization.[85] Changes in the endocrine system also lead to bone loss, which is significant in women after menopause. Increased or excess osteoclast activity occurs during aging, possibly as a result of vitamin D deficiency, leading to an imbalance in bone remodeling and ultimately weakening of cortical and trabecular bone.[37]

Neurologic

Increasing age is associated with decreased brain volume, frontal gray matter loss, and decreased cerebral blood flow. Cortical thinning occurs along with a shifting of brain activity from the posterior to the anterior regions.[66] Cognitive changes are discernible to many elderly patients and their caregivers and may give rise to concern for underlying disease processes, such as dementia. With age there is a decline in episodic memory, the long-term memory system that stores past events or "episodes" with personal context. Examples of episodic memory include: "what did you have for dinner last night?" and remembering "where" and "when" a specific trip to visit grandchildren occurred. By contrast, procedural and semantic memory is stable and may even improve with age. Learning new information (fluid intelligence), processing speed, multitasking, task shifting, and executive function may decrease with age.[83] Rates of cognitive decline vary between individuals and can affect the ability to live independently.[70]

Vision declines with age as a result of changes in all the tissues of the eye: retinal aging is associated with macular degeneration and loss of central vision; optic nerve damage can result in glaucoma and visual field loss; and lens aging may lead to cataracts with characteristic noncorrectable decrease in visual clarity, haloes, and poor night vision. Age-related hearing loss (AHL) is a common condition in elderly adults. AHL or presbycusis is a degenerative, bilateral, and symmetrical process driven by intrinsic (e.g., genetics, cochlear aging) and extrinsic factors (e.g., noise exposure, ototoxic drugs) that can affect multiple types of cells involved in hearing.[48] Olfaction may be impaired over time but is also associated with underlying processes, such as traumatic brain injury, Alzheimer disease, and Parkinson disease. Light touch sensation, vibration, and proprioception are also affected by age.

Cardiovascular

Maximal heart rate decreases approximately 6 to 10 beats per minute per decade and maximal oxygen consumption (VO_{2max}) decreases 5% to 15% per decade after the age of 25 years. With aging, the cardiovascular system has decreased arterial compliance, increased systolic blood pressure, left ventricular hypertrophy with impaired filling, decreased beta-adrenergic receptor stimulation response, decreased sinoatrial node automaticity, and a decreased number of myocytes.[43] The exercise-induced adaptations that occur in younger people, such as increased peripheral arteriovenous oxygen difference and increased cardiac size, stroke work, cardiac output, and left ventricular function,[1] are not as available to the elderly. Older patients with coronary artery disease have age-related increases in left ventricular and arterial wall stiffness and thickening, which limit some adaptations with conditioning.[1] In the operative setting, maintaining intravascular volume is important because the aged heart depends on preload more than in the younger person. Because afterload is increased by outflow tract stiffness, there is decreased sensitivity to catecholamines and impaired vasoconstrictive responses in the elderly.[68]

Pulmonary

In the lung, surface area decreases as the alveoli and ducts enlarge resulting in impaired pulmonary gas exchange and ventilation/perfusion (V/Q) mismatch. In addition, there is loss of elastic recoil and lung stiffening resulting in increased lung compliance and decreased thoracic wall mobility in the elderly.[36] Respiratory muscle strength also decreases. These changes lead to increased residual volume and functional residual capacity. Compensation during exertion can occur in healthy older adults to a limited extent.[78]

Gastrointestinal

Peripheral and central age-related changes in the gastrointestinal (GI) system can lead to decreased appetite and energy intake and possibly malnutrition, the "anorexia of aging."[12] Smell and taste sensation may decrease with age, leading to loss of enjoyment from eating and reduced food variety. Gastric compliance decreases with age causing early satiety and prolonged postprandial satiety. Aging is associated with decreased stomach acid production (hypochlorhydria) and subsequent impaired absorption of vitamin B_{12}, calcium, iron, zinc, and folic acid. Hypochlorhydria can also lead to bacterial overgrowth in the small intestine. The microbial flora of the GI tract forms a symbiotic relationship with the hosts and aids in food assimilation and provides a natural defense barrier. The change in GI flora with age is not fully understood, but the microbiome is affected by medications, such as antibiotics.

Cholecystokinin and leptin levels increase with aging and both have roles in suppressing appetite.[12]

Genitourinary

Renal mass and blood flow decrease with age. Glomerular filtration rate (GFR) may also decline after the age of 40 years, and GFR estimates in general are not reliable for elderly women and those with low body weight.[47] Aging also affects water balance as the kidneys are less capable of concentrating urine resulting in water loss. Urinary incontinence is common among elderly patients and more so in women, but is not a normal consequence of aging. Elderly individuals may continue to be sexually active. Although erectile dysfunction is common among older men, it is not a normal consequence of aging and underlying causes should be investigated.[34]

Endocrine

Aging results in reduced hormonal secretion as well as tissue responsiveness. Anabolic hormones including testosterone, growth hormone, and insulin-like growth factor decrease with age, resulting in impaired muscle fiber protein synthesis and changes in body composition. These changes can result in decreased glucose tolerance. Decrease in estrogen with age (menopause) leads to collagen loss and thinning of the skin.[19] Estrogen decline is also associated with bone loss, which may predispose postmenopausal women to osteopenia and osteoporosis. Change in tissue responsiveness to hormones and the complex interactions between hormonal systems may be part of the reason why hormone replacement therapy has not proven to be a straightforward approach to treat the effects of aging. Adrenal and thyroid levels may also change with age, but the clinical significance is not understood because the function of these systems appears to be robust throughout the life span, with the exception of disease processes.

Skin

Skin aging is caused by changes occurring during normal adult aging as well as insults from environmental factors. Age-related skin changes include thinning of the epidermis, decreased cell replacement, impaired immune response and wound healing, decreased moisture content, elasticity, blood supply, and sensory sensitivity.[19] These changes increase the risk of skin disorders and injury to the skin in the elderly. Noncosmetic moisturizers in combination with humectants are effective for treating excessively dry skin in the elderly.[51]

Medication Metabolism

Changes in pharmacokinetics and pharmacodynamics occur with age. Clinical drug trials are typically conducted with young and healthy age groups, and thus the reactions of the elderly to medications are not always the same as those of the population that was used to initially test the medication.[74] Adverse effects are more frequent[50] and may be more severe[65] in the elderly. The increase in adipose tissue that typically occurs with age causes a larger volume of distribution for fat-soluble drugs and prolongs their biologic half-life. Conversely, total body water decreases by as much as 15% between 20 and 80 years of age, which decreases the volume of distribution of water-soluble drugs and thus results in a higher drug serum concentration.[49] Hepatic drug clearance can be decreased up to 30% and renal clearance up to 50% in approximately 60% of elderly individuals.[49] Care must be taken when prescribing renally excreted drugs in older and frail individuals. Patients with low muscle mass may have low serum creatinine levels leading to an overestimation of GFR.

Gait

Locomotion in older people is affected by multiple factors that are under the influence of aging processes: vision, cognition, motor control, balance, peripheral sensation, strength, joint health, and metabolic demands. It is also becoming increasingly clear that gait, cognition, falls, and dementia are interdependent processes. Overall, gait in the elderly is characterized by decreased speed, increased double limb support, shorter stride length, and a broader base of support. These characteristics are also associated with falls and the fear of falling.

Studies have shown gait speed to be a predictor of survival and possibly a biomarker of health status in relatively healthy older adults. A walking speed of 1.0 m/sec has been considered a guidepost for relatively good function and 0.8 m/sec predicting median life expectancy for age and sex.[76] Baseline gait speeds vary among individuals, but are relatively stable until 65 years of age. The trajectory of gait speed decline varies among older adults.

In a longitudinal study of 2364 participants between the ages of 70 and 79 years, White et al.[86] found that gait trajectories could be categorized as slow, moderate, and fast decline. Compared with their baseline gait speeds, individuals in the slow decline trajectory experienced a gait speed decline of 11% over 8 years, the moderate decline trajectory dropped 14% in gait speed, and the fast decline trajectory showed a slowing of 22% during the study period. The fast decline group was associated with increased risk of mortality.[86] Therefore, age-related decrease in gait speed is not uniform and serial measurements of walking speed may be more informative because gait changes may indicate the presence of underlying pathologies.

Evaluation of the Elderly Patient

History Taking

When examining elderly patients, questions should be directed toward the patient and not the caregiver or family member. Time management will be of concern when taking the history of patients with complex problems, but spending sufficient time and showing patience will help develop the patient-physician relationship and improve care.

The review of systems in the geriatric patient may be complex if the patient is experiencing problems in multiple systems. Focusing on recent changes in constitutional symptoms including fatigue, sleep, weight loss/appetite, pain, and falls may be particularly informative. Fatigue has multiple causes and warrants a thorough evaluation for the underlying cause(s).[55] If sleep is impaired, what is the reason? Sleep management is different if the patient has pain, nocturia, or a mood disorder. Nocturia can result from the nighttime mobilization of peripheral edema. Urinary frequency, urgency, and subjective retention need to be identified and treated. Urinary incontinence should be excluded as a problem, and the examiner should bring up the topic because patients might be embarrassed about raising the problem. Is nutrition adequate? If not, is it because of a financial problem, being physically unable to get to a grocery store, being unable to carry food items back from the store, or being afraid of lifting hot items during cooking? When pain is a symptom, the history should specifically identify the sites and quality of the pain, as many older adults have multiple potential causes of pain.

Patients should be asked if they have fallen in the past year and about the circumstances regarding the fall. The frequency of falls, symptoms experienced at the time of the fall(s), and related injuries need to be determined. Those who report a fall within the past year are at higher risk for future falls. Questions about specific activities of daily living (ADLs) are important. Examples include: "Can you get in and out of a bathtub without assistance?" and "How often do you leave home?" Pain experiences or change in bowel or bladder function should be assessed because some elderly patients may assume new symptoms are as a result of "old age."

Alcohol use needs to be assessed because alcohol may play a role in nutritional deficiencies and falls. Recognize that elderly patients might be having unprotected sexual intercourse with exposure to sexually transmitted diseases and that age alone does not preclude the use of illicit drugs. Does the patient have informal support systems such as neighbors who can be relied on for some degree of assistance? The history should also include a discussion of advanced directives. The patient's goals and wishes should be a priority for the treatment plan and may be different from those of the patient's family and caregivers.

Medication Review

All medications should be reviewed and medicine reconciliation should be performed at each visit. This is especially important if the patient is complaining of new or worsening constitutional and neurologic symptoms. Sedation, confusion, visual problems, insomnia, dizziness, headaches, fatigue, muscle pain, or cramps are some of the many possible common adverse effects of medications. Although these symptoms might not be considered "serious" adverse effects, they do impact function and quality of life and predispose patients to misdiagnosis and adverse events.

Given the risk of falls in the elderly, special attention should be paid to medication with central nervous system activity, such as antidepressants, benzodiazepines, and those with anticholinergic effects. Sleeping pills, antihypertensives, metoclopramide, tricyclic antidepressants, and antiepileptic drugs can cause cognitive impairment. The necessity and efficacy of each medicine should be considered along with renal clearance and potential drug-drug interactions. Is the patient taking the medications as prescribed? Because of the risk for drug-drug interactions, the patient should also be asked if they are taking nonprescription medications, supplements, or vitamins.[65]

Physical Examination

In addition to the standard physiatric physical examination, there are some areas that physicians should be concerned with when evaluating elderly patients.

Neurologic disorders are particularly common causes of disability in elderly patients. Some neurologic changes are associated with normal aging, but abnormal examinations should not be automatically attributed to age-related changes, especially if they correlate with other symptoms or are a change from baseline. Psychomotor slowing, impaired balance, tremors, general loss of muscle or in myotomal distributions, sensory impairments, hypoactive deep tendon reflexes, impaired smell and taste, and change in bowel or bladder control may be difficult to assess in the context of preexisting conditions, and thus a patient and caregiver report is essential. Mental status assessment is a critical part of the geriatric examination and many different measures exist to assess functional status in the clinic setting, including the Mini-Mental State Examination. However, tests of executive function, such as the Executive Interview (Exit25), may correlate better with functional status and be more helpful for longitudinal tracking.[69]

Lower extremity function and performance has good predictive value for disability in community-dwelling adults without disability.[38] Tests of lower extremity function go beyond isolated manual muscle testing and should include balance measures (the Romberg balance test, single leg standing with eyes open or closed, tandem walking or standing, sitting balance); time to walk 8 ft; and rising from a chair five times. Formal balance testing may use the sensory organization test with dynamic posturography to determine whether deficits in the somatosensory, visual, or vestibular system are contributing to postural control problems.

The range of motion of the neck and shoulders should be thoroughly checked. Loss of shoulder internal rotation makes it difficult for the patient to get the hands to the back, as in attaching a bra strap. Loss of shoulder external rotation makes it difficult to get the hands to the top of the head for hair care. It is common to find limitations of hip extension and rotation in the elderly. This can have a negative impact on gait efficiency. In the patient with hip or low back complaints, the Ober test can be used to check for tightness in the tensor fasciae latae and iliotibial band. Limitations of knee extension and flexion should be identified because such losses of range of motion can have a major impact on the efficiency of gait. If decreased range of motion of the ankle is found, it should be determined whether it is caused by a joint capsule contracture, a bony block, or a tight gastrocnemius. Loss of ankle dorsiflexion range of motion that occurs only when the knee is extended is typically caused by tightness in the gastrocnemius. Ankle inversion and eversion range of motion is important for walking on uneven surfaces. Examination of the major joints for stability should be done.

Deformities of the feet are common in the elderly, such as a bunion (hallux valgus). Pes planus can also be present. Hallux rigidus can cause pain and interfere with gait efficiency. Hammer toes can be an incidental finding, a cause of pain, and a potential source of infection if skin integrity is not maintained. Skin calluses indicate the foot surfaces that are weight-bearing. Skin integrity is important in the feet for both prevention of infection and for comfort.

Conditions and Diseases in the Elderly

Frailty

Frailty can be defined as age- and disease-related loss of adaptation, such that events of previously minor stress result in disproportionate biomedical and social consequences. Fried et al.[29] defined frailty as "...an aggregate expression of risk resulting from age- or disease-associated physiologic accumulation of sub-threshold decrements affecting multiple physiologic systems." Or, more objectively, as the phenotype of a clinical syndrome in which three or more of the following are present: (1) unintentional weight loss of at least 10 lb over the past year; (2) self-reported exhaustion; (3) weakness (grip strength); (4) slow walking speed; and (5) low physical activity.[30] Frailty was held by the authors to be distinct from both disability and from comorbidity, although frailty can be a cause of disability. The authors postulated that one pathway in the development of frailty could be attributable to the physiologic changes of aging, with a separate pathway attributable to diseases and comorbidities. The authors also identified an intermediate group of individuals (prefrail) whose risk over 3 years was more than double those with no frailty characteristics at baseline.[30]

Other approaches assess the cumulative deficits in the frail individual with a frailty index, and several have been studied with different validities and predictive values.[79] Frailty, despite the variation in assessment approaches, is a concept that clinicians recognize as a category of patients at risk for adverse outcomes.

Age-related muscle wasting is associated with decreased anabolic function, suggesting that anabolic pathways may be a target for therapy. Studies with exogenous testosterone supplementation have shown improvements in lean body mass, but also increased risk of cardiovascular adverse events.[6] A phase II trial with a nonsteroidal, selective androgen receptor modulator (SARM) in healthy elderly men and postmenopausal women resulted in a dose-dependent improvement in total lean body mass and function.[22] However, the effects on function and risks vary with the SARM tested.[59] Stimulation of anabolic pathways increase cellular protein synthesis by upregulating the mammalian target of rapamycin (mTOR) pathway.[9] However, exogenously increasing anabolism may have negative consequences on life span because inhibition of the mTOR pathway with rapamycin resulted in lifespan extension in male and female mice.[41] Potential functional gains should be weighed with risks of cardiovascular events and decreased total life span in frail older adults.

Disuse and Immobilization

The overall decline in multiple body systems that comes with aging can be exacerbated by immobility.[60] The effects of bed rest and immobility have been studied for several decades and have parallels with the physical repercussions of space flight. These studies have shown that it is the combination of inactivity and lack of mechanical loading that produce the characteristic negative effects of bed rest.

Head down–bed rest studies have ranged from 7 to 120 days and show that loss of muscle mass from bed rest varies between muscle groups with lower extremity muscles being more affected than upper extremity muscles. Bed rest also leads to a loss of strength and power, which is even greater than loss of muscle mass. Other effects of immobilization include increased muscle insulin resistance; increased bone loss from increased calcium excretion and decreased calcium resorption; decreased pulmonary function and exercise capacity; orthostatic hypotension; and impaired balance and coordination.[60] Many of these conditions are already present in older adults, which suggest why immobility has more serious consequences for the elderly than for younger patients. Immobilization can combine with incontinence, skin fragility, and inadequate nutrition in the elderly to greatly increase the risk for pressure ulcers. Immobility from bed rest is a predictor of decline in ADLs, institutionalization, and death in hospitalized older patients.[13] Vigilance is needed to prevent or minimize the immobilization of elderly patients unless absolutely required by their medical condition.

Falls

Falls are common in the elderly and a major cause of morbidity. Falls cause the majority of the fractures of the forearm, hip, and pelvis in the elderly and increase the risk of placement in a skilled nursing facility. There are multiple risk factors for falls, of which the physician should be aware (Box 30-1).[82]

BOX 30-1

Risk Factors for Falls in the Elderly

- Age
- Physical impairments (gait dysfunction, muscle weakness, dizziness or balance impairment, visual impairment)
- Cognitive impairment, dementia, depression
- Previous falls
- Medications (psychoactive medications, total number of medications)
- Comorbid conditions (diabetes, Parkinson's disease)
- Chronic pain and arthritis
- Poor functional status

Adapted from Panel on Prevention of Falls in Older Persons, American Geriatrics Society and British Geriatrics Society: Summary of the updated American Geriatrics Society/British Geriatrics Society clinical practice guideline for prevention of falls in older persons, *J Am Geriatr Soc* 59:148-157, 2011; Stubbs B, Binnekade T, Eggermont L, et al: Pain and the risk for falls in community-dwelling older adults: systematic review and meta-analysis, *Arch Phys Med Rehabil* 95:175-187, 2014; Tinetti ME, Kumar C: The patient who falls: "it's always a trade-off," *JAMA* 303:258-266, 2010.

Cognitive impairment and dementia increase risk of falls, possibly as a result of decreased cognitive reserve and limited attentional resources that impair multitasking, such as walking while talking.[84] Impaired dual-tasking, as assessed with gait analysis, may be an objective marker of fall risk.[54] High-risk medications for falls are those with central nervous system activity including antidepressants, antipsychotics, antiepileptics, benzodiazepines, opioids, sedatives and muscle relaxants, antihistamines, and anticholinergics.

Age-related changes in gait are associated with falling and fear of falling in the elderly and include reduced stride length and speed; increased double-support time; and increased variability in stride length and speed. Chronic back, hip, knee, and foot, which also affect gait, can increase fall risk.[75] Pain is an important clinical sign that should raise concern for risk of falls, is usually assessed at each clinic visit, and can be linked to gait dysfunction by the rehabilitation specialist. Environmental conditions, such as dim lighting and high beds, can contribute to falls.

Fall prevention in the elderly has been studied in the acute care and community-dwelling settings with some distinctions between the two. Several systematic reviews of studies examining interventions to prevent falls or injuries related to falls have been performed.[17,20,35,58] Recommendations to prevent falls and fall-related injuries are summarized in Box 30-2.

Osteoarthritis

Osteoarthritis (OA) is a degenerative disease of the entire joint and involves all tissues of the joint. This is not simply an issue of wear and tear, but an end-stage phenotype of abnormal balance of breakdown and repair analogous to failure in other organs. Arthritis is common among older adults and those with multiple chronic conditions. Of those over 65 years of age, 50% were diagnosed with arthritis and 44% had limitations in activity related to this condition.[4]

BOX 30-2

Recommendations for Fall and Injury Prevention in the Elderly

- Fall risk assessment by qualified health care professionals or teams
- Individualized, group, and home-based exercise
- Balance, strength, and gait training exercise (e.g., tai chi)
- Home safety evaluations and modifications
- Medication review and reduction programs with family physician and patient involvement
- Careful, medically directed tapering of high-risk medications
- Addressing foot/ankle pain and dysfunction
- Treating vitamin D deficiency (at least 800 international units per day)
- Cataract surgery and dual chamber cardiac pacing if indicated

Adapted from Panel on Prevention of Falls in Older Persons, American Geriatrics Society and British Geriatrics Society: Summary of the updated American Geriatrics Society/British Geriatrics Society clinical practice guideline for prevention of falls in older persons, *J Am Geriatr Soc* 59:148-157, 2011.

Multiple joints are often affected in the same individual, but the most common sites are the hands and knees. The hips and spine are also frequently affected by OA and are significant sources of pain and disability. OA of the spine typically involves the back or neck at the synovial facet joints or the vertebral body with disk desiccation and can result in problems with structural integrity of the three-joint complex of the vertebral segment. Progressive degeneration can lead to spinal stenosis that affects the central canal and lateral recesses, which could cause spinal cord or nerve root impingement with neurologic signs.

Older adults and females have an increased risk of OA and evidence is increasing for genetic predisposition.[45] Other general risk factors include obesity and possibly diet that is inadequate in nutritional content. Modifiable risk factors for the joint include muscle strength. For example, knee extensor and flexor weakness may predispose the joint to OA or potentiate the process.[45]

Treatment decisions for OA include nonpharmacologic interventions (e.g., strengthening the musculature surrounding the joint and physical modalities for pain). Pharmacologic interventions include acetaminophen for pain and nonsteroidal antiinflammatory drugs for pain and swelling. However, these medications affect liver and renal function and may cause GI bleeding. Opioids including tramadol have modest pain-relieving effects, but have tolerance issues and side effect profiles that outweigh the benefits, especially in the elderly, making them inappropriate choices for OA treatment. Intraarticular corticosteroid injections have demonstrated short-term benefits for treating knee OA[8] and avoid the systemic complications of oral medications. Total hip arthroplasty (THA) and total knee arthroplasty (TKA) are frequently performed surgical interventions for hip and knee OA, respectively, with high patient satisfaction and good outcomes in older adults who are surgical candidates. Patients with poor physical fitness and health before surgery are at risk for increased perioperative morbidity and mortality and arthroplasty failure. In general, younger age is a risk factor for THA and TKA revision; however, older age may be associated with increased risk for THA revision as a result of dislocation.[63]

Osteopenia and Osteoporosis

The elderly have an increased incidence of osteopenia and osteoporosis affecting approximately 52 million people in the United States.[53] Low bone density in older adults increases risks of hand/wrist, hip, and vertebral body fractures, which can result in significant pain, immobility, and loss of functional independence.[24] Bone mineral density measurements with dual energy x-ray absorptiometry (DEXA) scans are typically used to diagnose and track low bone density and osteoporosis. Osteopenia is defined as bone mineral density with a T score between −1.0 and −2.5 where the normal young adult level is −1 or greater, and osteoporosis is present if the T score is −2.5 or less. Low bone density occurs in both genders, but is more common in postmenopausal women and increases risk of fractures. Risk factors for osteopenia and osteoporosis include increasing age, family history, glucocorticoid therapy, and smoking.

Intervention with the bisphosphonates (alendronate, risedronate, zoledronic acid) has been shown to reduce risk of hip, vertebral, and nonvertebral fractures in postmenopausal women with osteoporosis.[53] The risk of fracture is further decreased when alendronate is used in combination with calcium. Vitamin D levels show seasonal variation and decline with age. Oral supplementation with more than 800 units of vitamin D may reduce fracture risk and may be combined with calcium. Menopausal hormone therapy (MHT) reduces the risk of fracture in postmenopausal women, but not in women with osteoporosis. MHT with estrogen was used widely in the past, but because of negative side effects, selective estrogen receptor modulators, such as raloxifene, were developed. However, treatment with raloxifene is also associated with increased risk adverse reactions and events, such as pulmonary embolism, thromboembolisms, and muscle/limb pain.

There is currently insufficient evidence for type, frequency, or duration of exercise as an effective intervention or prevention for osteoporosis. The extensive knowledge about bone demineralization gained from bed rest studies and their correlates with aging,[60] however, suggests that more well-controlled clinical trials should be performed to determine the effect of exercise on prevention of these conditions.

Hip Fractures

Hip fractures are more common in older adults and are associated with increased morbidity, mortality, and health care use and costs.[24] These injuries result in long-term disability and increased functional dependence because many elderly never regain premorbid functional status after sustaining a hip fracture. Risk factors for hip fractures in elderly individuals include falls and the associated risks of fall, which usually occur from a standing position. Osteoporosis is also associated with increased risk of hip fractures, especially in women, which can be complicated by the increased rate of bone loss that occurs during the first year after hip fracture because of impaired mobility during recovery. The skeletal fragility after hip fracture increases risk of subsequent fractures.[24]

Prognosis for hip fractures in older adults is not encouraging and is likely to depend on the type and severity of fracture as well as the patient's premorbid health and comorbidities. Patients should be referred to an orthopedic surgeon to determine need and planning for surgical fixation. Because older patients typically have difficulty walking, with limited weight-bearing, the choices in surgical approach, fixation, and implants should allow weight-bearing as tolerated as soon as possible with overall goals of decreasing pain and returning patients to a prefracture level of function.

Fractures of the femoral neck are at risk for avascular necrosis because of the tenuous blood supply to the area. Most femoral neck fractures will require surgical fixation. Randomized controlled trials, systematic reviews, and metaanalysis have shown that for femoral neck fractures, arthroplasty has clear benefits over open reduction internal fixation (ORIF) in elderly patients.[16] THA and hemiarthroplasty (HA) have similar mortality rates with some studies showing decreased pain, increased function, and improved quality of life after THA; however, there is less risk of dislocation after HA.[15,16] Intertrochanteric fractures occur between the greater and lesser trochanters. The extracapsular region has good blood supply, and fractures in this region may heal better than femoral neck fractures with most treated with an ORIF. Subtrochanteric fractures occur distal to the lesser trochanter, although classification systems vary. Blood supply in this region is not as good as the intertrochanteric region and thus healing may be slower. Treatment of unstable subtrochanteric fractures is usually by ORIF, and increased force attributable to muscle attachments in this region may complicate recovery.

Rehabilitation of hip fractures should emphasize weight-bearing as soon as possible with goals of pain control and early loading while avoiding fracture dislocation or implant failure. Ideally, postfracture rehabilitation starts in the acute hospital setting and then continues at the appropriate postacute setting per individual needs. The multidisciplinary team approach to hip fracture rehabilitation may have better patient outcomes than approaches with usual care.[39] Multidisciplinary teams are composed of individuals from different clinical disciplines treating the same patient and in this case are led by physiatrists or geriatricians. Most rehabilitation programs aim to initiate mobilization early in the recovery course. However, the ideal time to initiate mobilization, setting, exercise, therapy types, and length of treatment course have not been conclusively determined by a metaanalysis because of the significant differences in clinical trials that investigated these issues.[40] Ideal rehabilitation programs are likely to depend on the individual patient's condition.

Stroke

Stroke is a leading cause of acute neurologic admissions to hospitals and death worldwide. Mortality rates from stroke have continued to decline during the twentieth century[52]; however, stroke survivors can be burdened with significant disability. Outcomes after stroke are worse among older adults because of other age-related comorbidities and frailty.

Patients who have access to advanced medical care benefit from improvements in stroke rehabilitation that begins in the acute setting and continues into the outpatient clinics where strengthening, range-of-motion, spasticity management, low-vision, cognitive, and urinary incontinence interventions can be performed. Most strokes are of the ischemic type and risk factors include previous stroke or transient ischemic attack, hypertension, hyperlipidemia, heart disease, and diabetes, which are common comorbid conditions among older patients.

Traumatic Brain Injury

Individuals over the age of 75 years have the highest incidence of hospitalizations and death as a result of traumatic brain injury.[80] The majority of these injuries are attributable to falls, followed by motor vehicle collisions. Poorer outcomes after head injury are associated with increasing age. Risk factors for traumatic brain injury attributable to falls in the elderly include physical and cognitive impairments along with having multiple medical conditions and medications (refer to the section on "Falls" discussed earlier).

Subdural hematomas (SDHs) among elderly are more common because age-related brain atrophy increases the subdural space, and vascular aging makes the bridging veins more fragile and susceptible to tears. The use of anticoagulant medication also increases the likelihood of an intracranial bleed. Concussions are common in the elderly and even mild head injuries can result in SDHs that develop slowly over weeks to months and go without detection until symptomatic, at which time surgical referral is required.

Spinal Cord Injury

Management of elderly patients with new spinal cord injury (SCI) or injury incurred when they were younger is complicated by the other pathophysiologic characteristics of this age group. Loss of bone mass and changes in body composition that occur with aging can increase the risk of SCI. Traumatic SCI in older adults is more likely to be from falls (even minor ones) followed by motor vehicle collisions. An elderly adult who sustains a SCI from a fall may have one or more preexisting condition(s) that increased their risk for fall (as discussed earlier in the section on "Falls"). Nontraumatic SCI in older adults may be attributable to cervical or lumbar spinal stenosis as a consequence of degenerative joint processes, disk herniation, or mass effect from hematomas or tumor growth that cause narrowing of the spinal canal.[44]

First-year survival after SCI is relatively good. However, mortality rates for those with SCI increase dramatically with age compared with the general population, depending on the level and severity of injury.[23] In elderly patients, those with incomplete and lower levels of SCI have mortality rates comparable to the general population.[23]

Dementia

Dementia is often equated with Alzheimer disease; however, the term is not synonymous with a single disease or etiology, but is a group of symptoms that affect the patient's daily function because of executive cognitive dysfunction, memory impairment, and mood, personality, and behavioral changes. There are several types and causes of dementing illnesses including those that are reversible with treatment, such as SDH, normal pressure hydrocephalus (NPH), depression, hormonal imbalances, drug and alcohol abuse, and vitamin deficiency.

Traditionally, the diagnosis of dementia has been used in those cases where the pathology and symptoms are not reversible such as those found with Alzheimer, Parkinson, and Huntington disease, AIDS, after repeated neurovascular insults, and severe or repetitive traumatic brain injuries. Alzheimer type dementia is thought to be the most common cause of progressive dementia in people over the age 65 years.

Because of the progressive and nonreversible nature of some dementing illnesses, early identification has been considered critical for determining appropriate treatment, planning long-term care, or developing interventional strategies. Mild cognitive impairment (MCI) is a clinical diagnosis used to designate an early, cognitive dysfunction in one or more cognitive domains that is not age-related. MCI is thought to be attributable to a neurodegenerative process that is differentiated from normal aging and lies on a spectrum between normal aging and dementia or Alzheimer disease. MCI is therefore considered a clinically identifiable precursor to Alzheimer disease. The conversion rate of MCI subjects to Alzheimer disease is accelerated compared with controls and the initial estimate was 12% per year.[61]

The effect of exercise on dementia has been studied extensively and the results of systematic reviews and meta-analyses are encouraging.[28,62] Exercise programs for cognitive impairment and dementia have varied in frequency between twice-weekly to daily and typically use aerobic exercise with positive effects on cognitive function and the ability to perform ADLs; however, these interventions had no significant effect on depression.[28,62]

Delirium

Delirium is an acute neurocognitive disorder that is transient and usually reversible, but can be persistent and disabling. Although patients in any age group can experience delirium, it occurs more commonly among the elderly and those with mental status impairments. Diagnostic criteria for delirium include: disturbance in attention and awareness that develops over a short period of time, is a change from baseline, and waxes and wanes during the course of the day; a disturbance in cognition; the disturbances in attention and cognition are not better explained by a preexisting neurocognitive disorder; there is evidence that the disturbance is directly due to a pathophysiologic process such as a medical condition or drug-induced toxicity.[3]

Workup of delirium should include a thorough review of potentially problematic medications, with attention to central nervous system–acting drugs, such as pain medications (particularly opioids), any medication prescribed for sleep, antihistamines, anxiolytics, muscle relaxants, and antidepressants.

Normal Pressure Hydrocephalus

The hallmark signs of NPH are dementia, gait disturbance, and urinary incontinence along with ventriculomegaly with normal cerebrospinal fluid pressures. Ataxia is an important clinical sign of NPH and early changes vary among patients, which can make differentiating these gait abnormalities from a Parkinsonian gait difficult. As NPH worsens, the patient may have difficulty initiating foot movement and clearance appearing as though the feet are attached to the floor by a magnet; a "magnetic gait." NPH can be idiopathic or related to previous meningitis or subarachnoid hemorrhage. It is one of the reversible causes of dementia and has been estimated to account for approximately 5% of dementia cases.[73] The reduced physical turgor of the brain tissue with aging is thought by some experts to allow even normal pressure to produce hydrocephalus and brain atrophy. In some cases, shunting to achieve a reduction in central nervous system fluid pressure can dramatically reverse the patient's condition. Most clinical trials of surgical treatment for NPH have compared shunting techniques, approaches, and shunt materials, but no randomized, blinded, placebo-controlled clinical trials have been performed to study efficacy of shunt placement in the treatment of NPH.[25]

Parkinson Disease

Parkinson disease is a progressive neurodegenerative disease present in up to 2% of people older than 60 years manifesting clinically with ataxia, bradykinesia, tremor, and cog-wheel rigidity. Patients with Parkinson disease may also have dementia. The tremor is present at rest and increases with stress. Voluntary movements are slow. Parkinsonian gait is characterized by small, shuffling steps without arm swing. It is difficult for the patient to initiate walking or other position changes, and turning is particularly difficult and unsteady. The gait can be festinating, in which gait speed increases as the patient attempts to prevent falling forward because of an abnormal center of gravity. Early in disease course, medications are prescribed to control symptoms, but eventually may necessitate the use of carbidopa-levodopa or dopamine agonists. Deep-brain stimulation has been effective in treating advanced Parkinson disease and shows promise in the early stages of disease.[72] Resistance training also appears to have positive effects on strength and function in those with mild to moderate Parkinson disease.[11]

Amputation

Most lower extremity amputations occur in older adults (over 65 years of age) and are usually attributable to vascular disease. Life expectancy in older adults after amputation is shorter and only 53% survive to be fitted with a prosthesis.[18] Prognosis for successful prosthetic rehabilitation is influenced by the number and types of comorbidities. Cardiovascular disease is usually present in patients who underwent dysvascular amputations, and the increased energy demands of patients who use a prosthetic may result in poor outcomes.[27] This is also true with comorbid respiratory disease, which may adversely affect gait retraining. Patients with end-stage renal failure may frequently miss rehabilitation times because of dialysis commitments and may experience frequent changes in limb volume that complicate prosthetic fit.[27]

Premorbid function is a more important predictor of successful prosthetic rehabilitation than age, although some older patients may have difficulty with gait retraining.[27] This is particularly true if the patient has cognitive impairment or dementia.

Cancer

Cancer is more prevalent among those over 65 years and increases exponentially with age. The cancer prevalence rates are expected to increase with the increasing elderly population. Multiple types of cancers contribute to mortality including prostate, bladder, colorectal, pancreas, stomach, lung, and uterus. Treating cancer in elderly patients is challenging because the geriatric oncologist must consider coexisting comorbidity and cognitive/functional status in addition to cancer type when considering treatment courses. Having multiple comorbid conditions increases the likelihood that the patient may die from non–cancer-related causes. The effects of treatment may compete with the patient's interests and wishes. Encouragingly, after cancer diagnosis is made, moderate physical activity of 150 minutes per week decreases total mortality risk by 24% among breast cancer survivors and 28% among colorectal cancer survivors.[71]

Polypharmacy

Polypharmacy, the use of multiple drugs by a patient, is a concern because the number of potential interactions increases as more medications are used. Older adults are at risk for adverse drug reactions (ADRs) resulting from multiple drug regimens and changes in drug metabolism associated with aging. Premarketing drug trials are commonly performed in younger adults and thus the side effects of these medications in elderly patients are not as well understood. Common ADRs include dizziness, insomnia, confusion, sedation, nausea, changes in bowel habits, and balance problems. Medication side effects can be confused as symptoms of a new illness rather than as an adverse reaction to medications. Prescribing new medications to treat symptoms that are as a result of an unrecognized ADR of an existing therapy is known as "the prescribing cascade."[67] This may further complicate the problem and increase the risk for adverse drug events, such as falls and delirium. One study[65] found that 29% of surveyed people between 57 and 85 years of age used at least five prescription medications and 46% of those with prescription medications also used over-the-counter medications. Four percent of individuals were at risk of a major potential drug-drug interaction and more than half of the major interactions involved nonprescription medications.[65] Many prescribers are wary of life-threatening ADRs or drug-drug interactions, but increased vigilance for common ADRs, which are by definition more likely to occur, may decrease the risk for iatrogenic adverse events.

Management Issues in the Elderly

The complex intermingling of comorbid conditions with frailty and disability can challenge the physician evaluating and treating older adults. Separating these issues into individual components is a helpful first step toward identifying treatment targets and developing treatment plans that improve function, decrease disability and mortality, and prevent adverse outcomes.[29] Rehabilitation specialists should realize that the presence of two or more chronic diseases/conditions increases the risk of disability and frailty.

Medication Management

Compliance with a medication program can be a problem because of the complexity of the regimen proposed, the cost of the medication, and the cognitive status of the patient. The treatment plan for an elderly patient has to be realistic and the prescriber must bear in mind that taking a medication multiple times per day challenges compliance for patients of all ages. It is better to work with the patient and caregivers to design a medication schedule that can actually be carried out rather than devise a plan that will work only under optimal conditions. This is particularly important if something completely new is being introduced to the patient, such as expecting a person with new diabetes and limited vision to learn to adjust insulin, check blood glucose levels four times a day, and change food preparation habits within a very short time. The inpatient rehabilitation setting affords the opportunity to consider feasibility of medication regimen concerns and monitor for ADRs.

Most clinical practice guidelines are developed with consideration of a single disease entity and do not apply to the older adult with complex comorbidities.[10] Treatment plans that approach diseases in isolation may not be the most effective or safest approach to use in an elderly patient with multiple comorbidities.[10,81] For example, prescribing an antihistamine for pruritus caused by xerosis in a patient who is also taking psychotropic medications for anxiety or depression increases the risk of sedation and falls. Because drug elimination is affected by age-related changes in hepatic and renal clearance, drug levels should be monitored closely.[49] Ideally, the physiatrist would partner with the referring geriatrician and a pharmacist in a multidisciplinary case conference to prioritize the patient's health care needs and goals to avoid ADRs or inappropriate prescribing.

Pain Management

Pain management in the elderly should include both pharmacologic and nonpharmacologic measures. Nonpharmacologic measures are even more important in the elderly than in the general adult population because of the increased risk for ADRs. The elderly frequently have less tolerance for pain medication, especially of the opioid type. Doses might need to be modified for those with impaired renal function or cognitive problems.

Nutrition

Weight loss and low body mass index are associated with higher mortality in the elderly and go hand in hand with poor nutrition. Some factors that are associated with increased likelihood of weight loss are possibly modifiable: depression, swallowing or chewing problems, inadequate oral intake, and feeding dependence.[77] Daily protein intake goals for adults older than 65 years should be 1.0 to 1.2 g/kg body weight per day.[7]

Adequate and appropriate nutrition guidelines for older patients may be dictated by their comorbid medical conditions (e.g., diabetes, cardiovascular or renal disease). Older adults with chronic disease may require increased protein intake (1.2 to 1.4 g/kg body weight per day), but those with severe renal disease, but not on dialysis, may need to limit protein intake.[7] Nutritional recommendations for sarcopenia are adequate protein and caloric intake, possibly obtained with a balanced protein/energy supplement. Overall, there should be an increase in protein intake, with goals of 1.0 to 1.5 g/kg body weight per day.[56] Leucine-enriched balanced essential amino acid mix and creatine supplements may help with sarcopenia.[56] Patients with sarcopenia should have vitamin D levels measured and treated accordingly. Patients who are prescribed anabolic therapeutics will also have increased dietary energy and protein needs.

Physical Exercise in the Elderly

Regular physical exercise in older adults can improve strength, range of motion, balance and coordination, reduce risk of cardiovascular disease, stroke, hypertension, obesity, type 2 diabetes, osteoporosis, and so on.[2] An exercise program may start with formal physical therapy individualized for the patient's diagnosis and condition, followed by a home program that the patient can perform independently.

Aerobic exercise can result in a lower resting heart rate, lower blood pressure, positive changes in muscle oxygen uptake, increased VO_{2max}, and cardioprotective effects[2] in healthy older adults after 3 to 4 months of moderate-intensity aerobic exercise. Other changes include improvements in body composition, improved glycemic control, postprandial lipid clearance, and slowing age-related decline in bone mass density.

Resistance training can lead to improved muscle force, power, muscle endurance, and increased bone mass density. Resistance training can also improve body composition: increased muscle cross-sectional area, muscle volume, and decreased body fat. Resistance training can be performed with machines or with callisthenic-based exercises, such as push-ups, squats, and sit-ups, that can be simplified for progressive loading and performed without equipment. Isometric exercises can activate muscles without joint involvement, which may be useful in patients with arthritis. However, care must be taken to avoid inadvertent Valsalva maneuvers. Weight-based training with machines, dumbbells, and barbells are also commonly used, but the latter two require much more balance, which may increase risk of injury.

Most research regarding balance and exercise in older adults has been with participants who were at risk for fall or fall-related injury.[42] Improved balance can come from dynamic standing balance training, computerized balance training and biofeedback, aerobic exercise, such as walking and cycling, resistance/strengthening exercise, and comprehensive activities, such as yoga and tai chi.[42]

It is possible to increase joint range of motion in older adults with dedicated stretching programs for the upper extremities, lower extremities, and spine. Some flexibility activities (yoga, tai chi, dancing) have components of strength, balance, and flexibility and may be useful choices of comprehensive exercise because the most effective type and duration of flexibility training has not been determined.[2]

For older adults with no limiting condition, an activity plan should be developed that includes the different recommended activities (Box 30-3).[57] Those individuals with chronic conditions should have plans that are both therapeutic and preventative, with emphasis on exercise most beneficial to the limiting condition (e.g., aerobic training for an individual with cardiovascular disease compared

BOX 30-3

Activity Recommendations in Older Adults With no Limitations

- Moderate-intensity aerobic activity: enough to result in noticeably increased heart rate and breathing, for at least 30 minutes 5 days a week.
- Resistance training (calisthenics, weight training): at least one set of 10 to 15 repetitions of an exercise that trains the major muscle groups on 2 or 3 nonconsecutive days each week.
- Flexibility: at least 10 minutes of stretching major muscle and tendon groups at least 2 days each week; 10 to 30 seconds of static stretches and three to four repetitions for each stretch. Ideally performed every day that aerobic and resistance training is performed.
- (Possibly) Balance exercise three times a week (ideal type, frequency, and duration has not been defined).

Adapted from American College of Sports Medicine, Chodzko-Zajko WJ, Proctor DN, Fiatarone Singh MA, et al: American College of Sports Medicine position stand. Exercise and physical activity for older adults, *Med Sci Sports Exerc* 41:1510-1530, 2009; Nelson ME, Rejeski WJ, Blair SN, et al: Physical activity and public health in older adults: recommendation from the American College of Sports Medicine and the American Heart Association, *Med Sci Sports Exerc* 39:1435-1445, 2007.

with weight-bearing/resistance training for someone with osteoporosis). A gradual increase in activity is recommended for sedentary, low fitness older adults new to an exercise program. This may mean several months of less than recommended intensity and volume. Barring any limiting condition, all exercise programs should have beneficial effects on lower extremity function (balance, walking speed, ability to rise from a chair), which are factors associated with possible future disability.[38]

Ambulatory Assistive Devices

Ambulation might require the use of assistive devices. A single-point or quad cane can be used to take some weight off a painful hip and provide additional stability for balance problems. For off-loading weight, it should be used in the hand opposite the painful extremity. Crutches are a poor choice in the elderly because of the increased demands on balance and energy. A walker provides stability and allows the person to convey items from place to place with a bag or basket on the walker. A platform walker can be used if hand or wrist function limits grip on a standard style. Wheelchairs allow for distance mobility in the community, even if not used within the home.

Orthoses and Footwear

Changes in footwear can improve stability with movement. Lower heels cause weight bearing to be spread over more of the foot than high heels, and change the work of the quadriceps. High-topped shoes that extend above the ankles give additional sensory feedback to foot position. Air stirrup devices can also serve this function and give additional ankle stability. Orthotic devices can help with pes planus. Over-the-counter shoe orthoses might provide adequate improvement, but many conditions require custom shoe insert orthoses to handle specific foot problems.

Psychosocial Support

The elderly have to deal with losses of family, friends, jobs, and function. These losses can lead to depression, even in people who never had depression earlier in life. Social work and psychology services are often critical in managing these life changes. Some problems can be addressed by facilitating access to services that an individual might not otherwise know about. For example, giving up a driver's license can lead to a difficult lifestyle change, but it can be made easier if the individual learns to use the available transportation services.

Modifying the Environment for the Elderly

Modifying the environment can have a positive impact on health, injury prevention, and quality of life. Chairs can be designed to ease the difficulty an elderly person has in changing position. No-slip rugs, improved lighting, lights along the running boards in the hallways for nighttime bathroom trips, and decreased bed height can prevent falls and fall-related injuries.[58] Design of larger spaces within the home, such as accessibility to the kitchen or bathroom while a rolling walker is used, can have a major impact on comfort and safety.

Modifying the environment can be carried out on a broader scale, such as when traffic lights are timed to allow adequate time for elderly persons to safely cross a street. Design of the community can encourage exercise in general and walking in particular. Street lighting should be sufficient to be safe for an elderly pedestrian. When elderly individuals can no longer safely drive because of visual problems, affordable and reliable alternative means of transportation are needed to ensure access to community centers and other places of activity for the elderly. One of the major effects of the Americans with Disabilities Act has been to make institutions and the individuals who run them more cognizant of the direct impact of architecture on mobility.

Summary

Physical medicine and rehabilitation emphasizes patient function and goals and is well suited to care for elderly individuals with complex medical needs. The holistic physiatric approach does not focus on single disease entities and thus may be the ideal strategy for promoting successful aging through increased independence, high-level functioning, overcoming disability and recovering from illness, and involvement in health-promoting activities.

KEY REFERENCES

1. Aggarwal A, Ades PA: Exercise rehabilitation of older patients with cardiovascular disease, *Cardiol Clin* 19:525–536, 2001.
2. American College of Sports Medicine, Chodzko-Zajko WJ, Proctor DN, Fiatarone Singh MA, et al: American College of Sports Medicine position stand. Exercise and physical activity for older adults, *Med Sci Sports Exerc* 41:1510–1530, 2009.
4. Barbour KE, Helmick CG, Theis KA, et al: Prevalence of doctor-diagnosed arthritis and arthritis-attributable activity limitation: United States, 2010-2012, *MMWR Morbid Mortal Wkly Rep* 62:869–873, 2013.

7. Bauer J, Biolo G, Cederholm T, et al: Evidence-based recommendations for optimal dietary protein intake in older people: a position paper from the PROT-AGE Study Group, *J Am Med Dir Assoc* 14:542–559, 2013.
8. Bellamy N, Campbell J, Robinson V, et al: Intraarticular corticosteroid for treatment of osteoarthritis of the knee, *Cochrane Database Syst Rev* (2):CD005328, 2006.
10. Boyd CM, Darer J, Boult C, et al: Clinical practice guidelines and quality of care for older patients with multiple comorbid diseases: implications for pay for performance, *JAMA* 294:716–724, 2005.
12. Britton E, McLaughlin JT: Ageing and the gut, *Proc Nutr Soc* 72:173–177, 2013.
14. Brunner F, Schmid A, Sheikhzadeh A, et al: Effects of aging on type II muscle fibers: a systematic review of the literature, *J Aging Phys Act* 15:336–348, 2007.
17. Cameron ID, Gillespie LD, Robertson MC, et al: Interventions for preventing falls in older people in care facilities and hospitals, *Cochrane Database Syst Rev* (12):CD005465, 2012.
19. Chang AL, Wong JW, Endo JO, Norman RA: Geriatric dermatology review: major changes in skin function in older patients and their contribution to common clinical challenges, *J Am Med Dir Assoc* 14:724–730, 2013.
20. Choi M, Hector M: Effectiveness of intervention programs in preventing falls: a systematic review of recent 10 years and meta-analysis, *J Am Med Dir Assoc* 13:188, e13–e21, 2012.
22. Dalton JT, Barnette KG, Bohl CE, et al: The selective androgen receptor modulator GTx-024 (enobosarm) improves lean body mass and physical function in healthy elderly men and postmenopausal women: results of a double-blind, placebo-controlled phase II trial, *J Cachexia Sarcopenia Muscle* 2:153–161, 2011.
28. Forbes D, Thiessen EJ, Blake CM, et al: Exercise programs for people with dementia, *Cochrane Database Syst Rev* (12):CD006489, 2013.
29. Fried LP, Ferrucci L, Darer J, et al: Untangling the concepts of disability, frailty, and comorbidity: implications for improved targeting and care, *J Gerontol A Biol Sci Med Sci* 59:255–263, 2004.
30. Fried LP, Tangen CM, Walston J, et al: Frailty in older adults: evidence for a phenotype, *J Gerontol A Biol Sci Med Sci* 56:M146–M156, 2001.
35. Gillespie LD, Robertson MC, Gillespie WJ, et al: Interventions for preventing falls in older people living in the community, *Cochrane Database Syst Rev* (9):CD007146, 2012.
38. Guralnik JM, Ferrucci L, Pieper CF, et al: Lower extremity function and subsequent disability: consistency across studies, predictive models, and value of gait speed alone compared with the short physical performance battery, *J Gerontol A Biol Sci Med Sci* 55:M221–M231, 2000.
39. Handoll HH, Cameron ID, Mak JC, Finnegan TP: Multidisciplinary rehabilitation for older people with hip fractures, *Cochrane Database Syst Rev* (4):CD007125, 2009.
40. Handoll HH, Sherrington C, Mak JC: Interventions for improving mobility after hip fracture surgery in adults, *Cochrane Database Syst Rev* (3):CD001704, 2011.
41. Harrison DE, Strong R, Sharp ZD, et al: Rapamycin fed late in life extends lifespan in genetically heterogeneous mice, *Nature* 460:392–395, 2009.
42. Howe TE, Rochester L, Neil F, et al: Exercise for improving balance in older people, *Cochrane Database Syst Rev* (11):CD004963, 2011.
46. Kalyani RR, Corriere M, Ferrucci L: Age-related and disease-related muscle loss: the effect of diabetes, obesity, and other diseases, *Lancet Diabetes Endocrinol* 2:819–829, 2014.
47. Karam Z, Tuazon J: Anatomic and physiologic changes of the aging kidney, *Clin Geriatr Med* 29:555–564, 2013.
49. Klotz U: Pharmacokinetics and drug metabolism in the elderly, *Drug Metab Rev* 41:67–76, 2009.
50. Kongkaew C, Noyce PR, Ashcroft DM: Hospital admissions associated with adverse drug reactions: a systematic review of prospective observational studies, *Ann Pharmacother* 42:1017–1025, 2008.
51. Kottner J, Lichterfeld A, Blume-Peytavi U: Maintaining skin integrity in the aged: a systematic review, *Br J Dermatol* 169:528–542, 2013.
53. Levis S, Theodore G: Summary of AHRQ's comparative effectiveness review of treatment to prevent fractures in men and women with low bone density or osteoporosis: update of the 2007 report, *J Manag Care Pharm* 18:S1–S15, discussion S13, 2012.
54. Montero-Odasso M, Verghese J, Beauchet O, Hausdorff JM: Gait and cognition: a complementary approach to understanding brain function and the risk of falling, *J Am Geriatr Soc* 60:2127–2136, 2012.
55. Morelli V: Toward a comprehensive differential diagnosis and clinical approach to fatigue in the elderly, *Clin Geriatr Med* 27:687–692, 2011.
56. Morley JE, Argiles JM, Evans WJ, et al: Nutritional recommendations for the management of sarcopenia, *J Am Med Dir Assoc* 11:391–396, 2010.
57. Nelson ME, Rejeski WJ, Blair SN, et al: Physical activity and public health in older adults: recommendation from the American College of Sports Medicine and the American Heart Association, *Med Sci Sports Exerc* 39:1435–1445, 2007.
58. Panel on Prevention of Falls in Older Persons, American Geriatrics Society and British Geriatrics Society: Summary of the updated American Geriatrics Society/British Geriatrics Society clinical practice guideline for prevention of falls in older persons, *J Am Geriatr Soc* 59:148–157, 2011.
59. Papanicolaou DA, Ather SN, Zhu H, et al: A phase IIA randomized, placebo-controlled clinical trial to study the efficacy and safety of the selective androgen receptor modulator (SARM), MK-0773 in female participants with sarcopenia, *J Nutr Health Aging* 17:533–543, 2013.
60. Pavy-Le Traon A, Heer M, Narici MV, et al: From space to Earth: advances in human physiology from 20 years of bed rest studies (1986-2006), *Eur J Appl Physiol* 101:143–194, 2007.
62. Potter R, Ellard D, Rees K, Thorogood M: A systematic review of the effects of physical activity on physical functioning, quality of life and depression in older people with dementia, *Int J Geriatr Psychiatry* 26:1000–1011, 2011.
63. Prokopetz JJ, Losina E, Bliss RL, et al: Risk factors for revision of primary total hip arthroplasty: a systematic review, *BMC Musculoskelet Disord* 13:251, 2012.
65. Qato DM, Alexander G, Conti RM, et al: Use of prescription and over-the-counter medications and dietary supplements among older adults in the United States, *JAMA* 300:2867–2878, 2008.
67. Rochon PA, Gurwitz JH: Optimising drug treatment for elderly people: the prescribing cascade, *BMJ* 315:1096–1099, 1997.
69. Royall DR, Palmer R, Chiodo LK, Polk MJ: Declining executive control in normal aging predicts change in functional status: the Freedom House Study, *J Am Geriatr Soc* 52:346–352, 2004.
70. Royall DR, Palmer R, Chiodo LK, Polk MJ: Normal rates of cognitive change in successful aging: the Freedom House Study, *J Int Neuropsychol Soc* 11:899–909, 2005.
75. Stubbs B, Binnekade T, Eggermont L, et al: Pain and the risk for falls in community-dwelling older adults: systematic review and meta-analysis, *Arch Phys Med Rehabil* 95:175–187, 2014.
76. Studenski S, Perera S, Patel K, et al: Gait speed and survival in older adults, *JAMA* 305:50–58, 2011.
78. Taylor BJ, Johnson BD: The pulmonary circulation and exercise responses in the elderly, *Semin Respir Crit Care Med* 31:528–538, 2010.
79. Theou O, Brothers TD, Mitnitski A, Rockwood K: Operationalization of frailty using eight commonly used scales and comparison of their ability to predict all-cause mortality, *J Am Geriatr Soc* 61:1537–1551, 2013.
80. Thompson HJ, McCormick WC, Kagan SH: Traumatic brain injury in older adults: epidemiology, outcomes, and future implications, *J Am Geriatr Soc* 54:1590–1595, 2006.
81. Tinetti ME, Bogardus ST, Jr, Agostini JV: Potential pitfalls of disease-specific guidelines for patients with multiple conditions, *N Engl J Med* 351:2870–2874, 2004.
82. Tinetti ME, Kumar C: The patient who falls: "it's always a trade-off,", *JAMA* 303:258–266, 2010.
83. Tucker-Drob EM, Johnson KE, Jones RN: The cognitive reserve hypothesis: a longitudinal examination of age-associated declines in reasoning and processing speed, *Dev Psychol* 45:431–446, 2009.
85. Vernikos J, Schneider VS: Space, gravity and the physiology of aging: parallel or convergent disciplines? A mini-review, *Gerontology* 56:157–166, 2010.
86. White DK, Neogi T, Nevitt MC, et al: Trajectories of gait speed predict mortality in well-functioning older adults: the Health, Aging and Body Composition study, *J Gerontol A Biol Sci Med Sci* 68:456–464, 2013.

The full reference list for this chapter is available online.

CHAPTER 31

RHEUMATOLOGIC REHABILITATION

Lin-Fen Hsieh, Carla P. Watson, Hui-Fen Mao

Introduction to Rheumatic Diseases

Rheumatic diseases manifest as painful conditions typically caused by inflammation, swelling, and pain in the joints or muscles. Because pain, swelling, and decline in functional status are the presenting symptoms, patients with rheumatic diseases can make up a large percentage of a physiatry practice (Table 31-1). There have been a growing number of people with rheumatic diseases who also largely contribute to the population of the permanently disabled. This has commanded the evolution and refinement of the treatment of these diseases. Thus, it is important to keep this chapter current and informative. Physiatrists can be the primary physicians for diagnosing and coordinating treatment for most of these diseases. To diagnose and treat these disorders, one must have an understanding of the joints and their components, as well as the nomenclature involved.

Structure and Components of Joints

All joints can be affected by rheumatic diseases. Joints are classified based on structure and function. Structure classification is based on the material that binds the bones together and the presence or absence of a joint cavity. Functional classification is based on the amount of movement allowed. There are three major types of joints in the body: fibrous joints (synarthroses), cartilaginous joints (amphiarthroses), and synovial joints (diarthroses). Fibrous joints (synarthroses) are immovable and do not have a joint cavity. An example would be the sutures of the cranium. For the purposes of this chapter as it relates to physiatry, the focus will be on cartilaginous joints and synovial joints.

The cartilaginous joints are distinguished by the connection between bones being entirely made of cartilage (fibrocartilage or hyaline). They are characterized by the amount of movement allowed across the joint. It is significantly less mobile than a synovial joint. It does not have a joint cavity. As a rule, amphiarthroses usually occur in the midline of the body. There are two types, synchondroses and symphyses. The manubrium and sternum are examples of synchondroses, whereas intervertebral disks and pubic symphysis are classified as symphyses.

The synovial joint (diarthrosis) is characterized by its joint mobility. These joints are able to move freely in multiple planes. It consists of two bony surfaces that articulate with one another. It is encompassed by a fibrous capsule with a synovial lining that contains fluid. The extracellular matrix consists of water and proteoglycans (glycosaminoglycan and hyaluronic acid). The viscoelastic properties of the synovial fluid and its inherent function as a lubricant and shock absorber are largely attributed to hyaluronic acid. The fibrous capsule has a rich network of substance P (neurotransmitter for pain) with nociceptive nerve fibers that can potentially generate pain. The limb joints are typically synovial joints (hip, knee, shoulder).

While inflammation ensues, fluid and polymorphonuclear leukocytes infiltrate the joint space. Vasodilation and venous congestion all contribute to pain-provoking capsular distention and neuronal sensitization of substance P nerve fibers. It is important to understand this cascade when educating patients on why they have joint pain and why treatment is aimed at limiting the damage from this cascade. If left untreated, the inflammatory cascade can destroy the integrity of a joint and permanently impair its function. This can lead to chronic pain and disability.

Kinematics plays an important role in the development and degradation of articular cartilage. Although joints with articular surfaces need a certain amount of load to maintain its integrity, excessive loading can lead to degradation of the joint.[4] Altered biomechanical values between two articular surfaces also influence disease formation in joints. Normal healthy cartilage responds positively to loading by increasing regional thickness. Diseased or injured cartilage degenerates in response to load and thus decreases regional thickness. Furthermore, disruption of normal gait mechanics whether from disease, acute injury, weight gain, or improper footwear shifts loading patterns during weight-bearing activity to cartilaginous regions not well adapted for that load.[4] Loading nonadapted areas can lead to cartilage fibrillation (softening) and degeneration.[32]

Although not a part of the synovial joint but frequently associated with them, bursae, tendon sheaths, and entheses are important to acknowledge during the physical examination and diagnostic stages of rheumatic diseases. They act to prevent friction on adjacent structures. Bursae are flattened fibrous sacs lined with a synovial membrane and contain a thin film of synovial fluid. They are common in sites where ligaments, muscles, skin, or tendons overlie and rub against bone. Tendon sheaths are elongated bursae that wrap around a tendon that is subject to friction. Entheses are the insertion sites of tendons to bones or ligaments to bones. They are functionally integrated with the synovial joint and can be involved in the rheumatic disease processes. The relationship of the surrounding soft tissue structures will be crucial for understanding the microanatomic basis for joint disease in seronegative

Table 31-1 Main Types of Rheumatic Diseases

Disease Group	Description	Examples
Degenerative and overuse syndromes	Diseases where repetitive trauma and "wear and tear" cause inflammation	Osteoarthritis, tendonitis, bursitis
Inflammatory arthropathies	Diseases with chronic inflammation of unknown cause; classified by pattern of joint involvement and associated features	Rheumatoid arthritis, psoriatic arthritis, spondyloarthropathies
Extraarticular rheumatism	Poorly understood disorders characterized by chronic pain with no evidence of inflammation	Fibromyalgia, nonspecific neck pain, nonspecific back pain
Connective tissue diseases	Autoimmune diseases of unknown etiology characterized by multisystem inflammation and damage	Systemic lupus erythematosus, polymyositis, dermatomyositis, scleroderma, vasculitis
Crystal-associated arthropathies	Diseases characterized by acute or recurrent inflammation caused by deposition of crystals in or around joints	Gout, calcium pyrophosphate crystals, hydroxyapatite crystals
Infectious arthropathies	Diseases caused by invasion of joint tissue by microorganisms	Viral, bacterial, tuberculosis, fungi
Postinfectious arthropathies	Diseases triggered by previous exposure to infectious agents	Poststreptococcal, postchlamydial, postviral

spondyloarthropathies and other rheumatic diseases, such as osteoarthritis (OA).[28]

Osteoarthritis

OA is one of the most common rheumatic diseases. OA has grown to affect 27 million people in the United States.[13] It is the leading cause of musculoskeletal pain and disability. It is predicted that with the increasing rates of obesity and the increase in the aging population, there will be an epidemic of OA in the next two decades.[13] It is more important now than ever to have a sound knowledge base for treating and preventing this disease.

OA is classified by its failure of the structure and function of synovial joints. It is characterized by its degradation of articular cartilage, subchondral bone alteration, meniscal degeneration, synovial inflammatory response, and overgrowth of bone and cartilage. The etiology of OA is multifaceted and can affect both weight-bearing and non–weight-bearing joints. OA can be initiated as a result of mechanical, structural, genetic, and environmental factors. When repeated exposure to physical activity is not offset with reciprocal time for tissue repair, bone resorption outweighs bone deposition.[32] This cycle over time is the precursor for degenerative joint disease. Other factors that influence bone resorption include hormone levels such as estrogen and vitamin D. Estrogen influences the rate of cell turnover. Vitamin D deficiency impairs bone deposition. Now that there is an increasing population of people that are vitamin D deficient, there is a link to OA prevalence, incidence, and progression. Most studies involving this link have been site specific to the knee.[32]

The risk of having OA is higher with age older than 45 years, women, obesity, bone deformities, joint injuries, and certain occupations with repetitive stress on particular joints. Advanced age is the strongest risk factor for the prevalence and incidence of OA. The estimates for influence of genetic factors in radiographic OA of the knee, hip, and hand are 39%, 60%, and 59%, with a similar range of estimates for cartilage volume change and progressive knee OA.[38]

Obesity is the primary modifiable risk factor that has the greatest potential for having an impact on treating the disease. Obese and overweight people have three times the risk of knee OA. By reducing the body mass index from more than 30 to less than 25, up to 29% of knee OA could be prevented.[38] The estimated risk of progression from symptomatic early OA to advanced OA for adults in the United States 60 to 64 years of age is 63% during a 10-year period in obese adults versus 37% in nonobese adults.[38] In contrast to knee OA, the association between obesity and incident of hip OA has been inconsistent.

Obesity has a systemic and a local mechanical effect on joints in OA. The radiographic findings in symptomatic OA of the hand emphasize the systemic factors in the link between obesity and OA, because unlike the knees or hips the hands are not primary weight-bearing joints. It is speculated that with excessive fat accumulation and intramuscular fat, there is some low-grade systemic inflammation.[38] This inflammation is now considered a hallmark of obesity with evidence in elevation in interleukins (IL-1beta, IL-6), tumor necrosis factor (TNF)-alpha, and the acute-phase reactant C-reactive protein (CRP).[38]

With advanced age and obesity being two of the major risk factors for having OA, it has to be mentioned that among the other joints the spine can be greatly affected. OA of the spine is a disorder of the synovial joints, the zygapophysial joints (z-joints), and the sacroiliac joint (SI joint). The z-joints function to support and stabilize the spine during loading, whereas the SI joint functions to transfer weight from the upper body to the lower extremities. OA does not account for all causes of z-joint and SI joint pain, but the relative percentage increases with age and obesity.[24,25] Intervertebral disc degeneration and loss of inherent structural integrity can predispose the lumbar z-joints to degenerate. The L4 to L5 and L5 to S1 levels (both weight-bearing and mobility) are the eminent explanation for the highest incidence of OA.[24] Degenerative arthrosis of SI joints may start at an earlier age and may predominantly affect the iliac cartilage. Blood vessels penetrate the subchondral bone plate of both the iliac and sacral facets and pass in close proximity to the articular cartilage. This may explain the high

Table 31-2 Kellgren-Lawrence Radiographic Grading Scale for Osteoarthritis of the Tibiofemoral Joint

Grade of Osteoarthritis	Description
0	No radiographic findings of osteoarthritis
1	Doubtful narrowing of joint space and possible osteophytic lipping
2	Definite osteophytes with possible narrowed joint space
3	Definite osteophytes with moderate joint space narrowing and some sclerosis
4	Definite osteophytes with severe joint space narrowing, subchondral sclerosis, and definite deformity of bone contour

incidence of SI joint involvement in systemic inflammatory diseases.[25]

There are various definitions of OA, both symptomatic and radiographic. Symptomatic OA usually includes pain, aching, and joint stiffness in the affected joint along with the presence of radiographic findings. Clinical criteria for diagnosis of knee and hip OA include pain, plus age older than 50 years old, stiffness for less than 30 minutes, and crepitus plus the radiographic finding of osteophytes. Knee OA may also include bony enlargement and bony tenderness.[13]

Kellgren-Lawrence is the most common radiologic grading system (Table 31-2). The Kellgren-Lawrence grading scale determines severity of knee OA on the presence and degree of osteophytosis, joint space narrowing, sclerosis, and deformity of the tibiofemoral joint.[6,21] It is key to note that symptoms can appear before any changes occurring on x-ray (Grade 0). Also, the presence of an abnormal x-ray is not a reliable identifier for pain.[6]

Treatment Options for Osteoarthritis

The treatment of OA has been expanding over the past few years. Treatments range from conservative and patient-driven to surgical interventions based on the severity of the disease process. Because pain and impaired function are typically the presenting symptoms, the treatment goals are directed at reducing pain and improving mobility. There is evidence that shows significant reduction in pain and improved physical performance and function in older adults after treatment that includes modest weight loss and moderate exercise. Resistance exercises to build the muscles that stabilize the involved joint have shown to reduce symptoms and improve functional mobility, even with severe OA. It has also been effective in the prehabilitation stage before a joint replacement to enhance postoperative recovery. The success of this treatment regimen, however, primarily lies in the patient's ability to comply with caloric adjustments and exercise. The specific modalities of physical and occupational therapy will be discussed later in the chapter but need to be mentioned as an option for conservative treatment.

For acute exacerbations of OA pain, the frontline treatment is going to be pharmaceutical agents. In mild OA, acetaminophen is used as a first-line agent because of a benign safety profile. Its mechanism of action is thought to be central via its inhibition on spinal nitric oxide mechanism and substance P receptors. Despite most experts' opinions that it does little for inflammation, it has demonstrated efficacy that is similar to that of nonsteroidal antiinflammatory drugs (NSAIDs).[10] NSAIDs are commonly used as second-line agents in patients with moderate to severe pain. The mechanism of action is through cyclooxygenase and leukotriene inhibition, which prevents the conversion of arachidonic acid to prostaglandins. Changes in the progression of the disease have not been documented with the use of NSAIDs, despite their efficacy in reducing synovial and systemic inflammation.[10] Long-term use of NSAIDs are associated with adverse side effects, particularly involving the gastrointestinal and renal systems. There have also been concerns regarding the cardiovascular effects of particular NSAIDs that are specific cyclooxygenase-2 inhibitors.[10]

The numerous side effects of oral NSAIDs have caused a boom in the use of topical NSAIDs and analgesics. Patches and gels can be applied directly to the painful joint. There has also been an emergence of compounding pain creams that include a combination of NSAIDs and anesthetics that can be tailored to the needs of each individual patient. They can be useful also as an adjuvant with other therapies.

Most oral medications that are used for peripheral joints with OA are used for spine OA. A notable exception would be muscle relaxants, which can be beneficial in treating neck and back pain associated with OA. This class of medication decreases muscle spasms associated with spine OA. It should also be noted, however, that there is no benefit to use muscle relaxants long term. A formal spine-focused, flexion-based therapy program remains the cornerstone of treating spine OA long term.[31] This should be used in conjunction with a home exercise program that addresses lumbar stabilization and core strengthening.

When oral medications are ineffective or if a patient has not been able to tolerate conservative treatment, intraarticular injections are considered. There are now various injectable medications including corticosteroids and viscosupplementation, such as hyaluronic acid. There are less traditional compounds that have gained a place in injectable treatment of OA, such as prolotherapy, NSAIDs, platelet-rich plasma, and botulinum toxin type A.[26] Intraarticular injections should also be considered in patients who are surgical candidates but are trying to delay total joint replacement. Interventional spine procedures include fluoroscopy-guided corticosteroid injections and image-guided nerve blocks, particularly of the medial branches that innervate the z-joint.[35] If this is successful in alleviating pain, the more expensive radiofrequency ablation of these branches can be considered.

Before considering surgical intervention, all nonoperative treatments should be exhausted. Total joint arthroplasty can offer some relief to those with severe refractory OA. Depending on the joint involved, there are proven long-term results. Hips and knees have the best outcome with pain relief and restoring function.[29] Shoulders, elbows, and ankles can improve pain and function, but are associated with higher complication rates. In the spine, fusion of the z-joints and SI joints can also be considered to reduce pain and stabilize and restore function.

Note that the majority of patients will respond to conservative therapy. As the treating physiatrist, the initial plan should include education on activity modification, dietary changes, weight loss, and exercise. Pharmacologic treatment can be initiated to control symptoms but should be tailored to each individual patient based on severity, chronicity, and other organ system comorbidities. Although tramadol and opioids are potent analgesics, they should not be routinely used to treat OA long term as a result of their central nervous system side effects and risk of addiction and tolerance.[10] Intraarticular injections should be used wisely because they have limitations in the frequency in which they are given depending on the medication being injected.[26] Joint replacement surgery is reserved for last resort treatment.[39]

Rheumatoid Arthritis

Rheumatoid arthritis (RA) is a chronic, systemic inflammatory disease of unknown etiology that primarily involves the joints. It also often involves soft tissues, such as tendon sheaths and bursae. In addition it may present with extraarticular manifestations. Inflammation and destruction of the joint and soft tissue may lead to joint deformity and loss of physical function. This can happen if left untreated or when the disease becomes unresponsive to treatment. The prevalence of RA varies from 0.3% to 1.5% of the population, with a female-to-male ratio of around 3 to 1.

Typically, the disease onset is insidious, with pain, stiffness, and swelling of the joints being the predominant symptoms. Morning stiffness, or stiffness after prolonged inactivity, often lasts more than an hour in the active inflammatory stage. Up to one third of patients with RA experience acute onset of polyarthritis associated with systemic symptoms including fatigue, myalgia, depression, low-grade fever, and weight loss. The most common joints involved in the early stage of the disease are the metacarpophalangeal (MCP) and proximal interphalangeal (PIP) joints of the fingers, the interphalangeal joints of the thumb, the wrists, and the metatarsophalangeal joints of the toes. Other joints, such as the shoulders, elbows, hips, knees, and ankles are also frequently affected. Over the whole course of the disease, the facet and atlantoaxial joints of the cervical spine, and the acromioclavicular, sternoclavicular, temporomandibular, and cricoarytenoid joints may also be involved. The distal interphalangeal (DIP) joints are rarely involved in RA, perhaps resulting from less synovium than the MCPs and PIPs. In addition to involvement of the joints, tenosynovitis is also common in patients with RA, and may cause trigger finger, De Quervain disease, carpal tunnel syndrome, tendon rupture, and even compression of the cervical cord resulting from narrowing of the space available for the upper cervical cord.

In the late stage of RA, joint deformities commonly occur. Buttonhole (or bouttonière) deformity is flexion of the PIP joints, with extension of the DIP joints (Figure 31-1, *A*). Because the central extensor tendon is destroyed by tenosynovitis, the PIP joints pop up dorsally, resulting in lateral and ventral displacement of the lateral bands of the extensor tendon. In this condition, the lateral bands of the extensor tendon act as flexors of the PIP joints and, with tendon shortening, hyperextension of the DIP joints develops. In contrast, the swan neck deformity is the opposite of the buttonhole deformity, with hyperextension of the PIP joints and flexion of the MCP and DIP joints (Figure 31-1, *B*). Shortening of the intrinsic muscle exerts tension on the dorsal tendon sheath, leading to hyperextension of the PIP joints. The lateral bands of the extensor tendon sublux dorsally as the PIP joints herniate in the ventral direction. In addition, shortening of the deep flexor tendons causes flexion of the DIP joints. Other deformities include ulnar deviation (Figure 31-1, *C*) of the MCP joints, palmar subluxation of the wrists, arthritis mutilans, hammer toe deformity, clawed toe deformity, flat feet, hallux valgus (Figure 31-1, *D*), metatarsal joint subluxation, and "Z" deformity of the thumb (hyperextension of the interphalangeal joint, flexion, and subluxation of the MCP joints).

As a result of the extraarticular foci of the immune response, patients with RA may have different types of extraarticular manifestations during the course of the disease. Common extraarticular features include fatigue, mild normocytic normochromic anemia, rheumatoid nodule (subcutaneous nodule, occurs in 15% to 20% of patients with RA), scleritis, episcleritis, myositis, vasculitis, neuropathy, pericarditis, interstitial pneumonitis and fibrosis, nodular lung disease, myocarditis, cardiac conduction defect, Felty syndrome (RA with neutropenia and splenomegaly), Sjögren syndrome, and amyloidosis. Vasculitis is a serious condition; it can present itself in five different clinical ways: distal arteritis, cutaneous ulceration, palpable purpura, arteritis of viscera, and peripheral neuropathy (mononeuritis multiplex or distal sensory neuropathy). Extraarticular features may be associated with poor prognosis, particularly vasculitis and rheumatoid lung disease. The presence of rheumatoid factor (RF) and anticitrullinated peptide antibodies (ACPAs) is also common in patients with RA.

Until 2010, the classification criteria for RA had been based on the 1987 American Rheumatism Association (ARA) revised criteria, which included four clinical criteria (morning stiffness, arthritis of ≥ 3 joint areas, arthritis of hand joints, and symmetrical arthritis), positive RF, the presence of rheumatoid nodules, and radiographic changes (Box 31-1). The four clinical criteria must have been present for 6 weeks.[5] These criteria may be useful for clinical study and can rule out some varieties of transient polyarthritis (e.g., acute viral polyarthritis). However, a major drawback of these criteria is their ineffectiveness in identifying some patients with early disease who subsequently have typical RA because rheumatoid nodules and radiographic erosive changes are usually not present in the early stage of disease. In addition, ACPA testing (which has a similar sensitivity for RF, but is much more specific for RA) was not previously available. In contrast, the ARA criteria did not require any exclusion, thus a patient could initially fulfill the diagnostic criteria of RA, but evolve into other diagnoses later, particularly Sjögren syndrome, scleroderma, psoriatic arthritis, crystalline arthritis, and systemic lupus erythematosus (SLE). To facilitate earlier diagnosis of RA and thus early effective treatment, The Joint Working Group of the American College of Rheumatology (ACR) and the European League Against Rheumatism (EULAR) developed new

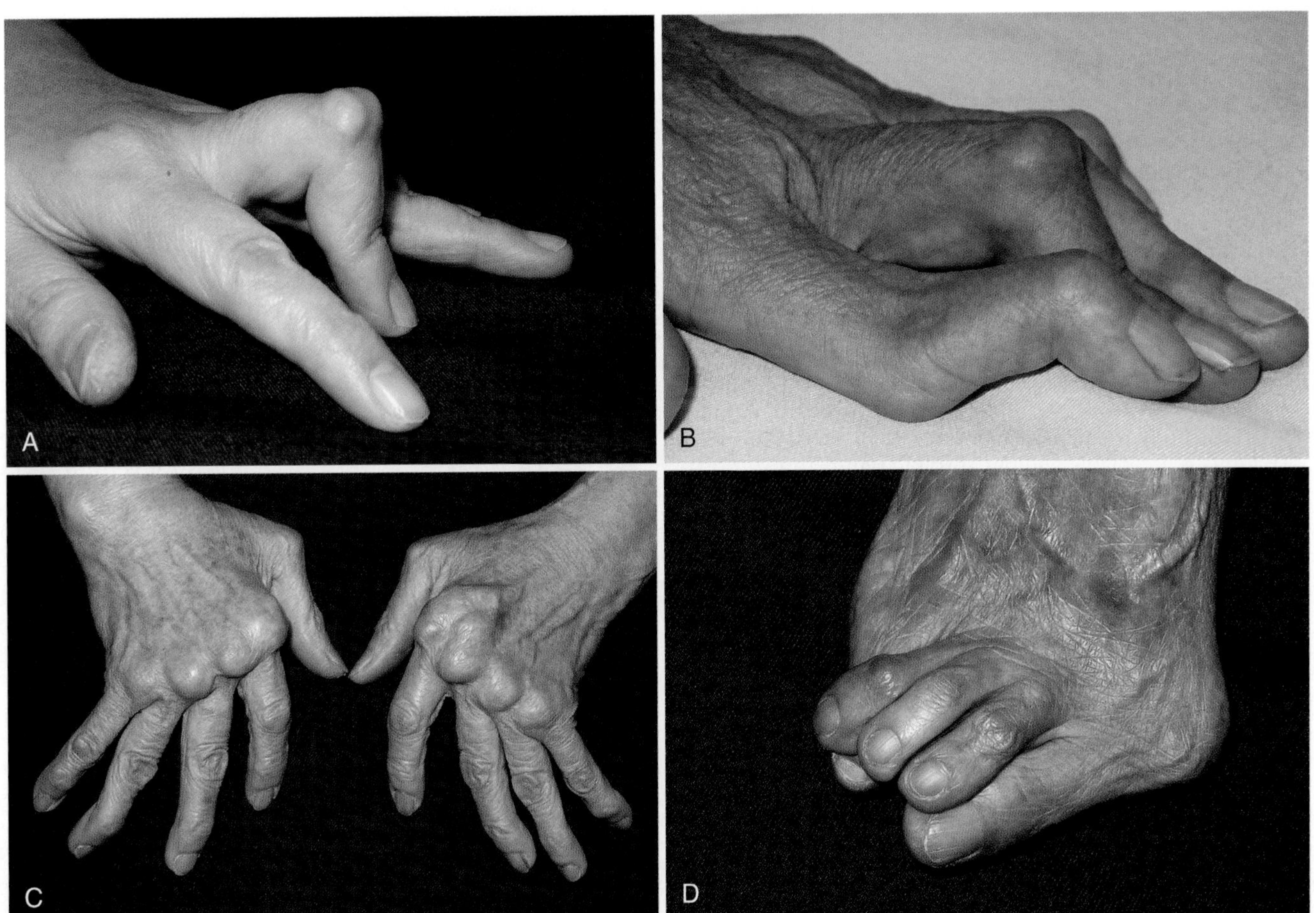

FIGURE 31-1 Typical deformities of the hands and foot in patients with rheumatoid arthritis. **A,** Buttonhole (the third finger) deformity. **B,** Swan neck (the second finger) deformity. **C,** Ulnar deviation. **D,** Hallux valgus and toes overriding.

classification criteria for RA in 2010 (Table 31-3).[2] The 2010 criteria comprises four domains: (1) type and number of affected joints, (2) RF and ACPA, (3) acute phase reactants (CRP and erythrocyte sedimentation rate [ESR]), and (4) the duration of symptoms. For evaluation of a patient with suspected RA, the highest category within each domain is taken and the four respective numbers are added. The maximum possible score is 10, where any score ≥6 indicates the presence of RA. The new criteria place a greater emphasis on serology and imaging studies (ultrasound and magnetic resonance imaging [MRI]), which can also be used to evaluate synovitis.

The comprehensive management of RA requires a combination of nonpharmacologic measures, medical interventions, and surgery. Nonpharmacologic measures include patient education, relative rest with appropriate exercise, physical therapy with modalities, occupational therapy, proper orthoses, shoes, and durable medical equipment. Nutritional counseling, psychosocial interventions, vocational training, and measures to prevent complications of drug therapy are also an integral part of treatment. Most of these measures are covered in the domain of rehabilitation management, which will be discussed later in this chapter.

Medical treatment of RA aims to control synovitis and prevent joint injury. Evidence suggests that significant, irreversible joint injury may occur as early as the first 2 years. Measures aimed at identifying early active RA and reducing inflammation are essential for improving disease outcomes. Over the past 3 decades, there has been a significant increase in the number of disease-modifying antirheumatic drugs (DMARDs) available. The 2010 ACR/EULAR classification criteria for RA facilitate recognition of patients with early arthritis, who are most likely to have progressive and erosive disease. The choice of treatment depends on the level of disease activity, stage of therapy (initial versus subsequent therapy), regulatory restrictions, and patient preference. Once the diagnosis of RA is established, antiinflammatory therapy with an NSAID or a glucocorticoid is suggested, and generally nonbiologic DMARD therapy begins, including methotrexate, hydroxychloroquine, sulfasalazine, or leflunomide (Table 31-4). Among the different nonbiologic DMARDs, methotrexate is most commonly used. Although NSAIDs are potent antiinflammatory drugs, they are not disease-modifying and have potential serious side effects; thus their use over time as monotherapy should be avoided. Combining NSAIDs with DMARDs is recommended. Glucocorticoids are also potent antiinflammatory drugs. They are particularly useful at the onset of disease. Glucocorticoids are used as a bridging strategy, during which they are tapered while the DMARDs take effect. They can also be used during disease flare or used as local injection agents when one or two joints or soft tissues are more inflamed.

BOX 31-1

1987 Revised American Rheumatism Association Criteria for Classification of Rheumatoid Arthritis*

Morning stiffness: Morning stiffness in and around the joints, lasting at least 1 hour, before maximal improvement.

Arthritis of three or more joint areas: Soft tissue swelling of fluid (not bony overgrowth alone) observed by a physician in at least three joint areas simultaneously. The 14 possible areas are right or left PIP, MCP, wrist, elbow, knee, ankle, and MTP joints.

Arthritis of hand joints: At least one area swollen (as defined above) in a wrist, MCP, or PIP joint.

Symmetrical arthritis: Simultaneous involvement of the same joint areas (as defined above for criterion 2) on both sides of the body (bilateral involvement of PIP, MCP, or MTP joints is acceptable without absolute symmetry).

Rheumatoid nodules: Subcutaneous nodules, over bony prominences, on exterior surfaces, or in juxtaarticular regions, observed by a physician.

Serum rheumatoid factor: Demonstration of abnormal amounts of serum rheumatoid factor by any method for which the result has been positive in less than 5% of normal controls.

Radiographic changes: Radiographic changes typical of rheumatoid arthritis on posteroanterior hand and wrist radiographs, which must include erosion or unequivocal bony decalcification localized in or most marked adjacent to the involved joints (osteoarthritis changes alone do not qualify).

From Arnett FC, Edworthy SM, Bloch DA, et al: The American Rheumatism Association 1987 revised criteria for the classification of rheumatoid arthritis, *Arthritis Rheum* 31:315-324, 1988.

*For classification purposes, patients have rheumatoid arthritis if they have satisfied at least four of these seven criteria. Criteria 1 through 4 must have been present for at least 6 weeks. Patients with two clinical diagnoses are not excluded. Designation as classic, definite, or probable rheumatoid arthritis is not to be made.

MCP, Metacarpophalangeal; *MTP*, metatarsophalangeal; *PIP*, Proximal interphalangeal.

Table 31-3 2010 American College of Rheumatology/European League Against Rheumatism Classification Criteria for Rheumatoid Arthritis Score-Based Algorithm for Classification in an Eligible Patient (cut-off point for rheumatoid arthritis: ≥6/10)

Joint Involvement*	**(0 to 5)**
1 medium to large† joint	0
2 to 10 medium to large joints	1
1 to 3 small‡ joints (with or without involvement of large joints)	2
4 to 10 small joints (with or without involvement of large joints)	3
>10 joints (at least one small joint)	5
Serology	**(0 to 3)**
Negative RF *and* negative ACPA	0
Low-positive RF *or* low-positive ACPA	2
High-positive RF *or* high-positive ACPA	3
Acute Phase Reactants	**1**
Normal CRP *and* normal ESR	0
Abnormal CRP *or* abnormal ESR	1
Duration of Symptoms	**(0 to 1)**
<6 weeks	0
≥6 weeks	1

Adapted, with permission, from Aletaha D, Neogi T, Silman AJ, et al: 2010 rheumatoid arthritis classification criteria: an American College of Rheumatology/European League Against Rheumatism collaborative initiative, *Ann Rheum Dis* 69:1580-1588, 2010.

*Joint involvement refers to any swollen or tender joint on examination, or evidence of synovitis on magnetic resonance imaging or ultrasonography. Distal interphalangeal joints, first carpometacarpal joint, and first metatarsophalangeal joint are excluded from assessment.

†Medium to large joints refer to shoulders, elbows, hips, knees, and ankles.

‡Small joints refer to the metacarpophalangeal joints, proximal interphalangeal joints, metatarsophalangeal joints 2 through 5, thumb interphalangeal joints, and wrists.

ACPA, Anticitrullinated protein/peptide antibody; *CRP*, C-reactive protein; *ESR*, erythrocyte sedimentation rate; *RF*, rheumatoid factor.

If patients show an inadequate response after several months of aggressive doses of a nonbiologic DMARD, adding a second nonbiologic DMARD (step-up combination) or a biologic DMARD is suggested. Several biologic DMARDs are FDA (U.S. Food and Drug Administration)-approved for the treatment of RA. Biologic DMARDs include TNF inhibitors (etanercept, infliximab, adalimumab, and golimumab), IL-1 inhibitor (anakinra), IL-6 inhibitor (tocilizumab), T-cell costimulation inhibitor (abatacept), and B-cell depletion therapy (rituximab, an anti-CD20 chimeric monoclonal antibody) (Table 31-5).[34,36] Several clinical trials have shown that TNF inhibitors, IL-1 or IL-6 inhibitors are efficacious as monotherapies for the treatment of RA. The pitfalls of biologic DMARDs are the high cost, possible side effects, and some serious adverse events (infection, tuberculosis, demyelinating syndromes, increased risk of certain malignancy, and drug-induced lupus). With regular assessment of disease activity and tight control of treatment strategies, many patients with RA remain in remission or in a state of low-disease activity; thus joint destruction and physical disability are avoided. In patients with intractable pain, severe joint destruction, or poor response to long periods of medical treatment and rehabilitation, surgery may be considered. Common surgeries for patients with RA are artificial joint replacement, synovectomy (for the hand, wrist, elbow, knee, and tendon sheath), tendon repair, osteotomy, and arthrodesis (for the wrist, ankle, or cervical spine).

Ankylosing Spondylitis

Seronegative spondyloarthropathy describes a type of chronic inflammatory arthritis involving the axial structures, manifested by chronic back pain and progressive stiffness of the spine. It can also involve the shoulders, hips, and other peripheral joints. It includes ankylosing spondylitis (AS), reactive arthritis, arthropathy of inflammatory bowel disease, psoriatic arthritis, undifferentiated spondyloarthropathy, and juvenile-onset AS. In addition to inflammation of the spine (including the sacroiliac joint), this disease is characterized by the absence of an RF, a tendency for familial aggregation, an association with the human leukocyte antigen (HLA)-B27, inflammation around the entheses (the site of tendon or ligament

Table 31-4 Nonbiologic Disease-Modifying Antirheumatic Drugs

Drug (Brand Name[s])	Response Rate; Onset of Action	Magnitude of Efficacy 0 to ++++	Dosage	Special Instructions	Common Side Effects	Comments
Hydroxychloroquine (Plaquenil)	30% to 50% 2 to 6 mo	++	200 to 600 mg/day in 1 or 2 doses	Take with milk or food, wear sunglasses in bright light	Blurred vision, headache, skin pigmentation changes, rash, anorexia, abdominal cramps, nausea, vomiting	Ophthalmologic examination, baseline and at 6-12 mo for retinal changes, complete blood count
Leflunomide (Arava)	50% 2 to 3 mo	++	10 to 20 mg daily, single dose	Loading dose of 100 mg/day for 3 days	Alopecia, headache, hypertension, skin rash	Avoid if pregnant; baseline hepatic function
Methotrexate	>70% 6 to 8 wk	+++	7.5 to 20 mg/wk in a single or divided doses	Avoid alcohol, folic acid intake; adequate hydration	Alopecia, headache, oral ulcers, photosensitivity, vasculitis, thrombocytopenia	Baseline hepatic function; white blood cell and platelet count every 4 wk, complete blood count, creatinine, liver function test every 3-4 mo
Minocycline (Minocin, Dynacin)			200 mg/day	Avoid antacid, iron, and dairy products	Photosensitivity, dizziness	Not FDA-approved for arthritis, check for tetracycline sensitivity
Sulfasalazine (Azulfidine)	>30% 2 to 3 mo	++	500 to 3000 mg daily; maximum 3 g in divided doses	Take after meals, can permanently stain soft contact lenses yellow	Headache, photosensitivity, diarrhea, vomiting, nausea, anorexia, reversible oligospermia	Inadequate fluid intake can cause urine crystals

FDA, U.S. Food and Drug Administration.

insertion into bone), uveitis, urethritis, and psoriatic skin lesion. AS is the prototypic form and is frequently encountered by physiatrists.

The prevalence of AS has been estimated to be 0.1% to 1.4% of the population (0.2% to 0.5% in the United States), and the male-to-female ratio is approximately 2 to 3. The prevalence of AS generally mirrors the frequency of HLA-B27 in the population, and the prevalence of AS is approximately 5% to 6% in people who are HLA-B27 positive.[33] The peak age of onset is between 20 and 30 years.

The most common presentation is chronic inflammatory back pain. The pain usually starts at the buttock or lower back level, with possible radiation to the posterior thigh. It is dull pain in nature, insidious in onset, and is chronic (lasting greater than 3 months). The pain is worse in the later part of the night and the early morning, with morning stiffness lasting more than 30 minutes, and often hours. It can be relieved with exercise or activity and worsened with rest (Table 31-6). It is usually improved with the use of NSAIDs. At first, buttock or lower back pain may be unilateral and intermittent; however, within a few months, pain becomes bilateral and persistent, and the lower back becomes stiff. Gradually, pain and stiffness may ascend from the lower back to the middle back, then the upper back and neck region.

Patients with AS may experience arthritis outside the spine, and peripheral arthritis occurs in approximately 35% to 50% of patients with AS over the course of the disease.[33] The most commonly affected joints, in order of frequency, are the shoulders, hips, and knees. Involvement of the ankles, sternoclavicular joints, and temporomandibular joints is also reported. Hip involvement is present in 25% to 35% of patients with AS and is associated with a high degree of physical disability and a poor prognosis.

Enthesitis, inflammation of the entheses, occurs in approximately 40% to 70% of patients with AS at some time during the course of the disease.[33] The most common location of enthesitis in patients with AS is the calcaneal attachments of the Achilles tendon. Other locations include the calcaneal attachments of the plantar fascia, the shoulders, the costochondral junctions, the sternoclavicular and manubriosternal joints, and the superior iliac crest. Dactylitis (or sausage digits) is characterized by diffuse swelling of the toes or fingers and is present in 6% to 8% of patients with AS.

Patients with AS may have extraarticular comorbidities including anterior uveitis, inflammatory bowel disease, psoriasis skin lesions, aortic regurgitation, cardiac conduction disturbance, restrictive lung disease, apical pulmonary fibrosis, immunoglobulin nephropathy, or renal amyloidosis. Among them, anterior uveitis (or iritis) is most common, occurring in 25% to 40% of patients with AS.[43] Anterior uveitis presents as acute eye pain, redness, photophobia, increased lacrimation, and blurring of vision. Treatment of acute uveitis should begin as early as possible to avoid complications such as glaucoma or vision loss.

Recent data suggest that the prevalence of osteoporosis and vertebral fractures in patients with AS is 25% and 10%, respectively. Approximately 65% of fractures are associated with a neurologic deficit. Spinal cord injury is 11 times

Table 31-5 Biologic Agents for Rheumatoid Arthritis

Drug (Brand Name)	Molecular Structures	Response Rate; Onset of Action	Dosage	Administration Instructions	Common Side Effects	Other Comments
Non-TNF						
Abatacept (Orencia)	Recombinant receptor-IgG Fc fusion protein; T-cell costimulation inhibition	50% to 70%; 4 wk	IV infusion, 500 to 1000 mg, repeat at 2 and 4 wk, and every 4 wk thereafter; or 125 mg SC once weekly	IV: Infuse over 30 min; administer through a 0.2 to 1.2 micron low-protein–binding filter SC: Allow prefilled syringe to warm to room temperature (for 30 to 60 min) before administration	Headache, dizziness, nausea, dyspepsia, abdominal pain, diarrhea, nasopharyngitis, upper respiratory tract infection, urinary tract infection, other infections, hypertension, skin rash	Higher incidences of infection and malignancy were observed in the older adult population; use caution with chronic obstructive pulmonary disease
Rituximab (Rituxan)	Chimeric monoclonal antibody specific to CD20 (B-cell depletion)	65% to 85%; 4 to 12 wk	IV infusion: 1000 mg on days 1 and 15 in combination with methotrexate; subsequent courses may be administered every 24 wk	Dilute to a concentration of 1 to 4 mg/mL in either 0.9% sodium chloride or 5% dextrose IV infusion: Start rate of 50 mg/hr; if there is no reaction, increase the rate by 50 mg/hr increments every 30 min, to a maximum rate of 400 mg/hr	Peripheral edema, hypertension, fever, fatigue, chills, headache, insomnia, pain, rash, nausea, neuropathy, abnormal liver function, hematologic abnormality	Risk of reactivation of hepatitis B virus infection; do not administer IV push or bolus; severe infusion-related reaction may happen
Tocilizumab (Actemra)	Anti–interleukin-6 receptor monoclonal antibody		IV: Initial: 4 mg/kg every 4 wk; may be increased to 8 mg/kg (maximum dose: 800 mg) SC: <100 kg: 162 mg every other week; increase to every week based on clinical response; ≥100 kg: 162 mg every wk	IV: Allow diluted solution for infusion to reach room temperature before administration; infuse over 60 min with a dedicated IV line SC: Administer the full amount in the prefilled syringe; rotate injection sites	Anaphylaxis/hypersensitivity reactions, elevated liver enzymes, fatal infection, gastrointestinal perforation, neutropenia, thrombocytopenia	Tuberculosis and malignancy have been reported; use is not recommended in patients with active hepatic disease or hepatic impairment; use with caution in patients with central nervous system demyelinating disease
Anti-TNF						
Adalimumab (Humira)	Human monoclonal antibody	46% to 73%	40 mg SC every 2 wk	Prefilled pens, syringes, and vials are available for use; inject into thigh or lower abdomen	Headache, skin rash, positive ANA titer, serious infection, local injection site reaction, increased creatinine phosphokinase, upper respiratory tract infection, sinusitis	Live vaccines should not be given concurrently; anaphylaxis, tuberculosis, malignancy, demyelinating disease, heart failure are rarely reported
Etanercept	Human recombinant receptor/Fc fusion protein	59% to 86%; 2 to 4 wk	25 mg SC on 2 different days, or 50 mg once weekly			
Infliximab	Chimeric monoclonal antibody					
Certolizumab pegol (Cimzia)	Humanized Fab fragment					
Golimumab (Simponi)	Humanized monoclonal antibody					

ANA, Antinuclear antibody; *IgG*, Immunoglobulin G; *IV*, intravenous; *SC*, subcutaneous; *TNF*, tumor necrosis factor.

Table 31-6 Differentiation of Inflammatory and Mechanical Low Back Pain

	Inflammatory Pain	Mechanical Pain
Age of onset	Younger than 40 years	Middle to old age
Type of onset	Insidious	Acute or insidious
Symptom duration	Greater than 3 months	Mostly less than 3 months
Night pain	Common	Rare
Effect of exercise	Improved	Usually worse (acute pain)
Sacroiliitis	Positive	Negative
Low back mobility	Limited in all motions	Limited in one or some motions
Neurologic deficits	Unusual	Possible

BOX 31-2

Radiograph Grading of Sacroiliitis

Grade 0: Normal

Grade 1: Suspicious changes

Grade 2: Minimal abnormality—small localized areas with erosions or sclerosis, without alteration in the joint width

Grade 3: Unequivocal abnormality—moderate or advanced sacroiliitis with erosions, sclerosis, widening, narrowing, or partial ankylosis

Grade 4: Total ankylosis

more common in patients with AS than in the general population and affects the cervical spine more often than the thoracic and lumbar spine. Spontaneous subluxation of the atlantoaxial joint and cauda equina syndrome may also occur in patients with AS.

Laboratory findings are generally nonspecific for AS. An elevated ESR or CRP is present in approximately 50% to 70% of patients who have AS with active disease. Normochromic normocytic anemia is occasionally seen, and HLA-B27 is present in 90% to 95% of patients with AS with European ancestry.

Plain radiography and MRI are the principal imaging techniques used to evaluate patients with AS, especially for sacroiliac joints. In general, radiographic changes need a few years to develop. Radiographic findings of sacroiliitis (pelvis anteroposterior view) include narrowing of the joint space, sclerosis, erosion, and bony ankylosis. These have been divided into five grades (Box 31-2, Figure 31-2). Other findings on plain radiograph of the pelvis include erosions and osteitis at the ischial tuberosity, femoral trochanter, iliac crests, and symphysis pubis. Radiographic change of the spine may show squaring of the vertebral bodies, syndesmophytes (Figure 31-3), ankylosis of the facet joints, and calcification of the anterior longitudinal ligament.

If the plain radiograph of the pelvis does not fulfill the criteria for sacroiliitis but the suspicion of AS remains high, the next step is MRI. In the case of active sacroiliitis, MRI can show bone marrow edema in the bones adjacent to the affected joints, as shown in STIR (short tau inversion

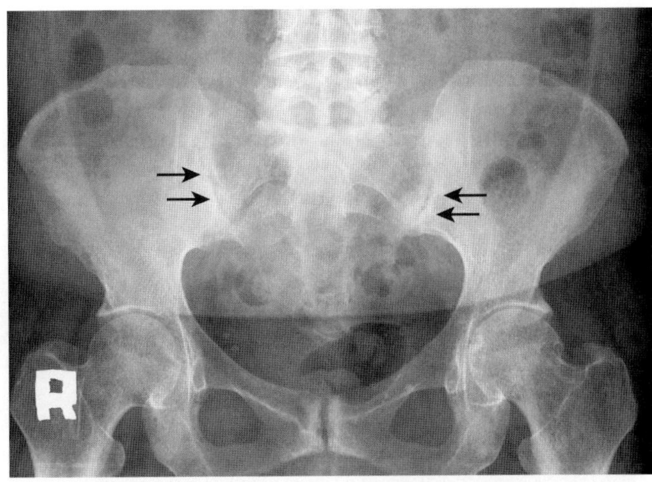

FIGURE 31-2 Anteroposterior view of the pelvis in a patient with ankylosing spondylitis shows grade 3 sacroiliitis bilaterally.

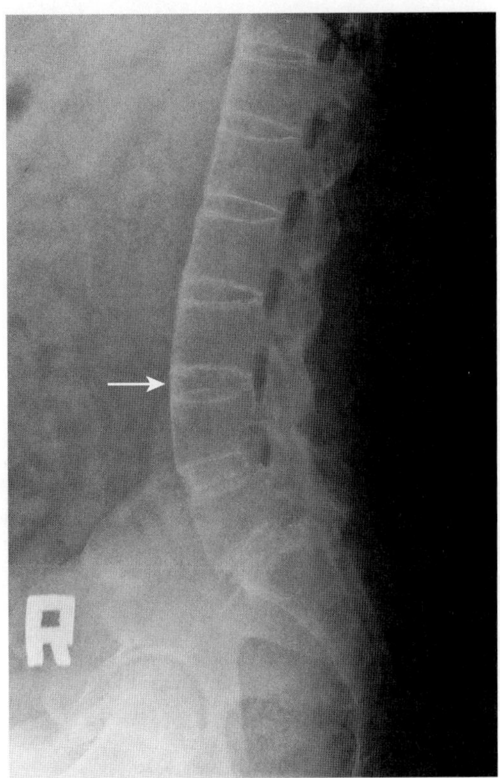

FIGURE 31-3 Lateral view of the thoracolumbar spine in a patient with ankylosing spondylitis shows syndesmophytes and a bamboo spine.

recovery) images (Figure 31-4) or T2-weighted images with fat suppression (not seen in T1-weighted images). MRI has been shown to be more sensitive than conventional radiography, bone scintigraphy, and computed tomography scans in the detection of sacroiliitis.[33]

Diagnosis (or classification) of classical AS is based on the 1984 modified New York criteria, which requires the symptoms of lower back pain, limited lumbar spine motion and chest expansion, and plain radiographs showing sacroiliitis (Box 31-3).[17]

The goals of management of patients with AS are: (1) symptom relief; (2) maintenance of function; (3) prevention of spinal disease complications; and (4) minimization

SERONEGATIVE SPONDYLOARTHROPATHY, SACROILIITIS

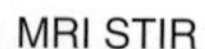

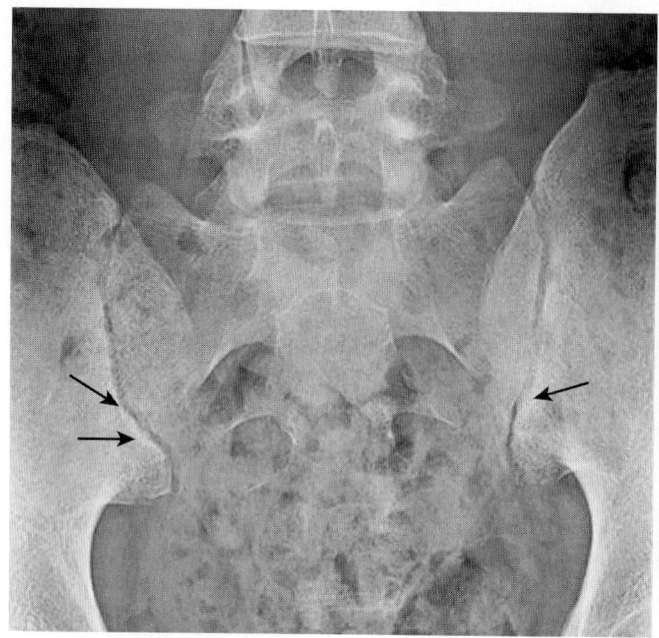

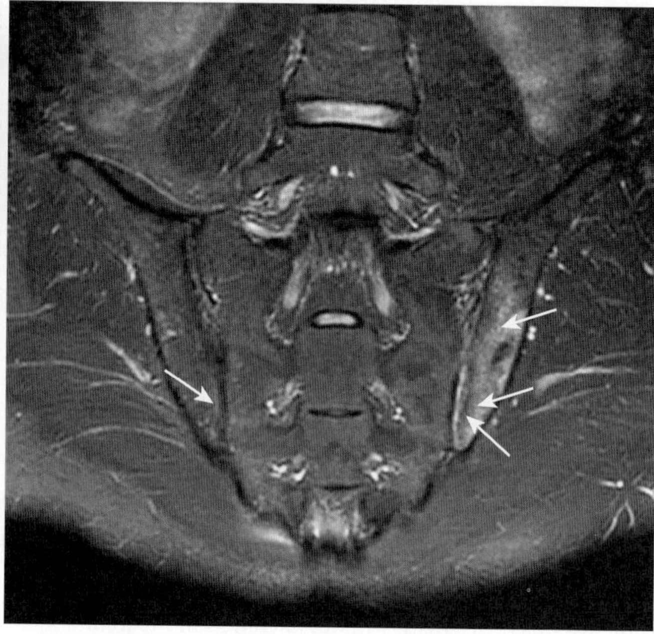

FIGURE 31-4 Comparison of anteroposterior view of the pelvis (*left*) and magnetic resonance imaging (MRI; short tau inversion recovery [STIR], *right*) of the sacroiliac joint in a patient with early ankylosing spondylitis. MRI shows left sacroiliitis, which is not shown on the plain film. (Courtesy Dr. Hung-Ta Wu.)

BOX 31-3

1984 Modified New York Criteria for Ankylosing Spondylitis

Clinical Variables

- Inflammatory back pain >3 months
- Limitation of motion of the lumbar spine in both the sagittal and frontal planes
- Limitation of chest expansion relative to normal values

Radiologic Variables (Plain Radiographs)

- Sacroiliitis grade ≥2 bilaterally
- Sacroiliitis grade 3 to 4 unilaterally

Definite Diagnosis

- At least one clinical variable plus at least one radiologic variable

of extraspinal and extraarticular comorbidities. Management includes a rehabilitation program (which will be discussed later), medication, and surgery. NSAIDs should be used for the initial therapy. Continuous NSAID use is suggested for patients who have AS with persistent active symptoms to lower the rate of radiographic progression in the spine. NSAIDs can be supplemented with a simple analgesic (acetaminophen) or low-potency opioids. For patients with axial disease who are not responsive to NSAIDs, an anti-TNF agent is recommended.[8] Anti-TNF agents are very effective for symptom relief, can stop bony destruction, and may have potential for disease modification. Reduction of acute spinal inflammation can be seen by MRI with anti-TNF agents.[33] In patients who have AS with predominantly peripheral arthritis, who are not responsive to NSAIDs, and for whom TNF inhibitors are not suitable, sulfasalazine and methotrexate are suggested. Local corticosteroid injections may be indicated for persistent peripheral arthritis, for sacroiliitis pain, or for enthesitis at sites other than the Achilles tendon (because this may cause tendon rupture). Systemic corticosteroids are not recommended. In patients with AS whose joints are destroyed, total joint replacement may be necessary. Wedge osteotomy of the spine is reserved for patients who have AS with severe spinal deformities (Figure 31-5). Fusion of the atlantoaxial joint is needed if there is significant neck or occipital pain, or evidence of spinal cord compression resulting from atlantoaxial subluxation.

Fibromyalgia

Fibromyalgia (FM) is a disorder characterized by widespread musculoskeletal pain. Although the etiology of FM is still unclear, it is agreed that the likely source of disturbance is within the central nervous system. Researchers believe the disorder amplifies pain by affecting the way the brain processes painful sensations. Women are more likely to have FM than men. It often presents as neck pain or back pain; upon physical examination, multiple tender points are found. Even though it is a disorder of the soft tissues, the tender points can be found at some joint lines; thus, when diagnosing this disorder, the history and physical examination can be key. FM is usually associated with constitutional symptoms such as fatigue, malaise, sleep disturbances, headaches, mood disturbances, memory loss, and irritable bowel symptoms. There is no cure for FM, but various treatment options are discussed in the Chapter 37.

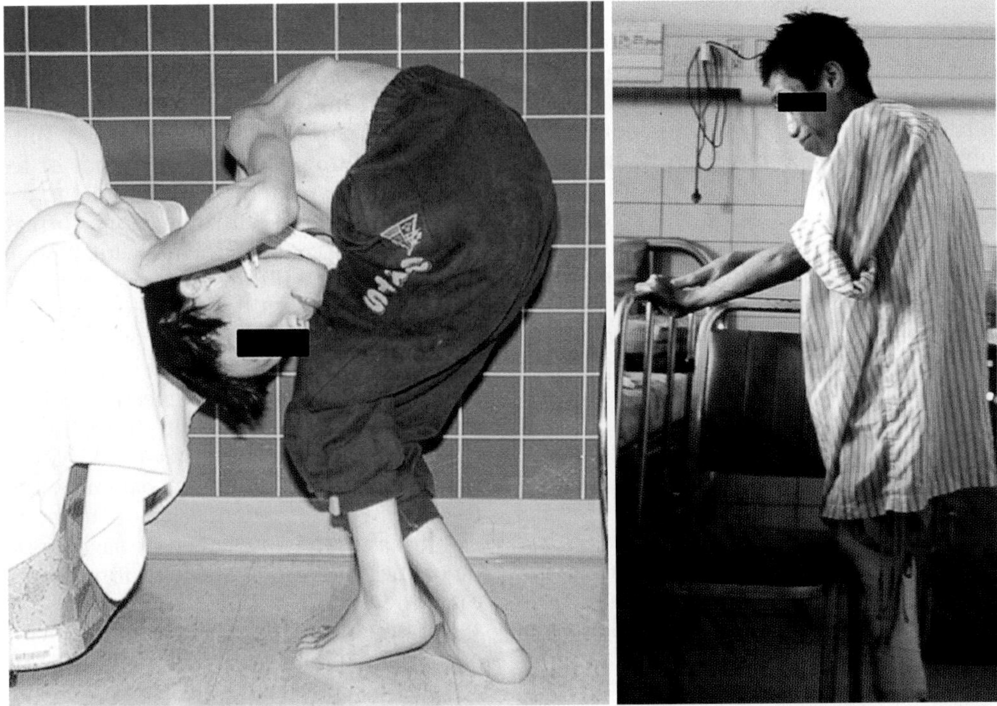

FIGURE 31-5 Severe deformity of the spine in a 29-year-old patient with ankylosing spondylitis. **A,** Before surgery. **B,** After surgery. Much improved after spinal osteotomy (90-degree correction) and total hip replacement (60-degree correction). (Courtesy Dr. Ing-Ho Chen.)

Arthritis Associated with Systemic Lupus Erythematosus

Systemic lupus erythematosus (SLE) is an autoimmune disease that can affect every organ system, because the immune systems attacks its own body. It is characterized by the production of antibodies to components of the cell nucleus. Because SLE affects every organ system, it can be difficult to diagnose initially. Joint pain is a prominent symptom that commonly causes an individual to seek medical attention. When diagnosing arthritis associated with SLE, RA must be ruled out because they can have very similar features. The etiology is still unclear. It is primarily a disease of young women with peak occurrence between ages 15 and 40 years. People of color are more affected than whites, particularly the African-American population. The joints most affected are the smaller peripheral joints, such as fingers, wrists, elbows, toes, ankles, and knees. Unlike RA, SLE is less likely to cause erosion and deformity of the joint. Muscles and soft tissues can be affected in SLE manifesting as myositis, tendonitis, or bursitis. The treatment of the musculoskeletal symptoms of SLE can be similar to those of other arthropathies. A formal physical therapy program with modalities in conjunction with appropriate pain medication tailored to not affect other involved organ systems is the key.

Crystal Deposition Arthropathies

Gout and pseudogout are the two most common crystal-induced arthropathies. Gout is caused by monosodium urate monohydrate crystals. Pseudogout is caused by calcium pyrophosphate crystals and is more accurately called calcium pyrophosphate deposition disease (CPPD). It is unclear why crystals deposit in the joints but the risk increases with age. Podagra is a common symptom in 50% of gout cases and can also be present in pseudogout. Podagra is a red, tender, swollen, hot joint usually the metatarsal-phalangeal at the base of the great toe. There can be arthritis in other sites, such as the instep, ankle, wrist, elbow, and ankle. The onset of gout is sudden with symptoms reaching maximum intensity within 8 to 12 hours. The course of pseudogout is more insidious gradually intensifying over several days. Without treatment, the symptom pattern can become polyarticular, resembling RA.

On physical examination, in addition to the inflamed joint, tophi in soft tissues can be found in the helix of the ear, fingers, olecranon, and prepatellar bursa. Patients can also have a fever. Diagnosis is made with joint aspiration and analysis of the synovial fluid for crystals. The blood uric acid level can be checked for gout; however, elevated uric acid level is not solely diagnostic. Plain x-ray films may show erosions over hanging edges in the joint space. These are pathognomonic findings in gouty arthritis. In CPPD, x-rays reveal the presence of calcium crystals. Ultrasound findings can show the "double-contour" sign, which is defined as a hyperechoic, irregular line of the monosodium urate crystals on the surface of the articular cartilage. "Wet clumps of sugar" can also be seen representing tophaceous material. This is defined by a hyperechoic and hypoechoic heterogeneous material with an anechoic rim. It might also show bony erosions adjacent to tophaceous deposits. Computed tomography scans can be complementary to the plain film. MRI with gadolinium is only recommended when tendon sheath involvement is a concern.

Treatment is usually done in three stages: treating the acute attack, providing prophylaxis to prevent acute flares, and lowering excess stores of uric acid crystals. The acute attack is treated with NSAIDs, such as indomethacin, or corticosteroids in both gout and CPPD. Colchicine is overlapped as a prophylactic medication but can be incorporated during the acute attack. If used early on, colchicine can abort a full blown gouty attack. Colchicine can be used to treat CPPD. Allopurinol is used to lower excess stores of uric acid crystals. Nonpharmacologic treatment includes abundant hydration, avoiding high-purine foods (meats and seafood) and high-fructose corn syrup (soft drinks and artificial fruit drinks), decreasing alcohol intake (especially beer), and weight reduction if obesity is an issue.

Psoriatic Arthritis

Psoriatic arthritis is a member of the seronegative spondyloarthropathy family and is defined as an inflammatory arthritis associated with psoriasis. It is usually negative for RF and affects women and men equally. The prevalence of psoriatic arthritis is approximately 1 to 2 per 1000, and the incidence is approximately 6 per 100,000 per year. It is estimated that 4% to 30% of patients with psoriasis have psoriatic arthritis.

Patients with psoriatic arthritis present with symptoms and signs of joint, entheseal, and spinal inflammation. Patients usually complain of pain and stiffness in the affected joints. Morning stiffness often lasts for longer than 30 minutes, and the stiffness is accentuated by prolonged immobility and is relieved by physical activity. Moll and Wright described five clinical patterns of psoriatic arthritis: (1) asymmetrical oligoarthritis (Figure 31-6); (2) polyarthritis; (3) predominant DIP joint involvement; (4) destructive arthritis (arthritis mutilans); and (5) predominant spondyloarthritis. Polyarthritis is the most common (63%), followed by oligoarthritis (13%), and predominant DIP involvement (less than 5%). Although spinal involvement is found in 40% to 70% of patients with psoriatic arthritis, spinal involvement alone occurs in only 2% to 4% of patients with psoriatic arthritis. Some patients present with more than one pattern, and the classification is not fixed. The pattern of disease may fluctuate. Other musculoskeletal features include dactylitis (sausage digit, resulting from inflammation of the soft tissue and joints), enthesitis, tenosynovitis, nail lesions (pits and onycholysis), and pitting edema in the hands or feet.

The most typical radiologic findings are the coexistence of erosive changes and new bone formation in the DIP joints. Other changes include fluffy periostitis with new bone formation at the site of enthesitis, lysis of the terminal phalanges, gross destruction of isolated joints, "pencil-in-cup" appearance, and the presence of both joint lysis and ankylosis. MRI may be more sensitive than conventional radiography in detecting articular, periarticular, and soft tissue inflammation. In recent years, the ClASsification of Psoriatic ARthritis (CASPAR) study developed new classification criteria for patients with psoriatic arthritis (Box 31-4). A patient with inflammatory musculoskeletal disease can be classified as having psoriatic arthritis if he or she has a total of at least three points out of the five categories.

Treatment for psoriatic arthritis includes therapy for both skin and joint disease. The treatment of psoriatic arthritis usually starts with NSAIDs. If the arthritis is not well controlled by the NSAIDs, the next step is a nonbiologic DMARD, preferably methotrexate, leflunomide, or sulfasalazine. For patients whose joint condition does not improve after 3 months of treatment, a TNF inhibitor may be added, usually etanercept, adalimumab, or infliximab. TNF inhibitors have been shown to reduce radiographic progression of disease and the effect is superior to methotrexate. Use of oral corticosteroids in patients with psoriatic arthritis should be avoided. Joint replacement may be suggested when psoriatic arthritis causes damage that limits movement and impairs function.

Inflammatory Myopathies

Idiopathic inflammatory myopathies are a heterogeneous group of autoimmune rheumatic disorders characterized by chronic muscle weakness and evidence of muscle

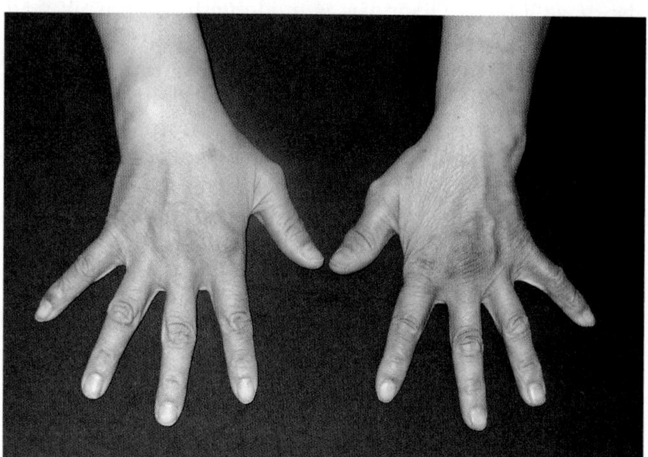

FIGURE 31-6 Swelling of right wrist and left third metacarpophalangeal in a patient with psoriatic arthropathy.

BOX 31-4

Classification Criteria for Psoriatic Arthritis (CASPAR Criteria)

- Inflammatory musculoskeletal disease (peripheral arthritis, spondylitis, or enthesitis) *and*
- At least 3 points from the following:
  - Current psoriasis (2 points), a personal history of psoriasis (1 point), or a family history of psoriasis (1 point)
  - Typical nail lesions (1 point): onycholysis, pitting
  - Dactylitis (1 point): present, or past, documented by a rheumatologist
  - Negative rheumatoid factor (1 point)
  - Juxtaarticular bone formation (1 point): on hand or foot radiographs

From Taylor W, Gladman D, Helliwell P, et al: Classification criteria for psoriatic arthritis: development of new criteria from a large international study, *Arthritis Rheum* 54:2665-2673, 2006.

inflammation. Of these, dermatomyositis (DM), polymyositis (PM), and inclusion body myositis (IBM) are the most common. The combined annual incidence of DM and PM is estimated at 2 per 100,000, and the prevalence ranges from 5 to 22 per 1,000,000. The mean age of onset in PM is 50 to 60 years, and in DM there are two peaks: 5 to 15 years and 45 to 65 years. IBM usually occurs in people over 50 years of age.

Painless muscle weakness is the most common feature of DM and PM. The distribution of weakness is usually symmetrical and proximal, typically in the neck, shoulder, pelvis, and thigh muscles. The onset is often subacute, developing over a few weeks, or insidious, occurring over several months. Patients often have difficulty walking uphill or upstairs, raising arms above the shoulders, or rising after sitting. If untreated, severe cases may become wheelchair bound. Some patients may have swallowing difficulty caused by weak pharyngeal muscles, and rarely, dyspnea as a result of involvement of the ventilatory muscles.

The most characteristic skin manifestations in patients with DM are Gottron papules and the heliotrope rash. Besides muscular and skin involvement, calcinosis, polyarthritis, interstitial lung disease, arrhythmia, gastrointestinal lesions, and kidney involvement may also be possible. These inflammatory myopathies may be associated with cancer and other rheumatic diseases, such as systemic sclerosis, mixed connective tissue disease, and SLE. Laboratory testing shows elevated muscle enzymes, including creatinine kinase and aldolase. Autoantibodies are also present, including antinuclear antibodies (ANAs), anti-Sjögren-syndrome-related antigen A (anti-Ro/SSA), anti-La/SSB, antiribonucleoprotein (anti-RNP), anti-Sm, anti-Jo-1, anti-signal recognition particle (anti-SRP), and antisynthetase antibodies. Electromyography is helpful in distinguishing myopathic causes of weakness from neuropathic disorders. Confirmation of diagnosis usually requires a muscle biopsy, which reveals the presence of mononuclear inflammatory cells in muscle tissue and degenerating, necrotic, and regenerating muscle fibers. In IBM, rimmed vacuoles are characteristic findings.

Treatment of PM and DM includes medication and physical exercise.[3] The initial medication for PM and DM is a high dose of glucocorticoids (prednisone): 0.75 to 2 mg/kg body weight per day for 4 to 12 weeks. After the disease is controlled, glucocorticoid is slowly tapered off. The total duration of glucocorticoid therapy is usually between 9 and 12 months. In cases of severe myositis, and in those with severe visceral organ involvement, intravenous methylprednisolone, 1 g/day for 3 consecutive days, is often used to achieve a more rapid response. Other treatments include a combination of glucocorticoid with immunosuppressive agents, intravenous immunoglobulin, and B-cell depletion therapy. There is a general consensus that glucocorticoid treatment improves strength and preserves muscle function in patients with DM or PM. Patients with IBM usually show poor response to glucocorticoids.

A combination of physical exercise and immunosuppressive agents has been shown to be safe and is beneficial to muscle function. Muscle biopsy studies have also revealed an increase of slow-twitch (type I) muscle fibers and reduction of muscle inflammation after exercise. To avoid worsening muscle inflammation, exercise should be submaximal and tailored to the patient's tolerance.

BOX 31-5

Rehabilitation Goals for Rheumatic Diseases

1. To increase or maintain functional performances
   - Including to develop problem-solving skills related to joint protection and energy conservation
2. To keep proper joint alignment and to prevent joint deformities
3. To relieve pain and inflammation
4. To increase or maintain mobility, strength, and endurance
5. To facilitate successful adaptation
   - To assist the patient to cope with the unpredictable nature of the disease
6. To achieve sense of self-efficacy and well-being

Rehabilitative Management of Rheumatic Diseases

The rehabilitation evaluation of the patient with a rheumatic disease can be a challenge because they probably will have comorbidities that need to be considered. The goal setting will need to accommodate those special considerations (Box 31-5). It requires an understanding of the disease process, specific conditions, potential deformities, how the arthritic condition has affected the individual's functioning, and the patient's individual needs. Holistic examination assists the professionals in appropriate goal setting and treatment planning. In addition to the medical treatments mentioned previously, the rehabilitative interventions should include patient education, improvement or maintenance of functional mobility, assessing the need for orthoses and durable medical equipment, appropriate physical modalities, and exercise.

Rehabilitation Evaluation of Patients with Rheumatic Diseases

To achieve the rehabilitation goals requires an understanding of the disease process, specific conditions, potential deformities, how the arthritic condition has affected the individual's functioning, and the patient's individual needs. Holistic examination assists the professionals in appropriate goal setting and treatment planning. The key components of the rehabilitation evaluation of patients with rheumatic diseases are described as follows (Box 31-6). In addition to the medical treatments mentioned earlier, the rehabilitative interventions should include the following.

Patient Education

Patients must understand that joint deformities cannot be prevented if the disease progresses without antiinflammatory or disease-modifying medication. Therefore, all interventions require teaching the patient and family about the disease, its symptoms, and how chronic synovitis can lead to irreversible destruction. They also need to know how to

BOX 31-6

Key Components of the Rehabilitation Evaluation of Patients with Rheumatic Diseases

Disease and Comorbidities
- Current diagnosis
- Current disease activity
- Cardiovascular comorbidities
- Depression
- Other

Body Function and Structure
- Pain
- Tender joint count
- Swollen joint count
- Nodules and nodes
- Range of motion
- Deformities
- Muscle strength
- X-ray, ultrasound, or MRI: erosions, loss of joint spaces, osteophytes

Activities: Execution of a Task or Action
- Reaching
- Manipulation
- Timed button test
- Hand function
- Six-minute walking test
- HAQ
- AIMS
- DAS 28
- WOMAC

Participation: Involvement in Life Situations
- Daily routines
- Self-care
- Domestic life
- Education
- Leisure
- Subscales of HAQ and AIMS
- WHODAS
- CHART
- Other

Environmental Factors: External Features of the Physical, Social, and Attitudinal World
- Occupation
- Home physical environment
- Workstation setup
- Broad-handle utensils
- Assistive devices and mobility aids
- Interpersonal environment
- Social support
- Societal policies and regulations

Personal Factors: Features of Individual and Not Part of Health Condition
- Personal identity
- Occupation
- Goal
- Beliefs about arthritis
- Coping style
- Self-efficacy
- Religious and spiritual beliefs

Adapted from Toledo SD, Trapani K, Feldbruegge E: Rheumatic diseases. In Braddom RL, editor: *Physical medicine and rehabilitation*, ed 4, Philadelphia, 2010, WB Saunders, pp 769–784.

AIMS, Arthritis Impact Measurement Scale; *CHART*, Caring Handicap Assessment Reporting Technique; *DAS 28*, Disease Activity Score Calculator for Rheumatoid Arthritis; *HAQ*, Health Assessment Questionnaire; *MRI*, magnetic resonance imaging; *WHODAS*, World Health Organization Disability Assessment Schedule; *WOMAC*, Western Ontario and McMaster Universities Osteoarthritis Index.

BOX 31-7

Principles of Joint Protection for Rheumatic Diseases

1. Respect pain as a signal to stop the activity.
2. Maintain muscle strength and joint range of motion.
   - Maintaining daily activities within the limitations of the patient's pain prevents disuse atrophy.
   - Strengthening around an unstable joint can increase stability and reduce pain.
3. Use each joint in its most stable anatomic and functional plane.
4. Avoid positions of deformity and forces in their direction.
   - For example: Turning resistive round doorknobs in an ulnar direction when the finger metacarpophalangeal joints are subluxed volarly and ulnarly should be avoided by use of a lever door opener.
5. Use the largest, strongest joints available for the job.
   - For example: Using a belted waist pack rather than holding purse with hook grasp.
6. Ensure correct patterns of movement.
   - For example: To push up when arising from a chair by using the flat surface of the palm rather than the dorsum of the fingers to prevent deforming forces toward metacarpophalangeal flexion; or cutting meat by holding the knife like a dagger.
7. Avoid staying in one position for long periods.
8. Avoid starting an activity that cannot be stopped immediately if it proves to be beyond capability.
9. Balance rest and activity.
10. Reduce the force.
    - Building up handles to avoid tight grasp.
    - Use of assistive devices, such as jar openers to reduce the stress of the hand and wrist joints.
    - For osteoarthritis, the cartilage is too thin to protect against repetitive use of force.
    - The patient should recognize the need to use alternative methods to accomplish the task. For example, the patient should use the handrail to reduce the impact load to involved knee joints while going up and down stairs.

Adapted from Cordery J, Rocchi M: Joint protection and fatigue management. In Melvin J, Jensen G editors. *Rheumatologic rehabilitation series, volume 1: assessment and management*, Bethesda, MD, 1998, American Occupational Therapy Association, pp 279–322.

use adaptive skills and environmental modifications and continue meaningful occupational functioning (Videos 31-1 to 31-7). In addition, exercises, weight loss (if obese), stress management/relaxation, and social support are usually included in the educational program. Fostering the patient's self-efficacy to follow treatment at home is important.[27]

Improve or Maintain Functional Mobility

Joint protection is a self-management technique widely taught to people with rheumatic diseases, especially RA (Box 31-7). Joint protection principles are ideally initiated early in the disease process to reduce loading to vulnerable joints, develop strategies with assistive devices and alternative movement patterns of affected joints to perform daily activities help preserve the present integrity of joint structures, relieve joint pain during activities, and relieve local inflammation.[11]

Research has provided strong evidence for the efficacy and long-term effect of joint protection programs.[18-20,30,37] Traditional teaching methods such as the use of written information, demonstrations, supervised practice, and visual aids have been successful in providing knowledge and skills. However, the behaviors of patients did not change and the efficacy was not significant. Following this, researchers emphasized that these principles require occupational therapists to apply teaching-learning techniques (i.e., skills practice, goal setting, and home programs) that will lead to these behavioral changes.

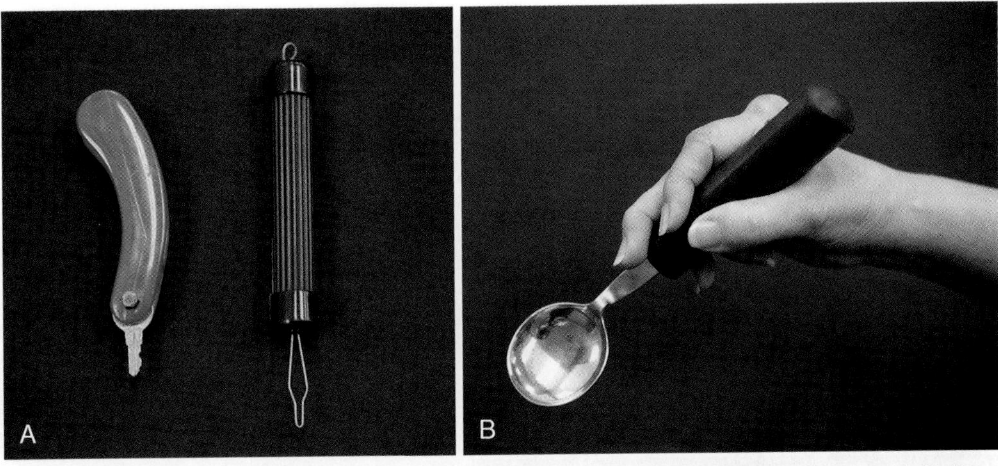

FIGURE 31-7 Assistive devices with built-up handles to avoid tight grasp. **A,** Broad key holder, buttoning and zipping aids. **B,** Easy-to-hold utensils.

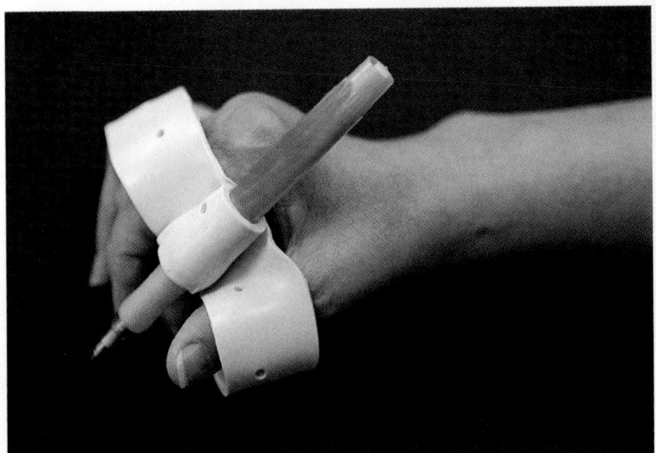

FIGURE 31-8 Writing aid.

Energy conservation principles are important to incorporate into the treatment intervention. Contributors to fatigue are multifactorial and include physiologic, behavioral, and environmental factors. To control the effects of fatigue on everyday activities, the therapist teaches the patient to analyze daily activities to determine what causes increased pain and fatigue. Taking short rest periods during a prolonged activity is often advised and is sometimes referred to as pacing.

Many devices and equipment can be applied to assist patients with rheumatic diseases, especially RA and OA. They are designed to limit stress to joints and to further achieve functional independence. For patients with limited range of motion (ROM) or pain in the hands, assistive devices such as a broad key holder, buttoning and zipping aids, and easy-to-hold utensils (Figure 31-7) were built with increased leverage or enlarged handles to decrease effort and dexterity demands.[12] Some devices, such as a writing aid (Figure 31-8), may enhance functional performance. Extended handle devices may be helpful for patients with limited ROM at shoulder, elbow, hip, or knee joints, such as long-handled comb, reacher, and sock aid (Figure 31-9). For patients with ambulation difficulties, mobility aids such as a walker, crutch, wheelchair, or scooter can be prescribed to accommodate different levels of difficulty or environmental requirements. An arthritic crutch with hand grip and forearm support is highly recommended for patients with arthritis to reduce the stress on hand or wrist joints during ambulation. Appropriate footwear or insoles may be considered to enhance comfort during ambulation. Some equipment can reduce the effort on the lower extremities (e.g., a lift chair, a shower chair, or elevated toilet seat) and may also help to reduce the stress placed on the hands. Generally, selection of these products requires professional advice.

Exercise

The purposes of exercise programs for patients with arthritis include: (1) increase and maintain ROM; (2) improve muscle strength and endurance; (3) increase aerobic capacity; (4) increase bone density; (5) improve functional ability; and (6) improve psychological function. In addition, through exercise programs, joints of patients with arthritis can function better biomechanically, and with improvement of aerobic capacity, cardiovascular morbidity and mortality is reduced.

Before exercise therapy is recommended, evaluating joint and periarticular conditions, as well as cardiopulmonary function and other systemic features is very important. Common exercise interventions for patients with arthritis include mobilization exercise, strengthening exercise, aerobic (or conditioning) exercise, and recreation exercise.

Mobilization exercise can be performed by ROM exercise, stretching exercise, proprioceptive neuromuscular facilitation (PNF) technique, or joint mobilization. In active inflamed joints, gentle active or active-assistive ROM through the possible range should be performed. Passive stretching should be applied with extreme caution, because it may be associated with rupture of the joint capsule with large effusion or may induce an inflammatory response in otherwise controlled joints. While inflammation subsides, the joint should be moved through the full range, possibly with assistance (active-assistive exercise). PNF techniques, such as hold-relax and slow reversal-hold-relax technique, could be applied to improve exercise efficiency.

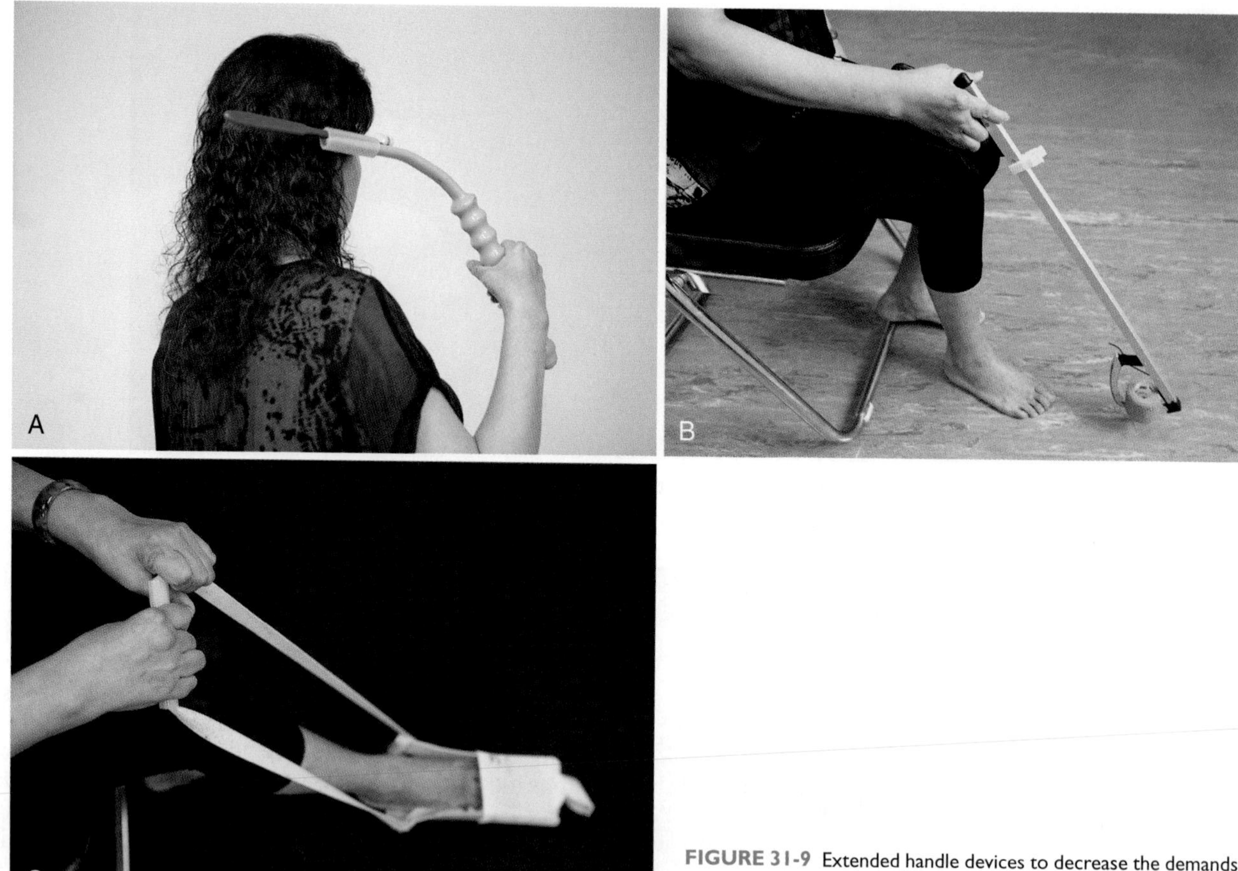

FIGURE 31-9 Extended handle devices to decrease the demands of range of motion at the shoulder and hip joints. **A,** Long-handled comb. **B,** Reacher. **C,** Sock aid.

Aquatherapy is also useful for mobilizing joints because buoyancy in water reduces the effect of gravity and thus unloads the joints. Mobilization exercise should commence in the early stages of arthritis, when just a few repetitions through the full range of motion is sufficient; if contracture or ankylosis of joints develops, it is difficult to restore the full range of motion.

The objective of strengthening exercise is to restore and maintain optimal muscle strength and endurance. There are three types of muscle contraction: (1) isometric or static contraction; (2) isotonic (dynamic) contraction; and (3) isokinetic dynamic contraction. During isometric contraction, there is no change in the muscle length and joint position. The advantage of isometric contraction is minimal joint stress during muscle contraction; thus it is suited to sufferers of arthritis with mechanically deranged joints. It may also be used in an acute inflammatory joint or immediately after surgery. During isotonic contraction, the load is fixed, but muscle length and joint position are changed. Isotonic contraction is suited for training of isotonic tasks and for patients without acute inflamed or biomechanically deranged joints, and should be avoided in patients with active arthritis, because isotonic contraction stresses the joint through its ROM. During isokinetic contraction, the velocity of muscle contraction is constant, but the muscle contraction force is changeable (accommodative resistance). Isokinetic contraction usually requires maximal force of contraction, which in most cases is not recommended for patients with arthritis (unless the joints are in very good condition).

The purpose of aerobic exercise is to increase aerobic capacity; it increases work capacity and promotes optimal function, and as such may reduce cardiovascular morbidity and mortality. Previous studies have showed that aerobic exercises increase aerobic capacity and functional ability in patients with RA, OA, AS, and FM. Before initiation of aerobic training, joint swelling and disease activity should be controlled. For patients with arthritis, the type of exercise should be low joint stress, such as walking, cycling, swimming, water aerobics, or low-impact aerobic dance. The exercise intensity, duration, and frequency could be adapted to those of cardiac rehabilitation. For water exercise, the temperature should be 83° F to 88° F (28° C to 31° C). Tai-chi exercise can also be used, but should be modified according to the patient's condition. Both land-based and water-based aerobic exercise programs 6 weeks to 3 months duration can have a positive effect on aerobic capacity, muscle strength, or functional ability.[23] During acute flares and periods of inflammation, strenuous exercises should be avoided. If joint pain persists for 2 hours after exercise and exceeds pain severity before exercise, the intensity and/or duration of exercise should be reduced.

Recreational exercise is often a combination of mobilization exercise, strengthening exercise, aerobic exercise, and also fun to do. It is usually a group exercise, that is, patients with a similar disease often exercise together.

Exercise programs may be a combination of land-based and water-based activities (Figure 31-10). Through recreational exercise, patients may improve muscle strength, aerobic capacity, as well as psychosocial well-being. It may provide social contact and have an antidepressant effect.

Orthoses

Orthotic positioning, especially hand splints, is usually considered and may have different benefits (decreasing inflammation and pain, function improvement, and minimizing deformity) for patients at different stages (Videos 31-8 to 31-14).[22,37] For example, it is very common to prescribe a resting hand splint to provide support and reduce pain for patients at the acute stage (Figure 31-11). To prevent undesirable position or motion, a three-point oval-8 splint (Figure 31-12) may be suggested to wear during occupational performance that allows flexion but prevents hyperextension of the finger PIP joints (swan neck deformity). The orthosis can be made of lightweight thermoplastics, or soft materials can be used to counteract the deforming forces.

There are indicative findings that splints are effective in reducing pain both immediately after provision of the splint and after splinting over a period of time.[42] A systematic review also indicated the temporary effectiveness in increasing grip strength while wearing a splint. However, there is no sufficient evidence to show that wearing a splint for a long time can decrease the severity of hand deformities or to preserve the hand function.[1,14,15,37]

Physical Modalities

Physical modalities such as thermotherapy (heat and cold therapy), electric therapy, and lower power laser are commonly used in rehabilitation practice to relieve pain and increase flexibility of joints and soft tissue in patients with rheumatic disorders.

Heat

Heat therapy (including superficial or deep heat) can increase both skin and joint temperature and increase the viscoelastic properties of collagen. Clinically, these two effects can relieve stiffness of joints and soft tissue, and

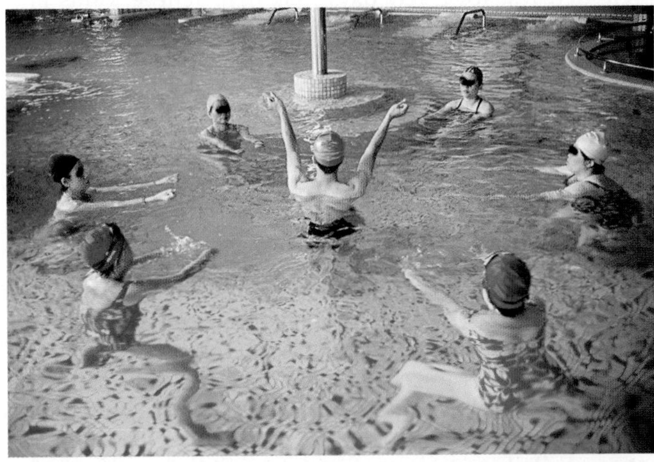

FIGURE 31-10 A group pool exercise for patients with rheumatoid arthritis.

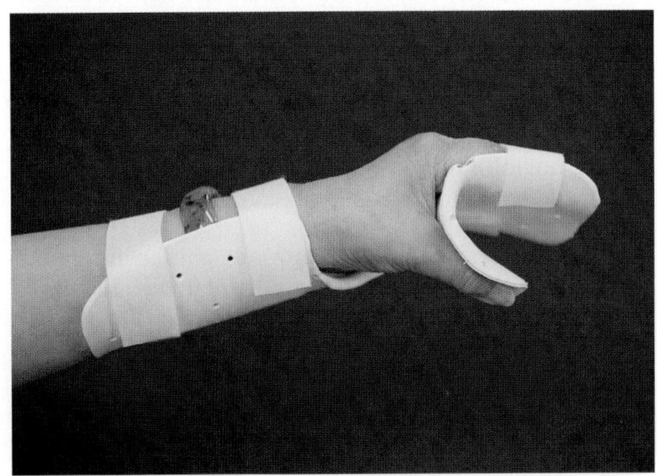

FIGURE 31-11 Resting splints (night splint).

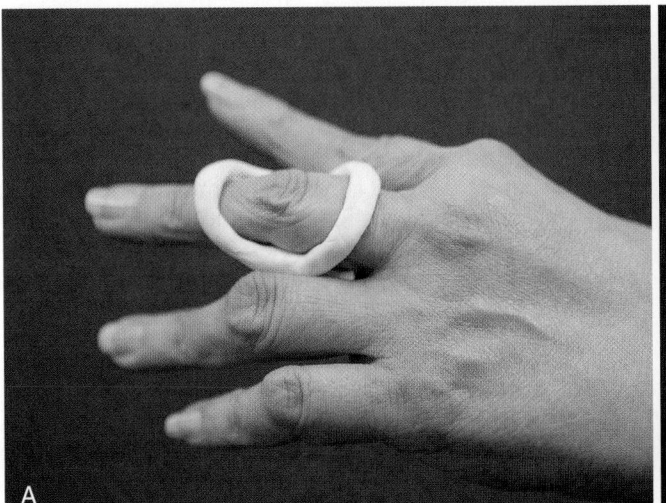

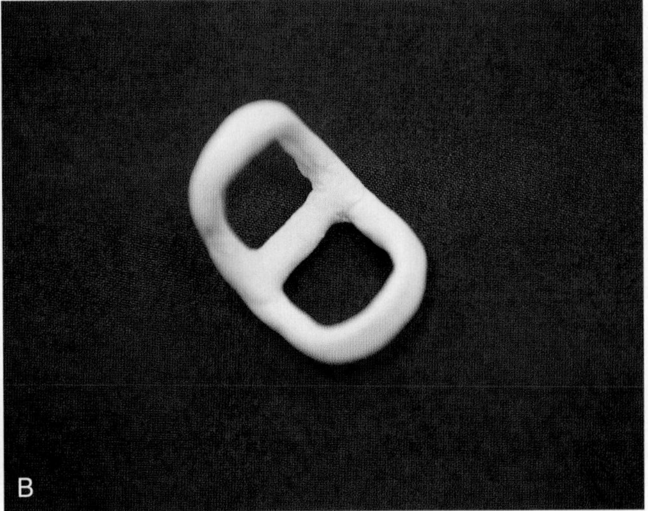

FIGURE 31-12 **A,** Orthotic positioning of a swan neck deformity. **B,** The oval-8 splint prevents proximal interphalangeal hyperextension and allows flexion.

thus enhance the efficacy of stretching. In addition, both superficial and deep heat can raise the pain threshold, producing analgesia and a sedation effect by acting on A-delta and C fibers and muscle spindles. Conversely, heat therapy can increase joint swelling, elevate leucocyte counts in the joint fluid of patients with arthritis, and may cause ischemic necrosis of the synovium by increasing its metabolic demand.

The most commonly used heat modalities in rheumatic diseases are moist heating pads, paraffin (Video 31-15), electric heating pads, infrared, ultrasound, and shortwave diathermy. Most studies conclude that heat modalities do not alter the disease process. There is also concern about the use of paraffin in systemic sclerosis, because microvascular pathology may create heat dissipation impairments. However, paraffin baths are recommended for short-term benefits for arthritic hands.

Cold

The effects of cold therapy are to reduce skin and joint temperature, reduce joint swelling and cell count in synovial fluid, decrease the metabolic demand of the synovium, and inhibit collagenase activity. It can also raise the pain threshold and inhibit muscle spindle activity. Therefore, it can provide pain relief and reduce inflammation in patients with acute arthritis. Common cold modalities include cold pack, cold air, ice pack, or cold bath. Cold should not be used in patients with cold hypersensitivity, Raynaud's phenomenon, cryoglobulinemia, or paroxysmal cold hemoglobinuria.

Electric Therapy

The purposes of electric therapy are pain control and muscle stimulation. There are different types, including transcutaneous electric nerve stimulation (TENS)[9] (Video 31-16) and middle frequency interferential therapy, and are commonly used in the treatment of rheumatic diseases. Electric therapy has been shown to have a clinically beneficial effect on grip strength for patients who have RA with hand atrophy. Another study showed that TENS may be more effective than hyaluronic acid intraarticular injection in patients with OA of the knee (Figure 31-13). Although evidence of the efficacy of electric therapy for rheumatic diseases is still lacking, electric therapy can reduce joint and soft tissue pain, thus it may reduce the dosage of pain medications.

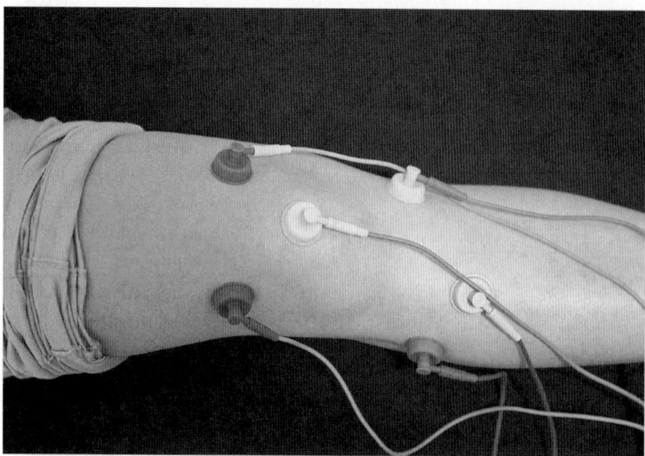

FIGURE 31-13 Transcutaneous electric nerve stimulation for arthritis of the knee. (Reprint with permission of *Archives of Physical Medicine and Rehabilitation.*)

Low-Level (or Low-Power) Laser Therapy

Low-level laser therapy has been used in the treatment of rheumatic diseases including RA, OA, lower back pain, and carpal tunnel syndrome for more than 20 years. Six studies of medium-quality tested over 220 patients with RA and showed that low-level laser therapy decreased pain and morning stiffness more than placebo laser therapy. No side effects were reported.

Rehabilitation Intervention for Rheumatoid Arthritis

Acute Stage

In the acute stage, patients with RA often have arthritis involving multiple joints, and this may be accompanied by fever, weight loss, anemia, and fatigue. In this stage, complete bed rest for a few days may help relieve joints and systemic symptoms. If one to two joints are more severe, resting splints are recommended. Application of a cold pack or TENS over the inflammatory joints may help reduce joint swelling and relieve joint pain. If there is severe spasm and pain in the nearby muscles, local hot packs or gentle massage would be beneficial. Bed rest should be as short as possible, because prolonged bed rest may lead to deconditioning.[41]

For prevention of joint and soft tissue contracture, actively inflamed joints should be moved gently through the possible range by the patient (active ROM) or with assistance from another person (active-assisted ROM). Three repetitions for each joint, once or twice daily, are suggested. As joint inflammation subsides, the range may be increased gradually to the full range, possibly with assistance. A PNF technique could be applied early on for selected muscle groups. Passive stretching is usually not performed in an inflammatory joint, and if performed it should be done with extreme caution, because it may worsen or prolong the inflammatory process, or lead to subluxation or rupture of a joint.

For minimizing muscle atrophy, isometric exercise at submaximal effort is recommended in the inflammatory condition. At first, a few nonresistive repetitions should be performed with a gradual increase in repetition and resistance. Isotonic exercise is not recommended in the acute inflammatory stage. Patient education (including joint protection and energy conservation techniques) should commence.[40]

Subacute and Chronic Stages

After the acute stage subsides, joint pain, morning stiffness, and joint swelling diminishes. Isotonic exercise can be added to the exercise program gradually, with increases in repetition and resistance. Local cold therapy can be changed to hot therapy if swelling of the joint subsides. Splints, foot orthoses, or assistive devices can be prescribed if indicated.

A forearm support crutch or cane is more preferable than a traditional wrist support device. If patient condition improves, endurance training, aerobic exercise, and recreational exercise can be added to the exercise program.

Rehabilitation Intervention for Ankylosing Spondylitis

The main symptoms of AS include chronic back pain, spinal deformity, limited chest excursion, and pain and contracture of the involved peripheral joints (especially the hips). The characteristic posture of patients with AS is loss of lumbar lordosis, increased thoracic kyphosis, compensatory extension of the cervical spine, and flexion of hip and knee joints. The center of mass of the trunk in the sagittal plane shifts forward and downward.[7] The main aims of management for patients with AS are pain relief, improvement of posture and mobility, and maintenance or improvement of respiratory function.

Pain relief may be achieved with the use of antiinflammatory drugs and physical modalities including hot or cold packs, hot baths, hydrotherapy, spa therapy, diathermy, electric therapy, and mobility exercise (Video 31-17). Maintenance of good mobility of the spine and peripheral joints not only relates to physical function but also affects relief of pain and stiffness. Before mobility exercise, a hot pack, or hot bath (shower), followed by 5 to 10 minutes of warm-up exercise is suggested. The target areas for stretching are the suboccipital muscles, pectoral muscles, hamstrings, hip flexors, and spinal rotators. The ROM exercise should include extension of all segments of the spine, as well as full ROM of the neck, shoulders, and hips. It is advisable for patients to perform the exercises at the time of a day when they feel the least pain or fatigue. PNF techniques provided by therapists are also suggested if available. Strengthening exercises for the major muscle groups including back extensors, shoulder retractors, hip extensors, and other postural muscles are also recommended (Videos 31-18 and 31-19). In addition, aerobic training with brisk walking, cycling (with upright handlebars), swimming, or other aquatic therapy can help increase muscle endurance and reduce cardiovascular morbidity and mortality.

Inflammation of the costochondral joints or costovertebral joints or entheses may cause chest pain and inhibit deep breathing. Treatment with antiinflammatory drugs and heat therapy may help relieve pain and improve breathing patterns. Daily deep-breathing exercises with an emphasis on full rib cage expansion are encouraged.

Education about correct posture is very important for patients with AS. Patients should be instructed how to check their postural alignment (e.g., measure body height, touch the occipital protuberance to the wall while standing), and avoid positions that encourage a stooped posture or spinal flexion for prolonged periods. A firm mattress and a small pillow or neck support are desirable for sleep. Lying on the side in a curved position should be avoided. Daily prone lying for 10 to 15 minutes or more is recommended.[16] Because patients with AS often have a fragile and osteoporotic spine, contact sports, cervical traction, or spinal manipulation should be avoided. Minor trauma that results in fracture or dislocation of the spine with spinal cord compression is not uncommon. For enhancing independence in activities of daily living, prism glasses, long-handled devices, or a cane may be needed.

Summary

With a growing number of patients with rheumatic diseases, research on prevention and treatment is evolving. Less invasive surgical options and expanding conservative treatment to combine allopathic and naturopathic medicine is the current trend. Physiatrists will continue to be an integral part of the management. The chronicity and disabling nature of these diseases will continue to challenge physiatrists to be innovative and creative.

REFERENCES

1. Adams J, Burridge J, Mullee M, et al: The clinical effectiveness of static resting splints in early rheumatoid arthritis: a randomized controlled trial, *Rheumatology* 47:1548–1553, 2008.
2. Aletaha D, Neogi T, Silman AJ, et al: 2010 rheumatoid arthritis classification criteria: an American College of Rheumatology/European League Against Rheumatism collaborative initiative, *Arthritis Rheum* 62:2569–2581, 2010.
3. Amato AA, Barohn RJ: Evaluation and treatment of inflammatory myopathies, *J Neurol Neurosurg Psychiatry* 80:1060–1068, 2009.
4. Andriacchi TP, Koo S, Scanlan SF: Gait mechanics influence healthy cartilage morphology and osteoarthritis of the knee, *J Bone Joint Surg Am* 91(Suppl 1):95–101, 2009.
5. Arnett FC, Edworthy SM, Bloch DA, et al: The American Rheumatism Association 1987 revised criteria for the classification of rheumatoid arthritis, *Arthritis Rheum* 31:315–324, 1988.
6. Barker K, Lamb SE, Toye F, et al: Association between radiographic joint space narrowing, function, pain, and muscle power in severe osteoarthritis of the knee, *Clin Rehabil* 18:798–800, 2004.
7. Bot SDM, Caspers M, van Royen BJ, et al: Biochemical analysis of posture in patients with spinal kyphosis due to ankylosing spondylitis: a pilot study, *Rheumatology* 38:441–443, 1999.
8. Braun J, van den Berg R, Baraliakos X, et al: 2010 update of the ASAS/EULAR recommendations for the management of ankylosing spondylitis, *Ann Rheum Dis* 70:896–904, 2011.
9. Chen WL, Hsu WC, Hsieh LF, et al: Comparison of intra-articular hyaluronic acid injection with transcutaneous electric nerve stimulation for the management of knee osteoarthritis, *Arch Phys Med Rehabil* 94:1482–1489, 2013.
10. Cheng D, Visco C: Pharmaceutical therapy for osteoarthritis, *PM&R* 4(Suppl 5):S82–S88, 2012.
11. Cordery J, Rocchi M: Joint protection and fatigue management, *Rheumatol Rehabil* 1:279–322, 1998.
12. Deshaies L: Arthritis. In Pendleton HM, Schultz-Krohn W, editors: *Pedretti's occupational therapy: practice skills for physical dysfunction*, ed 7, St Louis, 2011, Mosby Elsevier, pp 1003–1036.
13. Dillon CF, Rasch EK, Gu Q, et al: Prevalence of knee osteoarthritis in the United States: arthritis data from the Third National Health and Nutrition Examination Survey 1991–94, *J Rheumatol* 33:2271–2279, 2006.
14. Egan MY, Brousseau L: Splinting for osteoarthritis of the carpometacarpal joint: a review of the evidence, *Am J Occup Ther* 61:70–78, 2007.
15. Egan MY, Brousseau L, Farmer M, et al: Splints and orthoses for treating rheumatoid arthritis, *Cochrane Database Syst Rev* (4):CD004018, 2001.
16. Elyan M, Khan MA: Does physical therapy still have a place in the treatment of ankylosing spondylitis, *Curr Opin Rheumatol* 20:282–286, 2008.
17. Goie HS, Steven MM, van der Linden SM, et al: Evaluation of diagnostic criteria for ankylosing spondylitis: a comparison of the Rome, New York and modified New York criteria in patients with a positive clinical history screening test for ankylosing spondylitis, *Br J Rheumatol* 24:242–249, 1985.

18. Hammond A, Bryan J, Hardy A: Effects of a modular behavioral arthritis education program: a pragmatic parallel-group randomized controlled trial, *Rheumatology* 47:1712–1718, 2008.
19. Hammond A, Freeman K: The long term outcomes from a randomized controlled trial of an educational-behavioral joint protection program for people with rheumatoid arthritis, *Clin Rehabil* 18:520–528, 2004.
20. Hammond A, Jefferson P, Jones N, et al: Clinical applicability of an educational-behavioral joint protection program for people with rheumatoid arthritis, *Br J Occup Ther* 65:405–412, 2002.
21. Hannah MT, Felson DT, Pincus T: Analysis of discordance between radiographic changes and knee pain in osteoarthritis of the knee, *J Rheumatol* 27:1513–1517, 2000.
22. Harrell P: Splinting of the hand. In Robbins L, Burckhardt CS, Hannan MT, DeHoratius RJ, editors: *Clinical care in the rheumatic diseases*, ed 2, Atlanta, 2001, Association of Rheumatology Health Professionals, pp 191–196.
23. Hsieh LF, Chen SC, Chuang CC, et al: Supervised aerobic exercise is more effective than home exercise in female patients with rheumatoid arthritis, *J Rehabil Med* 41:332–337, 2009.
24. Laplante B, DePalma M: Spine osteoarthritis, *PM&R* 4(Suppl 5):S28–S36, 2012.
25. Lawrence JS, Bremner JM, Bier F: Osteoarthrosis: prevalence in the population and relationship between symptoms and x-ray changes, *Ann Rheum Dis* 25:1–24, 1966.
26. Leopold SA, Battista V, Oliverio JA: Safety and efficacy of intra-articular hip injection using anatomic landmarks, *Clin Orthop Relat Res* 391:192–197, 2001.
27. Marks R: Efficacy theory and its utility in arthritis rehabilitation: review and recommendations, *Disabil Rehabil* 23:271–280, 2001.
28. McGonagle D: The synovio-entheseal complex and its role in tendon capsular associated inflammation, *J Rheumatol Suppl* 89:11–14, 2012.
29. Mizner RL, Peterson SC, Stevens JE, et al: Preoperative quadriceps strength predicts functional ability one year after total knee athroplasty, *J Rheumatol* 32:1533–1539, 2005.
30. Niedermann K, deBie RA, Kubli R, et al: Effectiveness of individual resource-oriented joint protection education in people with rheumatoid arthritis: a randomized controlled trial, *Patient Educ Couns* 82:42–48, 2011.
31. Prather H: Physiatry serves an important role in the acute care of patients: disability prevention, *PM&R* 4:469–472, 2012.
32. Raisz L: Pathogenesis of osteoporosis: concepts, conflicts, and prospects, *J Clin Invest* 115:3318–3325, 2005.
33. Rudwaleit M, Baraliakos X, Listing J: at al: Magnetic resonance imaging of the spine and the sacroiliac joints in ankylosing spondylitis and undifferentiated spondyloarthritis during treatment with etanercept, *Ann Rheum Dis* 64:1305–1310, 2005.
34. Singh JA, Furst DE, Bharat A, et al: 2012 update of the 2008 American College of Rheumatology recommendations for the use of disease-modifying antirheumatic drugs and biologic agents in the treatment of rheumatoid arthritis, *Arthritis Care Res* 64:625–639, 2012.
35. Smith J, Hurdle MF: Office based ultrasound-guided intra-articular hip injection: technique for physiatric practice, *Arch Phys Med Rehab* 87:296–298, 2006.
36. Smolen JS, Landewé R, Breedveld FC, et al: EULAR recommendations for the management of rheumatoid arthritis with synthetic and biological disease-modifying antirheumatic drugs: 2013 update, *Ann Rheum Dis* 73:492–509, 2014.
37. Steultjens EM, Dekker J, Bouter LM, et al: Occupational therapy for rheumatoid arthritis: a systematic review, *Arthritis Care Res* 47:672–685, 2002.
38. Suri P, Morgenroth D, Hunter D: Epidemiology of osteoarthritis and associated comorbidities, *PM&R* 4:S10–S17, 2012.
39. Valle-Onate R, Ward MM, Kerr GS: Physical therapy and surgery, *Am J Med Sci* 343:353–356, 2012.
40. Vliet V, Theodora PM, van den Ende CH, Cornelia H: Nonpharmacological treatment of rheumatoid arthritis, *Curr Opin Rheumatol* 23:259–264, 2011.
41. Walker JM, Helewa A: *Physical rehabilitation in arthritis*, ed 2, St Louis, 2004, Saunders.
42. Weiss S, LaStayo P, Mills A, et al: Prospective analysis of splinting the first carpometacarpal joint: an objective, subjective, and radiographic assessment, *J Hand Surg* 13:218–227, 2000.
43. Zeboulon N, Dougados M, Gossec L: Prevalence and characteristics of uveitis in the spondyloarthropathies: a systemic literature review, *Ann Rheum Dis* 67:955–959, 2008.

SECTION 4

Issues in Specific Diagnoses

CHAPTER 32

COMMON NECK PROBLEMS

Michael J. DePalma, Justin J. Gasper, Curtis W. Slipman

Successful treatment of painful cervical spine disorders hinges on the accurate assessment of the underlying tissue injury, which can involve a broad range of biomechanical and biochemical disorders. The clinician needs to conceptualize a process of diagnosis and treatment that incorporates an understanding of the pathophysiology of cervical spine injury and the associated potential symptom manifestations, an awareness of the advantages and disadvantages of the myriad diagnostic tools, and knowledge of the potential therapeutic options. The initial step in this process is the history taking. It is important that one distinguish between cervical axial pain (neck pain) and upper limb pain. As eloquently stated by Bogduk,[29] the neck is not the upper limb, and the upper limb is not the neck. Pain in the upper limb is not pain in the neck, and vice versa.

Cervical axial pain must not be mistaken for cervical radicular pain. Cervical axial pain is defined as pain occurring in all or part of a corridor extending from the inferior occiput to the superior interscapular region, localizing to the midline or paramidline. The patient perceives it as stemming from the neck. Cervical radicular pain, defined as pain involving the shoulder girdle or distal areas, manifests as pain in the upper limb. The etiologies of these two different sets of symptoms vary, as does the diagnosis and management of each. Equating cervical axial and cervical radicular pain can result in misdiagnosis, inappropriate investigation, and institution of suboptimal treatment.[29] Such confusion can easily occur, because both disorders result from injury to the cervical spine. Each of these injuries or conditions differs in occurrence, mechanism, pathophysiology, treatment, and rehabilitation.

Epidemiologic reports have sometimes clustered neck and limb pain, but neck complaints are ubiquitous. The prevalence of neck pain with or without upper limb pain ranges from 9% to 18% of the general population,[131,147,242,253] and one out of three individuals can recall at least one incidence of neck pain in their lifetime.[131] Cervical pain is more frequently encountered in clinical practice than low back pain,[261] and traumatic neck pain becomes chronic in up to 40% of patients, with 8% to 10% experiencing severe pain.[55] The occurrence increases in the workplace, with a prevalence of 35% to 71% among Swedish forest and industrial workers.[99,101] The frequency of occupational cervical complaints increases with age. Approximately 25% to 30% of workers younger than 30 years of age report neck stiffness, and 50% of workers older than 45 years old report similar complaints.[100,242,253]

Cervical radiculopathy occurs less commonly, with an annual incidence of 83.2 per 100,000, and peaks at 50 to 54 years of age.[189] Five to ten percent of workers younger than 30 years old complain of pain referring into the upper limb, whereas 25% to 40% of those older than 45 years old experience pain in the upper limb.[100] Overall, 23% of working men have experienced at least one episode of upper limb pain.[100] Neck pain and cervical radicular pain are common complaints across different patient profiles.

Evaluating and treating common cervical spine disorders requires the completion of a probability analysis of what injured structure is most likely responsible for the patient's presentation. An astute spine clinician recognizes individual symptom composites to accurately diagnose and treat these injuries. This chapter is intended to be a foundation for approaching common painful cervical spine disorders, and provides a view of a tiered treatment algorithm that incorporates appropriate therapeutic interventions across a spectrum of care.

Pathophysiology and the Significance of Pain Referral Patterns

A working knowledge of the anatomic interrelationships within the cervical spine (Figure 32-1) is important to comprehend the pathomechanisms of cervical spine disorders. The cervical spine is a discrete segment of the axial skeleton (see Figure 32-1) and functions to support and stabilize the head; allow the head to move in all planes of motion; and protect the spinal cord, nerve roots, spinal nerves, and vertebral arteries.[177] There are seven cervical vertebrae and eight cervical nerve roots. The atlantooccipital (C0-C1) articulation permits 10 degrees of flexion and 25 degrees of extension. The C1-C2 level or the atlantoaxial joint (Figure 32-2) forms the upper cervical segment, and is responsible for 40% to 50% of all cervical axial rotation, demonstrated clinically by 45 degrees of rotation in either direction.[61,62,70,255] Below the C2-C3 level, lateral flexion of the cervical spine is coupled with rotation in the same direction. This spinal segment marks a transition where permitted motion changes from rotation to flexion, extension, and lateral bending.[70,247] This combined motion is facilitated by the 45-degree sagittal inclination of the cervical zygapophyseal joints (see Figure 32-1).[149] The zygapophyseal joints allow motion within the cervical spine, connect each vertebral segment,[220] and are innervated by medial branches from the cervical dorsal rami (Figure 32-3).[30] In addition, the C0-C1 joint is innervated by the C1 ventral ramus,[132] and the C1-C2 joint by the C2 ventral ramus laterally[132] and the sinuvertebral nerves of C1, C2, and C3 medially.[121] The greatest amount of flexion occurs at C4-C5 and C5-C6, whereas lateral bending occurs primarily at C3-C4 and C4-C5.[70,247] The lower cervical

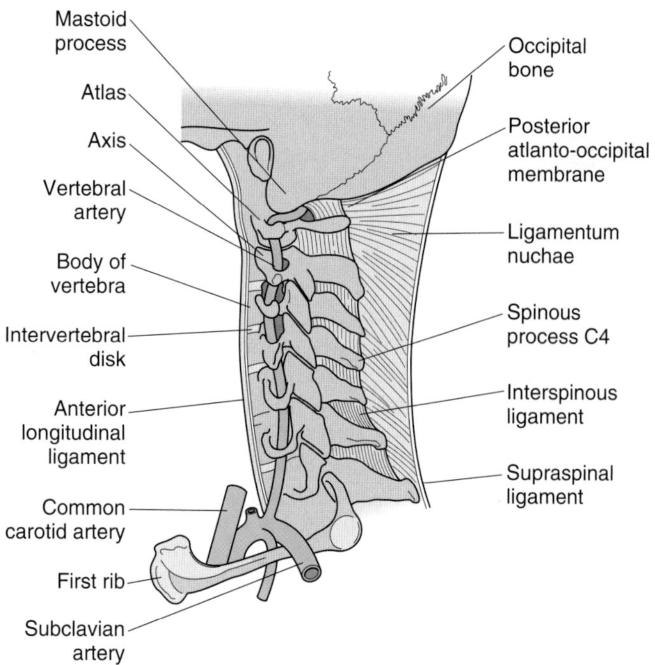

FIGURE 32-1 Anatomic relationship of cervical spine ligaments to other structures in the neck.

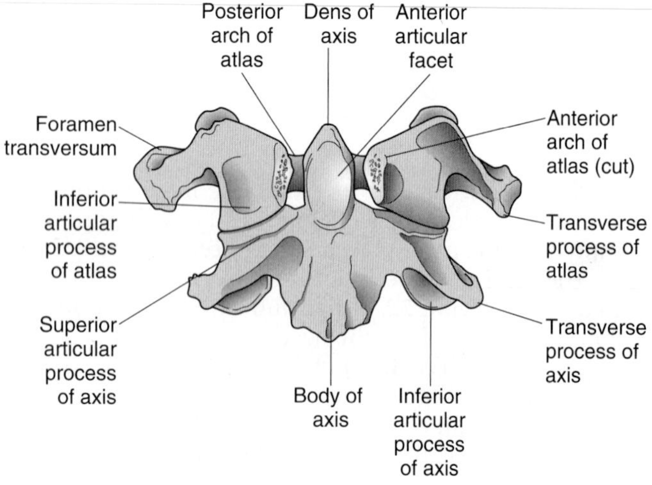

FIGURE 32-2 Anterior view of the atlas and axis. The anterior tubercle of the atlas has been removed to reveal the odontoid process of the axis.

vertebrae (C3-C7) have unique synovial jointlike articulations, uncovertebral joints, or joints of Luschka, located between the uncinate processes (Figure 32-4).[167] These joints commonly develop osteoarthritic changes, which can narrow the diameter of the intervertebral foramina (Figure 32-5).[81,98,238] These intervertebral foramina are widest at the C2-C3 level and progressively decrease in size to the C6-C7 level. The radicular complex of dorsal root ganglia, nerve roots, spinal nerve, and surrounding sheath accounts for 20% to 35% of the cross-sectional area of the intervertebral foramina.[81,98,238] The remaining intervertebral foramina volume is filled by loose areolar or adipose tissue, Hoffman ligaments, radicular artery, and numerous venous conduits that usually encircle the nerve roots.[220] The neuroforamina are bordered anteromedially by the uncovertebral joint, superiorly and inferiorly by successive pedicles, and medially by the edge of the vertebral end plate and intervertebral disk (Figure 32-5).[220]

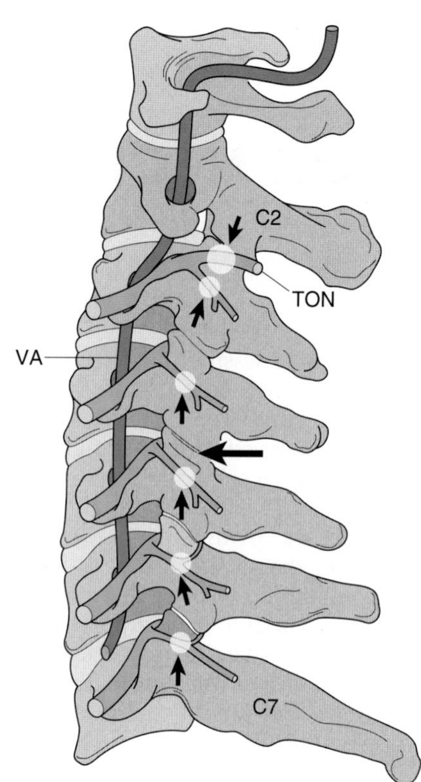

FIGURE 32-3 Target zones for cervical medial branch block. Lateral illustration of the cervical spine, showing target zones (*arrows* pointing to circles) located at the midportion of the C2 through C7 articular pillars. The third occipital nerve (TON) is a relatively large nerve branch that may require three separate blocks at the level of the C2 inferior facet-C3 superior facet and where it courses lateral to the C2-C3 facet joint. *VA*, Vertebral artery.

The intervertebral disks are located between the vertebral bodies of C2 through C7. Each is composed of an outer annulus fibrosus innervated posterolaterally by the sinuvertebral nerve, comprising branches from the vertebral nerve and ventral ramus, and innervated anteriorly by the vertebral nerve (Figure 32-6).[24] The inner portions of the disks comprise the gelatinous nucleus pulposus, providing transmission of axial loads to dissipate forces throughout various ranges of motion.[220] Each intervertebral disk is thicker anteriorly than posteriorly, which contributes to the natural cervical lordotic curvature.[220] Normal cervical spine anatomy can undergo degenerative or traumatic changes, leading to various cervical spine disorders.

Three essential requirements are needed for a structure to serve as a source of pain. It must be innervated, capable of producing pain similar to that seen clinically, and susceptible to disease or injury known to be painful.[28] Nonneural structures of the neck, such as the intervertebral disk, zygapophyseal joint, posterior longitudinal ligament, and muscles, can serve as a nidus for pain and produce somatic referral of pain into the upper limb.[38,69,117-119] Classic experiments have demonstrated that stimulation of these posterior midline structures produces local neck pain as well as somatically referred pain into the upper limb.[38,69,117-119,129] Kellegren[118,119] was first to investigate the pain referral patterns of nonneural spinal structures by stimulating periosteum, fascia, tendon, and muscle with

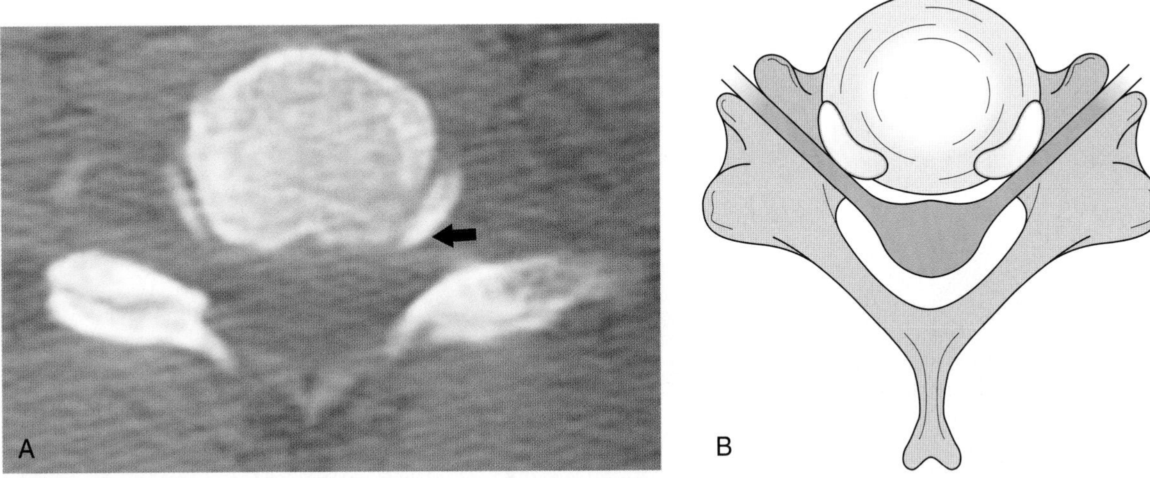

FIGURE 32-4 Luschka (uncovertebral) joints. **A,** The cervical spine, displaying Luschka joint (*arrow*). **B,** Proximity of uncovertebral joints to cervical nerve roots.

hypertonic saline. He hypothesized that a central nervous system phenomenon mediated the pain referral, because anesthetizing the corresponding peripheral nerve distal to the site of stimulation did not diminish the distally referred pain. These experiments were the first to demonstrate this phenomenon of somatically referred pain, and that cervical spinal disorders could produce pain in the upper limb as well as headache.[38,69,117-119,129] These symptoms were produced without irritation of neural tissue. Such pain referral has been termed *somatic,* previously labeled as sclerotomal, and occurs when a mesodermal structure such as a ligament, joint capsule, intervertebral disk annulus, or periosteum is stimulated, leading to symptoms referred into another mesodermal tissue structure of similar embryonic origin.[220] This mechanism of somatically referred symptoms involves convergence.[29] Afferents from both the cervical spine and the distal upper limb converge on second-order neurons within the spinal cord, allowing spine pain to be misperceived as arising from those distal limb sites.[29] It is via this mechanism that cervical intervertebral disks and zygapophyseal joints create upper limb symptoms.[220]

It is believed that biomechanical or biochemical insults to nonneural structures can trigger nociceptive nerve fibers, via compression or inflammation, causing pain referral.[220] Mechanical stimulation of the cervical zygapophyseal joints or their innervating nerves has been shown to produce head and neck pain with upper limb referral patterns (Figure 32-7).[10,59,63,73] Anesthetizing symptomatic joints has revealed similar patterns of symptomatic referral from the cervical joints.[22,223]

Pain emanating from the cervical zygapophyseal joints tends to follow relatively constant and recognizable referral patterns. The C1-C2 and C2-C3 levels refer rostrally to the occiput. The C3-C4 and C4-C5 joints produce symptoms over the posterior neck and C3-C4 can also refer into the occiput. Pain from the C5-C6 joint spreads over the supraspinatus fossa of the scapula, whereas pain from the C6-C7 joint spreads farther caudally over the scapula.*

*References 10, 22, 29, 59, 63, 73.

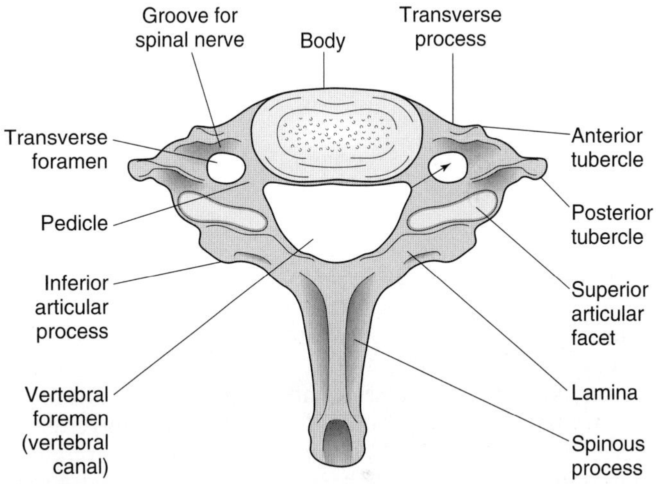

Groove for spinal nerve
Body
Transverse process
Transverse foramen
Anterior tubercle
Posterior tubercle
Pedicle
Inferior articular process
Superior articular facet
Lamina
Vertebral foremen (vertebral canal)
Spinous process

FIGURE 32-5 Axial view of the seventh cervical vertebrae, illustrating the intervertebral foramen (*black arrow*).

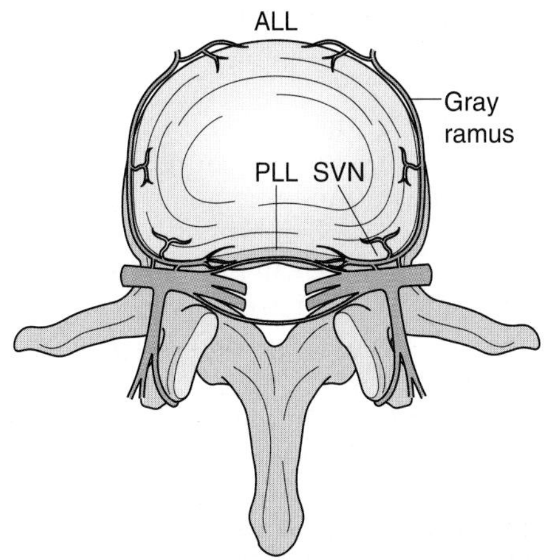

FIGURE 32-6 Nerve supply of the cervical intervertebral disk. *ALL,* Anterior longitudinal ligament; *PLL,* posterior longitudinal ligament; *SVN,* sinovertebral nerve. (From Bogduk N, Twomey LT: *Clinical anatomy of the lumbar spine,* New York, 1991, Churchill Livingstone, p 117.)

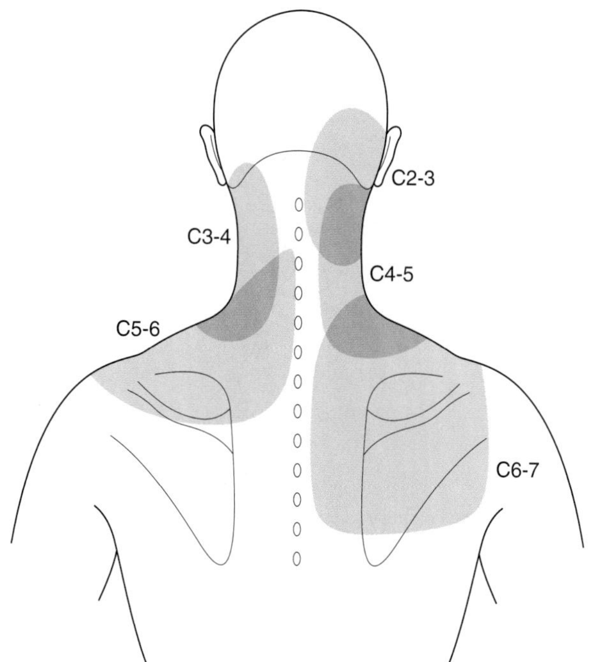

FIGURE 32-7 Pain referral from C2 to C3 through C6 to C7 facet joints. (From Dwyer A, Aprill C, Bogduk N: Cervical zygapophyseal joint pain patterns. I: a study in normal volunteers, *Spine* 15:453-457, 1990.)

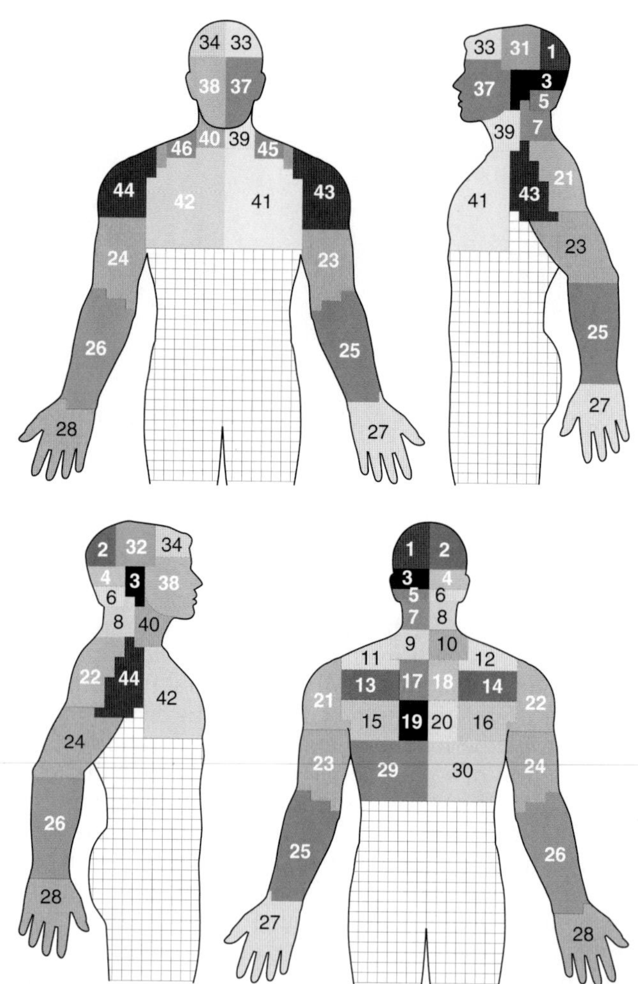

FIGURE 32-8 Dermatomal distribution of the cervical nerve roots. (From Ellis H: *Clinical anatomy: a revision and applied anatomy for clinical students*, ed 6, London, 1976, Blackwell, p 205.)

Additionally, C1-C2, C2-C3, C3-C4, and C4-C5 zygapophyseal joints can refer pain to the face, and C3-C4, C4-C5, and C5-C6 can refer symptoms to the head.[22] Each joint can produce unilateral or bilateral symptoms. It is not intuitive that a unilateral joint could trigger only contralateral pain, and this manifestation has never been formally investigated.[222]

Very similar pain referral patterns have been produced by mechanical stimulation of the cervical intervertebral disks (Figure 32-8).[45,79,205,228] In our experience, bilateral paramidline upper neck pain without associated headaches is commonly caused by cervical intervertebral disk disruption (CIDD) rather than zygapophyseal joint–mediated pain. Our observations are supported by Grubb and Kelly's[79] findings that 34% to 50% of cervical disks produced bilateral pain at each cervical disk level. Furthermore, a more detailed study from the Penn Spine Center[228] revealed that 30% to 62% of cervical disks produced bilateral pain during cervical diskography. When taken together, these findings support the notion that the pattern of pain stemming from a particular structure is a consequence of that structure's innervation rather than the structure itself.[29] In line with this logic is the finding that stimulation of the upper cervical musculature can produce pain in the head.[52] Discriminating CIDD-mediated pain from zygapophyseal joint pain or pain emanating from the cervical spine soft tissues requires systematic and meticulous interpretation of history and physical examination findings.

Cervical radicular pain is fundamentally a different clinical picture, because the presenting chief complaint is typically upper limb pain more severe than axial pain. The etiology of upper limb symptoms can be confusing when a nonradicular disorder creates symptoms in a radicular distribution, or when a usually radicular disorder causes pain in an uncharacteristic dynatomal pattern (pattern of referred symptoms).[229] Regardless, radicular pain is most consistent with upper limb symptoms that are more intense than axial complaints.[220] Upper limb pain caused by cervical radiculopathy can refer symptoms into the arm, forearm, or hand (Figure 32-9).[64] However, periscapular or trapezial pain greater than neck pain can be caused by upper cervical nerve root involvement such as C4 or C5.[229] Radicular pain from C5 tends to remain in the arm, but pain from C6, C7, and C8 extends into the forearm and hand. Nevertheless, pain that is primarily in the upper back with or without arm symptoms can emanate from the C4 through C6 roots. When experienced in the middle to lower aspect of the ipsilateral scapula, C7 or C8 roots could be the culprit.

Nerve vulnerability within the intervertebral foramina arises consequent to changes in one or more of three separate structures: the zygapophyseal joints, the uncovertebral joints, and the intervertebral disk. The most common cause of cervical radiculopathy is a herniated cervical intervertebral disk,[102] followed by cervical spondylosis[264] with or without cervical myelopathy (Box 32-1). The precise mechanism by which disk herniation or spondylosis causes radicular pain is still somewhat unclear. Direct

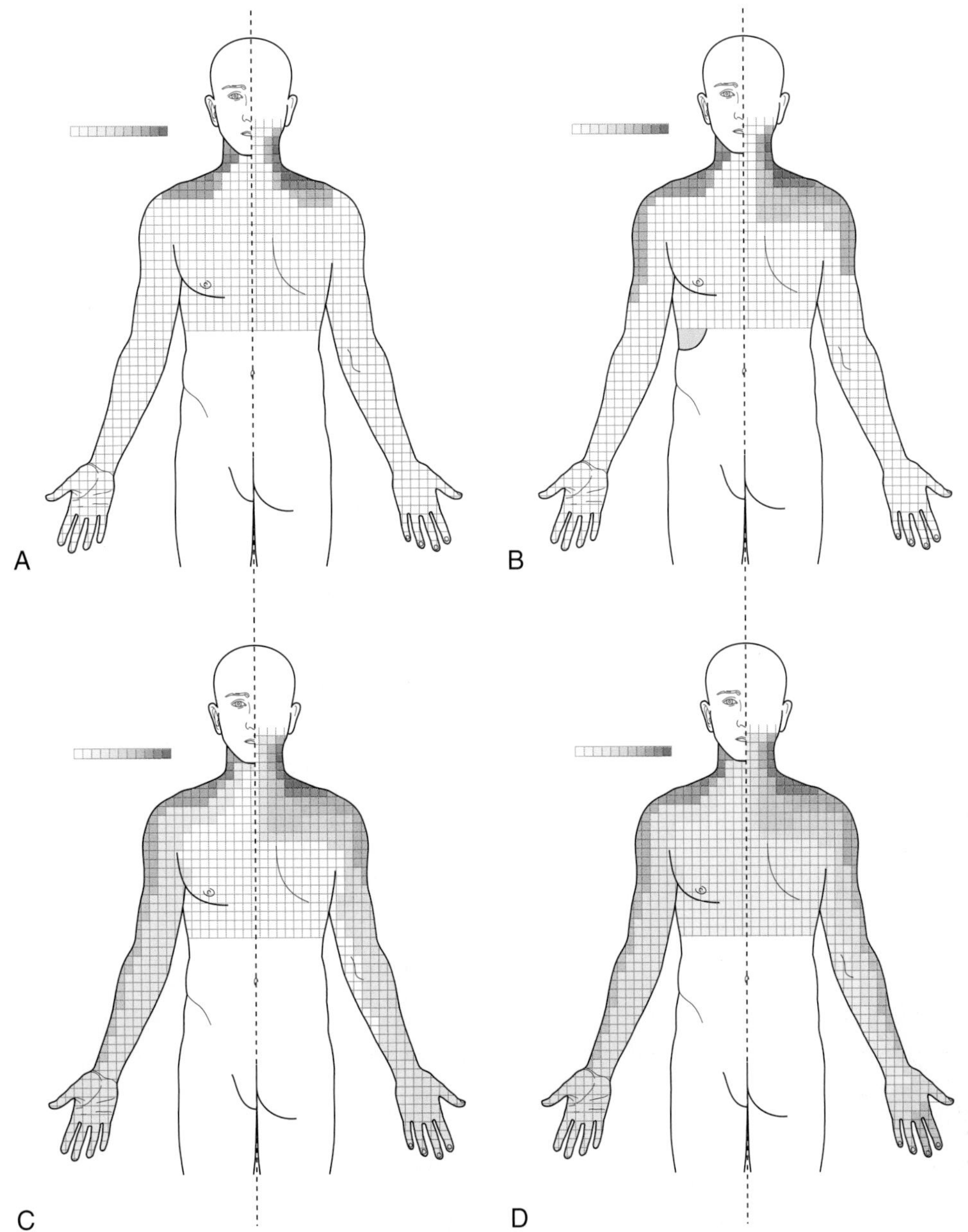

FIGURE 32-9 Dynatomal mapping of cervical radicular pain from mechanical stimulation of cervical nerve roots C4 **(A)**, C5 **(B)**, C6 **(C)**, and C7 **(D)**. (Courtesy C.W. Slipman, M.D.)

neurocompression of the nerve root does not necessarily cause pain,[97] and pure myotomal weakness can occur.[138] Proposed mechanisms for pain in cervical radiculopathy include nerve root inflammation,[29] increased discharge of the dorsal root ganglion, mechanosensitivity or chemosensitivity of the nerve root itself, or direct pressure on chronically injured axons or on a normal dorsal root ganglion.[97,191,265] Other potential causes of cervical radiculopathy include tumor,[250] trauma,[184] sarcoidosis,[11] arteritis,[202] and athetoid or dystonic cerebral palsy.[72]

Cervical intervertebral disk injury can be categorized into two broad categories: internal disruption and herniation. *Disk herniation* is a generalized term, which is further divided into protrusion, extrusion, and sequestration (Figure 32-10). A more thorough discussion of disk herniation follows later. Internal disk disruption is a descriptive phrase used to detail derangement of the internal architecture of the nucleus pulposus and/or annular fibers with little or no external deformation.[51] The process of disk degeneration occurs over a spectrum of disk abnormalities (Figure 32-11). Initially, circumferential outer annular tears secondary to repetitive microtrauma are associated with interruption in blood and nutritional supply to the disk. These tears eventually coalesce to form radial tears occurring concurrently with a decrement in the water-imbibing ability of the nucleus pulposus. The mechanical integrity of the intervertebral disk suffers as disk space narrows, more tears develop, and type 2 proteoglycans continue to degrade.[122] Biochemical insults have been purported to occur before these biomechanical alterations.[201] The result is a cervical disk that is biomechanically incompetent and prone to biochemical insult.

BOX 32-1

Disorders Affecting the Neck

Mechanical
- Cervical sprain
- Cervical strain
- Herniated nucleus pulposus
- Osteoarthritis
- Cervical spondylosis
- Cervical stenosis

Rheumatologic
- Ankylosing spondylitis
- Reiter syndrome
- Psoriatic arthritis
- Enteropathic arthritis
- Rheumatoid arthritis
- Diffuse idiopathic skeletal hyperostosis
- Polymyalgia rheumatica
- Fibrositis (fibromyalgia)

Infectious
- Vertebral osteomyelitis
- Diskitis
- Herpes zoster
- Infective endocarditis
- Granulomatous process
- Epidural, intradural, and subdural abscesses
- Retropharyngeal abscess
- AIDS

Endocrinologic and Metabolic
- Osteoporosis
- Osteomalacia
- Parathyroid disease
- Paget disease
- Pituitary disease

Tumors

Benign Tumors
- Osteochondroma
- Osteoid osteoma
- Osteoblastoma
- Giant cell tumor
- Aneurysmal bone cyst
- Hemangioma
- Eosinophilic granuloma
- Gaucher disease

Malignant Tumors
- Multiple myeloma
- Solitary plasmacytoma
- Chondrosarcoma
- Ewing sarcoma
- Chordoma
- Lymphoma
- Metastases

Extradural Tumors
- Epidural hemangioma
- Epidural lipoma
- Meningioma
- Neurofibroma
- Lymphoma

Intradural Tumors
- Extramedullary, intradural
  - Neurofibroma
  - Meningioma
  - Ependymoma
  - Sarcoma
- Intramedullary
  - Ependymoma
  - Astrocytoma

Others
- Arteriovenous malformations
- Syringomyelia

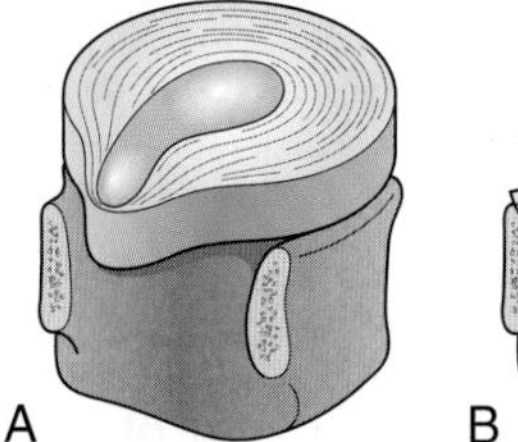

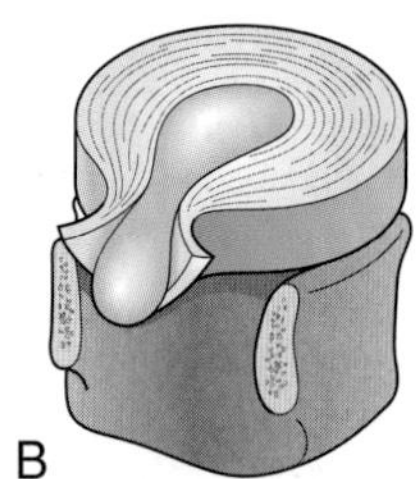

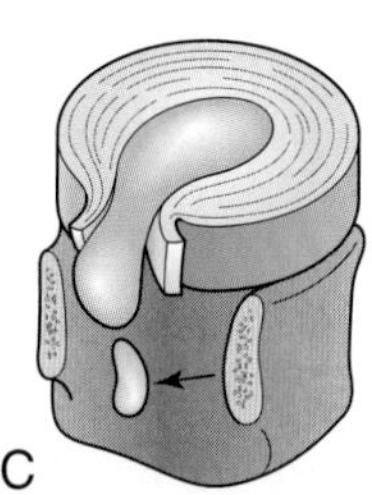

FIGURE 32-10 Cervical intervertebral disk herniations. **A,** Small subligamentous herniation or protrusion. **B,** Extrusion. **C,** Sequestered fragment (*arrow*).

Cervical zygapophyseal joint injury can occur because of osteoarthritis or trauma resulting from both macrotraumatic and microtraumatic events. Acceleration-deceleration zygapophyseal joint injuries can result in osseous injury to the articular pillars, articular surface, or subchondral bone; intraarticular hemarthrosis; contusion of the intraarticular meniscus; or tears of the zygapophyseal joint capsule (Figure 32-12).* We have successfully treated patients with cervical zygapophyseal joint synovitis, who had experienced the onset of symptoms on awakening after sleeping in an awkward position. Painful cervical zygapophyseal joint arthropathy can also result as a consequence of cervical intervertebral disk degeneration. Biochemical and biomechanical effects can both cause cervical zygapophyseal joint symptom manifestation.

Common Clinical Disorders

Cervical Strain and Sprains

Epidemiology

A cervical strain is a musculotendinous injury produced by an overload injury resulting from excessive forces imposed on the cervical spine.[38] In contrast, cervical sprains are overstretching or tearing injuries of spine ligaments.

*References 1, 2, 19, 43, 107, 130.

Muscular strains are seen most frequently because many cervical muscles do not terminate in tendons, but rather attach directly to bone via myofascial tissue that blends seamlessly with periosteum.[185] Cervical sprain and strain injuries account for approximately 85% of neck pain resultant from acute, repetitive, or chronic neck injuries.[106] These injuries are the most common type of injury to motor vehicle occupants in the United States,[187] and are one of the most common causes of pain after noncatastrophic sports injuries.[48] Approximately one third of motor vehicle accident victims develop neck pain within 24 hours of the injury.[210] Automobile-related cervical strain and sprain injuries are more common in Western societies and in metropolitan areas having higher densities of motor vehicles.[237] The incidence is higher in women and individuals aged 30 to 50 years old.[237]

Pathophysiology

Differing pathomechanisms are causal in cervical strain and sprain injuries, depending on the nature of the abnormal stress applied to the cervical spine. Acceleration-deceleration injuries result in excursions of the cervical spine that result in an S-shaped curvature approximately 100 ms after a rear-end impact.[114] By 200 to 250 ms after impact, the head initiates forward flexion of the neck after maximally extending to approximately 45 degrees.[156] Posterior neck muscle activation occurs by 90 to 120 ms[241] and coincides with the deceleration of the head moving forward.[156] As the head continues to move forward, the neck extensors eccentrically contract to decelerate the head, placing them at increased risk of injury (Figure 32-13).[170] These experimental findings lend support for a simple muscle or ligamentous strain injury during motor vehicle accidents. Partial and complete muscle tears and hemorrhage have been visualized by ultrasound[153] and magnetic resonance imaging (MRI),[182] and observed in postmortem examinations.[111] Tears of the anterior longitudinal ligament have been reported in surgical explorations[34] and identified at postmortem.[33] Anatomic studies have demonstrated that the anterior longitudinal ligament merges imperceptibly with the intervertebral disks and can be injured with injury to the cervical disk.[192]

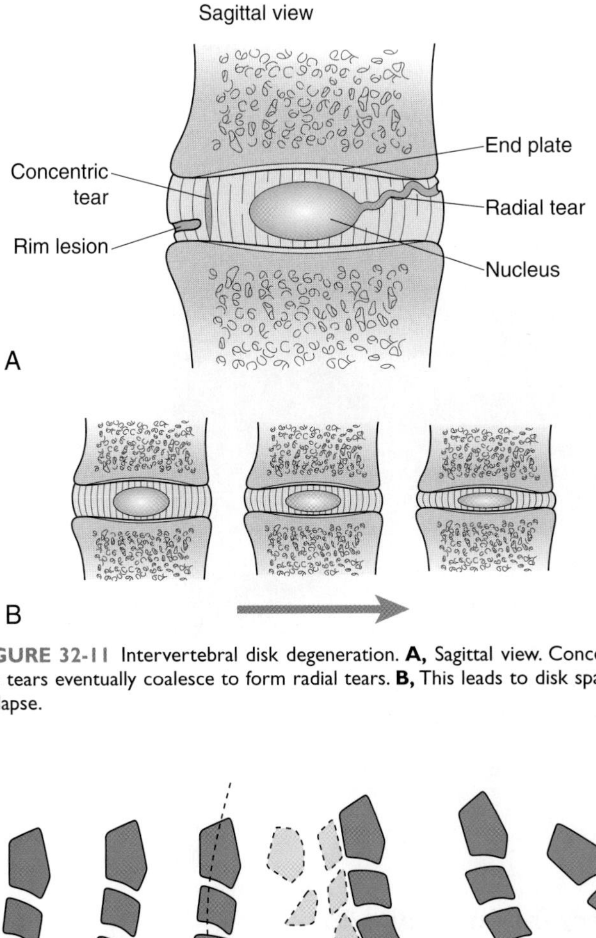

Sagittal view
Concentric tear
Rim lesion
End plate
Radial tear
Nucleus
A
B

FIGURE 32-11 Intervertebral disk degeneration. **A,** Sagittal view. Concentric tears eventually coalesce to form radial tears. **B,** This leads to disk space collapse.

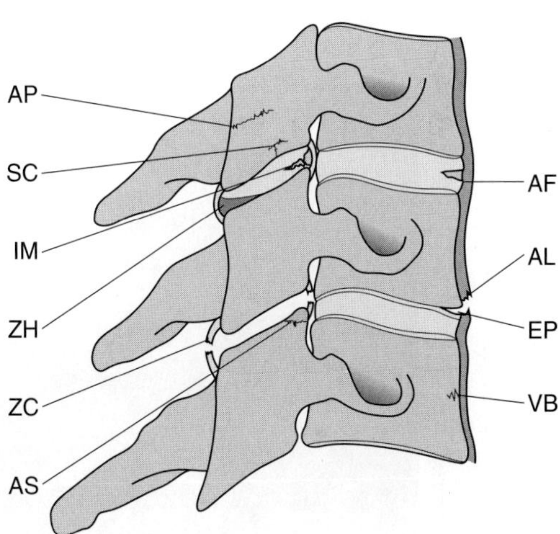

FIGURE 32-12 The more common lesions affecting the cervical spine following whiplash. *AF,* Tear of the annulus fibrosus of the intervertebral disk; *AL,* tear of the anterior longitudinal ligament; *AP,* articular pillar fracture; *AS,* fracture involving the articular surface; *EP,* end plate avulsion/fracture; *IM,* contusion of the intraarticular meniscus of the zygapophyseal joint; *SC,* fracture of the subchondral plate; *VB,* vertebral body fracture; *ZC,* rupture or tear of the zygapophyseal joint capsule; *ZH,* hemarthrosis of the zygapophyseal joint.

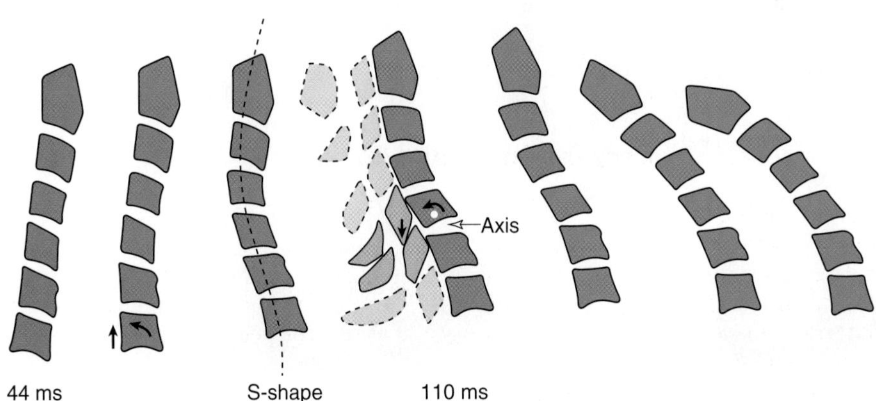

FIGURE 32-13 The appearance of sequential radiographs of the cervical spine during the extension phase of whiplash. At 110 ms, the C5 vertebra rotates about an abnormally high axis of rotation, causing the vertebral body to separate anteriorly from C6 (*white arrow*), and the inferior articular process of C5 to chisel into the superior articular process of C6 (*black arrow*). (From Kaneoka K, Ono L, Inami S, et al: Abnormal segmental motion of the cervical spine during whiplash loading, *J Jpn Orthop Assoc* 71:S1680, 1997.)

Physiologic forces acting on a relatively normal cervical spine result in typical soft tissue strain seen in nonathletes. In individuals with thoracic kyphosis and consequential cervical lordosis and extension, strain occurs in the levator scapulae, superior trapezius, sternocleidomastoid, scalene, and suboccipital muscles.[48] Traumatic blows often incurred in sporting injuries can result in a more acute cervical strain or sprain.[48] Repetitive motions that may occur in recreational activities can tax shortened and deconditioned cervical rotators, extensors, and lateral flexors that are frequently present in those with cervical spondylosis.[48]

Diagnosis

The history and physical examination findings guide the treating clinician in diagnosing cervical soft tissue injury. A thorough history of the mechanism of injury should be elicited from the patient. An acute event such as a motor vehicle accident, sports injury, fall, or industrial accident can create forces significant enough to injure cervical soft tissues. Details that should be sought are the exact onset of pain relative to a traumatic event, location of the symptoms, any referral pattern, or other associated symptoms. Cervical strain and sprain injuries can be associated with headaches. These headaches are typically sharp or dull and localize to the cervical or shoulder girdle musculature. The patient can also report neck fatigue or stiffness that lessens with gradual activity. Aggravating factors include passive or active motion.

Decreased cervical range of motion can be detected on gross examination. This is attributable to muscle guarding and splinting to avoid pain. Palpation of the involved region is usually uncomfortable or moderately painful. The most commonly involved areas are the upper trapezius and sternocleidomastoid muscles. Neurologic signs are typically absent, and neuroforaminal closure techniques should not elicit referral pain into the distal upper limb. Motor examination can reveal give-way weakness because of pain, but this pattern can be differentiated from true neuromuscular weakness.

Further diagnostic testing, such as imaging or electrodiagnostic evaluations, is not indicated unless neurologic or motor abnormalities are detected, or significant pain into the limbs is reported. Plain radiography would be ordered first to evaluate for bony malalignment or fractures. It is reasonable to examine cervical flexion and extension x-rays to evaluate for instability before prescribing functional restoration. In most instances, these images are normal or reveal nonspecific loss of cervical lordosis because of muscle splinting (Figure 32-14).

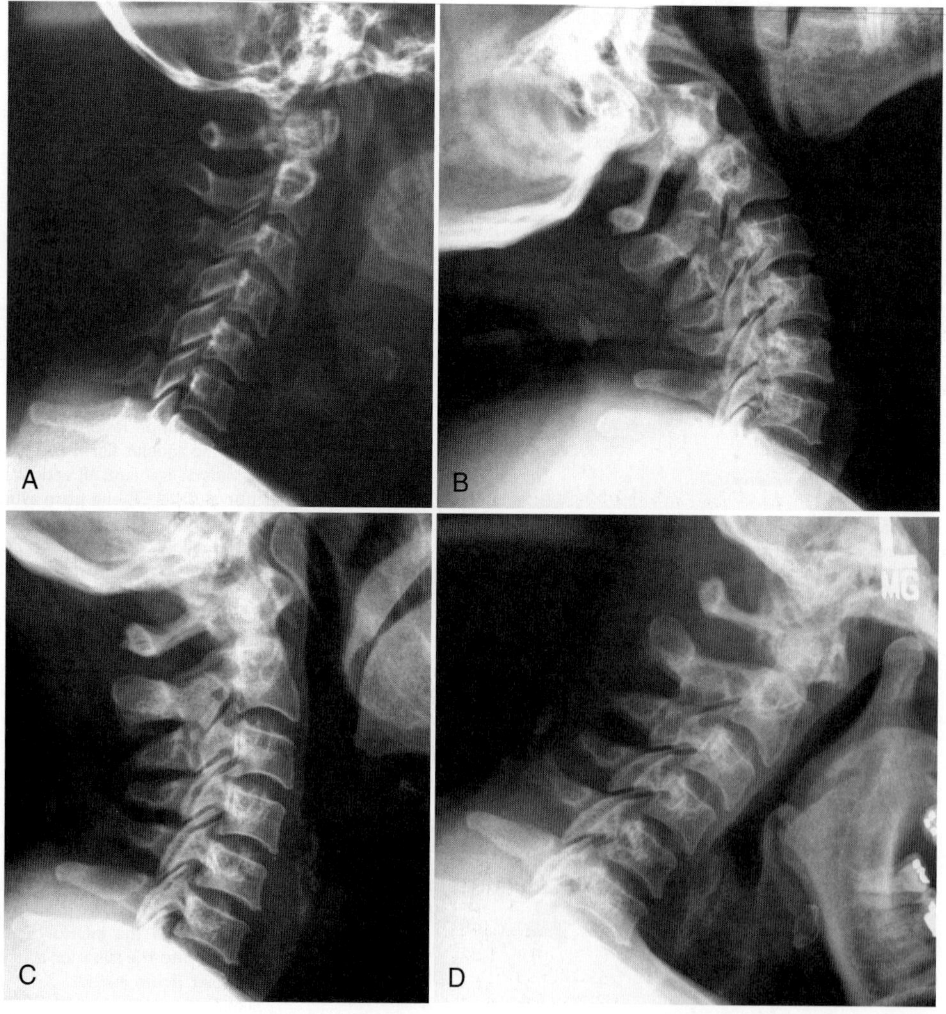

FIGURE 32-14 Lateral plain radiographs of the cervical spine, showing decreased lordosis **(A)**, extension **(B)**, neutral **(C)**, and flexion **(D)**.

Treatment

Initial care includes controlling pain and inflammation to curb the injury response, mitigate deconditioning, and facilitate active participation in a functional restoration program. Nonsteroidal antiinflammatory drugs (NSAIDs) and acetaminophen (paracetamol) aid in controlling pain and nurturing restorative sleep patterns. We do not typically prescribe muscle relaxants, but some clinicians use these medications for 5 to 7 days to improve sleep. If patients complain of substantial "spasm" not ameliorated by analgesics and proper positioning, tizanidine or tricyclic antidepressants may be helpful.

Physical modalities such as massage, superficial and deep heat, electrical stimulation, and a soft cervical collar can be used in the treatment program. Light massage causes sedation, reduction of adhesions, muscular relaxation, and vascular changes (see Chapter 16).[260] Superficial heat[133] and deep heat with ultrasound[67] produce analgesia and muscle relaxation, help resolve inflammation, and increase connective tissue elasticity (see Chapter 17)[194]. Transcutaneous electrical nerve stimulation (TENS) can also be effective in modulating musculoskeletal pain (see Chapter 17).[148] A soft cervical collar (see Figure 32-18) can be prescribed to ease painful sleep disturbances and reduce further neck strain. The collar can be worn while awake, but should be restricted to the first 72 hours after the injury to minimize interference with healing and prevent development of soft tissue tightening.[158] A gradual return to activities should be initiated by 2 to 4 weeks after injury, and should include a functional restoration program to address postural reeducation and functional biomechanical deficits.[48]

Once the acute pain has improved, proper spine biomechanics must be restored with the establishment of proper movement patterns. Healthy cervical segmental motion requires efficient stabilization throughout the cervical and thoracic spines. Proprioceptive retraining, balance, and postural conditioning should be incorporated into the exercise regimen. Flexibility and range of motion are improved by mobilization and stretching exercises. Proprioception is improved with visual feedback during exercises and functional tasks. These should be performed with simultaneous dynamic demands on the patient's base of support.[48,125] Such a program (Table 32-1) enhances the healthy dissipation of forces across the cervical spine with efficient myofascial efforts.

Table 32-1 Cervicothoracic Stabilization Exercises

	Cervicothoracic Stabilization Level		
Type of Exercise	**Level 2 (Basic)**	**Level 2 (Intermediate)**	**Level 3 (Advanced)**
Direct cervical stabilization	Cervical active range of motion Cervical isometrics	Cervical gravity Resisted isometrics	Cervical active Range gravity-resisted
Indirect Cervical Stabilization			
Supine, head supported	TheraBand chest press Bilateral arm raise Supported dying bug	Unsupported dying bug	Chest flies Bench press Incline dumbbell press
Sit	Reciprocal arm raise Unilateral arm raise Bilateral arm raise Seated row Latissimus pull-down	Swiss ball reciprocal Arm raises Chest press	Swiss ball bilateral Shoulder shrugs Supraspinatus raises
Stand	TheraBand reciprocal Chest press TheraBand straight arm latissimus pull-down TheraBand chest press TheraBand latissimus pull-down Standing rowing Crossovers Triceps press	Standing rowing Biceps pull-down	Upright row Shoulder shrugs Supraspinatus raises
Flexed hip-hinge position	0-30 degrees Reciprocal arm raise Unilateral arm raise Bilateral arm raise Interscapular flies	30-60 degrees Incline prone flies Reciprocal deltoid raise Cable crossovers	60-90 degrees Bilateral anterior Deltoid raises Interscapular flies
Prone	Reciprocal arm raise Unilateral arm raise Bilateral arm raise	Quadruped Head unsupported Swiss ball bilateral Anterior deltoid raises Swiss ball prone Rowing Swiss ball prone flies	Head supported Prone flies Latissimus flies
Supine, head unsupported	Not advised for level I	Partial sit-ups Arm raises	Swiss ball chest flies Swiss ball reciprocal

From Sweeney T, Prentice C, Saal JA, et al: Cervicothoracic muscular stabilizing technique, *Phys Med Rehabil State Art Rev* 4:335-360, 1990, with permission of Hanley & Belfus.

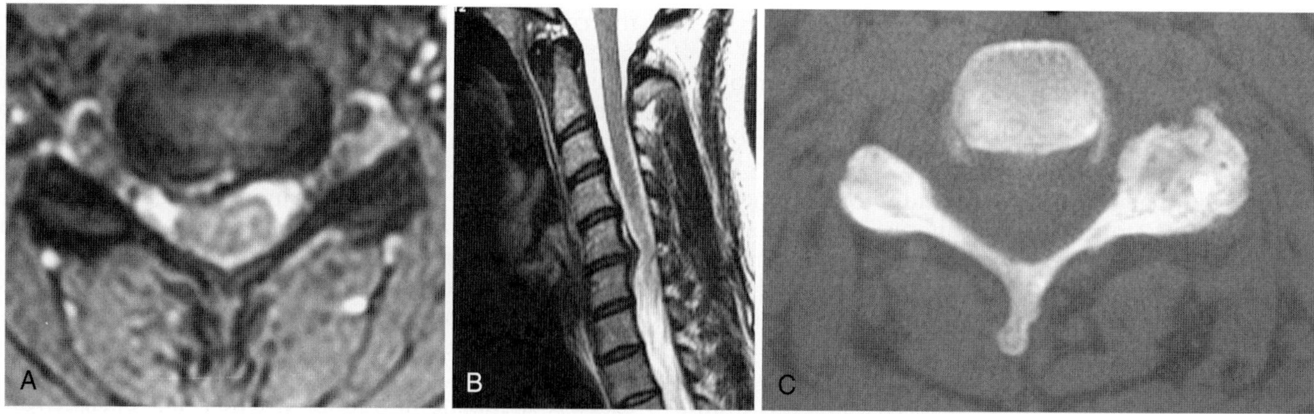

FIGURE 32-15 Axial **(A)** and sagittal **(B)** magnetic resonance imaging views revealing a central and rightward C5-C6 intervertebral disk extrusion. **C,** Axial computed tomography view of the C3-C4 segmental level, revealing moderate to severe left C4 foraminal stenosis caused by zygapophyseal joint arthrosis and uncovertebral joint hypertrophy.

Cervical Radiculopathy and Radicular Pain

Epidemiology

Cervical radiculopathy is a pathologic process involving neurophysiologic dysfunction of the nerve root.[64] Signs and symptoms of cervical radiculopathy include myotomal weakness, paresthesia, sensory disturbances, and depressed muscle stretch reflexes.[64] Cervical radicular pain represents a hyperexcitable state of the affected nerve root. Cervical radiculopathy, by contrast, involves reflex and strength deficits marking a hypofunctional nerve root as a result of pathologic changes in nerve root function.[29] Separating cervical radicular pain from cervical radiculopathy is important, because treatment strategies will vary depending on the presence or absence of the two conditions.

A large epidemiologic study of 561 patients in Rochester, Minnesota, found an average annual age-adjusted incidence of cervical radiculopathy of 83.2 per 100,000 for cervical radiculopathy.[189] The peak incidence occurred between the ages of 50 and 54 years in the study cohort.[189] A history of trauma or physical exertion preceding the onset of symptoms occurred in just under 15% of patients.[189] The order of decreasing frequency of involved levels was C7, C6, C8, and C5.[189]

Pathophysiology

Cervical nerve root injury is most commonly caused by cervical intervertebral disk herniation (CIDH),[102] with spondylitic changes the next most common cause (Figure 32-15).[264] The causal role of neural compression in CIDH-induced radiculopathy was first introduced by Semmes and Murphey[211] in 1943. Subsequent radiologic studies have demonstrated the existence of asymptomatic cervical disk abnormalities.[20,154,159,244] A growing body of evidence has emerged attesting to the etiologic role of an inflammatory response to a CIDH in some way triggering painful radicular signs and symptoms.[74,115,116] Animal studies have shown disrupted nerve root physiology caused by gradient pressure[199] and inflammation in the absence of compression.[174] Nerve roots are anatomically less resilient than peripheral nerves to both biomechanical and biochemical insults, and respond to each with the same pathologic sequence of events.[168]

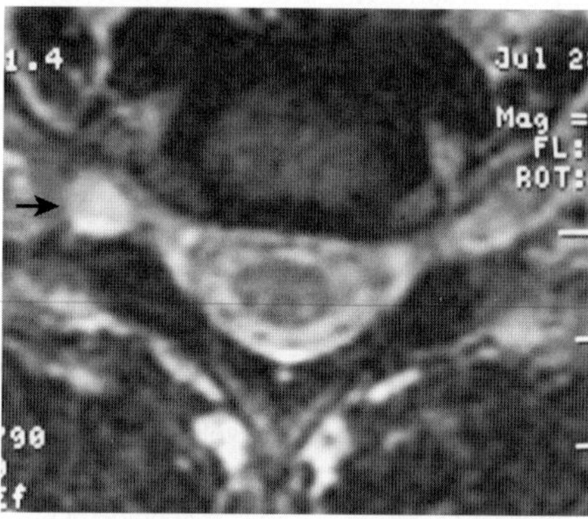

FIGURE 32-16 Axial view of the C7-T1 intervertebral disk, revealing an apparent zygapophyseal joint cyst (*black arrow*) emanating from the right C7-T1 joint.

Cervical spondylosis (or degenerative osteoarthritic changes) is manifested by ligamentous hypertrophy, hyperostosis (bony overgrowth), disk degeneration, and zygapophyseal joint arthropathy.[264] Hypertrophy of the zygapophyseal joints and uncovertebral joints results in intervertebral foramina stenosis and nerve root impingement.[220,264] Vertebral body osteophytes and disk material can form a "hard disk" that can also compress the adjacent nerve root.[189,264] Although cervical zygapophyseal joint cysts are rare,[143] patients with cervical zygapophyseal joint–induced radiculopathy have been treated at the Penn Spine Center (Figure 32-16). In these cases, it is not clear to what extent biochemical versus biomechanical influences affect the neural elements.

Diagnosis

History and Physical Examination. Patients with acute CIDH-related radiculopathy typically report a history of axial cervical pain that is then followed by an explosive onset of upper limb pain. In contrast, spondylitic radicular pain presents more gradually. Cervical radicular pain can masquerade as a deep dull ache or sharp lancinating pain. It can occur in a number of locations, including the medial scapular edge (C5, C6, or C7), superior trapezius (C5 or C6), precordium (C5 or C6), deltoid and lateral arm (C5 or C6), posteromedial arm (C7, C8, or T1), anterolateral

Table 32-2 Nerve Root Levels, Peripheral Nerves, and Muscles of the Upper Limb Commonly Evaluated in the Patient with Neck Pain

Nerve Root Level	Nerve	Muscle
C5, C6	Axillary	Deltoid
C5, C6	Musculocutaneous	Biceps brachii
C5, C6	Suprascapular Suprascapular	Supraspinatus Infraspinatus
C7	Radial Median	Triceps Pronator teres
C8, T1	Median Ulnar	Abductor pollicis brevis First dorsal interossei

forearm (C6 or C7), posterior forearm (C7 or C8), and any of the upper extremity digits (C6-C8 or T1).[64,229]

Exacerbating factors include activities that raise subarachnoid pressure, such as coughing, sneezing, or Valsalva maneuvers. If a significant component of stenosis is present, cervical extension can amplify the symptoms. Alleviation of the radicular pain by elevating the ipsilateral humerus is known as the shoulder abduction relief sign, which aids the diagnosis and can be used as a therapeutic maneuver.[54,68]

The physical examination begins with the clinical observation of neck position, as patients characteristically tilt toward the side of the disk herniation. Atrophy can be detected with more severe or long-standing lesions. Muscle wasting in the suprascapular or infrascapular fossae or deltoid suggests C5 or C6 involvement; triceps in C7 injury; thenar eminence in C8; and first dorsal interossei in T1.[189] Manual muscle testing has greater specificity than reflex or sensory abnormalities (Table 32-2),[262] and might need to be performed repetitively or with the muscle at a mechanical disadvantage to elicit subtle weakness. Severe weakness (<3/5 Medical Research Council) is less consistent with a single root lesion, and should alert the clinician to the presence of a possible multilevel radiculopathy, radiculomyelopathy, alpha motor neuron disease, plexopathy, or focal entrapment neuropathy. Sensation to light touch, pinprick, and vibration can be altered. The patient should be assessed for the presence of long tract signs such as Hoffman sign and Babinski response to ensure that there is no spinal cord involvement.

Provocative maneuvers such as neuroforaminal closure and root tension signs help localize the lesion to the cervical spine. Spurling maneuver,[235] cervical extension, lateral flexion, and ipsilateral axial rotation reproducing radicular symptoms are highly specific but not sensitive for cervical radiculopathy.[251] A positive Spurling maneuver increases the probability that nerve root compression is present on advanced imaging.[212] Nerve root tension, contralateral cervical axial rotation concurrent with ipsilateral glenohumeral abduction/extension with elbow and wrist extension, can help detect radicular pain. If this examination reveals radicular pain, presumably the imposed neural tension is provocative as a result of nerve root inflammation. Root tension–induced radicular pain may be more sensitive than Spurling maneuver but less specific,[197] and should be performed bilaterally to ensure absence of contralateral symptoms. Systematic studies comparing the utility of these two examination maneuvers have not been published. A L'hermitte sign,[136] which is rapid passive cervical flexion while the patient is seated, can produce an electric shock sensation down the spine and occasionally into the limbs in patients with cervical cord involvement as a result of tumor, spondylosis, or multiple sclerosis.[178]

Imaging Studies. Although plain radiography is not very sensitive in the detection of pathologic disk conditions, it remains the initial radiographic examination in almost every assessment of musculoskeletal injury.[165] Plain films of anteroposterior, lateral, open mouth, and flexion and extension views are indicated to evaluate spine stability in cases of rheumatoid arthritis or ankylosing spondylitis,[64] spondylolisthesis, postfusion, or after traumatic injury.[165] Computed tomographic myelography is regarded as the gold standard against which other imaging modalities should be judged in evaluating degenerative cervical spine conditions.[198] However, most clinicians reserve unenhanced computed tomography (CT) for the evaluation of osseous details such as foraminal stenosis,[165] bone tumors, and fractures.[113]

MRI is the imaging modality of choice in investigating cervical radiculopathy,[113,150] because it details diskal, ligamentous, osseous, and neural tissue very well.[166] MRI is noninvasive and does not expose the patient to radiation. Although it has become a widely prescribed imaging test, it is expensive, requires patient cooperation to minimize artifact, and is often not tolerated by patients who are claustrophobic. Patients with embedded metallic objects such as pacemakers or prosthetic heart valves cannot undergo MRI. Contrast-enhanced CT can accurately evaluate pathologic disk conditions[165] in these cases. Because cervical intervertebral disk abnormalities occur in patients who are asymptomatic,[20,94,154,159,244] the clinical findings have to be correlated with the imaging findings to accurately diagnose the lesion responsible for the patient's signs and symptoms.

Electrodiagnostic Evaluation. Nerve conduction studies and electromyography can be used to assess the neurophysiologic function of the nerve roots, plexus, and peripheral nerves. Electrodiagnostic examinations, if performed by an appropriately trained physician, can clarify or confirm the suspected diagnosis. Electrodiagnostic examination is also helpful in determining the prognosis of nerve injury. The American Association of Neuromuscular and Electrodiagnostic Medicine guidelines for the electrodiagnostic examination for a radiculopathy include abnormalities in two or more muscles innervated by the same root but different peripheral nerves, provided that normal findings are observed in muscles innervated by adjacent nerve roots.[257] At least one corresponding motor and sensory nerve conduction study should be performed in the involved limb to ensure the absence of a concomitant plexus or peripheral process. If abnormalities are found, the correlating contralateral muscle and nerves should be examined to exclude a generalized process such as peripheral neuropathy or motor neuron disease. A screening examination of six upper limb muscles in addition to the cervical paraspinals can identify 94% to 99% of cervical radiculopathies.[57] These studies can effectively exclude other diagnoses such

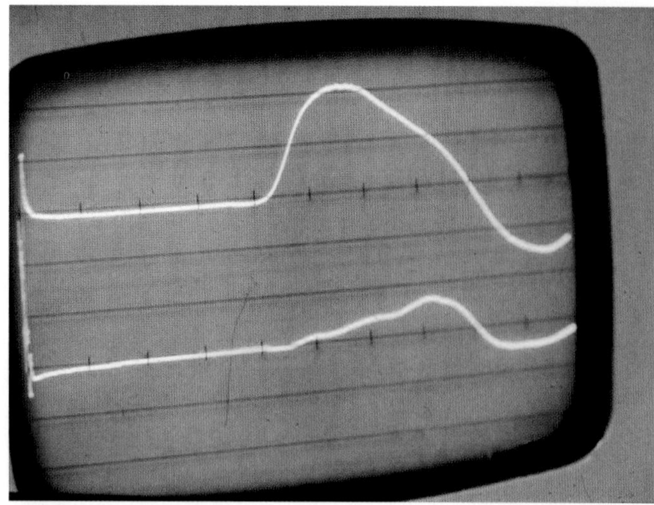

FIGURE 32-17 Oscilloscope screen waveform of bilateral abductor pollicis brevis compound muscle action potential (CMAP) amplitudes. The top trace demonstrates a healthy waveform with normal amplitude and duration. The bottom trace illustrates a 65% reduction of the CMAP amplitude of the contralateral muscle, with slightly increased duration.

as brachial plexus lesions (such as Pancoast tumor or Parsonage-Turner syndrome) and focal peripheral entrapments (such as carpal tunnel syndrome and ulnar entrapment at the elbow or wrist). If the amplitude of the clinically affected muscle's compound muscle action potential is reduced by less than 50% of that of the contralateral limb (Figure 32-17), functional motor recovery will probably return with conservative care, and repeat studies can be performed to document neurophysiologic healing (see Chapter 8).[109]

Treatment

Physical Medicine and Rehabilitation. The primary objectives of treatment of cervical radiculopathy include the resolution of pain, improvement in myotomal weakness, avoidance of spinal cord complications,[64,259] and prevention of recurrence.[259] Despite few outcome studies comparing surgical to medical rehabilitation and interventional (conservative) care, accumulated evidence supports the natural resolution of cervical radicular symptoms with conservative care.[53,88,200,221] The treatment approach must be molded to the individual patient. A definitive indication for a surgical approach is a progressive neurologic deficit. Otherwise, the patient's necessary level of posttreatment function can help dictate how aggressively to intervene. For example, a relatively sedentary patient might decide to tolerate a low level of discomfort after conservative care. An athlete, by contrast, might not want to settle for symptoms that are exacerbated by extreme physical activity. The design of the treatment plan has to take into account the individual and how he or she functions at home, at work, and in the community.

Modalities. Patient education, activity modification, and relief of pain are the initial treatment steps. The treating physician should explain to the patient the mechanism of how the injury occurred and the most likely treatment outcomes. This explanation should emphasize the importance of proper posture, biomechanics, and the utility of an ergonomic evaluation.[259]

Repetitive and heavy lifting must be avoided, as well as positioning the cervical spine in extension, axial rotation, and ipsilateral flexion. Severe pain can prohibit continued work or athletic activity, and restrict activities of daily living. Mild to moderate symptoms can usually be tolerated by the patient, allowing continued but restricted activities.

Thermotherapy is often used to modulate pain and to increase muscle relaxation.[135,163] No definitive guideline has been published to date regarding the role of thermal modalities in cervical radiculopathy.[193] Cold can be applied for 15 to 30 minutes one to four times a day, and superficial heat can be applied up to 30 minutes two to three times a day. The decision regarding which thermal agent to use is driven by the patient's perception of which provides the best pain relief.[134] Deep heating modalities such as ultrasound should be avoided in the treatment of cervical radiculopathy, because an increased metabolic response and subsequent inflammation can aggravate the nerve root injury.[135,193]

TENS is helpful in the management of various musculoskeletal and neurogenic disorders (see Chapter 17). It can be used early in the treatment course of cervical radiculopathy to help modulate pain and enable the patient to engage in other therapeutic modalities. TENS is believed to act via the gate theory. Stimulating large myelinated fibers presumably blocks nociceptive transmission in smaller fibers at the level of the spinothalamic tract neurons.[161] Although TENS has been shown to provide some relief of low back pain,[233] no studies have been published demonstrating conclusive evidence of its efficacy in cervical radicular pain.

Cervical orthoses function to limit painful range of motion and facilitate patient comfort during the acute injury phase (see Chapter 13).[193] Soft cervical collars limit flexion and extension by approximately 26%[110] and are prescribed as kinesthetic reminders of proper cervical positioning.[259] The narrower segment should be positioned anteriorly to maintain the neck in the neutral or slightly flexed position (Figure 32-18).[64,200,259] The exceptions to this include patients with a positive L'hermitte sign, and those with rheumatoid arthritis, or atlantoaxial subluxation. The use of a soft collar should be limited to the first week or two of symptoms[54,128] to minimize adverse outcomes related to further soft tissue deconditioning.

Cervical traction applies a distractive force across the cervical intervertebral disk space. It is commonly used by patients with cervical radiculopathy, despite a lack of proven efficacy.[64,259] It is presumed to work via the decompression of cervical soft tissues and intervertebral disks.[47,240] Superficial heat, massage, or TENS therapy can be performed before and during traction to relieve pain and to help relax the muscles.[46,47] A force of 25 lb is required to distract the midcervical segments when applied for 25 minutes at an angle of pull of 24 degrees.[46] Cervical traction can be executed with an intermittent heavy-weight or a continuous light-weight regimen in the therapy gym or home setting.[47] Traction is contraindicated in patients with myelopathy, positive L'hermitte sign, rheumatoid arthritis, or atlantoaxial subluxation (see Chapter 16).[47]

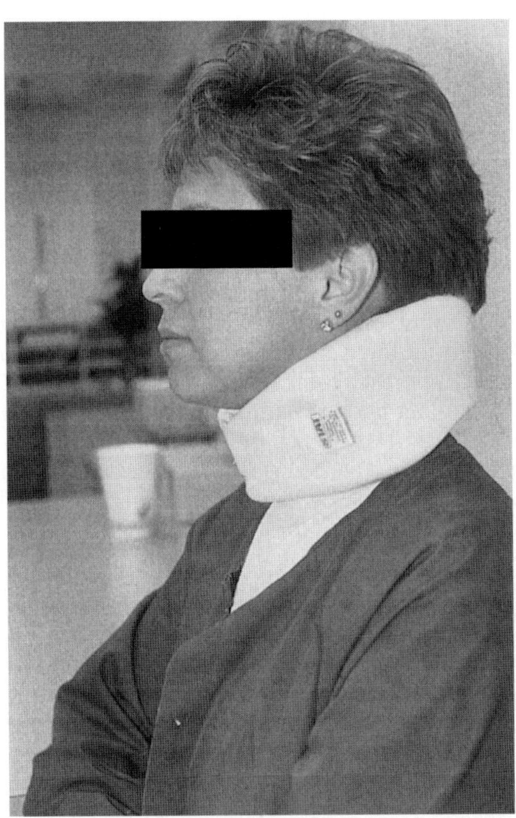

FIGURE 32-18 Cervical orthosis. A cervical soft collar with the widest side posteriorly and the narrowest side anteriorly.

Medications. A role for antiinflammatory medications is logical in light of the evidence of an inflammatory component to CIDH-related radiculopathy.[74,115,116] NSAIDs are the first line of pharmacologic interventions prescribed to treat cervical radiculopathy. At low doses, they provide an analgesic effect, and at high doses an antiinflammatory effect. Side effects associated with the use of NSAIDs relate to their irritation of the gastrointestinal mucosa, platelet inhibition, and renal function. Antiinflammatory agents that target the cyclooxygenase-2 pathway provide similar analgesia and antiinflammatory properties to those of their nonselective counterparts, but with better gastrointestinal tolerability and less antiplatelet effect.[86] For these reasons, these newer agents may be preferable to traditional NSAIDs for patients with cervical radiculopathy, and because diagnostic and therapeutic spinal injections can be performed without interrupting these therapeutic medications. However, some findings have emerged suggesting that caution should be exercised when prescribing celecoxib at high doses for an extended period, because of an increased cardiovascular risk (National Cancer Institute Adenoma Prevention with Celecoxib trial).

Adjunct medications are often used in conjunction with antiinflammatory medications and include muscle relaxants, tricyclic antidepressants, and antiepileptics. Muscle relaxers are sedating and secondarily relax skeletal muscle. They may be used to aid sleep for 5 to 7 days if disrupted by painful muscular guarding. Low-dose tricyclic antidepressant medications such as amitriptyline or nortriptyline, prescribed at 10 to 25 mg at bedtime, can be beneficial in decreasing radicular pain and aiding sleep.[64] Associated side effects are largely anticholinergic, such as dry mouth, urinary retention, drowsiness, and constipation. Antiepileptic medication such as gabapentin can be effective in modulating neuropathic pain. The therapeutic dose varies from 300 to 900 mg/day up to 3600 mg/day. The most common side effects are lethargy, fatigue, ataxia, and dry mouth. Hence, it is recommended to start at a low dose, 300 mg at bedtime, and titrate upward until either symptoms are controlled or side effects curtail the dosage curve. A newer agent, pregabalin (Lyrica), is an option and does not interfere with hepatic metabolism. Other options include tiagabine (Gabitril), zonisamide (Zonegran), and oxcarbazepine (Trileptal). Antiepileptic medications are typically reserved for patients with persistent radicular pain postoperatively or who are not appropriate surgical candidates after failure of other therapeutic interventions.

Opiate analgesics may be necessary at times when radicular pain is severe and disrupts sleep. Short-acting opioid-analgesic combination medications can be prescribed to facilitate restorative sleep patterns by controlling the radicular pain (sometimes in conjunction with the use of a soft cervical collar). Opiate medications typically should not be prescribed after the acute phase, and other interventions should be maximized before resorting to long-term use of opioids (see Chapter 37).

Stabilization and Functional Restoration. Rehabilitation requires approaching the patient as a whole, addressing both the psychological and behavioral consequences of injury, in addition to the physical impairments (E.W. Johnson, personal communication, Columbus, Ohio, 2002). Functional restoration includes biomechanical concerns, physical conditioning, and strength training. All of these are needed to facilitate injury healing and prevent injury recurrence.

Cervicothoracic stabilization is the functional restoration of spinal biomechanics, and is used to limit pain, maximize function, and prevent injury progression or recurrence.[48,239] Integral parts of this stabilization include restoration of spinal flexibility, postural reeducation, and conditioning. Normal range of motion and good posture are essential to prevent repetitive microtrauma to cervical structures caused by poor movement patterns.[36] The patient must be taught how to control activity throughout the kinetic chain. The stabilization program is initiated by establishing the pain-free interval of cervical range of motion, and then progressively adding motion outside this range as the symptoms subside. Any restriction of range of motion in the spine or soft tissues is aggressively treated to achieve full or functional range of motion. Proper cervical biomechanics are restored with passive range of motion, spine and soft tissue mobilization techniques, self-stretching, and correct posture. Improved neuromuscular control is developed first for static positions, and then advanced to dynamic and functional activities.[48]

Cervical strengthening begins with isometric exercises of the flexor, extensor, rotator, and lateral flexor muscles. The exercises are performed first in the supine position and then progressed to the seated and standing positions.[48] The patient is carefully progressed to concentric isotonic exercises, avoiding combined movements unless pain-free. Muscles that are stretched or weakened as a result of poor posture are targeted during this phase.[48] One of the main goals of the exercise program is improved muscular balance and flexibility of the cervicothoracic and capital muscle groups.[48]

Attention is also focused on the shoulder girdles and upper limb conditioning. Mid to upper cervical radiculopathies with myotomal weakness can disrupt scapulothoracic and glenohumeral stabilization. The trapezius, serratus anterior, rhomboids, and rotator cuff muscles must be strengthened.[48] Proper scapulothoracic kinetics and glenohumeral coupling allow mechanically efficient spinal posture, as well as efficient dissipation of energy by the upper limbs during functional activities.

Interventional Spine Care. Interventional spine care is a relatively young and developing subspecialty within the field of physiatry. The scope of this subspecialty involves the judicious use of precision, image-guided spine procedures to both diagnose and treat painful spine disorders. Interventional spine physiatrists rely on a knowledge-based algorithmic approach, which is a combination of evidence-based medicine and extensive clinical experience. The interventional spine care specialist, therefore, approaches patient care within the framework of a disease-based or specific structural injury medical model rather than a symptom-oriented medical model.

Diagnostic Selective Nerve Root Block. If imaging reveals a structural lesion at the nerve root level that corroborates the physical examination findings, and an electrodiagnostic evaluation confirms the clinical suspicion, therapeutic interventions can be pursued. However, if the physical examination and electrodiagnostic studies are equivocal in the setting of an abnormal MRI, the diagnosis can often be clarified with a fluoroscopically guided diagnostic selective nerve root block (SNRB) at the suspected segmental level (Figure 32-19). If the diagnostic block is negative, the next step in the diagnostic algorithm is investigated.[220] The specificity of cervical diagnostic SNRBs has been suggested to range from 87% to 100%,[6,120] and the sensitivity has been shown to be 100%.[6] The use of diagnostic lumbar SNRBs has been explored in the literature,* and the observed specificity and sensitivity values for lumbar diagnostic SNRBs closely mirror these values for their cervical counterparts. A diagnostic SNRB is a functional diagnostic test, because the patient's cooperation and understanding is imperative in gaining accurate and valid diagnostic information.[220] Because of a relative lack of methodological investigations configuring the sensitivity and specificity of cervical diagnostic SNRBs, we must extrapolate from the lumbar data.

Therapeutic Selective Nerve Root Injection. The natural history of radiculopathy caused by CIDH or spondylosis is a gradual resolution of symptoms with conservative care in 65% to 83% of patients.[88,189,200,225] Two of these studies,[200,225] however, incorporated fluoroscopically guided cervical epidural or selective nerve root injections (SNRIs) of corticosteroids. Heckman et al.[88] retrospectively observed that 65% of 60 patients with cervical radiculopathy (90% caused by CIDH, 10% caused by spondylosis) improved significantly with conservative care that did not involve spinal injections. Several studies have examined the use of cervical therapeutic SNRIs to treat cervical radiculopathy after failure of more conservative care.†‡ Good to excellent results have ranged from 50% to 83%, with follow-up intervals from 6 to 21 months.‡ More successful results have been obtained in the presence of CIDH[35,53,200] than with spondylotic changes.[17,53,226,248] Not surprisingly, traumatically induced cervical radiculopathy portends a poorer

*References 58, 85, 128, 208, 236, 249.
†References 17, 35, 53, 200, 226, 248.
‡References 16, 17, 35, 53, 200, 226, 248.

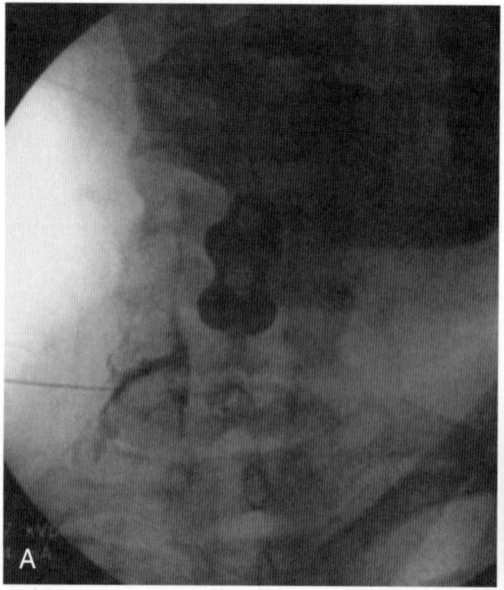

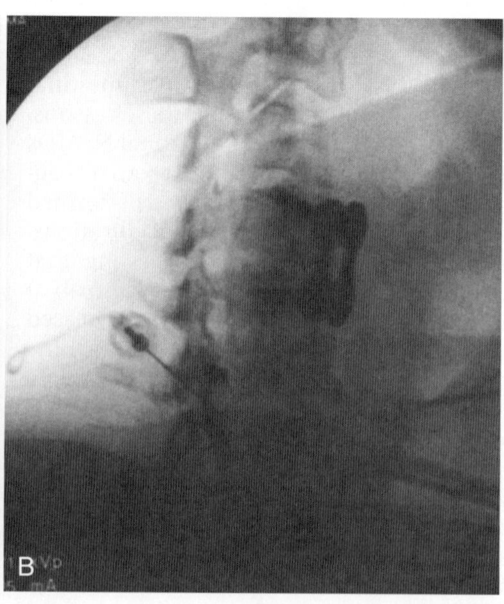

FIGURE 32-19 Fluoroscopic image of a right C7 selective nerve root block. **A,** Anterior posterior view depicting contrast within the foramen and along the medial edge of the right C7 pedicle extending toward the epidural space. **B,** Oblique view showing contrast around the nerve root in a semicircle pattern.

prognosis.[224,225] "Whiplash"-induced cervical radicular pain in the absence of concomitant foraminal stenosis and traumatic spondylotic cervical radicular pain are successfully treated with conservative care including up to two to four SNRIs in 14%[225] and 20%[224] of cases, respectively. In this patient profile, if an initial SNRI achieves no improvement in radicular pain, then further injections may not be warranted, as probably less than 20% of patients will respond to further injections.[224,225] Furthermore, injection of local anesthetic alone has demonstrated efficacy equal to anesthetic and steroid combined,[7] and equal reduction in avoiding surgery.[195]

Despite a growing concern regarding the safety of cervical SNRIs, when performed properly[25] they have been demonstrated to be safe[105] and offer a reasonable, minimally invasive treatment intervention to treat painful, nontraumatic cervical radicular symptoms. The goal of SNRI is to modulate the inflammatory response to the CIDH by injecting steroids close to the disk–nerve root interface. This is intended to control pain and to start the process of nerve root healing while the intervertebral disk herniation naturally resorbs or becomes inert tissue. A proportion of cases will eventually require decompression because of persistent intervertebral disk herniation volume and/or continuation of the inflammatory response.

Percutaneous Diskectomy/Disk Decompression. Percutaneous diskectomy has been investigated as a nonsurgical alternative for treating persistent cervical radiculopathy caused by a corroborative focal herniation.* Various technologies have been used to achieve cervical intervertebral disk decompression, including laser,[41,84,96,124,215] enzymatic,[90] and mechanical[41,43] decompression. The follow-up intervals have been relatively short[84,90,215] or unspecified.[96] The two studies with the longest outcome data demonstrated disparate results[41,124] and included a heterogeneous study cohort.[124]

Nucleoplasty is a technology that uses coblation energy to vaporize nuclear tissue into gaseous elementary molecules. It has also been developed and applied to the spine.[213] In a study conducted at the Penn Spine Center,[221] nucleoplasty was combined with SNRI to treat both the biomechanical and biochemical causes of CIDH-related cervical radicular pain that had been unresponsive to conservative care. These patients demonstrated a contained CIDH without stenosis and persistent radicular pain, and had been deemed appropriate surgical candidates. At 6 months, 91% to 95% of these 21 patients experienced an average 83% reduction in their pain level, with the greatest rate of reduction occurring within the first 2 weeks.[221] At 12 months, 17 of 21 had a good or excellent result. It should be noted that each of the 21 patients in this consecutive cohort had been considered candidates for surgery by a fellowship-trained spine surgeon, yet only two ultimately required surgery. No major complications were encountered, and the procedure was performed with light intravenous sedation on an outpatient basis. These findings have been corroborated by subsequent studies of nucleoplasty performed without an SNRI in which 81% to 85% of patients experienced good to excellent results at 6 to 12 months and significant reduction in radicular pain.[31,137] A randomized, controlled trial of 115 patients demonstrated significant reduction in pain and disability at 3, 6, and 12 months after nucleoplasty, compared with TENS, physical therapy, analgesics, and/or NSAIDs without complications.[39] Percutaneous diskectomy with coblation technology combined with or without SNRI can be safe and effective in relieving cervical radicular pain caused by a corroborative intervertebral disk protrusion. It can be offered as a nonoperative alternative to surgery if more conservative measures fail.

*References 41, 84, 90, 96, 124, 215.

Surgery. Indications for surgical treatment of CIDH or spondylotic-related cervical radiculopathy include intractable pain, severe myotomal deficit (progressive or stable), or progression to myelopathy. Surgical outcome studies have demonstrated good or excellent results in 80% to 96% of patients.[4,78,91,123] At 3 months postoperatively, surgical intervention such as anterior cervical diskectomy and fusion (Figure 32-20) or posterior foraminotomy has achieved quicker improvement in radicular pain, strength, and sensation than has conservative care.[181] These differences between conservative and surgical approaches equalize at 1 year.[181] Artificial cervical disk replacement has performed comparably to traditional anterior cervical diskectomy and fusion.[204] Our goal is to effectively modulate and enhance the body's natural response to a CIDH, beginning with conservative antiinflammatory measures, then moving to minimally invasive interventions, and culminating in open surgical decompression if necessary.

Cervical Joint Pain

Epidemiology

The prevalence of cervical facet joint–mediated pain in patients with complaints of neck pain ranges from 36% to 60%.[15,141,151,232] The most commonly symptomatic level, determined by controlled diagnostic blocks, is C2-C3 (36%), followed by C5-C6 (35%), and then C6-C7 (17%). Joints at C1-C2, C3-C4, and C4-C5 are each symptomatic in less than 5% of cases.[49] In patients with cervical facet

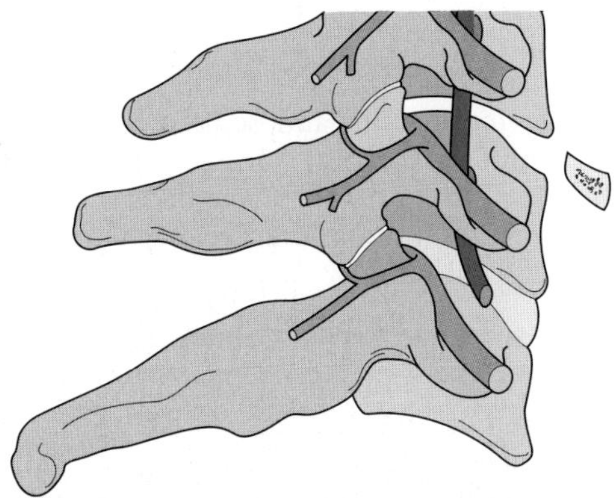

FIGURE 32-20 Anterior cervical diskectomy and fusion with the Smith-Robinson technique. The offending disk has been removed, and the block of bone graft is placed into the intervertebral level. The graft increases the disk height, thereby opening the foramen, and allows fusion. (From An HS, Simpson JM: *Surgery of the cervical spine*, London, 1994, Martin-Dunitz.)

joint pain, 52% have only one symptomatic joint and only rarely are two or more consecutive joints symptomatic.[49] Similarly, cervical zygapophyseal joints are a common source of chronic posttraumatic neck pain.[9] Chronic traumatic cervical zygapophyseal joint–mediated neck pain has an estimated prevalence of 54% to 64%.[15,21,141] Painful cervical zygapophyseal joints can occur concurrent with a symptomatic intervertebral disk at the same level.[21] In patients with chronic zygapophyseal joint pain, 58% to 88% complain of associated headaches.[15,141,142] The prevalence of C2-C3 zygapophyseal joint pain has been estimated to be 50% to 53% in patients whose chief complaint is posterior headaches after whiplash injury.[141,142] Traumatically induced lower cervical pain attributable to a zygapophyseal joint most commonly involves the C5-C6 level.[15,21,141] More than one structure can be injured in traumatically induced cervical zygapophyseal joint pain.[220] Spontaneous (nontraumatic) cervical zygapophyseal joint pain usually affects one joint and can be caused by spondylosis or improper biomechanics.

Diagnosis

History and Physical Examination. A detailed examination should be completed on any patient who sustains a whiplash injury to understand the mechanism of injury and to exclude spinal cord injury, plexopathy, or traumatic brain injury. Details of the accident, including the neck position at the time of impact, can help predict which structures are the most likely to be injured. However, the clinical history cannot provide pathognomonic findings to distinguish zygapophyseal joint–mediated pain from other sources of axial neck pain.[22] Traumatic upper zygapophyseal joint involvement such as at the C2-C3 joint is more likely to cause unilateral occipital headaches rather than neck pain.[49] Unilateral paramidline neck pain, with or without periscapular symptoms, that is more painful than any associated headaches, suggests zygapophyseal joint pain rather than disk or root injury.

The physical examination must assess neurologic function and cervical range of motion. The clinician should suspect zygapophyseal joint injury when the patient can pinpoint a localized spot of maximal pain, or define an area of pain typical for the referral distribution of a particular zygapophyseal joint. Focal tenderness to palpation posterolaterally over a joint lends further support for an underlying painful zygapophyseal joint.[112] Increased focal suboccipital pain that occurs or is exacerbated with 45 degrees of cervical flexion and sequential axial rotation suggests a painful C1-C2 joint.[59] Despite these suggestions, to date there have been no well-designed investigations of clinical examination findings that are diagnostic of cervical zygapophyseal joint pain.

Imaging Studies. Cervical zygapophyseal joint subluxation can be detected by plain radiography, and CT can better delineate joint fracture. Soft tissue injury, however, is largely undetected by advanced imaging. Imaging studies therefore have a limited role in determining the axial pain generator.[32,243] Nuclear imaging might demonstrate increased radiotracer uptake if there is an abnormality within the zygapophyseal joint, but it cannot discriminate between symptomatic and asymptomatic abnormalities.

Treatment

Physical Medicine and Rehabilitation. During the acute phase of injury, the treatment focuses on analgesia and antiinflammatory modalities. NSAIDs are indicated to provide pharmacologic control of pain and inflammation. If the pain is not controlled with these medications, opiates can be prescribed short-term to facilitate restorative sleep patterns and participation in functional restoration. Physical modalities should be used in the acute phase of injury to modulate pain and inflammation, and can be used to reduce or eliminate the need for opiates.

Superficial cryotherapy such as with ice application is preferred to superficial heat, because of its analgesic and antiinflammatory qualities. Although superficial heat has analgesic effects and relaxes muscles, its metabolic effects preclude its use in treating acute cervical zygapophyseal joint injuries. Cryotherapy should initially be applied for 20 minutes three or four times a day to cause vasoconstriction and decrease the release of pain and inflammatory mediators.[133] Soft tissue mobilization and massage can help break muscular guarding or splinting, but should not be the mainstay of treatment. Soft cervical collars can be worn for a short period of time, up to 72 hours after the initial injury. These are used for comfort, especially when sleeping. Patient education regarding proper positioning to avoid aggravating factors should occur concurrently with analgesic and antiinflammatory medications.

The restorative phase encompasses stabilization and functional restoration by normalizing the range of motion, soft tissue length, and biomechanical deficits, and strengthening the spinal musculature. Transition to this phase begins after there is a reduction in pain caused by the acute injury. Restoration of cervical spine motion helps achieve a balanced posture that decreases strain of the injured joints and also allows optimal strengthening to occur. Cervicothoracic stabilization addresses flexibility, posture reeducation, and strengthening, all of which reduce pain, improve function, and prevent recurrent injury.[239] Proprioceptive skills are implemented during strengthening exercises to achieve these goals.[48] The patient is discharged to a home exercise maintenance program to maintain mobility and strength.

Interventional Spine Care. The natural history of whiplash-induced neck pain is of gradual recovery in a majority of patients. It is imperative, however, that an accurate diagnosis is formulated to maximize treatment if a patient's pain is moderate or severe, or persists beyond this natural historical time frame. Determining precisely which joints are the source of symptoms requires the meticulous use of fluoroscopically guided target-specific injections.

Diagnostic Zygapophyseal Joint Blocks. The close anatomic relationship and overlapping referral patterns of spine structures necessitate the use of fluoroscopically guided diagnostic blocks to confirm a clinically suspected painful joint. Diagnostic blocks offer a definitive means by which to target symptomatic joints. Such blocks historically have been performed via the intraarticular injection of local anesthetic (Figure 32-21). Anesthetization of the medial branches innervating the suspected joint has been

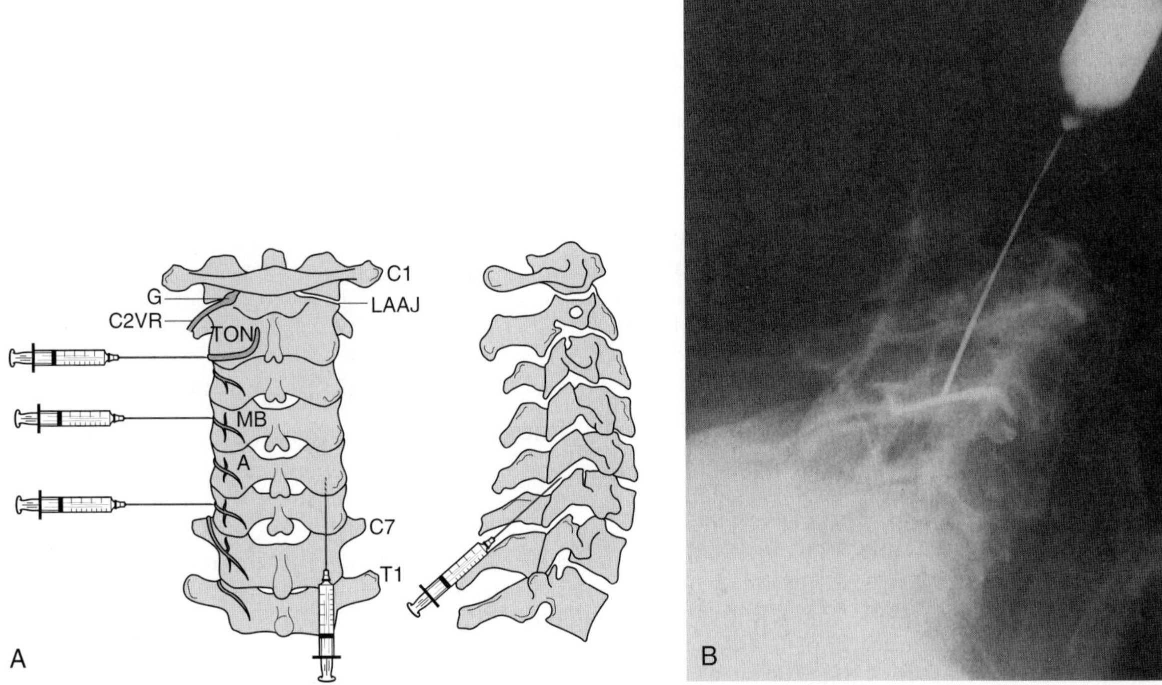

FIGURE 32-21 Cervical facet injections. **A,** Needle placement for medial branch nerve and intraarticular zygapophyseal injections. *Left,* Posterior view of the cervical spine, showing the location of the C2 ganglion (G) behind the lateral atlantoaxial joint (LAAJ), the C2 ventral ramus (C2VR), and the location of the medial branches of the cervical dorsal rami (MB), their articular branches (A), and the third occipital nerve (TON). Needles are positioned for injection of the C4 and C6 medial branches and the third occipital nerve. The articular pillar of C7 may be obscured by the shadow of the large C7 transverse process, in which case the C7 medial branch can be located midway between the lateral convexities of the C6-C7 and C7-T1 zygapophyseal joints. *Right,* Lateral view of the cervical spine, showing the course of the needle in the facet joint cavity of the C5-C6 facet joint, with a posterior approach. **B,** Lateral cervical radiograph showing precise needle placement into the zygapophyseal joint, producing a characteristic arthrogram. The joint was entered with a lateral approach to the cervical spine. (From Bogduk N: Back pain: zygapophyseal joint blocks and epidural steroids. In Cousins MJ, Bridenbaugh PO, eds: *Neural blockade in clinical anesthesia and pain management,* ed 2, Philadelphia, 1988, JB Lippincott, p 939.)

shown to predict treatment outcome after medial branch neurotomy.[139] The diagnosis is based on the concept that if the symptomatic structure is blocked, the patient's index pain will be relieved. If the pain is unrelieved, the tested joint is excluded as the source of the symptoms. Approximately one third of responders can represent false-positive results.[13] Consequently, comparative blocks[140] with anesthetics of varying duration of effect must be performed before treatment options are considered.

Therapeutic Zygapophyseal Joint Injections. Therapeutic intraarticular cervical zygapophyseal joint injections can be appropriate in individuals who have not improved from pharmacologic and physical modalities. Barnsley et al.[14] reported that single intraarticular steroid injections were not effective for the treatment of chronic whiplash-related cervical zygapophyseal joint pain. However, in this study the authors treated patients with only one therapeutic injection, used one outcome measure, and did not restrict physical therapy exercises.[14] Slipman et al.[227] demonstrated good to excellent results in 61% of patients who were having daily whiplash-related occipital headaches originating from the C2 to C3 joints. Patients who benefited from these injections underwent an average of two therapeutic injections.

Percutaneous Radiofrequency Ablation Medial Branch Neurotomy. If a patient's index neck pain is alleviated by two different medial branch blocks with local comparative anesthetic, then radiofrequency ablation of the joint's innervating medial branches is indicated. Lord et al.[139] established the efficacy of radiofrequency neurotomy in patients with chronic cervical zygapophyseal joint pain through a randomized, double-blind, placebo-controlled trial. The median time that elapsed before return of pain to preneurotomy level in the treatment group was 9 months, compared with 1 week in the sham control group. A subsequent study by McDonald et al.[157] observed that repeat neurotomy can provide the same pain relief if the patient's symptoms returned after an initially successful procedure. However, approximately 50% of patients may require over two repeat neurotomy procedures;[104] yet, repeat procedures achieve similar periods of symptom reduction as the initial treatment procedure.[104,157] There is currently no technique for denervating the atlantooccipital and atlantoaxial joints. Ablation of the third occipital nerve has been shown to successfully treat C2-C3 joint pain.[146] True randomized, controlled, patient-blinded studies of this technique are more challenging because of the adverse effect of suboccipital hypoesthesia from neurotomy of the third occipital nerve. We have successfully used radiofrequency neurotomy of the C2-C3 zygapophyseal joint, and most patients are not distressed by the suboccipital hypoesthesia. In short, medial branch radiofrequency ablation neurotomy is effective in reducing cervical zygapophyseal joint pain and associated disability in well-selected patients.

Cervical Internal Disk Disruption

Epidemiology

Internal disk disruption was first described by Crock[51] more than 30 years ago and indicates that an intervertebral disk has lost its normal internal architecture but maintains a preserved external contour in the absence of nerve root compression. In traumatically induced chronic neck pain, 20% of patients might have CIDD, and another 41% might have CIDD and a concomitant zygapophyseal joint injury.[21] Litigation might adversely affect treatment outcomes for CIDD,[56] but this potential litigation effect has not been substantiated in other investigations.[172,188,203] In nonlitigation cases, nonoperative and operative outcomes are similar to those for CIDD.[56]

Diagnosis

History and Physical Examination. The symptom complex of CIDD includes posterior neck pain, occipital and suboccipital pain, upper trapezial pain, interscapular and periscapular pain, nonradicular arm pain,[228] vertigo, tinnitus, ocular dysfunction, dysphagia, facial pain, and anterior chest wall pain.[75,207] Patients often report a history of preceding trauma such as a motor vehicle accident with acute onset. In the absence of a precipitating event, CIDD symptoms can start spontaneously and gradually, or explosively. If referral symptoms are present, the patient's chief complaint is primarily axial pain associated with nondescript upper limb symptoms. Exacerbating factors usually include prolonged sitting, and coughing, sneezing, or lifting. Lying supine or recumbent with head support typically alleviates the patient's symptoms.

The physical examination can show only subtle cervical range-of-motion restrictions, unless there has been previous cervical surgery. A thorough neuromusculoskeletal examination should be performed to exclude myelopathy or radiculopathy. If spondylosis is present, cervical extension and lateral bending are more restricted than flexion and axial rotation are. Palpation over the cervical spinous processes of the involved level can elicit pain in that region or a portion of the patient's axial pain. Separating these patients from those with nonorganic neck pain can be achieved by eliciting nonorganic signs, such as superficial or nonanatomic tenderness, pain with rotation of head and pelvis together, nonanatomic sensory loss, give-way weakness, and overreaction.[231]

Imaging Studies. Distinguishing painful from nonpainful cervical disks solely on imaging characteristics can be difficult. Disk abnormalities have been noted in patients who are asymptomatic,[20,154,244] and CIDD by definition displays an age-appropriate appearance on MRI.[51] Plain films can reveal hyperostosis and disk space collapse but frequently do not correlate with pain symptoms. Disk desiccation, loss of disk height, annular fissure, osteophytosis, and reactive end plate changes are markers of disk degeneration (Figure 32-22).[165] Decreased intradiskal signal on T_2-weighted images correlates well with histologic degeneration of the disk.[165] MRI features are not useful, however, in detecting symptomatic cervical disks.[205] Consequently, functional diagnostic testing such as provocation diskography is used to diagnose the painful disk level. Our understanding of pain distribution from affected disks has been expanded by studies of these functional diagnostic tests.[45,79,205,228]

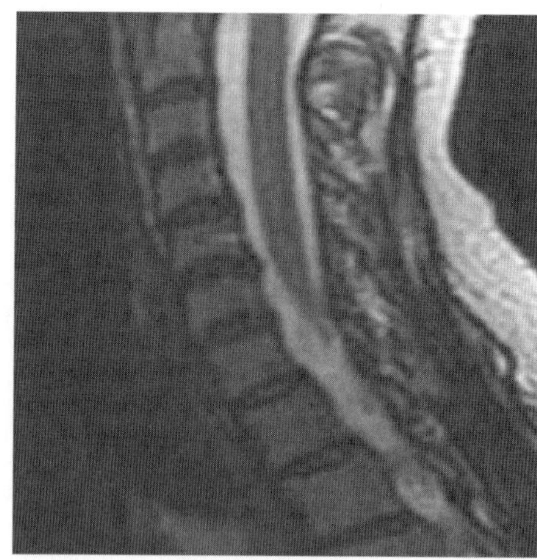

FIGURE 32-22 Magnetic resonance imaging scan depicting degenerative intervertebral disk space changes such as desiccation and mild loss of disk height.

Treatment

Physical Medicine and Rehabilitation. Treating cervical intervertebral disk injury without radiculopathy is similar to treating radicular symptoms. The initial step is to control pain and inflammation. NSAIDs can be used on a short-term basis unless contraindicated because of renal disease or gastrointestinal intolerance to NSAIDs. The American College of Rheumatology guidelines state that renal function in healthy patients should be checked at 6 weeks after initiating NSAIDs. If renal function is normal at 6 weeks, it should be checked again at 12 months. Adjunct medications such as tricyclic antidepressants can help modulate pain and aid in sleep regulation. Opiate analgesics are typically used sparingly and only for short periods.

Physical modalities could be prescribed to modulate pain and transition the patient from passive treatment to active functional restoration. Superficial modalities and TENS therapy can be used for pain. Heat modalities can also be used to increase soft tissue elasticity before and during cervical traction. In uncontrolled studies, electrical stimulation (TENS) has been found to be helpful in cervical pain. Traction might be beneficial by distracting painful intervertebral disks. However, traction should be used cautiously because distracting injured annular tissue can provoke painful symptoms. Cervical collars can help maintain comfortable positioning but should not be worn by the patient for more than 72 hours to minimize further deconditioning. These passive modalities should be used early in the treatment process and later on an as-needed basis, and should not replace activity-based therapies.

As with all other mechanical cervical spine disorders, CIDD requires a thorough evaluation of spine biomechanics. As the acute pain starts to subside, the patient is enrolled in an active stretching and flexibility program with transition to conditioning and stabilization. The independent effects of exercise and stabilization, specifically in the treatment of cervical disk injury, have not been scientifically validated.[234] However, a role for cervical spine stabilization rather than just stretching and strengthening is supported.[60,82] The effects can also be inferred from a lumbar stabilization research report that demonstrated a statistically significant reduction in pain and disability in a group of patients with spondylosis and spondylolisthesis.[175] The only methodologically correct way to study outcomes in patients with true cervical diskogenic pain would be to enroll and treat a cohort of patients after diskography-confirmed concordant axial neck pain. No such studies exist.

Interventional Spine Care

Provocation Diskography. Provocation diskography is a functional diagnostic test in which the accuracy of the investigation relies heavily on patient input. Smith and Nichols[230] first described cervical diskography in the early 1950s, and its utility has been contested ever since.[21] Provocation diskography is the only test that can assess whether a putatively painful disk is symptomatic, and is typically used when CIDD is in question. It is also used as a presurgical evaluation. A positive response requires structural evidence of internal derangement that corroborates production of the patient's usual cervical and referred pain (a concordant response).

Proponents of diskography suggest that healthy disks accept a finite volume of contrast and do not produce symptoms with mechanical stimulation.[209,256] Diskography should be considered valid only when an asymptomatic control disk injection accompanies a concordantly painful disk injection. Although false-positive results have been demonstrated in volunteers who are asymptomatic,[95] these findings can be dismissed because of technical insufficiencies. Cervical provocation diskography has not produced false-positive pain responses in volunteers who are asymptomatic.[205] On occasion, a provocative diskogram can produce a false-positive response in the presence of a painful cervical zygapophyseal joint.[21] Bogduk and April[21] warn that deducing that a positive cervical diskogram in traumatic chronic cervical pain is conclusive might be misleading, and recommends completing diagnostic zygapophyseal joint blocks at the level of the painful disk before pursuing treatment interventions. Cervical intervertebral disks have been shown to refer pain into the head and face both unilaterally and bilaterally,[228] and overlap pain referral patterns produced by painful zygapophyseal joints.[63]

Transforaminal Epidural Steroid Injections. Instillation of steroids into the anterior epidural space to bathe the posterolateral margins of annular surface of the intervertebral disks and posterior longitudinal ligament can address biochemically stimulated nociception.[220] A C7 transforaminal epidural steroid injection (TFESI) is performed if the symptoms are consistent with diskogenic pain and are primarily located at the base, or refer outward from the base, of the cervical spine. The identical procedure is performed at the C5 or C6 level to treat upper neck pain with or without headaches, facial, or upper limb symptoms.[220] If a steroid effect, defined as a 50% reduction in preinjection pain level lasting for 2 days within 7 days after the procedure, is not experienced by the patient, cervical diskography or diagnostic zygapophyseal joint blocks are typically pursued.

The effectiveness of TFESIs has not been systematically studied. Interlaminar epidural steroid injections have been investigated in a heterogeneous group of patients with axial and radicular pain.[42,186,196,214] Most of the patients in these studies had ill-defined symptoms of axial pain and/or radicular pain. The injections were completed posteriorly via the interlaminar approach without fluoroscopic guidance, with the loss-of-resistance technique. Outcomes were successful in approximately 40% to 84% of treated patients.[16,42,186,196,214] Medication injected posteriorly between the laminae might not diffuse anteriorly[127] to reach the potential pain generator. Despite the paucity of literature regarding the use of TFESIs in treating diskogenic cervical pain, the authors typically perform two injections initially before assessing the clinical response. In our experience, approximately 50% of patients experience significant and lasting relief. The more acute or subacute the symptom duration, the better the results, presumably because of a relatively acute inflammatory disk injury.

Surgery

Patients who have severe and recalcitrant axial cervical pain thought to be diskogenic in origin might be candidates for surgery. Our approach to patients with CIDD is to consider cervical diskography if the patient does not realize a pain-relieving steroid effect after two TFESIs. If the diskogram reveals one or two contiguous levels producing concordant pain, then the patient might be a surgical candidate. If three or more levels are concordant, two levels are noncontiguous, or any concordantly painful disks are lobular, then the patient requires a comprehensive chronic pain-modulation program.

The only surgical treatment for CIDD or symptomatic cervical degenerative disks is fusion,[77,103,254] which can be accomplished by anterior cervical diskectomy and fusion or by posterior fusion. The rationale is that, by fusing the bony vertebral elements, motion and the substrate for pain are eliminated, thereby reducing diskogenic pain. The use of provocation diskography to determine the level(s) to fuse is controversial. Some authors have reported "good or excellent" results in 70% to 96% of patients after cervical fusion of levels determined by diskography.[78,209,216,256,266] Seibenrock and Aebi[209] observed a pain reduction of greater than 75% in 96% of 27 patients who underwent cervical fusion of a total of 39 levels. The review was retrospective, and the authors might have included some patients who had primarily radicular complaints. Garvey et al.[76] found that 82% of 87 patients reported their self-perceived outcome as good, very good, or excellent at a mean of 4.4 years after fusion. Ninety-three percent of these patients reported greater than 50% reduction in their pain rating postsurgically. Interestingly, a statistically significant difference was obtained for patients who were treated based on a truly positive diskogram. An extensive literature review concluded that controlled cervical diskography improves surgical outcomes.[152]

Cervical Myelopathy and Myeloradiculopathy

Epidemiology

Cervical spondylitic myelopathy is the most common cervical cord lesion after middle age,[258] but it is not as common as spondylitic cervical radiculopathy.[3] The average age at onset is 50 years or older, and men predominate.[44] Other causes of myelopathy have to be ruled out, including multiple sclerosis, motor neuron disease, vasculitis, neurosyphilis, subacute combined degeneration, syringomyelia, and spinal tumors.[264] One of these other conditions can be present in up to 17% of patients having spondylitic myelopathy.[37]

Diagnosis

History and Physical Examination. Symptom onset is typically insidious, although a minority of patients can experience acute onset with or without a preceding traumatic event. Patients with myelopathy often complain of numbness and paresthesia in the distal limbs and extremities, weakness more often in the lower than upper limbs, and intrinsic hand muscle wasting.[264] Cervical axial pain can be the primary complaint in up to 70% of patients at one point in the disease course.[264] The natural history typically involves an initial deterioration, followed by a static period that can last several years.[173] Bladder function disturbances occur in approximately one third of cases and suggest more severe spinal cord injury.[264] Patients can concurrently complain of unilateral or bilateral radicular pain caused by nerve root involvement at the stenosed level. The combination of cord and radicular involvement is referred to as cervical spondylitic myeloradiculopathy.

A common examination finding is myelopathic weakness in the lower limbs and, to a lesser extent, in the upper limbs. The upper extremities will demonstrate intrinsic hand muscle weakness and wasting resulting from anterior horn cell damage.[264] Pain and temperature disturbances representing injury to the spinothalamic tracts appear as a level of sensory disruption in the thoracic or lumbar region, or "glove and stocking" distribution. Proprioception and vibratory deficits indicating posterior column malfunction are more common in the lower limbs than in the upper limbs.[264] Upper motor neuron signs such as Hoffman sign, brisk reflexes, and Babinski sign are often present. The signs and symptoms might or might not be symmetrical, and complete sparing of the upper limbs is rare. The clinical level of spinal involvement might not correlate with the radiologic level of maximum compression, and there can be a difference of one to two segments.[264] Asymmetrical reflexes in the upper limbs, or myotomal weakness, can indicate concomitant radiculopathy.

Imaging Studies. Radiographic evaluations typically demonstrate the cervical cord compression. Most are spondylitic in nature. Other causes include a superimposed CIDH impinging on the thecal sac, or ossification of the posterior longitudinal ligament (the etiology in 27% of middle-aged patients[246]). Plain radiography provides information regarding the osseous diameter of the central canal and decreased height of the intervertebral disk spaces, and the presence of posterior hyperostosis, foraminal encroachment, and subluxation. A central canal diameter less than 10 mm in a patient who is symptomatic supports the existence of myelopathy.[264] Asymptomatic central cervical spinal stenosis has been observed in 16% of individuals younger than 64 years.[244] A 30% reduction in the cross-sectional area of the cervical spine is the minimum decrement in patients who are symptomatic.[180] To accurately diagnose cervical spondylitic myelopathy, approximately one third of the central canal must be compromised, and objective central canal changes should be evident. These include a complete lack of cerebrospinal fluid flow, cord deformation, or intracord signal abnormalities. MRI allows detection of myelomalacia, which reflects progressive cord compression, signal alteration, atrophy,[190] and the amount of cerebrospinal fluid volume surrounding the cord (Figure 32-23). The preoperative transverse area of the spinal cord at the site of maximal compression tends to correlate with the eventual clinical outcome, whereas the postoperative dimension of the cord strongly correlates with clinical recovery.[168]

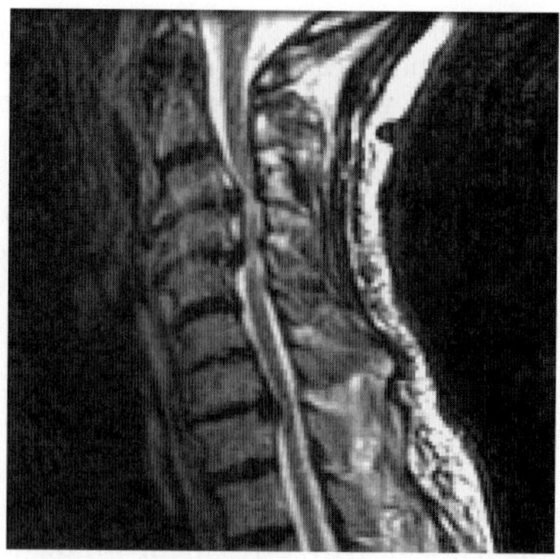

FIGURE 32-23 Sagittal magnetic resonance imaging scan of central spinal stenosis and myelomalacia. Note the lack of cerebrospinal fluid anterior and posterior to the cord at C3-C4 and C4-C5.

Electrodiagnostic Evaluation. Electromyography and nerve conduction studies can be performed to diagnose nerve root injury, as discussed in the section on cervical radiculopathy. In cases of cervical myelopathy, the needle electrode examination can reveal rate-coding abnormalities in muscles below the injured segment, in which the patient recruits normal-appearing motor unit potentials but in a less than full interference pattern at maximal effort, indicative of upper motor neuron injury.

The use of somatosensory evoked potentials to evaluate cervical myelopathy has been investigated.[40,263] Somatosensory evoked potentials with median, ulnar, and posterior tibial nerve stimulation are more sensitive in detecting posterior column dysfunction than clinical testing is. Somatosensory evoked potentials can be used to detect subclinical cord involvement, when the chief complaint is cervical axial or radicular pain. Cervical myelopathy can be distinguished from multiple sclerosis by the pattern of abnormalities obtained by somatosensory evoked potentials. Changes in peripheral nerve conduction studies, when combined with central slowing, are indicative of myeloradiculopathy.[40,263]

Treatment

Nonoperative Care. Conservative care can include physical therapy and cervical orthoses in patients with mild or static symptoms without hard evidence of gait disturbances or pathologic reflexes.[66,183] Improvement of sensory and motor deficits occurs in 33% to 50% of patients.[37,44,183]

Surgery. Surgery is indicated for patients with severe or progressive symptoms, or those for whom conservative measures failed.[108] If a CIDH alone is causing cord compression, then anterior cervical diskectomy and fusion at the appropriate level(s) is indicated.[92] In the case of impingement from degenerative spondylosis or ossification of the posterior longitudinal ligament, surgical intervention aims to remove either the offending anterior structures (such as osteophytes) or the calcified posterior longitudinal ligament (to decompress posteriorly). Both these interventions allow more space for the cord. Anterior decompression is frequently accomplished by corpectomy, in which a vertebral body is removed in addition to the adjacent intervertebral disks, and the segment is then fused with a fibula autograft or allograft of a bone cage.[18] Posterior decompression involves laminectomy with or without fusion,[80] or laminoplasty (Figure 32-24).[93] Extensive laminectomy without fusion can lead to postoperative deformity and kyphosis.[164] This has led to the frequent use of the technique of laminoplasty, in which deformity and kyphosis are much less common and motion is preserved because of absence of a fusion.[164]

The decision to decompress anteriorly or posteriorly is predicated on the number of stenotic levels and the contour of the cervical spine. If three or fewer levels are stenotic, anterior corpectomy and fusion is preferred.[92] In cases of three or more stenotic levels with lordosis preserved, laminoplasty is preferred.[5,92] If, however, three or more levels are involved, with loss of normal cervical lordosis, laminectomy and posterior fusion is performed to maintain cervical spinal stability.[238]

Effective treatment is afforded by anterior decompression, with symptomatic improvement in 85% to 99% of patients.[144,155] Performing corpectomy at more than two levels can result in a less stable construct, and is generally avoided because of complications arising from dislodgement of the graft[92] or nonunion.[89] Laminoplasty has been found to be more effective than laminectomy, with fewer complications in treating cervical myelopathy.[89]

Cervicogenic Headaches

Cervicogenic headaches are a constellation of symptoms that represent the common referral patterns of cervical spine structures. The term *cervicogenic headache* was first coined in 1983.[217] Its definition has been augmented or adjusted several times since.[87,160,162,218] This underscores the myriad pain generators and manifestations that make up cervicogenic headaches, and also points out the lack of consensus regarding the definition.

Epidemiology and Pathophysiology

The prevalence of cervicogenic headache has been reported to range from 0.4% to 2.5% in the general population,[219] to as high as 36.2% in patients with a complaint of

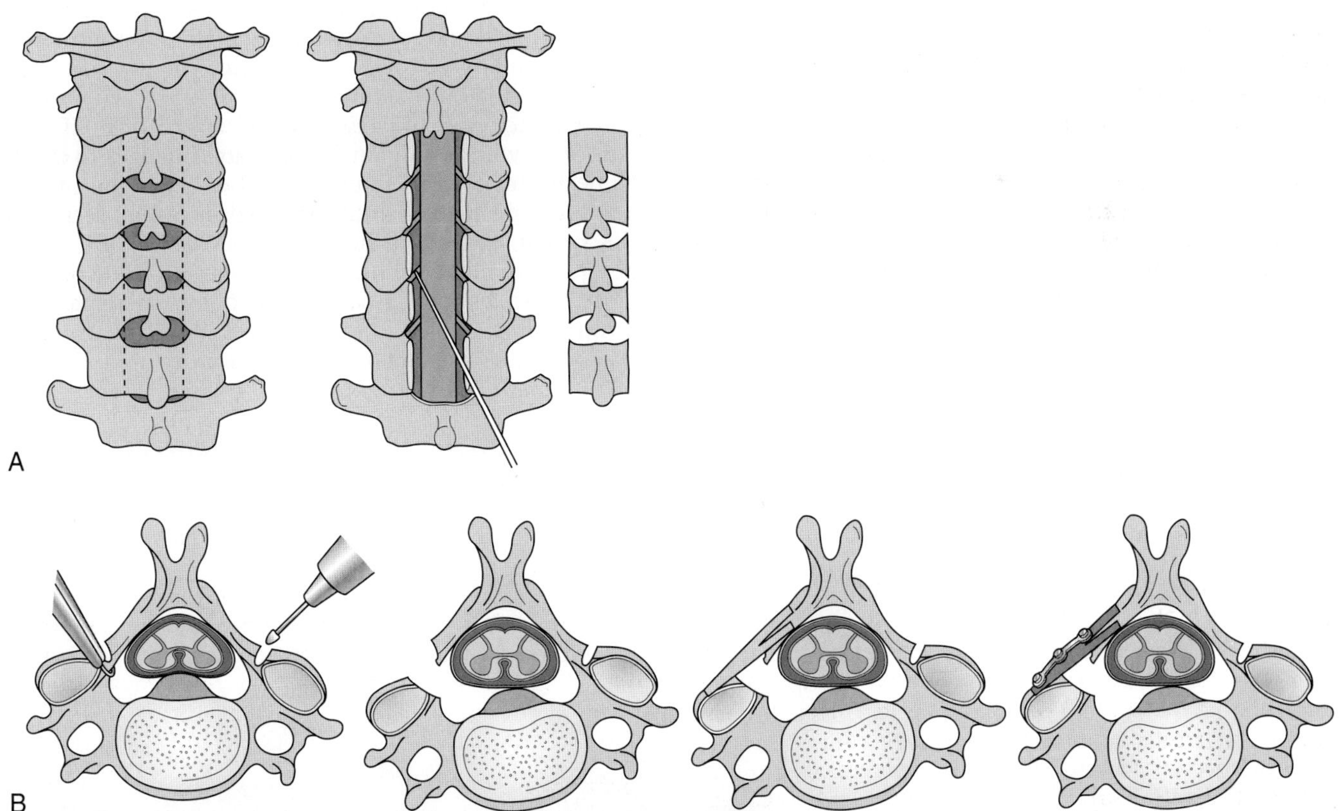

FIGURE 32-24 Laminectomy and laminoplasty. **A,** Laminectomy involves excision of the posterior elements laterally to the level of the pedicles. **B,** Laminoplasty is achieved by completely cutting the laminae on one side while burring the contralateral laminae, allowing this side to act as a hinge. The posterior elements will eventually heal with a widened canal as a graft is placed in the opening.

headaches.[8,171] Women are more commonly affected (79.1%) than men (20.9%)[252] with a mean age of 42.9 years and an average symptom duration of 6.8 years.[83]

Various spine structures have been implicated in cervicogenic headache, including nerve roots and spinal nerves, dorsal root ganglia, uncovertebral joints, intervertebral disks, facet joints, ligaments, and muscles.[217] Circumstantial evidence supports the convergence theory to explain why cranial symptoms can occur as a result of cervical spine pain generators. Convergence of two separate primary afferents derived from two different body regions on the same second-order intraspinal neurons allows the nociceptive activity of one afferent nerve to be perceived as pain in the distribution of the other afferent nerve.[27] The cervicogenic headache can be attributable to degenerative changes, a direct result of trauma, or occur without any underlying biomechanical insult to the various cervical spine structures subserved by cervical afferent fibers. The C2-C3 zygapophyseal joint[49,141,142] and the C2-C3, C3-C4, C4-C5, and C5-C6 intervertebral disks[228] have been primarily implicated as sources of cervicogenic headache.

Diagnosis

History and Physical Examination. Support for a structural source within the cervical spine as the etiology of the patient's headaches is obtained by eliciting any history of previous head or neck trauma such as a whiplash event.[218] Whiplash events such as motor vehicle accidents have been associated with injury to the cervical zygapophyseal joints, intervertebral disks, or nerve roots, either in isolation or in combination.[15,141,243] Cervicogenic headaches have been conceptualized as being primarily unilateral and stemming from the posterior occipital region. The referral of pain is toward the vertex of the scalp, ipsilateral anterolateral temple, forehead, midface, or ipsilateral shoulder girdle.[218,222,223,228] Symptoms can spread to involve the contralateral side,[222] but typically the side of the initial referral source remains most intense.[218] The character of the pain can vary from a deep ache to sharp and stabbing. The duration of the painful symptoms fluctuates from initial episodic bouts of pain, progressing to more chronic and constant pain. Patients often describe the pain as initiating in the cervical region, and traveling to the head and the neck as the pain becomes severe. The cervicogenic headache can then become the primary complaint, overshadowing the original cervical axial pain.

The duration of the symptoms ranges from a few hours to a few weeks, but characteristically lasts longer than that associated with migraine headaches. The pain intensity in cervicogenic headache is less excruciating than for cluster headaches, and is usually nonthrobbing in nature.[218] Autonomic complaints such as photophobia, phonophobia, and nausea are less apparent than in a migraine attack but can still occur.[71,218] Accompanying complaints of dizziness or vertigo sometimes associated with near-syncopal episodes have also been described but are not common.[71]

Physical examination of the patient with complaints of cervicogenic headache typically reveals reduced active range of motion because of muscle guarding, arthritic changes, or soft tissue inflexibility. If the cervicogenic headache is being produced by a cervical zygapophyseal joint, the patient can usually pinpoint with one finger or with the palm of the hand a unilateral area of maximal pain. Cervical intervertebral disk–induced cervicogenic headache typically begins as midline pain that spreads across the spine and into the head or face. However, unilateral occipital headache symptoms that are greater than the neck pain following a traumatic event are more suggestive of zygapophyseal joint pain than diskogenic symptoms.[15,141] Certain head and neck movements can precipitate painful symptoms, such as axial rotation or cervical extension. We have commonly seen patients report an onset after sleeping in an awkward position. Spurling maneuver does not reproduce upper limb radicular symptoms but usually aggravates the axial pain, and patients report reproduction of their paramidline zygapophyseal joint–mediated pain. This pain can also often be reproduced with deep palpation over the involved joint.

Imaging Studies. A history of trauma requires cervical flexion and extension lateral radiographs to detect abnormal segmental motion. It also requires anteroposterior views, including an open mouth view of the odontoid process, to rule out fractures (Figure 32-25).[165] Any suspicion for fracture mandates a subsequent cervical CT scan performed with multiplanar reformatted images to better delineate the osseous injury.[165] MRI is better than CT at evaluating the intervertebral disks for desiccation, decreased disk height, and frank herniation. However, MRI has a false-positive rate of 51% and a false-negative rate of 27% in detecting painful disks identified by diskography.[266] Abnormalities seen on imaging studies should be clinically correlated, because such findings can occur in lifelong asymptomatic individuals.[20,154,244]

Functional Diagnostic Tests and Treatment. Once the etiology of cervicogenic headache has been identified, the offending structure is treated in a similar manner as that outlined earlier. Cervicogenic headaches caused by

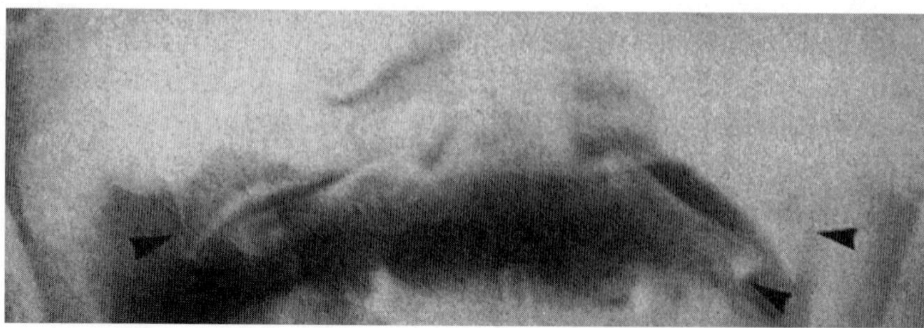

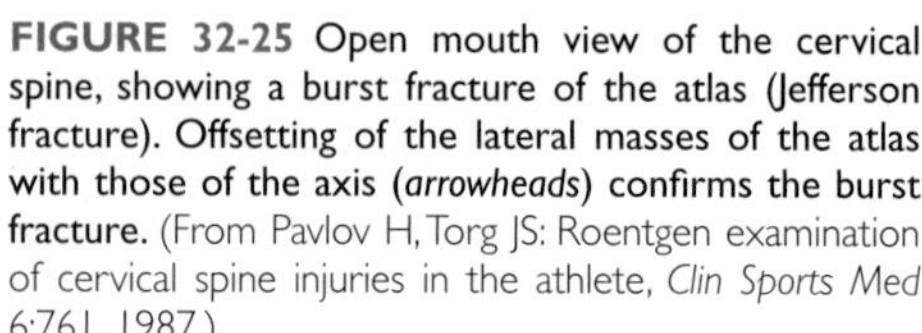

FIGURE 32-25 Open mouth view of the cervical spine, showing a burst fracture of the atlas (Jefferson fracture). Offsetting of the lateral masses of the atlas with those of the axis (*arrowheads*) confirms the burst fracture. (From Pavlov H, Torg JS: Roentgen examination of cervical spine injuries in the athlete, *Clin Sports Med* 6:761, 1987.)

upper cervical zygapophyseal joint pain can be studied with confirmatory diagnostic blockade. The traditional algorithm includes diagnostic blocks performed sequentially at C3-C4, and C1-C2 joints after assessing the C2-C3 joint by third occipital nerve blockade.[15] Following a zygapophyseal joint mapping study, we now also incorporate blockade of C4-C5 zygapophyseal joints if the headaches include anterior head or facial symptoms. Once the painful joint is identified, therapeutic procedures are performed as outlined in the section on treatment of cervical zygapophyseal joint pain for C1-C2 but medial branch neurotomy (or third occipital nerve neurotomy for C2-C3 joint) for other levels.

Whiplash Syndrome

Whiplash (hyperflexion-hyperextension) should be conceptualized as having three components. The *whiplash event* is the biomechanical effect incurred by the occupants of one vehicle when struck by another vehicle. The *whiplash injury* is the impairment, or injured structure, resulting from the whiplash event. The *whiplash syndrome* is the set of symptoms arising from the whiplash injury.[12] During a whiplash event, the head and neck do not suffer a direct blow, but each undergoes an excursion because of the inertial response of the body to forces imparted on it.[12] Rear-end collisions represent the most common pattern of whiplash-related injury, but injury caused by head-on and side collisions can also occur.[12]

Regardless of the direction of impact, whiplash is defined by the passive movement of the neck. Muscular control to stabilize the cervical spine does not react quickly enough to prevent injurious forces from occurring across the cervical functional spinal units. Both the lack of muscular pillaring and the generation of abnormal forces resulting in movements around abnormal axes of rotation subject the passive restraining structures to abnormal strain.[12,114] For example, at 110 ms after rear-end impact, the C5-C6 disk space widens anteriorly, causing abutment of the articular processes of the C5-C6 zygapophyseal joint[114] and posterior shear within the disk.[176] The anterior disk, anterior longitudinal ligament, posterior disk or annulus, and cervical zygapophyseal joints are all at risk of injury during a whiplash event.[12,114,176] Injury also occurs to the cervical soft tissues, resulting in strain and sprain injuries.[170] These injuries typically heal over a relatively short period, as would be expected for soft tissue injury. The most commonly reported symptoms of whiplash injury include neck pain and headaches, followed by shoulder girdle pain, upper limb paresthesia, and weakness. Less common symptoms include dizziness, visual disturbances, and tinnitus.[12]

Most patients with whiplash syndrome are destined to recover within the first 2 to 3 months after the injury, and after 2 years 82% are symptom-free.[188] Severely afflicted patients account for only 6% of all patients with whiplash at 3 months, and this percentage decreases minimally to 4% at 2 years.[188] Studies have demonstrated that chronicity of whiplash symptoms develops independent of litigation,[172] and litigation does not alter response to treatment.[203] The clinician should pursue evaluation and treatment of whiplash-related symptoms, rather than just assume that the pain is a result of mitigating circumstances such as secondary gain considerations.

Conclusion

Neck pain is one of the most common complaints of patients seeking medical attention. Knowledge of spinal biomechanics and pathophysiology helps determine the most likely pain generators in each case. A variety of spinal structures can produce overlapping or obscure symptoms. An accurate diagnosis provides the best opportunity for effective treatment. The building blocks for successful therapeutic interventions include controlling pain and inflammation while at the same time educating the patient about the injury, the treatment objectives, and the prognosis. As technology advances and our knowledge of cervical spine disorders grows, our clinical pathways for treatment of cervical problems will continue to evolve and improve. It is important to view the patient as a whole, and institute physical, pharmacologic, behavioral, and interventional treatments in the broad context of achieving what is best for the patient's physiologic and psychological well-being.

KEY REFERENCES

6. Anderberg L, Annertz M, Brandt L, et al: Selective diagnostic cervical nerve root block—correlation with clinical symptoms and MRI-pathology, *Acta Neurochir* 146:559–565, 2004.
7. Anderberg L, Annertz M, Persson L, et al: Transforaminal steroids injections for treatment of cervical radiculopathy: a prospective and randomised study, *Eur Spine J* 16:321–328, 2007.
9. Aprill C, Bogduk N: The prevalence of cervical zygapophyseal joint pain: a first approximation, *Spine* 17:744–747, 1992.
10. Aprill C, Dwyer A, Bogduk N: Cervical zygapophyseal joint pain patterns. II: a clinical evaluation, *Spine* 15:458–461, 1990.
15. Barnsley L, Lord SM, Wallis BJ, et al: The prevalence of chronic cervical zygapophyseal joint pain after whiplash, *Spine* 20:20–26, 1995.
20. Boden SD, McCowin PR, Davis DO, et al: Abnormal magnetic resonance scans of the cervical spine in asymptomatic subjects: a prospective investigation, *J Bone Joint Surg* 72:1178–1184, 1990.
21. Bogduk N, Aprill C: On the nature of neck pain, discography and cervical zygapophysial joint blocks, *Pain* 54:213–217, 1993.
22. Bogduk N, Marsland A: The cervical zygapophysial joints as a source of neck pain, *Spine* 13:610–617, 1988.
24. Bogduk N, Windsor M, Inglis A: The innervation of the cervical intervertebral discs, *Spine* 13:2–8, 1988.
25. Bogduk N, Dreyfuss P, Baker R, et al: Complications of spinal diagnostic and treatment procedures, *Pain Med* 9:S11–S34, 2008.
27. Bogduk N: Cervicogenic headache: anatomic basis and pathophysiologic mechanisms, *Curr Pain Headache Rep* 5:382–386, 2001.
29. Bogduk N: The anatomy and pathophysiology of neck pain, *Phys Med Rehabil Clin N Am* 14:455–472, 2003.
35. Bush K, Hillier S: Outcome of cervical radiculopathy treated with periradicular/epidural corticosteroid injections: a prospective study with independent clinical review, *Eur Spine J* 5:319–325, 1996.
46. Colachis S, Strohm B: A study of tractive forces angle of pull on vertebral interspaces in the cervical spine, *Arch Phys Med Rehabil* 46:820, 1965.
47. Colachis SC, Jr, Strohm BR: Effect of duration of intermittent cervical traction on vertebral separation, *Arch Phys Med Rehabil* 47:353–359, 1966.
49. Cooper G, Bailey B, Bogduk N: Cervical zygapophysial joint pain maps, *Pain Med* 8:344–353, 2007.
57. Dillingham TR, Lauder TD, Andary M, et al: Identification of cervical radiculopathies. Optimizing the electromyographic screen, *Am J Phys Med Rehabil* 80:84–91, 2001.
59. Dreyfuss P, Michaelsen M, Fletcher D: Atlanto-occipital and lateral atlanto-axial joint pain patterns, *Spine* 19:1125–1131, 1994.

63. Dwyer A, Aprill C, Bogduk N: Cervical zygapophyseal joint pain patterns. I: a study in normal volunteers, *Spine* 15:453–457, 1990.
68. Fast A, Parikh S, Marin E: The shoulder abduction relief sign in cervical radiculopathy, *Arch Phys Med Rehabil* 70:402–403, 1989.
73. Fukui S, Ohseto K, Shiotani M, et al: Referred pain distribution of the cervical zygapophyseal joints and cervical dorsal rami, *Pain* 68:79–83, 1996.
105. Huston CW, Slipman CW, Garvin C: Complications and side effects of cervical and lumbosacral nerve root injections, *Arch Phys Med Rehabil* 86:277–283, 2005.
109. Johnson EW, Melvin JL: Value of electromyography in lumbar radiculopathy, *Arch Phys Med Rehabil* June:239–243, 1971.
110. Johnson RM, Hart DL, Simmons EF, et al: Cervical orthoses: a study comparing their effectiveness in restricting cervical motion in normal subjects, *J Bone Joint Surg Am* 59:332, 1977.
112. Jull G, Bogduk NK, Marsland A: The accuracy of manual diagnosis for cervical zygapophysial joint pain syndromes, *Med J Aust* 148: 233–236, 1988.
116. Kang JD, Stefanovic-Racic M, McIntyre L, et al: Toward a biochemical understanding of human intervertebral disc degeneration and herniation: contributions of nitric oxide, interleukins, prostaglandins, and matrix metalloproteinases, *Spine* 22:1065–1073, 1997.
118. Kellegren JH: Observations on referred pain arising from muscle, *Clin Sci* 3:175–190, 1938.
119. Kellegren JH: On the distribution of pain arising from deep somatic structures with charts of segmental pain, *Clin Sci* 3:35–46, 1939.
139. Lord SM, Barnsley L, Bogduk N: Percutaneous radiofrequency neurotomy in the treatment of cervical zygapophysial joint pain: a caution, *Neurosurgery* 36:732–739, 1995.
140. Lord SM, Barnsley L, Bogduk N: The utility of comparative local anaesthetic blocks versus placebo-controlled blocks for the diagnosis of cervical zygapophysial joint pain, *Clin J Pain* 11:208–213, 1995.
141. Lord SM, Barnsley L, Wallis BJ, et al: Chronic cervical zygapophyseal joint pain after whiplash. A placebo-controlled prevalence study, *Spine* 21:1737–1745, 1996.
142. Lord SM, Barnsley L, Wallis BJ, et al: Third occipital nerve headache: a prevalence study, *J Neurol Neurosurg Psychiatry* 57:1187–1190, 1994.
146. MacVicar J, Borowczyk JM, MacVicar AM, et al: Cervical medial branch radiofrequency neurotomy in New Zealand, *Pain Med* 13:647–654, 2012.
181. Persson LC, Moritz U, Brandt L: Cervical radiculopathy: pain, muscle weakness and sensory loss in patients with cervical radiculopathy treated with surgery, physiotherapy or cervical collar. A prospective, controlled study, *Eur Spine J* 6:256–266, 1997.
188. Radanov BP, Sturzenegger M, Di Stefano G: Long-term outcome after whiplash injury: a 2-year follow-up considering features of injury mechanism and somatic, radiologic, and psychosocial findings, *Medicine* 74:281–297, 1995.
195. Riew DK, Kim Y, Gilula L: Can cervical nerve root blocks prevent surgery for cervical radiculopathy? A prospective, randomized, controlled, double-blind study, *Spine J* 6:2S–3S, 2006.
199. Rydevik B, Brown M, Lundborg G: Pathoanatomy and pathophysiology of nerve root compression, *Spine* 9:7–15, 1984.
200. Saal J, Saal J, Yurth E: Nonoperative management of herniated cervical intervertebral disc with radiculopathy, *Spine* 21:1877–1883, 1996.
203. Sapir D, Gorup J: Radiofrequency medial branch neurotomy in litigant and nonlitigant patients with cervical whiplash, *Spine* 26:E268–E273, 2001.
212. Shabat S, Leitner Y, David R, Folman Y: The correlation between Spurling test and imaging studies in detecting cervical radiculopathy, *Neuroimaging* 22:375–378, 2012.
220. Slipman CW, Chow DW, Isaac Z, et al: An evidence-based algorithmic approach to cervical spinal disorders, *Crit Rev Phys Med Rehabil Med* 13:283–299, 2001.
223. Slipman CW, Isaac Z, Thomas J, et al: Cervical zygapophyseal joint syndrome and referral to the head and face: preliminary data from 100 patients, *Arch Phys Med Rehabil* 83:1665, 2002.
226. Slipman CW, Lipetz JS, Jackson HB, et al: Therapeutic selective nerve root block in the nonsurgical treatment of atraumatic cervical spondylitic radicular pain: a retrospective analysis with independent clinical review, *Arch Phys Med Rehabil* 81:741–746, 2000.
228. Slipman CW, Plastaras C, Patel R, et al: Provocative cervical discography symptom mapping, *Spine J* 5:381–388, 2005.
229. Slipman CW, Plastaras CT, Palmitier RS, et al: Symptom provocation of fluoroscopically guided cervical nerve root stimulation: are dynatomal maps identical to dermatomal maps?, *Spine* 23:2235–2242, 1998.
231. Sobel JB, Sollenberger P, Robinson R, et al: Cervical nonorganic signs: a new clinical tool to assess abnormal illness behavior in neck pain patients: a pilot study, *Arch Phys Med Rehabil* 81:170–175, 2000.
235. Spurling RG, Scoville WB: Lateral rupture of the cervical intervertebral discs. A common cause of shoulder and arm pain, *Surg Gynecol Obstet* 78:350–358, 1944.
248. Vallee JN, Feydy A, Carlier RY, et al: Chronic cervical radiculopathy: lateral approach periradicular corticosteroid injection, *Radiology* 218:886–892, 2001.
249. Van Akkerveeken PF: The diagnostic value of nerve root sheath infiltration, *Acta Orthop Scand Suppl* 251:61–63, 1993.

The full reference list for this chapter is available online.

CHAPTER 33

LOW BACK PAIN

Karen P. Barr, Leah G. Concannon, Mark A. Harrast

Low back pain has become a costly burden to society and a leading cause of disability and loss of productivity. This chapter outlines the anatomy and biomechanics of the lumbar spine and our current understanding of the physiology of low back pain. The clinical evaluation and treatment of various etiologies of low back pain and leg pain caused by lumbar spine disease is also reviewed.

Epidemiology

Low back pain is a symptom, not a disease, and has many causes. It is generally described as pain between the costal margin and the gluteal folds. It is extremely common. Approximately 40% of people say they have had low back pain within the past 6 months,[237] and annually 15% report low back pain lasting longer than 2 weeks.[58] Studies have shown a lifetime prevalence as high as 84%.[244] Onset usually begins in the teens to early 40s. Most patients have short attacks of pain that are mild or moderate and do not limit activities, but these tend to recur over many years. Most episodes resolve with or without treatment and the great majority of people who have back pain do not seek medical care.[255] Approximately 10% to 15% of back pain becomes chronic and, for some of this group, it can cause substantial disability. In most studies, approximately half of the sick days used for back pain are accounted for by the 15% of people who are home from work for more than 1 month. Between 80% and 90% of the health care and social costs of back pain are for the 10% who develop chronic low back pain and disability. Just over 1% of adults in the United States are permanently disabled by back pain, and another 1% are temporarily disabled.[160]

Researchers have sought to determine what factors lead back pain to become chronic and disabling. Interestingly, unlike many other medical conditions, it does not appear to be related to the diagnosis or the cause of the back pain. Instead, the largest baseline predictors of persistent disabling back pain are maladaptive pain coping behaviors, the presence of nonorganic signs, presence of psychiatric disease, low physical function, and low general health.[51] The percentage of patients disabled by back pain, as well as the cost of low back pain, has steadily increased during the past few decades. This appears to be more from social causes than from a change in the conditions that cause low back pain. The two most commonly cited factors are the increasing societal acceptance of back pain as a reason to become disabled, and changes in the social system that pay disability benefits to patients with back pain.[242]

Public Health Perspective

Programs to decrease the incidence of back pain have been developed. Only exercise has been shown to be an effective intervention to prevent back pain. Interventions such as ergonomics, education, reduced lifting, and back supports have not shown to be effective.[23] Other public health interventions have focused on minimizing the chronicity and effects of low back pain. Public health campaigns throughout Europe, Canada, and Australia have attempted to use the media to elicit changes in beliefs and treatment seeking. This has been most effective in Australia, where it was shown to decrease disability behavior and work absences.[39]

Many countries have developed evidence-based guidelines to help practitioners manage this condition. Goals often include minimizing inappropriate interventions to decrease comorbidity associated with unnecessary treatments and control health care costs. The use of new and expensive technology to diagnose and treat back pain has not led to improved outcomes, but has caused greatly escalating costs and socioeconomic problems. The rate of expensive treatments such as injections and surgeries vary greatly by country and even regions within countries, without an associated improvement in outcomes in these regions. The trend of both increased cost of care and increasing comorbidities from these complex interventions continues, as does the trend of increasing disability from back pain.[16]

Anatomy and Biomechanics of the Lumbar Spine

General Concepts

The lumbar spine has a dichotomous role in terms of function, which is strength coupled with flexibility. The spine performs a major role in support and protection (strength) of the spinal canal contents (spinal cord, conus, and cauda equina) but also gives us inherent flexibility, allowing us to place our limbs in appropriate positions for everyday functions.

The strength of the spine results from the size and arrangements of the bones, as well as from the arrangement of the ligaments and muscles. The inherent flexibility results from the large number of joints placed so closely together in series. Each vertebral segment can be thought of as a three-joint complex: one intervertebral disk with vertebral end plates and two zygapophyseal joints. The typical lordotic framework of the lumbar spine assists with

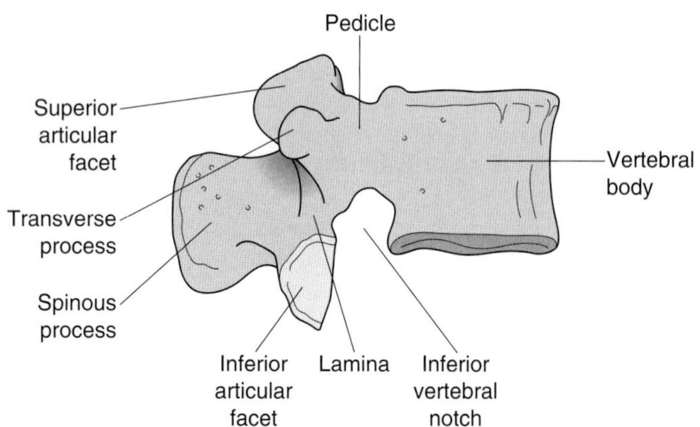

FIGURE 33-1 Lateral view of the lumbar vertebrae. (Modified from Parke WW: Applied anatomy of the spine. In Herkowitz HN, Garfin SR, Balderson RA, et al, editors: *Rothman-Simeone: the spine*, ed 4, Philadelphia, 1999, WB Saunders.)

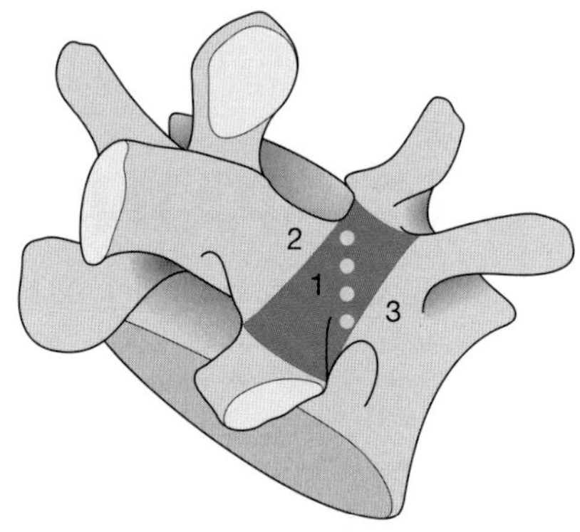

FIGURE 33-2 An oblique dorsal view of an L5 vertebra, showing the parts of the vertebral arch: *1*, pars interarticularis (*crosshatched area*); *2*, pars laminaris; and *3*, pars pedicularis. The dotted line indicates the most frequent site of mechanical failure of the pars interarticularis. (Modified from Parke WW: Applied anatomy of the spine. In Herkowitz HN, Garfin SR, Balderson RA, et al, editors: *Rothman-Simeone: the spine*, ed 4, Philadelphia, 1999, WB Saunders.)

this flexibility but also increases the ability of the lumbar spine to absorb shock.

Vertebrae

The bony anatomy of the lumbar spine consists of five lumbar vertebrae. A small percentage of the population has four (the fifth vertebra is sacralized) or six (the first sacral segment is lumbarized). The lumbar vertebrae are composed of the vertebral body, the neural arch, and the posterior elements (Figure 33-1). The vertebral bodies increase in size as you travel caudally in the spine. The lower three are typically more wedge-shaped (taller anteriorly), which helps create the normal lumbar lordosis. The structure of the vertebral bodies and the shock-absorbing intervertebral disks function together to withstand axially directed loads. The sides of the bony neural arch are the pedicles, which are thick pillars that connect the posterior elements to the vertebral bodies. They are designed to resist bending and to transmit forces between the vertebral bodies and the posterior elements. The posterior elements consist of the laminae, the articular processes, and the spinous processes. The superior and inferior articular processes of adjacent vertebrae create the zygapophyseal joints. The pars interarticularis is the part of the lamina between the superior and inferior articular processes (Figure 33-2). The pars is the site of stress fractures (spondylolysis) because it is subjected to large bending forces. This occurs as the forces transmitted by the vertically oriented lamina undergo a change in direction into the horizontally oriented pedicle.[27]

Intervertebral Disk

The intervertebral disk and its attachment to the vertebral end plate are considered a secondary cartilaginous joint, or symphysis. The disk consists of the internal nucleus pulposus and the outer annulus fibrosus. The nucleus pulposus is the gelatinous inner section of the disk. It consists of water, proteoglycans, and collagen. The nucleus pulposus is 90% water at birth. Disks desiccate and degenerate as we age and lose some of their height, which is one reason we are slightly shorter in our older adult years.

The annulus fibrosus consists of concentric layers of fibers at oblique angles to each other, which help to withstand strains in any direction. The outer fibers of the annulus have more collagen and less proteoglycans and water than the inner fibers.[22] This varying composition supports the functional role of the outer fibers to resist flexion, extension, rotation, and distraction forces.

The main function of the intervertebral disk is shock absorption (Figure 33-3). It is primarily the annulus, not the nucleus, that acts as the shock absorber because the liquid properties of the nucleus render it incompressible. When an axial load occurs, the increase in force in the incompressible nucleus pushes on the annulus and stretches its fibers. If the fibers break, then a herniated nucleus pulposus results.

Because flexion loads the anterior disk, the nucleus is displaced posteriorly.[121] If the forces are great enough, the nucleus can herniate through the posterior annular fibers. The lateral fibers of the posterior longitudinal ligaments are thinnest, however, making posterolateral disk herniations the most common (Figure 33-4). The posterolateral portion of the disk is most at risk when there is forward flexion accompanied by lateral bending (i.e., bending and twisting). The zygapophyseal joints cannot resist rotation when the spine is in flexion, thereby increasing torsional shear forces and putting the disks at risk.

The activity of the lumbar muscles correlates well with intradiskal pressures (i.e., when back muscles contract, there is an associated increase in disk pressure). These pressures change depending on spine posture and the activity undertaken. Figure 33-5 demonstrates the changes in L3 disk pressure under various positions and exercises.[158,159] Adding rotation to the already flexed posture increases the disk pressure substantially. Comparing lifting maneuvers, it has been shown that there is not a substantial difference in disk pressure when lifting with the legs (i.e., with the back straight and knees bent) versus lifting with the back (i.e., with a forward-flexed back and straight legs).[8,9] What decreases the forces on the lumbar spine is lifting the load close to your body. The farther the load

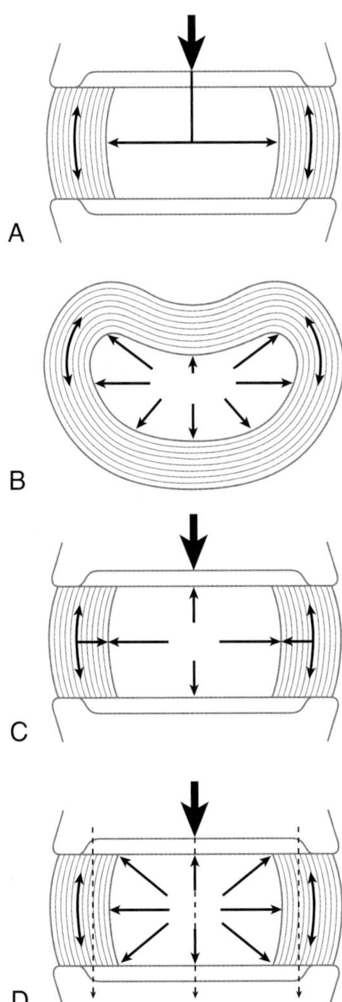

FIGURE 33-3 The mechanism of weight transmission in an intervertebral disk. **A,** Compression increases the pressure in the nucleus pulposus. This is exerted radially onto the annulus fibrosus, and the tension in the annulus increases. **B,** The tension in the annulus is exerted on the nucleus, preventing it from expanding radially. Nuclear pressure is then exerted on the vertebral end plates. **C,** Weight is borne, in part, by the annulus fibrosus and by the nucleus pulposus. **D,** The radial pressure in the nucleus braces the annulus, and the pressure on the end plates transmits the load from one vertebra to the next. (Modified from Bogduk N, editor: The inter-body joint and the intervertebral discs. In *Clinical and radiological anatomy of the lumbar spine and sacrum,* ed 5, Edinburgh, 2012, Churchill Livingstone.)

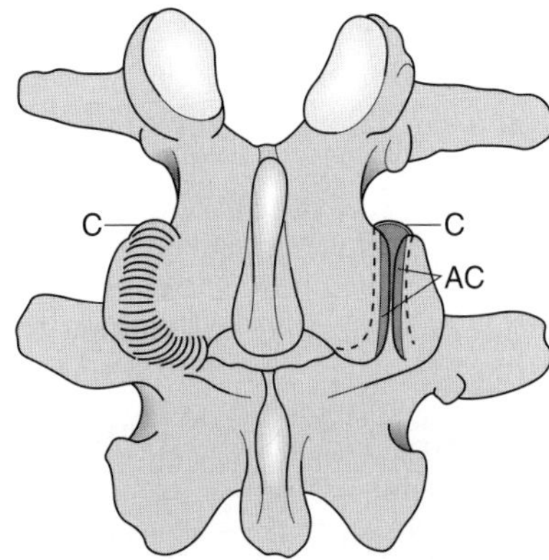

FIGURE 33-4 A posterior view of the L3-L4 zygapophyseal joints. On the left, the capsule of the joint (*C*) is intact. On the right, the posterior capsule has been resected to reveal the joint cavity, the articular cartilages (*AC*), and the line of attachment of the joint capsule (*dashed line*). The upper joint capsule (*C*) attaches further from the articular margin than the posterior capsule does. (Modified from Bogduk N, editor: The zygapophysial joints. In *Clinical and radiological anatomy of the lumbar spine and sacrum,* ed 5, Edinburgh, 2012, Churchill Livingstone.)

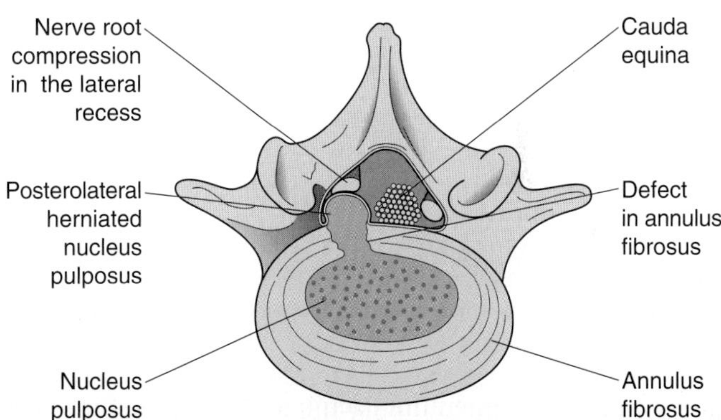

FIGURE 33-5 Posterolateral intervertebral disk herniation.

is from the chest, the greater the stress on the lumbar spine.[8]

Zygapophyseal Joints

The zygapophyseal joints (also known as Z joints and facet joints) are paired synovial joints with a synovium and a capsule (Figure 33-6). Their alignment or direction of joint articulation determines the direction of motion of the adjacent vertebrae. The lumbar zygapophyseal joints lie in the sagittal plane and thus primarily allow flexion and extension. Some lateral bending and very little rotation are allowed, which limits torsional stress on the lumbar disks. Rotation is more a component of thoracic spine motion. The majority of spinal flexion and extension (90%) occurs at the L4-L5 and L5-S1 levels, which contributes to the high incidence of disk problems at these levels.

Ligaments

The two main sets of ligaments of the lumbar spine are the longitudinal ligaments and the segmental ligaments. The two longitudinal ligaments are the anterior and posterior longitudinal ligaments. They are named according to their position on the vertebral body. The anterior longitudinal ligament acts to resist extension, translation, and rotation. The posterior longitudinal ligament acts to resist flexion. Disruption of either ligament primarily occurs with rotation rather than with flexion or extension. The anterior longitudinal ligament is twice as strong as the posterior longitudinal ligament.

The main segmental ligament is the ligamentum flavum, which is a paired structure joining adjacent laminae. It is the ligament that is pierced when performing lumbar punctures. It is a very strong ligament but is elastic enough to allow flexion. Flexing the lumbar spine puts this ligament on stretch, decreasing its redundancy and making it easier to pierce during a lumbar puncture.

The other segmental ligaments are the supraspinous, interspinous, and intertransverse. The supraspinous ligaments are the strong ligaments that join the tips of adjacent spinous processes and act to resist flexion. These ligaments,

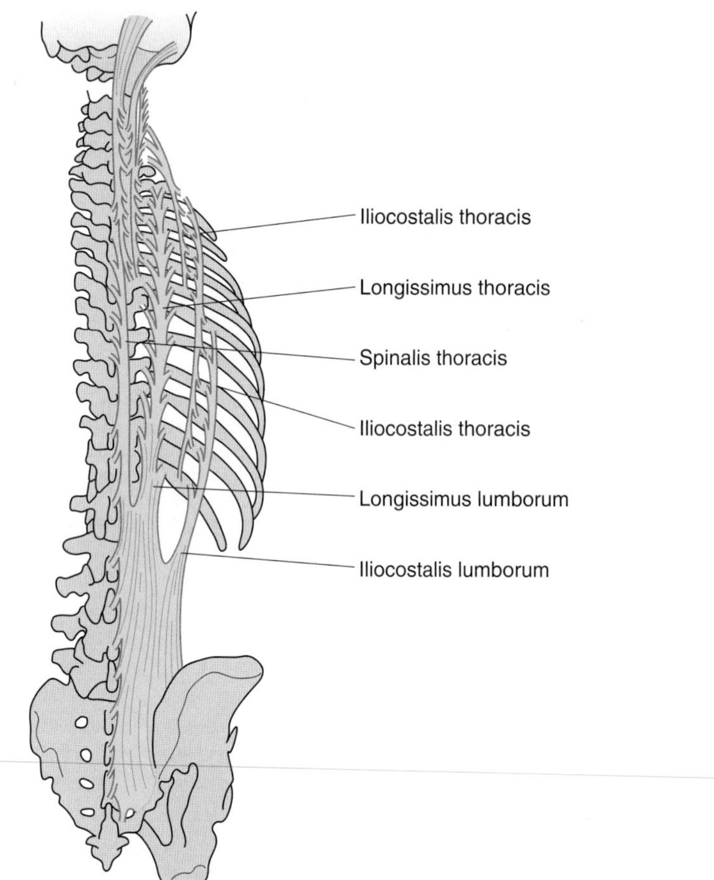

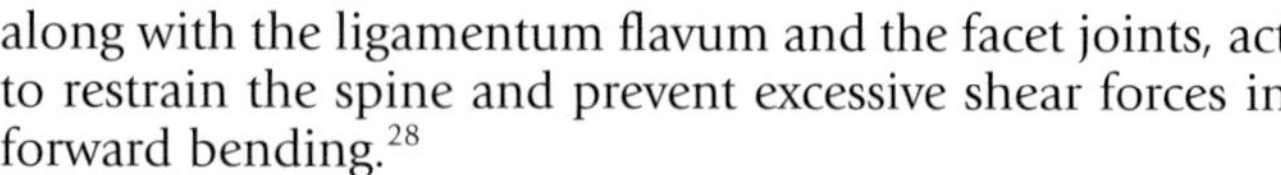

FIGURE 33-6 The intermediate layer of back muscles: the erector spinae.

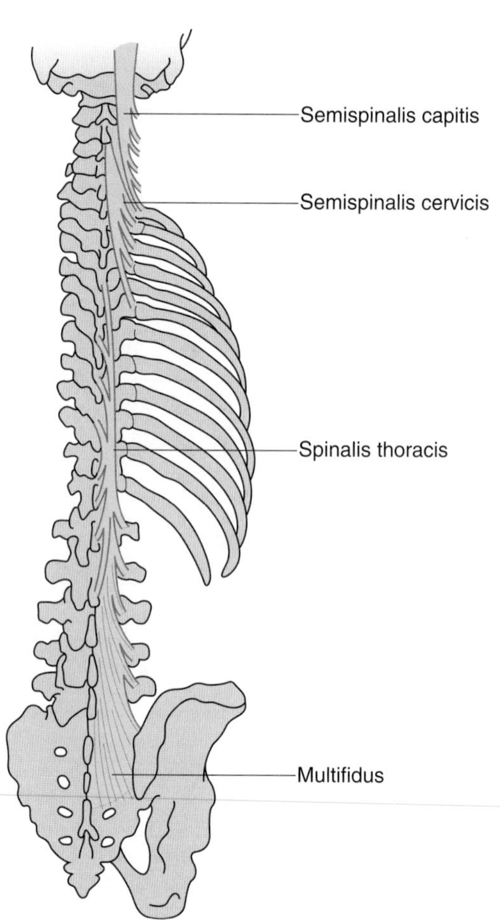

FIGURE 33-7 The deep back muscles: the multifidi.

along with the ligamentum flavum and the facet joints, act to restrain the spine and prevent excessive shear forces in forward bending.[28]

Muscles

Muscles with Origins on the Lumbar Spine

These muscles can be divided anatomically into posterior and anterior muscles. The posterior muscles include the latissimus dorsi and the paraspinals. The lumbar paraspinals consist of the erector spinae (iliocostalis, longissimus, and spinalis), which act as the chief extensors of the spine, and the deep layer (rotators and multifidi) (Figures 33-7 and 33-8). The multifidi are tiny segmental stabilizers that act to control lumbar flexion because they cannot produce enough force to truly extend the spine. Their most important function has been hypothesized to be that of a sensory organ to provide proprioception for the spine, given the predominance of muscle spindles seen histologically in these muscles.

The anterior muscles of the lumbar spine include the psoas and quadratus lumborum. Because of the direct attachment of the psoas on the lumbar spine, tightening this muscle accentuates the normal lumbar lordosis. This can increase forces on the posterior elements and can contribute to zygapophyseal joint pain. The quadratus lumborum acts in side bending and can assist in lumbar flexion.

Abdominal Musculature

The superficial abdominals include the rectus abdominis and external obliques (Figure 33-9, *A*). The deep layer consists of internal obliques and the transversus abdominis (see Figure 33-9, *B*). The transversus abdominis has been the focus of considerable attention recently as an important muscle to train in treating low back pain. Its connection to the thoracolumbar fascia (and consequently its ability to act on the lumbar spine) has probably been the major reason that it has received such attention of late.

Thoracolumbar Fascia

The thoracolumbar fascia, with its attachments to the transversus abdominis and internal obliques, acts as an abdominal and lumbar "brace," particularly when lifting. This abdominal bracing mechanism results from contraction of these deep abdominal muscles, which creates tension in the thoracolumbar fascia, which then creates an extension force on the lumbar spine without increasing shear forces.[86] The validity of this model has recently been called into question, however.[28]

Pelvic Stabilizers

The pelvic stabilizers are considered "core" muscles because of their indirect effect on the lumbar spine, even though they do not have a direct attachment to the spine. The gluteus medius stabilizes the pelvis during gait. Weakness

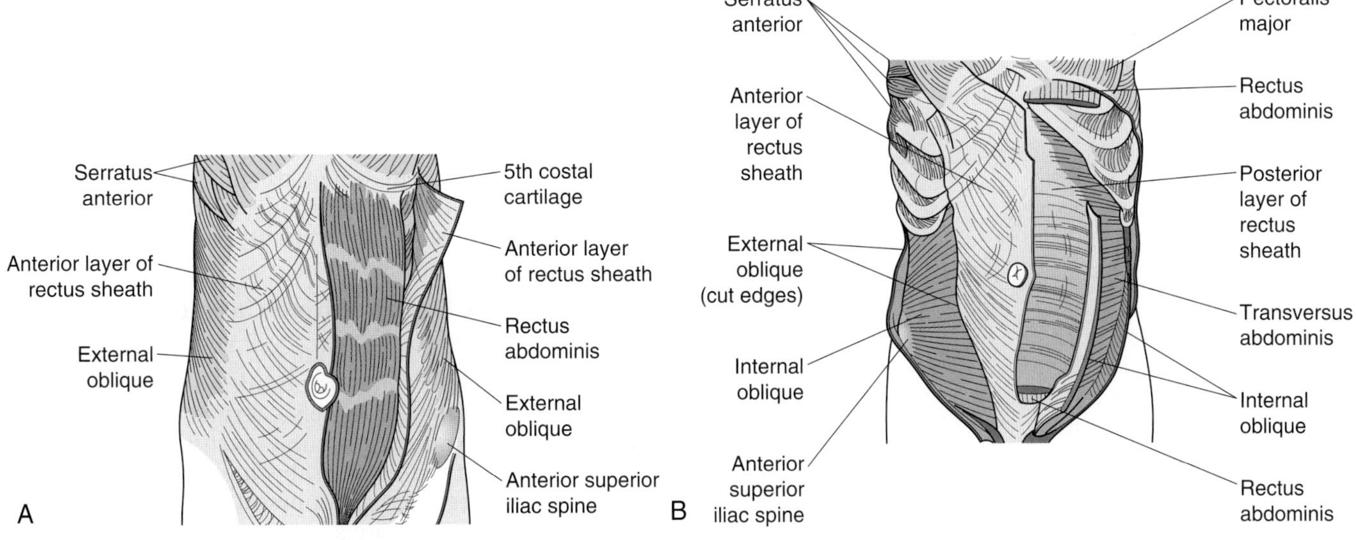

FIGURE 33-8 **A,** The superficial abdominal muscles. **B,** The deep abdominal muscles.

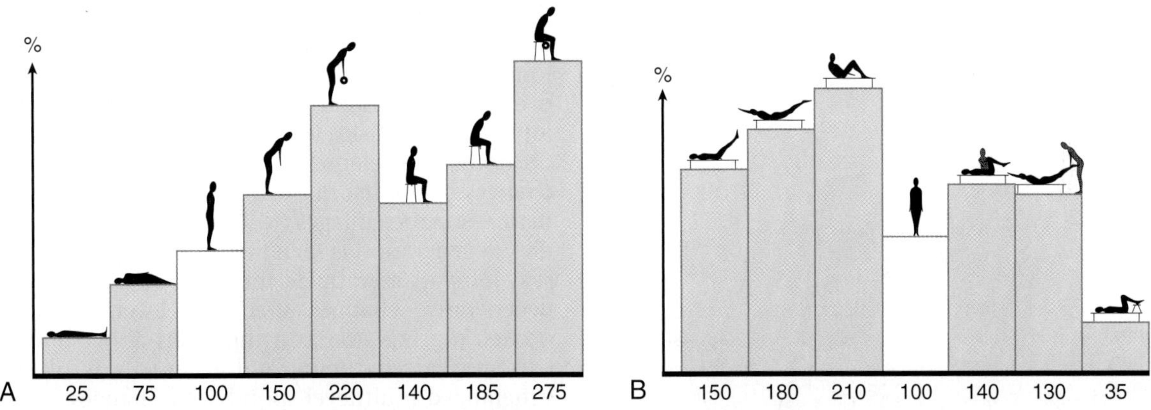

FIGURE 33-9 **A,** Relative change in pressure (or load) in the third lumbar disk in various positions in living individuals. **B,** Relative change in pressure (or load) in the third lumbar disk during various muscle-strengthening exercises in living individuals. Neutral erect posture is considered 100% in these figures; other positions and activities are calculated in relationship to this. (Modified from Nachemson AL, Morris JM: In vivo measurements of intradiscal pressure, *J Bone Joint Surg Am* 46:1077-1092, 1964.)

or inhibition of this muscle results in pelvic "instability," which introduces lumbar side bending and rotation, creating increased shear or torsional forces on the lumbar disks.

The piriformis is a hip and sacral rotator and can cause excessive external rotation of the hip and sacrum when it is tight. This can result in increased shear forces at the lumbosacral junction. Other pelvic floor muscles may also act to maintain proper positioning of the spine and are an important focus of some spine rehabilitation programs.

Nerves

The conus medullaris ends at about L2, and below this level is the cauda equina. The cauda equina consists of the dorsal and ventral rootlets, which join together in the intervertebral neuroforamen to become the spinal nerves (Figure 33-10). The spinal nerve gives off the ventral primary ramus. The ventral primary rami from multiple levels form the lumbar and lumbosacral plexus to innervate the limbs. The dorsal primary ramus, with its three branches (medial, intermediate, and lateral), innervates the posterior half of the vertebral body, the paraspinal muscles, and the zygapophyseal joints, and provides sensation to the back. The medial branch innervates the zygapophyseal joints and lumbar multifidi, and is the target during radiofrequency neurotomy for presumed zygapophyseal joint pain (Figure 33-11).[29]

Pain Generators of the Lumbar Spine

The low back is an anatomically diverse set of structures, and there are many potential sources of pain. One useful strategy to clarify these potential sources of pain is learning what low back structures are innervated (and can transmit pain through neural pain fibers) and what structures have no innervation (Box 33-1).

The sinuvertebral nerve innervates the anterior vertebral body, the external annulus, and the posterior longitudinal ligament. The posterior longitudinal ligament is a highly innervated structure and can play an important role in low back pain perception with lumbar disk herniations. The medial branch of the dorsal primary ramus innervates the

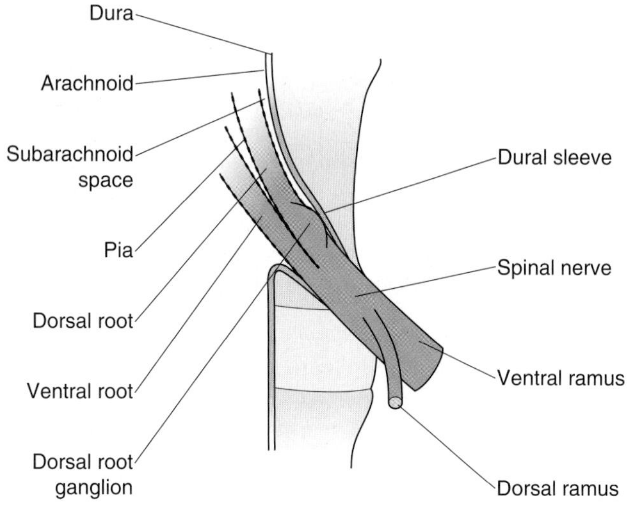

FIGURE 33-10 A lumbar spinal nerve, its roots, and meningeal coverings. The nerve roots are invested by pia mater, and covered by arachnoid and dura as far as the spinal nerve. The dura of the dural sac is prolonged around the roots as their dural sleeve, which blends with the epineurium of the spinal nerve. (Modified from Bogduk N: Nerves of the lumbar spine. In Bogduk N, editor: *Clinical and radiological anatomy of the lumbar spine and sacrum,* ed 5, Edinburgh, 2012, Churchill Livingstone.)

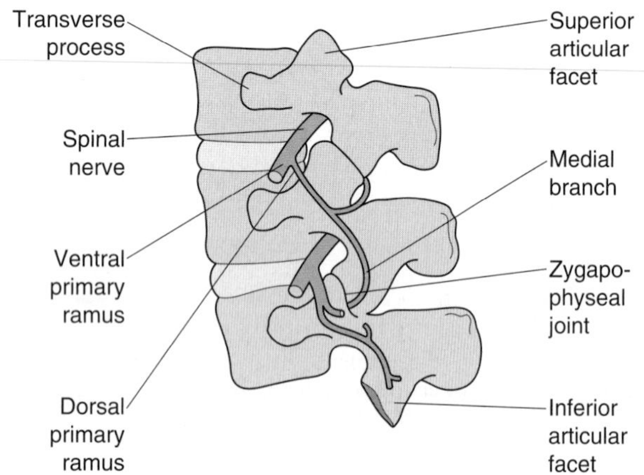

FIGURE 33-11 Observe that the innervation of the zygapophyseal joints derives from the medial branch off the dorsal primary ramus.

BOX 33-1

Potential Pain Generators of the Back

A useful classification system to understand the potential sources of low back pain depends on knowing what structures are innervated (and can transmit pain) and what structures have no innervation.

Innervated Structures

- Bone: Vertebrae
- Joints: Zygapophyseal
- Disk: Only the external annulus and potentially diseased disk
- Ligaments: Anterior longitudinal ligament, posterior longitudinal ligament, interspinous
- Muscles and fascia
- Nerve root

Noninnervated Structures

- Ligamentum flavum
- Disk: Internal annulus, nucleus pulposus

zygapophyseal joints and interspinous ligaments, as well as the lumbar multifidi. The other small branches of the dorsal primary ramus innervate the posterior vertebral body and other lumbar paraspinal musculature and fascia. The anterior longitudinal ligament is innervated by the gray rami communicans, which branch off the lumbar sympathetic chain. The internal annulus fibrosus and nucleus pulposus do not have innervation and therefore, in nondisease states, cannot transmit pain.

Aging Spine: A Degenerative Cascade

Kirkaldy-Willis et al.[118] have supplied us with the most accepted theory describing the cascade of events in degenerative lumbar spine disease that results in disk herniations, spondylotic changes, and eventually multilevel spinal stenosis. At the heart of this theory is the fact that, although the posterior zygapophyseal joints and the anterior intervertebral disks are separated anatomically, forces and lesions affecting one certainly alter and affect the other. For example, axial compressing injuries can damage the vertebral end plates, which can lead to degenerative disk disease, which eventually stresses the zygapophyseal joints, leading to the common degenerative changes seen over time. Torsional stress can injure the zygapophyseal joints and the disks, which in turn leads to increased stress on both these elements. It appears that commonly these changes begin first in the disks. By studying multiple magnetic resonance images (MRIs) of aging spines, evidence of disk degeneration is seen first, and can precede zygapophyseal joint disease by as much as 20 years.[76] When these degenerative changes affect one level, a chain reaction occurs, placing stress on the levels above and below the currently affected level, and eventually resulting in more generalized multilevel spondylotic changes.

To simplify discussion of the degenerative cascade, we will separate our discussion of the changes that occur in the zygapophyseal joints from those in the disk, fully realizing that they both can occur simultaneously and affect each other (Figure 33-12).

Tears in the annulus are thought to be the first anatomic sign of degenerative wear. When the annulus is weakened enough, typically posterolaterally, the internal nucleus pulposus can herniate. Internal disk disruption can occur without herniation, however, because age and repeated stresses acting on the spine cause the gelatinous nucleus to become more fibrous over time. Tears in the annulus can progress to tears in the fibrous disk material, resulting in "internal disk disruption" without frank herniation. All this results in a loss of disk height, which causes instability (because the end-plate connection to the disk is degenerated), as well as lateral recess and foraminal narrowing and potential nerve root impingement. The loss of disk height also places new stresses on the posterior elements, resulting in further instability of the zygapophyseal joints and further degeneration and nerve root impingement.

The degenerative changes that occur in the zygapophyseal joints from aging and repetitive microtrauma are similar to those that occur in the appendicular skeletal joints. The process begins with synovial hypertrophy, which eventually results in cartilage degeneration and destruction. With the resultant capsular laxity, the joint can

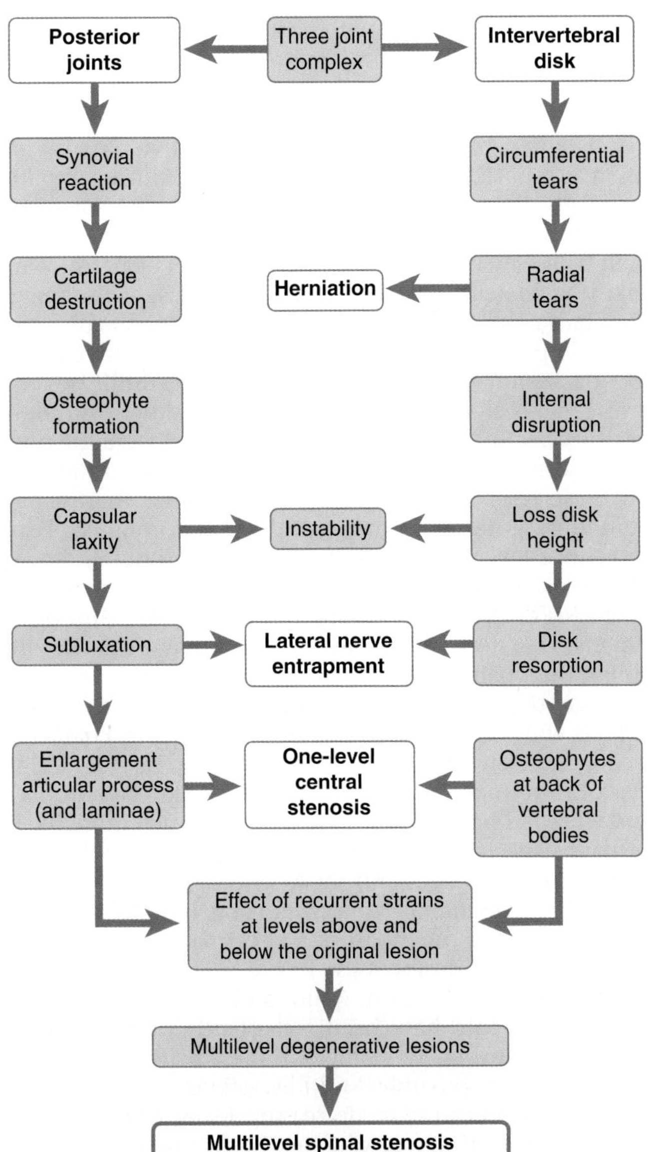

FIGURE 33-12 **The spectrum of degenerative change that leads from minor strains to marked spondylosis and stenosis.** (Modified from Kirkaldy-Willis WH, Wedge JH, Yong-Hing K, et al: Pathology and pathogenesis of lumbar spondylosis and stenosis, *Spine* 3:319-328, 1998, with permission of Lippincott Williams & Wilkins.)

become unstable, and with the subsequent repetitive abnormal joint motion, bony hypertrophy results, thus narrowing the central canal and lateral recesses and potentially impinging nerve roots.

These changes are commonly described clinically as segmental dysfunction. Segmental dysfunction can occur when either a segment is too stiff or too mobile. A segment encompasses the disk, the vertebrae on each side of the disk, and the muscles and ligaments that act across this area. Excessive mobility, also called instability, or potentially better termed "functional instability," can be the result of tissue damage, poor muscular endurance, or poor muscular control, and is usually a combination of all three. Structural changes from tissue damage, such as joint laxity, vertebral end-plate fractures, and loss of disk height, can lead to segmental dysfunction because of the altered anatomy. Muscles also provide a crucial component of spinal stability, and is one area of potential intervention through exercise. In normal situations, only a small amount of muscular coactivation (approximately 10% of maximal contraction) is needed to provide segmental stability. In a segment damaged by ligamentous laxity or disk disease, slightly more muscle coactivation might be needed. Because of the relatively gentle forces required to perform the activities of daily living, muscular endurance is more important than absolute muscle strength for most patients. Some strength reserve, however, is needed for unpredictable activities such as a fall, a sudden load to the spine, or quick movements. In sports and heavy physical work, both strength and endurance needs increase. This biomechanical model is particularly complex in the spine because of the presence of global movement patterns and segmental movement patterns. Two interrelated muscular tasks must be carried out at the same time: maintaining overall posture and position of the spine, and control of individual intersegmental relationships. Sufficient but not excessive joint stiffness is required at the segmental level to prevent injury and allow for efficient movement. This stiffness is achieved with specific patterns of muscle activity, which differ depending on the position of the joint and the load on the spine. The inability to achieve this stiffness, and the resulting segmental problems, is thought to be a factor in low back pain.[185] Alternatively, some segments are thought to be too stiff, because of osteoarthritis and ligamentous thickening in the spine, which is also considered to be a source of low back pain.

Although this theory offers an explanation as to how the spine ages, it is still unclear why there is such a marked disconnect between the occurrence of back pain and the anatomic changes in the spine associated with aging. Many patients with normal spine anatomy suffer from back pain, occasionally disabling pain, and many patients with marked degenerative changes on imaging are nearly or fully pain-free. One theory is that this is related to differences in muscular activation and neural control.

There appear to be consistent muscular problems in patients with chronic low back pain. Some of these factors might exist preinjury and make the spine more susceptible to injury, and some are adaptations to pain. Motor systems and their adaption to back pain appear to vary greatly between individuals and range from subtle changes in muscle activation to redistribute forces, to complete avoidance of activity. Studies have shown abnormal firing patterns in the deep stabilizers of the spine and transversus abdominis with activities such as limb movements, accepting a heavy load, and responding to balance challenges. Other researchers have found strength ratio abnormalities and endurance deficits in patients with low back pain, such as abnormal flexion to extension strength ratios and lack of endurance of torso muscles.[148] These motor adaptations may have persistent long-term consequences.[102]

Studies of lumbar paraspinals have found several abnormalities in patients with low back pain. Multiple imaging studies have demonstrated paraspinal muscle atrophy, particularly of the multifidi, in patients with chronic low back pain.[185] Recovery of the multifidi does not appear to occur spontaneously with the resolution of back pain.[101] Biopsies of multifidi in patients with low back pain also show abnormalities. Multifidi biopsies collected at the time of surgery for disk herniation showed type 2 muscle atrophy and type 1 fiber structural changes. On repeat biopsy repeated 5 years postoperatively, type 2 fiber atrophy was still found in all patients, in both those who had improved with surgery and those who had not. In the positive outcome group, however, the percentage of type 1 fibers with abnormal structures had decreased, and in the negative outcome group there was a marked increase in abnormal type 1 fibers.[183]

Centralization and Pain

The experience of nociception is processed by the body in complex ways. The theory that pain is a simple loop from injury to perception of injury is much too simplistic. Pain processing begins in the spinal cord and continues extensively in the brain, and the ultimate pain that someone experiences is the sum of multiple descending and ascending facilitatory and inhibitory pathways. Extensive evidence now supports the theory that persistent pain might be caused by central sensitization, which could help explain why often no pain generator is found in chronic low back pain.[54]

Psychosocial Factors and Low Back Pain

Pain is an individual experience, and biomechanical and neurologic factors alone do not explain much of the variance seen clinically in patients with back pain. Multiple psychosocial factors have been found to play a role in low back pain. This is briefly discussed here and more thoroughly discussed in the chapter on chronic pain (see Chapter 37), as these issues are shared by multiple painful conditions and not just low back pain.

Depression, Anxiety, and Anger

It appears that between 30% and 40% of those with chronic back pain also have depression.[125] This rate is so high because patients who are depressed are more likely to develop back pain and to become more disabled by pain, and also because some patients with persistent pain become depressed. Patients who are depressed are at increased risk of developing back and neck pain. In a recent analysis of factors leading to the onset of back and neck pain, those in the highest quartile for depression scores had a four-fold increased risk of developing low back pain than those in the lowest quartile for depression scores.[45] Strong evidence also shows that psychosocial factors are closely linked to the transition from acute pain to chronic pain and disability. In a study of 1628 patients with back pain seen at a pain clinic, those with a comorbid diagnosis of depression were more than three times more likely to be in the worst quartiles of physical and emotional functioning on the 36-Item Short-Form Health Survey than those who were not depressed.[79] Multiple other studies have found that depression, anxiety, and distress are strongly related to pain intensity, duration, and disability.[128]

Research has also shown a high correlation with anger measurements and pain, thought to be related to deficient opioid modulation in those with high anxiety, anger, and fear reactivity.[37] Patients with posttraumatic stress disorder also have a high incidence of chronic low back pain.[204]

Patient Beliefs About Pain and Pain Cognition

Beliefs about back pain can be highly individual and are often not based on facts. Some patients with back pain, especially those with chronic low back pain that keeps them from working, have a great deal of fear about back pain. These include fears that their pain will be permanent, that it is related to activity, and that exercise will damage their back. This set of beliefs is referred to as fear avoidance. For example, studies have found that patients with chronic low back pain who perform poorly on treadmill exercise tests,[196] walk slower on treadmill tests,[2] and perform more poorly on spinal isometric exercise testing,[3] were the ones with more anticipation of pain than those who did well on these tests. Fear-avoidance beliefs rather than actual pain during testing predicted their performance. Fear-avoidance levels explain self-reported disability and time off work more accurately than actual pain levels or medical diagnosis does.[136] This finding has led Waddell and other experts to state that "the fear of pain may be more disabling than pain itself."[238]

Large, population-based studies have found that individuals with high levels of pain catastrophizing, characterized by excessively negative thoughts about pain and high fear of movement and injury or reinjury (kinesiophobia), and who had back pain at baseline were much more likely to have especially severe or disabling pain at follow-up evaluation compared with those who did not catastrophize.[255] The presence of catastrophizing is not limited to back pain and is often part of a larger pattern of relationships and thought processes.

Patients' beliefs about pain and their approach to dealing with pain have been consistently found to affect outcomes. Fortunately, changes in these beliefs and cognitive patterns are possible. Multidisciplinary pain programs have proven effective in decreasing fear-avoidant beliefs and catastrophizing (see Chapter 37).[208] These changes in beliefs can also improve function. For example, a study in which a group of patients with chronic low back pain underwent a cognitive-behavioral treatment program found that, although there were not significant changes in pain intensity, those with reductions of fear-avoidance beliefs had significant reductions in disability. Changes in fear-avoidant beliefs accounted for 71% of the variance in reduction in disability in this study.[258]

History and Physical Examination of the Low Back

A complete history and physical examination is important in the evaluation of low back pain to determine the cause of the symptoms, rule out serious medical disease, and determine whether further diagnostic evaluation is needed.

History

As with any pain history, features of back pain that should be explored include location; character; severity; timing, including onset, duration, and frequency; alleviating and aggravating factors; and associated signs and symptoms. Each of these features can assist the clinician in obtaining a diagnosis and prognosis and determining the appropriate treatment. Elements of historical information that suggest a serious underlying condition as the cause of the pain such as cancer, infection, long tract signs, and fracture are called red flags (Box 33-2). When these are present, further workup is necessary (Table 33-1).

BOX 33-2

"Red Flags": Most Common Indications from History and Examination for Pathologic Findings Needing Special Attention and Sometimes Immediate Action (Including Imaging)

- Children <18 years old with considerable pain, or new onset in those >55 years old
- History of violent trauma
- Nonmechanical nature of pain (i.e., constant pain not affected by movement, pain at night)
- History of cancer
- Systemic steroid use
- Drug abuse
- HIV infection or other patients who are immunocompromised
- Unintentional weight loss
- Systemically ill, particularly signs of infection such as fever or night sweats
- Persisting severe restriction of motion or intense pain with minimal motion
- Structural deformity
- Difficulty with micturition
- Loss of anal sphincter tone or fecal incontinence, saddle anesthesia
- Progressive motor weakness or gait disturbance
- Marked morning stiffness
- Peripheral joint involvement
- Iritis, skin rashes, colitis, urethral discharge, or other symptoms of rheumatologic disease
- Inflammatory disorder such as ankylosing spondylitis is suspected
- Family history of rheumatologic disease or structural abnormality

Besides determining a diagnosis, a purpose of the history is to explore the patient's perspective and illness experience. Certain psychosocial factors are valuable in determining prognosis (Box 33-3). Factors such as poor job satisfaction, catastrophic thinking patterns about pain, the presence of depression, and excessive rest or downtime are much more common in patients in whom back pain becomes disabling. These are called yellow flags because the clinician should proceed with caution, and further psychological evaluation or treatment should be considered if they are present. Some of these psychosocial factors are addressed by specific questions, and some become evident through statements that patients make during the history as they describe their illness experience. Questions about, for example, what patients believe is causing the pain, their fear and feelings surrounding this belief, their expectations about the pain and its treatment, and how back pain is affecting their lives (including work and home life) can yield valuable information. Many of these yellow flags are better prognostic indicators than the more traditional medical diagnoses.[239]

BOX 33-3

Some Common "Yellow Flags" Associated with the Development of Chronic Disabling Pain, Suggesting Additional Attention May Be Necessary

- Presence of catastrophic thinking: there is no way the patient can control the pain, that disaster will occur if the pain continues, etc.
- Expectations that the pain will only worsen with work or activity
- Behaviors such as avoidance of normal activity and extended rest
- Poor sleep
- Compensation issues
- Emotions such as stress and anxiety
- Work issues, such as poor job satisfaction and poor relationship with supervisors
- Extended time off work

Table 33-1 Sensitivities and Specificities of Different Elements of the History and Examination for Some Specific Causes of Low Back Pain

Disease or Group of Diseases	Symptom or Sign	Sensitivity	Specificity
Spinal malignancy	Age >50 years	0.77	0.71
	Previous history of cancer	0.31	0.98
	Unexplained weight loss	0.15	0.94
	Pain unrelieved by bed rest	0.90	0.46
	Pain lasting >1 month	0.50	0.81
	Failure to improve with 1 month of conservative therapy	0.31	0.90
	Erythrocyte sedimentation rate >20 mm	0.78	0.67
Spinal infection	Intravenous drug abuse, urinary tract infection, skin infection	0.40	—
	Fever	0.27-0.83*	0.98
	Vertebral tenderness	"Reasonable"	"Low"
	Age >50 years	0.84	0.61
Compression fracture	Age >70 years	0.22	0.96
	Corticosteroid use	0.66	0.99
Herniated intervertebral disk	Sciatica	0.95	0.88

From Nachemson A, Vingard E: Assessment of patients with neck and back pain: a best-evidence synthesis. In Nachemson AL, Johnsson B, editors: *Neck and back pain: the scientific evidence of causes, diagnosis, and treatment*, Philadelphia, 2001, Lippincott Williams & Wilkins.

*The sensitivity of "fever."

Table 33-2 Physical Examination for Low Back Pain

Examination Component	Specific Activity	Reason for This Part of the Examination
Observation	Observation of overall posture	Determine whether structural abnormality or muscle imbalances are present
	Observation of lumbar spine	Further define muscle imbalance and habitual posture
	Observation of the skin	Search for diagnoses such as psoriasis, shingles, or vascular disease as cause of the pain
	Observation of gait	Screen the kinetic chain and determine whether muscular, neurologic, or joint problems are contributing to symptoms
Palpation	Bones	Search for bony problems such as infection or fracture
	Facet joints	Identify whether specific levels are tender
	Ligaments and intradiskal spaces	Determine whether these are tender
	Muscles	Search for trigger points, muscle spasms, muscle atrophy
Active range of motion	Forward flexion	Amount, quality if painful
	Extension	—
	Side bending	Same, also side to side differences
	Rotation	—
Neurologic examination	Manual muscle testing of L1-S1 myotomes	Determine weakness
	Pinprick and light touch sensation, L1-S1 dermatomes	Determine sensory loss
	Reflexes: patellar, hamstring, Achilles	Test injury to L4, L5, or S1 roots if diminished, upper motor neuron disease if brisk
	Balance and coordination testing	Signs of upper motor neuron disease
	Plantar responses	Same
	Straight leg raise	Neural tension at L5 or S1
	Femoral nerve arch	Neural tension at L3 or L4
Orthopedic special tests	Abdominal muscle strength	Determines weakness and deconditioning
	Pelvis stabilizer strength (i.e., gluteus medius, maximus, etc.)	Determines weakness and deconditioning
	Tightness or stiffness of hamstrings	Determines areas of poor flexibility
	Tightness or stiffness of hip flexors	—
	Tightness or stiffness of hip rotators	—
	Prone instability test	Signs of instability

Physical Examination

Table 33-2 outlines a thorough examination of the lumbar spine.

Observation

Observation should include a survey of the skin, muscle mass, and bony structures, as well as observation of overall posture (Figures 33-13 and 33-14, Table 33-3) and the position of the lumbar spine in particular. Gait should also be observed for clues regarding etiology and contributing factors.

Palpation

Palpation should begin superficially and progress to deeper tissues. It can be done with the patient standing. To ensure that the back muscles are fully relaxed, palpation is often done with the patient lying prone, perhaps with a pillow under the abdomen to slightly flex the spine into a position of comfort. It should proceed systematically to determine what structures are tender to palpation.

Range of Motion

Quantity of Range of Motion. Several methods can be used to measure spinal range of motion (ROM). These include using a single or double inclinometer; measuring the distance of fingertips to floor; and, for forward flexion, a Schober test (measuring distraction between two marks on the skin during forward flexion). Of these methods, the

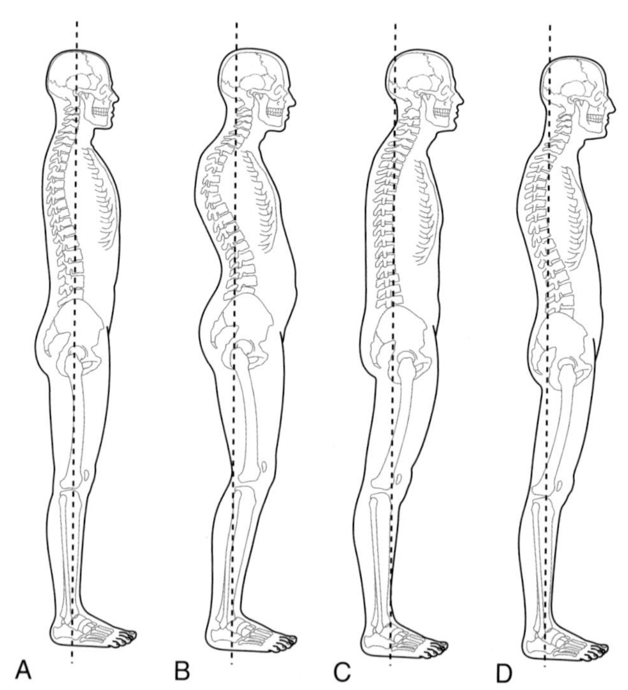

FIGURE 33-13 Four types of postural alignment. **A,** Ideal alignment. **B,** Kyphosis-lordosis posture. **C,** Flat back posture, **D,** Sway-back posture. (Modified from Kendall FP, McCreary EK: *Trunk muscles in muscle testing and function,* Philadelphia, 1983, Lippincott Williams & Wilkins.)

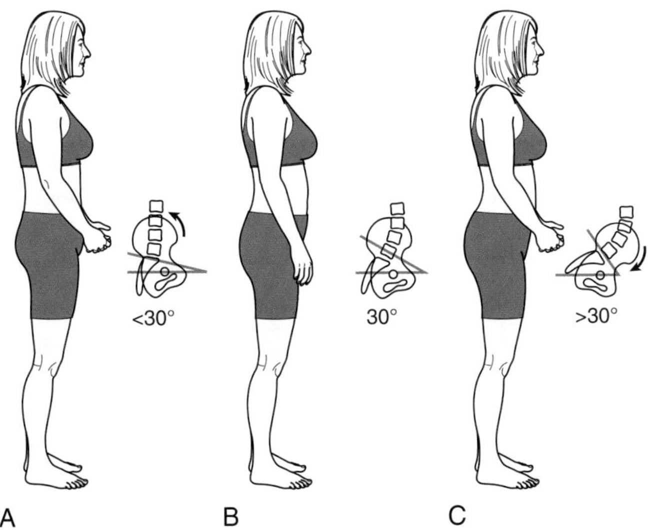

FIGURE 33-14 The effect of pelvic tilting on the inclination of the base of the sacrum to the transverse plane (sacral angle) during upright standing is shown. **A,** Tilting the pelvis backward reduces the sacral angle and flattens the lumbar spine. **B,** During relaxed standing, the sacral angle is about 30 degrees. **C,** Tilting the pelvis forward increases the sacral angle and accentuates the lumbar lordosis. (Modified from Sahrmann SA: *Movement impairment syndromes of the lumbar spine: diagnosis and treatment of movement impairment syndromes,* St Louis, 2002, Mosby.)

Table 33-3 Factors That Affect Posture

Reason for Abnormality	Clinical Example
Bone structure	Compression fractures Scheuermann disease
Ligamentous laxity	Hyperextension of the knees, elbows
Muscle and fascial length	Tight hamstrings that cause a posterior pelvic tilt Weak and long abdominal muscles that allow an anterior pelvic tilt
Body habitus	Obesity or pregnancy causes changes in force and increased lumbar lordosis
Neurologic disease	Spasticity causes an extension pattern of the lower limb
Mood	Depression causes forward slumped shoulders
Habit	Long-distance cyclists have increased thoracic kyphosis and flat spine from prolonged positioning while riding

double inclinometer has been shown to correlate the closest to measurements on radiographs.[88] Fingertip to floor has good interrater and intrarater reliability, but this takes into account the movement of the pelvis and is affected by structures outside the spine, such as tight hamstrings.[176] A Schober test is commonly used to assess a decrease in forward flexion in ankylosing spondylitis. It is sensitive for this condition but is not specific. General figures for normal ROM are forward flexion, 40 to 60 degrees; extension, 20 to 35 degrees; lateral flexion, 15 to 20 degrees; and rotation, 3 to 18 degrees. Studies to determine normal ROM in adults who are asymptomatic have found large variations.[172] The importance of decreased ROM in patients with back pain is unclear because many people without back pain also have limited range. ROM can also change depending on the time of day, the effort the patient expends, and many other factors.[263]

Quality of Range of Motion. The examiner should record whether there are abnormalities in the patient's movement pattern during ROM, such as a "catch" in the range or whether or not it causes pain. This might give clues to the diagnosis. For example, pain with forward flexion can signify disk disease, and pain with extension can indicate spondylolisthesis, zygapophyseal joint disease, or spinal stenosis.

Neurologic Examination

The neurologic examination of the lower limbs can rule out clinically significant nerve root impingement and other neurologic causes of leg pain (Table 33-4). The physical examination should logically proceed to discover whether or not a particular root level is affected by combining the findings of weakness, sensory loss, diminished or absent reflexes, and special tests such as the straight leg–raising maneuver. Upper motor neuron abnormalities should also be ruled out. The accuracy of the neurologic examination in diagnosing herniated disk is moderate. The accuracy can be increased considerably, however, with combinations of findings.[59] The sensitivity and specificity of different findings for lumbar radiculopathy have been well studied (Table 33-5).

Orthopedic Special Tests to Assess for Relative Strength and Flexibility

Back pain may be caused by deconditioning, poor endurance, and muscle imbalances. Identifying inefficient or abnormal movement patterns of muscles that control the movement of the spine and the position of the pelvis help direct the exercise prescription.

Because of its stabilizing effect on the spine, abdominal muscle strength and endurance is important. Several different methods can be used to measure abdominal muscle strength and control (Figures 33-15 and 33-16). One grading system assesses if the patient is able to maintain a neutral spine position while adding increasingly more challenging leg movements (Figure 33-17).

Besides determining the strength of the abdominals, strength testing of the back muscles and pelvic stabilizers, such as the hip abductors, can be useful. Assessing for areas of relative inflexibility is also important. Commonly performed tests are hip flexor flexibility, hamstring flexibility, other hip extensors' length, and gastrocnemius/soleus length. Balance challenges, such as the ability to maintain single-footed stance, the ability to lunge or squat, and other functional tests are also helpful to determine a patient's baseline status.

Orthopedic Special Tests for Lumbar Segmental Instability

Many clinicians and researchers believe that one cause of low back pain is segmental instability that responds to specific stabilization treatments. Therefore, accurately identifying this group from other forms of low back pain could be important. These special tests include passive intervertebral motion testing and the prone instability test.

Table 33-4 Lumbar Root Syndromes

Root	Dermatome	Muscle Weakness	Reflexes or Special Tests Affected	Paresthesias
L1	Back, over trochanter, groin	None	None	Groin
L2	Back, front of thigh to knee	Psoas, hip adductor	None	Occasionally front of thigh
L3	Back, upper buttock, front of thigh and knee, medial lower leg	Psoas, quadriceps—thigh wasting	Knee jerks sluggish, pain on full straight leg raise	Inner knee, anterior lower leg
L4	Inner buttock, outer thigh, inside of leg, dorsum of foot, big toe	Tibialis anterior, extensor hallucis	Straight leg raise limited, neck flexion pain, weak knee jerk, side flexion limited	Medial aspect of calf and ankle
L5	Buttock, back and side of thigh, lateral aspect of leg, dorsum of foot, inner half of sole, and first, second, and third toes	Extensor hallucis, peroneals, gluteus medius, ankle dorsiflexors, hamstrings—calf wasting	Straight leg raise limited to one side, neck flexion pain, hamstring reflex decreased, crossed leg–raising pain	Lateral aspect of leg, medial three toes
S1	Buttock, back of thigh, and lower leg	Calf and hamstrings, wasting of gluteals, peroneals, plantar flexor	Straight leg raise limited, decreased ankle jerk	Lateral two toes, lateral foot, lateral leg to knee, plantar aspect of foot
S2	Same as S1	Same as S1, except peroneals	Straight leg raise limited	Lateral leg, knee, heel
S3	Groin, inner thigh to knee	None	None	None
S4	Perineum: genitals, lower sacrum	Bladder, rectum	None	Saddle area, genitals, anus, impotence

From Maguire JH: Osteomyelitis. In Braunwald E, Fauci AS, Kasper DL, et al, editors: *Harrison's principles of internal medicine*, ed 15, New York, 2001, McGraw-Hill.

Table 33-5 Lumbosacral Radiculopathy in Patients With Sciatica*

Finding†	Sensitivity (%)	Specificity (%)	Positive Lumbosacral Radiculopathy	Negative Lumbosacral Radiculopathy
Motor Examination				
Weak ankle dorsiflexion	54	89	4.9	0.5
Ipsilateral calf wasting	29	94	5.2	0.8
Sensory Examination				
Leg sensation abnormal	16	86	NS	NS
Reflex Examination				
Abnormal ankle jerk	48	89	4.3	0.6
Other Tests				
Straight leg–raising maneuver	73-98	11-61	NS	0.2
Crossed straight leg–raising maneuver	23-43	88-98	4.3	0.8

From McGee SR: *Evidence-based physical diagnosis*, Philadelphia, 2001, Saunders.

*Diagnostic standard: For lumbosacral radiculopathy, surgical finding of disk herniation compressing the nerve root.

†Definition of findings: For ipsilateral calf wasting, maximum calf circumference at least 1 cm smaller than on contralateral side; for straight leg–raising maneuvers, flexion at hip of supine patient's leg, extended at the knee, causes radiating pain in affected leg (pain confined to back or hip is a negative response); for crossed straight leg–raising maneuver, raising contralateral leg provokes pain in the affected leg.

NS, Not significant.

Passive Intervertebral Motion Testing. The patient lies prone. The examiner applies a firm steady anteriorly directed pressure over the spinous process and assesses the amount of vertebral motion and whether pain is provoked.[100]

Prone Instability Test. The patient lies prone, with the torso on the examining table and the legs over the edge of the table with the feet resting on the floor. The examiner performs passive intervertebral motion testing at each level and notes provocation of pain. Then the patient lifts the legs off the floor, and the painful levels are repeated. A positive test is when the pain disappears when the legs are lifted. This is because the extensors are able to stabilize the spine in this position.[100,147]

Examining the Area Above and Below the Lumbar Spine

Similar to the evaluation of other joints, the areas above and below the lumbar spine should be evaluated to be sure nothing is missed. ROM of the hip joints should be assessed, and a quick screen of the knee and ankle joint can determine whether disease in these areas is contributing to the back problem. The thoracic spine can be quickly screened as well during ROM and palpation.

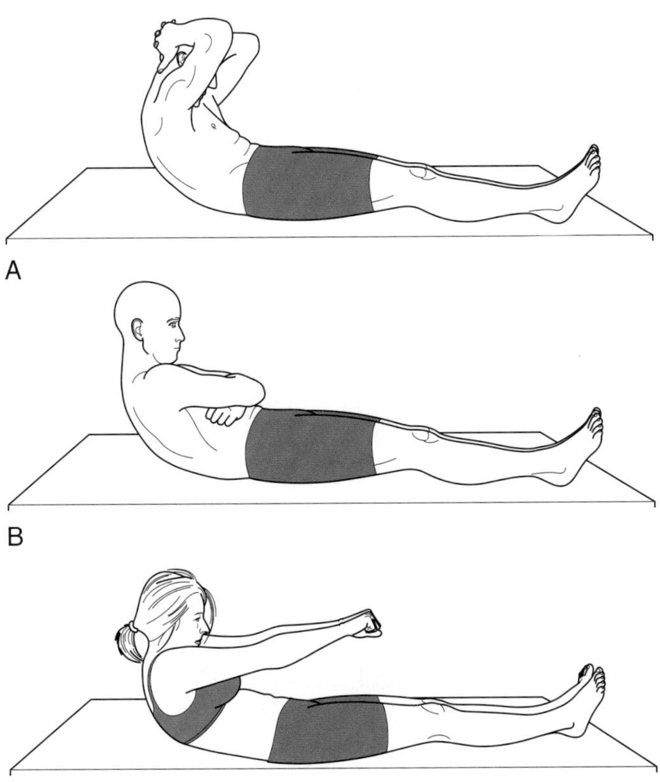

FIGURE 33-15 Trunk raising forward: grading. The curl trunk sit-up is performed with the patient lying supine and with the leg extended. The patient posteriorly tilts the pelvis and flexes the spine, and slowly completes a curled trunk sit-up. Kendall and McCreary[114] state that the "crucial point in the test for the abdominal muscle strength is at the moment the hip flexors come into strong action. The abdominal muscle at this point must be able to oppose the force of the hip flexors in addition to maintain the trunk curl." At the point where the hip flexors strongly contract, patients with weak abdominal muscles will tilt the pelvis anteriorly and extend the low back. **A,** A 100% or normal grade is the ability to maintain spinal flexion and come into the sitting position with the hands clasped behind the head. **B,** An 80% or good grade is the ability to do this with the forearms folded across the chest. **C,** A 60% or fair grade is the ability to do this with the forearms extended forward. A 50% or fair grade is the ability to begin flexion but not maintain spinal flexion with the forearms extended forward. (Modified from Kendall FP, McCreary EK: *Trunk muscles in muscle testing and function,* Philadelphia, 1983, Lippincott Williams and Wilkins.)

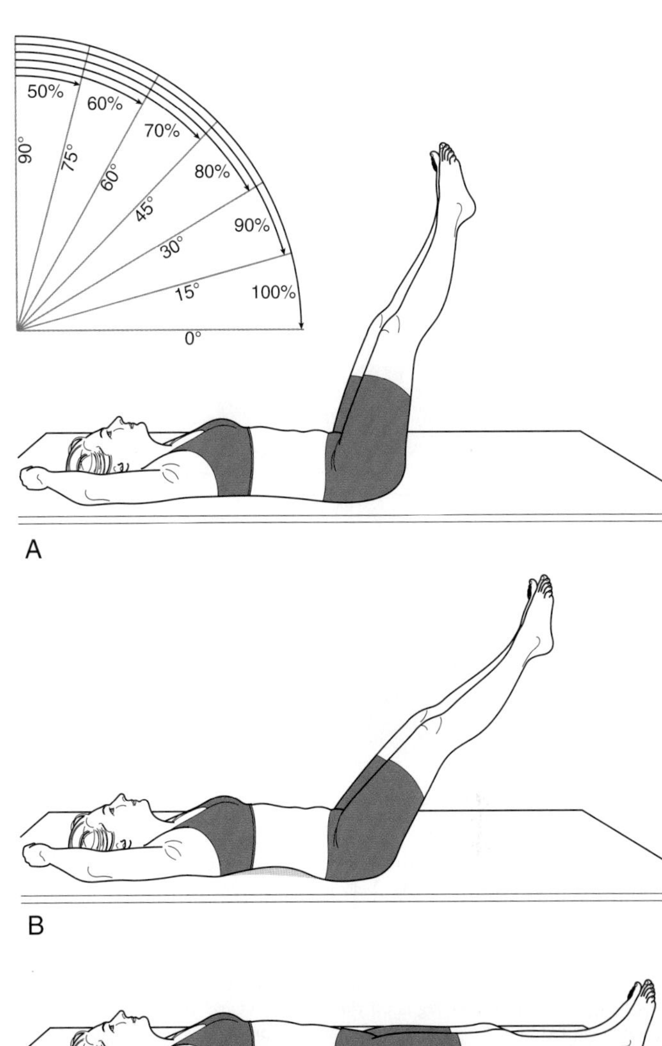

FIGURE 33-16 Leg lowering: grading. In the second test, the patient raises the legs one at a time to a right angle, and then flattens the low back on the table. The patient slowly lowers the legs while holding the back flat. A 100% or normal grade is the ability to hold the low back flat on the table as the legs are lowered to the fully extended position. An 80% or good grade is the ability to hold the low back flat and lower the legs to a 30-degree angle. **A,** A 60% or fair plus grade is the ability to lower the legs to 60 degrees with the low back flat. **B,** The pelvis tilted anteriorly and the low back arched as the legs were lowered. **C,** The final position. Kendall and McCreary[114] note that this second test is more important than the first (see Figure 33-15) in grading muscles essential to proper posture, and that often patients who do well on the first test do poorly on the second. (Modified from Kendall FP, McCreary EK: *Trunk muscles in muscle testing and function,* Philadelphia, 1983, Williams and Wilkins.)

Illness Behavior and Nonorganic Signs Seen on Physical Examination

Multiple reasons can explain why patients with back pain might display symptoms out of proportion to injury. Illness behaviors are learned behaviors and are responses that some patients use to convey their distress. Several studies have found that patients with chronic low back pain and chronic pain syndrome experience significant anxiety during the physical examination, even to the level experienced during panic attacks. This anxiety is generally manifest as avoidance behavior, such as decreased ROM or poor effort with muscle testing.[92] Other reasons for illness behavior include malingering and a desire to prove to physicians how disabling the pain is. One way to assess for illness behavior on physical examination is to perform parts of the examination to search for Waddell signs.[238] These may be seen with malingering, but are nonorganic findings that may also indicate psychological distress. They are as follows:

- Inappropriate tenderness that is widespread or superficial.
- Pain on testing that only simulates loading the spine, such as light pressure applied to the top of the head, which reproduces back pain, or rotating the hips and shoulders together to simulate twisting without actually moving the spine, which reproduces back pain.

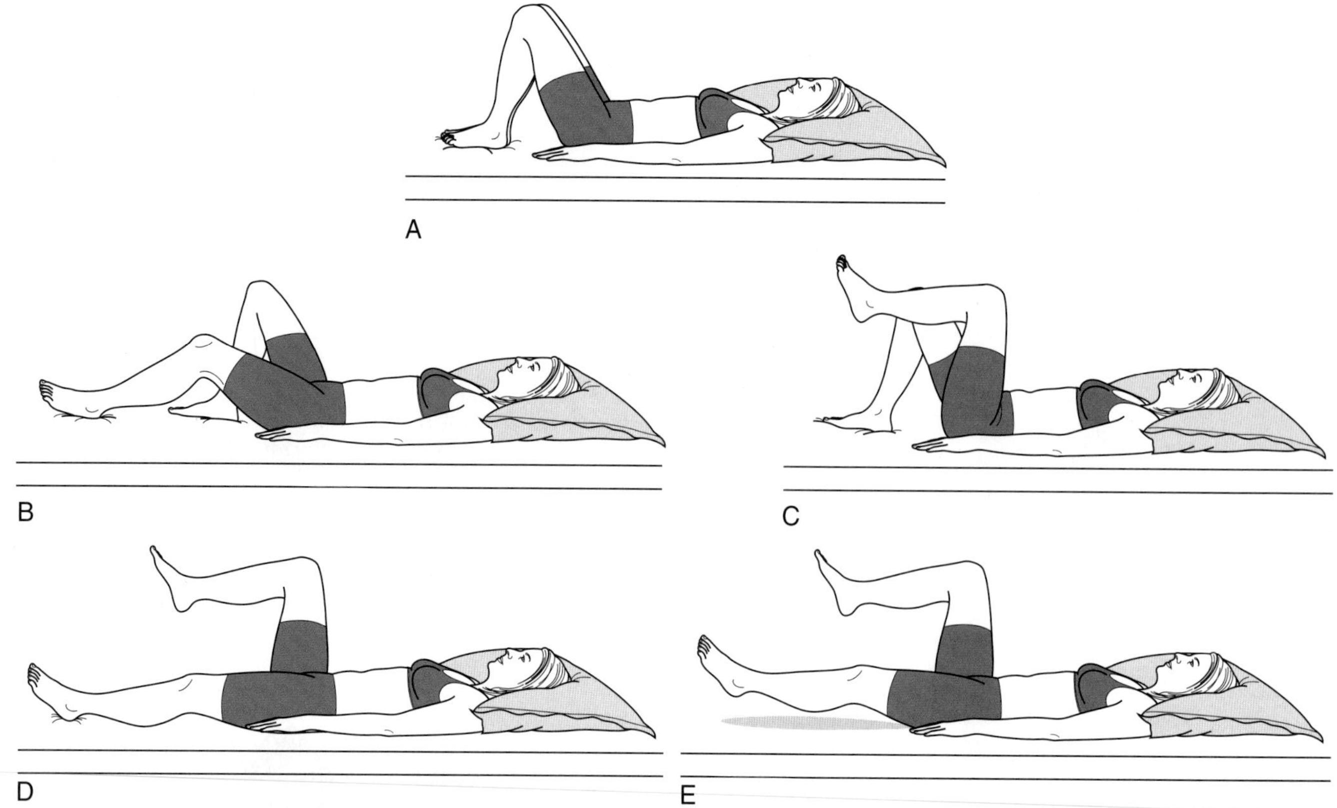

FIGURE 33-17 Abdominal strength grading. **A,** The patient lies supine with the knees bent (supine hook lying). The physician cues the patient to activate the transversus abdominis ("Pull your belly button toward your backbone"), and a very slight lumbar lordosis is maintained in a neutral position in which the spine is neither flexed nor extended. The ability to maintain the neutral spine is progressively challenged by loading the spine via lower extremity movements. Grading is as follows. **B,** Grade 1: The patient is able to maintain a neutral spine while extending one leg by dragging the heel along the table; the other leg remains in the starting position. **C,** Grade 2: The patient is able to maintain a neutral spine while holding both legs flexed 90 degrees at the hip and 90 degrees at the knee, and touching one foot to the mat and then the other. **D,** Grade 3: The patient is able to maintain a neutral spine while extending one leg by dragging the heel along the table. The other leg is off the mat and flexed 90 degrees at the hip and 90 degrees at the knee. E, Grade 4: The patient is able to maintain a neutral spine while extending one leg hovered an inch or two above the table, and the other leg is off the mat and flexed 90 degrees at the hip and 90 degrees at the knee. Grade 5: The patient is able to extend both legs a few inches off the mat and back again while maintaining the spine in neutral.

- Inconsistent performance when testing the same thing in different positions, such as a difference in outcome of the straight leg–raising test with the patient supine versus sitting.
- Regional deficits in strength or sensation that do not have an anatomic basis.
- Overreaction during the physical examination.

Findings in three of these five categories suggest psychological distress and also suggest that other parts of the physical examination that require patient effort or reporting of symptoms might be inaccurate.

Clinical Evaluation: Diagnostics

Imaging Studies

Imaging of the lumbar spine should be used in the evaluation of low back pain if specific pathology needs to be confirmed after a thorough history and physical examination.

Plain Radiography

Conventional radiographs are indicated in trauma to evaluate for fracture and to look for bony lesions such as tumor when red flags are present in the history. As an initial screening tool for lumbar spine pathology, however, they have very low sensitivity and specificity.[84] Anterior-posterior and lateral views are the two commonly obtained views. Oblique views can be obtained to examine for a spondylolysis by visualizing the pars interarticularis and the "Scottie dog" appearance of the lumbar spine (Figure 33-18). Lateral flexion-extension views are obtained to check for dynamic instability, although the literature does not support their usefulness.[64] They are potentially most helpful from a surgical screening perspective when evaluating a spondylolisthesis. They are commonly obtained in patients after trauma or surgery.

Magnetic Resonance Imaging

MRI is the preeminent imaging method for evaluating degenerative disk disease, disk herniations, and radiculopathy (Figure 33-19). On T2-weighted imaging, the annulus can be differentiated from the internal nucleus, and annular tears can be seen as high-intensity zones. These zones are of unclear clinical significance but are thought to be potential pain generators.

Adding gadolinium contrast enhancement helps to identify structures with increased vascularity. Contrast is always indicated in evaluating for tumor or infection or to determine scar tissue (vascular) versus recurrent disk herniation (avascular) in postsurgical patients with recurrent radicular symptoms.

The downside of MRI is that, although it is a very sensitive test, it is not very specific in determining a definite source of pain. It is well established that many people without back pain have degenerative changes, disk bulges, and protrusions on MRI. Boden et al.[25] demonstrated that one third of 67 individuals who were asymptomatic were found to have a "substantial abnormality" on MRI of the lumbar spine. Of the individuals younger than 60 years, 20% had a disk herniation, and 36% of those older than 60 years had a disk herniation and 21% had spinal stenosis. Bulging and degenerative disks were even more commonly found. In another study of lumbar MRI findings in people without back pain, Jensen et al.[108] demonstrated that only 36% of 98 patients had normal disks. They found that bulges and protrusions were very common in individuals who were asymptomatic, but that extrusions were not. In a study in 2001, Jarvik et al.[107] confirmed these findings.

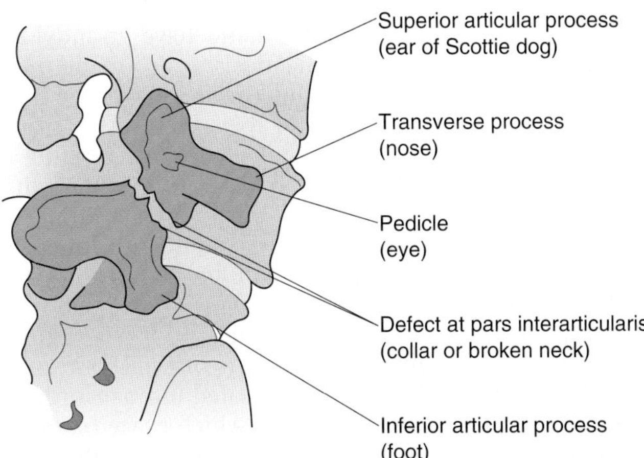

FIGURE 33-18 Oblique drawing of the lumbosacral junction, outlining the "Scottie dog" and the area of spondylolysis.

Computed Tomography

Because of the resolution of anatomic structures seen on MRI, it has essentially replaced computed tomography (CT) scanning as the imaging study of choice for low back pain and radiculopathy. CT scanning is still more useful than MRI, however, in evaluating bony lesions. CT scans are also useful in the postsurgical patient with excessive hardware that can obscure MRIs, and in patients with implants (aneurysm clips or pacemakers) that preclude MRI.

Myelography

In myelography, contrast dye is injected into the dural sac and plain radiographs are performed to produce images of the borders and contents of the dural sac (Figure 33-20). CT images can also be obtained after contrast injection to produce axial cross-sectional images of the spine that enhance the distinction between the dural sac and its surrounding structures. This is typically reserved as a presurgical screening tool but has been used less with the advancement of MRI.

Scintigraphy

Radionuclear bone scanning is a fairly sensitive but not specific imaging modality that can be used to detect occult fractures, bony metastases, and infections. To increase anatomic specificity, single-photon emission computed tomography (SPECT) bone scanning is used to obtain bone scans with axial slices. This allows the diagnostician to differentiate uptake in the posterior elements from more anterior structures of the spine. The diagnostic use of this study with regard to altering clinical decision-making is controversial. Studies have been published demonstrating that the use of SPECT can help identify patients with low back pain who might benefit from zygapophyseal joint injections.[179]

Electromyography

Electromyography is useful in evaluating radiculopathy because it provides a physiologic measure for detecting

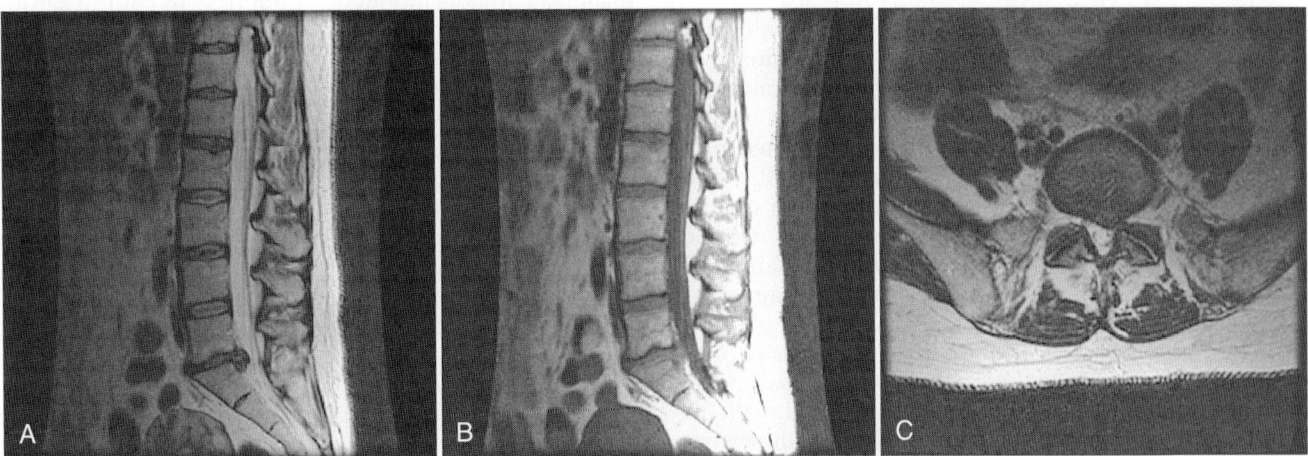

FIGURE 33-19 Disk extrusion in a 48-year-old woman with back and left leg pain. **A** and **B,** Sagittal T2-weighted and T1-weighted magnetic resonance image (MRI) showing L5-S1 disk extrusion with caudal extension. **C,** Axial T2-weighted MRI showing the extrusion is left paracentral in the lateral recess, occupying the space where the S1 root resides.

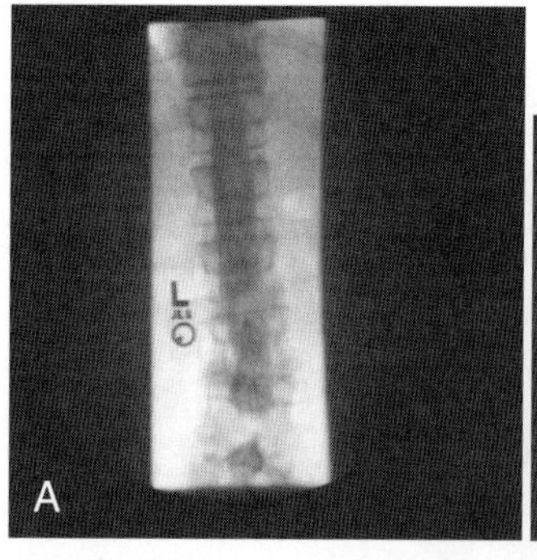
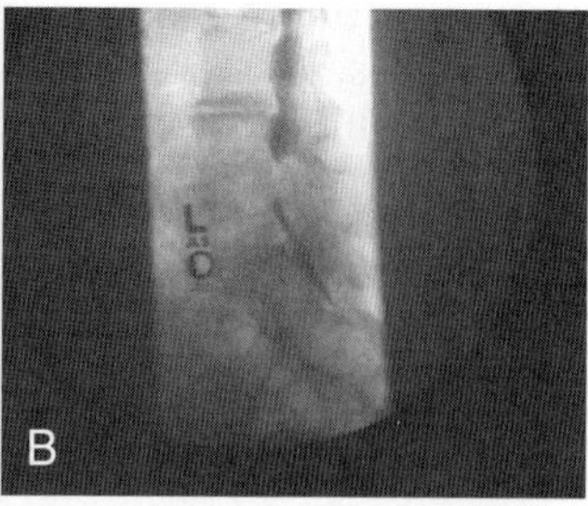

FIGURE 33-20 Anteroposterior (**A**) and lateral (**B**) myelograms of a 59-year-old woman with severe L4-L5 central stenosis caused by a large left L4-L5 zygapophyseal joint synovial cyst. Note the obvious filling defect at the L4-L5 level. She had symptoms of cauda equina syndrome and regained full neurologic function after decompression surgery.

neurogenic changes and denervation with good sensitivity and high specificity. It can help to provide information as to which anatomic lesions found in imaging studies are truly physiologically significant.[188] It is important to remember, and to educate referring physicians, that electromyography cannot diagnose a pure sensory radiculopathy. See Chapter 8 for further details.

Laboratory Studies

Blood tests are rarely used in isolation as a diagnostic strategy for low back pain. They may be helpful as an adjunct in diagnosing inflammatory disease of the spine (with markers of inflammation such as sedimentation rate and C-reactive protein), as well as some neoplastic disorders, such as multiple myeloma with serum and urine protein electrophoresis.

Differential Diagnosis and Treatment: Back Pain Greater Than Leg Pain

Nonspecific Low Back Pain

Nearly 85% of those who seek medical care for low back pain do not receive a specific diagnosis.[59] The majority of these patients are likely to have a multifactorial cause for back pain, which includes deconditioning; poor muscle recruitment; emotional stress; and changes associated with aging and injury such as disk degeneration, arthritis, and ligamentous hypertrophy. This type of back pain can be given many names; nonspecific low back pain, simple backache, mechanical low back pain, lumbar strain, and spinal degeneration are a few of the common names for this condition. By definition, the history and physical examination do not suggest a more specific diagnosis, and diagnostic tests used to exclude other likely causes of the symptoms are negative. Risk factors remain difficult to discern. So far, researchers have been able to show that obesity, smoking, a very sedentary lifestyle, very vigorous physical activity (i.e., both extremes of the activity continuum), and genetic effects have all been found to be risk factors for nonspecific low back pain. Interestingly, neither abnormalities on MRI nor work-related activities such as lifting, twisting, standing, and awkward positions have been found to be risk factors.[16] Treatment is discussed in a subsequent section.

Lumbar Spondylosis

In an attempt to arrive at a more specific diagnosis and to determine subgroups of patients who may respond to different treatments, rather than using the term *nonspecific low back pain,* the diagnosis of lumbar spondylosis is often used for older patients with back pain. Because degenerative disease of the zygapophyseal joints generally coexists with degenerative disk disease, it is difficult to separate the two entities. Both can cause axial back pain. Both can also cause referred pain into the buttocks and legs. Mooney and Robertson[187] and McCall et al.[144] have studied the sclerotomal distribution of zygapophyseal joint pain in detail. Zygapophyseal joint pain has even been reported to refer below the knee in some cases.

Delineating a degenerative zygapophyseal joint as the primary pain generator in axial low back pain, however, is difficult. Imaging studies are not particularly useful because many people who are asymptomatic have spondylotic changes in their spines. This diagnosis is also made more commonly in older patients. Older individuals have multiple findings in their history, in their physical examination, and on imaging studies that complicate arriving at specific diagnosis or specific pain generators as the cause of their complaints. Spondylotic zygapophyseal joints are seen commonly with other potential sources of low back pain, such as degenerative disks and lumbar stenosis. On physical examination, patients with these imaging findings commonly have postural abnormalities, poor pelvic girdle mechanics, and potentially multiple myofascial sources for pain. They typically have an accentuated lumbar lordosis, in part because of tight hip flexors, which exacerbates the problem by increasing stress on the posterior elements.

From biomechanical studies and knowledge of anatomy, we know that lumbar extension and rotation increase forces placed on the posterior zygapophyseal joints. This specific maneuver, however, has not been shown to be diagnostic for zygapophyseal joint pain in clinical settings (by either history or examination). No unique identifying features are found in the history, physical examination, or radiologic imaging that are diagnostic for zygapophyseal joint pain. The only diagnostic maneuvers for zygapophyseal joint pain are fluoroscopically guided zygapophyseal joint injections with local anesthetic and medial branch blocks (i.e., local anesthetic blocks of the medial branches of the dorsal primary rami that innervate the zygapophyseal joints).[61,139] With these injection techniques, the prevalence of facet-mediated pain in chronic low back pain sufferers has been estimated to be 15% in the younger population and 40% in older age groups.[197,198] In a study in 1994, Schwarzer et al.[197] demonstrated that the vast majority of lumbar zygapophyseal joint pain originates from the L4-L5 and L5-S1 zygapophyseal joints.

More conservative management options for the spondylotic spine and facet-mediated pain should be tried before resorting to invasive procedures such as intraarticular zygapophyseal joint corticosteroid injections or medial branch neurotomies. The conservative treatments are similar to treatments for osteoarthritic joints and can be categorized as lifestyle and activity modification, medications, and exercise, and are described in the section on treatment later.

Lumbar Disk Disease

Identifying diskogenic causes of low back pain is another attempt to separate patients from the nonspecific low back pain group. These can be divided into three categories: degenerative disk disease, internal disk disruption, and disk herniation. Diskogenic pain is classically described as bandlike and exacerbated by lumbar flexion, but this is not always the case. It can be unilateral, can radiate to the buttock, and can even be worsened by extension or side bending (depending on the site of disk pathology).

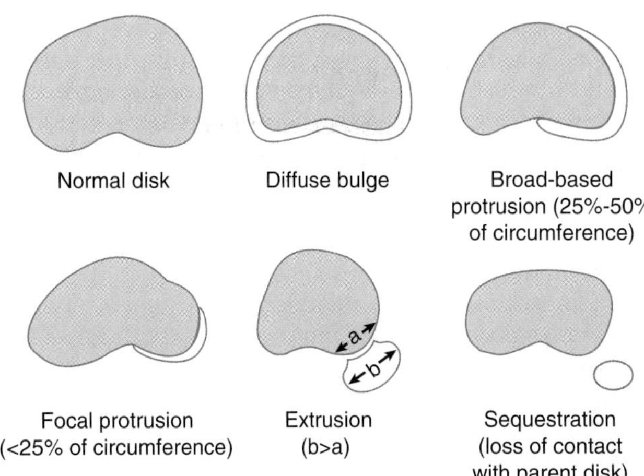

FIGURE 33-21 Disk herniation, protrusion, and extrusion. (Modified from Maus TP: Imaging of the spine and nerve roots, *Phys Med Rehabil Clin N Am* 13:487-544, 2002.)

Internal Disk Disruption

Bogduk[31] defines internal disk disruption as a condition in which the internal architecture of the disk is disrupted, but its external surface remains essentially normal (i.e., there is no bulge or herniation). It is characterized by degradation of the nucleus pulposus and radial fissures that extend to the outer third of the annulus (high-intensity zone areas on MRI).[11] Diagnosis requires reproduction of pain on diskography and annular fissure on postdiskography CT.[31] Although the use of diskography is controversial, most believe that annular tears (especially those that reach the outer third of the annulus, i.e., the innervated fibers) can be a source of low back pain. It must be remembered, however, that similar to most abnormalities on lumbar spine imaging, annular tears or high-intensity zones are seen commonly in individuals who are asymptomatic.

The proposed mechanisms for pain generation from internal disk disruption are chemical nociception from inflammatory mediators and mechanical stimulation.

Disk Herniation

The terminology used to describe disk material that extends beyond the intervertebral disk space is confusing. *Herniated disk, herniated nucleus pulposus, disk bulge, disk protrusion, ruptured disk,* and *prolapsed disk* are all commonly used terms, and sometimes are incorrectly used synonymously. Displaced disk material can be initially classified as a bulge (disk material is displaced greater than 50% of its circumference) or as a herniation (less than 50% of its circumference) (Figure 33-21[143]).[66] Disk herniations can then be subclassified into protrusions or extrusions. A disk protrusion is defined as a herniation with the distance of the edges of the herniated material less than the distance of the edges at its base. A disk extrusion occurs when the distance of the edges of the herniated material is greater than the distance of the edges at its base. A disk extrusion can be further subclassified as sequestrated if the extruded disk material has no continuity with the disk of origin. Disk herniations can also be described as contained or uncontained depending on the integrity of the outer annular fibers. If the outer annular fibers are still intact, it is described as a contained disk herniation. This classification has no relevance to the integrity of the posterior longitudinal ligament.

More than 95% of lumbar disk herniations occur at the L4-L5 and L5-S1 levels.[57,207] Next most common is L3-L4, followed by L2-L3. The most common lumbosacral radiculopathies are consequently L5 and S1. Posterolateral disk herniations are most common because the annulus fibrosus is weakest posterolaterally. Posterolateral disks can affect the nerve root as it descends in the lateral recess or just before it enters the neural foramen. Far lateral or extraforaminal herniations can affect the nerve root as it exits the neural foramen, and central disk herniations can affect any part of the cauda equina, depending on the level.

Disk herniations can cause an inflammatory response that can affect the nerve root, or there can be mechanical compression, both of which can cause radicular symptoms. Disk herniations, however, can also cause solely axial pain. Diagnosing diskogenic low back pain is a challenge because we know that individuals who are asymptomatic can have disk herniations present on MRI.[25,107,108] Diskography is a controversial diagnostic tool for diskogenic pain (see Chapter 32). Historically, it is typically used as a presurgical screening tool.

The mainstay of treatment for diskogenic back pain is conservative. Because of the difficulty of definitively diagnosing this as a source of low back pain, there are no proven specific treatments. Even when it is agreed that the etiology of low back pain is diskogenic, patients still respond differently to various exercise regimens, primarily because the location of the disk herniation typically dictates which lumbar spine movements can enhance pain and which do not. For example, posterolateral disks cause more pain with flexion, central disks are usually more painful in extension, and far lateral disks cause more pain with ipsilateral side bending. It is appropriate to individualize rehabilitation programs according to which movements patients can do with little pain, and slowly progress their exercise program or movement patterns to include more planes of motion to improve the patients' functioning with less pain.

Most patients with diskogenic pain do well with conservative management. However, there are still some patients who do not respond to these conservative measures. Over the past few years, there have been a number of interventional procedures used to tackle the problem of diskogenic back pain, aimed at preventing the need for surgical management. Growing literature supports epidural steroid injections as a pain management strategy for disk herniations with radiculitis. Because it is well accepted that a disk herniation can cause an inflammatory response, epidural steroid injections for diskogenic pain (i.e., without radicular symptoms) have been used and may be indicated, although there is no literature to prove this. Buttermann[43] has supplied us with some potential criteria for the role of epidural steroid injections in presumptively symptomatic degenerative disks. Many percutaneous disk procedures are in use, and new ones are continually being developed to treat patients with diskogenic pain that has failed to respond to more conservative management (Boxes 33-4 and 33-5).[180,206] None of these, however, has definitively been shown to have better results than a surgical microdiskectomy. The literature on surgical management for diskogenic pain is similar to that regarding epidural steroid injections, that is, surgery is most effective in improving radicular leg symptoms and is less impressive for axial back complaints. The most common surgical procedure is diskectomy. If there is concern for instability (i.e., in patients with significant multilevel degenerative disease), spinal fusion is sometimes also considered. Recently, prosthetic disk replacements have been considered as a replacement for spinal fusion. The literature, however, does not demonstrate better outcomes with disk arthroplasty compared with fusion, only equal outcomes[260] The potential complications with disk arthroplasty are significantly more concerning, however, and it is currently unclear who would benefit from a disk arthroplasty over lumbar fusion.

BOX 33-4

Procedures for Disk Herniations and Radiculopathy (Leg Pain >> Axial Pain)

- Epidural steroid injections
- Percutaneous disk decompression procedures
- Chemonucleolysis
- Thermal/Laser
- Mechanical
  - Intradiskal electrothermoplasty
  - Radiofrequency nucleoplasty/coblation
- Surgery
  - Microdiskectomy

BOX 33-5

Procedures for Diskogenic Low Back Pain (Internal Disk Disruption) (Axial Pain >> Leg Pain)

- Intradiskal steroids
- Annuloplasty
- Lumbar fusion
- Disk arthroplasty

Treatment of Low Back Pain

Most studies of the various treatments for low back pain, particularly chronic low back pain, unfortunately have shown limited efficacy. Even the most commonly prescribed treatments, such as medications, exercise, and manipulation, in large trials tend to show improvements of only 10 to 20 points on a 100-Point Pain Visual Analog Scale. For this reason, most clinicians use multiple treatments on a particular patient in the hope that their cumulative effect will provide sufficient pain relief and an improvement in symptoms. The most common treatments for low back pain are discussed as follows.

Reassurance and Patient Education

Given the prevalence of back pain as a source of disability, the complex interplay between pain and beliefs about pain, and the often inaccurate, profit-driven material ubiquitously available to patients about the causes and treatment of back pain, the importance of an expert physician providing accurate, understandable patient education cannot be overstated. Reassurance that there is no serious underlying pathology, that the prognosis is good, and that the patient can stay active and get on with life despite the pain can help counter negative thoughts and misinformation that the patient might have about back pain. Providing empathy and a strong therapeutic alliance will improve adherence to treatment and better outcomes.[239]

Strong evidence from systematic reviews indicates that the advice to continue ordinary activity as normally as possible fosters a quicker recovery and can lead to less disability than the advice to rest and "let pain be your guide."[240] It is controversial whether patients with low back pain fare better with a specific diagnosis or not. Education and explanations, however, should be adequate. Beyond a diagnosis, there is other information that patients want about low back pain. In a study of patients who had low back pain and went to their primary care physicians in a health maintenance organization setting, the information that patients wanted from their physician included the likely course of their back pain, how to manage their pain, how to return to usual activity quickly, and how to minimize the frequency and severity of recurrences. They ranked each of these areas of education a higher priority than finding a cause or receiving a diagnosis for their pain.[239] Providing this information in a way that patients can understand helps build a therapeutic physician-patient relationship and, it is hoped, helps reduce anxiety and speed recovery.

Back Schools

The term *back school* is generally used for group classes that provide education about back pain. The content and length of these classes varies a great deal, but generally they include information about the anatomy and function of the spine, common sources of low back pain, proper lifting technique and ergonomic training, and sometimes advice about exercise and remaining active. Studies have generally found back schools to be effective in reducing disability and pain for those with chronic low back pain.[228] They do not appear to prevent the occurrence of low back pain.[224]

Exercise

A metaanalysis that included over 1100 individuals failed to show that exercise is effective for the treatment of acute low back pain. Exercise for acute episodes appear to be no better than no care or advice to stay active,[225] although many practitioners believe that exercise is appropriate to prevent deconditioning.

Multiple high-quality studies have found, however, that exercise results in positive outcomes in the treatment of chronic low back pain.[230] This includes pain relief (although this relief is modest, with a metaanalysis of 43 trials showing a mean difference of 10 points on a 100-point scale), improvement in function, and slightly reduced sick leave.[49,98] It appears that the most effective exercise for low back pain includes an individualized regimen learned and performed under supervision that includes stretching and strengthening.[98] This is not surprising because it is generally believed that the purpose of exercises for the treatment of low back pain is to strengthen and increase endurance of muscles that support the spine and improve flexibility in areas where this is lacking. This is combined with motor retraining to establish normal patterns of muscle activity, and treatment of deficits of the kinetic chain that interfere with biomechanical efficiency. Despite multiple studies, there is no conclusive evidence that one form of exercise is better than another in the treatment of chronic low back pain.[224] One reason that studies have not been able to determine what exercises are best for patients with low back pain could be that multiple forms of exercise can achieve the goal of restoring function and regaining physical fitness.[126,229,243]

The exact amount of exercise, how exercises should be advanced, and the ideal length of supervised treatment are not known.[248] Because endurance is a significant problem with many patients with persistent back pain, activity levels should be increased in planned, fixed increments based on realistic goals rather than on symptoms. This is because it is normal in the course of low back pain that there will be temporary exacerbations of pain along the way. Beyond the physiologic benefits of exercise, increasing activity has positive effects on beliefs and behaviors about pain. Small amounts of exercise that are not sufficient to cause physiologic change have been found to increase function and decrease pain. When specifically studied, this appeared to be from decreased fear-avoidance beliefs and reduced anxiety. By exposing patients who are fearful to physical activity through gradually increasing activity levels despite pain, they receive positive reinforcement by meeting goals, and personal experience can reduce fear of movement, reinjury, and catastrophizing.[26] Adverse effects of exercise for low back pain are rarely reported, thus it is generally a very safe form of treatment.

The American College of Sports Medicine recommends that exercise as rehabilitation be incorporated into exercise guidelines for general health and fitness.[80] Therefore, for a patient with chronic low back pain, recommending 30 minutes of moderate aerobic exercise such as walking or water aerobics five times a week should be part of the exercise prescription. No particular type of aerobic activity has been found to be more effective than another for gaining fitness or decreasing pain for patients with back pain. A willingness to regularly participate in the activity at an intensity level to improve fitness is a more important factor than the specific type of exercise.[257]

If increasing aerobic fitness in a commonly used activity is the goal, then walking might be the best way to achieve this, despite pain complaints in patients with back pain. Patients with chronic low back pain tend to select a slower gait than those without pain. This is linked more with fear of pain and high scores on fear-avoidance and catastrophic thinking scales than with pain ratings.[3] Interestingly, a slow stroll reduces spine motion and causes almost static loading of tissues, overall higher spine loading, and therefore more pain than faster walking with arm swings. Faster walking causes cyclic loading of tissues and results in lower spine torques, muscle activity, and loading. Swinging the arms facilitates efficient storage and use of elastic energy, which reduces the need for concentric muscle contractions with each step.[148] Fast walking has been shown to be therapeutic for low back pain, as has other aerobic activity.[148,199]

In addition to aerobic exercise, various strengthening and stretching exercises, such as lumbar stabilization programs that focus on strengthening the abdominal, low back, and hip muscles, and increasing flexibility have been found to be effective in the treatment of low back pain.[224] Often, supervised exercise treatment is prescribed so that patients can learn how to do these exercises correctly and to improve adherence.[21] Lack of compliance is one of the main reasons why exercise treatments fail, and the physician should emphasize that exercise needs to become a daily habit.

Some programs emphasize beginning with training of the deep stabilizers, such as the multifidi and transversus abdominis. Typically, the exercise program is then progressed to include more complex dynamic and functional tasks. These are sometimes called motor control exercises because of the emphasis on precision of movement, rather than simply gaining global strength or flexibility. Multiple randomized controlled trials have shown that lumbar stabilization exercises, core strengthening, and motor control exercises are beneficial in reducing pain and improving function in patients with persistent low back pain. It is not clear whether these types of exercises are superior to other types.[131]

Extension-based exercises are often done with the principles of the McKenzie method of physical therapy and are commonly used particularly when back pain is accompanied by radicular leg pain. This therapy approach divides the diagnosis for back pain into three categories: derangement, dysfunction, and postural syndrome. The most common of these are derangements, and exercises are chosen that centralize the pain, that is, move the pain from the leg or buttock into the low back. Although early studies were very promising, later studies have found this type of physical therapy to be helpful for low back pain but no more effective than other types of exercise.[227]

Exercise has generally been found to be one of the most effective treatments for decreasing pain and increasing function in chronic low back pain. The many other health benefits of exercise, along with the low risk of causing harm, make it a first-line treatment.

Aquatic Exercises

Patients who have not tolerated land-based exercises are often able to participate in pool exercises. Exercising in water has several benefits. One is buoyancy and reduction of gravitational stress. The greater the amount of the body that is submerged the greater the effect. For example, there is a 90% reduction in gravitational stresses when exercising in the vertical position when the patient is immersed to the neck.[120] Water can also decrease pain via the gate theory, in which the sensory input from the water temperature, hydrostatic pressure, and turbulence cause the patient to feel less pain. Muscle guarding and muscle overactivity might also be decreased in warm water. For those patients fearful of movement and reinjury, moving in the pool can increase their confidence because they see they can progress without pain. The same principles for progressing therapy apply to aquatic exercise as to land-based exercise. Patients can learn neutral position, stabilizing, and other strengthening exercise, while walking, jogging (these can be done in deep water with a buoyancy belt or vest), or swimming can add an aerobic component.[120] Multiple studies have found a beneficial effect on pain and function for patients with low back pain who exercise in the water.[120,245]

Exercise After Spine Surgery

Most of the research in this area has been done on patients who have undergone lumbar disk surgery. One systematic review of this topic found no evidence that exercising after disk surgery increases injury rate or need to reoperate.[167] Overall, exercise appears to be effective in decreasing pain and increasing return to work rates. Those who used high-intensity exercise compared with low-intensity exercise resulted in significantly better short-term pain relief, functional status, and faster return to work. No difference was found, however, between the high-intensity and low-intensity groups at 1-year follow-up evaluation, perhaps because of long-term compliance issues with the high-intensity exercises. Home exercise programs have been found to be equally effective to a supervised exercise program when all patients are given the same exercises.[167]

Medication

Nonsteroidal Antiinflammatory Drugs. Multiple studies provide strong evidence that nonsteroidal antiinflammatory drugs (NSAIDs) prescribed at regular intervals provide pain relief for both acute and chronic low back pain. Studies comparing the effectiveness of NSAIDs have not found any particular NSAID to be superior to others.[229,233] NSAIDs are associated with some risk, including gastrointestinal bleeding, decreased hemostasis, and renal dysfunction or failure in patients with abnormal renal function or hypovolemia.[18] The cardiovascular risks of NSAIDs are also becoming more evident. Data on the long-term benefits and side effects associated with NSAIDs for low back pain are lacking. For example, of 51 trials included in the Cochrane Review on NSAIDs and low back pain, the longest trial evaluated only 6 weeks of therapy.[50]

Muscle Relaxants. The use of muscle relaxants remains controversial. One reason is that it is unclear what role muscle "spasms" play in low back pain. Some object to the term *muscle spasm* for skeletal muscle because only smooth muscles have the syncytial innervation pattern needed to actually spasm. They prefer the term *muscle guarding*. Other experts do not believe that pain in the low back is generally caused by muscles. Despite this controversy, 35% of patients who visit a primary care physician for low back pain are prescribed muscle relaxants.[232] These medications fall into three classes of drug: the benzodiazepines, the nonbenzodiazepines that are antispasmodics, and antispasticity medication.

The mechanism of action for benzodiazepines is the enhancement of gamma-aminobutyric acid (GABA) inhibitory activity. The limited research done on this class of medication has found them to be effective for both acute and chronic low back pain for short-term pain relief (trials generally lasted from 5 to 14 days). They have significant adverse effects, however, such as sedation, dizziness, and mood disturbances. Rapid withdrawal can cause seizures. These medications have serious abuse and addiction potential, and they are not recommended for low back pain except in unusual cases for a short time.[52,232] No evidence exists to support that they are more effective than other muscle relaxants such as cyclobenzaprine.[50,163]

Nonbenzodiazapine antispasmodics include medications with multiple mechanisms of action. Cyclobenzaprine has a structure similar to that of tricyclic antidepressants and is believed to act in the brainstem. Carisoprodol blocks interneuronal activity in the spinal cord and descending reticular formation. The mechanism of action of methocarbamol is not known but could be as a result of central nervous system depression.[10] Multiple high-quality studies show that these medications are effective for patients with acute low back pain for short-term pain relief (usually 2 to 4 days' duration). The most common side effects are drowsiness and dizziness. Currently, no evidence shows that one is more efficacious than another. Carisoprodol is metabolized to meprobamate, an antianxiety agent. It has significant potential for abuse and can result in psychological and physical dependence.[232] Because of this risk, and the fact that it is not more efficacious than other muscle relaxants, it should not be used except in rare cases. Little literature exists on the use of muscle relaxants for chronic pain. The drug manufacturers in this class state that they are not for long-term use.[52]

Antispasticity medication has also been used to treat low back pain. Baclofen is a GABA derivative that inhibits transmission at the spinal level and brain. One study has shown this medication to be effective for short-term pain relief in those with acute low back pain. Dantrolene works on the muscle, blockading the sarcoplasmic reticulum calcium channels. A small study of 20 patients found it to be effective for acute low back pain. It does not have the drowsiness side effect of the other muscle relaxants, but there is a risk of severe hepatotoxicity.[232] Tizanidine, a centrally acting alpha$_2$-agonist developed to treat spasticity, has been shown to be effective for acute low back pain in multiple trials. No studies support its use for chronic low back pain.[50]

Antidepressants. Tricyclic antidepressants are an effective treatment for many painful conditions, such as diabetic neuropathy, postherpetic neuralgia, fibromyalgia, and headaches. No adequate studies show whether they are effective for the treatment of acute low back pain. Multiple studies and reviews have shown their effectiveness, however, for chronic low back pain. Staiger et al.[209] did a best-evidence synthesis of randomized, placebo-controlled trials on this topic, which included 440 patients. They found that the tricyclics and tetracyclics had significant effects in reducing pain. These reductions were seen in studies in which patients who were depressed were excluded, thus the mechanism is independent of any treatment of underlying depression. The doses used in almost all these studies were within the Agency for Health Care Policy and Research guidelines for treatment of depression. The most common side effects seen with the use of tricyclic antidepressants are dry mouth, blurry vision, constipation, dizziness, tremors, and urinary disturbances.

The selective serotonin reuptake inhibitors and trazodone are not effective in treating chronic low back pain, which is consistent with the findings in studies for other painful conditions, such as diabetic neuropathy.[223] The selective serotonin and norepinephrine reuptake inhibitors are still undergoing evaluation for treatment of low back pain.

Opioids. Many providers use short-acting opioids to treat acute low back pain. The use of opioids for chronic nonmalignant pain is much more controversial. Opioid use for chronic back pain varies a great deal by treatment setting, ranging from 3% to 66%, with the highest numbers in specialty treatment centers.[141] Studies regarding the efficacy of opioids for chronic low back pain have not demonstrated that they are significantly better than placebo or other nonopioid medications.[46,56,141] Studies have also not been able to demonstrate improvements in function with opioid use for chronic low back pain.[141]

Opiate side effects are substantial, and in many studies occur in more than half the participants. These effects include nausea, constipation, somnolence, dizziness, and pruritus.[19] In studies that have compared long-acting with short-acting opioids, the long-acting medications appear to generally give better pain relief, are better tolerated, and are thought to have less abuse potential. Because of side effects, abuse potential, tolerance, unknown long-term effects on pain and neuronal functioning, and questionable efficacy, opioid medications are generally avoided, and a more global approach to nonspecific low back pain is used. As with other treatments, long-term opioid treatment should be used only after careful analysis of the positive and negative impacts on function and quality of life. Outcomes beyond simple pain reduction should be used, and a rational end point of treatment and criteria for tapering and discontinuing the medications should be determined. Opioid medications should not be used without regular follow-up evaluation (see Chapter 37).[18,19]

Anticonvulsants. The anticonvulsants, particularly gabapentin and pregabalin, are widely used for neuropathic pain. Large randomized controlled trials have not yet been conducted with these medications for the treatment of low back pain. One study of topiramate showed small improvement in chronic low back pain. Side effects include sedation and diarrhea.[116,156]

Tramadol. In a metaanalysis it was found to be helpful for short-term treatment of chronic low back pain. Small studies suggest it is probably equivalent to antidepressants, and may be slightly better than NSAIDS in decreasing pain, but the quality of the studies is not sufficient to make conclusions, and there is no evidence to show it improves function.[46]

Systemic Steroids. Multiple studies have found them not to be effective for axial low back pain.[50]

Herbal Medicines. Several herbal medicines are used in the treatment of low back pain. Literature studies in this area tend to be of low quality, but several herbal preparations seem to reduce pain more than placebo, including *Capsicum frutescens* (cayenne) in a topical preparation, *Salix alba* (white willow bark), and *Harpagophytum procumbens* (devil's claw). More research in this area is necessary.[78]

Antibiotics. A recent small randomized controlled trial[5] evaluated the use of amoxicillin-clavulanate versus placebo for 100 days for treatment of chronic low back pain in patients with previous disk herniation with evidence of Modic type 1 changes in adjacent vertebra on MRI. The antibiotic group had improved pain and less disability after treatment at 1 year follow-up, but further research is needed to confirm this finding.[5]

Topical Treatments. Lidocaine (lignocaine) patches have been found to be effective by some patients for the treatment of back pain. No large studies have proved or disproved its efficacy. A variety of creams and lotions are used by patients, including irritants and antiinflammatory creams. Some individuals find them effective, but they have not been subjected to extensive research. These treatments carry little risk and have a low incidence of side effects.

Injections and Needle Therapy for Low Back Pain

Myofascial Pain and Trigger Point Injections. The theory that irritable foci in skeletal muscle can cause both local and referred pain is generally accepted, although some physicians doubt the diagnosis of myofascial pain because, in general, the research supporting the biochemical and mechanical basis of trigger points is inconclusive. With regard to low back pain, it is thought that acute trauma or overload, chronic overwork and fatigue, or altered neurologic input causes trigger points to develop. They are treated by a combination of techniques, which include reducing biomechanical stress in the area by avoiding tissue overload, making postural changes, ischemic compression, stretching, and injections.[219,220] The injection component has been the most studied. A Cochrane Review of injection therapy for low back pain pooled the results of multiple studies that have found injections of trigger points to be effective in the treatment of low back pain. These included studies that evaluated dry needling, lidocaine (lignocaine) alone, and lidocaine with steroid injections. The reviewers concluded that trigger point injections are better than placebo injections for long-term pain relief based on these studies.[161] Repeated injection should be avoided, and the addition of corticosteroid or botulinum toxin does not improve results.[137]

Acupuncture. Acupuncture has been used for the treatment of pain conditions for thousands of years. From a Western medicine perspective, it appears to have multiple mechanisms of action, including effects on the endogenous opioid peptide system, an effect on the sympathetic nervous system, and alterations in pain processing in the spinal cord and brain.[99] The efficacy of acupuncture in the treatment of low back pain is difficult to determine. Similar to other physical treatments, it is difficult to perform blinded studies. When comparing acupuncture with other standard treatments for low back pain, such as exercise, the results are difficult to interpret because the placebo effect is thought to increase with more invasive procedures. Great variations exist in the diagnosis and treatment of low back pain by acupuncturists. Similar to other treatments for low back pain, such as physical therapy and medication regimens, treatments are patient-specific and provider-specific, and acupuncture treatments vary from one another by the points chosen, what type of needle stimulation is done, and the duration of the treatment.[103,110]

Despite these difficulties, the effectiveness of acupuncture to treat low back pain is increasingly being studied. There seems to be general consensus in multiple reviews that the evidence for acupuncture in relieving low back pain is either positive or inconclusive.[24]

A systematic review has also yielded mixed results with the consensus being that acupuncture can be a useful supplement to other forms of treatment.[262] A recent meta-analysis indicated that acupuncture is better than no treatment, but may be no better than sham acupuncture.[259] More high-quality definitive studies and clinical experience are obviously needed to reach a final conclusion in this area. Acupuncture is safe for the treatment of low back pain, with very low complication rates and few side effects. The most common side effects are bruising and pain at the site of needle insertion.[24]

Experimental Injection Procedures. Botulinum toxin injections are increasingly being used to treat low back pain. The mechanism of action could be through changes in sympathetic tone, reduction of muscle spasms, or another unknown mechanism. Studies in this area are currently small, and a Cochrane Review found that the currently available evidence is of low or very low quality. The results are inconclusive as to whether or not this will be an effective treatment for back pain.[247]

Prolotherapy is another controversial procedure gaining popularity in certain parts of the United States. It consists of a series of injections into spinal ligaments to cause inflammation and thickening of the ligaments. It has not been found to be effective for treatment of nonspecific low back pain.[49]

Steroid Injections and Other Spinal Procedures. See Chapter 32 for other specific spinal procedures used in the treatment of low back pain.

Manual Mobilization or Manipulation

Historical references to manual medicine go back more than 4000 years. In the nineteenth century, an increased interest in manual medicine began in Great Britain and the United States. Multiple theories exist as to how manual medicine works. One theory is that it restores normal motion to restricted segments. Another is that it changes neurologic control via reflex mechanisms, especially the interaction between the autonomic nervous system and the spinal cord.[87]

Multiple randomized controlled trials and systematic reviews have been done to assess the efficacy of manual therapy. In most countries with national guidelines for the treatment of low back pain, spinal manipulation is recommended for acute low back pain,[241,242] although this is not universal. The recommendations for chronic back pain are much more varied. Assendelft et al.[13] performed a meta-analysis of the effectiveness of this treatment for low back pain, which included a total of 5486 patients. For both acute and chronic low back pain, the authors found spinal manipulation to be more effective than placebo (which was either sham manipulation or treatments judged to be ineffective) for short-term pain relief. An improvement in function was noted, but this did not reach statistical significance. When spinal manipulation was compared with other treatments known to be effective, such as analgesics, exercise, and physical therapy, the authors could find no statistically significant benefits compared with other therapies. Results did not change when they looked at studies in which only manipulation and not mobilization was used. They also could not identify any particular subgroup of patients for whom manipulation was particularly effective, although they theorized that if such a group existed, it would be small (see Chapter 16). The authors also did not find other commonly used treatments, such as physical therapy and medication, to be statistically significantly more effective than spinal manipulation. Their conclusion was that spinal manipulation is more effective than placebo, and is one of several options of modest effectiveness for patients with low back pain.

Traction

The literature in this area has been criticized because of disagreement as to whether available studies have used the appropriate weight of traction, frequency of treatment, and length of treatment session. Many studies have been of traction used once per week, and some practitioners believe that traction should be done daily and that outcomes of studies with frequency less than this are invalid.[96] Multiple randomized controlled trials using different doses of traction have been done, however, and most have not found traction to be effective for the treatment of back pain. No well-done study has shown that a specific weight or frequency of traction is more effective than sham treatment.[229,233]

Lumbar Supports

Lumbar supports are used to both treat and prevent low back pain. Multiple types of lumbar support can be used. They vary from a simple elastic wrap to custom-molded plastic braces. High-quality studies comparing the effectiveness of different braces are generally lacking, although one study showed that patients who wore a lumbar support plus a rigid insert in the back had more subjective improvement than those who wore a brace without a rigid support.[152]

Several mechanisms of action have been proposed as to why lumbar supports would be effective, although none have been proven. One hypothesis is that they prevent excessive spinal motion, either by physically blocking extremes of motion or by providing sensory feedback to remind the patient not to bend excessively. Another theory is that they increase intraabdominal pressure without increasing abdominal muscle activity, and therefore could reduce muscle force, fatigue, and compressive loading on the spine.[226] In general, lumbar supports decrease ROM, but the results are not consistent. Decreases in ROM vary between individuals, with some individuals even showing increased range while wearing a brace. The plane of motion that is reduced also varies between individuals and the types of braces tested. Some types of brace reduce rotation, whereas others reduce flexion and extension. No evidence exists that lumbar supports actually increase intraabdominal pressure or decrease muscle forces and fatigue.[226] There is limited evidence that lumbar supports provide some pain relief for low back pain when compared with no treatment, but when compared with other treatments they are no more effective. Studies also have shown that generally there is poor compliance for individuals to consistently wear lumbar supports. No consistent evidence exists that lumbar supports prevent the occurrence of back pain (see Chapter 13).[230]

Transcutaneous Electrical Nerve Stimulation

The development of transcutaneous electrical nerve stimulation (TENS) was based on the gate control theory of pain of Melzack and Wall.[149a] In this theory, the stimulation of large afferent fibers inhibits small nociceptive fibers, causing the patient to feel less pain. Multiple types of TENS applications can be used, such as high frequency moderate intensity, low frequency high intensity, and burst frequency. Many patients find TENS helpful for temporary relief of low back pain. Evaluating the research in this area is difficult because of the difficulty of an equivalent placebo and the different types of TENS applications used between studies, and because most of the study designs are subject to recall bias.[35] Metaanalyses of TENS outcomes show trends toward better pain reduction, better function, and satisfaction with treatment compared with placebo, but do not reach statistical significance. Larger and methodologically sound studies are still needed to evaluate the efficacy of this treatment.[153]

Massage

Massage is one of the most commonly used complementary therapies for low back pain. The mechanism of action is thought to include relaxation, the therapeutic benefits of touch, and beneficial effects on the structure or function of tissues.[77] Research on massage has generally fallen into two categories: studies that measure the effect of massage and studies that assess the effectiveness of other interventions and use massage as a control with hands-on effects. In studies in which massage was used as the control, massage was not generally found to be more beneficial. This could be because of the effectiveness of both interventions, explaining why no differences were found, or it could have been as a result of publication bias. In studies in which massage was one of the main interventions, massage has been found to be effective for pain relief and in restoring function. For example, Cherkin et al.[47] performed an interesting study that compared massage, acupuncture, and self-care education for chronic low back pain. After 10 weeks in which up to 10 treatments were allowed, the massage group showed improvements on disability scales, had decreased medication use, and had less time with restricted activity than the control group. After 1 year, many of these gains were maintained.[47] Other high-quality studies have also found massage to be effective for improving symptoms and functions in those with subacute and chronic low back pain.[77] High-quality studies on the effects of massage on acute low back pain have not yet been done.

Complementary Movement Therapies

Many movement therapies are used in the treatment of low back pain. A few of the most commonly used therapies are listed as follows. These therapies have been found to be helpful in case series but have not been subjected to stringent randomized controlled trials.

- Yoga: This is both an exercise system and philosophy that promotes relaxation, acceptance, and breathing techniques while various stretching and strengthening exercises are done. Multiple studies have found this to be as effective for low back pain as other group exercise programs.[216]
- Pilates: This is a form of core-strengthening exercises that stresses alignment and proper form. Positive results from small studies suggest that this might be an effective type of treatment for low back pain.[154]
- Alexander technique: This is an educational approach to posture and normalizing movement patterns. One recent randomized controlled trial of this technique showed short-term and long-term effectiveness (up to 1 year) with this treatment.[129]
- Feldenkrais method: This is a combination of classes and hands-on work with therapeutic exercise to promote natural and comfortable movement patterns and improve body awareness.

Interdisciplinary Pain Treatment Programs

Strong evidence exists that an interdisciplinary program with a goal of functional restoration is helpful for severe chronic pain.[229] This is discussed further in Chapter 37 on chronic pain.

Treatment of Comorbidities

Multiple comorbidities are often seen with back pain. Issues commonly associated with low back pain include depression, anxiety, and sleep disturbances. Treating these conditions often decreases pain and increases function. Those who suffer from low back pain often also have other illnesses associated with an unhealthy and sedentary lifestyle, such as obesity, non–insulin-dependent diabetes, and cardiovascular disease. These comorbidities must be taken into account when formulating a rehabilitation plan.

Prognosis of Low Back Pain

Prognosis is difficult to fully ascertain for several reasons. One is that low back pain is a symptom caused by a vast spectrum of pathology with a variety of prognostic outcomes. Another is that the pain experience is individual, and treatment expectations vary. A large body of medical literature highlights the complex cultural, psychological, social support, and economic factors that influence pain and rehabilitation outcome.[127]

The much-quoted view that 90% of cases of acute low back pain will recover within 6 weeks does not include the entire story of low back pain, either in clinical practice or in reviews of the scientific literature. Most studies are performed with individuals who seek medical care for their low back pain, and this might be a select population not generalizable to all those who develop back pain. A metaanalysis of patients who sought medical care for back pain of less than 3 weeks' duration included both those in treatment arms of studies and in the placebo arms, so that both the natural course and the clinical course of back pain could be evaluated.[175] The study found that most patients rapidly improved within 1 month, and that most continued to have pain decrease, although more slowly, until approximately 3 months. From 3 months to 1 year, little change in pain was seen. The risk of a recurrence within 3 months varied between 19% and 34%, and the risk of a recurrence within 1 year was between 66% and 84%. This was a heterogeneous diagnostic population, although the vast majority of patients fell under the diagnosis of nonspecific low back pain. The remainder of this chapter discusses back pain that has a more specific diagnosis.

Spinal Fractures

Spondylolysis

Spondylolysis is a defect of the pars interarticularis, or the isthmus between the superior and inferior articular facets, and is a common cause of back pain in children and adolescents. The most common mechanism of injury is repetitive extension or rotation in the immature spine, and is commonly reported in adolescent gymnasts and football linemen.[69,105] Acute fracture from a severe hyperextension injury is also possible but less commonly reported.[68] Pars defects have also been reported in nonathletic individuals. Population-based studies suggest that spondylolysis is an acquired condition that occurs early in life, associated only with bipedal ambulation. The defect is not seen before walking begins and most commonly occurs at age 7 to 8 years.[162] An increase in incidence occurs during the adolescent growth spurt between ages 11 and 15 years. Young athletes have a higher prevalence of spondylolysis than nonathletes. In one cohort, active spondylolysis was found in 55% of athletes aged 10 to 30 years with low back pain.[142] The pars defect appears to result from a combination of hereditary dysplasia of the pars and repetitive stressing of the spine by walking and extension/rotation loading.[51] Unilateral or bilateral defects can occur, but bilateral involvement might result in spondylolisthesis. Ninety percent of these lesions occur at the L5-S1 level.

Patients typically have low back pain that is exacerbated by extension and alleviated by rest or activity limitation. Physical examination can demonstrate focal tenderness, pain with lumbar extension, and hamstring tightness. The neurologic examination is usually normal. If a spondylolisthesis is present, a palpable step-off with examination of the spinous processes might be evident. However, given the high prevalence of spondylolysis in adolescent athletes with low back pain, it is imperative for clinicians to maintain a high index of suspicion in any young athlete with low back pain regardless of positive or negative physical examination findings.

The ideal radiographic assessment of a suspected pars injury is debated. Plain radiographs are of limited use in diagnosing a symptomatic spondylolysis. Oblique views can show a pars defect well; however, the sensitivity of detection on plain films does not increase much, and the radiation exposure is significantly greater.[182] Standing anteroposterior and lateral radiographs can be obtained initially to identify a spondylolisthesis or any gross bony abnormalities.[210] SPECT is more sensitive than plain radiography and planar bone scans. A positive bone scan or SPECT scan correlates with a painful pars lesion.[97] In most retrospective analyses, however, increased uptake is present for approximately 1 year after the occurrence of the fracture.[182] If the SPECT study is consistent with an active pars injury, a thin-slice CT through the abnormal level can be helpful to confirm the diagnosis and stage the lesion. Staging the lesion according to chronicity is helpful to predict healing. The Tokushima classification grades defects by CT as acute, progressive, or terminal (Box 33-6).[75] In a metaanalysis using this classification system, 68% of acute defects healed, 28% of progressive lesions healed, and no terminal lesions healed.[119] Determining chronicity can help the clinician decide how quickly the athlete should progress through treatment. The use of MRI in diagnosing spondylolysis has garnered much attention in recent years. Standard magnetic resonance sequences identify only 80% of pars lesion seen on SPECT and should be used to look for other pathology.[142] Campbell et al.,[44] however, showed that nonstandard magnetic resonance sequences (oblique sagittal images) found 39 of 40 pars defects seen on CT and SPECT, but still only CT correctly staged the lesion.[33] Until more standard MRI protocols evolve and are adopted as usual practice, the discerning clinician should exercise caution when interpreting data or basing treatment decisions solely on MRI findings.

A number of successful management strategies for spondylolysis have been used. Conservative management is most common, typically beginning with relative rest and avoidance of activities that increase pain (especially repetitive extension). Patients typically are advised to rest for 3 months.[210] This is the shortest amount of time over which

BOX 33-6

Tokushima Classification for Grading Pars Defects

- Acute (early): Hairline defect
- Progressive: Moderately wide defect with round margins
- Terminal (chronic): Wide defect with sclerotic margins

healing of a pars lesion has been identified on serial imaging.[261] In a recent cohort of athletes treated for spondylolysis, those athletes who rested from sport for at least 12 weeks were 16.4 times more likely to have the most favorable outcome compared with athletes who returned early.[65]

Bracing, although a very commonly cited treatment, is not absolutely necessary. A metaanalysis demonstrated that 84% of 665 patients with a spondylolysis treated nonoperatively were able to return to pain-free unrestricted activity by 1 year. No statistically significant difference in clinical outcomes was seen between the braced and nonbraced groups.[119] A rigid brace might be considered after 2 weeks of rest if symptoms are not resolving.[210] A radiographically stable bony union is the obvious goal but is not an absolute necessity, given that many young athletes can become symptom-free in sports and everyday life even with a persistent pars defect. That same metaanalysis studied 847 defects and showed a 28% radiographic healing rate; 71% of the unilateral defects healed and only 18% of the bilateral defects healed.[119]

In any event, braced or not, the young athlete is at risk for deconditioning. When pain allows, the patient should be encouraged to begin aerobic conditioning and eventually enter a spinal rehabilitation program before return to a sport. Once the athlete has mastered a basic core stabilization program, functional progression back to the specific sport is appropriate, with a focus on neuromuscular proprioceptive control and sport-specific drills before full return to play. For the patient with chronic low back pain and spondylolysis, O'Sullivan et al.[166] demonstrated that a specific exercise program focused on training the lumbar multifidi and deep abdominals can be very effective. Surgical treatment is rarely indicated for the patient with spondylolysis alone but is more common in the setting of spondylolisthesis and/or radiculopathy.

The natural history of spondylolysis and low-grade (less than 2) spondylolisthesis is benign, that is, it is rare to have progressive slippage. Saraste[195] demonstrated this in a study of 225 patients with a 20-year follow-up period. Most cases of progressive slippage occur during the adolescent growth spurt, however, thus very young athletes should be monitored with lateral flexion-extension plain films every 6 to 12 months until skeletal maturity is reached. Besides the adolescent growth spurt, a listhesis greater than 50% is considered a risk factor for progressive slip.

Spondylolisthesis

Lumbar spondylolisthesis or anterior slippage of one vertebra on another can result from many causes. Spondylolisthesis can be grouped into six different categories by etiology. The most common is the isthmic spondylolisthesis (Figure 33-22). The isthmic slip occurs as a result of a spondylolysis or "stress fracture" of the pars interarticularis (as described earlier). The dysplastic spondylolisthesis is a congenital slip and is caused by dysplasia of the facet joints, leading to an inability to resist shear stresses and forward slippage. Degenerative spondylolisthesis is seen in the older spine and is related to long-standing intersegmental instability from degenerative facet or disk disease.

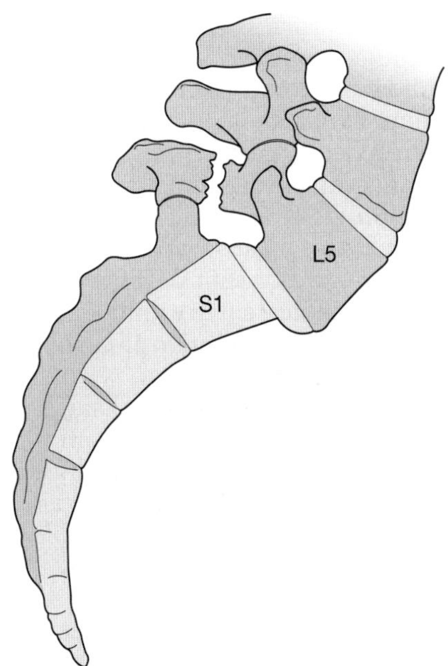

FIGURE 33-22 Grade I isthmic spondylolisthesis.

Table 33-6 Meyerding Grading System for Spondylolisthesis*

Grade	Percentage Slip
I	<25
2	25-49
3	50-74
4	75-99
5	≥100 (spondyloptosis)

*Meyerding divided the anterior-posterior diameter of the superior surface of the first sacral vertebral into quarters and assigned the grade accordingly.[256]

The most common level affected in a degenerative slip is the L4-L5 level. Traumatic spondylolisthesis is rare and is caused by acute fracture secondary to trauma. Pathologic spondylolisthesis is attributable to medical causes of generalized or local bone disease that can cause decreased bony strength. This form can present as an isthmic defect or an elongated, intact pars. The final category is postsurgical and is attributable to resulting instability from an extensive decompression, which is uncommon now because of the amount of hardware used for fusions after extensive decompressions.

The patient with spondylolisthesis typically presents with low back pain. Sometimes there is a complaint of intermittent radicular symptoms related to a dynamic radiculitis, that is, nerve root irritation caused by subtle instability at the listhetic segment. Physical examination is not different from that seen in spondylolysis. When imaging a patient with suspected spondylolisthesis, standing lateral flexion-extension views are helpful for presurgical screening. With lateral plain films, the degree of slip is graded 1 through 5 (Table 33-6).

The natural history of spondylolisthesis is spontaneous stabilization. It is generally accepted that significant slip progression rarely occurs in adults.[195,200] Some controversy exists regarding slip progression in adolescents. Harris and Weinstein[95] studied youths with grade 3 or 4 slips in a long-term follow-up study and noted that there was a higher incidence of progression of the slip until skeletal maturity was reached. Saraste[195] and Seitsalo[200] had similarly large long-term observational studies that demonstrated that slip progression in youths and adults was small overall. Possible factors positively correlating with slip progression include degree of slip, degenerative disk disease at the level of slip, adolescent age, and ligamentous laxity that manifests as hypermobility on imaging (i.e., motion on flexion-extension views).

Treatment for an isthmic spondylolisthesis in a young patient is similar to that for the athlete with spondylolysis, as described in the previous section. Fusion surgery is generally considered in adolescents if the slip is grade 3 or greater. For degenerative spondylolisthesis, nonoperative management with a rehabilitation program similar to that described in the section on degenerative zygapophyseal joint and disk disease is appropriate because both are typical findings with a degenerative slip. Operative intervention with fusion is generally considered only for recalcitrant pain after an appropriate rehabilitation program, persistent radiculopathy, or progressive instability.

Other Spinal Fractures

Many other types of spinal fracture can occur, the most common of which are briefly discussed in the following sections. Many are secondary to trauma. Evidence-based guidelines have not yet been developed for the treatment of traumatic spine fractures. Current literature in this area is mainly of retrospective case series. Outcomes appear to be most dependent on the amount of neurologic injury at the time of injury, and on the time elapsed between injury and surgery if a neurologic injury exists.[234]

The three-column structural concept of Denis is the most common method to classify spinal fractures. This concept divides the spine into anterior, middle, and posterior columns. The anterior column is made up of the anterior longitudinal ligament and the anterior half of the vertebral body and disk. The middle column is made up of the posterior longitudinal ligament and the posterior half of the vertebral body and disk. The posterior column is made up of the rest of the bony and soft tissues of the spine. If two of the three columns are intact, the spine is stable and treatment with pain management and rehabilitation is generally indicated.

Posterior Column Fractures

This includes transverse process and spinous process fractures. These are stable injuries. They are treated by pain management techniques and avoiding contact sports until the fractures have healed.

Anterior Column Fractures

These are compression fractures and are generally caused by flexion injuries. These fractures usually do not cause neurologic deficits and do not require surgery. If greater than 50% of the height of the vertebral body is lost, there is an increased chance that the fracture can be unstable because posterior injury might also be involved, and further investigation may be warranted. The treatment of traumatic compression fractures remains controversial.

Anterior and Middle Column Fractures

These are burst fractures and are usually the result of compression and flexion injuries. Instability and cord compression should be ruled out with plain films, a CT scan, and a thorough neurologic assessment. If patients are neurologically intact and there is no evidence of posterior instability, they can often be treated with a brace, usually a thoracic-lumbar-sacral orthosis for 12 weeks. If there is injury to the posterior longitudinal ligament, then surgery is usually required. Burst fractures in which there is loss of 50% or more of the height of the vertebral body, greater than 50% impingement into the spinal canal, or greater than 20 degrees of kyphosis require surgery to achieve stability.

Anterior and Posterior Column Fractures

These are caused by flexion and distraction injuries, and are called chance fractures. They are usually caused by seat belt injuries in high-impact motor vehicle accidents. They are unstable fractures and are sometimes treated with bracing but often require surgery.[173]

Osteoporotic Compression Fractures

Osteoporotic compression fractures are important to diagnose, both because they are a significant source of morbidity and because they can herald the risk for subsequent fractures, particularly hip fractures, which have high morbidity and mortality rates. Patients who have had a previous vertebral fracture have 3.8 times the risk of suffering a hip fracture compared with those who have not. The risk of compression fractures increases as bone density decreases. Genetic factors account for much of the risk, as well as female gender, nonexercisers, low calcium intake, smoking, alcohol use, and younger age at puberty (see Chapter 34).

Compression fractures can be a significant cause of pain and are generally the reason that there is a higher incidence of back pain in older adult women compared with men. Pain is especially prevalent if three or more fractures are present. These individuals have twice as much back pain as those without compression fractures.[74] Fractures can be asymptomatic or can present with sudden onset of severe pain. Pain can radiate anteriorly and usually gradually improves over several weeks.

Up to 30% of those with osteoporotic compression fractures have secondary osteoporosis. Common causes of secondary osteoporosis are use of oral steroids, hyperthyroidism, metastases, and multiple myeloma. Any underlying causes should always be ruled out. Bone mineral density measurements are useful to confirm the diagnosis of osteoporosis and to assess the efficacy of treatment.

Treatment. A balance should be found between alleviating pain and medication side effects. Calcitonin, either subcutaneous or intranasal, has been found in multiple studies to decrease pain without substantial side effects. Adjunct treatment and modalities such as TENS might be helpful. Intercostal nerve blocks are sometimes used to treat the pain.

Vertebroplasty is a procedure in which bone cement is injected into the bone for pain relief and to strengthen the bone. Vertebroplasty may be recommended for patients with severe pain not responding to conservative management.[7] Many of the randomized controlled trials to date have not been blinded, however. The complications can include compression of the spinal nerve roots and spinal cord, and pulmonary embolism.[74]

Osteoporosis requires treatment with a combination of medication, lifestyle modification, and exercise (see Chapter 34).

Cancer and Low Back Pain

Cancer is the second leading cause of death in the United States, and two thirds of patients with cancer develop metastases. The spine is the most common site for bony metastases, and vertebral body metastases are found in more than one third of patients with cancer. The most common cancers that involve the spine are lung, breast, prostate, and renal cell.[174]

Back pain is by far the most common symptom of metastatic disease. It is caused by stretching of the periosteum and tumor mass effect. The thoracic region of the spine is most commonly involved, although the lumbar spine is a more common site for colorectal cancer.[184] Pain can start gradually and increase as the bone is destroyed. It is a constant ache not exacerbated by movement. Sometimes the pain has a more sudden onset because of a pathologic fracture, and this type of pain can be worse with movement, especially if the spine is unstable. Deyo et al.[59] found that the most specific historical feature for malignancy as a source of back pain is a previous history of cancer (98% specific), and the authors considered it prudent to consider new-onset back pain in a patient with a history of cancer to be malignant disease until proven otherwise. This historical feature has a sensitivity of only 0.31, however, thus approximately only one third of patients with spinal malignant neoplasm have a history of cancer. Consequently, other features suggestive of malignancy must be explored in the history. Back pain unrelieved by bed rest is greater than 90% sensitive, thus if the pain is relieved by bed rest, malignancy is unlikely. This is not specific, however; therefore many patients without malignancy also complain that their pain is not relieved by bed rest. Other historical features related to cancer include unexplained weight loss and failure to improve with conservative care. New onset of back pain after age 50 years is suspicious for malignancy because many other common causes of back pain begin at an earlier age. These features can be combined to give the clinician confidence in determining whether or not cancer should be included in the differential diagnosis.[59] Neurologic deficits occur in 5% to 10% of patients with spinal metastases either from the mechanical pressure of the tumor or from bone extruded from a collapsed vertebral body.[222] Neurologic deficits often occur several months after the back pain began.[82] MRI is the imaging modality of choice for a full evaluation of spinal metastases. It is very sensitive and can show early changes in the bone marrow. It also shows both bony destruction and neural compression.[82,184]

Spinal Infections

Spinal infections include osteomyelitis, diskitis, pyogenic facet arthropathy, and epidural infections. These structures are often all infected at the same time. The incidence of spinal infections is increasing. Some of the causes of this include the growing numbers of immunocompromised patients who are at high risk, drug resistance of some infections, and recent increases in tuberculosis.[214] It is important to diagnose and treat spinal infections quickly to prevent increased morbidity and mortality, and to prevent complications such as epidural abscesses that can cause paralysis.[115] However, this is not always easy. In a review article on spinal infection, Tali[214] describes the "rule of 50" to assist in the diagnosis of spinal infections: 50% of the patients are older than 50 years, 50% will have a fever, and 50% will have an abnormal white blood count. The urinary tract is the source in 50%; *Staphylococcus aureus* is the organism in 50%; the lumbar spine is affected in 50%; and symptoms are present for greater than 3 months in 50% of cases.[214]

Vertebral osteomyelitis can occur from hematogenous spread or be secondary to a contiguous focus of infection. Hematogenous spread occurs via spinal arteries, and infection can quickly advance from the end plate of one vertebral body into the disk and then into the adjacent vertebral body. The most common source is urinary tract infections, often caused by *Escherichia coli* and other enteric bacilli. Hematogenous spread is also seen from other sources, such as infected intravenous lines or endocarditis. Patients with diabetes, those on hemodialysis, intravenous drug users, and other patients who are immunocompromised are at increased risk.[135,214] The most common location is the lumbar spine, and the most common symptom is back pain, although 15% of patients also have radicular pain. Symptoms can begin slowly and progress over months. Many patients do not have a fever or elevated white blood count. The erythrocyte sedimentation rate, however, is usually elevated. The infection can spread to surrounding tissues, and epidural, paraspinal, and psoas abscesses can also be present.

Plain films are usually normal the first 2 weeks, and then the first sign is a periosteal reaction. As the infection progresses, plain films show irregular erosions in the end plates of adjacent vertebral bodies and narrowing of the disk space. This appearance is nearly pathognomonic for infection because tumors and other causes of irregular erosions rarely cross the disk space. Bone scan shows changes as soon as 24 hours after symptoms begin but are not specific. MRI is as sensitive as bone scan and can give important anatomic information; therefore, it is generally the imaging technique that should be used.[115,118]

Treatment for spinal infections is usually a 4- to 6-week course of intravenous antibiotics. Sensitivity can often be determined by blood cultures, but if these are negative, samples from a bone biopsy might be necessary. Following the erythrocyte sedimentation rate is helpful to determine the effectiveness of treatment. Surgery is generally necessary only if the spine has become unstable, there are progressive neurologic deficits, or medical treatment fails. Spontaneous fusion of the infected segments often occurs after treatment.[115]

Osteomyelitis secondary to a contiguous focus of infection is seen after surgical procedures and with extension of infection from adjacent soft tissue. The most common organism is *S. aureus*.[135,214] Risk factors for development of postoperative osteomyelitis include history of smoking, obesity, poor nutrition, uncontrolled diabetes, administration of steroids, history of malignancy, and radiation treatment in the area of surgery.[115] These infections usually present about 14 to 30 days after surgery.[115] Diagnosis is sometimes difficult because symptoms such as pain or fever can be attributed to soft tissue infection or the surgical procedure. Imaging studies can also be less conclusive because of surgical or soft tissue changes. The erythrocyte sedimentation rate is usually elevated after surgery, thus it is not as useful in making the diagnosis in the first weeks after surgery.[115] Treatment for these types of infection usually requires surgical débridement and then a course of antibiotics.[135,214]

Diskitis can occur from contiguous spread of infection or iatrogenically from procedures such as diskectomy and diskography. The incidence of these types of infection is low, and studies report a 0% to 3% incidence with procedures, but morbidity if infection occurs is significant. One study found that 55% to 87% of patients were unable to return to their normal work after diskitis. One reason for this poor outcome is the difficulty of using antibiotics to treat the infection because of the relative avascularity of disks.[36]

Spondyloarthropathies

Spondyloarthropathies are a group of diseases associated with the *HLA-B27* allele. They are also termed *seronegative spondyloarthropathies* because patients generally have negative antinuclear antibodies and rheumatoid factor. They include ankylosing spondylitis, reactive arthritis (Reiter syndrome), psoriatic arthritis, enteropathic arthritis, and undifferentiated spondyloarthropathy. It is hypothesized that, in genetically susceptible individuals, an interplay of environmental and immunologic factors leads to clinical manifestations. Although the diseases are grouped together, each has unique features on clinical presentation.[112]

Ankylosing Spondylitis

Ankylosing spondylitis is the prototype for the spondyloarthropathies. It is three times more common in men than in women. Symptoms usually begin in the late teens or 20s. It generally first presents with morning stiffness and a dull ache in the low back or buttocks. On physical examination, there is decreased spinal mobility, decreased chest expansion, and tenderness of the sacroiliac joints with direct pressure and with maneuvers that stress the joints.[112]

Findings outside the spine are also common. Hip or shoulder arthritis is seen in approximately 30% of patients, and asymmetric peripheral joint arthritis is also seen in approximately 30% of patients. Bony tenderness and enthesitis at multiple sites, such as the heels, greater trochanters, iliac crests, and tibial tuberosities, are common. Systemic disease manifestations include anterior uveitis, heart disease, and inflammatory bowel disease.[215]

Radiographs of the lumbar spine may demonstrate squaring of the vertebral bodies, eventually forming syndesmophytes and the appearance of a bamboo spine. Sacroiliitis on radiographs can help to establish the diagnosis, but changes may not appear until late in the disease. Findings on MRI will appear much earlier in the course of the disease, and have more recently been accepted to aid in a clinical diagnosis of ankylosing spondylitis.[189] The *HLA-B27* gene is present in 90% of patients with ankylosing spondylitis. Most patients also have an acute phase response, with elevated erythrocyte sedimentation rate or C-reactive protein.

The initial treatment includes exercises that promote spinal extension. Evidence exists that exercise promotes mobility, improves function, and prevents severe deformity in many cases.[215] NSAIDs are helpful to relieve pain and inflammation so that the exercises can be done and function maintained. Indomethacin is particularly effective for this condition. Sulfasalazine and methotrexate are sometimes used, especially if there is peripheral arthritis. Disease-modifying agents such as the tumor necrosis factor inhibitors are also used to treat ankylosing spondylitis. They appear to be effective in controlling articular inflammation but do not appear to prevent joint ankylosis.[106] Sacroiliac injections under fluoroscopy can reduce symptoms acutely but do not have long-term benefit.[215]

Other Spondyloarthropathies

- Reactive arthritis (Reiter syndrome) can affect the spine. Asymmetric sacroiliitis and discontinuous spondylitis are seen. These usually begin after a genitourinary or gastrointestinal infection. Systemic symptoms are common, and conjunctivitis is seen in up to 50% of patients.
- Psoriatic arthritis can affect the spine, but an oligoarticular pattern of distal joints is much more common.
- Enteropathic spondyloarthropathies occur in approximately 20% of patients with inflammatory bowel disease and can be indistinguishable from ankylosing spondylitis.
- Undifferentiated spondyloarthropathies are said to occur if a patient has some features of, but does not fully meet, the diagnostic criteria for a well-defined spondyloarthropathy. Treatment of these conditions from a rehabilitation standpoint is similar to the treatment of ankylosing spondylitis.[112]

Differential Diagnosis and Treatment: Leg Pain Greater Than Back Pain

The differential diagnosis for those with leg pain greater than back pain is shorter than that for whom back pain predominates. Common causes of this are discussed in the following sections, as are common mimickers of radicular pain.

Lumbosacral Radiculopathy

Radicular symptoms can be the result of overt mechanical compression of a nerve root or a chemically mediated inflammatory process. Many patients with radicular pain have no neural impingement noted on MRI. Studies have shown that disk herniations can cause an inflammatory response.[140,145,193] The mechanism stems from the fact that the nucleus pulposus is highly antigenic as a result of being in an immunoprotected setting in nonpathologic states. When the fluid of the nucleus pulposus is exposed to neural tissue of the spinal canal and neuroforamen through a defect in the annular fibers, an autoimmune-mediated inflammatory cascade begins. The inflammatory mediators generated can cause swelling of the nerves. This can alter their electrophysiologic function, sensitizing these neurons and enhancing pain generation without specific mechanical compression.

The mechanism of mechanical compression of the nerve roots has also been studied.[14,191] Compression of nerve roots can induce structural and vascular changes as well as inflammation.[159] Neural compression can result in impairment of intraneural blood flow, with subsequent local ischemia and formation of intraneural edema. This can set off an inflammatory cascade similar to that described previously. Mechanical stimulation of lumbar nerve roots has also been shown to stimulate production of substance P, the neuropeptide known to modulate sensory nociceptive feedback.[14] With these biochemical reactions, the local structural effects of mechanical compression (demyelination and axonal transport block) compound the symptomatic response.

The most common compressing lesion by far is a disk protrusion. Fewer than 1% of patients who present with radicular symptoms have other causes, including infection, malignancy, or fracture.[55] Rare presentations of radiculopathy, that is, those with fever, weight loss, night pain, cancer history, or osteoporosis risk factors, certainly warrant special attention to evaluate for the less common but potentially more catastrophic causes of radiculopathy.

The most common levels of disk herniation are L4-L5 and L5-S1, with L5 and S1 being the most common nerve roots involved in radiculopathy. Multiple nerve roots can be affected by a single disk herniation, given the organization of the cauda equina. The affected nerve root level might not correlate with the level of the disk herniation. For example, a central L3-L4 disk herniation could impact the L5 or S1 rootlets as they descend through the thecal sac before exiting out of their expected neural foramen. True cauda equina syndrome occurs when the lowest sacral rootlets are affected, resulting in bowel, bladder, and sexual dysfunction. Up to 1% of all disk herniations present as cauda equina syndrome.[202] In the appropriate clinical setting, a large postvoid residual of urine is a good predictor of cauda equina syndrome.[55] Cauda equina syndrome is a surgical emergency. Recovery of neurologic deficits, including bowel and bladder dysfunction, is greatest if decompressive surgery is performed within 48 hours.[244]

The natural history of lumbosacral radiculopathy resulting from disk herniation tends to favor spontaneous resolution of symptoms over time.[42] Multiple reports have shown that disk protrusions and extrusions can regress without surgical treatment.[217] Conservative treatment is best used to decrease pain and improve the patient's level of functioning during acute management of radiculopathy. Even with some neurologic injury, conservative management should be considered because various studies have documented the same neurologic recovery in groups treated surgically and nonsurgically.[250]

The specifics of conservative management of lumbosacral radiculopathies, however, are still debatable. NSAIDs have not been found to be effective in patients with radiculopathy.[50,231] No definite support exists for oral steroids in the treatment of acute radiculopathy.[48] The neuropathic pain agents (anticonvulsants and tricyclic antidepressants) are often used for radicular pain.[48] Small studies have found gabapentin and topiramate to be associated with small improvements in pain scores.[50]

Although exercise therapy has not specifically been demonstrated to alter the course of acute radiculopathy, there is probably a role for exercise.[227] Saal et al.[192] reported very favorable outcomes using aggressive nonoperative care (an active exercise program potentially with epidural steroid injections) in the treatment of lumbar disk herniation with radiculopathy. Their protocol is the basis for many exercise programs used in the treatment of lumbar disk herniations with radiculopathy today.

Lumbar epidural steroid injections have become a common adjuvant for the treatment of lumbosacral radiculopathy. The more recent literature supports the use of fluoroscopically guided transforaminal epidural injections for short-term improvement in pain and potentially a reduced need for surgical intervention.[83,130,178,186] They are best used in combination with an active rehabilitation program and are commonly used to facilitate active therapy by decreasing pain and inflammation.

Surgical management of lumbosacral radiculopathy is best reserved for those patients who have significant persistent radicular symptoms despite 6 to 8 weeks of maximized conservative management, neurologic progression, or cauda equina syndrome. Common decompressive procedures with favorable outcomes include lumbar hemilaminotomy with diskectomy and lumbar hemilaminectomy.[211] The highly anticipated Spine Patient Outcome Research Trial was a randomized trial evaluating the effect of surgery over individualized nonoperative treatment involving 13 spine centers across the United States with 501 surgical candidates with lumbar radicular symptoms for at least 6 weeks caused by a disk herniation.[253] Individuals randomized to either surgery or nonoperative treatment improved substantially over the 2-year period of the study, and the primary outcomes were not statistically significantly different between groups. A secondary outcome of sciatica severity, however, did show statistical significance in favor of surgery. Patients need to be counseled regarding appropriate expectations after surgery for lumbar disk herniation with radiculopathy. Surgery might slightly accelerate the resolution of neurologic deficits for the typical radiculopathy; however, the major benefit of surgical intervention is pain relief.[57] Relief of leg pain should be expected; however, back pain relief is more difficult to predict. Patients should be counseled that they are likely to have recurrent back difficulties even after successful decompressive surgery. Figure 33-23 shows a useful algorithmic approach to the management of acute lumbosacral radiculopathy.

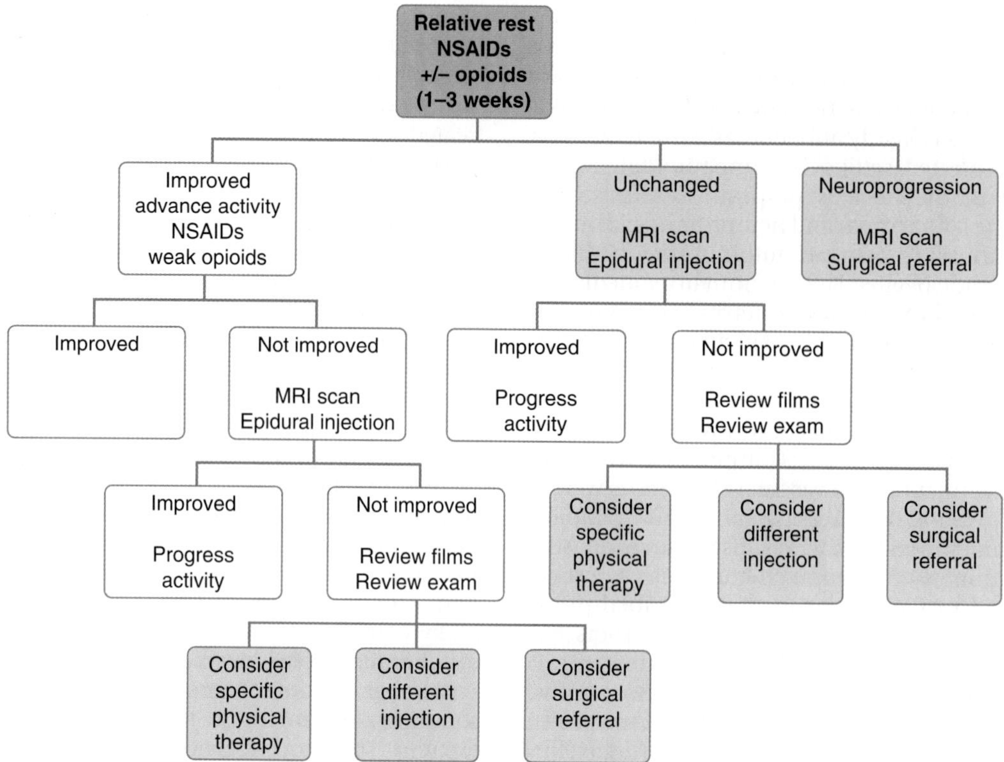

FIGURE 33-23 Algorithmic approach to acute lumbosacral radiculopathy (without cauda equina). (Modified from Chiodo A, Haig AJ: Lumbosacral radiculopathies: conservative approaches to management, *Phys Med Rehabil Clin N Am* 13:609-621, 2002.)

Lumbar Spinal Stenosis

The symptoms of spinal stenosis result from a complex series of changes within the lumbar spine.[81] These changes are generally related to aging. The narrowing of the spinal canal that occurs in stenosis results from the degenerative changes described by Kirkaldy-Willis et al.[118] Not all patients with substantial narrowing, however, have symptoms. If mechanical compression was the sole problem in spinal stenosis, decompressive surgeries would be the only needed cure for symptomatic neurogenic claudication. We know that this is untrue, and consequently alternative theories on the pathogenesis of symptomatic spinal stenosis have been studied. Two theories supporting a vascular component to symptoms of spinal stenosis are the venous engorgement and arterial insufficiency theories.[1]

In the venous engorgement theory, the spinal veins of patients with stenosis dilate, causing venous congestion and stagnating blood flow.[53] This pooling of blood in the spinal veins increases epidural and intrathecal pressures, leading to an ischemic neuritis, which in turn leads to the typical neurogenic claudication symptoms of stenosis.

The arterial insufficiency theory of spinal stenosis is based on the arterial dilatation of the lumbar radicular vessels during lower limb exercise to provide increased blood flow and nourishment to the nerve roots. In patients with spinal stenosis, this reflex dilatation might be defective.[15] Because patients with spinal stenosis are typically older adults, they are also at higher risk for atherosclerosis, which in turn amplifies the arterial insufficiency.

Box 33-7 gives a classification schema for spinal stenosis, and Table 33-7 outlines a radiologic grading scale.

BOX 33-7

Classification of Spinal Stenosis

- Congenital
  - Achondroplasia or dwarfism
  - Idiopathic
- Acquired
  - Degenerative
  - Iatrogenic or postsurgical
- Traumatic
- Combined

Table 33-7 Grading Lumbar Stenosis on Magnetic Resonance Imaging

Grade	Percentage of the Anteroposterior Canal Dimensions at a Normal Level
Mild	75-99
Moderate	50-74
Severe	<50

Electrodiagnostic studies are often performed in patients with spinal stenosis. In addition to ruling out other reasons for leg symptoms (such as peripheral neuropathy), they can be helpful in fully characterizing the stenosis. In one study, H reflexes and F waves were shown to correlate with anatomic changes on MRI of spinal stenosis, whereas limb electromyography did not.[48] This is consistent with the clinical observation that MRI findings and radicular complaints often do not correlate.

The variable symptoms of spinal stenosis are attributable to the fact that a single nerve or multiple nerve roots can be affected at one or multiple locations within the lumbar spine. Mechanical compression of the nerves can occur as a result of central canal narrowing, lateral recess narrowing, and intervertebral foraminal narrowing. This results in variable symptoms, from a monoradiculopathy to polyradiculopathy to the hallmark symptoms of neurogenic claudication.

Neurologic claudication is the most common presenting symptom of lumbar stenosis and results from central canal narrowing. It is classically described as bilateral leg pain initiated by walking, prolonged standing, and walking downhill (relative lumbar extension). It is typically relieved by sitting or bending forward. If foraminal or lateral recess stenosis is the primary pathologic issue, then patients can present with more standard radicular pain in the typical dermatomal distribution. Most patients default to a forward-flexed posture to widen the central canal, subsequently decreasing mechanical compression of the nerve roots. This can lead to substantial hip flexion contractures.

The natural history of lumbar spinal stenosis is fairly favorable overall. Johnsson et al.[109] followed patients with lumbar stenosis over a 4-year period with conservative treatment. Based on subjective patient reports, 70% remained unchanged, 15% improved, and 15% worsened. Walking capacity improved in 42% of patients, remained unchanged in 32%, and decreased in 26%. Amundsen et al.[6] reported on a 10-year study of patients randomly assigned to surgical or nonsurgical treatment. Nonsurgical treatment consisted of bracing for 1 month followed by physical therapy. They demonstrated that neurologic deterioration was rare, that delaying surgery (with conservative management) had no effect on postoperative outcomes, and that, at 4 years, half the conservative treatment group and four fifths of the surgical group had favorable outcomes. During the final 6 years of study, clinical deterioration of symptoms was rare. In general, most patients with symptomatic stenosis remain unchanged, whereas some improved and others worsened. It is impossible to predict which patients will fall into each of these categories. It is useful information that a diagnosis of lumbar stenosis does not mean rapid neurologic deterioration, and that conservative management for those with mild to moderate symptoms is warranted.

The primary goals of conservative management are pain control and reducing the functional limitations that result from the lessened activity and the pain of stenosis. Multiple facets are used in this management program, including oral medications, epidural steroids, and a comprehensive functional rehabilitation program. The oral medications are no different than what have been described previously for treatment of radiculopathy. Even more attention needs to be placed on side effects, however, because most patients with lumbar stenosis are older adults and potentially have multiple medical problems that already require multiple medications.

There may be a role for epidural steroid injections in the nonoperative treatment of symptomatic lumbar stenosis. A recent systematic review demonstrated short-term improvement in pain and walking tolerance following epidural steroid injections, while acknowledging the lack of available strong evidence in the literature.[34]

Although there is a paucity of studies examining specific rehabilitation protocols, there is certainly a role for a therapeutic exercise program in the management of lumbar spinal stenosis. The basis of any protocol should be flexion-based lumbar stabilization exercises. This includes strengthening the abdominals and pelvic girdle stabilizers, including the gluteals. Improving hip mobility through stretching, especially of the anterior muscles (iliopsoas and rectus femoris), is also key. Aerobic conditioning is the final component of a comprehensive rehabilitation program for stenosis. Bracing with an abdominal corset might be beneficial for overweight patients with a protuberant abdomen to lessen the forces creating an exaggerated lordotic posture. However, there are a lack of clear data supporting the role of lumbosacral orthoses in spinal stenosis.

Surgical consideration for lumbar stenosis should be given to patients with intractable pain resistant to nonoperative management, profound or progressive neurologic deficit, or lifestyle impairment. A study comparing surgical management of spinal stenosis versus "usual care" showed that by 3 months after surgery, the surgical group had better pain control than the conservative care group and that this improvement in pain persisted for years. No improvement, however, was seen in function in the surgical group compared with the conservative care group.[254] Of note, this was not a placebo-controlled study, and other studies involving surgery have shown profound placebo effects with surgery.[190] Age is not a contraindication to surgery, although the patient's general health status must be considered.[12] Laminectomies are the most common decompressive procedures.[190] Fusion is often performed when spinal stenosis is associated with instability, degenerative spondylolisthesis, deformity, or recurrent stenosis. Instrumentation often improves the fusion rate but does not influence the clinical outcome.[201] If selectively chosen, most patients with neurogenic claudication do well with surgical management. If the main symptomatic complaint is axial low back pain, however, the surgical outcome is generally poorer.[113]

Nonlumbar Spine Causes of "Radicular" Leg Symptoms

A number of nonspinal disorders mimic lumbar radiculopathy because they generate pain referral patterns similar to lumbosacral dermatomes. Their etiology is diverse and includes joint, soft tissue, vascular, and peripheral nerve sources. A thorough history and physical examination can typically help differentiate these disorders from lumbosacral radiculopathy; however, other diagnostic studies might be necessary.

Joint Disorders

The sacroiliac joint is now generally accepted as a potential pain generator that can refer pain into the lower limb. Other than true sacroiliitis (associated with the spondyloarthropathies), the exact pathologic structure or source of pain from the sacroiliac joint is still uncertain. In 2002, Vilensky et al.[235] reported that substance P can be found in the posterior sacroiliac ligament. It is still not known, however, whether it is the synovium, the articular cartilage, the capsule, the ligamentous structures, the muscular support of the sacroiliac joint, or a combination of these that is the primary source of pain referred to as sacroiliac joint pain.

Although there are multiple physical examination maneuvers created to stress the sacroiliac joint and reproduce pain, rigorous studies have demonstrated that no one physical examination maneuver (nor combination) correlates well with a diagnosis of sacroiliac joint pain confirmed with diagnostic local anesthetic injections into the joint.[62] The gold standard for diagnosing sacroiliac joint pain is a fluoroscopically guided injection of local anesthetic into the sacroiliac joint.

Guided injections have helped to delineate the sclerotomal referral pattern of pain emanating from the sacroiliac joint.[72,73] Sacroiliac joint pain generally does not radiate above the lumbosacral junction. It can radiate into the groin, thigh, and even below the knee, with substantial overlap of lumbosacral radicular pain patterns.

Disorders involving the hip joint generally refer pain into the groin and sometimes the anterior thigh. The prototypical disorder is osteoarthritis of the hip. This pain pattern is easily confused with L1-L2 to L3 nerve root involvement. Patients may also complain of posterior pelvic pain concomitantly with groin pain.[181] Plain films of the hip and hip ROM on physical examination are generally most helpful in differentiating an intraarticular hip source of pain from spinal referred pain.

Soft Tissue Disorders

Piriformis syndrome is thought to cause sciatica from local pressure on the sciatic nerve in the pelvis. Pain generally radiates into the posterior thigh but can refer below the knee in an L5 or S1 dermatomal pattern. The patient also describes buttock pain and typically has tenderness over the sciatic notch. Multiple examination maneuvers are used to reproduce sciatica resulting from piriformis syndrome.[20] The Pace maneuver is described as resisted abduction and external rotation of the thigh. The Freiberg maneuver is forceful internal rotation of the extended thigh. Beatty described his maneuver as deep buttock pain produced by the sidelying patient holding a flexed knee several inches off the table. Fishman and Zybert[71] described an electrophysiologic approach to diagnose piriformis syndrome using H waves.

Greater trochanteric pain syndrome is a descriptive term for a regional pain syndrome focused about the greater trochanter, buttock, and lateral thigh.[203] It is often initially diagnosed as trochanteric bursitis but is probably multifactorial in etiology. An association probably exists with gluteal muscle (medius and minimus) pathology, potentially tendinopathy, tears, or myofascial pain. Physical examination shows generalized tenderness in the region, and typically there is substantial gluteal muscle inhibition and deconditioning that can manifest as hip abductor weakness. A comprehensive rehabilitation program focusing initially on pain control and neuromuscular reeducation of the gluteal muscles is important before progressing to strength-building exercises for the gluteals.

Iliotibial band syndrome can be confused with an L4 or L5 radiculopathy. The iliotibial band is an extension of the tensor fasciae latae that traverses the lateral aspect of the thigh, attaching at Gerdy tubercle on the proximal lateral tibia. Iliotibial band syndrome typically presents as lateral knee pain, but it can also present with more proximal (lateral thigh) pain or radiate distally into the calf. When the iliotibial band is tight, it can also exacerbate greater trochanteric pain syndrome and be associated with lateral hip and buttock pain. Iliotibial band tightness is evaluated with the Ober maneuver.[134]

Myofascial pain syndromes are common and are thought to arise from active trigger points within a muscle or its fascia.[205] Activation of trigger points in various muscles have typical pain referral patterns that can mimic lumbosacral dermatomes.

Vascular Disorders

Vascular claudication from peripheral vascular disease can be difficult to differentiate from neurogenic claudication secondary to lumbar spinal stenosis, especially because both are common in older adult patients. Symptoms from both are exacerbated by walking. A major difference, however, is that spinal forward flexion or sitting is necessary to alleviate the symptoms of neurogenic claudication. The pain of intermittent vascular claudication typically resolves when walking is discontinued, even if the patient remains standing. Leaning forward on a grocery cart or walker while ambulating can also reduce neurogenic claudication but does not help with vascular claudication. The bicycle test can be used to differentiate between the two because any lower limb exercise should exacerbate vascular claudication, but stationary cycling (while sitting with lumbar flexion) should not exacerbate neurogenic claudication. A patient with neurogenic claudication also typically has more pain with downhill walking because of the relative lumbar extension and resultant narrowing of the spinal canal. Uphill walking is more strenuous and can rapidly bring on symptoms of vascular disease.

Peripheral Nerve Disorders

Peripheral polyneuropathy is a common cause of paresthesias in the distal lower limbs and feet that can mimic symptoms of lumbar stenosis. They are often seen together in older adult patients with diabetes. Electrodiagnostic studies can be used to diagnose a superimposed peripheral polyneuropathy in patients who have MRI findings of lumbar stenosis. Epidural steroid injections can sometimes be helpful in this situation to help determine how much of the patient's leg and foot symptoms are related to spinal stenosis over peripheral polyneuropathy. The reason for this is that an epidural steroid injection may improve the symptoms of spinal stenosis syndrome but has no impact on the symptoms of peripheral neuropathy.

Low Back Pain in Special Populations

Low Back Pain in Pregnancy

Low back pain is a common problem in pregnancy. Patients are generally divided into two categories: those with low back pain and those with pelvic girdle pain (pain below the iliac crest, such as sacroiliac joint–related pain). Multiple studies have estimated the prevalence of low back pain in pregnancy at 49% to 76%.[67,122,169,170,246] Risk factors include a history of previous back pain, previous pregnancy-related back pain, and low back pain during menses.[38,246] Low back pain can begin at any time during the pregnancy and generally reaches a peak at 36 weeks.[122,170,246] Pain decreases after this point and in most patients is substantially improved by 3 months postpartum.[170]

A small group of patients will have persistent pain even after postpartum recovery. Risk factors for persistent back pain after pregnancy include having both low back pain and pelvic girdle pain, pain occurring in early pregnancy, weakness of back extensors, older patients, and those with work dissatisfaction.[90]

The etiology of low back pain in the pregnant woman is hypothesized to be attributable to increased biomechanical strain or to an altered hormonal influence. The biomechanical alterations are as a result of changes in spine posture related to the anterior movement of the pregnant woman's center of gravity. An argument against purely biomechanical factors as the primary cause, however, is that the back pain often starts before substantial weight gain by the mother, and the incidence does not parallel the weight gain.[40] A hormonal influence probably exists in the etiology of low back pain in pregnancy. Hormonal changes during pregnancy may alter the lumbopelvic ligaments, which influences the stability of the lumbosacral spine and makes it more vulnerable to loading.[122] A direct correlation between circulating levels of the hormone relaxin and pelvic and back pain, however, is controversial.[4,93,123,133] The prevalence of disk abnormalities on MRI is the same for pregnant and nonpregnant women, thus this might be a source of pain for some pregnant women.[252] Only a few high-quality studies have evaluated therapeutic interventions in pregnancy-related low back pain, and there is not much evidence on which to base recommendations for management.[212] Individualized physical therapy, water aerobics, acupuncture, and massage therapy can be recommended to decrease pain.[70,117,165,251] Instruction on a home exercise program, use of a sacroiliac belt, and back school have not been shown to significantly decrease pain intensity.[63,138,150,164] No data support the use of lumbar-abdominal orthoses that are designed to support the pregnant woman's abdomen. A full discussion regarding the use of medication during pregnancy is beyond the scope of this chapter. In general, any medication use should be discussed with the patient's obstetrician. Even medications generally thought of as safe and well tolerated can have unexpected consequences during pregnancy. For example, the use of NSAIDs in late pregnancy can cause premature closure of the ductus arteriosus and neonatal renal failure.[177] Most antidepressants have not been approved for use during pregnancy, and for most antiseizure medications, such as gabapentin, there is evidence for increased incidence of birth defects in animals, and they have not been well studied in humans.[111]

Pediatric Low Back Pain

In the past, back pain in the pediatric population was considered to be relatively rare, and when present raised a concern for serious pathology. This belief is now known to be untrue. In a subset of studies involving more than 300 children each, the prevalence of back pain was cited between 30% and 51%.[17,85] Severe back pain, which is either relapsing or permanent, was reported in 3% to 15%.[17] An increase in back pain prevalence is noted as the child ages. In a Finnish cohort study, back pain prevalence was reported as 1% in children 7 years old, 6% in those 10 years old, and 18% when 14 years old.[213] Another reported the prevalence at 12% for children 11 years old and 50% for those 15 to 18 years old, which approaches the adult prevalence.[41] The same study reported that the pain is often recurrent but that the experience of back pain is frequently forgotten. Other studies demonstrate that the prevalence of low back pain has the greatest increase during puberty and the time of the maximum growth spurt.[124,236] Risk factors for nonspecific low back pain in the pediatric population include increase in age, female gender, parents with low back pain, hyperlordotic posture, history of spinal trauma, participation in competitive sports, a high level of physical activity, and depression.[17] The literature does not support the following as risk factors for pediatric back pain: being overweight, hamstring tightness, a low level of physical activity, and poor school performance.[17] Sitting appears to be the main exacerbating factor of low back pain in the pediatric population.[17] There also appears to be a positive correlation between low back pain in adolescence and the presence of pain as an adult.[94]

There has been more recent attention focused on the role of backpack use in the development of pediatric low back pain; however, there is still not a proven correlation. Carrying a backpack greater than 7.5% to 15% of the wearer's body weight increases the metabolic demands over what is required to move a person's body weight alone.[132,187] The general recommendation for a child's backpack weight is limited to 10% of body weight.[132] This limit is based on concerns of increasing metabolic costs and not on the risk of back pain development (there are conflicting reports in the literature regarding backpack weight and back pain).[91,132,221,249] Many new backpack designs improve ergonomic fit; however, there are no studies demonstrating their effectiveness in reducing back pain.[132]

Some of the specific causes of low back pain in the pediatric population are listed in Box 33-8. Spondylolysis and isthmic spondylolisthesis often present in young athletes with back pain and have been reported as the most common underlying cause of persistent low back pain

BOX 33-8

Etiology of Pediatric Low Back Pain

- Nonspecific
- Spondylolysis with or without spondylolisthesis
- Lumbar disk herniation
- Slipped vertebral apophysis
- Scheuermann disease
- Diskitis
- Vertebral osteomyelitis
- Neoplasm
- Rheumatic disease
- Somatization

among children and adolescents.[151] Most believe the etiology is from overuse, particularly during the growth spurt. The presence of isthmic defects in children in the Western world is between 2% and 7%, and as high as 30% in elite athletes.[168]

Scheuermann disease typically presents in the adolescent as painless exaggerated thoracic kyphosis. From a postural standpoint, the teenager typically presents with excessive thoracic kyphosis (which is demonstrated to be fixed in attempted hyperextension), with a compensatory lumbar hyperlordosis. Radiographic criteria for the diagnosis of Scheuermann disease include anterior wedging of at least three adjacent vertebrae, end-plate irregularities, Schmorl nodes, and disk-space narrowing.[89] These findings are present equally in the adolescent population without back pain, but there is a higher prevalence of concomitant degenerative disk changes in those with pain.[218]

The etiology of Scheuermann disease is uncertain. Some believe that it is attributable to repetitive loading of the immature spine that might have some preexisting abnormality of the cartilaginous end plate.[104] There does appear to be a familial link.[149] Scheuermann disease can have a benign course, although some untreated patients develop progressive structural kyphosis. Brace wearing is recommended until skeletal maturity is reached to help prevent the progressive kyphosis.

Idiopathic scoliosis is not generally painful. If associated with pain, often there is more serious underlying pathology such as tumor, infection, or spondylolisthesis. The curve direction in idiopathic scoliosis is typically right thoracic and left lumbar. If an atypical curve is encountered, further evaluation beyond plain films is generally warranted.

Neoplastic disease of the pediatric spine is fortunately rare. Most pediatric spinal tumors are primary (not metastatic) benign bone tumors arising from the vertebrae.[104] The most common tumors of the pediatric spine include osteoid osteoma, osteoblastoma, and aneurysmal bone cysts. The classic pain of osteoid osteoma is nocturnal pain that responds to aspirin. The most frequent malignant lesion affecting the pediatric spine is Ewing's sarcoma.

ACKNOWLEDGMENT: The authors would like to thank Mia Coleman for her assistance in preparing this manuscript.

KEY REFERENCES

1. Akuthota V, Lento P, Sowa G: Pathogenesis of lumbar spinal stenosis pain: why does an asymptomatic stenotic patient flare? *Phys Med Rehabil Clin N Am* 14:17–28, 2003.
6. Amundsen T, Weber H, Nordal HJ, et al: Lumbar spinal stenosis: conservative or surgical management? A prospective 10-year study, *Spine* 25:1424–1435, 2000.
8. Andersson GB, Johnsson B, Nachemson AL: Intradiscal pressure, intra-abdominal pressure and myoelectric back muscle activity related to posture and loading, *Clin Orthop* 129:156–164, 1977.
13. Assendelft WJ, Morton SC, Yu EI, et al: Spinal manipulative therapy for low back pain: a meta-analysis of effectiveness relative to other therapies, *Ann Intern Med* 138:871–881, 2003.
19. Bartleson JD: Evidence for and against the use of opioid analgesics for chronic nonmalignant low back pain: a review, *Pain Med* 3:260–271, 2002.
21. Beinart NA, Goodchild CE, Weinman JA, et al: Individual and intervention-related factors associated with adherence to home exercise in chronic low back pain: a systematic review, *Spine J* 13:1940–1950, 2013.
23. Bigos SJ, Holland J, Holland C, et al: High-quality controlled trials on preventing episodes of back problems: systematic literature review in working-age adults, *Spine J* 9:147–168, 2009.
25. Boden SD, Davis DO, Dina TS, et al: Abnormal magnetic-resonance scans of the lumbar spine in asymptomatic subjects: a prospective investigation, *J Bone Joint Surg Am* 72:403–408, 1990.
31. Low back pain. In Bogduk N, editor: *Clinical and radiological anatomy of the lumbar spine and sacrum*, ed 5, Edinburgh, 2012, Churchill Livingstone.
34. Bresnahan BW, Rundell SD, Dagadakis MC, et al: A systematic review to assess comparative effectiveness studies in epidural steroid injections for lumbar spinal stenosis and to estimate reimbursement amounts, *PM R* 5:705–714, 2013.
46. Chaparro LE, Furlan AD, Deshpande A, et al: Opioids compared with placebo or other treatments for chronic low back pain: an update of the Cochrane Review, *Spine (Phila Pa 1976)* 39:556–563, 2014.
48. Chiodo A, Haig AJ: Lumbosacral radiculopathies: conservative approaches to management, *Phys Med Rehabil Clin N Am* 13:609–621, 2002.
50. Chou R, Huffman LH: Medications for acute and chronic low back pain: a review of the evidence for an American Pain Society/American College of Physicians clinical practice guideline, *Ann Intern Med* 147:505–514, 2007.
51. Chou R, Shekelle P: Will this patient develop persistent disabling low back pain? *JAMA* 303:1295–1302, 2010.
59. Deyo RA, Rainville J, Kent DL: What can the history and physical examination tell us about back pain? *JAMA* 268:760–765, 1992.
62. Dreyfuss P, Michaelsen M, Pauza K, et al: The value of medical history and physical examination in diagnosing sacroiliac joint pain, *Spine* 21:2594–2602, 1996.
65. El Rassi G, Takemitsu M, Glutting J, Shah SA: Effect of sports modification on clinical outcome in children and adolescent athletes with symptomatic lumbar spondylolysis, *Am J Phys Med Rehabil* 92:1070–1074, 2013.
80. Garber CE, Blissmer B, Deschenes MR, et al: American College of Sports Medicine position stand. Quantity and quality of exercise for developing and maintaining cardiorespiratory, musculoskeletal, and neuromotor fitness in apparently healthy adults: guidance for prescribing exercise, *Med Sci Sports Exerc* 43:1334–1359, 2011.
98. Hayden JA, van Tulder MW, Tomlinson G: Systematic review: strategies for using exercise therapy to improve outcomes in chronic low back pain, *Ann Intern Med* 142:776–785, 2005.
106. Jacques P, Mielants H, De Vos M, et al: Spondyloarthropathies: progress and challenges, *Best Pract Res Clin Rheumatol* 22:325–337, 2008.
114. Kendall FP, McCreary EK: *Trunk muscles in muscle testing and function*, Philadelphia, 1983, Lippincott Williams & Wilkins.
118. Kirkaldy-Willis WH, Wedge JH, Yong-Hing K, et al: Pathology and pathogenesis of lumbar spondylosis and stenosis, *Spine* 3:319–328, 1978.
126. Liddle SD, Baxter GD, Gracey JH: Exercise and chronic low back pain: what works? *Pain* 107:176–190, 2004.
128. Linton SJ, van Tulder MW: Preventive interventions for back and neck pain. In Nachemson AL, Johnsson B, editors: *Neck and back pain: the scientific evidence of causes, diagnosis, and treatment*, Philadelphia, 2000, Lippincott Williams & Wilkins.
131. Macedo LG, Maher CG, Latimer J, et al: Motor control exercise for persistent, nonspecific low back pain: a systematic review, *Phys Ther* 89:9–25, 2009.
136. Main CJ, Waddell G: *Beliefs about back pain. The back pain revolution*, Edinburgh, 2004, Churchill Livingstone.
145. McCarron RF, Wimpee MW, Hudkins PG, et al: The inflammatory effect of nucleus pulposus: a possible element in the pathogenesis of low-back pain, *Spine* 12:760–764, 1987.
170. Ostgaard HC, Zetherstrom G, Roos-Hansson E: Back pain in relation to pregnancy: a 6-year follow-up, *Spine* 22:2945–2950, 1997.
175. Pengel LH, Herbert RD, Maher CG, Refshauge KM: Acute low back pain: systematic review of its prognosis, *BMJ* 327:323, 2003.
188. Robinson LR: Electromyography, magnetic resonance imaging, and radiculopathy: it's time to focus on specificity, *Muscle Nerve* 22:149–150, 1999.
194. Deleted in review.
208. Spinhoven P, Ter Kuile M, Kole-Snijders AM, et al: Catastrophizing and internal pain control as mediators of outcome in the multidisciplinary treatment of chronic low back pain, *Eur J Pain* 8:211–219, 2004.

212. Stuge B, Hilde G, Vollestad N: Physical therapy for pregnancy-related low back and pelvic pain: a systematic review, *Acta Obstet Gynecol Scand* 82:983–990, 2003.
223. Urquhart DM, Hoving JL, Assendelft WW, et al: Antidepressants for non-specific low back pain, *Cochrane Database Syst Rev* (1):CD001703, 2008.
224. van Middelkoop M, Rubinstein SM, Kuijpers T, et al: A systematic review on the effectiveness of physical and rehabilitation interventions for chronic non-specific low back pain, *Eur Spine J* 20:19–39, 2011.
248. Waterschoot FP, Dijkstra PU, Hollak N, et al: Dose or content? Effectiveness of pain rehabilitation programs for patients with chronic low back pain: a systematic review, *Pain* 155:179–189, 2014.
253. Weinstein JN, Lurie JD, Tosteson TD, et al: Surgical vs nonoperative treatment for lumbar disk herniation: the Spine Patient Outcomes Research Trial (sport) observational cohort, *JAMA* 296:2451–2459, 2006.
255. Wertli MM, Burgstaller JM, Weiser S, et al: Influence of catastrophizing on treatment outcome in patients with nonspecific low back pain: a systematic review, *Spine (Phila Pa 1976)* 39:263–273, 2014.
256. Wiltse LL, Winter RB: Terminology and measurement of spondylolisthesis, *J Bone Joint Surg Am* 65:768–772, 1983.

The full reference list for this chapter is available online.

CHAPTER 34

OSTEOPOROSIS

Mehrsheed Sinaki

Bone, to be maintained, needs to be mechanically strained—within its biomechanical competence.

Mehrsheed Sinaki, MD, MS

Osteoporosis consists of a heterogeneous group of syndromes in which bone mass per unit volume is reduced in otherwise healthy bone, resulting in fragile bone. The increment in bone porosity results in architectural instability of bone and increases the likelihood of fracture. The mineral/matrix ratio is normal in osteoporosis, but in osteomalacia the mineral content is markedly reduced.

Clinicians can add quality to the years of life of patients with osteoporosis through the use of an interdisciplinary approach. This condition is the most prevalent metabolic bone disease in the United States and is a major public health problem. The direct and indirect cost of osteoporosis in the United States alone is estimated to be more than $14 billion annually.[93] Much of this expense relates to hip fractures. In 15% to 20% of hip fracture cases, the outcome is fatal.

The World Health Organization has defined osteoporosis as bone mineral density (BMD) of 2.5 standard deviations below the peak mean bone mass of young healthy adults.[1] The T score shows the amount of one's bone density compared with a young adult (at the age of 35 years) of the same gender with peak bone mass. The Z score is calculated in the same way, but the comparison is made with someone of the same age, gender, race, height, and weight. The Z score is adjusted for an individual's age, and the T score is not. For example, a 75-year-old woman with a Z score of −1.0 is one standard deviation below the BMD of an average 75-year-old woman, but her T score may be −3.0 because she is three standard deviations below the BMD of an average 35-year-old woman. Normal BMD is a T score −1 or greater; osteopenia, a T score between −1 and −2.5; osteoporosis, a T score −2.5 or less; and severe osteoporosis, a T score −2.5 or less with fracture. In the asymptomatic stage, osteoporosis is characterized simply by decreased bone mass without fracture. Osteoporosis becomes clinically problematic only when the bone fractures.

Bone Function and Structure

Bone serves as a mechanical support for musculoskeletal structures, as protection for vital organs, and as a metabolic source of ions, especially calcium and phosphate. Despite its appearance, bone is an active tissue. To maintain its biomechanical competence, bone tissue undergoes continuous change and renewal so that older bone tissue is replaced by newly formed bone tissue. Approximately 20% of bone tissue is replaced annually by this cyclic process. There are two types of bone cells: osteoclasts, which resorb the calcified matrix, and osteoblasts, which synthesize new bone matrix.[57]

Osteoclasts are localized on the endosteal bone surfaces. Their origin is hematopoietic, and they share a common precursor with the monocyte macrophage. Osteoclasts are large multinucleated cells with an average of 10 to 20 nuclei. They have a special cell membrane with folds that invaginate at the interface with bone surface, called the *ruffled border*. To induce resorption of bone and the mineralized bone matrix, osteoclasts produce proteolytic enzymes in this ruffled border.

Osteoblasts are derived from mesenchymal cells. The role of osteoblasts is mineralization of the matrix through budding of vesicles from their cytoplasmic membrane. These vesicles are rich in alkaline phosphatase. Osteoblasts secrete all the growth factors that are trapped in the matrix.

Bone Remodeling

Bone remodeling is a process that allows removal of old bone and replacement with new bone tissue. This process allows maintenance of the biomechanical integrity of the skeleton, and it supports the role of bone in the provision of an ionic bank for body and mechanical support. Bone remodeling has five phases.

1. *Activation:* Osteoclastic activity is recruited.
2. *Resorption:* Osteoclasts erode bone and form a cavity.
3. *Reversal:* Osteoblasts are recruited.
4. *Formation:* Osteoblasts replace the cavity with new bone.
5. *Quiescence:* Bone tissue remains dormant until the next cycle starts.

This process is cyclical, starting with bone resorption and finishing with bone formation. In adult human bone, each cycle of remodeling lasts 3 to 12 months. The signal that stops osteoclastic activity is not yet completely defined. After bone resorption, the reversal phase starts, which involves osteoblastic activity. Osteoblasts start to fill the resorption cavity. During the process of osteoclastic activity, the growth factors that are stored in the bone matrix are released and subsequently stimulate osteoblastic proliferation.

This process of bone resorption and formation is called *coupling*. The ideal situation in the coupling process is equilibrated bone formation and resorption. In osteoporosis, however, there is disequilibrium between resorption and formation, as coupling favors resorption that results in bone loss.

The number of active remodeling units in trabecular bone is approximately three times greater than in cortical bone. The physical endurance of any bone is affected by the percentage of cortical bone involved in its structure. Trabecular bone is more active metabolically than cortical bone because of the considerable surface exposure areas. Consequently, more bone loss occurs at the trabecular areas when resorption is greater than formation. The vertebrae consist of 50% trabecular bone and 50% cortical bone, whereas the femoral neck consists of 30% trabecular bone and 70% cortical bone. When bone turnover increases, bone loss and osteoporosis occur in the vertebrae before they occur in the femoral neck.

Pathogenesis

Peak adult bone mass is achieved between ages 30 and 35 years. Bone mass at any point in life thereafter is the difference between the peak adult bone mass and the amount that has been lost since the peak was reached. Age-related bone loss is a universal phenomenon in humans. Any circumstances that limit bone formation or increase bone loss increase the likelihood that osteoporosis will develop later in life. Measures that can maximize peak adult bone mass are clearly desirable.

Trabecular (or cancellous) bone represents approximately 20% of skeletal bone mass and makes up 80% of the turnover media. The cortex makes up only 20% of the turnover media and is made of compact bone, which represents 80% of skeletal bone mass. In both cortical and trabecular bone, bone remodeling is initiated with the activation of osteoclasts. The resulting resorption sites are then refilled by osteoblastic activities, a process called *bone formation*. If the amount of bone resorbed equals the amount formed, the bone loss is zero. The remodeling process does not result in zero balance after age 30 to 35 years, however, and after this age the normal process of remodeling results in bone loss.[53]

Certain conditions, such as hyperparathyroidism or thyrotoxicosis, can increase the rate of bone remodeling. These conditions increase the rate of bone loss, which results in high-turnover osteoporosis. The secondary causes of osteoporosis are associated with an increased rate of activation of the remodeling cycle. Although factors such as calcium intake, smoking, alcohol consumption, physical exercise, and menopause are important factors in determining BMD, genetic factors are the major determinant and contribute to 80% of the variance in peak BMD.[16] Fracture incidence related to osteoporosis is lower in men than in women because the diameter of vertebral bodies and long bones is greater in men at maturity and bone loss is less (about half that of women) throughout life.[58]

Classification of Osteoporosis

Osteoporosis can be primary or secondary to other disorders that result in bone loss. The most common causes of osteoporosis are listed in Box 34-1. The most common type of osteoporosis is either postmenopausal or age-related.[46]

BOX 34-1

Common Causes of Osteoporosis

Hereditary, Congenital

- Osteogenesis imperfecta, neurologic disturbances (myotonia congenita, Werdnig-Hoffmann disease), gonadal dysgenesis

Acquired (Primary and Secondary)

Generalized

- Idiopathic (in premenopausal women and middle-aged or young men; juvenile osteoporosis)
- Postmenopausal
- Age-related
- Endocrine disorders: Acromegaly, hyperthyroidism, Cushing's syndrome (iatrogenic or endogenous), hyperparathyroidism, diabetes mellitus (?), hypogonadism
- Nutritional problems: Malnutrition, anorexia or bulimia, vitamin deficiency (C or D), vitamin overuse (A or D), calcium deficiency, high sodium intake, high caffeine intake, high protein intake, high phosphate intake, alcohol abuse
- Sedentary lifestyle, immobility, smoking
- Gastrointestinal diseases (liver disease, malabsorption syndromes, alactasia, subtotal gastrectomy) or small bowel resection
- Nephropathies
- Chronic obstructive pulmonary disease
- Malignancy (multiple myeloma, disseminated carcinoma)
- Drug use: Phenytoin, barbiturates, cholestyramine, heparin, excess thyroid hormone replacement, glucocorticoids

Localized

- Inflammatory arthritis, fractures and immobilization in cast, limb dystrophies, muscular paralysis

Primary osteoporosis is the rare disorder of idiopathic juvenile osteoporosis. This type of osteoporosis typically occurs before puberty (between ages 8 and 14 years), and patients present with osteoporosis that is progressive over 2 to 4 years in association with multiple axial or axioappendicular fractures. Remission usually occurs by the end of the 2- to 4-year course.[34] In this type of osteoporosis, the process of bone formation is normal but osteoclastic activity increases, resulting in increased bone resorption. Idiopathic juvenile osteoporosis is most evident in the thoracic and lumbar spine and needs to be distinguished from juvenile epiphysitis or Scheuermann disease. It is usually self-limiting, but the radiographic appearance might not return to normal. The laboratory values are typically normal, and the diagnosis is made by exclusion.

Hormones and Physiology of Bone

The rate of bone remodeling can be increased by parathyroid hormone (PTH), thyroxine, growth hormone, and vitamin D (1,25-dihydroxyvitamin D_3 [1,25$(OH)_2D_3$]) and decreased by calcitonin, estrogen, and glucocorticoids.[38]

The major hormone for calcium homeostasis is PTH. It is secreted by the parathyroid glands, which are located behind the thyroid glands. The level of plasma calcium is the major moderator of the secretion of PTH, which regulates the plasma calcium ion (Ca^{2+}) concentration in three ways:

1. In the presence of active vitamin D, PTH stimulates bone resorption and the release of calcium and phosphate.
2. Through production of calcitriol in the kidneys, it indirectly increases intestinal absorption of calcium and phosphate.
3. It increases active reabsorption of calcium ions in the renal distal tubal area.

PTH also reduces proximal tubular reabsorption of phosphate. In general, PTH increases serum calcium concentration and primarily tends to decrease serum phosphate concentration.

Calcitonin is a hormone secreted by the parafollicular cells of the thyroid gland. The major stimulus of calcitonin production is the serum level of calcium. Calcitonin directly prohibits calcium and phosphate resorption through inhibition of osteoclastic activity, lowering the serum calcium level.

The main regulators of vitamin D synthesis are the serum concentrations of $1{,}25(OH)_2D_3$, calcium, phosphate, and PTH. Vitamin D can also be synthesized through exposure to the sun and conversion in the liver. PTH is the major inducer of the production of the active form of vitamin D in the kidney. This function is accomplished through the effect of the enzyme 1-α-hydroxylase, which transforms the inactive form of vitamin D to the potent form. The active form of vitamin D increases intestinal absorption of calcium and phosphate. Vitamin D is also required for appropriate bone mineralization. The influence of the active form of vitamin D is both a direct effect through stimulating osteoblastic activity and an indirect effect through increasing the intestinal absorption of calcium and phosphorus.

Role of Sex Steroids

The main endocrine function that occurs at menopause is loss of secretion of estrogen and progesterone from the ovaries.[38,58] The premenopausal ovary produces primarily estradiol. Progesterone secretion, which occurs cyclically after ovulation in the premenopausal stage, also decreases to very low levels in the postmenopausal stage. These changes in circulating sex steroids are gradual in a woman's sexual reproductive life. The premenopausal ovary also produces androgens, especially testosterone. The circulating testosterone levels decrease after menopause. The major source of estrogen in postmenopausal women is conversion from dehydroepiandrosterone. The latter is then converted into androstenedione, which changes into estrone in fat cells. Estrone is the major source of estrogen in postmenopausal women.

Men do not have the equivalent of menopause, but in some elderly men bone mass decreases along with a decline in gonadal function. The testosterone level in men decreases with age as a result of a decreased number of Leydig cells in the testes. Male hypogonadism is typically associated with bone loss.[47]

Other Factors Affecting Bone Mass

Several other factors can contribute to the reduction of sex-related steroid levels. In hyperprolactinemia, which is attributable to a prolactin-secreting pituitary tumor, failure of the gonadal axis results in a substantial loss of bone. Amenorrheic athletes who exercise excessively, such as high-mileage runners or ballet dancers, who have lower-than-normal body weight, have lower circulating estradiol, progesterone, and prolactin levels. Their amenorrhea is associated with hypothalamic hypogonadism, which leads to excessive bone loss. This bone loss can be mostly reversed when training distances are decreased.[21] With weight gain and improvement in nutrition, these young women can facilitate resumption of menses and reversal of bone loss.[10,21,96] Reduction of sex steroid concentrations is not the only cause of bone loss. Other factors such as race, genetics, nutrition, physical exercise, and lifestyle can also contribute to the rate of bone loss after an ovariectomy or natural menopause.[61] It is well known that bone must be physically stressed to be maintained. A considerable body of data shows that the rate of change in strain also influences bone growth and remodeling.[43]

Effect of Aging on Bone Mass

In the normal aging process, there is an imbalance between resorption and formation because osteoblastic activity is not equal to osteoclastic activity. The result of the remodeling process is bone loss during each cycle of remodeling. Bone loss occurs even when the remodeling process is not increased. In fact, activation of skeletal remodeling is decreased as a result of the aging process. This decreased activation gives rise to the concept of low-turnover osteoporosis, which occurs concomitantly with the aging process.

Age plays a considerable role in the rate of bone turnover. It has been clearly determined that bone turnover increases in women at menopause, but bone turnover does not increase substantially in men with aging. Most studies have shown that plasma levels of the active form of vitamin D, $1{,}25(OH)_2D_3$, decrease with age by approximately 50% in both men and women.

Growth hormone stimulates renal production of $1{,}25(OH)_2D_3$. Growth hormone production decreases with age. Secretion of growth hormone is reduced in patients with osteoporosis. Growth hormone and insulin-like growth factor 1 have several positive effects on calcium homeostasis, including synthesis of $1{,}25(OH)_2D_3$, osteoblast proliferation, osteoclast formation, and bone resorption.

It appears that special forms of vitamin K therapy in elderly persons can be associated with a reduction in the rate of bone resorption, demonstrated by decreased excretion of urinary hydroxyproline. Further studies are needed in this area. Studies have shown that calcium absorption is less efficient in elderly people.[31] Bone loss has also been related to deficiencies in trace metal elements, such as copper, zinc, and magnesium, but this issue is not fully resolved.

Plasma calcitonin levels are higher in men than in women. Calcitonin levels do not change with age. Studies have shown that estrogens stimulate calcitonin secretion.[91] Thyroid hormone levels typically show no change or are slightly decreased with age. The PTH level increases with age, perhaps because of mild hypocalcemia and decreased $1,25(OH)_2D_3$ concentration. This reduction in the active form of vitamin D can be as a result of decreased consumption of dietary vitamin D, decreased exposure to sunlight, decreased skin capacity for vitamin D conversion, reduced intestinal absorption, and reduced 1-α-hydroxylase activity.

Several studies have shown that the level of physical activity decreases with aging.[64,69] This is important because physical strain and mechanical load also positively affect bone mass.[23] Female gymnasts, both children and college-aged athletes, reportedly have higher BMD than swimmers.[9,19] Exercise is known to stimulate the release of growth hormone or other trophic factors that can stimulate osteoblastic activity.[20] Optimal nutrition and physical activity are necessary to achieve the genetic potential for bone mass. The peak bone mass attained by early adulthood is a major determinant of bone mass in later life. Nutrition can also affect both bone matrix formation and bone mineralization. In general, in estrogen-deficient women, calcium intake of 1500 mg/day and 800 international units/day of vitamin D are recommended.

Clinical Manifestations of Osteoporosis

Osteoporosis is typically a "silent disease" until fractures occur. Osteoporotic vertebral fractures can go unnoticed until they are incidentally seen on a chest radiograph. Appendicular fractures, however, typically require immediate attention. The fact that a fracture resulted from osteoporosis should not affect the orthopedic method of management. The most common areas for osteoporotic fractures are the midthoracic and upper-lumbar spine (Figure 34-1),[84] hip (proximal femur), and distal forearm (Colles fracture). The highest incidence of fractures is in white women. The female/male ratio is approximately 7:1 for vertebral fractures, 2:1 for hip fractures, and 5:1 for Colles fractures. It has been estimated that after menopause, a woman's lifetime risk of sustaining an osteoporotic fracture is 1 in 2 or 3.[42]

Hip fracture is the greatest concern clinically because the risk of death with osteoporotic hip fracture is 15% to 20%. This is despite all the modern developments in surgical and nonsurgical intervention. The management of an osteoporotic spine fracture requires immobilization of the involved vertebral bodies and analgesia. Fortunately, these fractures heal through becoming more condensed and, unlike appendicular fractures, typically do not require any specific treatment. If there is nonunion of the appendicular fracture, one needs to look for conditions other than osteoporosis, such as osteomalacia or hyperparathyroidism. The duration of immobilization should be for only a limited time, sufficient to ensure the primary fracture-healing process. Prolonged immobilization is discouraged because it can contribute to additional osteoporosis.

The orthopedic management for most osteoporotic fractures is generally noncontroversial, except for the management of hip fracture. The management of femoral neck fracture creates a great deal of controversy because of the high complication rate. Efforts are ongoing to solve these controversies through prospective studies. Despite these efforts, the treatment of hip fracture remains a challenge, and each case creates an emergency situation. Shoulder fracture, especially fracture in the surgical neck of the proximal humerus, is not uncommon in elderly women. This type of fracture usually occurs from an impact force directly to the shoulder during a fall. A conservative treatment regimen typically suffices for this fracture.

Fractures and Management

The relationship between bone mass and spinal fractures has been extensively studied, and it is known that fracture risk increases as bone mass decreases. For every standard deviation of decrease in BMD, the risk of osteoporotic fracture of the spine increases 1.5- to 2-fold, and the risk

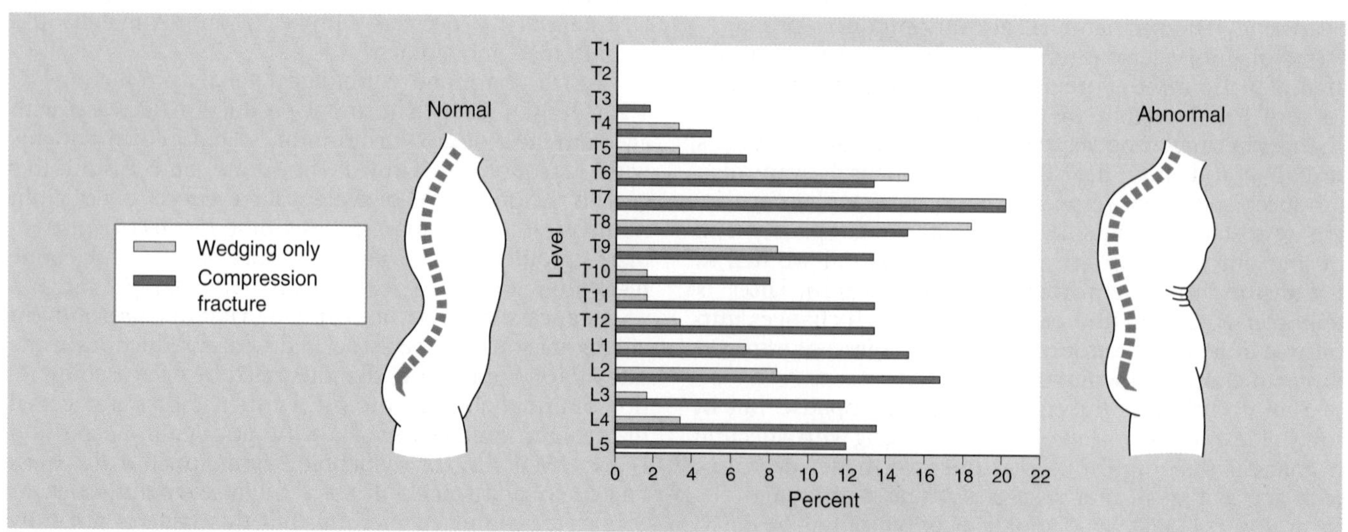

FIGURE 34-1 Incidence of wedging and compression fractures at various levels of the spine. (Modified from Sinaki M, Mikkelsen BA: Postmenopausal spinal osteoporosis: flexion versus extension exercises, *Arch Phys Med Rehabil* 65:593-596, 1984, with permission.)

BOX 34-2

Management of Acute Pain in Patients With Osteoporosis

- Bed rest (2 days): Substantial bone loss is not likely to occur with 2 days of bed rest
- Analgesics: Avoid constipating medicines, such as codeine derivatives
- Avoidance of constipation
- Physical therapy: Initially cold packs, then mild heat and stroking massage
- Avoidance of exertional exercises
- Knowledge of lifting and standing principles to avoid excessive spinal strain
- Back supports if needed to decrease pain and expedite ambulation
- Gait aids if needed

BOX 34-3

Factors Contributing to Risk for Falls

Extrinsic

- Environmental: Obstacles, slippery floors, uneven surfaces, poor illumination, stairs not well defined, pets, icy sidewalks
- Extraskeletal: Inappropriate footwear, obstructive clothing

Intrinsic

- Intraskeletal: Lower-extremity weakness (neurogenic or myopathic), balance disorder (vestibular dysequilibrium, peripheral neuropathy, hyperkyphosis), visual impairment, bifocal use, vestibular changes, cognitive decline, decreased coordination (cerebellar degeneration), postural changes, imbalance, gait unsteadiness, gait apraxia, reduced muscle strength, reduced flexibility, orthopnea, postural hypotension, cardiovascular deconditioning, iatrogenically reduced alertness

of hip fracture increases 2.6-fold.[29] Another predictor of fracture risk is age itself. The risk of fracture as a result of osteoporosis doubles every 5 to 7 years.[29] It is not clear whether age-related changes in bone density or bone quality are factors that increase the risk of fractures caused by falls.

Vertebral Fracture

The incidence of vertebral fractures is poorly understood because 50% of these fractures can be subclinical and the patient might not seek medical attention. Vertebral fractures can create both acute and chronic pain.

Acute pain that occurs in the absence of a previous fracture is usually as a result of compression fractures of the vertebrae. Sometimes, a minor fall or even an affectionate hug can cause a compression fracture. The compressed vertebrae might not be apparent on radiographs for up to 4 weeks after the injury.[46] Compression fractures usually result in acute pain that later resolves (Box 34-2).[65] The spinal deformity that can result from these fractures can produce chronic pain.[65]

Kyphotic postural change is the most physically disfiguring and psychologically damaging effect of osteoporosis.[77] The incidence of osteoporosis and kyphosis can be substantially decreased only by early detection and subsequent intervention in high-risk patients.

Disproportionate weakness in back extensor musculature relative to body weight or spinal flexor strength considerably increases the possibility of compressing the vertebrae in the fragile osteoporotic spine. Recognition and improvement of decreased back extensor strength can enhance the ability to maintain proper vertical alignment.[59] The geriatric population has an increased risk of debilitating postural changes because of several factors, the two most apparent being a greater prevalence of osteoporosis and an involutional loss of functional muscle motor units.[26,41] Development of kyphotic posture not only can predispose to postural back pain but can also increase the risk of falls.[40] Several other factors can also contribute to the risk for falls (Box 34-3).

Chronic spinal pain can be attributable to the deformity caused by vertebral wedging and compression, as well as

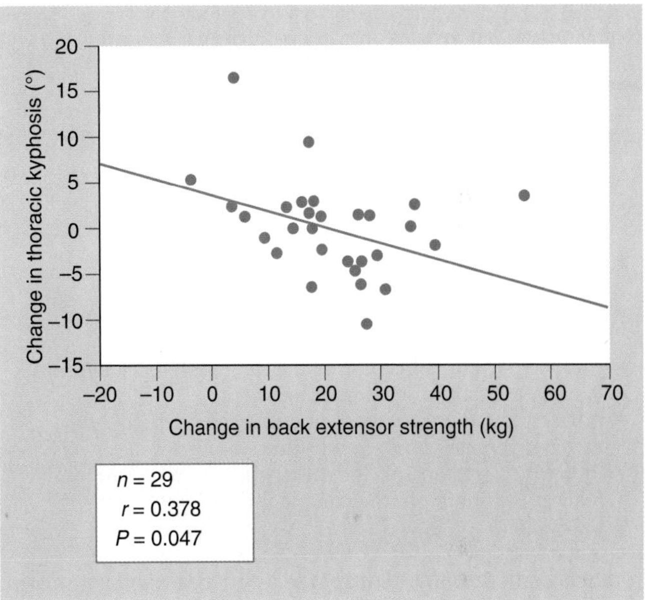

FIGURE 34-2 Correlation between change in back extensor strength and change in thoracic kyphosis in 29 healthy estrogen-deficient women with hyperkyphosis (≥34.1 degrees). A significant negative correlation was found. (Modified from Itoi E, Sinaki M: Effect of back-strengthening exercise on posture in healthy women 49 to 65 years of age, *Mayo Clin Proc* 69:1054-1059, 1994, with permission of Mayo Foundation for Medical Education and Research.)

by secondary ligamentous strain. These deformities are often difficult to distinguish from the usually associated disk deterioration. The intervertebral disks undergo the most dramatic age-related changes of all connective tissues.[2] With aging, there is an increase in the number and diameter of the collagen fibrils in the disk. This change is accompanied by a progressive decrease in disk resilience, and loss of distinction between the nucleus pulposus and the annulus fibrosus eventually occurs.

Chronic back pain secondary to osteoporosis is related to postural changes resulting from vertebral fractures.[77,80] Strong back muscles contribute to good posture and skeletal support (Figure 34-2).[32,89,90] One controlled study showed the long-term effects of back extensor resistance training 8 years after cessation of the exercise.[81,82] None of the women in either group in the study received hormone

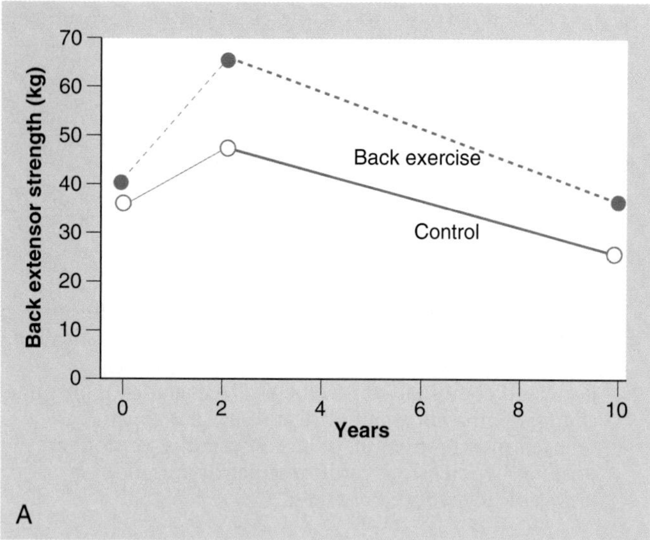

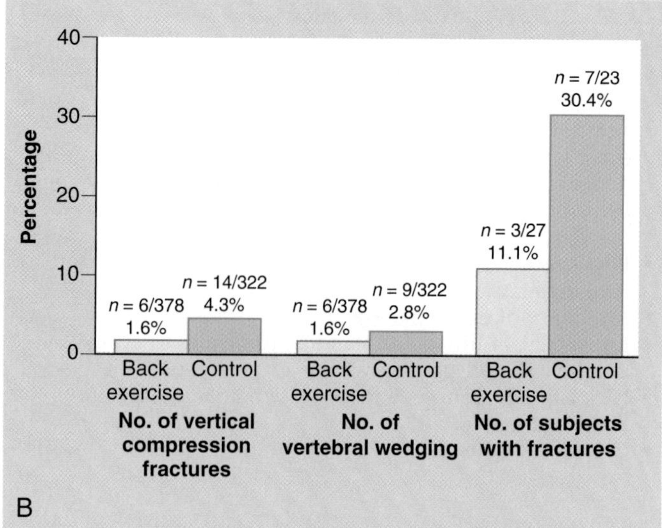

FIGURE 34-3 At 10-year follow-up evaluation, (**A**) back extensor strength and (**B**) vertebral compression fractures were found in 14 of 322 vertebral bodies examined (4.3%) in the control group and 6 of 378 vertebral bodies examined (1.6%) in the back extension exercise group (χ^2 test, $P = 0.029$). The number of control subjects with vertebral fractures was three times greater in the control group than in the back exercise group. (Modified from Sinaki M: Critical appraisal of physical rehabilitation measures after osteoporotic vertebral fracture, *Osteoporos Int* 14:773-779, 2003. Erratum: *Osteoporos Int* 17(11):1702, 2006, used with permission.)

BOX 34-4

Management of Chronic Pain in Patients With Osteoporosis

- Improve faulty posture; may need weighted kypho-orthosis
- Manage pain (ultrasound, massage, or transcutaneous electrical nerve stimulation)
- If cause of pain is beyond correction, apply back support to decrease painful stretch of ligaments
- Advise the patient to avoid physical activities that exert extreme vertical compression forces on vertebrae
- Prescribe a patient-specific therapeutic exercise program
- Start appropriate pharmacologic intervention

replacement therapy. Compared with the exercise group, the control group had a 2.7-times greater number of vertebral fractures at 10-year follow-up evaluation.[81] The pain and skeletal deformity associated with osteoporosis might secondarily reduce muscle strength. The reduction in muscle strength can further exacerbate the postural abnormalities associated with this condition (Figure 34-3).[32]

Chronic pain can also be attributable to microfractures that are visible only on bone scanning and can occur continuously. Management of chronic osteoporosis-related pain is outlined in Box 34-4. Prescription of opiate analgesics, such as codeine sulfate or its derivatives, should be undertaken judiciously, as their use can cause constipation.[65]

New Hypothesis on the Most Effective Exercise to Reduce the Risk for Vertebral Fracture

After a 10-year follow-up study,[81] the author developed the following hypothesis: "Back resistive exercises performed in a prone position (nonloading) rather than in vertical loading position can decrease risk of vertebral fractures through improvement of horizontal trabeculae."[68] The exercise needs to be progressive, resistive, and nonloading to avoid vertebral compression fracture.

Vertebroplasty and Kyphoplasty

Vertebroplasty and kyphoplasty procedures are used for the management of vertebral fractures.[35,78] These procedures involve the injection of acrylic cement (such as polymethylmethacrylate) into a partially collapsed vertebral body. Jensen et al.[33] found that 63% of patients with osteoporosis who underwent vertebroplasty decreased their use of opiates and analgesics for pain control, 7% increased their use, and 30% continued on the same use. More recently, two multicenter randomized controlled trials evaluating vertebroplasty demonstrated no significant difference in pain relief when compared with a sham procedure.[8,35] Vertebroplasty does not substitute for rehabilitative measures that are needed after fracture.[30,50] One study showed considerably fewer vertebral refractures after vertebroplasty in patients who received instruction for back extension exercises.[30] The author recommends a rehabilitation program, especially back extension exercises, for osteoporosis management.[78]

Hip Fracture

Falls and hip fractures can be life-threatening.[45,92] In addition to weakness of the lower limbs, one of the contributing factors to falls is disequilibrium of individuals with spinal kyphotic posture.[73] The kyphotic posture places the center of gravity closer to the limit of stability.[74] Measures that reduce instability, such as exercise programs for equilibrium, including tai chi, some yoga poses,[71] and use of a weighted kypho-orthosis (WKO), as in the Spinal Proprioceptive Extension Exercise Dynamic (SPEED) program, can reduce both the fear of falls and the risk of falls (Figure 34-4).[74]

Hip fracture is an emergency situation. In typical cases, the limb is rotated outward (externally rotated) and shortened. It is difficult to tell from the clinical evaluation whether the fracture is intracapsular (femoral neck fracture) or extracapsular (trochanteric fracture). Radiographs are necessary to make this distinction because the operative treatment and the outcome of intracapsular versus extracapsular hip fractures differ considerably. The consensus is that surgery is the treatment of choice for both femoral neck fracture and trochanteric hip fracture. In some unusual cases of impacted fracture, however, conservative treatment might be advisable. This is particularly true when the patient is severely debilitated and has impaired general health.

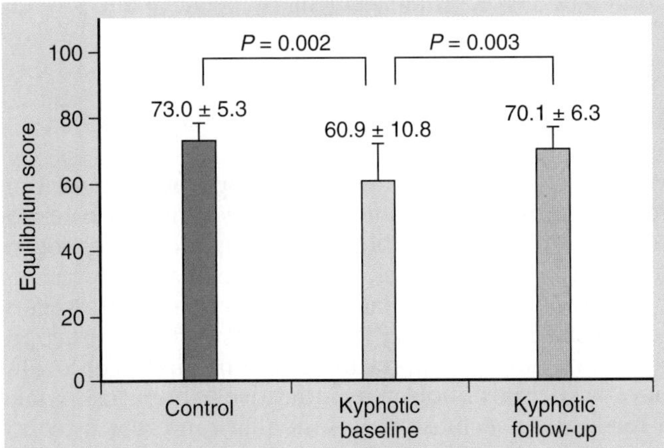

FIGURE 34-4 Composite score of computerized dynamic posturography in control subjects and subjects with osteoporosis-kyphosis at baseline and at follow-up evaluation. Patients with kyphosis improved significantly after a 4-week trial of a spinal proprioceptive extension exercise dynamic program and spinal weighted kypho-orthosis. Data are presented as mean ± standard deviation. A score of 68 or more is normal for age 60 years or older. (From Sinaki M, Brey RH, Hughes CA, et al: Significant reduction in risk of falls and back pain in osteoporotic-kyphotic women through a Spinal Proprioceptive Extension Exercise Dynamic (SPEED) program, *Mayo Clin Proc* 80:849-855, 2005, used with permission of Mayo Foundation for Medical Education and Research.)

Femoral neck fracture requires fixation, and the type of fixation differs among surgeons. Because of the high incidence of operative failures after internal fixation of these fractures, most orthopedists prefer arthroplasties. Some orthopedists prefer total joint replacement, whereas others prefer hemiarthroplasty only for the femoral neck and head. The rationale is that total hip arthroplasties are considered to stay intact longer than hemiarthroplasties. The hemiarthroplasty, however, is a considerably smaller surgical trauma for the patient and is advocated for the very old or frail patient with a prognosis of limited mobility.

The trochanteric hip fracture creates fewer problems, despite the fact that the fracture engages more bone than the femoral neck fracture. The operative treatment of choice is internal fixation (Figure 34-5). The postoperative course for all hip fractures, regardless of whether internal fixation or joint arthroplasty is done, is less eventful if physical therapeutic measures are used postoperatively, including the use of gait aids with partial weight-bearing on the operative side. Only for patients with severely comminuted fractures, or fractures in which the operative result has been unsatisfactory, is the restriction of weight-bearing to no weight-bearing needed.

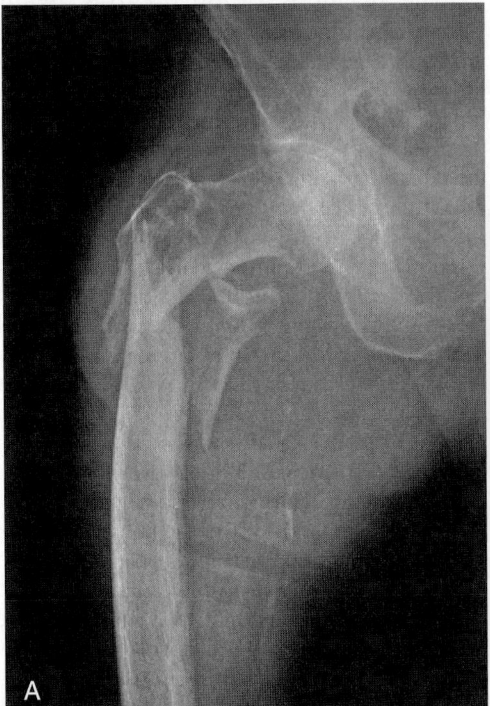

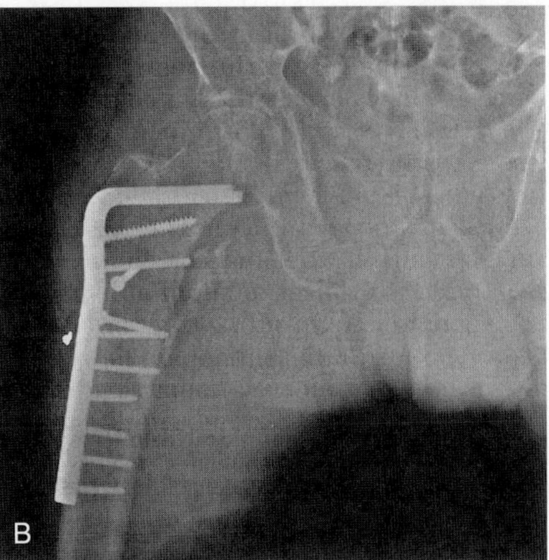

FIGURE 34-5 **A,** The right femur with medial displacement of a large fragment containing the lesser trochanter with lateral angulation across the fracture. **B,** Internal nail, plate, and screw fixation in the same patient.

Hip Pads for Fracture Prophylaxis

There is conflicting evidence as to whether hip protectors can reduce the incidence of hip fractures in the elderly, high-risk population. Compliance with use of the hip protectors has been a concern in the nursing home population. One study showed no substantial difference in the incidence of hip fractures, even in the participants who were compliant with the use of the hip protectors.[94] It appears that at-risk elderly individuals, especially those with a history of falls, impaired balance, and decreased cognition, would benefit from use of hip pads in addition to use of gait aids.[63] Also, rehabilitation for patients to learn how to fall and land safely can decrease the risk of hip fracture resulting from high-impact contact during a fall. Landing on the buttocks is less traumatic to hips than landing on the greater trochanters.[56]

Sacral Insufficiency Fracture

Other axial skeletal fractures, such as fractures of the sacral alae and pubic rami, can also occur (Figure 34-6). Pelvic fractures are particularly common in patients with osteoporosis. Fractures of the pubic rami can occur with minimal strain, and most patients can hardly recall having a traumatic event or an incident of severe strain. Healing typically occurs without invasive procedures. Ambulatory activities are reduced temporarily, and a wheeled walker is initially recommended to decrease pain. Later in the treatment, crutches and a cane can be used. Weight bearing is limited, as dictated by the level of pain in the pelvic area. Fracture of the sacrum with minimal trauma can also occur, and the goal of management is to decrease weight-bearing pain with use of proper assistive devices for ambulation.[65] For management of pelvic pain, physical therapeutic measures are recommended.

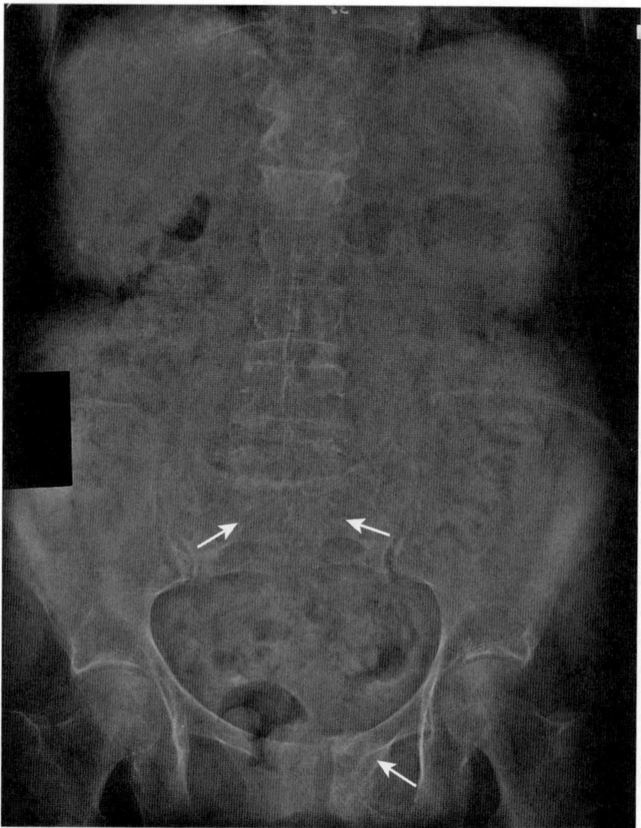

FIGURE 34-6 Insufficiency fractures (*arrows*) of the left pubic bone and both sacral alae in a 75-year-old woman with osteoporosis. (Modified from Sinaki M: Musculoskeletal challenges of osteoporosis, *Aging Clin Exp Res* 10:249-262, 1998, used with permission.)

Diagnostic Studies in Osteoporosis

Who is at risk? The National Osteoporosis Foundation recommends that individuals who are at risk for osteoporosis have a BMD evaluation. This group includes estrogen-deficient women with risk factors, women aged 65 years or older (regardless of risk factors), women in the postmenopausal stage who have at least one risk factor for osteoporosis including having fractured a bone, and people who have a vertebral abnormality indicative of bone loss or take a medication such as prednisone that can cause osteoporosis. This group also includes individuals who have type 1 diabetes mellitus, liver disease, kidney disease, thyroid disease, or family history of osteoporosis, as well as women who had early menopause. In addition to the above recommendations, it is thought that individuals who abuse alcohol or are cigarette smokers are at increased risk. A follow-up BMD study should be done after 2 years or longer, depending on the baseline T score and the patient's risk factors. Bone markers can also be used for additional information on follow-up evaluations, especially those for shorter intervals (i.e., <3 months).

The diagnosis of osteoporosis requires a thorough history and physical examination, including family history of osteoporosis, type and location of musculoskeletal pain, general dietary calcium intake, height and weight measurements, and level of physical activity (Table 34-1).

Several biochemical indices are also used in the differential diagnosis of metabolic bone disease or, in some instances, for therapeutic follow-up.[15] Biochemical markers for bone formation include calcium, phosphorus, PTH, bone-specific alkaline phosphatase, and serum osteocalcin. Resorption markers include 24-hour urinary calcium excretion (corrected by creatinine excretion), hydroxyproline, and pyridinium cross-links (in urine). Unfortunately, the interpretation of these tests is clouded in patients with osteoporosis because the intraindividual and interindividual variations are substantial for these parameters. Also, indices of bone turnover show seasonal and circadian variations (see Table 34-1).

Radiographic findings of osteoporosis consist of increased lucency of the vertebral bodies with loss of horizontal trabeculae, increased prominence of the cortical end plates, vertically oriented trabeculae, reduction in cortex thickness, and anterior wedging of vertebral bodies (Figure 34-7).[24] The degree of wedging that indicates a true fracture varies from a 15% to 25% reduction in anterior height relative to the posterior height of the same vertebra. Other morphologic changes occur, such as biconcavity

Table 34-1 Some of the Diagnostic Evaluations for Osteoporosis

Evaluation	Details
History and physical examination	Family history of osteoporosis, type and location of pain, general dietary calcium intake, level of physical activity, height and weight
Radiographs of chest and spine	To rule out lymphomas, rib fractures, compression fractures, etc.
Bone mineral density (spine and hip)	At menopause and every 2 years for high-risk patients and every 5 years for low-risk patients
Complete blood cell count	To rule out anemias associated with malignancy, etc.
Chemistry group (serum calcium, phosphorus, vitamin D, parathyroid hormone, bone-specific alkaline phosphatase, osteocalcin)	To assess the level of alkaline phosphatase, which may be increased in osteomalacia, Paget's disease, bony metastasis and fracture, intestinal malabsorption, vitamin D deficiency, chronic liver disease, alcohol abuse, phenytoin (Dilantin) therapy, hypercalcemia of hyperparathyroidism, hypophosphatemia of hyperparathyroidism and osteomalacia, malabsorption, or malnutrition
Erythrocyte sedimentation rate and seroprotein electrophoresis	To determine changes indicative of multiple myeloma or other gammopathies
Total thyroxine	Increased total thyroxine concentration may be a cause of osteoporosis because of increased bone turnover
Immunoreactive parathyroid hormone	Hyperparathyroidism (accompanied by hypercalcemia)
25-Hydroxyvitamin D and 1,25-dihydroxyvitamin D_3	Gastrointestinal disease, osteomalacia
Urinalysis and 24-h urine	To check for proteinuria caused by nephrotic syndrome and for low pH resulting from renal tubular acidosis; a 24-h urine test can exclude hypercalciuria (normal calcium value in men is 25-300 mg/specimen; in women, 20-275 mg/specimen)*
Optional: Bone scan, iliac crest biopsy	After tetracycline double-labeling for bone histomorphometry, bone marrow biopsy may be indicated to exclude multiple myeloma and metastatic malignancy
Biochemical markers of bone turnover (Eastell)	Formation: Serum osteocalcin, alkaline phosphatase (bone), procollagen type 1, C and N propeptides Resorption: Serum acid phosphatase, pyridinoline, deoxypyridinoline, hydroxyproline, cross-linked telopeptides of type 1 collagen, urinary calcium, or creatinine

*From Sinaki M: Effect of physical activity on bone mass, *Curr Opin Rheumatol* 8:376-383, 1996.

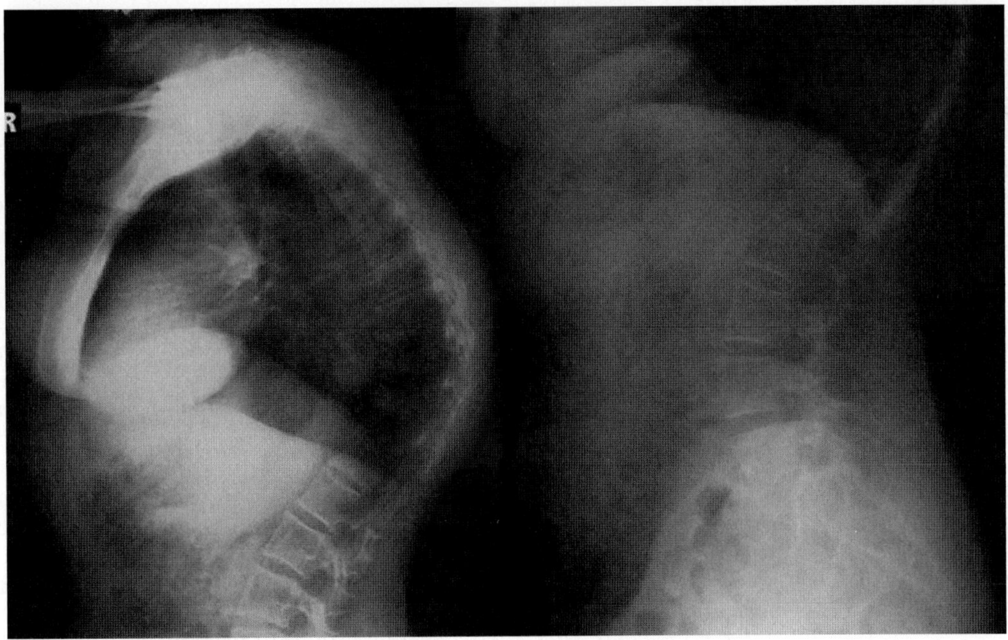

FIGURE 34-7 Thoracolumbar kyphoscoliosis. Osteoporosis. Compression of multiple thoracic vertebral bodies. Hypertrophic and degenerative changes in the thoracic spine.

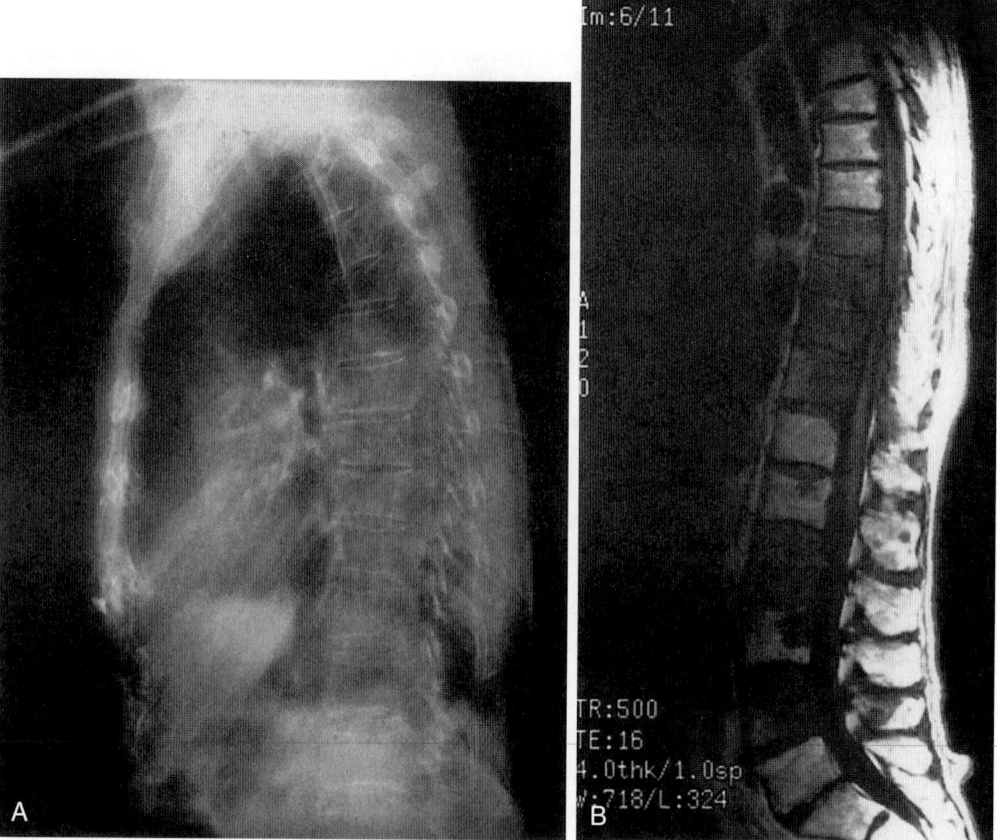

FIGURE 34-8 **A,** Lateral radiograph of the spine in a 77-year-old man with persistent back pain. No evidence of metastatic lesion was identified. **B,** Magnetic resonance image demonstrating extensive skeletal metastases from T3 through the lower lumbar spine, with involvement of nearly every vertebral body. The most extensive involvement is at T3, T8 through T11, T12, and L4.

of vertebral bodies and complete compression fractures (reduction in both anterior and posterior heights by at least 25% compared with adjacent normal vertebrae).[24] Bone scan and magnetic resonance imaging can further define the cause of bone loss (Figure 34-8), if needed.

Osteoporosis is typically not visible on conventional radiographs until at least 25% to 30% of bone mineral has been lost. Consequently, evaluation of BMD through absorptiometry techniques is recommended.[95] These measurements are also helpful in treatment because calculated bone loss or gain is required in therapeutic trials of agents affecting bone mass. The different methods for evaluation of bone mass have different levels of precision. Other available methods include photon absorptiometry (single or dual), finger x-ray spectrometry, ultrasound densitometry, qualitative computed tomography, and dual-energy x-ray absorptiometry. The most commonly used technique is dual-energy x-ray absorptiometry; it has high precision and is frequently used for research and clinical evaluations to measure the BMD of the spine and hips (Figure 34-9).

This can also be used to measure total-body bone mass. It is x-ray–based and has a precision of approximately 1%. The amount of radiation used is less than 3 mrad. More commonly measured is the BMD of the femoral neck,[95] because spinal bone density can be erroneously high as a result of osteoarthritis of the spine.

Treatment

Osteoporosis treatment is best done with a team approach because it is a multifactorial condition.[5] For the cause to be defined and proper pharmacotherapy and physical interventions to be initiated, endocrine consultation is needed, along with interventions from specialists in physical medicine and rehabilitation, pharmacology, psychology, and nutrition. The World Health Organization has defined osteoporosis as a T score of less than −2.5. Detailed definitions of normal BMD, osteopenia, and osteoporosis are provided earlier in the text of this chapter. These definitions facilitate decision-making for therapeutic trials. They are also helpful for prescription of a proper exercise program.

Fractures generally occur with falls; therefore, the prevention of falls decreases the risk of fracture. Falls are multifactorial.[63] A controlled trial showed that patients with osteoporosis who had kyphosis were substantially more at risk for falls than controls without osteoporosis/kyphosis.[73] A considerable improvement in risk for falls was demonstrated by the SPEED program. This program produced a decreased step width, improved steadiness of gait on gait laboratory testing, decreased risk for falls at obstacles, and increased velocity, cadence, and stride length in individuals.[74] Through use of a WKO and SPEED program, back pain decreased and the level of physical activity increased.

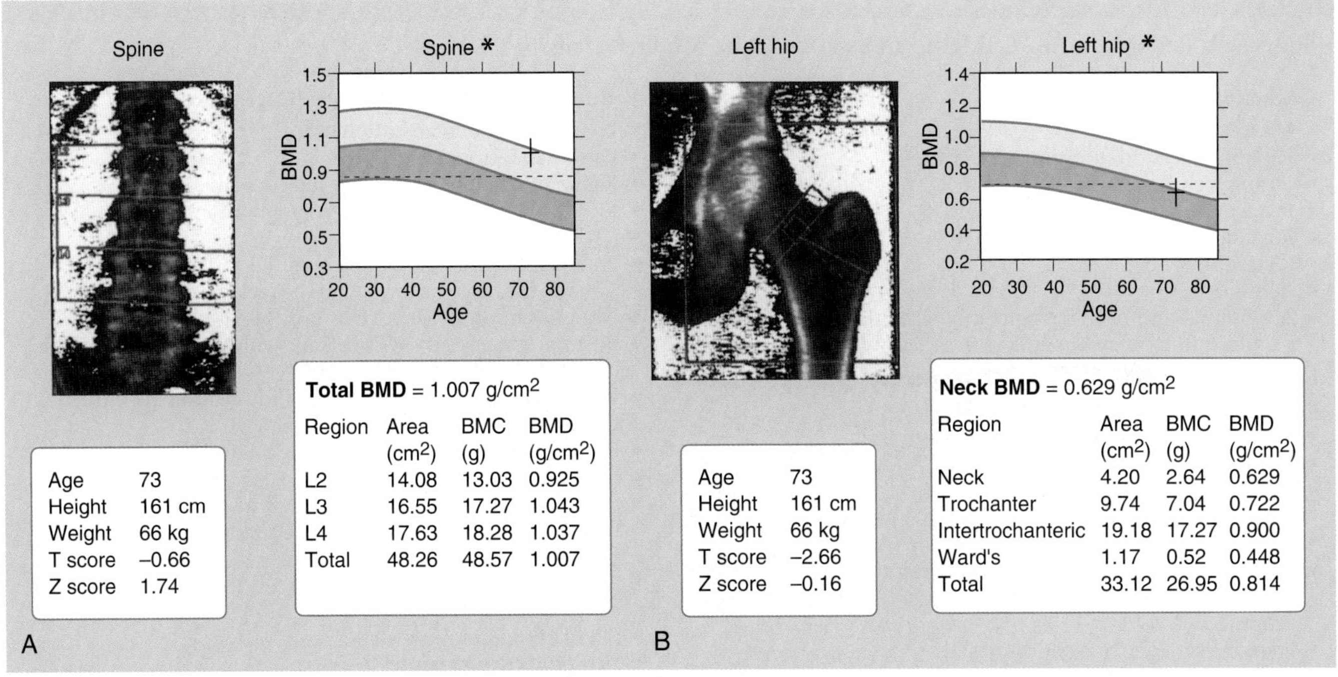

FIGURE 34-9 Reports of bone mineral density (BMD) studies with dual-energy x-ray absorptiometry of spine and hip in a patient with osteoporosis. **A,** Lumbar spine BMD. **B,** Femoral neck BMD. The BMD of the spine may be erroneously high because of osteoarthritis of the spine. *Age- and sex-matched. *BMC,* Bone mineral content; *T,* peak bone mass; *Z,* age-matched.

The SPEED program opens a new area of investigation for reducing risk for falls in kyphotic, osteoporotic individuals with balance disorder.[74]

Exercise

The efficacy of exercise for improving bone mass is supported by hormonal and nutritional factors (Box 34-5). To meet the challenge of mechanical load, skeletal tissue must have enough bone mass and proper architecture to withstand the physical strain that is imposed on it. Normal musculoskeletal structure is highly adaptable and can meet the challenge of usual mechanical loads. The challenge from mechanical load and strain might not be tolerated in those with osteopenia and osteoporosis without damage to the architecture of bone. A supervised, nonstrenuous, progressive resistive exercise program can improve bone mass in inactive individuals.[88] By understanding both the benefits and the shortcomings of nutritional and exercise approaches for musculoskeletal management of osteoporosis, we can create an improved prophylactic program for patients with osteoporosis.[79] Not all exercises that promote musculoskeletal health are safe for bone loss in osteoporotic, osteopenic spine. Some yoga position exercises can improve balance disorder and musculoskeletal health but could cause vertebral compression and undesirable side effects, such as vertebral fracture; the latter needs to be taken into consideration before prescribing an exercise program (Figures 34-10 and 34-11).[71]

High rates and magnitude of bone strain are produced during high-impact sports activities, such as gymnastics, badminton, tennis, volleyball, and basketball. The high-impact bone loading results in site-specific increases in BMD. One study showed a marked difference in BMD between gymnasts and volleyball players. The lower limbs are loaded differently in these two athletic activities.[19] Gymnasts had higher BMD than volleyball players, except in the pelvic bone. Swimming can improve muscle strength but not bone mass.[17] According to the theory of Frost,[22] a minimum threshold of mechanical loading is needed to evoke an increased level of BMD. This theory is referred to as that of the minimum effective strain stimulus. Lanyon[37] suggested that the greatest osteogenic effect from mechanical loading occurs when the strain is vigorous (high strain), repeated daily, short in duration, and applied to a specific bone site. Mechanical loading, when applied properly, can stimulate osteogenic activity. Axial loading of the skeleton during lifting activities at a person's job or in the care of children can be as osteogenic as mechanical-loading exercises in a gym (Figure 34-12).[76] Individuals with normal BMD can perform high-impact exercises, such as aerobics, jogging, and skiing. For persons with osteoporosis, nonstraining exercises are recommended, such as walking for 45 minutes three times a week or for 30 minutes daily. Aquatic exercises are recommended for patients who are unable to perform antigravity exercises because of pain or weakness. The nonstrenuous, low-resistance exercises can be advanced to antigravity and strengthening exercises as permitted by a patient's musculoskeletal status.[66,75]

Spinal extension exercises should be used along with exercises to reduce lumbar lordosis.[60,80] One study showed that progressive resistive back-strengthening exercises can improve back strength considerably.[89] A recent randomized controlled trial showed the most effective, safe back-strengthening exercise to be the original.[89] The most effective back-strengthening exercise continues to be progressive resistive back extension exercise.[28,72,87,89] Weakness

BOX 34-5

Suggested Rehabilitation Guidelines Based on Bone Mineral Density T Scores*

Reduction to −1 SD (Normal)

- No treatment
- Patient education, preventive measures
- Lifting techniques
- Proper diet (calcium and vitamin D)
- Jogging (short distances)
- Weight training
- Aerobics
- Abdominal and back-strengthening exercises†
- Conditioning of erector spinae muscles

Reduction to −1 to −2.5 SD (Osteopenia)‡

- Consultation for treatment
- Patient education, preventive interventions
- Pain management
- Back-strengthening exercises
- Limit load-lifting (≤10-20 lb)
- Aerobic exercises: Walking 40 min/day
- Strengthening exercises: Weight training three times a week
- Postural exercises: WKO combined with pelvic tilt and back extension
- Frenkel exercises, prevention of falls
- Tai chi, if desired
- Antiresorptive agents, if required

Reduction to −2.5 SD or More (Osteoporosis)‡

- Pharmacologic intervention
- Pain management
- Range of motion, strengthening, coordination
- Midday rest, heat or cold, stroking massage, if needed
- Back extensor strengthening
- Walking 40 min/day, as tolerated; Frenkel exercises
- Aquatic exercises once or twice a week
- Fall prevention program (see Box 34-3)
- Postural exercises: WKO program with pelvic tilt and back extension
- Prevention of vertebral compression fractures (orthoses, as needed)
- Prevention of spinal strain (lifting ≤5-10 lb)
- Evaluation of balance, gait aid
- Safety and facilitation of self-care through modification of bathrooms (grab bars) and kitchen (counter adjustment); occupational therapy consultation
- Start strengthening program with 1-2 lb and increase, as tolerated, to 5 lb in each hand
- SPEED program, if needed
- Hip protective measures

*T score: SD below peak normal bone mass in young adults.
†See Figures 34-10 and 34-11 for proper exercise program and posture.
‡*Osteopenia* or *osteoporosis* as defined by the World Health Organization.[1]
SD, Standard deviation; *SPEED,* Spinal Proprioceptive Extension Exercise Dynamic; *WKO,* weighted kypho-orthosis.

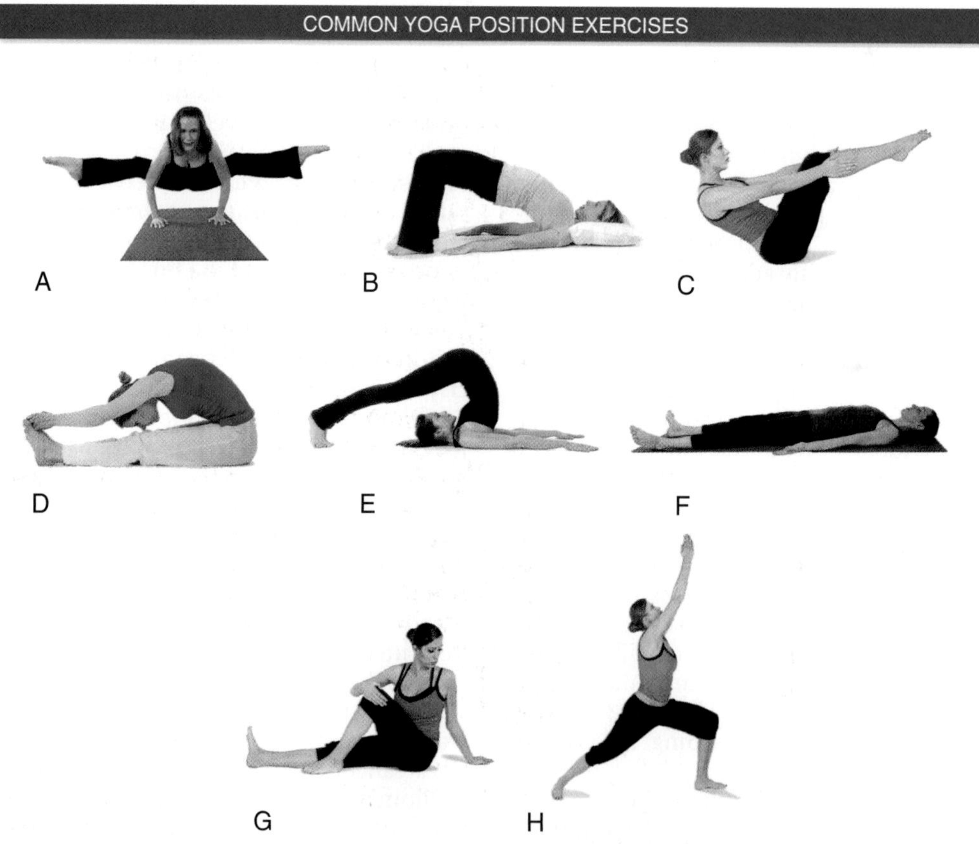

FIGURE 34-10 **A** to **H,** Common yoga positions. The various positions can cause extreme spinal flexion (**B, D, E**), extreme cervicothoracic strain (**B, E**), kinetic thoracic and shoulder strain (**A, G, H**), and kinetic low back strain (**H**).

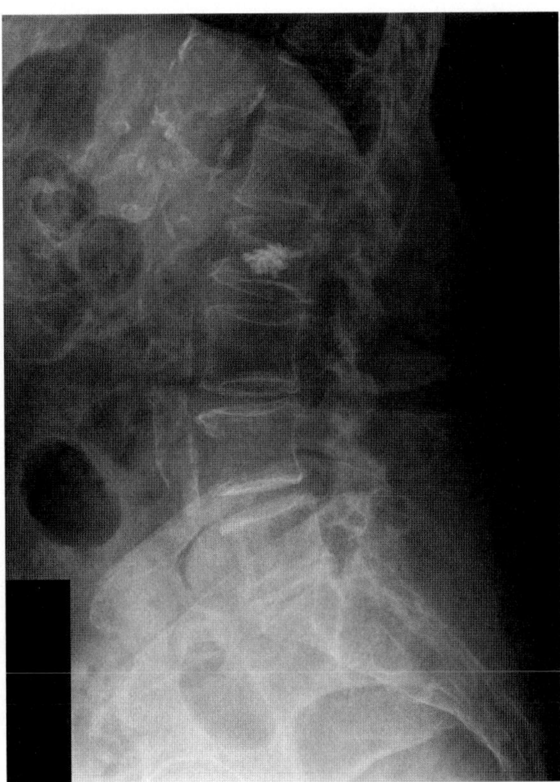

FIGURE 34-11 Acute back pain after yoga flexion position exercises. Spinal radiographs showed a vertebral compression fracture (VCF) at L2. Host vertebroplasty cement in place without aberrant cement in canal or evidence of impingement.

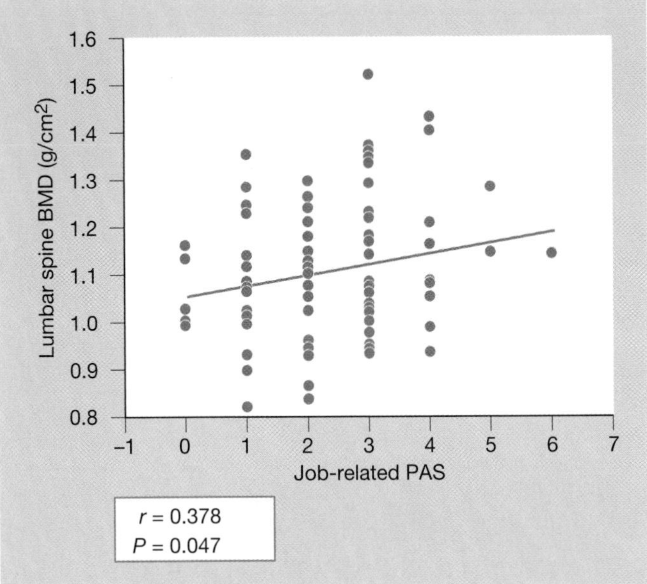

FIGURE 34-12 Job-related physical activity score (PAS) markedly correlated with spinal bone mineral density (BMD). (Modified from Sinaki M, Fitzpatrick LA, Ritchie CK, et al: Site-specificity of bone mineral density and muscle strength in women: job-related physical activity, *Am J Phys Med Rehabil* 77:470-476, 1998, used with permission.)

in abdominal muscles adds to the problems of poor posture and protruded abdomen. To complement a posture training exercise program, isometric abdominal muscle-strengthening exercises should be included (Figures 34-13 and 34-14). The author's osteoporosis back exercise program has been studied extensively through controlled trials, by other investigators, and has been proven to be safe and effective.[7,28,29,81,84]

Strenuous spinal flexion and spinal flexion exercises should be avoided in patients with osteoporosis (Figure 34-15).[84] In a study by Sinaki and Mikkelsen[84] comparing the effect of flexion and extension exercises on the spine, it was demonstrated that, even without pharmacotherapy, patients with osteoporosis who performed back extension exercises (see Figure 34-13, *K*) had a considerably lower rate of fracture than those who performed spinal flexion exercises or no exercise.[84] This issue was further substantiated after patients who were in good health and had osteopenia suffered vertebral compression fracture when they participated in yoga spinal flexion position exercises (see Figure 34-11).[71,73] Women with osteoporosis generally have weaker back extensors than healthy women of comparable age (Figure 34-16). The choice of physical activity is important and has to be individualized. Fitness programs, such as swimming or short periods of stationary biking, are not sufficiently osteogenic,[48] but can fulfill the need for cardiovascular fitness without straining the osteoporotic frame. Walking for 40 minutes at least three times a week is effective for maintaining lower-limb bone density. Knowledge of a person's BMD is helpful before recommending a weight-training or mechanically loading exercise program.[62,88]

Posture Training Program and the Osteoporotic Skeletal Frame

Any support that can improve posture and decrease pain-related paraspinal muscle cocontraction is desirable. The number and diameter of collagen fibrils of the intervertebral disks decrease with aging. This reduction results in loss of resiliency of the disks. The effect of aging on intervertebral disk is substantial. The disk collagens and proteoglycans undergo quantitative and qualitative changes.[2] This disk degeneration related to aging is clinically greater at L4/L5 than L2/L3 and could be clinically asymptomatic.[6] In addition, reduced paraspinal muscle strength[85] and forward tendency of head and trunk related to the effect of gravity can cause neck and upper-back pain as well as iliocostal friction syndrome and flank pain.[62] This pain does not respond to the use of conventional orthoses. Indeed, orthoses such as corsets can make the pain worse through pressure over the lower rib cage (Figure 34-17). Posture training programs that are intended to decrease kyphosis can also subsequently reduce iliocostal friction syndrome.[36,64,86a] One study showed that use of a WKO and back exercise increased back strength more significantly ($P < 0.02$) than back exercise alone.[36] The same study also showed that use of a thoracolumbar support interfered with improving back strength with exercise (Figure 34-18). Posture training programs, such as the application of a WKO for 20 minutes two to three times a day in cases of

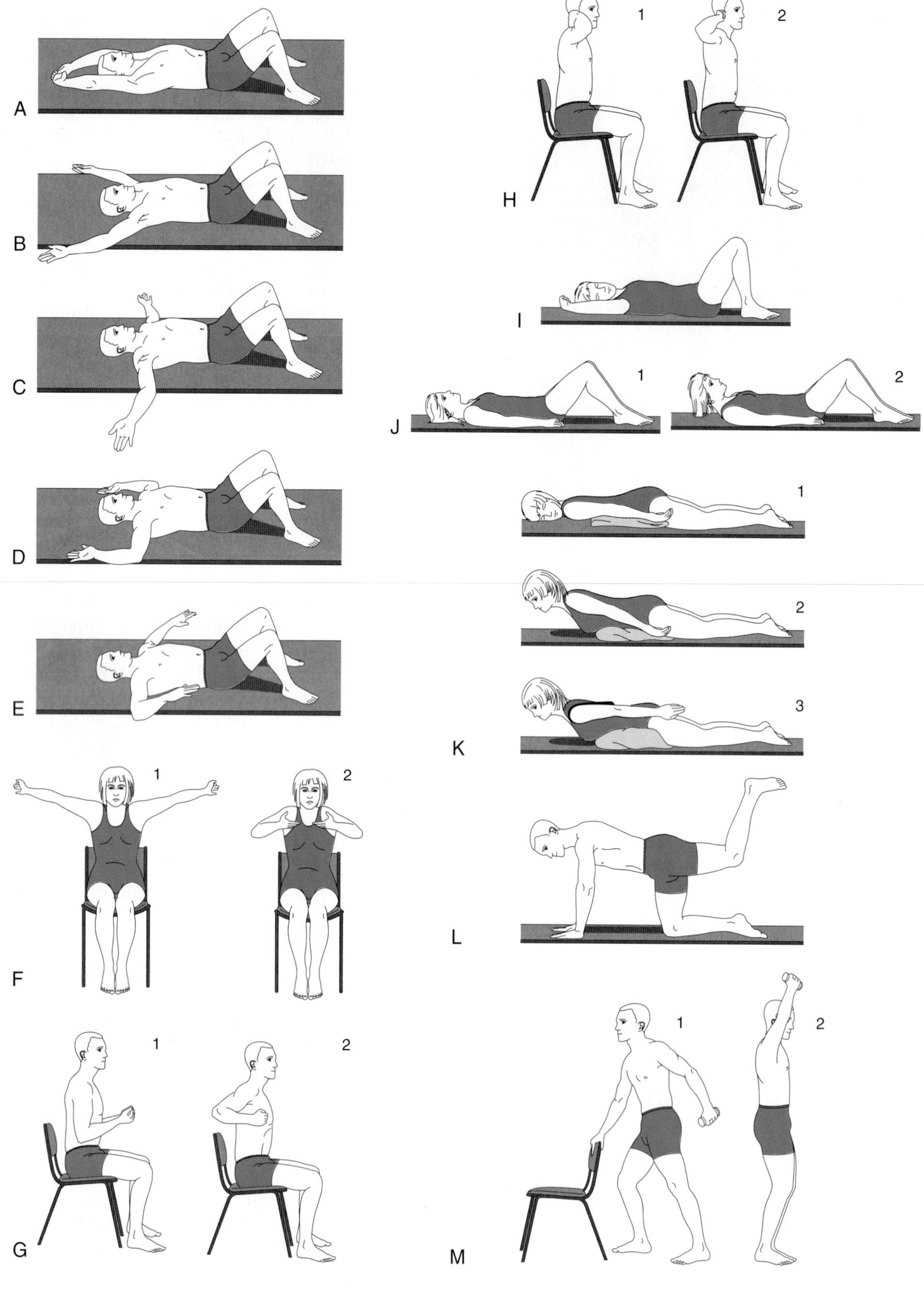
A
B
C
D
E
F
1
2
G
1
2
H
1
2
I
J
1
2
K
1
2
3
L
M
1
2

FIGURE 34-13 Nonstrenuous progressive exercises for patients with severe osteoporosis. **A** to **C,** Upper back and shoulder extension exercise performed with spine supported. **D** and **E,** Flexibility of the shoulder joint may contribute to improvement of upper-back posture. To avoid upper-back and neck strain in a fragile skeleton, shoulder rotation exercises can be performed in the supine position. **F1** and **F2,** Pectoral stretching exercise performed in the sitting position. This exercise is used to reduce kyphotic posturing. **G1** and **G2,** Back extension exercise in the sitting position. This position avoids or minimizes pain in patients with severe osteoporosis. **H1** and **H2,** Deep-breathing exercise combined with pectoral stretching and back extension exercise. The patient sits on a chair, places hands at head level, and inhales deeply while gently extending the elbows backward. While exhaling, the patient returns the arms to the starting position. This exercise is repeated 10 to 15 times. **I,** Exercise to decrease lumbar lordosis with isometric contraction of lumbar flexors. **J1** and **J2,** Isometric exercise to strengthen abdominal muscles. **K1** to **K3,** Extension exercises in the prone position with a pillow under the abdomen (to avoid hyperextension). Exercise (**K3**) helps to increase the effect of back extension strengthening, and weight is added. **L,** Exercise for improving strength in lumbar extensors and gluteus maximus muscles. **M1** and **M2,** Specificity of exercises is for muscle strengthening and weight-loading that may decrease bone loss. (These exercises were developed for the osteopenic spine by M. Sinaki through a grant from the Retirement Research Foundation. These techniques are designed to decrease strain on the spine despite weight-lifting.) Note: The amount of weight lifted is approximately 1 to 2 lb in each hand, not to exceed 5 lb in each hand. The amount of weight needs to be prescribed according to the patient's bone mineral density (status of osteoporosis) and the condition of the upper extremities. In exercise **M1**, shoulder extensors contribute to reduction of kyphotic posturing. Shoulder extensors can be strengthened with a proper combination of weight-lifting and weight-bearing exercises while balance is maintained. One knee is bent to avoid lumbar strain. To avoid spine strain and to maintain balance, leaning or holding onto a steady object for support is recommended. Exercise **M2** is a bilateral or unilateral spine and hip weight-loading exercise. When weight is lifted above the head, the knees should be bent slightly to avoid straining the lumbar spine. (**A** to **H2, L,** and **M,** Modified from Sinaki M: Metabolic bone disease. In Sinaki M, editor: *Basic clinical rehabilitation medicine,* ed 2, St Louis, 1993, Mosby, used with permission of Mayo Foundation for Medical Education and Research; **I, J, K1,** and **K2,** modified from Sinaki M: Exercise and physical therapy. In Riggs BL, Melton LJ 3rd, editors: *Osteoporosis: etiology, diagnosis, and management,* New York, 1988, Raven Press, used with permission of Mayo Foundation for Medical Education and Research; **K3,** modified from Sinaki M: *PTS: posture training support brochure,* Jackson, 1993, Camp International, used with permission of Mayo Foundation for Medical Education and Research.)

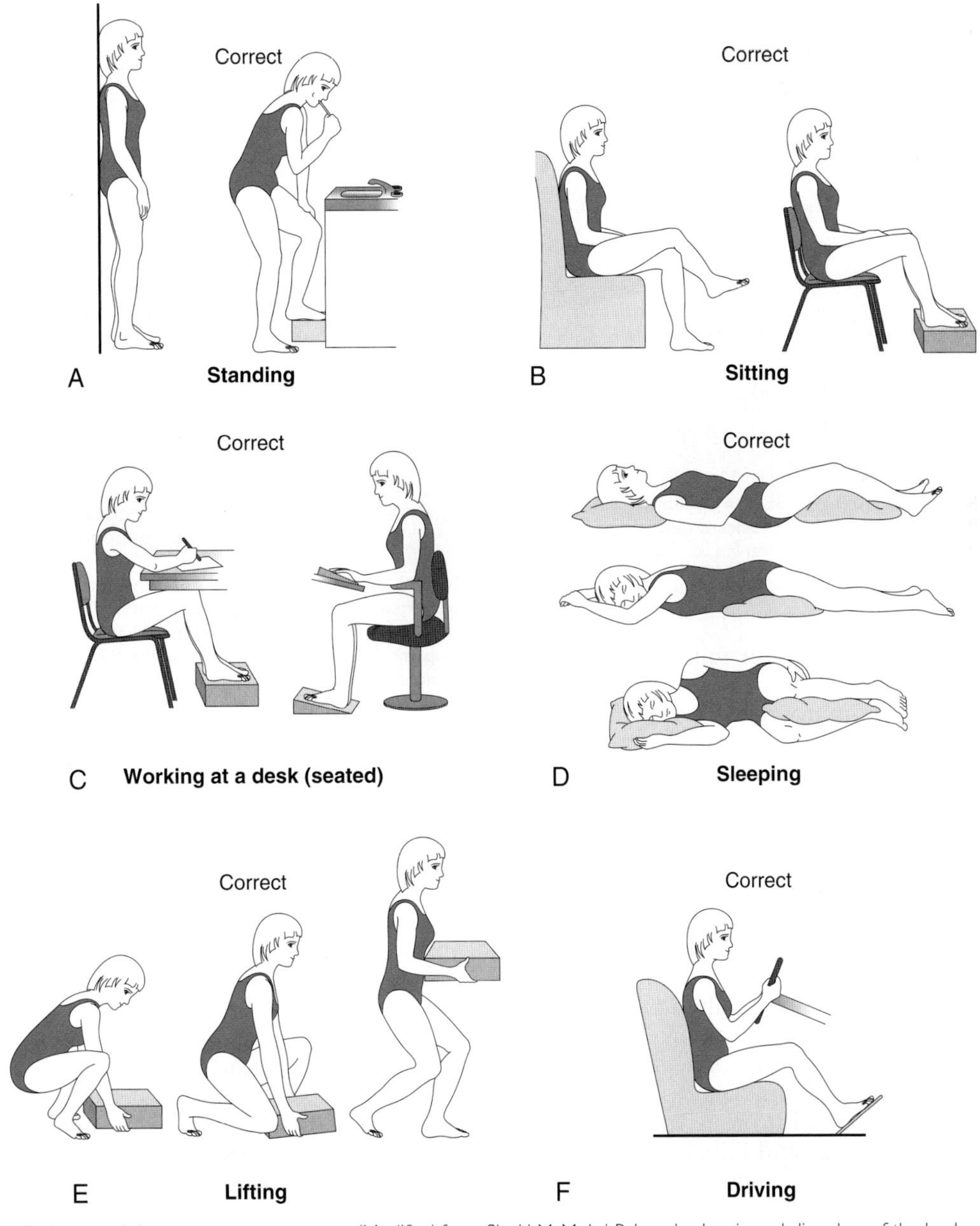

FIGURE 34-14 **A** to **F,** Static and dynamic correct postures. (Modified from Sinaki M, Mokri B: Low back pain and disorders of the lumbar spine. In Braddom RL, editor: *Physical medicine and rehabilitation,* Philadelphia, 1996, WB Saunders, used with permission.)

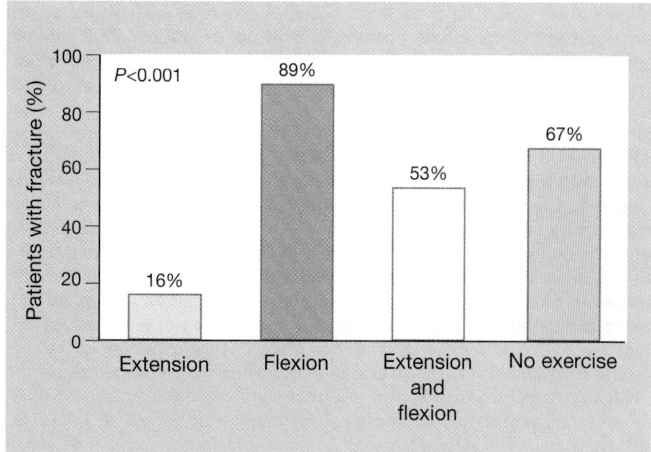

FIGURE 34-15 **Percentage of patients with new vertebral fracture after spinal extension exercise, spinal flexion exercise, extension and flexion exercise, and no exercise.** (Data from Sinaki M, Mikkelsen BA: Postmenopausal spinal osteoporosis: flexion versus extension exercises, *Arch Phys Med Rehabil* 65:593-596, 1984.)

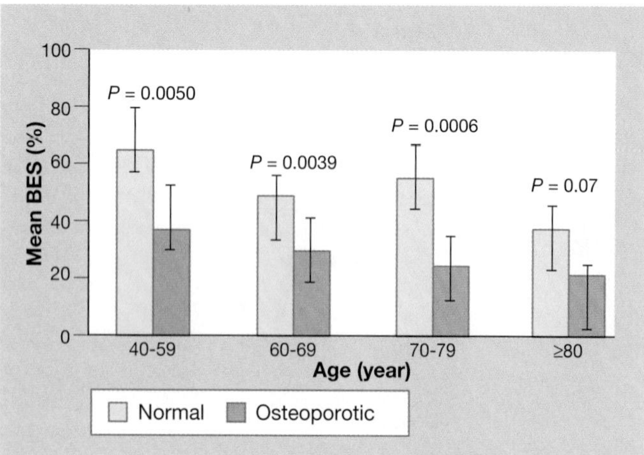

FIGURE 34-16 **Back extensor strength (BES) in healthy women versus women with osteoporosis. Error bars indicate standard deviation.** (Data from Sinaki M, Khosla S, Limburg PJ, et al: Muscle strength in osteoporotic versus normal women, *Osteoporos Int* 3:8-12, 1993.)

severe kyphosis or less frequently in milder cases while contracting the back extensors, can provide reeducation of the paraspinal muscles for improvement of kyphotic posturing and reduction of the risk of falls (Figure 34-19).[83] In some severe cases, back extension is not possible without use of a WKO. Furthermore, proper use of a WKO can decrease back and flank pain in osteoporosis.[36,49,64,67,86a]

Orthoses and the Osteoporotic Spine

Acute compression fracture usually results in severe pain and, if not managed well, can lead to prolonged immobility. The final outcome is creation of chronic pain behavior and subsequent psychological consequences. Acute pain needs to be actively managed with proper physical measures. Sedative stroking massage and initial application of cold, and later heat, and isometric muscle contractions of

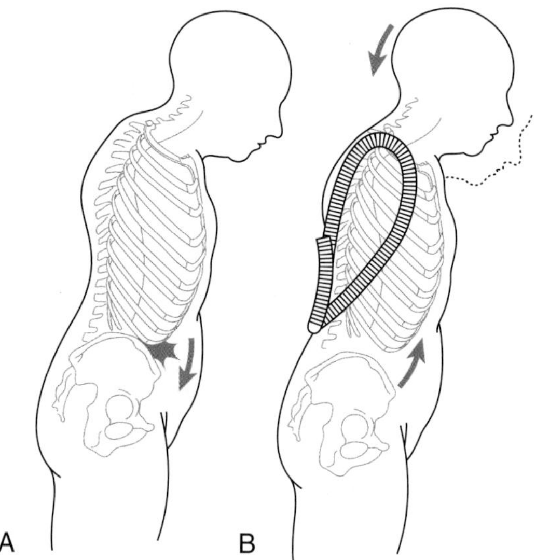

FIGURE 34-17 **A, Severe kyphosis can result in iliocostal contact or iliocostal friction syndrome. B, Application of a weighted kypho-orthosis provides counteracting forces, which enable users to contract their erector spinae muscles better and decrease kyphotic posturing.** (Modified from Sinaki M: The influence of exercise on bone and the rehabilitation of osteoporotic patients. In Passeri M, editor: *The opinion of the orthopedist and physiatrist,* Pavia, 1995, EDIMES Publishing, used with permission.)

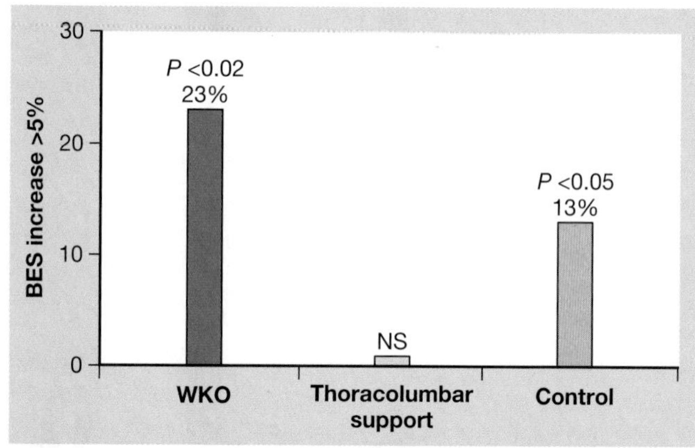

FIGURE 34-18 **Comparison of the three study groups that all performed back extensor strengthening (BES) exercise for 4 months. At the end of the study, stronger back was achieved in the weighted kypho-orthosis (WKO) group and the control group than in the thoracolumbar support group, who had no significant (NS) improvement in back strength.** (Data from Kaplan RS, Sinaki M, Hameister MD: Effect of back supports on back strength in patients with osteoporosis: a pilot study, *Mayo Clin Proc* 71:235-241, 1996.)

the paraspinal muscles can be helpful. Rigid thoracolumbar orthoses to promote extension of the spine are helpful (Figure 34-20) (also see Chapter 13).[49,67,83] If thoracolumbar orthoses are not tolerated because of postural changes, a thoracic WKO (Figure 34-21) or a combination of a kypho-orthosis and lower-back support (elastic abdominal support) might suffice. In some cases, long-distance ambulatory activities might require use of a cane or a wheeled walker. Temporary use of a wheelchair with a supportive back cushion is indicated in some cases. Every effort needs to be taken to prevent falls as well as immobility, including having the patient confined to one room or under prolonged bed rest. Immobility should be limited to avoid resulting reactive depression and bone loss. Safety during

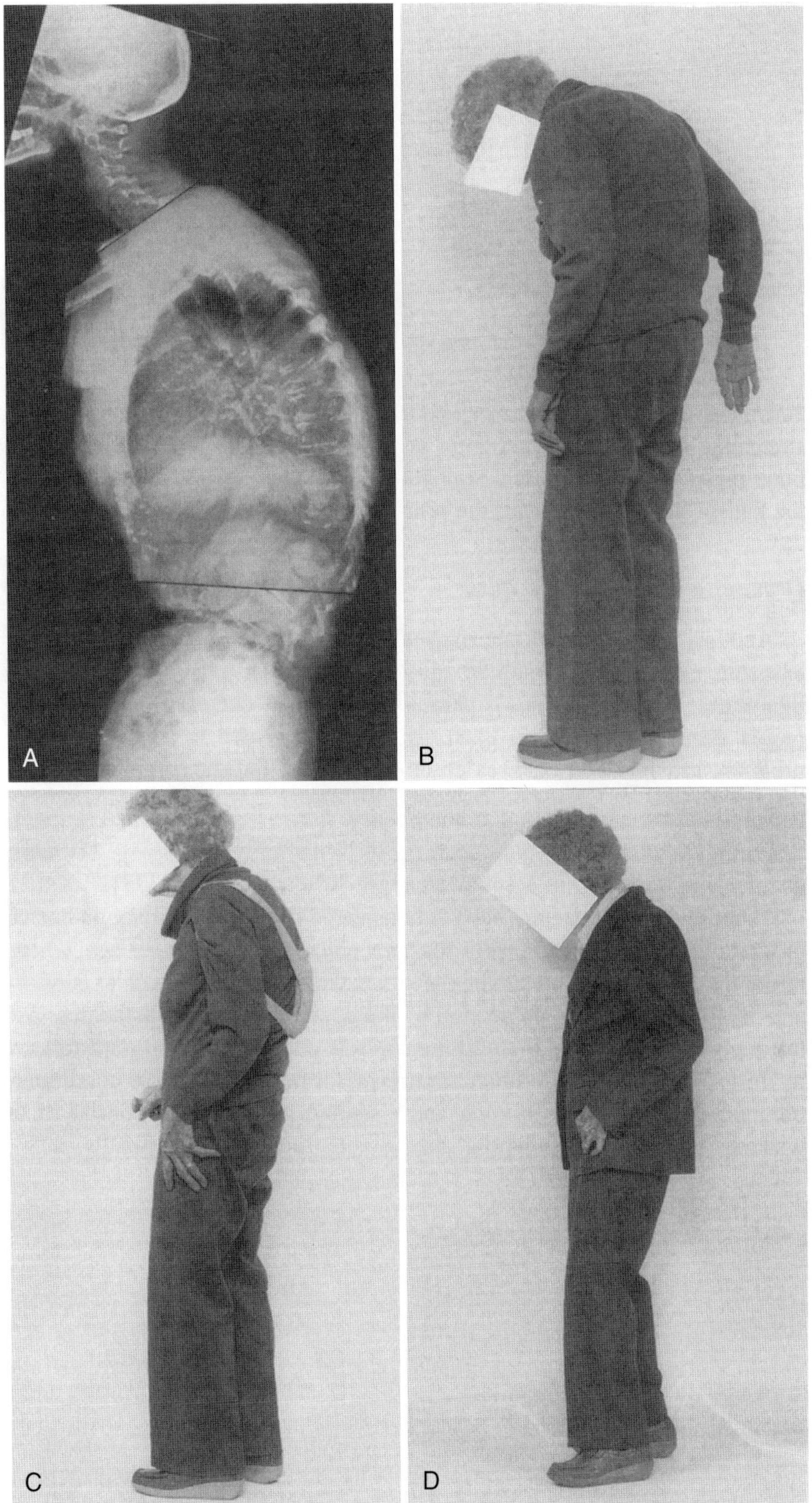

FIGURE 34-19 An 86-year-old woman with osteoporosis. **A,** Radiograph of the spine depicts osteoporotic and postural changes. **B,** Severe kyphotic posturing, which made ambulation difficult. **C,** The same woman wearing a weighted kypho-orthosis. **D,** The same woman's postural correction at age 92 after a 6-year trial with a weighted kypho-orthosis and posture training program; the patient is not wearing the kypho-orthosis. (**A** and **D,** Modified from Sinaki M: Musculoskeletal challenges of osteoporosis, *Aging Clin Exp Res* 10:249-262, 1998, used with permission; **B** and **C,** modified from Sinaki M: Rehabilitation of osteoporotic fractures of the spine, *Phys Med Rehabil* 9:105-123, 1995, used with permission.)

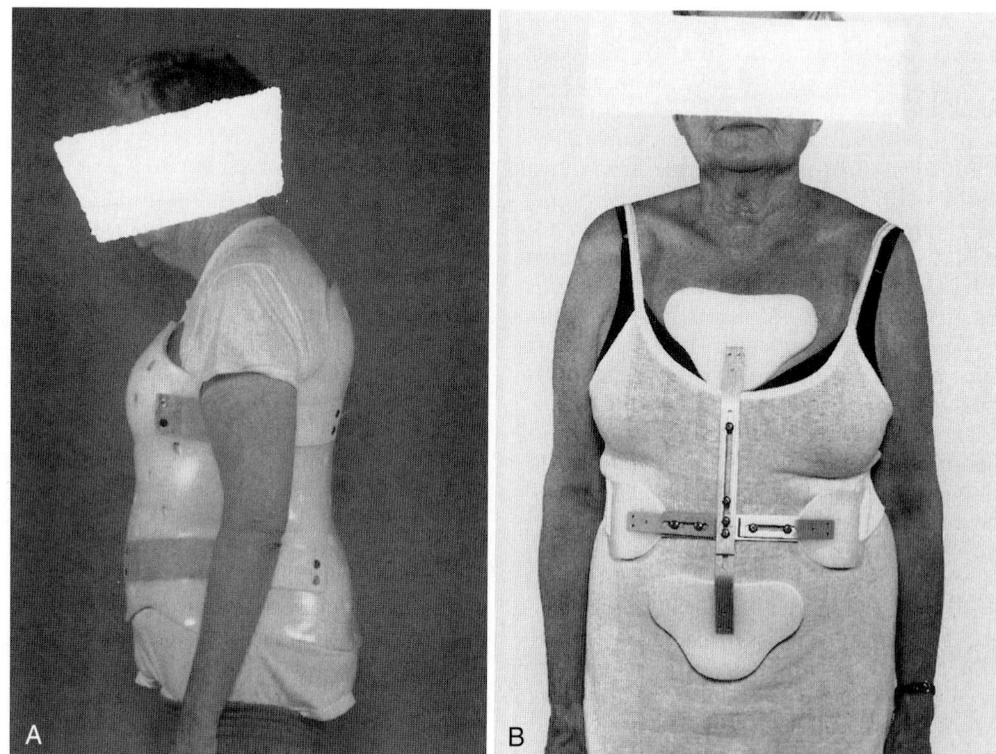

FIGURE 34-20 **A,** Rigid back support: bivalved body jacket. The brace is made of polypropylene and is custom-fitted. **B,** Cruciform anterior spinal hyperextension (CASH) brace. This patient with osteoporosis of the spine and compression fractures was unable to tolerate increased intraabdominal pressure with use of abdominal back support because of hiatal hernia. The patient was fitted with a CASH brace satisfactorily. (**A,** Modified from Sinaki M: Prevention of hip fracture: physical activity. In Ringe J, Meunier PJ, Baudoin C, editors: *Osteoporotic fractures in the elderly: clinical management and prevention,* Stuttgart, 1996, Georg Thieme Verlag, used with permission; **B,** modified from Sinaki M: Exercise and physical therapy. In Riggs BL, Melton LJ 3rd, editors: *Osteoporosis: etiology, diagnosis, and management,* New York, 1988, Raven Press, used with permission of Mayo Foundation for Medical Education and Research.)

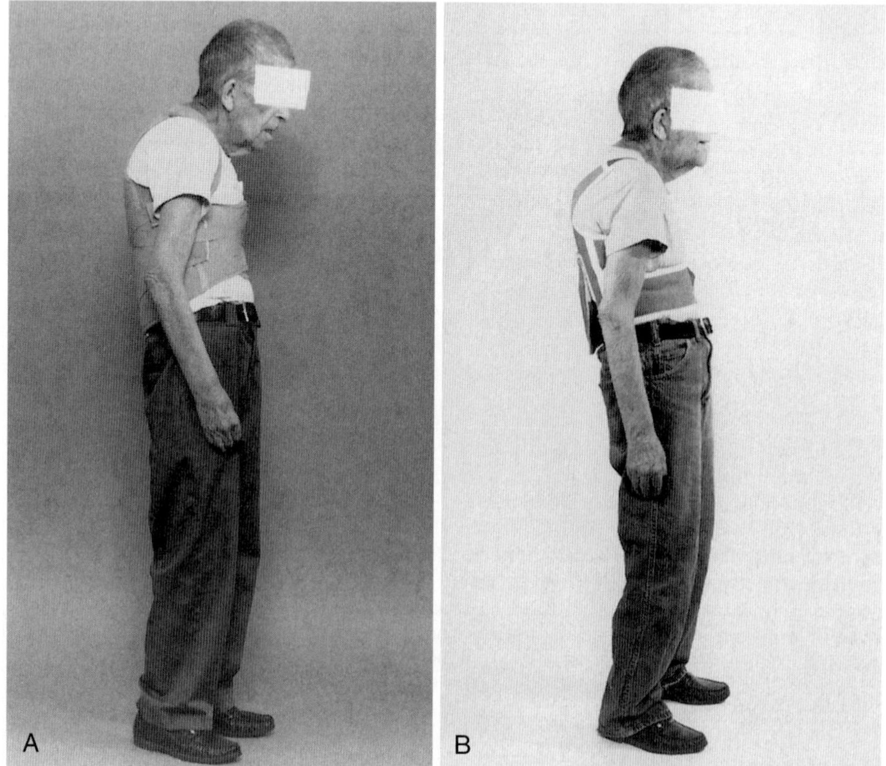

FIGURE 34-21 **A,** Thoracolumbar support (rigid stays). A problem with fitting was as a result of spinal deformities. **B,** Posture training support (weighted kypho-orthosis) vest sometimes is tolerated better than conventional thoracolumbar support. Weight in the pouch can range from 1 to 2.5 lb, as required.

ambulation is paramount, and prevention of falls and fracture should be taught in the rehabilitative program for patients with osteoporosis. Implementation of the SPEED program can decrease gait unsteadiness and posture-related back pain, and increase the level of physical activity.[74]

Pharmacologic Interventions

Pharmacotherapy is essential for improving bone mass, but its efficacy in prevention of skeletal deformities depends on musculoskeletal rehabilitation. Over the years, through many research studies, the efficacy of measures implemented in rehabilitation of osteoporosis has been substantiated. Of course, the best osteoporosis treatment is prevention of fall and vertebral fracture through improving muscle strength,[60,67,81] level of physical activity, and peak bone mass before the age of 30 years.[82] In addition, maintaining some level of physical activity[86] throughout life could reduce bone loss. Muscle strength and exercise play substantial roles in the prevention of vertebral fractures[81] and falls.[60] There are two categories of pharmacotherapy for management of osteoporosis: antiresorptive agents that slow bone loss and anabolic agents that contribute to bone formation. Antiresorptive agents include bisphosphonates, calcitonin, denosumab, estrogen, estrogen agonists, and androgens. Calcium, vitamin D, and bisphosphonates are the most commonly advocated pharmacologic treatments for involutional osteoporosis. Anabolic agents or osteoblast stimulator agents include fluoride and PTH. Fluoride is not approved by the U.S. Food and Drug Administration (FDA) at this time for the treatment of osteoporosis because of an increased risk of appendicular fractures (Table 34-2).

Table 34-2 FDA-Approved Medications for Use in Postmenopausal Osteoporosis

Medication	Prevention	Treatment (Dose)
Bone-Antiresorptive Agents*		
Estrogen	?	No
Alendronate (Fosamax)	Yes	10 mg/day or 70 mg/wk orally
Risedronate (Actonel)	Yes	5 mg/day or 35 mg/wk orally
Ibandronate sodium (Boniva)	Yes	150 mg/mo orally or 3 mg intravenously every 3 mo
Zoledronic acid (Reclast)	No	5 mg intravenously (over 15-min infusion) every 12 mo
Raloxifene (Evista)	Yes	60 mg/day orally
Calcitonin (Miacalcin) (not commonly used)	No	200 international units/day intranasally
Denosumab (Prolia)	No	60 mg subcutaneously every 6 mo
Bone-Forming Agent		
Teriparatide (Forteo)	No	20 μg/day subcutaneously
Also Required		
Calcium	Yes	1200-1500 mg/day† (food and/or supplement)
Vitamin D	Yes	800-1000 international units/day†

*Side effects. *Estrogen:* Breast cancer, endometrial cancer, etc., if used without progestin therapy. *Bisphosphonates:* Esophagitis, rare occurrence of jaw osteonecrosis. *Raloxifene:* Deep vein thrombosis, hot flashes, nausea, leg cramps, cerebrovascular accident. *Calcitonin:* See chapter text.

†Includes food and supplements.

FDA, U.S. Food and Drug Administration.

Teriparatide, a form of PTH, is currently the only bone-forming agent approved by the FDA. PTH(1-34) can decrease the risk of vertebral fractures and increase BMD of vertebral, femoral, and total body.[93] PTH is self-administered through subcutaneous injections (20 μg/day). To maintain PTH-induced gains after an 18- to 24-month drug therapy course, antiresorptive agents need to be considered.[44] There can reportedly be a 9% to 13% increase in BMD of the spine and a 65% to 69% reduction in risk of new vertebral fractures in patients receiving the treatment compared with those receiving placebo.[44] PTH therapy is contraindicated in patients who have a history of cancer; adverse effects include nausea, dizziness, leg cramps, headache, and hypercalcemia. Investigators are currently evaluating new agents that might improve bone mass. In one randomized study, receipt of a 15-minute infusion of zoledronic acid (5 mg in 100 mL) or placebo once yearly showed reduced incidence of vertebral fracture by 70% and hip fracture by 41% in the treatment group compared with the placebo group over the 3-year trial.[4] Zoledronic acid is approved for the prevention and treatment of osteoporosis in postmenopausal women. It is also approved to increase bone mass in men.[39,47,93] Osteonecrosis of the jaw has been reported to occur in patients taking bisphosphonates, and a warning regarding this adverse effect has recently been added to the labeling of all bisphosphonates.

Cessation of tobacco and alcohol abuse is necessary. An adequate calcium intake is required to permit normal bone development and, potentially, to decrease bone loss. Adequate calcium and vitamin D intake appears to have only a modest effect on bone loss after menopause. Inadequate intake of calcium and vitamin D is common, especially in elderly residents of nursing homes. One study showed the efficacy of supplementation of calcium and vitamin D for reduction of the risk of hip fracture in elderly patients.[11] Typical recommendations for women with hormone deficiency are 1200-1500 mg of elemental calcium daily in divided doses and between 800 and 1000 international units of vitamin D daily. The recommended dose of vitamin D varies and depends on the patient's exposure to the sun and dietary intake of vitamin D. Combining calcium and vitamin D into one supplement may increase adherence and efficacy.[55] It is necessary to determine the serum level of $1,25(OH)_2D_3$ in some cases (normal levels are at least 30 to 35 ng/mL and preferably 30 to 50 ng/mL), and serum levels below 20 ng/mL are considered a serious deficiency. These values can differ in different laboratories and locations in the United States.

Antiresorptive agents are numerous. Estrogen acts directly on bone cells and is an antiresorptive agent that has been shown to decrease the rate of bone loss and fractures in postmenopausal women, whether their menopause is natural or surgical. Estrogen is not as commonly used now because of the alarming results of the Women's Health Initiative studies.[3,18,25] When a patient with an intact uterus is treated with estrogen, progesterone should also be used under a proper regimen to prevent endometrial hyperplasia and possibly endometrial carcinoma. There are several regimens for estrogen and progesterone use. These agents may be used concurrently (combination pills) or cyclically. The proper regimen needs to be individualized.

Minimal effective doses of some form of oral estrogen are usually used (conjugated equine estrogens, 0.3 mg/day; estradiol, 50 mg/day). Parenteral estrogens can be administered as patches, implants, or gels. Implants are not popular in the United States. Estrogen patches deliver estradiol through the skin and are changed once or twice weekly. The advantage of parenteral estrogen is that metabolism in the liver is bypassed, making smaller doses sufficient. The strength of the commonly used transdermal estradiol-17 (patch) can vary from 0.05 mg (usual dose) to 0.1 mg (high dose). In some instances, a dose as low as 0.025 mg is used.

Contraindications to estrogen replacement therapy include liver or gallbladder disease, recent history of thromboembolism or thrombophlebitis, and suspected breast or endometrial carcinoma. Estrogens can also have an adverse effect on existing hypertension, hyperlipidemia, migraine headaches, chronic thrombophlebitis, and endometriosis. Administration of progestins can result in uncomfortable adverse effects, such as fatigue, depression, breast tenderness, bloating, menstrual cramps, and headaches.[51] Other potential adverse effects are weight gain, depression or mood change, increased serum triglyceride and glucose levels, and abnormal vaginal bleeding. The role of hormone replacement therapy for prevention and treatment of osteoporosis has been modified extensively.

Estrogen protects against both osteoporosis and cardiovascular disease. However, many postmenopausal women discontinued their use of hormone replacement therapy after the results of the Women's Health Initiative studies became available.[13,51] Of all breast cancer cases, 78% occur in women after age 50 years. There are reports that hormone replacement therapy increases the risk of breast cancer by 2.3% per year, and this risk increases to 3.5% per year after 5 years. Women who have cardiovascular disease should not use hormone replacement therapy for prevention. Estrogen therapy should also be discontinued if a woman has an acute cardiovascular event. In general, decision making for use of the therapy is better based on noncoronary benefit. The patient's preference is important for management of menopausal symptoms. Prevention of osteoporosis is no longer considered an indication for use of estrogen therapy.

Calcitonin, an antiresorptive agent, is not used as a first choice and acts directly on the osteoclasts. Calcitonin has a few disadvantages that limit its use[52] and it is not commonly recommended. It is most effective in patients whose rate of bone turnover is high. Calcitonin is approved for treatment of established osteoporosis, but the long-term fracture-reducing efficacy of calcitonin has not been clearly demonstrated. The subcutaneous or intramuscular injection of 50 to 100 units of salmon calcitonin or 0.5 mg of human calcitonin, given every other day, is commonly used. Use of nasal calcitonin might improve a patient's compliance; the adverse effects of parenteral use, such as flushing and nausea, and development of antibodies may limit its use. The nasal spray may cause nasal irritation, crusting, and ulcerations, which usually require discontinuation of its use.

Ibandronate sodium (Boniva) is approved for prevention and treatment of osteoporosis in postmenopausal women. It can reduce the incidence of vertebral fractures by approximately 50% over 3 years.[93] Ibandronate is taken orally once monthly as 150-mg tablets or as an intravenous injection (over 15-30 seconds) of 3 mg every 3 months.[93] Bisphosphonates affect trabecular bone, especially in the lumbar spine, where BMD increases of 5% to 10% occur during the first 2 years of treatment (see Table 34-2). Alendronate sodium, an aminobisphosphonate, has been shown to normalize the rate of bone turnover and increase bone mass.[12] Alendronate (10 mg/day or a once-a-week dose of 70 mg) must be taken with a full glass of water on awakening. The patient should not eat or recline for 30 to 45 minutes after taking the medication because of the risk of esophageal irritation. Patient education and compliance are important for the proper use of alendronate. Risedronate sodium or Actonel also increases bone density and reduces risk of spine and nonspine fractures by 35% to 45% over 3 years. Risedronate is another bisphosphonate that has been used for the treatment of osteoporosis. Treatment with risedronate (5 mg/day or a once-a-week dose of 35 mg) has been shown to considerably decrease the incidence of vertebral and nonvertebral fractures in postmenopausal osteoporosis.[27] Weekly doses of bisphosphonates are commonly recommended. One potential adverse effect of oral bisphosphonates is esophageal irritation, particularly in patients with reflux or other esophageal dysfunction.[93] Anabolic androgenic steroids (e.g., testosterone) can increase bone and muscle mass in women with hypogonadism,[93] but can produce unacceptable adverse effects. Low-dose testosterone therapy has been used by some women. Anabolic steroids have an osteoblastic effect. They are used only under the most extreme circumstances, however, because they can have marked androgenic effects and induce liver function abnormalities. Thiazide diuretics inhibit urinary excretion of calcium and can retard bone loss and reduce the rate of fractures in patients with osteoporosis.

Sodium fluoride stimulates osteoblastic activity and is used as a therapeutic measure for osteoporosis in some European countries but is not used as a routine form of treatment in the United States. It can increase bone density annually by up to 8% in the lumbar spine and 4% in the proximal femur; however, it decreases cortical bone density in the radius by approximately 2% per year. There also have been reports of an increased rate of nonvertebral fractures in patients treated with fluoride.

Denosumab (Prolia) is approved by the FDA to use in the treatment of osteoporosis in postmenopausal women at high risk of fracture and to increase bone mass in men with osteoporosis at high risk of fracture. It is a RANK ligand inhibitor/human monoclonal antibody. Denosumab is to be taken as a single subcutaneous injection of 60 mg every 6 months. A health care professional should administer the injection for better adherence. Patients need to have a blood test before each dose to confirm that the blood calcium level is normal. It is important to get enough calcium and vitamin D and to perform proper exercises every day.

Denosumab does have some adverse effects. It may lower calcium levels in the blood. If blood calcium levels are low before denosumab is received, this must be corrected before medication is injected, or it may become worse.

Newer medications are becoming available, and numerous studies are in progress. Some of these new medications include anabolics such as antisclrostin (Romosozumab) and an antiresorptive cathepsin K inhibitor (Odanacatib). I suggest that readers review upcoming literature updates and results of new studies related to the benefits and adverse effects of these medications before recommending them to their patients.

The estrogen receptor mixed agonist-antagonists tamoxifen and raloxifene protect against bone loss in ovariectomized rats. They have an antiestrogenic effect on breast tissue. These agents are also known as selective estrogen receptor modulators (SERMs).[14] The mechanism by which these compounds affect bone is not completely defined. Raloxifene appears to decrease the risk of estrogen-dependent breast cancer by 65% over 8 years and is approved for prevention and treatment of osteoporosis in postmenopausal women.[93] One of the adverse effects related to tamoxifen treatment is uterine hyperplasia, but this effect is not a concern with raloxifene treatment. Raloxifene decreases serum total cholesterol and low-density-lipoprotein cholesterol levels. Raloxifene (60 mg/day orally) is currently used only in the postmenopausal stage of osteoporosis. Potential adverse effects are leg cramps, hot flashes, and deep vein thrombosis. Raloxifene should not be given to women at increased risk for stroke.

Treatment of osteoporosis in men includes the usual supplementation with calcium (1200 to 1500 mg/day) and vitamin D (1000 international units/day), limitation of alcohol use, and cessation of smoking. In cases of hypogonadism in men, endocrine consultation is necessary, and testosterone replacement therapy is a possibility. Bisphosphonates have also been helpful as antiresorptive agents for management of osteoporosis in men. Zoledronic acid is also approved for increasing bone mass in men.[47]

Management of steroid-induced osteoporosis requires calcium and vitamin D supplementation, use of oral antiresorptive agents, such as alendronate sodium (70 mg once a week) or risedronate (35 mg once a week), and implementation of a proper weight-bearing and weight-training exercise program. In advanced stages of bone loss and muscle weakness, when fragility occurs, use of assistive devices or a wheelchair might be necessary.[65] If hyperparathyroidism or thyrotoxicosis is present, proper management should be implemented. In the case of hyperparathyroidism, surgical removal of the parathyroid adenoma is recommended.

A balanced diet is needed for maintenance of musculoskeletal health. Excessive dietary intake of sodium and phosphorus should be avoided. Studies of young women with malnutrition caused by anorexia nervosa have demonstrated irregularity of menstrual periods, estrogen deficiency, poor muscle strength, and marked loss of bone mass.

With regard to osteoporosis, the distinct effects of nutrition, exercise, hormones, and lifestyle cannot be separated.[67-69] There are genetic controls of bone, including gender, race, and nongender (environmental) factors (i.e., hormone status, nutrition, age, level of physical activity, and lifestyle changes).[54] A patient's quality of life can certainly be affected by musculoskeletal challenges related to osteoporosis. Practical treatment of patients with osteoporosis requires pharmacologic interventions, physical and rehabilitative measures, and good nutrition. It also requires consideration of the psychological consequences and reactions experienced by the patient. Public education can contribute to prevention, better understanding, and management of the consequences of osteoporosis. For up-to-date information, the National Osteoporosis Foundation[93] and the International Osteoporosis Foundation are excellent educational sources.

KEY REFERENCES

2. Adams MA, McNally DS, Dolan P: "Stress" distributions inside intervertebral discs. The effects of age and degeneration, *J Bone Joint Surg Br* 78:965–972, 1996.
7. Borgo M, Sinaki M: Back progressive resistive exercise program to reduce risk of vertebral fractures, *J Mineralstoffwechs* 17:66–71, 2010.
17. Emslander HC, Sinaki M, Muhs JM, et al: Bone mass and muscle strength in female college athletes (runners and swimmers), *Mayo Clin Proc* 73:1151–1160, 1998.
19. Fehling PC, Alekel L, Clasey J, et al: A comparison of bone mineral densities among female athletes in impact loading and active loading sports, *Bone* 17:205–210, 1995.
20. Felsing NE, Brasel JA, Cooper DM: Effect of low and high intensity exercise on circulating growth hormone in men, *J Clin Endocrinol Metab* 75:157–162, 1992.
21. Fredericson M, Kent K: Normalization of bone density in a previously amenorrheic runner with osteoporosis, *Med Sci Sports Exerc* 37:1481–1486, 2005.
22. Frost HM: A determinant of bone architecture. The minimum effective strain, *Clin Orthop Relat Res* 175:286–292, 1983.
24. Genant HK, Vogler JB, Block JE: Radiology of osteoporosis. In Riggs BL, Melton LJ 3rd, editors: *Osteoporosis: etiology, diagnosis, and management*, New York, 1988, Raven Press.
28. Hongo M, Itoi E, Sinaki M, et al: Effects of reducing resistance, repetitions, and frequency of back-strengthening exercise in healthy young women: a pilot study, *Arch Phys Med Rehabil* 86:1299–1303, 2005.
30. Huntoon EA, Schmidt CK, Sinaki M: Significantly fewer refractures after vertebroplasty in patients who engage in back-extensor-strengthening exercises, *Mayo Clin Proc* 83:54–57, 2008.
32. Itoi E, Sinaki M: Effect of back-strengthening exercise on posture in healthy women 49 to 65 years of age, *Mayo Clin Proc* 69:1054–1059, 1994.
35. Kallmes DF, Comstock BA, Heagerty PJ, et al: A randomized trial of vertebroplasty for osteoporotic spinal fractures, *N Engl J Med* 361:569–579, 2009.
36. Kaplan RS, Sinaki M, Hameister MD: Effect of back supports on back strength in patients with osteoporosis: a pilot study, *Mayo Clin Proc* 71:235–241, 1996.
37. Lanyon LE: Using functional loading to influence bone mass and architecture: objectives, mechanisms, and relationship with estrogen of the mechanically adaptive process in bone, *Bone* 18:37S–43S, 1996.
40. Lynn SG, Sinaki M, Westerlind KC: Balance characteristics of persons with osteoporosis, *Arch Phys Med Rehabil* 78:273–277, 1997.
47. Orwoll ES, Bilezikian JP, Vaneerschueren D, editors: *Osteoporosis in men: the effects of gender on skeletal health*, Boston, 2010, Elsevier.
49. Pfeifer M, Begerow B, Minne HW: Effects of a new spinal orthosis on posture, trunk strength, and quality of life in women with postmenopausal osteoporosis: a randomized trial, *Am J Phys Med Rehabil* 83:61–66, 2004.
50. Pfeifer M, Sinaki M, Geusens P, et al: Musculoskeletal rehabilitation in osteoporosis: a review, *J Bone Miner Res* 19:1208–1214, 2004.
54. Rizzoli R, Bonjour JP, Ferrari SL: Osteoporosis, genetics and hormones, *J Mol Endocrinol* 26:79–94, 2001.

56. Robinovitch SN, Inkster L, Maurer J, et al: Strategies for avoiding hip impact during sideways falls, *J Bone Miner Res* 18:1267–1273, 2003.
58. Seeman E: The dilemma of osteoporosis in men, *Am J Med* 98:76S–88S, 1995.
59. Sinaki M: Beneficial musculoskeletal effects of physical activity in the older women, *Geriatr Med Today* 8:53–59, 1989.
60. Sinaki M: Critical appraisal of physical rehabilitation measures after osteoporotic vertebral fracture, *Osteoporos Int* 14:773–779, 2003.
62. Sinaki M: Exercise for patients with osteoporosis: management of vertebral compression fractures and trunk strengthening for fall prevention, *PM R* 4:882–888, 2012.
63. Sinaki M: Falls, fractures, and hip pads, *Curr Osteoporos Rep* 2:131–137, 2004.
64. Sinaki M: Musculoskeletal challenges of osteoporosis, *Aging Clin Exp Res* 10:249–262, 1998.
66. Sinaki M: Musculoskeletal rehabilitation in patients with osteoporosis: rehabilitation of osteoporosis program-exercise (ROPE), *J Mineralstoffwechs* 17:56–61, 2010.
67. Sinaki M: Nonpharmacologic interventions. Exercise, fall prevention, and role of physical medicine, *Clin Geriatr Med* 19:337–359, 2003.
68. Sinaki M: The role of physical activity in bone health: a new hypothesis to reduce risk of vertebral fracture, *Phys Med Rehabil Clin N Am* 18:593–608, 2007.
70. Deleted in review.
71. Sinaki M: Yoga spinal flexion positions and vertebral compression fracture in osteopenia or osteoporosis of spine: case series, *Pain Pract* 13:68–75, 2013.
72. Sinaki M, Borgo MJ, Itoi E: An effective progressive resistive exercise program from prone position for paravertebral muscles to reduce risk of vertebral fractures, *J Bone Miner Res* 23:S495, 2008.
73. Sinaki M, Brey RH, Hughes CA, et al: Balance disorder and increased risk of falls in osteoporosis and kyphosis: significance of kyphotic posture and muscle strength, *Osteoporos Int* 16:1004–1010, 2005.
74. Sinaki M, Brey RH, Hughes CA, et al: Significant reduction in risk of falls and back pain in osteoporotic-kyphotic women through a Spinal Proprioceptive Extension Exercise Dynamic (SPEED) program, *Mayo Clin Proc* 80:849–855, 2005.
75. Sinaki M, Canvin JC, Phillips BE, et al: Site specificity of regular health club exercise on muscle strength, fitness, and bone density in women aged 29 to 45 years, *Mayo Clin Proc* 79:639–644, 2004.
76. Sinaki M, Fitzpatrick LA, Ritchie CK, et al: Site-specificity of bone mineral density and muscle strength in women: job-related physical activity, *Am J Phys Med Rehabil* 77:470–476, 1998.
78. Sinaki M, Huntoon E: Back pain in the osteoporotic individual: a physiatric approach, *Tech Reg Anesth Pain Manage* 15:64–68, 2011.
80. Sinaki M, Itoi E, Rogers JW, et al: Correlation of back extensor strength with thoracic kyphosis and lumbar lordosis in estrogen-deficient women, *Am J Phys Med Rehabil* 75:370–374, 1996.
81. Sinaki M, Itoi E, Wahner HW, et al: Stronger back muscles reduce the incidence of vertebral fractures: a prospective 10 year follow-up of postmenopausal women, *Bone* 30:836–841, 2002.
82. Sinaki M, Limburg PJ, Wollan PC, et al: Correlation of trunk muscle strength with age in children 5 to 18 years old, *Mayo Clin Proc* 71:1047–1054, 1996.
83. Sinaki M, Lynn SG: Reducing the risk of falls through proprioceptive dynamic posture training in osteoporotic women with kyphotic posturing: a randomized pilot study, *Am J Phys Med Rehabil* 81:241–246, 2002.
84. Sinaki M, Mikkelsen BA: Postmenopausal spinal osteoporosis: flexion versus extension exercises, *Arch Phys Med Rehabil* 65:593–596, 1984.
85. Sinaki M, Nwaogwugwu NC, Phillips BE, et al: Effect of gender, age, and anthropometry on axial and appendicular muscle strength, *Am J Phys Med Rehabil* 80:330–338, 2001.
86. Sinaki M, Offord KP: Physical activity in postmenopausal women: effect on back muscle strength and bone mineral density of the spine, *Arch Phys Med Rehabil* 69:277–280, 1988.
86a. Sinaki M, Pfeifer M: Treatment of vertebral fractures due to osteoporosis, *Osteologie* 24:7–10, 2015.
87. Sinaki M, Pfeifer M, Preisinger E, et al: The role of exercise in the treatment of osteoporosis, *Curr Osteoporos Rep* 8:138–144, 2010.
88. Sinaki M, Wahner HW, Bergstralh EJ, et al: Three-year controlled, randomized trial of the effect of dose-specified loading and strengthening exercises on bone mineral density of spine and femur in nonathletic, physically active women, *Bone* 19:233–244, 1996.
89. Sinaki M, Wahner HW, Offord KP, et al: Efficacy of nonloading exercises in prevention of vertebral bone loss in postmenopausal women: a controlled trial, *Mayo Clin Proc* 64:762–769, 1989.
90. Sinaki M, Wollan PC, Scott RW, et al: Can strong back extensors prevent vertebral fractures in women with osteoporosis?, *Mayo Clin Proc* 71:951–956, 1996.
93. National Osteoporosis Foundation: *Clinician's guide to prevention and treatment of osteoporosis*, Washington, 2013, National Osteoporosis Foundation. Available at: http://nof.org/.
94. van Schoor NM, Smit JH, Twisk JW, et al: Prevention of hip fractures by external hip protectors: a randomized controlled trial, *JAMA* 289:1957–1962, 2003.

The full reference list for this chapter is available online.

CHAPTER 35

UPPER LIMB PAIN AND DYSFUNCTION

Jonathan T. Finnoff

"The whole is greater than the sum of its parts." This statement is surely reflected in the upper limb. Through the complex interplay of neuromusculoskeletal elements in the upper limb, activities as dichotomous as playing a piano and throwing a shot put can be achieved. The diversity of functional roles performed by the upper limb is reflected by the multitude of injuries that can occur in this anatomic region.

Upper Limb Physical Examination

Shoulder Special Tests

Anterior Apprehension and Relocation Tests

These are tests for anterior glenohumeral joint instability. The patient is placed in the supine position. The examiner abducts the patient's shoulder 90 degrees and flexes the elbow 90 degrees. The examiner then uses one hand to slowly externally rotate the patient's humerus, using the patient's forearm as the lever. At the same time, the examiner's other hand is placed posterior to the patient's proximal humerus and exerts an anteriorly directed force on the humeral head. The test result is considered positive if the patient indicates a feeling of impending anterior dislocation. If the examiner removes the hand from behind the proximal humerus and places it over the anterior proximal humerus and then exerts a posteriorly directed force, and the patient subsequently reports a reduction in apprehension, then a positive relocation test has occurred.[73]

Posterior Apprehension Test

This test evaluates posterior glenohumeral joint stability. The patient's affected shoulder is forward flexed to 90 degrees and then maximally internally rotated. A posteriorly directed force is then placed on the patient's elbow by the examiner. A positive test result causes a 50% or greater posterior translation of the humeral head or a feeling of apprehension in the patient.[73]

Sulcus Sign

The sulcus sign is used to evaluate inferior glenohumeral joint instability. The patient is seated or standing with the arm relaxed in shoulder adduction. The patient's forearm is grasped by the examiner, and a distal traction force is placed through the patient's arm. In the presence of inferior instability, a sulcus will develop between the humeral head and the acromion.[73]

O'Brien Test

This test evaluates for acromioclavicular (AC) joint and labral abnormalities. The shoulder is flexed to 90 degrees with the elbow fully extended. The arm is then adducted 15 degrees, and the shoulder is internally rotated so that the patient's thumb is pointing down. The examiner applies a downward force against the arm that the patient is instructed to resist. The shoulder is then externally rotated so that the patient's palm is facing up, and the examiner applies a downward force on the patient's arm that the patient is instructed to resist. A positive test result is indicated by pain during the first part of the maneuver with the patient's thumb pointing down that is then lessened or eliminated when the patient resists a downward force with the palm facing up. Pain in the region of the AC joint indicates AC pathology, whereas pain or painful clicking deep inside the shoulder suggests labral pathology.[89,112]

Horizontal Adduction Test

The shoulder is passively flexed to 90 degrees and then horizontally adducted across the chest. Pain located in the region of the AC joint suggests AC joint pathology, whereas posterior shoulder pain suggests posterior capsular tightness.[75]

Speed Test

This test is for biceps tendonitis. The patient's shoulder is forward flexed to 90 degrees with the elbow fully extended and the palm facing up. The examiner applies a downward force against the patient's active resistance. Pain in the region of the bicipital groove suggests bicipital tendonitis.[73]

Yergason Test

With the patient's arm at the side, the elbow is flexed to 90 degrees and the forearm is pronated. The patient then tries to simultaneously supinate the forearm and externally rotate the shoulder against the examiner's resistance. This test can provoke bicipital region pain in patients with bicipital tendonitis and a painful "pop" in patients with bicipital tendon instability.[73]

Neer-Walsh Impingement Test

The patient's shoulder is internally rotated while at the side. The examiner passively forward flexes the patient's shoulder to 180 degrees while maintaining internal rotation. Pain in the subacromial area suggests rotator cuff tendonitis.[73]

Hawkins-Kennedy Impingement Test

The patient's shoulder and elbow are each passively flexed to 90 degrees, respectively. The examiner then grasps the patient's forearm, stabilizes the patient's scapulothoracic joint, and uses the forearm as a lever arm to internally rotate the glenohumeral joint. A positive test result is indicated by pain in the subacromial region occurring with the internal rotation.[73]

Drop Arm Test

The examiner passively abducts the patient's shoulder 90 degrees. The patient is then asked to slowly lower the arm back to the side. A positive test result is indicated by pain and an inability to slowly lower the arm to the side, suggesting a rotator cuff tear.[73]

Elbow Special Tests

Cozen Test

The patient is asked to fully extend the elbow, pronate the forearm, and make a fist. The examiner then resists the patient's attempt to extend and radially deviate the wrist. Pain over the lateral epicondyle represents a positive test result and suggests the presence of lateral epicondylitis.[71]

Ligamentous Instability Test

The examiner flexes the patient's elbow 20 to 30 degrees and stabilizes the patient's arm by placing a hand at the elbow and a hand on the distal forearm. Varus and valgus forces are placed across the elbow by the examiner to test the stability of the radial and ulnar collateral ligaments (UCL), respectively.[71]

Wrist and Hand Special Tests

Finkelstein Test

This test is used to detect tenosynovitis of the extensor pollicis brevis and abductor pollicis longus tendons (de Quervain tenosynovitis). The patient makes a fist with the thumb inside the fingers, and the examiner passively deviates the wrist in an ulnar direction. A positive test result causes pain in the affected tendons.[72]

Watson Test

This test assesses scapholunate stability. The patient's wrist begins in an ulnarly deviated position. The examiner places a dorsally directed force against the proximal volar pole of the scaphoid. The examiner then radially deviates the wrist while continuing to place the same force against the scaphoid. A "pop" or subluxation of the scaphoid indicates a positive test result.[72]

Rehabilitation Principles of Upper Limb Injury

The importance of making the correct diagnosis in planning an appropriate treatment program cannot be overemphasized. A complete diagnosis includes whether the injury is acute, chronic, or an acute exacerbation of a chronic injury. Understanding the mechanism of injury is important. Tissues that are overloaded by the injury, as well as those directly injured, must be identified. Functional biomechanical deficits such as strength and flexibility imbalances are frequently present. The patient often tries to compensate for the injury by altering movement patterns and using muscle substitutions, which leads to a reduction in functional performance and secondary injuries at distant sites in the kinetic chain.

Once an accurate diagnosis has been made with a thorough history, physical examination, and appropriate diagnostic testing, an effective treatment program can be developed. Kibler[58] has proposed three broad stages of rehabilitation: the acute stage, the recovery stage, and the functional stage. The acute stage of rehabilitation focuses on reducing the patient's symptoms and facilitating tissue healing. In specific circumstances, immobilization through splinting or casting might be used during the acute stage of rehabilitation.

RICE (*r*est, *i*ce, *c*ompression, and *e*levation) is frequently used in this phase of rehabilitation. Rest should not be absolute. It is important for the patient to maintain cardiovascular fitness, strength, and flexibility during this phase. In fact, core strengthening and aerobic conditioning should be emphasized during this phase of rehabilitation. The patient should be instructed on appropriate activities that can be performed during the acute stage of rehabilitation that will not aggravate symptoms nor be detrimental to tissue healing. For example, if a volleyball player has rotator cuff tendonitis, activities that could be done include passive glenohumeral joint range-of-motion (ROM) exercises to maintain flexibility and glenohumeral joint health, riding a stationary bicycle for cardiovascular fitness, and performing scapular stabilizing exercises in preparation for more advanced rehabilitative exercises of the shoulder. Kinetic chain deficits should be identified and treated during the acute rehabilitation stage.

During the acute phase of rehabilitation, cryotherapy can be used for acute injuries to decrease pain, inflammation, muscle guarding, and edema.[47,57] Heat increases blood flow, reduces muscle "spasm," reduces pain, and can be used in the acute phase of rehabilitation for chronic injuries.[57] High-frequency electrical stimulation is often used during the acute phase of rehabilitation to reduce muscle guarding and increase local circulation.[124]

Opioid and nonopioid analgesics might be required for pain control during the acute phase of rehabilitation. Nonsteroidal antiinflammatory drugs (NSAIDs) are often used for their analgesic and antiinflammatory properties. Randomized, placebo-controlled trials have demonstrated reduced pain, edema, and tenderness, and a faster return to activity in NSAID-treated athletes than in those treated with placebo.[4,122] It is important to remember, however, that NSAIDs are not entirely benign and can cause significant gastrointestinal, renal, cardiovascular, hematologic, dermatologic, and neurologic side effects.[21,38,115] Because of these concerns, NSAIDs should be used only if local physical modalities and less toxic medications such as acetaminophen are not effective.

Oral and injected corticosteroids have also been used for pain control and reduction of inflammation during the acute phase of rehabilitation. Because of the possibility of significant systemic and localized consequences of corticosteroid use, however, their use should be limited to very select cases.[33,104] Potential complications include suppression of the hypothalamic-pituitary-adrenal axis, osteoporosis, avascular necrosis, skin depigmentation, fat atrophy, infection, tendon or ligament rupture, delayed healing, and worsening of the underlying condition.[24]

The patient can advance to the recovery phase of rehabilitation when the pain has been adequately controlled and tissue healing has occurred.[58] This is indicated by full pain-free ROM and the ability to participate in strengthening exercises for the injured limb. The emphasis of the recovery phase of rehabilitation involves the restoration of flexibility, strength, and proprioception in the injured limb. Strength and flexibility imbalances and maladaptive movement patterns and muscle substitutions should be corrected in this phase of rehabilitation. Open kinetic chain exercises can be beneficial when correcting strength imbalances, whereas closed chain exercises are frequently used to provide joint stabilization through muscle cocontraction. Cardiovascular and general fitness should be maintained with progression to functional activities toward the end of this phase.

The patient can begin the functional stage of rehabilitation when the injured limb has regained 75% to 80% of normal strength compared with the uninjured limb, and when there are no strength and flexibility imbalances.[58] The patient's rehabilitation needs to continue to address maladaptive movement patterns and muscle substitutions, and full strength should be obtained. Functional activities should be incorporated into the rehabilitation program with a vocational/avocational-specific progression that eventually leads to a return to normal activities.

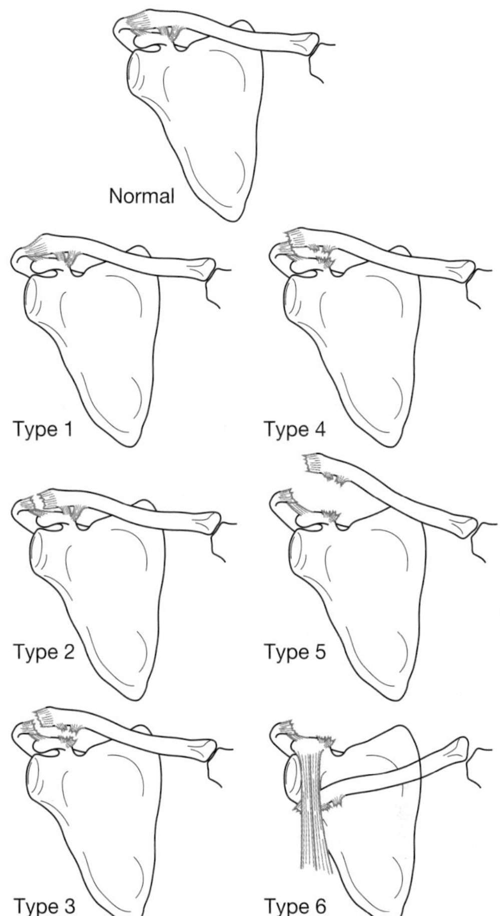

FIGURE 35-1 The Rockwood classification of acromioclavicular joint sprains.

Musculoskeletal Problems of the Upper Limb

Conditions of the Shoulder

Acromioclavicular Joint Sprains

AC joint sprains account for only 9% of all shoulder injuries, are most frequent in men in their third decade of life, and are usually partial rather than complete sprains.[75] Most injuries occur as a result of direct trauma from a fall or blow to the acromion. Physical examination demonstrates point tenderness, a positive horizontal adduction test, and a positive O'Brien test.

Rockwood[105] classified AC joint sprains into six types (Figure 35-1). Type 1 sprains involve a mild injury to the AC ligaments, and radiologic evaluation is normal. Type 2 injuries involve the complete disruption of the AC ligaments but with intact coracoclavicular ligaments. Radiographs might demonstrate clavicular elevation relative to the acromion but less than 25% displacement. Type 3 sprains result in the complete disruption of the AC and coracoclavicular ligaments, but the deltotrapezial fascia remains intact. Radiographs reveal a 25% to 100% increase in the coracoclavicular interspace relative to the normal shoulder. Type 4 sprains involve complete disruption of the coracoclavicular and AC ligaments, with posterior displacement of the distal clavicle into the trapezius muscle. In type 5 sprains, the coracoclavicular and AC ligaments are fully disrupted along with a rupture of the deltotrapezial fascia. This results in an increase in the coracoclavicular interspace to greater than 100% of the normal shoulder. Type 6 sprains involve complete disruption of the coracoclavicular and AC ligaments, as well as the deltotrapezial muscular attachments, with displacement of the distal clavicle below the acromion or the coracoid process.

Radiographic evaluation of the AC joint should include anteroposterior and lateral views of the AC joint and a Zanca view (anteroposterior projection with 15-degree cephalic tilt). Stress views do not provide additional clinically useful information.[75]

Type 1, 2, and 3 AC joint sprains are usually treated nonoperatively, with the previously described principles of rehabilitation. A brief period of sling immobilization might be required for pain control. Indications for surgical intervention for type 3 sprains include persistent pain or unsatisfactory cosmetic results. Some authors advocate operative treatment of type 3 sprains in heavy laborers and athletes who participate in sports that place a high demand on the upper limbs,[19,62,96] but the current literature favors nonoperative treatment for type 3 sprains.[116] Type 4, 5, or 6 sprains require surgical treatment.[75]

Rotator Cuff Tendonitis and Impingement

Injuries to the rotator cuff are common. Although macrotrauma can cause rotator cuff injuries, repetitive

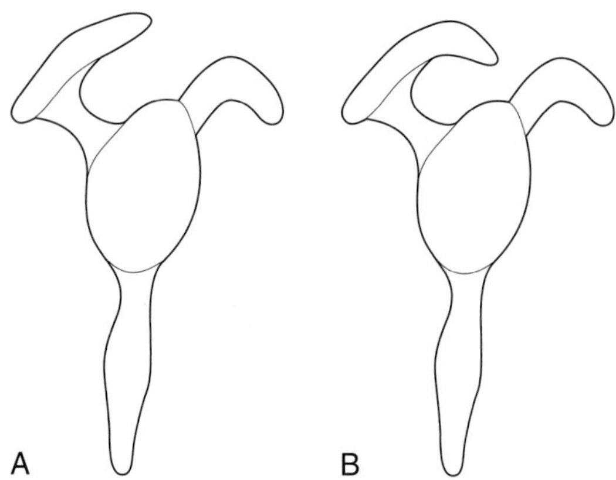

FIGURE 35-2 **A,** Type I acromion. **B,** Type 3 acromion.

microtrauma and outlet impingement between the acromion and greater tuberosity of the humerus are more common.[80] On cadaveric examination, Bigliani et al.[15] found a relation between the acromial shape and the presence of rotator cuff tears. He classified the acromions into three types (Figure 35-2). Type 1 acromions were relatively flat, whereas type 2 acromions demonstrated a curve, and type 3 acromions were hooked. The incidence of rotator cuff tears increased as the acromion progressed from a type 1 to a type 3 shape. This was presumably related to the greater outlet impingement of the rotator cuff caused by an increasing acromial curve.

Microvascular studies of the rotator cuff have found a hypovascular zone in the articular surface of the leading edge of the supraspinatus tendon.[70,100] This hypovascular area has been implicated as a cause of rotator cuff degeneration and correlates with the higher incidence of articular-sided partial-thickness tears in the anterior aspect of the supraspinatus tendon.

Subacromial, or "outlet," impingement can be primary or secondary. Examples of causative factors leading to primary impingement include a hooked acromion or a thick coracoacromial ligament. Secondary impingement has many causes, including glenohumeral joint instability, weak scapular stabilizers, scapulothoracic dyskinesis, and instability.[44,45] Lack of adequate scapular control or weakness in the scapular stabilizers can lead to inadequate acromial retraction during overhead activities, creating secondary impingement. Regardless of whether the impingement is primary or secondary, the underlying cause must be determined to formulate an appropriate treatment program.

Another form of impingement, internal impingement, can occur in overhead athletes.[27,121] When the arm is abducted 90 degrees and maximally externally rotated, there is contact between the undersurface of the rotator cuff and the posterosuperior glenoid rim. This is augmented by anterior glenohumeral joint instability and posterior glenohumeral joint capsular tightness. Internal impingement causes pathologic changes to the undersurface of the rotator cuff.

Patients with rotator cuff injuries frequently note anterior or lateral shoulder pain that occurs with overhead activity and also at night while trying to sleep. Symptoms such as stiffness, weakness, and catching might also be present. It is important to try to elicit any symptoms of underlying glenohumeral joint instability such as numbness, tingling, feelings of subluxation, or previous "dead arm" episodes.

The physical examination of patients with suspected rotator cuff pathology should include an evaluation of the cervical spine because problems originating in the cervical spine frequently refer symptoms to the shoulder. During inspection, the examiner should be sure to assess for proper scapulothoracic mechanics. Strength testing of the rotator cuff muscles can detect weakness as a result of a rotator cuff tear or pain inhibition caused by tendonitis or tendinosis. The Neer-Walsh and Hawkins-Kennedy impingement tests should be performed. Elimination of the pain provoked by impingement testing after injection of 10 mL of 1% lidocaine into the subacromial space confirms the diagnosis of impingement.

The examination of individuals with suspected rotator cuff pathology should also include maneuvers to detect underlying glenohumeral joint instability. The anterior apprehension test can be used to detect both anterior instability of the glenohumeral joint and also internal impingement. If the patient has a sensation of anterior apprehension during the test that is relieved with the relocation test, then there is likely anterior instability. If, however, there is pain in the posterior aspect of the shoulder during the anterior apprehension test that is relieved with the relocation test, then internal impingement is occurring.

Radiographic evaluation of patients with suspected rotator cuff pathology should include anteroposterior, supraspinatus outlet, and axillary radiographs. Anteroposterior radiographs should be performed in the neutral, external, and internal rotation positions to adequately visualize the glenohumeral joint and the greater and lesser tuberosities. Large rotator cuff tears can be indicated by an acromiohumeral distance of less than 7 mm and sclerosis on the undersurface of the acromion. The supraspinatus outlet view allows for categorization of the acromion type and will reveal AC joint osteophytes. Double-contrast arthrograms identify full-thickness rotator cuff tears, partial-thickness articular surface tears, and biceps tendon pathology. Bursal surface and intrasubstance partial-thickness rotator cuff tears are poorly evaluated with this technique. Ultrasound and magnetic resonance imaging (MRI) have higher levels of sensitivity and specificity for rotator cuff pathology than radiographs.[9,50]

Nonoperative treatment should include application of the previously described rehabilitation principles. Strengthening exercises for the scapular stabilizing muscles rather than the rotator cuff should be emphasized in the acute rehabilitation stage. Specifically, strengthening muscles that retract and depress the scapula (e.g., serratus anterior and inferior trapezius) and stretching muscles that protract and elevate the scapula (e.g., pectoralis minor and upper trapezius) reduce impingement. Posterior glenohumeral joint capsular tightness should be corrected, particularly in patients with internal impingement. It is imperative to reestablish normal scapulothoracic kinematics through neuromuscular retraining. This can begin once shoulder ROM is pain-free. Rotator cuff muscle strengthening should begin with closed chain exercises to promote stability and proprioception. Open chain exercises can be used to correct strength imbalances, such as weakness of the shoulder external rotators relative to the internal rotators. Some patients benefit from a subacromial corticosteroid injection, although studies of corticosteroid injections have shown mixed results.[46,77,78,84] Patients recalcitrant to these measures might benefit from extracorporeal shock-wave therapy or, if calcific tendonitis is present, ultrasound-guided percutaneous lavage and aspiration of the calcification.[28,90] If the patient fails to respond to the above measures, surgical evaluation should be considered.

Patients who have sustained an acute full-thickness rotator cuff tear should receive early surgical intervention to maximize their postoperative recovery potential. If the rotator cuff tear is chronic or degenerative, an initial trial of nonoperative rehabilitation measures can be used with the goal of restoring the patient to a functional level. In the young or active subgroups, however, nonoperative measures frequently fail to restore the patient to an adequate level of function, and surgical intervention is required.

Glenohumeral Joint Instability

Glenohumeral joint stability is provided by a combination of static and dynamic stabilizers. The static stabilizers of the glenohumeral joint include the bony congruence between the humeral head and the glenoid fossa, the glenoid labrum, the negative intraarticular pressure, the glenohumeral joint capsule, and the glenohumeral ligaments.[1] The dynamic stabilizers of the glenohumeral joint include the scapular stabilizing and rotator cuff muscles, and the long head of the biceps.[63] The importance of optimal scapular function for glenohumeral joint stability cannot be overemphasized. The scapular stabilizing muscles orient the scapula properly in relation to the humerus for optimal static and dynamic stability of the glenohumeral joint and stabilize the scapula during glenohumeral joint movements.[32] The primary scapular stabilizing muscles include the serratus anterior, trapezius, pectoralis minor, rhomboideus minor and major, latissimus dorsi, and levator scapulae.[32]

The rotator cuff muscles include the supraspinatus, infraspinatus, subscapularis, and teres minor. These muscles contribute to dynamic glenohumeral joint stability through a number of mechanisms. Concavity compression, first described by Lippitt et al.,[68] refers to the compressive forces placed on the glenohumeral joint during rotator cuff muscle cocontractions. These forces press the humeral head into the glenoid fossa, center the humeral head within the glenoid fossa, and help resist glenohumeral translation. Because the glenohumeral ligaments are lax in the midranges of glenohumeral joint motion, coordinated rotator cuff muscle contraction and concavity compression are particularly important mechanisms for glenohumeral joint stability in these ranges.[63]

At the distal insertion of the rotator cuff muscles on the humerus, there is an intertwining of the joint capsule with the rotator cuff tendons. With rotator cuff muscle contraction, it is possible that the glenohumeral joint capsule develops tension and increases in stiffness, consequently acting as a dynamic musculoligamentous stabilizing system.[63]

The rotator cuff muscles also provide glenohumeral joint stability through passive muscle tension and act as barriers to glenohumeral joint translation during active motion.[17,20] The subscapularis appears to be an especially important stabilizer for both anterior and posterior glenohumeral joint stability.[16,29]

Proprioception and neuromuscular control refer to the mechanism by which the position and movements of the shoulder girdle are sensed (proprioception), processed, and result in an appropriate motor response (neuromuscular control).[83] Glenohumeral joint instability is often associated with a concomitant decrement in proprioception.[66] The abnormal proprioception is restored after surgical correction of the joint instability, suggesting that one of the mechanisms causing proprioceptive deficits in unstable glenohumeral joints is a lack of appropriate capsuloligamentous tension.[67]

The classification of glenohumeral joint instability includes the degree, frequency, etiology, and direction of instability.[10] The degree includes dislocation, subluxation, or microinstability. A dislocation implies that the humeral head is disassociated from the glenoid fossa and often requires manual reduction. A subluxation occurs when the humeral head translates to the edge of the glenoid, beyond normal physiologic limits, followed by self-reduction. Microinstability is attributable to excessive capsular laxity, is multidirectional, and is frequently associated with internal impingement of the rotator cuff.[10]

The frequency of instability can be either acute or chronic.[10] Acute instability involves a new injury resulting in subluxation or dislocation of the glenohumeral joint. Chronic instability refers to repetitive instability episodes.

The etiology of glenohumeral joint instability can be traumatic or atraumatic.[10] Unidirectional instability is frequently caused by a traumatic event resulting in disruption of the glenohumeral joint. Atraumatic instability is attributable to congenital capsular laxity or repetitive microtrauma. Atraumatic instability can be subclassified into voluntary and involuntary categories. Voluntary instability refers to an individual who volitionally subluxes or dislocates his or her glenohumeral joint, whereas those with involuntary instability do not. Some patients with voluntary instability have associated psychological pathology, which often portends a poor outcome if surgical stabilization is performed.[106]

Glenohumeral joint instability can be unidirectional or multidirectional. Unidirectional instability refers to instability only in one direction. The most frequent type of unidirectional instability is traumatic anterior instability.[10] Multidirectional instability is instability in two or more directions and is usually caused by congenital capsular laxity or chronic repetitive microtrauma.[10]

Traumatic anterior glenohumeral dislocation frequently tears the anterior inferior glenohumeral joint capsule (e.g., the middle glenohumeral ligament and/or anterior band of the inferior glenohumeral ligament [IGHL]) and avulses the anterior inferior glenoid labrum with or without some underlying bone from the glenoid rim.[63] The latter of these two entities is frequently referred to as a Bankart lesion.[11] Acute anterior glenohumeral joint dislocations are also frequently associated with a compression fracture of the posterolateral aspect of the humeral head, referred to as a Hill-Sachs defect.[107]

Inferior glenohumeral joint instability typically does not occur in isolation. Causes of inferior glenohumeral joint instability include capsuloligamentous laxity or injury and absence of the glenoid fossa upward tilt.

Congenital glenoid hypoplasia or excessive glenoid or humeral retroversion has been reported to contribute to posterior glenohumeral joint instability. The more common lesions that lead to posterior glenohumeral joint instability, however, include excessive capsuloligamentous laxity or injury, or injury to the subscapularis tendon.[6] A tear of the posterior inferior glenoid labrum causing separation from the glenoid fossa rim, often referred to as a "reverse Bankart lesion," or a fracture of the posterior inferior glenoid fossa rim can also cause posterior glenohumeral joint instability.[6,98] A "reverse Hill-Sachs defect" can also be present, representing an impaction fracture of the anterior humeral head.[6,98]

Multidirectional instability can be caused by primary or secondary capsuloligamentous laxity. It is frequently seen bilaterally and can be accompanied by generalized ligamentous laxity.[10] Recurrent unilateral joint instability occasionally stretches the glenohumeral capsuloligamentous structures to the point that multidirectional instability develops secondarily.[10] Another possible cause for secondary multidirectional instability is the presence of an underlying connective tissue disorder such as Marfan or Ehlers-Danlos syndromes.[10]

Although many patients with glenohumeral joint instability have vague symptoms, common complaints of patients with shoulder instability include pain, popping, catching, locking, an unstable sensation, stiffness, and swelling.[12] A history of acute trauma or chronic, repetitive microtrauma should be obtained. Some patients might have a history of glenohumeral joint dislocation, and the examiner should find out the direction of dislocation, the duration of the dislocation, whether it has recurred, and whether it required manual reduction or spontaneously reduced. Subluxation episodes are commonly associated with a burning or aching dead feeling in the arm. Repetitive overhead activities such as baseball pitching can cause enough microtrauma to lead to symptomatic laxity.[12] Patients should be asked whether they or their family members have a history of generalized ligamentous laxity or connective tissue disorders.

The physical examination should include inspection, palpation, glenohumeral joint ROM, analysis of scapulothoracic kinesis, upper limb strength, sensation (including proprioception), reflex evaluations, and special tests for glenohumeral joint instability.

The most common initial radiographic views for the evaluation of glenohumeral joint instability include the anteroposterior shoulder view, axillary lateral view, and scapular "Y" view.[10] The anteroposterior view allows visualization of the osseous structures of the shoulder, including the scapula, clavicle, upper ribs, humeral head, and glenoid rim.[107] With internal rotation, the anteroposterior view can also allow visualization of a Hill-Sachs defect.[107] The scapular Y view can help in the assessment of glenohumeral joint alignment after acute dislocations.[107] The axillary lateral view can assess anterior or posterior subluxation or dislocation, as well as fractures of the anterior or posterior glenoid rim.[107] Other specialized views include the Garth view and the West Point view, both of which are useful in the detection of Bankart fractures. The Stryker Notch view can be used for evaluation of Hill-Sachs defects and stress views for the documentation of the degree of glenohumeral joint instability.[107] Magnetic resonance arthrography provides optimal visualization of the labrum, cartilage, and joint capsule. Imaging of nondisplaced injuries to the IGHL and anteroinferior glenoid labrum is improved by placing the arm in an abducted and externally rotated position.

The treatment options for glenohumeral joint instability and dislocation include nonoperative and operative approaches. After glenohumeral joint subluxation episodes and in patients with multidirectional instability or unidirectional posterior or inferior instability, a comprehensive rehabilitation program that addresses kinetic chain deficits, scapulothoracic mechanics, and shoulder girdle strength, flexibility, and neuromuscular control is appropriate. Operative intervention should be considered only in those patients who have failed to improve after a comprehensive nonoperative treatment program.

For patients with glenohumeral joint instability, the strengthening program should begin with closed chain exercises that promote cocontraction of the glenohumeral joint–stabilizing musculature. The patient can eventually progress to functional open chain exercises as stability is achieved. Proprioceptive closed and open chain exercises are also important to recoordinate the stabilizing shoulder girdle musculature and attain engrams that respond appropriately to a dynamically changing environment.

For patients who have suffered a first-time traumatic anterior glenohumeral joint dislocation, the decision between a trial of nonoperative treatment versus immediate surgical stabilization is more controversial. In the older, less active patient, nonoperative management frequently is successful.[3] In the younger, more active patient involved in contact sports, studies have shown a very high redislocation rate in those treated nonoperatively compared with those receiving early operative intervention.[7,8,59,113]

Regardless of whether or not a patient opts for early surgical intervention, closed reduction confirmed by radiologic examination should be performed on all patients who sustain an acute glenohumeral joint dislocation that does not spontaneously reduce. Radiologic studies should be performed in two planes, such as anteroposterior and axillary lateral views, to confirm relocation and exclude an associated fracture.[107] Sensory testing over the deltoid muscle is important to rule out an associated axillary nerve injury.[10]

Standard sling immobilization can be used for comfort but does not change future redislocation rates.[48,49,110] Immobilization in shoulder external rotation does not appear to reduce redislocation rates.[52-55] The previously described shoulder instability rehabilitation program can be used to treat patients who opt for nonoperative treatment of their shoulder dislocation.

Adhesive Capsulitis

Adhesive capsulitis, or "frozen shoulder," is characterized by painful, restricted shoulder ROM in patients with normal radiographs.[39,85] Adhesive capsulitis occurs in approximately 2% to 5% of the general population, is 2 to

Table 35-1 Stages of Adhesive Capsulitis

Stage	Symptom Duration	Signs and Symptoms
1	1-3 mo	Painful shoulder movement, minimal restriction in motion
2	3-9 mo	Painful shoulder movement, progressive loss of glenohumeral joint motion
3	9-15 mo	Reduced pain with shoulder movement, severely restricted glenohumeral joint motion
4	15-24 mo	Minimal pain, progressive normalization of glenohumeral joint motion

4 times more common in women than men, and is most frequently seen in individuals between 40 and 60 years of age.[18,23]

Adhesive capsulitis is usually an idiopathic condition but can be associated with diabetes mellitus, inflammatory arthritis, trauma, prolonged immobilization, thyroid disease, cerebrovascular accident, myocardial infarction, or autoimmune disease. Pathologic evaluation can reveal perivascular inflammation, but the predominant abnormality is fibroblastic proliferation with increased collagen and nodular band formation.[18]

Adhesive capsulitis has been divided into four stages (Table 35-1).[42] Stage 1 occurs for the first 1 to 3 months and involves pain with shoulder movements but no significant glenohumeral joint ROM restriction when examined under anesthesia. In stage 2, the "freezing stage," symptoms have been present for 3 to 9 months and are characterized by pain with shoulder motion and progressive glenohumeral joint ROM restriction in forward flexion, abduction, and internal and external rotation. During stage 3, or the "frozen stage," symptoms have been present for 9 to 15 months and include a significant reduction in pain but maintenance of the restricted glenohumeral joint ROM. In stage 4, frequently referred to as the "thawing stage," symptoms have been present for approximately 15 to 24 months and ROM gradually improves.

Routine radiographic evaluation is usually normal, but glenohumeral joint arthrography typically shows a significant reduction in the capsular volume.

Treatment during stages 1 and 2 of adhesive capsulitis includes physical modalities, analgesics, and activity modification to reduce pain and inflammation. Up to three intraarticular corticosteroid injections can be used during stages 1 and 2 of adhesive capsulitis to reduce inflammation and pain, facilitate rehabilitation, and shorten the duration of this condition.[42,109] Postural retraining to reduce kyphotic posture and forward humeral positioning should be undertaken. Passive joint glides and passive and active assisted ROM exercises should be initiated. Early scapular stability exercises and closed chain rotator cuff exercises can be instituted. As the patient's symptoms improve, active ROM activities can be added, along with open chain and proprioceptive exercises. Most patients will have restoration of normal function over a 12- to 14-month period.[41,81] In patients who do not improve after 6 months of nonoperative treatment, more aggressive treatments such as capsular hydrodilatation, manipulation under anesthesia, and arthroscopic lysis of adhesions can be considered.*

Conditions of the Elbow

Lateral Epicondylitis

Lateral epicondylitis is a common tendinopathy of the lateral elbow and is frequently referred to as tennis elbow. This malady dates back to 1883, when it was described as an injury resulting from lawn tennis,[26] and it is reported to occur in up to 50% of tennis players.[88] Any activity that places excessive repetitive stress on the lateral forearm musculature, however, can cause this condition.

Lateral epicondylitis is more common in patients older than 35 years of age and peaks in those between 40 and 50 years old.[56,87] It is more common in male than in female tennis players but does not display a gender predilection in the general population.[25] When lateral epicondylitis results from a work-related injury, conservative measures are less successful, and surgical intervention occurs more frequently.[36]

Lateral epicondylitis is a misnomer for this condition because the pathologic changes (i.e., angiofibroblastic hyperplasia) are not inflammatory but rather degenerative.[87,101] A more appropriate term for this condition is lateral epicondylosis rather than epicondylitis. The degenerative changes occur most commonly in the origin of the extensor carpi radialis brevis but also involve the extensor digitorum communis origin in 30% of cases.[87] The origins of the extensor carpi radialis longus or extensor carpi ulnaris are only rarely involved.

Patients with lateral epicondylosis frequently report a gradual onset of symptoms, which usually occur after specific activities. Traumatic or sudden onset of symptoms can also occur. The backhand swing in tennis frequently exacerbates the symptoms, as does gripping and activities that require repetitive wrist extension and forearm pronation and supination. Physical examination can reveal point tenderness over the lateral epicondyle and a positive Cozen test. Entrapment of the posterior interosseous branch of the radial nerve can mimic lateral epicondylosis, but the tenderness associated with this condition is 3 to 4 cm distal to the lateral epicondyle rather than directly over it.[123]

Although standard anteroposterior and lateral radiographs are usually normal, an oblique view of the lateral epicondyle might reveal punctuate calcifications in the extensor tendon origin.[25]

Treatment involves discontinuation of provocative activities, oral analgesics, physical modalities, and bracing (e.g., lateral counter-force strap or neutral wrist splint). It is important to correct kinetic chain deficits, training errors, and inappropriate tennis racquet grip size and string tension. Eccentric strengthening of the wrist extensors appears to be the most effective exercise regimen for the treatment of lateral epicondylosis.[117] Peritendinous corticosteroid injections are occasionally used, but their long-term efficacy is questionable.[5,86] Promising new treatments include ultrasound-guided percutaneous needle tenotomy, autologous blood injections, and platelet-rich plasma

*References 14, 23, 40, 42, 91, 97, 99, 118.

injections.[31,79,82] Extracorporeal shock-wave therapy for lateral epicondylosis has been reported to be successful in 48% to 73% of cases recalcitrant to other nonoperative measures.[90] Recalcitrant cases can also be treated with surgical débridement of the degenerative tissue with approximately 85% of surgically treated patients reporting good to excellent results and only 3% reporting no improvement.[30,88]

Medial Epicondylitis

Medial epicondylitis, frequently referred to as golfer's elbow, has the same degenerative pathologic changes as those described in lateral epicondylitis and is more correctly termed medial epicondylosis.[92] This condition occurs 3 to 7 times less frequently than lateral epicondylosis, and the degenerative changes are most frequently found in the pronator teres and flexor carpi radialis origins.[92] Risk factors for medial epicondylosis include training errors, faulty equipment, repetitive activities requiring wrist flexion and forearm pronation, and biomechanical abnormalities (such as poor strength, flexibility imbalances, and joint instability).

Patients often report a gradual onset of pain over the medial epicondyle that is exacerbated by activities that require repetitive gripping, wrist flexion, and forearm pronation and supination. The patient might report a feeling of grip strength weakness. This condition occasionally occurs traumatically as a result of an acute rupture of the UCL of the elbow. Symptoms of a concomitant ulnar neuropathy can also be present. Physical examination demonstrates tenderness to palpation over the medial epicondyle, weakness in grip strength, pain when a tight fist is made, and pain with resisted wrist flexion and forearm pronation.

Oblique radiographs of the medial epicondyle can reveal punctuate calcifications in the region of the flexor tendon origins.[25] It is also important to rule out degenerative changes in the posterior medial aspect of the olecranon, because this condition can cause symptoms similar to those seen with medial epicondylosis.

Nonoperative treatment should include discontinuation of aggravating activities and use of analgesics, physical modalities, bracing (e.g., medial counter-force strap and neutral wrist splint) for pain control, and correcting kinetic chain deficits and training errors. Eccentric exercises can be used for the treatment of tendinopathy. Corticosteroid injections have been used to treat this condition but can lead to further tendon degeneration and a predisposition to tendon rupture. Autologous blood injections might be beneficial.[116] Medial epicondylosis can also be responsive to extracorporeal shock-wave therapy.[90] Operative treatment can be warranted for those who fail to improve with conservative measures.

Olecranon Bursitis

The olecranon bursa lies subcutaneously over the olecranon process. Olecranon bursitis can be septic or aseptic. Aseptic bursitis is either acute hemorrhagic bursitis resulting from a macrotraumatic insult to the bursa or chronic bursitis caused by repetitive microtrauma. Aseptic bursitis is frequently seen in athletes who participate in football or hockey.[61]

Aseptic bursitis can begin with a direct blow to the area, but some patients report an insidious onset of symptoms after a small abrasion or laceration to the area. If the injury is chronic and recurrent, the patient can experience an initial period of swelling that feels like a small liquid pouch. This pouch eventually organizes into a permanently thickened bursa with intrabursal bands.

Septic bursitis can occur as a result of a localized or systemic infection. It is associated with significant edema, erythema, and hyperthermia in the area of the infected bursa, and is frequently accompanied by systemic symptoms of infection. Physical examination reveals an edematous area over the olecranon that is usually tender to palpation. Elbow ROM can be limited because of tissue tightness and pain. If the bursa is infected, the area can feel warm, and the patient can have an increased white blood cell count.

Radiographic evaluation should be performed to determine whether the patient has an osteophyte over the tip of the olecranon or calcification within the bursal sac.

The initial treatment of an acute traumatic aseptic bursitis includes sterile aspiration of the bursa followed by application of a compressive dressing. The patient should begin an NSAID medication and frequently apply ice to the area. The olecranon should be protected from further insult with an elbow pad.

For those with chronic bursitis, treatment should include ice, intermittent NSAIDs, and protection of the area from further insult. If edema is present, a compressive dressing should be applied. An intrabursal injection of corticosteroid medications can be helpful. For aseptic bursitis that is recalcitrant to standard treatment, sclerotherapy with a tetracycline injection into the bursa has been advocated.[43] Surgical excision is also an option for patients who do not obtain relief with the above measures.

For patients with septic bursitis, the bursa should be aspirated for symptomatic relief and to obtain a fluid sample for laboratory analysis, including Gram stain, culture and sensitivity, and crystal analysis. The area should then be wrapped in a compressive dressing, and the patient should be instructed to elevate the arm. Intravenous antibiotics are warranted in patients with systemic symptoms, but oral antibiotics might be adequate for those experiencing only localized symptoms. If the patient does not improve with the above measures, referral for incision and drainage should be made.

Ulnar Collateral Ligament Sprain

Injuries to the UCL of the elbow are a result of valgus stress to the elbow. This can be caused by a single traumatic episode but frequently is seen with the repetitive microtrauma associated with throwing. The late cocking phase of overhead throwing is characterized by a valgus torque of approximately 64 N-m across the elbow.[34] During the acceleration phase of overhead throwing, the valgus forces across the elbow are increased, leading to further stress on the UCL.

The UCL is composed of an anterior, posterior, and transverse bundle. It is primarily stabilized by the anterior bundle.[119] The anterior bundle has a thin superficial and thick deep layer, and the superficial or deep layer can be torn individually or as a unit.[120]

Patients with UCL injuries complain of medial elbow pain exacerbated by the late cocking and acceleration phases of throwing. If the injury was acute, an audible pop might have been heard. More frequently, however, the symptoms have an insidious onset. Throwing athletes can experience a decrement in throwing velocity and accuracy. Ulnar nerve traction and neuritis can occur because of the increased laxity of the elbow. Physical examination frequently shows a 5-degree elbow flexion contracture, UCL tenderness, and pain with or without laxity during UCL instability testing.

Anteroposterior, lateral, and oblique radiographs of the elbow should be obtained. Calcification of the UCL can occur, and avulsions from the humeral or ulnar attachments should be ruled out.[108] Computed tomography (CT) or MRI arthrograms can further define the injury, particularly if the injury is a partial tear of the UCL that only involves the deep fibers.[108] MRI has the advantage of excellent soft tissue visualization.

Partial UCL injuries should be initially treated with nonoperative measures. Conservative treatment includes discontinuation of throwing activities for 3 to 6 weeks and initiation of gentle elbow ROM, modalities, and analgesics. Progressive strengthening of the medial forearm musculature should be done because these muscles are dynamic stabilizers of the medial elbow against valgus stress. Occasionally, a hinged elbow brace is used for initial support and comfort. Taping the medial elbow to resist valgus stress can be helpful. When the patient has full pain-free ROM and symmetric strength, an interval throwing program can be initiated with the overhead-throwing athlete (Box 35-1). Proper throwing mechanics should be ensured. Patients who fail to improve after conservative management can be candidates for UCL reconstruction.

Patients with full-thickness UCL injuries are less likely to respond favorably to nonoperative measures, and ligament reconstruction is often required for definitive treatment.

BOX 35-1

Interval Throwing Program

Athletes are allowed to progress from one phase to the next as soon as they are able to complete the phase pain-free.

45-ft Phase

- Step 1: Warm up, 25 45-ft throws × 2 with 15-min rest between sets
- Step 2: Warm up, 25 45-ft throws × 3 with 15-min rest between sets

60-ft Phase

- Step 1: Warm up, 25 60-ft throws × 2 with 15-min rest between sets
- Step 2: Warm up, 25 60-ft throws × 3 with 15-min rest between sets

90-ft Phase

- Step 1: Warm up, 25 90-ft throws × 2 with 15-min rest between sets
- Step 2: Warm up, 25 90-ft throws × 3 with 15-min rest between sets

120-ft Phase

- Step 1: Warm up, 25 120-ft throws × 2 with 15-min rest between sets
- Step 2: Warm up, 25 120-ft throws × 3 with 15-min rest between sets

150-ft Phase

- Step 1: Warm up, 25 150-ft throws × 2 with 15-min rest between sets
- Step 2: Warm up, 25 150-ft throws × 3 with 15-min rest between sets

180-ft Phase

- Step 1: Warm up, 25 180-ft throws × 2 with 15-min rest between sets
- Step 2: Warm up, 25 180-ft throws × 3 with 15-min rest between sets
- Step 3: Begin throwing off of the mound or return to the athlete's respective positions

Conditions of the Forearm, Wrist, and Hand

De Quervain Syndrome

The first dorsal compartment of the wrist contains the abductor pollicis longus and extensor pollicis brevis tendons. These tendons run beneath a sheath over the dorsal aspect of the radial styloid process, along the inferior portion of the anatomic snuff box. Shear and repetitive microtrauma in this area can result in a stenosing tenosynovitis referred to as de Quervain syndrome.[103] De Quervain syndrome is the most common tendonitis of the wrist and is most frequently seen in patients who perform activities requiring forceful gripping with ulnar deviation of the wrist or repetitive use of the thumb.[22,69]

Patients with this condition present with insidious onset of pain over the dorsal radial aspect of the wrist aggravated by activities such as racquet sports, golf, or fly fishing. Patients can also report a sensation of wrist crepitus. Physical examination frequently demonstrates mild edema localized to the dorsal radial wrist and tenderness to palpation over the first dorsal compartment. Finkelstein test is pathognomonic for the diagnosis.[103] A Finkelstein test is performed by placing the patient's elbow in extension, with the forearm in neutral rotation and the wrist in radial deviation. The patient should be asked to place the thumb in the palm and grip the thumb with the fingers. The examiner should then passively bring the wrist into ulnar deviation. A positive test results in pain provocation in the first dorsal wrist compartment tendons.

Treatment for de Quervain syndrome includes rest, modalities, analgesics, and a thumb spica splint. First dorsal compartment peritendinous corticosteroid injection reduces symptoms in 62% to 100% of cases.[60,125]

Scapholunate Instability

Scapholunate instability resulting from ligamentous injury is the most common type of wrist ligament injury.[74] This can occur when a person falls on a pronated outstretched hand with the wrist in extension and ulnar deviation. After scapholunate ligament disruption, the scaphoid moves into a flexed position, whereas the lunate and triquetrum become extended. This pattern is referred to as dorsal intercalated segmental instability, or a "DISI" pattern (Figure 35-3).[65] If this injury is not diagnosed early and treated properly, joint stress will ultimately lead to progressive wrist arthrosis and scapholunate advanced collapse.[102]

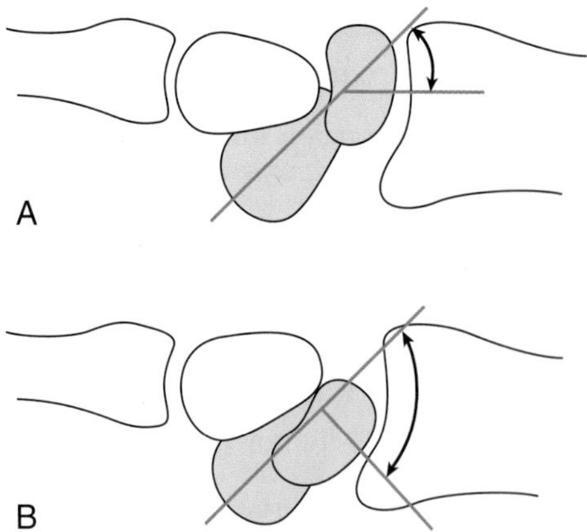

FIGURE 35-3 **A,** Normal scapholunate angle between 30 and 60 degrees. **B,** Scapholunate angle greater than 60 degrees indicating a dorsal intercalated segmental instability (DISI) pattern suggestive of scapholunate dissociation.

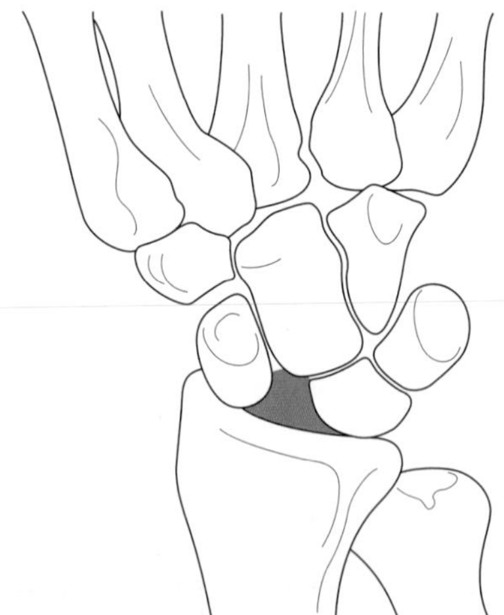

FIGURE 35-4 A gap between the scaphoid and lunate on anteroposterior radiographs indicates scapholunate dissociation.

Patients who sustain a scapholunate injury typically report falling on their outstretched hand with subsequent wrist edema, ecchymosis, and restricted ROM. Physical examination shows tenderness over the scapholunate joint, particularly on the dorsum of the wrist. The patient typically has a positive result on the Watson test.[72] To perform the Watson test, the patient's wrist should be placed passively into ulnar deviation. The examiner should place his or her thumb over the scaphoid tubercle, located on the volar surface of the wrist. The patient's wrist should be brought passively from ulnar to radial deviation while the examiner places a dorsally directed force against the scaphoid tubercle with his or her thumb. A positive test result is indicated by a painful click and dorsal shift of the scaphoid bone relative to the lunate bone during this movement.

Radiographic evaluation should include anteroposterior, anteroposterior with a clenched fist, lateral, and oblique radiographs.[102] The presence of associated fractures should be assessed. The lateral radiograph can reveal the presence of a DISI pattern injury (see Figure 35-3). This is characterized by a scapholunate angle of more than 60 degrees.[102] A gap of more than 3 mm between the scaphoid and lunate on anteroposterior radiographs is also diagnostic for scapholunate instability (Figure 35-4).[102]

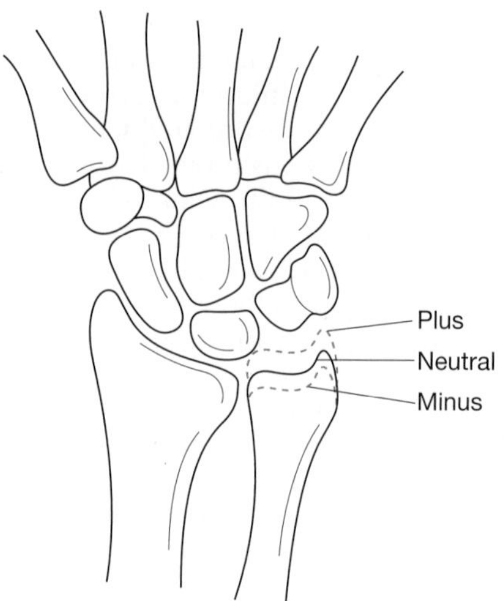

FIGURE 35-5 Ulnar-minus variant.

The clenched fist view exaggerates this finding. Radiographic evaluation should include comparison studies with the opposite wrist.

If standard radiographs are not diagnostic, further studies including arthrography or MRI can be obtained. The sensitivity and specificity of these studies, however, are variable.[102] Wrist arthroscopy has become the gold standard for diagnosing this entity.

Acute scapholunate ligament injuries should be treated surgically. Chronic scapholunate injuries are more difficult to treat but also require surgical intervention. Partial wrist arthrodesis can improve chronic scapholunate instability, and a proximal row carpectomy frequently is used to treat advanced scapholunate collapse.[102]

Triangular Fibrocartilage Complex Injuries

The triangular fibrocartilage complex (TFCC) is composed of an avascular central articular disc and vascular dorsal and palmar radioulnar ligaments.[102] The TFCC is the primary stabilizer of the distal radioulnar joint and can be injured in an acute traumatic event such as falling on an outstretched hand or through repetitive microtrauma such as in gymnastics. Axially loading the wrist results in 18% of the load being born through the TFCC and the remaining 82% through the radiocarpal joint.[95] A positive ulnar variance results in an increase in the load-bearing function of the TFCC, which results in a higher incidence of TFCC injuries (Figure 35-5).[95]

Patients who sustain a TFCC injury might report either an insidious onset or a single traumatic event. Traumatic tears occur more frequently in young athletes, whereas degenerative tears are more common in older patients. Patients with acute injuries often report an axial load to the wrist associated with rotational stress.[102] The patient can also report wrist catching and locking. Physical examination can show tenderness to palpation in the hollow between the flexor carpi ulnaris tendon and the extensor carpi ulnaris tendon, just distal to the ulnar styloid process.[102]

Radiographic evaluation of the wrist can reveal an ulnar-plus variant on the anteroposterior view. Tricompartment

Table 35-2 Ligamentous Injury Grading Scale

Grade	Signs
1	Tenderness to palpation without joint laxity
2	Tenderness to palpation with joint laxity but a good end point
3	Tenderness to palpation with significant joint laxity and no end point

wrist arthrogram, MRI, and MRI arthrogram can provide more specific information regarding TFCC pathology.[102]

When the central articular disc of the TFCC has been acutely injured, surgical débridement is the treatment of choice. A 90% good-to-excellent result with this treatment was reported by Bednar and Osterman.[13] Peripheral tears of the TFCC also respond well to surgical intervention, but the postoperative recovery process is slower than for central articular disc injuries.[102] Patients with degenerative tears of the TFCC should be evaluated for an ulnar-plus variant, and if this is present, an ulnar shortening procedure should be considered along with surgical débridement of the TFCC.[102]

First Metacarpophalangeal Joint Ulnar Collateral Ligament Sprain

Radially directed forces across the first metacarpophalangeal (MCP) joint can result in a UCL injury. This injury, often referred to as "gamekeeper's thumb," is frequently seen in skiers and athletes who participate in sports such as basketball and football.[103] UCL injuries to the first MCP joint can be categorized into a three-grade severity scale of ligament sprains (Table 35-2).

When a grade 3 UCL sprain of the first MCP joint occurs as a result of avulsion of the distal end of the ligament from the base of the first proximal phalanx, there is the possibility of interposition of the adductor pollicis aponeurosis between the base of the first proximal phalanx and the ruptured end of the UCL.[114] This is called a Stener lesion and can prevent adequate healing of this injury, leading to chronic joint pain and instability.

Patients who sustain first MCP joint UCL injuries report a radially directed force across the first MCP joint. They might report an associated "pop" and a feeling of instability in the joint. Physical examination reveals tenderness to palpation over the UCL. If a Stener lesion is present, a palpable mass on the ulnar side of the first MCP joint might be present, representing the avulsed UCL.[2]

UCL stress examination should be performed after local anesthesia via a wrist block, although an initial examination without local anesthesia can be attempted. The stress examination should be performed with the joint in both full extension and 30 degrees of flexion. A complete tear is indicated by an angular difference between the injured and uninjured first MCP joint during stress examination of greater than 15 to 30 degrees.[51,94] A lack of an end point during stress examination also suggests complete UCL disruption.

Radiologic evaluation should include anteroposterior, lateral, and oblique radiographs to detect the presence of fractures or joint subluxation. MRI allows better visualization of the soft tissue injuries, but its sensitivity and specificity for this condition is still being examined.

Treatment of partial tears involves modalities, analgesics, and immobilization in a thumb spica cast for 10 to 14 days, followed by a wrist-hand-thumb spica orthosis for 2 weeks and a hand-based thumb spica orthosis for 2 to 4 more weeks.[37] Patients who participate in contact sports should continue to wear a thumb spica splint during competition for the remainder of the season. Local taping for stability during activity can be used after the period of splinting is completed. Gentle progressive ROM exercises should begin after cast immobilization by removing the splint twice daily, and activity should be progressed as tolerated.

Early surgical repair has been advocated for complete ruptures of the UCL, particularly if a Stener lesion is present.[35,64,76,93,111] Surgery is also indicated for individuals with an avulsion fracture of the base of the proximal phalanx with angulation and displacement greater than 3 mm, or with chronic recurrent instability.[79]

Conclusion

There are many common upper limb injuries and syndromes. Although most can be treated nonoperatively, some require surgical intervention. Accurate diagnosis and initiation of appropriate treatment will enhance the patient's recovery.

KEY REFERENCES

1. Abboud J, Soslowsky LJ: Interplay of the static and dynamic restrains in glenohumeral instability, *Clin Orthop* 400:48–57, 2002.
3. Abrams J, Savoie FH, 3rd, Tauro JC, et al: Recent advances in the evaluation and treatment of shoulder instability: anterior, posterior, and multidirectional, *Arthroscopy* 18:1–13, 2002.
5. Altay T, Gunal I, Ozturk H: Local injection treatment for lateral epicondylitis, *Clin Orthop* 398:127–130, 2002.
6. Antoniou J, Harryman DT: Posterior instability, *Orthop Clin North Am* 32:463–473, 2001.
9. Awerbuch M: The clinical utility of ultrasonography for rotator cuff disease, shoulder impingement syndrome and subacromial bursitis, *Med J Aust* 188:50–53, 2008.
10. Backer M, Warren RF: Glenohumeral instabilities. In DeLee J, Drez D, Miller MD, editors: *DeLee and Drez's orthopaedic sports medicine: principles and practice*, Philadelphia, 2003, Saunders.
12. Beasley L, Faryniarsz DA, Hannafin JA: Multidirectional instability of the shoulder in female athletes, *Clin Sports Med* 19:331–349, 2000.
14. Bell S, Coghlan J, Richardson M: Hydrodilatation in the management of shoulder capsulitis, *Australas Radiol* 47:247–251, 2003.
19. Clark H, McCann P: Acromioclavicular joint injuries, *Orthop Clin North Am* 31:177–187, 2000.
24. Coombes BK, Bisset L, Brooks P, et al: Effect of corticosteroid injection, physiotherapy, or both on clinical outcomes in patients with unilateral lateral epicondylalgia. A randomized controlled trial, *J Am Med Assoc* 309:461–469, 2013.
28. del Cura J, Torre I, Zabala R, et al: Sonographically guided percutaneous needle lavage of calcific tendinitis of the shoulder: short- and long-term results, *Am J Roentgenol* 189:W128–W134, 2007.
30. Dunn J, Kim JJ, Davis L, et al: Ten to 14-year follow-up of the Nirschl surgical technique for lateral epicondylitis, *Am J Sports Med* 36:261–266, 2008.
31. Edwards S, Calandruccio JH: Autologous blood injections for refractory lateral epicondylitis, *J Hand Surg [Am]* 28:272–278, 2003.
32. Ellen M, Gilhool JJ, Rogers D: Scapular instability: the scapulothoracic joint, *Phys Med Rehabil Clin N Am* 11:755–770, 2000.
37. Graham T, Mullen DJ: Athletic injuries of the adult hand. In DeLee J, Drez D, Miller MD, editors: *DeLee and Drez's orthopaedic sports medicine: principles and practice*, Philadelphia, 2003, Saunders.

39. Griffin L: The female athlete. In DeLee J, Drez D, Miller MD, editors: *DeLee and Drez's orthopaedic sports medicine principles and practice*, Philadelphia, 2003, Saunders.
40. Hamdan T, Al-Essa KA: Manipulation under anaesthesia for the treatment of frozen shoulder, *Int Orthop* 27:107–109, 2003.
41. Hand C, Clipsham K, Rees JL, et al: Long-term outcome of frozen shoulder, *J Shoulder Elbow Surg* 17:231–236, 2008.
42. Hannafin J, Chiaia TA: Adhesive capsulitis, *Clin Orthop* 372:95–109, 2000.
46. Hay E, Thomas E, Paterson SM, et al: A pragmatic randomised controlled trial of local corticosteroid injection and physiotherapy for the treatment of new episodes of unilateral shoulder pain in primary care, *Ann Rheum Dis* 62:394–399, 2003.
52. Itoi E, Hatakeyama Y, Kido T, et al: Immobilization in external rotation after dislocation reduces the risk of recurrence: a randomized controlled trial, *J Bone Joint Surg Am* 89:2124–2131, 2007.
53. Itoi E, Hatakeyama Y, Kido T, et al: A new method of immobilization after traumatic anterior dislocation of the shoulder: a preliminary study, *J Shoulder Elbow Surg* 12:413–415, 2003.
55. Itoi E, Sashi R, Minagawa H, et al: Position of immobilization after dislocation of the glenohumeral joint, *J Bone Joint Surg Am* 83:661–667, 2001.
62. Lemos M: The evaluation and treatment of the injured acromioclavicular joint in athletes, *Am J Sports Med* 26:137–144, 1998.
63. Levine W, Flatow EL: The pathophysiology of shoulder instability, *Am J Sports Med* 28:910–917, 2000.
66. Liphart S, Henry TJ: The physiological basis for open and closed kinetic chain rehabilitation for the upper extremity, *J Sport Rehabil* 5:71–87, 1996.
75. Mazzocca A, Sellards R, Garretson R, et al: Injuries to the acromioclavicular joint in adults and children. In DeLee J, Drez D, Miller MD, editors: *DeLee and Drez's orthopedic sports medicine principles and practice*, Philadelphia, 2003, Saunders.
77. McInerney J, Dias J, Durham S, et al: Randomised controlled trial of single, subacromial injection of methylprednisolone in patients with persistent, post-traumatic impingement of the shoulder, *Emerg Med J* 20:218–221, 2003.
78. McShane J, Shah VN, Nazarian LN: Sonographically guided percutaneous needle tenotomy for treatment of common extensor tendinosis in the elbow: is corticosteroid necessary, *J Ultrasound Med* 27:1137–1144, 2008.
79. Melone C, Beldner S, Basuk RS: Thumb collateral ligament injuries: an anatomic basis for treatment, *Hand Clin* 16:345–357, 2000.
81. Miller M, Wirth MA, Rockwood CA, Jr: Thawing the frozen shoulder, the "patient" patient, *Orthopedics* 19:849–853, 1996.
82. Mishra A, Pavelko T: Treatment of chronic elbow tendinosis with buffered platelet-rich plasma, *Am J Sports Med* 34:1774–1778, 2006.
83. Myers J, Lephart SM: Sensorimotor deficits contributing to glenohumeral instability, *Clin Orthop* 400:98–104, 2002.
84. Naredo E, Cabero F, Beneyto P, et al: A randomized comparative study of short term response to blind injection versus sonographic-guided injection of local corticosteroids in patients with painful shoulder, *J Rheumatol* 31:308–314, 2004.
86. Newcomer K, Laskowski ER, Idank DM, et al: Corticosteroid injection in early treatment of lateral epicondylitis, *Clin J Sport Med* 11:214–222, 2001.
89. O'Brien S, Pagnani MJ, Fealy S, et al: The active compression test: a new and effective test for diagnosing labral tears and acromioclavicular joint abnormality, *Am J Sports Med* 26:610–613, 1998.
90. Ogden J, Alvarez RG, Levitt R, et al: Shock wave therapy (orthotripsy) in musculoskeletal disorders, *Clin Orthop* 387:22–40, 2001.
96. Payvandi S, Jeong J, Seitz WH, Jr: Treatment of complete acromioclavicular separations with a modified Weaver and Dunn technique, *Tech Hand Up Extrem Surg* 12:59–64, 2008.
97. Pearsall A, Speer KP: Frozen shoulder syndrome: diagnostic and treatment strategies in the primary care setting, *Med Sci Sports Exerc* 30(Suppl 4):S33–S39, 1998.
98. Petersen S: Posterior shoulder instability, *Orthop Clin North Am* 31:263–283, 2000.
99. Quraishi N, Johnston P, Bayer J, et al: Thawing the frozen shoulder: a randomised trial comparing manipulation under anesthesia with hydrodilatation, *J Bone Joint Surg Br* 89:1197–2000, 2007.
102. Rettig A: Athletic injuries of the wrist and hand. I. Traumatic injuries of the wrist, *Am J Sports Med* 31:1038–1048, 2003.
103. Rettig A: Athletic injuries of the wrist and hand. II. Overuse injuries of the wrist and traumatic injuries to the hand, *Am J Sports Med* 32:262–273, 2004.
107. Sanders T, Morrison WB, Miller MD: Imaging techniques for the evaluation of glenohumeral instability, *Am J Sports Med* 28:414–433, 2000.
109. Shah N, Lewis M: Shoulder adhesive capsulitis: systematic review of randomised trials using multiple corticosteroid injections, *Br J Gen Pract* 57:662–667, 2007.
112. Spencer E: Treatment of grade III acromioclavicular joint injuries: a systematic review, *Clin Orthop* 455:38–44, 2007.
113. Stein D, Jazrawi L, Bartolozzi AR: Arthroscopic stabilization of anterior shoulder instability: a review of the literature, *Arthroscopy* 18:912–924, 2002.
115. Stollberger C, Finsterer J: Nonsteroidal anti-inflammatory drugs in patients with cardio- or cerebrovascular disorders, *Z Kardiol* 92:721–729, 2003.
116. Suresh S, Ali KE, Jones H, et al: Medial epicondylitis: is ultrasound guided autologous blood injection an effective treatment?, *Br J Sports Med* 40:935–939, 2006.
117. Svernlov B, Adolfsson L: Non-operative treatment regime including eccentric training for lateral humeral epicondylalgia, *Scand J Med Sci Sports* 11:328–334, 2001.
118. Tasto J, Elias DW: Adhesive capsulitis, *Sports Med* 15:216–221, 2007.

The full reference list for this chapter is available online.

CHAPTER 36

MUSCULOSKELETAL DISORDERS OF THE LOWER LIMB

Pamela A. Hansen, A. Michael Henrie, George W. Deimel, Stuart E. Willick

This chapter reviews musculoskeletal disorders of the lower limb, including soft tissue, bone, and joint disease. The chapter is organized by anatomic region within diagnostic categories. Although the authors acknowledge that this organizational scheme is somewhat arbitrary, it was chosen to decrease redundancy in describing certain conditions that can occur in multiple anatomic locations, such as osteoarthritis or stress fractures. The authors also acknowledge that space does not permit a comprehensive discussion of all musculoskeletal disorders of the lower limbs. The conditions of primary interest to the practitioner of musculoskeletal and sports medicine are covered in greater detail.

The first section of this chapter discusses disorders of muscle and tendon groups in the lower limb, with a special focus on kinetic chain considerations. The second section of the chapter reviews disorders of the joints of the lower limbs. The final section discusses the spectrum of bone overload conditions.

Over the past 15 years, a new lexicon has evolved among practitioners of musculoskeletal rehabilitation. There are several terms that are used throughout the chapter that might not be familiar to all readers. For the sake of clarity, we would like to first define some of these terms.

First and foremost, the term *kinetic chain* refers to the model of human motion that analyzes and treats dysfunction along connected anatomic regions, rather than focusing only on a single location of pain. This model recognizes that dysfunction in one anatomic region can cause dysfunction in other anatomic regions that are linked to the first region during motion. Treatment plans that address only the painful site, and ignore underlying pathology at other sites along the motion chain, have less chance of success than a treatment plan that restores proper function along the entire motion chain. Kinetic chain considerations are most relevant when discussing muscle and tendon pathology, but should not be ignored when addressing bone and joint pathology.

The term *biomechanical deficits* refers to any deficiencies in range of motion, flexibility, strength, endurance, or motor control. The term *muscle imbalance* refers to the divergence from normal function of different muscle groups that work as agonists or antagonists to stabilize a body part or create motion. Muscle imbalances often occur between muscles on the anterior versus posterior side of a joint, such as the hip flexors versus the hip extensors, or the medial versus lateral side of a joint, such as the hip adductors versus the hip abductors. The literature has suggested that these types of muscle imbalances predispose to injury.[47]

The term *functional exercise* refers to exercise movements that stimulate muscle groups to work in a way that they normally work during functional or athletic activities. Functional exercise is distinguished from more conventional types of exercise that tend to isolate muscle groups, rather than have various muscle groups within a kinetic chain working together. For example, a previously accepted method to strengthen the peroneal muscles after a lateral ankle sprain was to have the patient evert the foot against the resistance of a TheraBand. Although this method is effective in strengthening the peroneal muscles, it is not a motion that people normally perform in an isolated manner during everyday activities or athletic activities. A more sophisticated and functional ankle rehabilitation exercise program might have the patient standing on the affected leg while performing movements with the other leg, or standing on the affected leg while performing movements with the upper limbs and torso in patterns that the body uses during real life activities. "Sport-specific" exercises are functional exercises that use motion patterns that athletes must perform in their athletic events. Finally, the terms *tendonitis* and *tendinosis*, although sometimes used interchangeably, more correctly refer to acute and chronic overload conditions of tendons, respectively.

Disorders of Muscle-Tendon Groups of the Lower Limb

Disorders of the Iliotibial Band, Including Trochanteric Bursitis

The iliotibial band (ITB) is a strong fascial band that runs along the lateral aspect of the thigh from the level of the greater trochanter to the proximal, anterolateral tibia (Figure 36-1). ITB motion is controlled proximally primarily by the gluteus maximus and tensor fascia lata, the two muscles that insert into it at its origin and therefore are primarily responsible for control of it. The ITB inserts distally onto a bony prominence at the proximal, anterolateral tibia called the Gerdy tubercle. The ITB can therefore exert forces at the hip and at the knee. Conversely, alterations in various lower limb mechanics, such as genu valgum, pes planus, and tibial internal or external rotation, can affect ITB function. There are three clinically important bursae related to the ITB. The proximal bursa is positioned to decrease friction between the ITB and the greater trochanter of the femur. Another site of potential friction is where the ITB runs over the lateral epicondyle of the femur.

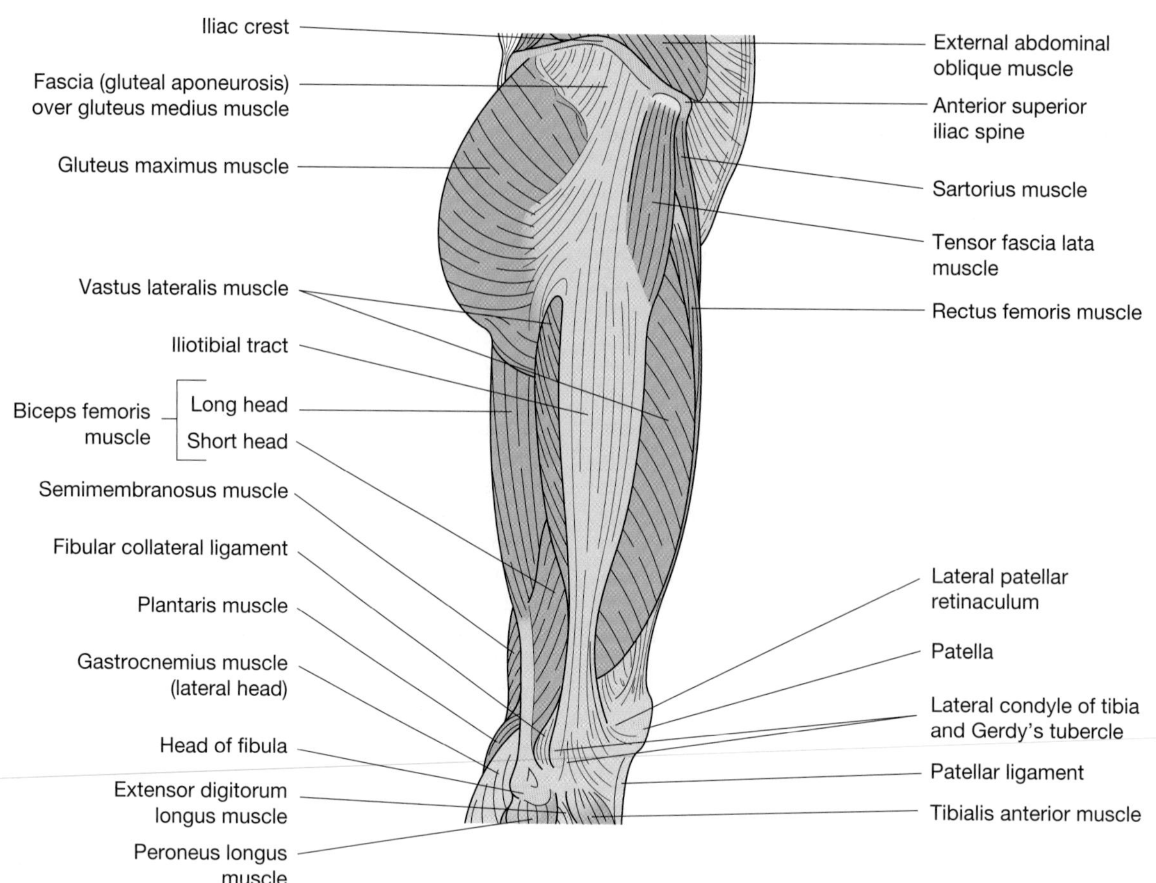

FIGURE 36-1 The iliotibial band is a strong fascial band that runs from the lateral hip to the lateral knee.

The third lies at the distal attachment of the ITB on the tibia.

Although a bursa can become inflamed from direct trauma, it is far more common for a bursa to become gradually inflamed as a result of improper training techniques or abnormal biomechanics. In these cases, the bursal inflammation is not a primary process, but rather secondary to muscle imbalance around the hip girdle or other abnormalities along the kinetic chain. The purpose of a bursa is to allow for low-friction gliding of soft tissues over a bony prominence. Any imbalance or dysfunction of the hip muscles can result in abnormal ITB motion and trochanteric bursitis. Patients with trochanteric bursitis can usually localize pain to the lateral hip. The pain is sometimes felt along the path of the ITB in the lateral thigh. On examination, there is tenderness to palpation directly over the greater trochanter or immediately posterior to it. There is often weakness of the gluteus medius and the hip external rotators, which can be detected with manual resistance testing. A typical hip girdle muscle imbalance seen in the setting of trochanteric bursitis includes tensor fascia lata tightness and gluteus maximus inhibition or weakness. The modified Thomas test is an excellent physical examination maneuver to assess for inflexibility around the hip girdle. One should always check the function of the deep hip external rotators as well as muscle function along the entire kinetic chain, from the core region to the ankle (Video 36-1). The function of the hip external rotators can be tested statically and dynamically. In runners and cyclists with ITB symptoms, it is important to perform a biomechanical assessment while the patient is running or riding. Occasionally, an audible snap can be heard as the ITB rubs over the greater trochanter. This is sometimes referred to as lateral snapping hip syndrome. This condition is contrasted with the so-called internal snapping hip syndrome, in which a deeper, more medial snap is appreciated by the patient. Internal snapping hip is thought to be attributable to the iliopsoas tendon rubbing over the iliopectineal eminence or the femoral head. The same kinetic chain abnormalities that can cause ITB pain at the lateral hip can also cause pain and tenderness where the ITB passes over the lateral epicondyle of the femur, or at its insertion onto the Gerdy tubercle. Symptoms are exacerbated by repetitive activities such as running or cycling.

Regardless of the location of symptoms related to ITB dysfunction, the treatment principles remain the same. The patient should reduce or eliminate the exacerbating activities. Ice is helpful for reducing pain and inflammation, and for facilitating a stretching program. The exercise prescription should be based on the patient's relevant biomechanical deficits, which are determined by the office examination and a functional examination of the patient while she or he is participating in activities. Providing standardized exercise handouts or prescribing nonspecific rehabilitation protocols can result in failure to improve. One common example of prescribing nonspecific exercises for an ITB problem is to prescribe ITB stretches, when the primary deficit is hip abductor weakness. Another common mistake is to focus on hip abductor strengthening if the most relevant biomechanical deficit is impaired eccentric control of the hip external rotators. Because all the hip girdle muscles originate on the pelvis, the core musculature must be able to adequately stabilize the pelvis for the hip girdle muscles to perform their functions during dynamic activities. Other interventions, such as ITB massage, myofascial release, or ultrasound (US) may facilitate the patient's rehabilitation program. Off-the-shelf and custom-made foot orthoses can be helpful in reducing impact and improving subtalar positioning and tibial rotation. If errors in training technique are thought to have contributed to the onset of symptoms, then appropriate training regimens should be discussed with the patient.

Disorders of the Hamstring Muscle Group

Strains of the thigh muscles are common in individuals participating in ballistic activities. The most commonly strained muscle group in the thigh is the hamstring group. The hamstring group includes semimembranosus, semitendinosus, and the short and long heads of biceps femoris. Hamstring strains most commonly occur with forceful eccentric contraction of the hamstring muscles, especially when the muscle is at a mechanical disadvantage near full flexion or full extension (Figure 36-2). The patient will usually be able to describe an appropriate, acute overload mechanism. On examination, hamstring pain can be reproduced by passive stretch of the muscle, by resistance testing of the muscle, and by direct palpation of the injured area. The strain can occur near the hamstring origin at the ischial tuberosity, in the belly of the muscle, or in the region of the distal musculotendinous junction. Severe hamstring strains will produce visible ecchymosis at and distal to the site of injury. A large muscle tear might produce a palpable defect. Imaging is usually not necessary to establish the diagnosis. If needed, US or magnetic resonance imaging (MRI) can help determine the severity of the injury.[51] Acute treatment consists of relative rest, ice, early gentle range-of-motion exercises, and gently progressive strengthening exercises as tolerated. Exercises should be progressed to higher weight and include more ballistic and sport-specific movements when tolerated. It is not uncommon for an acute hamstring strain to keep an individual from their usual athletic activities for 6 weeks or more.

With proximal hamstring injuries, occasionally the bone fails before the muscle or tendon fails, resulting in an ischial avulsion injury. The most common age group for ischial avulsion fractures is 15 to 25 years of age. The most common activities that cause ischial avulsion fractures include gymnastics, hurdling, and dance. The patient can usually describe sudden onset of pain at the ischial tuberosity after a forceful movement involving hamstring contraction, while the muscle was at maximum length with full hip flexion and knee extension. On physical examination, there is typically point tenderness at the ischial tuberosity, pain with passive hamstring stretch, and pain with knee flexion or hip extension against resistance. Plain films are usually adequate to visualize the avulsion (Figure 36-3, *A*, *B*). These fractures usually do not need surgery and can be treated similar to other hamstring injuries, although the period of relative rest might be longer to allow for bone healing. If initial symptoms are severe enough to prevent comfortable ambulation, crutches can be used for a few days. Ice should be applied frequently over the first few days to decrease pain and swelling. Nonsteroidal antiinflammatory drugs (NSAIDs) can be taken for the same reasons. Although surgical intervention is rarely needed, orthopedic consultation should be obtained if the avulsion fragment is displaced greater than 2 cm, or

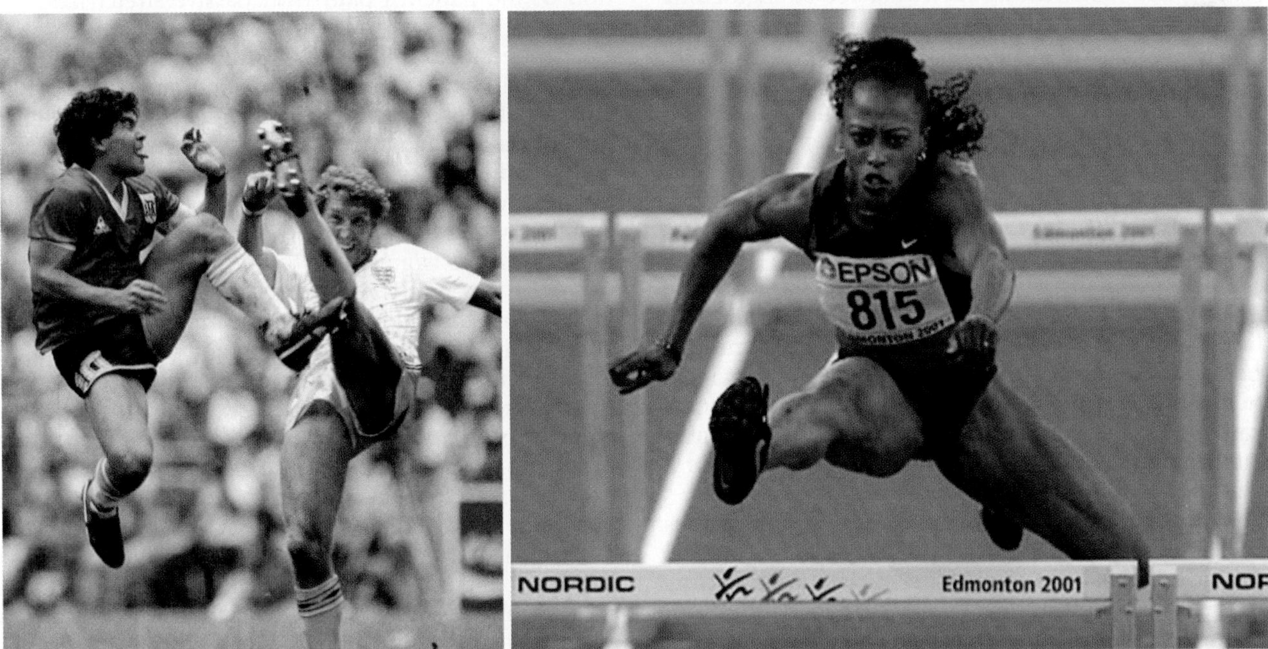

FIGURE 36-2 The primary function of the hamstring muscle group is to slow down knee extension during open kinetic chain movements. This muscle group is at risk for acute overload during ballistic activities.

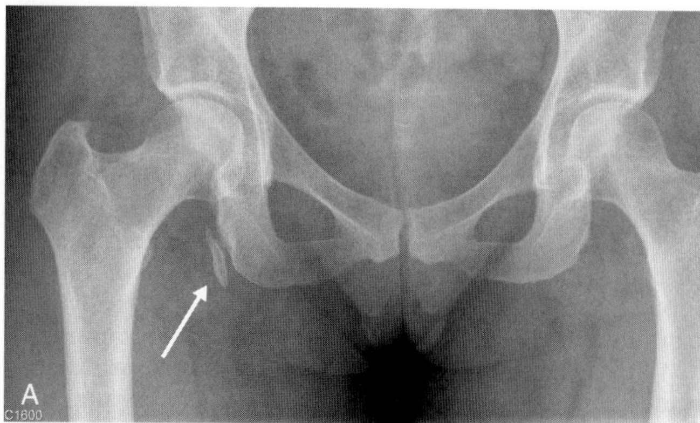

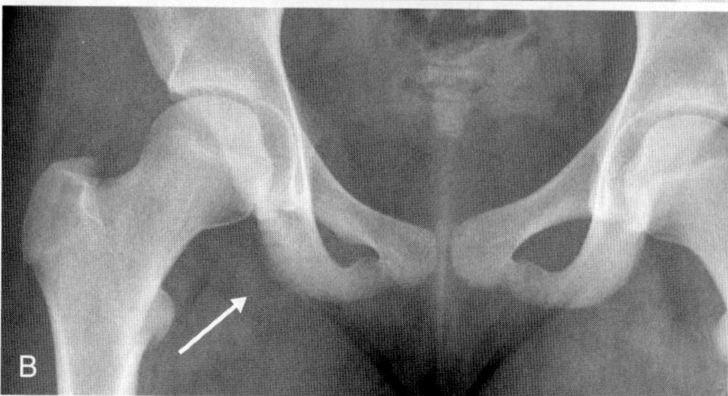

FIGURE 36-3 Examples of ischial avulsion fractures. **A,** Anteroposterior radiograph of the pelvis, showing an old ischial avulsion fracture (*arrow*). The patient was a 17-year-old female cheerleader who had sudden onset of buttock pain with a high-kicking maneuver 9 months before presentation. **B,** Anteroposterior radiograph of the pelvis, showing irregularity of the right ischial tuberosity (*arrow*). The patient was a 14-year-old cheerleader with acute onset of right buttock pain after a high-kicking maneuver. In both cases, symptoms resolved completely after a period of relative rest followed by progressive rehabilitation.

if resolution of symptoms does not occur in the expected time period. As pain decreases over the first 1 to 3 weeks, slowly progressive hamstring stretching and strengthening should be started. The rehabilitation program must be undertaken very cautiously during the first several weeks to avoid further displacement of the avulsion. There is no predetermined amount of time, however, that one should wait before starting a stretching and strengthening program for the hamstring muscle group after this injury.[11] A general guideline is that the patient should experience no discomfort or only mild discomfort with the rehabilitation program.

In older (skeletally mature) individuals, the proximal hamstring tendon might avulse because in these individuals the weakest link is the tendon rather than the bone. The mechanism of injury is the same as described earlier. In high-demand athletes, surgical reattachment is usually indicated. Although late repair is feasible, early identification and surgical intervention usually produce the best outcomes.

Hamstring muscle disorders can also have an insidious onset. Hamstring tendinopathy can occur at the ischial tuberosity or distally in the medial or lateral hamstring tendons. In addition to pain with activities, a careful history often reveals a change in the patient's activity level, such as a recent, rapid increase in running. The physical examination findings are similar to, but usually less dramatic than, those seen with an acute hamstring strain. In addition to the usual rehabilitation protocols such as relative rest, ice, NSAIDs, and hamstring stretching and strengthening, one should try to identify and correct errors in training technique, running gait, cycling or jumping mechanics, and relevant biomechanical deficits. Eccentric training of the hamstring group helps the muscle to absorb more loading force, and restoring as much balance as possible to the quadriceps-hamstring force couple is also important. A local injection of steroid in the region of the ischial bursa might help facilitate the active exercise program during rehabilitation, but potential side effects need to be kept in mind, including weakening of the tendon.

Disorders of the Adductor Muscle Group

The adductor muscle group consists of adductor magnus, adductor longus, adductor brevis, sartorius, gracilis, and pectineus. As with other muscle or tendon injuries, strains of the hip adductor muscles usually occur with forceful activation of the muscles, especially when in a lengthened position. Adductor strains can be caused by acute or repetitive overload. These injuries can occur in anyone, but are particularly common in athletes involved in soccer, hockey, and skiing. Strains of the adductor group most commonly occur at or near their origin of the inferior pubic ramus. Intramuscular strains also occur. The adductor longus is most commonly involved. Isolated sartorius muscle strains can also occur. A sudden, forceful contraction of sartorius can result in an avulsion fracture at the proximal attachment of the muscle at the anterior superior iliac spine. This injury is treated similarly to other acute tendon strains, although a longer period of relative rest might be required before progressing the patient to stretching and strengthening exercises.

The physical examination is most notable for reproduction of the patient's pain with passive stretch and active resistance testing of the adductor group. Radiographs are not needed to establish a diagnosis of adductor strain, but are useful when looking for bone injuries such as avulsion factures. If needed, MRI can frequently show signal change in the area of injury (Figure 36-4, *A, B*). Treatment includes early, gradually progressive range-of-motion exercises and careful strengthening exercises, with return to sport-specific exercises when tolerated. If the rehabilitation program is performed too aggressively in the early stages, there is a risk of further injury. Although the rehabilitation program focuses on the adductor muscle group, one needs to address the entire kinetic chain and the hip adductor-abductor force couple to decrease the chance of recurrent injury. Because the adductors arise from the pelvis, the pelvis must be stabilized with a core exercise program. In the groin, the adductor muscle group lies in close proximity to the iliopsoas. Therefore, symptoms of iliopsoas overload can overlap symptoms of adductor overload. This needs to be kept in mind during the workup and treatment of groin pain. The rehabilitation program should seek to maximize flexibility, strength, motor control, and endurance of the hip flexors, hamstrings, hip abductors, and hip extensors, in addition to the adductor muscle group. One should also check for and correct tightness of

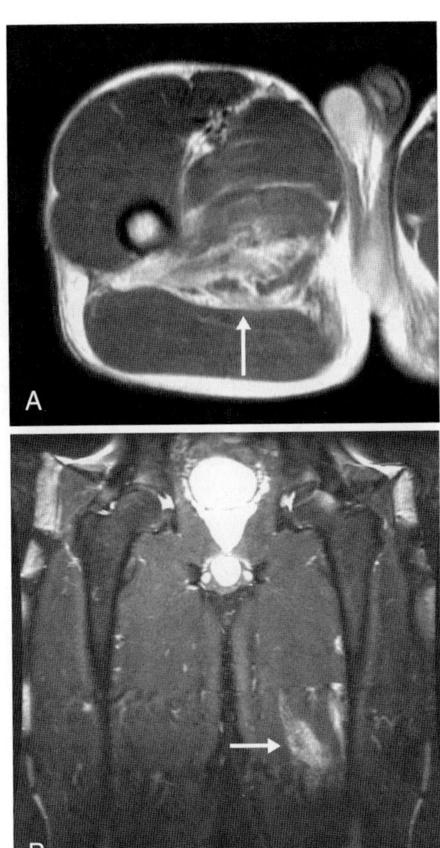

FIGURE 36-4 Examples of adductor strains. **A,** T2-weighted axial magnetic resonance imaging (MRI) of the proximal thigh, showing a hemorrhagic tear in the proximal adductor muscle group (*arrow*). The patient was an Olympic hockey player who got checked from the right side while the right leg was in an abducted position. **B,** T2-weighted coronal MRI of the thighs, showing a more distal, less severe strain of the left adductor muscle group than that seen in **A** (*arrow*). This patient was also a hockey player.

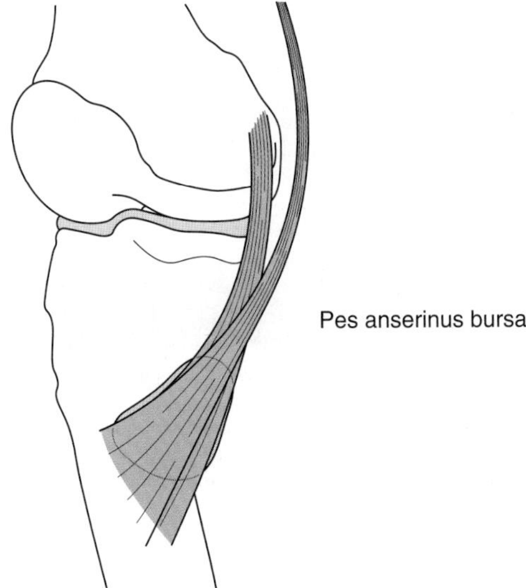

FIGURE 36-5 The semitendinosus, sartorius, and gracilis tendons form a conjoined tendon on the anteromedial aspect of the proximal tibia referred to as the pes anserinus.

the ITB, which if present can inhibit strengthening of the adductors.

Combined Muscle Group Injuries

Pes Anserine Tendonitis or Bursitis

One hamstring muscle (semitendinosus) and two adductor muscles (sartorius and gracilis) course together along the medial aspect of the knee to insert on the proximal, anteromedial tibia (Figure 36-5). The anatomist who coined the name pes anserinus thought that the insertion of these three tendons looked like a goose's foot. Acute inflammation of one or more of these three tendons near their insertion is called pes anserine tendonitis. Subacute or chronic irritation of one or more of these tendons near their tibial attachment is called pes anserine tendinosis. Inflammation of the bursa that lies just under the tendons near their insertion is termed pes anserine bursitis. Clinical differentiation between primary tendon pain versus primary bursal pain can be challenging, and the two conditions often coexist. Bursal pathology is usually secondary to dysfunction of the overlying tendons. The patient typically complains of pain in the region of the pes anserine insertion. The patient sometimes provides a history of a sudden increase in activity level. On palpation, there is usually local tenderness at the pes anserine insertion. Common biomechanical deficits that are associated with this condition include a weak core, weak medial hamstrings, and weak hip adductors. Initial treatment includes ice and NSAIDs to decrease pain and swelling. Although the rehabilitation program focuses on maximizing flexibility, strength, endurance, and motor control of the pes anserine muscles, the entire kinetic chain must be addressed. Core control should be maximized to allow for proper hamstring and hip adductor function. Anterior to posterior and medial to lateral muscle imbalances should be identified and rehabilitated. Impaired subtalar motion and abnormal tibial rotation should also be addressed. In runners and cyclists, running gait and cycling mechanics need to be analyzed, and modified if necessary. Running shoes and inserts need to be appropriate for each individual's biomechanical characteristics. Imaging is usually not indicated unless there is suspicion for stress fracture or intraarticular pathology, such as an injury to the medial meniscus. Underlying bone and joint injuries can sometimes cause secondary dysfunction of the pes anserine tendons. The pes anserine tendons and bursa can be visualized with both US and MRI. A local steroid injection can help facilitate the active exercise program if pain limits the patient's ability to exercise, although risks and benefits of a steroid injection should be weighed appropriately.

Athletic Pubalgia and Sportsman's Hernia

Athletic pubalgia and sportsman's hernia refer to a spectrum of disorders that cause pain in the lower abdomen and groin. Pain generators can include overload of one or more of the lower abdominal muscles near the superior pubic ramus, a strain of the hip flexors or hip adductors, stress response or stress fracture of the pubic rami, and pubic symphysitis (Figure 36-6, *A, B, C*).[13] A defect in the fascia of the lower, anterior abdominal wall has also been described. Overload injury in this region is most commonly seen in football, soccer, and hockey. There can be a delay in accurate diagnosis, and rehabilitation is often

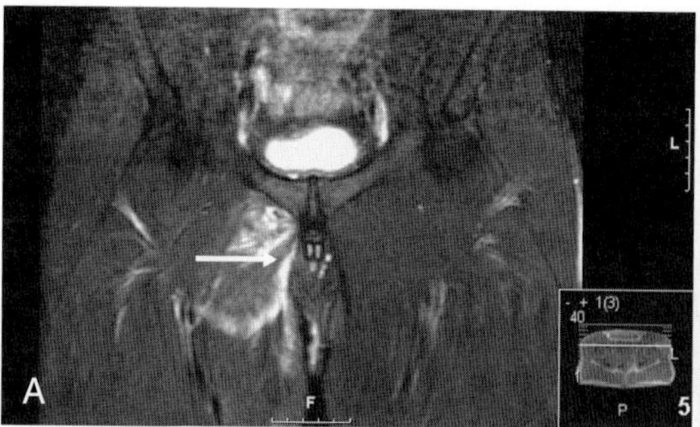

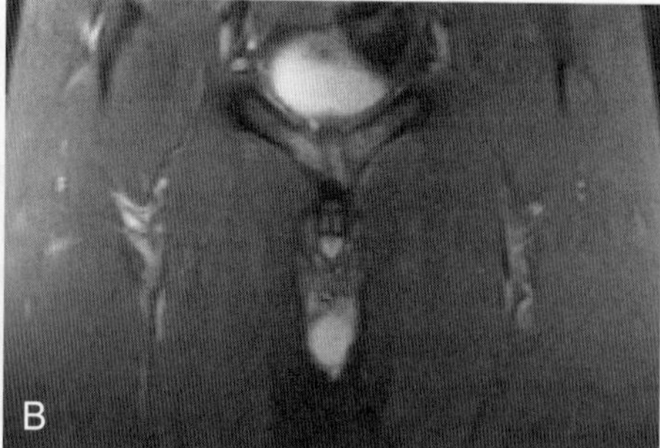

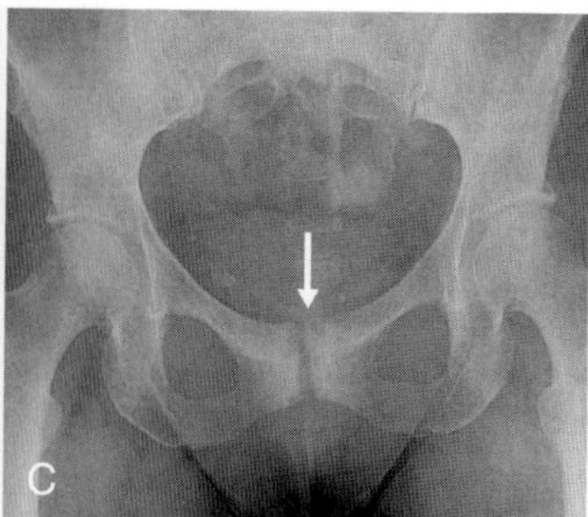

FIGURE 36-6 Examples of the spectrum of conditions seen in athletic pubalgia. **A,** T2-weighted, short tau, inversion recovery, coronal magnetic resonance imaging (MRI) of a college football place kicker, showing a hemorrhagic tear (*arrow*) of the right hip adductor muscles of the pubic ramus. **B,** T2-weighted, fat suppression, coronal MRI of the pelvis of a collegiate pole vaulter, showing increased signal intensity of both pubic rami and the pubic symphysis, consistent with stress responses of the superior pubic rami and pubic symphysitis. **C,** Anteroposterior radiograph of the pelvis, showing irregularity, subchondral cyst formation, and subchondral sclerosis of the symphysis pubis (*arrow*), consistent with symphysitis. The patient was a 22-year-old soccer player with chronic, bilateral groin pain.

incomplete. Because symptoms of athletic pubalgia can easily become chronic, it is imperative to establish an accurate and complete diagnosis and to institute comprehensive rehabilitation as early as possible. Maximizing core stability and restoring full range of motion, strength, endurance, and motor control of the core muscles, hip flexors, and adductors are key to successful rehabilitation. Functional exercises to retrain these muscle groups should be started as soon as the patient is able to tolerate them. Surgical consultation should be considered if there is a suspicion for a fascial defect of the anterior abdominal wall or a true inguinal hernia.[43] Impact or repetitive loading activities should be avoided in the setting of bone overload, such as pelvic stress response or stress fracture.

Injuries to the Quadriceps Muscle Group

Patellar Tendinopathy

A common term for patellar tendinopathy is jumper's knee. Symptoms of patellar tendon overload most commonly start insidiously. When the patient is able to localize a point of maximum pain, it is usually at the inferior pole of the patella. The pain, however, can occur anywhere along the course of the tendon or at the distal insertion on the tibial tubercle. Individuals at risk for patellar tendon overload include those who participate in repetitive knee flexion and extension activities, such as basketball players, volleyball players, bicyclists, rowers, and mogul skiers. The diagnosis is primarily made by history. Patients may or may not have tenderness along the course of the tendon. The examiner should look for biomechanical deficits that can lead to unequal distribution of forces along the links in the kinetic chain that are most involved with jumping. For example, the knee extensor mechanism can become overloaded during repetitive flexion and extension if more proximal muscle groups, such as the lumbar and hip extensors, are not adequately activating. Distally, the knee extensor mechanism can be placed at a biomechanical disadvantage if the individual lacks adequate ankle dorsiflexion, which is a necessary motion for squatting. Ankle dorsiflexion is also necessary for maximum activation of the calf muscles, which assist the quadriceps in jumping and eccentrically controlling the landing motion. The muscle groups involved in the jumping motion should be evaluated for eccentric as well as concentric function

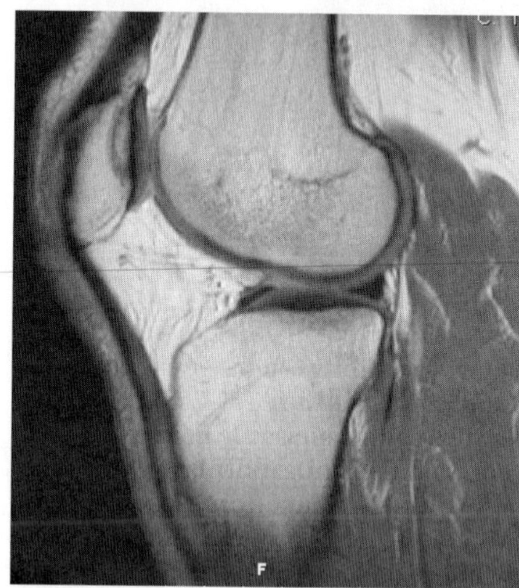

FIGURE 36-7 T1-weighted sagittal magnetic resonance imaging of the knee, showing extensive signal change within the distal patellar tendon, consistent with patellar tendonosis. The patient was a 37-year-old ultramarathoner whose symptoms failed to improve with cessation of running, appropriate physical therapy, various nonsteroidal antiinflammatory drugs, and modalities including extracorporeal shock wave treatment. He ultimately underwent surgical débridement of the tendon and was able to return to running 6 months later.

because both types of muscle action are involved in jumping and landing. Imaging is usually not necessary to make the diagnosis. For refractory cases, or when the clinical diagnosis is in question, MRI and US both provide adequate visualization of the tendon (Figure 36-7 and Figure 36-8, *A, B, C*).

Treatments include ice, NSAIDs, cross-friction massage, modalities, quadriceps stretching, and strengthening exercises, and addressing relevant biomechanical deficits. Some patients gain symptomatic relief from a patellar tendon (or "Cho-Pat") strap. Identifying and correcting errors in training technique can prevent recurrence. For long-standing, refractory cases that will not respond to an appropriate rehabilitation program, surgical débridement of the tendon might be of benefit.

Osgood-Schlatter Disease and Sinding-Larsen-Johansson Disease

When a young adolescent presents with pain at the tibial tuberosity that is exacerbated with activities and direct

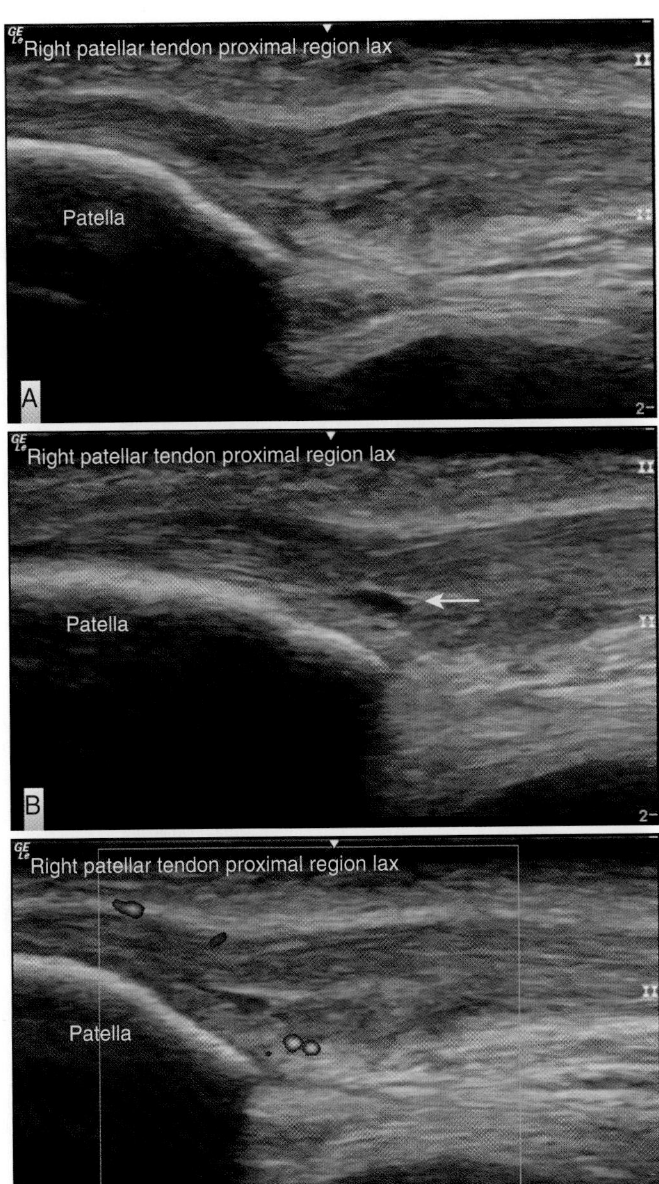

FIGURE 36-8 Longitudinal gray scale 12 to 5 MHz ultrasound images of the proximal patellar tendon demonstrates **(A)** a thickened, ill-defined hypoechoic tendon representing tendinopathy and **(B)** a hypoechoic, intrasubstance, longitudinal tear with **(C)** color Doppler imaging showing areas of intratendinous hyperemia.

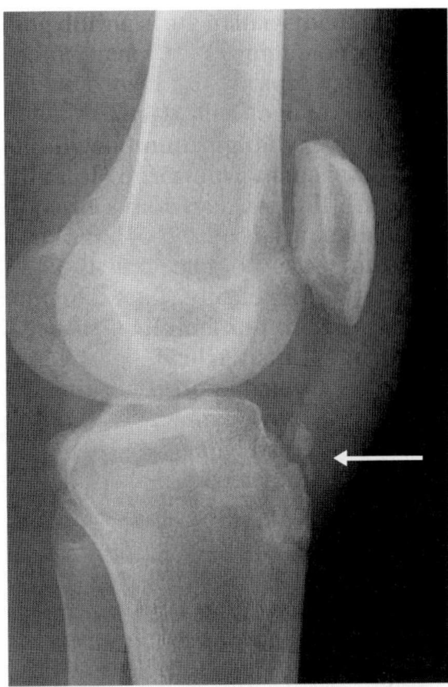

FIGURE 36-9 Lateral radiograph of the knee, showing the typical appearance of Osgood-Schlatter disease. There is irregularity and fragmentation of the tibial tuberosity (*arrow*). The patient was a 16-year-old wrestler with a 3-month history of increasing anterior knee pain. His other knee and his brother's knees all had a similar radiographic appearance.

contact, Osgood-Schlatter disease should be considered. The underlying cause of this relatively common condition is not clear, but repetitive overload at the patella tendon insertion can cause inflammation, irregularity, or partial avulsions of the secondary ossification center of the tibial tuberosity. Clinically, the diagnosis is made when there is significant pain and tenderness at the tibial tubercle. The radiographic hallmark of Osgood-Schlatter disease is irregularity and fragmentation of the tibial tuberosity (Figure 36-9). Although far less common than Osgood-Schlatter disease, similar findings can be seen at the origin of the patella tendon at the inferior pole of the patella In this case the condition is called Sinding-Larsen-Johansson disease. For both conditions, the mainstays of treatment include ice, judicious use of NSAIDs, gently progressive quadriceps stretching, careful pain-free quadriceps strengthening, and activity modification. Activity modification is sometimes the most difficult part of the treatment regimen because the individuals who suffer from these conditions are usually very active adolescents. Realistically, activity modification can mean encouraging the patient to participate in one sport per season rather than two or three. Symptoms might be intermittent or persistent until the growth plates close, at which point symptoms usually resolve spontaneously.

Quadriceps Strain, and Quadriceps and Patella Tendon Rupture

Forceful quadriceps contraction with the foot planted can cause injury to the quadriceps muscle itself or failure of either the quadriceps or patella tendon (Figure 36-10). The patient can usually describe an appropriate mechanism of injury, and might describe a sense of having an unstable knee. On examination, there is anterior knee swelling and a palpable defect just proximal or just distal to the patella. The patient will be unable to extend the knee. When asked to do so, the patella will not move if there is a quadriceps tendon rupture, but will elevate without causing knee extension with a patella tendon rupture. A careful musculoskeletal and neurovascular examination should be performed to assess for associated injuries such as anterior cruciate ligament (ACL) tear and femoral neuropathy. A patient with an acute quadriceps or patella tendon rupture should be placed in a knee immobilizer and made non-weight bearing with crutches. Rupture of the quadriceps or patella tendons requires surgical repair within a few days for optimal results.

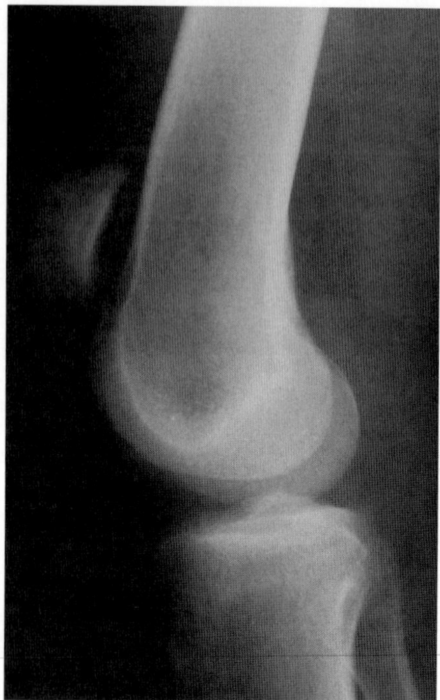

FIGURE 36-10 Lateral radiograph of the knee, showing an abnormally high-riding patella after an acute patella tendon rupture. The patient was a 40-year-old airline pilot who described "landing a little aft of center" while alpine skiing. A sudden forceful quadriceps contraction while attempting to regain balance resulted in this injury.

Rectus Femoris Avulsion from the Anterior Inferior Iliac Spine

A forceful contraction of rectus femoris can result in an avulsion fracture of the anterior inferior iliac spine. This diagnosis is distinguished from a simple muscle strain by radiographs, but treatment follows the same rehabilitation guidelines, with ice, relative rest, and gently progressive stretching and strengthening exercises when tolerated. Surgery is indicated only for dramatically displaced avulsion fragments, which are uncommon.[32]

Quadriceps Contusions and Myositis Ossificans

Contusions of the quadriceps muscle group resulting from a direct and forceful blow to the area are fairly common (Figure 36-11, *A, B*). The patient can usually provide a history of direct trauma to the front of the thigh. The patient typically reports pain at the site of the injury, and might report stiffness and difficulty with weight bearing. An antalgic gait is usually noted, along with tenderness, ecchymosis, and swelling in the anterior thigh. Knee flexion can be severely restricted (Video 36-2). Extension is often preserved. Radiographs should be obtained to look for an underlying femur fracture. Ice should be applied aggressively to decrease swelling and pain. Early range of motion should be started as soon as it is tolerated to decrease muscle stiffness, which invariably ensues. Some practitioners advocate immobilizing the knee in flexion for a few days to decrease contracture of the quadriceps muscle.

Following a severe quadriceps contusion, the intramuscular hematoma can undergo calcific transformation, resulting in myositis ossificans. Myositis ossificans occurs in up to 10% to 20% of all thigh contusions, and the quadriceps is the most common location for myositis ossificans to occur.[27] Aspirin and standard antiinflammatory medications should be avoided in the first few days because of the theoretically increased risk of promoting additional bleeding into the injury site. Cyclooxygenase-2 inhibitors, which do not interfere with platelet function, can be used. If pain and stiffness persist or worsen after several weeks of appropriate care, consideration should be given to repeating radiographs and obtaining advanced imaging with a bone scan, MRI, or US to look for calcification in the muscle. Bone scan and MRI are more sensitive in the early stages of myositis ossificans than plain films.

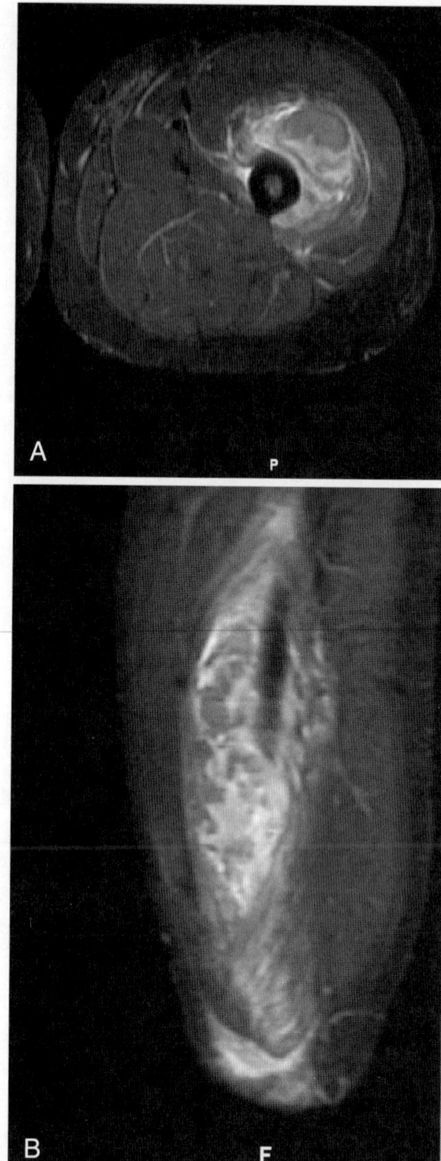

FIGURE 36-11 Quadriceps contusion. T2-weighted axial **(A)** and sagittal **(B)** magnetic resonance images of the thigh, showing a massive contusion of the vastus intermedius muscle. The patient was a female Olympic hockey player who was struck by the knee of a male player during a scrimmage. The forces were efficiently transferred through the superficial quadriceps muscles, which were spared injury, to the deep quadriceps muscle. With aggressive rehabilitation, the athlete was able to compete during the Olympics and led her team in scoring. She did not develop myositis ossificans, demonstrating the capricious nature of the condition.

If myositis ossificans develops, first-line treatment includes progressive range of motion and medication. Radiation therapy can be tried for recalcitrant symptoms, although this works to prevent further bony formation rather than to treat the existing lesion. Surgical resection of the calcified tissue is indicated for unresponsive cases that are impinging nerves or restricting functional range of motion, but in general it is thought that this should not be undertaken before maturation of the mass because of the high risk of recurrence. Radiation after surgery may help prevent recurrence. A cold bone scan provides evidence that osteoblastic activity has ceased.

Patellofemoral Arthralgia

As its name implies, the term *patellofemoral arthralgia* refers to pain in the joint between the patella and the femur. Other terms that have been used to refer to this condition include patellofemoral pain syndrome and chondromalacia. The latter term is discouraged because it lacks specificity. Patellofemoral arthralgia is the most common cause of knee pain seen in the younger population. Although patellofemoral pain can arise from an acute traumatic event, such as a fall onto the knee with injury to the cartilage or subchondral bone, it is more commonly gradual in onset.

As the knee goes through flexion and extension, the patella normally tracks proximally and distally within the trochlear groove. Abnormal mechanics along the kinetic chain can cause improper tracking of the patella. There are several typical biomechanical abnormalities that one should look for during a comprehensive assessment. A tight quadriceps muscle can cause the patella to ride high within the trochlear groove, and therefore create abnormal forces on the retropatellar cartilage (see Video 36-2). A tight ITB, via fibers that attach to the lateral retinaculum of the patella, can cause the patella to track laterally. An ineffective oblique portion of the vastus medialis will not be able to oppose the lateral pull of a tight ITB. Pes planus is associated with tibial internal rotation, which may position the patella medially within the trochlear groove through the pull of the patella tendon. On the proximal side of the kinetic chain, ineffective eccentric function of the hip external rotators might fail to adequately control femoral internal rotation during running, which can also cause abnormal patellofemoral tracking, and weak hip abductors can place increased load on the ITB.

The patient with patellofemoral arthralgia can usually localize the pain to the anterior knee, or even say that the pain is "under the kneecap." At times, one can elicit a history of a recent increase in activity, such as putting in a new floor without using knee pads, or a rapid increase in running. A mainstay of clinical diagnosis is tenderness to palpation under the medial and lateral aspects of the patella. Pain or apprehension with medial-lateral glide and tilt maneuvers of the patella also supports the diagnosis (Video 36-3). The functional examination should look for all the biomechanical deficits listed in the previous paragraph. Conditions such as patellar tendonitis that share predisposing biomechanical risk factors can coexist with patellofemoral arthralgia. The differential diagnosis includes infrapatellar or suprapatellar bursitis, synovial plica, quadriceps tendonitis, patellar tendonitis, Sinding-Larson-Johansson disease, and intraarticular pathology such as a meniscus tear.

Initial treatment protocols use the usual principles of musculoskeletal rehabilitation, including ice, NSAIDs, strengthening weak or imbalanced muscle groups in the core and lower limbs, and stretching tight structures such as the ITB. Activity modification, such as temporarily substituting swimming for running, is important. Many advocate the use of patellofemoral taping techniques to improve patellofemoral tracking and decrease pain. Specific patellofemoral control braces can also decrease pain and improve muscle activation in up to 50% of patients.[36] Improving quadriceps strength strongly correlates with symptomatic improvement. Patellofemoral forces can be minimized during quadriceps strengthening by performing closed kinetic chain strengthening exercises between 0 degrees and 30 degrees of flexion.[45]

Despite the best efforts of the patient and the treatment team, patellofemoral symptoms can become refractory. Although there is not sufficient literature to support their use, consideration should be given for trials of steroid injection, hyaluronate injections, acupuncture, and arthroscopy if a patient fails to respond to noninterventional measures. In very carefully selected patients, surgical release of the lateral retinaculum and tightening or reconstruction of the medial patellofemoral ligament can improve patellar positioning within the groove and improve symptoms.

Injuries to the Anterior Leg Muscle Group

Tibialis Anterior, Extensor Hallucis Longus, and Extensor Digitorum Longus

Overload injuries to these muscles are less common than overload injuries to other muscle-tendon groups of the lower limbs. A common history for overload of the tibialis anterior is onset of anterior leg pain following an increase in downhill running. During downhill running, the ankle dorsiflexors can become overloaded as they work eccentrically during and just after heel strike to slow down ankle plantar flexion. Pain can be experienced in the belly of the muscle, at the musculotendinous junction, or at the insertion of tibialis anterior on the anteromedial midfoot. On examination, symptoms are usually reproduced with resisted ankle dorsiflexion. If symptoms are mild, the sensitivity of the examination may be increased if performed after the patient has run to fatigue. Treatment consists of ice, a short course of NSAIDs, strengthening the ankle dorsiflexors, stretching the heel cord, and a period of relative rest without running downhill followed by a slower progression of hill running and other activities. The differential diagnosis includes stress fracture and anterior compartment syndrome.

Injuries to the Posterior Leg Muscle Group and Associated Soft Tissue Structures

Gastrocnemius, Soleus, Tibialis Posterior, Flexor Hallucis Longus, and Flexor Digitorum Longus

Any of the muscles of the deep or superficial compartments of the posterior leg can become acutely or insidiously overloaded. As with other overload injuries, these muscles are

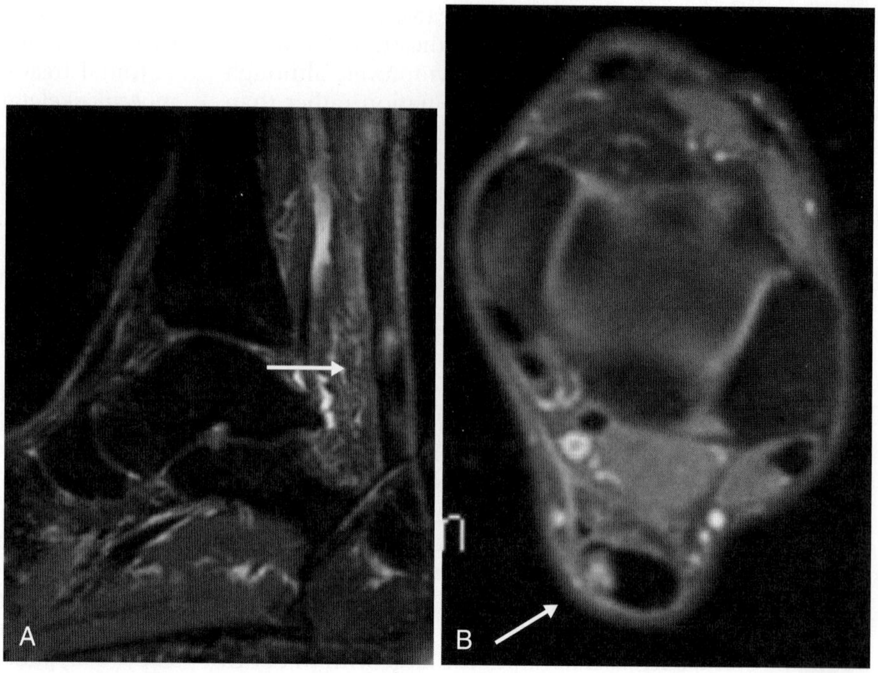

FIGURE 36-12 Achilles tendinopathy. T2-weighted, fat suppression, sagittal **(A)** and axial **(B)** magnetic resonance imaging of the ankle, showing diffuse thickening and increased signal in the Achilles tendon consistent with Achilles tendonosis. The patient was a 42-year-old ultradistance runner who had acute and chronic posterior heel pain.

more prone to sudden or repetitive eccentric overload. Achilles tendon overload is common, and can be either chronic or acute. In the chronic setting, typical changes of tendinosis can be seen clinically by way of a swollen, nodular, tender Achilles tendon. Although not usually necessary for diagnosis, US and MRI show typical changes that correspond to microscopic features of breakdown in the normal collagen orientation, vacuole formation, and microscopic tearing (Figure 36-12, *A, B*). Treatment consists of ice, NSAIDs, activity modification, stretching, and strengthening exercises. Eccentric strength training has been shown to be especially effective in the rehabilitation of chronic Achilles tendinopathy.[3] Muscle groups along the kinetic chain that work synergistically with the ankle plantar flexors must also be tested and rehabilitated, if indicated. For example, in the running, jumping, and cycling motions, the ankle plantar flexors work synergistically with the knee and hip extensors. Additionally, one must address errors in training technique, such as increasing the volume of running or jumping too rapidly. Technique issues, such as toe running should also be addressed as toe running can place excessive eccentric demands on the ankle plantar flexors. Some newer treatment modalities such as platelet-rich plasma injections are being investigated for treatment of Achilles tendinopathy. However, the data published in the current scientific literature are inconsistent and show mixed outcomes.

A sudden, powerful eccentric force can cause an acute rupture of the Achilles tendon. Patients can almost always describe such a mechanism, usually during ballistic sporting activities such as basketball. The event is sometimes accompanied by an audible pop, with inability to continue the activity. Patients commonly relate that they feel as if they were "kicked in the calf." On examination, there will be swelling in the region of the Achilles tendon, and often the examiner can appreciate a palpable defect in the tendon. The patient typically has difficulty with plantar flexion, although some plantar flexion activity might be provided by the other posterior leg muscles. This compensation limits the sensitivity of the Thompson test, in which the examiner squeezes the calf muscles of the prone patient and looks for passive plantar flexion in response. The treatment of acute Achilles tendon rupture includes surgical reconstruction followed by immobilization and then aggressive rehabilitation, versus immobilization followed by aggressive rehabilitation. The period of immobilization can be as long as 3 months. Which treatment to pursue depends on multiple factors, including the age, health, and activity level of the patient; the presence of a partial versus complete tear; the amount of retraction of the torn ends; and the preference of the patient and practitioner. Although good outcomes have been reported with and without surgery, the incidence of a repeat Achilles tendon rupture is lower following surgical reconstruction.[52]

Sever Disease

Sever disease is a traction apophysitis of the Achilles tendon insertion on the posterior calcaneus. Similar to Osgood-Schlatter disease, it is most commonly seen in active adolescents at a time of rapid growth, during which muscles and tendons become tighter as bones become longer. The primary symptom is pain at the Achilles insertion that is exacerbated with activities and improved with rest. The primary physical examination finding is tenderness at the Achilles insertion. The gastrocnemius-soleus complex can be tight. Radiographs are usually not necessary to make the diagnosis but can reveal irregularity of the posterior calcaneus apophysis. Treatment includes ice; relative rest; gentle, progressive heel cord stretching; and gentle, progressive, pain-free calf-strengthening exercises. A heel lift can be used for a short period to unload the area. Symptoms resolve with skeletal maturity.

Flexor Hallucis Longus Overload

Overload of the flexor hallucis longus tendon is seen in dancers, gymnasts, and other active individuals who

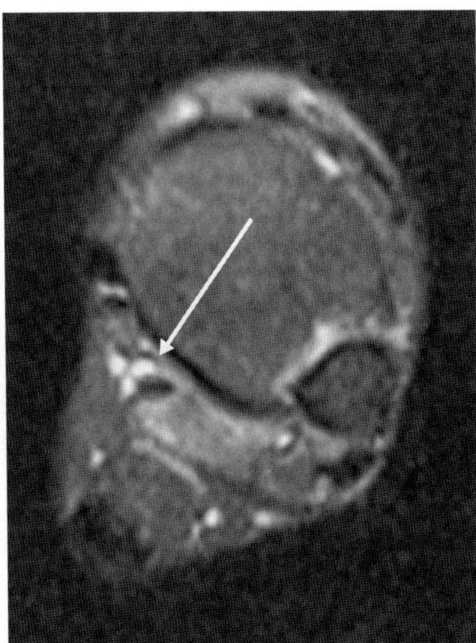

FIGURE 36-13 T2 axial magnetic resonance imaging of the ankle, showing increased signal around the flexor hallucis longus tendon (*arrow*). The patient was a professional dancer.

perform repetitive and forceful toe flexion. The patient can present with pain anywhere along the course of the flexor hallucis longus muscle-tendon unit. Symptoms are reproduced with flexion of the great toe against resistance and direct palpation of the tendon. Passive stretch of the muscle-tendon does not reproduce symptoms as reliably as with some other injuries, such as hamstring strains. Imaging studies are not initially indicated, but when necessary, MRI is the study of choice (Figure 36-13). US performed by a physician skilled in musculoskeletal sonography can also be used and provides some advantages over MRI. As with other muscle and tendon overload conditions, treatment consists of ice, judicious use of NSAIDs, activity modification, and strengthening exercises. In some circumstances, local injection of anesthetic and corticosteroid around the tendon can decrease pain and inflammation, and facilitate progress with the exercise program.

Tibialis Posterior Overload or Medial Tibial Stress Syndrome

Dysfunction of the tibialis posterior muscle is common. The muscle serves many roles. It functions concentrically as an ankle inverter and weak plantar flexor. It creates a force couple with tibialis anterior to support the medial longitudinal arch. It can easily be placed at a biomechanical disadvantage in the setting of anatomic abnormalities such as pes planus and calcaneal eversion. Certain conditions, most notably rheumatoid arthritis, are associated with dysfunction and pathologic rupture of the tibialis posterior tendon. One can assess for tibialis posterior function by performing a resistance test of ankle inversion combined with plantar flexion, and by viewing calcaneal motion from behind as the patient performs slow heel raises. A normally functioning tibialis posterior tendon will permit the calcaneus to rise in line with the leg or in slight calcaneal varus. A dysfunctional tibialis posterior allows the calcaneus to rise in valgus.

There is a spectrum of overload pathology in the medial leg that is collectively referred to as medial tibial stress syndrome. The common term is shin splints. There are several tissues that can be involved when a patient presents with medial or posteromedial leg pain. As mentioned earlier, tibialis posterior can hurt along its origin at the posteromedial border of the tibia. Overload of medial gastrocnemius or medial soleus can also cause pain in this region. Persistent stress can cause progression of pathology to involve the periosteum of the tibia, a condition called periostitis. When further stress is placed on the bone, frank breakdown of the osseous microarchitecture ensues, resulting in stress reaction in the bone and finally stress fracture.

Patients with medial tibial stress syndrome have pain and tenderness along the medial or posteromedial border of the tibia. One can often elicit a history of a rapid increase in running or other athletic activities. Walking and running gait evaluations can show that the patient is a toe walker or a toe runner, which can cause excessive eccentric overload to the ankle plantar flexors. One should look for static and dynamic pes planus, which can place the tibialis posterior at a biomechanical disadvantage. Conversely, if tibialis anterior is weak or inhibited, it may be unable to perform its function as a supporter of the medial longitudinal arch of the foot. A kinetic chain evaluation should focus on other muscle groups that work synergistically with tibialis posterior during functional activities.

It can be difficult or impossible to clinically distinguish exactly which of the tissues mentioned earlier are involved in the overload process when a patient presents with medial leg pain. Clinically, one often proceeds with a course of rehabilitation at the time of the initial evaluation. Usual rehabilitation principles apply, including ice, activity modification, tibialis posterior strengthening, and kinetic chain functional exercises. Off-the-shelf or custom-made foot orthoses can be helpful to provide shock absorption and accommodate for a pes planus. A gradual return to higher level activities is prescribed. If the patient fails to adequately improve with an appropriate rehabilitation program, consideration should be made for imaging to look for periostitis, stress reaction, or stress fracture. These bone overload conditions are rarely appreciated with plain films. MRI has replaced bone scan in most centers as the study of choice to look for stress reaction and stress fracture. If the patient initially presents with point tenderness or risk factors for stress fracture, such as the female athlete triad, one should proceed with imaging at the time of the initial visit. The differential diagnosis also includes compartment syndrome. Further discussion of compartment syndromes and bone overload conditions in the lower limbs is presented later in the chapter.

Injuries to the Lateral Leg Muscle Group

Fibularis Longus and Brevis

The correct anatomic name for the peroneus muscle has been changed to fibularis. However, for the purpose of this discussion we will refer to this muscle group in terms of its widespread usage, which is peroneus. The peroneal muscles can be injured either from a sudden, forceful contraction or from repetitive overload. Acute injuries

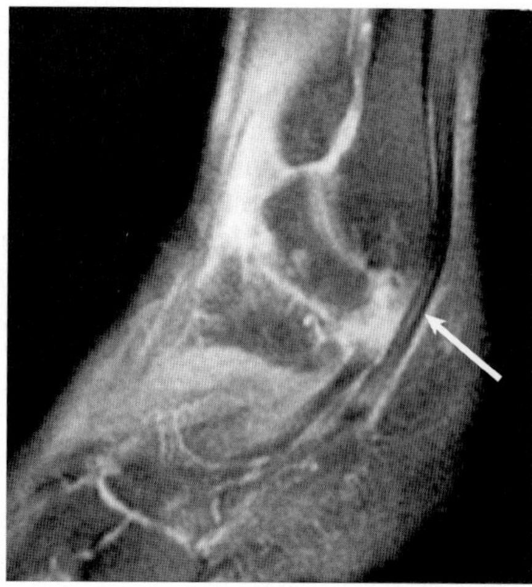

FIGURE 36-14 T2-weighted sagittal short inversion time–inversion recovery magnetic resonance imaging of the ankle, showing a longitudinal split tear of the peroneus brevis tendon (*arrow*).

sometimes occur at the time of a lateral ankle sprain, when the peroneal muscles will activate eccentrically to counteract the inversion moment.[35] On physical examination, there is tenderness over the lateral leg, usually approximately 12 cm proximal to the medial malleolus at the level of the musculotendinous junction. On MRI or US, a longitudinal tear of peroneus longus, peroneus brevis, or both can be seen (Figure 36-14). Although many of these injuries respond well to ankle rehabilitation, persistent cases can require surgical intervention.

Two other conditions of the peroneal muscles should be familiar to the musculoskeletal physician. The peroneal muscles are held in place behind the lateral malleolus of the ankle by the superior peroneal retinaculum. An incompetent retinaculum allows for subluxation of a peroneal tendon around the lateral malleolus. Damage to the retinaculum that causes peroneal tendon subluxation can occur with a severe ankle sprain. If subluxation is recurrent, symptoms are often best addressed with a surgical procedure entailing peroneal tendon groove deepening and retinacular repair. Rarely, the peroneus longus muscle herniates through a fascial defect on the lateral aspect of the leg, usually near the junction of the middle and distal thirds. This is usually a benign condition and infrequently requires surgical consultation.

Compartment Syndrome

The term *compartment syndrome* refers to a condition in which the pressure within a given muscle compartment is abnormally elevated. There are two types of compartment syndrome: acute and chronic. Acute compartment syndrome is usually caused by significant trauma, such as a fracture or crush injury, and is a surgical emergency. Chronic exertional compartment syndrome (CECS) of the lower extremity is seen most commonly in high-volume runners. Symptoms can mimic those of tendinopathy or stress fracture. Patients with CECS complain of recurrent leg cramping or pain with activities. Symptoms usually come on at a predictable time point in their exercise routine. Occasionally, the patient can localize the cramping to a particular compartment of the leg (anterior, lateral, superficial posterior, and deep posterior). More often, however, the cramping is difficult to localize. Neurologic symptoms, such as temporary foot drop during activities, can occur when high compartment pressures cause ischemia to the tibial or peroneal nerves. Definitive diagnosis is by intramuscular compartment pressure testing. In addition to a history and physical examination that are consistent with CECS, one or more of the following criteria must be met to formally establish the diagnosis:

- Preexercise pressure ≥ 15 mm Hg;
- 1-minute postexercise pressure ≥ 30 mm Hg; or
- 5-minute postexercise pressure ≥ 20 mm Hg.

Newer MRI imaging techniques that measure increased T2 signal in a specific compartment after exercise might provide a noninvasive way of documenting selective compartment pressure increase.[29] Treatment can be challenging. The primary nonsurgical treatment is avoiding the inciting activities. Massage therapy can sometimes be helpful. If prolonged activity modification and rehabilitation are unsuccessful, fasciotomy or fasciectomy should be considered, and in the carefully selected patient can be very effective.[46]

Injury to the Plantar Foot Muscles and Plantar Fascia; Plantar Fasciitis

Four plantar foot muscles take their origin from the volar calcaneus: adductor hallucis, quadratus plantae, flexor digitorum brevis, and abductor digiti minimi quinti. Overload of these muscles can result in an enthesopathy at the calcaneus, causing volar heel pain. The same process can cause inflammation and pain in the plantar fascia. This condition is referred to as plantar fasciitis. Patients with plantar fasciitis present with volar heel pain that is often, but not always, worse with their first few steps in the morning. Tenderness to palpation is present at the volar aspect of the heel, usually slightly medial to midline. Imaging studies are usually not indicated, unless there is a history of acute trauma or symptoms become recalcitrant. The presence or absence of a calcaneal traction spur correlates poorly with symptoms of plantar fasciitis.[24]

As with other musculotendinous injuries, a similar biomechanical approach should be taken when treating plantar fasciitis. The rehabilitation plan should focus on restoring range of motion, strength, endurance, and motor control of the heel cord and foot intrinsic muscles. If pain with the first few steps in the morning is a prominent symptom, then a resting night splint can be very helpful in preventing overnight tightening of the heel cord and plantar structures (Figure 36-15). A kinetic chain evaluation might reveal predisposing biomechanical deficits. If the patient is a toe runner, then the foot intrinsic muscles can become eccentrically overloaded. Similarly, a tight heel cord or a tight hamstring can prevent proper heel strike and result in excessive forces being placed on the plantar foot muscles. If tibialis posterior or tibialis anterior tendons are not doing their assigned job of supporting the medial longitudinal arch, the plantar foot muscles can become overloaded as they try to compensate for their more proximal agonists. More proximally still, the dynamic function of the hip external rotators should be assessed. The hip external rotators eccentrically control femoral internal rotation during the weight-bearing phase of running, and

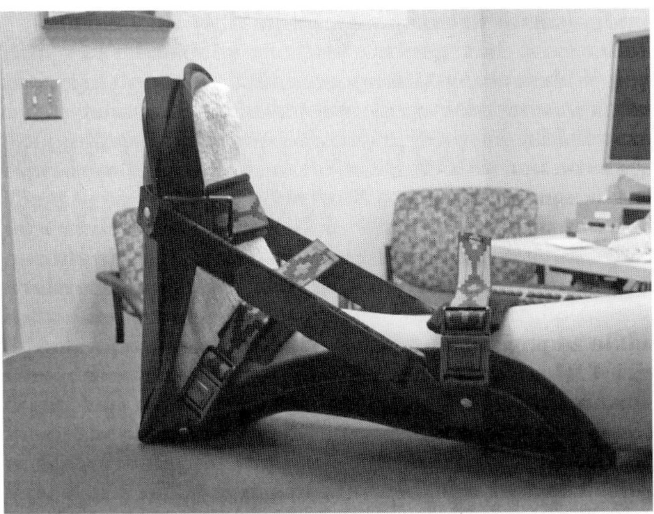

FIGURE 36-15 Resting night splint.

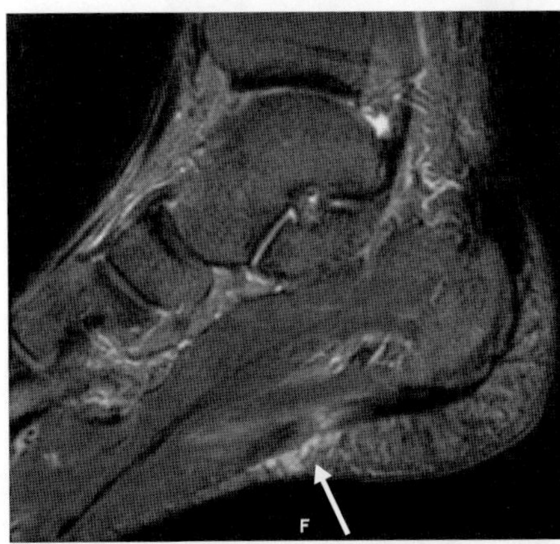

FIGURE 36-16 T2-weighted fat suppression magnetic resonance imaging of the foot, showing increased signal in the midportion of the plantar fascia (*arrow*), indicating an acute rupture of that structure. The patient was an Olympic bobsledder who was unable to compete with this injury.

therefore have an indirect effect on tibial rotation and subtalar pronation. Local injection of corticosteroid can assist in decreasing local inflammation and pain, but the patient must be cautioned that corticosteroid can increase the risk of rupture of the plantar fascia (Figure 36-16).

Disorders of the Joints of the Lower Limb

Osteoarthritis

Osteoarthritis in the weight-bearing joints of the lower extremities is very common. Osteoarthritis was previously thought to be a purely degenerative condition associated with aging. More recently, links between biomechanical factors, developmental abnormalities of the femur and acetabulum, local biochemical processes, and genetic predisposition have also been identified as contributing factors in the development of osteoarthritis. Additionally, joint trauma and obesity are known risk factors for developing osteoarthritis in the weight-bearing joints. Pain or functional limitations are the usual presenting complaints in patients with osteoarthritis. Pain and stiffness are common first thing in the morning, typically lasting less than 1 hour. This is in contrast to inflammatory arthropathies, where the pain often lasts greater than 1 hour. Patients with lower limb osteoarthritis typically complain of joint pain that is worse with weight bearing and improved with rest. Because the principles of diagnosis and treatment are similar, osteoarthritis of the hip, knee, ankle, and foot are discussed together.

Pain from hip osteoarthritis can refer to the groin region or into the anterior thigh down to the knee. Pain is less commonly described as being posterior or lateral. The differential diagnosis of hip osteoarthritis includes referred pain from the lumbar spine, anterior hip muscle pathology, and hernia. The physical examination is most notable for an antalgic gait on the affected side and reproduction of groin pain with passive hip internal rotation. Loss of internal rotation is one of the earliest physical examination findings. Knee osteoarthritis can affect the medial tibiofemoral compartment, the lateral tibiofemoral compartment, the patellofemoral joint, or all three compartments. The medial compartment is often involved first, with varus alignment noted on inspection. Other findings can include joint line tenderness, crepitus, effusion, and palpable osteophytosis. Ankle and foot arthritis often occurs years after trauma to these joints or with malalignment that loads joints abnormally. Frequent locations of osteoarthritis include the ankle joint, subtalar joint, and the first metatarsophalangeal joint of the great toe. Ankle arthritis is characterized by pain, swelling, and stiffness in the anterior ankle. Pain from subtalar arthritis is appreciated when walking on uneven surfaces and is often especially painful. Osteoarthritis of the first metatarsophalangeal joint (hallux rigidus) results in loss of dorsiflexion, joint swelling, and pain. Plain radiographs are the study of choice to assess for osteoarthritis. The radiologic hallmarks of osteoarthritis include joint space narrowing, marginal osteophytosis, subchondral sclerosis, and subchondral cyst formation (Figure 36-17, *A, B, C, D*).[7]

There are many treatment options for lower limb osteoarthritis. The primary focus is on symptom management and maintenance or restoration of functional capacity through a combination of nonpharmacologic and pharmacologic interventions. An individualized, patient-centered approach is recommended. The American College of Rheumatology recently published recommendations for the treatment of hip and knee osteoarthritis based on a systematic review of the existing literature.[19] In general for patients with osteoarthritis in the weight-bearing joints, regular exercise and weight loss were strongly recommended. Strength training and aerobic exercise can improve joint control and decrease pain. Strategies aimed at reducing loads on joints include weight loss, cushioned shoes, and walking aids such as a cane. Activity modification can help decrease symptoms such as switching from higher impact activities such as basketball to lower impact activities such as bicycling or swimming. Acetaminophen, oral NSAIDs, and tramadol were conditionally recommended to reduce joint pain in hip and knee osteoarthritis. Topical NSAIDs were conditionally recommended for patients with knee osteoarthritis. Although a few previous studies

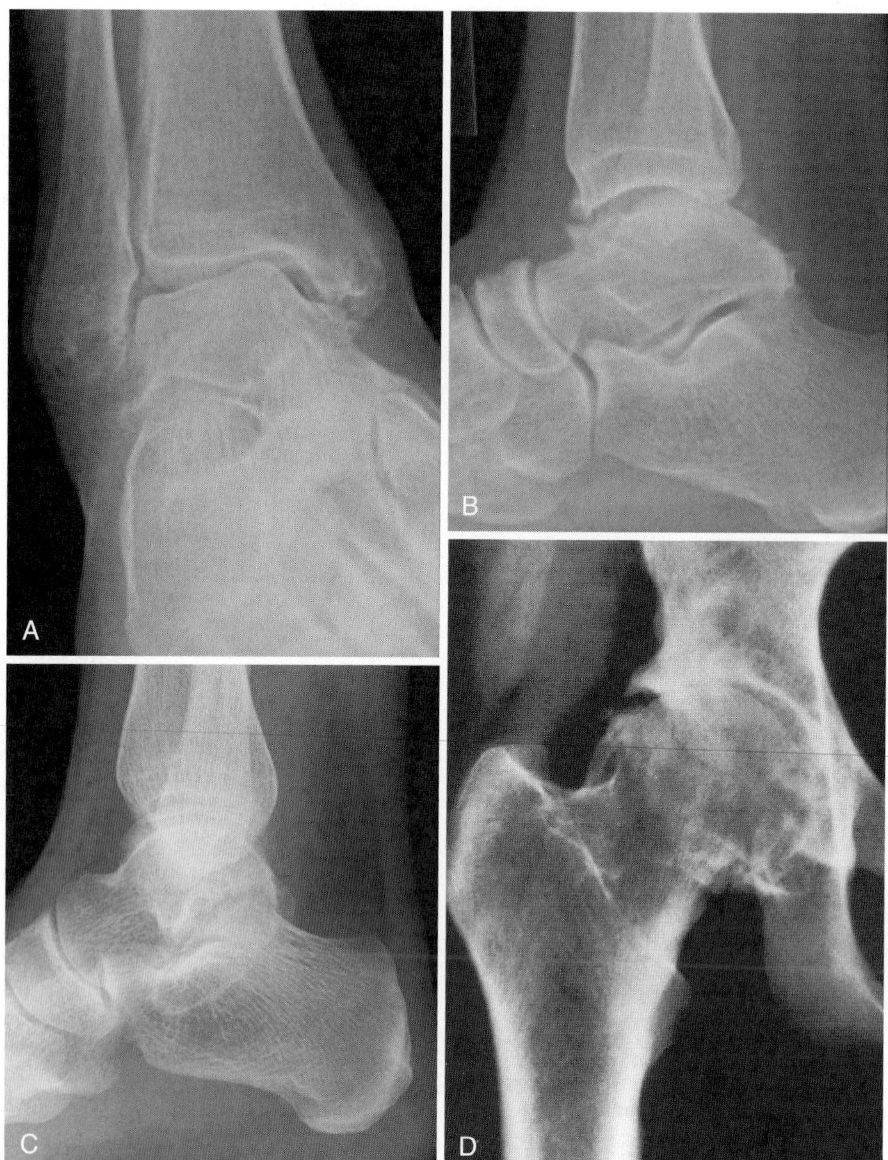

FIGURE 36-17 Examples of osteoarthritis. Anteroposterior **(A)** and lateral **(B)** radiographs of the ankle, showing advanced osteoarthritis in the ankle joint. There are large dorsal spurs, small intraarticular calcific bodies, and varus alignment is present at the joint, with widening of the joint space laterally, consistent with chronic ligamentous laxity. **C,** Lateral radiograph of the ankle, showing advanced osteoarthritis of the posterior subtalar joint. There is significant irregularity of the joint margins, with subchondral sclerosis and cyst formation. **D,** Anteroposterior radiograph of the hip, showing very severe osteoarthritis, with near-complete obliteration of the joint space and extensive remodeling of the femoral head.

have demonstrated efficacy of glucosamine and chondroitin sulfate supplementation, the most recent American College of Rheumatology guidelines conditionally recommend that patients with hip and knee osteoarthritis not use these products. Intraarticular corticosteroid injections were conditionally recommended for both hip and knee osteoarthritis. Previously, injections of the foot, ankle, and hip joints were best performed under fluoroscopic guidance with contrast confirmation. However, with the emergence of musculoskeletal US, image-guided intraarticular anesthetic injections can be done in the office setting and can assist in cases where there might be diagnostic uncertainty.[44,54] Research into the efficacy of intraarticular hyaluronate injections is ongoing. Several investigations have concluded that intraarticular hyaluronate injections relieve pain and improve function in patients with mild and moderate knee osteoarthritis. The guidelines did not provide recommendations based on a lack of high-quality studies, and the evidence regarding intraarticular viscosupplementation into other lower extremity weight-bearing joints for treatment of osteoarthritis is also limited.[2,31] For patients with recalcitrant pain or severe functional limitations, arthroplasty can provide substantial improvement in pain and function.

Disorders of the Hip Joint

Avascular Necrosis

Avascular necrosis, also called osteonecrosis, is caused by ischemia to a bone with resultant death of osteocytes and surrounding marrow, which can lead to microfractures and eventual collapse of the affected segment. The femoral

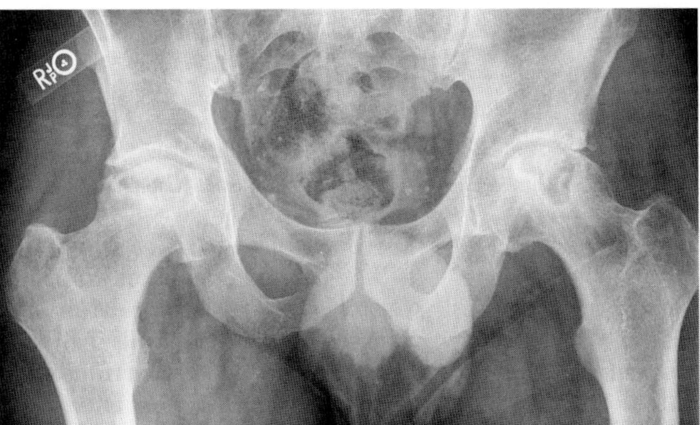

FIGURE 36-18 Anteroposterior radiograph of the pelvis, showing advanced avascular necrosis of both femoral heads.

head is the most common location resulting from a tenuous blood supply at baseline. Disruption of blood flow to the femoral head can be caused by various conditions, including trauma; high doses of corticosteroids; alcohol abuse; and systemic illnesses such as diabetes, systemic lupus erythematosus, and sickle cell anemia.[22] The severity of symptoms with avascular necrosis is usually related to the degree of articular surface disruption.[34] Symptoms are similar to those experienced with hip osteoarthritis, including groin pain that increases with weight bearing. Often, there is limited motion and pain with internal rotation, flexion, and abduction of the hip. Radiographs can reveal sclerosis of the femoral head, or in severe cases, collapse of the femoral head (Figure 36-18). In mild cases, the plain films can be normal. MRI and computed tomography (CT) can detect the condition in its earlier stages. Conservative treatments include keeping weight off the affected joint and use of pain medications. Once collapse occurs, joint replacement surgery is indicated to improve pain and function.

Legg-Calvé-Perthes Disease

Legg-Calvé-Perthes disease is an idiopathic osteonecrosis of the femoral head that occurs in children, typically boys between the ages of 4 and 10 years. The disease can be bilateral in up to 10% of cases. The child may complain of groin or thigh pain and present with antalgic gait and limited hip range of motion, especially abduction and internal rotation. Because of the potential for revascularization of the femoral head and bone remodeling in children, the prognosis in children is significantly better compared with adults with avascular necrosis. Despite this, a recent prospective long-term study demonstrated high rates of ongoing hip dysfunction, including pain and premature arthritis in patients with Legg-Calvé-Perthes disease who were followed into early adulthood. Age of onset, degree of deformity, and percent involvement of the femoral head are important prognostic factors.[25] Good outcomes have been shown in children younger than 6 years of age who are treated nonsurgically with physical therapy, protected weight bearing, and femoral head containment with the use of bracing (Scottish Rite Orthosis), or casting in an attempt to maintain the femoral head in a spherical state. Osteotomy is often performed in older children.[26]

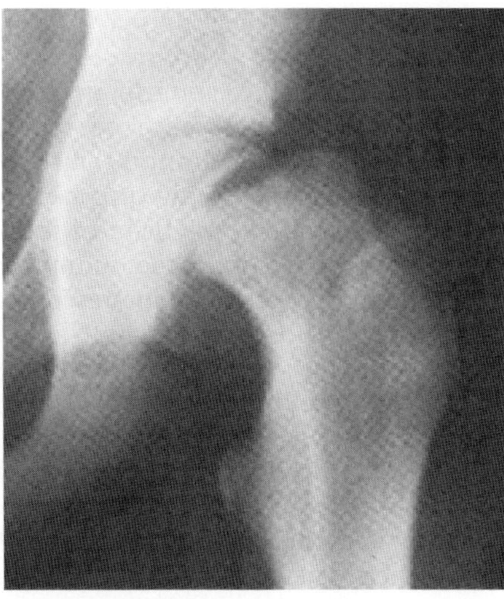

FIGURE 36-19 Anteroposterior radiograph of a severe, acute slipped capital femoral epiphysis.

Slipped Capital Femoral Epiphysis

Slipped capital femoral epiphysis (SCFE) refers to the displacement of the capital femoral epiphysis from the metaphysis, secondary to disruption of the physis in the immature hip. Injury to the physeal plate of the proximal femur with medial displacement of the femoral head relative to the femoral shaft can be caused by acute trauma or repetitive microtrauma. SCFE is the most common hip disorder in adolescent populations, affecting boys 1.5 to 2 times more than girls. Age of presentation ranges from 8 to 15 years old with the average age of diagnosis being 12 years old in girls and 13.5 years old in boys.[15] SCFE occurs bilaterally in approximately 50% of patients. It is strongly associated with obesity and there has been evidence linking it to endocrinopathies and renal osteodystrophy.

An adolescent with hip pain and difficulty walking necessitates clinical and radiographic evaluation. Clinically, an adolescent with an acute slip presents with severe hip, groin, or thigh pain that is exacerbated with any motion. Loss of internal rotation and obligatory external rotation (external rotation with passive hip flexion) are helpful physical examination findings. Radiographic evaluation should include anteroposterior views and lateral views (frog leg lateral or cross-table lateral) to assess for widening of the physis, decreased epiphyseal height, or Klein line (Figure 36-19).

The goal of treatment is to stabilize the slip in an attempt to prevent further progression and hopefully avoid subsequent long-term complications such as avascular necrosis of the femoral head, rotational deformity, and osteoarthritis. Attempts at closed reduction increase the risk of osteonecrosis and should be avoided. It is recommended that SCFE is treated as an orthopedic emergency with prompt referral to an orthopedic surgeon for immediate internal fixation. Following surgery, gentle range of motion can be started within a few days, followed by protected weight bearing for 6 to 8 weeks. After this time period, gradually progressive strengthening and functional exercises are advanced with return to advanced activities (i.e., sports) once they have regained full strength and can participate without pain.

Hip Dislocation

Because of the depth of the acetabulum, dislocation of the femoroacetabular joint requires significant trauma. In children, hip dislocation is more common than hip fractures. In adults, fractures of the acetabulum often accompany hip dislocations. Most commonly, the head of the femur dislocates posteriorly relative to the acetabulum. The patient with an acute posterior hip dislocation presents with severe hip pain and tends to hold the hip in flexion, internal rotation, and adduction. With the less common anterior dislocations, the hip is held in an extended, abducted, and externally rotated position. On physical examination, there will be an obvious deformity. The patient will not tolerate range-of-motion or resistance testing as a result of pain. A complete neurologic examination should be performed to assess for lumbosacral plexopathy, sciatic neuropathy, and femoral neuropathy. One should always assess for associated injuries, in particular spine and ipsilateral knee trauma, which can be masked by hip pain. Radiographs (anterior posterior pelvis and a 15 degree oblique lateral) are indicated to confirm the clinical diagnosis and look for associated injuries. At times, CT or MRI is obtained if further characterization of associated injuries is needed.

Hip dislocations are considered an orthopedic emergency, and closed reduction under anesthesia should be performed as soon as possible. Postreduction radiographs are obtained to confirm anatomic alignment. Surgery is indicated if attempts at closed reduction are unsuccessful, and to repair displaced or comminuted fractures and remove intraarticular loose bodies. Most clinicians recommend non–weight bearing for 3 to 4 weeks, followed by protected weight bearing for an additional 3 weeks. Gradually, progressive rehabilitation can start a few days to a couple of weeks after reduction, depending on the patient's comfort level and whether or not surgery was performed. The most concerning complications of hip dislocation include sciatic nerve injury, posttraumatic osteoarthritis, and avascular necrosis, which occur in up to 10% of patients.

Labral Injuries

The acetabular labrum has many functions including acting as a shock absorber and providing stability of the femoroacetabular joint. Injuries to the acetabular labrum can result from acute or repetitive trauma, hypermobility of the hip joint, and dysplasia. More recently, labral injuries have been associated with patients who have underlying morphologic abnormalities of the femoral head or acetabulum.[17] The diagnosis of acetabular labral pathology can be challenging. Historical features and physical examination maneuvers lack specificity. Pain is typically located in the groin. Patients with acetabular labral tears can also present with painful clicking and catching of the hip, especially when the hip is at a particular angle. Anterior hip impingement tests are most consistent at provoking symptoms as well as femoral-acetabular grind maneuvers. Magnetic resonance arthrography with intraarticular contrast is the imaging study of choice to assess for these injuries (Figure 36-20). Definitive diagnosis is by arthroscopy or open surgery. Treatment options include physical therapy, NSAIDs, relative rest, intraarticular steroid injections, and arthroscopic débridement and repair.

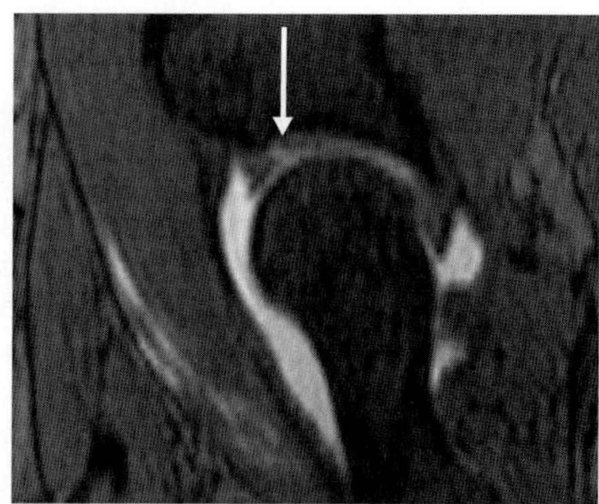

FIGURE 36-20 Gadolinium-enhanced sagittal magnetic resonance imaging of the hip, showing an anterior labrum tear (*arrow*).

Impingement Syndromes

In recent years, there has been greater attention given to the concept of hip impingement. Impingement about the hip can be caused by a variety of conditions but the two main causes are morphologic variants of the acetabulum or femoral head and neck resulting in abnormal and potentially damaging mechanical contact between these two structures. The term *femoroacetabular impingement* has been added to the medical lexicon and refers to a clinical syndrome of limited hip range of motion and pain in the setting of the anatomic abnormalities mentioned earlier.

Femoroacetabular impingement can be classified into two types: CAM and Pincer. CAM morphology refers to anatomic variation at the femoral head-neck junction with a so-called bump. Pincer type describes morphologic changes with the acetabulum caused by acetabular overcoverage of the femoral head or abnormal orientation (retroversion) of the acetabulum. Although two distinct types are described, epidemiologic studies have demonstrated that most patients have features of both CAM and Pincer type morphology. The result of these anatomic abnormalities is abnormal contact between the femoral head and neck and the superolateral acetabulum leading to pain and restricted range of motion. Aside from the functional limitations associated with this condition, there has also been a link to early chondrolabral injury and hip joint degeneration.

Patients with femoroacetabular impingement typically present with insidious onset groin pain that is worse with activity. They may notice pain with end range of motion, particularly hip flexion and internal rotation and describe limitations in activities that involve squatting or getting into a crouched position. Radiographs can assist in the diagnosis and include anterior posterior pelvis and frog leg lateral, cross-table lateral, false profile, or Dunn lateral views. Clinical correlation is important because recent studies have demonstrated a high prevalence of radiographic abnormalities in patients who are asymptomatic. Advanced imaging, including MRI or magnetic resonance arthrography, may be indicated to assess for other injuries or evidence of degenerative joint changes.[48] Treatments range from conservative management, including physical therapy, NSAIDs, and activity modification, to a variety of surgical interventions ranging from open surgical dislocation to arthroscopy, with the focus of these interventions on hip preservation.[21,37]

Disorders of the Knee Joint

Knee Ligament Injuries

Four ligaments provide static stability to the knee. The most commonly injured knee ligaments are the medial collateral ligament (MCL) and the ACL. The MCL courses from the medial femoral condyle to the proximal, medial tibia, and provides restraint against valgus force. Patients presenting with an MCL sprain will often be able to describe sustaining a sudden valgus force with the foot planted. They will often be able to localize the pain to the medial side of the knee. The physical examination will be most notable for tenderness along the course of the MCL and a positive valgus stress test (Video 36-4). If the patient is apprehensive with valgus stress testing but a firm end feel is appreciated, then the injury is most likely a grade 1 sprain with no gross tearing of the ligament (Figure 36-21). If the medial joint line opens up without apparent restraint, the injury is a grade 3 sprain, representing complete disruption of the ligament. Depending on the degree of ligament injury, medial knee swelling may be present, but an intraarticular effusion is absent in isolated MCL sprains because the MCL is extraarticular. Although plain films are usually unremarkable in an isolated MCL injury, anteroposterior and lateral radiographs are useful to rule out an associated bony injury. MRI is the imaging study of choice to evaluate the MCL, but is usually obtained only if other injuries are suspected or if the patient is an elite athlete. Initial treatment most commonly consists of aggressive use of ice and elevation to decrease swelling and pain. A knee immobilizer may be used for 1 to 2 weeks to provide joint stability and allow reparative scar tissue to begin forming. Early, gentle knee flexion and extension exercises are initiated in the first 1 to 2 weeks, and gradual return to full activities as tolerated is progressed over 1 to 4 weeks, depending on the severity of the injury. Isolated MCL tears, even grade 3, rarely if ever require surgery.

Tears of the ACL are the most functionally devastating because of the crucial role of the ACL in the dynamic stability of the knee, especially during activities involving side-to-side or cutting maneuvers. The ACL courses from the medial wall of the lateral femoral condyle anteromedially to the anterior spine of the tibial plateau. The ACL restrains anterior displacement of the tibia relative to the femur, and internal rotation of the tibia relative to the femur. ACL tears can occur as a result of contact or noncontact injuries. Although different mechanisms can place the ACL at risk, the individual is often rotated on a planted foot with the knee in flexion and the quadriceps activating strongly. The patient will often report hearing or feeling a "pop." The patient will also describe a sense of knee instability, especially with twisting activities such as changing direction when walking. Return to sports participation is usually impossible or associated with repeated episodes of instability. In the acute setting, pain might not be a prominent symptom. When significant pain is present acutely, it can suggest the presence of an associated injury, such as a bone contusion or meniscus tear. On physical examination, an effusion is usually present, and the anterior drawer and Lachman tests reveal increased anterior displacement of the tibia relative to the femur. The Lachman test is reported to have greater sensitivity for detecting ACL insufficiency compared with the anterior drawer test (Videos 36-5 and 36-6).[50] Plain films can show an effusion. The presence of a small capsular avulsion fracture of the lateral tibial plateau is termed a Segond fracture, and is considered pathognomonic of the presence of an ACL tear (Figure 36-22). An MRI is often obtained to confirm the clinical diagnosis and look for associated injuries, such as meniscal tears, capsular injuries, other ligament injuries, bone bruises, and muscle/tendon injuries (Figure 36-23, *A, B, C, D*).

The management of acute ACL tears includes aggressive use of ice, elevation, and compression. A knee immobilizer or hinged knee brace can be used initially to provide

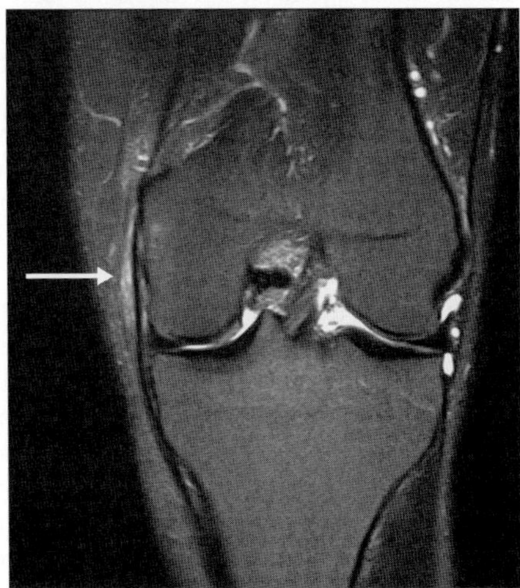

FIGURE 36-21 T2-weighted, fat suppression, coronal magnetic resonance imaging of the knee, showing increased signal surrounding the medial collateral ligament with intact fibers of the ligament, consistent with grade 1 strain (*arrow*). The patient was a football player who sustained a valgus injury to the knee with his foot planted on the ground.

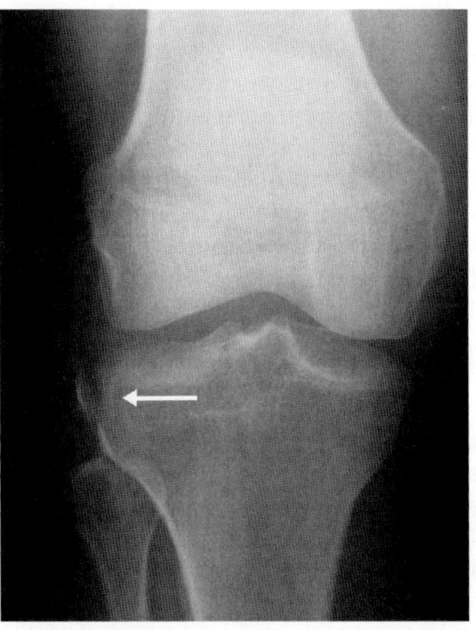

FIGURE 36-22 Anteroposterior radiograph of the knee, showing a large Segond fracture (*arrow*), indicating the likely presence of an anterior cruciate ligament tear.

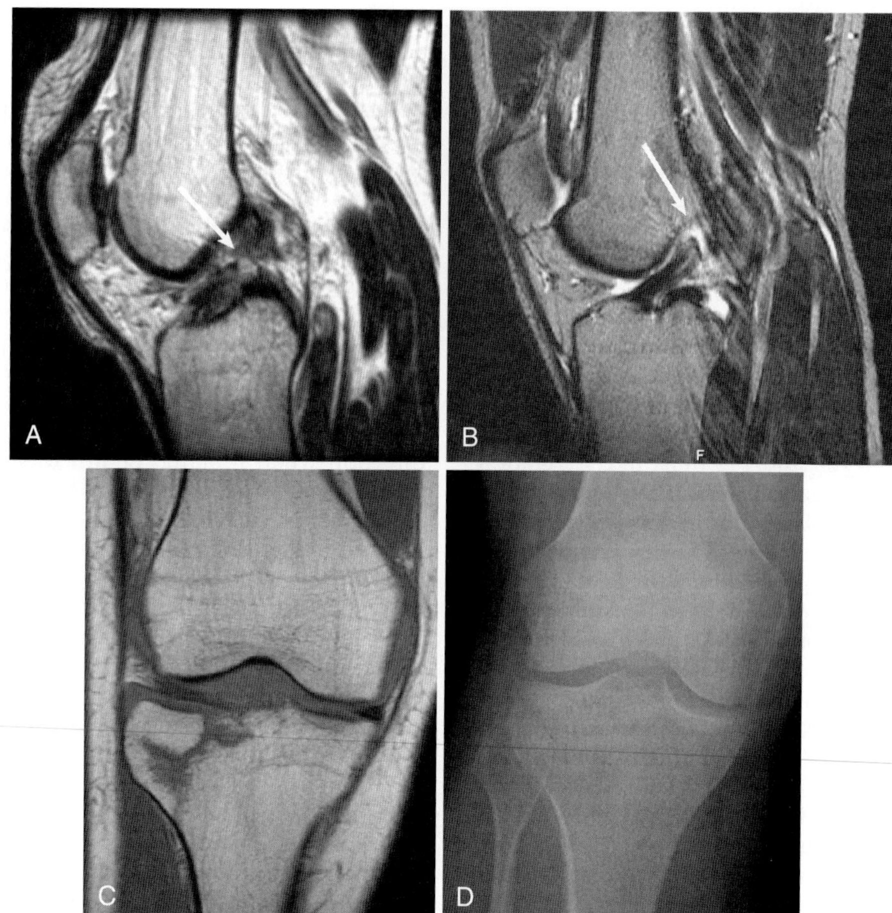

FIGURE 36-23 Examples of anterior cruciate ligament (ACL) tears and associated injuries. **A,** T1 sagittal magnetic resonance imaging (MRI) showing a midsubstance tear of the ACL (*arrow*). **B,** T1 sagittal MRI showing an ACL tear from the proximal attachment site on the femur (*arrow*). **C,** Coronal T1-weighted MRI showing a nondisplaced tibial plateau fracture that was associated with an ACL injury. **D,** The fracture was not appreciated on initial radiographs, which were normal.

stability. Crutches can also be used if needed. Early, gentle knee flexion and extension exercises can minimize the development of stiffness. Quadriceps inhibition is almost ubiquitous after ACL tears, and atrophy in this muscle group can be fairly dramatic even within a few weeks of injury. Straight leg raises performed in the knee immobilizer promote safe quadriceps activation and decrease atrophy. The longer term treatment of ACL tears depends primarily on the patient's desired activity level. Young healthy individuals who participate in cutting sports should strongly consider ligament reconstruction to increase knee stability and decrease the chance of developing posttraumatic osteoarthritis from a chronically unstable knee. Sedentary individuals or individuals participating primarily in straight ahead activities such as walking and cycling might opt for aggressive rehabilitation to maximize muscular control of the joint. It is also reasonable for patients to pursue aggressive rehabilitation and defer surgical reconstruction if they are not experiencing episodes of instability and are willing to avoid impact and aggressive cut-pivot activities. Most knee surgeons recommend waiting at least 2 to 3 weeks before reconstruction, to allow time for swelling and stiffness to decrease. The use of functional knee braces in patients who are ACL-deficient seems to provide some benefit in moderate activities and appears to limit subluxation events, although the mechanism for this is unclear. There is no evidence to show that these braces prevent ACL injury.[8]

The posterior cruciate ligament (PCL) courses posteriorly and inferiorly from the femoral intercondylar notch to the posterior tibial spine. It serves to restrain posterior displacement of the tibia relative to the femur. A common mechanism for PCL disruption is a forceful blow to the proximal, anterior leg. This can drive the tibia posterior relative to the femur. PCL disruptions have occurred in soccer goalkeepers who get kicked in the shin when sliding to make a save, in individuals who fall on to their shins, and in motor vehicle accidents when a front seat passenger has the shin driven into the dashboard (the so-called dashboard injury). Injuries of the PCL are less common than injuries of the ACL. Isolated PCL deficiency generally results in less significant functional limitations compared with the ACL-deficient knee. The clinical diagnosis of a PCL tear is primarily based on a positive posterior drawer test (Video 36-7). Plain films are usually negative in isolated PCL injuries. MRI can be obtained to confirm the diagnosis and look for associated injuries including possible posterolateral corner injuries (discussed later). Acute management includes ice, elevation, pain control if needed, and early gentle range-of-motion exercises. If the individual is having difficulty with walking, a knee immobilizer and crutches can be used for 1 to 2 weeks. Most individuals with isolated PCL injuries can return to full activities, including athletics, with functional rehabilitation. On rare occasions, surgical reconstruction of an isolated PCL injury is undertaken if the individual continues to experience instability symptoms or functional limitations.

The lateral collateral ligament, also called the fibular collateral ligament, courses from the lateral femoral condyle to the fibular head, and resists varus forces at the knee. The lateral collateral ligament is rarely injured in isolation but can be torn in multiligament injuries and knee dislocations.

Posterolateral Corner Injuries

The posterolateral corner is a complicated anatomic region that includes the lateral collateral ligament, popliteus tendon, posterolateral joint capsule, biceps femoris tendon, peroneal nerve, lateral head of gastrocnemius, lateral meniscus, and posterior meniscofemoral ligament. It provides support to the PCL in restraining tibial external rotation. Injury to any or all of these structures can accompany a severe knee sprain such as an ACL tear, PCL tear, or a knee dislocation with multiligamentous injury, with the most common mechanism of injury being a strong hyperextension and varus force.[30]

Accurate diagnosis of injuries to the posterolateral corner of the knee can be difficult, but is important to ensure complete management of these types of injuries. MRI is helpful to determine the extent of structural involvement. Treatment options range from nonoperative management to surgical reconstruction. Early surgical evaluation is recommended to optimize outcomes.

Meniscal Injuries

Injuries to the menisci are common. They can be the result of acute trauma or gradual degeneration. A sudden or forceful twisting motion on a planted foot is the most common mechanism of injury for acute meniscus tears. The patient typically reports a slow onset of swelling after the injury, and pain with weight bearing and twisting maneuvers. Sometimes there is clicking within the knee. Locking of the knee suggests the presence of a bucket handle meniscus tear that has flipped up into the intercondylar notch (Figure 36-24). The hallmarks of the physical examination include medial or lateral joint line tenderness, effusion, and a positive McMurray test (Video 36-8). MRI is the study of choice to evaluate meniscus tears.

Initial treatments include ice, elevation, NSAIDs, and bracing. Additional treatments depend on healing potential and the patient's goals. Simple tears have a greater chance of healing than complex tears. Tears in the outer portion of the meniscus, referred to as the vascularized "red zone," have greater healing potential than tears located centrally in the avascular "white zone." Vascular zone tears in younger individuals can be amenable to arthroscopic meniscal repair procedures. In older athletes, if there are no mechanical symptoms present, it is reasonable to allow 3 to 6 weeks of relative rest and rehabilitation to see if symptoms improve. Referral for consideration of arthroscopic intervention is indicated if the patient remains limited in function, has persistent mechanical symptoms, or has recurrent episodes of pain and swelling. Patients who need to return to full activities quickly,

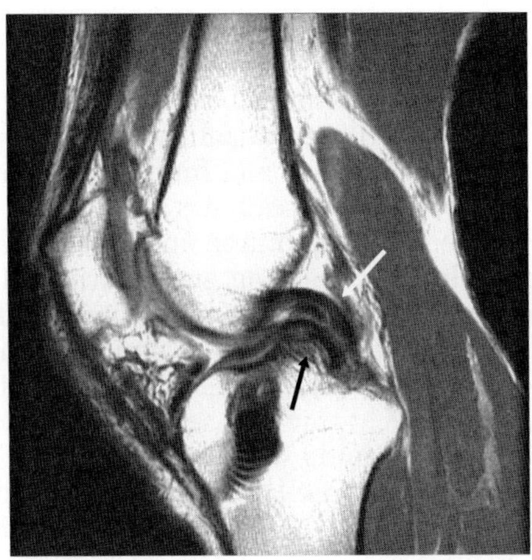

FIGURE 36-24 T1 sagittal magnetic resonance imaging of a knee, showing a bucket handle meniscus tear that flipped up into the notch, creating the so-called double posterior cruciate ligament (PCL) sign. The patient was an Olympic alpine ski racer who had a previous anterior cruciate ligament (ACL) reconstruction and who sustained this meniscus injury during competition. The tibial tunnel and screw were not placed anterior enough in the tibia, essentially creating a nonfunctional ACL graft and leaving the knee unstable. The superior black line, denoted by the white arrow, is the real PCL. The inferior black line, denoted by the black arrow, is the bucket handle meniscus tear that displaced into the notch.

such as elite athletes, often proceed with arthroscopy sooner. Arthroscopic treatment options include repair of the meniscus tear versus débridement of the meniscus with partial meniscectomy.

Osteochondral Lesions (Osteochondritis Dissecans)

Osteochondritis dissecans (OCD) is a lesion of subchondral bone that can progress to secondarily affect the overlying articular cartilage. The underlying mechanism is poorly understood but is likely to be multifactorial with contributions from constitutional, hereditary, vascular, and traumatic factors. Although OCD can affect any joint, the knee is the most common location. Within the knee, the most common site for OCD lesions to occur is the lateral aspect of the medial femoral condyle, but they can also be seen in the lateral femoral condyle or retropatellar cartilage. Adolescent (10 to 15 years old) boys are the most commonly affected group.[10]

OCD lesions of the knee are classified based on the location of the lesion and degree of fragmentation or displacement. Grade 1 lesions involve compression of subchondral trabeculae with preservation of the cartilage. Grade 2 involves incomplete detachment of an osteochondral fragment. Grade 3 involves complete avulsion of an osteochondral fragment without dislocation. Grade 4 involves complete avulsion of an osteochondral fragment with dislocation (loose body).[10] Symptoms include recurrent swelling and pain with activity that is lessened with rest. The Wilson test, which involves extending the knee the last 30 degrees with the foot internally rotated, can be positive. Because these symptoms might be caused by other injuries, such as meniscus tears and articular cartilage defects, formal diagnosis usually awaits imaging studies or direct arthroscopic visualization. Treatment depends on the grading and stability of the lesion, age of the patient, status of the physes, and severity of symptoms. Options vary from relative rest to surgery.

Prepatellar Bursitis

Prepatellar bursitis, also known as housemaid's knee, is a common cause of swelling and pain anterior to the patella. The term *housemaid's knee* comes from its association with individuals whose work necessitates kneeling for extended periods of time and is common in professions such as carpet laying, plumbing, mining, and gardening. It can also be seen in wrestlers secondary to irritation or friction from the wrestling mat. The diagnosis is typically made based on clinical and physical examination, although differentiation between acute/chronic and septic/aseptic will sometimes be needed to guide treatment decisions. For most cases, treatment of prepatellar bursitis begins with avoiding the aggravating activities. Ice, compression, and NSAIDs are useful to decrease swelling and pain. Aspiration followed by instillation of corticosteroid can be helpful, but a septic bursitis should be ruled out first with culture and gram stain. In rare, recalcitrant cases, surgical excision of the bursa might be indicated.[1]

Disorders of the Ankle and Subtalar Joints

Sprains

Ankle sprains are the most common musculoskeletal injury in the lower limb. They account for 25% of all sports injuries. The strongest predictor of ankle sprains is a history of previous sprain. The most commonly injured ligament is the anterior talofibular ligament, which has the weakest tensile strength of the lateral ankle ligament complex. The most common mechanism for ankle sprains is inversion, usually combined with plantar flexion. Syndesmotic and medial ankle sprains are uncommon and are more severe injuries. Syndesmotic injuries involving the thick ligaments connecting the tibia and fibula are often referred to as "high" ankle sprains; they require more time to heal (5 to 10 weeks) and are more likely to require surgical stabilization. Sprains of the deltoid ligament on the medial aspect of the ankle are far less common than lateral ankle sprains, accounting for approximately 10% of ankle sprains. These occur during forceful and sudden ankle eversion and are associated with a fracture the majority of the time, usually in the distal fibula or medial malleolus.

Ankle injuries are graded from simple distortion or partial tear in the ligament with no instability (grade 1) to partial or complete tear of the ligament with instability (grades 2 and 3, respectively). Accurate diagnosis can be difficult immediately after an injury because of the presence of diffuse pain and swelling. Grading the degree of ligament damage with the physical examination is sometimes more reliable a few days after the injury. The combination of pain over the anterior talofibular ligament, hematoma discoloration, and a positive anterior drawer test has a sensitivity of 96% and specificity of 84% for diagnosing a grade 2 or grade 3 sprain (Videos 36-9 and 36-10).[12] A positive squeeze test (Video 36-11) (compressing the tibia and fibula at midcalf) and external rotation test (externally rotating the dorsiflexed foot) are suggestive of a syndesmotic injury. When tenderness is present over the distal fibula, ankle joint, syndesmosis, base of the fifth metatarsal, or other bony structures, radiographs should be obtained to rule out fracture. Avulsion fractures of the

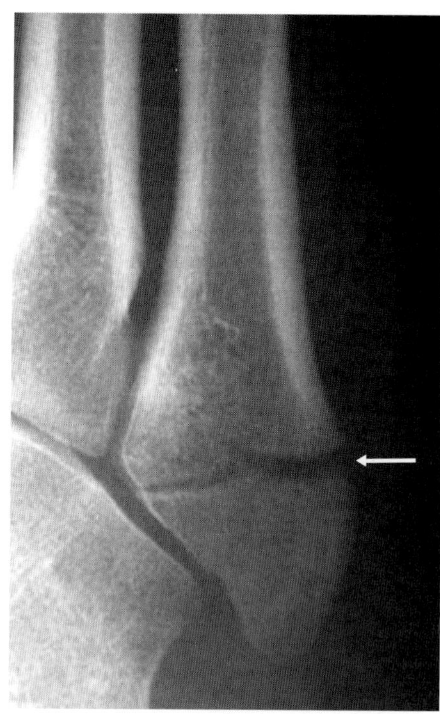

FIGURE 36-25 Anteroposterior radiograph of the foot, showing a minimally displaced avulsion fracture of the base of the fifth metatarsal (*arrow*). The patient was a division I cross-country runner who sustained an inversion ankle sprain during a race. This injury is usually treated nonoperatively with short-term immobilization and progressive ankle rehabilitation.

base of the fifth metatarsal can occur from the pull of peroneus brevis (Figure 36-25). If nondisplaced or mildly displaced, these fractures can usually be treated nonoperatively with use of an orthopedic shoe for 1 to 2 weeks or until pain subsides. Greater displacement of the avulsion fragment might require screw or pin fixation.

Acute treatment includes icing and compressive wrapping of the ankle. Icing and elevation can help minimize swelling, and early mobilization and use of a brace for support can be helpful initially. Crutches are used only when pain precludes full weight-bearing. Sensorimotor control is reduced in persons with persistent instability complaints after injury. Balance and proprioceptive training improves sensorimotor control and can reduce the risk of future injury. As a patient progresses in therapy, dynamic strengthening and sport-specific functional drills should be incorporated into the exercise program. Functional tests to determine readiness to return to activity include "shuttle runs" and single-leg hopping. In returning to sport, taping or bracing have been shown in some studies to be helpful in reducing the risk of recurrent ankle sprains. These effects are probably as a result of mechanical restriction as well as neuromuscular and sensory mechanisms. Bracing is often favored over taping because it better restricts ankle motion without affecting performance, it retains its restrictive property longer, and it is more cost-effective in the long term. Medial ankle sprains and syndesmotic injuries require longer healing times than lateral sprains. A walking boot can be used during the course of healing for stable injuries. Approximately one third of patients have mild to moderate residual pain with activity.

In cases of a complete syndesmotic injury, screw fixation is indicated. Most other ankle injuries heal without complication. With a functional rehabilitation program, the patient can return to full activity within a few days to weeks, depending on the severity of the sprain. Residual symptoms are more likely if the rehabilitation is incomplete. It has been reported that up to 40% of ankle sprains lead to persistent problems with pain and instability.[14] Occult injuries must be suspected in these individuals. The most commonly overlooked injuries include fractures (talus or anterior process of calcaneus), osteochondral lesions, injuries to the subtalar joint or syndesmosis, peroneal tendinopathy or rupture, proprioceptive deficit, and impingement syndrome. Pain is the most common cause of subjective or "functional" instability. In these patients, physiologic range is not exceeded on examination. A few of the common causes include peroneal muscle weakness, proprioceptive deficit, and subtalar instability. If pain is not present between episodes of instability, there might be true mechanical instability. These patients have ankle mobility beyond the physiologic range of motion, with abnormal laxity on examination. Studies have shown that balance exercises and peroneal strengthening can restore functional stability to even the mechanically unstable ankle. Surgery can be indicated after failure of an extended period (6 months or so) of appropriate aggressive ankle strength and stability treatment in patients with symptomatic mechanical instability.

Osteochondral Lesions of the Ankle

The talus ranks third in location after the knee and elbow for osteochondral lesions. Osteochondral lesions occur in approximately 6.5% of all ankle sprains and there is a history of trauma in approximately 80% of these cases.[49] Patients present with deep ankle pain that is worse with weight bearing and improved with rest. Tenderness can sometimes be elicited with palpation in the region of the subtalar joint and with subtalar joint play maneuvers. MRI is more sensitive than plain films for visualizing the lesion and assessing soft tissue structures (Figure 36-26). Osteochondral lesions can affect the medial or lateral talus. Medial lesions usually occur following a compressive force with an inversion-flexion movement. Medial lesions are less commonly related to acute trauma, tend to be less severe, and are more likely to undergo spontaneous healing. Lateral talus osteochondral lesions often occur following forced eversion and dorsiflexion. Symptoms are more pronounced and self-healing occurs less frequently. Osteoarthritic changes may develop earlier in these patients. Nonoperative treatment of symptomatic osteochondral lesions of the talus fails in 30% to 40% of patients. Generally, stage 1 disease is treated nonoperatively. Stage 4 is treated operatively. Stages 2 and 3 are treated conservatively on the medial side and surgically on the lateral side.[49]

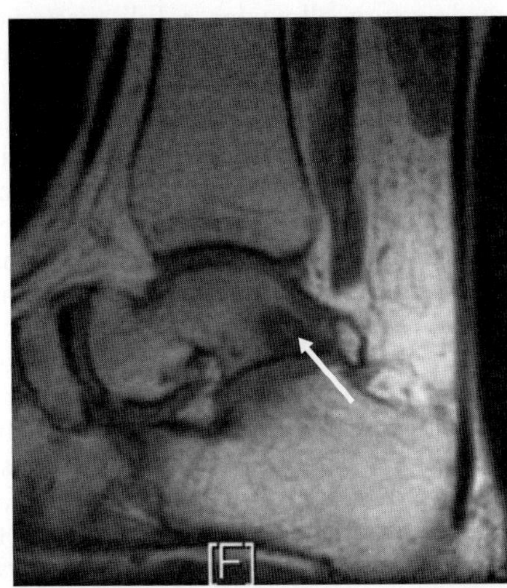

FIGURE 36-26 Sagittal T1-weighted magnetic resonance imaging of the ankle, showing a large osteochondral lesion (*arrow*) in the inferior posterior talus.

Miscellaneous Disorders of the Ankle and Foot

Several miscellaneous disorders of the ankle and foot deserve mention. Tarsal coalition involves the bridging of two or more tarsal bones. It can occur in three types: fibrous, cartilaginous, or osseous. It occurs in less than 1% of the population and is oftentimes bilateral. It can present in children or adolescents with a painful flat foot. The union in children is thought to be mobile and fibrous and may become more symptomatic as the union becomes cartilaginous or osseous. The two most common types are calcaneonavicular and talocalcaneal. Less common are calcaneocuboid, talonavicular, and cuboideonavicular. Treatment may be conservative with nonsteroidal antiinflammatories, steroid injections, orthotics, and physical therapy for strengthening and mobilization. Surgical treatment consists of interposing fat, tendon, or muscle at the coalition site.

Os trigonum involves an ossicle arising from the posterior talar process that is present in approximately 10% of the population. In athletes who perform frequent and forceful plantar flexion, this can become a source of pain. Resolution of symptoms occurs in most cases with relative rest and NSAIDs. Surgical excision may be required for failure with conservative management.

Lisfranc ligament injury is an injury to the tarsometatarsal joint. This is most often seen with high energy trauma but can be seen in athletes with lower energy mechanisms. The second metatarsal is connected to the medial cuneiform by the strong Lisfranc ligament. If there is no instability (diastasis), non–weight bearing with a cast for 6 weeks is appropriate. Displaced or unstable injuries are treated with stabilization with screws or percutaneous wires.

Morton Interdigital Neuroma, Metatarsalgia, and Sesamoiditis

Although distinct clinical entities, these conditions are reviewed jointly because they have similar presentations. Morton neuroma is caused by irritation of one of the interdigital nerves of the foot as it passes below the transverse ligament of the metatarsal heads. The most common location for an interdigital neuroma is between the third and fourth metatarsal heads, but it can also occur between the other metatarsal heads. Symptoms usually start insidiously. The patient typically presents with pain in the region of the metatarsal heads. There can be referral of pain or paresthesias into the two toes innervated by the interdigital nerve in question. Patients sometimes describe a sensation of having a pebble in their shoe or a wrinkle in their sock. Pain is exacerbated with forefoot weight bearing, narrow toe boxes, and high heels, all of which can load the region of the metatarsal heads and interdigital nerves. If there are no neurologic symptoms referred to the toes, the challenge of the physical examination is to distinguish between pain coming from between two metatarsal heads versus pain coming from the metatarsal heads themselves, which would be more consistent with metatarsalgia. Occasionally, the examiner appreciates a click when palpating a larger or firmer neuroma, especially when palpation is combined with squeezing the metatarsal heads together from the medial and lateral sides. Metatarsalgia, as its name implies, is pain coming from the metatarsal heads. Jumping, toe running, and high heels can all cause overload of the metatarsal heads, just as they can cause entrapment or irritation of the interdigital nerve beneath the transverse metatarsal ligament. The second metatarsal head is the most commonly involved.

When the pain is in the region of the first metatarsal head, the differential diagnosis includes injury to the sesamoid bones in the flexor hallucis tendon, such as stress response or stress fracture. Pain coming from an injured sesamoid bone is sometimes referred to as sesamoiditis. Distinguishing between metatarsalgia, sesamoid stress response, and sesamoid fracture can be clinically challenging. A bipartite sesamoid seen on plain films can be a normal variant, and advanced imaging with MRI or bone scan might be required to diagnose a fracture of the sesamoid.

For interdigital neuromas, metatarsalgia, and sesamoiditis, first-line interventions aim to unload the forefoot. Avoiding high heels is recommended. Shoes that have larger toe boxes can also be helpful. Gel inserts are effective at distributing forces more evenly. Custom-made foot orthoses with premetatarsal pads, or simply with premetatarsal pads alone, can transfer forces from the region of the metatarsal heads to slightly more proximal and therefore unload the painful area. Local injection with anesthetic and steroid is often useful both diagnostically and therapeutically for interdigital neuroma. There is no role for injections for metatarsalgia. For recalcitrant neuroma symptoms that are unresponsive to these measures, surgical excision can be considered, with the understanding that recurrence can occur.

Apophysitis of the fifth metatarsal base, or Iselin disease, is an overuse osteochondrosis seen in growing children. Although amenable to treatment, it is a self-limiting disorder, disappearing spontaneously with completion of growth. Osteonecrosis of the foot includes Freiberg disease and Kohler disease. Freiberg disease affects the metatarsal heads (most commonly the second metatarsal). Its typical presentation is an adolescent who presents with forefoot pain. Radiographic findings may include flattening of the metatarsal head and fragmentation of growth plates. MRI may be necessary. If caught early, conservative treatment with relative rest, metatarsal padding, and orthotics may be successful. Later stages may require surgical referral. Kohler disease affects the tarsal navicular and is usually seen in young boys who may present with a limp and pain over the navicular. They often walk on the outside of the foot to avoid pressure over the arch. Radiographs may show fragmentation of the navicular. Treatment is symptomatic with a cast or walking boot. Most children grow out of the condition within a year.

Turf Toe

Sudden and forceful hyperextension (or less commonly hyperflexion) of the first metatarsophalangeal joint can cause a sprain of the joint capsule and ligaments, with subsequent swelling and pain. The incidence of this injury has increased since the advent of artificial turf. Radiographs should be obtained to exclude fracture. Initial treatment consists of ice and stiff-soled shoes to protect the joint. Although many of these injuries resolve within 3 to 4 weeks, some can result in functional limitations for a much greater period of time.

Bone Injuries of the Lower Limb

A comprehensive discussion of acute fractures of the lower limbs is beyond the scope of this chapter. Many acute fractures of the lower limb can be successfully treated without surgical intervention. Examples include nondisplaced pubic rami fractures, pelvic avulsion fractures, many nondisplaced or minimally fibular fractures, and nondisplaced or minimally displaced foot fractures. The most important take home point for the nonsurgeon who is treating fractures is to consult with orthopedic colleagues frequently to make sure that a surgical injury is not being undertreated. The final section of this chapter focuses on the spectrum of repetitive overload injuries of the bones of the lower limb.

Stress Reactions and Stress Fractures

Injuries to bone can be caused by acute trauma, chronic repetitive overload, metabolic disorders, and neoplasm. Although a musculoskeletal physician must be able to recognize and appropriately treat or triage any of these conditions, space does not allow for a full discussion of all disorders of bone. This section focuses on repetitive overload injuries to the bones of the lower limb.

These types of injury are common in individuals who are physically active, especially those who participate in endurance activities such as distance running. In cases of repetitive stress, or in the setting of impaired bone metabolism, bone strain occurs on a continuum from "stress response" or "stress reaction" to overt stress fracture. Bone overload can occur in any location in the lower limb (Figure 36-27, *A, B, C, D*). The ability of bone to withstand repetitive forces without breaking down depends on several factors. The stronger the bone is before being subjected to repetitive loading, the better it is able to withstand the loads applied to it. Both intrinsic and extrinsic factors are important to consider in determining the risk for stress reactions or stress fractures. Intrinsic risk factors include poor dietary habits, altered menstrual status, and biomechanical abnormalities that do not allow for proper distribution of forces along the kinetic chain. Extrinsic factors

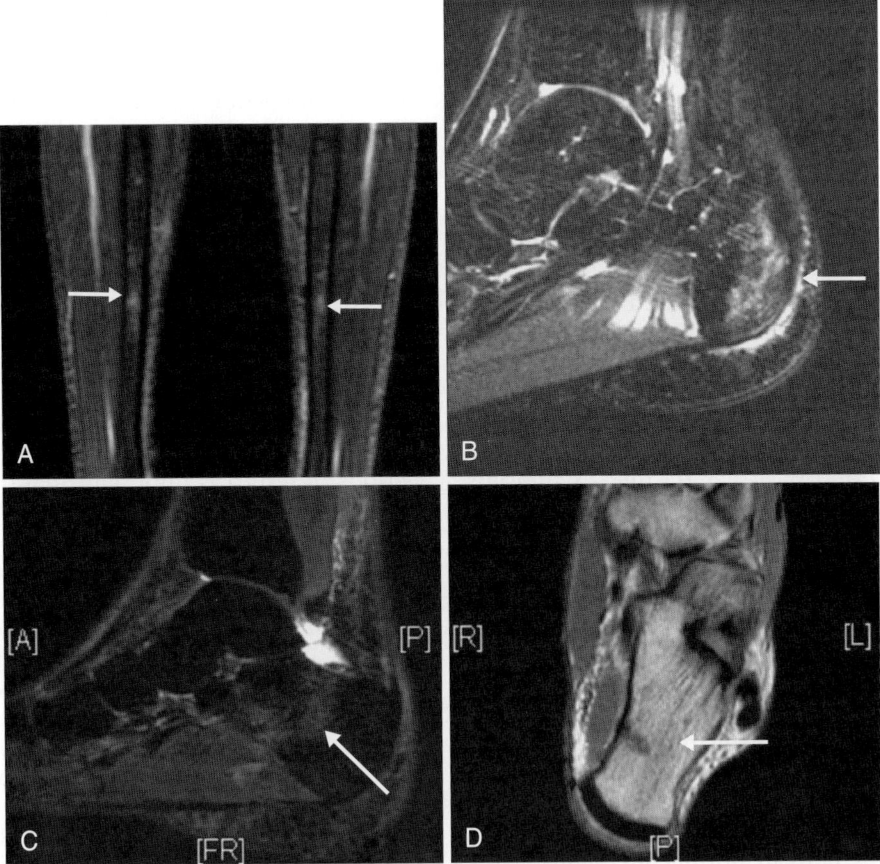

FIGURE 36-27 Examples of stress responses and stress fractures. **A,** T2-weighted, fat suppression, coronal magnetic resonance imaging (MRI) of the legs shows increased signal in the medullary cavity of both tibiae (*arrows*), consistent with stress response or stress reaction. There is no discrete line indicative of a stress fracture. The patient was a division I cross-country runner with oligomenorrhea and disordered eating. **B,** T2-weighted, fat suppression MRI of the foot, showing increased signal in the calcaneus (*arrow*), consistent with a stress response. The patient was an Olympic freestyle skiing aerialist who had bilateral heel pain. The contralateral heel MRI had a similar appearance. T2-weighted, fat suppression, sagittal **(C)** (*arrow*) and T1-weighted, axial **(D)** magnetic resonance images showing a calcaneal stress fracture (*arrow*). The patient was a 29-year-old ultramarathoner.

can include training surface type, training errors, footwear, and insoles.

Athletes report a greater frequency of disordered eating patterns than the general population, especially in sports emphasizing leanness. Individuals with disordered eating can have insufficient dietary intake of calories, protein, calcium, and other nutrients to achieve optimal bone quality. The triad of disordered eating, amenorrhea, and osteopenia that occurs in athletic females has been referred to as the female athlete triad. Restrictive eating behaviors increase the likelihood of stress fractures in women.[6] Low caloric intake with negative protein balance has been hypothesized as one of the mechanisms for menstrual disturbances in female athletes.[56] There is evidence that menstrual and hormonal disturbances increase the risk of stress fracture and lead to premature bone loss, particularly at trabecular sites.[33]

Skeletal alignment affects the amount of force absorbed by the foot, and how much force is transferred to proximal structures during ground contact. A rigid pes cavus foot is less able to absorb shock during and just after heel strike, and can therefore transmit greater forces to proximal bones than a foot that is able to undergo normal pronation. Similarly, a pes planus foot does not allow the normal pronation mechanism to properly absorb forces. Either foot alignment can increase the risk of a stress fracture, the location of which can vary depending on the foot type and activity.[42] Other studies looking at alignment have suggested that leg length discrepancy and increased Q angle can increase the risk of stress fracture.[9]

Although it is clear that training errors contribute to stress fractures, there is limited research identifying the contribution of various training components. Furthermore, appropriate training regimens vary greatly among individuals. Athletes should be encouraged to keep training logs documenting type of training, volume, intensity, and rest periods. A rapid increase in training volume and intensity often precedes a stress fracture, just as it might precede a muscle-tendon overload injury. Articles about training in military situations have shown that elimination of running and marching on concrete, preentry physical conditioning, and inclusion of rest periods were thought to reduce stress fracture risk.[40]

Shoes and insoles can be an important component in minimizing stress fracture risk. Proper shoe fit that matches an individual's foot type, as well as adequate support and shock absorption, are essential. Studies looking at the effect of insoles or other footwear modifications on the prevention of stress fractures have shown a reduction in the number of stress fractures by greater than 50%.[16] Adequate support with good cushioning and replacing shoes every 300 to 500 miles has been a recommendation over the years. This is an interesting topic with the current trend of minimalist shoewear in running. Some maintain by altering one's running gait (reducing heel strike), it may lead to fewer injuries. It begs the question whether hindfoot injuries may be reduced at the expense of forefoot injuries or fractures in these runners.

The patient presenting with a suspected stress fracture usually provides a history of a recent acceleration in the intensity or duration of training before the onset of symptoms. The patient most frequently complains of insidious onset of focal pain that is exacerbated with weight-bearing activities. In cases of certain stress fractures, such as femoral neck and navicular fractures, symptoms can be vague, thus increasing the time to diagnosis. The differential diagnosis usually includes tendinopathy, enthesopathy, and CECS.

Imaging studies are not always necessary. A 6-week period of relative rest with nonimpact rehabilitation and alternative training methods such as pool running can be instituted. Imaging can be reserved for individuals who remain symptomatic and are unable to return to full activities. In these cases, or when complete diagnosis is required sooner, the initial imaging study of choice is radiographs. It should be kept in mind, however, that plain films are relatively insensitive and detect less than 50% of stress fractures.[28] When radiographs are normal but the suspicion for stress fracture remains high, advanced imaging studies are appropriate. Bone scans are sensitive for detecting stress fractures but lack anatomic definition. They can also remain positive long after symptoms have resolved. This limits the ability of bone scans to aid in return to sport decisions. MRI provides excellent anatomic information, and can be more useful in grading lesions and assessing soft tissue structures. CT provides optimal definition of bony architecture.

Multiple factors influence the length of time required to safely return to full activities following a stress fracture. These include duration of symptoms, stage of stress reaction, site of stress fracture, and level of activity or competition. Most stress fractures heal without complication with activity modification and allow gradual return to sports in 4 to 8 weeks. There are a few high-risk stress fractures, however, that require more aggressive treatment (these are discussed later).

Initial treatment includes pain management, activity modification, strengthening, fitness maintenance, and risk factor modification. Once healing is well underway and pain is minimum, the gradual resumption of the impact-loading phase of rehabilitation begins.

Pain can be a problem mainly during weight bearing with lower extremity stress fractures. It might be appropriate to minimize weight bearing for the first 7 to 10 days. Modalities such as ice can also be helpful. Analgesics such as acetaminophen are appropriate. There is some debate about the use of NSAIDs after a stress fracture. On a theoretical basis at least, the mode of action of these medications might prevent optimal repair of the stress fracture, with reduction in the bone-remodeling process.

Activity modification includes eliminating impact activities for a period of time until daily ambulation is pain-free. During this time, it is important to continue muscle strengthening and cross-training to keep the cardiopulmonary system fit.

Reduced muscle size and strength have been shown to predispose to stress fractures.[20] In endurance events, muscle fatigue can increase the strain on bone.[55] Muscle mass is important to build and maintain because the load placed on bone can be reduced at sites when muscles are better able to absorb repetitive impact.[39] A strengthening program should therefore begin immediately after a diagnosis of stress fracture is made. The exercises prescribed should not cause pain at the fracture site.

Inactivity has negative impacts on the cardiovascular system, metabolism, and skeletal muscle after even brief periods of rest. It is important that the physician and the patient understand that fitness should be maintained in ways that avoid overloading the bone. The most common cross-training activities include cycling, swimming, water running, rowing, and StairMaster. The more sport-specific the cross-training is, the better the carryover effect of the training. It is for this reason that deep water running has become so popular among runners with stress fractures. Studies have shown no significant differences in maximal oxygen uptake, anaerobic threshold, running economy, stride length, and 2-mile performance after 4 to 8 weeks of land versus deep water running training.[53] In sports requiring specific skills, the neuromuscular adaptations are not easily duplicated with cross-training, and it is important to find appropriate ways to resume these isolated sport-specific skills as soon as possible.

When walking is pain-free, the graduated impact phase of rehabilitation should progress on an individualized basis according to fracture site and symptoms. A progressive increase in load is necessary to allow bone to adapt with increases in strength. Resumption of activity should not be accompanied by pain, but it is not uncommon to have some mild discomfort at the fracture site. If bony pain occurs, then activity should be stopped for 1 to 2 days. When the individual is pain-free while walking, the activity is resumed at a level prior to where symptoms occurred. When training resumes, it is important to allow adequate recovery time after hard sessions or hard weeks of training. Progress should be monitored clinically by the presence or absence of symptoms and local signs. It is not necessary to monitor progress by imaging studies. Radiologic healing lags behind clinical healing.

Although most stress fractures heal without incident with the treatment strategies mentioned earlier, there are particular stress fractures that tend to develop complications and therefore require specific treatment. These include femoral neck, anterior cortex of the middle third of the tibia, navicular, and proximal fifth metatarsal fractures.

In femoral neck stress fractures, symptoms are often vague, and one should have a high index of suspicion to catch this diagnosis early and avoid complications such as displacement or avascular necrosis. If suspicion is present, an MRI should be obtained (Figure 36-28). Fractures on the tension side (lateral) are less common and require immediate surgical referral. Fractures on the compression

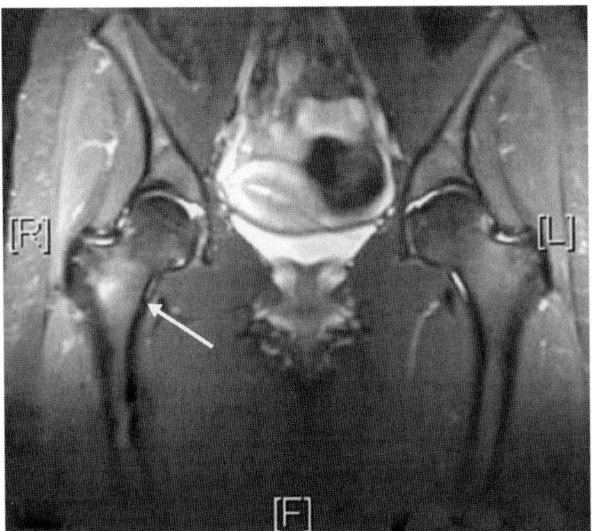

FIGURE 36-28 T2-weighted, fat suppression, coronal magnetic resonance imaging of the pelvis, showing increased signal in the right femoral neck (*arrow*), consistent with stress fracture. The patient was an elite cross-country ski racer who had onset of symptoms after "bounding" exercises, which involve running uphill on one leg.

side (medial) are more common. If the fracture line extends greater than 50% of the width of the femoral neck, percutaneous fixation should be considered because the likelihood of displacement is higher.[41] When the fracture line is less than 50% of the width of the femoral neck, strict non–weight-bearing status is necessary for approximately 4 to 6 weeks until the patient is pain-free. This should be followed by functional rehabilitation with progressive weight bearing over the next 4 to 8 weeks according to symptoms. If the athlete is not progressing as expected, additional radiologic evaluation should be considered.

Navicular fractures have a higher likelihood of delayed union, nonunion, or avascular necrosis. There is evidence that continued weight bearing on a tarsal navicular fracture is associated with a 74% failure rate of healing.[23] Therefore, early diagnosis and treatment are important. Radiographs are often normal, and an MRI or bone scan can confirm the diagnosis. If positive, a CT scan is often the most appropriate study to optimally visualize the bone. Navicular fractures involving a cortical break at the dorsal aspect of the navicular alone have the best prognosis, typically healing by 3 months. With propagation of the fracture into the navicular body, healing time is slightly longer. Initial management of these fractures consists of non–weight-bearing, with boot immobilization for 6 to 8 weeks. If symptoms persist, one should consider use of a bone stimulator or surgical fixation.[18] Navicular fractures that propagate across the body and involve another cortex have a significantly higher risk of complication, and early surgical intervention should be considered.[38]

The "dreaded black line" is a tension-type stress fracture of the anterior cortex of the middle third of the tibia. These fractures are well known for their progression to nonunion or complete fracture. With continued activity, the risk of complete fracture is 60%.[5] Even with appropriate activity modification for 9 to 12 months, nonsurgical treatment fails in 25% to 60% of cases.[4] Initial treatment may consist

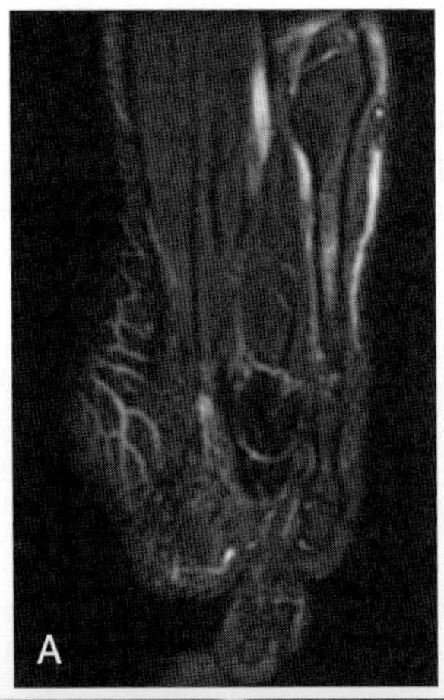

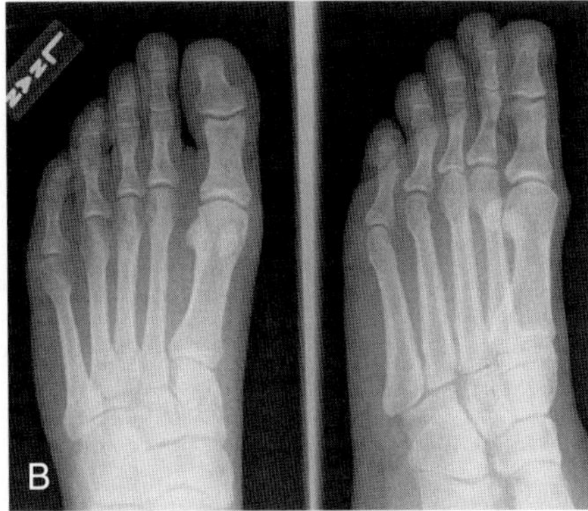

FIGURE 36-29 **A,** T2-weighted, short inversion time–inversion recovery, fat suppression, axial magnetic resonance imaging of the foot, showing increased signal in the fifth metatarsal consistent with stress fracture. **B,** No lesion in the bone was appreciated on the initial radiographs.

of activity modification and pneumatic leg splints. Intramedullary fixation, however, can also be considered as an appropriate initial treatment.

Stress fractures of the fifth metatarsal are prone to nonunion and refracture (Figure 36-29, *A, B*). Early stress fractures (bony edema only) are typically treated with non–weight-bearing immobilization for 6 weeks, followed by 6 weeks of protected weight bearing. If healing still has not occurred, surgical fixation is appropriate. Surgery is usually considered as first-line treatment in cases where a clear fracture line is present or in elite athletes.

Stress fractures of the lower limbs are common and should be recognized and treated early to maximize successful outcome. Although most individuals go on to heal with an appropriate functional rehabilitation program, there is a subset of fractures that are at high risk of complications and need to be identified early and managed appropriately.

Summary

Having a sound understanding of anatomy and kinetic chain biomechanics, in conjunction with fundamental history and physical examination skills, permits a practitioner to establish appropriate diagnoses for patients presenting with soft tissue, bone, and joint disorders of the lower limbs. Ancillary testing, such as imaging studies, can help confirm or disprove clinical diagnoses and establish the severity of injury. The majority of lower limb injuries can be successfully treated with nonoperative measures that include medications, activity modification, and intelligent exercise strategies. The practitioner should be able to recognize injuries that require surgical consultation.

REFERENCES

1. Aaron DL, Patel A, Kayiaros S, et al: Four common types of bursitis: diagnosis and management, *J Am Acad Orthop Surg* 19:359–367, 2011.
2. Abate M, Pelotti P, De Amicis D, et al: Viscosupplementation with hyaluronic acid in hip osteoarthritis (a review), *Ups J Med Sci* 113:261–277, 2008.
3. Alfredson H, Pietila T, Jonsson P, et al: Heavy-load eccentric calf muscle training for the treatment of chronic Achilles tendinosis, *Am J Sports Med* 26:360–366, 1998.
4. Batt ME, Kemp S, Kerslake R: Delayed union stress fractures of the anterior tibia: conservative management, *Br J Sports Med* 35:74–77, 2001.
5. Beals RK, Cook RD: Stress fractures of the anterior tibial diaphysis, *Orthopedics* 14:869–875, 1991.
6. Bennell KL, Malcolm SA, Thomas SA, et al: Risk factors for stress fractures in track and field athletes: a 12-month prospective study, *Am J Sports Med* 24:810–818, 1996.
7. Boegart T, Jonsson K: Radiography in osteoarthritis of the knee, *Skeletal Radiol* 28:605–615, 1999.
8. Cawley PW, France E, Paulos LE: The current state of functional knee bracing research. A review of the literature, *Am J Sports Med* 19:226–233, 1991.
9. Cowan DN, Jones BH, Frykman PN, et al: Lower limb morphology and risk of overuse injury among male infantry trainees, *Med Sci Sports Exerc* 28:945–952, 1996.
10. Crawford DC, Safran MR: Osteochondritis dissecans of the knee, *J Am Acad Orthop Surg* 14:90–100, 2006.
11. Croisier J, Forthomme B, Namurois MH, et al: Hamstring muscle strain recurrence and strength performance disorders, *Am J Sports Med* 30:199–203, 2002.
12. van Dijk CN, Lim LS, Bossuyt PM, Marti RK: Physical examination is sufficient for the diagnosis of sprained ankles, *J Bone Joint Surg Br* 78:958–962, 1996.
13. Fricker PA: Management of groin pain in athletes, *Br J Sports Med* 31:97–101, 1997.
14. Gerber JP, Williams GN, Scoville CR, et al: Persistent disability associated with ankle sprains: a prospective examination of an athletic population, *Foot Ankle Int* 19:653–660, 1998.
15. Gholve PA, Cameron DB, Millis MB: Slipped capital femoral epiphysis update, *Curr Opin Pediatr* 21:39–45, 2009.
16. Gillespie WJ, Grant I: Interventions for preventing and treating stress fractures and stress reactions of bone of the lower limbs in young adults, *Cochrane Database Syst Rev* (2):CD000450, 2000.
17. Groh MM, Herrera J: A comprehensive review of hip labral tears, *Curr Rev Musculoskelet Med* 2:105–117, 2009.
18. Harmon KG: Lower extremity stress fractures, *Clin J Sports Med* 13:358–364, 2003.
19. Hochberg MC, Altman RD, April KT, et al: American College of Rheumatology 2012 recommendations for the use of nonpharmacologic and pharmacologic therapies in osteoarthritis of the hand, hip, and knee, *Arthritis Care Res* 64:465–474, 2012.
20. Hoffman JR, Chapnik L, Shamis A, et al: The effect of leg strength on the incidence of lower extremity overuse injuries during military training, *Mil Med* 164:153–156, 1999.
21. Hunt D, Prather H, Harris Hayes M, et al: Clinical outcomes analysis of conservative and surgical treatment of patients with clinical indications of prearthritic, intra-articular hip disorders, *PM&R* 4:479–487, 2012.
22. Kerachian MA, Seguin C, Harvey EJ: Glucocorticoids in osteonecrosis of the femoral head: a new understanding of the mechanisms of action, *J Steroid Biochem Mol Biol* 114:121–128, 2009.
23. Khan KM, Fuller PJ, Bruckner PD, et al: Outcome of conservative and surgical management of navicular stress fracture in athletes: eighty-six cases proven with computerized tomography, *Am J Sports Med* 20:657–666, 1992.
24. Kibler WB, Goldberg C, Chandler TJ: Functional biomechanical deficits in running athletes with plantar fasciitis, *Am J Sports Med* 19:66–71, 1991.
25. Kim HK: Legg-Calve-Perthes disease, *J Am Acad Orthop Surg* 18:676–686, 2010.
26. Kim HK: Pathophysiology and new strategies for the treatment of Legg-Calve-Perthes disease, *J Bone Joint Surg Am* 94:659–669, 2012.
27. King JB: Post-traumatic ectopic calcification in the muscles of athletes: a review, *Br J Sports Med* 32:287–290, 1998.
28. Kiuru MJ, Pihlajamaki HK, Hietanen HJ, et al: MR imaging, bone scintigraphy, and radiography in bone stress injuries of the pelvis and the lower extremity, *Acta Radiol* 43:207–212, 2002.
29. Lauder TD, Stuart MJ, Amrami KK, et al: Exertional compartment syndrome and the role of magnetic resonance imaging, *Am J Phys Med Rehabil* 81:315–319, 2002.
30. Levy BA, Stuart MJ, Whelan DB: Posterolateral instability of the knee: evaluation, treatment, results, *Sports Med Arthrosc* 18:254–262, 2010.
31. Migliore A, Giovannangeli F, Bizzi E, et al: Viscosupplementation in the management of ankle osteoarthritis: a review, *Arch Orthop Trauma Surg* 131:139–147, 2011.
32. Miller ML: Avulsion fractures of the pelvis, *Am J Sports Med* 13:349–358, 1985.
33. Myburgh KH, Bachrach LK, Lewis B, et al: Low bone mineral density at axial and appendicular sites in amenorrheic athletes, *Med Sci Sports Exerc* 25:1197–1202, 1993.
34. Nam KW, Kim YL, Yoo JJ, et al: Fate of untreated asymptomatic osteonecrosis of the femoral head, *J Bone Joint Surg Am* 90:477–484, 2008.
35. Patterson MJ, Cox WK: Peroneus longus tendon rupture as a cause of chronic lateral ankle pain, *Clin Orthop Relat Res* 365:163–166, 1999.
36. Powers CM: The effects of patellar bracing on clinical changes and gait characteristics in subjects with patellofemoral pain [abstract], *Phys Ther* 30:S48, 1998.
37. Sankar WN, Matheney TH, Zaltz I: Femoroacetabular impingement: current concepts and controversies, *Ortho Clin North Am* 44:575–589, 2013.
38. Saxena A, Fullem B, Hannaford D: Results of treatment of 22 navicular stress fractures and a new proposed radiographic classification system, *J Foot Ankle Surg* 39:96–103, 2000.
39. Scott SH, Winter DA: Internal forces at chronic running injury sites, *Med Sci Sports Exerc* 22:357–369, 1990.
40. Shaffer RA, Brodine SK, Almeida SA, et al: Use of simple measures of physical activity to predict stress fractures in young men undergoing a rigorous physical training program, *Am J Epidemiol* 149:236–242, 1999.
41. Shin AY, Gillingham BL: Fatigue fractures of the femoral neck in athletes, *J Am Acad Orthop Surg* 5:293–302, 1997.
42. Simkin A, Leichter I, Giladi M, et al: Combined effect of foot arch structure and an orthotic device on stress fractures, *Foot Ankle* 10:25–29, 1989.
43. Simonet WT, Saylor HL, III, Sim L: Abdominal wall muscle tears in hockey players, *Int J Sports Med* 20:31–37, 1995.
44. Smith J, Hurdle MF, Weingarten TN: Accuracy of sonographically guided intra-articular injections in the native adult hip, *J Ultrasound Med* 28:329–355, 2009.
45. Steinkamp LA, Dillingham MF, Markel MD: Biomechanical considerations in patellofemoral joint rehabilitation, *Am J Sports Med* 21:438–444, 1993.
46. Styf JR, Korner LM: Chronic anterior-compartment syndrome of the leg: results of treatment by fasciotomy, *J Bone Joint Surg Am* 68A:1338–1347, 1986.
47. Taimela S, Kujalu U, Osterman K: Intrinsic risk factors and athletic injuries, *Sports Med* 9:205, 1990.
48. Tannast M, Siebenrock KA, Anderson SE: Femoroacetabular impingement: radiographic diagnosis—what the radiologist should know, *Am J Roentgenol* 188:1540–1552, 2007.
49. Tol JL, Struijis PA, Bossuyt PM, et al: Treatment strategies in osteochondral defects of the talar dome: a systematic review, *Foot Ankle* 21:119–126, 2000.
50. Tria AJ, editor: *Ligaments of the knee*, New York, 1995, Churchill Livingstone.
51. Verrall GM, Slavotinek JP, Barnes PG, et al: Diagnostic and prognostic value of clinical findings in 83 athletes with posterior thigh injury—comparison of clinical findings with magnetic resonance imaging

documentation of hamstring muscle strain, *Am J Sports Med* 31:969–973, 2003.
52. Weber M, Niemann M, Lanz R, et al: Nonoperative treatment of acute rupture of the Achilles tendon: results of a new protocol and comparison with operative treatment, *Am J Sports Med* 31:685–691, 2003.
53. Wilber RL, Moffatt RJ, Scott BE, et al: Influence of water-run training on running performance [abstract], *Med Sci Sports Exerc* 26:S4, 1994.
54. Yoong P, Guirguis R, Darrah R, et al: Evaluation of ultrasound-guided diagnostic local anaesthetic hip joint injection for osteoarthritis, *Skeletal Radiol* 41:981–985, 2012.
55. Yoshikawa T, Mori S, Santiesteban AJ, et al: The effects of muscle fatigue on bone strain, *J Exp Biol* 188:17–33, 1994.
56. Zanker CL, Swaine IL: Relation between bone turnover, estradiol, and energy balance in women distance runners, *Br J Sports Med* 32:167–171, 1998.

CHAPTER 37

CHRONIC PAIN

Steven P. Stanos, Mark D. Tyburski, R. Norman Harden

There are among us those who haply please to think our business is to treat disease.

And all unknowingly lack this lesson still 'tis not the body, but the man is ill.

S. Weir Mitchell (cited by Schofield 1902)

Historical Overview

Pain Defined

Pain is a subjective and entirely individually personal experience influenced by learning, context, and multiple psychosocial variables.[100] Pain is not merely the end product of peripheral receptor stimulation and afferent signaling, but a complicated dynamic process of neural interplay with the noxious environment along ascending and descending peripheral, spinal cord, and brain networks. The International Association for the Study of Pain (IASP) defines pain as "an unpleasant sensory and emotional experience associated with actual or potential tissue damage, or described in terms of such damage."[102] Pain serves an adaptive function, a warning system designed to protect the organism from harm. With chronicity and neuraxial pathology, however, the nociceptive system can become maladaptive and reflect endogenous pathology instead of an exogenous state.[130] Acute pain is usually a response to a "noxious" event (i.e., a mechanical, thermal, or chemical insult) causing depolarization of the nonspecialized transducers (the nociceptors). It is time-limited, and treatment should be aimed at removing the underlying pathologic process. Concurrent behaviors will be designed to avoid or remove the offending noxious stimulus. In contrast, chronic pain is designated 3 to 6 months after the initiating event and in many cases might not be associated with any obvious ongoing noxious event or pathologic process. Behavior can become pathologic as attempts to avoid the noxious element fail, fight or flight responses escalate to no purpose, and so on. Chronic pain can differ from acute pain conditions in that underlying tissue pathology or injury begins to less directly correlate with levels of pain report. Whereas acute pain can be considered a physiologic response to tissue trauma or damage, chronic pain involves a more dynamic interplay of additional psychological and behavioral mechanisms (Table 37-1).[26] Chronic pain is often associated with disrupted sleep and declining function and eventually can cease to serve any protective role. At this point, pain can become a source of dysfunctional behaviors, suffering, and disability, often completely perplexing to the patient as well as to the unprepared physician.

Environmental and affective factors can contribute to the persistence of pain and subsequent illness behaviors. The individual's subjective response to chronic pain is shaped by the cognitive repertoire involved in attending to and anticipating noxious sensory signals as well as in appraising events associated with those signals (Figure 37-1). Chronic painful conditions, when left untreated, can result in multiple problems, including unnecessary personal suffering for the patient, increased medical care use, overuse or misuse of psychoactive medications, iatrogenic complications secondary to inappropriate surgeries, excess disability, comorbid emotional problems (including increased risk of suicide), and increased economic and social costs. A multidisciplinary approach that addresses psychosocial and biological factors and focuses on functional restoration in all areas of life is *sine qua non.*

The prepared physiatrist can offer a unique perspective and skill set to the assessment and management of chronic pain and the psychosocial sequelae. The rehabilitative interdisciplinary team approach, a model for the treatment of other chronic disability conditions (e.g., spinal cord injury, stroke-related disorders, and amputee-related conditions), is focused on maximizing independent physical function, improving psychosocial state, and returning patients to work and previous leisure pursuits, as well as maximizing patients' reintegration into the community and subsequent improvement of general quality of life. To achieve these ambitious goals, as well as adding the goal of decreasing the pain to tolerable levels, the physiatrist must thoroughly understand and appreciate the biological, psychological, and socioeconomic implications of pain and pain-related disability. A list of pain terminology and definitions is included for review (Table 37-2).

This chapter offers the foundation for comprehensive pain management skills; a review of historical aspects that shaped the field of pain management and research; a review of our current understanding of both physiologic and pathophysiologic mechanisms of pain, the impact of psychosocial factors on the experience of pain, and their role in pain assessment and treatment; and a review of multidisciplinary treatment options that pertain to various chronic pain conditions. A multidisciplinary approach will be proposed as unequivocally the best model for successful and comprehensive chronic pain management.

Prevalence

Chronic pain and related suffering and disability represent an accelerating public health concern with considerable impact on the U.S. economy. Prevalence rates of chronic pain vary widely, from 2% to 55% in general population

Table 37-1 Basic Differentiation of Major Temporal Pain Classifications

Characteristic	Acute	Subchronic	Chronic
Duration	Seconds	Hours to days	Months to years
Temporal features	Instantaneous and simultaneous to cause	Resolves on recovery	Persistent, long-term disease; may exceed resolution of tissue damage
Major characteristics	Proportional to cause	Primary and secondary hyperalgesia, allodynia, spontaneous pain	Subchronic characteristics plus paresthesias, dysesthesias, pronounced affective component
Class	Nociceptive	Principally nociceptive, neuropathic	Principally neuropathic, nociceptive
Source of pain	Transient nociceptive activation	Peripheral and central mechanisms	Peripheral and central mechanisms
Adaptive value	High, preventive	Protective, recovery	None, maladaptive
Adaptive response	Withdrawal, escape	Quiescence, avoidance of contact with injured tissue	Cognitive behavioral, catastrophizing, pain-related anxiety and fear, helplessness
Examples	Contact with hot surface	Inflamed wound	Chronic low back pain, muscle pain syndromes

From Millan MJ: The induction of pain: an integrative review, *Prog Neurobiol* 57:1-164, 1999, with permission.

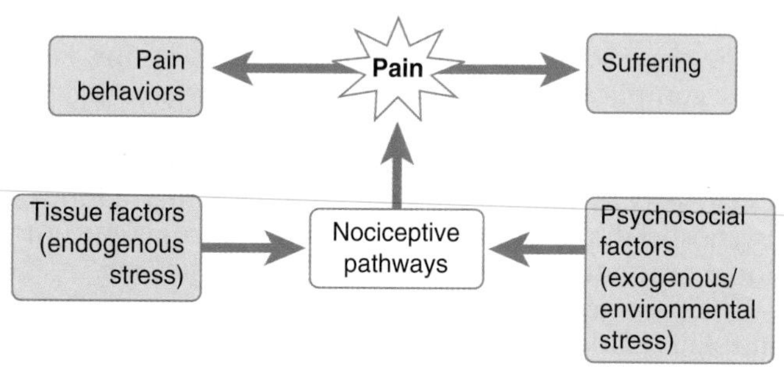

FIGURE 37-1 Processes of chronic pain. (Modified from Kidd BL, Urban LA: Mechanisms of inflammatory pain, *Br J Anaesth* 87:3-11, 2001, with permission.)

studies,[154] and many pain-related conditions (i.e., osteoarthritis and spine-related conditions) accounting for a large proportion of reported pain and correlate with a high concurrent risk for disability.

Reviews of chronic pain as a secondary problem in patients with a primary disability, such as spinal cord injury, amputation, cerebral palsy, and multiple sclerosis, have demonstrated even higher prevalence rates of intolerable pain (greater than 70%), which can substantially add to disability. Pain associated with rehabilitation diagnoses is often reported in multiple sites, not just the focal site of the primary injury,[39] and can contribute to a more generalized loss of function and related disability.

Cost of Chronic Pain

The progression from acute to chronic pain inevitably includes a greater impact in related psychological and social functioning. Chronic pain-related impairment and disability have significant socioeconomic consequences as a result of high health care costs, lost wages and productivity, and the growing costs of disability benefits and other compensation.[152] Chronic pain is responsible for 90 million physician visits, 14% of all prescriptions, and 50 million lost workdays per year.[12] Stewart et al.[140] found that 75% of pain-related productivity loss was on the job, not a result of absence from work.

Early History of Pain Theory: A Peripheral Perspective

The development of pain medicine as a more formal science has been closely related to advancements in pain theory. Understanding historical factors related to the works of scientists and physicians can help the clinician better understand the complexities of the multidimensional experience of pain and suffering. The following is an overview of key factors related to pain theory, beginning with specificity theory up through and including contemporary theories.

The dualistic or mind-body controversy started with the biomedical theories of René Descartes (1596-1650) and can be seen as a precursor to specificity theory. He likened the pain system to a bell-ringing mechanism. The individual on the ground pulls the rope, ringing the bell in the tower. Similarly, placing the foot next to a burning flame would set particles in the foot in motion, traveling up the leg, back, and to the head, causing activation of pain. This theory, traditionally ascribed to Descartes, actually has earlier antecedents of Galen, based on the central position of the pineal gland, the center of the soul, and the sensory motor system.[98]

The specificity theory remained somewhat unchallenged until the nineteenth century, with the emergence of physiology as a more formal scientific field of study. Claude Bernard (1813-1878) was the first to publish observations about the relationship of the autonomic nervous system to pain, and one of his students, the American Civil War surgeon Silas Weir Mitchell, would go on to elucidate what he called *causalgia* (now called complex regional pain syndrome type 2). The qualities of pain experience were thought to be associated with properties of sensory nerves. Johannes Müller was the first to elaborate on more specific neural pathways for pain in his theory of *specific nerve energies* (1842) as well as a distinction of four major cutaneous modalities (i.e., touch, warmth, cold, and pain), each with its own projection system to the brain.[98]

With the evolution of the microscope, Max von Frey proposed the presence of cutaneous sensitivity maps on the skin, and although later disproved, described specific pain receptors. Today, his legacy includes von Frey

Table 37-2 Terminology Used in the Discussion of Pain

Term	Definition
Addiction	A chronic biopsychosocial disease characterized by impaired control over drug use, compulsive use, continued use despite harm, and craving
Allodynia	Pain caused by a stimulus that does not normally provoke pain
Analgesia	Absence of pain in response to stimulation that would normally be painful
Central pain	Pain initiated or caused by a primary lesion or dysfunction in the central nervous system
Dependence	A maladaptive pattern of drug use marked by tolerance and a drug class–specific withdrawal syndrome that can be produced by abrupt cessation, rapid dose reduction, decreasing blood levels of drug, or administration of an antagonist
Dysesthesia	An unpleasant abnormal sensation, whether spontaneous or evoked
Hyperalgesia	An increased response to a stimulus that is normally painful
Hyperesthesia	Increased sensitivity to stimulation, excluding the special senses
Neurogenic pain	Pain initiated or caused by a primary lesion, dysfunction, or transitory perturbation in the peripheral or central nervous system
Neuropathic pain	Pain initiated or caused by a primary lesion or dysfunction in the nervous system*
Nociception	A receptor preferentially sensitive to a noxious stimulus that would become noxious if prolonged
Noxious stimulus	A noxious stimulus is one that is damaging to normal tissues
Pain	An unpleasant sensory and emotional experience associated with actual or potential tissue damage
Paresthesia	An abnormal sensation, whether spontaneous or evoked, that is not unpleasant
Peripheral neurogenic pain	Pain initiated or caused by a primary lesion, dysfunction, or transitory perturbation in the peripheral nervous system
Peripheral neuropathic pain	Pain initiated or caused by a primary lesion or dysfunction in the peripheral nervous system
Psychogenic pain	Pain not caused by an identifiable, somatic origin and that may reflect psychological factors
Tolerance	A state of adaptation in which exposure to a drug induces changes that result in diminution of one or more of the effects of the drug over time

From Merskey H, Bogduk N: *IASP Task Force on Taxonomy classification of chronic pain: description of chronic pain syndromes and definition of pain terms*, Seattle, 1994, IASP Press, with permission.

*See also neurogenic pain and central pain. Peripheral neuropathic pain occurs when the lesion or dysfunction affects the peripheral nervous system. Central pain may be retained as the term when the lesion or dysfunction affects the central nervous system.

filaments and von Frey hairs, important bedside sensory testing modalities.

In the 1870s, in a movement away from specificity theories, Erb proposed the intensive (summation) theory, in which individual sensory transducers were capable of producing pain only if the stimulus reached a sufficient intensity.[14] Goldscheider later (1894) refined the stimulus intensity and summation theories and proposed the pattern theory. In pattern theory, pain results after total output at the cellular level reaches a critical level, either by stimulation by nonnoxious stimuli or by pathologic conditions that enhance summation. The theory centered on the contention that all nerve fibers are alike, and that pain is produced by spatiotemporal patterns of neuronal impulses versus activity on "specific" nerve fibers.

Central Theories of Pain

Until the late 1800s, pain theory was based primarily on peripheral mechanisms and failed to explain persistent pain states. The work of William Livingston with injured soldiers in World War II, and later in chronic work-related injuries, suggested that some portion of chronic pain mechanisms might be related to more specific central nervous system dysfunction.[81] The summation theory by Livingston stated that pathologic stimulation of sensory nerves after nerve injury could lead to reverberating circuits in neuron pools of the spinal cord, which could later be triggered by peripheral nonnoxious inputs. This volley of nerve impulses could lead to a vicious cycle between central and peripheral processes.

Although debate continued among three basic pain theories, specificity ultimately prevailed and was universally accepted and practiced. An appreciation for cognitive and psychological aspects of pain processing, although secondary, slowly emerged within the fourth theory of pain, proposed by Hardy, Wolff, and Goodell. Pain was separated into two components: the perception of pain (afferent) and the reaction to pain (efferent). Pain perception was thought as a more hardwired physiologic process, whereas reaction to pain was under the influence of complex psychological and physiologic processes influenced by past experiences, the environment, and emotional state.[61]

The Dutch surgeon Willem Noordenbos suggested that pain transmission was not a one-to-one synaptic transmission system but rather involved a multisynaptic modification process with complex interactions (such as convergence) between synapses. The sensory interaction theory of Noordenbos (1959) proposed two systems involving transmission of pain and other sensory information: a slow system (unmyelinated and thinly myelinated fibers) and a fast-acting system (large myelinated fibers). Large fibers could inhibit transmission of impulses from small fibers. This set the stage for the seminal work of Melzack and Wall on the gate control theory of pain modulation in 1965. Although controversial then and now, it brought an emphasis to a more convergent view of central pain processing at the spinal cord and cerebral levels.

The gate control theory by Melzack and Wall championed a more convergent view of pain processing. The spinal cord is not just a passive conduit for pain transmission but also an active modulator of pain signals. Activity in large myelinated afferent fibers theoretically activates dorsal horn encephalitogenic interneurons that inhibit cephalad transmission in small unmyelinated primary afferent nociceptive fibers and the secondary transmission cells in the lateral spinothalamic tracts.[101] Somatic afferents activate convergent wide dynamic range cells deep in the dorsal horn (lamina V), which project in the spinothalamic tract to higher somatosensory processing in the thalamus and cortex. In theory, inhibiting pain by rubbing the skin activates large-diameter afferents inhibiting small-diameter fiber activation of wide dynamic range cells—that is, "closing the gate."

Additional work 3 years later by Melzack and Casey emphasized motivational, affective, and cognitive aspects of the pain experience. Neural pathways could activate both sensory discriminative information about the location and intensity of pain, as well as more emotional and motivational effects of pain experience. Descending inhibition from cortical structures could also influence pain. Descending modulation of the gate theoretically could block nociceptive signals at the dorsal horn and provide the basis for behavioral-induced reduction of pain. In turn, psychological processes such as depression could potentially increase pain by "opening" gating mechanisms at the dorsal horn. This modulation, carried down to the dorsal horn in the dorsolateral funiculus and ramifying throughout the entire neuraxis, provides a way for the central nervous system to actively modulate the afferent input at multiple levels of the central nervous system. This affects all aspects of the pain experience, including affective, subjective, and evaluative components. The gate control theory offered a new model for the successful integration of experimental and clinical observations related to the study of pain. The gate control theory, although challenged as somewhat incomplete, has remained the core of contemporary pain science. It has spurred the development of new clinical treatments, including neurophysiologically based procedures (transcutaneous electrical nerve stimulation, spinal cord stimulation), and pharmacologic, cognitive, and behavioral treatments.

Melzack has extended his work with the gate control theory to include the more central *neuromatrix* theory based on concepts from cognitive neuroscience network theory. Dimensions of the pain experience are considered as output of the neuromatrix, which proposes a *neurosignature* of pain experience that is unique to each individual and is influenced by sensory, psychosocial, and genetic factors. This pattern is modulated by various sensory inputs from the environment and by cognitive events such as psychological stress. In turn, these multiple parallel processing inputs contribute to the sensory, affective, and cognitive dimensions of the pain experience and subsequent behavior.

Recent advances in neuroimaging and the exploding field of neuroscience networking have offered greater insight into higher-level cerebral plasticity related to acute and chronic pain. Apkarian et al.[4] studied brain morphologic changes with the use of high-resolution magnetic resonance imaging in a group of patients with chronic low back pain. Significant evidence of discrete central nervous system degeneration (gray matter atrophy) in the chronic pain patient group was demonstrated. Discrete thalamic and prefrontal cortex atrophy was reported at a rate approximately 5 to 10 times greater than that of normal age-related atrophy. This underscores the importance of appropriate and aggressive treatment of pain as a means of preventing possible long-term or permanent central nervous system changes. In addition, these findings add to the ongoing developments in neural plasticity of pain because these changes are not plastic but are perhaps permanent (Figure 37-2). The use of positron emission tomography and functional magnetic resonance imaging has offered accelerating insight into the main cerebral components of human nociceptive processing and networking at the brain and spinal cord levels.[69]

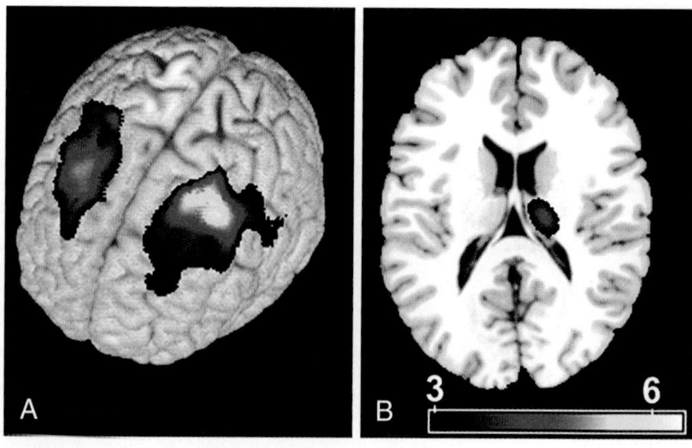

FIGURE 37-2 **Regional gray matter density decreases in patients with chronic low back pain.** (From Apkarian AV, Sosa Y, Sonty S, et al: Chronic back pain is associated with decreased prefrontal and thalamic gray matter density, *J Neurosci* 24:10410-10415, 2004, with permission.)

History of Contemporary Advancements in Psychological Aspects of Pain

The twentieth century also provided significant growth in the fields of psychiatry and psychosomatic medicine. Sigmund Freud emphasized the potential link between psychological and physical factors in a number of medical conditions. Later, disenchantment with Freud's psychoanalytic principles led to the development of the field of psychosomatic medicine and the subsequent rapid development of the fields of health psychology and behavioral medicine in the 1970s.[52] Physicians such as George Engel (1959) challenged the biomedical model of disease as inadequate, in that it failed to include the social, psychological, and behavioral dimensions of illness. A classic article by Engel, "'Psychogenic' Pain and the Pain-Prone Patient," discussed various contextual meanings of persistent pain and the importance of an individual's interpretation of his or her pain. Sternbach argued that physiologic and affective perceptions of pain should be understood as learned responses under the control of environmental forces and addressed psychophysiologic pain syndromes, including "stress-induced pain disorders."[138] Wilbert Fordyce later proposed an operant conditioning model of chronic pain based on an ends approach of identifying and treating pain behaviors. More recently, higher cognitive functioning in pain states (such as memory and emotive components) were embraced in the cognitive behavioral approach, led by health psychologists such as Dennis Turk and Frances Keefe, emphasizing the role of attributions, efficacy, personal control, and problem solving. Thoughts and beliefs could influence, and be influenced by, emotional and physiologic responses.[150] This has contributed to the evolution of a more clinically pragmatic school of pain assessment and treatment: the biopsychosocial model. This model incorporates the physical, cognitive, affective, and behavioral components related to ongoing pain experience. In this context, biological factors can initiate a physical disturbance, but psychosocial factors often influence pain perception, pain behavior, and the ongoing pain experience.[149]

Physiology and Pathophysiology of Pain

In a normal homeostatic state, cutaneous, visceral, and musculoskeletal pain serve as an alarm system to the body that indicates damage or potential damage in the environment. The purpose of nociception is to alert the organism to this potential damage so that avoidance behavior can be initiated. In contrast, chronic pain states might represent an alteration involving damage or injury to the central nervous system that serves no real protective role, reflecting a pathologic as opposed to physiologic state. The complex interaction between the initial stimulus of tissue injury and the subjective experience of nociception and acute and chronic pain can be described by four general processes known as transduction, transmission, modulation, and perception (Table 37-3).

Normal pain, or nociception, is characterized primarily by the processes of transduction and transmission, with minimal emphasis on modulation and a "normal" perception process. With chronic or persistent pain states, there is a shift of focus to the processes of modulation and perception. These four general processes are reviewed in the following sections and serve as an important foundation for a more clear understanding of complex pain mechanisms and possible rational pharmacotherapeutic, interventional, and cognitive behavioral treatment approaches.

Transduction

The principal receptors for pain are the branched endings of C and Aδ fibers (Table 37-4) in the skin, muscles, and joints. Damaging (or potentially damaging) energy in the cellular environment impacts the free nerve endings, and the complicated cellular processes of nociceptive transduction occur. Inflammatory cascades are concurrently activated (e.g., prostaglandin, leukotriene) and immediately become principal players in the transduction process. Recent histochemical studies have revealed two broad categories of C fibers: peptidergic and isolectin B_4 binding. Peptidergic fibers contain a variety of peptide neurotransmitters, including substance P and calcitonin gene-related peptide (CGRP), and express tyrosine receptor kinase A receptors, which show high affinity for nerve growth factors. Peptidergic neurons appear to be key players in neurogenic inflammation (where the transduction cells themselves become active participants in the local

Table 37-3 Signal Processing

Stage	Description
Transduction (receptor activation)	One form of energy (thermal, mechanical, or chemical stimulus) is converted electrochemically into nerve impulses (action potentials) in primary afferents
Transmission	Coded information is transferred from primary afferent fibers to spinal cord dorsal horn and onto brainstem, thalamus, and higher cortical structures
Modulation	Involves activity- and signal-induced dorsal horn neural plasticity, which includes altered receptor and channel function (i.e., wind-up and central sensitization), gene expression,[165] and changes in brain-mediated descending inhibition and facilitation
Perception	Begins with activation of sensory cortex. The cortex is in intimate communication with motor and prefrontal cortices, which initiate efferent responses, as well as more primitive structures involved in the emotive aspects of pain

Table 37-4 Nerve Fiber Classification

Sensory and Motor Fibers	Sensory Fibers	Diameter (μm)	Myelinated	Velocity (m/s)	Motor Function	Sensory Function
Aα	Ia Ib	10-20 10-20	Yes Yes	0-120 50-120	α-Motor neurons —	Muscle spindle afferents Golgi tendon organs, touch, pressure
Aβ	2	4-12	Yes	25-100	Motor neurons to intrafusal and extrafusal muscle fibers	Secondary muscle spindle afferents, touch, pressure, vibration
Aγ		2-8	Yes	10-50	Motor neurons to intrafusal muscle fibers	—
Aδ (types 1 and 2)	3	1-5	Lightly	3-30	—	Touch, pain, and temperature
B		1-3	No	3-15	Preganglionic autonomic fibers	—
C	4	<1	No	0.5-2	Postganglionic autonomic fibers	Pain and temperature

inflammatory process) and other chronic inflammatory states.[166] The other class, isolectin B_4 binding, contains few neuropeptides but expresses a surface carbohydrate group selectivity binding to the plant lectin isolectin B_4 and is supported by glial-derived neurotrophic factor.[142] Isolectin B_4 expresses P2X3 receptors, a subtype of ATP-gated ion channels.[72] Differences in supporting trophic factors might be responsible for differing functional responses to painful stimuli between these distinct C-fiber types. Neurotrophins have emerged as potential factors for activity-dependent changes at the synapse and possibly subsequent central nervous system plasticity.

Multiple arachidonic acid residue receptors are probably involved (e.g., prostaglandin, leukotriene), and the "chaos" level of complexity is further complicated by the very active presence of the support cells (glia and myelin) and the efferent input by the central nervous system itself, primarily via the sympathetic nervous system. Noradrenergic receptors are on the transduction cell, and these can be "uncovered" or activated in inflamed tissue.

Aδ nociceptors (also responders to noxious, thermal, and chemical stimuli) are most easily classified on functional grounds. Type 2 Aδ exhibit short response latencies to heat and are activated at relatively higher thresholds (43° C). Type 2 Aδ are responsible for the initial sensation of a burn stimulus. Type 1 Aδ exhibit longer response latencies and are activated at much higher temperatures (greater than 50° C). Type 1 Aδ and nociceptive C fibers are more commonly associated with persistent painful sensations.[24]

Transmission

Cutaneous peripheral afferent neurons can be classified into three types based on diameter, structure, and conduction velocity of action potentials. In general, C fibers (thin, unmyelinated, slowly conducting; 0.5 to 2.0 m/s) and Aδ fibers (medium, thinly myelinated, rapidly conducting; 12 to 30 m/s) carry noxious stimuli, and Aβ fibers (large, myelinated, and fast; 30 to 100 m/s) carry innocuous stimuli (touch, vibration, and pressure), except in situations of peripheral or central sensitization (see Table 37-4). The percentage of distribution of nociceptors in the skin is roughly proportioned 70%, 10%, and 20%, respectively. With peripheral and central neuroplastic changes in Aβ fibers, innocuous stimuli might be perceived as painful, resulting in allodynia. Aδ nociceptors respond to intense mechanical and temperature stimuli, and with sensitization contribute to the process called hyperpathia, in which noxious stimuli become frankly more painful and the pain perception can last longer, even after the initial stimulus is removed. Most C fibers are polymodal transducers. Aβ fibers demonstrate encapsulated nerve endings involved in nonnociceptive function. Aδ fibers mediate the fast, prickling quality of pain, whereas C fibers mediate the slow, burning quality of pain. An additional class of nociceptors, the so-called silent or sleeping nociceptors, makes up approximately 10% to 20% of C fibers in the skin, joints, and viscera, and is normally unresponsive to acute noxious stimuli. With inflammation and tissue injury, these "silent" nociceptors are sensitized via activation of second-messenger systems and the release of a number of local chemical mediators (i.e., bradykinin, prostaglandins, serotonin, and histamine) and can contribute to temporal and spatial summation, increasing afferent input at the dorsal horn.[53]

Peripheral Sensitization

C fibers and Aδ receptors undergo changes in response to tissue injury such as inflammation, ischemia, and compression. These changes are marked at the peripheral terminals by the release of chemical mediators from damaged and inflammatory cells. The so-called inflammatory soup, rich in analgesic substances, causes a lowering of threshold for activation and subsequent evoked pain. Algogenic substances also activate second-messenger systems, which induce gene expression in the cell. Excitatory amino acids and neuropeptides (substance P, CGRP, and neurokinins) are released by peripheral and central nociceptive C fibers, inducing neurogenic inflammation. Neurogenic inflammation involves retrograde release of algogenic substances, which in turn excites other nearby nociceptors, creating local feed-forward loops of sensitization and activation.

Modulation

Primary afferents subserving distinct input from cutaneous, muscle, and visceral tissues converge at the dorsal horn. Several ascending pathways are involved in transferring and modulating this nociceptive input. At the cellular level, the influx of sodium is fundamental to electrical signaling and subsequent generation of action potentials and excitatory postsynaptic potentials. This is followed by calcium channel opening, contributing to more prolonged depolarization, as well as second-messenger molecular changes involved in more permanent neuroplastic central nervous system changes. At the synaptic terminal of the axon, action potentials lead to the release of neurotransmitters. Neurotransmitter release depends on specific ion channels, which are either ligand-gated, opening in response to binding of ligands to receptors, or voltage-gated, opening in response to changes in membrane potentials. Other targeted receptor and ion channels include vanilloid (capsaicin) receptor, heat-activated, ATP-gated purinergic receptor (P2X), proton-gated or acid-sensing ion channels, and voltage-gated sodium channels. The vanilloid receptor is a nonselective cation channel (vanilloid receptor 1) activated by elevated temperature (greater than 43° C) and acidification.

Aδ and C fibers convey nociceptive information primarily to superficial laminae (I and II) and deep laminae (V and VI) of the dorsal horn. Lamina I plays an important role in relaying information on the current state of tissues, including damaging mechanical stress, heat and cold, local metabolism (acid pH, hypoxia), cell breakdown (ATP, glutamate), mast cell activation (serotonin, bradykinin), and immune activity (cytokines).[30] Aβ fibers transmit innocuous, mechanical stimuli to deeper laminae (III to VI). Lamina I cells are activated by nociceptive-specific neurons, whereas lamina V cells respond to wide dynamic range neurons of "wide" stimulus intensities. Wide dynamic range neurons receive input from mechanoreceptive Aβ fibers and nociceptive (Aδ and C) fibers (Figure 37-3).

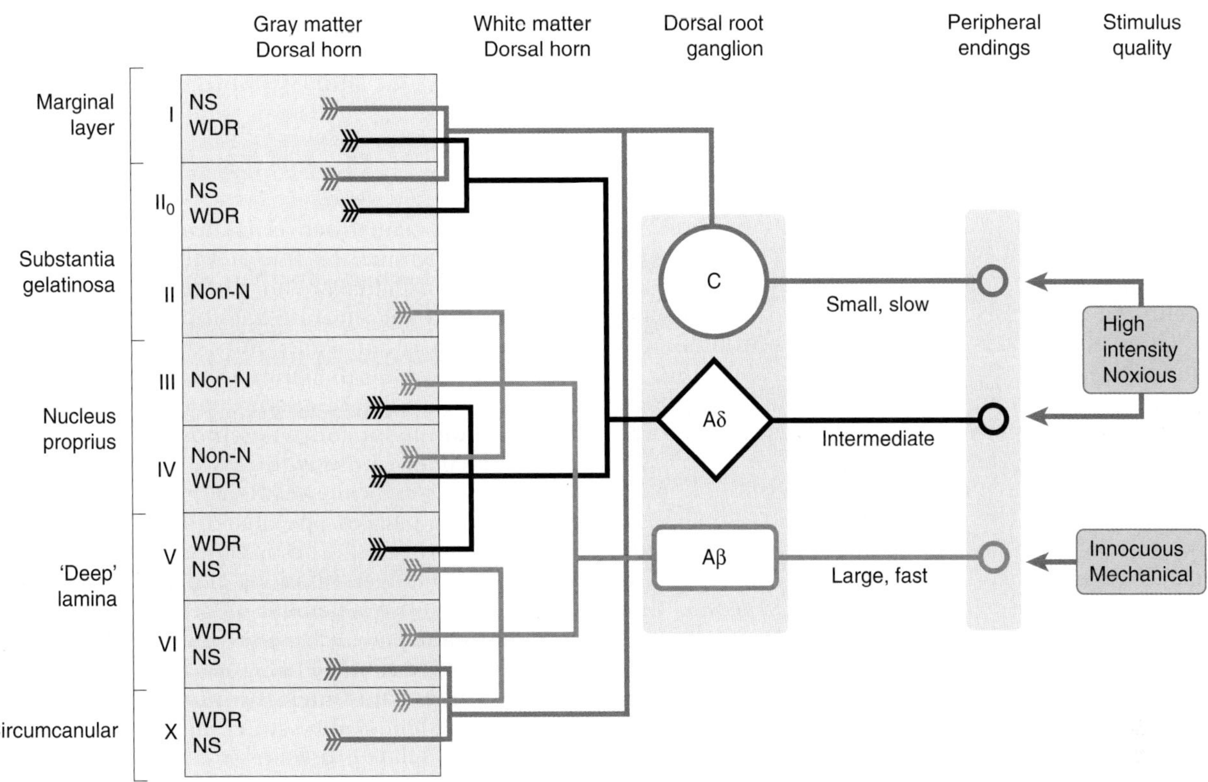

FIGURE 37-3 Organization of cutaneous, primary afferent input to the dorsal horn of the spinal cord. *Non-N,* Nonnoxious; *NS,* nociceptive-specific; *WDR,* wide dynamic range. (Modified from Millan MJ: The induction of pain: an integrative review, *Prog Neurobiol* 57:1-164, 1999, with permission.)

Normal synaptic transmission conduction of action potentials at the dorsal horn initiates neurotransmitter release. Low-intensity stimulations (i.e., brush, touch, or vibration) activate Aβ fibers only, releasing fast, glutamate-mediated postsynaptic currents. Fast excitatory transmission glutamate is coreleased presynaptically with neuropeptides such as substance P, CGRP, cholecystokinin, proteins (brain-derived neurotrophic factor), and glial-derived factors.[86] Glutamate acts on a range of transmission cell receptors, such as *N*-methyl-D-aspartate (NMDA) (slow current), α-amino-3-hydroxy-5-methyl-4-isoxazolepropionic acid (AMPA) (fast current), metabotropic glutamate receptors, and kainate ligand-gated ion channels. With normal transmission, sodium flows only through the AMPA receptor, whereas the NMDA receptor is blocked by magnesium. Prolonged depolarization of the postsynaptic cell causes voltage-dependent magnesium removal, opening the channel and allowing additional sodium and calcium to enter the cell. This amplified evoked response to subsequent input describes the process of wind-up.[86]

Central Sensitization

The term *central sensitization* describes a complex set of activation-dependent posttranslational changes occurring at the dorsal horn, brainstem, and higher cerebral sites. For example, at the dorsal horn, nociceptors release neurotransmitters (glutamate, substance P, and brain-derived neurotrophic factor) onto the transmission cells, which results in changes in activation of related receptors and channels (as described earlier). This results in an increase in calcium influx (and efflux from cytoplasmic organelles), contributing to potentiation of the cell by activation of calcium-dependent enzyme protein kinases (e.g., protein kinase C, cyclic AMP, and tyrosine receptor kinase). Posttranslational changes also include phosphorylation of NMDA and AMPA receptors, activation of second messengers such as nitric oxide, and central prostaglandin production.[165]

Ascending and Descending Modulation

Melzack & Casey's classic descriptions of neuroanatomic pathways make a distinction between the lateral and medial pain systems corresponding to their relationship with the thalamus.[100] The two systems are highly interdependent, the lateral (neospinothalamic) system generally representing sensory-discriminative dimensions versus the medial (paleospinothalamic) system involving more motivational-affective and cognitive-evaluative dimensions of the pain experience. Additional ascending pathways, including the spinothalamic, spinomesencephalic, spinoreticular, spinolimbic, spinocervical, and dorsal column pathways, are described elsewhere.

The lateral system projects to the ventral posterolateral and ventral posteromedial thalamic nuclei before projecting to the somatosensory and premotor cortices. The motor input is nearly as large as the sensory input, and this theoretically prepares the recipient of the painful input for the appropriate efferent (behavioral) response. The more medial pathway projects to the medial thalamic nuclei and limbic cortices, which include the anterior cingulated cortex, orbitofrontal cortex, and amygdala. The medial system involves important connections with periaqueductal gray, a key area involved in modulating nociceptive inhibition and behavioral responses to potentially threatening stimuli. Animal and human studies have identified the anterior cingulated cortex in regulating avoidance behaviors and the perception of pain unpleasantness. Only a small proportion of these action potentials normally reach the thalamus and higher brain centers as a result of significant modulating or filtering effects at the spinal cord and brainstem. Of course, with prolonged disease and inflammation these filters "break down," contributing to central sensitization.

In addition to descending inhibition, the endogenous inhibitory system also includes local endogenous opioids (from periaqueductal gray), biogenic amines (serotonin and noradrenaline [norepinephrine]), and γ-aminobutyric acid (GABA), which generally act to inhibit pain signals. Important excitatory transmitters in this system include glutamate and substance P.[164] Besides descending inhibition from cortical areas, recent studies have suggested that descending facilitatory pathways might link brainstem and spinal cord areas via pronociceptive serotonergic[136] and opioid mechanisms.[42] These pronociceptive pathways could help explain the possible mechanism of persistent pain signs and symptoms, such as allodynia and hyperalgesia, that are common to chronic pain conditions.

Pathways originating from the spinal cord dorsal horn activate brain structures involved in rudimentary aspects of the autonomic system response (i.e., escape, arousal, and fear), including the medulla and midbrain reticular formation, amygdala, hypothalamus, and thalamic nuclei.[114] Activation of somatosensory cortices (S1 to S2) provides information regarding the quality and intensity of pain. Affective aspects of the pain experience, such as pain unpleasantness, reflect more of the aversive qualities of the pain experience, such as the suffering component. Higher processing involves parietal and insular regions, contributing to an overall sense of intrusion and unpleasantness.[117] Finally, convergence of these pathways with more frontal regions, such as the anterior cingulate cortex, is responsible for attention and emotional valence of the overall pain experience.

Although cutaneous and visceral pain share common cortical and subcortical networks, differences in response pattern, frequency, and processing might underlie differences in quality, affect, and resultant behavioral responses.[141] Visceral pain has a more indistinct quality, poor localization, and in general is associated with autonomic markers such as bradycardia and hypotension. Cutaneous nociceptive reactions more classically involve protective reflexes such as tachycardia and hypertension.

Psychological Issues Related to Chronic Pain

The physiatric approach to chronic pain conditions must include an understanding of the wide array of important psychological (affective and cognitive) factors that affect the multidimensional experience of pain. Psychological factors can serve to decrease or increase the subjective perception of pain and adjustment to ongoing pain-related disability. Affective factors usually include more negative emotions, such as depression, pain-related anxiety, and anger. Cognitive factors include catastrophizing, fear, helplessness, decreased self-efficacy, pain coping, readiness to change, and acceptance.

Affective Factors

Depression

A strong association between chronic pain and depression has been suggested.[53,119] The prevalence estimates of major depression in patients with chronic pain conditions vary from 5% to 87%, and this variation could be attributable to a number of analytic factors, including the diagnostic criteria used, type of pain studied, and selection bias.[50] Somatic symptoms of major depressive disorder can also be common in patients with chronic pain (i.e., change in appetite, change in weight, loss of energy, and sleep disturbance). The incidence of depression among patients with chronic pain can be higher than with other chronic medical conditions.[6] The presence of chronic pain might be related to longer durations of depressive symptoms.[108b] In general, most systematic reviews on the relationship between pain and depression suggest that chronic pain precedes depression.[44] Predictors of depression in chronic pain include pain intensity, number of painful areas reported, frequency the severe pain is experienced, and a number of related psychosocial factors. Patients with depression can report higher levels of pain, be less active, report greater disability and life interference related to pain, and are more likely to display overt pain behaviors.[75] Brown et al.[18] examined the mediating factors of the relationship between chronic pain in patients with rheumatoid arthritis and decreased cognitive functioning, which included measures of inductive reasoning and working memory. Elevated depression mediated the relationship between higher levels of pain and reduced cognitive functioning,[18] underscoring the importance of the complex relationship among depression, chronic pain, and functional impairment.

Anxiety

Anxiety related to pain is an important factor involved in maladaptive responses, behavioral interference, and affective distress. Heightened pain-related anxiety has been described as one of the most disabling aspects of ongoing chronic pain. It is closely related to avoidance activities (discussed later), which serve to promote ongoing pain, physical deconditioning, and social isolation.[60] Anxiety as a psychological construct in chronic pain has been developed by McCracken et al.[91] as pain-related anxiety. Pain-related anxiety encompasses fear reactions across the cognitive, behavioral, and physiologic dimensions of pain. In chronic pain, it has been found to be a significant predictor of pain severity, disability, and pain behaviors.[91]

Anger

Ongoing failure to achieve pain relief and repeated unsuccessful attempts to escape pain have been shown to be associated with increased levels of anger and physiologic responses to pain, independent of pain intensity.[2] In a study of patients presenting for chronic pain management, Okifuji et al.[109] reported 70% of participants with angry feelings, most commonly with themselves (74%) and health care professionals (62%). In this study, anger toward oneself was associated with pain and depression, whereas "only anger" was related to perceived disability.

Conceptualizations of anger in chronic pain vary. A more classic definition of anger has been described as a "feeling involving a belief that a person one cares for has, intentionally or through neglect, been treated without respect, and a want to have that respect reestablished."[133] Anger as a construct has also been considered to be related to personality dispositions associated with unconscious conflicts, or as a reaction to the presence of ongoing unrelieved pain.[41] Others have suggested that chronic pain might develop as a conversion-like symptom to suppress feelings of anger, and suppressed anger could be negatively related to adjustment to ongoing chronic pain.[76] In contrast, "anger out" has also been linked to poor adjustment. These styles of anger management, suppression (anger in) and expression (anger out), are distinguished from overt hostility. Hostility has been defined as "an attitude of cynical mistrustfulness, resentment, and interpersonal antagonism."[134] Burns[19] has demonstrated how anger management style and hostility can affect maintenance and exacerbation of chronic low back pain via symptom-specific physiologic responses (i.e., increased muscle stress reactivity in lumbar paraspinals in patients with low back pain). This work was based on the studies of Flor et al.,[45] who showed that patients with chronic low back pain exhibited greater stress-induced increases in electromyogram readings in lower paraspinal muscles compared with normal individuals. Anger and related physiologic responses are additional targets for pharmacologic and behavioral treatments, including relaxation training and other mind-body treatments.

Cognitive Factors

Many patients with chronic pain demonstrate a reduction in goal-directed activities and assume a more passive sedentary lifestyle. This further contributes to a downward spiral of inactivity, deconditioning, and increased somatic focus. Individual responses to pain are recognized as important variables of the pain experience and can be associated with a greater risk of maintaining pain-related disability. Patients who frequently have excessively negative thoughts about themselves, others, and the future are more likely to experience high levels of depression, low levels of activity, and increased tension.[54,144] Pain beliefs (pain-related fear and self-efficacy), anger, and passive coping are important affective factors, which can significantly affect pain response, behavior, and function. Other neurocognitive factors, unique to each patient, including attention, expectation or anticipation, and appraisals, can contribute to maladaptive behaviors and can represent important targets for cognitive and behavioral interventions.

Learning Factors

Operant Learning

Fordyce's operant conditioning approach to pain serves as one of the earliest psychological models for chronic pain.[46] The model focuses primarily on observable behavioral manifestations of pain, which are subject to both reinforcement and avoidance learning. When an individual is exposed to a stimulus that causes tissue damage, an immediate response occurs that involves withdrawal or attempts to escape the stimulus. By successfully avoiding pain (i.e., "punishment"), the individual achieves a reduction in pain, thus rewarding the avoidance behavior. The acquisition of pain behaviors can be determined initially by the history of learned avoidance behaviors. In these cases, pain becomes a discriminating stimulus signaling behaviors that are pain reducing, such as rest and analgesic medication consumption. With time, pain-eliciting situations such as movement and activity cause anticipatory fear and are avoided. Over time, pain avoidance behaviors can generalize to other potentially painful stimuli, contributing to more inactivity and passivity.[80,157] In a similar way, verbal expression of pain (e.g., complaining) and nonverbal pain behaviors (e.g., limping and grimacing) can be maintained by external reinforcement contingencies such as subtle rewards by significant others or family members who respond to these behaviors.

Waddell et al.[158] identified a set of "nonorganic" signs that can be used as a simple clinical screening tool to help identify signs and symptoms of pain behavior (tenderness, simulation, distraction, and regional sensory and motor impairments). Although controversial, a study of nonorganic signs in a group of patients with low back pain found that demonstration of at least three of the five signs correlated with psychological distress.[158]

Fear of Movement

Kinesophobia, a term that describes an irrational and excessive fear of movement, physical activity, and reinjury, is exhibited by many patients with chronic pain. Fear of movement can be initially induced by classical conditioning but is reinforced through operant learning; by avoiding the conditioned anxiety and fear associated with movement, the patient never extinguishes the fear. It has been shown in studies to strongly correlate with other responses, such as catastrophic thinking and subsequent increased fear and avoidance behaviors, in patients with chronic low back pain. In this way, increased levels of fear and disability can occur independently of the experienced pain intensity.[156] McCracken et al.[92] found that increased fear and anxiety in patients with low back pain correlated with decreased range of motion and increased expectation of pain. Other studies in chronic low back pain have found pain-related fear and fear-avoidance beliefs as predictors of disability, decreased activities of daily living, and lost work time.[95]

A cognitive behavioral model emphasizes two opposing behavioral responses: confrontation and avoidance. The conclusion of Waddell et al. that "fear of pain and what we do about pain can be more disabling than pain itself"[159] underscores the importance of identifying and treating such maladaptive thinking and behavior in a physiatric approach to effectively managing chronic pain.

Behavioral Treatment Approaches

Operant Behavioral Techniques

Operant behavioral therapy refers to interventions focused on the observed behavior of the patient. As proposed by Fordyce,[46] operant models of pain are based on both positive and negative reinforcement contingencies. Environment and social factors serve to maintain pain behaviors. For example, the verbal expression of pain and nonverbal pain behaviors (e.g., grimacing and guarding) can be maintained by both positive (attention from others, potential monetary gain) and negative reinforcement (nonoccurrence of aversive stimuli, avoidance of activity).[73] Once identified, these behaviors serve as targets for treatment. Many times these behaviors need to be reinforced only intermittently. Operant behavioral therapy can be most useful and practical with patients demonstrating excessive pain behaviors despite limited tissue pathology, poor insight into the relationship of their own behavior and subjective experiences of pain, and operant-related issues (secondary gain).

Goals of operant behavioral therapy include encouraging the development and acquisition of more adaptive pain management strategies, which include establishing wellness behaviors and discouraging or reducing reinforcement of pain behaviors.[29] The theory suggests that both wellness and pain behaviors can be shaped. Management techniques target unlearning these behaviors and serve as the basis of most functional restoration-based programs developed by Mayer and Gatchel.[89] Operant behavioral therapy techniques are provided to patients in individual and group settings, focusing on helping patients to master and apply multiple strategies including pacing and graded exercise, scheduling and/or limiting pain medications and passive treatments, and counseling regarding negative and positive social reinforcement via spouse and family training.

Cognitive Behavioral Techniques

Cognitive therapy techniques are based on the notion that one's cognitions can have an impact on mood, behavior, and physiologic function.[9] Techniques used in pain management are designed to help patients notice and modify the negative thought patterns that contribute to ongoing pain and affective distress. These include cognitive restructuring, problem solving, distraction, and relapse prevention.[160] Five primary assumptions underlie all cognitive behavioral therapy interventions (Box 37-1).[15] Cognitive behavioral therapy is a flexible, viable, and empirically validated approach for effectively treating patients with persistent pain.[106]

BOX 37-1

Five Primary Assumptions That Underlie All Cognitive Behavioral Therapy Interventions

1. Individuals actively process information regarding internal stimuli and environmental events.
2. Cognitions interact with emotional and physiologic reactions as well as with behavior.
3. Reciprocal interactions occur between an individual's behavior and environmental responses.
4. Effective treatment interventions must address the cognitive, emotional, and behavioral dimensions of the presenting problem.
5. It is necessary to help individuals become active participants in learning adaptive methods of responding to their problems.

Sleep and Chronic Pain

Sleep is a dynamic, complex physiologic process that is required for survival. During sleep there is decreased sensitivity to the external environment and increased activity of the parasympathetic nervous system. Sympathetic nervous system activity is similar to that in wakefulness, except for during periods of rapid eye movement (REM). Breathing is irregular, and control of body temperature is altered. Sleep comprises alternating REM and non-REM (NREM) states that cycle at an ultradian rhythm of approximately 90 minutes.[121]

Sleep of 8 to 8.5 hours is considered restorative in adults. Sleep is entered through NREM, and the NREM-REM cycle occurs three to six times during a normal 8-hour sleep period. The determinants of sleep are numerous and include homeostasis, the circadian rhythm, control via the ventrolateral preoptic nucleus, age, drugs, external temperature, medical and psychiatric disease, and other environmental factors.[121] The ventrolateral preoptic nucleus has been shown to contain GABAergic and galaninergic neurons that are necessary for normal sleep.[128] Lesions to this region have been shown to decrease both REM and NREM sleep by 55%, verifying their function in inhibiting the firing of cells involved in wakefulness. These inhibited neurons contain the neurotransmitters histamine, norepinephrine, serotonin, hypocretin, and glutamate. Age represents a strong determinant of sleep, as time spent in stages 3 and 4 decreases by 10% to 15%, latency to fall asleep increases, and the number and duration of overnight arousal periods increase in older adults compared with young adults.[124]

The interrelationship between disturbed sleep and chronic pain conditions is well documented for both adults and adolescents.[105,110] Prevalence estimates of disturbed sleep range from approximately 50% to 90% depending on the clinical study population under evaluation.[105] Although the nature of the relationship between pain and disturbed sleep is not well understood, a reciprocal association is suggested.[1] Current research suggests a multifactorial relationship including depression, fear-avoidance behaviors, catastrophizing, and even treatments such as benzodiazepines and chronic opioid therapy.[85] Patients with chronic pain can display frequent sleep fragmentation, longer sleep latency, and decreased overall quality of sleep. Sleep fragmentation is characterized by repetitive short interruptions in sleep and is a recognized factor in the cause of excessive daytime sleepiness. This inability to maintain sleep can be the most important factor in the treatment of disturbed sleep in individuals with chronic pain. The strength of this relationship between disturbed sleep and chronic pain cannot be underestimated.

Assessment

The assessment of chronic pain involves a thorough physical examination and a comprehensive evaluation of pain intensity and psychosocial factors related to ongoing pain experience and interference with sleep, daily activities, family life, and employment. Subjective reports of pain intensity are an important part of the initial assessment and subsequent visits and can include pain intensity numeric rating scales, visual and verbal analogue scales, and pain drawings. Self-monitored pain intensity ratings are both reliable and valid.[66] Patient variability remains, however, when interpreting self-report measurement scales. A significant area of study has examined the level of change that best represents a clinically important improvement with the use of the numeric rating scale in monitoring pain response with drug treatment trials. Farrar et al.[40] found that a reduction of approximately 30% represented a clinically important difference. A commonly used comprehensive measure of pain intensity, the McGill Pain Questionnaire Short Form, measures three dimensions of pain: sensory, affective, and evaluative. It uses 20 subclasses or groupings of pain adjectives, including sensory (e.g., "sharp," "dull," and "heavy") and affective (e.g., "annoying," "tiring," and "exhausting"); it also includes pain drawings and the visual analogue scale.[99]

Additional psychometric measures can also be included in the initial assessment focusing on psychosocial factors such as mood (depression, anxiety, and anger), attitudes, beliefs, functional capacity, activity interference, and personality traits (Table 37-5). The use and combination of these different methods depend largely on the goal of the

Table 37-5 Psychometric Assessment Tools

Psychometric Measure	Psychometric Assessment Tool	Description	Reference
Pain intensity	Numeric Rating Scale Visual Analogue Scale Verbal Rating Scale	0-10, 0-100, "no pain" to "worst pain" Straight line, 0-10 cm List of adjectives or descriptors	—
Pain affect	McGill Pain Questionnaire-Short Form (MPQ-SF)	20 descriptors (sensory, affective, evaluative), pain drawing, visual analogue scale; 4-point Likert scale from 0 (none) to 3 (severe)	Melzack[99]
	Brief Pain Inventory (BPI) and Brief Pain Inventory-Short Form (BPI-SF)	Measures the impact of pain on everyday activities and mood	Cleeland and Ryan[28]
Anxiety and coping	Pain Anxiety Symptoms Scale (PASS)	40 items; anxiety related to pain on 6-point scale, subscales: cognitive anxiety symptoms, escape and avoidance, fearful appraisals, physiologic symptoms	McCracken et al.[95]
	Spielberger State-Trait Anxiety Inventory (STAI)	40 items; differentiates between the temporary condition of "state anxiety" and the more general and long-standing quality of "trait anxiety"	Spielberger et al.[136]
	Survey of Pain Attitudes (SOPA)	57-item, 5-point scale assessing control, disability, medical cures, solicitude, medication, emotion, and harm	Jensen et al.[67]
Depression	Beck Depression Inventory (BDI)	21-item, 4-point scale assessing mood and neurovegetative dimensions of depression	Beck and Steer[10]
	Center for Epidemiologic Studies Depression Scale (CES-D)	Less compromised validity by somatic symptoms compared with the Beck Depression Inventory, more sensitive to changes in severity of depression	Radloff[116]
	Zung Self-Rating Depression Scale	20-item, rapid assessment tool for severity of depression	Zung[170]
Mood and personality	Minnesota Multiphasic Personality Inventory (MMPI)	567 true-false items, 60-90 min to administer	Butcher et al.[20]
	Symptom Checklist 90 (SCL-90-R)	90-item, 5-point scale, global index score, and 9 subscales of general emotional distress	Derogatis[35]
	Millon Behavioral Health Inventory	150 true-false items, assesses styles of relating to providers, psychosocial stressors, and response to illness	Millon et al.[103]
Functional capacity and activity interference	Sickness Impact Profile (SIP)	136 items, 12 dimensions of function	Bergener et al.[11]
	36-Item Short-Form Health Survey (SF-36)	Eight scales to measure limitations in physical and social activities caused by physical and emotional problems, bodily pain, vitality, and general health perceptions	Ware and Sherbourne[160]
	West Haven-Yale Multidimensional Pain Inventory (WHYMPI or MPI)	52-item, 7-point scale, 12 dimensions (pain experience, perceptions of others, common daily activities), classifies patients primarily into three classes (dysfunctional, interpersonally distressed, and adaptive copers)	Kerns et al.[76a]
	Pain Disability Index (PDI)	7 questions: degree of interference with functioning, home, recreation, social activities, occupations, sexual behavior, self-care, and life support	Trait et al.[147]
	Oswestry Disability Questionnaire	10 sections, assesses the effect of back and leg pain on activities of daily living and patient's everyday life	Leclaire et al.[79]
Coping and beliefs	Coping Strategies Questionnaire (CSQ)	50 items, cognitive and behavioral coping strategies assessed	Rosenstiel and Keefe[120]
	Survey of Pain Attitudes (SOPA)	57 items, subscales (control, disability, medical cures, solicitude, medication, emotion, and harm)	Jensen et al.[67]

assessment. A semistructured interview by an experienced psychologist is the most comprehensive means of evaluating the psychological state of the patient. A pack of self-reported questionnaires completed by the patient before the evaluation, measuring a wide spectrum of the multidimensional factors related to pain, can be used in isolation or as an adjunct to the psychological and medical interview.

The comprehensive evaluation should include a complete medical history and physical examination identifying related impairments, pain behaviors, and postural and soft tissue abnormalities (i.e., regional myofascial pain). The psychological interview, administered by a psychiatrist or pain psychologist (structured or semistructured), can lead to the diagnosis according to the *Diagnostic and Statistical Manual Fifth Edition* (DSM-V) criteria. The DSM-V no longer classifies the manifestations of the chronic pain experience into a "pain disorder" in which just pain is predominant. The pain disorder criteria include the following:

- Pain is in one or more anatomic sites.
- Pain causes clinically significant distress or impairment.
- Psychological factors are judged to play an important role.
- Symptoms are not intentionally produced.
- Pain is not better accounted for by another condition.

Pain disorder can be associated with a psychological and/or a general medical condition.[3]

Treatment

The ultimate goal of a rehabilitation-based approach to chronic pain is the reduction of pain and the restoration of function. The physiatrist plays a critical role in the assessment and management of chronic pain conditions and leads the team of health care professionals in achieving this goal of maximal functional recovery. The treatment of chronic pain conditions has been practiced according to a number of different patient care models. Regardless of the setting, recent data suggest that chronic pain management is best addressed with a biopsychosocial assessment and approach to treatment.[94,148] The traditional biomedical model fails because it focuses on the identification and treatment of a specific anatomic pain generator without accounting for the psychological determinants involved in the pain experience. The treatment goals of chronic pain management encompass the acceptance and reduction of pain, maximal restoration of functional mobility, restoration of sleep, improvement in mood, return to leisure activity, and return to work (Box 37-2).

Pain Treatment Programs

The IASP classifies four types of pain treatment programs (Table 37-6).[82] In general, multidisciplinary treatment centers or clinics might or might not include a formal

BOX 37-2

Chronic Pain Management: Goals of Treatment

- Maximize and maintain physical activity and function.
- Reduce the misuse or abuse of dependency-producing medications, invasive procedures, and passive modalities, fostered by a change toward active patient self-management.
- Return to previous levels of activity at home, in the workplace, and in leisure pursuits.
- Reduce subjective reported pain intensity and maladaptive pain behaviors.
- Assist patients in obtaining resolution and/or closure of contentious work-related or litigation aspects of the pain condition.

Table 37-6 Classification of Pain Treatment Centers

	Multidisciplinary Pain Center	Multidisciplinary Pain Clinic	Pain Clinic	Modality-Oriented Clinic
Comprehensive assessment and management	Yes	Yes	Yes	No
Physicians	Multispecialty	Multispecialty	Single specialty	Single specialty
Psychologists	Yes	Yes	Variable	No
Other health care professionals	Physical, occupational, recreation therapists; nurses; biofeedback, relaxation specialists; movement-based therapy practitioners; vocational counselors; other specialists	Physical, occupational, recreation therapists; nurses; biofeedback, relaxation specialists; movement-based therapy practitioners; vocational counselors; other specialists	Variable	No
Therapeutic modalities	Multiple	Multiple	Variable	Focused
Affiliation	Major health science institutions	Variable	Variable	Variable
Research and educational activity	Yes	Variable, not typical	Variable, not typical	Variable, not typical
General or specific focus of care	Comprehensive, acute and chronic pain	Comprehensive, chronic pain	Specific, chronic pain (i.e., regional focus such as headaches)	Specific, acute and chronic pain (i.e., nerve block clinics)

interdisciplinary collaboration model. Although the terms *multidisciplinary* and *interdisciplinary* are many times used interchangeably, multidisciplinary more formally refers to collaboration with members of different disciplines (including various medical specialists and therapists) managed by a leader who directs a range of ancillary services. Team members assess and treat patients independently and then share information. Interdisciplinary describes a deeper level of a consensus-based collaboration in which the entire process (i.e., evaluation, goal setting, and treatment delivery) is orchestrated by the team, facilitated by regular face-to-face meetings, and primarily delivered within a single facility. Many multidisciplinary and interdisciplinary program facilities can be accredited by the Commission on Accreditation of Rehabilitation Facilities, with established treatment standards and ongoing outcome measurement. The interdisciplinary team is commonly led by a physiatrist or other pain specialist and includes physical and occupational therapists, pain psychologists, relaxation training experts, vocational rehabilitation and therapeutic recreational specialists, social workers, and nurse educators (Box 37-3). A key process in multidisciplinary treatment is the comprehensive evaluation. This usually incorporates a thorough musculoskeletal evaluation, psychological assessment, and, in patients with work-related injuries, a vocational rehabilitation interview. The evaluation enables the team to assess patient motivation and realistic goals for return to function and/or work. Those patients accepted for treatment are placed in a structured outpatient environment with one-on-one and group-based treatments.

Interdisciplinary and Multidisciplinary Approaches

Interdisciplinary Treatment

Interdisciplinary biopsychosocial rehabilitation-based programs have been increasingly and successfully used in the treatment of patients with chronic pain and related psychosocial dysfunction.[59,118] Comprehensive reviews of the clinical and cost-effectiveness of interdisciplinary programs have demonstrated significant improvements in return to work, function, reduced health care use, and closure of disability claims.[148] Positive functional results have been shown in patients classified as having both short-term and long-term disability at the onset of care.[70] These comprehensive programs have also shown clear benefits over conventional management with regard to decreasing pain behavior and improving mood.

Scope and intensity varies, with most outpatient-based centers offering part-time (2 days per week) or full-time (5 days per week, 6 to 8 hours per day) programs lasting 4 to 6 weeks in total duration. The interdisciplinary model provides ongoing communication for all members of the treatment team, helping to facilitate patient progress while they progress the behavioral, cognitive, and active therapy treatments. Patients are discussed individually in a team conference format on a weekly basis, enabling ongoing communication of progress and adjustment of treatment goals. Physician follow-up visits two or three times per week are ideal for ongoing pharmacologic trials (targeted for improving mood, disturbed sleep, and analgesia) and encouraging progress across the multiple therapy domains. Desirable attributes of interdisciplinary treatment programs have been described by multidisciplinary associations, including the American Pain Society.[151] At completion of treatment, patients are encouraged to continue with their own individually structured home exercise, aerobic, and stretching program. They should also be independent in their own use of various relaxation and pacing techniques. The identification of a chronic pain condition as a chronic *disease* imparts an important facet into the continued care of these patients. As with a chronic disease such as diabetes or hypertension, self-control and self-management of symptoms are crucial for successful treatment. It logically follows that chronic pain should be treated as any other chronic disease or illness, in that regular follow-up evaluation and reassessment of psychosocial and physical function be performed.[77]

BOX 37-3

Interdisciplinary Pain Team Members

- Physiatrist
- Physical therapist
- Occupational therapist
- Pain psychologist
- Social worker
- Recreational therapist
- Biofeedback specialist
- Nursing educator
- Vocational counselor

Multidisciplinary Team

Physical Therapy and Occupational Therapy. Physical and occupational therapists use active and passive therapeutic exercises, manual techniques, and passive physical modalities (Table 37-7) to address deficits in flexibility, strength, balance, neuromuscular control, posture, functional mobility, locomotion, and endurance. Both types of therapists help patients to overcome fear of movement. Although there is some crossover between the skill sets of physical and occupational therapists, they possess established core competencies that are fairly universal. Physical therapists specialize in gait training and locomotion, core stability, lower extremity biomechanics, and functional mobility, as well as activities of daily living such as bed mobility and transfers. They are also experts in the development of aerobic conditioning programs aimed at improving cardiopulmonary health and endurance. Occupational therapists typically concentrate on educating patients regarding proper posture and ergonomics related to upper limb functional activities such as lifting and computer usage. They address upper extremity-related activities of daily living including feeding, hygiene, grooming, bathing, and dressing. Physical and occupational therapists also play a primary role in the education of patients, family members, and other caregivers.

Physical and occupational therapists involved in interdisciplinary chronic pain treatment programs must be adept in their ability to assess initial levels of functional ability and then monitor and progressively increase the

Table 37-7 Modalities Used in the Treatment of Chronic Pain

Modality	Superficial or Deep	Mechanism of Action	Example	Indication	Precautions and Contraindications
Heat	Superficial	Conduction	Hydrocollator packs	Pain, contracture, hematoma, muscle spasm, arthritis, before stretching program to increase collagen extensibility	Acute trauma, hemorrhage, bleeding diathesis, impaired sensation, altered thermal regulation, malignancy, ischemia, cognitive deficits, or inability to report pain
		Conduction	Paraffin baths		
		Convection	Whirlpool baths		
		Convection	Fluid therapy		
	Deep	Conversion	Ultrasound		
		Conversion	Shortwave diathermy		
		Conversion	Microwave		
Cold	Superficial	Conduction	Ice	Pain, acute trauma, acute inflammation, joint effusion, hemorrhage, muscle spasm, spasticity	Cold hypersensitivity, ischemia, impaired sensation, cognitive deficits, areas over superficial peripheral nerves, Raynaud phenomenon or disease, cryoglobulinemia, arterial vascular disease
		Conduction	Cold packs		
		Conduction	Cryotherapy-compression units		
		Convection	Whirlpool baths		
		Evaporative	Vapocoolant spray		
Electrical stimulation	Superficial	Gate control, endogenous opioid release, direct peripheral effects	Transcutaneous electrical nerve stimulation	Rheumatoid arthritis, osteoarthritis, deafferentation pain syndromes, visceral pain, sympathetically mediated pain, tension headache, acute postoperative pain, Raynaud disease, ischemic pain, urogenital dysfunction	Demand-type cardiac pacemaker; carotid sinus, laryngeal or pharyngeal muscles, eyes, and mucosal membranes; cognitive deficits; abdominal, lumbosacral, or pelvic areas of pregnant women; edema; open wounds or skin irritation
		Direct stimulation of muscle fibers	Interferential current therapy		

level and complexity of therapeutic exercises. The majority of patients with chronic pain have secondary impairments in addition to their primary pain-related diagnoses (i.e., general inflexibility, deconditioning, myofascial pain, and other postural abnormalities), which are important focuses of treatment. A functional cognitive behaviorally mediated therapeutic approach might be necessary to maximize outcomes. This approach can help foster patient optimism, decrease fear of reinjury, and maximize patient compliance.

Psychology. Pain psychology assessment and therapeutic interventions focus on both cognitive and behavioral factors related to pain. As noted earlier, key psychological factors involved in the development of and adaptation to chronic pain include anxiety and fear-avoidance behavior,[74] pain catastrophizing,[143] and helplessness. Factors identified with improvement in adjustment to chronic pain include self-efficacy, pain-coping strategies, readiness to change, and acceptance. Psychological intervention focuses on unlearning maladaptive responses and reactions to pain, while fostering self-efficacy, wellness, improved coping, perceived control, decreased catastrophizing, and acceptance (Figure 37-4).[74] Phases of individual and group-based treatment include education, skills training, application, and relapse prevention.

Relaxation training can be provided by a number of team disciplines, including psychology, physical therapy, nursing, or certified biofeedback specialists. Formal techniques include guided relaxation response training (guided imagery, visual or auditory guided biofeedback), meditation, and hypnosis. These techniques help to encourage the patient's role as an active participant in ongoing self-management (see the section on mind-body medicine in this chapter).

Vocational Rehabilitation. The Centers for Medicare and Medicaid Services define vocational rehabilitation as "the process of facilitating an individual in the choice of or return to a suitable vocation."[25] Title I of the Rehabilitation Act of 1973 describes the goods or services provided to render an individual with a handicap employable. Vocational rehabilitation counselors should be involved with patient care early in the process of chronic pain management to ensure identification of employment as a long-term goal for the patient.

Vocational counselors participate in the analysis of current or previous job descriptions, provide suggestions for work accommodation or modification and, if necessary, facilitate vocational testing and targeted retraining. At the end of the rehabilitation process, vocational rehabilitation can help coordinate functional capacity evaluation

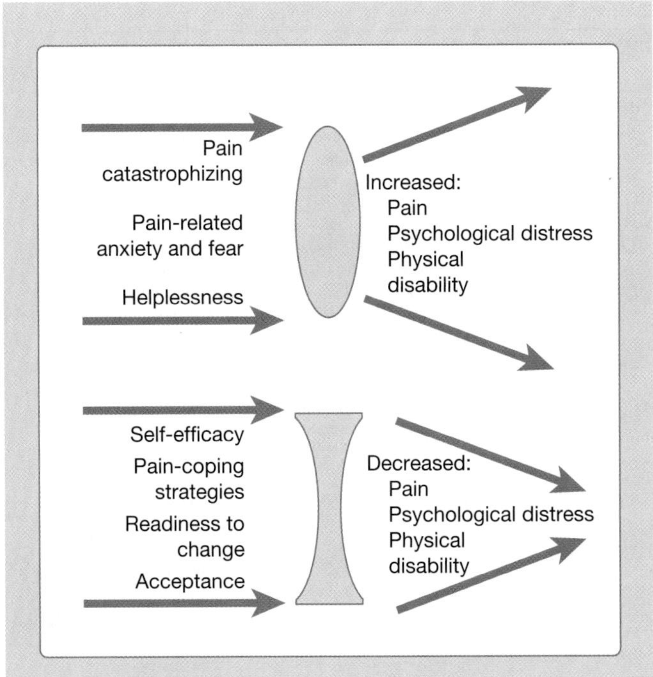

FIGURE 37-4 **Factors associated with adjustment to pain.** (Modified from Keefe FJ, Rumble ME, Scipio CD, et al: Psychological aspects of persistent pain: current state of the science, *J Pain* 5:195-211, 2004, with permission.)

testing and finalize return to work issues (i.e., restrictions and level of work). Vocational rehabilitation counselors acquire information from the physical therapists, occupational therapists, and physicians to address instructions as to limitation of duty (full or limited) and the functional restrictions or modifications that might be required. These restrictions or modifications include sitting or standing tolerance, walking, pushing, pulling, stair usage, bending at the waist, sustained postures, hot or cold tolerance, data entry or other repetitive tasks, grip, tool usage, and vibration factors.

Nurse Facilitator. The program nurse or nursing staff member plays an essential role in coordinating patient progress and care during evaluation, treatment, and ongoing follow-up evaluation. Nursing plays a crucial role in educational aspects of treatment, including basic instruction on pain pathways, pharmacology, nutrition, and sleep hygiene. The nurse facilitator can also serve as a patient advocate in ongoing communication with all team members.

Medications

Pharmacotherapy is a crucial component in the treatment of chronic pain conditions. The importance of specific treatment targets can vary considerably from those addressed in acute pain treatment paradigms. Whereas acute pain treatment primarily focuses on analgesia and control of inflammation, drug therapy in chronic pain states requires a more comprehensive focus including mood and sleep disturbances. A mechanistic approach to rational pharmacology is an important component of the practitioner's armamentarium for managing the diverse nature of chronic pain. This approach incorporates the use of oral and topical medications, including traditional and newer-generation antidepressants, anticonvulsants, sleep agents, nonopioid analgesics, antiinflammatories, and, in selected cases, chronic opioid therapy.

This section reviews current updates in pharmacotherapy because it applies to a broad range of chronic pain conditions, including neuropathic pain and manifestations of chronic pain conditions (e.g., pain, affective distress, and sleep disturbance). The section includes an overview related to controversies in the use of cyclooxygenase-2 (COX-2) inhibitors and pharmacologic use of opioids, tricyclic antidepressants (TCAs), novel antidepressants, anticonvulsant medications, sleep-related drugs, and topical analgesics.

Nonsteroidal Antiinflammatory Drugs and Cyclooxygenase-2 Inhibitors

Conventional (i.e., nonspecific) nonsteroidal antiinflammatory drugs (NSAIDs) have been a first-line treatment for analgesia and the treatment of inflammatory conditions, including osteoarthritis, rheumatoid arthritis, and the various musculoskeletal-related conditions.[153] COX-1 and COX-2 isoforms catalyze the conversion of arachidonic acid to prostaglandins. More recent classification of NSAIDs is as follows:

- Conventional or nonselective NSAIDs; those that inhibit both the COX-1 isoenzyme and the COX-2 isoenzyme.
- NSAIDs that are more selective for the COX-2 isoenzyme (COX-2 inhibitors).

Conventional nonselective NSAIDs were found to offer effective analgesic responses but are limited by potential upper gastrointestinal bleeding and ulceration, renal toxicity, and platelet dysfunction (Table 37-8). The isolation of the COX-2 protein in the early 1990s led to the development and release of a new class of NSAIDs, the COX-2 inhibitors. Pharmacologic studies suggested that COX-1 was constitutively expressed in most tissues, being responsible for homeostatic functions such as platelet aggregation and the maintenance of upper gastrointestinal mucosa integrity by producing protective prostaglandins. COX-2, a largely "inducible" constitutive isoenzyme, was proposed to be primarily responsible for producing inflammation and pain. Additional studies suggested that COX-2 was induced in early inflammation and neuropathic pain states and was related to both peripheral and central sensitization. Major studies of specific COX-2 inhibitors have demonstrated significant safety benefits of these agents as compared with nonselective NSAIDs, including reduced incidence of symptomatic gastric ulcers and renal toxicity.[13,34] Reevaluation of these studies, however, has demonstrated possible greater toxicity of COX-2 agents, leading to voluntary removal of many of the compounds from the market.[107] In response to a greater appreciation for possible cardiac, gastrointestinal, and bleeding effects of COX-2 inhibitors and "nonselective NSAIDs," the U.S. Food and Drug Administration (FDA) established class effect warnings in 2004 for all NSAID-related compounds (i.e., COX-2 inhibitors, NSAIDs, aspirin). Today, package inserts for all NSAIDs (oral and topical, prescription, and

Table 37-8 Commonly Prescribed Nonsteroidal Antiinflammatory Medications

Class	Generic Name (Trade Name)	Dose (Older Adult/Adult)	Half-Life (Onset)	Mechanism of Action	Other
Cyclooxygenase-2 (COX-2) inhibitors	Celecoxib (Celebrex)	100/100-200 mg twice daily or 200 mg daily	9-10 hr (<60 min)	Suppresses prostaglandin synthesis; selective COX-2 inhibition; analgesic, antipyretic, and antiinflammatory actions	Does not inhibit platelet aggregation; crosses placenta; sulfonamide moiety
Oxicam derivatives	Meloxicam (Mobic)	7.5/7.5-15 mg daily	15-20 hr	Prostaglandin synthetase inhibition; some selectivity for COX-2; analgesic, antipyretic, and antiinflammatory actions	Does not generally affect platelet counts, prothrombin time, or partial thromboplastin time; patients with coagulation disorders or patients receiving anticoagulants should be carefully monitored
Propionic acid derivatives	Ibuprofen (Motrin, Advil, Ibuprin, Nuprin, Rufen, Saleto)	200/200-800 mg four times daily	2-4 hr (30 min)	Reversible nonselective COX inhibitor—inhibits formation of prostaglandin and thromboxane A_2; various effects on leukotriene production; inhibition of platelet aggregation	Analgesic action at doses <1600 mg/day; doses >1600 mg/day needed for antiinflammatory action; available in over-the-counter preparation
	Naproxen (Anaprox, Naprelan, Naprosyn, Aleve)	250/250-500 mg twice daily; acute pain 1.5 g/day in divided doses	12-15 hr (60 min)	Reversible nonselective COX inhibitor—inhibits formation of prostaglandin and thromboxane A_2; various effects on leukotriene production; inhibition of platelet aggregation	Available in over-the-counter preparations
Acetic acid derivatives	Etodolac (Lodine)	400/400-600 mg twice daily	7.3 hr (30 min)	Reversible nonselective COX inhibitor—inhibits formation of prostaglandin and thromboxane A_2; various effects on leukotriene production; inhibition of platelet aggregation	Relative COX-2 activity
	Ketorolac (Toradol, Acular [ophthalmic])	Intramuscular single dose 30/60 mg; intramuscular multidose (maximum 5 days) 15/30 mg every 6 hr (maximum 120 mg/day)	2.4-8.6 hr (10 min intramuscularly)	Reversible nonselective COX inhibitor—inhibits formation of prostaglandin and thromboxane A_2; various effects on leukotriene production; inhibition of platelet aggregation	Also available in intravenous, ophthalmic, and oral formulations; oral indicated only for continuation of parenteral therapy; not for chronic use—total treatment should exceed 5 days
	Diclofenac (Cataflam, Voltaren, Solaraze; with misoprostol, Arthrotec)	50 mg twice daily/50 mg 2 to 4 times daily, or 75 mg twice daily	2 hr (30 min)	Reversible nonselective COX inhibitor—inhibits formation of prostaglandin and thromboxane A_2; various effects on leukotriene production; inhibition of platelet aggregation	Alternate formulation; diclofenac with misoprostol (Arthrotec)
Salicylate derivatives	Aspirin (Aspirin CR, Easprin, Ascriptin, Bayer, Ecotrin, Empirin, Bufferin)	325/325-650 mg/day (maximum 4 g/day)	3-6 hr (15-30 min)	Inhibition of prostaglandin synthesis and release, formation of thromboxane A_2; inhibition of platelet aggregation	Therapeutic response may take 2 weeks for arthritis treatment
	Salsalate (Amigesic, Disalcid, Argesic-SA, Salflex, Mono-Gesic, Salsitab)	500/500-750 mg 2 or 3 times daily (maximum 3 g/day)	7-8 hr	Inhibition of prostaglandin synthesis	Does not inhibit platelet aggregation; onset of antiinflammatory action in 3-4 days

Table 37-8 Commonly Prescribed Nonsteroidal Antiinflammatory Medications (Continued)

Class	Generic Name (Trade Name)	Dose (Older Adult/Adult)	Half-Life (Onset)	Mechanism of Action	Other
Para-aminophenol derivatives	Acetaminophen (Tylenol, Panadol, Neopap, Apacet, Acephen)	325-1000 mg every 4-6 hr (4 g daily maximum)	3-4 hr (10-30 min)	COX inhibitor in central nervous system, analgesic and antipyretic, no antiinflammatory properties	Several adverse effects include hepatic and renal failure; available in alternate forms (rectal, drops, elixir)
Barbituric acid derivatives	Butalbital compounds (butalbital plus acetaminophen or aspirin plus caffeine); with acetaminophen and caffeine (Fioricet, Medigesic, Endolor, Americet); with codeine (Fioricet with codeine); with acetaminophen (Phrenilin, Triaprin); with acetylsalicylic acid and caffeine (Fiorinal, Farbital); with codeine (Fiorinal with codeine)	1 or 2 tablets every 4 hr (maximum 6 tablets/day)	3-4 hr	Analgesic properties of acetaminophen, aspirin, caffeine; anxiolytic and muscle relaxant properties of butalbital	Risk of psychological or physical dependence

over-the-counter products) include a boxed warning to highlight the potential increased risk of cardiovascular events and the risk of serious and potentially life-threatening gastrointestinal bleeding.[145]

A number of topical diclofenac preparations have been approved in the United States for the management of sprains and strains (diclofenac epolamine [Flector] patch 1.3%), pain related to osteoarthritis in joints amenable to topicals (diclofenac sodium [Voltaren] gel 1%), and pain related to osteoarthritis of the knee (diclofenac sodium solution 1.5%). These topical preparations and over-the-counter products all carry the identical black box warning, although systemic effects of topical agents are much less than oral preparations (5% to 10%). Physicians need to assess relative risks versus potential benefits (analgesia, decreased stiffness, and improved function) on a case-by-case basis. Ongoing monitoring of blood pressure, cardiac, and renal status is recommended with acute and chronic use of both nonselective NSAIDs and selective COX-2 inhibitors.[113]

Opioid Analgesics

Opioid and opioid-like medications are potent analgesics (Table 37-9). Opioids work by binding to three receptor types (μ, δ, and κ) belonging to a G-protein receptor family. Presynaptic effects of opioids decrease calcium into the cell, inhibiting subsequent release of excitatory neurotransmitters (serotonin, norepinephrine, substance P, and glutamate). Postsynaptic effects include increasing potassium efflux, resulting in hyperpolarization of the neuron, decreasing synaptic transmission. At the brainstem level, opioids inhibit GABAergic transmission, leading to excitation of descending inhibition.[63]

Because of the potential risk of abuse, misuse, addiction, diversion, and fatal adverse effects, a "universal precautions" approach should be applied to the management plan for chronic prescribing of opioid analgesics (Box 37-4). Further discussion on opioid management strategies is beyond the focus of this chapter.

BOX 37-4

Universal Precautions in Pain Medicine

1. Diagnosis with appropriate differential.
2. Psychological assessment, including risk of addictive disorder.
3. Informed consent.
4. Treatment agreement.
5. Preintervention and postintervention assessment of pain level and function.
6. Appropriate trial of opioid therapy with/without adjunctive medications.
7. Reassessment of pain score and level of function.
8. Regularly assess the four A's of pain medicine (Analgesia, Activities of daily living, Adverse effects, and Aberrant behavior).
9. Periodically review pain diagnosis and comorbid conditions, including addictive disorders.
10. Documentation.

Anticonvulsant Medications as a Treatment for Neuropathic Pain Conditions

Neuropathic pain has been defined as "pain caused by a lesion or disease of the somatosensory nervous system."[62] Neuropathic pain manifests as spontaneous pain (stimulus-independent, i.e., paresthesia and dysesthesia) or pain hypersensitivity caused by a stimulus after damage or changes in the sensory neurons (stimulus-evoked pain, i.e., allodynia and hyperalgesia).[37] Peripheral mechanisms include sensitization of nociceptors by local chemical inflammatory changes (including substance P, serotonin, bradykinin, histamine, and COX and lipoxygenase pathways); ectopic activity from damaged, demyelinated, or regenerating nerve sprouts; noradrenergic sensitivity; lowering of neuronal threshold for firing at ectopic areas by accumulation of sodium and calcium channels; and changes at the more proximal dorsal root ganglion (i.e.,

Table 37-9 Commonly Prescribed Opioid Analgesics

Class	Name (Trade Name)	Dose (Older Adult/ Adult)	Half-Life (Onset)	Mechanism of Action	Other
Natural opium alkaloids	Morphine (Avinza, Duramorph, Infumorph, Kadian, MS Contin, MSIR, Oramorph SR, RMS, Roxanol)	Oral: 5-30 mg every 4 hr Subcutaneous/ intramuscular: 4-15 mg in 4-5 mL of H_2O for injection over 5 min Rectal: 10-20 mg every 4 hr Oral, sustained release: 15-60 mg every 8-12 hr (based on 24-hr requirements of immediate-release oral MSO_4)	2.5-3 hr (subcutaneous/ intramuscular, 10-30 min; intravenous, rectal or oral suspension)	Opioid agonist activity at multiple receptors; μ (supraspinal analgesia and euphoria), κ (spinal analgesia and sedation), and δ (dysphoria, psychotomimetic effects)	Sustained-release oral form available; epidural or intrathecal injectable solution available: treat overdose with naloxone 0.2-0.8 mg intravenous
	Morphine/naltrexone [sequestered] (Embeda)	Oral (mg morphine/mg naltrexone): 20/0.8, 30/1.2, 50/2; 60/2.4, 80/3.2, 100/4	28.8 hr (T_{max}, 7.5 h)	Opioid agonist activity at multiple receptors: μ, κ, δ	Controlled-release morphine, if crushed, rapid release of morphine and naltrexone may cause decrease liking
	Codeine (with acetaminophen or acetylsalicylic acid) (Tylenol #2, #3, #4; Empirin #3, #4; Robitussin AC; Capital, Aceta, Phenaphen, Fioricet with codeine, Fiorinal with codeine)	Oral: 15-60 mg every 4 hr (maximum daily acetaminophen/ acetylsalicylic acid dose 4 g)	2.5-3.5 hr (orally 30-60 min)	Opioid agonist activity at multiple receptors: μ (supraspinal analgesia and euphoria), κ (spinal analgesia and sedation), and δ (dysphoria, psychotomimetic effects)	Compared with MSO_4: decreased analgesia, constipation, respiratory distress, sedation, emesis, and physical dependence; increased antitussive effects
(Pyridomorphinan)	Oxymorphone ER (Opana ER)	Oral: 5, 7.5, 10, 15, 20, 30, 40 mg	9-11 hr (orally 30 min)		
	Oxymorphone (Opana)	Oral: 5, 10 mg	7-9 hr (orally 30 min)		
Phenanthrene derivatives	Hydrocodone (with acetylsalicylic acid or acetaminophen) (Lortab, Lortab ASA, Vicodin, Norco, Vicoprofen, Entuss-D, Z-Tuss, S-T Forte, P-V-Tussin, Tussanil, Tussafed HC)	Oral: 5-10 mg every 4-6 hr (maximum daily acetaminophen/ acetylsalicylic acid dose 4 g)	3.8 hr (10-30 min)	Opioid agonist activity at multiple receptors: μ (supraspinal analgesia and euphoria), κ (spinal analgesia and sedation), and δ (dysphoria, psychotomimetic effects)	Compared with MSO_4: decreased analgesia, respiratory depression, and physical dependency; equivalent antitussive effects
	Oxycodone (±acetaminophen or acetylsalicylic acid) (OxyContin [CR], Oxy IR, Percolone, OxyFast, Roxicodone); with acetylsalicylic acid (Percodan, Endodan, Roxiprin); with acetaminophen (Percocet, Endocet, Tylox, Roxicet, Roxilox)	Oral: 5 mg every 6 hr (4 g maximum dose of acetylsalicylic acid or acetaminophen) Controlled release: 10, 15, 20, 30, 40, 50, 60, 70, 80 mg every 12 hr	2-5 hr (10-15 min)	Opioid agonist activity at multiple receptors: μ (supraspinal analgesia and euphoria), κ (spinal analgesia and sedation), and δ (dysphoria, psychotomimetic effects)	Compared with MSO_4: equivalent analgesia, constipation, antitussive effects, respiratory depression, sedation, emesis, and physical dependence
	Hydromorphone (Dilaudid) Hydromorphone hydrochloride-ER (Exalgo)	Oral: 1-4 mg every 4-6 hr ER: 8, 12, 16 mg every 24 hr Rectal: 3 mg every 6-8 hr	2.6 hr (<15 min) Exalgo: median T_{max} 12-16 hr	Opioid agonist activity at multiple receptors: μ (supraspinal analgesia and euphoria), κ (spinal analgesia and sedation), and δ (dysphoria, psychotomimetic effects)	Compared with MSO_4: equivalent analgesia, constipation, sedation, respiratory depression; decreased emesis; available in intravenous, intramuscular, and subcutaneous formulations; sustained-release preparation recently FDA-approved with 24-h dose schedule

Table 37-9 Commonly Prescribed Opioid Analgesics (Continued)

Class	Name (Trade Name)	Dose (Older Adult/ Adult)	Half-Life (Onset)	Mechanism of Action	Other
Diphenylheptane derivative	Methadone (Dolophine)	Oral: 2.5-10 mg every 6 hr Subcutaneous/ intramuscular: 2.5-10 mg every 3-4 hr Maintenance of dependency, oral: 20-120 mg/day	13-47 hr (orally 30-60 min; subcutaneously/ intramuscularly 10-20 min)	Opioid agonist activity at multiple receptors: μ (supraspinal analgesia and euphoria), κ (spinal analgesia and sedation), and δ (dysphoria, psychotomimetic effects); NMDA receptor antagonist	Compared with MSO_4: equivalent analgesia, antitussive effects, respiratory distress, and constipation; less sedation, emesis, physical dependence; commonly used for the detoxification and maintenance of opiate dependence; possibly NMDA antagonist effects of reduced central sensitization and reduced opioid tolerance
	Propoxyphene (±acetaminophen) (Darvon, Dolene; Darvon-N); with acetaminophen (Darvocet, Propacet, Wygesic)	Oral: 65 mg every 4 hr (maximum 390 mg/ day) Napsylate: 100 mg every 4 hr (maximum 600 mg/day)	6-12 hr (15-60 min)	Opioid agonist activity at multiple receptors: μ (supraspinal analgesia and euphoria), κ (spinal analgesia and sedation), and δ (dysphoria, psychotomimetic effects)	Compared with MSO_4: less analgesia, sedation, emesis, respiratory depression, and physical dependence
Phenylpiperidine derivative	Fentanyl (Sublimaze); transdermal (Duragesic); transmucosal (Actiq, Oralet)	Transdermal: 25/25-100 μg/h every 72 hr Transmucosal: 200, 400, 600, 800, 1200, 1400, 1600 μg	2.5-4 hr (orally 5-15 min; intramuscularly, 7-15 min; intravenously, 1-2 min) Transdermal: half-life 17 hr after patch removal, steady state at 24 hr	Opioid agonist activity at multiple receptors: μ (supraspinal analgesia and euphoria), κ (spinal analgesia and sedation), and δ (dysphoria, psychotomimetic effects)	Compared with MSO_4: equivalent analgesia; less respiratory depression and emesis; transdermal delivery for use in chronic pain—other forms used for perioperative anesthesia
Other	Tapentadol (Nucynta)	Oral: 50, 75, 100 mg	4 hr (orally T_{max} 1.2 hr)	Opioid agonist activity at multiple receptors and norepinephrine reuptake inhibition	

ER, Extended release; *FDA*, U.S. Food and Drug Administration; *NMDA*, N-methyl-D-aspartate; T_{max}, time after administration of drug when maximum plasma concentration is reached.

spontaneous activity).[7] Peripheral changes can also lead to loss of central GABAergic inhibition, opioid receptor downregulation, and interneuron cell death.[162] Central nervous system changes are primarily caused by phenotypic changes of Aβ and C fibers, sprouting of nerve fibers in deeper layers of dorsal horn laminae,[167] and effects of central sensitization. Central sensitization is primarily mediated by the release of neurotransmitters (e.g., substance P, glutamate, CGRP, neurokinin A, and GABA), increased calcium flux, and activation of NMDA receptors.[137]

Understanding the basic physiologic neurotransmitter changes can help target the use of a single or a number of anticonvulsants in the management of chronic neuropathic pain states, including postherpetic neuralgia, diabetic peripheral neuropathy, spinal radiculopathy, trigeminal neuralgia, human immunodeficiency virus (HIV)-related neuropathic pain states, and small-fiber neuropathy. Recent treatment recommendations highlight the importance of a mechanistic approach to diagnosis and treatment, as well as to proposed first-line medications (i.e., gabapentin, 5% lidocaine [lignocaine] patch, opioid analgesics, tramadol, and TCAs) based on positive results from multiple randomized trials, and to second-line agents based on positive results from a single randomized controlled trial or inconsistent finding. Second-line agents in some cases have shown greater efficacy but are awaiting future randomized controlled trials.[37]

First-generation anticonvulsants include phenytoin, phenobarbital, carbamazepine, and valproic acid. Phenytoin and carbamazepine exert membrane-stabilizing effects by blocking sodium channels and reducing neuronal excitability, presumably in sensitized C nociceptors.[36] The use of newer-generation anticonvulsants has made their incorporation into outpatient management more practical, given their more favorable metabolic and interaction profiles compared with traditional anticonvulsants. Most of the anticonvulsant agents have been used off-label, except those with FDA approval: The 5% lidocaine patch (Lidoderm) and gabapentin (Neurontin) are approved for postherpetic neuralgia. Pregabalin (Lyrica) is approved for postherpetic neuralgia, neuropathic pain associated with diabetic peripheral neuropathy or spinal cord injury, and fibromyalgia. Carbamazepine (Tegretol) is approved for the treatment of pain associated with trigeminal neuralgia.

Gabapentin has also found wide off-label use for a number of chronic neuropathic pain conditions. Randomized, double-blind, placebo-controlled studies have demonstrated efficacy with analgesia in diabetic peripheral neuropathy (titrated from 900 to 3600 mg/day)[5] and postherpetic neuralgia.[122] Gabapentin enacarbil extended release tablets are indicated for the management of postherpetic neuralgia. Gabapentin, although structurally related to GABA, is an $\alpha_2\delta$ ligand. The $\alpha_2\delta$ receptor is a protein associated with neuronal voltage-gated calcium channels. Binding to this channel reduces presynaptic calcium influx into the cell at the dorsal horn, reducing the release of several neurotransmitters (glutamate, substance P, norepinephrine, and CGRP). A number of indirect GABAergic mechanisms have also been proposed. Multiple studies have demonstrated significantly reduced pain and improved sleep, mood, and quality of life at doses between 1800 and 3600 mg/day. Side effects include somnolence and dizziness. The unique pharmacokinetics of gabapentin lend to the necessity of using higher doses compared with other newer-generation anticonvulsants. With escalating dose titration, the intestinal active transport absorption system becomes saturated, decreasing the percentage of bioavailability, resulting in a nonlinear relationship between serum concentration and dose.

Pregabalin is also an $\alpha_2\delta$ ligand and is structurally related to gabapentin but with no intrinsic GABA activity. Studies have demonstrated efficacy in the management of postherpetic neuralgia,[125] diabetic peripheral neuropathy,[47] general peripheral neuropathy,[64] and generalized anxiety disorder[38] with doses between 150 and 600 mg/day. Pregabalin demonstrates linear pharmacokinetics and has a rapid onset of actions (within 1 hour), stable bioavailability independent of dose (approximately 90%), and an affinity for the $\alpha_2\delta$ subunit that is six times greater than that of gabapentin. Pregabalin appears to work by modulating voltage-gated calcium channels, decreasing calcium influx into the cell, and limiting release of excitatory neurotransmitters (substance P, glutamate, aspartate, and norepinephrine).[43] The relatively increased potency, linear pharmacokinetics, and stable bioavailability of pregabalin, compared with gabapentin, might diminish the need for prolonged dose titration.

Lamotrigine blocks voltage-dependent sodium channels and N-type calcium channels, and inhibits glutamate release.[58] Doses range from 50 to 400 mg/day. Efficacy has been demonstrated in studies of patients with trigeminal neuralgia[168] and central poststroke pain[155] resistant to other therapies. A recent Cochrane review of Lamotrigine for acute and chronic pain suggested that Lamotrigine at doses of approximately 200 to 400 mg daily was not effective in treating acute or chronic pain.[168]

Oxcarbazepine is an analogue of carbamazepine, without the epoxide metabolite. It is thought that the epoxide metabolite is a possible contributor to drug interactions and adverse events associated with carbamazepine use.[96] Oxcarbazepine has shown efficacy in patients with postherpetic neuralgia, trigeminal neuralgia, and diabetic peripheral neuropathy at doses averaging between 600 and 1200 mg/day. Side effects may be prohibitive to treatment in a large percentage of patients.[23] Tiagabine is a novel selective GABA reuptake inhibitor, indicated for partial seizures, that has also been used off-label for chronic neuropathic pain, anxiety, and insomnia. Theoretically, increasing GABA levels at the synaptic cleft (dorsal horn and brain) might help to increase the inhibitory effects of GABA on neuronal excitability. Increased GABA levels have been associated with improved sleep, characterized by increasing time in NREM stage 3 and 4 sleep.[87]

Topiramate and zonisamide are broad-spectrum anticonvulsants with a number of proposed mechanisms, including inhibition of voltage-gated sodium channels, potentiation of GABAergic inhibition, and blocking excitatory glutamate activity and voltage-gated calcium channels. Inhibition of carbonic anhydrase and antiglutamate effects have been considered as mechanisms responsible for the clinically significant weight loss associated with these medications.[16,48] The mechanism of levetiracetam, an agent with a chemical structure unrelated to that of other anticonvulsants, remains unclear but might include calcium channel effects.[83] It is similar to gabapentin, having minimal drug-drug interactions, and is easily renally excreted.

Antidepressants

Antidepressants have demonstrated mixed efficacy in a number of chronic pain-related conditions (i.e., nociceptive, neuropathic, inflammatory, poststroke pain conditions, central pain states, and headache) and chronic pain-related disorders (i.e., depression, anxiety, and insomnia).[31] Antidepressants can be divided into general classes: TCAs, selective serotonin reuptake inhibitors (SSRIs), selective serotonin-norepinephrine reuptake inhibitors (SNRIs), and triazolopyridines (i.e., trazodone and nefazodone). Analgesic effects of antidepressants have primarily been associated with peripheral and central norepinephrine and serotonin effects, but might also involve binding to opioid and NMDA receptor complexes, reducing intracellular Ca^{2+} accumulation, as well as binding to α-adrenoceptors and a number of ion channels (i.e., Na^+, Ca^{2+}, and K^+).[129] Emotional and painful symptoms of depression might be regulated by overlapping pathways for serotonin and norepinephrine at the brain and spinal cord, affecting mood, sleep, coping, and painful symptoms. A more divergent view of transmitter effects has also suggested that the noradrenergic system is involved with motivational activities, including energy, interest, and concentration, compared with serotonergic systems influencing behavioral activity (i.e., sexual function, appetite, and impulsiveness).[33]

Tricyclic Antidepressants and Selective Serotonin Reuptake Inhibitors. Tricyclic antidepressants have been found to be effective in controlled trials for a variety of chronic pain conditions.[84] Their use as both potent antidepressants and sedating medications can fit into a number of therapeutic targets related to symptom management of chronic pain syndrome (e.g., pain, depression, and disturbed sleep) (Table 37-10). Doses of these medications initially at night can be of benefit for the relatively potent serotonergic, noradrenergic, and antihistaminergic effects. Noradrenergic side effects can be associated with

Table 37-10 Commonly Used Medications for the Treatment of Disturbed Sleep

Class	Drug	Typical Dose (Older Adult/ Adult)	Half-Life	Mechanism of Action	Comments
Nonbenzodiazepine hypnotics	Zaleplon (Sonata)	5/10 mg	1 hr	Interacts with GABA-benzodiazepine complex to facilitate GABA transmission	Especially suitable for sleep initiation disorders
	Zolpidem (Ambien)	5/10 mg	2-4 hr	Interacts with GABA-benzodiazepine complex to facilitate GABA transmission	Useful for initiation of sleep; few residual effects with doses up to 30 mg
	Eszopiclone (Lunesta)	2/3 mg	4-6 hr	Exact mechanism unknown; interacts with GABA-benzodiazepine complex to facilitate GABA transmission	Binds BZD-I receptor with greater affinity than benzodiazepines; FDA-approved for long-term management of insomnia
Benzodiazepines	Triazolam (Halcion)	0.125/0.25 mg	1.5-5.5 hr	Enhances inhibitory action of GABA	Useful for initiation of sleep; anterograde amnesia with higher doses; no active metabolites
	Temazepam (Restoril)	7.5-15/15-30 mg	8-15 hr	Enhances inhibitory action of GABA	Useful for initiation of sleep; intermediate duration; no active metabolites
	Lorazepam (Ativan)	0.5-1/1-2 mg	12-15 hr	Enhances inhibitory action of GABA	No active metabolites; not marketed as a hypnotic
	Flurazepam (Dalmane)	7.5-15/15-30 mg	30-100 hr	Enhances inhibitory action of GABA	Risk of significant accumulation, especially in the older adult population
Tricyclic antidepressants: tertiary amines	Doxepin (Sinequan, Adapin)	25/50-100 mg	8-24 hr	Serotonin > noradrenaline (norepinephrine) reuptake inhibition, strong anticholinergic effect, antagonize α_2 and H_1 receptors, Na^+ channel blockade	Sedative effect at lower doses than antidepressant effect
	Amitriptyline (Elavil); with chlordiazepoxide (Limbitrol); with perphenazine (Triavil)	25/50-100 mg	10-28 hr (nortriptyline metabolite 18-60 hr)	Serotonin > noradrenaline (norepinephrine) reuptake inhibition, strong anticholinergic effect, antagonize α_2 and H_1 receptors, Na^+ channel blockade	Beneficial for patients with depression and early morning awakening; neuropathic pain; strong anticholinergic action; sedative effect at lower doses than antidepressant effect
	Imipramine (Tofranil, Tofranil PM)	10/25-75 mg	6-20 hr	Serotonin > noradrenaline (norepinephrine) reuptake inhibition, strong anticholinergic effect, antagonize α_2 and H_1 receptors Na^+ channel blockade	Sedative effect at lower doses than antidepressant effect
Tricyclic antidepressants: secondary amines	Nortriptyline (Aventyl, Pamelor)	10/25 mg	28-31 hr	Serotonin > noradrenaline (norepinephrine) reuptake inhibition, anticholinergic effects, antagonize α_2 and H_1 receptors, Na^+ channel blockade	Less sedation and fewer anticholinergic effects
	Desipramine (Norpramin)	10/25 mg	14-62 hr	Noradrenaline (norepinephrine) > serotonin reuptake inhibition, anticholinergic effects, antagonize α_2 and H_1 receptors, Na^+ blockade	Less sedation and fewer anticholinergic effects
Triazolopyridine derivatives	Trazodone (Desyrel)	25/50-100 mg	Biphasic (3-6 h, 5-9 hr)	Serotonin receptor antagonist, serotonin reuptake inhibition	Shorter half-life than tricyclic antidepressants; lower anticholinergic profile
Nonprescription antihistamines	Diphenhydramine (Benadryl, Banaril, Dytuss, Hyrexin), with acetaminophen (Excedrin PM, Tylenol PM, Sominex Pain Relief)	12.5/25-50 mg	3.5-17.5 hr	Antihistamine, H_1 receptor	Mild sedation; effect may be lost after 3-4 days of use; strong anticholinergic effects

BZD-I, Benzodiazepine-I; *GABA*, γ-aminobutyric acid, *FDA*, U.S. Food and Drug Administration.

autonomic (i.e., orthostatic hypotension, dizziness, and urinary retention), cardiac (i.e., tachycardia), and ocular (i.e., blurred vision) disturbances. Serotonergic effects can include increased gastric distress, agitation, and headaches.[112] Antihistamine-mediated effects can include decreased gastric acid secretion and sedation. The so-called serotonin syndrome[139] is a rare, reversible clinical syndrome and medical emergency associated with toxic serum and cerebrospinal fluid levels of serotonin. The syndrome is characterized by mental state dysfunction and autonomic and neurologic symptoms, and can occur with concomitant use of TCAs and other medications, including SNRIs, SSRIs,[104] and tramadol (a synthetic codeine analogue with noradrenergic and serotonergic effects).[55]

Analgesic effects of TCAs can be evident within 1 week of dose initiation, followed later by antidepressant effects with escalating dose titration.[84] Although SSRI use has surpassed the use of traditional antidepressants because of a more tolerable side effect profile, analgesic effects of these compounds have been mixed in a number of controlled studies, including diabetic peripheral neuropathy[88,132] and fibromyalgia.[163] Studies involving the use of triazolopyridines, which are compounds with similar chemical properties to those of TCAs (including trazodone and nefazodone), have demonstrated little to no analgesic effects, although they can be beneficial in restoring sleep.[32] A more rational polypharmacy approach can include the use of SSRIs with doses in the morning in conjunction with a more sedating TCA or TCA-like medication at night for pain-related insomnia.

Serotonin-Norepinephrine Reuptake Inhibitors. The newest class of antidepressants, dual monoamine reuptake inhibitors, was developed for the treatment of depression with a goal of providing shorter onset of antidepressant effects and fewer side effects as a result of their relative serotonin and norepinephrine selectivity. Mirtazapine is a potent antagonist of central α_2-adrenergic receptors, an antagonist of 5-HT_2 and 5-HT_3 receptors, and an enhancer of norepinephrine and serotonin neurotransmission. Mirtazapine is indicated for the treatment of depression and can be used to enhance the efficacy of SSRIs. Its relatively sedating effects can have additional benefits for improving sleep in patients with chronic pain. Venlafaxine is a potent dual reuptake inhibitor of serotonin (at lower doses) and of norepinephrine and possibly dopamine (at higher doses), without binding to cholinergic, histaminic, or α_1-adrenergic receptor sites. Analgesic effects have been found in animal models[78] and in human studies, including a number of case reports and case series of heterogeneous chronic pain conditions,[135] neuropathic pain states,[146] and fibromyalgia.

Duloxetine is a potent balanced reuptake inhibitor of both serotonin and norepinephrine and demonstrates a higher affinity for monoamine transporters compared with venlafaxine.[21] In the United States, duloxetine is indicated for major depressive disorder, diabetic peripheral neuropathy, and management of fibromyalgia. Efficacy has been reported in double-blind, placebo-controlled trials of various pain etiologies (diabetic peripheral neuropathic pain, fibromyalgia, chronic pain resulting from osteoarthritis, and chronic low back pain).[132a] Milnacipran (Savella), an SNRI, is approved for the management of fibromyalgia in the United States. Studies in patients with fibromyalgia (100 mg in divided doses) demonstrated clinically meaningful improvement in pain reduction, patient global impression of change, and physical function.[27]

Medication for Insomnia

Pain is an important factor related to sleep problems in community-based studies[56] and can reflect a bidirectional relationship in which pain might interrupt onset and quality of sleep, whereas pain intensity might be exacerbated by insufficient or nonrestorative sleep patterns.[1] Pain clinic studies report that more than 70% of patients report disturbed sleep.[111] Severity of sleep disturbance has also been correlated with greater pain, depression, and disability.[93] To complicate this relationship further, the effects of chronic opioid therapy on disordered sleep reveal conflicting results. Whereas multiple studies have noted that effective opioid analgesia results in improved sleep measures,[17] in a study of patients on chronic methadone, long-term opioid therapy correlated with sleep apnea and apnea severity.[161] Multiple classes of medications with a number of differing mechanisms are available for pain-related insomnia and can be incorporated into a rational polypharmacy approach (see Table 37-10).

During the past decade, the use of benzodiazepines for pain-related insomnia has decreased with the introduction of the nonbenzodiazepine hypnotics, zolpidem, zaleplon, and eszopiclone.[131] Similar to the benzodiazepines, the Z drugs facilitate $GABA_A$ transmission by preferential binding at the 1a receptor subunits (corresponding to benzodiazepine receptor subtype 1), and therefore are devoid of the significant muscle relaxant, anxiolytic, and anticonvulsant activity of traditional full-agonist benzodiazepines.[127] A third nonbenzodiazepine hypnotic, eszopiclone, is approved by the FDA for the long-term management of insomnia and retains a greater half-life (5 to 5.8 hours), with evidence of greater sleep maintenance efficacy compared with the current relatively shorter half-life Z drugs.[169] Some evidence suggests that eszopiclone (3 mg) might also have a positive effect on depression, anxiety, and quality of life. In addition to medications that affect the benzodiazepine receptor complex, there are a number of other drugs that have profound effects on sleep and wakefulness. Medications such as the TCAs and trazodone are especially useful in patients with disturbed sleep that is present with concurrent chronic conditions such as elevated anxiety levels, depression, and myofascial or neuropathic pain. These drugs increase total sleep time and NREM stage 2 sleep. They act by inhibition of norepinephrine and serotonin uptake and block histamine and acetylcholine. When choosing a medication to address disturbed sleep, the half-life of the medication should be considered to ensure that the medication is appropriate for the particular sleep disturbance. Patients with trouble initiating sleep might require shorter-acting medications, whereas those with fragmented sleep and frequent awakenings could more ideally benefit from medications with an intermediate to long half-life.

Little evidence supports the long-term use of benzodiazepines for the management of insomnia and anxiety in chronic pain.[57] Some have suggested that chronic use might simply prevent rebound insomnia rather than promote restorative sleep.[126] Chronic benzodiazepine use can lead to associated cognitive impairment, and it can increase risk for falls, produce rebound insomnia with prolonged use, disrupt normal sleep architecture, and promote misuse and abuse in patients with histories of substance-related disorders.[123] Medications with other secondary sedating qualities might also be considered as part of this approach (i.e., muscle relaxers, TCAs and tricyclic-like antidepressants, and novel antidepressants). Older- and newer-generation anticonvulsants have been shown to decrease sleep latency and to increase total sleep time and slow-wave sleep.[115] In general, opiates tend to produce sedation and have the effect of increasing sleep fragmentation and decreasing REM and stage 2 sleep. Antidepressants in the SSRI class are associated with both insomnia and somnolence, depending on the specific medication. They generally tend to decrease total sleep time and are less sedating than the TCAs. SSRIs can reduce REM sleep. A complete sleep history can help determine behavioral issues affecting insomnia as well as the excessive use of nicotine and alcohol before bedtime. Nicotine use can lead to delayed sleep onset. The relatively sedating qualities of alcohol might facilitate sleep by increasing slow-wave and reducing REM sleep, but it also might cause a rebound increase in sleep fragmentation later in the sleep cycle.

Novel mediation treatments for insomnia are currently in development. Orexin receptor antagonists target the orexin peptides produced by lateral hypothalamic neurons that are prominently involved in the maintenance of wakefulness.

Topical Analgesics

The use of over-the-counter and prescription topical analgesics continues to grow. An increased understanding of nociceptor physiology, including a greater understanding of thermosensation, has been spurred by identification of proteins called vanilloid receptors, detectors of noxious heat, and subsequent identification of a new family of thermosensation receptors, the transient receptor protein vanilloid (TRPV) channel family.[71] The vanilloid receptor (TRPV1) is a nonselective cation receptor activated by capsaicin, the pungent agent found in chili peppers. Another TRPV receptor, the cold- and menthol-sensitive receptor, has been identified and might contribute to a better understanding of cold thermosensation and the possible development of targeted cold-producing analgesics. Pharmacologic studies of menthol have suggested a possible κ-opioid receptor effect, providing additional analgesic properties to the substance.[49] A number of prescription and over-the-counter topical therapies are available for the treatment of musculoskeletal and neuropathic pain states, including the lidocaine (lignocaine) patch, topical TCAs, capsaicin creams, and topical NSAIDs.

Prescription medications include lidocaine 5% patches that are indicated for postherpetic neuralgia. Lidocaine acts peripherally by blocking sodium channels. Randomized placebo-controlled studies have demonstrated analgesic efficacy in postherpetic neuralgia[122] and focal peripheral neuropathic pain syndromes.[97] Safety and decreased risk for systemic effects with multiple patches worn up to 24 hours at a time has more recently been reported.[51]

More widely used in Europe, topical TCAs such as doxepin and amitriptyline have demonstrated efficacy in a number of neuropathic pain states.[90] Topical capsaicin, which depletes substance P and CGRP to produce a pharmacologic desensitization of nociceptors, has demonstrated efficacy in a number of trials, including diabetic peripheral neuropathy, HIV-associated neuropathic pain, and painful distal polyneuropathy.[22]

Greater use in those with chronic pain is limited by poor patient tolerability of the necessary desensitization application process.

Over-the-counter topical analgesics include NSAIDs, capsaicin, and menthol-based products. Compounding pharmacies can serve a unique service in providing customized compounding of various creams and gels for topical use, including ketamine, gabapentin, cyclobenzaprine, and various NSAIDs.[68]

Mind-Body Medicine

Mind-body medicine describes a subset of medical care that attempts to tie together methods of ancient traditional Eastern healing techniques with the modern biopsychosocial model of health care. Therapies that fall under the guise of mind-body medicine include but are not limited to relaxation therapy, biofeedback, meditation, hypnosis, guided imagery, yoga, and T'ai Chi. Two of the more commonly used mind-body medicine techniques, relaxation training and biofeedback, are described in the following sections.

Relaxation Training

Relaxation techniques are incorporated to some extent as an element of almost all mind-body medicine therapies, most notably in meditation, guided imagery, hypnosis, and biofeedback. The technique of progressive muscle relaxation as developed by Jacobson in 1938[65] is perhaps the most popular form of relaxation training, although it has been modified and abbreviated by various practitioners. Progressive muscle relaxation teaches the patient to sequentially voluntarily contract and then relax various muscle groups. Through this voluntary cycle, the patient gains insight into the sensation of muscle tension, which can then facilitate subsequent muscular relaxation.

Progressive muscle relaxation has been studied in various chronic conditions, with strong support for its use in the treatment of anxiety, depression, headache, and insomnia, as well as chronic pain.[8,108a]

Biofeedback

Biofeedback is a therapeutic technique that uses various forms of auditory and visual physiologic monitoring to teach patients to modify physiologic functions that are not normally under conscious control. Common target responses include heart rate, blood pressure, skin temperature, and muscle tension. Clinical approaches used during biofeedback training are similar to those used in relaxation therapy and include diaphragmatic breathing, imagery, progressive muscle relaxation, and autogenic training.

It is an important form of therapeutic training for chronic pain conditions because it allows and encourages the patient to achieve an improved sense of self-control and self-efficacy. A number of movement-based therapies may be of additional value for patients and include a wide range of interventions including aquatic therapy, Pilates, yoga, Feldenkrais Method, and T'ai Chi.

Summary

The quest to relieve pain and suffering has challenged humankind for centuries. Treatment and a better understanding of the complex multidimensional experience of pain have historically evolved with the growth in understanding of anatomy and physiology, psychology, and behavioral and cognitive aspects of human behavior. A crude understanding of basic pain pathways as a peripheral specific mechanism has evolved into a more central comprehensive understanding of the nature of complicated pain pathways, cellular mechanisms of pain transmission (peripheral and central sensitization), complex interactions of cerebral inputs into pain processing, and effects of previous experiences in shaping the experience of pain and pain-related suffering.

A biopsychosocial physiatric approach to understanding and treating pain (acute or chronic) can be the most pragmatic one. Psychological factors, including levels of affective distress, maladaptive beliefs, operant issues, fears, and level of social support, can be important contributors to the subjective experience of pain and are therefore appropriate targets for treatment. A thorough pain assessment and likelihood of a more accurate clinical diagnosis can be achieved with the incorporation of related psychometric measures and diagnostic tests in conjunction with a comprehensive history and physical examination.

A rational approach to treatment incorporates goals for achieving realistic levels of analgesia, improvement of mood and sleep, and restoration of function with the use of one or a number of medications with complementary pharmacologic activity at different sites along the pain pathway. Successful use of a rational polypharmacy approach (i.e., TCAs, NSAIDs, novel antidepressants, and opioids) is based on appropriate patient selection, understanding mechanisms of action of medication, pharmacokinetics, pharmacodynamics, side effect profiles, and risks for potential aberrant use, addiction, and diversion. Appropriate goal-oriented treatment can include active and passive therapies, cognitive behavioral therapy, relaxation training, and other mind-body therapies. Formal multidisciplinary and/or interdisciplinary functional restoration treatment programs might be necessary for those patients who have failed more unimodal approaches. The physiatrist is encouraged to approach all patients with persistent pain from a diagnostic and therapeutic perspective in a multidisciplinary biopsychosocial manner as a means of improving psychosocial function, decreasing pain, and improving quality of life.

KEY REFERENCES

1. Affleck G, Urrows S, Tennen H, et al: Sequential daily relations of sleep, pain intensity, and attention to pain among women with fibromyalgia, *Pain* 68:363–368, 1996.
4. Apkarian AV, Sosa Y, Sonty S, et al: Chronic back pain is associated with decreased prefrontal and thalamic gray matter density, *J Neurosci* 24:10410–10415, 2004.
6. Banks SM, Kerns RD: Explaining high rates of depression in chronic pain: a diathesis-stress framework, *Psychol Bull* 119:95–110, 1996.
8. Barrows KA, Jacobs BP: Mind-body medicine. An introduction and review of the literature, *Med Clin North Am* 86:11–31, 2002.
9. Beck AT, Rush AJ, Shaw BF, et al: *Cognitive therapy of depression*, New York, 1979, Guilford Press.
12. Berry PH, Chapman CR, Covington EC, et al: *Pain: current understanding of assessment, management, and treatments*, Oakbrook Terrace, 2001, Joint Commission on Accreditation of Healthcare Organizations.
13. Bombardier C, Lain L, Reicin A, et al, for VIGOR Study Group: Comparison of upper gastrointestinal toxicity of rofecoxib and naproxen in patients with rheumatoid arthritis, *N Engl J Med* 343:1520–1528, 2000.
24. Caterina MJ, Julius D: Sense and specificity: a molecular identity for nociceptors, *Curr Opin Neurobiol* 9:525–530, 1999.
27. Clauw D, Mease P, Palmer R, et al: Milnacipran for the treatment of fibromyalgia in adults: a 15-week, multicenter, randomized, double-blind, placebo-controlled, multiple-dose clinical trial, *Clin Ther* 30:1988–2004, 2008.
30. Craig AD: Pain mechanisms: labeled lines versus convergence in central processing, *Annu Rev Neurosci* 26:1–30, 2003.
37. Dworkin RH, Backonja M, Rowbotham MC, et al: Advances in neuropathic pain: diagnosis, mechanisms, and treatment recommendations, *Arch Neurol* 60:1524–1534, 2003.
38. Dworkin RH, Corbin AE, Young JP, et al: Pregabalin for the treatment of postherpetic neuralgia: a randomized, placebo-controlled trial, *Neurology* 60:1274–1283, 2003.
40. Farrar JT, Young JP, Jr, LaMoreaux L, et al: Clinical importance of changes in chronic pain intensity measured on an 11-point numerical pain rating scale, *Pain* 94:149–158, 2001.
41. Fernandez E, Turk DC: The scope and significance of anger in the experience of chronic pain, *Pain* 61:165–175, 1995.
46. Fordyce WE: *Behavioral methods of chronic pain and illness*, St Louis, 1976, Mosby.
47. Frampton JE, Scott LJ: Pregabalin: in the treatment of painful diabetic peripheral neuropathy, *Drugs* 64:2813–2820, 2004.
52. Gatchel RJ: Perspectives on pain: a historical overview. In Gatchel RJ, Turk DC, editors: *Psychosocial factors in pain*, New York, 1999, Guilford Press.
53. Gebhart GF: *Visceral pain*, Seattle, 1995, IASP Press.
55. Gilliam PK: Serotonin syndrome: history and risk, *Fundam Clin Pharmacol* 12:482–491, 1998.
59. Guzman J, Esmail R, Karjalainen K, et al: Multidisciplinary rehabilitation for chronic low back pain: systematic review, *BMJ* 322:1511–1516, 2001.
61. Hardy JD, Wolff HG, Goodell H: *Pain sensations and reactors*, New York, 1952, Williams & Wilkins.
66. Jensen MP, Karoly P: Self-report scales and procedures for assessing pain in adults. In Turk DC, Melzack R, editors: *Handbook of pain assessment*, New York, 2001, Guilford Press.
71. Julius D: The molecular biology of thermosensation. In Dostrovsky JO, Carr DB, Koltzenburg M, editors: *Proceedings of the 10th World Congress on Pain: progress in pain research and management*, vol 24, Seattle, 2003, IASP Press.
72. Julius D, Basbaum AI: Molecular mechanisms of nociception, *Nature* 413:203–210, 2001.
73. Keefe FJ, Lefebvre JC: Behavior therapy. In Melzack R, Wall P, editors: *Textbook of pain*, London, 1999, Churchill Livingstone.
75. Keefe FJ, Wilkins RH, Cook WA, et al: Depression, pain and pain behavior, *J Consult Clin Psychol* 54:665–669, 1986.
76. Kerns RD, Rosenberg R, Jacob MC: Anger expression and chronic pain, *J Behav Med* 17:57–67, 1994.
77. Lanes TC, Gauron EF, Spratt KF, et al: Long-term follow-up of patients with chronic back pain treated in a multidisciplinary rehabilitation program, *Spine* 20:801–806, 1995.
81. Livingston WK: *Pain and suffering*, Seattle, 1998, IASP Press.
82. Loeser JD: *Desirable characteristics for pain treatment facilities*, Seattle, 1992, IASP Press.
84. Lynch ME: Antidepressants as analgesics: a review of randomized controlled studies, *J Psychiatry Neurosci* 261:30–36, 2001.
85. MacDonald S, Linton SJ, Jansson-Frojmark M: Avoidant safety behaviours and catastrophizing: shared cognitive-behavioral processes and consequences in co-morbid pain and sleep disorders, *Int J Behav Med* 15(3):201–210, 2008.
86. Mannion RJ, Woolf CJ: Pain mechanisms and management: a central perspective, *Clin J Pain* 16:S144–S156, 2000.
88. Max MB, Lynch SA, Muir J, et al: Effects of desipramine, amitriptyline, and fluoxetine on pain in diabetic neuropathy, *N Engl J Med* 326:1250–1256, 1992.

89. Mayer TG, Gatchel RJ: *Functional restoration for spinal disorders: the sports medicine approach*, Philadelphia, 1988, Lea & Febiger.
90. McCleane G: Topical application of doxepin hydrochloride, capsaicin and a combination of both produces analgesia in chronic human neuropathic pain: a randomized, double-blind, placebo-controlled study, *Br J Clin Pharmacol* 49:574–579, 2000.
91. McCracken LM, Gross RT, Aikens J, et al: The assessment of anxiety and fear in persons with chronic pain: a comparison of instruments, *Behav Res Ther* 34:927–933, 1996.
94. McCracken LM, Turk DC: Behavioral and cognitive-behavioral treatment for chronic pain. Outcome, predictors of outcome, and treatment process, *Spine* 27:2564–2573, 2002.
95. McCracken LM, Zayfert C, Gross RT: The Pain Anxiety Symptom Scale: development and validation of a scale to measure fear of pain, *Pain* 50:67–73, 1992.
97. Meier T, Wasner G, Faust M, et al: Efficacy of lidocaine patch 5% in the treatment of focal peripheral neuropathic pain syndromes: a randomized, double-blind, placebo-controlled study, *Pain* 106:151–158, 2003.
98. Melzack R: *The puzzle of pain*, New York, 1973, Basic Books.
99. Melzack R: The Short Form McGill Pain Questionnaire: major properties and scoring methods, *Pain* 1:277–299, 1975.
102. Merskey H, Bogduk N: *IASP Task Force on Taxonomy classification of chronic pain: description of chronic pain syndromes and definition of pain terms*, Seattle, 1994, IASP Press.
105. Moldofsky H: Management of sleep disorders in fibromyalgia, *Rheum Dis Clin North Am* 28:353–365, 2002.
106. Morley S, Eccleston C, Williams A: Systematic review and meta-analysis of randomized controlled trials of cognitive behavior therapy and behavior therapy for chronic pain in adults, excluding headache, *Pain* 80:1–13, 1999.
108b. Ohayon MM, Schatzberg AF: Using chronic pain to predict depressive morbidity in the general population, *Arch Gen Psychiatry* 60:39–47, 2003.
110. Palermo TM, Fonareva I, Janosy NR: Sleep quality and efficiency in adolescents with chronic pain: relationship with activity limitations and health-related quality of life, *Behav Sleep Med* 6:234–250, 2008.
114. Price DD: Psychological and neural mechanisms of the affective dimension of pain, *Science* 288:1769–1772, 2000.
118. Robbins H, Gatchel RJ, Noe C, et al: A prospective one-year outcome study of interdisciplinary chronic pain management: compromising its efficacy by managed care policies, *Anesth Analg* 97:156–162, 2003.
119. Romano JM, Turner JA: Chronic pain and depression: does the evidence support a relationship?, *Psychol Bull* 97:18–34, 1985.
122. Rowbotham MC, Davies PS, Verkempinck C, et al: Lidocaine patch: double-blind controlled study of a new treatment method for post-herpetic neuralgia, *Pain* 65:39–44, 1996.
123. Rush CR, Griffiths RR: Zolpidem, triazolam, and temazepam: behavioral and subject-rated effects in normal volunteers, *J Clin Psychopharmacol* 16:146–157, 1996.
125. Sabatowski R, Galvez R, Cherry DA, et al: Pregabalin reduces pain and improves sleep and mood disturbances in patients with post-herpetic neuralgia: results of a randomized placebo-controlled clinical trial, *Pain* 109:26–35, 2004.
126. Salzman C, Watsky E: Rational prescribing of benzodiazepines. In Hallstrom C, editor: *Benzodiazepine dependence*, Oxford, 1993, Oxford University Press.
128. Saper CB, Chou TC, Scammell TE: The sleep switch: hypothalamic control of sleep and wakefulness, *Trends Neurosci* 24:726–731, 2001.
131. Scharf MB, Roth T, Vogel GW, et al: A multicenter, placebo-controlled study evaluating zolpidem in the treatment of chronic insomnia, *J Clin Psychiatry* 55:192–199, 1994.
135. Songer DA, Schulte H: Venlafaxine for the treatment of chronic pain, *Am J Psychiatry* 153:737, 1996.
142. Stucky CL, Gold MS, Zhang X: Mechanisms of pain, *Proc Natl Acad Sci USA* 98(21):11845–11846, 2001.
143. Sullivan MJ, Stanish W, Waite H, et al: Catastrophizing, pain, and disability in patients with soft tissue injuries, *Pain* 77:253–260, 1998.
148. Turk DC: Clinical effectiveness and cost effectiveness of treatment for patients with chronic pain, *Clin J Pain* 18:355–365, 2002.
149. Turk DC, Flor H: Chronic pain: a biobehavioral perspective. In Gatchel RJ, Turk DC, editors: *Psychosocial factors in pain: critical perspectives*, New York, 1999, Guilford Press.
157. Vlaeyen JW, Seelen HA, Peters M, et al: Fear of movement/(re)injury and muscular reactivity in chronic low back pain patients: an experimental investigation, *Pain* 82:297–304, 1999.
158. Waddell G, McCulloch JA, Kummel E, et al: Nonorganic physical signs in low-back pain, *Spine* 5:117–125, 1980.
164. Woolf CJ: Pain: moving from symptom control toward mechanism-specific pharmacologic management, *Ann Intern Med* 140:441–451, 2004.
165. Woolf CJ, Costigan M: Transcriptional and posttranslational plasticity and the generation of inflammatory pain, *Proc Natl Acad Sci USA* 96:7723–7730, 1999.

The full reference list for this chapter is available online.

CHAPTER 38

PELVIC FLOOR DISORDERS

Sarah M. Eickmeyer, Kelly M. Scott, Jaclyn Bonder, Sarah Hwang, Colleen Fitzgerald

Pelvic floor disorders are a wide-ranging group of potentially disabling, embarrassing, and often painful conditions that can greatly affect a person's quality of life. The pelvic floor consists of the muscles, fascia, and ligaments that support the pelvic organs and help to provide control for bodily functions. Pathology within the musculoskeletal and neurologic structures of the deep pelvis can lead to the development of pelvic pain, dyspareunia, voiding dysfunction including urinary incontinence or urinary urgency, fecal incontinence (FI), constipation, and pelvic organ prolapse.

Both women and men can develop pelvic floor disorders, although women are at increased risk compared with men because of their unique anatomy and biomechanics. A more broad and shallow female pelvis requires greater muscular and ligamentous stiffness to provide support to the bony pelvic girdle.[106] Women are also more likely to have injury to the pelvic floor as a result of pregnancy and childbirth. As a result, abnormal biomechanics of the pelvic floor muscles (PFMs) may lead to changes in contraction, relaxation, muscle strength, and myofascial pain. In a 2008 study, the prevalence of symptomatic pelvic floor disorders in the United States was estimated to be approximately 24%.[100]

People with pelvic floor disorders often benefit from an interdisciplinary rehabilitation approach to improve function and reduce pain. Physiatrists, with experience in acute and chronic pain, neurologic and musculoskeletal conditions, and neurogenic bowel/bladder management, are well suited to direct the patient's care. The role of the physiatrist is to summarize the musculoskeletal findings of the history, physical examination, and diagnostic testing and to provide a specific physical therapy (PT) prescription.[106] This prescription allows the physiatrist to convey impressions and suggest specific interventions for the pelvic floor as well as other related musculoskeletal structures (e.g., lumbar spine, pelvis, and hip). The rehabilitation provider must be aware of when to consult obstetrics-gynecology, urogynecology, urology, colorectal surgery, gastroenterology, and psychology specialists to provide additional specialist care (Table 38-1). In this chapter, we will review the anatomy and physical examination of the pelvic floor, discuss the definitions and epidemiology of pelvic floor disorders, and explain the rehabilitation approach to treating these common disorders.

Pelvic Floor Neuromusculoskeletal Anatomy

The pelvic floor is composed of muscles, ligaments, and fascia that act as a sling to support the bladder, reproductive organs, and rectum. This sling of soft tissue is enclosed by the bony scaffolding of the pelvis, formed from the ilium, ischium, and pubis, which articulate with the sacrum posteriorly and each other anteriorly (Figure 38-1). Extending from the sacrum is the coccyx, which acts as an important ligamentous and tendinous anchor.

The stability of the articulating surfaces of the pelvis is thought to arise through mechanisms termed "force closure" and "form closure." Force closure is achieved through the interlocking of the ridges and grooves of the bony joint surfaces in the pelvis, whereas form closure is achieved through the compressive forces of the muscles, ligaments, and fascia providing passive stability.[104,137] In the posterior pelvic ring there are two sacroiliac joints (SIJs). The anterior sacroiliac ligaments, comprising the anterior longitudinal ligament, the anterior sacroiliac ligament, and the sacrospinous ligament, stabilize the joint by resisting upward movement of the sacrum and lateral movement of the ilium. The posterior sacroiliac ligaments are made up by the short and long dorsal sacroiliac ligaments, the supraspinous ligament, the iliolumbar ligament, and the sacrotuberous ligament. These ligaments function to resist downward and upward movement of the sacrum and medial motion of the ilium. Anteriorly, the pubic symphysis is a cartilaginous joint between the two pubic bones reinforced by superior, inferior, anterior, and posterior ligaments. Functionally it resists tension, shearing, and compression, and is subject to great mechanical stress as it widens during pregnancy.

The superficial PFMs are the bulbospongiosus, ischiocavernosus, and superficial and deep transverse perineal muscles. The deep PFMs that line the inner walls of the pelvis are the levator ani and coccygeus, which along with the endopelvic fascia comprise the pelvic diaphragm (Table 38-2). The levator ani is composed of three muscles: the puborectalis, pubococcygeus, and iliococcygeus (Figure 38-2). The pubococcygeus is located most anteriorly. It originates from both the posterior pubic bone and the anterior portion of the arcus tendineus; it inserts into the anococcygeus ligament and the coccyx. The iliococcygeus is the posterior part of the levator ani. It originates from the posterior part of the arcus tendineus and ischial spine and attaches along the anococcygeal raphe and coccyx. Lastly, the puborectalis is located below the pubococcygeus and forms a U-shaped sling around the rectum. Its sphincterlike action pulls the anorectal junction forward, contributing to continence. The coccygeus muscle is triangular in shape, reinforcing the posterior pelvic floor by arising from the ischial spine and inserting on the lower sacral-coccygeal bones and is contiguous with the sacrospinous ligament. The perineal body or central perineal tendon is located between the vagina and anus. This is a site where the pelvic

Table 38-1 Possible Etiologies of Pelvic Floor Pain or Dysfunction by Medical Specialty

Gynecologic	Gastrointestinal/Genitourinary	Musculoskeletal	Psychological
Vulvodynia	Interstitial cystitis	Low back pain	Anxiety
Dysmenorrhea	Urgency/frequency syndrome	Lumbar radiculopathy	Depression
Endometriosis	Levator ani syndrome	Sacroiliac joint dysfunction	History of abuse
Fibroids	Bowel/bladder incontinence	Coccydynia	
Organ prolapse		Hip disorders	

Table 38-2 Pelvic Floor Musculature Anatomic Origins, Insertions, Innervation, and Function

Muscle	Origin	Insertion	Innervation	Function
Puborectalis	Pubic symphysis	Pubic symphysis	S3 to S5, direct innervation from sacral nerve roots	Raises the pelvic floor
Pubococcygeus	Posterior pubic bone and arcus tendineus	Anococcygeus ligament and coccyx	S3 to S5, direct innervation from sacral nerve roots	Maintains floor tone in upright position
Iliococcygeus	Ischial spine and arcus tendineus	Anococcygeal raphe and coccyx	S3 to S5, direct innervation from sacral nerve roots	Voluntary control of urination
Coccygeus	Ischial spine	Lower sacral and upper coccygeal bones	S3 to S5, direct innervation from sacral nerve roots	Support of fetal head
Piriformis	Anterior sacrum	Posterior surface of greater trochanter	S1 to S2 via nerve to piriformis	Lateral rotation, abduction of thigh; retroversion of pelvis
Obturator Internus	Pelvic surface of ilium, ischium, and obturator membrane	Posterior surface of greater trochanter	L5, S1 to S2 via nerve to obturator internus	Lateral rotator of thigh

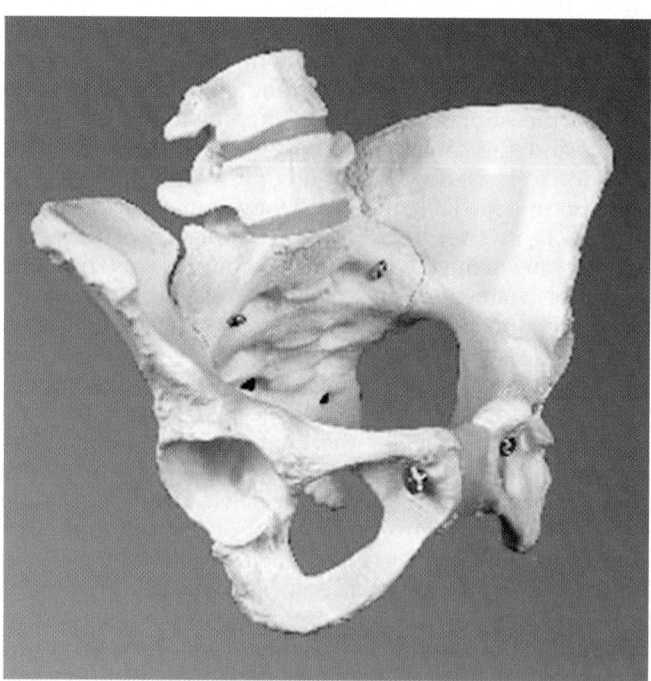

FIGURE 38-1 The bony pelvic girdle consists of the two innominate bones and the sacrum, which are connected by two posterior sacroiliac joints and one anterior pubic symphysis joint.

muscles and sphincters converge to provide support to the pelvic floor. Rupture of this entity during childbirth can lead to pelvic organ prolapse. The PFMs function to support the pelvic organs by coordinated contraction and relaxation.[94] At rest, the pelvic floor provides active support through muscular activity and passive support from the surrounding connective tissue and fascia. With an increase in intraabdominal pressure, the PFMs contract with upward movement and closure of the vagina, urethral, and anal sphincters. This action is important for maintaining continence. Pelvic floor relaxation returns the muscles to their resting state and allows for normal micturition and defecation. Lining the lateral walls of the pelvis, the piriformis arises from the anterior sacrum, with the sacrotuberous ligament and attaches on the superior border of the greater trochanter. When the sacrum is fixed, the piriformis laterally rotates an extended thigh or abducts a flexed thigh. If the femurs are fixed it can retrovert the pelvis. The obturator internus, another lateral rotator of the thigh, arises from the pelvic surfaces of the ilium, ischium, and obturator membrane. It also attaches just distally to the piriformis on the greater trochanter.

The PFMs receive innervation through somatic, visceral, and central pathways. Skin innervation of the lower trunk, perineum, and proximal thigh is mediated through the iliohypogastric, ilioinguinal, and genitofemoral nerves (L1 to L3). Perhaps the most clinically relevant nerve to this chapter is the pudendal nerve and its branches (Figure 38-3). Arising from the ventral branches of S2 to S4 of the sacral plexus, the pudendal nerve passes between the piriformis and coccygeal muscle as it traverses through the greater sciatic foramen, over the spine of the ischium, and back into the pelvis through the lesser sciatic foramen. It courses along the lateral wall of the ischiorectal fossa, where it is contained in a sheath of the obturator fascia termed the pudendal (or Alcock) canal.[5] There are three main terminal branches of the pudendal nerve: the inferior rectal nerve (which typically originates proximal to the Alcock canal), the perineal nerve, and the dorsal nerve of the penis/clitoris. The pudendal nerve innervates the penis/clitoris, the bulbospongiosus and ischiocavernosus muscles, the anterior portions of the levator ani muscles,

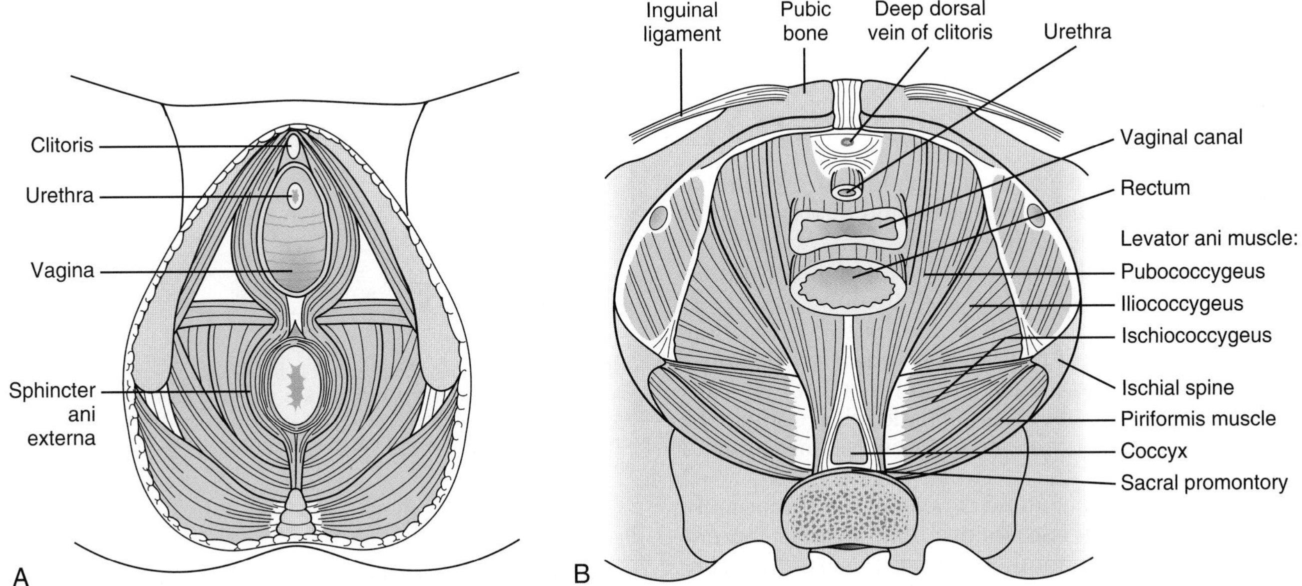

FIGURE 38-2 **The muscles of the (A) superficial pelvic floor and (B) deep pelvic floor. Illustration by Elijah Leonard.** (Redrawn from Prather H, Dugan S, Fitzgerald C, Hunt D: Review of anatomy, evaluation, and treatment of musculoskeletal pelvic floor pain in women, *PM R* 1:346-358, 2009.)

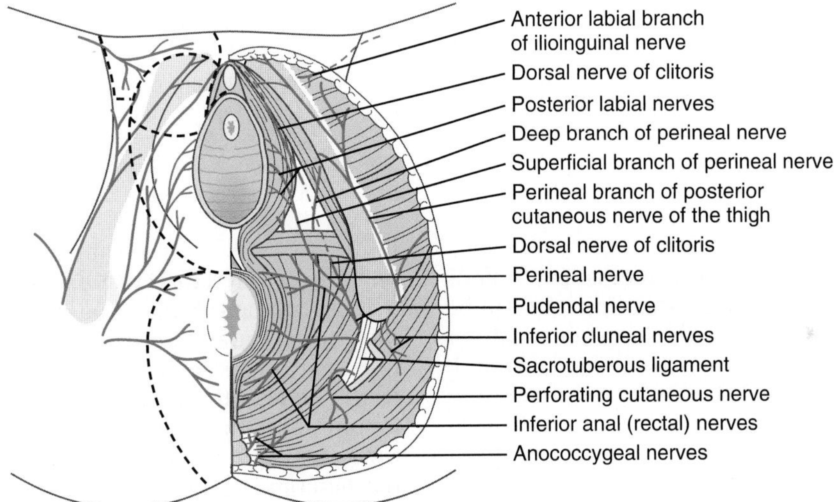

FIGURE 38-3 **Innervation of the pelvic floor.** (Redrawn from Prather H, Dugan S, Fitzgerald C, Hunt D: Review of anatomy, evaluation, and treatment of musculoskeletal pelvic floor pain in women, *PM R* 1:346-358, 2009.)

the perineum, the anus, the external anal sphincter, and the urethral sphincter. This nerve contributes to external genital sensation, continence, orgasm, and ejaculation. Muscles of the levator ani are thought to have direct innervation from sacral nerve roots S3 to S5.[10]

Overview of Terminology

In 2005, the International Continence Society (ICS) presented a standardized terminology for PFM function and dysfunction.[94] The PFMs function by coordinated contraction and relaxation as a unit. *Voluntary contraction* occurs when the patient can contract the PFMs on demand; *voluntary relaxation* occurs when the patient can relax the PFMs on demand after a contraction. *Involuntary contraction* of the PFMs occurs during a rise in intraabdominal pressure to prevent incontinence, such as during a cough. *Involuntary relaxation* occurs during a strain or Valsalva maneuver to allow for normal micturition or defecation.

Contraction and relaxation can be observed during the pelvic floor physical examination, as described later in this chapter. Based on examination of the PFMs, the following conditions have been defined by the ICS: *Normal PFMs* refer to muscles that can voluntarily and involuntarily contract with normal strength and relax completely. *Overactive PFMs* (also termed nonrelaxing PFMs) do not relax and may paradoxically contract when relaxation is needed, such as during micturition or defecation. *Underactive PFMs* (also called noncontracting PFMs) cannot voluntarily contract when desired. *Nonfunctioning PFMs* refer to no palpable PFM action and can be based on a noncontracting, nonrelaxing pelvic floor where the muscles are both weak and hypertonic. These categories can be helpful for generating a differential diagnosis for possible etiologies of pelvic floor dysfunction (see Table 38-1).

Pelvic Floor Physical Examination

A thorough musculoskeletal examination of the lumbar spine, hips, pelvic girdle, lower limbs, and PFMs will guide the differential diagnosis. The pelvic floor examination consists of vaginal and rectal examination of the PFM function and a neurologic examination of the lower sacral segments. A musculoskeletal pelvic floor examination does not obviate the need for gynecologic, urologic, or colorectal evaluation because visceral structures are not typically evaluated. Verbal consent from the patient is required. The examination should occur in a private examination or treatment room.

The examination begins with external inspection for swelling, cysts, scars, and lesions that may necessitate appropriate referral to another specialist. Next, the examiner visualizes the lift of the perineal body with a voluntary contraction (termed a Kegel contraction) and involuntary contraction (cough), as well as normal descent of the perineal body with voluntary relaxation and then involuntary relaxation (Valsalva maneuver). In women, the vaginal vestibule is evaluated for any visible organ prolapse. The Q-tip test for vulvodynia is performed by lightly touching a cotton swab inside the vestibule to elicit any pain or allodynia. The examiner proceeds to an external sensory examination of the S2 to S5 sacral dermatomes (see Figure 38-3). An anal wink reflex is obtained near the anus to test the sacral reflex arc. The superficial PFMs are palpated for any tenderness.

Next, the examiner moves on to the internal pelvic floor examination; both vaginal and rectal examinations can be performed. It is best to use a flat examination table without stirrups. The vaginal examination is performed in hook lying position, supine with the knees bent, and ankles hip-width apart. The rectal examination is typically performed in a left lateral decubitus position.

One lubricated, gloved finger is inserted into the vaginal introitus or anal canal to palpate the PFMs internally. A clock face diagram is useful to correctly identify the anatomic positions of the PFMs with the pubic bone at 12 o'clock and the anus and coccyx at 6 o'clock (Figure 38-4). The levator ani can be palpated on both vaginal and rectal examinations from 1 to 5 o'clock on the left and 7 to 11 o'clock on the right, with the pubococcygeus located more anteriorly and the iliococcygeus located more posteriorly. The obturator internus is located just above 3 o'clock on the left and 9 o'clock on the right, and is separated from the levator ani by locating the arcus tendineus, which feels similar to a guitar string on palpation (see Figure 38-2). The obturator internus can also be identified by having the patient externally rotate the hip to activate the muscle causing it to bulge medially, which can be appreciated with internal digital palpation. Rectal examination affords the ability to additionally assess anal sphincter tone as well as the coccygeus, piriformis, and puborectalis muscles. The puborectalis can be easily appreciated, forming the innermost portion of the anal canal. The coccyx can be examined intrarectally to assess for tenderness, mobility, and anterior or lateral deviation. The PFMs are palpated for tenderness, taut bands, and referring trigger points. The presence of intramuscular scar tissue should be noted. PFM tone can be assessed as either an increased or decreased resting state of the muscle. A Tinel sign can be obtained by tapping over the pudendal nerve as it courses inferior to the ischial spine and may provoke pelvic floor or perineal paresthesias.

Voluntary contraction of the PFMs is felt as a tightening, lifting, and squeezing action under the examining finger that occurs upon demand.[94] Voluntary contraction is graded with the Modified Oxford scale.[42] Similar to manual muscle testing for limb muscles, the scale ranges from 0/5 signifying "absent" contraction to 5/5, which implies that the patient is able to "lift, tighten, and maintain for 10 seconds" (Table 38-3). Strength testing should be performed in four quadrants, especially in patients with neurologic deficits, such as hemiplegia. *Voluntary relaxation* of the PFMs is felt as a termination of the contraction as the muscles return to their resting state. The examiner then has the patient cough to look for presence or absence of *involuntary contraction*, and then perform a Valsalva maneuver to look for presence or absence of *involuntary relaxation*. It is important to assess for dyssynergia or inappropriate contraction of the PFMs during attempts at Valsalva. Endurance is tested by asking the patient to hold a full contraction for 10 seconds. Coordination is tested by performing "quick flicks" or asking the patient to contract and relax the PFMs rapidly.

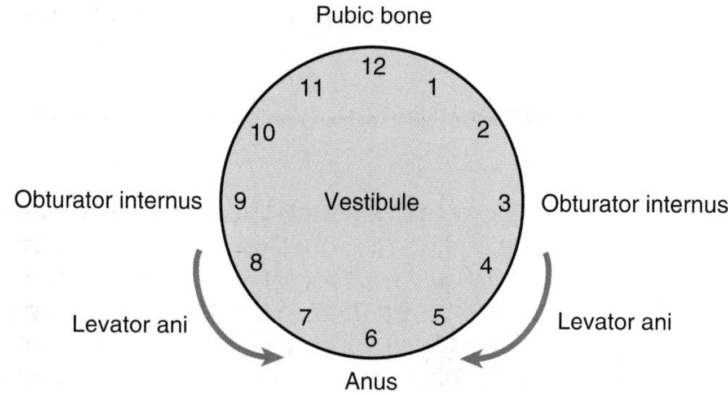

FIGURE 38-4 A clock face diagram can be useful for locating the pelvic floor muscles during examination. 12 o'clock is the pubic bone and 6 o'clock is the anus. Levator ani is located from 3 to 5 o'clock on the left and 7 to 9 o'clock on the right. Obturator internus is located just above 3 o'clock on the left and 9 o'clock on the right.

Table 38-3 Modified Oxford Scale Used to Grade Internal Manual Muscle Testing of the Pelvic Floor Muscles

Grading	Contraction	Lift or Tighten
0/5	No	No
1/5	Flicker	No
2/5	Weak	No
3/5	Moderate	Some lifting/tightening, contraction visible
4/5	Good	Holds for 5+ seconds
5/5	Strong	Holds for 10+ seconds

Types of Pelvic Floor Dysfunction

Urinary Incontinence

Definitions and Etiology

Urinary incontinence, defined as the involuntary leakage of urine,[56] can be divided into three main types. Stress urinary incontinence (SUI) is the loss of urine with increased intraabdominal pressure, such as during coughing, laughing, sneezing, or physical exertion. SUI occurs where there are deficiencies in the PFMs, urethra, bladder, and/or sphincter such that it is difficult to maintain urethral closure pressures. The etiology is multifactorial and has been shown to be related to pregnancy, vaginal delivery, pelvic surgery, pelvic organ prolapse, neurologic causes, active lifestyle, obesity, and aging. Urge urinary incontinence (UUI) is involuntary leakage accompanied by or immediately preceded by the sudden onset of an urge to void that cannot be deferred easily. UUI can be caused by an involuntary detrusor contraction that overcomes the sphincter mechanism or poor bladder compliance that results from loss of the viscoelastic features of the bladder. The cause of UUI may be neurogenic or idiopathic. Neurologic processes that can cause low bladder compliance include spinal cord injury, spinal stenosis, multiple sclerosis, and stroke. Nonneurogenic etiologies are usually processes that change the bladder tissue, such as radiation. Mixed urinary incontinence (MUI) occurs when a patient experiences both SUI and UUI symptoms.

Epidemiology

Urinary incontinence is by far more common in women. A survey of 45,000 households in the United States with a mixed respondent population (82% women) found a 34% prevalence of urinary incontinence.[71] The prevalence of urinary incontinence has been shown to increase in both men and women with age. Prevalence rates by age group were found to be 15% for ages 18 to 24 years and 46% for ages 60 to 64 years.[64] Reported risk factors for urinary incontinence include race, hormonal status, obesity, history of pregnancy or childbirth, and chronic disease, such as diabetes.[92] The prevalence of urinary incontinence also increases with smoking, body mass index, and increased parity.[33] One study, which looked at vaginal delivery and its effect on the prevalence of different types of urinary incontinence in women, found a 15.3% rate of SUI, a 6.1% rate of UUI, and a 14.4% rate of MUI.[49] High-level female athletes are also at an increased risk of developing incontinence; one recent study indicated an SUI prevalence in this population of 41.5%.[68] Other risk factors not consistently reported include constipation and family history.

Diagnosis and Physical Examination

Physiatrists often discover urinary incontinence as part of screening questions for back pain or on review of systems. This is essential because fewer than 50% of those suffering from this condition will seek out treatment. If a patient admits to this condition, it is important to review their medical history, noting any neurologic disease. The physician should determine whether the patient has SUI, UUI, or MUI with questions regarding timing of accidents and relation to activity and urgency symptoms. If a patient with urinary incontinence has presented to the office because of back pain, it is necessary to rule out surgical emergencies, such as cauda equina syndrome. Patients who do not have neurologic deficits should be further examined by a physiatrist who is comfortable performing a pelvic floor examination or referred to a urologist for additional workup.

A thorough neurologic, lower extremity, and pelvic floor physical examination can help distinguish between neurogenic causes and PFM contributions to incontinence. For urinary incontinence, pelvic floor examination should focus on inspection of the vulva and perineum, sensory testing of S2 to S5 dermatomes, tone and strength testing of the PFMs, and assessment for a gross pelvic organ prolapse (POP). It is important to note POP in a patient with back pain and incontinence because this may be a source of vague, achy low back pain. The PFMs are usually found to be *underactive* and weak in SUI and *overactive* in UUI. The integrity of the vaginal mucosa should also be noted because menopausal hypoestrogenic state has been associated with urinary incontinence.[79] Determination of when to refer for advanced testing, such as cystoscopy, postvoid residuals, and urodynamics, should be made on an individual basis.

Treatment

Management for urinary incontinence includes pharmacologic, surgical, behavioral, and exercise-based treatments. Conservative treatment for urinary incontinence often results in improvement of symptoms, but the initial severity usually dictates the amount of success. Treatment options vary for SUI and UUI, but both respond well to behavioral modifications and rehabilitation interventions.

Behavioral and lifestyle alterations include changes in diet, regulating fluid intake, and bladder training. Reduction of more than 5% body weight has led to a 47% decrease in incontinence episodes versus 28% with education alone.[126] Bladder training usually consists of two parts, timed voiding and urge suppression techniques, and can take approximately 12 weeks to see improvement. The overall goals of bladder training are to prolong the time between voids and to void before experiencing a sense of urgency or UUI. Using a bladder diary to identify the shortest interval between voids, patients are instructed to increase this time by approximately 15 to 30 minutes until there is approximately 3 hours between voids. Urge suppression can temporarily reduce the intensity of a bladder contraction by causing reflex inhibition of the parasympathetic nerves acting on the detrusor muscle. When one feels an urge, they should stop and/or sit, perform five to six quick voluntary PFM (or Kegel) contractions, take a deep breath, relax until the urge passes, and then walk to the restroom normally.

PFM contraction (or Kegel) exercises can be used to strengthen the PFMs and reduce episodes of SUI. The majority of people who try to perform a proper PFM (or Kegel) contraction are unable to do so. As such, patients should be taught how to perform these exercises with a pelvic floor expert. Biofeedback therapy with or without electrical stimulation is often used to improve a patient's ability to perform a PFM contraction (Figure 38-5). A strengthening program for the PFMs increases support for

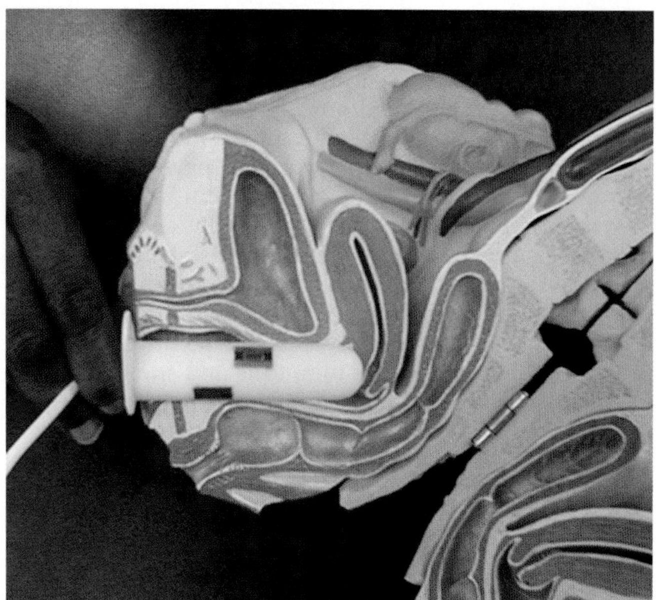

FIGURE 38-5 Intravaginal biofeedback may be used during physical therapy to provide objective feedback to the patient about pelvic floor muscle activation and relaxation.

the bladder and urethra and helps maintain the urethral closure pressures. As strength improves, patients can be taught to make a PFM contraction an automatic response when anticipating increase in intraabdominal pressure (such as with a sneeze), and to perform them during functional activities. The long-term effect of PFM strengthening for SUI symptom improvement ranges from 41% to 85%.[14]

Pharmacologic management of UUI focuses on medications for overactive bladder (OAB) (see the following section). There are currently no approved drugs for SUI in the United States. The mainstay of pharmacologic management of OAB and UUI are anticholinergic medications that decrease urgency and detrusor instability by blocking parasympathetic nerves of the bladder. However, their use and efficacy are often limited by side effects, such as constipation, drowsiness, and dry mouth.

When conservative measures have failed, botulinum toxin and neuromodulation can be used to decrease detrusor muscle contractility and treat UUI. When botulinum toxin is injected into the detrusor muscle, daily frequency, urgency, and incontinence can be reduced by 29%, 3%, and 59%, respectively.[87] Neuromodulation by stimulation of S3 sacral nerve root can lead to effective control of UUI and symptoms of urgency and frequency.

Other forms of therapy for SUI include urethral bulking agents and surgery. Urethral bulking agents increase the compressive force on the urethral lumen by augmenting the submucosal layer. The most common surgery for SUI has become the placement of midurethral slings. These slings are thought to improve urethral support, create resistance to increases in abdominal pressure, and restore the normal forces on the urethra.

Urinary Urgency and Frequency

Definitions and Etiology

Urinary urgency is defined as "the complaint of a sudden compelling desire to pass urine which is difficult to defer" by the ICS. Frequency of urination more than every 2 to 3 hours can be considered abnormal. The symptoms of urgency and frequency are similar to those of UUI that were discussed earlier. Urinary urgency associated with or without incontinence, daytime frequency, and nocturia is termed OAB. As its name describes, the diagnosis of OAB should be reserved for cases that are clearly of bladder origin, namely detrusor muscle overactivity. There are also neurogenic, medical, and muscular causes of urgency/frequency symptoms.

The pathophysiology of neurogenic urgency and frequency is usually attributable to detrusor overactivity as a result of disruption to the complex micturition reflex at the cerebral, pons or corticospinal level. Such neurologic causes include stroke, Alzheimer disease, Parkinson disease, or multiple sclerosis.[107] Lower motor neuron causes or peripheral neuropathies can also cause voiding dysfunction.

Medical causes of urinary urgency and frequency include urinary tract infections in which increased inflammation in the bladder leads to sensory afferent upregulation, ultimately causing detrusor muscle instability. Similarly, estrogen deficiency can lead to vaginal and urethral irritation, which may bring on increased infections and OAB. The normal aging process also leads to increased bladder contractility and decreased bladder compliance resulting in urgency and frequency, respectively.

Patients with urinary urgency and frequency in the absence of bladder or neurologic pathology may have these symptoms as a result of *overactive* PFMs. Those in this category will have dysfunctional voiding with a sense of urgency and/or frequency resulting from increased external pressure around the urethra. Patients can describe a constant need or an exaggerated urge to void. Patients with hypertonic PFMs can have difficulty with voluntary relaxation or can have involuntary contractions during voiding. Other symptoms of pelvic floor dysfunction resulting from *overactive* PFMs includes postvoiding pain, urethral pain, hesitancy, or incomplete bladder emptying. Patients with functional constipation or bowel impaction (discussed later) should be screened for urinary urgency and frequency because both can be a result of *overactive* pelvic floor dysfunction. Development of *overactive* PFMs with urinary dysfunction is often attributable to holding behaviors developed during childhood or as a result of circumstances that may cause one to suppress the urge to void for many hours (such as working as a taxi driver, teacher or nurse, or having a fear of voiding in public restrooms). *Overactive* pelvic floor dysfunction is also associated with a history of sexual abuse or those with severe anxiety disorders.[103]

Diagnosis and Physical Examination

Patients presenting with pure urinary urgency and frequency symptoms need to be initially evaluated by a urologist for a complete workup of their voiding dysfunction, including postvoid residuals and urodynamic testing. Men should have a thorough prostate examination. As with urinary incontinence, a thorough evaluation of patients with urinary frequency and urgency includes a full medical history and physical examination to assess for medical or neurogenic causes. Diagnosis of *overactive* PFMs can be made during a musculoskeletal pelvic floor examination.

Externally, minimal movement of the perineal body when patients are asked to do voluntary PFM contraction or relaxation should lead the examiner to consider a hypertonic state. On the internal (vaginal or rectal) assessment, attention is focused on the stiffness and length of the levator ani muscles. Patients are likely to have shortened levator ani muscles that feel weak when tested for strength. These patients often have pain in the PFMs as a result of chronic hypertonicity. Again, minimal movement of the muscles during the internal part of the examination will help diagnose hypertonic or *overactive* PFM dysfunction.

Treatment

The underlying etiology of the voiding dysfunction should be treated, if possible. Patients who have idiopathic or pure muscular causes of urinary frequency and urgency can be treated conservatively with pelvic floor PT. The goal of this treatment program is to teach patients how to relax the PFMs during voiding. PFM training focuses first on developing an awareness of muscle contraction versus relaxation with biofeedback. The focus should then turn to teaching volitional relaxation of the PFMs in the context of voiding. Perineal, rectal, or vaginal biofeedback can be especially useful for bringing muscle tension to a conscious level. In addition, to facilitate relaxation patients can be taught to relax the muscle for a longer period of time compared with a contraction, usually in a 1:2 ratio. Patients with urgency and frequency voiding dysfunction should be taught urge suppression techniques with bladder training (as described earlier). Lifestyle modifications and education about fluid management, bladder irritants, and weight loss should also be stressed.

Fecal Incontinence

Definitions and Etiology

Fecal incontinence (FI) is defined as the involuntary loss of liquid or solid stool that is a social or hygienic problem.[98] A related term is anal incontinence (AI), which is defined as the involuntary loss of liquid or solid stool, mucus, or flatus. FI is strongly associated with aging.[98] Other risk factors include nursing home residence, obesity, poor general health, physical limitations, and neurologic disease. Patients with gastrointestinal disorders, such as irritable bowel syndrome or inflammatory bowel disease, have a higher likelihood of FI. FI is more common in patients who have weakness or injury to the anal sphincter. Obstetric factors are likely to play a large role: sphincter laceration, use of forceps, midline episiotomy, and intrapartum pudendal nerve damage have all been shown to contribute to the development of subsequent FI. Pelvic surgeries can also predispose to the development of this disorder. FI has been reported as a complication in 33% of hemorrhoidectomies, 11% of sphincterotomies, and 9% to 32% of radical prostatectomies.[98] Pelvic radiation can lead to the development of FI in 14% to 46% of patients.[98]

Epidemiology

Prevalence has been reported at 2% to 24% of the adult population,[15] with 1% to 2% experiencing significant impact on daily activities.[101] A survey study of over 10,000 respondents found that 5.7% of women and 6.2% of men over 40 years of age report some degree of FI, with prevalence increasing with age.[101] FI is also prevalent in high-level athletes, although to a lesser extent than SUI. One study of 393 female athletes found a prevalence of AI of 14.9% and reported that 8% of all high-level athletes needed to wear a pad for protection as a result of significant FI.[135] It is estimated that less than 30% of the people who struggle with FI discuss the problem with their health care providers.[98]

Diagnosis and Physical Examination

As with urinary incontinence, it is important for the physician to enquire about the presence of FI, because patients are often reluctant to discuss the subject. It is important to determine whether there is loss of liquid or solid stool, mucus, or flatus. The timing and frequency of episodes, the volume of stool loss, and the ability of the patient to sense the involuntary passage of anal contents are all necessary elements of the history. The physical examination should include a thorough neurologic and spine examination, as well as a digital rectal examination to assess for sphincter tone, sphincter defects, PFM tone, strength, and endurance are important. Diagnostic tools for FI include anorectal manometry, which measures the strength and endurance of the anal sphincter at rest and with contraction. Pudendal nerve terminal motor latency testing can be performed as part of electrodiagnostic testing. Endoanal ultrasound is a very effective tool for the evaluation of the integrity of the internal and external anal sphincters.

Treatment

Treatments include conservative measures such as dietary modifications, medications, and pelvic floor rehabilitation, as well as more invasive approaches such as the use of perianal injectable bulking agents, sacral nerve stimulation, or surgery.[127] Many patients prefer to avoid the risk of interventions, and a stepwise approach to treatment has been advocated to minimize injury to patients.[13]

Pelvic floor rehabilitation has been used successfully in the treatment of FI and can produce significant functional and quality of life benefits for patients.[97] Most of the reported literature in this area has been in the form of case reports and nonrandomized prospective trials. In fact, more than 70 such uncontrolled studies have been published, with the majority reporting a response range of 50% to 90%.[97] There have been a smaller number of randomized controlled trials (RCTs) on pelvic floor rehabilitation for FI, less than 30 in total of high quality, according to two recently published Cochrane reviews on the topic.[61,97] Most RCTs also demonstrated successful improvement of FI symptoms in 50% to 80% of participants.[36,61,97]

Pelvic floor rehabilitation techniques for the treatment of FI include bowel management education and retraining, PFM training, biofeedback therapy, the use of electrical stimulation, manual myofascial release, and connective tissue mobilization techniques. The different rehabilitation techniques can be used independently, but more frequently are used in conjunction with one another in a multimodal approach to produce the maximum benefit for the patient.[116] The primary goal of all forms of pelvic floor rehabilitation is to improve pelvic floor and anal sphincter muscle strength, tone, endurance, and coordination to effect a positive change in function with a decrease in symptoms. Additional goals include increasing the patient's awareness of their own muscles, improving rectal sensitivity, and reducing scar burden to allow for improved muscle function.

There are three main approaches for the use of biofeedback as a part of pelvic floor rehabilitation for FI.[97] Biofeedback therapy is most commonly used to improve strength and endurance of the PFMs and/or external anal sphincter. It has been theorized that this training is effective because it enables the patient to hold the stool within the rectal vault for a longer period of time, allowing them to make it to the restroom with less accidents. The second treatment modality is to use biofeedback to improve rectal sensitivity or compliance. This type of treatment is typically done with sequentially inflated rectal balloons.[25] The rationale behind sensory retraining is to allow the patient to detect smaller volumes of stool at an earlier time, again making it possible for them to reach the restroom before an accident occurs. The third biofeedback approach deals with coordination training for the anal sphincter.

The incorporation of lifestyle education into the therapeutic treatment program is of vital importance for patients with FI. It is important to instruct patients about optimal fluid intake; dietary adjustments can be important in certain patient populations.[95] Patients with irritable bowel syndrome and FI, for example, often find that regulating dairy, gluten, and fiber can be an important component of controlling their stool leakage.[54] It is generally recommended that all patients with FI increase their fiber intake, as Bliss et al.[12] were able to demonstrate that fiber supplementation significantly reduced the rate of FI. Behavior modification can also be explored with patients, including training on the establishment of a predictable pattern of bowel evacuation, timing of defecation relative to activities to limit incontinent episodes, techniques to reduce straining, proper defecation posture when sitting on the toilet, and fecal urge suppression techniques.[95,98,124] Weight reduction is typically encouraged.

There have only been a few studies that have looked at which types of patients will most likely benefit from a rehabilitation approach to treatment for FI. Good sphincter function and mild to moderate symptomatology are considered as more favorable prognostic factors.[16] Disruption of the anal sphincter, spinal cord injury or other neurogenic disorders, severe impairment of rectal sensory function, cognitive impairments, severe depression or other mental illness, and age less than 6 years are all thought to be predictors of poor response to biofeedback and other rehabilitation treatments.[25]

Functional Constipation

Definitions and Etiology

Functional constipation, as defined by the Rome III diagnostic criteria must include two or more of the following: straining during at least 25% of defecations, lumpy or hard stools in at least 25% of defecations, sensation of incomplete evacuation for at least 25% of defecations, sensation of anorectal obstruction/blockage for at least 25% of defecations, manual maneuvers to facilitate at least 25% of defecations (e.g., digital evacuation, support of the pelvic floor), and fewer than three defecations per week.[81] Loose stools are rarely present without the use of laxatives and patients should not meet the criteria for irritable bowel syndrome.

Functional constipation is further subdivided into normal transit constipation, slow transit constipation, and outlet constipation.[69] Normal transit constipation occurs when there is a self-reported perception of constipation with normal stool movement through the colon. Slow transit constipation occurs when there is prolonged transit time through the colon, confirmed with a motility study. Outlet constipation (also called dyssynergia, disordered defecation, or nonrelaxing puborectalis syndrome) occurs as a result of pelvic floor dysfunction, when there is a defect in the coordination that is needed for stool evacuation. Most often, this incoordination occurs because of the failure of the PFMs to relax appropriately during evacuation efforts. Other causes of outlet dysfunction constipation may include rectocele, enterocele, peritoneocele, and intrarectal intussusception. Common features of outlet constipation include prolonged or excessive straining, soft stools that are difficult to pass, and rectal discomfort.[69] The etiology of outlet constipation is unclear.

Epidemiology

Chronic constipation has been reported to affect approximately 15% of the general population, including all ages and both sexes, with estimates ranging from 2% to 27%.[60] Constipation significantly decreases the quality of life of those affected.[65]

Diagnosis and Physical Examination

When taking a history from a patient with constipation, it is important to ask about the number of bowel movements per week, stool consistency, the presence of straining, and the presence of bleeding or mucus. Hard, small, pellet-shaped stools are indicative of poor colonic transit or significant time in the rectal vault. Pencil-shaped stools are a common finding with a nonrelaxing puborectalis syndrome, also termed *overactive* PFMs. The physician should ask about the use of manual maneuvers to facilitate defecation and the use of over-the-counter laxatives and fiber. The physical examination should include abdominal examination and digital rectal examination to assess the sphincter tone and the PFMs. When asked to strain as if having a bowel movement or to attempt to expel the examiner's finger, the examiner should appreciate relaxation of the anal sphincter and relaxation of the puborectalis muscle with decent of the perineum. Additionally, when the patient contracts the PFMs, the examiner should appreciate a lift of the PFMs. Absence of these findings suggests pelvic floor dysfunction.

Diagnostic testing for functional constipation includes anorectal manometry, Sitz study, and defecography.[76] Anorectal manometry can be used to determine if anal sphincter pressures rise with attempts at defecation or rectal balloon expulsion, hallmarks of dyssynergia. Digital rectal examination is reasonably accurate relative to manometry for assessing anal resting tone and squeeze function and for identifying dyssynergia.[128] A Sitz study can be performed to assess colonic motility. The patient is asked to swallow a capsule containing 25 radiopaque markers and an abdominal plain film is obtained 5 days later at which time a majority of the markers should no longer be visible. Sitz markers scattered throughout the colon indicate a problem of slowed colonic transit. Sitz markers clustered in the rectum and sigmoid colon indicate a problem of outlet dysfunction or dyssynergia. Defecography is another important tool in the diagnosis of constipation, because it can distinguish between the many causes of outlet dysfunction constipation including PFM dyssynergia, rectocele, and intrarectal intussusception. Defecography can be done via plain films but magnetic resonance (MR) defecography is emerging as the modality of choice because of its superior image quality.

Treatment

The treatment of functional constipation depends greatly on the cause. Slow transit constipation can benefit from increasing fluid intake, fiber supplementation, magnesium supplementation, and stool softener or laxative use. Nonstimulant laxatives, such as polyethylene glycol, are preferred to stimulant laxatives, such as bisacodyl and senna, because stimulant laxatives have been shown to cause dependency and decreased bowel function over time. Prescription medications for constipation include lactulose, lubiprostone, and linaclotide. Laxative enemas and intrarectal suppositories can also be of benefit. If such measures are not effective for severe slow transit constipation, surgical options include subtotal or total colectomy with ileoanal anastomosis or colostomy.

Dyssynergia is ideally treated with pelvic floor PT. Treatment should include biofeedback and pelvic floor relaxation training.[81,128] Biofeedback therapy can be used to teach the patient how to perform evacuation by relaxing and paring outward the abdominal and PFMs.[80] Protocols of five to six training sessions lasting 30 to 60 minutes, spaced 2 weeks apart, have been shown to be beneficial.[108] The goals of therapy include education about disordered defecation, coordination of increased intraabdominal pressures with pelvic floor relaxation during evacuation, and therapist-assisted practiced defecation simulation with an intrarectal balloon. Techniques employed may also include diaphragmatic breathing, intrarectal and intravaginal myofascial release, visceral mobilization, abdominal wall and colonic massage/stimulation techniques, or the use of anal dilators. The therapist will typically ensure that the patient is using proper defecatory posture while sitting on the toilet, and often will instruct the patient to prop their feet up on a stool and lean forward slightly during defecation to allow for maximum relaxation of the PFMs. Options are limited for patients with severe dyssynergia or anismus who do not respond to pelvic floor PT. Botox to the puborectalis (typically done under endoanal ultrasound guidance) can be considered, but the risk of development of subsequent FI must be taken into careful consideration.[76] The only surgical option is colostomy.

Patients with a symptomatic rectocele can be taught to splint intravaginally with their thumb pressing backward to facilitate stool expulsion. Patients with a significant enterocele, peritoneocele, or intrarectal intussusception often need surgical intervention such as a resection rectopexy.

Pelvic Floor Myofascial Pain

Definitions and Etiology

Pelvic floor myofascial pain is characterized by muscular pain, taut bands, and trigger points that cause pain referral with pressure, usually resulting from underlying overuse or weakness.[29] Myofascial trigger points can develop from functional events through overuse, repetitive strains, motion injuries, or dysfunctional posturing as well as a result of a viscerosomatic reflex.[120] Pelvic floor myofascial dysfunction refers to abnormal muscle activation patterns of the PFMs.[38] Pelvic floor myofascial pain and dysfunction can contribute to the symptom of dyspareunia, or painful sexual intercourse, and to chronic pelvic pain (CPP), but there are many other causes of these conditions with significant overlap.

Epidemiology

PFM pain was found on vaginal physical examination in 22% of women with CPP (ages 14 to 79 years),[132] 70% of women with pregnancy-related pelvic girdle pain (PGP) in the second trimester,[38] and 52% of postpartum women with chronic lumbopelvic pain that began during pregnancy.[104] CPP affects 25% of community-dwelling adult women.[78]

Diagnosis and Physical Examination

The diagnosis of pelvic floor myofascial pain and dysfunction is made clinically by a combination of a focused history and pelvic floor physical examination. Patients with pelvic floor myofascial pain will report pain that is "deep" and internal. They may report associated symptoms of dysuria, dyschezia, dysmenorrhea, or dyspareunia, but often must be prompted with direct questioning because of the intimate nature of pelvic floor pain. Pelvic floor myofascial pain and dysfunction are often related to painful bladder syndrome/interstitial cystitis, urinary urgency/frequency syndrome, vulvar vestibulitis, and chronic prostatitis. A history of related pelvic visceral disorders, such as infection, endometriosis, or fibroids, should be ascertained as these can be related to pelvic floor pain and dysfunction via the viscerosomatic reflex. History of birth trauma, instrumentation (forceps), prolonged labor, or perineal tears during vaginal delivery may point to injury to the PFMs. A history of abuse (physical, sexual, or emotional) can manifest later in life as pelvic pain with PFM overactivity. Finally, a poor response to traditional therapy and treatments for hip and low back pain can often indicate an underlying pelvic floor disorder.

During internal examination of the PFMs, myofascial pain is identified by pain on palpation of the levator ani and obturator internus muscles with taut bands and trigger points that refer pain with pressure. Making note of *underactive* and *overactive* PFM tone is useful to direct further intervention. A complete neurologic and musculoskeletal examination of the spine and lower extremities is important to evaluate for other contributing spine, pelvis, or hip pathology.

Diagnostic imaging can also be useful to aid in ruling out other musculoskeletal causes of lumbopelvic pain.[136] Typically, a conventional pelvic and lumbar radiograph is useful to evaluate the structural integrity of the spine and pelvis; based on physical examination findings, the physician may consider the addition of hip radiographs. Magnetic resonance imaging (MRI) of the spine, hip, or pelvis may be useful to rule out serious causes of pelvic pain, including herniated lumbosacral disk or sacral fracture. Ultrasound is an emerging imaging technique, with increasing musculoskeletal applications to evaluate soft tissue, superficial joints, and neural structures.

Treatment

Pelvic floor PT is a mainstay of rehabilitation treatment for pelvic floor myofascial pain and dysfunction. The goals of pelvic floor PT are to restore muscle imbalances, improve function, and reduce pain. Therapeutic options for myofascial pain are based on myofascial release techniques combined with neuromuscular reeducation to inactivate trigger points.[67] Soft tissue mobilization can address adhesions, diminish trigger points, and desensitize tissue. Manual techniques for myofascial trigger points include manual release, acupressure, muscle energy, and strain-counterstrain. Because the PFMs are intimately related to the anatomic structures of the pelvic girdle, hip, spine, and core musculature, exercises are also prescribed to restore normal movement patterns, joint range of motion, and muscle strength.[106] Adjuvant treatments include the use of biofeedback to improve muscle firing patterns in both *underactive* and *overactive* PFMs by providing the patient with objective feedback about muscle activation at rest and with activities of daily living (see Figure 38-5). Electrical stimulation can be used to increase PFM activity in underactive muscles or provide pain relief in overactive muscles by the use of surface electrodes or vaginal/rectal probes.

Medication use in pelvic floor myofascial pain and dysfunction is aimed at reducing pain, treating anxiety, and restoring restful sleep. Medications, such as nonsteroidal antiinflammatory drugs (NSAIDs), are often used for acute pain but are limited from long-term use by gastrointestinal side effects and the risk of bleeding. Tricyclic antidepressants (TCAs) (e.g., nortriptyline) and related mediations, such as trazodone and cyclobenzaprine, may be used to address pain, mood, and sleep in myofascial pain syndromes, but can cause anticholinergic side effects, such as dry mouth, constipation, or urinary retention. If there is a neurogenic or central sensitization component, antiepileptics (e.g., gabapentin or pregabalin) or serotonin norepinephrine reuptake inhibitors (SNRIs) (e.g., duloxetine or venlafaxine) may also be useful. SNRIs may be better tolerated than antiepileptics because of less sedating side effects. Muscle relaxants (e.g., cyclobenzaprine) may be helpful, especially for painful nighttime muscle spasms, but are limited by the side effect of sedation and are not recommended for long-term use. Care should be taken to avoid long-term use of narcotic pain medications. Topical medications are often a helpful adjuvant treatment option, including estrogen creams and topical anesthetics (e.g., lidocaine cream). Antispasmodic medications, such as valium or baclofen, may be used as an intravaginal suppository or made into a compounded cream. It is often helpful to use intravaginal valium or baclofen before pelvic floor PT, before sexual intercourse, or before going to sleep at night.

When the previously mentioned rehabilitation treatment interventions do not provide adequate relief from pelvic floor myofascial pain, injections can be used to reduce pain and increase participation in therapeutic exercises. Combining trigger point injections with manual techniques in PT may provide additional, longer lasting relief. Specific medical management techniques for myofascial trigger points include local anesthetic, botulinum toxin, corticosteroid injections, as well as dry needling.[67] The use of botulinum toxin for trigger point injections remains an off-label indication. If the patient also complains of posterior pelvic pain, a trial of an ultrasound-guided piriformis muscle trigger point injection may be indicated. Cadaveric studies demonstrate that the piriformis and obturator internus muscles are fused in approximately 40% of people,[141] and the combination of piriformis and obturator internus injection provided substantial relief in patients with posterior pelvic pain.[31] Additionally, fluoroscopic-guided SIJ, pubic symphysis, or hip intraarticular steroid injections may be additional targets to reduce pain and improve function, given the anatomic relationships described earlier. Injection treatment should be guided by a detailed history and musculoskeletal physical examination to identify potential pain generators. Injection interventions should not be used in isolation, but as part of a comprehensive rehabilitation plan to aid in diagnosis, progress goals in therapy, reduce pain, and improve function.

Pregnancy and Postpartum Pelvic Floor Dysfunction

Definitions and Etiology

Many musculoskeletal changes occur during pregnancy to accommodate for the growing fetus and prepare the woman's body for childbirth.[41,46] In addition to the increase in body mass, the abdominal muscles lengthen, there is an increase in lumbar lordosis, an increase in the anterior pelvic tilt, an increase in the pelvic width, and the center of gravity shifts anteriorly as the fetus grows. Hormonal changes also increase joint laxity. All of these changes lead to an increased demand being placed on the hip extensors, hip abductors, ankle plantar flexors, and the PFMs.

Musculoskeletal pain during pregnancy can arise from numerous areas, including the pelvic girdle, lumbar spine, hip, and PFMs. It is important to remember that anything that occurs in the nonpregnant woman can also occur during pregnancy. Although pain can arise from multiple locations, PGP is the most common cause of back and pelvic pain in pregnancy.[136] PGP is pain experienced between the posterior iliac crest and the gluteal fold, particularly in the region of the SIJs.[136] The pain may radiate to the posterior thigh. PGP may include pubic symphysis pain, which may radiate to the anterior thigh. Women with PGP have a diminished endurance capacity. To diagnose PGP, lumbar causes of pain must be excluded and the pain must be reproducible by specific clinical tests.

Several etiologies have been proposed with regard to PGP, including mechanical, hormonal, inflammatory, collagen abnormalities, and neural. It has been shown that women with PGP are more likely to have deep PFM tenderness in both the levator ani and obturator internus.[38] Joint laxity has also been studied in patients with PGP.[32] No relationship has been shown between increased SIJ laxity and pelvic pain during pregnancy; however, there was a correlation between asymmetric laxity of the SIJs and pain during pregnancy.

Relaxin, a hormone produced by the corpus luteum that relaxes the uterine musculature and allows for an increase in pelvic expansion, has been studied in PGP. Relaxin elevates during the first trimester of pregnancy and then remains stable throughout the rest of the pregnancy. The levels then decline sharply after delivery. There have been multiple studies showing a correlation between relaxin levels and PGP,[72,73,85] whereas other studies have shown no correlation.[53,88,117] These differences may be explained by study method variation because different studies had different methods of measuring joint laxity, some measured laxity in nonpelvic joints and used varying definitions of PGP. Marnach et al.[88] looked at several different hormone levels in pregnancy and found that cortisol, estradiol, and progesterone all substantially increase with each trimester. Women with joint complaints were more likely to have higher levels of estradiol and progesterone and lower levels of relaxin. Hormones may change the elasticity of ligaments by affecting collagen metabolism, which may contribute to the laxity of the joints during pregnancy. Kristiansson et al.[72] demonstrated that serum concentrations of a collagen turnover marker were significantly correlated with pelvic pain in pregnancy.

Epidemiology

PGP is estimated to affect approximately 20% of pregnant women.[136] Risk factors for development of PGP include a history of low back pain and previous trauma to the pelvis. Probable risk factors include parity and workload. The use of oral contraceptive pills, time interval since last pregnancy, height, weight, smoking, and age are not risk factors.

PGP can be further subdivided into four groups of pain patterns, defined by the locations of the painful joint(s) in the pelvis.[3] Double-sided SIJ syndrome, the most common of the four groups, affects approximately 6.3% of pregnant women.[3] Pelvic girdle syndrome affects approximately 6% of pregnant women and is diagnosed in women with daily pain in all three pelvic joints. One-sided SIJ syndrome is the next most common, affecting 5.5% of pregnant women, and finally, symphysiolysis or pubic symphysis pain affects 2.3% of pregnant women.

Diagnosis and Physical Examination

History and physical examination are the primary diagnostic tools for evaluation of the pregnant patient. A pain history should focus careful attention to previous history of low back pain or pelvic trauma. PGP is typically unilateral or bilateral posterior pelvic pain near the SIJs, but may also involve the lower abdominal area near the pubic symphysis. Radicular leg pain or paresthesias, groin pain, difficulty with weight bearing, and new onset bowel or bladder symptoms may be red flags of other underlying pathology.

Physical examination should include a general examination, neurologic examination of the lower extremities, and musculoskeletal examination of the pertinent areas of the patient's complaints, generally including the spine, pelvis, and hips. The external pelvic examination should focus on the SIJs and the pubic symphysis. The external pelvic examination should include palpation of the long dorsal ligament and pubic symphysis.[136] Provocative pain testing for the SIJs should include the Patrick (FABER) test, posterior pelvic pain provocation (P4 or PPPP), and the Gaenslen test. Pain provocation testing of the pubic symphysis can be done using the modified Trendelenburg test. Functional stability testing should also be performed with the active straight leg raise test. Rectal examination can be performed if there is concern for coccydynia or pelvic floor disorder; however, vaginal examination of the pelvic floor should be avoided during pregnancy unless approved by the patient's obstetrician.

Treatment

The mainstay of treatment for PGP is individualized PT that includes realignment and stabilizing exercises.[136] Pelvic floor PT, especially with external biofeedback or intrarectal treatments, can be performed with the obstetrician's permission if the patient has PFM overactivity. Pelvic manipulations and SIJ belts have been beneficial for symptomatic relief but do not alter the course of the disease.[93] There is no evidence for massage, specific pillow use, education apart from PT treatment, or bed rest in the treatment of PGP. Ice and acetaminophen are also often used in this patient population. Lidoderm patches and cyclobenzaprine are pregnancy class B and can be used for symptomatic relief. Low-dose opioids are generally considered safe and may be necessary when severe pain does not respond to other rehabilitation treatments. NSAIDs are not thought to be safe for use during pregnancy, but may be resumed in the postpartum period, even when breastfeeding. Approximately 6 weeks after delivery, the postpartum patient can be further evaluated and treated with both pelvic girdle and pelvic floor PT if there is remaining pelvic floor myofascial pain and/or dysfunction (as discussed earlier).

Pelvic Nerve Injuries

Definitions and Etiology

Neural injury can be a source of CPP and can coexist with pelvic floor dysfunction and pelvic floor myofascial pain. The iliohypogastric, ilioinguinal, genitofemoral, and pudendal nerves most commonly contribute to pelvic pain symptoms. Pudendal neuropathy has also been implicated as a potential cause of urinary incontinence and FI, as well as sexual dysfunction. The anatomy of these nerves has been reviewed earlier.

The iliohypogastric and ilioinguinal nerves are particularly susceptible to injury if a Pfannenstiel or low transverse incision is dissected too far laterally beyond the edge of the rectus abdominis muscles.[17,83] Neuroma formation is common after such nerve damage and can be a source of chronic pain.[82] The genitofemoral nerve can be damaged via compression during gynecologic surgery, often by poor placement of self-retaining retractors.[17] All three of these nerves are thought to be common causes of chronic groin pain after surgery for inguinal hernia repair.[50]

Injury to the pudendal nerves during vaginal delivery has been well reported in the literature, and pudendal neuropathy has been implicated as a possible contributing factor to new onset postpartum urinary incontinence and FI.[27,45] The pudendal nerve can also be injured in pelvic surgeries (particularly with the use of vaginal mesh), in cases of pelvic trauma, with bicycle riding, with chronic straining to defecate, and during anal intercourse.[58]

Epidemiology

Overall incidence of ilioinguinal and/or iliohypogastric nerve injury after a Pfannenstiel incision has been estimated at 2% to 4%.[82-84] The incidence of chronic groin pain after hernia repair attributable to injury of one of these three nerves is thought to be as high as 16%, with 6% to 8% of all patients after herniorrhaphy having moderate-to-severe, disabling symptoms.[24,110]

Reported incidence of pudendal neuralgia in the general population has ranged from 1% to 4%.[58] Allen et al.[4] recruited a group of 75 women who agreed to pudendal nerve terminal motor latency testing and needle electromyography (EMG) of the external anal sphincter at 36 weeks' gestation and again at 2 months' postpartum. While pregnant, pudendal neurophysiology testing was normal, but EMG evidence of pelvic floor reinnervation potentials were seen in 80% of the postpartum women.

Diagnosis and Physical Examination

Having a high index of suspicion is the key to diagnosing a pelvic nerve injury. The history is often more helpful than the physical examination. The symptoms of iliohypogastric and ilioinguinal neuralgia typically include pain in the lower abdomen, groin, or pubis. There can be accompanying numbness. Genitofemoral neuralgia is also often described as pubic or groin pain, but can also be appreciated as labial or scrotal/testicular pain. If the femoral branch of the genitofemoral is involved, there can be pain in the upper anterior thigh. Symptoms of pudendal neuralgia include perineal pain and pain medial to the ischial tuberosity. Symptoms are most often unilateral. The pain is most often described as burning, with occasional numbness or paresthesia. Pain is worse with sitting, dyspareunia is common, and patients may report a sensation of a foreign body in the rectum or perineum.

Many patients with pelvic nerve injury will also have pelvic floor myofascial dysfunction; it can be difficult to determine on physical examination whether the muscles or the nerves are the source of the pain. Many patients with pudendal neuralgia are thought to have significant PFM overactivity, which in turn compresses the small, infiltrating branches of the pudendal tree, producing the characteristic burning sensation even in the absence of a true pudendal nerve lesion or entrapment.[58] It should be noted that, despite the anatomic function of the pudendal nerve, in many cases of pudendal neuralgia, there is no objective sensory loss and anal sphincter tone, and other neurologic examination testing may be normal in all but the most severe cases.[58] The Nantes criteria are a validated set of clinical conditions which, when met, make it likely that the patient has pudendal neuralgia.[75]

The iliohypogastric, ilioinguinal, genitofemoral, and pudendal nerves can be evaluated electrophysiologically via a number of different methods.[74] Unfortunately, these nerves are technically difficult to study; therefore these studies are not routinely used. Pudendal nerve terminal motor latency can be obtained through the use of a St. Mark electrode, with nerve stimulation at the ischial spine and recording of muscle contraction response at the external anal sphincter.[27] The usefulness of pudendal nerve terminal motor latency has been questioned, because it has been shown to have a high rate of interobserver and intraobserver variability.[59] Needle EMG of the external anal sphincter or bulbospongiosus muscles can be performed.[4] The bulbocavernosus reflex latency can also be obtained by stimulating at the clitoris or penis.[66] Electrodiagnostic testing for pudendal neuropathy may be less well tolerated than standard nerve conduction studies and needle EMG of the extremities.

Diagnostic nerve blocks are a potentially good option for diagnosis. A positive response to infiltration of a local anesthetic around the iliohypogastric, ilioinguinal, and genitofemoral nerves is thought to be a reliable indicator of etiologic correlation.[123] It is less clear that a positive response to a pudendal block is definitively correlated with true pathology.[75] It is always preferable to use ultrasound, pulsed radiofrequency, or ideally computed tomography (CT) guidance for better accuracy when performing these diagnostic injections.[59]

Ultrasound, in general, is not particularly useful for evaluating nerve injuries about the hip and pelvis, because these nerves are typically too deep to allow for long segment exploration and good visualization.[89] MR neurography technology is rapidly becoming recognized as one of the most effective diagnostic tools for nerve injury and is thought to be far superior for nerve visualization than standard MRI.[102,121] MR neurography of the lumbosacral plexus is often able to demonstrate injury to the iliohypogastric, ilioinguinal, genitofemoral, and pudendal nerves. Figure 38-6 shows MR neurography images of a left genitofemoral neuropathy.

Treatment

The first line of treatment for pelvic nerve injuries may include pelvic floor PT or medications. Neuropathic pain medications, such as gabapentin pregabalin, SNRIs, or TCAs, may be of benefit. Compounded neuropathic pain creams and vaginal/rectal suppositories are being prescribed more frequently in recent years, although data on their effectiveness are scarce. These creams often consist of a mixture of various neuropathic medications (e.g., gabapentin or amitriptyline), but the key ingredient is typically ketamine at a concentration of 5% to 10%.[105] Systemic absorption is thought to be low and side effects are typically minimal when used externally.

Therapeutic injections of corticosteroid mixed with local anesthetic, delivered either as a single intervention or as an injection series, have been reported to be helpful for ilioinguinal, iliohypogastric, genitofemoral, and pudendal neuropathies.[59,123,133] As with diagnostic injections, therapeutic injections should ideally be performed under ultrasound or CT guidance. Radiofrequency ablation and pulsed radiofrequency treatments for some of these nerves have also been described.[111,114] There have been a few descriptions of successful treatment of ilioinguinal or pudendal neuropathic pain via neuromodulation either at the level of the spinal cord, sacral plexus, or of the individual nerves themselves, but at this time neuromodulation has not been studied extensively enough to recommend its use in this patient population.[21,57,109,112]

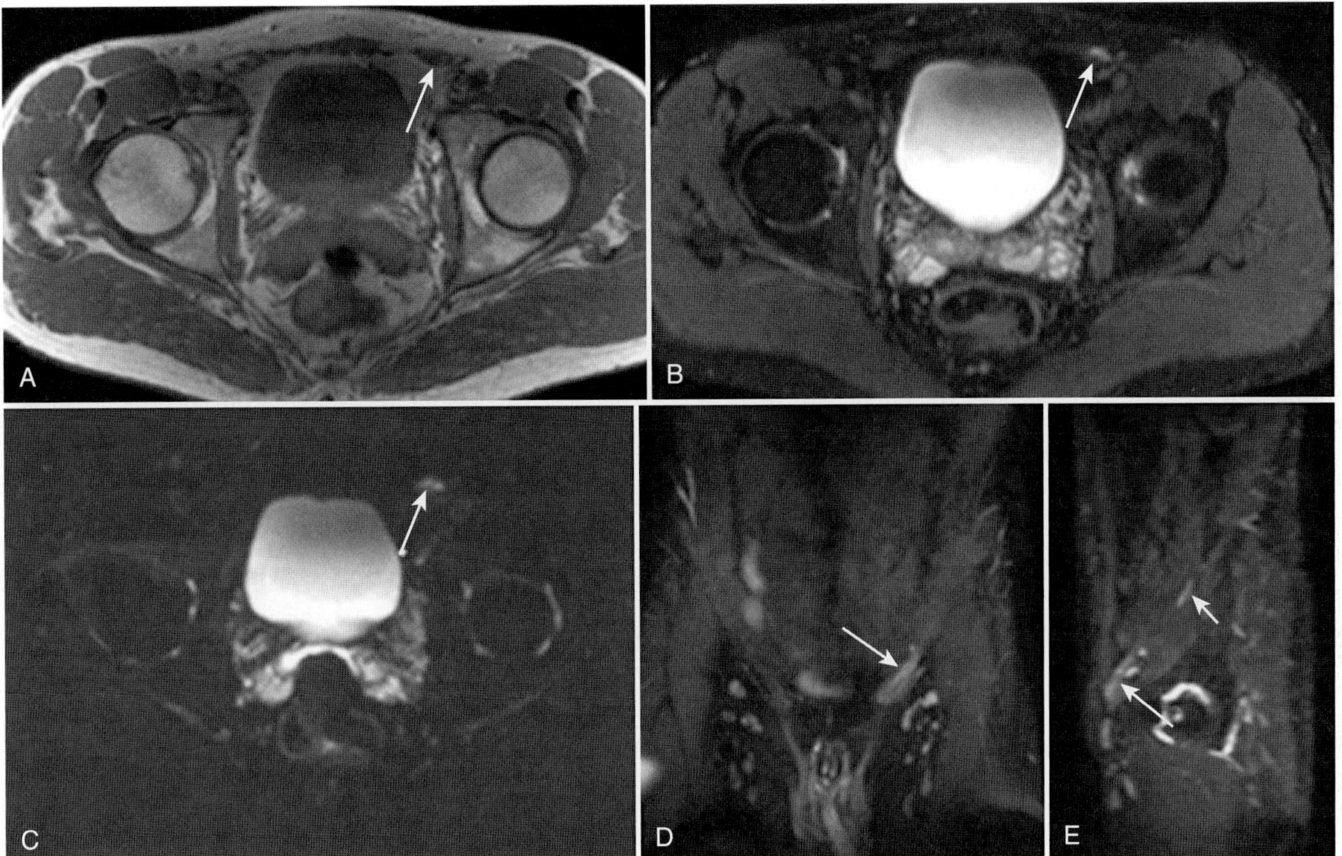

FIGURE 38-6 A to E, Left genitofemoral neuropathy as seen on magnetic resonance neurography. (Courtesy Dr. Avneesh Chhabra, used with permission.)

Surgery can be an effective solution in some cases, particularly for chronic iliohypogastric, ilioinguinal, and genitofemoral neuralgia.[24,83,123] Neurectomy, also known as nerve resection or transection, is the preferred surgical option for these three nerves. Increasingly, a "triple neurectomy" of all three nerves is performed at the same time for patients with severe groin pain.[24] Rates of complete or moderate pain relief after neurectomy of the iliohypogastric, ilioinguinal, and genitofemoral nerves have been reported in the range of 66% to 100% of patients.[24,83,142]

Various approaches have been described for decompression (or neurolysis) of the pudendal nerve in cases of entrapment.[59] Outcomes for pudendal decompression surgeries have not been uniformly good, perhaps because many patients with pudendal neuralgia do not have actual pudendal nerve entrapment. Short-term improvement of some degree has been seen in 50% to 70% of patients after 3 to 12 months, but 50% to 66% of all patients undergoing surgery have no long-term benefit.[90,113] Appropriate patient selection and a high level of surgeon experience seem to be the key to successful outcomes with higher satisfaction rates.[58]

Overlap of Pelvic Floor Disorders and Chronic Pelvic Pain

Chronic pelvic pain (CPP), defined as noncyclic pain of 6 or more month's duration that localizes to the anatomic pelvis, anterior abdominal wall at or below the umbilicus, the lumbosacral back or the buttocks that is severe enough to cause some disability,[62] affects 25% of women ages 18 to 50 years and can also affect men.[78] There are numerous stakeholders involved in caring for patients with these chronic symptoms including those in primary care, gynecology, gastroenterology, urology, neurology, physical medicine and rehabilitation, psychology, and PT. Although CPP includes several visceral and somatic causes (see Table 38-1), many patients undergo surgical interventions for presumed visceral origins before musculoskeletal causes are considered, which delays diagnosis and treatment of musculoskeletal pelvic pain.[18,34] It is important to correctly understand the anatomic basis and differences between these conditions, and to identify musculoskeletal causes of pelvic pain, such as pelvic floor myofascial pain, PGP, and pelvic nerve injuries (as described in more detail earlier), to provide appropriate rehabilitation treatments in a timely manner. CPP subtypes are comorbid with other CPP and nonpelvic pain conditions.[70] Several subtypes of CPP will be reviewed to provide an appropriate differential diagnosis for the rehabilitation provider, guide conservative management, and direct appropriate referrals.

Chronic Pelvic Pain Subtypes

Interstitial Cystitis/Painful Bladder Syndrome

Interstitial cystitis/painful bladder syndrome (IC/PBS) is a urologic diagnosis characterized by suprapubic pain and urinary urgency and frequency. It is commonly diagnosed in the fourth decade,[119] is nine times more prevalent in women,[30] and appears to be comorbid with fibromyalgia, vulvodynia, and endometriosis.[26,138] The current mechanistic understanding of IC/PBS remains elusive. Proposed etiologies have included neurogenic inflammation, epithelial dysfunction, autoimmune, infectious, and peripheral/central sensitization.[2] On history, patients should be queried for risk factors for bladder visceral sensitivity, such as previous instrumentation as a child, recurrent urinary tract infections, and history of sexual abuse. Patients should be ruled out for urinary tract infection, nephrolithiasis, and underlying malignancy. On abdominal examination, suprapubic tenderness is the hallmark. On pelvic examination, anterior vaginal wall, bladder base, and PFM tenderness is often found. Further diagnostic testing may include maximum cystometric capacity with a retrograde filling test and an intravesical anesthetic challenge.

Endometriosis

Endometriosis is defined as the presence of endometrial glands and stroma outside the endometrial cavity and uterine musculature. Women with endometriosis also appear to have generalized pain sensitivity not just regional pelvic pain sensitivity.[9] Symptoms of endometriosis may include disabling menstrual cramps, CPP or low back pain, pain during or after intercourse, painful bowel movements, painful urination during menstrual periods, heavy menstrual periods, premenstrual spotting or bleeding between periods, and/or a history of infertility. The role of diagnostic laparoscopy is to rule out endometriosis or pelvic adhesions.[63] Laparoscopic excision of the implants with histologic confirmation is now considered diagnostic standard of care.

Irritable Bowel Syndrome

Irritable bowel syndrome is defined as at least 3 months of continuous or recurrent symptoms including pain relieved by defecation and/or associated with change in frequency of stool or consistency of stool.[122] Patients may have constipation or diarrhea predominant symptoms. No structural or biochemical abnormality is present to explain the symptoms. Approximately 15% of the general population in Western countries have this diagnosis. Symptoms suggestive of irritable bowel syndrome are present in approximately 50% to 80% of patients with CPP. Potential mechanisms contributing to irritable bowel syndrome include abnormal motility, heightened visceral perception, pelvic floor dysfunction, psychological distress, and intraluminal factors irritating the bowel, such as lactose, other sugars, and bile acid.[19] Patients with irritable bowel syndrome will typically have a normal general physical examination but may have an abnormal pelvic floor examination. Diagnostic studies should include a complete blood count with differential, electrolytes, stool for occult blood, white blood cells, ova and parasites, *Clostridium difficile* toxin, and screening for celiac sprue, lactose intolerance, and colon cancer. Treatment ranges from regulating diet to optimizing the use of nonirritant oral agents (e.g., bulk agents, natural laxatives) to psychological interventions to manage stress.

Vulvodynia

Vulvodynia is defined as focal chronic nonmalignant urogenital pain characterized by chronic vulvar discomfort without any visual abnormality.[8] Symptoms of itching, burning, stinging, or stabbing in the area around the opening of the vagina predominate. The pain may be provoked with attempts at penetration with intercourse or unprovoked. The pain may also be localized or generalized vulvar dysesthesia. The main physical finding is a positive Q-tip test suggestive of vulvar allodynia.[99] This subtype appears to have a 16% lifetime prevalence[55] and 61% of women have symptoms during their reproductive years, whereas 25% of women have symptoms postmenopause.[52] Oral contraceptives may contribute to the development of localized vulvodynia.[8] Patients with vulvar pain appear to have higher systemic pain perception, autonomic abnormalities, such as low diastolic blood pressure, and higher anxiety traits.[48] This diagnosis is often comorbid with irritable bowel syndrome, fibromyalgia, and IC/PBS.[47]

Rehabilitation Treatment for Chronic Pelvic Pain

A Cochrane review recommends that overall treatments for CPP should include hormonal treatments, counseling after negative ultrasound, multidisciplinary approach to pain management including PT, psychotherapy, diet, and environmental factors.[125] Selected medication options are suggested but not well studied and include NSAIDs, acetaminophen, and tramadol. Other medication options include TCAs (e.g., amitriptyline), antiepileptics (e.g., gabapentin, pregabalin), benzodiazepines, anticholinergics, antispasmodics, and ovarian cycle inhibitors for patients with hormonally driven pain.[134] Medical pelvic floor treatments including compounded vaginal diazepam suppositories and topical compounded ointments have varied effects or lack adequate study in CPP.[22,28]

First-line treatment for IC/PBS should be general relaxation, stress and pain management, patient education, and self-care.[51] Second-line treatment is manual pelvic floor PT[40] along with consideration for amitriptyline, cimetidine, hydroxyzine, and intravesical treatments, such as heparin or lidocaine. Patients with IC/PBS are advised to avoid citrus, chocolate, caffeine, sodas, alcohol, and heavily seasoned foods.[43] Medical treatment for irritable bowel syndrome ranges from laxatives and prokinetics to antibiotics, probiotics, and neuropathic pain medications.[91] Vulvodynia treatments have included dietary modifications, PT, and vulvar care measures.[77] Vestibulectomy, or surgical removal of the vestibule (tissue containing the opening of the urethra) and hymen, has been shown to have reasonable long-term efficacy.[6,130]

Rehabilitation addresses behavioral management as well as multiple biomechanical factors. This includes treatment of the pelvic joints, motor control of core musculature including the pelvic floor, along with body awareness and function. Pelvic floor PT includes manual therapy (vaginal and rectal) with soft tissue and joint mobilization (as described earlier in further detail). Biofeedback therapy or real-time ultrasound can be an excellent adjunct to manual therapy. Electrical stimulation and vaginal dilators are tools that can also be used in pain management, particularly as a home exercise program.

Therapeutic injections are widely used clinically but are not well supported in the literature for CPP. This includes pelvic floor trigger point injections, pelvic joint injection under fluoroscopy, nerve blocks, neurolysis, and botulinum toxin.[1] Other treatments for CPP including acupuncture, electrical stimulation, Chinese herbal medicine, and psychological therapies have also been described.[20,23] Sacral nerve stimulation for CPP has gained promise.[129]

Conclusion

In summary, pelvic floor disorders are generally not life-threatening but can greatly effect one's quality of life. The prevalence of these disorders is likely to be higher than reported because many individuals are embarrassed by their symptoms and do not report them to health care providers. Diagnosis of pelvic floor disorders can often be made with history and physical examination. Treatment should include a trial of conservative therapies that can often provide significant symptom reduction and improved quality of life.

KEY REFERENCES

3. Albert H, Godskesen M, Westergaard J: Prognosis in four syndromes of pregnancy-related pelvic pain, *Acta Obstet Gynecol Scand* 80:505–510, 2001.
4. Allen R, Hosker G, Smith A, et al: Pelvic floor damage and childbirth: a neurophysiological study, *Br J Obstet Gynecol* 97:770–779, 1990.
14. Bø K, Hilde G: Does it work in the long term?—A systematic review on pelvic floor muscle training for female stress urinary incontinence, *Neurourol Urodyn* 32:215–223, 2013.
25. Chiaroni G, Whitehead W: The role of biofeedback in the treatment of gastrointestinal disorders, *Nat Clin Pract Gastroenterol Hepatol* 5:371–382, 2008.
29. Cummings M, Baldry P: Regional myofascial pain: diagnosis and management, *Best Pract Res Clin Rheumatol* 21:367–387, 2007.
37. Fall M, Baranowski AP, Elneil S, et al: European Association of Urology: EAU guidelines on chronic pelvic pain, *Eur Urol* 57:35–48, 2010.
39. Deleted in review.
42. Frawley H: Pelvic floor muscle strength testing, *Aust J Physiother* 52:307, 2006.
56. Haylen BT, de Ridder D, Freeman RM, et al: An International Urogynaecological Association (IUGA)/International Continence Society (ICS) joint report on the terminology for female pelvic floor dysfunction, *Int Urogynecol J* 21:5–26, 2010.
58. Hibner M, Castellanos M, Desai N, et al: Pudendal neuralgia, *Glob Libr Womens Med* 2011. doi: 10.3843/GLOWM.10468.
59. Hibner M, Desai N, Robertson L, et al: Pudendal neuralgia, *J Minim Invasive Gynecol* 17:148–153, 2010.
61. Hosker G, Cody J, Norton C: Electrical stimulation for faecal incontinence in adults, *Cochrane Database Syst Rev* (3):CD001310, 2007.
62. Howard FM: Chronic pelvic pain, *Obstet Gynecol* 101:594–611, 2003.
67. Itza F, Zarza D, Serra L, et al: Myofascial pain syndrome in the pelvic floor: a common urological condition, *Actas Urol Esp* 34:318–326, 2010.
70. Jarrell JF, Vilos GA, Allaire C, et al: Consensus guidelines for the management of chronic pelvic pain, *J Obstet Gynaecol Can* 27:781–826, 2005.
75. Labat J, Riant T, Robert R, et al: Diagnostic criteria for pudendal neuralgia by pudendal nerve entrapment (Nantes criteria), *Neurourol Urodyn* 27:306–310, 2008.
80. Liu LW: Chronic constipation: current treatment options, *Can J Gastroenterol* 25:(Suppl B):22b–28b, 2011.
81. Longstreth GF, Thompson WG, Chey WD, et al: Functional bowel disorders, *Gastroenterology* 130:1480–1491, 2006.
94. Messelink B, Benson T, Berghmans B, et al: Standardization of terminology of pelvic floor muscle function and dysfunction: report from the pelvic floor clinical assessment group of the International Continence Society, *Neurourol Urodyn* 24:374–380, 2005.
97. Norton C, Cody J: Biofeedback and/or sphincter exercises for the treatment of faecal incontinence in adults, *Cochrane Database Syst Rev* (7):CD002111, 2012.
103. Peters KM, Carrico DJ: Frequency, urgency, and pelvic pain: treating the pelvic floor versus the epithelium, *Curr Urol Rep* 7:450–455, 2006.
106. Prather H, Dugan S, Fitzgerald C, Hunt D: Review of anatomy, evaluation, and treatment of musculoskeletal pelvic floor pain in women, *PM R* 1:346–358, 2009.
107. Rahn DD: Pathophysiology of urinary incontinence, voiding dysfunction, and overactive bladder, *Obstet Gynecol Clin North Am* 36:463–474, 2009.
125. Stones RW, Mountfield J: Interventions for treating chronic pelvic pain in women, *Cochrane Database Syst Rev* (4):CD000387, 2000.
128. Tantiphlachiva K, Rao P, Attaluri A, et al: Digital rectal examination is a useful tool for identifying patients with dyssynergia, *Clin Gastroenterol Hepatol* 8:955–960, 2010.
134. Vercellini P, Vigano P, Somigliana E, et al: Medical, surgical and alternative treatments for chronic pelvic pain in women: a descriptive review, *Gynecol Endocrinol* 25:208–221, 2009.
136. Vleeming A, Albert HB, Ostgaard HC, et al: European guidelines for the diagnosis and treatment of pelvic girdle pain, *Eur Spine J* 17:794–819, 2008.
142. Zacest A, Magill S, Anderson V, et al: Long-term outcome following ilioinguinal neurectomy for chronic pain, *J Neurosurg* 112:784–789, 2010.

The full reference list for this chapter is available online.

CHAPTER 39

SPORTS MEDICINE AND ADAPTIVE SPORTS

Mark A. Harrast, Scott R. Laker, Erin Maslowski, Arthur J. De Luigi

Physiatrists are uniquely qualified to serve as sports medicine physicians and care for the recreational and competitive athlete as well as those who exercise for health-related benefits. Physiatrists are trained extensively in musculoskeletal medicine and injury, functional rehabilitation, and coordinating and leading a team of professionals to optimize care of patients. The sports medicine team includes the athlete, his or her family, specialty and primary care physicians, athletic trainers, physical and massage therapists, chiropractors, dieticians, psychologists, and coaches. Physiatrists are also skilled in prehabilitation, or preventive rehabilitation, which is an important aspect of care for any athlete involved in routine physical training.

Exercise physiology, emergency medical care, and more routine medical care are also important to any well-rounded sports medicine physician. This chapter covers the breadth of sports medicine for the physiatrist, including the general role and medicolegal aspects of being a team physician, sporting event administration with a particular focus on emergency preparedness, athletic conditioning and training principles, injury prevention and functional rehabilitation, biomechanics of sports, pharmacology in sports, emergency assessment and care of the athlete, common medical and neurologic conditions in athletes, and a review of specific populations of athletes and their common ailments, including a special focus on athletes with disabilities and adaptive sports medicine. This chapter is not intended to be a musculoskeletal medicine chapter because other chapters in this text cover in-depth musculoskeletal issues that overlap with the musculoskeletal injuries seen in athletes.

Role of the Team Physician

The team physician has multiple, overlapping roles within the framework of the team itself, the individual athletes and their families, the school or overseeing organization, and the community. The primary responsibility is caring for the health and well-being of the individual athlete. The chief duties are to determine initial medical eligibility, provide care for the injured athlete, facilitate and determine return to play, create and maintain emergency preparedness, oversee the healthfulness of the team's overall training program, supervise the personnel providing health care for the team, and protect against institutional and personal liability.[148] The role of intermediary for each of these groups is both challenging and rewarding. The team physician is responsible for conveying information to other medical specialists, allied health professionals, athletic trainers, and coaches, as well as for creating and coordinating health care plans for the athletes.[3]

These multiple roles can at times be in conflict, and it is essential to recognize that the primary obligation is always to the athlete as patient. The specific details of confidentiality and the flow of information are defined by the Health Information Privacy and Portability Act. Specifically, the components of consent for treatment and the authorization to release information are most pertinent to the team physician. It is prudent to review this document and the applicable state law as well as to discuss these matters with all involved parties (e.g., athletes, coaches, families) before issues arise.

Beyond the medical obligation to the athlete, the team physician has an assumed medicolegal responsibility. Physicians receiving financial or other obvious remuneration for services are bound by normal medicolegal responsibilities. The physician might be held legally liable if injury occurs as a result of negligence or treatment below the professional standard of care. Those physicians who volunteer their services may not be covered by Good Samaritan laws, particularly if they are the "designated" medical provider for an event, regardless of whether or not they are remunerated for their services. Preparticipation physical evaluations (PPEs) are not covered under Good Samaritan laws. In some cases, athletes might be legally allowed to participate despite a disqualifying PPE.

The team physician is also responsible for the final decision regarding clearance to play or return to play (RTP) after injury. These issues can be complex, and several fundamentals must be met before the athlete should be cleared. When recovering from an injury, the athlete must have completed appropriate rehabilitation; a health care professional must document the athlete's recovery; and the risks of return must be discussed and documented. The team physician must obtain the appropriate consultant opinions when dealing with conditions or injuries outside the scope of his or her practice. Although some states have determined that athletic participation implies assumed risk, this is not universal. Team physicians have been held liable for injury occurring after full RTP has been granted. In cases of differing opinions of the team physician and a consultant, the final responsibility typically lies with the team physician.

The traveling team physician presents a unique issue given that licensure and malpractice coverage are state-specific. There is currently a bill (Sports Medicine Licensure Clarity Act of 2015) before the 114th Congress that could protect sports medicine physicians who travel across state lines and provide care for athletes in states in which they are not licensed.

Event Administration

The two most common competition venues where the sports medicine physician practices are on the sidelines of a sporting event (e.g., football, soccer, gymnastics) and at mass participation endurance events (e.g., marathons, road races, triathlons). These are unique venues that require appropriate planning, organization, rehearsal, and communication to provide optimal medical care.

Both require significant preseason or preevent planning.[88] From an administrative perspective, it is essential that the team physician or chief medical officer develops a chain of command that defines the responsibilities of the medical providers, emergency medical services, event officials, and other parties involved. Establishing and regularly rehearsing an emergency action plan (EAP) are critical. Reviewing the medical equipment that will be available at the event as well as the protocols for attending to an injured athlete are standard components of preparation. The team physician must also assess environmental concerns and playing conditions and have a policy to modify or suspend practice or competition if adverse conditions exist.

Administering care at a mass participation endurance event such as a marathon requires unique planning given the sheer number of participants, the unique medical illnesses encountered, the length of the course, the number of medical sites needed, and the large medical team required to staff such an event. Given its size, the potential impact of the event on the community and its resources needs to be accounted for in planning and implementation. These large mass participation events require the coordination of public, private, and medical agencies, as well as effective communication among them during race planning and race day.

Although any marathon has a known number of people requiring medical assistance (2% to 20% of participants, depending on event size, duration, and weather conditions), if these numbers should increase unexpectedly, there is a potential for the community resources to become overwhelmed if not allocated appropriately.[34,159] For this reason, communication among the medical team, race officials, emergency medical services, local hospitals, and participants is crucial to help prevent and respond to incidents during the race. It is the role of the chief medical officer to coordinate these effective lines of communication.

Medical staff need to be familiar with the more common ailments that runners can present with during or after the race and to have the appropriate equipment available in advance. Exercise-associated collapse, a common medical entity seen in marathon medical tents, has a broad differential diagnosis, which includes fairly benign to potentially life-threatening disorders (see later). Appropriate medical equipment for a marathon includes devices for rapid electrolyte blood testing, cardiac monitoring capabilities, automated external defibrillators (AEDs), rectal thermometers, rapid warming and cooling protocols and equipment, and personnel and equipment for starting intravenous therapy.

Prevention of medical tent encounters is an even better way to enhance safety. Preventing race day maladies in marathoners requires educating racers and properly coordinating appropriate resources (aid and fluid replacement stations) along the course. Educate the runners in the months, weeks, and even the day before and day of the event to "listen to their bodies," train adequately, determine/estimate fluid needs before the race and stick to a plan during the race, and adjust race/time expectations if the weather conditions are adverse. Education is an important strategy to lessen morbidity (and potentially mortality) during and after the race.

Principles of Conditioning and Training

Effective training programs require a fundamental understanding of strength, flexibility, and endurance development, as well as the basic principles of specificity, individuality, periodization, overload, and tapering. Please refer to Chapter 15 for an overview of strength, flexibility, and endurance training.

The body's adaptation to physical training is metabolically and neuromuscularly specific to the exercise performed. The principle of sport specificity highlights the importance of training in the same sport the athlete will be competing in. For example, although cycling and cross-country skiing are valuable forms of aerobic exercise, an athlete who is training to run a marathon needs to focus on running as the major component of training to ultimately maximize running performance. It must be realized, however, that individuals respond differently to the same training stimulus. For example, a less-conditioned athlete will make larger gains in fitness than a more conditioned athlete who embarks on a training program.

The principle of overload requires that the training stimulus be greater than how the athlete normally performs in competition. Exercise frequency, duration, and intensity are manipulated to produce overload. These specific training variables (frequency, duration, and intensity) must be periodically increased for an athlete to progress (Box 39-1).

Periodization

Periodization is one structured training approach that highlights this concept. It was developed by a Russian physiologist in the 1960s but has had a significant resurgence in today's training programs (Figure 39-1). In periodization, training is divided into defined "periods" to allow buildup of training stresses, time for rest and adaptation to training, and continual progression of fitness. These periods include macrocycles (commonly lasting 1 year),

BOX 39-1

Training Program Design Variables: FITT

F Frequency of training
I Intensity of training
T Type of exercise mode
T Time of exercise duration

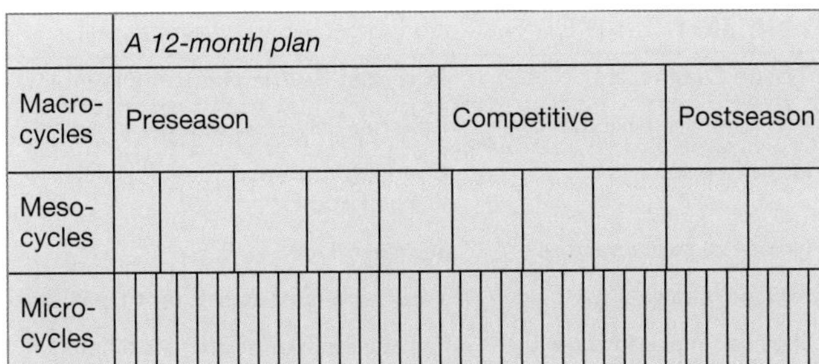

FIGURE 39-1 A template for a periodized training program. (From Bachl N, Baron R, Smekal G: Principles of exercise physiology and conditioning. In Frontera WR, et al, editors: *Clinical sports medicine: medical management and rehabilitation*, Philadelphia, PA, 2007, Saunders.)

which are divided into shorter mesocycles (commonly lasting 1 month), which are then subdivided into microcycles (commonly lasting 1 week). Microcycles are generally the weekly training programs. Each mesocycle can be made up of 4 weekly microcycles with a gradual buildup of training frequency and intensity over the first 3 weeks and then a slight decrease in the fourth week to allow for rest and the subsequent metabolic training adaptations to occur. The athlete is then ready to enter the next 4-week mesocycle and progress through another 4 weekly microcycles. The amount and intensity of training in each mesocycle depend on where the athlete is in relationship to the competitive season, which is how macrocycles are structured.

A typical year-long training program will have three macrocycles: preseason or "buildup phase," competitive season or "maintenance and fine-tuning phase," and finally a postseason or "recovery phase." The preseason macrocycle is typically the longest, occurring before the competitive season. It is designed to develop fitness in anticipation of the more intense training to follow.[195] During the preseason macrocycle the athlete generally focuses on higher volume and lower intensity exercise.

The competitive season macrocycle follows the preseason period. The focus here is to develop and maintain peak fitness with a focus on high-intensity training and sport-specific technique drills.[195] Because of the higher intensity training, the volume must be significantly reduced.

Finally, the postseason macrocycle is a time for the athlete to recover from the previous year's training and physically and mentally prepare for the next year of training and competition.[195] The early portion of this period necessitates "active rest." The athlete generally participates in unstructured, non–sport-specific recreational activities to allow for recovery from the stresses of the competitive season. This is an important period for the athlete to adequately recover from injuries, prevent overtraining, and take a "mental break" from the competitive season.

During the competitive season, a typical microcycle includes a tapering period just before competition. The taper is a short period of reduced training before an important competition with the goal of optimizing performance. Although it is well recognized that a reduction in training before competition improves performance, it is not definitively known what is the most ideal taper strategy regarding altering training volume, intensity, and frequency.[7,93,135] A recent metaanalysis demonstrated that the most efficient strategy to maximize performance gains appears to be a 2-week taper during which training volume is exponentially reduced by 41% to 60%.[21] This study found that the ideal taper for endurance athletes kept training intensity and frequency stable, with only volume being progressively reduced.

Overtraining Syndrome

An important set of symptoms to be aware of for any athlete, coach, or sports medicine physician is that related to overtraining syndrome. When prolonged, excessive training occurs concurrently with insufficient recovery, the athlete might have unexplainable performance decrements resulting in chronic maladaptations leading to overtraining syndrome.[128] Common symptoms of overtraining syndrome in addition to an unexplained performance decrement include generalized fatigue, mood disturbance, poor sleep, and increased rates of illness and injury. By definition, these symptoms persist despite more than 2 weeks of rest.[188] The treatment is rest, from weeks to months, with gradual resumption of training. Prevention, however, is the best treatment, and following a periodized training program is one method to ensure adequate rest from more intense bouts of training.

Altitude Training

Altitude/hypoxic training is a controversial area of research and sports performance. Many elite endurance athletes incorporate altitude training into their typical training program in hope of enhancing performance in competition. For those athletes who do not live in mountainous areas, there are a variety of "altitude tents" on the market that can be used to simulate living at high altitude. Some controversy arose in 2006 when the World Anti-Doping Agency (WADA) considered placing "artificially-induced hypoxic conditions" on the Prohibited List of Substances/Methods.[199] Another area of controversy is the uncertain primary physiologic mechanism(s) responsible for the effect of altitude training on sea-level performance. The proposed mechanisms include accelerated erythropoiesis (increased erythrocyte volume) as the primary hematologic effect, as well as nonhematologic factors such as improved muscle efficiency at the mitochondrial level, glucose transport alterations, and enhanced muscle-buffering capacity via pH regulation.[75]

Most scientists agree that the most effective form of altitude/hypoxic training is the "live high–train low" method whereby athletes "live high" to stimulate erythropoietin and subsequently increase erythrocyte volume and "train low" at a higher intensity with improved oxygen flux to induce beneficial metabolic and neuromuscular training adaptations.[200] The controversy here comes from not knowing what the optimal "dose" of altitude training truly is. So far, the research suggests that for athletes to derive the most beneficial hematologic effects while using natural altitude, they need to live at an elevation of 2000 to 2500 meters for 22 hours a day for 4 weeks. For those using simulated altitude environments, 12 to 16 hours of hypoxic exposure might be necessary but at a higher elevation (2500 to 3000 meters).[200]

Injury Prevention and Rehabilitation

Injuries that occur in the course of an athlete's life will be because of a multitude of causes. These include acute trauma, overuse, and injuries secondary to poor technique. Certain injuries are predictable and even preventable in many cases.

Kinetic Chain Assessment

The kinetic chain model is based on the idea that each complex, athletic movement is the summation of its constituent parts. For example, a quarterback's throwing motion is created through the action of feet on the playing surface, loading of the lower limbs, rotation of the hips and abdominal muscles, activation of the latissimus dorsi, stabilization of the glenohumeral joint by the periscapular muscles, loading of the throwing arm through the deltoid and biceps, and finally from the upper limb motion of elbow extension and wrist flexion. The upper limb acts as a "funnel" for the energy generated by the core and lower limbs.[101] Each of the "links" in the chain must function well to optimize performance and minimize potential tissue trauma.

"Catch-up" occurs when an athlete tries to compensate with one segment for a deficiency in a separate segment. This phenomenon puts higher stress on the tissues of the distal segment and predisposes it to injury.[101] For example, a runner might present with patellofemoral pain for a variety of reasons. It could simply be an overtraining phenomenon, or it might be caused by weak or inhibited hip musculature, abnormal foot and ankle biomechanics, or poor running technique.[123] Relief can be achieved through temporary resting, but the pain might consistently return unless the causative issue is corrected. The experienced sports medicine physician will identify the tissue diagnosis and treat it appropriately and will also identify and correct all predisposing factors. It is important that the physician is able to explain these concepts to the athlete and the treatment team to achieve optimal results.

Rather than view all similar overuse injuries as the same issue, the sports medicine physiatrist is able to break down the complex motions of the athlete into the constituent parts, identify the maladaptive pattern, and create a rehabilitation program that will prevent the injury from recurring. When examining the injured athlete, it is vital to make a biomechanical diagnosis rather than to focus exclusively on the injured tissue. Although it is easy to focus exclusively on the painful tissue, it is essential to assess the entire athlete and his or her mechanics to make appropriate tissue and biomechanical diagnoses (Table 39-1).

Evaluating an injured athlete involves a thorough discussion of the current problem, previous athletic injuries in the same area, as well as other seemingly unrelated injuries. Discussion of training patterns, including intensity and volume, as well as competition details is important. Proper equipment fit and technique should also be assessed. Differentiating between a slowly worsening insidious process and a more acute injury is key to creating an appropriate treatment plan. These subtle distinctions can frequently reveal the underlying cause of the current injury.

Table 39-1 Tissue Diagnosis and Biomechanical Diagnosis

Tissue Diagnosis	Potential Biomechanical Diagnosis
Lateral/medial epicondylitis	Posterior deltoid weakness
Hamstring strain	Overly tight hamstring, weak gluteal musculature
Metatarsal stress fracture	Supinated foot
Athletic pubalgia	Weak core musculature, tight hip girdle
Shoulder impingement with rotator cuff strain	Periscapular weakness or inhibition
Patellofemoral syndrome—patellar cartilage irritation or chondromalacia	Quadriceps and gluteal weakness or inhibition, overpronation
Repetitive ankle sprains—anterior talofibular ligament FL laxity	Weak peroneals, proprioceptive dysfunction

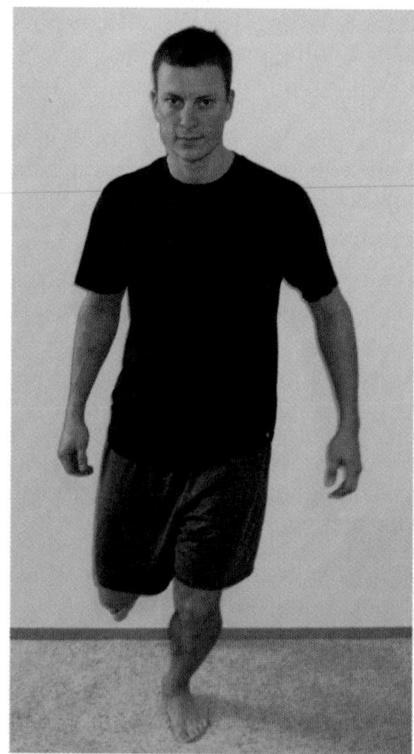

FIGURE 39-2 Single leg squat.

The physical examination of the athlete must be focused on finding the biomechanical culprit, rather than focusing solely on the painful tissue. The athlete must be examined in detail to fully assess the possible causes of the injury. Select upper limb tests that help determine the role of the scapula in upper limb injuries include the scapular assistance test and the scapular retraction test.[103] Core muscle function must be assessed dynamically and addressed as part of the rehabilitation plan.[104] Examples of physical examination maneuvers to evaluate core muscular function in the athlete are demonstrated in Figures 39-2 to 39-5. The kinetic chain assessment is designed to assess flexibility, strength, and functionality of the affected limb. The examination essentially assesses multiplane sports-specific dynamics rather than single-plane, solitary joint movements.

Proprioception and neuromuscular control are vital, and often unrecognized, components of athletic activity, and loss of these is increasingly noted as a predisposing factor for injury. Commonly called "muscle memory," these abilities help an athlete control the limbs throughout the full spectrum of motion. Deficits here can be subtle and difficult to assess in the typical office visit. Testing must be multiplanar and mimic the athlete's typical motion patterns.

It is vital for the examining physician to have a thorough understanding of the motions involved in the athlete's sport to make the appropriate changes; for example, a difference of 10 degrees in knee extension during the cocking phase of a tennis serve increases the valgus load at the elbow by 21%.[60] When necessary, this can be accomplished through discussion with the athlete, parent, coach, and/or trainer.

Prehabilitation

Prehabilitation is based on the concept that many sports injuries can be prevented if the athlete engages in an appropriate preseason prehabilitation program. Most of the scientific literature regarding prehabilitation programs focuses on noncontact anterior cruciate ligament tears.[89,90,116] Poor form is also linked to numerous athletic injuries. Balance perturbation, plyometric training, and stretching programs all have a role in the prehabilitation of the athlete. Ideally, some of these issues can be assessed during the preseason physical examination and corrected before the start of the season. A large proportion of sports injuries are related to overuse, and it is wise to have a discussion of these issues with athletes and coaches in the preseason. Off-season cross-training, core muscle work, and cardiovascular preparation are generally considered key to a healthy season.

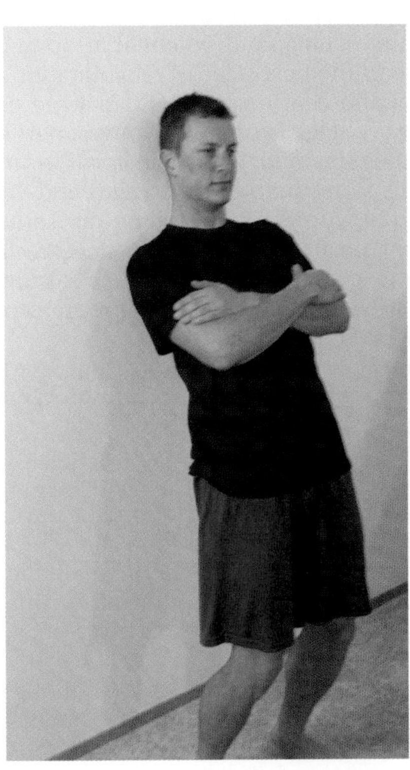

FIGURE 39-3 Sagittal plane evaluation.

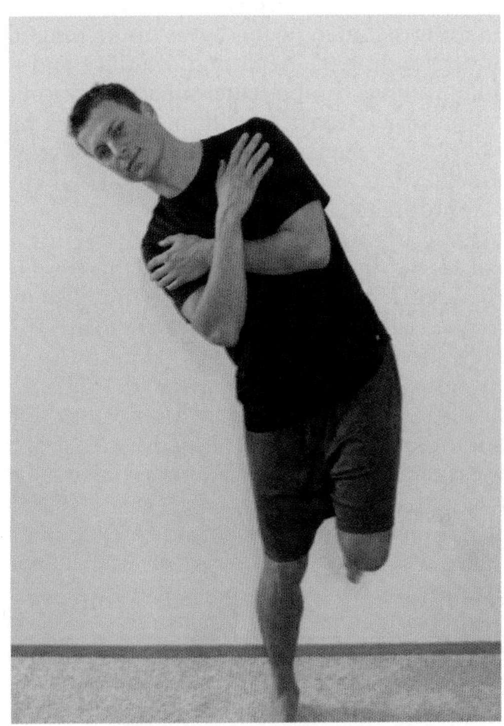

FIGURE 39-4 Frontal plane evaluation.

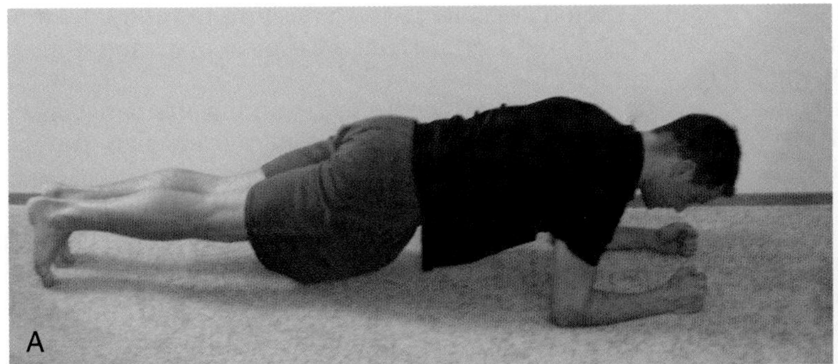

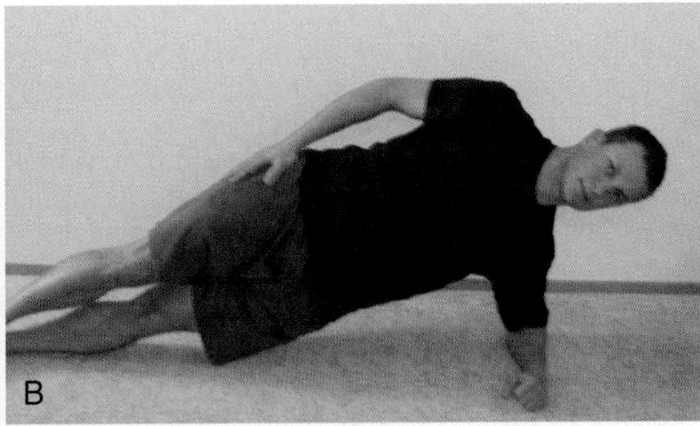

FIGURE 39-5 (**A**) Plank. (**B**) Side plank evaluation.

Prehabilitation can be viewed as an injury prevention program. These programs are sport specific, and often position specific, but always address the basic components of all athletic movements and the potential "breaks" in the kinetic chain: (1) flexibility, (2) strength, and (3) endurance. These programs can be used preseason, postseason, or during the season to treat previous injury or to prevent future injuries. For example, a soccer prehabilitation program could involve daily postactivity stretching, strength and plyometric training three times per week, and cardiovascular exercise three times per week. A thrower's prehabilitation program might involve a focus on daily postexercise range of motion (ROM), strength training two times per week, and daily technique practice, with pitch/throw volumes increasing weekly. Additional focus can be placed on any component based on the individual athlete's needs.

Injury Phases

Rehabilitation is guided by the status of the injured tissue, so an understanding of the timing of injury and recovery is essential. Injuries can be acute, subacute, chronic, or an exacerbation of a chronic condition. A detailed history is required because athletes will present at varying points of their tissue healing, and the treatment plan will have to be created appropriately. Four general phases are typically seen in tissue injury and repair. The physician caters the treatment to the individual tissue and the timing of the injury. The first phase involves the initial injury and the subsequent inflammation, edema, and pain. This phase is typically short, lasting days, depending on the severity of the injury. The reparative phase of the injured tissue might last from 6 to 8 weeks. It involves cell proliferation, granulation tissue formation, and neovascularization. The last phase is remodeling, which occurs as the tissue matures and realigns.

Excessive inflammatory response or exuberant repair can result in poor outcomes. For example, problems experienced during the remodeling phase can result in excessive scar tissue formation and development of recurrent/chronic injury. Many athletes return before the tissue itself is adequately healed and experience reinjury or an exacerbation of their previous symptoms. This likely occurs if the injured tissue is not fully healed or if the new tissue has not adapted to tolerate the desired motion or inherent stresses of the sport.

Stages of Rehabilitation

Rehabilitation can be viewed as a 3-stage spectrum from acute to recovery, and then to the final functional stage through return to full play (Table 39-2).[102] Each stage has individual goals that lead to the overall goal of RTP. The acute stage of rehabilitation is focused on managing the symptoms and signs of the injury. The classic PRICE (protection, rest, ice, compression, and elevation) approach is often followed. Medications, manual therapy, and physical modalities are also used during this phase. If necessary, bracing, injection, or surgery is performed to facilitate protection and future healing. ROM, strength, and cardiovascular fitness must be maintained as much as possible and tolerated. This can be accomplished by exercising the upper body of an athlete with a lower body injury. Passive ROM must be viewed with caution in the acute to subacute injury phase because it might injure the tissue, leading to increased pain and inflammation. Isometric strength exercises can be prescribed during this stage, if tolerated, to decrease pain, edema, and potential atrophy. The athlete can advance to the next stage of rehabilitation if adequate pain control and near-normal ROM is achieved.

Table 39-2 Typical Return-to-Play Phases

Phase	Goal	Timing
Phase I (acute)	Allow injured tissue time to heal, decrease symptoms, maintain range of motion.	<72 hr
Phase 2 (recovery)	Increase demands on the athlete; flexibility, strength, endurance training; kinetic chain corrections; maintain cardiovascular fitness through cross-training.	Variable
Phase 3 (functional)	Advance toward full return to play, advance cardiovascular fitness.	2 to 4 wk

The recovery stage is often the longest part of the rehabilitation program and shifts the focus from symptom management to restoration of strength and endurance as it applies to function. Tissue healing can continue at this time and will dictate the type of treatments recommended. Therapies move from passive to active during this stage. Flexibility, strength, symmetry, and proprioception are all addressed at this time.

Strength exercises advance from isometric to isotonic, including both concentric and eccentric movements. Open-chain exercises are ones in which the distal segment is free, whereas closed-chain exercises are ones in which the distal segment is fixed. Closed-chain activities are designed to stabilize an injured segment or to decrease the force passing across a joint. They also allow for a stepwise approach to kinetic chain rehabilitation. The rehabilitation program should typically focus on correcting erroneous movement patterns rather than creating completely new patterns for the athlete to learn.

In the case of an athlete with a shoulder injury, the rehabilitation program moves from predominantly closed-chain exercises, to axial-loaded exercises, to open kinetic chain exercises, to full sport-specific rehabilitation.[127] Kinetic chain rehabilitation is modified to the individual athlete's symptoms and dysfunction. Rather than view this type of rehabilitation as a series of discrete steps, the physiatrist should consider it as a transition from dysfunction to function and adjust the treatment plan and timing accordingly.[94]

The parameters of the strength training program (repetitions, resistance, speed, multijoint movements) can be adapted during this time, depending on the clinical scenario. Preexisting kinetic chain issues or tissue overload issues from the current injury are addressed at this time as well. As the rehabilitation program continues, increasingly athletic maneuvers (running, jumping, cutting) are used. Neuromuscular control (NMC) involves proprioception, muscle control, and the interplay between them. Without sufficient NMC, the athlete might continue to be predisposed to future injury. This recovery phase is the most variable and has the highest potential for reinjury, as the tissue is actively remodeling. The athlete must be reevaluated frequently during this phase because setbacks are common and can require modification of the rehabilitation plan. The athlete can advance to the final stage once pain-free ROM is achieved and strength is 75% to 80% or greater (compared with the noninjured side).

During the final functional stage of rehabilitation, the focus remains on kinetic chain issues and technique errors. Strength balance, power, endurance, functional ROM, and NMC are aggressively addressed. Sport-specific drills are used during this stage and advanced to include practice. Full RTP is achieved when the injury is no longer painful; when there is normal flexibility, strength, and proprioception; and when appropriate sport-specific mechanics and sport-specific skills are achieved and reproducible. In many cases, this rehabilitation phase becomes the maintenance program.[70]

Biomechanics of Sports

Throwing

Pitching a baseball is a classic example of the body acting as a kinetic chain of motion where foot placement and ankle ROM will affect how the pitcher uses his or her shoulder girdle and subsequently throws the ball. If there is a "weak link" in the pitcher's kinetic chain, there can be a predisposition to injury because of the repetitive nature of pitching. Whole body activity is involved in transferring momentum from the body to the ball. The momentum begins with a drive from the large leg muscles and rotation at the hips, progressing through segmental rotation of the trunk and shoulder girdle, transferring energy through elbow extension, next through the small forearm and hand muscles, and finally to the ball. This transfer of momentum and subsequent energy is related to a series of body segment accelerations and decelerations. When an initial segment of the body (e.g., trunk) accelerates, the next segment (e.g., arm) within the kinetic chain is left behind. When the trunk decelerates, the momentum is transferred to the arm with an increased velocity of the arm that is accentuated by the forces acting on the shoulder/arm. This motion and the forces are ultimately transferred to the ball.

Approximately 50% of the velocity of a pitch results from the step and body rotation (from the potential energy stored in the large leg and trunk musculature).[184] The other 50% comes from the smaller muscles of the shoulder, elbow, wrist, and hand. When forward stride is not allowed, the peak velocity of a pitched ball decreases to 84%. When the lower body is restricted, it decreases to 64%. Peak velocities in water polo are approximately 50% that of baseball because of the lack of a ground reaction force.

The baseball pitch is composed of six phases (Figure 39-6). Understanding these phases is critical to understanding, diagnosing, preventing, and treating throwing injuries.

Windup begins when the pitcher initiates motion and ends with maximum knee lift of the lead leg when the ball is removed from the glove. Push-off of the stride leg allows the center of gravity of the body to move forward. Few injuries occur in this early phase because the shoulder musculature is relatively inactive and most forces arise in the lower half of the body.

Early cocking is next and is often called the stride phase.[129] The stride leg extends toward the batter, as does the knee and hip of the pivot leg, propelling the body forward into the stride. As the hips rotate forward, the trunk follows and subsequently, the throwing shoulder abducts, extends, and externally rotates, leaving the shoulder in a "semicocked" position. Again, in this early phase, there is less risk of injury because most forces are still being generated in the trunk and lower limbs; however, shoulder activity does become more evident. The trapezius and serratus anterior demonstrate moderate to high activity to protract and upwardly rotate the scapula. The middle deltoid generates the abduction force, and the supraspinatus fine-tunes humeral head positioning within the glenoid.

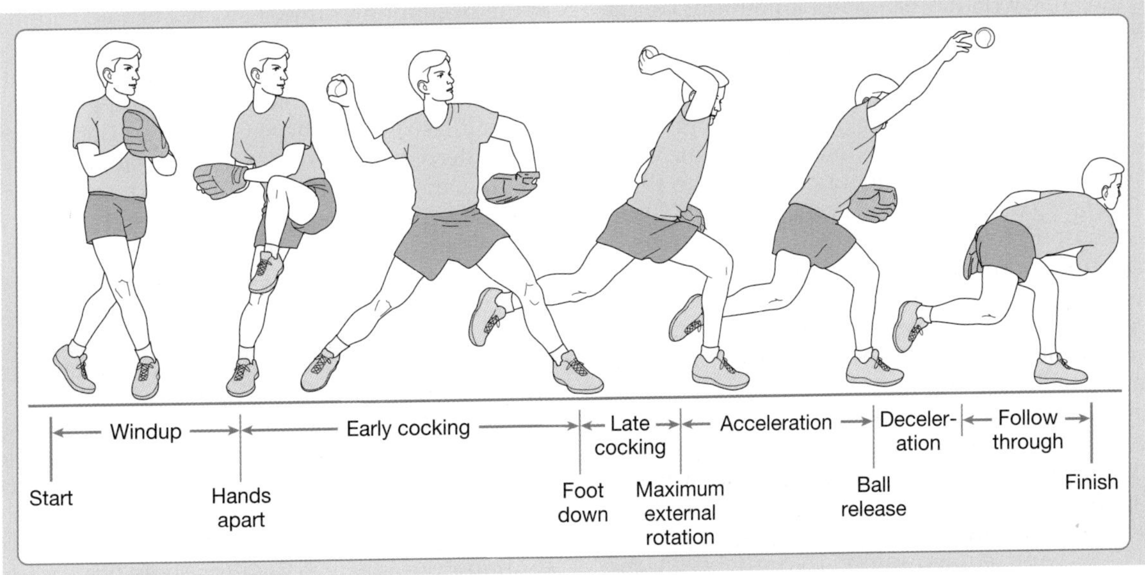

FIGURE 39-6 The six phases of the baseball pitch.

BOX 39-2

Common Injuries in the Late Cocking Phase of Pitching

- Anterior instability
- Internal (posterior-superior) impingement
- Type II SLAP lesion
- Articular surface rotator cuff tears
- Bicipital tendinopathy
- Medial tension injuries at the elbow
- Ulnar collateral ligament injury

SLAP, Superior labrum, anterior to posterior.

The next phase is late cocking. The hallmark of this phase is when maximal shoulder external rotation is obtained. The shoulder begins this phase in approximately 50 degrees of external rotation and ends in about 175 degrees at maximal external rotation. This extreme amount of rotation allows the greatest accelerating force to the ball over the greatest possible distance. The amount of external rotation obtained correlates with the speed of the pitched ball. A majority of injuries occur in the late cocking and deceleration phases of throwing (Box 39-2).[145] For late cocking, this is caused by the forces needed to stabilize the shoulder in this extreme ROM. The dynamic stabilizers of the anterior shoulder (long head of the biceps, subscapularis, and pectoralis major) are very active in this phase. The static stabilizers (glenohumeral ligaments, capsule, and labrum) are active as well. The glenohumeral ligaments and capsule increase in laxity because of the extreme ROM in the overhead athlete. This laxity is necessary for performance; however, overstretching these ligaments enhances the work of the dynamic stabilizers with a resultant potential for injury.

During the acceleration phase, the shoulder is powerfully internally rotated from 175 degrees of external rotation to 90 to 100 degrees at ball release. Shoulder abduction is relatively fixed in all throwers at 90 degrees. Trunk lateral flexion (and not shoulder abduction) generally determines what position the arm is in relative to the vertical plane. "Over the top" throwers have a greater amount of contralateral trunk flexion, and "sidearm" throwers have less. If there is less than 90 degrees of abduction as a result of fatigue, weakness, or just poor form, the common observation is a "dropped elbow." "Hanging" or dropping the elbow results in a reduced pitch velocity and an increased risk of injury to the shoulder (rotator cuff) and the elbow (ulnar collateral ligament injury). Another common injury in the acceleration phase, particularly in older pitchers, is from subacromial impingement as they internally rotate and adduct the abducted arm during acceleration.

The deceleration phase is manifested by large eccentric muscular forces of the posterior shoulder girdle to decelerate that rapid internal rotation of the acceleration phase.[24] Deceleration begins after ball release and ends when the arm reaches 0 degrees of internal rotation. The posterior shoulder girdle is active in this phase, including the scapular muscles, rotator cuff external rotators (particularly the teres minor), and the posterior deltoid. Because of these large eccentric contractions, injury is common in this phase (Box 39-3).

BOX 39-3

Common Injuries in the Deceleration Phase of Pitching

- Posterior instability
- Isolated rotator cuff tears
- SLAP lesions

SLAP, Superior labrum, anterior to posterior.

Table 39-3 Age-Based Pitch Counts

Age	Pitches Per Game	Per Week	Per Season	Per Year
9-10	50	75	1000	2000
11-12	75	100	1000	3000
13-14	75	125	1000	3000

Modified from USA Baseball Medical and Safety Advisory Committee, 2006.

The final phase of pitching is the follow-through phase. This is a "passive" phase in which the body is merely catching up with the throwing arm. Low-grade eccentric loading of the shoulder musculature and little risk of injury are noted during this phase.

Because of the high risk of overuse injury in the young pitcher's throwing arm, age-based pitch count guidelines have been developed to decrease this risk (Table 39-3).[99] For similar reasons, curve balls and sliders should not be pitched until the athlete reaches puberty. It is also recommended that young pitchers not compete in baseball more than 9 months per year. During those 3 "off" months, they should not compete in other overhead arm sports, such as competitive swimming or javelin throwing.

Running

Notable differences are observed between a walking gait cycle and a running gait cycle.[143] One in particular is a third phase in running called the float phase. Float is a period when neither foot is in contact with the ground. It occurs at the beginning of initial swing and the end of terminal swing (Figure 39-7).

The walking gait cycle has a period of double limb support, which is not present in running; it occurs in the first and last 10% of the stance phase. The stance phase of gait is decreased from 60% while walking to 30% while running and 20% while sprinting. Consequently, as speed increases, the stance phase decreases. As speed increases, the velocity and range of lower limb motion increase, which in turn serve to minimize vertical displacement and improve efficiency. The body lowers its center of gravity by increasing hip flexion, knee flexion, and ankle dorsiflexion; consequently, the major kinematic difference between walking and running occurs in the sagittal plane of motion.

Faster running also changes foot contact.[201] In slower running and walking, contact is typically heel to toe. As running speed increases, foot strike occurs with the forefoot and heel simultaneously, or the forefoot strikes initially followed by the heel lowering to the ground. In sprinting, the athlete maintains weight bearing on the forefoot from loading response to toe-off.

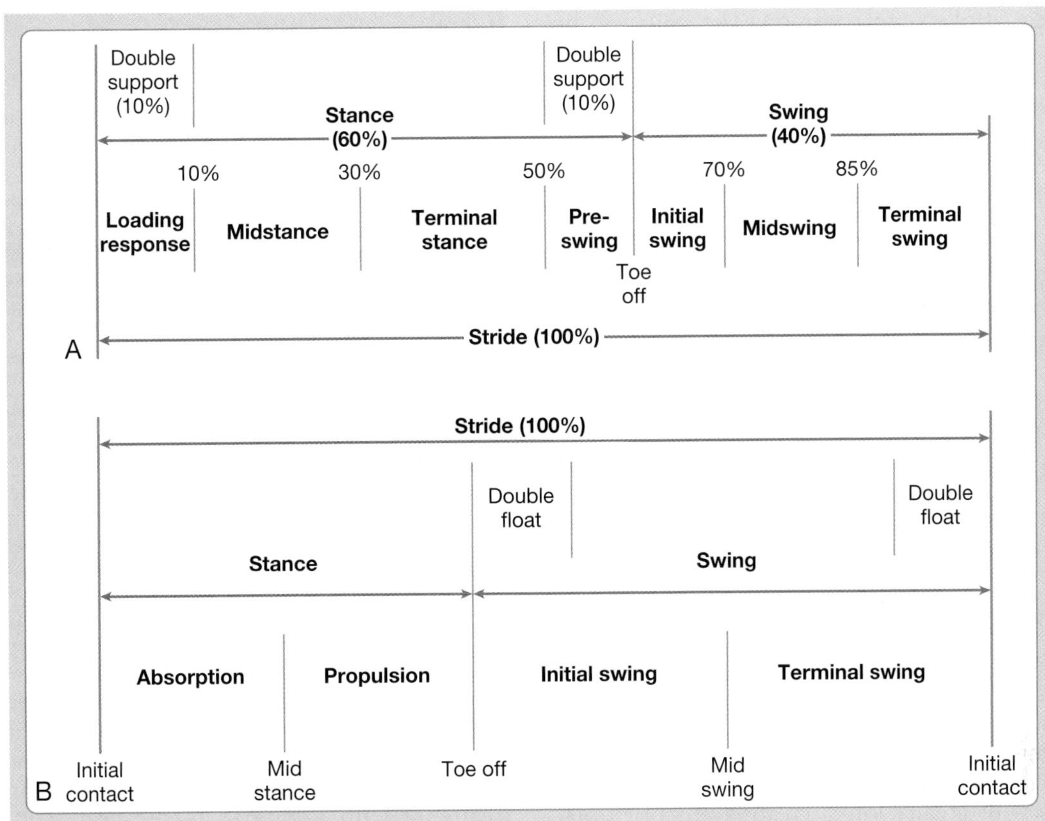

FIGURE 39-7 A comparison of the walking (**A**) and running (**B**) gait cycles. (Modified from Ounpuu S: The biomechanics of walking and running, *Clin Sports Med* 13:843-863, 1994.)

The angle of gait is different between walking and running. This is the angle between the longitudinal bisection of the foot and the line of progression. This angle is 10 degrees in walking. In running, it approaches 0 degrees as foot strike is on the line of progression to allow more efficient locomotion by limiting deviation of the center of gravity.

Barefoot running, simulated by running in minimalist shoes, has gained popularity over the past decade. Minimalist shoes are generally defined (and considered different from conventional running shoes) by less heel cushioning and a "zero drop" from heel to toe, meaning that the shoe's heel contour is not built-up so that the heel is at the same level as the forefoot. Running in minimalist shoes tends to move initial contact to the forefoot and lessens impact forces, which could potentially lessen overuse injuries in runners (though this has not been proven). Runners who run in minimalist shoes tend to forefoot strike and have an increased stride cadence. However, it is not known if the shoes or if changing a runner's stride (increased cadence with a shortened stride and running "light and quiet"), which minimalist shoes facilitate, is the driving factor for lessening impact forces and thus potentially lessening injury rate.

Swimming

Four competitive strokes are used in swimming: freestyle (crawl), backstroke, butterfly, and breaststroke. Four phases of the swim stroke are common to freestyle, backstroke, and butterfly. The first phase is the entry or catch. This encompasses hand entry into the water until the beginning of its backward movement. The propulsive phase is divided into two separate phases: pull and push. The pull phase ends as the hand arrives in the vertical plane of the shoulder. During the push phase, the hand is positioned below the shoulder and pushes through the water until its exit from the water historically at the level of the greater trochanter. The final phase is the recovery phase, which entails the aerial return of the hand.

During the propulsive phases of swimming, the arm is moved through adduction and internal rotation starting from a stretched position of abduction and external rotation. The pectoralis major and latissimus dorsi are the major contributors to this motion; however, the serratus anterior and the internal rotator function of the subscapularis and teres provide a major assist.[186]

During the recovery phase, scapular retraction is provided by the rhomboids and middle trapezius, whereas shoulder external rotation is provided by the posterior deltoid, teres minor, and infraspinatus. In preparation for hand entry during midrecovery, the serratus anterior and upper trapezius upwardly rotate the scapula for shoulder stabilization.

Kick patterns are also an important part of swimming mechanics. In the flutter kick for the freestyle stroke, the knees should flex only about 30 to 40 degrees, and hip flexion should be minimal. The breaststroke kick is a whip-kick that creates a significant valgus moment at the knee. Because of this increased knee valgus, medial knee injuries in breaststrokers are common. The pain can be from a medial collateral ligament sprain or a medial plica/synovitis.

General rehabilitation and prehabilitation principles have been established for swimmers with shoulder pain, and all sports medicine clinicians should be familiar with them. The overarching principle is that most shoulder pain in swimmers (impingement and rotator cuff tendinopathy) is caused by dynamic muscle imbalances, weakness, and biomechanical faults, and not hard anatomic factors. A major tenet of shoulder rehabilitation for the swimmer is scapular stabilization, with a prime focus on endurance training of the serratus anterior and lower trapezius. The serratus anterior is a muscle of particular focus because it has been demonstrated to function at 75% of its maximum test ability in swimming and is active throughout the swim stroke cycle.[169] Other tenets of shoulder rehabilitation in swimmers include stretching the internal rotators and posterior capsule and cervical and thoracic mobilization.

BOX 39-4

History of Doping and Drug Monitoring

- World War II—Steroids used in the belief that male hormones could benefit the emaciated prisoners rescued from concentration camps
- 1950s-1960s—Amphetamines and anabolic steroids widely used by athletes
- 1962—International Olympic Committee passed a resolution against doping, banned steroid use
- 1967—Medical commission started medical controls in 1968 Olympics
- 1976—Anabolic steroids controlled for the first time in Olympics
- 1988—First gold medal stripped in track and field because of doping
- 1990—The Anabolic Steroid Act passed
- 1998—The World Anti-Doping Agency formed in Montreal, Quebec, Canada
- 2003—The World Anti-Doping Code is passed

Jumping and Landing

The biomechanics of jumping and landing in sports is particularly well researched in the setting of noncontact anterior cruciate ligament (ACL) injuries of the knee. Noncontact ACL injuries occur more frequently with the knee in less flexion.[205] In this position there are greater knee extensor loads with greater forces creating anterior tibial translation and subsequent ACL injury. A well-defined gender difference observed in jumping and landing mechanics is likely one reason for the higher rate of noncontact ACL injuries in female athletes.[33] Female athletes land more erect with less knee and hip flexion. They land with less hip external rotation and abduction. They also generally have an imbalance of increased quadriceps to hamstrings activation ratio, creating greater knee extension and lesser knee flexion forces. One goal of ACL injury prevention programs is to improve jumping and landing technique by increasing knee and hip flexion during landing and balancing the quadriceps to hamstring activation ratio.

Pharmacology in Sports

"Doping" refers to any substance or method used to increase performance, possibly to the detriment of the health of the athlete or the ethics of the competition.[50] WADA was created to unify the fight against doping. WADA rulings are accepted by all National Olympic committees, the International Olympic Committee (IOC), International Paralympic Committee (IPC), national governments, and international sports federations. The agency, based in Montreal, Canada, consists of government representatives from all continents and members of the Olympic movement. The World Anti-Doping Code was developed in 2003 and enforced in 2004, with a complete listing of banned substances and methods.[50] A brief history of doping in sports is presented in Box 39-4.

A summarized list of substances banned by WADA is available online. Banned substances are divided into those that are banned in and out of competition and those that are banned in competition only.[202] The lists of drugs and supplements banned by the National Football League (NFL), National Collegiate Athletic Association (NCAA), and other organizations are also available online.[136]

When an athlete has an illness or condition that requires treatment with a banned medication, a therapeutic use exemption (TUE) can provide the authorization to take the needed medicine. Per WADA, all international federations and national antidoping organizations must have a process in place whereby athletes with documented medical conditions can request a TUE.[81]

The following is a brief overview of therapeutic and performance-enhancing drugs and supplements, all of which are given careful consideration by these agencies.

Therapeutic Drugs

Analgesics

Acetaminophen can be linked to decreased muscle building after exercise (to an extent similar to that of ibuprofen). Prostaglandins are normally released after eccentric resistance exercise. This response might be blunted after consumption of maximal doses of ibuprofen or acetaminophen, profoundly influencing the anabolic response of muscle to this type of exercise.[185]

Antiinflammatories

One study found that 15% of high school football players used nonsteroidal antiinflammatory drugs (NSAIDs) daily.[193] Although the pain relief provided by NSAIDs might enhance performance, NSAIDs are not considered ergogenic. NSAIDs can mask pain and interrupt a natural defense mechanism for preventing injury. Because of their antiinflammatory effects, NSAIDs likely inhibit the production of prostaglandin E2, which is known to play a role in bone healing.[149] Consequently, in those with suspected or known fractures, NSAIDs might be contraindicated.

Corticosteroids are potent antiinflammatories. In general, when given orally, rectally, intravenously, or intramuscularly, their use is prohibited by WADA. Topical preparations for skin, eye, ear, nose, or buccal cavity or for iontophoresis are allowed. For applicable athletes, epidural and intraarticular steroid injections, as well as inhaled steroids, require a TUE.[201]

Antihypertensives

Experts recommend diuretics as first-line treatment of hypertension in the general population, possibly with early addition of a β-blocker or angiotensin-converting enzyme inhibitor (ACE-I).[179] ACE-I or calcium channel blockers can be considered first-line agents for treatment of hypertension in athletes because diuretics and β-blockers have side effects that may hinder performance. The detection and management of hypertension and the efficacy of various agents are beyond the scope of this chapter. Rather, this discussion will focus on the aspects of these medications that affect athletes.

Diuretics can decrease plasma volume, cardiac output, and peripheral vascular resistance. Dehydration and electrolyte alterations might result in cramps or even heat stroke. For amateur athletes, the benefits of antihypertensive therapy with diuretics likely outweigh the risks. In the case of elite athletes, diuretics are banned in part for their theoretical ability to increase urine output and mask use of other banned agents (although this method rarely works optimally).[149]

β-Blockers can reduce exercise tolerance by increasing perceived effort. They can also inhibit glycolysis and glycogenolysis with resulting hypoglycemia after exercise. The negative chronotropic effects of β-blockers can decrease heart rate recovery after exercise. β-Blockers are banned in certain sports because of their anxiolytic effects.[149]

Diabetes Drugs

Insulin doses might need to be adjusted for persons with insulin-dependent diabetes starting a new exercise program. A 20% to 40% reduction is typical because of increased insulin sensitivity with exercise. High-intensity exercise (i.e., greater than 80% maximum oxygen consumption [VO_{2max}]) can cause a temporary increase in blood glucose secondary to increased sympathoadrenal activation. In that situation, supplemental insulin, if used, should be given at a smaller dose than that given for hyperglycemia at rest.[15,95]

Intramuscular injections of insulin should be avoided because muscle contraction can accelerate insulin absorption. Heat can increase absorption rates of insulin, although cold can decrease them. Therefore athletes with insulin-dependent diabetes mellitus should avoid modalities that use extremes of temperature, such as hot or cold whirlpools. Extreme ambient temperature can also reduce insulin action in athletes.[95]

Asthma Drugs

Exercise-induced bronchospasm (EIB) can be treated effectively with a short-acting β-agonist, such as albuterol, within 15 minutes before exercise.[179] If not sufficient to prevent symptoms, cromolyn (a mast cell stabilizer) can be added. Inhalation of either cromolyn sodium or a β-agonist, or both, 15 minutes before exercise is almost always successful in blocking EIB and airway inflammation.[112]

For patients who have chronic persistent asthma (forced expiratory volume in 1 second less than 80% of predicted and symptoms greater than twice a week), inhaled corticosteroids are standard treatment. Inhaled corticosteroids do not appear to have ergogenic or anabolic effects.[149]

Performance-Enhancing Drugs

Anabolic Steroids

It is estimated that 1 to 3 million athletes in the United States alone have used anabolic steroids (ASs),[174] with annual market sales well in excess of $100 million.[182] The Centers for Disease Control and Prevention found an overall prevalence of lifetime steroid use in females, grades 9 to 12, to be 3.2%.[122] As many as 1 in 10 steroid users is a teenager.[113] One study found that 6.3% of high school varsity football players were current or former AS users.[78]

ASs have three general effects that enhance athletic performance. By binding androgen receptors, ASs stimulate messenger RNA synthesis, increasing structural and contractile protein synthesis[113,182] and producing an anabolic state.[26] ASs are also anticatabolic via competitive inhibition of the glucocorticoid receptor, inhibiting the catabolic effects of cortisol[182] and preserving muscle mass.[26] Finally, ASs have emotional effects, pushing athletes to train more intensely and more often.[26]

Because ASs are illegal, studying their health risks and side effects is a challenge. Inconsistent formulations, dose administrations, and training habits make it difficult to derive statistically sound conclusions. Some studies show minimal effects on body composition and strength; although others show that supraphysiologic doses of testosterone (or its derivatives) can lead to an increase in lean mass and muscle size in humans (Table 39-4).[182] Typical users of steroids can take 10 to 40 times the prescribed dosage for disease states.[78,94,122,182] Users often share needles, at a rate of up to 25% in adolescents, with reports of HIV, hepatitis B and C, and abcesses.[182] Premature deaths have resulted from AS use, most commonly as a result of suicide and acute myocardial infarction.[94]

The Anabolic Steroid Control Act of 1990 prohibited the use of steroids for any use other than disease treatment, thereby classifying ASs as schedule III drugs within the Controlled Substances Act. ASs are banned by all major sporting leagues,[122] the IOC, and the NCAA.[94]

Erythropoietin and Blood Doping

Endurance athletes are particularly sensitive to the oxygen-carrying capacity in their blood. For years, athletes sought a competitive advantage by training at altitude or sleeping in altitude tents. This effect can be reproduced by blood doping, blood transfusion, or administration of the drug recombinant human erythropoietin (rhEPO).[31,182]

Erythropoietin (EPO) is a glycoprotein hormone produced mainly in the kidney in response to tissue hypoxia. EPO is part of a negative feedback cycle that controls tissue oxygen delivery by controlling the number of erythrocytes in the blood.[162] Both rhEPO and transfusions have been shown to increase VO_{2max}.[18,182]

The risks of artificially elevated hemoglobin/hematocrit include stroke, myocardial infarction, and pulmonary embolism. Blood transfusions, even conducted according

Table 39-4 Negative Effects of Anabolic Steroids

System	Effects
Cardiovascular	Increases in total LDL Decreases in HDL Hypertension Myocardial ischemia (imbalance between myocardial oxygen supply and demand) Myocardial infarction Cerebrovascular accident
Hepatic	Hepatocellular dysfunction (abnormal liver function tests) Peliosis hepatis (benign intrahepatic vascular disorder) Hepatocellular carcinoma
Male reproductive	Oligospermia, azoospermia Gynecomastia Decreased testicular size
Female reproductive	Decreased LH, FSH Decreased progesterone Menstrual irregularities Male pattern alopecia Hirsutism (irreversible) Clitoromegaly (irreversible) Deepening voice (irreversible)
Skeletal	Premature closure of the epiphyses
Skin	Acne (increased number of sebaceous glands) Striae
Psychologic	Decreased libido Mood swings Hypermania/hypomania Aggressive behavior ("roid rage") Withdrawal Depression Addiction

FSH, Follicle-stimulating hormone; *HDL*, high-density lipoprotein; *LDL*, low-density lipoprotein; *LH*, luteinizing hormone.

From Laos C, Metzl JD: Performance-enhancing drug use in young athletes, *Adolesc Med Clin* 17:719-731, abstract xii, 2006.

to hospital procedures, carry risks for infection, including HIV and hepatitis, as well as transfusion reaction.[182]

Stimulants

Stimulants might be the most common and underrecognized supplement used by high school athletes. Common stimulants include caffeine, ephedrine (ephedra or ma huang), pseudoephedrine, phenylephrine, amphetamines, and methamphetamines.[78] Stimulants increase arousal, respiratory rate, heart rate, and blood pressure. Side effects include dizziness, insomnia, agitation, restlessness, anxiety, confusion, paranoia, hallucinations, dyskinesias, gastrointestinal disturbances, heat intolerance, stroke, myocardial infarction, arrhythmia, and death.[78]

Pseudoephedrine (Sudafed) is a commonly used drug in this class. Although improved cycling power output[12] and pace in a 10-km run[13] have been demonstrated in studies of this drug, other trials contradict these findings.[74] Pseudoephedrine is a chemical precursor in the illicit manufacture of methamphetamine. Federal policies now restrict sales by limiting purchase quantities to consumers of a minimum age.[67] Pseudoephedrine is monitored in competition but is not included on the prohibited list.[137]

The herbals ephedra and ma huang have similar structural properties and physiologic effects to pseudoephedrine.[67] Ephedra and ephedra-containing products were taken off the market in 2004.[122] Ephedra is banned by the NCAA, IOC, and major league organizations.[122]

Caffeine is an adenosine receptor antagonist with stimulant properties.[67] Studies have shown that caffeine is ergogenic in most, if not all, exercise situations, with few negative effects during exercise.[77] Caffeine acts by binding to adenosine receptors in most tissues, including brain, heart, smooth muscle, fat, and skeletal muscle, with a wide spectrum of interacting responses. Caffeine also stimulates the secretion of epinephrine[77] and the central nervous system and enhances peripheral neuromuscular transmission and muscle contractility.[67] Side effects of caffeine include nausea, heart palpitations, headache, and muscle tension. Caffeine might also act as a diuretic, although no studies have shown a risk for dehydration in athletes.[67] Caffeine is monitored in competition but has not been prohibited by WADA since 2004.[202]

Supplements

A drug is any substance that exerts an effect on a body system, but a supplement is defined as a substance taken to augment the diet. Regulatory bodies within the U.S. government handle drugs and supplements differently, and supplement manufacturers are not held to the same standards as drug companies. Supplement manufacturing is overseen by the U.S. Food and Drug Administration (FDA) and treated as food as long as no drug claims are made.[78]

Most experts agree that a well-balanced, isocaloric diet of commonly available food is sufficient to guarantee basic nutritional requirements for most athletes, including macronutrients (carbohydrates, proteins, and lipids) and micronutrients (vitamins, minerals, and trace elements).[53] Despite this, many athletes take megadoses of essential nutrients as dietary supplements (amino acids, vitamins, minerals), at times above tolerable levels.[53] The supplement industry has been estimated to earn $1.2 to $3 billion per year.[113] Surveys have found that 25% to 38% of high school athletes used supplements.[78] A 2002 metaanalysis found that, of more than 250 dietary products available, only β-hydroxy-β-methylbutyrate and creatine supplements have sufficient scientific evidence to conclude that they significantly augment lean body mass and strength with resistance training.[140]

Creatine

According to one source, 90% of weightlifters and bodybuilders in the United States are regular users of creatine (Cr). They tend to be male, have an average age of 32 years, attended college, and have a substantial income.[151] In a survey of NFL trainers and team physicians, all teams had players actively taking the supplement, with estimated usage 33% to 90%.[182]

Cr, a naturally occurring compound made from amino acids glycine, arginine, and methionine, is the most popular nutritional supplement on the market.[113,182] It is proposed that Cr phosphate supplementation benefits short-duration, high-intensity, repetitive exercise by enhancing adenosine triphosphate regeneration.[113,149]

Cr appears to be most effective for activities that involve repeated short bouts of high-intensity physical activity,[78,182] such as jumping, sprinting, and cycling.[14] When maximal force or strength is the outcome measure, Cr has consistently been found to significantly affect force production regardless of sport, sex, or age.[182]

Common side effects of Cr include muscle cramping and gastrointestinal distress.[151] A number of cases of renal failure have been reversed by withdrawal of Cr supplementation.[113,182] It is notable that most studies in the literature were short term with healthy subjects. Also, there are insufficient data on the possible effects of Cr on other Cr-containing tissues, such as the brain, cardiac muscle, or testes.[182]

Because it is not classified as a drug, Cr is not under direct regulation by the FDA and is widely available over the counter.[182] The NCAA does not allow member teams to provide Cr to its players. According to one survey, 40% of NFL teams provided Cr for their players.[182]

For a summary of drugs and supplements used in sports, see Table 39-5.

Preparticipation Examination

The primary goals of the PPE are to (1) identify life-threatening conditions, (2) identify conditions that can limit competition, (3) identify factors that predispose the athlete to injury, and (4) meet the legal requirements of the institution and state. Added opportunities are to discuss preventative health and high-risk behaviors, establish rapport with the athlete, and evaluate the general health of a potentially underserved population. The preparticipation physical evaluation (PPE) is a consensus publication by the major sports medicine associations and is an excellent guide for the team physician.[3] It encourages safe participation and disqualifies less than 1% of high school athletes and 0.2% of college athletes. However, 14% of athletes have been found to require further evaluation.[76] The PPE should be performed with enough lead time to allow appropriate subsequent investigation before the season begins.

The PPE is not intended as a substitute for a comprehensive visit with a primary care physician. It typically does not allow for extended time for individual education, but it is a potential opportunity for the sports medicine physician to identify factors that are associated with future injury. When appropriate, the athlete should have an extended musculoskeletal examination assessing flexibility, strength, technique, and neuromuscular control. If abnormalities are found, the athlete should be referred to physical therapy for a prehabilitation program.

The most common settings for the PPE include individual examinations performed in the physician's office, station-based examinations, and group locker room examinations. Although individual examinations are the most commonly performed, station-based examinations might lead to more effective identification of musculoskeletal issues.[57] Individual examinations have the advantages of privacy and more opportunity to discuss other general health and safety issues.

Current reviews of systems, medical history, surgical history, injury history, gynecologic history, family history, and vaccination history are recorded. Screening questions

Table 39-5 Summary of Drugs and Supplements Used in Sports

Drug/Supplement (Street Name in Parenthesis)	Postulated Effect	Evidence of Effectiveness	Adverse Effects	Legal Status
Anabolic steroids (testosterone or "T," designer steroids)	Increase lean muscle mass	Effective	Significant, multiple systems	Illegal unless prescribed for disease state
Androstenedione and DHEA (Andro)	Increase testosterone and lean muscle mass	No effect with androstenedione; DHEA with some benefits in patients >70 years old	Possible cardiovascular effects	Prohibited by WADA, NFL, and NCAA; androstenedione is illegal.
β-Hydroxy-β-methylbutyrate (HMB)	Decrease protein breakdown; increase synthesis	Mixed	None, but long-term data lacking	Legal
Blood transfusion or erythropoietin (doping, EPO)	Increase endurance and oxygen delivery	Effective	Significant cardiovascular risks	Prohibited by WADA, NFL, and NCAA
Caffeine	Increases energy, systemic effects not fully known	Effective	Minimal	Legal
Creatine	Increase muscle mass and strength	Effective	Few case reports of renal failure; proposed risk of dehydration	Legal
Ephedrine, pseudoephedrine (Ma huang, guarana)	Increases energy, metabolism, decreases fatigue	Mixed	Significant cardiovascular, psychiatric risks, and others	Prohibited by WADA, NFL, and NCAA
Human growth hormone	Increase muscle protein synthesis and strength	Lack of evidence	Significant	Illegal unless prescribed for disease state

DHEA, Dehydroepiandrosterone; *NCAA*, National Collegiate Athletic Association; *NFL*, National Football League; *WADA*, World Anti-Doping Agency.

Modified from Bemben MG, Lamont HS: Creatine supplementation and exercise performance: recent findings, *Sports Med* 35:107-125, 2005; Fields J, Turner JL: Performance-enhancing sports supplements. In *Sports medicine and rehabilitation: A sport specific approach.* ed 2, Philadelphia, PA, 2009, Wolters Kluwer Lippincott Williams & Wilkins; Jenkinson DM, Harbert AJ: Supplements and sports, *Am Fam Physician* 78:1039-1046, 2008.

regarding performance-enhancing drugs/supplements, nutrition, drug, alcohol, and medication (including over the counter and supplement) use are also reviewed.

Height, weight, vital signs, hearing examination, and visual examination are performed and recorded. Normal values for blood pressure in the adolescent and pediatric population should be available for the examiner. The physical examination can be performed by different providers but must include the head, ears, eyes, nose, throat, cardiovascular system, pulmonary auscultation, abdomen, genitalia (males only), hernia palpation, skin, and neurologic and musculoskeletal systems (Figure 39-8). The female genitourinary examination is deferred to the primary care physician.

Many subspecialties might be involved in the PPE. The lead physician must be determined before the decision-making process begins. It is also vital for individual providers to be able to identify suspicious findings outside their own area of specialty and refer to the appropriate specialists when necessary. A provider who is unsure of a finding should always refer to a specialist for further investigation or consultation on final clearance to play, rather than make the decision on his or her own.

Clearance to Play

The lead physician must make the determination to clear the athlete without restrictions or with recommendations for further evaluation or treatment. Alternatively, athletes might not be cleared for participation in certain sports or might not be cleared for participation in any sport.

Cardiovascular Screening

Sudden cardiac death (SCD) is a rare and devastating condition seen at all levels of sport. The American Heart

Blood pressure	Heart rate	Respirations	Height	Weight	Vision	Hearing

System	**Normal**	**Abnormal findings**
HEENT		
Cardiovascular		
Pulmonary		
Abdomen		
Extremities		
Musculoskeletal		
Neurological		
Skin		

☐ Full-clearance, no restrictions

☐ Cleared with the following restrictions ______________________

☐ Not cleared for participation.

Recommend further consultation with ______________________

☐ Not cleared for participation.

FIGURE 39-8 Example of a preparticipation examination form.

BOX 39-5

American Heart Association Recommendations for Cardiovascular Screening of Competitive Athletes

Medical History

Personal medical history

1. Exertional chest pain/discomfort
2. Unexplained syncope/near syncope
3. Excessive exertional and unexplained dyspnea/fatigue
4. Previous recognition of heart murmur
5. Elevated systemic blood pressure

Family history

1. Premature death (sudden and unexpected, or otherwise) before 50 years as a result of heart disease, in ≥1 relative
2. Disability from heart disease in a close relative <50 years of age
3. Specific knowledge of certain cardiac conditions in family members: hypertrophic or dilated cardiomyopathy, long QT syndrome, or other ion channelopathies, Marfan syndrome, or clinically important arrhythmias

Physical Examination

1. Heart murmur
2. Femoral pulses to exclude aortic coarctation
3. Physical stigmata of Marfan syndrome
4. Brachial artery blood pressure (sitting position)

Association's (AHA) recommendations for cardiovascular screening include specific questions regarding family history, personal history, and a thorough physical examination (Box 39-5). Controversy exists in sports medicine regarding screening electrocardiograms (ECG) and echocardiography. The AHA currently does not recommend a screening 12-lead ECG, echocardiograms, or exercise stress testing for athletes without risk factors.[120] The IOC and the European Society of Cardiology recommend a screening ECG as part of the PPE, in part because of different etiologies of SCD between the United States and Europe.[42] The AHA decision is based on the low prevalence of SCD, limited resources, impracticality of mass screening, and lack of a physician base to interpret the ECG, as well as the consequences of false-positive test results.[42,120] Hypertrophic cardiomyopathy (HCM) is the most common cause of SCD in athletes in the United States. It is an autosomal dominant disease, and detailed family history might detect premature cardiac death and lead to further diagnostic testing in the athlete. Echocardiography is the most effective way of diagnosing HCM but would require the screening of 200,000 athletes before finding one with the condition.[61]

Medicolegal Aspects of the Preparticipation Evaluation

The majority of the responsibilities of a volunteer team physician are covered by Good Samaritan laws. The PPE is a notable exception. A physician might be held liable for malpractice if an athlete is cleared to play despite the presence of a medically contraindicated condition. Liability waivers and similar documentation are not acceptable in the presence of medically contraindicated conditions. Athletes can legally challenge physician nonclearance decisions and have occasionally won the right to participate despite medical judgment. In the presence of a life-threatening condition, physicians are advised to follow their medical judgment and not clear the athlete for play.

Emergency Assessment and Care

The first tenet of care for a sports medical emergency is preparing, developing, and rehearsing an EAP. The EAP is designed to develop comfort and control in the potential chaos of an emergency. The plan must be reviewed and practiced at least annually with all members of the sports medicine team. Those designated as "first responders" should be adequately trained in cardiopulmonary resuscitation (CPR) and AED use. One goal is to have access to early defibrillation, defined as the first shock given within 3 minutes of collapse. During the initial evaluation and triage, rapid recognition to determine whether the EAP or routine management should be enacted is critical. Having the sports medicine physician on the sidelines of an event is crucial to be able to witness the mechanism of injury. Being an eyewitness allows one to determine whether there was contact or a collision involved in the collapse and whether the collapse occurred during activity or after the play was over. Quickly determining whether additional providers or transport is necessary through emergency medical services is important at this stage as well. This section presents the basics of emergency assessment and care, including a review of CPR guidelines and sudden cardiac arrest in athletes. It then discusses specific emergency scenarios, including the initial assessment of the athlete with a cervical spine injury in contact sports and exercise-associated collapse in athletic endurance events.

The primary goal of CPR is to maximize blood flow by provision of effective and uninterrupted chest compressions for longer periods. Recent clinical studies have demonstrated improved survival when 90 to 120 seconds of CPR is used before shock delivery when the rescuer's arrival to the patient is greater than 5 minutes.[198] Perfusing the myocardium with oxygenated blood before defibrillation improves survival. If the collapse is witnessed (and the victim is down for less than 5 minutes), immediate defibrillation is still indicated. The emphasis of CPR has moved away from ventilation and placed further on chest compressions. In some locations, ventilations have been completely dismissed in favor of chest compressions only, begging a name change from CPR to CCR (cardiocerebral resuscitation).[62]

CPR guidelines are reviewed and updated every 5 years; therefore it is important for the sports medicine physician to stay abreast of current guidelines.

Sudden Cardiac Arrest in Athletes

The leading cause of death in young athletes is sudden cardiac arrest (SCA), typically as a result of a structural cardiac abnormality. In a cohort of 387 young athletes, HCM was the most common cause of SCA, accounting for 26% of deaths; commotio cordis was second at 20%; and coronary artery anomalies were third at 14%.[118] Coronary artery anomalies are the most common cause of SCA in young female athletes. In athletes over the age of 35, coronary artery disease is by far the most common cause of SCA at 75%. Nonstructural causes, such as inherited arrhythmia syndromes and ion channel disorders, are much less common sources of SCA in young athletes, making up only 2% of deaths in that cohort.

The incidence of SCA in high school–aged athletes is 1:100,000 to 1:200,000, and in college-aged athletes it is 1:65,000 to 1:69,000. A higher incidence is seen in males (5:1, males/females). Vigorous exercise appears to be a trigger for lethal arrhythmias because 90% of SCA occurs during training or competition. It is unfortunately very difficult to prevent given that most athletes are asymptomatic until the fatal event. Most patients with SCA are found in asystole of pulseless electrical activity (PEA), both nonshockable rhythms. The next most common are ventricular fibrillation (VF) and ventricular tachycardia (VT) (both shockable rhythms). It is likely that most victims start in VF or rapid VT at the time of collapse, but the rhythm has already deteriorated to asystole or PEA before the first rhythm analysis. The probability of successful defibrillation from VF decreases rapidly over time, with survival rates declining 7% to 10% for every minute defibrillation is delayed, which emphasizes the importance of AEDs and a well-rehearsed EAP.

Survival after SCA is dismal. In a cohort of 486 young athletes (ages 5 to 22), the survival rate was only 11%.[55] Besides the inherently poor prognosis, another factor affecting survival in SCA is delayed early recognition and consequently delayed defibrillation. Three main factors are known to delay treatment in SCA, and all medical personnel need to understand them. The first is agonal or occasional gasping mistaken for breathing. Second, many lay rescuers falsely identify the presence of a pulse; consequently, the updated CPR guidelines eliminate lay rescuer assessment of pulse and recommend assuming cardiac arrest if the victim does not demonstrate normal breathing. Finally, the third factor is myoclonic activity falsely identified as seizure and not cardiac arrest. Seizure activity is present in approximately 20% of patients with cardiogenic collapse.[56]

Cervical Spine

Cervical spinal cord injuries are one of the most catastrophic injuries in all of sports medicine. They have the potential to occur in any sport but are predominantly seen in football, gymnastics, and ice hockey. The data are most robust for high school and collegiate football, where the annual incidence of cervical spinal cord injury is 6:100,000 and 4:100,000, respectively.[134] Advances in helmet technology have decreased the incidence of intracranial hemorrhage but paradoxically increased the incidence of cervical spine injury. Rule changes, including the banning of spear tackling, have been effective at decreasing this rise. The risk of injury can never be fully avoided in contact sports, but the minutes that follow the injury itself are vital to prevent secondary neurologic or cardiopulmonary sequelae.

As with all injuries, the athlete should be assessed for the need of basic life support (BLS). If BLS will be needed, emergency personnel should be contacted and the EAP activated. Any athlete who is unconscious or unable to move must be treated as having a spinal cord injury or unstable fracture until proven otherwise. The athlete should not be moved unless absolutely essential to maintain the airway, breathing, or circulation. If the athlete must be moved, the spine should be kept in a neutral position, and the athlete should be placed supine. Athletes found prone must be moved safely into a supine position by a minimum of four trained individuals. These transfers are stressful, not intuitive, and must be practiced by the team physician and training staff to be performed safely and correctly.

Removal of the facemask must be done as soon as is prudent to ensure access to the airway, regardless of the patient's current respiratory status. Current recommendations advise against removal of an athlete's helmet or shoulder pads in an uncontrolled environment because of the amount of cervical movement that is created.[107]

Any athlete having significant spine pain, neurologic deficit, or diminished level of consciousness should be transported in the appropriate manner for further observation and testing. A written plan must be established for the care and transfer of an athlete with a potential spinal cord injury to a medical facility. Coaches and athletic trainers should have BLS skills and should be active participants in preparing a plan to stabilize an injured player. The athlete's equipment must be properly maintained, and the medical personnel that will assess players on the field must have the ability, skills, and tools necessary to remove the athlete's equipment if necessary.

Exercise-Associated Collapse in Athletic Endurance Events

Exercise-associated collapse (EAC) in the endurance athlete has a broad differential diagnosis (Box 39-6). Given space constraints, this section focuses on benign EAC, exercise-associated hyponatremia, cardiogenic collapse, and heat-related illnesses. In general, when an athlete collapses before the finish line in a race while still running, the diagnosis is more ominous. The assessment of a collapsed athlete starts with assessing the level of responsiveness and checking airway, breathing, and circulation (ABC). Depending on the severity of the presentation, specific symptoms, and vital signs, a diagnostic workup can include an assessment of cardiac rhythm, rectal temperature, and blood glucose and sodium levels.

BOX 39-6

Differential Diagnosis of Exercise-Associated Collapse

- Benign exercise-associated collapse
- Cardiac arrest*
- Heat-related illness
- Heat stroke*
- Hypoglycemia*
- Hyponatremia*
- Hypothermia
- Muscle cramps
- Other medical/neurologic conditions

*Medical emergency.

The most common cause of collapse in a marathon runner after crossing the finish line is benign EAC. This is generally considered a form of postural hypotension. While running, the leg muscles act as a venous pump to improve blood flow return to the central circulation. When the athlete stops running, venous pooling of blood in the legs can occur, resulting in a decrease in blood pressure and a subsequent collapse. This is exacerbated in warm environments because blood flow is shunted from the core to the skin to facilitate cooling. It is important to keep the athlete walking after crossing the finish line to keep the muscular venous pump engaged. Treating EAC means treating the primary cause of collapse and providing supportive care. If the underlying cause of the collapse is determined to be benign EAC, oral rehydration and lying the athlete down on a stretcher with legs and pelvis elevated above heart level are typically all that is needed. If the athlete does not improve within 15 to 30 minutes, a search for a more ominous cause of collapse should be undertaken, including orthostatics, if possible, and an electrolyte assessment, followed potentially by administration of intravenous fluids. It is rare to definitively need intravenous fluids after running a marathon.

Exercise-associated hyponatremia (EAH) was first reported in the 1981 Comrades Run (90-km ultramarathon) in South Africa; it received national and international media attention after the death of a 28-year-old female runner in the 2002 Boston Marathon. It is a hypervolemic hyponatremia causing early symptoms of lightheadedness, a nauseated feeling, later a progressive headache, vomiting, confusion, and finally obtundation, seizures, and death. The pathophysiology is fluid shifts from low osmotic pressure in the blood causing cerebral edema and then neurogenic pulmonary edema. Further research into this condition demonstrates similarities to the syndrome of inappropriate antidiuretic hormone (SIADH), which has an impact in understanding the pathophysiology underlying EAH. The early symptoms of EAH are nonspecific, so medical providers must have an index of suspicion in any marathoner who is not feeling well after the race. Risk factors for EAH include weight gain during the race, marathon race time more than 4 hours, and body mass index extremes.[2] Those at risk are runners who ingest too many fluids on the race course and subsequently gain weight. Slower runners have more of an opportunity to drink excessively, and smaller runners generally need less fluid to dilute their serum sodium levels.

Once the diagnosis is made, treatment is indicated according to the severity of presentation and serum sodium level. For those runners who are fluid overloaded with low serum sodium but have minimal symptoms, close observation and fluid restriction are indicated as a natural diuresis occurs. If the sodium level is low or is not reversing, hospital observation might be indicated. If the same athlete has progressive encephalopathic symptoms, treatment would include high-flow oxygen, a bolus of hypertonic saline (3% NaCl), and quick transport to an emergency facility.

Prevention of EAH should be the ultimate goal for any medical director of an endurance athletic event such as a marathon. Prevention starts with educating athletes about the risk of overdrinking on the course and teaching them to use their training in the months before the event to determine their individual fluid needs. Emphasizing individual differences and reminding the athletes to replace what they need (sweat losses) and not necessarily more is appropriate (Box 39-7). The mantra "drink when you are thirsty" is generally safe for slower and at-risk runners. Only if the athlete is a very salty sweater or if the competition lasts more than 6 hours should sodium or electrolyte replacement be necessary. Spacing the water/aid stations about every 1.5 miles along the course is another way to limit excessive drinking and potentially prevent EAH.

BOX 39-7

General Fluid Replacement Guidelines in a Marathon

- Drink when you are thirsty
- 400-800 mL (14-27 oz) per hour of racing
- The low end is for smaller, slower runners
- The high end is for larger, faster runners

Given the continued popularity of marathons and other mass participation endurance events, deaths are commonly reported in the media. With more events and more press coverage, there is an appearance of an increase in marathon-related deaths. The often-quoted risk of SCA in a marathon is 1:50,000. This is an old statistic from a study evaluating cardiac-related deaths in the Twin Cities Marathon and Marine Corp Marathon from 1976 to 1994.[119] When follow-up data from these marathons from 1995 to 2004 were analyzed, the new rate of cardiac-related deaths was 1:220,000.[160] The London Marathon also had a rate of 1:80,000 from 1981 to 2006.[187] Even though there are more marathons and marathoners, the rate of SCA has improved during the past 10 to 15 years. This could be related to earlier recognition, better preparation, and AED use.

Heat-related illness is another etiology of EAC. Heat exhaustion is the inability to continue to exercise in the heat but is not related to body temperature. It represents the failure of the cardiovascular response to workload, high environmental temperatures, and dehydration. No chronic or harmful effects are known. In contrast, heat stroke is a medical emergency. Heat stroke is defined as multiorgan system failure secondary to hyperthermia. The rectal core temperature in an athlete with heat stroke is generally more than 39° C. Treatment is immediate total body cooling. Disagreement exists on which cooling method is most efficient. Ice bath/cold water immersion, the "taco method" using wet sheets and ice, and finally administering ice to the head, neck, axilla, and groin are all common cooling methods used in the field (at races and in the military). Whatever method is used, it should be simple and safe, provide adequate cooling, and not restrict other forms of treatment, including CPR, defibrillation, and intravenous cannulation.[22] The mortality rate and extent of organ damage in athletes with heat stroke are proportional to the length of time between core temperature elevation and onset of cooling therapy. Finally, it is important to note that heat stroke can occur in cool environments and might be more of a genetic predisposition to excessive endothermy (i.e., endogenous heat production) and not just a factor of extreme environmental conditions.[156]

Specific Diagnoses in Sports Medicine

Sports Concussion

Concussions are mild traumatic brain injuries sustained as a result of direct blows to the head or forces transmitted through the head and neck. The Centers for Disease Control and Prevention estimates that 1.6 to 3.8 million sports- and recreation-related traumatic brain injuries occur each year. They occur in all sports but are most common in contact and collision sports. Concussions can result in symptoms, physical signs, behavioral changes, cognitive impairment, and sleep disturbance (Box 39-8). These symptoms are typically caused by a functional disturbance of the brain rather than a true structural injury. It is vital to recognize that concussions rarely result in a loss of consciousness. Concussion symptoms are generally transient, although chronic sequelae might occur.

Pathophysiologically the concussed brain exhibits increased metabolic needs combined with decreased cerebral blood flow.[15] This mismatch of "supply and demand" creates a state of tissue vulnerability. Second-impact syndrome is a rare and catastrophic outcome of concussion that might be caused by this mismatch. This phenomenon is seen when a youth athlete receives a second impact before the symptoms of the first concussion have subsided. These rare injuries have been reported only in youth athletes and result in severe brain injury and even death from malignant cerebral swelling.

The most vital component of concussion care is the prompt recognition of the injury itself. Athletes, coaches, trainers, and family members should have some degree of education regarding the most common signs and symptoms. An athlete with a suspected concussion should be removed from play immediately and evaluated on the sideline. The Standardized Assessment of Concussion, Pocket Sport Concussion Assessment Tool 3, and Maddocks questions are commonly used sideline tools. They do not replace the value of a more thorough assessment to detect more subtle abnormalities.[125] The current consensus is that athletes should not RTP on the same day as a concussion. In certain professional athletic settings, adult athletes can RTP on the same day once cleared by a health care provider.[125]

Imaging is initially reserved for situations in which an intracranial abnormality is suspected, including prolonged loss of consciousness, focal neurologic deficit, or progressive decline in neurologic status. In athletes with prolonged or severe symptoms, magnetic resonance imaging (MRI) can be used to evaluate for other intracranial abnormalities. Newer imaging protocols, such as functional and diffusion-weighted MRI, positron emission tomography, and diffusion tensor imaging, are emerging but are not yet part of current concussion management.

Neuropsychologic (NP) testing is a useful component in the management of concussions. Cognitive and somatic symptoms typically improve in parallel but often completely resolve at different times. As such, NP testing can give added information that cannot be gained in a typical clinical setting. Neuropsychologists are best suited to interpret these data, but in situations where no neuropsychologist is available, other medical professionals can be trained to perform the interpretation.[58] NP testing is only one component of concussion management, however, and the decision to RTP is ultimately a medical one.

In the first several days to weeks after an injury athletes with concussions are managed with both physical and mental rest. This includes limiting activities that require concentration and attention such as scholastic activity, video games, computer use, and text messaging. These activities often exacerbate the athlete's symptoms and can prolong the final resolution of symptoms. Youth athletes might require individualized schoolwork adaptations and the cooperation of school administration (e.g., extended test-taking time, tutors, limited class schedules). Section 504 of the Americans with Disabilities Act, part of a federal law that protects students with disabilities, is often used to create plans to help concussed athletes continue to participate in school.

Early data suggest that athletes with prolonged recoveries are safe to begin subthreshold exercise programs and that this may speed recovery. The optimal timing and type of exercise are unclear, but beginning exercise several weeks after the injury has proven safe in study protocols. Resistance and interval training has not yet been studied. Vestibular rehabilitation has been shown to aid athletes suffering from dizziness, vertigo, or impaired balance after concussion. Optimal timing and duration of these programs are not known.[168] Prognosis after concussion is typically excellent with 80% to 90% of athletes free of symptoms within 7 to 10 days.[124] Children and adolescents are notable exceptions and might have a longer recovery time.[125] RTP decisions can be challenging and must be made by practitioners familiar with concussion management. No athlete should RTP until all the symptoms of the concussion have resolved. Once the athlete is asymptomatic at rest, a stepwise approach RTP protocol must be completed before competition is resumed (Table 39-6). The athlete will need a 24-hour symptom-free period before advancing to the next step in the protocol. No athlete should be returned to competition while still symptomatic.

Athletes with repeated concussions must be evaluated on an individual basis. These athletes typically have a

BOX 39-8

Symptoms Reported After Concussion

- Headache
- Neck pain
- Nausea and/or vomiting
- Vision changes
- Balance problems
- Sensitivity to light
- Sensitivity to noise
- Feeling "slowed down"
- Feeling "in a fog"
- "Don't feel right"
- Difficulty concentrating
- Difficulty remembering
- Fatigue
- Confusion
- Drowsiness
- Trouble falling asleep
- Changes in emotionality
- Irritability
- Sadness
- Nervousness or anxiety

Table 39-6 Return-to-Play Protocol

Rehabilitation Stage	Functional Exercise at Each Stage of Rehabilitation	Objective
1. No activity	Complete physical and mental rest	Recovery and resolution of symptoms
2. Light aerobic exercise	Walking, swimming, or stationary cycling; low intensity, no resistance training	Increase heart rate.
3. Sport-specific exercise	Drills, no head impact activities	Add movement to test coordination and more complex motor skills.
4. Noncontact training drills	Progression to more complex training drills, add resistance exercise	Exercise, coordination, and cognitive load
5. Full contact practice	After medical clearance, participation in normal training	Restore confidence and assess functional skills.
6. Return to play	Normal game play	

Modified from McCrory P, Meeuwisse W, Johnston K, et al: Consensus statement on concussion in sport—The 3rd international conference on concussion in sport held in Zurich, November 2008, *Phys Med Rehabil* 1:406-420, 2009.

prolonged recovery course and might have higher symptom severity.[40,41,43,176] An increasing body of literature suggests concussions are an independent risk factor for long-term deficits in executive function and processing speed.[41,81] The phenomenon of athletes suffering increasingly severe concussions with decreasing impact severity should raise significant concerns for the physician. These athletes might need to consider giving up contact sports and might not be cleared to participate.[27]

There is a burgeoning field of knowledge regarding chronic traumatic encephalopathy (CTE), a disease thought to be caused by repeated concussive or subconcussive blows to the head. CTE typically presents many years after the last report of head injury. The symptoms include mood changes, memory deficits, impulse control problems, confusion, and eventual dementia. Pathophysiologically, the brain shows deposition of abnormal Tau protein and neurofibrillary tangles.[126] Most CTE cases have been reported in adults, though the youngest confirmed case is that of a 17-year-old high school football player who died from second impact syndrome. Physiatrists have a unique expertise in brain injury, sports medicine, and the complexities of managing the expectations of multiple involved parties in the care of a concussed athlete. Concussion is being increasingly recognized as a significant public health concern that can result in significant long-term deficits in a young, vulnerable patient population. The Zackery Lystedt Law was the first concussion management law, passed by the state of Washington in 2009. It requires that all youth athletes with suspected concussion must be removed from play, evaluated, and cleared by a medical professional before returning to play. All 50 states have concussion laws and sports medicine physicians need to educate themselves on the details of their individual state's laws.

Stingers

The stinger, sometimes termed a burner, is probably one of the most common but least understood peripheral nerve injuries in sports. Stingers are nerve injuries that occur within the peripheral neural axis at a specific but variable point from the nerve root to the brachial plexus. The true incidence of stingers is unknown; however, it is estimated that more than 50% of collegiate football players sustain a stinger each year.[38]

A great deal of controversy exists regarding the pathophysiology of stingers. The symptoms can result from a tensile (stretch) or compressive injury to the cervical nerve root or brachial plexus. Of the two, the cervical nerve root appears to be at greater risk for both tensile and compressive injury than the brachial plexus. However, the literature slightly favors brachial plexus tensile overload[1] over nerve root stretch,[178] nerve root compression,[150,163,196] and direct brachial plexus compression[51,117] as the primary mechanism of injury in stingers. The pathomechanics of each injury vary by the age and experience of the athlete as well as by specific sport. Tensile injuries typically occur in younger athletes with less experience who have weaker neck and shoulder girdle musculature, leaving them vulnerable to forceful contralateral neck lateral bending with ipsilateral shoulder and arm depression. Cervical root compression is likely to occur in the older, stronger, and more experienced athlete during forceful cervical extension and rotation, narrowing the neuroforamen. This scenario is more commonly seen in professional football defensive backs and offensive lineman. Least commonly, a compressive blow to the brachial plexus can result from equipment issues such as padding.

The patient with a stinger classically presents with sudden onset of a lancinating, burning pain in one upper limb after a traumatic event. The symptoms typically follow a single* dermatomal distribution, most commonly in a C5, C6, or C7 pattern. The pain usually lasts seconds to minutes, with the sensory disturbance usually resolving quickly; in contrast, weakness can be more persistent. Simultaneous, bilateral stingers are very uncommon; therefore any athlete with bilateral upper limb paresthesias or dysesthesias should be evaluated for a spinal cord injury. With the first occurrence of a stinger, symptoms generally resolve quickly and no medical attention is sought. With each subsequent recurrence, more distinct neurologic sequelae might result, including persistent motor weakness. Motor impairment (particularly in the deltoid and biceps, i.e., C5 myotome) is the more common residual neurologic symptom of an athlete with a stinger.[84]

The initial sideline evaluation includes determining the specific mechanism of injury and the precise distribution and duration of symptoms. The sideline physical examination includes cervical active ROM to assess pain

*References 6, 28, 48, 68, 116, 151.

provocation and rigidity, palpation for tenderness, and a detailed neurologic examination with close attention to the C5–C7 myotomes.

The duration of any given episode can vary from seconds to hours, much less commonly lasting for days or longer. Serial assessments are critical for RTP and management decisions. If symptoms progressively worsen over the first few days or if weakness persists more than 10 to 14 days, additional ancillary testing and specialty consultation would be indicated to precisely determine the site of injury and the degree of axonal damage.

If the athlete's symptoms resolve very quickly (within seconds to minutes) and physical examination demonstrates no abnormality (including full pain-free cervical ROM), then no additional testing might be necessary. Persistent symptoms or signs and recurrent stingers are indications for further workup.

Although plain radiographs of the cervical spine provide limited information in this setting, they can reveal clues to pathoanatomy contributing to the symptoms. A higher incidence of degenerative changes (creating central canal and neuroforaminal stenosis concomitantly) is noted in more experienced athletes who sustain stingers.[114] Levitz et al.[114] studied a cohort of football players with chronic stingers and demonstrated that 93% had significant cervical disk disease or neural foraminal narrowing.

Advanced imaging with MRI or computed tomography is indicated if the athlete experiences severe unrelenting pain, persistent symptoms, or abnormal neurologic findings on examination. Electrodiagnostic testing (EDX) is complementary to imaging studies. EDX can provide quantification of neural dysfunction and can help to determine the site of nerve injury. EDX is most useful in the athlete with persistent or progressive weakness beyond 2 weeks postinjury or in the setting of recurrent stingers. As with other nerve injuries, 7 to 10 days may be required for the axonal damage to manifest on electromyography (EMG), so this is not a test used immediately postinjury.

Treatment of stingers includes pain control, antiinflammatories, strengthening, and rehabilitation of postural faults and muscle imbalances that might have contributed to the athlete's risk of sustaining the stinger. Persistent symptoms can be treated with fluoroscopically guided epidural steroid injections, surgical decompression of neuroforaminal stenosis, or even anterior cervical diskectomy and fusion. Equipment modifications should be considered for prevention of recurrent injury, although research is lacking to support their effectiveness.[84]

Well-established guidelines do not exist for when athletes with stingers should return to competition. The following is an approach based on a combination of clinical experience, neurophysiologic principles, and extrapolation of information from other peripheral nerve injuries. After an initial stinger, if full recovery is demonstrated within 15 minutes, return to same game competition is allowed. If full recovery occurs within 1 week after the initial stinger, then return to competition that next week is allowed. A limited rehabilitation program to address postural dysfunction and relative weaknesses should be prescribed during the in-season strength and conditioning program, followed by a more comprehensive program in the off-season. If the athlete has sustained recurrent stingers, a general rule is to hold the player from competition for the number of weeks that corresponds to the number of stingers sustained in a given season (e.g., 2 weeks for a second stinger). If more than three stingers occur in a season, ending the season should be considered, especially if there is significant weakness, axonopathy on EMG, or focal disk herniation or foraminal stenosis noted on MRI.[83]

Exercise-Induced Bronchospasm

EIB describes airway narrowing that occurs in association with exercise. EIB can be present with chronic asthma but generally is a separate entity. The prevalence of EIB is significantly higher in athletes than the general population. A diagnosis based solely on clinical symptoms is often inaccurate, and pulmonary function testing and consultation with an asthma specialist are important to definitively diagnose and optimally treat EIB.[164]

Symptoms can include breathlessness with or without coughing and wheezing or even solely the vaguer symptom of decreased performance during vigorous endurance training or competition. Cross-country skiers and other winter sport athletes most often present with EIB, although runners are not far behind. EIB is much less common in swimmers. Cold, dry air is much more likely than warm, humid air to precipitate symptoms.

The mechanism of EIB is not fully understood but is certainly different from that of chronic asthma, which is caused by inflammation resulting from overly reactive airways to inhaled stimulants. EIB is thought to result from water loss and cooling in the airway that occurs with hyperventilation, which subsequently trigger bronchoconstriction.[29]

Several diagnostic testing options are available when EIB is suspected by history but the physical examination is normal (Box 39-9).[29] Once a diagnosis of EIB is made, treatment is multifaceted. An adequate warm-up has been demonstrated to reduce the severity of EIB. Some recommend inducing a refractory period by briefly precipitating symptoms with short, vigorous bursts of exercise lasting 15 to 20 minutes before the competitive endurance event. The mainstay of pharmacologic therapy is a short-acting

BOX 39-9

Diagnostic Testing for Exercise-Induced Bronchospasm

- Spirometry
- Formal PFTs
- Challenge testing
- Eucapnic voluntary hyperventilation challenge
  - Breathe in 4.5% CO_2 for eucapnia, then measure FEV_1
  - Any decrease in FEV_1 is diagnostic for EIB
- Exercise challenge in the field or laboratory
  - Useful because it simulates the sport-specific temperature/environment
- Methacholine challenge
  - Good to classify the severity of asthma
- Not specific for EIB

CO_2, Carbon dioxide; *EIB*, exercise-induced bronchospasm; *FEV_1*, forced expiratory volume in 1 second; *PFT*, pulmonary function test.

β-agonist 15 minutes before exercise. If this is ineffective, adding cromolyn, a mast cell stabilizer, is indicated first, then inhaled corticosteroids as the last addition to preexercise therapy. If EIB is refractory to this treatment, daily chronic asthma therapy should be added to the regimen. This includes inhaled corticosteroids first, and then long-acting β-agonists and leukotriene receptor antagonists can be added.[30]

Anemia

The three most common causes of anemia in the athlete are iron-deficiency anemia (IDA), physiologic anemia (pseudoanemia), and foot-strike hemolysis.

IDA is most common in menstruating women, and female athletes can be more prone to developing it. The etiology is either blood loss or poor iron intake. Many athletes consume restrictive diets that can have too little iron to meet daily needs. A complete history and physical examination are still important, however, to evaluate for "nonathletic" causes such as significant gastrointestinal or genitourinary blood losses. Usually a serologic workup is diagnostic and includes complete blood count (CBC), serum ferritin, and total iron binding capacity (TIBC). The CBC will show a microcytic anemia.[105] Serum ferritin levels that are less than 30 ng/mL in athletes are considered suggestive of IDA.[63] The TIBC will be elevated. If IDA is diagnosed, a trial of oral iron supplementation (typically ferrous sulfate or ferrous gluconate, 325 mg three times daily) is undertaken.[39] Iron is best absorbed in an acidic environment, so it is concomitantly administered with vitamin C, usually for a 2- to 3-month course.

Physiologic anemia is considered a pseudoanemia seen commonly in endurance athletes. Endurance athletes tend to have a lower hemoglobin concentration than the general population because of plasma volume expansion with a dilutional effect. It is an adaptation to exercise and is not considered to inhibit athletic performance. It generally normalizes with training cessation of 3 to 5 days. If IDA is ruled out, there is no necessary treatment.

Foot-strike hemolysis refers to red blood cell destruction in the feet from running impact. However, intravascular hemolysis is seen in swimmers, cyclists, and runners, but whether or not actual mechanical red blood cell trauma is the source is questionable. Possible reasons are intramuscular destruction, osmotic stress, and membrane lipid peroxidation caused by free radicals released by activated leukocytes. Intravascular hemolysis can even be regarded as a physiologic means to provide heme and proteins for muscle growth in athletes.[161] Generally the hemolysis is mild, and treatment is rarely required.

Specific Populations

Women in Sports

Until puberty, boys and girls are similar in body size, shape, and physiology.[20] On average, women have a larger surface area-to-mass ratio, lower bone mass, and a wider, shallower pelvis than men. Because of these differences, women might tolerate heat better than men, might be more prone to osteoporosis, and might develop knee problems more frequently.[20] The following discussion highlights one issue unique to the female athlete: the female athlete triad.

Female Athlete Triad

The female athlete triad is a constellation of interrelated findings of inadequate eating, menstrual abnormalities, and skeletal demineralization.[143] The definition of the triad does not require the simultaneous occurrence of all three components. Each facet, in isolation or combination, needs to be considered and treated.[139]

Inadequate eating describes women who eat insufficient calories for the amount of calories burned, as well as women with frank anorexia or bulimia (Box 39-10). Diminished athletic performance often results, and a vicious cycle develops in which psychologic distress and depression can develop.[138] A higher incidence of eating disorders has been reported in female athletes compared with the general population.[20,79] Female athletes are also more likely to have disordered eating than their male counterparts.[79] A higher rate of eating disorders has been reported among athletes in sports emphasizing leanness, such as gymnastics, figure skating, dancing, distance running, diving, and swimming.[10,20,138,139]

Athletic women are 3 times as likely to develop primary or secondary amenorrhea as their nonathletic counterparts.[153] Menstrual irregularities range from reduction in luteal phase length and suppression of luteal function to amenorrhea.[20] Women with athletic amenorrhea present

BOX 39-10

Diagnostic and Statistical Manual of Mental Disorders—-IV. Definitions of Anorexia, Bulimia Nervosa, and Eating Disorders Not Otherwise Specified[5]

Anorexia
- Body weight 15% below expected
- Morbid fear of fatness
- Feeling fat when thin
- Amenorrhea

Bulimia Nervosa
- Binge eating twice per week for at least 3 months
- Loss of control over eating
- Purging behavior
- Overconcern with body shape

Eating Disorders not Otherwise Specified
- All criteria for anorexia nervosa are met except amenorrhea, or the individual's current weight is within the normal range
- All criteria for bulimia nervosa are met except that binge and purge cycles occur at a frequency less than twice a week for a duration of <3 months
- An individual of normal body weight uses purging behaviors after eating small amounts of food
- An individual repeatedly chews and spits out, but does not swallow, large amounts of food

Modified from American Psychiatric Association: *Diagnostic and statistical manual of medical disorders, IV.* Arlington, VA, 1994, American Psychiatric Association.

with a reduction in luteinizing hormone pulse frequencies, which depend on energy availability.[138] Dietary supplementation (i.e., providing adequate energy sources) can prevent or eliminate menstrual disturbances.[20,79]

Skeletal demineralization is the third component of the triad and can lead to premature osteoporosis. The prevalence of osteopenia in female athletes has been reported to be 22% to 50%, whereas the prevalence of osteoporosis remains relatively low.[100] Bone undergoes continual resorption and formation, a process called remodeling. Hormonal status, weight-bearing physical activity, and dietary intake (particularly calcium) influence remodeling. Stress fractures pose a health risk to amenorrheic athletes as a result of reduced bone mass. The relative risk for stress fractures is 2 to 4 times greater for amenorrheic athletes compared with those with regular menses.[139]

Peak bone mass is achieved during the first 3 decades of life, with Tanner stages II and III (early to midpuberty) as the maturational stage in which physical activity has the strongest impact on bone.[139] Young athletes with primary amenorrhea might be unable to build bone during formative years, with the end result being that peak bone mass might never be achieved.[20]

Dual-energy x-ray absorptiometry is the most widely used and validated technique to assess bone mineral density (BMD).[98,139] The WHO defines osteoporosis as a BMD greater than 2.5 standard deviations (SDs) below the youthful mean (T score ≤–2.5 SDs).[98] Osteopenia is defined as a BMD between 1.0 and 2.5 SDs below the youthful mean (T score 1.0 to 2.5) (Table 39-7).[98] Notably, normative data for adolescent girls are not available to definitively define pathologic bone loss in this group; hence Z scores are best used in the skeletally immature athlete because the Z score is age-matched while the T score is compared with a 35-year-old person.[10,20]

Randomized controlled trials have shown that oral contraceptive pills might increase lumbar and total body BMD in patients with hypothalamic amenorrhea.[87,194] In addition, 1200 to 1500 mg of calcium and 400 to 800 IUs of vitamin D/day are recommended.[79] More recently, attention has turned to the cardiovascular risks associated with the hypoestrogenic state in women with hypothalamic amenorrhea. Estrogen has cardioprotective effects, such as increasing high-density lipoprotein and decreasing low-density lipoprotein cholesterol.[191] Estrogens also stimulate the production of nitric oxide (NO), a potent vasodilator and inhibitor of platelet aggregation, leukocyte adhesion, and vascular smooth muscle proliferation and migration, all of which are part of the atherosclerotic process. Flow-mediated vasodilatation (FMD) results from NO release in response to shear stress and increased blood flow.[92] Athletic amenorrhea is associated with decreased endothelium-dependent dilation of the brachial artery (a measure of FMD)[157,206] and unfavorable lipid profile.[157] Treatment with oral contraceptive pills has been associated with improved FMD.[158] Female athletes presenting with features of the female athlete triad require appropriate workup and referrals (Figure 39-9). Although referrals to a nutritionist, psychologist/therapist, and other medical specialists, such as endocrinologists, cardiologists, and gastroenterologists, might be necessary, a primary treatment focus should be to restore energy balance by improving caloric intake and potentially decreasing energy expenditure (limiting aerobic exercise). Finally, pregnancy should be excluded in any amenorrheic female of childbearing age.

Pediatric and Adolescent Athlete

According to one estimate, 30 million children and adolescents participate in organized sports activities in the United States.[1] As athletic involvement increases, the incidence of sports-related injuries also increases.[108,177]

Physically active adults had better standardized fitness scores as children,[49] suggesting that an active lifestyle as a child promotes continued lifelong physical fitness. Physical activity in children and adolescents prevents osteoporosis, improves self-esteem, and reduces anxiety and depression.[16,32] Furthermore, there is a positive relationship between physical fitness and academic achievement in English and mathematics.[35] High school athletes are more likely to engage in positive health behaviors and less likely to engage in negative health behaviors compared with nonathletes.[147]

When advising pediatric athletes about their training program, the physiologic and anatomic differences between children and adults must be considered. Strength training has been historically discouraged in the pediatric population because of concerns of growth disturbance and potential for other injuries.[108] According to a position statement

Table 39-7 Current Recommendations for the Diagnosis of Low Bone Mineral Density and Osteoporosis in Premenopausal and Postmenopausal Women and Young Athletes

	World Health Organization	International Society of Clinical Densitometry	International Olympic Committee
Targeted population	Postmenopausal women	Premenopausal women	Young, premenopausal athletes
Terminology	Osteopenia	BMD below expected range for age	BMD below expected range for age
Proposed cutoff score	T score: –1 to –2.5	>20 years of age: Z score* ≤ –2	>20 years of age: Z- or T score ≤ –1 should be of concern
Terminology	Osteoporosis	Low BMD for chronologic age or below expected range for age	Osteoporosis in athlete with amenorrhea
Proposed cutoff score	T score: ≤ –2.5	<20 years of age: Z score* ≤ –2	>20 years of age: Z score* –2.5

Modified from Beals KA, Meyer NL: Female athlete triad update, *Clin Sports Med* 26:69-89, 2007.
*Z score and T score might be similar in young women older than 20 years. *BMD*, Bone mineral density.

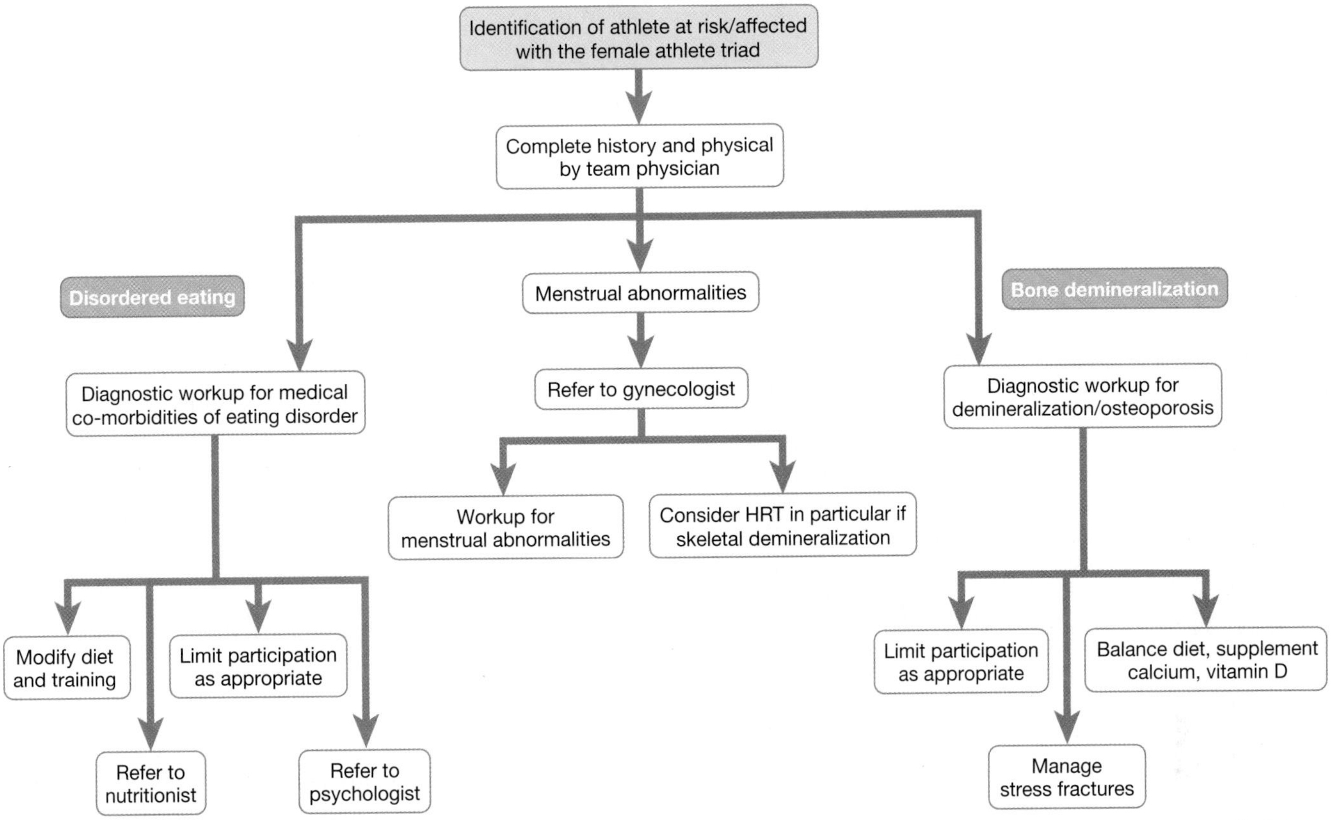

Identification of athlete at risk/affected with the female athlete triad

→ Complete history and physical by team physician

- **Disordered eating** → Diagnostic workup for medical co-morbidities of eating disorder
  - Modify diet and training
  - Refer to nutritionist
  - Limit participation as appropriate
  - Refer to psychologist
- Menstrual abnormalities → Refer to gynecologist
  - Workup for menstrual abnormalities
  - Consider HRT in particular if skeletal demineralization
- **Bone demineralization** → Diagnostic workup for demineralization/osteoporosis
  - Limit participation as appropriate
  - Manage stress fractures
  - Balance diet, supplement calcium, vitamin D

FIGURE 39-9 Overview of the management of the female athlete triad. *HRT,* Hormone-replacement therapy. (Modified from Borg-Stein J, Dugan SA, Solomon JL: Special considerations in the female athlete. In Frontera WR, Micheli LJ, Herring SA, et al, editors: *Clinical sports medicine: medical management and rehabilitation*, Philadelphia, PA, 2007, Saunders.)

by the American Academy of Pediatrics Committee on Sports Medicine, "short-term programs in which prepubescent athletes are trained and supervised by knowledgeable adults can increase strength without significant injury risk."[4] Although growth plate disturbances have been reported, these have been attributed to poor lifting techniques, lifting maximal weights, and lack of adult supervision.[82]

Training programs for pediatric athletes should include stretching routines. Children tend to lose flexibility with age, with the greatest losses occurring at puberty because of muscle-tendon imbalances that occur with rapid growth.[111] Loss of flexibility can make the athlete vulnerable to acute and overuse injuries involving the low back, pelvis, and knee.[131] Excessive flexibility, however, is associated with increased risk of sports-related injury, especially in sports that necessitate rapid change of direction or acceleration.[131]

The pediatric skeletal system is distinguished from that of adults by the presence of the active growth plate, or physis. The physis is situated between the epiphysis and metaphysis. Two types of epiphyses exist: traction and pressure.[25] The traction epiphysis, also known as the apophysis, is the point of attachment of a tendon to bone.[1] Because apophyses contribute to bone shape, but not bone length, acute or chronic injuries involving apophyses are not usually associated with growth disturbance. Osgood-Schlatter disease, Sever disease, and medial epicondylopathy are examples.[1,25]

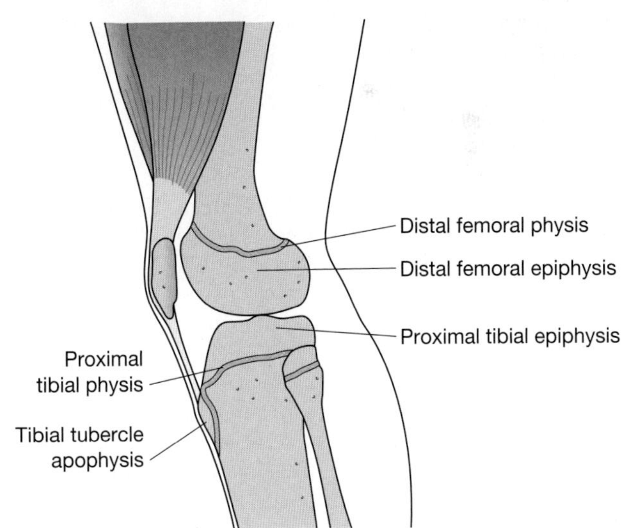

FIGURE 39-10 Physes of the distal femur and proximal tibia. (Modified from Caine D, DiFiori J, Maffulli N: Physeal injuries in children's and youth sports: reasons for concern? *Br J Sports Med* 40:749-760, 2006.)

Pressure epiphyses are found at the end of long bones such as the distal femur and proximal tibia (Figure 39-10). In contrast to apophyseal injuries, injuries to active pressure epiphysis can result in limb-length discrepancies or angular deformities.[25,175] The most common cause of acute injury to the pressure epiphysis is a fall. Acute physeal injuries are widely described using the system described by

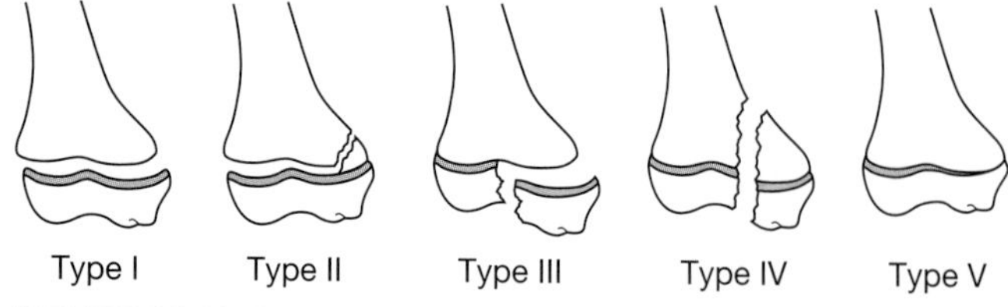

FIGURE 39-11 Growth plate injuries as described by Salter and Harris. (Modified from Caine D, DiFiori J, Maffulli N: Physeal injuries in children's and youth sports: reasons for concern? *Br J Sports Med* 40:749-760, 2006.)

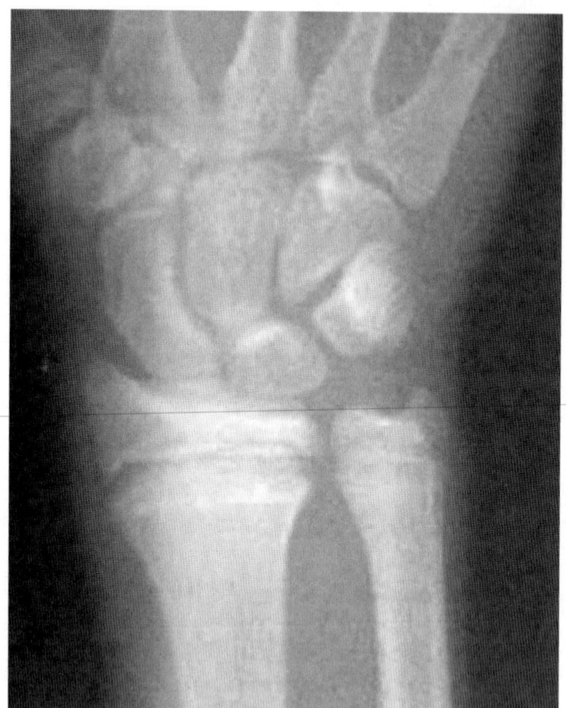

FIGURE 39-12 Radiograph of a chronic distal radius injury resulting from ongoing stress to the physis.

Salter and Harris (Figure 39-11). Chronic injuries result from ongoing stress to the physis, as is seen in distal radial injuries in young gymnasts (Figure 39-12).[25]

Older Athlete

According to the *Healthy People 2000* report, 60% of adults 65 and older engage in leisure-time physical activity.[91] Popular activities among seniors include gardening, dancing, golf, hunting, fishing, woodworking, tennis, bowling, biking, and swimming. Masters athletes have achieved impressive improvements in peak exercise performance. In fact, athletes older than 70 years of age have surpassed the winning time at the first modern Olympic Games held in Athens in 1896 in running events from 100 meters to the marathon.[181]

Benefits of Exercise in Older Adults

The benefits of exercise in older persons are many, although not entirely understood. Higher levels of physical activity are associated with lower rates of many afflictions associated with aging, including coronary heart disease and cancer, although the underlying mechanisms for these findings are largely unknown.[116] One theory is that exercise might reduce inflammation and oxidative stress, both of which are known to increase with aging.[37] Even short bouts of exercise might boost immune function, decreasing the likelihood of acute infection.[122] Weight-bearing exercise increases BMD.[139] A 2009 Cochrane Review found that exercise programs focusing on strength, balance, flexibility, and endurance were effective in reducing falls in elderly individuals living in the community.[73]

Together, these benefits confer a lower risk of mortality to the older individual. A 2006 study of healthy older adults living in the community found that for every 287 kcal/day in activity energy expenditure, there is an approximately 30% lower risk of mortality.[116] Exercise also provides a sense of psychologic well-being and enhanced quality of life. In one survey, 68% of athletic seniors regarded their quality of life as much better than that of their sedentary friends.[172]

The observed benefits are not limited to the very healthy in this age group. A 2002 systematic review of randomized controlled trials of exercise training in elderly, institutionalized adults found strong evidence that exercise increases strength and mobility in this population.[165] Moderate evidence was found for an effect on ROM, and contradictory evidence was seen regarding gait, activities of daily living, balance, and endurance. The authors concluded that more research is necessary to know the extent of possible advantages of exercise in this population. Notably, there were no ill effects reported as a result of exercise.[165]

Adaptive Sports Medicine

Athletes with impairments have been among the groups with the most rapidly increasing levels of sports participation over the past few decades. With advances in medicine and an emphasis on maintaining physical fitness, the disabled athlete population is growing. It is estimated that the disabled population in the United States is approximately 55 million according to the U.S. Census Bureau.[189] Although the number of people with a disability who participate in sporting activities is increasing, there are still only about 2 million recreational and competitive disabled athletes in the United States. Despite an increase in the development of a number of recreational and competitive sports programs, about 60% of people with a disability do not participate in any regular physical activity or sports.[203]

Although many opportunities exist for individuals with impairments, the two most limiting factors for participation in athletics are awareness and access.[203] Health care practitioners should make every effort to inform individuals of the multiple opportunities and encourage their safe participation. International organizations such as the IPC as well as National Governing Bodies (NGBs) for specific sports and regional and local organizations have been critical in providing the organization and inspiration to increase the numbers of athletes and sporting options in this population. Legislation that has advanced the rights of those with impairments has also greatly improved access to sports participation opportunities. Growth is best exemplified through the phenomenal rise of the Paralympic Games. The 1960 Paralympics in Rome had 400 athletes from 23 countries; the 2012 London Games had approximately 4200 athletes from 164 countries (www.paralympic.org/london-2012-overview). More countries competed at the Beijing 2008 Paralympics (3951 athletes, 146 countries) than in the Munich 1972 Olympic Games. In the 2014 Sochi Winter Games, the degree of media coverage was unprecedented, and it is widely anticipated that this trend will continue. There is a growing interest in and acceptance of sport for persons with a disability, and expansion of the Paralympics is most likely to continue.

This growth in participation has been accompanied by a concomitant increase in awareness of opportunities that has been supported by the medical community. Similar to any other athlete, sports participation among persons with impairments can have significant benefits in terms of general state of health, functionality, life skills, self-esteem, and overall quality of life.[22,59,171,180,190] It is imperative that medical providers promote activity among all their patients, including those with disability. However, the clinician should also be cognizant of the various complications associated with different disabilities and sports-specific activities to maximize patient safety and health.

There are multiple benefits to encouraging persons with impairments to participate in recreational and competitive sports and exercise. Athletes with impairments demonstrate increased exercise endurance, muscle strength, cardiovascular efficiency, and flexibility. They also demonstrate improved balance and better motor skills compared with individuals with disabilities who do not participate in athletics. In addition to physical benefits, the psychologic benefits of exercise include enhanced self-image, body awareness, motor development, and mood. Athletes with disabilities have fewer cardiac risk factors and higher high-density lipoprotein cholesterol levels and are less likely to smoke cigarettes than those who are disabled and nonactive.[68,46] Individuals with limb deficiencies who participate in athletics have improved proprioception and increased proficiency in the use of prosthetic devices.[197] Additionally, wheelchair athletes with paraplegia are less likely to be hospitalized, have fewer pressure ulcers, and are less susceptible to infections than nonactive individuals with paraplegia.[180]

Classifications

The IPC is the global governing body of the Paralympic Movement and organizes the Summer and Winter Paralympic Games. It was founded on September 22, 1989, in Dusseldorf, Germany, and was preceded by the International Coordination Committee of World Sports Organizations for the Disabled. The IPC serves as the International Federation for nine sports including track and field, skiing (Alpine, Nordic, biathlon), and sled hockey.

Athletes with impairments are an inherently heterogeneous group with highly variable profiles of sports capacity, depending on type, location, and severity of the disability. Similar to the weight classes used in boxing and wrestling, classification systems have been developed to maintain a measure of fairness in competition between those with both similar and different impairments. One of the first classification systems was used at the Stoke-Mandeville Games to avoid competition between athletes with dissimilar disadvantages resulting from their type of disability, e.g., a paraplegic individual competing against a tetraplegic individual. These classifications systems have been formalized over the years by the IPC and its member federations and NGBs and are continually revised to reflect advancements in sports and medicine.

Although many systems exist and are used depending on the NGB, number of participants, and available resources, the common purpose is to determine eligibility for participation and ensure that athletes are not precluded from success in competition on the basis of their disability.

To be eligible for Paralympic sports an athlete must have one of ten types of permanent impairments: ataxia, athetosis, hypertonia, leg length difference, limb deficiency, loss of muscle strength, loss of range of movement, short stature, low vision, or intellectual impairment. Athletes are placed more generally into six main disability categories: amputee, wheelchair, cerebral palsy, vision impaired, intellectual disability, or "les autres" (a French term meaning "the others" referring to those who do not fit well within any other category).[47]

Athletes are given a specific designation based on their disability category and functional ability. For example, athletes are classified based on different combinations of functional strength, truncal stability, ROM of arms and legs, use of a wheelchair, quality of ambulation and balance, and distribution and severity of muscle spasticity. Direct observation of the athlete during exercise and while participating in the activity is also often involved with some categories able to use more objective measures. This is of particular importance for evaluation of visual perception and field of view in the visually impaired category.

Because there are significant variances among the different sports, the sporting event also greatly influences the classification process. Within each sport, there are different types and severities of disability, which affect the performance to varying levels. Depending on the sport, designations may be condensed into fewer classes based on a wider range of disability. Additionally, some sports may have competition between athletes from different general disability categories who maintain similar functional levels. Team sports such as wheelchair basketball often incorporate a wide range of disabilities in direct competition via the use of point systems in which athletes with less disadvantageous levels of disability are assigned higher point values and the team is not permitted to exceed a given total point value for its players in the game.

An athlete's classification is always in evolution as there may be progressive worsening or improvement of the disease process, as well as the ability to adapt and overcome impairments. Thus, classifications are not permanently assigned. An athlete may change classifications throughout his or her life depending on the system and changes in functionality experienced over time. However, this also means that athletes with impairments that are responsive to training may be classified in one category in one training state only to compete later in a different state of training, thus gaining a competitive advantage. Therefore, it is imperative for the classifiers to be cognizant of this dynamic and evaluate for any intentional minimization of function during the evaluation process. These classification systems have also been criticized for a lack of peer-reviewed research supporting the limits and distinction of one designation from another and the use of objective criteria. Additionally, the rapid advancement of technology and materials, particularly within the amputee category, has also given rise to significant concerns regarding the level of competitive fairness given often-asymmetric levels of resources among competitors. In light of these issues, the IPC has committed to a vision of classification that is evidence-based and equitable to promote participation and competitive fairness. As such, continued assessment and revisions of these systems can be anticipated in years to come.

Adaptive Sports Equipment

When the physician is evaluating the athlete with limb deficiency for adaptive equipment, it is pertinent to consider several aspects. Compared with the prosthetic device for everyday use, there are various modifications that should be considered for specialized use. Of particular importance is the weight of the prosthesis, particularly in sports where increased weight may affect speed. Also, when prescribing an adaptive prosthesis, the clinician should consider alignment, prosthetic foot dynamics, shock absorption, and possible need for transverse rotation.

There are numerous sporting events that can incorporate adaptive sports equipment for the athlete who is limb deficient. The details, however, are beyond the scope of this chapter because of the exceedingly high volume of prosthetic modifications that can be made to various prostheses and other sporting equipment in various Paralympic sports and other recreational activities.

Medical advances in rehabilitation and in development of prosthetic devices has led to some controversy in competition against other athletes with disability. Access to different types of technology and materials can differ greatly depending on the athlete's socioeconomic status and country of origin, creating the potential for significant competitive imbalance between similarly disabled and conditioned athletes. These advances have also been cause for controversy in competition against able-bodied athletes, with continued improvements in prosthesis weight and energy-storage capabilities being a potential source of a competitive imbalance. However, many of these comparisons do not take into effect the increased energy cost of ambulation for the limb-deficient athlete. Therefore, to fully assess the energy-storing advantages in the prosthetic limb, the additional energy needs for the limb-deficient athlete to ambulate with the prosthetic device must be considered. Determining the most appropriate methods for assessing and rectifying any potential competitive imbalance will likely be an area of considerable evolution in the near future.

There are also numerous adaptations that can be made to traditional wheelchairs, which can aid participation in various sports. Of note, adjustments can be made in seating systems, leg rests, wheel type, wheel position, wheel angulation, and length to enhance athletic performance in any specific sport. Many advances in manual wheelchairs trace their origins to wheelchair sports. Sporting wheelchair adjustments that were used for racing and basketball approximately 25 years ago have become integral to the manual wheelchairs that people now use every day. Frame materials such as aluminum, titanium, and composite materials were all first introduced in sports wheelchairs. However, instead of solely improving sports performance, they help to increase the ability to independently perform activities and reduce repetitive strain injuries. In addition, the principles used in frame design of sports wheelchairs make them lighter and stiffer but ultimately faster and more responsive. They also, in general, make the chairs easier to propel, allow for easier transport of the wheelchair in a vehicle, and reduce upper limb strain in athletes and nonathletes alike. These materials and principles are now used widely in the design of ultralight manual wheelchairs.

Given the vast modifications that can be made to a wheelchair to facilitate participating in sports, the full extent of discussion is beyond the scope of this chapter.

Injury Patterns in Adaptive Sports Medicine

Injury rates for athletes with disability are similar to those for athletes without disability; however, location of injuries appears to be disability- and sport-dependent. Lower limb injuries are more common in ambulatory athletes (visually impaired, amputee, cerebral palsy), whereas upper limb injuries are more frequent in athletes who use a wheelchair.[66] Athletes with lower limb deficiency are at risk for injuries in both the intact and residual limbs. The distal residual limb is often the site of skin trauma caused by the prosthesis. Asymmetry is also commonly noted at the ipsilateral hip, as well as the pelvis and lumbar spine, as a result of increased hip power, pelvic rotation and obliquity, and spine lateral flexion and extension to improve clearance of the prosthesis during swing phase and to increase excursion and propulsion.[155] Such asymmetries may predispose athletes with these limb deficiencies to hip, sacroiliac, and lumbar spine pain.[69,133] Alternatively, the intact limb may experience significantly elevated forces compared with the residual limb from increased reliance by the athlete. This may increase the risk for overuse injuries such as tendinopathies and stress fractures of the intact limb, as well as long-term degenerative changes such as osteoarthritis.[141,166,170]

Similarly, significantly altered use patterns and loads on the intact side in upper limb deficiency can result in pain and injury to either limb or axial structures. Overuse injuries such as shoulder impingement, rotator cuff tears, epicondylitis, and peripheral nerve entrapments are common in the intact limb of upper limb amputees.[45,97,142,28] Differences in weight and swing excursion between the upper limbs, as well as the need to compensate at the shoulder for lost distal joint function, may cause significant asymmetry in the demands of the thoracic and cervical spines and paraspinal musculature and the periscapular stabilizing musculature, resulting in pain and dysfunction.[142,8]

Injuries and Complications by Cause of Disability

Disabled athletes are subject to many of the same injuries and complications from physical exertion as the able-bodied population. In addition, some specific diagnoses that result in disability also lead to increased risk of particular injuries and complications. There is certainly overlap between the categories of diagnoses resulting in disability. For example, many patients with spinal cord injuries are wheelchair users; however, athletes with limb deficiency may compete seated or standing depending on the level of deficiency. For the purposes of this discussion, the injuries and complications discussed will be broken down into the wheelchair-bound athlete and the limb-deficient athlete.

Wheelchair Athlete

Improvements in societal mindset, accessibility, and wheelchair technology have greatly increased the breadth and quality of athletic opportunities for the wheelchair user. Sports participation by wheelchair users has been found to be associated with improved functional outcomes, fewer physician visits, fewer hospitalizations, and fewer medical complications, while serving as a powerful means for improving inclusion and equality within society.[44,47,48,72,96] Most athletes in this category have spinal cord injuries, but eligibility may also extend to individuals with multiple amputations or neurologic disorders such as polio, spina bifida, and cerebral palsy.[47,48] Most of the discussion on wheelchair athletes will focus on considerations for the participation of athletes with spinal cord injuries; however, these considerations may be generalized to other wheelchair athletes, depending on the amount of trunk and upper extremity function, level of sensation, and preservation of bowel and bladder function.

Given the degree to which wheelchair users rely on their upper limbs for mobility and activities of daily living, the importance of recognizing, treating, and preventing upper limb injuries is magnified when compared with the able-bodied population. Because relative rest of the upper limb may be impossible or nearly impossible in this population, other measures should be considered. They may include splinting and orthotic prescriptions, admission to an inpatient setting if rest is required, home modifications, or additional assistance (e.g., Paralyzed Veterans of America).[47,48]

Shoulder Injuries. Wheelchair users are at increased risk for shoulder pathology including pain, rotator cuff injuries, subacromial bursitis, acromioclavicular joint abnormalities, coracoacromial ligament thickening, subacromial spurs, distal clavicle osteolysis, and impingement syndrome.[9,23,47,48,68] There are several factors contributing to the increased risk in this population including repetitive motion, increased pressure in the shoulder joint during wheelchair propulsion, and muscle imbalances in the shoulder girdle caused by weakness.[9,54,173,192] In wheelchair users, upper limb injuries including shoulder injuries are particularly disabling because these patients rely on their upper limbs for weight bearing, transfers, and ambulation in addition to all of the demands placed on the upper limbs in the able-bodied population. Despite increases in repetitive use and high-intensity activity, wheelchair athletes do not have a higher incidence of shoulder pain than nonathletic wheelchair users.[47,48] In fact, participation in athletic competition appears to be protective from shoulder pain.[71] This is likely because of increased strength and endurance in the athletic population. Shoulder complaints among wheelchair users can be reduced by appropriate wheelchair design and the use of ideal propulsion techniques.

Elbow Injuries. The elbow is another common site of both acute and chronic injuries in the wheelchair athlete. The most common sources of elbow pain are lateral epicondylitis, osteoarthritis, and olecranon bursitis.[47,48,144] The most frequently reported elbow-related injury is ulnar neuritis. Wheelchair users are an increased risk for ulnar neuropathy at the elbow.[80] There is no evidence to suggest that wheelchair athletes are at a greater risk than nonathlete wheelchair users.

Treatment of elbow pain and injuries in wheelchair users must be tailored to the individual needs of the patient, keeping in mind that many wheelchair users will be nonmobile if the individual is required to restrict weight bearing or otherwise limit activity involving their upper limb.[47,48,68]

Wrist Injuries. The wrist is another frequent site of both acute and chronic injuries in the wheelchair athlete. The most common sources of wrist symptoms are carpal tunnel syndrome (CTS), ulnar nerve entrapment in Guyon canal, osteoarthritis, tendinitis, and De Quervain tenosynovitis.[47,48,68,80,144,204]

The carpal tunnel is the most common site of nerve entrapment in able-bodied and disabled persons. Long-term wheelchair users have a 49% to 73% prevalence of CTS.[204] Wheelchair users with symptoms and physical examination findings of CTS have lower functional status compared with wheelchair users without CTS.[204]

Upper Limb Fractures. The incidence of upper limb fractures in wheelchair athletes or wheelchair users is not known. Wheelchair athletes may be at greater risk for upper limb fractures caused by repetitive falls associated with many wheelchair sports, propulsion requiring positioning the hand in a location that is susceptible to injury from nearby wheelchairs or collisions, and relatively high speeds achieved during certain wheelchair sports. Fractures should be treated as in the able-bodied population. Restricted upper limb weight bearing in a wheelchair user may result in a significant impact on ambulatory status.[47,48,68]

Thermoregulation. Following spinal cord injuries, there is disruption of neuroregulatory systems that are involved in control of body temperature. Below the level of the lesion, athletes with spinal cord injury have impaired shivering (to produce heat) and impaired sweating and vasodilation (to dissipate heat). Athletes with tetraplegia are at increased risk compared with athletes with paraplegia.[154]

It is expected that paraplegic and tetraplegic athletes will have greater increases in body temperature with exertion and greater decreases in temperature with exposure to cold weather. Prevention of temperature-related injuries requires heightened awareness and monitoring and the use of appropriate clothing and equipment, availability of rehydration, and avoidance of extremes of temperature when possible. Frostbite is of particular concern during cold weather events. Athletes with spinal cord injuries have impaired sensation and require frequent visual monitoring to prevent cold injuries.[47,48,68]

Autonomic Dysreflexia. Autonomic dysreflexia (AD) is a condition occurring from sympathetic outflow in response to a noxious stimulus being unregulated because of interruption of neural pathways after spinal cord injury. Spinal cord injuries at the level of T6 and above are at risk for AD. Symptoms of AD include paroxysmal hypertension, bradycardia, facial flushing, and headache. If the athlete with a spinal cord injury develops hypertension caused by AD, which continues to increase without treatment, stroke or death may occur.[146] For acute blood pressure control, chewable nifedipine or topical nitroglycerin paste can be used. It is imperative to immediately assess for the noxious stimulus. The most common noxious stimuli that lead to AD include tight clothing, urinary or fecal retention, renal or bladder stones, pressure ulcers, infections, or intraabdominal pathology (e.g., appendicitis). Treatment involves sitting the patient upright with loosened clothing and is directed at alleviating the source of the AD after identification of the noxious stimulus.[47,48,68]

"Boosting" is the practice of intentionally inducing AD by athletes with a spinal cord injury at or above the level of T6 for the purpose of improving athletic performance.[18,85] Boosting has been shown to confer up to a 9.7% improvement in race time. Additionally, to compete in a hazardous dysreflexic state, whether intentional or unintentional, is an extreme health risk. This dangerous practice should be discouraged and may be life-threatening. For these reasons, the IPC strictly bans the practice of boosting, and it has developed a protocol to test for it. The IPC has also been working on the development of biomarkers that would be able to identify athletes who have been boosting. Blauwet et al. reviewed the current testing policy and practices that were used at three major international Paralympic events.[18] Key parameters included the athlete's demographics, classification, and blood pressure measurements. An extremely elevated blood pressure was considered to be a proxy marker for AD, and a systolic blood pressure of at least 180 mm Hg was considered a positive test result. A total of 78 tests for the presence of AD were performed during the three games combined. However, at this point no athlete has tested positive with this testing method.[18]

Skin Breakdown. Following spinal cord injury, the patient will lose sensation below the level of the injury. This area of insensate skin leads to a risk of skin breakdown or pressure ulcer. Regardless of the level of the injury, the skin over the sacrum, coccyx, and ischial tuberosities is frequently insensate. These areas represent the highest risk for skin breakdown in athletes with spinal cord injuries. Specific athletic events may result in increased risk of skin breakdown in additional areas. For example, wheelchair racers may have increased risk of skin breakdown if the medial surface of the arm and forearm rubs against the wheelchair during propulsion. This may require customized equipment and padding to prevent skin breakdown in activity-specific high-risk areas. Athletic wheelchairs commonly sacrifice pressure relief for higher performance. This should cause the athlete and caregivers to increase vigilance in monitoring for skin breakdown, changing position frequently, and limiting time in the wheelchair. This is particularly important when an athlete is transitioning to a new piece of equipment (e.g., a new wheelchair). Prevention is of paramount importance in this population.[47,48,68]

At the first sign of skin breakdown or pressure ulcer, weight-bearing and athletic activities should be modified or restricted to prevent further injury. Pressure ulcers can be a significant cause of morbidity and mortality in persons with spinal cord injuries regardless of athletic ability.[47,48,68]

Heterotopic Ossification. The development of ectopic bone formation, heterotopic ossification (HO), in soft tissues surrounding major joints can occur following traumatic brain injury, spinal cord injury, burns, total joint arthroplasty, and even in the residual limbs of traumatic amputees.[152] The most common site of HO after spinal cord injury is the hip, but the knee, elbow, and shoulder may also be affected, depending on the level of injury. In contrast, following amputation, HO occurs in injured tissues in the residual limb and may not be in the vicinity of a joint. In the wheelchair athlete with spinal cord injury, the initial presentation may mimic deep venous thrombosis or joint infection. Diagnostic testing is often required to exclude other diagnoses. Diagnosis of HO may be made by x-rays, bone scan, or trends in alkaline phosphatase levels. HO in residual limbs may increase the risk of skin breakdown or cause pain with weight bearing, edema, fever, restricted range of motion, and activity limitations.[47,48,68]

HO typically develops within the first 6 to 12 months after amputation during the time of the amputee's prosthetic training. Prevention of HO involves frequent ROM exercises. Given that most amputees are still learning how to use their prosthesis when HO typically develops, most HO cases are known before the amputee engages in athletic competition. It would be rare for development of new HO during competition. Recognition of HO in residual limbs allows for modifications in the design of a prosthetic socket to accommodate for the ectopic bone. Furthermore, monitoring for skin breakdown should be increased in amputees with HO. Treatment of HO is no different in the athlete than in the nonathlete.

Spasticity. Spasticity is velocity-dependent increase in muscle tone that occurs after injury to the upper motor neuron. It is a common complication of persons with upper motor neuron injuries such as spinal cord injury, traumatic brain injury, and stroke. Spasticity may limit athletic participation by interfering with voluntary movements and restricting ROM. An increase in spasticity may be an indicator of a systemic or otherwise asymptomatic condition. For example, infections, intraabdominal pathology (e.g., appendicitis), skin breakdown, or bladder distension may have few symptoms that are sensed by a patient with spinal cord injury. Therefore, a sudden increase in spasticity should lead to a search for underlying pathology. Treatment for spasticity consists of oral medications, including baclofen, dantrolene, tizanidine, benzodiazepines; injectable medications such as botulinum toxin; and intrathecal medications such as baclofen. If spasticity is resistant to conservative treatment, surgery for tendon lengthening may improve hygiene, activities of daily living, and functional activities including participation in athletics.

Osteoporosis. Osteoporosis is a nearly universal complication of spinal cord injury. Patients will now have decreased weight bearing, which predisposes this population to osteoporosis; nevertheless, many risk factors are independent of alterations in weight bearing. They include severity of the injury, spasticity, and time since injury.[94a] Osteoporosis results in increased fracture risk of athletes with spinal cord injury. Because of impaired sensation below the level of the injury, athletes with spinal cord injury may not immediately complain of pain after a fracture. Thus, it is imperative for the physician to be aware of other warning signs, which may include increases in spasticity or AD. Prevention of osteoporosis should include calcium and vitamin D supplementation for all athletes with spinal cord injury. Bisphosphonates may also be used for prevention.[47,48,68]

Orthostatic Hypotension. Orthostatic hypotension is a frequent complication in many individuals with spinal cord injury. Orthostatic hypotension occurs after spinal cord injury because of decreased sympathetic efferent activity in vasculature below the level of the injury and also because of decreased reflex vasoconstriction. The result is venous pooling in dependent areas (lower limbs or abdomen) that occur with changes in position.[109] Symptoms include lightheadedness and dizziness, and syncope may occur if uncorrected. Prevention includes the use of lower limb compression stockings and abdominal binders, maintenance of hydration, and salt supplementation. If these measures are insufficient, pharmacologic treatment with midodrine, fludrocortisone, or ephedrine may be helpful.[109] Each of these medications is considered a stimulant and is currently banned by the WADA and the U.S. Anti-Doping Agency as performance-enhancing drugs. (www.globaldro.com). Therefore, in athletes with spinal cord injury who experience orthostatic hypotension, nonpharmacologic prevention should be attempted before the use of pharmacologic agents is considered.[47,48,68]

Acute Mountain Sickness. Acute mountain sickness (AMS) is thought to be caused by alterations in the blood-brain barrier and cerebral vasculature that occur at high altitudes.[52] AMS involves a constellation of symptoms including headache, nausea, weakness, and shortness of breath and occurs with exposure to high altitudes. The incidence of AMS increases with increasing altitude, and therefore there is an increased incidence in many winter sports because of competition at high altitudes. Given their altered neurophysiology and anatomy, athletes with spinal cord injury may be at higher risk of AMS.[52] Acetazolamide may be used as prophylaxis in high-risk scenarios. Treatment may include return to low altitude, acetazolamide, or dexamethasone.[47,48,68]

Limb-Deficient Athletes

Individuals with partial or full loss of limbs are eligible to compete under the classification of amputee athlete. Limb loss may be congenital or traumatic and involve the upper limbs, lower limbs, or both. Depending on the specific sport, the limb-deficient athlete may compete as a standing or seated competitor. Given the significant variance in the location and length of the amputated limb, the functionality of the participant also has significant variance. Medical conditions and injuries that are unique to limb-deficient athletes are discussed later.

Skin Disorders. Following amputation of the limb and subsequent prosthetic fitting, the skin of the distal portion of the residual limb takes on the new role of being a weight-bearing surface. As a result, the distal residual limb is at increased risk for skin breakdown and other skin disorders. Common skin problems associated with prosthetic use include ulcers, inclusion cysts, calluses, contact dermatitis, hyperhidrosis, verrucous hyperplasia, lichenification, and infections.[110,130,167]

Rashes are commonly encountered in persons using a prosthetic device and are frequently seen in amputee athletes, because of issues related to increased perspiration (www.amputeeprosthetist.com). Bacteria, fungi, allergic reaction, or chemicals on the skin can form a rash. General principles of treating a rash include cleaning the residual limb more often and using a hypoallergenic soap, and decreasing prosthesis use until the rash resolves. For bacterial or fungal rashes, antibacterial or antifungal medication is usually required. The rash may also be caused by an allergic reaction and may improve with the use of a mild corticosteroid cream. Such a rash should spur investigation as to the type of liner used with consideration of switching to a less irritating material or one that will allow greater perfusion of sweat away from the skin. Rash can be prevented by cleaning the residual limb and prosthesis as indicated.[47,68] All persons with limb deficiency will have certain adaptations to skin changes with the residual limb regardless of whether or not they use a prosthesis for sports, and skin breakdown is always a concern. At present there is no literature that the effect of traditional preventative remedies for skin breakdown, such as additional liners, padded sleeves, or socks, has any consequences on athletic performance. It is speculated that skin breakdown may be more prevalent in athletes in competition secondary to increased perspiration. Some athletes may prophylactically treat their residual limb with an antiperspirant to decrease the amount of perspiration. Environmental conditions may also play a role, particularly for marine sports (swimming, kayaking, and rowing) and participation in hot weather. In amputee athletes, increased frequency and intensity of weight bearing associated with athletic training and competition also increase the risk of skin breakdown. Identification of the functional demands the activity places on the residual limb will help determine the design of the prosthetic socket. Some sports such as running require quick movement and many steps for a limited amount of time, whereas other sports such as golf require many more steps over a period of several hours. Both running and golf could be considered high-activity levels; however, there is a significant difference between the duration of these activities. Therefore, it is imperative to understand the functional demands of each sport. The runner's prosthesis must absorb the impact of loading response, support body weight through midstance to allow a long stride length on the sound side, and provide a measure of propulsive thrust at the end of stance. In contrast, the golfer using a prosthesis endures long periods of standing, maintains overall stability when twisting during swings, and ambulates safely over uneven terrain, slopes, and inclines.

Overall, the best treatment of dermatologic issues is prevention, which can be achieved through education, close monitoring of prosthesis fit, strategic timing of donning a prosthesis, considerations of the time out of the prosthesis and liner, and responding to environmental factors.

Neuroma. A neuroma occurs at the distal end of a transected nerve in the residual limb of an amputee. When a neuroma is exposed to pressure, it creates paresthesias, dysesthesias, and radiating pain in the phantom distribution of the transected nerve. When a neuroma occurs at or near a weight-bearing structure, it can create severe pain with ambulation and weight bearing, limiting an athlete's ability to train and compete.

Treatment may involve prosthetic modifications to relieve pressure on the neuroma, oral medications including antiepileptics and tricyclic antidepressants, injection of corticosteroids and local anesthetic into the neuroma, and radiofrequency ablation.[106] Unfortunately, many of the medications commonly used to treat neuromas may be restricted in competition by WADA; thus, it behooves the sports medicine physician to be aware of the list of restricted medications (Global Drug Reference at www.globaldro.com), which is modified annually.

KEY REFERENCES

9. Bayley JC, Cochran TP, Sledge CB: The weight-bearing shoulder: the impingement syndrome in paraplegics, *J Bone Joint Surg Am* 69:676–678, 1987.
10. Beals KA, Meyer NL: Female athlete triad update, *Clin Sports Med* 26(1):69–89, 2007.
13. Bemben MG, Lamont HS: Creatine supplementation and exercise performance: recent findings, *Sports Med* 35:107–125, 2005.
18. Blauwet CA, Benjamin-Laing H, Stomphorst J, et al: Testing for boosting at the Paralympic games: policies, results and future directions, *Br J Sports Med* 47:832–837, 2013.
19. Boden BP, Tacchetti RL, Cantu RC, et al: Catastrophic cervical spine injuries in high school and college football players, *Am J Sports Med* 34:1223–1232, 2006.
22. Bragaru M, Dekker R, Geertzen JH, et al: Amputees and sports: a systematic review, *Sports Med* 41:721–740, 2011.
24. Burkhart SS, Morgan CD, Kibler WB: The disabled throwing shoulder: spectrum of pathology. Part I. Pathoanatomy and biomechanics, *Arthroscopy* 19:404–420, 2003.
34. Chiampas G, Jaworski CA: Preparing for the surge: perspectives on marathon medical preparedness, *Curr Sports Med Rep* 8:131–135, 2009.
41. Collins MW, Grindel SH, Lovell MR, et al: Relationship between concussion and neuropsychological performance in college football players, *JAMA* 282:964–970, 1999.
42. Corrado D, Pelliccia A, Bjornstad HH, et al: Cardiovascular preparticipation screening of young competitive athletes for prevention of sudden death: proposal for a common European protocol. Consensus Statement of the Study Group of Sport Cardiology of the Working Group of Cardiac Rehabilitation and Exercise Physiology and the Working Group of Myocardial and Pericardial Diseases of the European Society of Cardiology, *Eur Heart J* 26:516–524, 2005.
53. Di Luigi L: Supplements and the endocrine system in athletes, *Clin Sports Med* 27:131–151, 2008.
56. Drezner JA, Courson RW, Roberts WO, et al: Inter-association Task Force recommendations on emergency preparedness and management of sudden cardiac arrest in high school and college athletic programs: a consensus statement, *J Athl Train* 42:143–158, 2007.
62. Ewy GA: Cardiocerebral resuscitation: a better approach to cardiac arrest, *Curr Opin Cardiol* 23:579–584, 2008.
65. Ferrara MS, Palutsis GR, Snouse S, et al: A longitudinal study of injuries to athletes with disabilities, *Int J Sports Med* 21:221–224, 2000.
66. Ferrara MS, Peterson CL: Injuries to athletes with disabilities: identifying injury patterns, *Sports Med* 30:137, 2001.
71. Fullerton HD, Borckardt JJ, Alfano AP: Shoulder pain: a comparison of wheelchair athletes and nonathletic wheelchair users, *Med Sci Sports Exerc* 35:1958–1961, 2003.
81. Guskiewicz KM, McCrea M, Marshall SW, et al: Cumulative effects associated with recurrent concussion in collegiate football players: the NCAA Concussion Study, *JAMA* 290:2549–2555, 2003.
82. Guy JA, Micheli LJ: Strength training for children and adolescents, *J Am Acad Orthop Surg* 9:29–36, 2001.
84. Harrast M, Weinstein S: The Cervical Spine. In Kibler B, editor: *OKU orthopaedic knowledge update: sports medicine 4*, Rosemont, IL, 2009, American Orthopaedic Society for Sports Medicine.
89. Hewett TE, Ford KR, Myer GD: Anterior cruciate ligament injuries in female athletes: part 2, a meta-analysis of neuromuscular interventions aimed at injury prevention, *Am J Sports Med* 34:90–498, 2006.
90. Hewett TE, Myer GD, Ford KR: Anterior cruciate ligament injuries in female athletes. Part 1. Mechanisms and risk factors, *Am J Sports Med* 34:299–311, 2006.
103. Kibler WB, McMullen J: Scapular dyskinesis and its relation to shoulder pain, *J Am Acad Orthop Surg* 11:142–151, 2003.
104. Kibler WB, Press J, Sciascia A: The role of core stability in athletic function, *Sports Med* 36:189–198, 2006.
107. Kleiner DM: Prehospital care of the spine-injured athlete: monograph summary, *Clin J Sport Med* 13:59–61, 2003.
109. Krassioukov A, Eng JJ, Warburton DE, Teasell R: A systematic review of the management of orthostatic hypotension after spinal cord injury, *Arch Phys Med Rehabil* 90:876–895, 2009.
115. Mandelbaum BR, Silvers HJ, Watanabe DS, et al: Effectiveness of a neuromuscular and proprioceptive training program in preventing anterior cruciate ligament injuries in female athletes: 2-year follow-up, *Am J Sports Med* 33:1003–1010, 2005.
124. McCrea M, Guskiewicz K, Randolph C, et al: Effects of a symptom-free waiting period on clinical outcome and risk of reinjury after sport-related concussion, *Neurosurgery* 65:876–882, discussion 882–883, 2009.
125. McCrory P, Meeuwisse WH, Aubry M, et al: Consensus statement on concussion in sport—the 4th International Conference on Concussion in Sport, Zurich, November 2012, *J Athl Train* 48:554–575, 2013.
127. McMullen J, Uhl TL: A kinetic chain approach for shoulder rehabilitation, *J Athl Train* 35:329–337, 2000.
129. Meister K: Injuries to the shoulder in the throwing athlete. Part one: biomechanics/pathophysiology/classification of injury, *Am J Sports Med* 28:265–275, 2000.
133. Morgenroth DC, Orendurff MS, Shakir A, et al: The relationship between lumbar spine kinematics during gait and low-back pain in transfemoral amputees, *Am J Phys Med Rehabil* 89:635–643, 2010.
135. Mujika I, Padilla S: Scientific bases for precompetition tapering strategies, *Med Sci Sports Exerc* 35(7):1182–1187, 2003.
139. Nichols DL, Sanborn CF, Essery EV: Bone density and young athletic women: an update, *Sports Med* 37:1001–1014, 2007.
142. Ostlie K, Franklin RJ, Skjeldal OH, et al: Musculoskeletal pain and overuse syndromes in adult acquired major upper-limb amputees, *Arch Phys Med Rehabil* 92:1967–1973, 2011.
145. Park SS, Loebenberg ML, Rokito AS, et al: The shoulder in baseball pitching: biomechanics and related injuries, Part 1, *Bull Hosp Joint Dis* 61:68–79, 2002.
148. Pearsall AW, Kovaleski JE, Madanagopal SG: Medicolegal issues affecting sports medicine practitioners, *Clin Orthop Relat Res* 433:50–57, 2005.
149. Phillips GC: Medications, supplements, and ergogenic drugs. In *Clinical sports medicine*, Philadelphia, PA, 2006, Mosby.
154. Price MJ, Campbell IG: Effects of spinal cord lesion level upon thermoregulation during exercise in the heat, *Med Sci Sports Exerc* 35:1100–1107, 2003.
155. Prinsen EC, Nederhand MJ, Rietman JS: Adaptation strategies of the lower extremities of patients with a transtibial or transfemoral

amputation during level walking: a systematic review, *Arch Phys Med Rehabil* 92:311–1325, 2011.

159. Roberts WO: Administration and medical management of mass participation endurance events. In Mellion E, Walsh WM, Madden C, et al, editors: *Team physician's handbook*, Philadelphia, PA, 2002, Hanley & Belfus.
160. Roberts WO, Maron BJ: Evidence for decreasing occurrence of sudden cardiac death associated with the marathon, *J Am Coll Cardiol* 46:1373–1374, 2005.
166. Sagawa Y, Jr, Turcot K, Armand S, et al: Biomechanics and physiological parameters during gait in lower limb amputees: a systematic review, *Gait Posture* 33:511–526, 2011.
168. Schneider KJ, Iverson GL, Emery CA, et al: The effects of rest and treatment following sport-related concussion: a systematic review of the literature, *Br J Sports Med* 47:304–307, 2013.
169. Scovazzo ML, Browne A, Pink M, et al: The painful shoulder during freestyle swimming: an electromyographic cinematographic analysis of twelve muscles, *Am J Sports Med* 19:577–582, 1991.
177. Soprano JV: Musculoskeletal injuries in the pediatric and adolescent athlete, *Curr Sports Med Rep* 4:329–334, 2005.
181. Tanaka H, Seals DR: Endurance exercise performance in Masters athletes: age-associated changes and underlying physiological mechanisms, *J Physiol* 586:55–63, 2008.
199. Wilber RL: Application of altitude/hypoxic training by elite athletes, *Med Sci Sports Exerc* 39:610–1624, 2007.

The full reference list for this chapter is available online.

CHAPTER 40

MOTOR NEURON DISEASES

Shawn Jorgensen, W. David Arnold

Definition

A floppy infant, painless foot drop, and a paralyzed child are all potential manifestations of motor neuron disease (MND). Few diseases in medicine cause as much concern as these iconic presentations of spinal muscular atrophy (SMA), amyotrophic lateral sclerosis (ALS), and poliomyelitis. Few diseases as rare as ALS are a household name, yet Lou Gehrig's disease (synonymous with ALS or simply MND) is widely known even by those who never saw the "Iron Horse" play baseball or even know the full story of the great man after which the disease is named.

MNDs include a heterogeneous clinical spectrum of conditions associated with dysfunction and degeneration of motor neurons. A common thread of MNDs, the selective and relentless degeneration of motor neurons, invokes a remarkable yet often rational degree of fear in patients and providers alike. ALS is the prototypical MND and the most common form in adulthood. The objective of this chapter is to provide an overview of the spectrum of MNDs, predominantly focusing on the impact of ALS. The general approach to MNDs with regard to evaluation, diagnosis, and management will be reviewed.

Classification

MNDs can be broadly grouped into inherited and acquired causes. The main acquired or sporadic causes include poliomyelitis and ALS and ALS variants. Rarely implicated acquired causes may include immune-mediated, endocrine, traumatic, nonpoliomyelitis infections, and paraneoplastic etiologies. The most common inherited causes include SMA, familial ALS, and X-linked bulbospinal muscular atrophy (Kennedy disease [KD]). MNDs can also be divided into groups of disorders based on selectivity for loss of upper motor neurons (UMNs; corticospinal and corticobulbar tracts) or lower motor neurons (LMNs; spinal anterior horn cells and cranial nerve LMNs) (Box 40-1).

Amyotrophic Lateral Sclerosis and Variants

Amyotrophic Lateral Sclerosis

ALS has an incidence of 1.4/100,000.[111] It typically begins in the sixth to seventh decade of life. Men are affected somewhat more than women, with a ratio of 1.6 : 1.[105] An important and distinctive feature of ALS is the selectivity of degeneration of both the UMNs and LMNs, with relative sparing of other neurons in most cases. Although our understanding of ALS is ever expanding, the pathogenic mechanisms underlying the disease remain surprisingly undefined. The identification of numerous pathogenic gene mutations in association with familial ALS (fALS) has been an important factor contributing to progress within the field. There is remarkable clinical similarity between sporadic ALS and the numerous forms of fALS, suggesting that ALS may be a common disease pathway related to numerous upstream causes.[11] One of the most important recent discoveries was the identification of a hexanucleotide repeat expansion in the *chromosome 9 open reading frame 72* (*C9ORF72*) gene in a large proportion of patients with sporadic and fALS. This finding compels consideration of a pathogenesis related to that of other repeat diseases, such as myotonic dystrophy type 1.[106] In a manner similar to myotonic dystrophy type 1, accumulation of transcribed repeats may bind and sequester RNA-binding proteins and lead to abnormal RNA metabolism and processing. This could be one possible mechanistic explanation for motor neuron loss and a potential target for therapy.[66,106] Despite the relative selectivity of ALS for degeneration of both UMNs and LMNs, degeneration does occur in other cell types and evidence is mounting that non–cell-autonomous factors, such as astrocyte toxic gain of function, may have a contributory role in the development of motor neuron loss in both sporadic and familial forms.[97]

ALS by definition involves both the upper and lower neurons, but some variants may be restricted to only UMNs or LMNs, or certain body regions. Such variants include primary lateral sclerosis (PLS) and progressive muscular atrophy (PMA) where neuron loss is restricted to the UMNs or LMNs, respectively (Figure 40-1). Similarly, there are regional variants including progressive bulbar palsy affecting the cranial nerve nuclei of the bulbar musculature, brachial amyotrophic diplegia (BAD) affecting the upper limbs in a proximal predominant manner, and leg amyotrophic diplegia (LAD) predominantly affecting the distal lower limbs.[44,80] Restriction to certain motor neuron pools or regions is often associated with a different prognosis. Importantly, in many, if not most, cases there is subsequent progression to generalized involvement of both UMNs and LMNs typical of classic ALS. The relationship between ALS and other variants is not entirely clear, but there is strong evidence that these disorders are at a minimum tightly related. Phenotypic variability between genetically defined cases of fALS related to single mutations suggests that variants of ALS may be merely different faces of the same underlying pathogenic process.

Although the true pathologic relationship between ALS and ALS variants remains debatable, the distinction between these variants is helpful for the clinician. All restricted variants, with the unfortunate exception of

BOX 40-1

Classification of Motor Neuron Diseases

Mixed Upper and Lower Motor Neurons

Amyotrophic lateral sclerosis (ALS)
ALS-Plus

Upper Motor Neuron

Primary lateral sclerosis

Lower Motor Neuron

ALS-related variants with predominant lower motor neuron loss
- Progressive muscular atrophy
- Progressive bulbar palsy
- Brachial amyotrophic diplegia (flail arm syndrome)
- Leg amyotrophic diplegia (flail leg syndrome)

Acute poliomyelitis and postpolio syndrome
Spinal muscular atrophy
- Proximal
- Distal (hereditary motor neuropathy)

Scapuloperoneal SMA (Davidenkow syndrome)
Kennedy disease (X-linked spinobulbar muscular atrophy)
Hirayama disease (monomelic spinal muscular atrophy)

Less Common or Less Well-Defined Syndromes

Paraneoplastic
Non–polio-related infections
Electrical injury
Hereditary metabolic disorders
Hereditary bulbar syndromes

progressive bulbar palsy (PBP), have a better prognosis than more typical ALS. Patients with PLS, PMA, and PBP are not usually candidates for clinical trials as a result of lack of ALS diagnostic criteria because of absence of either UMN or LMN involvement. Thus, despite their similarities, it is still helpful to the clinician and the patient to cautiously use one of these labels if appropriate.

Primary Lateral Sclerosis

PLS is a disorder associated with progressive spasticity and weakness of limb and bulbar muscles related to degeneration of UMNs. It is rare and typically seen in the fifth decade. Similar to other sporadic MNDs, the etiology is not known. PLS is defined as having little or no LMN involvement clinically or by electromyography (EMG). In spite of this, most patients with PLS eventually have fasciculations and cramps,[88] some evidence of LMN on examination or EMG, and pathologic evidence of LMN involvement. Although there are clear similarities with ALS, PLS progresses much more slowly than ALS—studies show an average life span of between 8 and 15 years after diagnosis.[121,132] Thus, although it may not be entirely clear that ALS and PLS are different diseases, because of the different clinical features and prognosis, as Charcot wrote, "the clinical description deserves to exist alone."[25]

Most patients with PLS have unilateral leg spasticity, later involving the other leg approximately 1 to 2 years after, then progressing to the upper limbs 3 to 4 years later, and eventually showing pseudobulbar involvement 1 to 2 years later.[149] Mills syndrome, a hemiplegic variant of PLS

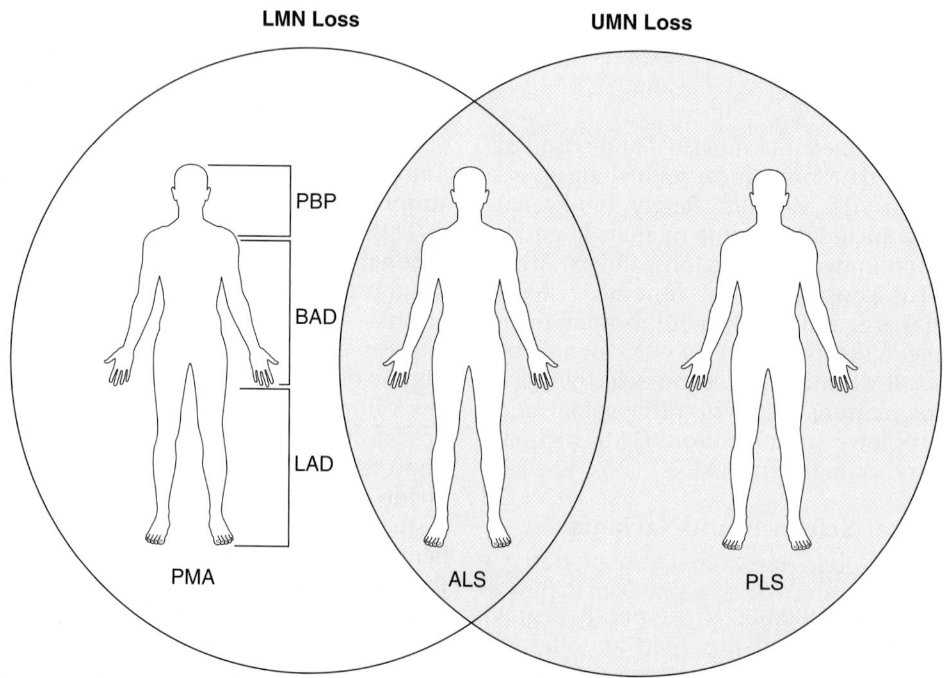

FIGURE 40-1 Spectrum of amyotrophic lateral sclerosis (*ALS*) and ALS variants. Progressive muscular atrophy (*PMA*) is associated with lower motor neuron (*LMN*) features of hypotonic muscle weakness, atrophy, fasciculations, flaccid dysarthria, and absent or reduced reflexes. Primary lateral sclerosis (*PLS*) is associated with weakness with incoordination or slowness of movements, brisk reflexes, spasticity, pathologic reflexes, and spastic dysarthria. ALS has features of both upper motor neuron (*UMN*) and LMN loss. PMA can be further divided into disorders that are restricted to certain regions including progressive bulbar palsy (*PBP*) affecting the bulbar muscles, brachial amyotrophic diplegia (*BAD*) affecting the upper limbs, and leg amyotrophic diplegia (*LAD*) affecting the lower limbs. (Figure design: courtesy Chad Myers.)

originally described in 1900, is associated with a unilateral presentation of UMN signs in the upper and lower limbs.[102] The primary findings on examination and the cause of disability in PLS are spasticity and clumsiness rather than weakness, consistent with a UMN syndrome.[88,149] Eventually, bulbar dysfunction is seen in nearly all patients. Unlike ALS, symptoms of bladder dysfunction are common late in the disease.[88,149]

The diagnosis of PLS is established clinically, but testing can be helpful to exclude other possible diagnoses. Evaluation with magnetic resonance imaging (MRI) should be performed primarily to exclude central nervous system disorders, such as multiple sclerosis; however, cortical atrophy and increased T2 signal intensity of the pyramidal tracts are often seen.[88,121] Transcranial magnetic stimulation (TMS) may be the confirmatory test, with nearly all patients showing severe abnormalities or absent potentials, but TMS is not widely available.[84,88,121] By definition, electrodiagnostic studies should not show significant LMN loss but minor changes can be seen. The differential diagnosis for PLS includes other central nervous system disorders; ALS and hereditary spastic paraparesis are two important conditions. Consideration should be given to genetic analysis for hereditary spastic paraparesis, particularly in patients with relatively symmetrical lower limb involvement. Electrodiagnostic studies should be performed to exclude LMN involvement and should be carried out on all patients. There is no disease-modifying treatment for PLS, and no studies have shown efficacy of riluzole.[132] Symptomatic treatment is similar to that of ALS for spasticity, pseudobulbar affect, and sialorrhea.[132]

Progressive Muscular Atrophy

PMA is an MND causing progressive weakness and muscular atrophy attributable to LMN degeneration. It is thus the LMN analogue of PLS. By definition, patients with PMA have no clinical evidence of UMN dysfunction at onset, but importantly as many as 70% of patients with PMA will eventually demonstrate signs of UMN degeneration.[141] PMA is a rare disease that usually affects older men. Techniques such as TMS and MRI spectroscopy can show subtle corticospinal tract involvement in over 50% of patients with PMA, and in one autopsy series nearly every patient showed ubiquitinated inclusions in LMNs, a pathognomonic sign of ALS.[74] It remains controversial whether PMA represents a disease separate from ALS. Nevertheless, the general approach to PMA is similar to ALS, but because of the different presentation, treatment, and prognosis it should be considered as a related but possibly distinct group of disorders.

Patients show atrophy and weakness, beginning in the hands in nearly 50% of cases, less commonly in the lower limbs, shoulder girdle, and rarely bulbar musculature.[28] Fasciculations are usually evident on examination. Reflexes are reduced or absent, and features of UMN dysfunction are absent. Similar to ALS, EMG abnormalities consist of fibrillation potentials, positive sharp waves, fasciculation potentials, large motor unit action potentials, and normal to decreased motor unit action potential recruitment. The differential diagnosis includes LMN-predominant ALS, other MNDs, and multifocal motor neuropathy (MMN). MMN is particularly important to exclude because this is a relatively treatable disorder with immunomodulatory treatment, such as immunoglobulin therapy.

PMA has not been shown to respond to riluzole. Treatment is supportive and similar to ALS without the complicating issues resulting from UMN involvement, such as spasticity and pseudobulbar affect. Prognosis is better than ALS, with a 5-year survival rate of over 50%, with patients living an average of 1 year longer than with ALS.[28,83] Older age, lower forced vital capacity (FVC), lower ALS-functional rating scale score, and widespread involvement are poor prognosticators.[28,83]

Regional Amyotrophic Lateral Sclerosis Variants

The typical onset and progression of ALS is that of focal onset and subsequent regional spread over time. Importantly, it is not uncommon for patients to not recognize mild or even moderate motor deficits, and at presentation disease may be more widespread on examination than acknowledged by the patient. During the natural course of ALS, most patients will develop generalized disease, but certain variants of ALS may remain restricted to certain regions or populations of motor neurons. Some of these variant syndromes include PBP, BAD, and LAD. PBP is an ALS variant with exclusively bulbar symptoms.[111] As mentioned, some patients may develop significant limb involvement and be characterized as bulbar-onset ALS, but this is a less common transition (7.5%) than in PLS or PMA.[70] It comprises almost 10% of all MNDs, primarily affecting women. The age of onset is significantly older than ALS and has a poorer prognosis.[23] BAD is an LMN syndrome closely related to ALS that has been defined differently by various groups.[80] Patients typically have proximal prominent upper limb weakness that starts unilaterally and spreads to the contralateral limb. Distal upper limb muscles are relatively spared and usually finger extensor muscles are more severely affected compared with finger flexors. Muscles of the bulbar, thoracic, and lumbar regions may remain unaffected for a decade or more, although in some cases there is more rapid progression. LAD is a lower limb correlate of BAD, but weakness tends to start in an asymmetrical, distal-predominant manner with subsequent spread to the contralateral lower limb. Similar to BAD, LAD may have delayed progression to other spinal regions and therefore improved prognosis. Interestingly, patients with genetically defined ALS may have clinical features of these variant syndromes, further supporting a close relationship between ALS and ALS variants.[142]

Familial Amyotrophic Lateral Sclerosis

There has been dramatic progress in the ALS field with regard to genetic understanding of the disease. There are a rapidly increasing number of causative genes identified that are related to a phenotype of ALS. *Superoxide dismutase 1* (*SOD1*) mutations were the first to be identified as a causative etiology of fALS.[125] Mutations in *SOD1* represent approximately 10% of fALS and are seen in approximately 1% of sporadic ALS. Even within the spectrum of *SOD1*-related ALS there is considerable phenotypic variability. For instance, the *D90A* mutation of *SOD1* portends an indolent course with ventilatory failure often occurring 10 years after onset, whereas *A4V* mutation is typically associated with rapid decline and death within a year of onset.[5,32]

Since the identification of *SOD1* mutations over 20 years ago, there have been numerous other ALS-related genes identified. More recently, a genome-wide association study in Finland demonstrated a peak on the short arm of chromosome 9.[86] This finding was vital for subsequent identification of a hexanucleotide repeat expansion in the *C9ORF72* gene, which are now known to be responsible for approximately 40% of fALS and approximately 5% of sporadic ALS.[40,94,123] There are currently over 20 gene mutations associated with the clinical syndrome of fALS, and because of rapid advances in genetic technology, the molecular understanding of sporadic ALS and fALS is constantly expanding. Continued identification of causative genes will help further the understanding of pathogenesis, guide determination of prognosis, and help design future therapeutic strategies. Currently, studies are under way that are targeting genetic mutations in patients with fALS related to *SOD1* mutations using antisense oligonucleotide therapy to knock-down expression of the *SOD1* gene.[101]

Amyotrophic Lateral Sclerosis-Plus Syndromes

Although ALS is usually associated with isolated motor deficits, involvement outside of the motor system can occur. By definition, ALS-Plus syndromes meet clinical and electrodiagnostic criteria for ALS, but also have associated nonmotor neuron features that may include parkinsonism, frontotemporal dementia, ocular motility abnormalities, extrapyramidal signs, autonomic dysfunction, or sensory loss.[9,129] Certain forms of fALS have been associated with development of nonmotor features. For instance, patients with *TAR DNA-binding protein* (*TARDBP*) gene mutations, known to cause fALS, have been reported with clinical features of parkinsonism.[56] Both frontotemporal dementia and fALS are seen in isolation and combination in patients and families with *C9ORF72* gene mutations.[40,123] The association of nonmotor features in some patients with sporadic and fALS strongly suggests that ALS is a multisystem disease with predilection for UMN and LMN involvement.

Other Motor Neuron Diseases

Spinal Muscular Atrophy

Spinal muscular atrophy includes a group of genotypically and phenotypically diverse disorders associated with features of LMN loss. The most common form, proximal SMA (also called SMN-related SMA, 5q-SMA, or simply SMA) is an autosomal recessive LMN disorder with a frequency of 1/11,000 births.[117,122] Carrier frequency is approximately 1/50.[134] Importantly, proximal SMA is the most common genetic cause of death in infants.[124] There is a spectrum of disease associated with SMA with regard to onset of disease and severity. Proximal SMA can be classified into five subtypes of disease (Figure 40-2).[6,47,119,148] The most severe form, type 0, has onset of very severe weakness before birth often with joint contractures resulting from diminished intrauterine movement (not shown in Figure 40-2). Type 1 is the most common form of the disease representing 60% to 70% of patients with SMA and is associated with onset before 6 months of age and inability to sit independently. Approximately 95% of patients with type 1 die by the age of 2 years without ventilatory and nutrition support.[14] Onset in patients with type 2 is between 6 and 18 months, and the ability to sit upright independently is achieved but ambulation is not. Patients with type 3 have an onset after 18 months of age and are able to walk independently. Type 4 is the mildest form, with onset in adulthood and relatively mild proximal limb weakness.[119]

SMA is related to homozygous deletion or mutation of the *survival motor neuron 1* (*SMN1*) gene.[89] In approximately 95% of cases, patients have a homozygous deletion of the *SMN1* gene, but the remaining 5% of patients will be compound heterozygotes with deletion of one *SMN1* allele and a missense mutation of the other *SMN1* allele. Importantly, a second closely related gene, *SMN2*, is retained in varying copy numbers within the population. Both the *SMN1* and *SMN2* genes make SMN protein, but because of the effects of a single nucleotide C-T transition in exon 7, the *SMN2* gene predominantly produces a shortened, unstable isoform of SMN that does not function normally and is rapidly degraded. Therefore, when there is loss of both alleles of the *SMN1* gene by deletion or mutation, there remains some reduced amounts of SMN protein from the *SMN2* gene.[6] Consequently, SMA is not related to absent SMN protein, but rather reduced levels. The mechanism of how motor neuron dysfunction is related to reduced SMN levels remains unknown.[6] The most likely cause is related to the loss of the action of SMN protein to assemble of Sm proteins onto small nuclear ribonucleic acids (snRNAs) and therefore disruption of normal RNA splicing.[6] Because there are varying copy numbers of the *SMN2* gene in the general population, this leads to variable levels of full-length SMN protein production. In cross-sectional studies, the copy number correlates inversely with severity of SMA. In general, SMA type 1 is associated with two copies of *SMN2*. It is important to note that *SMN2* copy number cannot precisely predict severity in an individual patient.

The clinical presentation of SMA is that of proximal predominant weakness and hypotonia. Reflexes may be absent or reduced in the setting of milder weakness, therefore mimicking a muscle disease. Sensory examination is typically normal. Most cases of SMA, approximately 60% to 70%, will have onset of weakness and hypotonia after birth but before 6 months of age and will not gain the ability to sit independently, therefore falling within the classification of type 1 disease. Other characteristic clinical features may include a fine tremor, often called polyminimyoclonus, and tongue fasciculations. The diagnosis of proximal SMA should be suspected in any infant developing hypotonia and weakness. The most efficient strategy for diagnosis is gene testing for homozygous deletion of the *SMN1* gene, which is seen in 95% of patients. In the other 5%, patients may be compound heterozygotes with a single deletion and a missense mutation. In such cases, dosage testing for a single *SMN1* deletion and sequencing of the remaining *SMN1* gene is required to confirm the diagnosis of SMA. Other testing strategies include electrodiagnosis and muscle biopsy, but following availability of molecular diagnosis such strategies are reserved for atypical cases or SMN not related to *SMN1* gene loss.

Electrodiagnostic testing, at one time a critical tool in the evaluation of suspected 5q-SMA, is less commonly necessary during the workup since the availability of genetic testing. Electrodiagnosis shows variable features of motor loss consistent with loss of motor neuron function

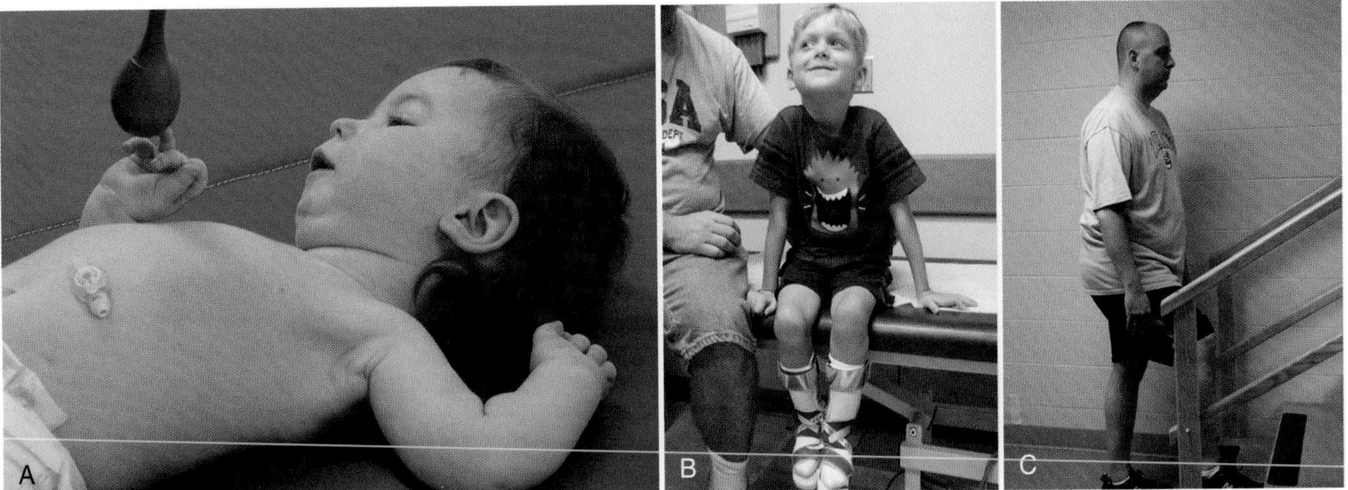

FIGURE 40-2 Subtypes of proximal spinal muscular atrophy (SMA) related to *SMN1* deletion. **A,** SMA type 1, the most common form, has onset before 6 months of age and the ability to sit upright is never achieved. **B,** SMA type 2 has onset between 6 and 18 months and the ability to sit independently, but not stand, is achieved. SMA type 3 is associated with onset after 18 months and patients are able to stand or walk at least temporarily. **C,** SMA type 4 is the mildest subtype with onset after 30 years of age. Type 0 with onset before birth is not shown.

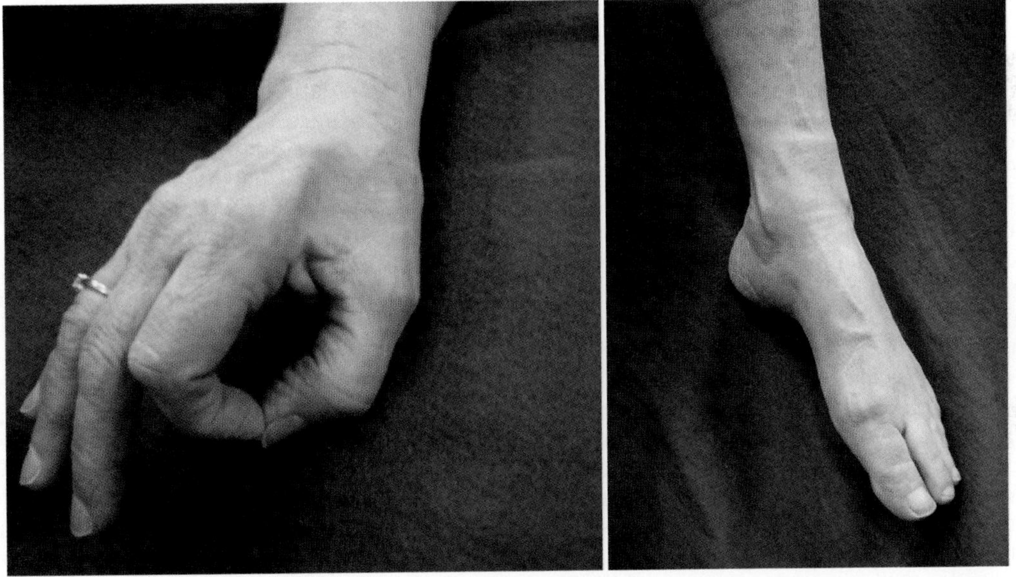

FIGURE 40-3 Distal predominant limb muscle atrophy in a patient with distal hereditary motor neuropathy mimicking that of Charcot-Marie-Tooth disease.

in correlation with clinical severity and age.[22,69,135] Sensory involvement is usually lacking, but exceptional cases have been reported with an association sensory neuropathy or sensory ganglionopathy.[48] Although electrodiagnosis is not usually a necessary part of the evaluation for most cases of SMA, it is still important in atypical cases and non–5q-related SMA.

Other gene mutations have been associated with a clinical pattern of proximal SMA. Autosomal recessive disorders include *IGHMP2*, causing SMA with respiratory distress (SMARD), and *Gle1*, causing severe lethal congenital contracture syndrome 1 resulting from fetal loss of motor neurons.[35] Autosomal-dominant proximal SMA has been associated with mutations in VAPB, TRPV4, LMNA, and recently *BICD2*.[35,108,114,118] X-linked recessive SMA is associated with *Ube1* mutations causing X-linked SMA.[10] Some forms of SMA are associated with a distal predominant patter of weakness, and therefore have been described with the term *distal SMA* (Figure 40-3). Importantly, there is significant phenotypic and genotypic overlap between distal SMA and other hereditary neuropathies (i.e., Charcot-Marie-Tooth disease); therefore, distal hereditary motor neuropathy (dHMN) is more frequently used. An ever-expanding number of genes have been found to be mutated in association with dHMN, including GARS, DCTN1, HSPB8, HSPB1, BSCL2, SETX, HSPB3, DYNC1H1, REEP1, and SLC5A7.[35,72] Distal SMA or dHMN have clinical features of distal weakness and atrophy with reduced to absent reflexes. Sensory function, by definition is preserved, but some patients will have features of sensory loss closely mimicking axonal forms of Charcot-Marie-Tooth disease. A more rare form of SMA called scapuloperoneal SMA or Davidenkow syndrome is associated with features of motor neuron and axonal loss in a periscapular and distal leg distribution, mimicking the pattern of facioscapulohumeral muscular dystrophy (Figure 40-4). This syndrome

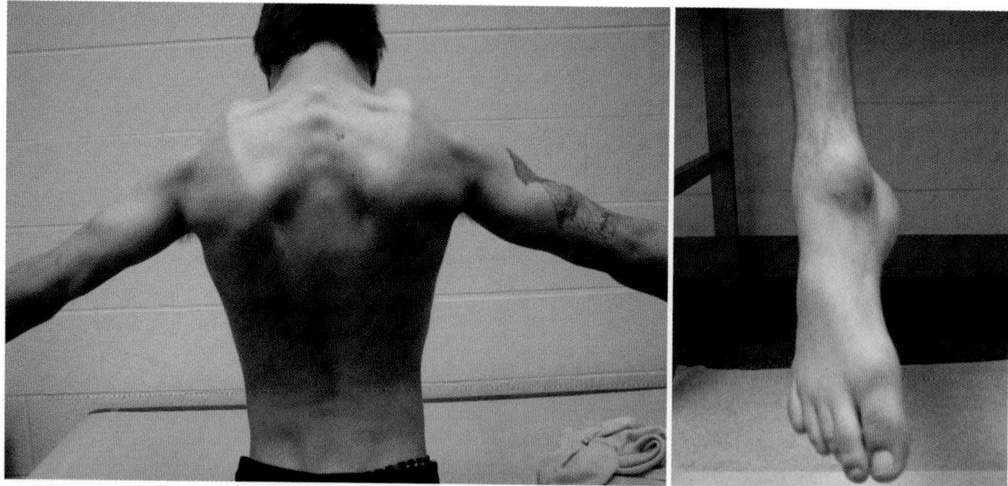

FIGURE 40-4 A patient with the unusual pattern of periscapular and distal leg muscle atrophy associated with the scapuloperoneal form of spinal muscular atrophy (Davidenkow syndrome) with striking similarity to that seen in facioscapulohumeral muscular dystrophy.

has been linked to chromosome 12q24.1-q24.31.[75] Chronic or adult-onset hexosaminidase deficiency, sometimes called late-onset Tay-Sachs disease, can cause a clinical syndrome of motor neuron loss similar to that of proximal SMA, sometimes associated with atypical features of cerebellar degeneration, dystonia, and psychosis.[116]

There are no effective therapies for any form of SMA, but supportive care can effectively reduce disease impact and burden. Type 0 is associated with disease onset before birth. The natural history of the remaining subtypes of 5q-SMA, although not fully defined, typically follows three main clinical phases. During the presymptomatic phase, before onset of motor neuron loss, function is relatively preserved even in infants with severe or type 1 SMA.[52] There is rapid onset of weakness at disease onset, which progresses for a period of time, and thereafter patients often have a plateau in the rate of strength loss. Standards of care are established and can alter the natural history in patients with 5q-SMA.[145] Such treatments are designed to address the primary and secondary effects of muscle weakness and include management of pulmonary complications, nutritional and gastrointestinal support, rehabilitative interventions, and end-of-life care. Restrictive lung disease is a major issue that should be aggressively managed similar to other MNDs. During the progressive phase of the disease ventilatory muscle strength may fall rapidly, whereas there is stability thereafter. Importantly, although motor neuron loss does stabilize, strength and vital capacity can often decrease during periods of growth.[55] Pulmonary disease is the main source of mortality and includes complications of muscle weakness leading to impaired ventilation and secretion management or secondary complications, such as pneumonia related to aspiration. Establishing a therapeutic relationship with an experienced pulmonary specialist familiar with the management of SMA is critical and should occur at the time of initial diagnosis to anticipate future needs and prevent complications. Pulmonary complications are related to severity of disease, and thus more severe disease burden requires closer monitoring and more frequent intervention. Determining the appropriate mechanism of ventilator support should be a combination of what is best for the patient and the wishes of the patient and family.

Scoliosis is common in SMA, and progression of scoliosis and the associated impact on pulmonary function is less severe in patients with SMA type 3 compared with type 2. A corset brace has been shown to be unable to halt scoliosis progression but may help provide seating stability and delay surgical need. Surgical treatment is well established in nonambulatory patients with progressive scoliosis at age 10 to 12 years. Bulbar weakness is common in severe forms of SMA predisposing to inadequate nutritional intake. Therefore, nutritional support is an important aspect of supportive care. The goals of nutritional support include adequate nutritional intake, avoiding undernutritional or overnutritional supplementation, and the reduction of the risk of aspiration pneumonia.

X-Linked Spinobulbar Muscular Atrophy (Kennedy Disease)

KD (or X-linked spinobulbar muscular atrophy) is an X-linked recessive disorder that leads to progressive limb and bulbar weakness, testicular atrophy, gynecomastia, muscle cramps, and fasciculations.[81] KD is related to an expanded cytosine-adenine-guanine (CAG) trinucleotide repeat in the q arm of the X chromosome within the first exon of the androgen receptor gene.[85] Healthy individuals have 10 to 36 repeats in this region, whereas patients with KD have 40 to 62 repeats. Usually female carriers are unaffected, but some investigations have suggested subclinical features in manifesting female carriers, including mainly muscle cramps and tremor, and electrodiagnostic or muscle biopsy evaluation may show features of denervation.[63] Early stages of the disease are associated with symptoms of muscle cramps, fasciculations, and tremor as the only manifestation, whereas progressive muscle loss and weakness are evident later. KD typically has an onset of more overt symptoms by the fourth or fifth decade. KD is a slowly progressive disorder, and therefore life span is not usually dramatically reduced. As a result of bulbar involvement, aspiration pneumonia can be a concern later in the disease course.

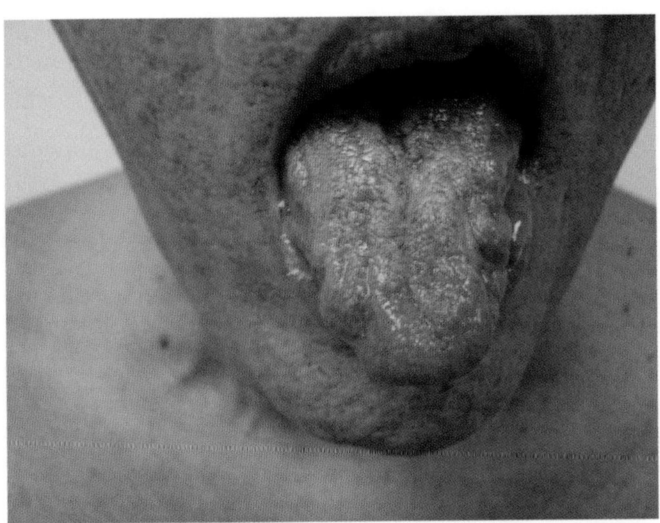

FIGURE 40-5 Typical features of atrophy seen in bulbar and tongue muscles in a patient with Kennedy disease.

Clinical examination demonstrates proximal predominant and bulbar muscular weakness and atrophy, but distal involvement and asymmetry can occur. This variability can sometimes complicate the clinical evaluation and more closely mimic the presentation of ALS. Reflexes are absent or reduced. Features of mild asymptomatic sensory loss are usually present. There may be features of androgen insensitivity such as gynecomastia and reduced fertility. Patients with KD often have prominent bulbar involvement with profound atrophy and perioral fasciculations (Figure 40-5).

Genetic testing for CAG repeats in the androgen receptor gene is diagnostic of KD, but because of a significant overlap with other MNDs, electrodiagnostic testing is often obtained. EMG shows features of active and chronic denervation with fibrillation potentials, fasciculations, and enlarged motor unit action potentials with decreased recruitment in a generalized distribution.[51] Facial muscle investigation usually shows features of fasciculations and myokymia, as well as fibrillations and neurogenic motor unit action potential changes. The nerve conduction studies may show reduced compound muscle action potential amplitudes and relatively preserved conduction velocities. A distinctive feature of KD is a superimposed sensory neuronopathy.[51] Importantly, this neuropathy is non–length-dependent in distribution, which is in contrast to typical neuropathy that may be occasionally seen incidentally in patients with ALS. The electrodiagnostic findings of non–length-dependent sensory neuropathy is consistent with the fact that KD is associated with both sensory and motor neuronopathy, but the features of LMN involvement in KD are more clinically evident and relevant. Creatine kinase (CK) is moderately elevated in the majority of patients with KD, and on average is approximately 5 times normal but can range up to 15 times normal.[54]

There is no curative treatment for KD. Mouse models of KD have shown improvement with treatment with androgen receptor antagonists.[77] Supportive treatment is similar to ALS without the need to treat complications of UMN dysfunction, such as spasticity and pseudobulbar affect. Respiratory and secretion management is particularly important given the high incidence of bulbar dysfunction.

Poliomyelitis and Postpolio Syndrome

Poliomyelitis is an MND caused by viral infection of the central nervous system resulting in loss of anterior horn cells and cranial nerve nuclei. Poliomyelitis results from infections with the poliovirus, a human enterovirus of the Picornaviridae family. Other enteroviruses and flaviviruses such as West Nile virus are also associated with poliomyelitis, but the poliovirus is the most widespread and well-known cause.[73,128] There are three serotypes of the poliovirus, and immunity is not conferred between serotypes as a result of differing capsid proteins and antigenicity.[103] There has been a dramatic reduction in the annual number of cases of polio as a result of the development of vaccination strategies in the 1950s, and in 1988 the World Health Assembly formulated plans for worldwide efforts to eradicate polio. These efforts have led to a dramatic reduction from over 300,000 cases worldwide to only 223 cases being reported in 2012, culminating in India and 10 other Asian countries declared polio-free in 2014. A continued possibility of resurgent disease remains as a result of persistent cases.[146]

Following exposure via the fecal-oral route, the poliovirus has a variable incubation period of a few days to over a month. During this period the virus replicates in the gastrointestinal tract. Infection can subsequently lead to a continuum of severity from asymptomatic infection to severe paralysis and death. Before the availability of vaccination, polio represented the most common cause of acute flaccid paralysis. In addition to wild-type poliovirus infection, vaccine-derived poliovirus can very rarely cause paralytic disease and spread to nonimmunized individuals.[45] Poliovirus infection may be associated with headache, fever, stiffness, and pain but is often asymptomatic.[73] Less than 5% of infections result in irreversible paralysis, and in these affected individuals mortality can be as high as 10% related to features of autonomic dysfunction, circulatory collapse, and ventilatory muscle failure.[73]

Symptoms of asymmetrical flaccid paralysis and subsequent atrophy are typically more common in limb muscles but may also affect bulbar muscles. It is rare that transverse myelitis associated with features of autonomic, sensory, and sphincter dysfunction can occur. The clinical presentation of poliomyelitis can be closely mirrored by other disorders of the spinal cord, muscle, and nerve.[73] Therefore, the approach to diagnosis should be directed toward the differential associated with acute flaccid paralysis. Electrodiagnostic testing shows features of asymmetrical or multifocal denervation. Cerebrospinal fluid analysis demonstrates elevated protein levels but in contrast to acute immune-mediated, such as Guillain-Barré syndrome, there is evidence of pleocytosis. MRI can show features of increased T2 signal intensity in the region of the ventral horn of the spinal cord.[95] Molecular testing with polymerase chain reaction can confirm viral serotype and can determine whether the infection is vaccine-derived or is a wild-type strain. Management of acute poliomyelitis is supportive and is similar to other disorders of flaccid paralysis.

Following paralytic poliomyelitis, the surviving motor neurons can compensate and through collateral reinnervation expand their territories to provide some functional recovery.[34] This phase usually maximizes within 2 years of disease, and thereafter motor system function stabilizes. For yet-to-be determined reasons, approximately 50% of patients with poliomyelitis develop late features of declining motor function, usually 30 or more years after onset.[34] Onset may be gradual or abrupt. Thorough evaluation is critical to exclude other disorders that may contribute to decline in function, and treatment is designed to maximize and maintain function. Therapeutic rehabilitation typically includes strategies to allow for energy conservation with both modification of the environment and the delivery of appropriate equipment needs similar to other disorders of the motor neuron.

Hirayama Disease

Hirayama disease (HD) is a relatively benign disorder associated with muscle weakness and atrophy of the distal upper limb muscles. Several names have been used to describe HD including monomelic amyotrophy, distal muscular atrophy of the distal upper extremity, and oblique amyotrophy. HD was first described in 1959 by Hirayama.[71] The pathogenesis of HD has been attributed to this anterior displacement of the dural wall causing impaired microcirculation of the lower cervical spinal cord and loss of motor neurons.[30,49] The disorder primarily affects males during the teenage years or early twenties, and the onset of weakness is insidious and slowly progressive. The natural history of the disease is associated with progression for 5 years or less.[60,61] Involvement may be unilateral or bilateral, but is usually more prominent in one limb (Figure 40-6). Interestingly, preponderance for right side involvement has been noted.[61] The phenomenon of worsening weakness with exposure to cold, termed cold paresis, has been frequently described in patients with HD.[61] Features including upper motor neuron signs, cranial nerve abnormalities, or incontinence of bowel or bladder are not seen, and sensory disturbance is usually absent or minimal.

Electrodiagnostic assessment demonstrates active and chronic denervation in muscles innervated by the C7-T1 myotomes with features of fibrillation potentials and enlarged motor unit action potentials with decreased recruitment. Fasciculations are not apparent on clinical or electrodiagnostic examination. MRI with neck flexion is used to assess for forward displacement of the posterior dural sac.[27,49,82]

As a result of insidious onset and slow progression and the overall uncommon nature of the disorder, there is typically a significant delay in recognition of HD. Although HD is an overall benign and self-limited disorder, early diagnosis is critical to avoid delay in treatment and avoid unnecessary loss of upper limb function. Treatment may include using a cervical collar to limit neck flexion, and in patients with continued progression despite conservative management cervical spine surgery for decompression and stabilization may be indicated.[137] Early treatment can demonstrate significant efficacy, supportive of a structural origin rather than a true degenerative process.[60]

Rare or Less Well-Defined Etiologies of Motor Neuron Disease

Disorders of the motor neuron are rare disorders. Beyond the more common forms of MND, there are myriad other unusual and atypical forms that are less well defined and preclude a detailed description within this chapter. Some of the uncommon forms have been attributed to paraneoplastic and idiopathic immune dysregulation, other infectious agents, hereditary metabolic disorders, electrical injuries, and other idiopathic processes. Fortunately, most of these are exceedingly uncommon. Because of the sheer rarity of MNDs as a whole, investigation of cause and effect versus chance association is at times difficult. A search of the literature often reveals confusing data in this regard. One such association is that of disorders of the endocrine system and MNDs. Primary hyperparathyroidism may lead to a condition of motor neuron dysfunction, but in relation to the pathogenesis of ALS, most data suggest that this association is coincidental.[76]

Paraneoplastic

Paraneoplastic degeneration of the UMNs and LMNs has been uncommonly reported as a cause of MNDs. In most cases reported, the link between MNDs and paraneoplastic degeneration is purely that of coincidental association. In some cases, an etiologic link has been suspected based on

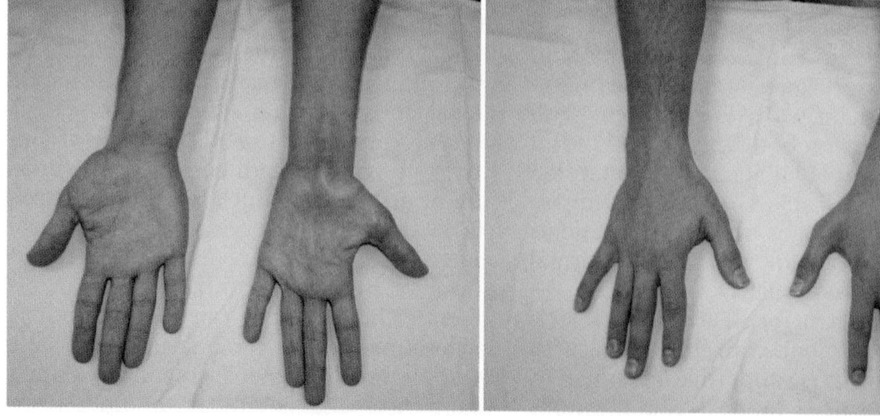

FIGURE 40-6 Asymmetrical left hand and forearm muscle atrophy in a patient with Hirayama disease.

a temporal relationship between the onset of MNDs and cancer, the presence of autoantibodies, and response to immunomodulation with treatments such as intravenous immunoglobulin or corticosteroids. The causative relationship between cancer and the development of motor neuron degeneration is thought to be unlikely in most cases of cancer and MNDs.[53] Some authors have even suggested that paraneoplastic processes could unmask fALS or increase penetrance underlying fALS-related gene mutations.[43,58] One of the best-defined paraneoplastic syndromes associated with MNDs is an anti-Hu syndrome.[53] The spectrum of anti-Hu–related paraneoplastic disorders include sensory neuronopathy, cerebellar ataxia, limbic encephalitis, overlapping syndromes of multifocal involvement, and a syndrome of motor neuron or motor axonal loss often with sensory involvement.[62] The presence of an anti-Hu MND-like phenotype is infrequent at less than 5%.[62] Anti-Hu antibodies are not thought to be pathogenic but appear to be a marker of autoimmunity against Hu antigens.[62] Treatment includes management of the underlying neoplasm and in some cases immunomodulation.

Nonpoliomyelitis Infections

Infections, other than poliomyelitis, have been more rarely implicated in the pathogenesis of MNDs.[67,110,126] Of these infections, the rare association of human immunodeficiency virus (HIV) infection with MNDs is well established.[3,93] Isolated UMN or LMN involvement may be seen with HIV infection, but patients predominantly have mixed UMN and LMN features. The disease may present at varying stages of HIV infection. A clinical pattern of progressive motor neuron degeneration over weeks rather than months and pathologic features of vacuolar myelopathy and inflammation suggest an immune pathogenesis distinct from ALS.[126] Recognition of this syndrome is important because at least 50% of cases will respond with adequate antiretroviral therapy, further supporting a link to HIV infection and pathogenesis.[3,115] Other infectious agents that have been suggested as possible etiologies of MNDs including Lyme disease (*Borrelia burgdorferi*), Herpes zoster, Creutzfeldt-Jakob disease, and human T-lymphotropic virus type 1 (HTLV-1) are more controversial. HTLV-1 infections are typically associated with a UMN-predominant syndrome of myelopathy called tropical spastic paraparesis or HTLV-1 association myelopathy (HAM).[59,147] This disorder is distinct from MNDs as a result of the presence of symmetrical lower limb involvement, sensory loss, and bowel and bladder changes. HAM occurs in approximately 1% to 3% of individuals infected with HTLV-1.[147] HTLV-1 infection is endemic in certain areas and therefore serologic evidence of previous infection should not be used to prove a causative relationship. Herpes zoster can result in segmental weakness and atrophy, with features that overlap with MNDs. It is not usually considered an isolated disorder of the motor neuron but affects the root, plexus, nerve, brain, and rarely the spinal cord.

Electrical Injury

There are sparse reports of electrical injury preceding syndromes of motor neuron loss.[1] The clinical features of such disorders are associated with variable delay of days to years following electrical injury and the epicenter of motor neuron degeneration loss occurs at the site of the electrical entry or exit in 90% of cases.[1] Myelopathic features can also be present in some cases including sensory symptoms, pain, and bowel and bladder dysfunction.

Hereditary Bulbar Syndromes

Brown–Vialetto–Van Laere syndrome 1 (BVLS1) and Fazio-Londe syndrome are two closely related and extremely rare childhood syndromes caused by autosomal recessive mutations in the *solute carrier family 52 (riboflavin transporter), member 1, 2,* and *3* (*SLC52A1, SLC52A2,* and *SLC52A3*) genes, which encode riboflavin transport proteins.[16] BVLS1 and Fazio-Londe syndrome both cause progressive motor neuron loss with prominent bulbar and respiratory involvement. Usually, BVLS1 is distinguished from Fazio-Londe syndrome as a result of the universal presence of hearing loss, but the two syndromes are now usually considered synonymous. Onset of both syndromes typically occurs in the first 2 decades of life. The pathogenesis of both syndromes is related to riboflavin deficiency; treatment therefore includes high-dose riboflavin supplementation.

Diagnosis

History

A thorough history and physical examination is vital when assessing a patient with a possible MND. The history should begin by focusing on when the patient (or family member) first noticed symptoms and the distribution and characteristics of these symptoms. Establishing the rate of progression is very helpful—a nonprogressive or very slowly progressive course may suggest particular entities such as inherited disorders. Patients are often uncertain about the duration and rate of progression, and asking about difficulty with specific tasks is helpful. A thorough family history is essential to assess for any clues of an underlying hereditary process, and sometimes examination of family members is necessary to identify similar but unrecognized clinical features. Associated features such as prominent sensory symptoms or complaints attributable to sphincter or autonomic dysfunction are unusual in pure motor neuron processes and should prompt consideration of an alternative process. Respiratory or bulbar involvement may be subtle and may take some probing by the provider to identify; features such as orthopnea or morning headaches may suggest diaphragm paralysis or nocturnal hypoventilation, respectively. The past medical history and review of systems can identify a systemic process that may be related to motor neuron dysfunction. The functional and social history will be critical in prescribing orthotics, assistive devices, and therapy, as well as eventually modifying the patient's living situation as the disease progresses. Physicians should expect to become familiar with family support and living conditions to anticipate transitional challenges with disease progression.

Patients with ALS or other MNDs usually have painless weakness. In ALS, often foot drop or hand weakness will bring a patient to their physician, and then signs of more generalized weakness or features of fasciculations or hyperreflexia are noticed on examination. Patients may not clearly articulate complaints of weakness, but rather may describe difficulties with certain activities such as climbing stairs, tripping while walking, or inability to open a jar. Focal painless weakness and atrophy without sensory loss should immediately raise red flags and ALS is an important consideration. The initial location of the weakness in ALS roughly divides into thirds: one third in the bulbar region, one third in the upper limb, and one third in the lower limb.[23] In the limbs, weakness usually starts in an asymmetrical and distally predominant manner.[70] It is not infrequent that close examination may disclose more generalized features of motor system involvement than recognized by the patient.

Bulbar involvement at presentation is twice as common in women as men and more common in older patients.[29,70] Although around one third of patients have bulbar symptoms as a chief complaint, the majority have such symptoms at presentation when specifically asked.[29] Patients with bulbar symptoms nearly always have dysarthria.[70] Dysphagia is a rare presenting complaint but is expected during the course of disease. Nearly a quarter of patients acknowledge respiratory symptoms when specifically addressed.[29] These may include sleep apnea, dyspnea on exertion, or orthopnea. Isolated respiratory insufficiency at presentation is exceedingly rare and when respiratory involvement is noted at presentation there are usually other generalized deficits also apparent on examination.[23,29] Presenting with isolated complaints of fasciculations is similarly rare, but it is not rare for fasciculations to be present on initial examination.[65] Pain and other sensory symptoms are rare at the time of diagnosis and suggest an alternative diagnosis. An exception is cramping, which is a presenting complaint in around 10% of patients.[65]

Physical Examination

A detailed physical examination with particular attention to the neurologic examination is mandatory in the evaluation of a patient suspected of having MND. Focal atrophy, weakness, and fasciculations are the primary features of LMN injury that should be sought. Fasciculations may be obvious on casual observation or may require prolonged inspection of various muscle groups. Tongue fasciculations are the most readily identified evidence of LMN injury in the bulbar muscles. Evidence of UMN degeneration in the upper limbs includes spasticity, clumsiness, increased muscle stretch reflexes, and UMN signs. A normal reflex in an atrophic limb is considered the equivalent of an exaggerated reflex. Increased reflexes are seen on presentation in approximately 50% of patients with ALS.[65] The Hoffmann sign in the upper limb and Babinski sign in the lower limb are useful signs of UMN pathology. In one series, 94% of patients with ALS and a positive Hoffman sign had evidence of corticospinal tract pathology at autopsy.[90] The Babinski sign is less reliable, with only a quarter of patients with ALS having a positive response bilaterally on presentation.[65] An exaggerated jaw jerk, pseudobulbar affect, positive snout, or palmomental reflexes can help establish UMN dysfunction in bulbar musculature.

Fasciculations (and fasciculation potentials on EMG) are most often of concern when a patient is suspected of having MND. Friends and family of patients with ALS as well as those with a medical background will often seek a medical opinion because of fasciculations, concerned about the possibility of ALS. Fasciculations near the surface of the muscle are often seen on examination, but in some cases fasciculations may occur deep within the muscle and can only be seen with needle EMG or with muscle ultrasound.[104] The implications of fasciculations depend almost entirely on the clinical context. In isolation, fasciculations are not pathognomonic for MND and can be seen in normal individuals, as well as numerous other conditions of the peripheral nervous system. Fasciculations should be interpreted in light of whether there are coexistent findings of active and chronic denervation. Findings of fasciculations in a patient with weakness and denervation on EMG are suggestive of MND. Patients without other physical examination or EMG abnormalities can be reassured that they have virtually no chance of developing ALS.[15]

Laboratory Studies

Laboratory testing may be utilized to help confirm clinically suspected MND or in other cases help exclude mimicking disorders. In particular, genetic testing can effectively confirm the diagnosis of hereditary MNDs and other testing may not be warranted. Such examples may include testing for homozygous deletion or mutation of the *SMN1* gene for proximal SMA or testing for CAG trinucleotide repeat number in the q arm of the X chromosome for possible KD. Owing to incomplete availability of molecular testing for many disorders of the motor neuron and the high cost for such testing, genetic testing requires a targeted analysis and a high suspicion for a particular disorder or gene mutation.[7] As genetic testing technologies and understanding of genetic etiologies of MNDs are improved, reliance on an a priori approach to testing will be less critical. Unfortunately for the majority of MNDs, including ALS, there are no laboratory tests that can establish the diagnosis. Similarly, in a patient whose clinical and electrophysiologic profile is strongly suggestive of ALS, there is no laboratory study that can effectively rule it out.[20]

The laboratory approach to the patient with possible MND should be guided by features on history and clinical examination. Laboratory evaluation is generally used to help exclude alternate diagnoses when the diagnosis is uncertain. Additionally, genetic testing can be helpful to determine the presence of a pathogenic mutation attributable to fALS. Importantly, some laboratory testing may show nonspecific abnormalities in patients with ALS, and in such cases diagnostic testing can cause confusion. For instance, CK is often elevated, but typically less than 10 times the upper limit of normal.[20] This can easily be misinterpreted as evidence for myopathy in a patient with a pure motor neuron syndrome. Cerebrospinal fluid protein may also be elevated, but rarely over 60 mg/dL.[70] Anti-monosialotetrahexosylganglioside antibodies (anti-GM1 antibodies) show that MMN is an important disorder in the differential of focal/multifocal weakness without sensory loss or pain. The presence of these antibodies can help support the diagnosis of MMN but have been shown to be positive in up to 10% of patients with ALS.[70] This can pose a problem in patients without UMN signs, in whom MMN is an important consideration.

Muscle biopsy is not normally necessary in patients with a suspected MND unless the presentation is atypical or myopathy is suspected. If a muscle biopsy is performed, it will be abnormal in nearly all patients with ALS if a weak muscle is biopsied. Signs of denervation are almost universal and evidence of reinnervation are seen in approximately 50% of biopsies.[70] Although rarely necessary, the high sensitivity of muscle biopsy to identify denervation can also be used to document LMN pathology where none can be confirmed clinically or on EMG.[20] Historically, before the availability of genetic testing in SMA, muscle biopsy (in addition to EMG) was an important diagnostic tool, but because of the wide availability of molecular testing muscle biopsies are uncommon and should not be performed before genetic testing.

Imaging studies may not be required in the evaluation of patients with suspected MND, but are very useful and sometimes of vital importance to help exclude mimicking or confounding diagnoses to explain UMN or LMN involvement. Corticospinal tract abnormalities can be seen in patients with ALS and PLS on brain MRI but are nonspecific and not usually helpful diagnostically. MRI of the cervical spine can help to rule out structural lesions associated with cord compression or syringomyelia. It is worth noting that incidental findings of mild-to-moderate cervical spondylosis on imaging is not infrequent, and features of ALS should not be mistakenly attributed to clinically insignificant focal structural lesions. Furthermore, lack of sensory symptoms to corroborate myelopathy or radiculopathy may help. MRI of the brain is also commonly performed, particularly in a patient with bulbar or pseudobulbar symptoms or signs. Similar to cervical spine and brain MRI, approximately 10% of patients will have incidental findings of nonspecific ischemic changes.[70] In circumstances of focal cervical spine disease and mild ischemic changes identified on MRI, features of LMN loss (outside of the cervical region in the case of cervical spine disease) support the diagnosis of ALS as opposed to another process affecting the central nervous system.

Electrodiagnosis

Electrodiagnostic testing is the primary diagnostic modality to confirm loss or dysfunction of the peripheral nervous system. Studies in patients with suspected MND are designed to identify LMN involvement and to exclude other mimicking disorders of the peripheral nervous system. Needle EMG is the most pertinent aspect of the electrodiagnostic examination for identification of LMN loss, but nerve conduction studies are equally important to help exclude other diagnostic possibilities within the peripheral nervous system. In the case of ALS, using current criteria, abnormalities on needle EMG have the same significance as clinical evidence of LMN disease. Usually needle EMG features of LMN involvement, such as fibrillation potentials, fasciculation potentials, or neurogenic changes in motor unit action potential characteristics, are more readily apparent than clinical features of LMN involvement. Motor nerve conduction studies may remain normal until there is sufficient motor axonal loss to result in diminished compound muscle action potential amplitudes. In general, measurements of action potential propagation including distal latencies and conduction velocities will be relatively normal. By definition, sensory conduction studies are usually normal. Coexistent sensory abnormalities can occur in ALS as frequent as 12% of cases, but in such cases findings are usually very mild compared with motor involvement.[70] Incidental findings of an asymptomatic or minimally symptomatic neuropathy with symptoms occurring over a different time frame should not distract from findings of a prominent motor process. Some MNDs are associated with characteristic concomitant sensory involvement, although this is less severe in comparison with motor axonal loss. One example in particular includes KD, which is usually associated with non–length-dependent sensory amplitude loss consistent with coexistent sensory ganglionopathy. Other measurements of nerve conduction, including the latencies of F-waves and Hoffmann reflexes, are relatively preserved in proportion to the motor axonal loss.

One particular entity that deserves attention during electrodiagnostic evaluation is MMN. MMN is an autoimmune disorder of the peripheral nerve that is associated with multifocal conduction block. Focal areas of conduction block in motor studies (but not sensory studies) outside of areas prone to entrapment can be seen in MMN. The distribution of motor abnormalities in MMN are typically more prominent in the upper greater than lower and distal greater than proximal limb. Multiple motor studies with multiple stimulation sites may be needed in some patients with suspected ALS to exclude subtle areas of conduction block. Importantly, some patients with otherwise typical MMN will not have features of conduction block but still have favorable response to immunomodulatory treatment. Another distinctive feature of MMN is neurogenic involvement in the distribution of peripheral nerves rather than the myotomal distribution typical of motor neuron loss.

Neuromuscular junction (NMJ) disorders also result in clinical phenotypes of pure motor deficits and should be high in the differential of a patient with a suspected MND. Clinical features of prominent ocular, bulbar, and proximal limb weakness with fatigability are characteristic of a primary NMJ transmission defect. Myasthenia gravis can most closely mimic MND with bulbar and LMN predominant involvement such as PBP. Electrodiagnostic studies to identify failure of NMJ transmission including repetitive nerve stimulation or single-fiber EMG (SFEMG) should be considered. This is particularly true in cases with evidence of fatigability on examination. Unfortunately, findings of NMJ transmission failure are not specific to primary NMJ disorders. Abnormal decrement may be seen on repetitive nerve stimulation studies in almost 20% of patients with ALS.[70] Similarly, SFEMG abnormalities of jitter and blocking can be seen in muscles that are normal on standard needle EMG, but such findings are usually associated with increased fiber density. The repetitive nerve stimulation and SFEMG abnormalities seen in MNDs are related to the inability of failing motor neurons to maintain sufficient synaptic output and reduced safety facture at newly formed, immature synapses following sprouting and collateral reinnervation. This can make distinguishing between NMJ disorders and MNDs more difficult, but other findings on needle EMG usually clarify these findings. Neurogenic changes in motor unit action potential size or recruitment are seen in MNDs but are absent in NMJ disorders. Fibrillations that are typically present in MNDs can also occur in some NMJ disorders including botulism and only rarely in other NMJ disorders.

The diagnosis of ALS is made primarily by clinical findings and by needle EMG. A combination of signs of active denervation (fibrillation potentials, positive sharp waves, and fasciculations) and chronic denervation (high amplitude and wide duration motor unit action potentials) are seen in most patients. Unstable motor unit action potentials on triggered analysis are considered evidence of chronic denervation and immature synapse formation. Reduced recruitment is expected. The distribution of these findings correlates with the clinical deficits and usually progression over time. Therefore, targeting clinically involved muscles increases yield. Needle EMG is particularly useful to show subtle evidence of LMN disease in areas where it is not clinically evident. Two muscles of different root or peripheral nerve supply must be involved to be considered evidence of LMN degeneration in a given region.[19] Early in the course of disease there is focal LMN degeneration. The majority of muscles on clinical and EMG assessment are often normal, making the diagnosis of ALS more challenging or impossible. Therefore, a high index of suspicion is needed to identify the disease earlier in the course.

Other less common electrodiagnostic techniques are sometimes utilized and can be helpful. Techniques such as macro-EMG and motor unit number estimation (MUNE) are specialized techniques that can investigate motor unit function. Although usually utilized more in the research setting, MUNE has shown promise as an outcome measure in preclinical and clinical trials of different types of MNDs including SMA, ALS, and KD.

BOX 40-2

Revised El Escorial Criteria with Awaji Modification

1. Principles

The diagnosis of amyotrophic lateral sclerosis (ALS) requires:

(A) The presence of

(1) Evidence of *lower motor neuron (LMN) degeneration* by clinical, electrophysiologic, or neuropathologic examination,

(2) Evidence of *upper motor neuron (UMN) degeneration* by clinical examination, *and*

(3) *progressive spread of symptoms or signs* within a region or to other regions, as determined by history, physical examination, or electrophysiologic tests

Together with:

(B) The absence of

(1) *Electrophysiologic or pathologic evidence of other disease processes* that might explain the signs of LMN and/or UMN degeneration, and

(2) *Neuroimaging evidence of other disease processes* that might explain the observed clinical and electrophysiologic signs.

2. Diagnostic Categories

Clinically definite ALS is defined by *clinical or electrophysiologic* evidence by the presence of LMN as well as UMN signs in the bulbar region and at least two spinal regions or the presence of LMN and UMN signs in three spinal regions

Clinically probable ALS is defined on *clinical or electrophysiologic* evidence by LMN and UMN signs in at least two regions with some UMN signs necessarily rostral to (above) the LMN signs

Clinically possible ALS is defined when *clinical or electrophysiologic* signs of UMN and LMN dysfunction are found in only one region; or UMN signs are found alone in two or more regions; or LMN signs are found rostral to UMN signs. Neuroimaging and clinical laboratory studies will have been performed and other diagnoses must have been excluded.

Modified from de Carvalho M, Dengler R, Eisen A, et al: Electrodiagnostic criteria for diagnosis of ALS, *Clin Neurophysiol* 119(3):497–503, 2008.

Amyotrophic Lateral Sclerosis: Diagnosis and Criteria

Criteria have been developed to assist clinicians and researchers in identifying patients with ALS. The original El Escorial criteria were created in 1994 and later revised in 1998. Even after the changes, the revised El Escorial criteria were criticized for lack of sensitivity; in one series, 22% of patients died of ALS without ever formally meeting the "Clinically Definite" or "Probable" ALS category.[141] The Awaji diagnostic algorithm is an attempt to fix this problem. These changes improve the ability to diagnose patients earlier in the disease, especially those with bulbar complaints, without sacrificing specificity. The revised El Escorial criteria with the Awaji modification form the diagnostic criteria generally used today (Box 40-2).[26,39]

A major change the Awaji modification creates is that EMG evidence of LMN loss is now considered equivalent to clinical findings of LMN loss. Also, unstable fasciculation potentials are considered evidence of active denervation in the setting of already established chronic denervation. Chronic denervation itself could be established with an unstable motor unit action potential on triggered analysis in this modification. The ability to use fasciculation potentials in bulbar muscles to show LMN injury was particularly helpful because previous studies had shown that the majority of patients with established ALS in fact had no identifiable fibrillation potentials or positive sharp waves in bulbar muscles and nearly half of those with bulbar onset had none in limb muscles.[38]

Three main clinical features are required to make the formal diagnosis of ALS: evidence of LMN degeneration, UMN degeneration, and involvement of different regions (bulbar, cervical, thoracic, and lumbar). EMG, pathologic, or neuroimaging evidence of another disease process excludes the diagnosis of ALS. Clinical evidence of LMN degeneration includes weakness, wasting, and fasciculations. Electrophysiologic evidence required for documentation of LMN degeneration has been outlined earlier and in Box 40-2. This evidence must be found in two muscles with different peripheral nerve and root supply in both the cervical and lumbar region, and one muscle in the bulbar or thoracic region to qualify. Neuropathologic proof of LMN degeneration requires evidence of chronic denervation/reinnervation on muscle biopsy. Clinical evidence of UMN involvement includes increased or clonic reflexes, spasticity, pseudobulbar features, the Hoffmann reflex, and extensor plantar response. Currently, UMN pathology can only be established clinically, although there is some evidence that TMS is helpful to document UMN pathology and may be included in criteria in the future.[20,39]

Findings of UMN and LMN dysfunction are grouped into four regions: bulbar, cervical, thoracic, and lumbar. If more regions are involved the patient is given a more certain diagnosis. "Clinically Definite" ALS requires that three regions show both UMN and LMN signs in the same region. "Clinically Probable" ALS requires that two regions show both UMN and LMN signs in the same region, but with the caveat that some UMN signs must be rostral to the LMN signs. "Clinically Possible" ALS requires one region with both UMN and LMN in the same region. Other ways a patient may qualify for "Clinically Possible" ALS are by having UMN findings in two or more regions or two regions with both UMN and LMN findings but with no UMN findings rostral to the LMN findings (which would otherwise qualify as "Clinically Probable"). The essence of the criteria is that finding both UMN and LMN findings in the same area is rare and suspicious for ALS. The more areas where these findings are identified, the more likely the diagnosis is ALS and the less likely it could be realistically explained by any other disorder.

General Approach

The overall approach to a patient with suspected ALS is complex and begins by establishing which type of motor neurons and which body regions are involved. A pragmatic approach is to first assess if there is clinical bulbar or pseudobulbar involvement. If so, an MRI of the brain should be obtained. If cervical, thoracic, and lumbar regions are involved, spinal MRI should be pursued or at least considered. This can help exclude the most common alternate diagnoses that are usually evident on neuroimaging. The differential can then be narrowed by the type of motor neurons that are clinically involved. Almost all patients should have an EMG performed. This helps determine the pattern of LMN involvement more accurately and makes the diagnostician more confident about the group of diagnoses to pursue.

The possible causes of both UMN and LMN injury in the same patient is a short list of rare conditions. A relatively common exception is cervical radiculomyelopathy related to degenerative cervical spine disease. A patient with this condition will have LMN injury and findings at the level of the radiculopathy, and UMN signs caudal to this level attributable to the myelopathy. A representative patient could have C6 cord compression from spondylosis. The resultant radiculopathy could lead to weakness and atrophy in the C6 myotome and diminished biceps and brachioradialis reflexes. The myelopathy would cause an increase in the triceps and lower limb reflexes, Hoffmann and Babinski signs, and lower limb weakness or clumsiness without atrophy. This is a reasonably common and treatable finding in clinical practice, making it important to exclude. A syrinx could cause a similar syndrome but is much less common. Key findings that can identify these syndromes and distinguishing from ALS are often the prominent sensory complaints that often overshadow the motor deficits. Also, it is very important to recognize that all UMN signs are caudal to the LMN signs. "Clinically Probable" ALS requires some UMN signs rostral to the LMN signs for this very reason. Another common combination is a cervical myelopathy associated with cervical spine degeneration and superimposed length-dependent neuropathy. The myelopathy would cause UMN findings in the upper limbs, but in the lower limbs the neuropathy often blunts reflexes to make them normal or hyporeflexic. In this case, the LMN findings are distal to the UMN findings and the rule for rostral findings of UMN signs is not helpful. In both situations, the sensory complaints and findings are often clearly evident. These clinical possibilities are both easily excluded with MRI of the cervical spine. The other possible causes of a combined UMN/LMN presentation include spinal dural arteriovenous malformations, hereditary motor neuropathy, and hereditary spastic paraparesis (see Box 40-5).

A patient with signs, symptoms, and testing consistent with LMN injury has a greater number of possible causes that need to be excluded. Myasthenia gravis and other NMJ disorders as well as MMN are important possibilities that are treatable and thus ruling them out is paramount. PMA, adult-onset SMA, inclusion body myositis, HD, and KD are other possibilities. Electrodiagnostic testing is usually needed with inclusion of multiple motor nerve conduction studies and multiple stimulation sites for each to rule out subtle areas of conduction block seen in MMN. Repetitive stimulation and occasionally SFEMG may be considerations. Although repetitive stimulation, anti-GM1 antibodies, and a CK are all worth obtaining, the clinician needs to be wary of false positives in all of these tests in patients with ALS (as described earlier).

A patient with primarily or exclusively UMN signs has a rather different list of possible diagnoses. These include inflammatory conditions such as multiple sclerosis and neuromyelitis optica. These should both be excluded easily by the rate of progression, sensory complaints, and MRI of the brain and spinal cord. Other myelopathies must be considered including compressive, malignant, vitamin B_{12} deficiency, copper deficiency, and syringomyelia—all excluded with imaging and laboratory testing. When imaging and laboratory testing is negative, PLS is high in the differential, but hereditary causes such as a female carrier of the X-linked adrenoleukodystrophy/adrenomyeloneuropathy, hereditary spastic paraparesis, or Silver syndrome (hereditary motor neuropathy V) are possibilities.

Patients with predominantly bulbar symptoms have a short list of alternate diagnoses. Myasthenia gravis, KD, and myopathies, particularly oculopharyngeal muscular dystrophy, are primary considerations. EMG testing is critical and needs to include repetitive stimulation of facial muscles and possibly SFEMG.

Making the diagnosis of ALS must be done with caution and usually confirmed by a clinician with expertise in MNDs (Box 40-3). There is a high price for both missing the diagnosis as well as giving it falsely. In many cases, a second opinion is warranted. Although patients should be left with hope, there is a great emotional burden linked with the perceived possibility that the doctor is wrong. Eliminating this burden justifies the second opinion by itself. Giving the diagnosis of ALS incorrectly (a false-positive diagnosis) is estimated to occur in 5% to 10% of

BOX 40-3

Key Points in the Diagnosis of Amyotrophic Lateral Sclerosis

History

- Focal weakness without pain or sensory complaints is suspicious for amyotrophic lateral sclerosis (ALS)
- Patients with sensory complaints or isolated fasciculations rarely have or develop ALS

Physical Examination

- Upper motor neuron (UMN) and lower motor neuron (LMN) findings in the same limb are very suspicious for ALS
- Fasciculations in isolation are common in healthy patients and in many LMN processes
- In combination with an abnormal examination or electromyography (EMG), fasciculations are highly suspicious for ALS or other motor neuron diseases (MNDs)
- When seen with otherwise normal examination findings and EMG, fasciculations are almost always benign

Testing

- Electrodiagnostic testing is the cornerstone of identification of LMN loss in all MNDs, but diagnosis of ALS requires clinical correlation with examination features of UMN involvement
- No laboratory or imaging test can make the diagnosis of ALS in isolation, but genetic testing can identify pathogenic gene mutations associated with familial ALS and in some cases of sporadic ALS
- In a patient with clinical features of ALS, no diagnostic test can rule out ALS
- Most patients suspected of having ALS should undergo testing to exclude mimicking conditions
- Some testing results can be nonspecific. For example, patients with ALS often have mildly elevated creatine kinase and occasionally elevated anti-monosialotetrahexosylganglioside antibodies (anti-GM1 antibodies)
- In most patients, imaging of the brain and cervical spine are particularly important to exclude other causes of UMN or LMN dysfunction

cases.[36,140] Approximately 50% of these cases had a treatable diagnosis, usually MMN or a cervical spondylotic myelopathy.[36,140] KD was missed in nearly 15% of false-positive ALS diagnoses. Facial fasciculations and a family history were both evident in 75% of cases and were keys in making the ultimate diagnosis. Gynecomastia and tremor were both only seen in approximately 50% of these patients and were less reliable than might be expected.[140] Clinicians should be on the lookout for red flags that the diagnosis of ALS is incorrect, including development of atypical symptoms or a failure to progress as expected.[36,140] This caution should occur during the initial diagnosis and continue over the course of the disease.

Missing the diagnosis of ALS (a false-negative diagnosis) also has consequences and is significantly more common. Nearly 50% of patients who are ultimately diagnosed with ALS were initially misdiagnosed.[12] These were most commonly lumbar and cervical stenosis. As mentioned earlier, spondylosis is very common in this age group and seen to some extent in most patients who are ultimately thought to have ALS. The provider must therefore be cautious to avoid quickly assuming a causal relationship. Unfortunately, around 10% of patients ultimately diagnosed with ALS have spinal surgery before they are diagnosed—an example of the cost of this mistake.[13] Other common misdiagnoses include cerebrovascular disease in approximately 10% and "nothing wrong" in around 15%.[13] A total of approximately 30% of patients have an unnecessary surgery.[13] An estimated cost for misdiagnosis is $30,000.[13] A loss of faith in the medical system and the emotional toll for patients and families is harder to quantify.

It is therefore difficult to decide when exactly the suspected diagnosis of ALS should be given. A level of certainty needs to be established, and a particularly high degree of certainty that a treatable diagnosis is not being missed is critical. Waiting until there is absolutely no question of the diagnosis can also have negative consequences. Giving the diagnosis early has psychological, economic, and medical benefit.[4] The manner in which the diagnosis is given is also important and has lasting consequences to the patient. Experts recommend that a doctor who knows the patient gives the diagnosis in person with distractions, such as a cell phone and incoming interruptions from staff, eliminated and with 45 to 60 minutes available. It is helpful to begin with what the patient knows to determine the best way to communicate with the patient. If family is available for the clinic visit and the patient is agreeable to having family be part of the discussion, this is usually very beneficial. The diagnosis and what it will mean to the patient should be rolled out in a stepwise manner, making sure each step is understood before moving on. Providing more information in writing or a recommended website is important. It is most important that the patient is assured in words and in actions that he or she will not be abandoned. Setting up a follow-up visit in 2 to 4 weeks before the patient leaves the office reinforces this. Common mistakes include withholding the diagnosis, delivering it without empathy, and not giving enough information. The patient needs to be left with hope, and phrases such as "there is nothing we can do" are inaccurate and unproductive. Giving the diagnosis with improper technique can lead to a sense of abandonment, erode the patient-physician relationship, and even affect the patient's psychological adjustment to bereavement.[4]

Treatment

General

Currently, there are no treatments that can dramatically counteract the effects or stop progression of most MNDs. Treatment strategies are generally designed to reduce the symptomatic impact on patients with MNDs (Box 40-4). Once the diagnosis of ALS is given, treatment should begin without delay. Although there is no cure for ALS, early treatment is recommended and is of proven benefit. It is important to avoid giving the impression that the medical community has nothing to offer. Not only is this incorrect but undermines the ability to improve survival and quality

BOX 40-4

Summary of Key Recommendations in the Treatment of Amyotrophic Lateral Sclerosis

Exercise

- Some form of therapeutic exercise should be offered to every patient with amyotrophic lateral sclerosis (ALS)
- Range-of-motion and stretching exercises should be offered to every patient
- A gentle aerobic exercise program should be offered to ambulatory patients
- A resistance exercise program of mild-to-moderate resistance exercise for 15 minutes
- A resistance exercise program of mild-to-moderate resistance exercise for 15 minutes twice daily should be offered to all high-functioning patients
- Patients should avoid
  - Exercising to fatigue
  - Exercising to dyspnea
  - Eccentric exercise
- Patients should scale back their program if they have
  - Muscle cramping
  - Excessive overuse weakness afterward

Nutrition

- Monitor weight every 3 months
- Percutaneous endoscopic gastrostomy (PEG) or radiologically inserted gastrostomy (RIG) tube
- Discuss with patients with indications:
  - Decreased caloric intake (specifics)
  - Dehydration
  - Meals limited by dysphagia and choking
  - Weight loss greater than 10% of body weight
  - Not aspiration pneumonia
- Ensure all patients have accurate information regarding risks and survival advantage of PEG or RIG
- Refer willing patients for PEG or RIG before forced vital capacity (FVC) drops below 50% predicted
- Refer willing patients with FVC between 50% and 30% for RIG
- Inform patients that no vitamins, minerals, or nutritional supplements have been shown to help patients with ALS

Medications

Riluzole

- Should be offered to every patient with ALS
- Dosage is 50 mg twice daily
- Treatment should be initiated as soon as possible
- Physicians should ensure patients have accurate information regarding riluzole
- Patients on riluzole should have liver function tests monitored
  - Alternative medications
- Patients should be advised that no other medication, nutritional supplement, or alternative medication has been shown to help patients with ALS

Multidisciplinary Clinics

- Extend survival and should be pursued when feasible

Mood Disorders

- Are common and should be treated to improve quality of life

Spasticity

- Intrathecal baclofen has been shown to work, but oral baclofen has not
- Botulinum toxin can be used but can lead to generalized weakness

Respiratory

- Respiratory measurements (usually FVC and maximal inspiratory pressure [MIP]) should be measured at every visit regardless of symptoms
- Noninvasive ventilation (NIV)
  - Extends survival, slows respiratory decline, and improves quality of life
  - Commonly begun when FVC <50% predicted and MIP $\leq$60 cm H_2O or a $PaCO_2$ of $\geq$45 mm Hg, although early NIV prolongs life
- Supplemental O_2 suppresses respiratory drive and can worsen symptoms and lead to respiratory arrest and should only be used for palliation of symptomatic hypoxia
- A mechanical insufflator-exsufflator (MI-E) improves secretion clearance and can be used in patients with a peak cough flow <300 to 350 L/min

Communication

- Is a major determinant of quality of life and should be optimized
- Patients should be routinely monitored by a speech-language pathologist

Palliative Care

- Discuss the patient's wishes and involve a palliative care team as early as possible
- Patient's distressing symptoms are often undertreated, and benzodiazepines and opioids titrated to clinical effect will almost never cause life-threatening respiratory depression

of life with proper nutrition, noninvasive ventilation (NIV), riluzole, and coordinated care. Multidisciplinary clinics have been shown to extend survival and if located within a reasonable distance can help simplify and improve care.[138] Members of the team include a physician with neuromuscular expertise (either a physiatrist or neurologist), gastroenterologist, pulmonologist, physical therapist, occupational therapist, speech therapist, dietician, counselor, and a physician with experience in palliative care. A physiatrist is a key member of a multidisciplinary team, but if necessary can individually help manage the multifaceted impact on patients with ALS to whom these clinics are unavailable.

Medication

There are no medications available with major disease-modifying capacity in the field of MNDs. The holy grail of ALS research is a safe medication that will cure or have a major disease-modifying effect. A great number of drugs have been studied and are being studied, but as of today riluzole is the only medication shown to slow the progression of ALS. Multiple studies have shown it to be safe and effective in slowing the progression of the disease.[99] The mechanism of effect of riluzole is unclear. Riluzole inhibits presynaptic release of glutamate, and glutamate toxicity is thought to contribute to neuronal death in ALS. Riluzole reduces mortality 23% at 6 months and 15% at 12 months, and appears to prolong survival by around 4 months.[139] There is a clear dose effect.[4] The best benefit-to-risk ratio is achieved at the standard dose of 50 mg twice daily. There are few serious side effects. The most common adverse reactions are dizziness, asthenia, and gastrointestinal disorders. Liver function test elevation is common but usually mild and elevations greater than five times the normal limit is seen in less than 5% of patients.[87] Monitoring of liver function tests is therefore recommended. Riluzole should be given as early as possible, as the life-prolonging effect seems to be greater when started earlier.[4]

Riluzole is currently the only pharmaceutical way to curb the progression of the disease, yet approximately 40% of patients do not use it.[18] Expense is the most common reason. Other barriers are a perceived lack of efficacy, lack of information about the drug, concern about side effects, and in some cases the treating physician recommended against it.[18] It is paramount that proper information is provided so that patients can make well-educated decisions. This is particularly true given that almost 80% of patients with ALS will use nonapproved vitamins and supplements that have no benefit and are nearly 50% of the cost of riluzole.[18]

Rehabilitation

Strategies for rehabilitation must be designed to the targeted patient population depending on disease impact and natural history. In particular, the progression of ALS makes prescribing rehabilitation interventions for patients difficult because of rapidly changing functional status. Additionally, the combination of spasticity and severe focal weakness creates a challenge for those trying to maximize their function and ease care. Patients with primarily spinal involvement tend to progress over six stages with common clusters of rehabilitation needs in each, although individuals can vary considerably and straddle stages rather than fall neatly into one.[131] Outlining these stages and their challenges helps the provider anticipate the rehabilitation treatments they will likely be discussing at the next visit.

Stage 1 includes patients who are ambulatory and fully independent, with mild weakness or clumsiness. They need only to maintain active range of motion, carry on with normal activities of daily living, but can benefit from strengthening unaffected muscle. Strengthening all muscles, including affected muscles, with caution for overwork damage is reasonable.

Patients in stage 2 remain ambulatory and independent but have moderate weakness. Functional impairment may be severe in some areas despite preserved overall function (Figure 40-7). They often benefit from ankle-foot orthoses to compensate for foot drop. If the patient has plantar flexion spasticity, a dorsiflexion assist can encourage clonus and should be avoided. Anterior trim lines add weight but can provide medial-lateral stability for those who require it. A wrist-hand orthosis to assist with wrist drop is often needed. An opponens splint can be used to accommodate lack of thumb opposition from thenar muscle weakness (Figure 40-8). Hand weakness also commonly makes buttoning difficult, and assistive devices to ease this task are helpful. Focal weakness of the cervical extensor muscles leading to head drop or chin-on-chest deformity is a

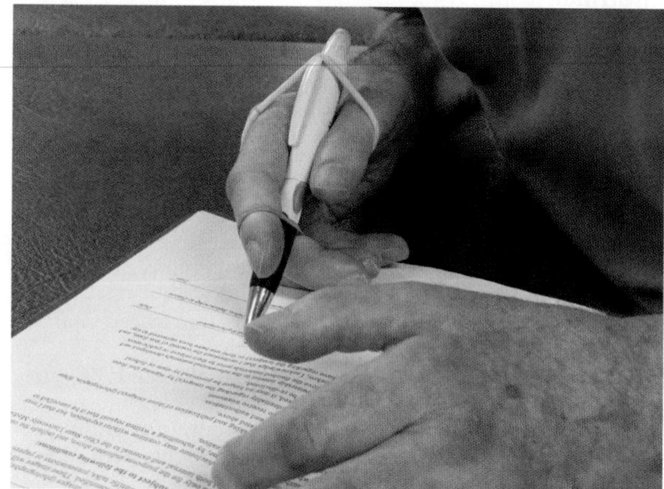

FIGURE 40-7 Profound intrinsic hand muscle weakness in a patient diagnosed with amyotrophic lateral sclerosis who has otherwise relatively retained bulbar and ambulatory function. The patient is unable to voluntarily grip the pen to sign a consent form.

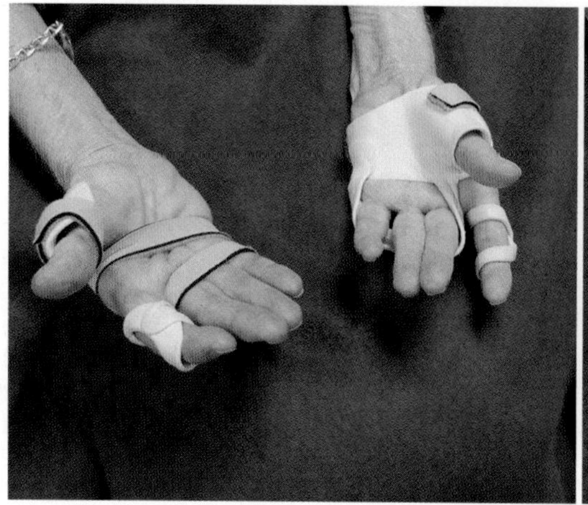

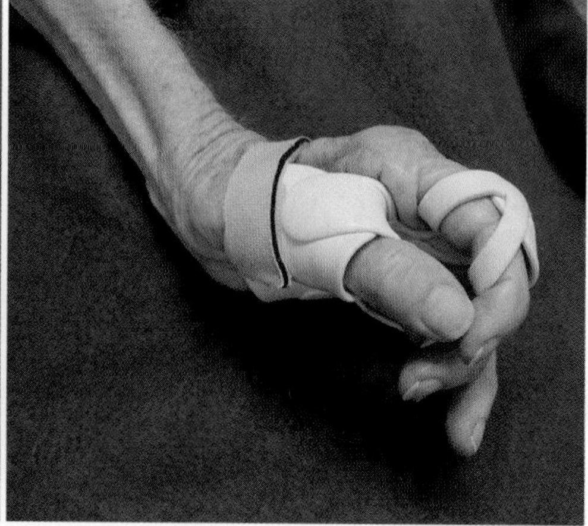

FIGURE 40-8 Orthotic intervention for severe intrinsic hand muscle weakness and impaired thumb opposition in a patient with amyotrophic lateral sclerosis.

common problem in ALS. Cervical orthoses to stabilize the cervical spine may help provide some relief but are sometimes poorly tolerated. Work simplification can be useful at this stage. Input from an occupational therapist is particularly important at this stage. Exercise prescription is similar to stage 1.

Stage 3 includes patients who remain ambulatory but have severe weakness in selected muscle groups. A common problem that arises at this stage is the inability to rise from a chair. Lift chairs and elevated toilet seats can mitigate this problem. Ambulation aids, such as a walker, can be helpful and a manual wheelchair for long trips is often necessary and facilitates socialization. This should be custom-fitted so as to provide pressure relief and support the spine, but financial and insurance constraints must be closely considered when determining the most appropriate type of durable medical equipment. At this stage, deep breathing exercises are helpful for those who develop mild respiratory muscle weakness.

Stage 4 includes patients who are nonambulatory but remain independent. Electrically powered chairs are usually appropriate. Exercise is usually limited to any unaffected muscles but utilization of range-of-motion exercises is still useful. A hospital bed facilitates bed mobility.

Stage 5 is entered when the patient is no longer independent. Transfer assistance, with devices such as Hoyer lifts, is generally required. Family education is a large part of the care of the patient. A wheeled shower chair is often helpful for these patients. A lack of mobility makes pressure relief measures in the wheelchair and bed higher priorities.

At stage 6 patients are completely bedridden, dependent, and requiring maximal assistance. Proper positioning is important to keep patients as comfortable as possible. Pressure relief and skilled caregivers are critical. Palliative care becomes the focus of treatment.

Exercise

Exercise in ALS and other progressive neuromuscular diseases is the subject of controversy. There is currently a lack of high-quality research in this area. Despite theoretical concerns of worsening weakness from overtaxing already struggling motor units, no controlled outcome study has shown worsening after exercise in patients with ALS. As most patients with ALS decline over time, a noncontrolled trial lacks the potential to show a greater decline in strength or function than might otherwise be seen over time. Conversely, the benefits of exercise have been established in controlled but small, often nonrandomized trials. The physician should therefore be looking for opportunities to allow patients the benefit of exercise when not contraindicated.

Range of motion and stretching are considered safe and should be prescribed for all patients with ALS. This is especially helpful in preventing contractures that could be a source of pain later in the disease.[37] There are no randomized trials to assess the benefits and risks of aerobic exercise, but the cardiovascular response of patients with ALS to aerobic conditioning is similar to healthy patients.[37] One small, nonrandomized trial has shown some benefit in ventilator-dependent patients using bilevel positive airway pressure (BiPAP) before and after treadmill training.[120] Resistance training has been shown to improve function and spasticity.[46] This was demonstrated in a trial that used a home exercise program with "modest" resistance for 15 minutes twice per day. Overall, at this point in time there is insufficient data to establish the benefit (or harm) of exercise in patients with ALS with a high degree of certainty.[33]

With the data available, it is reasonable to have patients or caregivers apply range-of-motion and stretching exercises to all patients with ALS, and encourage the patients who are more functional to engage in aerobic and mild resistance training. The latter can consist of mild-to-modest resistance exercises for 15 minutes twice daily. The potential for overwork weakness can be avoided by some common sense precautions such as avoiding resistance exercise to fatigue or cramping, aerobic exercising to the point of significant dyspnea, eccentric exercises, or exercising muscles with significant weakness. An unusual amount of delayed-onset muscle soreness is a sign to decrease the intensity of the program going forward. Care must be taken to avoid falls and injuries. Stationary cycling or pool therapy can reduce this risk. Overall, although a definitive evidential basis is lacking, exercise remains one of the few modalities that can improve the function of a patient with ALS. Some form of exercise should be discussed with every patient with ALS. In addition to the benefits in function a reasonable exercise program can offer, it allows the patient to exert some control over their disease in an active manner.

Specific Disease-Related Impact

Spasticity

Spasticity can have a significant impact on function of patients with significant UMN involvement. Treatment of spasticity in patients with ALS is similar to other disease states but with some important differences. Physical therapy has been shown to reduce spasticity; oral baclofen is commonly used but has not been shown to have clear benefit.[46,112] Intrathecal baclofen has been used successfully in patients with ALS.[96] Not all patients with ALS would be appropriate candidates, specifically patients with rapid progression or very advanced disease. Botulinum toxin can be useful in treating specific muscle groups as in other disorders, but can lead to generalized weakness that can be more problematic in a patient with ALS than someone with a traumatic brain injury or stroke might experience.[98] Tizanidine, dantrolene, gabapentin, and benzodiazepines are commonly used but have not been specifically studied in ALS.[4] Benzodiazepines carry the additional benefit of helping treat anxiety, but also carry the additional risk of respiratory depression. Dantrolene does not share this risk but some advocate avoiding it in patients with ALS.

Communication

Patients with ALS typically have a slow progression of communication difficulties, eventually leading to the inability to communicate independently. The first development is usually dysarthria, initially at the end of the day, then progressively worse, and more constant as the disease progresses.[107] Dysarthria is a result of both UMN and LMN dysfunction. Other barriers that patients with ALS face in effective communication include hypernasal speech as a result of air leaking through the nose, hypophonia, and cognitive impairments, such as frontotemporal dementia.

Effective communication is a major factor in the quality of life in patients with ALS and should be managed aggressively.[4,107] Many patients elect to withdraw support when they become "locked-in" and unable to communicate, rather than when they lose a given physical function. This underscores the importance of communication to patients. In addition to the inability to indicate needs, the main loss patients with impaired communication experience is of social closeness with their partner and family.[107] Given this, patients should be routinely monitored by a speech-language pathologist to optimize communication and monitor changing needs during the course of the disease.[4]

Treatment options include palatal lift or palatal augmentation prosthesis to decrease hypernasality.[4] As verbal communication becomes more limited, augmentative and alternative communications systems (AACs) are useful. These substantially improve the patient's quality of life.[4] AAC devices range from pointing boards to more complex eye-gaze devices or brain-computer interfaces.

Dysphagia

Dysphagia is rarely noted by patients with ALS at presentation but becomes a prominent and troubling symptom as the disease progresses. It contributes to malnutrition, poses a risk for aspiration, and can be a major source of anxiety. Dysphagia usually begins with thin liquids, and using thickener is a simple early solution. When dysphagia with solids begins, smaller, more frequent meals can be helpful. Moistening and softening solids can also make swallowing easier.[130] A speech therapist is a valuable team member and can teach and reinforce helpful strategies, such as supraglottic swallowing, postural changes, and using a chin tuck.[4] Ultimately, with disease progression the failing swallowing mechanism needs to be bypassed if the patient is going to get safe and adequate nutrition.

Nutrition

Improved nutritional status can have major impact of various MNDs. In fact, proper management of nutrition is one of the most important jobs of a physician managing a patient with ALS. Without intervention, eventually patients with ALS will not get enough calories and this problem magnifies as the disease advances.[78] This is attributable to a combination of factors: bulbar and masticatory muscle weakness, dysphagia, and fatigue and slow eating. Weight loss is therefore common in patients with ALS. Almost three quarters of ambulatory patients consume less than the recommended daily allowance of calories, and a quarter lose more than 10% of their body weight.[133] Malnutrition is proportional to the degree of dysphagia and is a major predictor of death in patients with ALS.[133] Recruiting the help of a dietician can help physicians maintain calorie intake for patients with ALS. Calorie intake and weight loss should be a part of every follow-up visit. The initial strategies mentioned earlier can relieve these symptoms in some patients with early ALS, but eventually to get proper nutrition and prolong survival more definitive measures need to be taken.

A nasogastric tube can provide greater nutrition to patients with dysphagia but is uncomfortable and can lead to aspiration if improperly placed. A percutaneous endoscopic gastrostomy (PEG) tube is a permanent solution, and there are excellent data to support the use of PEG tubes in patients with ALS. Use of a PEG tube helps to stabilize body weight and probably prolongs survival, although it is not clear if it improves quality of life.[79,100] Indications for placement of a PEG tube in a patient with ALS include decreased caloric intake with weight loss greater than 10% of baseline, dehydration, and meals limited by dysphagia or taking greater than 30 minutes.[130] Studies show a decreased risk of PEG placement if performed before the FVC drops below 50% of the predicted value.[79] PEG tubes do not reduce the rate of aspiration pneumonia and this is not an indication for placement. Risks of PEG tube placement include tube dislodgement, benign pneumoperitoneum, parietal hematoma, peritonitis, gastrointestinal bleeding, gastrocolic fistula, and death.[41] The overall risk of mortality for PEG tube placement in patients with ALS is 6% to 10%.[79] An alternative is a radiologically inserted gastrostomy (RIG) tube. The risks and survival benefits are the same as a PEG tube, but because it can be performed under local or light sedation (as opposed to deep sedation or general anesthesia), it can be done safely in patients with a lower FVC.[41]

Despite the benefits of a PEG or RIG tube, most patients with severe dysphagia do not use them.[18] There are a variety of barriers between appropriate patients with ALS and PEG or RIG tube. Physicians recommend a PEG tube in less than half of the patients in whom it is indicated.[18] Less than half of the patients to whom it is recommended actually elect to have it placed.[18] When the physician brings up PEG tube placement to a patient with ALS, it is often received as a sign that things are going badly and death is near. This often leads to a delay in the discussion until after the risk of placing the PEG increases. Although many patients ultimately decline a PEG tube because they are uncomfortable with the idea, over one third of patients who did not receive it either lacked information or erroneously believed their swallowing was adequate.[18] There is clearly an information gap that prevents appropriate patients from receiving one of the few significant benefits the medical system can offer them. Ultimately, many patients will refuse a PEG or RIG tube even with all the proper information, but the provider owes the patient the opportunity to make an informed decision.

Patients with ALS frequently look to alternative medicine for solutions that allopathic medicine is not providing. This is particularly true regarding nutrition. Nearly 80% of patients use nutritional supplements or high-dose vitamins.[18] Unfortunately, none have shown benefit. Vitamin E and creatine have been studied most extensively and are not recommended to patients with ALS.[99]

Sialorrhea

Sialorrhea in patients with ALS can be socially disabling and encourage oral infections.[4] It is attributable to impaired handling of saliva rather than overproduction, and patients with ALS actually salivate less than healthy patients.[24] A home suction machine is something most patients find helpful. Multiple medications are commonly used in ALS. Amitriptyline is cheap and effective and can be helpful in treating a concomitant mood disorder or pseudobulbar affect. Typical dose is 25 to 50 mg two to three times daily.[4]

Atropine drops 0.25 to 0.75 mg three times daily can also be used. Other treatments include nebulized or intravenous glycopyrrolate, oral or transdermal scopolamine, and benzatropine.[4] Side effects include constipation, urinary retention, confusion, and sedation. Treatment can also lead to excessive drying of the nasopharynx and thickening of the mucous deep in the throat. Botulinum toxin type A given every 3 months at a dose of 7.5 to 20 units into each parotid gland has been used effectively[144] Serious side effects including jaw dislocation have been reported.[136] Radiation treatment is a fast, safe, inexpensive, and effective option, but is not frequently used.[4] Side effects are mild and temporary. Surgical treatments are available but not generally recommended.[4]

Respiratory Insufficiency

Respiratory muscles may be affected by motor neuron loss similar to other muscles. Inevitably, this leads to symptomatic respiratory insufficiency, and if respiratory function is not supported, eventually respiratory failure. In addition to being the main source of mortality in patients with ALS and other MNDs, the choices and method of compensating for respiratory insufficiency ultimately may have the most impact on the lives of patients. Patients that choose tracheostomy and long-term ventilation will generally survive much longer but must consider the eventual possibility of a locked-in, non-communicative state.

Respiratory insufficiency is very rarely a presenting complaint for patients with ALS. Symptoms are present on presentation in around 25% of patients when specifically sought. For the remaining majority, no respiratory symptoms are noted for some time after diagnosis. These symptoms can include fatigue, dyspnea, orthopnea, and morning headaches. In spite of many patients having no symptoms, subclinical respiratory insufficiency is frequent. Up to 85% of patients with ALS will have an abnormal FVC at presentation.[50,64] The majority of patients with a less than 50% predicted FVC, for whom NIV is both advantageous and covered by Medicare, will have mild or no respiratory symptoms.[64] For this reason, experts recommend routine assessment of respiratory physiologic measurements in patients with ALS every 2 to 4 months, regardless of the presence of symptoms.[64]

There are several different measurements that can be used to assess and monitor respiratory function. FVC is the most commonly utilized measurement.[99] The difference between the upright and supine FVC correlates best with orthopnea, which in turn is the symptom most closely associated with quality of life.[64,143] The maximal inspiratory pressure (MIP) has the advantage of decreasing earlier than upright FVC.[64] The sniff transdiaphragmatic pressure (sniff Pdi) is most accurate at predicting hypercapnea (90% sensitive, 87% specific).[99] The sniff nasal pressure (SNP) is useful in a number of ways. It has greater predictive power and is more reliably recorded at later stages of disease than both FVC and MIP.[99] At a threshold of less than 32%, predicted SNP is 81% sensitive and 85% specific for predicting hypercarbic respiratory failure.[64] In spite of this, FVC and MIP are the most established respiratory measurements and are used by most experts and Medicare to justify NIV. Unfortunately, no measurements can predict respiratory insufficiency in the many patients with ALS and bulbar dysfunction.[4,92]

At some point, patients with ALS will need to decide if they wish to use respiratory support or not. This can be a difficult discussion, for although there are advantages to adopting it early, even reassurances to the patient usually cannot hide the milestone it represents. This is true even for patients that are not in denial. For this and other reasons, many patients are never offered NIV.[18] Approximately one third of patients who use NIV will start it emergently. This is not ideal, and yet the benefit of NIV can still be achieved when started emergently.[64] Those who choose respiratory support usually begin NIV. NIV is delivered through a mask or mouthpiece, without the need for a tracheostomy. This can be delivered with either a BiPAP machine or a portable ventilator connected to a mask. Both are portable and serve basically the same purpose. Portable ventilators have many more settings and can be used when and if the patient decides to undergo a tracheostomy and invasive ventilation.

NIV has many advantages to offer. It has been shown to improve quality-of-life measurements including energy, vitality, dyspnea, somnolence, depression, sleep quality, physical fatigue, concentration problems, and cognitive function.[17,99,109,130] It was shown in one study to prolong survival 205 days, although it is not clear if this applies to those with severe bulbar involvement.[17] It also slows the rate of respiratory decline from −2.2% per month before treatment to −1.1% after initiation.[17] NIV delays the need for a tracheostomy and mechanical ventilation but does not appear to add additional burden to caregivers.[4] Most patients who have undergone NIV would choose it again and recommend it to other patients with ALS.[99]

Thresholds for beginning NIV vary. Medicare requires an FVC of <50%, and MIP ≤60 cm H_2O, or a $PaCO_2$ of ≥45 mm Hg. The American College of Chest Physicians adds a criteria of nocturnal oximetry ≤88% for 5 consecutive minutes.[31] "Early" NIV, beginning with nocturnal oximetry with >15 desaturation events per hour, has been shown in nonrandomized trials to confer an 11-month benefit compared with controls using NIV at thresholds listed earlier.[99] Use of NIV for >4 hours per day offers a survival advantage of 7 months and a slower rate of respiratory decline when compared with those using it for less.[99] A typical initial prescription for NIV would include the ICD-9 335.20 diagnosis for ALS and would include documentation of an FVC <50% or MIP ≤60 cm H_2O or $PaCO_2$ ≥45mm Hg.[64]

In spite of the benefits of NIV, eventually all patients will require more respiratory support and secretion management, and the decision to undergo a tracheostomy and invasive ventilation (IV) with a mechanical ventilator will be faced. This decision is often made urgently, when a patient is intolerant of NIV or unable to clear secretions.[64] Triggers to consider IV on a nonurgent basis include use of NIV >12 hours or intolerance of NIV with an FVC <50% or symptoms of dyspnea.[64] A tracheostomy and IV can substantially prolong life—in one series, 47% of patients survived more than 5 years.[130] Much of this time was in a locked-in state, losing the ability to communicate.[130] Yet patients report an 80% positive perception and would have it again and would recommend it to another patient with ALS.[64] Unlike NIV, there is a significant burden of IV on caregivers, many of whom would not endorse IV so strongly or at all. Only 50% of caregivers would consider it for themselves if they were to need it, and 30% of caregivers report a worse quality of life than the patient.[64] IV via a tracheostomy is also costly, imposing an estimated over $150,000 per year on the health care system.[130]

Diaphragmatic pacers have been studied in patients with ALS, and additional controlled studies are ongoing. In one study, a PEG and diaphragmatic pacer were placed simultaneously. The rate of FVC decline dropped from −2.4% (per month) to −0.9% after surgery.[64] Oxygen therapy should almost never be used in patients with ALS. It worsens respiratory symptoms as well as hypercapnea and can lead to hypercapnic coma or respiratory arrest.[8] Flow rates as low as 0.5 to 2 L/min can worsen CO_2 retention in patients with neuromuscular disease.[64] The possible exception to this rule is patients in the terminal phase who may need oxygen for palliative relief of air hunger.

Bronchial secretions are often problematic in patients with ALS and a major source of anxiety. First-line treatments include a portable home suction device and room humidifier. Mucolytics, such as *N*-acetylcysteine, 200 to 400 mg three times daily, can also be helpful. Nebulized saline, beta-antagonists, anticholinergic bronchodilators, and mucolytics have been used in various combinations with success. Surgical cricopharyngeal myotomy has been used to relieve cricopharyngeal spasm and severe bronchial secretions.[4] High-frequency chest wall oscillation, used effectively in cystic fibrosis, has been shown not to work in two randomized trials, and the American Academy of Neurology indicates that there is insufficient data to support or refute use in patients with ALS.[64,99] Breath stacking is a technique that involves multiple sequential inhalations before an exhalation. It can increase inspiratory volume up to 20% and increase the peak cough flow (PCF) significantly.[64] Patients can do this without assistance if they can close their glottis between inspiratory efforts; otherwise, a caregiver can use a resuscitation bag connected to a mask. A manual cough assist can be performed by a caregiver. This consists of a caregiver leaning over a partially supine patient and applying downward pressure on the chest with one forearm while thrusting on the abdomen with the other hand during expiration.[64] The combination of manual cough assist and breath stacking is more effective than breath stacking alone.[64] Manual cough assist should be avoided in patients with a Greenfield filter and used with caution in patients with recent abdominal surgery, abdominal feeding tubes, and those at high risk of rib fracture.[64] If a patient has a vital capacity of less than 340 mL or peak cough flow less than 90 L/min, they will typically need to transition to mechanical insufflation-exsufflation.[64]

A mechanical cough assisting device (mechanical insufflator-exsufflator or MI-E) can be very effective via a face mask and has been shown to be effective in uncontrolled trials.[68,127] It works by providing positive airway pressure for a few seconds, then suddenly switching to negative pressure to simulate the pressures created in a healthy cough. Treatments usually consist of four to six insufflation-exsufflation cycles in a sequence. Sequences are separated by 30 seconds of rest. Four to six sequences make up a treatment, and patients usually receive three to four treatments per day.[64] This can increase to one to two treatments per hour in the setting of a respiratory tract infection.[64] The combination of NIV and MI-E has been shown to reduce hospitalization and improve oxygen saturation in patients with neuromuscular disorders including ALS.[64] A typical prescription would read: cough assist device, four treatments per day and as needed, five coughing cycles per sequence followed by 30 seconds of rest, with five sequences for each treatment, beginning at +15 cm H_2O insufflation pressure/−15 cm H_2O exsufflation pressure, increased in 5 to 10 cm H_2O increments, to a target +40/−40 cm H_2O and oxygen saturation greater than 94%.[64] It is covered by Medicare for patients with ALS and a PCF of less than 300 to 350 L/min (5 to 6 L/s).[64] It is less effective for patients with significant bulbar dysfunction, in whom a tracheostomy is often a better solution for secretion management. Contraindications include bullous emphysema, pneumothorax, and pneumomediastinum.[64]

Mood and Cognitive Disorders

Mood disorders are common in ALS. It is important for treating providers to discuss symptoms of mood disorders with patients (and families of patients) with ALS, as they are associated with a lower quality of life.[91] Tricyclic antidepressant and selective serotonin reuptake inhibitors are often used. Tricyclic antidepressants have the added benefit of treating sialorrhea and insomnia but are complicated by many side effects. Insomnia is common and zolpidem and nonpharmacologic sleep hygiene can be helpful. Anxiety can be a particular problem when respiratory insufficiency develops and benzodiazepines are commonly used. They are effective but can contribute to suppressing respiratory drive. Counseling is helpful to many patients and is an integral part of most multidisciplinary clinics. Support groups through an organization such as the Muscular Dystrophy Association or others specific to ALS should be encouraged to patients who are open to the idea. Approximately 50% of patients with ALS will develop at least mild-to-moderate impaired cognition, and around 15% of patients develop features of frontotemporal dementia.[2] Symptoms of frontotemporal dementia may include apathy, change in emotional reactivity, sleep disturbances, stereotypical or repetitive behaviors, poor insight or judgment, and loss of expressive language with relative preservation of comprehension. Treatment is supportive, and no medication therapy has been shown to improve cognition, but selective serotonin reuptake inhibitors can be used to help with behavioral changes.

Pseudobulbar Affect

Pseudobulbar affect is pathologic weeping, laughing, and yawning that is inappropriate or excessive to the emotional state of the patient. It can consist of laughing or crying spontaneously when there is no apparent reason and can be alarming and distressing to those around the patient. The underlying mechanism is unknown but may be as a result of loss of frontal lobe inhibition of spontaneous brain stem–generated emotional responses. Pseudobulbar affect is seen in over 50% of patients with ALS, with or without bulbar motor signs.[57] It is not a mood disorder and often does not reflect the emotional state of the patient. Caregivers are often more concerned than patients themselves, and if educated on the true nature of the expression it can often be ignored. Multiple antidepressants and even levodopa and lithium have been used.[130] A combination of dextromethorphan and quinidine has been approved by the U.S. Food and Drug Administration for treatment of pseudobulbar affect and has been shown to improve both symptoms and quality of life.[21] It is not clear how this combination helps pseudobulbar affect, but dextromethorphan is a known *N*-methyl-D-aspartate antagonist. Approximately 25% of patients discontinued the combination, with common but mild side effects including nausea, dizziness, and somnolence. There were increases in the QT interval seen in trials that were not thought to be clinically significant.[21]

Pain and Cramps

Cramps are common in patients with various forms of MNDs. In KD, cramps are an early feature of the disease and are thought to be related to axonal hyperexcitability and may occur before symptoms of motor deficits. Cramps are a common source of discomfort in patients with ALS and are fairly common early in the disease. Empirical treatments include massage, physical therapy, magnesium, carbamazepine, phenytoin, verapamil, and gabapentin, although none have been studied in ALS.[4] Pain is a common feature of ALS in later stages, and contractures and prolonged immobilization may contribute to this. Immobility seems to be the other most common cause of pain in ALS. Treatment therefore should begin with range-of-motion exercises. Physical modalities such as ice and heat can be used. If these are ineffective, acetaminophen or nonsteroidal antiinflammatory medications and antispasticity agents are commonly used. Opioids are often necessary in time. They are effective nearly 75% of the time and have the advantage of relieving air hunger and anxiety.[113] Respiratory depression, loss of airway protection and cough, and constipation need to be monitored and dosing adjusted accordingly.

Prognosis and End-of-Life Care

End-of-life issues need to be addressed early in the management of every patient with ALS and other severe MNDs. Delaying uncomfortable end-of-life conversations may be tempting for both provider and patient alike. The alternative to a potentially uncomfortable conversation includes critical decisions during a crisis with family members who may be unaware of the patient's true wishes. Establishing a health care proxy, living will, and do-not-resuscitate order help avoid this. Clear and repeated communication of the patient's wishes to caregivers and family is still important, even if all of these listed arrangements are in place. Palliative care specialists should be involved early.[4] It is helpful to review the patient's wishes every 6 months to ensure that documentation is current and compatible with the patient's recent state of mind.

Providers often soften the blow of the initial diagnosis by making a promise: that everything will be done to keep the patient comfortable. The actual medical treatment of distressing symptoms in the last months of life is often done too conservatively. One survey found that in the last month of life, on a scale of 1 to 6 (6 representing constant suffering, 1 representing no suffering), caregivers gave an average rating of 4, and nearly half rated this final month as a 5 or 6.[130] It appears that more needs to be done to deliver on this promise. There may not be a more important task that a physician must undertake.

Common complaints in the last month of life are dyspnea, difficulty sleeping, choking episodes, pain that was often severe, anxiety, confusion, and depression.[130] The initial management of many of these issues has been discussed earlier. Symptomatic treatment of intermittent dyspnea can consist of lorazepam 0.5 to 2.5 mg sublingually and morphine 2.5 mg orally or subcutaneously.[4] Chronic dyspnea of a moderate degree can be treated with this same morphine regimen four to six times daily.[4] Severe dyspnea can be treated with morphine intravenously or subcutaneously at 0.5 mg/h and titrated to effect.[4] Midazolam or diazepam can be used for nocturnal symptoms.[4] Pain can be treated with nonnarcotic medications but generally requires opioids, which have many cross-benefits for dyspnea and anxiety. Benzodiazepines are usually used for anxiety as well as dyspnea.

Providers are often concerned about overtreating the patient, but palliative care experts assert that titrating doses of benzodiazepines and opioids to clinical symptoms will almost never result in life-threatening respiratory depression.[4] Supplemental oxygen, however, can suppress respiratory drive and cause hypercarbic respiratory failure. It should only be given to patients with palliation when symptomatic hypoxia is present. Restlessness and confusion as a result of hypercapnea can be treated with neuroleptics such as chlorpromazine 12.5 mg every 4 to 12 hours per os, intravenously, or per rectum. Patients and caregivers can be reassured that death itself is peaceful. Surveys have found that 91% of deaths resulting from ALS in the United States and Canada were considered peaceful by caregivers.[130]

The prognosis of MNDs may vary from a benign process with favorable outcome to very poor depending on the underlying pathophysiology. The prognosis for ALS is grim (Box 40-5). There is a small (10%) subset of patients with longevity for reasons that are unclear. A fortunate 50% of these have a more benign course; the other 50% have prolonged but severe involvement.[111] Overall survival from the onset of symptoms averages between 2 and 3 years, and

BOX 40-5

Important Statistics in the Prognosis in Amyotrophic Lateral Sclerosis

Average survival from onset of symptoms: 2 to 3 years
Average survival from diagnosis: 15 months
Three year survival rate (from diagnosis): 41%
Five year survival rate (from diagnosis): 20%
Factors negatively impacting prognosis at diagnosis:
- Female sex
- Increasing age
- Bulbar onset
- Rapid early progression
- More definite diagnostic category

Treatment factors impacting prognosis:
- Percutaneous endoscopic gastrostomy
- Noninvasive ventilation
- Riluzole
- Participation in multidisciplinary clinics

survival after the diagnosis is 15 months, with significant variability between individual patients.[65,111] The prognosis is worse with age and bulbar involvement. Men survive longer than women, possibly because of their lower incidence of bulbar involvement.[23] Malnutrition causes a nearly eightfold increase in the risk of death.[42] Those with more diffuse involvement and a more rapid rate of decline have a shorter survival. Treatment with a PEG tube, NIV, riluzole, and participation in multidisciplinary clinics improves survival.[29,138]

Conclusions

MNDs represent a diverse group of disorders with the common feature of motor neuron loss and associated deficits within the motor system. The goal of this chapter is to provide a general framework to the approach to patients with suspected MND. The spectrum of disorders reviewed, although not all encompassing, includes the more common of these relatively uncommon disorders. The effects of MNDs are often devastating, and there is generally no cure. Yet, there is a surprising difference that an attentive and educated physician can make on extending and improving the life of patients with MNDs, and there is real hope. At the same time as polio is being steadily eradicated, treatments for halting or reversing SMA and ALS are tantalizingly close, and could impact patients receiving the diagnosis of MND even today. In the meantime, a physiatrist's view of the entire function of the patient, ability to coordinate with multiple disciplines, and focus on quality of life are ideal when treating a patient with MND. Proper diagnosis and management of MNDs has never been more important. A multidisciplinary approach is usually the most effective to address the complexities of diagnosis, prognosis, and management, and physiatrists have key roles in the detailed evaluation, accurate and timely diagnosis, and treatment of patients with MNDs. Although there are no current therapies that offer a cure, there are many therapeutic interventions that can lessen disease impact on patients and families.

ACKNOWLEDGMENTS: We gratefully thank Wendy King, P.T., and John T. Kissel, M.D., for their assistance with the clinical images for the figures presented in this chapter, J. Chad Hoyle, M.D., for reviewing this chapter and providing helpful suggestions, and Donna Winkelman, B.S., M.L.S., for her invaluable research assistance.

KEY REFERENCES

1. Abhinav K, Al-Chalabi A, Hortobagyi T, Leigh PN: Electrical injury and amyotrophic lateral sclerosis: a systematic review of the literature, *J Neurol Neurosurg Psychiatry* 78(5):450–453, 2007.
2. Achi EY, Rudnicki SA: ALS and frontotemporal dysfunction: a review, *Neurol Res Int* 2012:806306, 2012.
4. Andersen PM, Borasio GD, Dengler R, et al: Good practice in the management of amyotrophic lateral sclerosis: clinical guidelines. An evidence-based review with good practice points. EALSC Working Group, *Amyotroph Lateral Scler* 8(4):195–213, 2007.
6. Arnold WD, Burghes AH: Spinal muscular atrophy: the development and implementation of potential treatments, *Ann Neurol* 74(3):348–362, 2013.
7. Arnold WD, Flanigan KM: A practical approach to molecular diagnostic testing in neuromuscular diseases, *Phys Med Rehabil Clin N Am* 23(3):589–608, 2012.
15. Blexrud MD, Windebank AJ, Daube JR: Long-term follow-up of 121 patients with benign fasciculations, *Ann Neurol* 34(4):622–625, 1993.
16. Bosch AM, Stroek K, Abeling NG, et al: The Brown-Vialetto-Van Laere and Fazio Londe syndrome revisited: natural history, genetics, treatment and future perspectives, *Orphanet J Rare Dis* 7(1):83, 2012.
17. Bourke SC, Bullock RE, Williams TL, et al: Noninvasive ventilation in ALS: indications and effect on quality of life, *Neurology* 61(2):171–177, 2003.
18. Bradley WG, Anderson F, Gowda N, et al: Changes in the management of ALS since the publication of the AAN ALS practice parameter 1999, *Amyotroph Lateral Scler Other Motor Neuron Disord* 5(4):240–244, 2004.
19. Brooks BR: El Escorial World Federation of Neurology criteria for the diagnosis of amyotrophic lateral sclerosis. Subcommittee on Motor Neuron Diseases/Amyotrophic Lateral Sclerosis of the World Federation of Neurology Research Group on Neuromuscular Diseases and the El Escorial "Clinical limits of amyotrophic lateral sclerosis" workshop contributors, *J Neurol Sci* 124(Suppl):96–107, 1994.
20. Brooks BR, Miller RG, Swash M, et al: El Escorial revisited: revised criteria for the diagnosis of amyotrophic lateral sclerosis, *Amyotroph Lateral Scler Other Motor Neuron Disord* 1(5):293–299, 2000.
22. Buchthal F, Olsen PZ: Electromyography and muscle biopsy in infantile spinal muscular atrophy, *Brain* 93(1):15–30, 1970.
26. Chen A, Weimer L, Brannagan T, 3rd, et al: Experience with the Awaji Island modifications to the ALS diagnostic criteria, *Muscle Nerve* 42(5):831–832, 2010.
28. Chiò A, Brignolio F, Leone M, et al: A survival analysis of 155 cases of progressive muscular atrophy, *Acta Neurol Scand* 72(4):407–413, 1985.
29. Chiò A, Mora G, Leone M, et al: Early symptom progression rate is related to ALS outcome: a prospective population-based study, *Neurology* 59(1):99–103, 2002.
33. Dal Bello-Haas V, Florence JM: Therapeutic exercise for people with amyotrophic lateral sclerosis or motor neuron disease, *Cochrane Database Syst Rev* 5:Cd005229, 2013.
34. Dalakas MC, Elder G, Hallett M, et al: A long-term follow-up study of patients with post-poliomyelitis neuromuscular symptoms, *N Engl J Med* 314(15):959–963, 1986.
36. Davenport RJ, Swingler RJ, Chancellor AM, Warlow CP: Avoiding false positive diagnoses of motor neuron disease: lessons from the Scottish Motor Neuron Disease Register, *J Neurol Neurosurg Psychiatry* 60(2):147–151, 1996.
37. de Almeida JP, Silvestre R, Pinto AC, de Carvalho M: Exercise and amyotrophic lateral sclerosis, *Neurol Sci* 33(1):9–15, 2012.
39. de Carvalho M, Dengler R, Eisen A, et al: Electrodiagnostic criteria for diagnosis of ALS, *Clin Neurophysiol* 119(3):497–503, 2008.
40. DeJesus-Hernandez M, Mackenzie IR, Boeve BF, et al: Expanded GGGGCC hexanucleotide repeat in noncoding region of *C9ORF72* causes chromosome 9p-linked FTD and ALS, *Neuron* 72(2):245–256, 2011.
49. Elsheikh B, Kissel JT, Christoforidis G, et al: Spinal angiography and epidural venography in juvenile muscular atrophy of the distal arm "Hirayama disease, *Muscle Nerve* 40(2):206–212, 2009.
51. Ferrante MA, Wilbourn AJ: The characteristic electrodiagnostic features of Kennedy's disease, *Muscle Nerve* 20(3):323–329, 1997.
64. Gruis KL, Lechtzin N: Respiratory therapies for amyotrophic lateral sclerosis: a primer, *Muscle Nerve* 46(3):313–331, 2012.
65. Gubbay SS, Kahana E, Zilber N, et al: Amyotrophic lateral sclerosis. A study of its presentation and prognosis, *J Neurol* 232(5):295–300, 1985.
69. Hausmanowa-Petrusewicz I: Karwanska A: Electromyographic findings in different forms of infantile and juvenile proximal spinal muscular atrophy, *Muscle Nerve* 9(1):37–46, 1986.
70. Haverkamp LJ, Appel V, Appel SH: Natural history of amyotrophic lateral sclerosis in a database population. Validation of a scoring system and a model for survival prediction, *Brain* 118(3):707–719, 1995.
71. Hirayama K, Toyokura Y, Tsubaki T: Juvenile muscular atrophy of unilateral upper extremity: a new clinical entity, *Psychiatr Neurol* 61:2190–2197, 1959.
73. Howard RS: Poliomyelitis and the postpolio syndrome, *BMJ* 330(7503):1314–1318, 2005.

80. Katz JS, Wolfe GI, Andersson PB, et al: Brachial amyotrophic diplegia: a slowly progressive motor neuron disorder, *Neurology* 53(5): 1071–1076, 1999.
81. Kennedy WR, Alter M, Sung JH: Progressive proximal spinal and bulbar muscular atrophy of late onset. A sex-linked recessive trait, *Neurology* 18(7):671–680, 1968.
83. Kim WK, Liu X, Sandner J, et al: Study of 962 patients indicates progressive muscular atrophy is a form of ALS, *Neurology* 73(20):1686–1692, 2009.
85. La Spada AR, Wilson EM, Lubahn DB, et al: Androgen receptor gene mutations in X-linked spinal and bulbar muscular atrophy, *Nature* 352(6330):77–79, 1991.
86. Laaksovirta H, Peuralinna T, Schymick JC, et al: Chromosome 9p21 in amyotrophic lateral sclerosis in Finland: a genome-wide association study, *Lancet Neurol* 9(10):978–985, 2010.
89. Lefebvre S, Bürglen L, Reboullet S, et al: Identification and characterization of a spinal muscular atrophy-determining gene, *Cell* 80(1):155–165, 1995.
97. Meyer K, Ferraiuolo L, Miranda CJ, et al: Direct conversion of patient fibroblasts demonstrates non-cell autonomous toxicity of astrocytes to motor neurons in familial and sporadic ALS, *Proc Natl Acad Sci U S A* 111(2):829–832, 2014.
99. Miller RG, Jackson CE, Kasarskis EJ, et al: Practice parameter update: the care of the patient with amyotrophic lateral sclerosis: multidisciplinary care, symptom management, and cognitive/behavioral impairment (an evidence-based review): report of the Quality Standards Subcommittee of the American Academy of Neurology, *Neurology* 73(15):1227–1233, 2009.
100. Miller RG, Rosenberg JA, Gelinas DF, et al: Practice parameter: the care of the patient with amyotrophic lateral sclerosis (an evidence-based review): report of the Quality Standards Subcommittee of the American Academy of Neurology: ALS Practice Parameters Task Force, *Neurology* 52(7):1311–1323, 1999.
101. Miller TM, Pestronk A, David W, et al: An antisense oligonucleotide against *SOD1* delivered intrathecally for patients with *SOD1* familial amyotrophic lateral sclerosis: a phase 1, randomised, first-in-man study, *Lancet Neurol* 12(5):435–442, 2013.
107. Murphy J: Communication strategies of people with ALS and their partners, *Amyotroph Lateral Scler Other Motor Neuron Disord* 5(2):121–126, 2004.
111. Norris F, Shepherd R, Denys E, et al: Onset, natural history and outcome in idiopathic adult motor neuron disease, *J Neurol Sci* 118(1):48–55, 1993.
119. Piepers S, van den Berg LH, Brugman F, et al: A natural history study of late onset spinal muscular atrophy types 3b and 4, *J Neurol* 255(9):1400–1404, 2008.
122. Prior TW, Snyder PJ, Rink BD, et al: Newborn and carrier screening for spinal muscular atrophy, *Am J Med Genet A* 152A(7):1608–1616, 2010.
123. Renton AE, Majounie E, Waite A, et al: A hexanucleotide repeat expansion in *C9ORF72* is the cause of chromosome 9p21-linked ALS-FTD, *Neuron* 72(2):257–268, 2011.
125. Rosen DR, Siddique T, Patterson D, et al: Mutations in *Cu/Zn superoxide dismutase* gene are associated with familial amyotrophic lateral sclerosis, *Nature* 362(6415):59–62, 1993.
128. Sejvar JJ, Haddad MB, Tierney BC, et al: Neurologic manifestations and outcome of West Nile virus infection, *JAMA* 290(4):511–515, 2003.
130. Simmons Z: Management strategies for patients with amyotrophic lateral sclerosis from diagnosis through death, *Neurologist* 11(5):257–270, 2005.
132. Singer MA, Kojan S, Barohn RJ, et al: Primary lateral sclerosis, *Muscle Nerve* 35(3):291–302, 2007.
135. Swoboda KJ, Prior TW, Scott CB, et al: Natural history of denervation in SMA: relation to age, *SMN2* copy number, and function, *Ann Neurol* 57(5):704–712, 2005.
140. Traynor BJ, Codd MB, Corr B, et al: Amyotrophic lateral sclerosis mimic syndromes: a population-based study, *Arch Neurol* 57(1):109–113, 2000.
148. Zerres K, Rudnik-Schoneborn S: Natural history in proximal spinal muscular atrophy. Clinical analysis of 445 patients and suggestions for a modification of existing classifications, *Arch Neurol* 52(5):518–523, 1995.

The full reference list for this chapter is available online.

CHAPTER 41

REHABILITATION OF PATIENTS WITH NEUROPATHIES

Anita Craig, James K. Richardson, Rita Ayyangar

Disorders of the peripheral nervous system are common but are often a challenge to diagnose. Further, inaccurate diagnosis often leads to incremental anxiety for patient and health care practitioner. Given the physiatrist's electrophysiologic expertise and familiarity with musculoskeletal syndromes, which often mimic or accompany peripheral neurologic diseases, physicians in physical medicine and rehabilitation are ideally positioned to accurately diagnose peripheral neuropathies and provide rational advice regarding prognosis and therapy. Peripheral nerve disorders also often accompany, as well as complicate, rehabilitation diagnoses. For example, patients with stroke and spinal cord injury can develop nerve compression syndromes from overuse in their less impaired limbs. Familiarity with the peripheral nerves and their areas of vulnerability is critical in identifying injuries that may accompany severe musculoskeletal trauma and surgical interventions. Conversely, peripheral neurologic disease can predispose to musculoskeletal disorders such as rotator cuff dysfunction in the setting of a C5/C6 radiculopathy. Although most focal disorders of the peripheral nervous system do not affect mortality or longevity, they clearly affect quality of life and function in work and daily living. This makes their diagnosis and effective treatment worthy goals. In contrast, the systemic neuropathies not only influence function and quality of life but also are usually signs of an underlying disease process that demands diagnosis and treatment. When the generalized peripheral neurologic disorder is also the presenting manifestation of the underlying disease, accurate diagnosis of the neuropathy can influence quantity and quality of life. The patient is well served when the physiatrist has a solid understanding of the diagnosis and treatment of peripheral neurologic disorders.

Anatomy and Physiology

The peripheral nervous system is made up of 12 cranial nerves and 31 spinal nerves, which innervate specific sensory distributions (dermatomes) (Figure 41-1) and muscle groups (myotomes). In the cervical and lumbosacral regions, the spinal nerves intermingle to create plexuses, which then form individual peripheral nerves. In disease, the distribution of motor and sensory abnormalities characterizes particular spinal nerve, plexus, or peripheral nerve disorders.

The basic neural structure is the neuron and its associated axon, or nerve fiber. The axon is enclosed within a Schwann cell. A Schwann cell can encircle multiple axons, in which case they are referred to as unmyelinated. An axon that is invested solely by a Schwann cell wrapping around it several times is known as a myelinated fiber. The myelinated axon is invested by a series of Schwann cells that are separated by small sections of uncovered axon known as nodes of Ranvier (Figure 41-2). Nerve depolarization "jumps" from node to node, a process known as salutatory conduction. Impulse propagation in this manner is far more rapid (50 to 60 m/s) than that in unmyelinated axons (1 to 2 m/s).

Each nerve fiber and its associated Schwann cells are surrounded by an endoneurium. Several of these axons are grouped together in fascicles that are enclosed in a perineurium (although individual axons can cross from one fascicle to another along the course of a nerve). The fascicles are bundled together within the epineurium, which sheaths the entire peripheral nerve (Figure 41-3).

Classification of Neuropathies

Pathology of the peripheral nervous system can be caused by generalized processes or focal injury, or a combination of the two. Generalized neuropathies are typically caused by systemic processes that are often toxic, metabolic, or immunologic in nature. Focal neuropathies are usually the result of localized compression, traction, or trauma to a specific nerve.

Generalized peripheral neuropathies can be characterized by their location along three major axes based on whether the process affects (1) the axon (axonal) or the myelin (demyelinating) or has features of both; (2) the motor or sensory fibers; or (3) the peripheral nerves in a symmetrical fashion, typically in a distal to proximal gradient, or in an asymmetrical or multifocal pattern (Box 41-1). Neuropathies can also preferentially affect specific nerve types, such as large fiber or small fibers, the latter often including autonomic involvement. For example, alcoholic neuropathy tends to be predominantly axonal, sensorimotor, and symmetrical, whereas classic Guillain-Barré syndrome (GBS) is demyelinating, with greater motor than sensory involvement and a multifocal pattern.

Localized nerve injuries, or mononeuropathies, are classified by the degree of axonal and supporting structure involvement. The main classification schemes are the Seddon system[143] and the Sunderland system.[155] Neurapraxia in the Seddon system refers to focal injury to the myelin causing conduction block without axonal injury. Axonotmesis in the Seddon system refers to axonal damage with resultant Wallerian degeneration, but with the supporting endoneurium and perineurium still intact. Neurotmesis is the most severe insult and involves injury to the

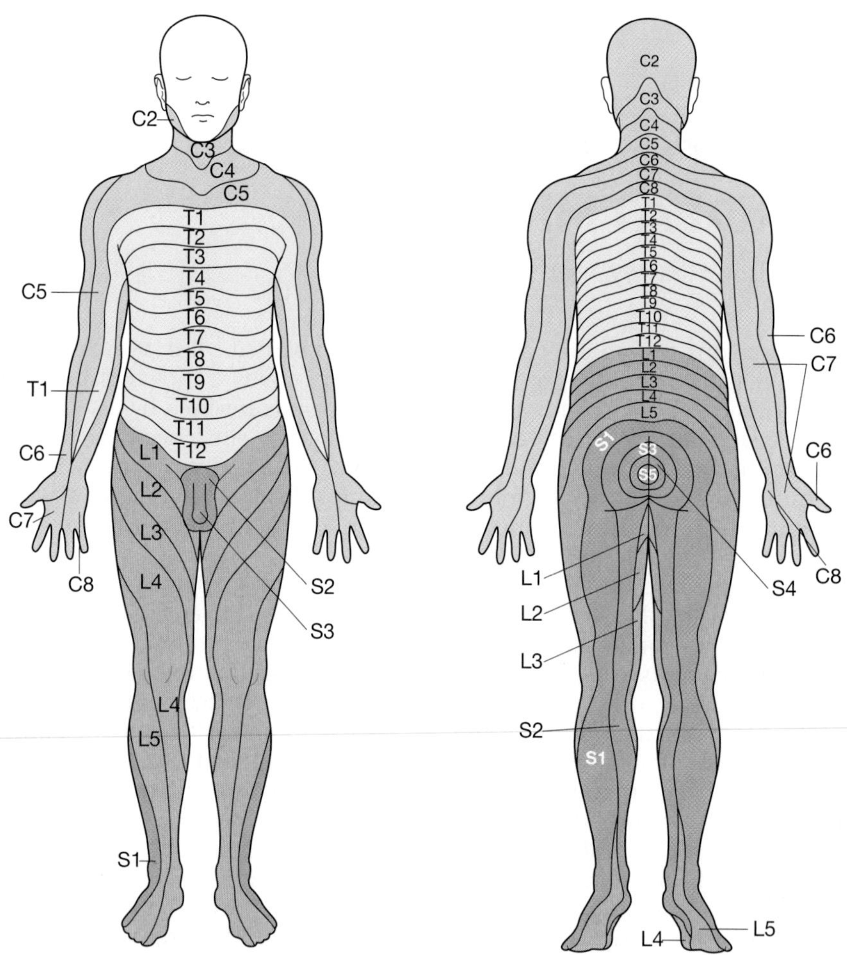

FIGURE 41-1 Dermatomal innervation of spinal nerves. (Modified from Hockberger RS, Kaji AH: Spinal injuries. In Marx JA editor: *Rosen's emergency medicine* ed 6. Philadelphia, PA, 2006, Mosby.)[69]

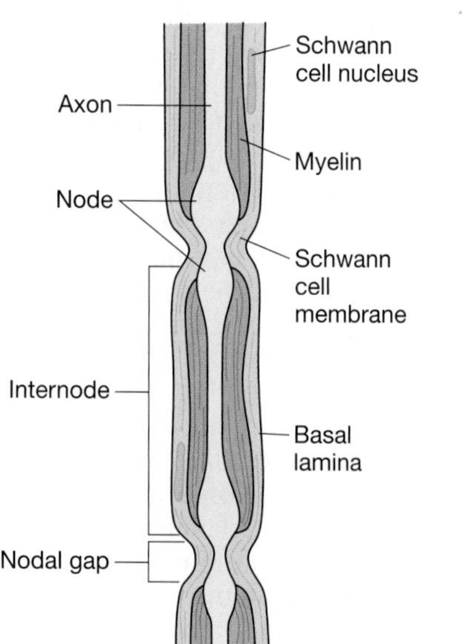

FIGURE 41-2 Myelinated axon invested by Schwann cells separated by nodes of Ranvier. (Modified from Jobe MT, Martinez SF: Peripheral nerve injury. In: Canale ST, Beaty JH, editors: *Campbell's operative orthopaedics,* ed 11. Philadelphia, PA, 2009, Mosby.)[80]

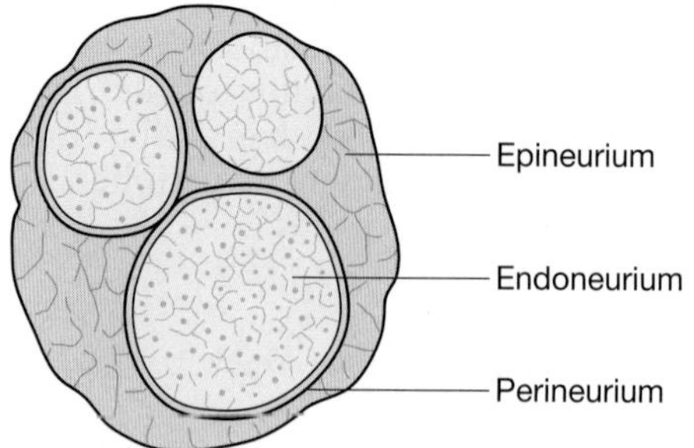

FIGURE 41-3 Anatomy of a nerve. Each axon is surrounded and associated Schwann cell enclosed by endoneurium. Multiple axons grouped in fascicles surrounded by perineurium. Fascicles are enclosed in epineurium to form the peripheral nerve. (Modified from Miller RD: Anatomy of the peripheral nerve. In Miller RD, editor: *Miller's anesthesia,* ed 6. Philadelphia, PA, 2005, Elsevier.)[108]

BOX 41-1

Classification of Peripheral Neuropathies and Common Etiologies

Demyelinating Mixed Sensory and Motor, Diffuse
- Hereditary motor and sensory neuropathies (1,3, and 4)

Demyelinating Mixed Sensory and Axonal, Multifocal
- Acute inflammatory demyelinating polyneuropathy (AIDP)
- Chronic inflammatory demyelinating polyneuropathy (CIDP)
- Leprosy

Demyelinating Motor > Sensory, Multifocal
- Multifocal motor neuropathy

Axonal, Mixed Motor, and Sensory, Diffuse
- Alcohol neuropathy
- Acquired immune deficiency syndrome (AIDS) neuropathy
- Amiodarone

Axonal, Mixed Motor and Sensory, Multifocal
- Mononeuritis multiplex

Axonal, Motor > Sensory, Diffuse
- Lead neuropathy
- Dapsone toxicity
- Hereditary motor and sensory neuropathies (HMSN) type 2 and 5

Axonal, Motor > Sensory, Multifocal
- Axonal Guillain-Barré
- Porphyria
- Diabetic amyotrophy

Axonal, Sensory > Motor, Diffuse
- Carcinomatous neuropathies (oat cell)
- Vitamin B_6 toxicity
- Vitamin E deficiency
- Drugs: vincristine, cisplatin, isoniazid

Axonal, Sensory > Motor, Multifocal
- Miller Fisher variant of AIDP
- Sjögren syndrome

Axonal and Demyelinating, Motor and Sensory, Diffuse
- Diabetes
- Uremia

axon, myelin, and supporting structures of the nerve (typically the nerve is no longer in anatomic continuity). In the Sunderland system, first-degree injury and second-degree injury correspond to neurapraxia and axonotmesis, respectively. The Sunderland system subdivides neurotmesis into third-degree injury (which involves the axon and endoneurium), fourth-degree injury (which affects the perineurium as well), and fifth-degree injury (which reflects damage to all supporting structures of the nerve) (Table 41-1).

Table 41-1 Classification of Nerve Injury: Seddon and Sunderland Systems

Seddon	Sunderland	Description
Neurapraxia	First-degree	Focal conduction block without axonal damage
Axonotmesis	Second-degree	Axon damage with Wallerian degeneration, supporting structures intact
Neurotmesis	Third-degree	Damage to axon and endoneurium
	Fourth-degree	Damage to perineurium and endoneurium
	Fifth-degree	Damage to axon and all supporting structures

Evaluation of Generalized Neuropathies

Overview

The goal of the evaluation is to develop a description of the neuropathy, with reference to the three axes described above. If this is achieved, then the likelihood that a specific etiologic diagnosis can be determined is markedly enhanced.

History

Evaluation of neuropathies begins with a detailed history of symptoms, functional impairments, medical comorbidities, and family history. Detailed characteristics of the symptoms should be elicited, including duration, rate of progression, and distribution. Symptoms can involve a variety of sensory modalities, such as pain, pressure, proprioception, and temperature. Pain is prominent in small fiber neuropathies, whereas sensory symptoms are rarely significant in those with hereditary neuropathies. In contrast to these "positive" symptoms, some patients might describe "negative" symptoms; that is, they have an awareness of the absence of sensation. Such patients might describe their feet as feeling like "wood" or that the plantar surface of their feet feels indistinct when walking. Motor symptoms might be more easily overlooked by the patient but can manifest as gait difficulties or a decrease in fine motor skills. Impaired balance (and even falls) can be the initial presenting complaint and has significant functional consequences. In fact any patient, particularly the older adult, who presents with repeated falls or an injury associated with a fall, warrants a careful clinical examination for peripheral neuropathy (PN). Children with neuropathy often present because of the parents' concerns that they are not meeting normal developmental milestones. Older children may be noted to be clumsier than their peers or have difficulty with coordination and participation in normal childhood activities. Typically, children, particularly younger ones, do not express positive symptoms associated with PN. A slow, insidious onset would suggest an inherited neuropathy. A more acute or fluctuating course, particularly in an older child, favors an acquired neuropathy.

Neuropathies can be associated with many medical comorbidities, including diabetes, renal failure, and HIV. Possible toxic exposure should be investigated, as well as search for any medications that might be associated with neuropathy (Box 41-2). A careful family history might reveal known hereditary neuropathies or similar symptoms and findings, such as gait problems or pes cavus, suggesting a previously undiagnosed familial condition.

BOX 41-2

Medications Associated with Peripheral Neuropathy

Amiodarone	Hydralazine
Amitriptyline	Isoniazid
Chloramphenicol	Lithium
Cisplatin	Misonidazole
Colchicine	Nitrofurantoin
Dapsone	Phenytoin
Disulfiram	Pyridoxine
Halogenated hydroxyquinolones	Thalidomide
	Vincristine

BOX 41-3

Examination Findings Predictive of Electrodiagnostically Confirmed Peripheral Neuropathy

- Loss of Achilles reflex
- Perceive less than 8 of 10 movements at great toe
- Less than 8 seconds detection of 128-Hz tuning fork vibration at great toe

Physical Examination

A general inspection can reveal clues to the presence of a neuropathic condition. Atrophy might be noted, especially involving the intrinsic muscles of the hands and feet. Foot deformities, such as pes cavus, can be seen in those with hereditary neuropathies. Other foot deformities, such as hammer toes and even deformity and collapse of the midfoot architecture, are seen in advanced neuropathic disease. Autonomic dysfunction can result in decreased sweating and dry, cold feet. Small fiber neuropathy can result in increased blood flow and "hot foot." Skin lesions or ulceration might be seen in an insensate foot. Fasciculations are occasionally observed.

Sensory testing should assess multiple sensory modalities with attention paid to the distribution of abnormalities, particularly the presence of a distal to proximal gradient if a diffuse process is suspected. Light touch (with a 10-gauge monofilament), pinprick, proprioception, and vibratory sensation should be evaluated. Proprioception can be tested by assessing the patient's ability to perceive 8 to 10 small (1-cm) movements at the great toe. Vibration is assessed with a 128-Hz tuning fork placed at the great toe. In those with pure small fiber neuropathies, pinprick and temperature sensation are usually affected, although large fiber-mediated proprioception and vibration can be relatively preserved.

Muscle stretch reflexes are diminished in a distal to proximal gradient in the setting of a symmetrical neuropathy although deviation from this pattern suggests a multifocal process. The Achilles reflex is the most commonly affected in a diffuse neuropathy and can be obtained either by direct percussion over the tendon or by plantar strike technique, which might be more reliable in older persons. Facilitation might be needed, such as gentle plantar flexion. Distinguishing the "normal" distal decrement in neuromuscular function associated with aging from that resulting from disease can be difficult. The physical findings that are predictive of electrodiagnostic confirmation of PN in this population is loss of the Achilles reflex, inability to perceive at least 8 of 10, 0.5- to 1.0-cm movements, or inability to detect a vibrating 128-Hz tuning fork for at least 8 seconds at the great toe[126] (Box 41-3).

Motor deficits can also be found in a distal to proximal gradient or in a multifocal distribution, and are often characterized by easy fatigability. Detection of weakness might be improved by testing the muscle in question multiple consecutive times. Pain, poor cooperation, and poor understanding of instruction can interfere with full muscular effort. In such circumstances, the examination is augmented by observing the patient performing functional tasks. For example, unipedal stance time is a sensitive test of balance impairment. Not only is a markedly decreased unipedal stance time associated with a diffuse PN in young and middle-aged men,[74] but unipedal stance time also strongly correlates with frontal plane sensory and motor function at the ankle among older persons with neuropathy.[60,151] Clinicians should observe the patient walking and look carefully for increased variability of lateral foot placement and frank crossover steps. These suggest instability during single-limb stance and increase the risk of foot collisions during ambulation. The distal upper extremity sensorimotor function can be evaluated by assessing the ability to do fine motor tasks, such as buttoning a shirt without visual input.

Careful observation of the distribution of motor and sensory deficits can offer clues to the nature of the neuropathy and where it lies on the three axes. For example, weakness without significant atrophy can suggest a demyelinating etiology, whereas atrophy in proportion to the weakness is more consistent with a primarily axonal neuropathy. The relative impairments in sensory compared with motor function provide clues to the second axis, and the presence of side-to-side asymmetries and/or proximal sensorimotor dysfunction greater than distal suggests a multifocal rather than diffuse neuropathy. These features can then be delineated further with electrodiagnostic testing.

Electrodiagnostic Studies

Electrodiagnostic studies quantify and refine what is learned after a thorough physical examination and are useful in detecting, characterizing, and assessing the severity of PN. Sensory nerve conduction studies assess the number of axons excited and the speed of conduction of the axons. The amplitude, measured from baseline to peak, correlates with the number of axons excited, and a decrement usually suggests axon loss. In a demyelinating process, dyssynchrony of the axons measured can cause temporal dispersion of the sensory response, with decreased amplitude without true axon loss. Reduced sensory amplitude with relatively normal distal latency and conduction velocity suggests axon loss. If the sensory nerve response is completely absent, it is not possible to characterize whether it is an axonal or demyelinating process; consequently an intact sensory response elsewhere should be sought.

Motor nerve conduction studies assess the amplitude of the compound muscle action potential (CMAP), distal latency, and conduction velocity with proximal and distal stimulation sites. Reduction in CMAP usually reflects axon loss; however, it can also be seen when stimulating across areas of demyelination. Focal demyelination can be found by stimulation proximal and distal to the site, with stimulation at the proximal site resulting in lower amplitude, temporal dispersion, and conduction slowing compared with the distal site. In severe demyelination the action potential can fail to conduct entirely, which is referred to as conduction block. Acquired demyelinating neuropathies often present with nonuniform demyelination and focal conduction block, whereas hereditary neuropathies usually result in uniform demyelination but without focal block. Late responses (F waves) are useful for assessing more proximal segments and can be particularly sensitive for demyelinating processes, such as early GBS.

Neuropathies caused by demyelinating processes will demonstrate prolonged distal and F wave latency, slowed conduction velocity, and conduction block (see Box 41-4 for demyelinating criteria). Amplitudes are generally preserved, although some decrease can be seen as a result of conduction block. Axonal neuropathies will result in amplitude loss without significant prolongation of distal latency or conduction slowing; however, loss of the fastest conducting fibers often results in mild slowing.

Although nerve conduction studies are the most useful component of the electrodiagnostic examination in the evaluation of neuropathies, it is important to be attentive to their limitations. For example, nerve conduction studies predominantly test large fiber nerves and so will likely be unrevealing in pure small fiber neuropathies. It is also important to be aware of conditions that can distort the results, such as limb temperature, superimposed focal neuropathies such as carpal tunnel syndrome (CTS), and chronic pressure on foot intrinsic muscles caused by shoes or distorted foot anatomy. Studies should assess at least one motor and one sensory nerve in the upper and lower limb. If abnormalities are found, the contralateral side should be examined to document symmetry. If a multifocal neuropathy is suggested from history and physical examination, a more extensive study is required, assessing the clinically affected nerves. Late responses (F waves) should be obtained, particularly if a demyelinating process is suspected. If a mild distal neuropathy is clinically suspected but sural sensory responses are normal, the plantar sensory responses might reveal abnormalities.[1]

Needle electromyography (EMG) is typically normal in purely demyelinating processes; however, when axonal involvement positive waves and fibrillation potentials are seen, ongoing axon loss and denervation of the sampled muscle are indicated. If the denervating process is slow, collateral sprouting can keep pace with the axon loss, and little spontaneous activity may be appreciated. In that setting voluntary motor unit changes occur, reflecting the process of collateral sprouting reinnervating affected motor units. Initially decreased recruitment is seen as the motor units are lost. As collateral sprouting begins, the motor unit shows increased duration and polyphasia as a result of the dyssynchronous conduction along poorly myelinated, immature sprouts. As the remodeled motor unit matures, an increase in motor unit amplitude is seen. Proximal and distal muscles in the upper and lower limbs, as well as clinically weak muscles, should be evaluated. If an abnormality is found, the contralateral muscle should be assessed to document symmetry. A distal to proximal gradient of abnormalities is seen in diffuse neuropathies. In a suspected multifocal neuropathy, the clinically affected muscles, as guided by a detailed physical examination, should be well sampled. In purely demyelinating neuropathies, the needle examination is normal, although decreased recruitment can result from conduction block.

BOX 41-4

Electrodiagnostic Criteria for Demyelinating Peripheral Neuropathy[2]

- Conduction velocity slowed to <80% of the lower limit of normal (LLN) if the compound muscle activated potential (CMAP) is more than >80% of LLN and <70% if CMAP is <70% of lower limit of normal (LLN)
- Distal latency is prolonged more than 125% of the upper limit of normal (ULN) if CMAP is >80% of LLN and more than 150% of ULN if CMAP is <80% of LLN
- F wave latency more than 120% of ULN if CMAP amplitude was >80% of LLN and more than 150% of ULN if CMAP is <80% of LLN, or absence of F wave response
- Partial conduction block with a >30% decrease in amplitude between stimulation of proximal and distal sites.

Complications of Neuropathies

Foot Complications

Foot ulceration is a major complication in patients with PN, particularly in those with diabetes mellitus, who manifest a lifetime risk of 15%.[51] The presence of neuropathy is associated with an 8- to 18-fold increased risk of foot ulcer and a 2- to 15-fold greater risk of amputation.[115] Loss of protective sensation in PN can lead to unrecognized foot trauma and skin breakdown. Motor neuropathy causes muscle atrophy and weakness, distorting normal foot architecture, and leads to abnormal pressure distribution and overloaded plantar areas.

Autonomic dysfunction causes decreased sweating, resulting in skin dryness and cracking, further compromising skin integrity. The detrimental impact of autonomic dysfunction is accentuated by arteriovenous shunting, which leads to alteration of perfusion with secondary osteopenia caused by bone resorption and impaired healing. In addition to skin breakdown, neuropathy can also lead to Charcot changes. Charcot neuroarthropathy is characterized by destruction of the joints of the foot, with pathologic fracture and joint dislocation often in the midfoot region. It can result in severe deformity (Figure 41-4).

Patients with neuropathy should be educated on the importance of daily inspection of their feet using a mirror. Properly protective socks and appropriate shoe wear, including extra depth toe boxes and custom orthoses, should be used to offload high pressure areas. Feet should be kept dry and the skin well moisturized, with caution to

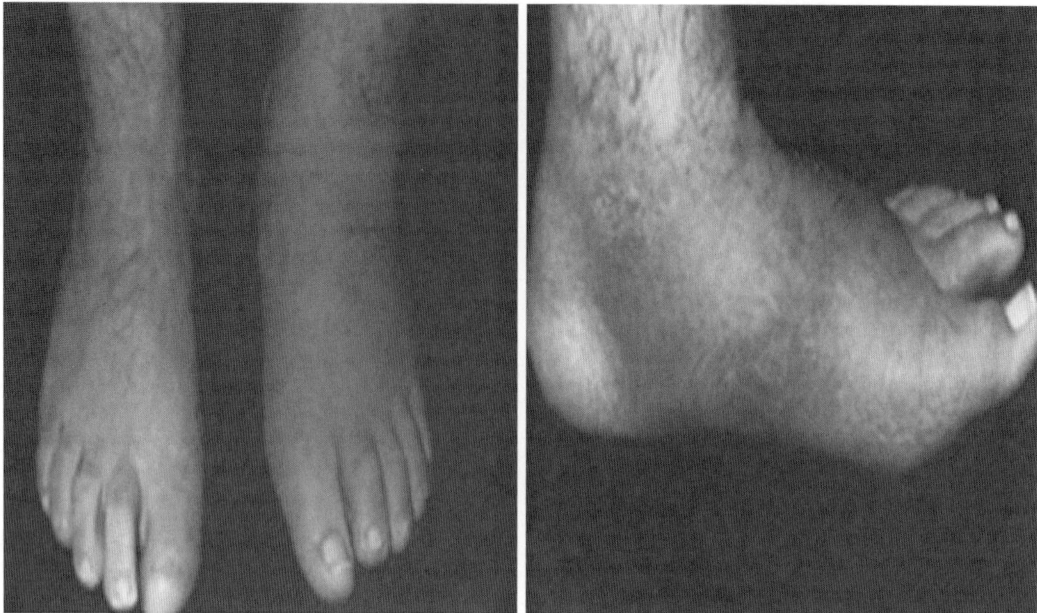

FIGURE 41-4 **Charcot neuropathy causing pathologic fracture, dislocation, and deformity of the midfoot.** (From Ishikawa SN: Diabetic foot. In Canale ST, Beaty JH, editors: *Campbell's operative orthopaedics*, ed 11. Philadelphia, PA, 2009, Mosby.)[75]

avoid extreme temperatures, particularly hot water. Nail care and callus management are important and might necessitate care by a podiatrist or diabetic foot clinic. Prompt management of skin breakdown and aggressive management of infection are important to avoid progression to amputation. Acute Charcot foot can present similarly to cellulitis, as a warm, erythematous, and swollen foot. Radiographs can be normal acutely, before showing the fractures and joint dislocation later in the course of the disease. The bone scan, however, is often positive early. Strict immobilization with a total contact cast is used to manage acute Charcot arthropathy. Immobilization is maintained until clinical signs of warmth and tenderness have significantly decreased and the bone scan has negative findings is or less active, indicating that bone remodeling is near complete. At this point careful weaning from the orthosis can begin. This is often done in association with physical therapy with a gradual resumption of weight bearing and strengthening foot and ankle musculature. Prevention and treatment programs can significantly reduce lower extremity breakdowns and amputations.

Pain

Neuropathic pain is common and can be incapacitating. Large fiber neuropathies often manifest with dull, deep, toothache-like, or cramping pain. Small fiber neuropathies affect small unmyelinated C fibers that control thermal perception, pain, and autonomic function, and frequently initially manifest with significant pain in the feet. Small fiber neuropathy is commonly perceived as superficial, burning, and hypersensitive. Other sources of foot pain should be considered and excluded before treatment of presumed neuropathic pain occurs. Among the alternative diagnoses for painful feet are lumbar radiculopathy, vascular claudication, tarsal tunnel syndrome, plantar fasciitis, osteoarthritis, and Morton neuroma. It should also be kept in mind that each of these diagnoses can coexist with symptomatic painful neuropathy.

Treatment of neuropathic pain can be challenging, and the side effects of the medications used can be problematic, particularly in older patients. A topical agent such as capsaicin cream has the advantage of having no systemic side effects, but its use can be cumbersome (requiring application 3 to 4 times/day) and can cause initial irritation. Transdermal lidocaine patches are more easily applied and can be useful in those with a relatively discrete distribution of pain. Transcutaneous electrical stimulation might also be of benefit. Tricyclic antidepressant medications were the first class of medications to show efficacy in the management of neuropathic pain. Amitriptyline use is limited by anticholinergic effects, including sedation, dry mouth, urinary retention, and orthostatic hypotension, as well as potentially dangerous arrhythmias. Low-dose nortriptyline, 10 to 50 mg at bedtime, might be better tolerated and has been shown to be equivalent to amitriptyline on some types of neuropathic pain[179] with fewer side effects. Gabapentin, at doses up to 3600 mg/day, has been shown to reduce pain.[144] Gabapentin can cause somnolence and dizziness, particularly on initiation of treatment. It can exacerbate gait and cognitive problems in older patients, but it is generally well tolerated and lacks significant drug-drug interactions. Gabapentin should be initiated at low doses, 100 to 300 mg at night, and slowly titrated up to 3 times a day. Duloxetine (Cymbalta) and pregabalin (Lyrica) are two newer drugs that have been approved by the United States Food and Drug Administration for the treatment of neuropathic pain. Duloxetine use can be limited by gastrointestinal side effects. Pregabalin, like gabapentin, can cause sedating and cognitive side effects. Tramadol has been shown to have beneficial effects on the allodynia associated with diabetic PN.[149] It binds to μ-opioid receptors and is a weak norepinephrine and serotonin reuptake inhibitor. Tramadol can cause cognitive impairment, and serotonin syndrome might occur with concomitant use of other serotonergic medications. Opioid analgesics have been shown to improve pain and sleep but not function or mood.[124] Because opioids can cause cognitive side effects, physiologic dependency, and addiction, they should be used judiciously. Second-line medications for the treatment of neuropathic pain include lamotrigine, carbamazepine, other selective serotonin reuptake inhibitors, and clonidine.

Functional Impairment

Peripheral neuropathy can have significant impact on functional mobility and quality of life. Patients with PN are approximately 20 times more likely to fall than those without neuropathy.[128,133] Neuropathy impairs proprioceptive sensation at the ankle, and those with neuropathy are less able to rapidly develop ankle torque to correct for lateral lean.[60] Therefore, patients with neuropathy are doubly penalized when their center of mass is displaced as a relatively greater displacement occurs before loss of balance is perceived, and then there is a delay in corrective ankle torque generation. As a result, the patient with neuropathy experiences dynamic postural instability, particularly on uneven surfaces and in dim lighting, where visual cues cannot assist in compensating for proprioceptive loss. Both a perceived and real risk of instability can lead to increasingly limited physical activity, physical deconditioning, isolation, and depression.[10,174]

Although neuropathy-related impairments in ankle sensory and motor function have been recognized for some time and can be accurately estimated with the fibular motor amplitude recording at the extensor digitorum brevis,[127] an understanding of the relationship between suboptimal distal neuromuscular function and proximal strength has only recently developed. It appears that the ratio of proximal strength at the hip to ankle proprioceptive precision predicts unipedal stance time[6] (Figure 41-5), falls, and fall-related injury in older patients with diabetic neuropathy.[129] Of interest, nether age nor neuropathy severity were predictors of these outcomes when the ratio was taken into account. The clinical relevance of the ratio relates to the concept that increased hip strength can compensate for imprecise ankle proprioceptive precision, and there is evidence to support this. Of note, patients with neuropathy caused by type 2 diabetes mellitus respond well to resistance training.[121] Aside from proximal strengthening, other interventions can improve gait and balance. Vision should be regularly tested, and corrective eyewear should be used as needed. Patients should consider using glasses for walking that correct distance vision only, because the use of bifocals has been independently associated with falls.[99] Patients should be taught to use proper lighting, particularly when getting up at night. Balance can be improved with proper shoes that have a wide base of support and thin soles. A cane can stabilize gait, but to achieve maximal benefit, patients should be able to support up to 25% of their body weight on the cane to prevent a fall.[7] The cane should be brought down with each contralateral footstep. Acceptance of the use of a cane can be improved if presented as a substitute for the loss of a special sense, much like eyeglasses, and used only as

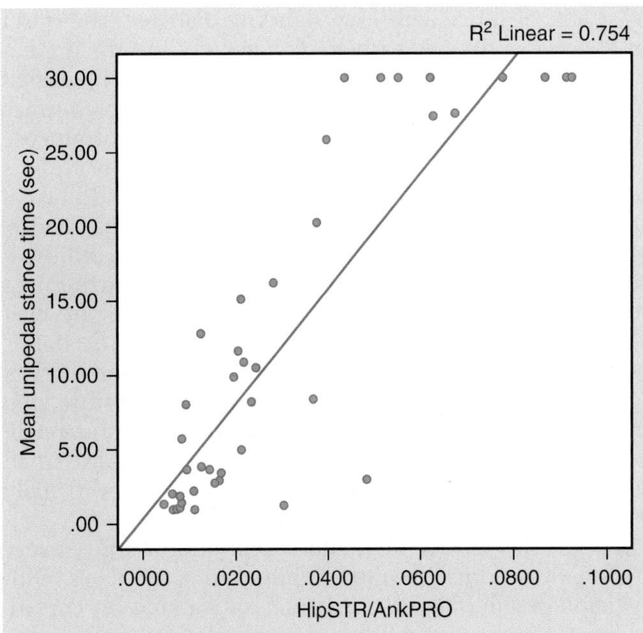

FIGURE 41-5 Scatterplots illustrating the relationship of hip to ankle proprioception to unipedal stance time.

needed on uneven surfaces and in unfamiliar areas. A disadvantage of canes, however, is that they can be associated with decreased walking speed. Use of ankle orthoses with medial and lateral support has been shown to improve gait and stability parameters.[136] They also have the advantages of allowing both hands to be free and better walking speed than a cane, but the skin in contact with the orthoses must be monitored for breakdown. A recent exercise trial involving older subjects with neuropathy demonstrated that Tai Chi and functional balance training showed improvement in clinical measurements of balance.[135,123] Specific exercises aimed at strengthening hip abductors and possibly more importantly the adductors and abdominals can improve frontal plane hip and trunk stability. Strengthening of grip, shoulder depression, and elbow extension can improve support when using a cane or other means of upper limb stabilization.

Specific Neuropathies

Diabetic Neuropathies

Diabetes is one of the most common causes of neuropathy. Neuropathy causes significant morbidity and mortality in diabetic patients and leads to more hospitalizations for diabetic patients than any other complication. Diabetes can cause a number of patterns of neuropathy. They can be classified into symmetrical, asymmetrical, and focal:

- Symmetrical: Chronic sensorimotor distal, acute sensory, autonomic
- Asymmetrical: Proximal motor
- Focal: Mononeuritis, entrapment neuropathies

Distal Symmetrical Sensorimotor Polyneuropathy

A distal symmetrical sensorimotor polyneuropathy is the most common type of diabetic neuropathy and affects at least half of those with long-standing diabetes. The onset of PN may occur very early in diabetes, even in the prediabetic state. Impaired glucose tolerance has been identified in up to 56% of patients with idiopathic PN, three times the prevalence of matched controls with normal glucose tolerance.[150] A major risk factor for development of PN is the severity and duration of hyperglycemia.[55] Additional risk factors include hypertension, elevated triglycerides, tobacco use, obesity, microvascular disease, and cardiovascular disease.[158] Onset is usually insidious, occurring first in the toes and forefeet and progressing proximally over time. Symptoms are usually only perceived in the hands when the lower limb symptoms have reached the level of the knees. If upper limb symptoms develop before that time, then an entrapment neuropathy should be suspected. Most patients have involvement of both large and small nerve fibers, although large fiber involvement usually predominates.

Large fiber involvement affects both motor and sensory nerves. Symptoms are often minimal in early stages, with patients describing odd sensations of walking on cotton, vague unsteadiness, or difficulty manipulating small objects such as buttons. Pain is less frequent but when present is described as a dull, cramping ache. Often these complaints are only elicited with a specific inquiry. Physical examination often reveals abnormalities before symptoms are perceived. Decreased vibratory sensation and position sense loss are some of the earliest findings, along with depressed Achilles reflexes. The use of a tuning fork for detection of vibratory sensation loss can detect neuropathy even when monofilament testing is normal.[114] Muscle wasting, particularly of the intrinsic foot muscles, is found as the neuropathy progresses. Electrodiagnostic studies can demonstrate findings consistent with both axon loss and demyelination. Sensory abnormalities usually occur first, with the sural sensory studies showing the earliest changes on routine studies. If suspicion is high in a patient younger than 60, however, medial plantar nerve conduction studies may be more sensitive given the abnormalities' more distal location.[1] Motor nerve conduction abnormalities occur later in the course of the disease. EMG needle examination typically shows neuropathic abnormalities in a symmetrical pattern, with a distal to proximal gradient. This often occurs before there is any clinical weakness, although quantified strength testing often demonstrates reduced strength. With regard to the three descriptive axes mentioned previously, diabetic neuropathy is symmetrical, with features of both demyelination and axon loss and sensory greater than motor involvement.

Involvement of small unmyelinated C fibers can occur early in diabetes and presents with significant pain and hyperalgesia. Later there is loss of thermal sensation and autonomic abnormalities, with loss of sweating, dry feet, and vasomotor changes. This leads to increased risk of foot ulceration and infections. Later in the course of the neuropathy the pain might subside, but this is a sign of progression rather than regression of the disease. When small fiber disease occurs in isolation from large fiber involvement, there can be minimal physical examination findings despite significant symptoms. Additionally, electrodiagnostic studies are not as sensitive for small fiber nerves and can be normal.[70] Galvanic skin responses might be abnormal but are unreliable. Skin biopsy can be definitive, with quantification of small fibers, but it is not done routinely. Management of distal PN has been addressed previously; however, it is important to emphasize the role of controlling blood sugars to prevent diabetic PN. Strict glycemic control is shown to reduce the prevalence of PN by almost 70% and autonomic dysfunction by over 50%.[34] Tight glycemic control has not as yet been shown to reverse PN.[36,118] Therefore it is important to counsel patients with newly diagnosed type 2 diabetes about the importance of early initiation of good glycemic control to reduce risk of PN.

Proximal Neuropathy

Diabetic proximal neuropathy, also known by the term *diabetic amyotrophy*, is typically seen in older patients with type 2 diabetes. It classically presents acutely or subacutely with severe pain that is unilateral or bilateral. The pain tends to attenuate over weeks to months, an event often accompanied by marked atrophy of the thigh muscles; particularly the quadriceps, adductors, and iliopsoas, with relative sparing of gluteal and hamstring muscles. Sensory abnormalities are seen in the femoral distribution and sometimes in the saphenous distribution. Patients with diabetes can also develop proximal neuropathy affecting the thoracic dermatomes, presenting with severe abdominal or chest pain, associated with weight loss, often prompting concern for malignancy. Proximal diabetic neuropathy is almost invariably seen in diabetic patients with preexisting distal neuropathy. A variant of this condition can present with acute and debilitating pain in a younger patient with early, mild diabetes (or previously undiagnosed diabetes), with no evidence of distal neuropathy. Electrodiagnostic studies reveal a pattern of lumbosacral plexopathy sometimes combined with multilevel radiculopathy on EMG needle examination. Femoral nerve conductions reveal predominantly axonal involvement, with reduced CMAP but relatively spared distal latency. Distal nerve conduction studies often show evidence of a concomitant distal neuropathy, even in patients without clinical complaints of distal neuropathic symptoms. The mechanism of injury is thought to be an immune-mediated microvasculitis affecting the nerve roots and plexus. Management of diabetic amyotrophy consists of tight glycemic control and aggressive management of neuropathic pain. Corticosteroids, plasmapheresis, and intravenous immunoglobulin (IVIG) have not been shown to be efficacious. Although extremely debilitating, the prognosis for improvement is good, with recovery typically occurring over a 12- to 24-month period.[160] Differential diagnosis includes spinal stenosis and chronic inflammatory demyelinating polyneuropathy (CIDP). Spinal stenosis is common in older adults, and although compression is most common at the L5 level, when occurring at higher levels it can mimic symptoms of diabetic amyotrophy. CIDP is also common in this age group, and it is important to diagnose because it is amenable to steroids, IVIG, plasmapheresis, and other immune-modulating agents.

Focal Mononeuropathies

Mononeuropathies typically occur in older individuals with diabetes and are usually acute in onset and associated with pain. Recovery is spontaneous and occurs over 6 to 8 weeks. Cranial nerves III, VI, and VII and median, ulnar, and peroneal nerves are most commonly affected, and the neuropathies are caused by microvascular infarction. Patients with diabetes are also predisposed to entrapment neuropathies at common sites, such as the median, ulnar, and peroneal nerves. Carpal tunnel syndrome is 3 times more common in individuals with diabetes than in the general population.[84]

Autonomic Neuropathy

Diabetic autonomic neuropathy is a significant cause of morbidity and even mortality in persons with diabetes. This can affect the cardiovascular, gastrointestinal, genitourinary, and thermoregulatory systems.

Involvement of the cardiovascular system limits activity tolerance and can have life-threatening consequences. Patients with cardiac autonomic neuropathy have 40% greater mortality compared with those without.[79] Causes include silent ischemia, lethal arrhythmias, and prolongation of QT interval. Patient with cardiac involvement have resting tachycardia greater than 100 beats per min (bpm), orthostasis, and a decrease of systolic blood pressure greater than 20 mm Hg on standing, which occurs without appropriate heart rate response. This limits exercise tolerance and increases the risk of sudden death and silent myocardial ischemia. Both hypotension and hypertension can develop after exercise. Orthostasis is the most common clinical complaint in the setting of cardiac autonomic neuropathy. Initial management includes education regarding the need for slow postural changes, elevation of the head of the bed, and use of compression garments, such as compressive stockings and abdominal binders. If these are inadequate, mineralocorticoids such as fludrocortisone or the α-agonist midodrine can be used.

Autonomic dysfunction of the gastrointestinal system can lead to esophageal dysmotility, gastroparesis, constipation or diarrhea, and bowel incontinence.[17] Gastroparesis causes a sensation of bloating, nausea, heartburn, early satiety, and erratic glycemic control. These symptoms are typically managed with metoclopramide.

Diabetic autonomic neuropathy can lead to erectile dysfunction and is usually irreversible.[44] Treatment consists of assessing for secondary causes of erectile dysfunction, counseling, medications, suction erectile devices, and penile implants. Neurogenic bladder leads to overflow incontinence, recurrent urinary tract infection, and pyelonephritis. If retention is suspected, it can be diagnosed with postvoid residuals and might need more formal urodynamic studies to determine the severity. In mild cases the patient can be instructed to void every 2 to 3 hours while awake. In more severe cases, intermittent catheterization may be necessary.

Abnormalities in sweating and thermoregulation necessitate counseling about adequate hydration and caution with exertion in hot or cold environments. Lack of sweating can lead to dryness and cracking and fissuring of the feet, creating conditions susceptible to foot ulceration and infection. Patients should be taught to keep the feet well moisturized.

Guillain-Barré Syndrome

GBS was first described almost a century ago by French neurologists Guillain, Barré, and Strohl. With the eradication of polio, it is now the most common cause of acute neuromuscular paralysis in the Western world, with an annual incidence of 1 to 2 per 100,000.[122] GBS is a progressive, symmetrical weakness of the limbs, with hyporeflexia or areflexia, with or without sensory abnormalities. Maximal weakness occurs within 4 weeks, although typically peaks by 2 weeks. GBS is now recognized to be a group of disorders, with various subtypes. The most common is the acute demyelinating polyradiculoneuropathy (AIDP) affecting both motor and sensory nerves. This type accounts for 95% of all cases of GBS in Europe and North America.[63] Purely axonal forms are rare (<5%). They can occur as an acute motor axonal neuropathy (AMAN) or acute motor and sensory axonal neuropathy (AMSAN). The axonal forms of GBS are more common in Asia and South America, making up 30% of the cases in those populations.[116] The Miller Fisher variant is a triad of ataxia, areflexia, and ophthalmoplegia, although bulbar abnormalities, ptosis, facial weakness, and papillary dysfunction can be seen (Table 41-2).[49]

Clinical Features

GBS presents with progressive onset of limb weakness both proximally and distally that is typically symmetrical, with strength nadir in 2 to 4 weeks. Reflexes are typically lost early in the disease; although reflexes can be retained or even brisk with axonal forms.[91] Sensory loss is variable. The cranial nerves can be affected, with facial palsy and bulbar weakness. Muscles of respiration are frequently affected with decline of vital capacity and ventilatory support is required in 25% of cases. The autonomic system can be affected, causing tachycardia, hypertension, and cardiac arrhythmias. Pain can be a significant complaint and might even precede onset of clinical weakness. In the acute stages the pain is often described as deep and aching, affecting the back, buttocks, and posterior thighs. This might be caused by nociceptive pain from inflammation. Later neuropathic pain can be described with degeneration and regeneration of sensory nerves. Fatigue is a common complaint, even after good neurologic recovery from GBS. Amantadine and other pharmacologic agents have not been shown to help, but bicycle exercise training has been

Table 41-2 Variants of Acute Inflammatory Demyelinating Polyradiculoneuropathy

	Clinical Features	Antibodies
Acute inflammatory demyelinating polyradiculoneuropathy	Symmetrical weakness of all limbs Hyporeflexia, areflexia Mild sensory symptoms Respiratory involvement Facial nerve palsy	Anti-GM1
Axonal (AMAN, ASMAN)	Symmetrical weakness Reflexes may be normal or increased Variable sensory symptoms Respiratory involvement	Anti-GM1, GD1a, GalNac-GD1a
Miller Fisher	Ophthalmoplegia Ataxia Areflexia Minimal weakness	Anti-GQ1b

AMAN, Acute motor axonal neuropathy; *ASMAN*, acute motor sensory axonal neuropathy; *GalNac*, N-acetylgalactosaminyl.

shown to reduce fatigue and improve functional outcome and quality of life.[54]

Pathophysiology

Two thirds of patients with GBS have an antecedent infection with 3 weeks of onset of weakness. The most commonly identified infectious agent is *Campylobacter jejuni*. Other causative agents are cytomegalovirus (CMV), Epstein-Barr virus, *Mycoplasma pneumoniae*, and *Haemophilus influenzae*.[64] Studies of the swine flu vaccine during the 1976 epidemic demonstrated an increased risk of 1 excess case of GBS for every 100,000 people vaccinated.[141] Little strong evidence is known to link GBS with other vaccines, including newer influenza vaccines.[62] The strong association with antecedent infection suggests that at least in some cases there is an immune response to these infectious agents that triggers damage to peripheral nerves. The preceding infectious agent is also associated with the subtype of GBS that develops. Patients with *C. jejuni* infection are more likely to develop axonal forms of GBS, and those with CMV infections tend to have more cranial nerve, respiratory, and severe sensory involvement. Epstein-Barr virus infection usually confers milder disease.[122] The infectious agents share localized regions capable of eliciting an immune response (epitopes) with antigens in peripheral nerve tissue, triggering antibody-mediated damage to the peripheral nerves. Various antiganglioside antibodies have been identified in the subtypes of GBS. Nerves are affected at the root level initially, followed by distal segments, and the intervening areas later in the course of the disease.[11]

Diagnosis

Required clinical features for the diagnosis of GBS are progressive weakness in both arms and legs, and areflexia. Supportive features include progression of weakness over days to 4 weeks, symmetry of symptoms, mild sensory symptoms, cranial nerve involvement, autonomic involvement, pain (which can be prominent), high protein concentration in the cerebrospinal fluid (CSF), and typical electrodiagnostic findings. A number of features raise doubts about the diagnosis of GBS (Box 41-5).

Lumbar puncture is routinely performed in the workup of patients presenting with rapidly progressive weakness. In GBS the characteristic finding is an elevated CSF protein with normal white blood cell (WBC) count (<5 to 10 × 10⁶ cells/L), often referred to as albuminocytologic dissociation.

Electrodiagnostic testing is the most useful confirmatory test for GBS and can differentiate between the more common demyelinating form (AIDP) and axonal forms, AMAN, and AMSAN. Early in the course of AIDP, the nerve conduction studies can be normal. Because the nerve roots are typically affected first, prolongation of the F wave latencies are often the earliest abnormality seen as they measure conduction in the proximal nerve segments.[4] Nerve conduction studies demonstrate a demyelinating pattern with motor involvement occurring earlier and more extensively than sensory abnormalities. Sensory changes tend to be patchier in distribution, and median and ulnar sensory responses tend to be affected to a greater extent than the sural response. Temporal dispersion and partial conduction block, findings consistent with an acquired demyelinating disease, can be seen between proximal and distal stimulation sites. Needle examination typically shows decreased firing of motor units on maximal contraction. An axonal variant of GBS is suggested if there is significant reduction in CMAPs and early and significant findings of abnormal insertional activity on needle examination. CMAPs that fall below 20% of LLN predict poor functional outcome.[109] Electrodiagnostic findings usually lag behind clinical severity.

BOX 41-5

Features not Consistent with Guillain-Barré Syndrome

- Severe pulmonary involvement early, without significant weakness
- Bowel or bladder involvement at onset
- Severe sensory symptoms with minimal weakness
- Fever
- Well delineated sensory level
- Slow progression, limited weakness, no respiratory involvement
- Marked asymmetry
- Increased mononuclear cell in cerebrospinal fluid ($>50 \times 10^6$/L)
- Polymorphonuclear cells in cerebrospinal fluid

Management of Guillain-Barré Syndrome

Management of GBS consists of supportive care, disease-modifying treatment, and rehabilitation. Most patients require admission to the hospital for close monitoring. Mortality for GBS is 10%, with infections, pulmonary embolus, and cardiac arrhythmia the most common causes of death. Deep venous thrombosis prophylaxis should be initiated, particularly in nonambulatory patients. Vital capacity should be sequentially monitored every 2 to 4 hours initially, and mechanical ventilation should be initiated when vital capacity falls below 20 mL/kg.[94] Autonomic involvement can result in labile blood pressure and cardiac arrhythmias and can require monitoring in the intensive care unit. Serious bradyarrhythmias can develop, requiring atropine or transcutaneous pacemaker.[184] In some patients pain can be difficult to treat, requiring opioids, gabapentin, and other agents for this neuropathic pain. Prevention of pressure ulcers with proper positioning and turning, as well as range of motion and splinting to prevent contractures, should be instituted. Swallowing function should be monitored, particularly in those with signs of facial or bulbar involvement.

Immunotherapy has been proven to be of benefit in patients with GBS. Plasma exchange administered five times over the course of 2 weeks is beneficial when started within 4 weeks of onset of weakness but is most effective within the first 2 weeks.[59] IVIG has been shown to be as effective as plasma exchange[173] and is usually the preferred treatment because of greater convenience and availability. It is administered at 0.4 g/kg daily for 5 consecutive days. Combining plasma exchange and IVIG has not been shown to be superior to monotherapy.[120] Five to 10% of patients develop neurologic deterioration after initial improvement after treatment. It is common practice to administer a second course of IVIG in these patients. Oral or intravenous steroids have not been shown to be effective in altering the course or functional outcome of GBS.[73]

Rehabilitation of patients begins in the acute phase with prevention of contractures with proper range of motion, positioning, and splinting. Early mobilization as the patient's medical condition permits is essential in minimizing the effects of bed rest. Aggressive pulmonary hygiene reduces risk of atelectasis and pneumonia. The inpatient rehabilitation stage is usually initiated when immunotherapy has been completed, and the neurologic deterioration has reached its nadir. The patient should be autonomically stable. Pulmonary status should be stabilized, and the patient should either be weaned from the ventilator or transferred to a facility that has ventilator capabilities. Orthostasis is a common problem, and use of a tilt table to help overcome postural hypotension might be necessary before standing and gait training. Lower extremity orthoses are usually indicated when initiating ambulation. Functional and weight-training exercises are also used for upper extremity strengthening, and assistive devices might be needed for self-care activities. Exercise in GBS patients should be nonfatiguing because they can be prone to declines in strength if exercise is advanced too rapidly (particularly in muscles with less than antigravity strength).

Prognosis of GBS is typically good, especially given the often marked initial degree of weakness. Persistent disability, however, occurs in 20% of patients who will remain nonambulatory or require an assistive device to walk at 6 months.[72] Poor outcome is associated with advanced age, male gender, axonal involvement, antecedent diarrhea, and CMV infection.[122] Relapse is rare, at a rate of 3% to 5%.[64]

Chronic Inflammatory Demyelinating Polyneuropathy

The electrodiagnostic features of CIDP were first described in 1975[41]; however, since then, several variants have been recognized. CIDP is an immune-mediated disorder of the peripheral nervous system. The classic form of CIDP is symmetrical neuropathy that affects motor function predominantly, both proximally and distally. Variants include a multifocal, asymmetrical form and both a motor and symmetrical form known as Lewis-Sumner syndrome. Variants also exist that are purely sensory forms, as well as forms associated with IgG and IgA paraproteins, CNS demyelination, and various systemic disorders (Box 41-6). A number of conditions also are important to differentiate from CIDP variants, especially because they respond differently to treatment. These include multifocal motor neuropathy and IgM-related neuropathies such as POEMS (*p*olyneuropathy, *o*rganomegaly, *e*ndocrinopathy, *M* protein, and *s*kin changes).

Clinical Features

CIDP progression occurs over at least 2 months, a feature that differentiates it from GBS. Motor symptoms generally predominate, and both proximal and distal muscles are affected. Because CIDP is a primarily demyelinating disorder, muscle atrophy is not a significant feature. Muscle stretch reflexes are reduced or absent. Cranial involvement can occur in 10% to 20% of cases, and a small number of patients have painful dysesthesias. Sensory involvement typically affects large fiber nerves, consequently preferentially affecting vibration and proprioception. Sensory symptoms generally progress from distal to proximal, although hand involvement is often perceived as early as that in the feet. The classic course of CIDP is one of recurrence and remittance (polyphasic), a pattern that tends to occur in younger patients. Older adults are more likely to have a progressive form of CIDP (monophasic).[140] Given the low childhood prevalence of CIDP (0.5 per 100,000), best information about the disease may be obtained from a recent metaanalysis by McMillan et al.[105] Their report of a large cohort of 30 children and children from 11 other case studies (for a total number of 143) revealed that CIDP in children is relapsing in nature with a slow, chronic onset of symptoms (i.e., more than 8 weeks) and no gender predilection. A small number (20%) may have a subacute onset (4 to 8 weeks) or an acute "GBS-like" symptom onset before it eventually evolves into a relapsing form.

BOX 41-6

Chronic Inflammatory Demyelinating Polyneuropathy Variants

- Lewis-Sumner syndrome, multifocal acquired demyelinating sensory and motor neuropathy
- Demyelinating neuropathy associated with IgG or IgA gammopathy
- Sensory predominant demyelinating neuropathy
- Chronic inflammatory demyelinating polyneuropathy (CIDP) with central nervous system demyelination
- Demyelination associated with systemic disorder
- Diabetes mellitus
  - Systemic lupus erythematosus
  - Collagen vascular disorders
  - Human immunodeficiency virus (HIV) infection
  - Sarcoidosis
  - Thyroid disease
  - Chronic active hepatitis
  - Lymphoma
  - Organ and bone marrow transplant
  - Inflammatory bowel disease
  - Nephrotic syndrome
- CIDP in patients with hereditary neuropathy

Diagnosis

Electrodiagnostic studies are essential for confirmation of CIDP. Nerve conduction studies demonstrate primary demyelination in multiple segments. Findings consistent with demyelination include conduction block, conduction slowing that is greater than can be explained by axon loss, prolonged F wave and H reflex latencies, and temporal dispersion of CMAP between proximal and distal stimulation points. Sural nerve biopsy can show demyelination or findings pointing to other disorders that can mimic CIDP, such as vasculitis or amyloidosis. Because CIDP is multifocal and motor predominant, however, sural biopsy can be normal and therefore is not routinely done. Lumbar puncture will show albuminocytologic dissociation in 90% of patients. Magnetic resonance imaging (MRI) with

BOX 41-7

Clinical Criteria of Chronic Inflammatory Demyelinating Polyneuropathy

Typical

- Symmetrical proximal and distal weakness and sensory abnormalities in all extremities
- Reduced or absent reflexes
- Progressive over 2 months, stepwise or recurrent
- Cranial nerves may be affected

Atypical (One of the Following)

- Predominantly distal findings
- Pure motor or sensory presentation
- Asymmetrical presentation
- Focal presentations
- Central nervous system involvement

Diseases Commonly Associated with Chronic Inflammatory Demyelinating Polyneuropathy

- Diabetes mellitus
- IgG or IgA monoclonal gammopathy of undetermined significance
- IgM monoclonal gammopathy without antibodies to myelin-associated glycoprotein
- Systemic lupus erythematosus
- Other connective tissue diseases
- Human immunodeficiency virus (HIV) infection
- Sarcoidosis
- Thyroid disease
- Chronic active hepatitis

From Joint Task Force of the EFNS and PNS: European Federation of Neurological Societies/Peripheral Nerve Society guideline on management of chronic inflammatory demyelinating polyradiculoneuropathy, *J Peripher Nerv Syst* 10:220-228, 2005.

BOX 41-8

Electrodiagnostic Criteria of Chronic Inflammatory Demyelinating Polyneuropathy

(Criteria based on assessment of median, ulnar, peroneal, and tibial nerves tested on one side)

Definite (At Least One of the Following)

- Distal motor latency >150% of upper limit of normal in two nerves
- Motor conduction <70% of lower limit of normal in two nerves
- F wave latency >120% of upper limit of normal in two nerves
- Absence of F waves in two nerves if compound muscle activated potential (CMAP) amplitude <80% of lower limit of normal and at least one other demyelinating parameter in one other nerve
- Partial conduction block (at least 50% reduction in CMAP amplitude of proximal stimulation compared with distal) in two nerves, or in one nerve plus other demyelinating parameter in one other nerve
- Abnormal temporal dispersion in at least two nerves
- Distal CMAP duration >9 ms in at least one nerve plus other demyelinating criteria in at least one other nerve

Probable

- At least 30% reduction in CMAP amplitude between proximal and distal stimulation in at least two nerves, or in one nerve with other demyelinating parameter in one other nerve

Possible

- Definite demyelinating criteria in only one nerve

From Joint Task Force of the EFNS and PNS: European Federation of Neurological Societies/Peripheral Nerve Society guideline on management of chronic inflammatory demyelinating polyradiculoneuropathy, *J Peripher Nerve Syst* 10:220-228, 2005.

gadolinium of the brachial and lumbar plexi and cauda equina can reveal enhancing or enlarged nerves.

The European Federation of Neurological Societies/Peripheral Nerve Society proposed diagnostic criteria for CIDP based on review of available evidence and expert consensus.[82] Diagnostic probability is based on presence of typical or atypical clinical features (Box 41-7), electrodiagnostic findings of demyelinating disease (Box 41-8), and supportive evidence. Supportive evidence includes MRI abnormalities, CSF findings, nerve biopsy, and response to immunomodulating treatment. These recommendations permit the description of CIDP as typical or atypical, with or without concomitant disease, and definite, probable, or possible.

Treatment

Like GBS, CIDP is responsive to IVIG and plasma exchange. CIDP also responds to corticosteroids, although GBS does not. In severe attacks, IVIG and plasma exchange can be used to produce rapid improvement in symptoms; however, they rarely result in complete remission, and most patients require repeated treatment at intervals of 2 to 6 weeks to prevent relapse.[96] IVIG is usually favored over plasma exchange. Corticosteroids are more likely than IVIG or plasma exchange to produce remission of disease in the more common demyelinating form; however, corticosteroids are not effective and can even be detrimental to pure motor variants of CIDP. Randomized clinical trials of treatment are lacking in children, but metaanalysis[105] showed that the children have an 80% to 100% response rate to standard treatments of IVIG and corticosteroids, and complete functional recovery is seen in most. Overall, plasma exchange is used less frequently and appears less efficacious in childhood CIDP than in adult-onset CIPD (often caused by issues surrounding vascular access) but still has a role in situations in which steroids and IVIG have not been adequately effective.[105]

After stabilization of initial onset or recurrence of CIDP, appropriate physical and occupational therapy, orthotic management, and treatment of neuropathic pain should be addressed. A course of inpatient rehabilitation might be appropriate.

Infectious Neuropathies

Infections are the most common cause of neuropathy in the world, with leprosy being the most common cause. HIV is responsible for a number of neuropathic syndromes, and the agents used to treat HIV can also be responsible for PN. Lyme disease, a tick-borne infection common in the United States and Europe, is also responsible for PN. Infection can cause neuropathy either through the inflammatory reactions induced by the infectious agent or through the body's immune reaction to the organism.

Leprosy (Hansen Disease)

Leprosy is caused by *Mycobacterium leprae,* which is found primarily in tropical and subtropical developing countries. Three clinical presentations exist, which are determined by the host immune response to the bacillus: tuberculoid, lepromatous, and borderline leprosy. Tuberculoid leprosy causes single or multiple well-circumscribed cutaneous lesions. High levels of cell-mediated immunity kill the bacilli and cause destruction of nerves that travel through the granulomatous tuberculoid lesions. The most commonly involved nerves are the ulnar, median, common peroneal, facial, superficial radial, digital, posterior auricular, and sural nerves.[138] The bacillus tends to proliferate in areas of lower temperature. The lepromatous form occurs in the setting of deficient cell-mediated immune response. No granulomas are formed, and nerve destruction is thought to occur from direct nerve invasion of the bacillus, particularly affecting the Schwann cell. Nerve destruction is typically diffuse and symmetrical. In both forms the predominant finding is sensory loss affecting nerves in areas of lower temperature such as extensor surfaces, earlobes, and over the maxilla. The soles of the feet and the palms are characteristically spared. Motor weakness is a late development, only after there is significant sensory loss. Leprosy is treated with dapsone, which itself can cause neuropathy. Dapsone primarily causes a progressive motor neuropathy that can preferentially affect the hip girdle muscles or both hand and foot muscles in a symmetrical fashion.[175]

Lyme Disease

Lyme disease is a tick-borne illness that is caused by the spirochete *Borrelia burgdorferi*. The disease has three stages: early infection, characterized by a local erythematous lesion (erythema migrans); disseminated infection; and finally late-stage infection. Meningitis is the most common neurologic abnormality in Lyme disease. A variety of peripheral nerve abnormalities can also occur and vary with the stage of the disease.[38] Cranial mononeuropathies occur in stage 2, most commonly affecting the facial nerve (bilaterally in 50% of cases). Radiculoneuritis that progresses to a mononeuritis multiplex pattern, or a plexopathy, is also reported. The lower limbs are affected more than the upper limbs. In stage 3, about half of patients develop a distal symmetrical neuropathy, presenting with a stocking glove distribution of paresthesia and sensory loss. Other presentations can also occur, including mononeuropathies, acute polyradiculoneuropathies, and asymmetrical distal neuropathies. Although the clinical presentation of peripheral nerve dysfunction is broad, the underlying injury is an irregular axonal neuropathy. Treatment of Lyme disease with neurologic involvement consists of intravenous ceftriaxone for 2 to 4 weeks. Improvement in acute neurologic symptoms is fairly good with antibiotic treatment; however, chronic neuropathies respond more slowly and can result in residual deficits.[159]

HIV-Associated Neuropathies

HIV infection is associated with a number of neurologic disorders that can occur at any stage of the disease. Early in the course of HIV infection these neurologic insults are often caused by immune dysregulation. AIDP can occur at the time of seroconversion, whereas CIDP manifests later, usually with a CD4 count less than 50 cells/mm^3.[53] The clinical features are identical to those in HIV-negative patients and are treated in the same manner and respond similarly to patients without HIV. Immune-mediated vasculitic neuropathies, cranial mononeuropathies, brachial plexopathies, and multiple mononeuropathies are also seen early in HIV infection. In mid- to late-stage infection, neuropathies that are caused by the HIV replication can be seen, most commonly a sensory polyneuropathy or an autonomic neuropathy. Later-stage disease brings neuropathies associated with opportunistic infection, such as CMV, syphilis, and zoster. Neuropathies associated with malignancy and nutritional deficiency can also occur. The drugs used to treat HIV infection also are known to cause neuropathy. For example, nucleoside reverse transcriptase inhibitors cause a distal sensory neuropathy that is clinically and electrodiagnostically identical to that associated with primary HIV infection. The use of antiretroviral therapy (ART) can also lead to exaggerated immune response to an already present opportunistic infection such as *Mycobacterium leprae*. This is known as the immune reconstitution inflammatory response (IRIS) and is associated with CD4 count lower than 50 cells/μL at initiation of ART. IRIS is associated with greater morbidity and mortality and is usually managed by discontinuation of ART and use of corticosteroids or thalidomide.[102] Diffuse infiltrative lymphocytosis (DILS) can be seen in HIV-positive patients with a persistent CD8 hyperlymphocytosis and Sjögren-like syndrome. In these individuals nerve biopsy will show CD8$^+$ infiltration causing a painful sensorimotor axonal neuropathy that responds to ART and steroids.[24] It is believed to be an exaggerated immune response to HIV (Box 41-9).

Distal Sensory Polyneuropathy

A symmetrical distal sensory polyneuropathy can be seen either as a result of HIV (HIV-DSP) or antiretroviral drug toxicity (ARV-DSP). Since the introduction of highly active ARV treatment (HAART), the incidence of clinical DSP is estimated to be 30%, although on autopsy close to 100% of patients demonstrated histologic evidence of DSP.[71] Risk factors for HIV-DSP are older age, CD4 count less than 50 cells/mm^3, coexisting diabetes mellitus or nutritional deficiency, and use of neurotoxic drugs and alcohol.[28] DSP causes distal axonal degeneration of small unmyelinated fibers. Pain and uncomfortable sensory symptoms are present, first in the soles of the feet and progressing in a "stocking-glove distribution." Symptoms are typically symmetrical, although a unilateral presentation can occur initially. Physical examination is consistent with abnormalities of small fiber sensory nerves, with abnormal pain and temperature perception distally, but with relatively preserved proprioception and strength. Achilles reflexes are absent or decreased. Electrodiagnostic studies, which are relatively insensitive to small fiber dysfunction, might be normal or demonstrate a length-dependent sensory axonal neuropathy. Needle EMG examination is typically normal, although it occasionally can show chronic denervation and reinnervation in foot intrinsic muscles. Skin biopsy with epidermal nerve fiber density is useful in the detection of

BOX 41-9

Neuropathies Associated with Human Immunodeficiency Virus (HIV)-1

Immune Mediated

- Acute inflammatory demyelinating polyradiculoneuropathy
- Chronic inflammatory demyelinating polyradiculoneuropathy
- Cranial mononeuropathies
- Vasculitic neuropathy
- Brachial plexopathy
- Multiple mononeuropathies
- Immune reconstitution inflammatory response
- Diffuse infiltrative lymphocytosis

Human Immunodeficiency Virus (HIV)-1 Replication Associated

- Distal sensory polyneuropathy
- Autonomic neuropathy

Drug Related

- Antiretroviral, nucleoside reverse transcriptase inhibitors; ddI, ddC, d4T
- Other drugs, ethambutol, vincristine, isoniazid

Opportunistic Infection/Malignancy

- Cytomegalovirus (CMV) progressive polyradiculopathy
- CMV mononeuritis multiplex
- Syphilitic polyradiculopathy
- Tuberculous polyradiculomyelitis
- Zoster
- Lymphomatous polyradiculopathy

Nutritional

- Acquired immune deficiency syndrome (AIDS) cachexia neuropathy
- Nutritional deficiency, vitamin B_6, B_{12}

small fiber neuropathy and correlates with severity of painful symptoms.[147] It is important to differentiate between HIV-DSP and ARV-DSP because discontinuation of the drug can reverse ARV-DSP. The differentiation is usually made on historic grounds based on a close temporal relationship between drug initiation and onset of symptoms. Discontinuation or reduction of dose leads to improvement within 8 weeks, although there can be a period of worsening initially after stopping the drug.[56]

Children with HIV infection in Africa are often affected by PN, which may be the result of infection, HIV treatment, an immune response, or associated factors such as malnutrition. Although various types of neuropathy may be seen, the typical distal symmetrical polyneuropathy is more common in adult patients with HIV-1 infection than children. Peripheral neuropathy in children with HIV has not been extensively studied, but it occurs often in the form of AIDP at the time of seroconversion as an immune reconstitution phenomenon, and in relation to secondary infection with CMV. Children with AIDP who are not infected with HIV will have albumin–cytologic dissociation in contrast to those with HIV seroconversion, which will demonstrate pleiocytosis. The AIDP in HIV-infected children has a similar clinical phenotype to distal symmetrical polyneuropathy, and children may have severe sensory features of intense distal burning affecting the hands and the feet, as well as distal weakness. Peripheral neuropathy can occur as an adverse side effect of therapy with the nucleoside reverse transcriptase inhibitors, stavudine and, to a lesser extent, didanosine.[183]

Cytomegalovirus-Related Progressive Polyradiculomyelopathy

CMV infection can cause a severe, rapidly progressive polyradiculomyelopathy that is a true neurologic emergency. It presents with symptoms of cauda equina syndrome developing over days to weeks. Initially there is low back pain with unilateral lower limb radiation and urinary incontinence, followed quickly by progressive leg weakness and saddle anesthesia. Flaccid paraplegia develops if untreated, with onset of weakness and death within weeks. Examination of CSF reveals CMV infection by culture, polymerase chain reaction assay, elevated protein, low glucose, and polymorphonuclear pleocytosis. Electrodiagnostic studies are consistent with an axonal loss in the lumbosacral roots. Sural nerve biopsy is generally unremarkable or might show a minimal amount of inflammation.[27] MRI might show enhancement of the lumbosacral roots. CMV-associated polyradiculoneuropathy is treated with ganciclovir or other antiviral agents. A similar clinical picture can be seen in syphilitic, tubercular, or cryptococcal infection, lymphoma, and concurrent HTLV1 infection, as well as in IRIS and DIL.[53]

Toxic Neuropathies

Although toxins are a less common cause of PN, diagnosis is important because prompt identification of a chemical insult can lead to improvement if withdrawal of the offending agent occurs. Recognition of a source of chronic exposure in the household or workplace can also prevent development or progression of similar disease in others at risk. Toxic exposure can be occupational, as occurs with industrial solvents and glues; environmental as in lead exposure; secondary to abuse as seen in alcohol abuse or "huffing" of household solvents; the result of intentional poisoning (suicide or homicide attempts); or iatrogenic from medications used to treat a variety of diseases (Table 41-3).

Toxic exposure is often suspected when standard historic clues and laboratory tests are unrevealing in the workup of PN. With any neuropathy evaluation a careful exposure history should be obtained, which includes understanding the patient's workplace and any chemicals to which he or she might be exposed. Recreational activities are another source of exposure, particularly ones that involve glues or solvents or exposure to pesticides. In the case of children, especially those with pica, exposure to toys containing lead-based paint may be a particular hazard. A recreational drug history can be revealing, particularly involving alcohol and intentional inhalation of glues and aerosols (huffing). Toxic neuropathies also frequently present with other systemic effects, which range from subtle to severe and life-threatening. Gastrointestinal complaints are reported in arsenic, lead, and thallium poisoning. A variety of cutaneous findings can be seen, such as Mees lines in the fingernails in lead and arsenic poisoning; gingival abnormalities in phenytoin, lead, and mercury

Table 41-3 Features of Toxic Neuropathies[38,98]

Agent	Clinical Symptoms	Systemic Effects	Diagnostic Findings
Sensory and Sensory Greater than Motor, Axonal			
Nitrofurantoin	Pain, paresthesias, gait dysfunction, can progress to profound quadriparesis		Electromyography (EMG): absent or severely decreased sensory and motor amplitudes, relatively preserved conduction velocity (when obtained), significant neuropathic changes on needle electrodiagnostic examination (NEE)
Ethyl alcohol	Distal symmetrical sensory loss, affects hands late	Dementia/ophthalmoplegia/ataxia (Wernicke syndrome), cirrhosis, cerebellar degeneration	
Colchicine	Mild decrease in touch, vibration, and proprioception, pinprick and temperature sensation less affected, proximal weakness (caused by severe myopathy)		EMG: ↓ sensory and motor amplitudes, normal distal latency; myopathic changes proximally on needle examination
Amitriptyline	Stocking glove distribution (rare)		Significantly decreased sensory nerve action potential (SNAP), motor conduction velocity (CV) 80% or lower limit of normal (LLN), neuropathic changes on NEE
Lithium	Distal sensory loss, weakness	Tremor, confusion, seizure	Absent SNAP and compound muscle activated potential (CMAP) in lower extremity (LE), markedly reduced amplitude in upper extremity (UE) with normal CV
Phenytoin	Mild sensory symptoms in stocking glove distribution, with toxicity numbness, tingling, gait difficulties with mild weakness	Gingival hyperplasia, cerebellar ataxia	Mildly reduced SNAP, mildly reduced motor CV, NEE normal or mildly neuropathic distally
Cisplatin	Affect dorsal root ganglion and large myelinated sensory nerves, numbness, painful paresthesias, ↓ proprioception, ↓ deep tendon reflexes (DTR)	Nephrotoxicity, ototoxicity, nausea, vomiting, myelosuppression	Reduced or absent SNAP in UE and LE, mildly prolonged latency, motor conductions and NEE normal
Pyridoxine	Gait dysfunction, L'hermitte sign, decreased/absent DTR, normal strength, affects dorsal root ganglion		Significantly decreased to absent SNAP with normal CV, CMAP normal to borderline low, NEE-decreased recruitment
Thallium	Small fiber predominant, painful dysesthesias, preserved reflexes	Gastrointestinal symptoms, cardiac and respiratory failure, renal insufficiency, encephalopathy, alopecia, and Mees lines (late findings)	EMG: Can be normal initially as a result of small fiber loss, sensory axonal findings late
Motor and Motor Greater than Sensory, Axonal			
Lead	Early upper extremity weakness, preferential involvement of radial nerve, atrophy of hand and foot intrinsics, sparing all sensory modalities	abdominal pain, constipation, gingival discoloration	Nerve conduction study: mildly decreased amplitude and CV, NEE with neuropathic motor unit changes and fibrillation potentials and positive sharp waves
Organophosphates	Length-dependent weakness followed by proximal weakness, spasticity and upper motor neuron signs resulting from corticospinal tract involvement	Symptoms of cholinergic excess, myasthenia-like syndrome, pulmonary edema, dermatitis, corticospinal tract dysfunction	EMG: sensorimotor axonal neuropathy with conduction slowing
Vincristine	Early pain and small fiber sensory loss, distal symmetrical weakness	Autonomic dysfunction	EMG: ↓ motor and sensory amplitude

Continued on following page

Table 41-3 Features of Toxic Neuropathies—cont'd

Agent	Clinical Symptoms	Systemic Effects	Diagnostic Findings
Motor and Motor Greater than Sensory with Conduction Slowing			
Amiodarone	Symmetrical, distal sensorimotor neuropathy Rapidly progressive motor predominant (mimic acute inflammatory demyelinating polyneuropathy [AIDP])	Action tremor, myopathy, optic neuropathy, encephalopathy, basal ganglia dysfunction, pseudotumor cerebri	EMG: Varies from predominant conduction slowing to predominant sensory amplitude reduction Sural nerve biopsy: either axonal or demyelinating findings
Arsenic	High dose: mimics AIDP, flaccid quadriparesis, facial weakness, respiratory failure Chronic: dermatologic symptoms first, length-dependent painful neuropathy, fewer motor symptoms	Gastrointestinal symptoms, hyperpigmentation, Mees lines, hyperkeratosis, desquamation of hands and feet, hepatomegaly, cardiomyopathy, and renal failure, anemia, basophilic stippling of red blood cells	EMG: ↓ amplitude, motor > sensory, borderline low CV, prolonged F waves, partial conduction block Laboratory: urine arsenic >25 μg/24 hr, hair and nail levels (chronic)
Hexacarbons "huffing"	Length-dependent distal sensory loss, weakness, atrophy, absent Achilles reflex, cranial nerve involvement Massive exposure: more cranial and motor involvement Chronic: degeneration of distal corticospinal tract and dorsal columns	Autonomic dysfunction, impairment of color vision (chronic)	Marked decreased SNAP, mildly prolonged latency, significantly decreased CMAP with CV 70% to 80% of LLN, NEE with fibrillation potential and positives waves, fasciculations
Mononeuritis Monoplex			
Dapsone	Motor predominant, asymmetrical, occurring with chronic (years of) exposure		Asymmetrical, motor without conduction slowing or increased latencies
Trichloroethylene	Cranial mononeuropathies, with ptosis, facial and bulbar weakness, extraocular muscle dysfunction, trigeminal involvement	Dermatitis, cirrhosis, cardiac failure	Normal standard limb peripheral nerve conduction studies

AIDP, Acute demyelinating polyradiculoneuropathy; *CV,* conduction velocity; *DTR,* deep tendon reflex; *EMG,* electromyography; *LE,* lower extremity; *LLN,* lower limit of normal; *NEE,* needle electrodiagnostic examination; *SNAP,* sensory nerve action potential; *UE,* upper extremity.

exposure; and irritant dermatitis with acrylamide, thallium, and toluene exposure.[98] Cardiovascular, hepatic, and renal abnormalities are also associated with many toxic exposures. Exposure to organophosphates causes symptoms of cholinergic excess, such as bradycardia, sweating, excess salivation, miosis, bronchospasm, and diarrhea. The CNS can be affected, as well as the peripheral nervous system. Chronic alcohol abuse can cause midline cerebellar degeneration and a triad of ataxia, dementia, and ophthalmoplegia known as Wernicke syndrome. Some toxins produce different syndromes depending on whether the exposure is high dose and acute or low dose and chronic. Arsenic presents with a syndrome of flaccid quadriparesis that resembles AIDP with high-dose exposure.[58] By contrast, chronic arsenic poisoning presents with more dermatologic abnormalities and a painful length-dependent neuropathy with less motor involvement.[47] Although most toxin-related PN has a distal symmetrical distribution, lead poisoning has a predilection for the radial nerve, and patients can present with wrist extension weakness or frank wrist drop. Although the CNS is vulnerable to the effects of lead poisoning in both children and adults, the developing brain is particularly vulnerable, and cognitive, learning, and behavioral impairments may be seen in children even with blood lead levels around 10 μg/dL. The CDC now recommends further investigation and public health actions when levels are 5 μg/dL or more.[3] Peripheral neuropathy is a more frequent occurrence in adults with lead toxicity but has been reported in children especially those with concomitant sickle cell disease. Lead levels between 20 and 30 μg/dL have been implicated in peripheral nerve dysfunction. Early diagnosis and removal from continuing lead exposure is important with initiation of chelation therapy for levels greater than or equal to 45 μg/dL recommended to enhance chances of clinical and neurophysiologic improvement in lead poisoning and acute neuropathy, although effects on subacute or chronic PN remain unclear.[89]

The patient's medication list should always be reviewed as a number of pharmaceutical agents can cause nerve toxicity. Factors that may increase risk of medication-induced PN include impaired renal or hepatic function causing decreased drug metabolism or clearance and the presence of an unrelated neuropathy such as Charcot-Marie-Tooth (CMT). Many chemotherapeutic drugs can cause treatment-limiting neuropathies. Onset of PN can be either acute or subacute and symptoms of neuropathy can appear or progress for up to 2 months after cessation of the agent, known as the "coasting phenomenon."[61] Dose reduction, longer infusion times, or longer periods between doses may improve symptoms, but sometimes treatment must be ceased and recovery can be incomplete. Amiodarone is an agent used to manage ventricular arrhythmias and can cause encephalopathy, basal ganglia dysfunction, optic neuropathy, pseudotumor cerebri, and action tremor. Concomitant myopathy is present with colchicine-induced neuropathy. Lipid-lowering agents such as simvastatin are well recognized to be associated with myopathies. They have also been implicated in causing PN although it is infrequent and in some settings may be neuroprotective.[181]

Electrodiagnostic Classification of Toxic Neuropathies

Most toxin-induced neuropathies are distal sensorimotor neuropathies without conduction slowing but with predominant axon loss. These include many therapeutic drugs such as metronidazole, amitriptyline, lithium, nitrofurantoin, phenytoin, vincristine, hydralazine, and isoniazid. It is also seen in chronic alcohol abuse, as well as chronic arsenic, carbon monoxide, and mercury poisoning. Motor-predominant neuropathies without conduction slowing are seen with organophosphates and vincristine. Pure sensory axonal neuropathies have been associated with cisplatin, nitrofurantoin, thalidomide, alcohol, pyridoxine (vitamin B_6), and thallium. Some toxins produce neuropathies with significant conduction slowing, often resembling AIDP. Acute arsenic poisoning, amiodarone, and hexacarbons (particularly in "huffers" who inhale large quantities) produce a motor-predominant demyelinating neuropathy. A sensory greater than motor neuropathy with conduction slowing is seen in the neurotoxin saxitoxin caused by shellfish poisoning associated with red tide, as well as tetrodotoxin from ingestion of the puffer fish. A rare toxin-associated presentation is multiple mononeuropathies (referred to clinically as *mononeuritis multiplex*) seen with the antimycobacterial drug dapsone and with trichloroethylene (which produces a cranial mononeuritis multiplex) (Table 41-4).[142] Lead neuropathy will have different presentations depending on the length of exposure. Lead-induced neuropathy following about 5 years of sustained exposure usually presents as a subacute motor neuropathy (with minimal sensory involvement) with segmental demyelination and axonal degeneration, with predominantly upper limb involvement at onset (wrist drop) but also involving the lower extremities in due course (foot drop). A more indolent and slowly progressive sensorimotor neuropathy may be seen after 10 to 20 years of low-level exposure. A monophasic high-intensity exposure may also result in an acute neuropathy without other systemic features.[162]

Table 41-4 Typical Electrodiagnostic Classifications of Toxic Neuropathies

Neuropathy	Toxin
Distal sensorimotor, axonal	Metronidazole, lithium, nitrofurantoin, phenytoin, vincristine, hydralazine, isoniazid Alcohol abuse Chronic arsenic poisoning Carbon monoxide Mercury
Motor, axonal	Organophosphates Vincristine
Sensory, axonal	Cisplatin, nitrofurantoin, thalidomide, pyridoxine (vitamin B_6) Thallium Alcohol
Motor, with conduction block	Acute arsenic poisoning Amiodarone Hexacarbons
Sensory greater than motor, with conduction block	Saxitoxin (shellfish), tetrodotoxin (puffer fish)
Multiple mononeuropathies	Dapsone Trichloroethylene

Vasculitic and Connective Tissue Disease Neuropathies

Neuropathies associated with the vasculitides and connective tissue diseases can have varied presentations. Although distal symmetrical neuropathy and single mononeuropathies are possible, the prototypical neuropathy caused by vasculitic and connective tissue disorders is an asymmetrical mixed motor and sensory pattern, often referred to as a mononeuritis multiplex. Typical presentation begins with vasculitic ischemia and acute onset of pain in the distribution of the affected nerve, followed by sensory disturbance. Occasionally the symptoms progress in a more gradual fashion, although it is typically asymmetrical. The lower extremity nerves are more commonly affected, with the peroneal nerve being involved 63% of the time, followed by the tibial, ulnar, and median nerves.[139] The cranial nerves are rarely affected. Affected nerves are more likely to have injury at more proximal sites than those seen with compression neuropathies.

The vasculitic disorders that commonly cause PN include polyarteritis nodosa, Churg-Strauss syndrome, microscopic polyangiitis, and Wegner granulomatosis (Box 41-10). Nerves can also be affected by a nonsystemic vasculitis of the peripheral nerves, that is, a vasculitis without other organ or system involvement. The vasculitic injury to the peripheral nervous system usually results in the asymmetrical mononeuritis multiplex pattern. Connective tissue disorders such as rheumatoid arthritis (RA), systemic lupus erythematosus (SLE), and Sjögren syndrome more frequently cause a diffuse symmetrical PN. The distal neuropathy in both RA and SLE tends to be mild, late presentation in the disease. RA can progress to rheumatoid vasculitis, causing multiple mononeuropathies. Compression neuropathies, especially CTS, are more common in both SLE and RA. Sjögren syndrome, which can affect the nervous system in a variety of ways, can also present as a pure sensory neuropathy.

The hallmark of mononeuritis multiplex on physical examination is weakness or sensory loss that represents a side-to-side asymmetry of the same peripheral nerve, or an instance in which there is greater proximal than distal involvement of different peripheral nerves in sites that are not typical sources of anatomic compression. Electrodiagnostic testing in mononeuritis multiplex shows decreased sensory nerve action potentials in affected nerves, with normal-to-borderline low conduction velocity. The findings are similar for motor conductions. There can be marked asymmetry between the same nerves on the right and left sides. Nerves in the lower extremities are usually more affected. Conduction block can be seen in affected nerves, in segments not typically involved in compression. F waves can be prolonged. Needle EMG shows positive waves and fibrillation potentials with reduced recruitment and neuropathic motor unit changes in the territory of the affected nerves. As the disease progresses and involves more nerves, the findings can coalesce and the confluence of findings makes differentiation from a diffuse, symmetrical pattern difficult. In patients with known vasculitic or

BOX 41-10

Neuropathies Associated with Vasculitic and Connective Tissue Disease

Polyarteritis Nodosa (PAN)
- 50% with peripheral neuropathy (PN)
- Mononeuritis multiplex 57%
- Distal symmetrical PN 25%
- Single mononeuropathy 17%

Churg-Strauss Syndrome
- PN more common than in PAN
- Similar distribution as in PAN

Microscopic Polyangiitis
- PN less likely (14% to 36%)

Wegner Granulomatosis
- PN less common (<15%)

Mixed Cryoglobulinemia
- 30% to 60% with PN
- Distal symmetrical sensory or sensorimotor neuropathy

Giant Cell Arteritis
- Carpal tunnel syndrome

Rheumatoid Arthritis
- Compression neuropathies, carpal tunnel syndrome
- Mild distal symmetrical sensory neuropathy, late complication
- Mononeuritis multiplex in rheumatoid vasculitis

Sjögren Syndrome
- 10% to 50% with PN
- Sensorimotor neuropathy
- Pure distal sensory
- Trigeminal sensory neuropathy
- Autonomic neuropathy
- Carpal tunnel syndrome

Systemic Lupus Erythematosus
- 25% to 50% with PN
- Symmetrical diffuse sensory or sensorimotor axonal PN-late
- Carpal tunnel syndrome

Systemic Sclerosis
- PN uncommon

connective tissue disease, the occurrence of new findings of PN can indicate more active disease and the need for more aggressive management. Peripheral neuropathy can also be the presenting sign of these disorders. In those without known systemic disease, the finding of mononeuritis multiplex requires a search for systemic involvement and might require nerve or muscle biopsy.

Prompt identification of a vasculitic-associated neuropathy is important because management with immunomodulators such as corticosteroids and cyclophosphamide can halt progression. Specific rehabilitation recommendations vary based on the specific nerves affected and will follow those provided later in the sections on mononeuropathies.

Charcot-Marie-Tooth Disease

Charcot-Marie-Tooth disease is the most common inherited PN with a prevalence of 17 to 40 per 100,000.[104] CMT is a genetically heterogeneous disorder characterized by

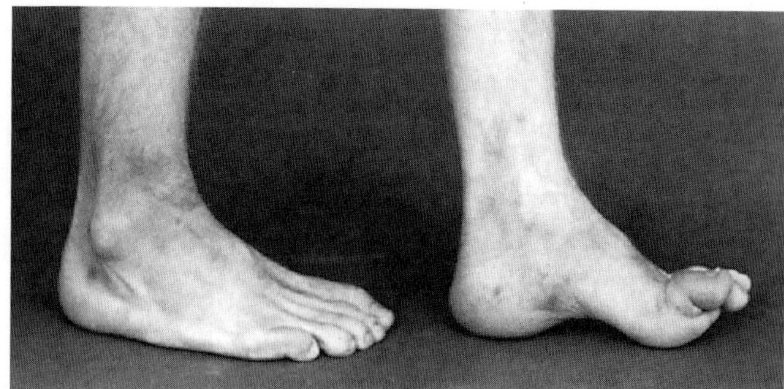

FIGURE 41-6 Pes cavus deformity and hammer toes associated with Charcot-Marie-Tooth disease. (From Warner WC: Neuromuscular disorders. In Canale ST, Beaty JH, editors. *Campbell's operative orthopaedics*, ed 11. Philadelphia, PA, 2009, Mosby.)

wasting of the distal limb muscles, particularly the peroneal innervated muscles, with distal sensory loss, decreased or absent muscle stretch reflexes, and skeletal deformity. CMT is often referred to as a hereditary motor and sensory neuropathy (HMSN) and has been subclassified as HMSN types I through VI. HMSN I is now known as CMT1 and is characterized by slow conduction velocities and diffuse demyelination. HMSN II/CMT2 is the axonal form with evidence of axonal degeneration and preserved or only mildly slowed conduction velocities. HMSN III is now more commonly known as Déjèrine-Sottas neuropathy and is characterized by early onset with severe "hypertrophic" demyelination. HMSN IV, HMSN V, and HMSN VI describe various motor-only forms now referred to as distal hereditary motor neuropathies. At least 40 different genetic forms of CMT have been identified, and any one genotype can have variable penetrance and phenotypical expression.[78] The most common phenotype seen is CMT1 (74%)[66] with the most common genotype being CMT1A. CMT usually has autosomal dominant transmission, although in up to 10% of cases it can be cross-linked. Autosomal recessive forms, causing severe, early-onset demyelinating disease, are classified under CMT4. Patients with sporadic mutations are uncommon.

The typical pattern for CMT is a slow progression of onset, starting in the first 2 decades of life. Children and teenagers might first present with steppage gait, associated with weakness of the peroneal innervated muscles and the development of pes cavus (Figure 41-6). Weakness of the ankle plantar flexors is less severe, and atrophy of the lower limbs is often described as resembling an inverted champagne bottle. Upper limb involvement occurs much later in the course of the disease, with claw hand being the most common deformity. Although gait is affected, loss of independent ambulation is rare.[67] Sensory symptoms are less prominent than motor symptoms. Loss of sensation for pain, touch, and vibration is seen in the feet, with clinical proprioception relatively preserved. Positive sensory symptoms, such as pain or paresthesias, are less common and less severe, but complaints of cold feet and muscle cramps might be noted. Muscle stretch reflexes are decreased to absent in the demyelinating CMT1 but are less affected in CMT2. Skeletal deformities are seen in 66% of all CMT patients, with pes cavus and hammer toes the most common abnormality and scoliosis occurring less frequently. Foot deformities can occur as a result of the imbalance in strength of the foot intrinsic and leg muscles. Late-onset CMT tends to result in more subtle foot abnormalities or even no foot abnormalities.[117]

From an electrodiagnostic standpoint, nerve conduction tests are the primary diagnostic tests for CMT. CMT1, the demyelinating form of CMT, is characterized by marked slowing of nerve conduction studies as defined as median nerve conduction values <38 m/s.[67] Discriminating hereditary from acquired neuropathies can be challenging when the onset of noticeable signs and symptoms does not appear until the adult years. It has been recognized that nerve conduction slowing in hereditary neuropathies tends to be uniform and diffuse, whereas in acquired demyelinating neuropathies (such as CIDP), the demyelination is patchy and asymmetrical with temporal dispersion and partial conduction blocks occurring away from common points of entrapment.[97] Although this distinction is useful, there is an exception in that cross-linked CMT1 might present with nonuniform demyelination and temporal dispersion, and can be misdiagnosed as CIDP.[22] CMT2 demonstrates normal or mildly slowed conductions velocities (>38 m/s) with reduced motor and sensory amplitudes. Needle examination demonstrates signs of chronic denervation greater distally than proximally in all types of CMT, and fibrillation potentials and positive waves are present in severe or rapidly progressing forms.

There is a growing body of evidence demonstrating the merits of exercise for people with CMT and showing that not only will it not hurt, it actually has the potential to improve functional ability, independence, and quality of life. Since function is likely highest in children with CMT compared with adults, regular exercise and activity may help preserve physical ability into adulthood. Progressive strengthening of the hip flexors improves hip flexor fatigue resulting in improved walking duration, and strengthening of the ankle musculature results in improved muscle strength, walking speed, cadence, step time, and stride length. Similar to adults with CMT, children have shown responsiveness to progressive strength training with improvement in muscle strength and walking speed, cadence, step time, and stride length.[21,125]

Mononeuropathies

Focal mononeuropathies are more common than generalized peripheral neuropathies and affect otherwise healthy individuals, although those with a generalized neuropathy may be less tolerant of focal injury. Mononeuropathies are usually caused by local trauma or compression of a specific nerve, often in a location where it is anatomically vulnerable to compression (such as a constrictive structural canal or where it passes superficially and is susceptible to external compression). Mononeuropathies can occur by repetitive motion, direct forceful trauma, or prolonged compression caused by positioning or use of bracing or assistive devices. The general assessment begins with a detailed description of the distribution of sensory and motor symptoms.

The history of onset can be revealing, such as a change in occupational demands, hobbies, association with medical procedures, or traumatic injury. A detailed vocational and avocational history should be obtained, with the pattern of exacerbating and relieving factors. An understanding of the anatomic distribution of specific nerves, their course and areas of mechanical vulnerability, and the specific muscles and sensory distribution they supply is critical in localizing the patient's lesion and formulating strategies for treatment.

Brachial Plexopathy

The brachial plexus arises from C5–C8 and T1 ventral rami, whose fibers intermingle to form the nerves that supply the upper limb. The roots join to form the trunks (upper, middle, and lower), which then divide to form the cords (lateral, posterior, and medial). The posterior cord continues into the arm as the radial nerve; the medial cord terminates in the ulnar nerve; and the median nerve is formed from the medial cord and part of the lateral cord. Smaller nerves arise at various levels along the plexus, including the dorsal scapular nerve that supplies the rhomboid from the C5 ventral ramus, the long thoracic nerve from the C5–C7 rami, the suprascapular nerve from the upper trunk, the musculocutaneous nerve from the lateral cord, and the axillary nerve from the posterior cord along with the thoracodorsal nerve (Figure 41-7).

Trauma is the most common cause of brachial plexus injury. Closed injury can occur from traction when the head and neck are forcibly bent away from the shoulder, or in association with fractures of the clavicle or shoulder. Open injuries can occur with knife or missile wounds. Often a patient has other serious injuries, which can delay identification of the brachial plexus injury. Traumatic injuries usually affect multiple trunks or cords, or even avulsion injuries to the roots and individual nerves. The large number of possible types and patterns of injury make localization particularly challenging. Milder plexus injuries have been associated with sports, particularly American football. Players can experience a sharp burning pain in

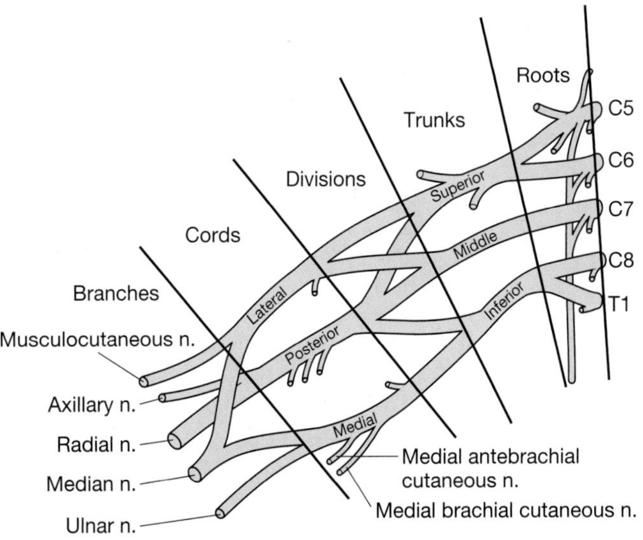

FIGURE 41-7 Brachial plexus. (Modified from Wedel DJ, Horlocker TT: Nerve Blocks. In: Miller RD, editor: *Miller's anesthesia*, ed 7. Philadelphia, PA, 2010, Elsevier.)[180]

the shoulder with transient weakness after a blow to the head, neck, or shoulder, known as a "stinger" or a "burner." Weakness, particularly of the biceps and shoulder muscles, rarely lasts beyond a few days to weeks. Injuries can also occur during operative procedures, especially with median sternotomy. Brachial plexus injuries can occur in newborns during delivery, with the upper trunk being most commonly affected, causing weakness of shoulder abduction and elbow flexion, as well as forearm supination known as Erb palsy. Erb palsy is often recognized after a difficult delivery with shoulder dystocia, forceps delivery, and prolonged labor. Masses can also affect the brachial plexus. Lung, breast, and lymphoma are the most common metastatic tumors that affect the plexus. Involvement of the brachial plexus is usually a later manifestation of the cancer and might need to be differentiated from radiation-induced plexopathy, particularly in treated breast cancer. A Pancoast tumor arises from the superior pulmonary sulcus at the apex of the lung and affects the lower trunk of the brachial plexus, often with an associated Horner syndrome.

Electrodiagnostic studies of the affected limb show abnormalities in the distribution of the affected portions of the plexus. Sensory nerve potentials are reduced in affected nerve distribution unless the lesion is at the root level. Effort should be made to obtain a reliable sensory response originating from each of the major components of the plexus (Table 41-5). In this way the rostral/caudal distribution of the plexus injury can be evaluated. Similarly, needle electromyography can be used to determine the proximal/distal injury location within each plexus component, as well as confirm the presence/absence of residual axonal continuity. In plexus injuries that do not involve the roots, the cervical paraspinal muscles should be normal. Imaging studies might be indicated to evaluate for underlying tumor, mass, or disruption of the plexus.

Management of brachial plexopathy includes proper positioning with orthoses to stabilize affected joints and improve function. Range-of-motion exercises and physiotherapy are important to reduce contractures and strengthen recovering motor function. Medication management is appropriate for neuropathic pain, which can be prominent. Surgical treatment can consist of neurolysis or primary nerve repair. Tendon or nerve grafting and transfer can be used if there is no improvement or if there is a plateau in recovery.

Acute Brachial Neuritis

Acute brachial neuritis (often referred to as Parsonage-Turner syndrome) typically presents with acute onset of severe pain in the shoulder blade and upper arm or neck, followed days to 2 weeks later by weakness of the muscles of the shoulder girdle and/or upper limb. Antecedent events such as immunizations, infections, surgery, and pregnancy are common. Because of the severe pain at onset, it is frequently misdiagnosed as an acute shoulder injury. Weakness is bilateral in one third of cases, although one side usually predominates.[39] The upper trunk of the brachial plexus is preferentially affected, although focal involvement of individual nerves is also seen (with the long thoracic, suprascapular, axillary, radial, anterior interosseous, and phrenic nerves most commonly involved).[153]

Initial treatment of acute brachial neuritis consists of management of the initial severe pain with analgesics.

Table 41-5 Localization of Focal Brachial Plexus Lesions

Plexus Lesion	Nerves Affected	Muscles Affected	Sensory Nerve Conduction Studies Affected
Trunks			
Upper	Suprascapular Lateral pectoral Musculocutaneous Lateral portion median Portion of radial Axillary	Supraspinatus, infraspinatus Upper portion pectoralis major Biceps Pronator teres, flexor carpi radialis Brachioradialis Deltoid	Lateral antebrachial cutaneous (LAC) median radial
Middle	Thoracodorsal Subscapular Radial Lateral portion median	Latissimus dorsi Teres major All radial muscles (except brachioradialis) Pronator teres, flexor carpi radialis	Median Radial
Lower	Medial Pectoral Ulnar Medial portion median	Lower pectoralis major All ulnar muscles All median muscles except pronator teres and flexor carpi radialis	Ulnar to fifth digit Medial
Cords			
Lateral	Musculocutaneous Lateral portion median	Biceps Pronator teres Flexor Carpi Radialis	LAC Median to first digit
Posterior	Thoracodorsal Subscapular Axillary Radial	Latissimus dorsi Teres major Deltoid All radial muscles	Median to third digit Radial to first and third digits
Medial	Ulnar Medial half of median	All ulnar muscles All median muscles excepts pronator teres and flexor carpi radialis	Ulnar to fifth digit MAC

Systemic corticosteroids might also help with the acute pain but do not alter the course of the disease.[166] Shoulder range of motion should be maintained, and orthoses should be used as appropriate to assist function. Prognosis is generally good; however, recovery might occur over several years, with 85% recovering over 3 years.[167] Residual weakness can lead to musculoskeletal disorders later in life, as commonly occurs when postbrachial neuritis scapular stabilizer weakness predisposes to rotator cuff pain.

Thoracic Outlet Syndrome

Neurogenic thoracic outlet syndrome (TOS) is far more common than vascular TOS.[19] Neurogenic TOS occurs from compression of the brachial plexus as it passes through and exits the thoracic outlet. The brachial plexus typically travels posterior and superior to the subclavian vein, passing over the rib, between the medial and anterior scalene muscles, referred to as the interscalene triangle (Figure 41-8). At its midcourse the plexus runs between the first rib and the clavicle. Distally, as it enters the axilla, it passes beneath the pectoralis muscle close to its insertion on the coracoid process. The plexus can become compressed at any of these points. A common cause of TOS is the presence of a cervical rib, with fibrous bands, accessory and hypertrophied scalene muscles, anatomic variations in the course of the muscle, and postural factors also described. The lower trunk is most commonly affected. The typical presentation is a thin female with long neck, kyphotic posture, and protracted shoulders, complaining of symptoms of paresthesias along the medial aspect of the arm and hand with neck and shoulder pain. Weakness and atrophy of the hand intrinsic muscles may be seen. X-ray, computed tomography, and MRI may reveal a cervical rib, fibrous band, or abnormal anatomy. Electrodiagnostic studies will reflect lower trunk involvement, with the T1-originating fascicles most affected. Therefore, a typical pattern is an absent medial antebrachial cutaneous response, low median motor and ulnar sensory responses, and relatively normal median sensory response. Needle study will likewise demonstrate abnormalities in lower trunk muscles predominantly, with the T1-innervated thenar eminence muscles more affected than the C8-innervated ulnar hand intrinsics. Management will be directed by the severity and cause of the TOS. In mild cases therapy can alleviate postural strain on the plexus. The use of botulinum toxin injection to the scalene, subclavius, and/or pectoralis minor muscles has been found to helpful in many cases.[164] Surgical management, including scalenectomy with or without first rib resection, is required in some.

Neoplastic-Induced and Radiation-Induced Plexopathies

Both neoplasm and late effects of radiation treatment can involve the brachial plexus. Neoplastic plexopathy is most commonly seen with lung and breast cancer and most commonly involves the lower plexus. Less commonly head and neck cancers will preferentially affect the upper portion of the plexus, although lymphatic metastasis will demonstrate a more patchy distribution. The most common early symptom of neoplastic plexopathy is pain in the shoulder and axilla with dermatomal involvement of the medial arm and hand and weakness involving muscles supplied by the lower plexus (C8-T1). If the mass is adjacent to the first thoracic vertebrae it may affect the sympathetic ganglia causing a Horner syndrome. Radiation-induced plexopathy is a late effect of treatment, presenting 0.5 to 20 years after treatment[77] and is dose related. The etiology of injury is caused by both direct toxic effects on the axon and damage to the vasa vasorum of the nerve causing ischemia. In a patient presenting with plexopathy after radiation treatment for cancer it is important to differentiate between radiation effects compared with recurrent tumor (Table 41-6). Radiation plexopathy tends to present with numbness, sensory changes, and weakness, with less initial pain, and gradual progression.[46] Radiation is more likely to be bilateral, and less likely to solely affect the lower trunk.[77]

MRI or computed tomography may detect tumor recurrence, with enhancement of the affected nerves and T2-weighted hyperintensity seen in neoplastic plexopathy. Positron emission tomography can also detect recurrent neoplasm, although it will be negative in radiation

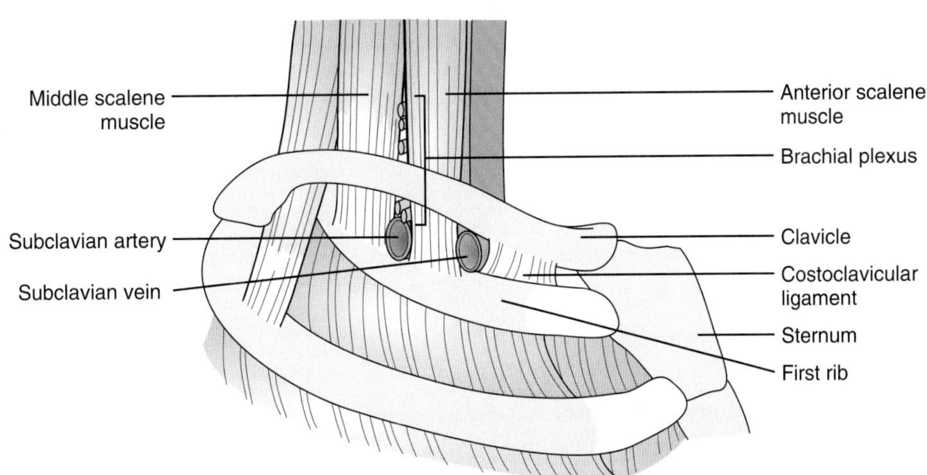

FIGURE 41-8 Neurogenic thoracic outlet syndrome occurs from compression of the brachial plexus as it passes through and exits the thoracic outlet. The brachial plexus typically travels posterior and superior to the subclavian vein, passing over the rib, between the medial and anterior scalene muscles, referred to as the interscalene triangle.[172]

plexopathy. EMG may show more widespread denervation than clinically suspected. The presence of myokymia is very characteristic of radiation plexopathy, seen in up to 75% of cases[42] and not seen in neoplasm.

Pain from neoplastic plexopathy may be relieved with radiation treatment; however, it can be very severe and require aggressive management. If pharmacologic treatment is inadequate, regional blocks, sympathectomy, rhizotomy, or other measures may be required. Management of both neoplastic and radiation plexopathy is largely supportive with therapy to maintain range of motion and prevent contractures, adaptive measures, and management of lymphedema and prevention of skin breakdown. Occasionally nerve transfer or reconstruction has been utilized in select patients with radiation plexopathy.[168]

Proximal Upper Limb Mononeuropathies

The median, ulnar, and radial nerves are the major terminal branches supplying the upper limb. Multiple smaller nerves arise directly from the brachial plexus to supply the muscles of the shoulder girdle and proximal arm muscles. These are summarized in Table 41-7.

Table 41-6 Differentiating between neoplastic and radiation brachial plexopathy

	Neoplasm	Radiation
Location	Unilateral, lower plexus	May be bilateral, upper plexus
Presenting symptoms	Prominent pain	Sensory changes, weakness
Associated symptoms	Horner syndrome	Upper extremity edema
EMG	No myokymia	Myokymia
MRI	Nerve enhancement, T2 hyperintensity	No nerve enhancement, T2 hyperintensity may be seen
PET scan	Positive	Negative

PET, Positron emission tomography.

Median Mononeuropathies

The median nerve is formed from the medial and lateral cords of the brachial plexus just distal to the axilla. In the upper arm the nerve courses parallel to the intermuscular septum, then passes under the bicipital aponeurosis (lacertus fibrosis) before entering the antecubital fossa medial to the biceps tendon and anterior to the brachialis muscles. In a small percentage of people there is a small bone spur that is proximal to the medial epicondyle that is spanned by a ligament called the ligament of Struthers, which crosses over the nerve. The median nerve usually courses between the superficial and deep heads of the pronator teres and then between the humeroulnar and radial portions of the flexor digitorum superficialis, supplying these muscles along with the flexor carpi radialis. About 4 cm distal to the medial epicondyle of the humerus, the median nerve gives off the anterior interosseous nerve, which supplies the lateral portions of the flexor digitorum profundus, flexor pollicis longus, and the pronator quadratus muscles. Just before entering the wrist the median nerve gives off the palmar cutaneous branch, which supplies the skin over the thenar eminence. At the wrist the median nerve passes through the carpal canal, which is made up of the carpal bones and the transverse carpal ligament. The carpal canal contains the four tendons, each of the flexor digitorum superficialis and profundus, the flexor pollicis longus, and the median nerve (Figure 41-9). After exiting the carpal tunnel in the hand, the median nerve supplies the first and second lumbricals, opponens pollicis, abductor pollicis brevis, and the digital cutaneous branches, which supply the palmar surface of the thumb and second, third, and lateral portion of the fourth fingers (Figure 41-10). The median nerve is vulnerable to injury at a number of sites,

Table 41-7 Neuropathies of the Shoulder Girdle and Proximal Arm

Nerve	Clinical Presentation	Causes
Long thoracic Serratus anterior	Winging of the medial scapular border at rests Shoulder abduction and flexion limited to 90° Sensory normal	Traumatic Surgery: thoracotomy, radical mastectomy, axillary node resection, first rib resection Acute brachial plexitis Idiopathic
Suprascapular Supraspinatus Infraspinatus	Weakness of abduction and external rotation Tenderness at suprascapular notch May be difficult to differentiate from rotator cuff tear	Trauma: blunt, scapular fracture Compression at suprascapular notch or spinoglenoid notch Sports: baseball, volleyball Acute brachial plexitis
Axillary Deltoid	Weakness abduction (intact supraspinatus may compensate) Small area of sensory loss over deltoid	Trauma: Shoulder dislocation, fracture neck of humerus, blunt trauma Injections, shoulder surgery Positional (prone with arms over head) Acute brachial plexitis
Musculocutaneous Biceps Brachialis	Weakness of elbow flexion Sensory loss radial aspect of forearm	Trauma-humerus fracture, stab, gun shot Strenuous exercise, violent elbow extension
Spinal accessory (cranial nerve 11) Sternocleidomastoid Trapezius	Shoulder depressed, weakness of shoulder shrug, flexion, abduction Lateral winging of scapula	Cervical lymph node dissections, radical neck dissection, carotid endarterectomy Blunt injury to posterior neck, compression from slings Heavy lifting with turning of head

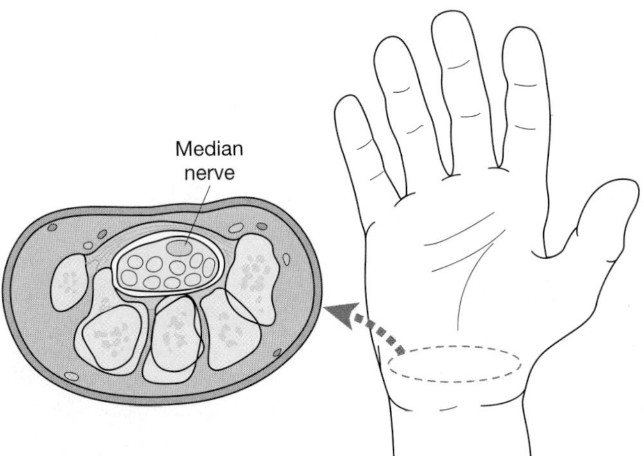

FIGURE 41-9 The carpal canal is formed by the carpal bones and the flexor retinaculum. The contents include the median nerve, flexor pollicis longus tendon, and four tendons each of the flexor digitorum profundus and superficialis muscles. (Modified from Moeller JL, Hutchinson MR: Carpal tunnel. In Rakel RE, editor: *Textbook of family medicine*, ed 7. Philadelphia, PA, 2007, Saunders.)

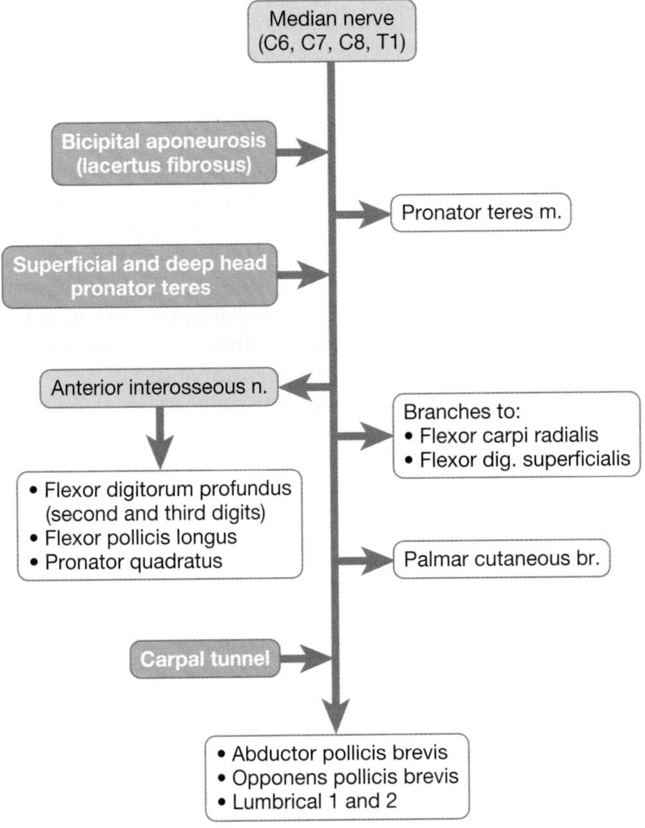

FIGURE 41-10 Median nerve.

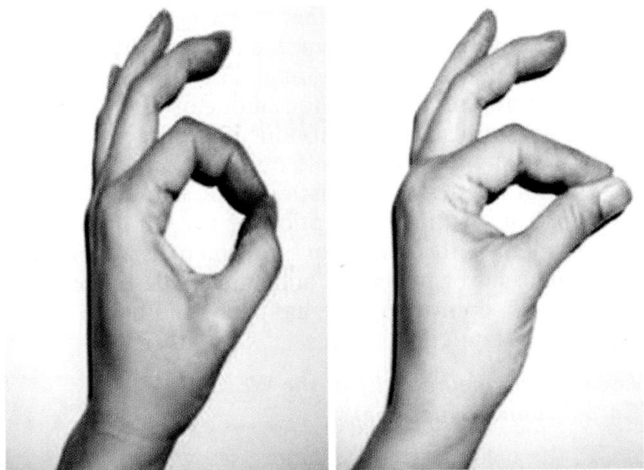

FIGURE 41-11 Anterior interosseous syndrome causes weakness of flexors to distal joints of the fingers and inability to form the "OK" sign (*right*).

with compression at the wrist (CTS) being the most common compressive neuropathy. Other sites of median nerve compression occur at the anterior interosseous nerve and the pronator muscle.

Anterior Interosseous Syndrome

The anterior interosseous nerve can be compressed at the fibrous arch formed by the flexor digitorum superficialis and the pronator teres. The nerve can also be injured from repetitive forearm flexion or pronation, elbow or forearm fracture, or in association with brachial neuritis. Anterior interosseous injury is a purely motor syndrome resulting in weakness of flexion of the interphalangeal joint of the thumb and distal interphalangeal joints of the index and middle fingers. This can be assessed by asking the patient to make the "OK" sign. Because of weakness of the flexors of the distal joints of the fingers, they will substitute with a key pinch (Figure 41-11). Weakness of the pronator quadratus is typically less apparent because of intact strength of the pronator teres. Testing pronation with the elbow in flexion will better isolate the action of the pronator quadratus. Patients often complain of an aching pain in the forearm, but there is no sensory loss. On electrodiagnostic studies, typical nerve conduction studies are normal, and needle examination might demonstrate denervation in the muscles supplied by the interosseous nerve.

Conservative treatment is usually initiated with a trial of nonsteroidal antiinflammatory drugs (NSAIDs) and avoidance of repetitive elbow flexion, pronation, or forced gripping. A posterior elbow splint can be applied. Spontaneous improvement has been reported from 3 to 24 months after symptom onset.[57] Surgical decompression can be indicated if there is no motor recovery.

Pronator Syndrome

Pronator syndrome occurs when the median nerve is compressed as it passes between the two heads of the pronator teres, a fascial band from the flexor digitorum superficialis, or the biceps aponeurosis. Patients present with pain and paresthesias in the first three fingers of the hand, often mimicking CTS. There will also be involvement of the skin over the thenar eminence, which is usually spared in CTS. Nocturnal awakening as a result of pain is a common feature of CTS but not of pronator syndrome. Weakness and easy fatigue can be seen in all the muscles innervated by the median nerve, except for the pronator teres, which is innervated proximal to the site of entrapment. Pain might be provoked by resisted elbow flexion and pronation and resisted finger flexion. Tenderness over the nerve at the area of compression or a Tinel sign might be elicited.

On electrodiagnostic studies, median sensory amplitudes are diminished or absent. Median sensory latencies, when present, are typically normal. The amplitude of the median motor response in the abductor pollicis brevis muscle is diminished, and conduction velocity over the forearm can be slowed. Needle examination can demonstrate abnormalities in all muscles supplied by the median nerve, usually with the exception of the pronator teres. Improvement with conservative treatment is reported in more than half of patients,[81] and surgical decompression in those who do not improve has been reported to have a high success rate.[166]

Median Mononeuropathy at the Wrist (Carpal Tunnel Syndrome)

In CTS the median nerve is compressed within the carpal canal, approximately 1 to 2 cm beyond the distal wrist crease. It is more common in women and is often bilateral but more severe in the dominant hand.[145] Repetitive hand and wrist movement, such as with keyboarding or use of vibratory tools, has been associated with CTS. A number of medical conditions are associated with CTS, including diabetes, hypothyroidism, and RA,[152] as well as obesity[13] and pregnancy. Infrequently CTS can be caused by a mass lesion at the wrist, such as a ganglion cyst or neurofibroma, or associated with acute trauma to the wrist. The great majority of cases of CTS are idiopathic.

The typical presentation of CTS includes paresthesias and numbness of the second and third digits and variably the thumb and lateral fourth digits, although often the patient will have more diffuse complaints of the entire hand being numb. Usually the thenar eminence will be spared any sensory abnormalities because the palmar cutaneous branch comes off proximal to the carpal tunnel. Symptoms are classically worse at night, causing nocturnal wakening, and relieved by flicking the hands and placing them in a dependent position. Other exacerbating activities include driving or holding objects, such as a telephone, book, or steering wheel, with a flexed or extended wrist. Occasionally patients complain of pain that radiates up the forearm or even to the shoulder. Weakness of the median innervated muscles of the hand can be perceived as difficulty opening jars, buttoning, or dropping objects. Weakness involves primarily thumb abduction and opposition. When severe, atrophy of the thenar eminence can be seen. Long finger flexor strength should be normal, as should be ulnar innervated finger abduction. A Tinel sign can be elicited, usually 1 to 2 cm distal to the wrist crease, reproducing symptoms in the median distribution. A Phalen sign reproduces paresthesias in the second and third fingers by holding the wrist in a flexed position by pressing the dorsum of both hands together for 30 to 60 seconds (Figure 41-12). This test might be overly sensitive for other causes of pain, such as joint pain at the wrist or even eliciting pain in the ulnar nerve distribution from the associated flexion at the elbow. Muscle stretch reflexes are unaffected in CTS.

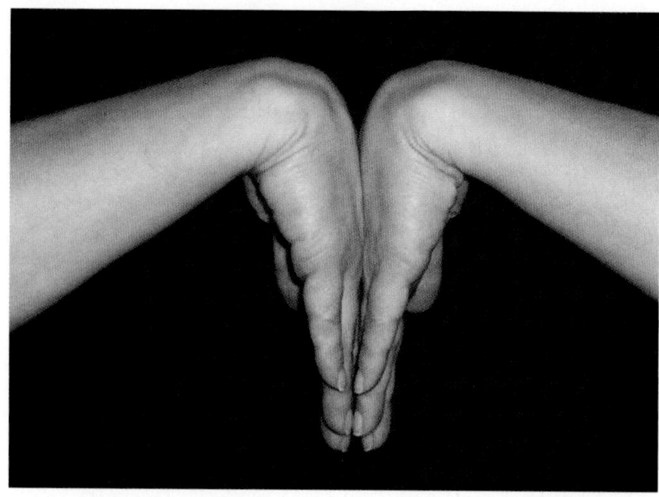

FIGURE 41-12 The Phalen test for median nerve compression.

The differential diagnosis of CTS includes proximal median nerve injury (pronator syndrome), C6 or C7 radiculopathy, and brachial plexopathy. An alternative diagnosis should be suspected if there is weakness of non-median-innervated muscles or proximal median-innervated muscles, or if there is asymmetry of muscle stretch reflexes or prominent neck pain. Electrodiagnostic studies are useful in confirming the diagnosis of CTS and assessing the severity, as well as excluding other neurologic diagnoses. Median sensory abnormalities are typically seen earlier than motor abnormalities. Median sensory latencies are prolonged, particularly compared with ulnar sensory latency on the same hand, with a difference of more than 0.5 ms significant (assuming the same distance is used for the stimulation to recording electrode). Midpalmar stimulation might be more sensitive because it records over a shorter segment across the carpal tunnel.[37] Median motor responses are affected in more severe disease and can show decreased compound motor amplitude and prolonged distal latency, with normal conduction velocity across the forearm. Needle EMG can demonstrate acute or chronic denervation in the abductor pollicis brevis or opponens pollicis muscles in moderate to severe CTS and is also useful in excluding alternative or concomitant disease, such as cervical radiculopathy or plexopathy. The role of ultrasonography (US) in the diagnosis and management of CTS is evolving. It appears unlikely that US is superior to electrodiagnostic techniques in evaluating CTS, and it may actually be inferior.[26]

Mild to moderate CTS usually responds to conservative measures. Exacerbating activities, such as those associated with repetitive or excessive wrist flexion and extension and gripping, should be avoided. The wrist should be splinted in 0 to 5 degrees of extension. Wrist splints are widely available but frequently hold the wrist in greater than 30 degrees of extension. In this case the patient should be instructed in reducing the wrist extension angle of the metal plate along the dorsum of the wrist, which is typically easily done. The splint is worn at night and as tolerated during the day. NSAIDs are often used, but there is no evidence of their usefulness. One study suggests that they are ineffective; in contrast, oral steroids are often helpful.[25] Local corticosteroid injections into the carpal tunnel have been shown to be superior to surgical decompression for clinical symptoms at 3 months and similar at 1 year. Two injections can be required if nocturnal paresthesia persists after the initial treatment.[100] Surgical decompression is indicated in patients with severe or rapidly progressive weakness and atrophy, or for those who fail to respond to conservative measures, or if there is a mass lesion causing the median nerve compression. A recent review of the treatment of CTS emphasized that surgery is far from uniformly effective, and that liberalization of the use of injections might be indicated.[15] The authors' experiences and recent research findings support this view, given that injections yield a high rate of success and are often associated with improvement in nerve conduction study parameters, as well as symptoms.[9,65] A trial comparing US-guided versus palpation-guided carpal tunnel injection techniques found that both methods provided clinically significant improvements in symptoms and hand function. One symptom scale favored the US technique at 12 weeks, but not 6 weeks, and there were no group differences in hand function. Moreover, the palpation technique used an ulnar approach rather than the more midline and proximal approach used in most studies.[100] At this point, practitioners can be assured that carpal tunnel injection, regardless of technique used, provides reliable improvement in symptoms and hand function.

Ulnar Mononeuropathies

The ulnar nerve originates from the C8 and T1 nerve roots, which merge to form the lower trunk of the brachial plexus. The lower trunk continues on as the medial cord and then as the ulnar nerve after giving off the medial antebrachial cutaneous branch. This anatomic relationship has diagnostic significance in that ulnar nerve lesions do not cause sensory changes to the medial aspect of the forearm, whereas T1 radiculopathy and lower trunk plexopathy can do so. The ulnar nerve courses along the medial aspect of the upper arm in close proximity to the median nerve. Just proximal to the elbow the nerve runs relatively superficially in the groove made by the medial epicondyle and the olecranon, and then dives between the tendons of the flexor carpi ulnaris (which originate from the same two structures). The ulnar nerve innervates the flexor carpi ulnaris, usually distal to the elbow, and travels distally along the medial aspect of the forearm, giving branches in the distal third to the palmar and dorsal aspects of the medial hand. This arrangement also has clinical relevance in that elbow lesions can cause numbness of the entire medial aspect of the hand; in contrast, wrist injuries primarily affect the digits. The nerve enters the Guyon canal in the wrist between the hook of the hamate and the pisiform bone. Although the nerve is accompanied by an artery, the canal includes no tendons, possibly explaining why injuries to it are more likely related to external compression than overuse. After entering the hand the ulnar nerve branches to supply the structures indicated in Figure 41-13, terminating in the adductor pollicis and flexor pollicis brevis within the thenar eminence. The nerve is most vulnerable to injury at the elbow and wrist, and these are explored further below.

Ulnar Neuropathy at the Elbow

CTS is the only focal neuropathy more common than ulnar neuropathy at the elbow (UNE). UNE incidence rates are estimated to be 25.2 to 32.7 for men and 17.2 to 18.9 for women per 100,000 person-years.[93,110] Risk factors for UNE have been less studied than those for CTS. Recent work suggests that UNE preferentially affects the left side regardless of hand dominance and, in addition to mechanically demanding events, such as repetitive elbow flexion, gripping, or external pressure over the ulnar groove,[33] older age, male gender, and smoking cigarettes increase the risk of UNE.[12,50,131,132] With regard to smoking as a modifiable risk factor, two studies have found that pack-years of smoking correlate negatively with electrophysiologic ulnar parameters across the elbow[131,134] and a third showed that likelihood of UNE increased with tobacco exposure.[50] These findings have clinical relevance with reference to patient teaching, and in the resolution of worker compensation cases involving ulnar nerve injuries. Moreover, prevention of UNE is of clinical relevance, given that results of therapy are often disappointing[48] and hand function is significantly compromised absent normal ulnar innervation.

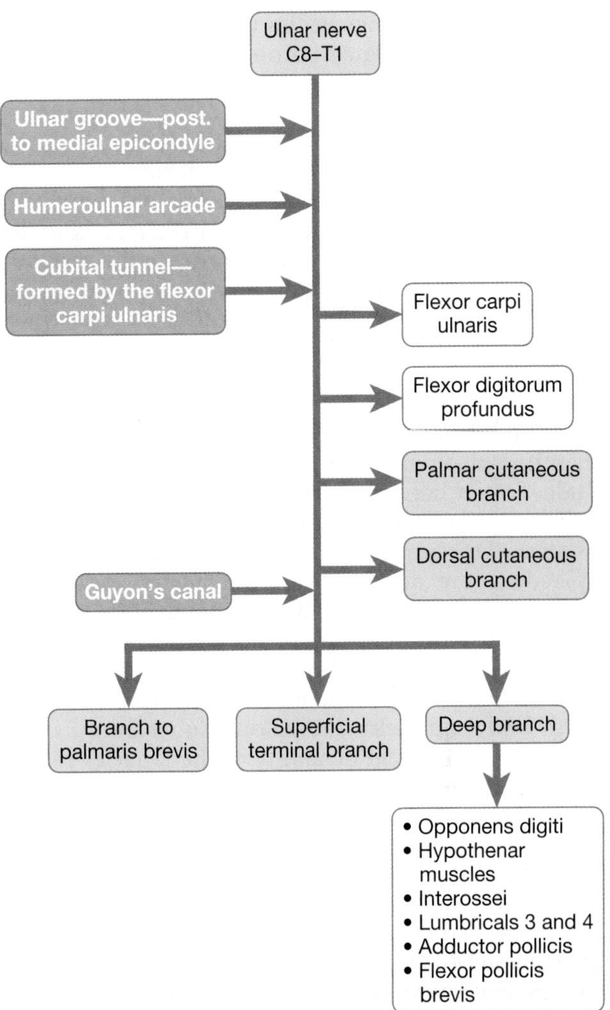

FIGURE 41-13 Ulnar nerve.

Patients with UNE typically present with dysesthesia and sensory change over the ulnar aspect of the hand. In contrast to CTS, patients less frequently report that the entire hand feels numb. Patients might also report pain or discomfort over the medial aspect of the forearm. As the disease advances, patients report loss of dexterity and grip strength and difficulty with eating and dressing. Examination reveals altered sensation in the ulnar distribution of the hand, including the segment from wrist to proximal interphalangeal joints, with sparing of the medial forearm. A Tinel sign is often elicited over the nerve in the retroepicondylar region or slightly distally, where the nerve dives between the twin head origin of the flexor carpi ulnaris tendons, although its diagnostic utility has been questioned.[14] Strength of the interossei is reduced, and with advanced cases, scalloping of the region over the first dorsal interosseous muscle is noted (often in association with some "clawing" of the hand as a result of intrinsic muscle weakness).

Electrodiagnostic studies are usually able to differentiate UNE from other diagnostic considerations. C8–T1 radiculopathy and lower trunk plexopathy are usually associated with minimal ulnar nerve slowing across the elbow and include EMG changes in nonulnar innervated muscles such as opponens pollicis, flexor pollicis longus, and extensor indices. Lower trunk and medial cord lesions also typically reduce the amplitude of the medial antebrachial cutaneous response. More difficult, however, is localizing an ulnar lesion to the region of the elbow. Nerve conduction studies across the elbow are fraught with difficulty related to elbow position, elbow temperature, segment length, body habitus, anomalous innervation in the forearm, differential vulnerability of the fascicles that run within the nerve, and slowing of the forearm segment of the nerve as a result of axonal degeneration. Typical, but not universal, handling of these concerns is by: (1) maintaining the elbow at 90 degrees flexion and the wrist in neutral during nerve conduction studies; (2) warming the elbow as needed to keep it more than 31.0° C (87.8° F); (3) testing an 80- to 100-mm segment across the elbow; (4) measuring carefully in patients with large upper limbs so as to not falsely increase the nerve conduction velocity in that segment; (5) evaluating median nerve stimulation in the antecubital fossa and recording over an ulnar innervated hand intrinsic muscle, to make certain that a median to ulnar contribution in the forearm is not responsible for an apparent conduction block; and (6) considering nerve conduction studies to the first dorsal interosseous muscles and the more standard abductor digiti quinti muscle. Lastly, if technical factors remain a concern, then performing a mixed nerve study recording over the median and ulnar nerves in the medial humerus and stimulating distally over the same nerves eliminates concerns regarding temperature, body habitus, and elbow positioning.[106] The absence of prolongation of the ulnar response onset of more than 1.4 ms compared with the median onset suggests that no ulnar lesion is present.[106] If the ulnar response is prolonged, then reasonable criteria for localizing the problem to the elbow include: (1) conduction velocity across the elbow less than 50 m/s; (2) a decrement in conduction velocity across the elbow, compared with that in the forearm, of more than 10 m/s; and (3) conduction block across the elbow of more than 20%. Because of the technical challenges, it is likely that using just one criterion for UNE will be overly sensitive. Therefore, it is recommended that UNE be considered likely in the correct clinical setting if two of three criteria are met, or definite if three of three criteria are met. The first dorsal interosseous is the muscle most likely affected during EMG needle examination, with the abductor digit quinti and flexor carpi ulnaris, respectively, less involved. If there is diagnostic uncertainty in the setting of presumed UNE, diagnostic ultrasonography is reasonable to consider with nerve enlargement the most robust diagnostic finding.[23]

The results of therapy for UNE, both surgical and nonsurgical, are variable. Typical strategies include avoiding power gripping at work or in avocation, preventing prolonged or repetitive elbow flexion (using a splint as necessary to enforce this restriction), cushioning of the posterior–medial elbow to prevent compression, and educating patients. In the absence of clinical or electrodiagnostic improvement within 2 to 3 months, surgical evaluation and transposition of the nerve or release of the fascia associated with the twin heads of the flexor carpi ulnaris are often performed. Given that smoking appears to be an independent risk factor for UNE and reduces patient satisfaction after surgery,[112] avoidance of tobacco is a reasonable recommendation.

Ulnar Neuropathy at Wrist

Ulnar neuropathy at the wrist (UNW) is rare compared with UNE and CTS and has a more varied presentation. The nerve in the hand and wrist has four sites of potential injury. When the nerve is compressed within the Guyon canal, the patient has altered sensation in the fourth and fifth digits, with sparing of the dorsal ulnar region of the hand, and weakness of all the ulnar innervated hand muscles. The superficial sensory branch arises just distal to Guyon canal so that with injury distal and medial to the canal, the same pattern of weakness will be present but without sensory loss. With a more distal injury, usually related to a penetrating wound or a ganglion, there is sparing of hypothenar musculature and sensation, with weakness in the interossei. On rare occasions there can be injury to the superficial sensory branch only, leading to sensory loss without weakness. When UNW is suspected, the electromyographer should stimulate the ulnar nerve and record from the first dorsal interosseous and the hypothenar eminence, and consider performing a dorsal ulnar cutaneous study as well. With these studies, as well as needle EMG of these same muscles, the site of most lesions can be determined. Although lesions within Guyon canal resulting from prolonged wrist radial deviation or pressure over the ulnar aspect of the wrist, as occurs with distance cycling, can respond to activity modification, most patients with these injuries are best referred to a qualified hand surgeon for consultation.

Radial Mononeuropathies

The radial nerve is the largest terminal branch off the brachial plexus, with contribution from C5–C8 nerve roots. It continues from the posterior division of the plexus and runs along the lateral wall of the axilla, supplies the triceps muscles, and then winds around the spiral groove of the humerus. It then pierces the intermuscular septum below the deltoid and supplies the brachioradialis muscle and extensor carpi radialis longus and brevis above the elbow. It then enters the forearm between the biceps and brachioradialis muscles and divides into the posterior interosseous nerve and superficial radial nerve at the level of the elbow

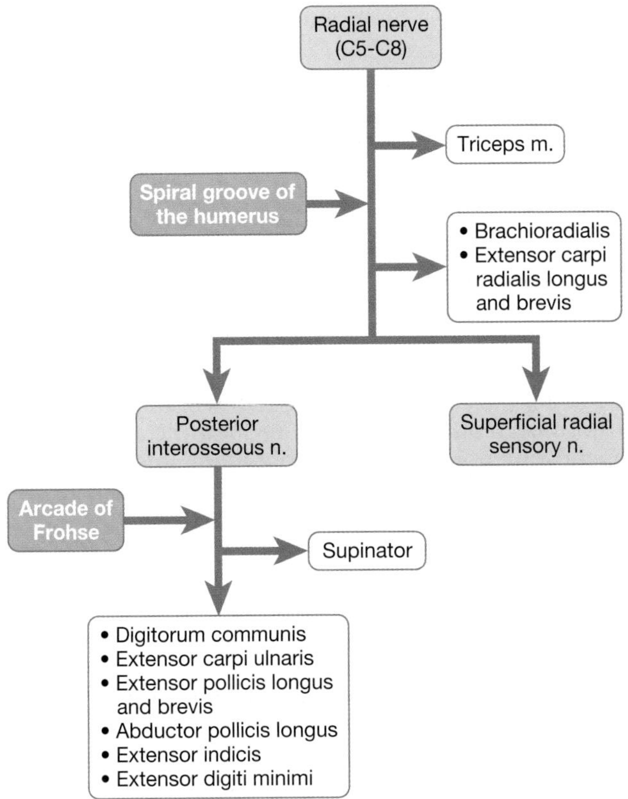

FIGURE 41-14 Radial nerve.

joint. The posterior interosseous nerve courses around the neck of the radius passing through the arcade of Frohse, which is made up of the proximal border of the supinator muscle. The posterior interosseous nerve innervates the supinator muscle before entering the extensor compartment of the forearm, where it supplies the extensor digitorum communis, extensor carpi ulnaris, extensor pollicis longus and brevis, abductor pollicis longus, extensor indicis, and extensor digiti minimi. The superficial radial nerve traverses the forearm to supply sensation to the dorsolateral portion of the hand and first three digits (Figure 41-14). The radial nerve is less commonly injured than the median and ulnar nerves, and less susceptible to compression. The nerve is usually injured proximally at the spiral groove or at the level of the posterior interosseous nerve. Occasionally the superficial radial branch will be injured at the wrist, causing purely sensory abnormalities on the dorsolateral aspect of the hand. This is encountered with use of handcuffs, tight wristwatches, or even wrist braces used for other conditions such as CTS.

Radial Neuropathy at the Spiral Groove

The most common injury to the radial nerve occurs at the radial groove from fracture of the humerus as a result of the nerve's close association with the humerus in the spiral groove. The radial nerve can also be injured in this area as a result of external compression from tourniquets. It can also be injured during prolonged sleep or unconsciousness. This can occur with persistent pressure from a sleeping partner's head on the patient's outstretched arm (so-called honeymooner's paralysis). It more commonly occurs when the patient's arm is draped over a chair for a long period (so-called Saturday night palsy when associated with inebriation). The radial nerve can also be injured in the proximal arm from poorly placed injections. Occasionally delayed radial nerve palsy can occur after humeral fracture as a result of compression or entrapment within the healing callous. Radial injury at the spiral groove typically presents with wrist drop and inability to extend the fingers. Extension of the elbow is usually spared because the triceps is innervated before the spiral groove. Elbow flexion might be mildly weak as a result of involvement of the brachioradialis. Median and ulnar innervated muscles should be strong; however, finger abduction can falsely appear weak unless the metacarpophalangeal joints of the hand are held in passive extension. In radial nerve injury in the region of the spiral groove of the humerus, sensation is abnormal in the lateral aspect of the dorsum of the hand and the dorsum of digits one through four. The brachioradialis reflex is diminished or absent, whereas the triceps and biceps reflexes are spared. Differential diagnosis for hand and wrist drop includes more proximal radial injury, usually in the axilla, C7 or C8 radiculopathy, or posterior lesion of the brachial plexus. Weakness involving the triceps and diminished triceps reflex would suggest that the radial lesion is more proximal than the region of the spiral groove. Involvement of median or ulnar innervated C7 and C8 muscles and the cervical paraspinals is consistent with radiculopathy. A posterior cord lesion would also cause weakness of the deltoid muscle. Motor nerve conduction studies can be performed recording over the extensor indicis and stimulating over the radial nerve at the elbow, spiral groove, and more proximally either at the Erb point or in the axilla. Conduction block is diagnosed with a more than 50% decrease in amplitude of the motor response when stimulating proximally compared with distally to the site of the lesion. The superficial radial sensory nerve can also be assessed. Needle EMG can also be helpful in localizing the level of radial injury and ruling out other causes.

Treatment of proximal radial nerve injuries depends on the cause of the injury. Weakness that is caused by external compression is typically a neurapraxic injury that usually recovers spontaneously within 2 months.[165] Radial nerve injury caused by a humeral fracture can have a poorer outcome. Radial lesions caused by closed fractures have better recovery than with more complex fractures. If any response can be recorded from the extensor indicis, there is a 90% chance that antigravity wrist strength will develop.[101] If there is no recovery within 8 to 10 weeks, surgical exploration is indicated, and if there is no return of function after 1 year, tendon transfer is considered to improve upper limb functioning. During the recovery period a "cock-up" splint is used to maintain the wrist and fingers in an extended position.

Posterior Interosseous Neuropathy

The most common cause of posterior interosseous neuropathy (PIN) is entrapment at the arcade of Frohse (also known as supinator syndrome).[30] The nerve can also be injured from elbow fractures, laceration, or compression from soft tissue masses such as lipomas,[182] neurofibromas, schwannomas, hematomas, and elbow synovitis from RA.[107] Onset is usually insidious and can be associated with strenuous use of the forearm, particularly pronation and supination. Weakness is seen in the finger extensors and the extensor carpi ulnaris. The brachioradialis and radial wrist extensors are spared. When the patient is asked to extend the wrist, radial deviation is seen. The supinator muscle is variably affected. Sensation in the radial distribution is spared because the posterior interosseous nerve has no sensory fibers. Nerve conduction studies to the extensor indicis are abnormal, whereas radial sensory conductions are preserved. The EMG needle examination typically localizes the lesion. Treatment for idiopathic PIN involves avoidance of provocative activities, use of oral NSAIDs, and splinting. Resolution of symptoms is seen in up to 80% with conservative treatment.[83] If no improvement is seen after 4 to 12 weeks, or if there is progressive or severe weakness and atrophy, surgical treatment brings good to excellent recovery of function in up to 90% of patients.[68] If a mass lesion is present, surgical exploration is usually required. In the unlikely event that there is no return of strength, tendon transfers can be used to improve function.

Concept of Double Crush

On closing the section of upper limb focal neuropathies, it is appropriate to address the "double-crush" hypothesis. This appealing concept suggests that when peripheral nerves are compressed proximally, they are predisposed to a distal compression to a greater degree than if the proximal injury was not present, presumably as a result of a disruption in axoplasmic flow. The most commonly cited and originally hypothesized example is that of cervical radiculopathy predisposing to CTS.[111,148,170] No clear reason is known, however, why a lesion proximal to the dorsal root ganglion, as occurs with cervical radiculopathy, should affect distal sensory nerve function, as commonly occurs with CTS (because axoplasmic flow within the sensory nerve is not disrupted). Adding to this deductive line of thought, careful neurophysiologic analyses of CTS in the setting of different levels of cervical radiculopathy, as well as radiculopathy level and frequency in the setting of more distal lesions, do not support the double-crush hypothesis.[130] A neurophysiologic rationale, therefore, for the double-crush hypothesis is unlikely. Because of the high coincidence of median neuropathy at the wrist in a large group of patients with electrodiagnostically confirmed cervical radiculopathy,[130] it is possible that there are intrinsic or extrinsic conditions that predispose patients to both diagnoses. Possibilities include repetitive upper limb usage, a subclinical predisposition to pressure injury or a tendency to generate thickened or hypertrophied ligamentous or other connective tissue, or presence of a systemic disease that can affect nerves, such as diabetes, all of which would increase patient risk for both diseases. This possibility aside, the words of John D. Stewart[153] are insightful regarding this controversial concept: "In summary, it seems highly unlikely that proximal focal neuropathies such as radiculopathies lead to, or worsen, more distal focal neuropathies in the same limb. The term *double-crush syndrome* and the admittedly attractive concept it embodies should be dropped from use. The disconcerting trend of performing several surgical procedures on a limb to decompress allegedly double- or multiple-crush sites should be discontinued."[153]

Lumbosacral Plexopathies

The lumbosacral plexus can be divided into the lumbar plexus and the sacral plexus. The lumbar portion is formed within the psoas muscle from the L1-L3 nerve roots with contributions from T12 and L4. The lumbar plexus provides direct branches to the psoas. The terminal branches are the ilioinguinal, iliohypogastric, genitofemoral, femoral, lateral femoral cutaneous, and obturator nerves, which will be discussed in detail in subsequent sections. The sacral plexus forms within the pelvis anterior to the piriformis. Terminal branches include the nerves to the superior/inferior gemelli, the obturator internus, piriformis, the superior and inferior gluteal, posterior femoral cutaneous, and the sciatic (Figure 41-15).

The plexus can be injured by trauma, usually associated with pelvic or hip fractures. This preferentially affects the sacral plexus because of direct compression or laceration from bony fragments or from traction injury. Concurrent root avulsion can occur, usually in association with separation of the sacroiliac (SI) joint. Incomplete lesions commonly occur and are often overlooked in the acute phase because of pain and immobility from the orthopedic injury or from altered mental status from concurrent brain injury or intubation. It is not uncommon to detect these injuries during consultation in the trauma unit, or after the patient has begun the rehabilitation course. Therefore, have a high index of suspicion for plexus and other peripheral nerve injury in the setting of trauma.

The plexus is susceptible to compressive lesions. Tumor can injure the plexus through direct extension to adjacent tissues, commonly seen with colorectal, gynecologic, and prostate cancer. Metastatic deposit near the plexus occurs most commonly with breast and thyroid cancer or sarcoma. Direct deposit to the plexus itself can occur. Lymphoma has also been implicated. Plexopathy caused by malignancy usually presents with pain as the predominant symptoms, with weakness and sensory loss occurring later. The lumbar plexus is preferentially affected by compression because of retroperitoneal hemorrhage, usually in association with anticoagulation, blood dyscrasias such as hemophilia, and leaking aortic aneurysm. An important cause of nontraumatic plexopathy is radiation-induced plexopathy. This typically presents years to decades after treatment for malignancy. It is important to distinguish this from plexopathy caused by cancer recurrence. Radiation plexopathy will often present painlessly, with predominantly insidious weakness. It is often bilateral. Obstetric injury can occur, with risk factors including cephalopelvic disproportion, abnormal fetal presentation, and use of forceps during delivery. Diabetes can also cause a lumbosacral plexitis as previously discussed in this chapter.

Electrodiagnosic testing is helpful in confirming a plexopathy and documenting the severity and extent of the lesion. It may also be useful in differentiating between plexopathy, radiculopathy, and individual mononeuropathy. MRI and CT are important to evaluate for injuries in the setting of trauma or compressive lesions in nontraumatic cases.

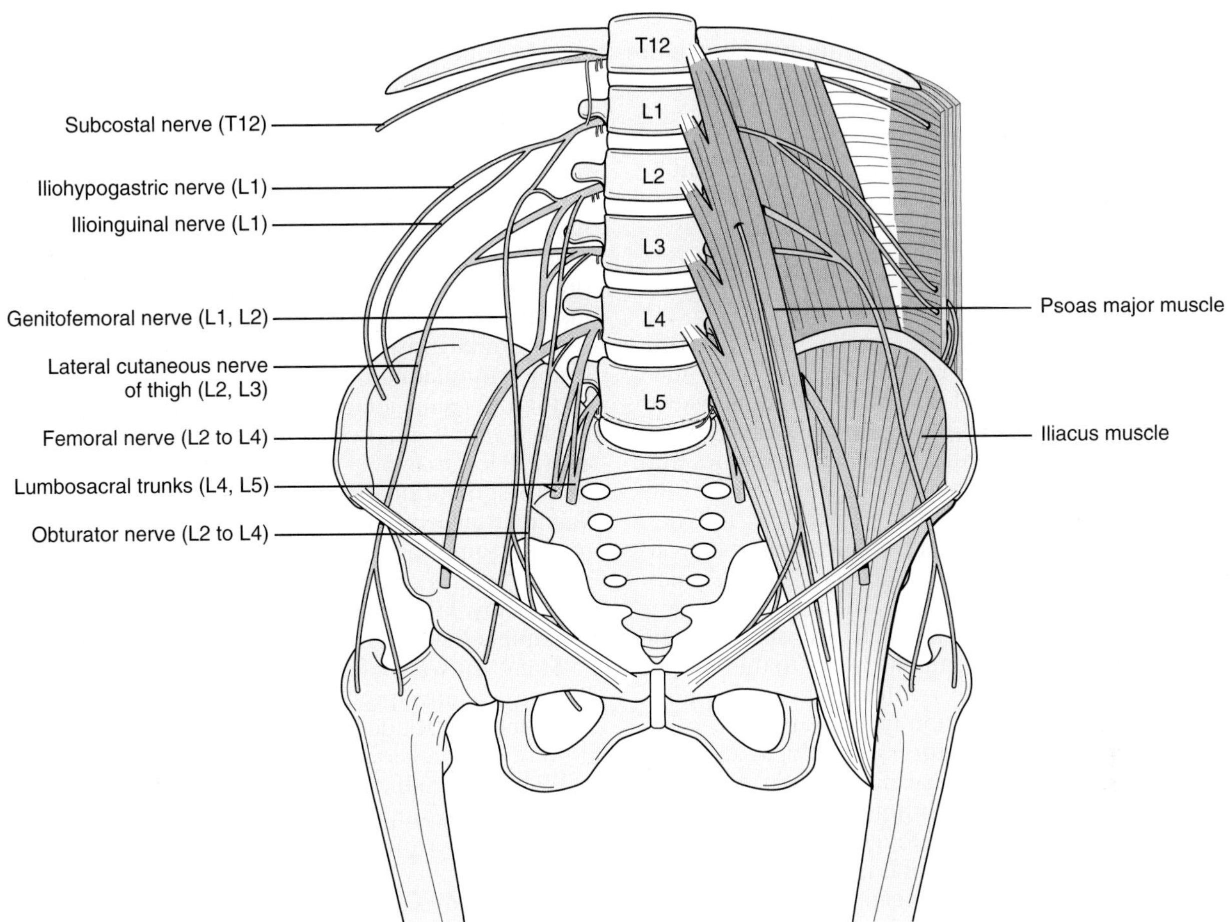

FIGURE 41-15 The lumbosacral plexus.

Table 41-8 Anatomic Pattern of the Lower Abdominal Muscles

Nerve	Root Level	Course	Typical Innervation Pattern
Ilioinguinal	L1 (variable T12)	Lateral border psoas, along iliac crest, pierces transversus abdominis near anterior superior iliac spine (ASIS), accompanies spermatic cord/round ligament in inguinal canal	Upper portion inner thigh, base of penis and upper scrotum, mons pubis and lateral labia
Iliohypogastric	L1 (variable T12)	Passes over lateral border of psoas, along inner surface of ilium, between transversus and external oblique.	Posterolateral gluteal and abdomen above pubis
Genitofemoral	L1 and L2	Travels through psoas. Femoral branch passes under inguinal ligament. Genital branch passes through the inguinal ligament.	Round ligament, labia majora, base of scrotum, and cremasteric muscle

Lower Abdominal Neuropathies

Pain affecting the lower abdomen and genital region can be a manifestation of injury to the ilioinguinal, iliohypogastric, and genitofemoral nerves. This can be a diagnostic challenge and patients may present after unfruitful gastroenterologic, urologic, or gynecologic workup. Localization can be challenging as these nerves have overlapping and variable patterns of innervation (Table 41-8). Generally these neuropathies will present with pain or abnormal sensation in their dermatomal distribution. Weakness of the anterior abdominal muscle can contribute to hernia formation. A Tinel sign can sometimes be elicited near the anterior superior iliac spine (ASIS). The cremasteric reflex may be lost. Extension of the spine puts tension on the nerves, and patients may adopt a forward flexed posture.

Frequent areas of entrapment or injuries to these nerves include the psoas muscle, the transverse abdominis muscle, and the inguinal ligament and canal. Most of these injuries are iatrogenic and associated with Pfannenstiel incisions, placement of lateral trochars in inguinal hernia repairs, and in surgeries with low transverse incisions such as abdominoplasty and C-section. The nerves may be compressed by space-occupying lesions of the psoas muscle, entrapment in the transversus abdominus near the ASIS, or blunt trauma in this area. Scar tissue entrapment after surgery in the inguinal region could also occur. These nerves cannot be directly visualized on imaging; however, imaging can reveal a compressive space-occupying lesion if clinically suspected. EMG does not directly assess these nerves but can rule out a high lumbar radiculopathy or plexopathy. If the neuropathic pain cannot be managed conservatively, nerve blocks can be both therapeutically and diagnostically useful. The use of US or nerve stimulation for localization can increase accuracy.[161] Finally neurolysis or resection can be successful in recalcitrant cases.

Femoral Neuropathy

The L2–L4 spinal roots form the femoral nerve, which supplies the psoas muscles within the pelvis. The nerve then travels between the psoas and iliacus muscles, innervating the iliacus just before it passes under the inguinal ligament. After emerging under the inguinal ligament, it divides into its terminal branches, which supply the four heads of the quadriceps muscle, the sartorius and pectineus muscles, and the medial and intermediate cutaneous branches to the anterior thigh, and the saphenous nerve, which innervates the medial leg (Figure 41-16). The femoral nerve is usually injured within the retroperitoneal space in the pelvis or under the inguinal ligament. Injury to the femoral nerve is most commonly the result of iatrogenic causes such as intraabdominal and intrapelvic surgeries, often caused by self-retaining retractors, gynecologic and urologic procedures, and ilioinguinal nerve blocks and catheterization procedures.[35] The lithotomy position, with extreme hip flexion and external rotation, has been implicated in compression of the femoral nerve at the inguinal ligament.[5] Thin individuals have greater risk of injury from retractors and the lithotomy position,[178] although obese patients are at greater risk of femoral nerve injury from high energy pelvic trauma.[95] Hematomas caused by anticoagulant therapy and blood dyscrasias are also common causes of femoral neuropathy.

Femoral neuropathy presents with unilateral thigh weakness and numbness of the anterior thigh and leg. Lesions caused by lithotomy positioning can occasionally present bilaterally. Often a sensation of instability around the knee and buckling, with particular difficulty with stairs and inclines, is noted. The patellar reflex can be depressed or absent. If the nerve is compressed within the pelvis, hip flexion can also be affected. Adduction and abduction of the thigh should be normal, as should knee flexion and strength around the ankle. Pain with extension of the hip (the so-called reverse leg raise) can be seen with femoral nerve injury. Sensory changes are seen in the anterior thigh and medial lower leg in the saphenous nerve distribution.

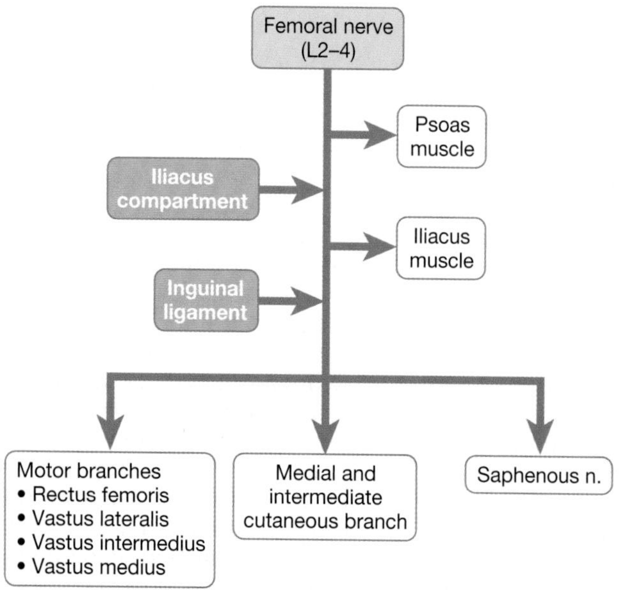

FIGURE 41-16 Femoral nerve.

Electrodiagnosis includes femoral motor conduction studies stimulating the groin. If the CMAP is at least 50% of the opposite side, the prognosis is good for improvement within 1 year, whereas fewer than half of those with a CMAP less than 50% will improve.[90] Needle examination can assist in localizing the site of the lesion to the inguinal ligament or pelvis based on involvement of the iliopsoas muscle. Sampling of the hip adductor muscles and paraspinal muscles can exclude high lumbar radiculopathy or plexopathy. MRI and CT are indicated if there is suspicion for a mass lesion.

Many causes of femoral neuropathy are preventable. During operative procedures, extremes of flexion, external rotation, and abduction of the hip should be avoided to prevent compressions as the nerve passes under the inguinal ligament. Self-retaining retractors are also a source of injury during surgeries, and care should be taken with placement to avoid compressing the nerve as it passes the psoas muscle.[20] When a femoral neuropathy is suspected, imaging studies can assess for compression caused by hematoma, masses, or pseudoaneurysm. If a correctable cause is found, immediate surgical intervention might be indicated. Incomplete lesions usually improve significantly on their own. Early physical therapy for strengthening and range of motion should be initiated. The patient can be trained to activate the gluteal muscles and/or plantar flexors in stance phase to augment weakened knee extension. With mild to moderate weakness, an ankle-foot orthosis with dorsiflexion stop can create an extension moment at the knee to compensate for quadriceps weakness. If the weakness is severe, knee-ankle-foot orthosis may be indicated; however, these are often poorly tolerated. A walker to keep the ground reaction force anterior to the knee's axis of rotation during stance is often more functional. Serial clinical and electrodiagnostic examinations should be performed. If there is no improvement after 3 to 6 months, either clinically or electrodiagnostically, surgical intervention might be indicated.[35] As the quadriceps is such a large muscle, it is important to extensively sample the muscle for signs of reinnervation, as early recovery in the more proximal portions may be missed if only sampled in the more typically studied middistal portions.

Lateral Femoral Cutaneous Neuropathy

Mononeuropathy of the lateral femoral cutaneous nerve, also known as meralgia paresthetica, is a common and benign cause of anterolateral thigh numbness.[52] The lateral femoral cutaneous nerve is a purely sensory nerve arising from the L2 and L3 nerve. There are a number of anatomic

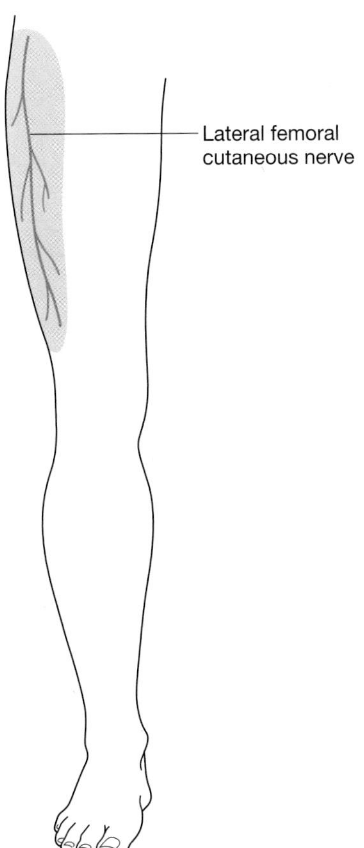

FIGURE 41-17 The sensory territory of the lateral femoral cutaneous nerve. (Modified from Craig EJ, Clinchot DM: Lateral femoral cutaneous neuropathy. In Frontera WR, Silver JK, Rizzo TD, editors: *Essentials of physical medicine and rehabilitation: musculoskeletal disorders, pain, and rehabilitation.* Philadelphia, PA, 2008, Saunders.)

variations as the nerve exits the pelvis most commonly in close relationship with the ASIS and the inguinal ligament, making the nerve vulnerable to compression in this area.[8] The nerve then divides into anterior and posterior divisions and supplies the sensory territory of the anterolateral thigh (Figure 41-17). Meralgia paresthetica is usually idiopathic and associated with obesity, pregnancy, and diabetes.[76] External sources of compression include heavy tool belts, habitually leaning against a table, or wearing tight waist bands. Occasionally injury can occur during surgery, particularly during hernia repair, renal transplantation, harvesting of iliac bone graft, hip surgery, and aortic valve and coronary bypass surgery.[145] Tumor involving the iliac crest can also compress the nerve at the anterior superior iliac spine, or more proximally it can be affected by an abdominal aneurysm or other pelvic mass.

Patients with a lateral femoral cutaneous nerve dysfunction present with numbness and pain in a generally well-circumscribed distribution on the anterolateral thigh. These symptoms can be exacerbated by walking or extension of the hip and by wearing tight clothing or undergarments. No weakness of the lower limb is noted because this is a purely sensory nerve. On physical examination, in addition to numbness or hyperesthesia in the territory of the lateral femoral cutaneous nerve, Tinel sign might be elicited by percussing just medial and inferior to the ASIS. Manual motor testing and muscle stretch reflexes should not be affected. Symptoms consistent with meralgia paresthetica must be differentiated from femoral neuropathy, lumbar plexopathy, and high lumbar radiculopathy. In those with femoral neuropathy and lumbar radiculopathy, the sensory abnormalities are more widespread, involving the entire thigh and extending into the medial lower leg. Femoral and lumbar radiculopathies, unlike meralgia paresthetica, can also cause weakness of thigh muscles and a depressed patellar reflex.

Nerve conduction studies of the lateral femoral cutaneous nerve can reveal asymmetry when comparing the symptomatic side with the unaffected side. It should be noted, however, that this is a technically difficult sensory response to obtain, even in healthy, nonobese individuals.[92] Although not routinely performed in EMG laboratories, ultrasound can improve the ability to obtain a response by visualizing the nerve.[16] Needle EMG is normal in those with meralgia paresthetica. Anesthetic nerve block of the lateral femoral cutaneous nerve can help confirm the diagnosis, although the anatomic variability of the nerve may lead to a negative block.

Meralgia paresthetica is usually benign and self-limiting and improves with conservative treatment over a few months. Eliminating any exacerbating factors, such as tight clothing or tool belts, and weight loss will often resolve the symptoms. When painful paresthesia is present, topical agents such as capsaicin cream and Lidoderm patches can be helpful, particularly because the distribution of symptoms is localized. Oral agents used for neuropathic pain such as tricyclic antidepressants or antiseizure medications such as gabapentin, pregabalin, or carbamazepine can also control symptoms. Local corticosteroid injections might bring temporary relief.[40] Because of anatomic variability, ultrasound can improve localization. In refractory cases, surgery might be indicated, with high success rates reported for both decompression and neurectomy,[88] although patients will be left with a persistent area of numbness with the latter procedure.

Obturator Neuropathy

The obturator nerve forms within the psoas from the L2-4 nerve roots and runs anterior to the sacroiliac joint. Following the wall of the lateral pelvis the nerve passes through a fibro-osseous canal between the obturator muscles and the obturator sulcus of the pubic bone. It supplies the adductor longus and brevis, gracilis, pectineus, obturator externus, and a portion of the adductor magnus, which is dually innervated with the sciatic nerve. It also gives off articular branches to the hip and knee joint, as well as sensation to the distal two thirds of the medial thigh. Pelvic trauma, especially when involving disruption of the sacroiliac joint, rarely injures this nerve in isolation but is usually accompanied by damage to other nerves of the lumbar plexus or nerve roots. A number of iatrogenic injuries have been reported in association with the lithotomy position and in childbirth, caused by compression of the fetal head against the pelvis.[29,176] Entrapment in the fascia overlying the adductor brevis has been described in athletes, resulting in deep aching pain and weakness with exercise.[18]

Obturator neuropathy will present with loss of sensation of the medial thigh and weakness of adduction and internal rotation of the hip. A circumducted gait may be appreciated. In the case of trauma or surgery, pain may initially mask this weakness, delaying recognition of a nerve injury. EMG is most useful for detecting this injury. There is no nerve conduction study to evaluate this nerve, however needle examination will detect denervation in obturator innervated muscles.

Most obturator injuries recover well with conservative management. In those with compression at the obturator canal surgical release can be useful, particularly in those who fail conservative treatment and respond to a diagnostic block, especially athletes.[163]

Fibular (Peroneal) Mononeuropathies

The fibular nerve arises from the L4–S1 nerve roots and runs with the tibial nerve in the posterior thigh as part of the sciatic nerve. Before dividing from the tibial nerve at the popliteal fossa, it gives off a muscular branch to the short head of the biceps femoris, the only muscle of the thigh that is innervated by the peroneal (fibular) division of the sciatic nerve. Within the popliteal fossa it sends off a cutaneous branch to join a branch from the tibial nerve to form the sural sensory nerve. After dividing from the tibial nerve it courses around the fibular head, where it is firmly tethered by a fibro-osseous band; it then forms its terminal branches, the superficial and deep peroneal nerves. The superficial fibular nerve innervates the peroneus longus and brevis muscles, and it also supplies sensory innervation to the lower two thirds of the lateral leg and the dorsum of the foot, but not the first web space. In 12% to 35% of the population the superficial fibular nerve will give off an accessory peroneal nerve, which will contribute motor innervation to the extensor digitorum brevis.[169] The deep fibular nerve supplies the anterior tibialis, extensor hallucis longus, peroneus tertius, extensor digitorum brevis, and skin of the first web space (Figure 41-18).

Fibular neuropathy is the most common nerve injury in the lower extremity.[86] Lesions to the common fibular nerve frequently occur at the fibular head, where it is vulnerable because of its superficial location and because it is relatively tethered by a fibrous band that makes it susceptible to traction. Injury can result from compression from prolonged positioning during surgery or bed rest, particularly in cachectic patients. Splints, braces, and casts that are improperly placed can cause direct pressure over the nerve at the fibular head. Prolonged squatting can place excessive traction on the nerve. The nerve can be acutely injured by trauma to the knee, particularly with fractures of the fibular head.[85] Space-occupying lesions such as callous formation from healed fractures, Baker cysts, and tumor can cause compression. Anterior compartment syndrome preferentially injures the deep fibular nerve. Inversion sprains of the ankle can cause injury from traction and tearing of the vasa vasorum.[154] The deep fibular nerve can be compressed at the talonavicular joint deep to the extensor hallucis longus tendon or the superior and inferior extensor retinaculum. This is also known as anterior tarsal tunnel syndrome.

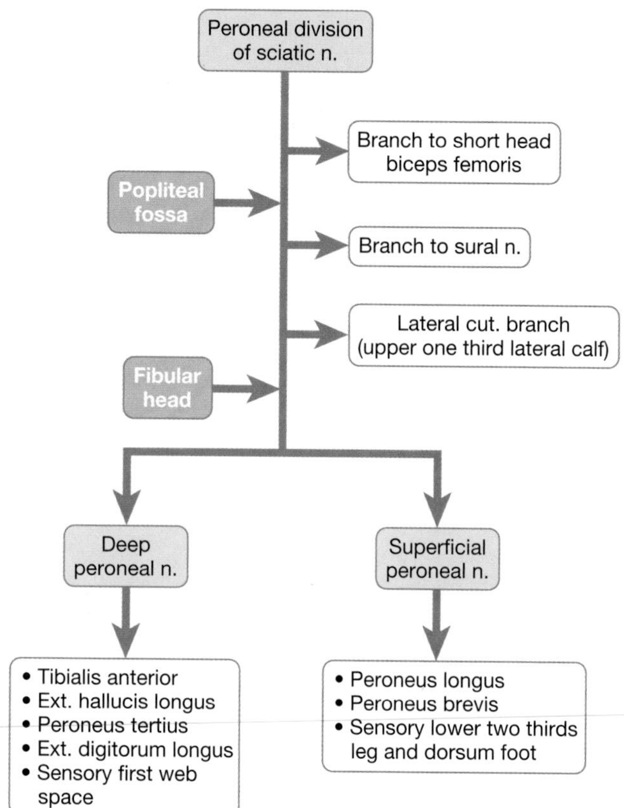

FIGURE 41-18 Peroneal nerve.

The most striking clinical finding is weakness of ankle dorsiflexion. In severe injury complete foot drop can result in a steppage gait, which allows the patient to clear the toe during the swing phase of gain. With more subtle weakness, premature foot flat or "foot slap" can be seen after heel strike on the affected side. Often the deep fibular branch is more affected than the superficial branch, with foot eversion less impaired. Sensation is diminished in the lower two thirds of the lateral leg and dorsum of the foot. A Tinel sign may be produced by tapping over the common fibular nerve as it courses around the fibular neck.

The clinical presentation of foot drop can be an interesting diagnostic challenge because several neurologic problems can present in a similar manner. The differential diagnosis includes L5 radiculopathy, lumbosacral plexopathy, and sciatic neuropathy. The presence of back pain, prominent leg pain, and depressed hamstring reflex would suggest radiculopathy. Weakness affecting hamstring muscles or weakness of plantar flexion would suggest sciatic or plexus involvement. Electrodiagnosis is the most helpful test for evaluating foot drop. The fibular motor study should be evaluated with conduction above and below the fibular head. The fibular motor response can be recorded over either the extensor digitorum brevis (EDB) in the foot or the anterior tibialis. Although the EDB is routinely used, it is frequently atrophic as a result of local trauma and might be less reliable. Focal conduction block, with greater than 20% drop in motor amplitude above to below the fibular head, is 99% specific in localizing fibular lesions at the knee.[119] The presence of any compound action potential response to the anterior tibialis (AT) or EDB on nerve conduction studies is associated with

Table 41-9 Electromyographic Evaluation of Foot Drop

	Superficial Peroneal Sensory Nerve Conduction	Anterior Tibialis	Peroneus Longus	Gluteus Medius	Medial Gastrocnemius	Biceps Femoris (Short Head)	Lumbar Paraspinals
Deep peroneal	Nl	Abnl	Nl	Nl	Nl	Nl	Nl
Common peroneal at fibular head	Decreased	Abnl	Abnl	Nl	Nl	Nl	Nl
Sciatic neuropathy	Decreased	Abnl	Abnl	Nl	Abnl	Abnl	Nl
L5 radiculopathy	Nl	Abnl	Abnl	Abnl	Nl	Nl	Abnl
Lumbosacral plexopathy	Decreased	Abnl	Abnl	Abnl	Abnl	Abnl	Nl

Abnl, Abnormal; *Nl*, normal.

recovery of good (grade 4 to 5) strength compared with absent responses.[32] Sural sensory and tibial motor conductions should be normal in those with fibular nerve injury and radiculopathy. Needle EMG is particularly useful in the evaluation of foot drop. Muscles supplied by both the superficial and deep fibular nerves should be sampled. The short head of the biceps femoris muscle is particularly useful for ruling out a sciatic lesion because it is the only muscle innervated by the fibular division before it separates from the tibial portion above the knee, and the tibial innervated muscles might be spared in a mild sciatic lesion. Nonfibular L5 innervated muscles such as the gluteus medius proximally or the posterior tibialis distally can exclude L5 radiculopathy. S1 innervated tibial muscles are also sampled to exclude a sciatic mononeuropathy (Table 41-9).

If symptoms are associated with a trauma, x-rays may demonstrate a fracture around the fibular head. MRI can visualize a space-occupying lesion as well as directly visualize the fibular nerve in the popliteal fossa and denervated muscles. Ultrasound can also visualize the nerve as it passes near the fibular head.

Treatment of fibular neuropathy starts with prevention. Because many cases of fibular neuropathy are caused by improper positioning during prolonged hospitalization or surgery, care should be taken to offload the lateral aspect of the knee with pillows and pressure-relieving ankle–foot orthoses. Casts and braces should be carefully evaluated and reevaluated for pressure points at the fibular head. Atraumatic outpatients with fibular neuropathy should be quizzed regarding prolonged knee flexion, severe weight loss, and habitual leg crossing. Ankle–foot orthoses are often needed when the foot drop is severe. Surgical management includes neurolysis and decompression, nerve repair, and nerve or posterior tendon transfers.

Tibial and Plantar Mononeuropathy

The tibial nerve arises from the L5–S2 nerve roots and forms the tibial division of the sciatic nerve. As part of the sciatic nerve it innervates all the hamstring muscles, with the exception of the short head of the biceps femoris. It also partially innervates the adductor magnus muscle. Within the popliteal fossa it contributes to the sural sensory nerve, innervating the lateral lower leg and foot, and continues on to supply the muscles of the posterior compartment of the lower leg. At the ankle it passes posterior to the medial malleolus through the tarsal tunnel, which is formed by the flexor retinaculum that spans the space between the medial malleolus and the calcaneus. Accompanying the tibial nerve is the posterior tibial artery, posterior tibialis, flexor digitorum longus, and flexor hallucis longus tendons. The tibial nerve then divides into its three terminal branches: the calcaneal branch and medial and lateral plantar nerves (Figure 41-19).

Proximal tibial neuropathies are unusual but can occur with injury to the popliteal space or with space-occupying lesions such as Baker cysts or hemorrhage. Blunt trauma or fracture of the distal femur of proximal tibia can also damage the nerve at this level. Lesions at this level would result in weakness of plantar flexion and inversion of the ankle, as well as sensory abnormalities in the sole of foot and sural nerve distribution. Midshaft injuries are very uncommon as the nerve is well protected in the posterior compartment, and in the absence of trauma would raise suspicion for a space-occupying lesion.

Lesions at the ankle occurring under the flexor retinaculum are referred to as tarsal tunnel syndrome. The compression can involve any of the three terminal branches.[113] Most cases are idiopathic, but other causes include ankle trauma, arthritis, deformity of the heel, talocalcaneal coalition,[157] vascular compression, and masses such as ganglion cysts or lipomas. Typical presentation of tarsal tunnel syndrome includes paresthesias and pain in the sole of the foot and heel, exacerbated by standing and walking. Physical examination might reveal sensory loss in the lateral or medial plantar distribution, although it will often spare the heel. A Tinel sign might be elicited by percussion over the flexor retinaculum at the medial malleolus. The interdigital nerves can become entrapped under the intermetatarsal ligament and form a Morton neuroma with chronic compression. These most commonly form in the second and third intermetatarsal spaces.

The differential diagnosis for tarsal tunnel syndrome includes diffuse PN, proximal tibial mononeuropathy, and S1 radiculopathy. Typically, tarsal tunnel syndrome is unilateral, whereas the symptoms of PN are usually bilateral and symmetrical and a Tinel sign is not present. Proximal tibial mononeuropathies can be differentiated by the presence of plantar flexion and inversion weakness and a depressed or absent Achilles reflex. S1 radiculopathies usually present with back, buttock, and posterior thigh pain and weakness in plantar flexors, knee flexors, and the gluteus maximus.

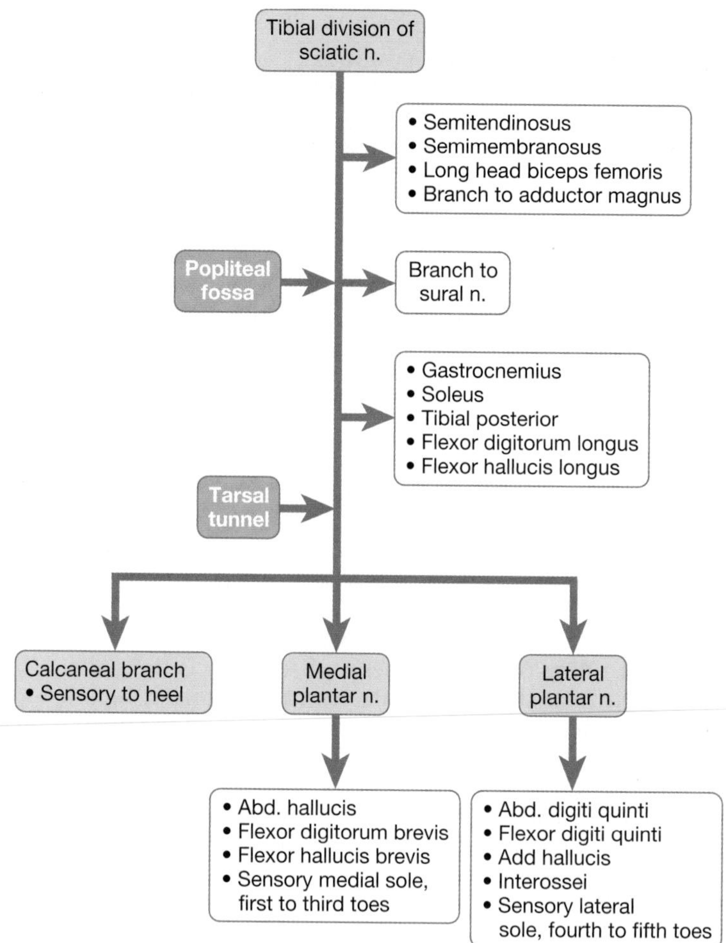

FIGURE 41-19 Tibial nerve.

X-rays are indicated if there is history of trauma to evaluate for fracture. MRI or US can demonstrate compressive masses and also can directly visualize the tibial nerve in the popliteal fossa. At the ankle MRI is useful in assessing the tarsal tunnel and evaluating for tenosynovitis, structural abnormalities, hypertrophied or accessory muscles, or other mass lesions. Nerve conduction studies will demonstrate variably affected sural responses if the lesion is proximal to the branch at the popliteal fossa. Tibial motor response from the abductor hallucis will be low. Needle examination is useful in localizing the level of the tibial lesion. Electrodiagnosis of tarsal tunnel syndrome includes nerve conduction studies of the medial and plantar nerves, which should be compared with those of the unaffected side,[31] particularly as abnormalities of the plantar responses can be seen in very early PN. Assessment of the plantar nerves can also be limited by technical factors such as thick foot calluses, foot and ankle deformity, and ankle edema. Needle examination of the abductor hallucis for the medial plantar nerve, and the abductor digiti quinti for the lateral plantar nerve might demonstrate abnormalities consistent with denervation; however, these muscles are painful to examine and can be denervated from local trauma in asymptomatic individuals.[45]

Treatment consists of NSAIDs, local corticosteroid injections, and orthoses to correct biomechanical abnormalities such as overpronation or excessive supination. An ankle-foot orthosis (AFO) with dorsiflexion stop can partially compensate for weakness of the medial gastrocnemius. Surgical release can be indicated for those who do not respond to conservative management but might be more effective in those with space-occupying lesions as the source of compression, in those with a positive Tinel sign, and when decompression occurs within 10 months of onset of symptoms.[171]

Sural Mononeuropathy

The tibial and fibular nerves both contribute sensory branches to the sural nerve. Occasionally a purely tibial innervated sural nerve occurs, and even less commonly purely fibular.[137] The sural nerve provides the sensory innervation to the posterolateral aspect of the distal third of the lower leg and the lateral aspect of the foot. Proximal injury is rare but has been reported in hemorrhage of the gastrocnemius muscle and masses within that muscle such as heterotopic ossification as well as Baker cysts within the popliteal fossa. Compression by a thickened gastrocnemius aponeurosis that is characterized by pain with exercise has been reported in athletes.[43] Iatrogenic injury can occur with ankle surgery or Achilles tendon repair, or deliberately sacrificed for graft harvesting in repair of fibular nerve or brachial plexus injuries. Distally the nerve is vulnerable to injury to the Achilles tendon, the ankle, and with fracture of the fifth metatarsal.

Treatment is directed at alleviating compressive sources and symptomatic management. In athletes with suspected compression at the aponeurosis neurolysis, an incision of the gastrocnemius fibrous arch can relieve symptoms if conservative measures fail.

Sciatic Mononeuropathy

As discussed previously, the sciatic nerve is made up of fibers from the L4–S2 nerve roots, forming the two divisions of the sciatic nerve, the tibial and fibular divisions. These divisions run as distinctly separate nerves that do not interchange fascicles. The fibular division is much more susceptible to injury than the tibial division. This is caused by two main factors. The fibular nerve is tethered at two points, the sciatic notch and at the fibular head, making it more vulnerable to traction than the tibial nerve, which is not similarly restricted. The fascicular pattern of the fibular nerve contains less supporting tissues and has larger and fewer fascicles than the tibial nerve, which is more invested with elastic epineurial tissue and is therefore more tolerant of external pressure.[156] The propensity for greater injury to the fibular division of the sciatic nerve can make it challenging to differentiate a sciatic lesion from a common fibular lesion. The tibial innervated hamstring and plantar flexor muscles are powerful, making subtle weakness less obvious than with muscles innervated by the fibular nerve. Common causes of sciatic nerve injury include hip fracture, posterior hip dislocation, and hip surgery, particularly total hip arthroplasty. Poorly placed gluteal injections, knife or gunshot wounds, compression resulting from positioning during hospitalization in patients with thin body habitus, and the lithotomy position[177] can also injure the nerve. Space-occupying lesions such as tumors, hematoma, aneurysm, and heterotopic ossification can cause compression of the nerve.

As discussed with fibular neuropathy, electrodiagnostic studies are designed to differentiate between sciatic neuropathy, common fibular or tibial mononeuropathy, L5 or S1 radiculopathy, and lumbosacral plexopathy. In severe sciatic neuropathy, all the fibular and tibial motor conduction studies are absent or reduced, as are the sural and superficial fibular sensory responses. In mild cases, side to side asymmetry of sensory and motor nerve conduction amplitudes are evaluated. On needle examination both fibular and tibial innervated muscles show abnormalities consistent with denervation, usually with fibular muscles more affected. Occasionally the fibular division can be exclusively injured in a sciatic lesion, in which case sampling of the short head of the biceps femoris is useful to differentiate it from a more distal common fibular lesion.[87] Gluteal and paraspinal muscles are spared in sciatic lesions. MRI can demonstrate compressive lesions and, along with CT scan, characterize traumatic injury. The sciatic nerve itself can be well visualized with MRI, showing focal enlargement and abnormal signal intensity. Ultrasound is not of use to evaluate the nerve within the pelvis; however, it may be useful to evaluate the nerve below the piriformis muscle.[103]

Treatment of sciatic nerve injury is largely supportive, with more specific management directed at the cause of the injury. If a compressive lesion such as tumor or hematoma is identified, decompression may be indicated. Nerve grafting outcomes are guarded caused by the size and length of the sciatic nerve.

KEY REFERENCES

3. Advisory Committee on Childhood Lead Poisoning Prevention of the Centers For Disease Control and Prevention: Guidelines for measuring lead in blood using point of care instruments. Retrieved from: www.cdc.gov/nceh/lead/ACCLPP/20131024_POCguidelines_final.pdf. Accessed 06/29/2014.
7. Ashton-Miller JA, Yeh MWL, Richardson JK, et al: A cane reduces loss of balance in patients with peripheral neuropathy: results from a challenging unipedal balance test, *Arch Phys Med Rehabil* 77:446–452, 1996.
11. Barohn RF, Saperstein DS: Guillain-Barré syndrome and chronic inflammatory demyelinating polyneuropathy, *Semin Neurol* 18:49–61, 1998.
15. Bland JDP: Treatment of carpal tunnel syndrome, *Muscle Nerve* 36:167–171, 2007.
16. Boon AJ, Bailey PW, Smith J, et al: Utility of ultrasound-guided surface electrode placement in lateral femoral cutaneous nerve conduction studies, *Muscle Nerve* 44:525–530, 2011.
17. Boulton AJM, Vinik AI, Arezzo JC, et al: Diabetic neuropathies: a statement by the American Diabetes Association, *Diabetes Care* 28:956–962, 2005.
19. Brantigan CO, Roos DB: Etiology of neurogenic thoracic outlet syndrome, *Hand Clinic* 20:17–22, 2004.
23. Cartwright MS, Walker FO: Neuromuscular ultrasound in common entrapment neuropathies, *Muscle Nerve* 48:696–704, 2013.
30. Cravens G, Kline DG: Posterior interosseous nerve palsies, *Neurosurgery* 27:397–402, 1990.
32. Derr JJ, Mickelsen PJ, Robinson LR: Predicting recovery after fibular nerve injury: which electrodiagnostic features are most useful?, *Am J Phys Med Rehabil* 88:547–553, 2009.
35. Ducic I, Dellon L, Larson EE: Treatment concepts for idiopathic and iatrogenic femoral nerve mononeuropathy, *Ann Plast Surg* 55:397–401, 2005.
39. Dumitru D, Zwarts M, Amato A: Peripheral nervous system's reaction to injury. In Dumitru D, Amato A, Zwarts M, editors: *Electrodiagnostic medicine*, ed 2, Philadelphia, PA, 2002, Hanley & Belfus.
53. Gabbai AA, Castelo A, Bulle Oliveria AS: HIV peripheral neuropathy. In Said G, Krarup C, editors: *Handbook of Clinical Neurology*, vol 115, ed 3, 2013, Elsevier.
55. Genuth S: Insights from the Diabetes Control and Complications Trial/Epidemiology of Diabetes Interventions and Complications Study on the use of intensive glycemic treatment to reduce the risk of complications of type 1 diabetes, *Endocr Pract* 12(Suppl 1):34–41, 2006.
56. Gonzalez-Duarte A, Robinson-Papp J, Simpson DM: Diagnosis and management of HIV-associated neuropathy, *Neurol Clin* 26:821–832, 2008.
61. Guitiérrez-Guitiérrez G, Sereno M, Miralles A, et al: Chemotherapy-induced peripheral neuropathy: clinical features diagnosis, prevention and treatment strategies, *Clin Transl Oncol* 12:81–91, 2009.
67. Harding AE, Thomas PK: The clinical features of hereditary motor and sensory neuropathy (types I and II), *Brain* 103:259–280, 1980.
71. Hoke A, Cornblath DR: Peripheral neuropathies in human immunodeficiency virus infection, *Suppl Clin Neurophysiol* 57:195–210, 2004.
77. Jaeckle KA: Neurologic manifestations of neoplastic and radiation-induced plexopathies, *Semin Neurol* 30:254–262, 2010.
78. Jani-Acsadi A, Krajewski K, Shy ME: Charcot-Marie neuropathies: diagnosis and management, *Semin Neurol* 2:185–194, 2008.
81. Johnson RK, Spinner M, Shrewsbury MM: Median nerve entrapment syndrome in the proximal forearm, *J Hand Surg [Am]* 4:48–51, 1979.
82. Joint Task Force of the EFNS and PNS: European Federation of Neurological Societies/Peripheral Nerve Society guideline on management of chronic inflammatory demyelinating polyradiculoneuropathy, *J Peripher Nerv Syst* 10:220–228, 2005.
88. Khalil N, Nicotra A, Rakowicz W: Treatment for meralgia paresthetica, *Cochrane Database Syst Rev* 3:1–14, 2008.
90. Kuntzer T, van Melle G, Regli F: Clinical and prognostic features in unilateral femoral neuropathies, *Muscle Nerve* 20:205–211, 1997.

96. Lewis RA: Chronic inflammatory demyelinating polyneuropathy, *Neurol Clin* 25:71–87, 2007.
98. London Z, Albers JW: Toxic neuropathies associated with pharmacologic and industrial agents, *Neurol Clin* 25:257–276, 2007.
103. Martinoli C, Miguel-Perez M, Padua L, et al: Imaging of neuropathies about the hip, *Eur J Radiol* 82:17–26, 2013.
105. McMillan HJ, Kang PB, Royden Jones H, et al: Childhood chronic inflammatory demyelinating polyradiculoneuropathy: combined analysis of a large cohort and eleven published series, *Neuromuscular Disord* 23:103–111, 2013.
115. Paola LD, Faglia E: Treatment of diabetic foot ulcer: an overview. Strategies for clinical approach, *Curr Diabetes Rev* 2:431–447, 2006.
117. Pareyson D, Scaioli V, Laurà M: Clinical and electrophysiological aspects of Charcot-Marie-Tooth disease, *Neuromolecular Med* 8:3–22, 2006.
120. Plasma Exchange/Sandoglobulin Guillain-Barré Syndrome Trial Group: Randomised trial of plasma exchange, intravenous immunoglobulin, and combined treatments in Guillain-Barré syndrome, *Lancet* 349:225–230, 1997.
123. Quigley PA, Bulat T, Schulz B, et al: Exercise interventions, gait, and balance in older subjects with distal symmetric polyneuropathy: a three-group randomized trial, *Am J Phys Med Rehabil* 93:1–16, 2014.
124. Raja SN, Haythornthwaite A, Pappagallo M, et al: Opioids versus antidepressants in postherpetic neuralgia: a randomized, placebo-controlled trial, *Neurology* 59:1015–1021, 2002.
126. Richardson JK: The clinical identification of peripheral neuropathy among older persons, *Arch Phys Med Rehabil* 83:205–209, 2002.
129. Richardson JK, DeMott T, Allet L, et al: The hip strength: ankle proprioceptive threshold ratio predicts falls and injury in diabetic neuropathy, *Muscle Nerve* 50:437–442, 2014.
130. Richardson JK, Forman G, Riley B: An electrophysiologic exploration of the double crush hypothesis, *Muscle Nerve* 22:71–77, 1999.
133. Richardson JK, Hurvitz EA: Peripheral neuropathy: a true risk factor for falls, *J Gerontol Ser A Biol Sci Med Sci* 50A:211–215, 1995.
136. Richardson JK, Thies SB, DeMott TK, et al: Interventions improve gait regularity in patients with peripheral neuropathy while walking on an irregular surface under low light, *J Am Geriatr Soc* 52:510–515, 2004.
138. Said G: Infectious neuropathies, *Neurol Clin* 25:115–137, 2007.
139. Said G: Necrotizing peripheral nerve vasculitis, *Neurol Clin* 15:835–848, 1997.
143. Seddon HJ: Three types of nerve injury, *Brain* 66:237–288, 1943.
150. Singleton J, Smith A: Neuropathy associated with prediabetes: what is new in 2007?, *Curr Diab Rep* 7:420–424, 2007.
151. Son J, Ashton-Miller JA, Richardson JK: Frontal plane ankle proprioceptive thresholds and unipedal balance, *Muscle Nerve* 39:150–157, 2009.
153. Stewart JD: Brachial plexus. In Stewart JD, editor: *Focal Peripheral Neuropathies*, Philadelphia, PA, 2000, Lippincott Williams & Wilkins.
158. Tesfaye S, Chaturvedi N, Eaton SEM, et al: Vascular risk factors and diabetic neuropathy, *N Engl J Med* 352:341–350, 2005.
159. Thaisetthawatkul P, Logigia EL: Peripheral nervous system manifestations of Lyme borreliosis, *J Clin Neuromusc Dis* 3:165–171, 2002.
162. Thomson RM, Parry GJ: Neuropathies associated with excessive exposure to lead, *Muscle Nerve* 33:732–741, 2006.
163. Tipton JS: Obturator neuropathy, *Curr Rev Musculoskel Med* 1:234–237, 2008.
165. Trojaborg W: Rate of recovery in motor and sensory fibres of the radial nerve: clinical and electrophysiological aspects, *J Neurol Neurosurg Psychiatry* 33:625–638, 1970.
169. Tzika M, Paraskevas GK, Kitsoulis P: The accessory deep peroneal nerve: a review of the literature, *Foot* 22:232–234, 2012.
171. Urguden M, Bilbasar H, Ozdemir H, et al: Tarsal tunnel syndrome-the effect of the associated features on outcome of surgery, *Int Orthop* 26:253–256, 2002.
177. Warner MA, Warner DO, Harper M, et al: Lower extremity neuropathies associated with lithotomy position, *Anesthesiology* 93:938–942, 2000.
181. Weimer LH, Sachdev N: Update on medication-induced peripheral neuropathy, *Curr Neurol Neurosci Rep* 9:69–75, 2009.

The full reference list for this chapter is available online.

CHAPTER 42

MYOPATHY

Carl D. Gelfius

Considering that movement, balance, coordination, circulation, respiration, speech, and swallowing all require adequate and appropriate force generation by muscle fibers, it is not surprising the wide-ranging impact a myopathy may have on an individual's function. A key role of the physiatrist includes appropriately diagnosing the specific myopathy because the clinical severity, rate of progression, and associated comorbidities vary greatly with the different muscle disorders. In addition, having an understanding of the etiology and natural history of muscle diseases provides the physiatrist a basis from which to work with the patient and the interdisciplinary team to institute treatments and interventions to limit morbidity and mortality while maximizing independence and quality of life. "Myopathies" encompass a large group of generally pure motor syndromes with symmetrical proximal greater than distal weakness. A small number of muscle diseases also include sensory or autonomic involvement. Successful identification and classification of a myopathic disease entails obtaining a detailed history and physical examination accompanied by the judicious use of diagnostic strategies. Box 42-1 presents a suggested guide for evaluating a patient with a myopathy, which is expanded upon in the following section. This approach should be tailored based on the specific individual and his/her clinical scenario.

Evaluation of the Patient with a Suspected Myopathy

Disease History

Successfully diagnosing, or ruling out, a myopathy begins with obtaining a detailed medical history. Weakness and hypotonia are common presenting concerns of parents of children with suspected muscle disease. Additionally, early feeding, respiratory difficulties, and delayed developmental milestones might prompt referral for evaluation. Although many muscle disorders have a genetic basis, clinical symptoms and physical findings may not become apparent until later in life. For some myopathies, the accumulation of muscle fiber injury may result in progressive weakness with characteristic periods of clinical disease onset. For other diseases, the limited force generation potential of the muscles becomes apparent as a child grows, causing the center of mass to elevate, and thereby increasing the force required to maintain posture and mobility. An adolescent or adult is more likely to have symptoms that include weakness, pain, muscle cramps, decreased endurance, difficulty keeping up with peers, and muscle atrophy.

For an infant or a child, a complete pregnancy and birth history are necessary. Questions should be asked to determine the quality of fetal movements, the presence of any complications during the pregnancy, and if any perinatal issues were present. Perinatal concerns, including respiratory distress, need for intubation or supported ventilation, and feeding difficulties, may raise suspicion for a myopathy. Timing of developmental milestones, including bringing hands to mouth, independent sitting, crawling, cruising, independent walking, and talking, may provide insight to disease progression.

For the adolescent and older patient, a more detailed history may be obtained, including the distribution of weakness, rate of progression, exacerbating factors, and ameliorating factors, to help narrow the differential diagnosis. In addition to functional limitations related to the suspected myopathy, a broad review of systems should be taken. Systemic information, including history of difficulty breathing, recurrent pneumonia, coughing with meals, respiratory impairment, daytime somnolence, morning headache, syncope, irregular heartbeat, exertional chest pain, rashes, weight loss, muscle atrophy, fatigue, academic performance, and previous issues with anesthesia (e.g., malignant hyperthermia), aid in determination of the breadth of the disease. Questions regarding sensation change or loss may suggest an alternative diagnosis.

Family History

Given the genetic origin of most muscle diseases, a careful family history of myopathy should be elicited. Completing a family pedigree may demonstrate a potential genetic transmission pattern of the muscle disorder. Autosomal dominant disorders may demonstrate nearly one half of siblings having the disorder without sexual predilection. By contrast, X-linked recessive disorders, such as Duchenne muscular dystrophy, will have nearly one half of males being affected on the maternal side. Increasing phenotypic severity in subsequent generations suggests genetic anticipation as may occur in myotonic muscular dystrophy.

Physical Examination

A comprehensive physical examination is the initial step in a myopathy evaluation. Information obtained from direct examination of the patient will guide the selection and interpretation of subsequent diagnostic testing, including laboratory studies, genetic testing, electrodiagnosis, and muscle biopsy.

Although it may be tempting to focus on the muscular examination, a thorough assessment of the entire body is essential to narrow the differential diagnosis of myopathic

BOX 42-1

Evaluation of the Patient with a Suspected Myopathy

Disease History
- Presenting symptom(s)
- Age of onset
- Birth history
- Developmental history
- Rate of disease progression
- Exacerbating/ameliorating factors
- Review of systems

Family History
- Known neuromuscular diseases
- Family with similar impairments

Physical Examination
- Craniofacial
- Cardiovascular
- Respiratory
- Abdominal
- Dermatologic
- Musculoskeletal
- Neurologic

Laboratory Workup
- Creatine kinase (CK)
- Alanine aminotransferase (ALT)
- Aspartate aminotransferase (AST)
- Aldolase
- Lactate
- Pyruvate

Molecular Genetics
- Gene mutation/deletion analysis
- Gene sequencing

Electrodiagnostic Studies (If Indicated)
- Nerve conduction studies
  - Sensory
  - Motor
- Repetitive nerve stimulation
- Electromyography

Muscle Biopsy
- Immunohistochemistry
- Western blot analysis

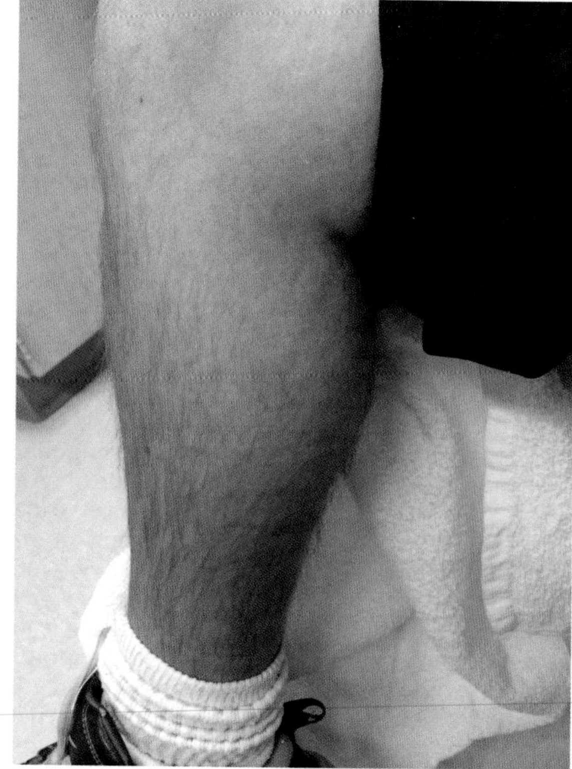

FIGURE 42-1 Calf pseudohypertrophy in a patient with limb-girdle muscular dystrophy 2C.

disease. The craniofacial examination may reveal a high arched palate or dental malocclusion that can be found in congenital myopathies and congenital muscular dystrophies. Macroglossia may be noted in certain limb-girdle muscular dystrophies. Temporal wasting and tenting of the upper lip are seen in myotonic muscular dystrophy. Some muscular dystrophies, such as Duchenne muscular dystrophy, sarcoglycanopathy, and Emery-Dreifuss muscular dystrophy, may have cardiac muscle involvement with resultant muscle fiber injury and endomysial fibrosis that alter conduction pathways, making cardiac evaluation imperative. Cardiac examination should include auscultation to evaluate for murmurs that may be related to a dilated cardiomyopathy. A shifted point of maximal impulse may suggest cardiac dilatation. Palpation of the distal pulse may reveal an irregular rhythm caused by a second or third degree heart block. Evaluation of the pulmonary system may demonstrate poor aeration of lung fields and restricted rib excursion from fibrosis of intercostal muscles. Accessory respiratory muscle use and nasal flaring may be markers of global weakness and compromised respiratory function. Hepatomegaly may be palpated in individuals with certain metabolic myopathies, such as acid maltase deficiency (Pompe disease, glycogen storage disease type II). In dermatomyositis, skin examination may be remarkable for a heliotrope rash around the eyes and erythema of extensor joint surfaces.

Evaluation of the musculoskeletal system may start with assessment of muscle bulk. Identifying muscles with atrophy, persevered size, and pseudohypertrophy may suggest a pattern common to a specific disease. For example, individuals with Duchenne muscular dystrophy may have pseudohypertrophy of the deltoid and infraspinatus causing a posterior axillary depression sign on examination. Pseudohypertrophy of the calves may be seen in Duchenne muscular dystrophy and sarcoglycanopathy (Figure 42-1). Preferential atrophy of the biceps and triceps is noted in individuals with facioscapulohumeral muscular dystrophy and Emery-Dreifuss muscular dystrophy. Scapular winging may be observed in cases of calpainopathy and sarcoglycanopathy (Figure 42-2). The presence, distribution, and timing of contractures are other important examination points. Congenital myopathies and congenital muscular dystrophies may have such profound weakness that the joints do not develop normally in utero resulting in arthrogryposis noted at birth. Some myopathies have characteristic contractures, such as early elbow flexion contractures in Emery-Dreifuss muscular dystrophy. Ullrich congenital muscular dystrophy has a unique combination of proximal joint contractures (i.e., knees, elbows) with distal joint hypermobility (i.e., wrists, ankles). Progressive muscle fiber injury and fibrosis, as occurs in several muscular dystrophies, may result in increasing contractures as strength declines. Evaluation of the spine may demonstrate scoliosis that may be observed in patients with central core myopathy, nemaline myopathy, multiminicore myopathy, and Duchenne muscular dystrophy.

The neurologic examination in patients with suspected myopathy should include cognitive assessment. Cognitive impairment may be present in individuals with Duchenne muscular dystrophy, congenital muscular dystrophy,

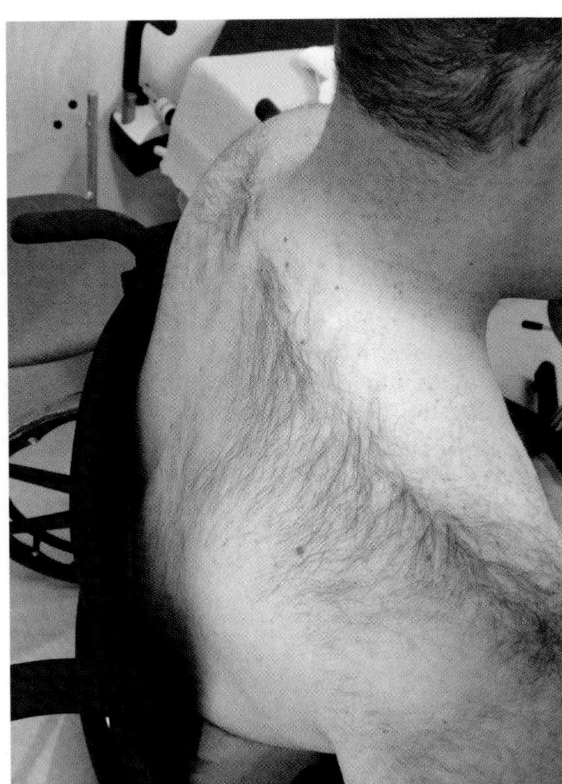

FIGURE 42-2 Scapular winging in a patient with limb-girdle muscular dystrophy 2C.

congenital myotonic muscular dystrophy, and mitochondrial myopathies. Evaluation of strength will aid in differentiating myopathic disorders. After 5 years of age, most cognitively intact children will be able to fully participate in manual muscle testing. For patients unable to comprehend the instructions for strength testing, attempting to have them reach for an object, kick an object, or mirror the examiner's movements can provide insight to which muscle groups have at least antigravity strength. Facial weakness is not universally seen with myopathies and may suggest specific disorders, such as facioscapulohumeral muscular dystrophy, congenital fiber-type disproportion, and myotonic muscular dystrophy. Similarly, ophthalmoparesis may help narrow potential disorders to centronuclear myopathy, multiminicore myopathy, congenital fiber-type disproportion, and mitochondrial myopathy. Most myopathies have proximal greater than distal weakness; however, exceptions with greater distal weakness, including inclusion body myositis, myotonic muscular dystrophy, and some variants of multiminicore myopathy, may stand out. Depending on the severity of weakness, muscle stretch reflexes may be normal or diminished. Percussion myotonia may be elicited in individuals with myotonic muscular dystrophy. Functional assessment, including transitions from supine to sit and sit to stand, may demonstrate neck flexion weakness, core weakness, and limb-girdle weakness. Myopathies associated with pelvic girdle weakness may demonstrate a Gower sign, in which the upper limbs are used to generate hip extension moments by "walking" up the lower limbs.

Gait may be altered for many reasons in myopathic diseases. Hip extension weakness may result in increased lumbar lordosis that shifts the weight line posterior to the hip. In this situation, the extension of the femurs will be limited by the Y ligaments of Bigelow and will require minimal hip extension strength to maintain. As knee extension becomes weaker, individuals may develop an equinus gait pattern that causes an extension moment at the knee and moves the weight line anterior to the knee. Both of these biomechanical changes help stabilize the knee in extension preventing knee buckling. Hip abductor weakness, involving gluteus medius in particular, may contribute to a drop of the pelvis such that the lower limb in swing phase will be lower as the contralateral hip abductors have insufficient strength to maintain a level pelvis. Compensation for gluteus medius weakness includes lateral bending of the torso toward the weak side (compensated Trendelenburg gait pattern) to functionally limit the pelvic drop.

Laboratory Workup

Initial laboratory screening tests typically include serum creatine kinase (CK), alanine aminotransferase (ALT), aspartate aminotransferase (AST), and aldolase. CK reversibly catalyzes creatine and adenosine triphosphate (ATP) to phosphocreatine and adenosine diphosphate (ADP) with energy release. Although CK is found predominantly in muscle, the liver contains high amounts of ALT, AST, and aldolase. In myopathies where muscle fibers are injured, these enzymes are released into the serum. Gamma-glutamyl transferase (GGT) is found mainly in the liver and can be evaluated to help differentiate muscle and liver disease. An elevated CK level may suggest a muscle disease but lacks sensitivity and specificity. In Duchenne and Becker muscular dystrophies, a marked elevation in CK (up to 100 times the upper limit of normal for Duchenne and up to 20,000 for Becker) is typical, with a normal CK level excluding these diagnoses.[29] Inflammatory myopathies, limb-girdle muscular dystrophy, facioscapulohumeral muscular dystrophy, and Emery-Dreifuss muscular dystrophy may also demonstrate elevated CK levels. CK levels, however, may be elevated after strenuous exercise in normal individuals. Myopathic disorders with structural abnormalities that affect contractility without causing fiber breakdown may have normal to slightly elevated CK values. Congenital myopathies such as central core myopathy, nemaline myopathy, and centronuclear myopathy represent such conditions. Additionally, CK level does not correlate with disease severity because chronic myopathies with significant atrophy may have a normal or even a low value. Because needle electromyography causes a transient increase in CK, testing should occur before electrodiagnostic evaluation or at least 72 hours afterward.[25]

Clinical scenarios suggestive of metabolic myopathies may benefit from further testing. The respiratory chain abnormalities seen in mitochondrial myopathies may cause elevated lactate and pyruvate levels.[4,33] Ischemic forearm exercise testing without at least a 3-fold increase in lactate level from baseline may support further evaluation for a glycogen storage disease.[48] Serum uric acid may be elevated in acid maltase deficiency (Pompe disease, glycogen storage disease type II), whereas myoglobinuria may be noted in myophosphorylase deficiency (McArdle disease, glycogen storage disease type V).[4] Quantification of urine amino and organic acids in addition to plasma amino acids further aids in the differentiation of some metabolic myopathic disorders.[42]

Molecular Genetics

Progress in molecular genetics has tremendously improved the understanding of many myopathies, especially muscular dystrophies. Because the phenotypic presentation of familial myopathies can vary, understanding of the pathophysiologic etiology has allowed clarification of inheritance patterns and refined classification schemata.[18] Additionally, identification of specific genetic mutations and deletions has fundamentally changed the diagnostic approach in some areas. For example, dystrophin gene sequencing may detect nearly 100% of mutations causing Duchenne and Becker muscular dystrophies, eliminating the need for electrodiagnostic studies and muscle biopsy for these cases.[18] Genetic heterogeneity seen with certain myopathic disorders necessitates multimodal diagnostic evaluations, when such diseases are being evaluated. Nemaline myopathy, multiminicore myopathy, and congenital fiber-type disproportion are a few examples of muscles diseases with multiple gene loci and inheritance patterns. A challenge to molecular genetic testing includes cost, notably in situations where multiple genes may underlie the disorder. A further limitation of genetic studies is that allelic variation may result in different clinical diseases being associated with the same gene. Lamin A/C mutations may result in autosomal dominant limb-girdle muscular dystrophy 1B, autosomal dominant Emery-Dreifuss muscular dystrophy 2, and autosomal recessive Emery-Dreifuss muscular dystrophy 2.[34,49]

Electrodiagnostic Studies

Because an electrodiagnostic study is considered an extension of the physical examination, in clinical cases in which a myopathy is strongly suspected, an electrodiagnostic evaluation may not be indicated because the study will rarely provide a specific diagnosis.[35] In these situations, pursuing genetic studies and muscle biopsy are more likely to yield the myopathic diagnosis. Electrodiagnosis may be of utility when the underlying pathologic process is unclear.[3] Neuromuscular junction disorders, motor neuropathies, and motor neuron diseases may be excluded from the differential diagnosis based on electrodiagnostic findings. Electromyography may provide information regarding the distribution of muscle involvement that can aid in the selection of muscle biopsy sites.[16]

Sensory nerve conduction studies should have normal peak latencies and normal amplitudes in myopathic diseases. Motor nerve conduction studies of individuals with a myopathy are typically normal; however, with increasing muscle injury and atrophy the compound motor action potential amplitude may be reduced.[26] Repetitive nerve stimulation studies are usually normal in myopathic disease, but could be included if a neuromuscular junction disorder, such as myasthenia gravis, is clinically suggested.[35]

Of the components that comprise an electrodiagnostic study, needle electromyography will provide the greatest information about a muscle disorder. Insertional activity is variable depending on the underlying disease process. Although many myopathies will have normal insertional activity, disorders that lead to muscle fibrosis, such as Duchenne muscular dystrophy, may have decreased insertional activity. Acid maltase deficiency (Pompe disease) may have increased insertional activity. The motor unit morphology may demonstrate the characteristic short duration, low amplitude, polyphasic motor unit action potentials with increased or "early" recruitment. These findings are not absolute because myopathic disorders can have normal-appearing motor units. Steroid myopathy, which predominantly affects type II fibers, may appear normal on electromyography because type I fibers are the first recruited muscle.[35] An electrodiagnostic evaluation may also reveal unique features of the myopathy. Spontaneous electrical activity, such as fibrillation potentials, positive sharp waves, complex repetitive discharges, and myotonic discharges, may be present depending on the underlying myopathy (Box 42-2).[26,35] Muscle fiber necrosis may result in effectively denervating some fibers through the loss of the motor end plate. Similarly, muscle fiber splitting may denervate muscle, as the fibers will not be in continuity, thereby blocking fiber-to-fiber depolarization. Fibrillation potentials and positive sharp waves may be generated from these denervated fibers. Myotonic muscular dystrophies will often have the characteristic "dive

BOX 42-2

Myopathies with Spontaneous Electrical Activity

Fibrillation Potentials/Positive Sharp Waves
- Polymyositis/dermatomyositis
- Inclusion body myositis
- Duchenne muscular dystrophy/Becker muscular dystrophy
- Facioscapulohumeral muscular dystrophy (+/–)
- Emery-Dreifuss muscular dystrophy
- Myotonic muscular dystrophy
- Nemaline myopathy (+/–)
- Centronuclear myopathy
- Acid maltase deficiency (Pompe disease)
- Myophosphorylase deficiency (McArdle disease) (late)
- HIV infection

Complex Repetitive Discharges
- Inclusion body myositis
- Duchenne muscular dystrophy/Becker muscular dystrophy (+/–)
- Centronuclear myopathy
- Acid maltase deficiency (Pompe disease)
- Myophosphorylase deficiency (McArdle disease) (late)

Myotonic Discharges
- Polymyositis/dermatomyositis (+/–)
- Inclusion body myositis
- Duchenne muscular dystrophy/Becker muscular dystrophy (+/–)
- Myotonic muscular dystrophy
- Myotonia congenita
- Paramyotonia congenita
- Schwartz-Jampel syndrome
- Centronuclear myopathy (+/–)
- Acid maltase deficiency (Pompe disease)
- Myophosphorylase deficiency (McArdle disease) (late)

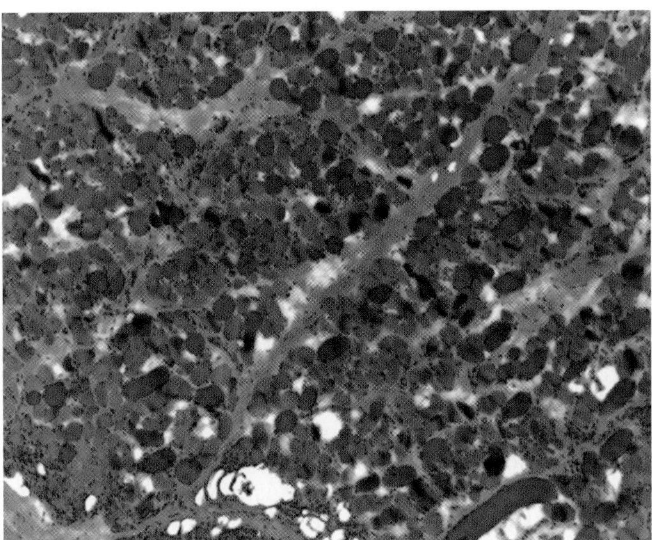

FIGURE 42-3 Muscle biopsy from a patient with Duchenne muscular dystrophy, demonstrating increased fiber size variability (including fiber atrophy and hypertrophy) and a small cluster of basophilic regenerating fibers (just left of center).

bomber" sound of waxing and waning motor unit frequency and amplitude from myotonic discharges.

Muscle Biopsy

Muscle biopsy allows for direct examination of structural changes caused by a myopathic process. A tissue specimen may be obtained via open or needle biopsy. Although a needle muscle biopsy is less invasive, this technique yields smaller tissue samples and does not allow direct inspection of the tissue before a sample is taken.[20,30] In suspected myopathies that will require histochemistry studies or may have focal involvement, open biopsy would be a preferred procurement method. For any muscle biopsy, close coordination between the individual obtaining the tissue specimen, the processing laboratory, and the pathologist will maximize the utility of the endeavor. Selection of the biopsy site will often be guided by clinical and electrodiagnostic examination. A weak muscle is typically selected; however, one with marked atrophy or profound weakness is best avoided because fibrotic and fatty replacement may limit diagnostic information that can be obtained.[3] Electromyography should only be performed on one side, with the biopsy obtained from the contralateral side, to minimize needle injury of the muscle, confounding histologic findings.[20] Because most myopathies involve proximal musculature, biopsies are commonly obtained from the biceps, triceps, deltoid, and quadriceps.[30]

The histology and histochemistry evaluations of the muscle identify structural alterations, including fiber size change, fiber splitting, fiber necrosis, inflammatory infiltration, and fibrosis (Figure 42-3). Congenital myopathies, including central core myopathy, nemaline myopathy, and multiminicore myopathy, are classified based on structural characteristics.[40] Mitochondrial myopathies with defective oxidative phosphorylation may demonstrate accumulations of abnormal mitochondria resulting in the ragged-red fibers.[33] The presence of rimmed vacuoles may suggest the diagnosis of inclusion body myositis. Immunohistochemical staining and quantification of proteins may further elucidate the etiology of the myopathic disorder (Table 42-1).[20,30]

Table 42-1 Immunohistochemical Staining Target Proteins and Related Myopathies

Protein	Disease
Dystrophin	Duchenne and Becker muscular dystrophies
Sarcoglycan	Sarcoglycanopathies (limb-girdle muscular dystrophy 2C to 2F)
Dysferlin	Dysferlinopathy (limb-girdle muscular dystrophy 2B)
Collagen VI	Ullrich congenital muscular dystrophy
Emerin	Emery-Dreifuss muscular dystrophy

Specific Myopathic Disorders

Classification of Myopathies

The term myopathy encompasses a large heterogeneous collection of diseases defined by muscle abnormality. Myopathic diseases may be separated into two large categories: acquired and hereditary. Acquired myopathies include inflammatory myopathies, toxic myopathies, and systemic disease associated myopathies. The pathology of an acquired myopathy involves alteration of normal muscle fibers by extrinsic factors. Inflammatory cells, toxins, endocrinopathies, and infections are examples of external mediators that may impact the function and survival of muscle fibers.

Hereditary myopathies are inherited disorders with genetic mutations that compromise the muscle fiber structure, physiology, or both. Myopathies with muscle fiber destruction are classified as muscular dystrophies. Phenotypic characteristics, electromyographic findings, and genetic variations have been utilized to further group subtypes of muscular dystrophies. Although the genetic basis for hereditary myopathies is present at birth, individuals with these diseases may not clinically manifest weakness or functional change initially. Myopathic disorders that are clinically symptomatic at birth or during the perinatal period are referred to as congenital. Metabolic and mitochondrial myopathies represent hereditary myopathies classified by the mechanism underlying the muscle fiber physiologic dysfunction.

Inflammatory Myopathies

Dermatomyositis. Dermatomyositis is an inflammatory myopathy that may affect adults and children. Dermatomyositis is a rare disease affecting 4 to 10 per 1 million annually.[22] The clinical findings of dermatomyositis include heliotrope rash around the eyelids; erythematous macular rash of the face, neck, or chest; Gottron papules on the extensor surfaces of joints; and nailfold telangiectasias.[13,22] Juvenile dermatomyositis may have a preceding fever and skin changes in addition to multisystem involvement.[13] Symmetrical weakness of proximal muscles and pharyngoesophageal musculature may occur with or without associated myalgia. Although both juvenile and adult dermatomyositis may be associated with interstitial lung disease, only the adult form is generally associated with malignancy (ovarian for women and small cell lung cancer in men),[13] thus malignancy screening should be included in the workup of this disease. Cardiac involvement, ranging from arrhythmias to heart failure, is commonly found in individuals with dermatomyositis.[22]

CK is usually elevated in cases of dermatomyositis, but may be normal. Electromyography demonstrates increased insertional activity, fibrillation potentials, positive sharp waves, and short-duration low-amplitude motor units.[22,35] Muscle biopsy to evaluate for deposition of the complement membrane attack complex around small blood vessels is highly sensitive and specific for dermatomyositis.[13,49] Other biopsy findings may include perifascicular atrophy and decreased capillary density.[20]

Pharmacologic treatment of dermatomyositis typically involves immunosuppression. If the myopathy is associated with a malignancy, treatment of the cancer may improve the weakness. Although corticosteroids are frequently the first line of therapy, adjunctive treatment with methotrexate, azathioprine, or other immunomodulating drugs may be needed for resistant cases.[13]

Polymyositis. Polymyositis is an inflammatory myopathy of individuals over 20 years old. Polymyositis is a rare disease affecting 4 to 10 per 1 million annually.[22] Often a diagnosis of exclusion, polymyositis has a female predilection with neck flexor and symmetrical proximal limb involvement.[13] The weakness may be associated with myalgia and muscle tenderness.[22] Cardiac involvement may be seen in polymyositis and has been reported as a cause of death in up to 20% of cases.[22] Interstitial lung disease and malignancy are more closely associated with dermatomyositis, but may also occur in polymyositis.[13] Malignancy screening should be considered as part of the workup of this disease.

CK is elevated in cases of active polymyositis and may be used as a marker of treatment response.[13] Electromyography demonstrates increased insertional activity, fibrillation potentials, positive sharp waves, and short-duration low-amplitude motor units.[22,35] Muscle biopsy may demonstrate characteristic findings such as partial invasion of nonnecrotic muscle fibers with activated macrophages and $CD8^+$ cytotoxic T cells.[13,20,22] Major histocompatibility complex class 1 (MHC-1) may be expressed on the surface of myocytes even after immunosuppressive treatment in both polymyositis and inclusion body myositis.[13,22]

Similar to dermatomyositis, the pharmacologic management of polymyositis involves immunosuppression. Corticosteroids are typically the first line of therapy. They may be combined with adjunctive treatments such as methotrexate, azathioprine, or other immunomodulating agents.[13]

Inclusion Body Myositis. Sporadic inclusion body myositis is an inflammatory myopathy that predominantly affects individuals over the age of 30 years old and is the most common inflammatory myopathy in individuals over 50 years old. The incidence of sporadic inclusion body myositis has been reported to range between 4.9 and 9.3 per 1 million.[43] Patients often have asymmetrical weakness including finger flexors and knee extensors.[43] The finger flexor weakness gives the unusual "intrinsic positive" hand posterior, with marked difficulty making a fist. Distal lower limb weakness resulting in foot drop and pharyngeal weakness causing dysphagia may also occur.

CK may be elevated in individuals with sporadic inclusion body myositis but typically not exceeding 12 times the upper limit of normal.[43] Electrodiagnostic studies demonstrate increased insertional activity and short-duration polyphasic motor units on electromyography and in some cases a peripheral neuropathy may be noted on nerve conduction studies.[35] Muscle biopsy may demonstrate rimmed vacuoles, cytoplasmic inclusions, and mononuclear cell invasion in endomysial fibers.[20,43]

The pathogenesis of sporadic inclusion body myositis continues to be studied. Research is exploring both degenerative and immune-mediated etiologies for this myopathy.[43] Functional decline in individuals with sporadic inclusion body myositis is often slow; however, no pharmacologic interventions have been found efficacious in halting or reversing the progressive weakness.[43] Although some patients may have inflammatory cells on biopsy, this condition is not steroid-responsive.

Toxic Myopathies

Steroid Myopathy. Steroid myopathy refers to the mild generalized weakness typically sparing neck flexors associated with steroid exposure. Hyperadrenocorticalism and chronic steroid use may result in atrophy of type II muscle fibers; however, an acute quadriplegic form may occur in the setting of critical illness in which the patient is receiving high-dose corticosteroids and being mechanically ventilated.[11] The chronic type occurs with high doses of corticosteroid (≥20 mg daily) given for more than 2 weeks with a high cumulative dose (≥186 mg).

The pathogenesis of steroid myopathy has not been fully elucidated. CK levels are normal, and because type II fibers are selectively involved, there are little to no abnormalities noted on electromyography.[11,35] Muscle biopsy may demonstrate type II fiber atrophy with normal type I fibers.[3,20] Treatment includes decreasing or discontinuing the corticosteroids and exercise.[3]

Muscular Dystrophies

Dystrophinopathies. Dystrophinopathies are X-linked recessive muscular dystrophies caused by mutation of the dystrophin gene found at locus Xp21.2.[8,9,15,37] The 427-kDa dystrophin protein functions as a plasma membrane stabilizer, preventing fiber damage from the mechanical stress associated with muscle contraction.[9,15] Without the dystrophin protein to link the intracellular cytoskeleton with transmembrane glycoproteins, the skeletal muscle may have membrane rupture, cellular damage, and fiber necrosis.[37] Dystrophin is also expressed in the central nervous system, peripheral nerves, cardiac muscle, and smooth muscle.[37] The 2.4-megabase dystrophin gene comprises 79 exons and is the largest identified human gene.[9,15,18] Up to 70% of dystrophinopathy mutations are deletions that may change the reading frame of the gene.[15,37] Frame-shift mutations will prevent dystrophin protein expression, resulting in the more severe Duchenne phenotype.[15,37]

Mutations with a persevered reading frame will yield a truncated dystrophin protein and the milder Becker phenotype.[15,37]

Duchenne muscular dystrophy has an incidence of 1 in 3600 to 6000 live male births and a prevalence of nearly 2.5 per 100,000.[8,37] Duchenne muscular dystrophy may be suspected in males with hypotonia, delayed developmental milestones, limb-girdle weakness, difficult climbing stairs and running, and frequent falls.[8,15] Examination of individuals with Duchenne muscular dystrophy typically reveals calf pseudohypertrophy, compensatory toe walking, and the use of a Gower maneuver to facilitate transition to standing.[8,15] Most children with Duchenne muscular dystrophy are diagnosed by 5 years of age.[8,15]

Becker muscular dystrophy is much less common compared with Duchenne muscular dystrophy, with an incidence of 1 in 18,000 live male births and a prevalence of approximately 0.5 per 100,000.[37] Becker muscular dystrophy shares a similar limb-girdle weakness pattern with the allelic Duchenne muscular dystrophy but with less severity and often presenting after 7 years of age.[9,15,37] Individuals with Becker muscular dystrophy may have muscle atrophy and pseudohypertrophy similar to Duchenne muscular dystrophy; however, joint contractures occur less frequently in cases of Becker muscular dystrophy.[15,37]

The initial workup for dystrophinopathies usually starts with CK that is elevated up to 100 times the normal level in both individuals with Duchenne muscular dystrophy and Becker muscular dystrophy.[8,15] AST and ALT are expressed in liver and muscle cells. Both AST and ALT may be elevated in dystrophinopathies and further workup for Duchenne muscular dystrophy and Becker muscular dystrophy should be considered in young males being evaluated for increased transaminases to prevent unnecessary liver biopsy.[8,15] Dystrophin gene mutation testing of a blood sample is the next step in the evaluation for a dystrophinopathy. Current testing techniques include multiplex polymerase chain reaction, multiplex amplifiable probe hybridization, multiplex ligation-dependent probe amplification, and single-condition amplification/internal primer.[8,18,34] Open muscle biopsy may be considered in cases in which no genetic mutation has been genetically identified but the clinical findings strongly suggest a dystrophinopathy.[8,15] Immunocytochemistry and immunoblotting may be used to determine the presence, quantity, and molecular size of dystrophin.[8,49] Electromyography has been supplanted by genetic testing for Duchenne muscular dystrophy and Becker muscular dystrophy and generally is not indicated.

The natural history of Duchenne muscular dystrophy is progressive weakness resulting in loss of ambulation between 7 and 12 years of age and death at the start of the third decade.[3,15] Becker muscular dystrophy progresses slower, with ambulation preserved until after 16 years of age or later.[3,8] Scoliosis and limb contractures typically progress around the time ambulation is lost in patients with Duchenne muscular dystrophy resulting from overall weakness.[41] Bracing does not slow scoliosis progression and timing for spinal fusion must take into consideration the individual's respiratory function. Monitoring of respiratory function is critical in patients with Duchenne muscular dystrophy. Although ambulatory, individuals with Becker muscular dystrophy usually do not have the rapid changes in scoliosis and decline in respiratory muscle strength noted in Duchenne muscular dystrophy. Duchenne muscular dystrophy and Becker muscular dystrophy have cardiac involvement in up to 90% of cases that range from conduction abnormalities to severe systolic and diastolic dysfunction.[14] Because up to 50% of carriers have cardiac involvement, cardiology evaluation and monitoring is necessary for patients with Duchenne muscular dystrophy and Becker muscular dystrophy and mutation carriers.[14,18]

Corticosteroid therapy has been shown to improve strength and slow functional decline in Duchenne muscular dystrophy.[8,15] Preservation of ambulation for up to 3 years may occur with prednisone 0.75 mg/kg/day or deflazacort 0.9 mg/kg/day.[8,15] Steroid therapy is usually initiated when motor function plateaus; however, the timing of initiation and duration of treatment has not been universally established.[8] Studies continue to explore alternative dosing regimens. Chronic steroid use increases the risk of obesity, behavior changes, immune suppression, cataracts, and bone demineralization requiring regular monitoring.[8,15] Investigational treatments are exploring mechanisms to induce exon skipping to change a Duchenne muscular dystrophy genotype into a Becker muscular dystrophy phenotype.[15] Gene transfer studies have been attempted to utilize adeno-associated virus to deliver microdystrophin constructs into muscle cells.[15]

Limb-Girdle Muscular Dystrophies. Limb-girdle muscular dystrophies are a large group of myopathic diseases with predominantly proximal limb-girdle weakness. This genetically diverse collection of myopathies is classified into dominant (LGMD1) and recessive (LGMD2) types (Table 42-2).[7,9,46] Each type is further divided based on gene discovery, approximately following subtype frequency. Most limb-girdle muscular dystrophies are slowly progressive, presenting from early childhood for LGMD2 to the start of the third decade of life for LGMD1.[46] Outside of founder effects, limb-girdle muscular dystrophy is rare, and other myopathies should be considered and excluded first.[7] Family history with passage of limb-girdle muscular dystrophy from parent to child may suggest LGMD1-dominant inheritance; however, spontaneous mutations may confuse interpretation of inheritance.[46] One clinical phenotype of LGMD2 that deserves special attention is severe childhood autosomal recessive muscular dystrophy (SCARMD). Mutations of any of the four muscle sarcoglycans can result in SCARMD that may mimic Duchenne muscular dystrophy, but has an autosomal rather than X-linked inheritance pattern and spares cognitive function.[7,49]

Evaluation for limb-girdle muscular dystrophy typically begins with measurement of CK, which is generally elevated. Some subtypes, including caveolinopathy (LGMD1C), dysferlinopathy (LGMD2B), and sarcoglycanopathies (LGMD2C-2F), frequently have marked CK elevations.[46,49] Electrodiagnostic studies reveal small-amplitude polyphasic motor units with early recruitment.[46] Muscle biopsy may demonstrate evidence of muscle fiber degeneration, regeneration, fiber splitting, and fibrosis.[46] Immunohistochemistry and immunoblotting may help narrow the differential diagnosis if specific proteins are

Table 42-2 Limb-Girdle Muscular Dystrophies

LGMD Type	Locus	Protein	Clinical Characteristics
1A	5q31	Myotilin	Proximal then distal weakness, dysarthria, myalgia, cardiomyopathy
1B	1q11-21	Lamin A/C	Variable phenotype, contractures, cardiomyopathy
1C	3p25	Caveolin 3	Proximal or distal weakness, rippling muscle, calf hypertrophy
1D	7q	Desmin	Lower more than upper limb involvement, dysphagia, cardiac conduction defects
1E	6q23	DNAJB6	Proximal or distal weakness, cardiomyopathy
2A	15q15.1	Calpain 3	Scapular winging, proximal weakness with adductor and hip extensor sparing, contractures, scoliosis
2B	2p13	Dysferlin	Deltoid and calf pseudohypertrophy, contractures
2C	13q12	γ-Sarcoglycan	Calf pseudohypertrophy, scapular winging, cardiomyopathy, respiratory involvement
2D	17q21	α-Sarcoglycan	Calf pseudohypertrophy, scapular winging, cardiomyopathy, respiratory involvement
2E	4q12	β-Sarcoglycan	Calf pseudohypertrophy, scapular winging, cardiomyopathy, respiratory involvement
2F	5q33	δ-Sarcoglycan	Calf pseudohypertrophy, scapular winging, cardiomyopathy, respiratory involvement
2G	17q12	Telethonin	Calf pseudohypertrophy, cardiomyopathy
2H	9q31	TRIM32	Lower more than upper limb involvement, slowly progressive
2I	19q	FKRP	Calf pseudohypertrophy, cardiomyopathy, mild to severe variants
2J	2q24.2	Titan	Severe progressive proximal weakness, no cardiac or respiratory involvement
2K	9q34	POMT1	Calf pseudohypertrophy, contractures
2L	11p13-p12	Anoctamin 5	Quadriceps atrophy, myalgia

LGMD, Limb-girdle muscular dystrophy.

absent or reduced in quantity.[7,15,46] DNA analysis for mutations is the mainstay of diagnosis for limb-girdle muscular dystrophy.[3,7] Genetic overlap between limb-girdle muscular dystrophy and other types of myopathies, however, may limit the clinician's ability to make a diagnosis based solely on molecular genetic testing.

Merosin-Deficient Congenital Muscular Dystrophy. Merosin-deficient congenital muscular dystrophy, also known as MDC1A, was previously reported to comprise up to 40% of congenital muscular dystrophies; however, advances in diagnostic testing has decreased this estimate to 22%.[31] Merosin refers to the group of laminins that contain the laminin α2 chain, which comprises the structural framework of basement membranes.[9,49] The laminin α2 chain (*LAMA2*) gene is located on chromosome 6q22-23.[31] Although complete absence of merosin is related to mutations of the *LAMA2* gene, partial merosin deficiencies may be related to other gene mutations.[5] Patients with MDC1A present from birth to the first month of life with symptoms including hypotonia, weakness, and respiratory impairment.[31] Some individuals with MDC1A achieve unsupported sitting.[31] By contrast, nearly all cases will have dysphagia and progressive respiratory decline requiring ventilatory support by the start of the second decade.[5,31] Thirty percent of patients with merosin-deficient congenital muscular dystrophy have associated seizures.[5]

Elevated CK more than five times the normal level may be noted early in the patient's life.[5,15] Electrodiagnostic studies may demonstrate myopathic findings on electromyography and a mild demyelinating motor peripheral neuropathy on nerve conduction studies.[31,46] Muscle biopsy with immunohistochemical staining allows quantification of merosin content. Muscle fibers typically demonstrate changes consistent with degeneration and regeneration with associated increase in fatty and connective tissue.[46] Magnetic resonance imaging (MRI) of the brain characteristically reveals increased T2-weighted and fluid attenuation inversion recovery (FLAIR) signal of the white matter with sparing of the cerebellum, corpus callosum, and internal capsule.[5,49]

α-Dystroglycanopathies. α-Dystroglycanopathies (ADGpathies) are a group of congenital muscular dystrophies characterized by hypoglycosylation of α-dystroglycan (ADG).[5,15,31] Mutations in at least six genes have been associated with or suspected to cause ADGpathies.[5,15] Genes involved in the ADG glycosylation pathway include protein-O-mannosyltransferase 1 (*POMT1*), protein-O-mannosyltransferase 2 (*POMT2*), protein-O-mannose β-1,2-*n*-acetylglucosaminyltransferase 1 (*POMGnT1*), fukutin (*FKTN*), fukutin-related protein (*FKRP*), and *LARGE*.[5,15,31] Despite progress in understanding the pathophysiology of ADGpathies, currently identified genes are only associated with 50% of clinical cases.[5,31] This group of congenital muscular dystrophies typically has central nervous system involvement and occasional eye defects in association with a myopathic process involving the proximal limbs.[5,49]

Because many ADGpathies have brain abnormalities on MRI, an elevated CK may guide the evaluation of a neonate with hypotonia toward congenital muscular dystrophy rather than a primary central nervous system etiology. Myopathic changes are noted on electromyography.[46] Muscle biopsy is necessary in most cases and reduction in glycosylated ADG staining may direct evaluation to this class of myopathies.[15] Muscle fibers typically demonstrate changes consistent with degeneration and regeneration with fibrosis and increased connective tissue.[46] Early classification of ADGpathies divided these myopathies based on clinical phenotypes.[31] With the discovery of genetic heterogeneity between clinical phenotypes and that some mutations could underlie multiple contrasting phenotypes, diagnostic panels to evaluate for multiple mutations may be indicated.[15] Clinical phenotypes may still have a role in helping to prioritize genetic testing. Individuals with muscle-eye-brain (MEB) disease usually have brain involvement (including cerebellar cysts and cognitive impairment), ocular involvement (including cataracts, congenital glaucoma, ocular hypoplasia, and retinal hypoplasia), and prominent weakness.[5,15,46] MEB phenotype should be evaluated for mutations of *POMGnT1*, *FKRP*, *FKTN*, and *LARGE* genes.[5] Patients with Walker-Warburg syndrome (WWS) typically have ocular malformations (including coloboma and microphthalmia), cortical migration deficits, lissencephaly, and profound cognitive impairment.[5,46] *POMT1* and *POMT2* gene mutations should be obtained in the workup of WWS.[5]

Ullrich Congenital Muscular Dystrophy. Ullrich congenital muscular dystrophy is one of the most common congenital muscular dystrophies, second only to merosin-deficient congenital muscular dystrophy.[49] Ullrich congenital muscular dystrophy is associated with *COL6A1* and *COL6A2* genes on chromosome 21q22 and *COL6A3* gene on chromosome 2q37.[5,31,46] Mutation of these genes results in absence or a significant decrease in collagen VI, which is a major component of the basal lamina.[5,34] Both recessive and dominant inheritance patterns have been reported. Newborns with Ullrich congenital muscular dystrophy have hypotonia, proximal contractures, and distal joint hypermobility.[5,31] Hip dysplasia, kyphoscoliosis, and torticollis may also be present at birth.[5,31] Developmental delay and respiratory insufficiency may also prompt evaluation and workup.[31] Findings similar to other collagen diseases such as keloids and hypertrophic scarring frequently occur.[31]

Mild elevation of CK may be found on serum studies. Muscle biopsy findings may vary from severe dystrophic changes with fatty replacement to moderate myopathic fibers.[31] Staining for collagen VI reveals absence or decreased quantity in the basal membrane.[5] Because respiratory involvement is nearly universal, forced vital capacity should be monitored on a routine basis.

Most individuals with Ullrich congenital muscular dystrophy have a steady decline in function with aging. Nearly 70% of patients with Ullrich congenital muscular dystrophy will require wheelchairs for mobility after the first decade of life and nearly all will require noninvasive ventilation by age 15 years.[31]

Facioscapulohumeral Muscular Dystrophy. Facioscapulohumeral muscular dystrophy is the third most common muscular dystrophy, after Duchenne and myotonic muscular dystrophies, with a prevalence between 1 per 15,000 and 1 per 20,000.[15,45] This autosomal dominant myopathy has been linked to a contraction of D4Z4 repeats on chromosome 4q35 from 11 to 100 units to 1 to 10 units in 95% of cases.[18,45] The protein encoded by this sequence has not been identified nor has the mechanism of muscle wasting and weakness been clarified. Interestingly, at least one unit of D4Z4 must be present for an individual to develop facioscapulohumeral muscular dystrophy.[45] Most patients with facioscapulohumeral muscular dystrophy will demonstrate asymmetrical weakness by 20 years of age, often presenting with inability to reach overhead. Individuals may first notice facial weakness, typically more severe in the lower face.[3,15] Biceps, triceps, and abdominal muscles are frequently involved, whereas deltoids and forearm musculature are spared.[45] The trapezius muscle is spared, causing superior displacement of the scapulae with shoulder forward flexion, whereas rhomboid weakness results in lateral winging with shoulder abduction.[3] Ankle dorsiflexion weakness may be present; however, respiratory compromise and extraocular involvement are not found in facioscapulohumeral muscular dystrophy.[45] Weakness of the pelvic girdle with loss of ambulation may occur in nearly a quarter of patients.[15]

Facioscapulohumeral muscular dystrophy may have a number of extramuscular findings. Nearly 5% of cases with facioscapulohumeral muscular dystrophy have cardiac conduction abnormalities. A majority of patients have high-frequency sensory neural hearing loss, which is often asymptomatic.[15,45] Retinal telangiectasias are present in more than half of individuals with facioscapulohumeral muscular dystrophy and in rare cases may cause retinal detachment.[45]

Serum CK levels range from normal to moderately elevated and electromyography is consistent with a myopathic process.[3,15] Muscle biopsy may have inflammatory findings but is generally nonspecific.[34,45] Molecular genetic testing allows quantification of D4Z4 repeats to aid in confirmation of a diagnosis of facioscapulohumeral muscular dystrophy.[18] Audiology, cardiology, and ophthalmology referrals should be a routine component of care for patients with facioscapulohumeral muscular dystrophy.

Emery-Dreifuss Muscular Dystrophy. Emery-Dreifuss muscular dystrophy encompasses mutations of the emerin and lamin A/C genes.[9,18,34] The emerin (*EMD*) gene, located on Xq28, encodes for a protein that bridges the nuclear lamina and inner nuclear membrane.[28] The lamin A/C (*LMNA*) gene on 1q21.2-q21.3 undergoes alternative splicing producing two proteins that interact with the emerin protein.[28] X-linked Emery-Dreifuss muscular dystrophy is less common than the autosomal dominant form. Autosomal dominant Emery-Dreifuss muscular dystrophy may present earlier than the X-linked type; however, both demonstrate weakness, elbow flexion contractures, ankle plantar flexion contractures, and limb atrophy.[6,41] Both forms of Emery-Dreifuss muscular dystrophy have humeroperoneal weakness, whereas the autosomal dominant type also has scapular involvement.[6,46]

Laboratory analysis may demonstrate mildly elevated CK.[46] Electromyography may show myopathic motor units, early recruitment, and occasionally changes of denervation.[46] Muscle biopsy rarely demonstrates necrotic fibers and increased connective tissue.[6] Type I fibers may be slightly reduced in size with an increased predominance.[6] Gene sequencing of the *LMNA* and *EMD* genes will detect most mutations.[18] Cardiac involvement may lead to arrhythmia, complete heart block, and cardiomyopathy.[9,46] Autosomal dominant Emery-Dreifuss muscular dystrophy generally has more severe cardiac conduction deficits; however, most patients with Emery-Dreifuss muscular dystrophy will have abnormalities by early adulthood.[6] Female carriers of X-linked Emery-Dreifuss muscular dystrophy may also have cardiac involvement despite absence of clinical weakness.[46] For these reasons, early cardiac evaluation and ongoing monitoring are important to decrease mortality associated with Emery-Dreifuss muscular dystrophy.

Myotonic Myopathies

Myotonic Muscular Dystrophy. Myotonic muscular dystrophy includes genetically and clinically different entities. Myotonic dystrophy type 1 (DM1), also known by the eponym Steinert disease, is caused by an unstable CTG trinucleotide expansion of the dystrophia myotonica protein kinase (*DMPK*) gene on chromosome 19q13.3.[18,19,47] Myotonic dystrophy type 2 (DM2), or proximal myotonic myopathy, is caused by a CCTG nucleotide expansion of the zinc finger protein 9 on chromosome 3q21.[18,19,47]

DM1 is the most common adult-onset muscular dystrophy with a prevalence of 3 to 15 per 100,000, but may be higher in certain regions.[47] This autosomal dominant disorder has genetic anticipation between generations that is molecularly related to expansion of the CTG sequence during cellular replication. Clinical manifestation of DM1 is related to the number of CTG repeats with normal being less than 37. Large CTG expansions are often maternally transmitted possibly related to the increased DNA size effects on sperm viability and motility.[47] Congenital DM1, associated with greater than 1000 CTG repeats, may have decreased fetal movement, hypotonia, respiratory insufficiency, and weakness. Facial weakness with a tented upper lip makes feeding difficult. Cognitive impairment coupled with weakness results in delayed developmental milestones.[47] Classic DM1 with onset between late adolescents and early adulthood is correlated with 100 to 1000 repeat sequences.[47] Repeat numbers ranging from 50 to 150 may result in mild, late-onset DM1 that may not be diagnosed until the seventh decade of life.[47]

Individuals with classic DM1 have predominantly distal muscle weakness.[18] Other clinical findings may include facial weakness with a tented upper lip, frontal balding, temporal muscle atrophy, cognitive impairment, and learning disabilities.[19] Clinical myotonia may be observed in the forms of eye closure myotonia, handgrip myotonia, and percussion myotonia. Individuals with DM1 may demonstrate the "warm-up phenomenon" where repeated muscle contractions may decrease myotonia and improve strength.[47] Ophthalmologic examination may reveal cataracts in patients under the age of 50 years.[18]

CK levels may be elevated but are typically normal in DM1. Electromyography may demonstrate predominantly distal limb electrical myotonia.[35] Genetic testing for CTG repeat number has replaced electrodiagnostic testing and muscle biopsy in the diagnosis of DM1.[18,47] Cardiac conduction abnormalities are common in individuals with DM1 and are associated with increased mortality. Electrocardiographic monitoring and referral to a cardiology should be considered with this diagnosis.[18,19] Patients with DM1 also have an increased incidence of constipation, dysphagia, gallstones, hypothyroidism, pneumonia, and sleep apnea.[19,47] Managing physicians should monitor for signs and symptoms of these frequent issues and investigate appropriately. Glucose tolerance testing often demonstrates insulin insensitivity; however, the incidence of diabetes mellitus is not increased in DM1.[47]

DM2 is also inherited in an autosomal dominant manner, but does not demonstrate anticipation like DM1. Onset of DM2 ranges from 8 to 60 years, without correlation to CCTG repeat number.[47] Individuals with DM2 typically have symptoms in adulthood of proximal muscle weakness, including neck flexors, hip extensors, and hip flexors that may be associated with pain.[3,19] Clinical myotonia similar to DM1 may be observed in individuals with DM2. Mild cognitive impairment and daytime somnolence may also be present.

Patients with DM2 may have serum CK levels elevated to four times the upper limit of normal.[3] Electrodiagnostic studies often demonstrate electrical myotonia distally in the upper limbs but throughout the lower limbs.[35] Muscle biopsy commonly reveals myopathic changes.[3] As with DM1, the diagnosis of DM2 has shifted to genetic evaluation of nucleotide repeat frequency. DM2 should be considered in individuals clinically suspected to have DM1 but with normal CTG repeat numbers. CCTG repeats exceeding 75 confirms the diagnosis of DM2.[19] DM2 is associated with increased incidence of cardiac arrhythmias, cataracts, dysphagia, hypogonadism, and insulin insensitivity. Screening and monitoring of these issues should be considered in patients with DM2.

Myotonia Congenita. Myotonia congenita includes an autosomal dominant form (Thomsen disease) and an autosomal recessive form (Becker disease). Skeletal muscle chloride channel 1 (*CLCN1*) gene mutations underlie both disorders. These channelopathies result in nondystrophic myopathies associated with clinical myotonia, muscle hypertrophy, the "warm-up" phenomenon, and exacerbations with cold and emotional stimuli.[19,39] Thomsen disease typically presents as painless myotonia in childhood that is exacerbated by muscle contraction after rest.[19] Becker disease presents after the second decade with more severe myotonia that can cause "transient paresis."[19] The Becker subtype of myotonia congenita may have pain and weakness, which are not typically seen in the Thomsen form.

Electrodiagnostic testing of both forms of myotonia congenita demonstrates diffuse myotonic discharges.[35] Becker disease may demonstrate a short-duration low-amplitude "myopathic" pattern on electromyography. Short exercise testing may demonstrate compound muscle action potential decrement after exercise in both subtypes but is generally more notable in the recessive form.[19]

Paramyotonia Congenita. Paramyotonia congenita is a sodium channelopathy associated with an *SCN4A* gene mutation on chromosome 17q23.[19] This autosomal dominant disease has the "paradoxical" finding of increased myotonia with exercise.[39] Children usually present for evaluation of face, neck, and upper limb weakness worsened or triggered by cold exposure, exercise, and fasting.[19,39] Muscle hypertrophy is common but usually less than that seen with myotonia congenita.

Myotonic discharges may be found in all muscles but most commonly in distal musculature. Myotonia and fibrillation potentials increase as strength declines with cooling. Below 28° C, fibrillation potentials cease. Further cooling below 20° C results in electrical silence with no spontaneous or voluntary activity on electromyography.[19]

Congenital Myopathies

Central Core Myopathy. Central core myopathy is a rare predominantly autosomal dominant disorder typically associated with the ryanodine receptor (*RYR1*) gene on chromosome 19q13.[32,40] More severe phenotypes have been associated with an autosomal recessive variant. As with most congenital myopathies, the initial presentation is of a floppy infant with hypotonia and proximal weakness. Individuals may have cardiac involvement, skeletal abnormalities including scoliosis, and facial weakness without ophthalmoplegia.[32,40] The proximal weakness associated with central core myopathy can vary from static to mildly progressive.[32]

Similar to other congenital myopathies, CK measurement is often of little benefit with normal to mildly elevated values noted. Electrodiagnostic studies are consistent with a myopathic process. Muscle biopsy usually leads to a diagnosis based on the presence of unstained "cores" found predominantly in the center of type I muscle fibers.[20,32,40] The mechanism by which the cores form has not been fully elucidated. Limb MRI may support the diagnosis of central core myopathy with selective involvement of the adductor magnus, sartorius, vasti, gastrocnemii, fibular musculature, and soleus muscles. Genetic testing may evaluate for the more than 80 mutations that have been reported in the 106-exon *RYR1* gene.[40]

Because the *RYR1* gene mutations alter specific calcium channels also connected to malignant hyperthermia, individuals with central core myopathy must be provided education about avoiding inhaled anesthetic gases.

Nemaline Myopathy. Nemaline myopathy is a rare myopathy with six different clinical phenotypes. Nemaline myopathy is associated with autosomal dominant and recessive mutations including the genes encoding actin $\alpha 1$ (*ACTA1*), nebulin (*NEB*), and tropomyosin-3 (*TPM3*).[32,40] The presentation of nemaline myopathy varies with the severity of the subtype. Severe forms may have no movement, arthrogryposis, and respiratory insufficiency on examination.[32] Intermediate subtypes present in childhood and adolescence. Mild subtypes may not have clinical weakness noted until adulthood. Individuals with nemaline myopathy may have extraocular and facial muscle weakness. Dilated and hypertrophic cardiomyopathy is associated with nemaline myopathy.

CK and electromyographic findings are similar to those found in central core myopathy. Muscle biopsy reveals multiple threadlike inclusions on Gomori trichrome staining.[20,40] Nemaline comes from the Greek word "*nema*" meaning thread. The quantity of rods does not relate to or predict disease severity.[32] Genetic testing may be used to identify *NEB* gene mutations that account for up to 50% of cases, *ACTA1* gene mutations that cause 20% of cases, and *TPM3* gene mutations that result in up to 10% of cases.[40]

Centronuclear Myopathy. Centronuclear myopathy is a rare myopathy inherited both in autosomal dominant and recessive patterns. Mutations of the *DNM2* gene have been related to dominant types of centronuclear myopathy.[32] Dynamin 2, a GTPase, has a role in cytoskeletal and membrane dynamics.[32,40] Recessive mutations in the amphiphysin 2 gene are correlated with centronuclear myopathy. Amphiphysin 2 affects the function of dynamin 2 that together regulate skeletal muscle fiber organization.[40] Centronuclear myopathy may have symptoms neonatally such as poor cry, weak suck, and hypotonia. In childhood, a milder form may have symptoms including hypotonia, proximal weakness, ptosis, facial weakness, and ophthalmoplegia.[32,40]

Although CK levels are similar to other congenital myopathies, electromyographic findings are unique in that there is characteristically an abundance of fibrillation potentials and positive sharp waves as well as the early recruitment of short-duration low-amplitude motor unit action potentials. Muscle biopsy includes findings of centrally located nuclei, type I fiber predominance, and type I fiber atrophy.[20,32,40]

Multiminicore Myopathy. Multiminicore myopathy is a rare myopathy that has been associated with autosomal recessive mutations of the ryanodine receptor (*RYR1*) and selenoprotein N (*SEPN1*) genes.[40] The *RYR1* and *SEPN1* mutations genetically overlap with central core myopathy and congenital muscular dystrophy with spinal rigidity, respectively. A significant proportion of cases with multiminicore myopathy still have undetermined genetic associations. The classic multiminicore myopathy phenotype includes proximal and axial muscle weakness, respiratory weakness, scoliosis, and spinal rigidity.[32,40] Some individuals with multiminicore myopathy may have arthrogryposis, external ophthalmoplegia, or predominantly distal weakness. Despite progressive respiratory decline in some, most patients with multiminicore myopathy achieve and maintain ambulation ability.[32]

Mild elevations of CK may be found and electromyography may demonstrate short-duration low-amplitude motor unit action potentials with early recruitment. Multiple small unstructured cores and sarcomeric disruption of type I and type II fibers are found on muscle biopsy. As the multiminicores may be seen in healthy individuals after exercise and other pathologic processes, the constellation of clinical findings and biopsy results is necessary to make a diagnosis of multiminicore myopathy.

Congenital Fiber-Type Disproportion. Congenital fiber-type disproportion is a diagnosis of exclusion because fiber-type disproportion may be seen in many congenital myopathies.[40] Individuals with congenital fiber-type disproportion often have symptoms in childhood, including proximal greater than distal weakness, hypotonia, delayed developmental milestones, facial weakness, and ophthalmoplegia. Clinical findings may also include joint contractures, high arched palate, and kyphoscoliosis. This myopathy is nonprogressive and generally has a good prognosis.[40] Some cases have been related to mutations in the *ACTA1* gene, which has also been associated with nemaline myopathy.

CK and electrodiagnostic findings are nonspecific and similar to other congenital myopathies. Muscles biopsy is notable for type I fiber predominance on histology.[40] In congenital fiber-type disproportion, the type I fibers are more than 12% smaller than type II fibers. Evaluation should exclude findings consistent with nemaline myopathy or centronuclear myopathy because these diseases may also have fiber-type disproportion.

Metabolic Myopathies

Acid Maltase Deficiency (Pompe Disease, Glycogen Storage Disease Type II). Pompe disease is a rare autosomal recessive disorder caused by a mutation of the acid α-glucosidase (*GAA*) gene. The GAA enzyme breaks down glycogen into glucose in lysosomes. The infantile form of Pompe disease includes cardiomegaly, hepatomegaly, hypotonia, weakness, and death by 1 year of age from cardiorespiratory failure.[2] The late-onset form of Pompe disease presents after 1 year of age with slowly progressive proximal more than distal muscle weakness. Other symptoms of late-onset Pompe disease include muscle cramps, fatigue, myalgia, and respiratory insufficiency.[2]

Serum CK levels vary from normal to 15 times the upper limit of normal in late-onset Pompe disease.[35] Electromyography may demonstrate early recruitment of low-amplitude short-duration motor units with complex repetitive discharges, fibrillation potentials, myotonic discharges, and positive shape waves.[2,3] Thoracic paraspinal musculature may be the only site of membrane irritability and should be included in the electrodiagnostic assessment.[35] Nerve conduction studies, by contrast, are normal. Muscle biopsy demonstrates muscle vacuoles containing glycogen.[2,20] GAA enzyme activity analysis can be performed on blood or tissue samples. GAA gene sequencing of chromosome 17q may reveal the specific mutation of this highly polymorphic sequence.[2] Given the known respiratory involvement, pulmonary function tests should be monitored. Treatment with recombinant human GAA enzyme replacement may limit disease progression.

Myophosphorylase Deficiency (McArdle Disease, Glycogen Storage Disease Type V). McArdle disease is a rare autosomal recessive disorder caused by a *PYGM* gene mutation altering the structure of myophosphorylase.[42] This enzyme is required for glycogenolysis within skeletal muscle. The prevalence of McArdle disease is estimated to be 1 per 100,000.[3] Late in childhood, patients with McArdle disease have symptoms including myalgia, weakness, and exercise intolerance after vigorous exercise.[3,42] In extreme cases, rhabdomyolysis may occur. Individuals with McArdle disease may experience a "second wind" phenomenon in which muscle stiffness, painful cramps, and exercise tolerance improve after a brief rest.[3,4]

Laboratory testing is remarkable for elevated serum CK and uric acid levels in addition to myoglobinuria.[4,42] Forearm exercise testing reveals elevated ammonia levels without concomitant lactate and pyruvate increases.[3,42] Although electromyography is usually normal, histochemical analysis of muscle biopsy shows reduction or absent myophosphorylase.[20] Molecular genetic testing may diagnose nearly 90% of patients with McArdle disease.[3,42]

There is no proven treatment for McArdle disease. Symptoms can be decreased by eating 40 g of fructose or sucrose before strenuous physical activity. Additionally, maintaining a diet including complex carbohydrates with consistent aerobic exercise has been recommended to limit functional impairment.[3,42]

Mitochondrial Myopathies

Kearns-Sayre Syndrome. Kearns-Sayre syndrome (KSS) is a mitochondrial myopathy with symptom onset before the age of 20 years.[33,36] A sporadic single, large deletion of mitochondrial DNA (mtDNA) results in abnormalities of the respiratory chain complexes.[33] Clinically, individuals with KSS have progressive external ophthalmoplegia and pigmentary retinopathy.[33] Other associated findings include ataxia, cardiac conduction abnormalities, diabetes mellitus, myopathy, and sensorineural hearing loss.[36]

Laboratory studies, such as CK, are often normal or only slightly increased. A serum lactate level may be increased, especially after exercise.[33] Electromyography may be normal but may reveal a proximal myopathic pattern in some cases.[33] Muscle biopsies of clinically weak muscles are evaluated with histochemical functional assays.[36] Genetic analysis of mtDNA may identify the causative deletion. Given the high incidence of cardiac involvement even in patients who are asymptomatic, screening electrocardiograms and echocardiograms should be obtained.[36]

Because there is no treatment for KSS, management focuses on addressing complications related to the disease. Many nutritional supplements, including CoQ_{10}, have been studied without evidence of efficacy in controlled, blinded studies.[36] Despite these findings, many patients with mitochondrial myopathies are prescribed CoQ_{10}, vitamin C, vitamin K_3, riboflavin, and thiamin, based on anecdotal reports of improvement without significant side effects.

Mitochondrial Encephalomyopathy, Lactic Acidosis, and Strokelike Episodes (MELAS). Mitochondrial encephalomyopathy, lactic acidosis, and strokelike episodes (MELAS) is a mitochondrial myopathy with symptom onset generally in childhood but may occur as late as 40 years old.[36] Nearly 80% of MELAS is related to a point mutation of A3243G in the tRNA-encoding mtDNA gene.[33] In addition to the encephalopathy and strokelike episodes, individuals with MELAS may have ataxia, cardiomyopathy, deafness, diabetes mellitus, migraines, myopathy, seizures, and, rarely, progressive external ophthalmoplegia.[36]

The workup and findings for MELAS are similar to those noted previously for KSS. Additionally, muscle biopsy may demonstrate blood vessels that stain positive for succinate dehydrogenase. Urine testing can be used to detect the mtDNA A3243G mutation; however, this mutation is associated with multiple mitochondrial syndromes.[36] Cardiac evaluation should be pursued even in patients who are asymptomatic.[36]

Although there is no curative treatment for MELAS, small studies have suggested that L-arginine may be used to acutely manage the strokelike episodes.[36] Valproic acid should be avoided in individuals with mitochondrial diseases because it interferes with mitochondrial function exacerbating clinical symptoms.[33,36]

Myoclonic Epilepsy With Ragged-Red Fibers. Myoclonic epilepsy with ragged-red fibers (MERRF) is a mitochondrial myopathy with symptom onset generally occurring in childhood.[36] MERRF is frequently associated with a point mutation of A8344G in the tRNA-encoding mtDNA gene.[33] Ataxia, cardiomyopathy, and occasionally progressive external ophthalmoplegia may be noted in addition to defining generalized seizures and myoclonus of MERRF.[36]

The workup and findings for MERRF are similar to those noted previously for KSS and MELAS. Additionally, muscle biopsy may demonstrate subsarcolemmal accumulation of mitochondria on Gomori trichrome stain commonly referred to as "ragged-red fibers."[3,36] If genetic testing for the A8344G point mutations is normal, full mtDNA sequencing can be pursued.[33] Similar to KSS and MELAS, cardiac screening is recommended as a result of the frequency occurrence of dilated or hypertrophic cardiomyopathy.[36]

Supportive management is the mainstay of care because there is currently no curative agent. Similar to other mitochondrial myopathies, valproic acid should be avoided as a result of its negative mitochondrial effects.[33,36]

Systemic Disease Associated Myopathies

Thyroid Disorders. Muscular dysfunction has been associated with hypothyroidism and hyperthyroidism. Although most patients with either abnormality do not have clinically significant weakness, some may have mild proximal limb and neck flexor weakness. Reports of subjective weakness and muscle cramps, by contrast, are common for both.

Hypothyroid myopathy may have a CK increase to 1500 international units per liter; however, hyperthyroid myopathy usually has a normal CK level.[44] Similarly, electromyography is typically normal for both myopathies only demonstrating myopathic units in 33% of hypothyroid and 10% of hyperthyroid cases.[44] Muscle biopsy in hypothyroid myopathy demonstrates loss of myofibrils, loss of striations, decreased oxidative enzyme activity, type I fiber hypertrophy, and type II fiber atrophy.[44] Hyperthyroid myopathy does not have any characteristic findings on muscle biopsy.

Treatment of the underlying thyroid endocrinopathy improves the individual's symptoms. Correction of the thyroid level has been reported to normalize strength within 3 months for hypothyroidism and 3.5 months for hyperthyroidism.[44]

Human Immunodeficiency Virus Infection. Human immunodeficiency virus type 1 (HIV-1) may cause multiple neuromuscular disorders in infected individuals. Up to 50% of patients who are HIV positive may have some manifestation of neuromuscular pathology, which can be the presenting sign of infection.[24] With regard to muscle involvement, individuals with HIV may have painless CK elevation, myalgia and fatigue, or proximal weakness of the lower more than upper limbs. These muscle disorders can occur at any time in the disease process. Clinically, patients may develop widespread muscular wasting associated with HIV infection.[24]

Laboratory findings may include elevated serum CK and myoglobinuria. Electromyography may demonstrate low-amplitude short-duration motor units with fibrillations and positive shape waves. Some cases may also have evidence of an HIV-associated neuropathy. Muscle biopsy commonly reveals muscle fiber degeneration with variable macrophage and $CD8^+$ infiltration. Rarely, muscle fibers may contain inclusion bodies that mimic nemaline rods.[24]

If the myopathy in the patient who is HIV positive has evidence of inflammation, treatments including intravenous immunoglobulin, plasmapheresis, or steroids may be considered.[24] Because zidovudine (AZT) may cause a myopathy itself, individuals receiving AZT treatment should be carefully evaluated to differentiate the origin of their symptoms. AZT myopathy improves with discontinuation of the medication.

Rehabilitation of Individuals with Myopathies

Exercise

The fundamental impairment in myopathies is muscular weakness. Most myopathic diseases do not have a treatment to limit or reverse the underlying pathology; however, research is ongoing seeking new treatment strategies. For this reason, optimization of the remaining muscular function is desired to minimize an individual's disability and handicap. Progressive resistive exercise, although the primary means of maintaining and increasing strength and endurance in the nonmyopathy population, has been controversial in its application for addressing such issues in myopathy populations. Strength training may involve concentric (muscle shortening during the contraction) or eccentric (muscle lengthening during the contraction) movement of a weight. These forces induce microinjuries to the muscle fibers that start a cascade of pathways ultimately resulting in increased muscle fiber size and force generation potential.[1] Especially in muscular dystrophies in which sarcolemma breakdown occurs, exercise-induced increase in muscle fiber injury has been feared to potentially further weakness and disease severity.[1] The limited quality studies, wide array of myopathies, inconsistent outcome measures, and variety of exercise protocols have prevented reported research from clarifying the efficacy of resistive exercise in patients who are myopathic.[10]

Despite lack of definitive evidence regarding efficacy, small studies and case series have demonstrated that low to moderate intensity exercise may increase strength with little to no muscle injury even in dystrophinopathies, limb-girdle muscular dystrophies, facioscapulohumeral dystrophy, and myotonic muscular dystrophy.[1] General guidelines for a myopathy exercise prescription are to avoid muscle damage and include not exercising to exhaustion, not overworking the muscle (avoiding weakness 30 minutes after exercising), and not causing delayed muscle soreness (pain 1 to 2 days after exercising).

Exercise interventions for individuals who are myopathic may also include aerobic endurance training. Aerobic training includes walking, stationary bike, arm cycle ergometer, and swimming. Through activation of large muscle groups with adequate duration and intensity, aerobic training may increase cardiac output and improve oxygen utilization by muscles. Clinically, such adaptations may result in a decrease in fatigue and an increase in endurance. A review of research on aerobic exercise in muscle disorders suggested that such activity might have a positive effect on body function, patient activity, and patient participation.[10] Although aerobic exercise may be of benefit to many people with a myopathy, marked muscle weakness should be considered a contraindication as a result of the greater risk for muscle damage with training.[1]

Bracing and Adaptive Equipment

Maximizing the independence of an individual with a myopathy often involves the use of bracing and adaptive equipment. Considerations for improving a patient's quality of life, minimizing risk of injury to both the patient and caregiver, and minimizing caregiver burden may also prompt exploration for assistive devices. Understanding of expected myopathic disease and impairment progression is critical for anticipating potential activity limitations and participating restrictions. Providing anticipatory education to the patient and caregiver facilitates the acceptance and use of such equipment.

Bracing in myopathies may be incorporated to help maintain joint range of motion. Especially in dystrophic myopathies, such as Duchenne muscular dystrophy, fibrous replacement of muscle tissue coupled with increasing weakness limiting full-joint extension predisposes the individual to joint contractures. Most myopathies have proximal greater than distal weakness; however, as more severe diseases advance, nighttime bracing of the wrists, fingers, and ankles may be of benefit to minimize flexion contracture progression. Although finger flexion, wrist flexion, and ankle plantar flexion contractures are typically the most functionally limiting contractures, elbow flexion contractures, a hallmark of Emery-Dreifuss muscular dystrophy, may also impair an individual's independence when more than 30 degrees of extension is lost. Maintaining ankle dorsiflexion range of motion in Duchenne muscular dystrophy has not been demonstrated to prolong ambulation; however, having adequate range of motion to obtain at least neutral foot position will allow for shoe wearing and possibly minimize skin pressure issues on the plantar aspect of the forefoot.[41]

Lower limb bracing in myopathic disorders with ankle-foot orthoses (AFOs) and knee-ankle-foot orthoses (KAFOs) is often used to provide stability to compensate for muscular weakness. The selection of the appropriate level of bracing will be determined by the underlying disease pathology and distribution of involvement. In myotonic muscular dystrophy, some limb-girdle muscular dystrophies, and Emery-Dreifuss muscular dystrophy, distal lower limb musculature is affected and bracing may improve foot position during gait, improving gait efficiency. In myopathies such as Duchenne muscular dystrophy, proximal and distal weakness may be better stabilized through the use of KAFOs. The use of lower limb braces is affected by multiple factors, including acceptance of bracing by the patient, available range of motion of joints to be braced, and residual strength.[41] Custom-molded braces will maximize fit and comfort of the braces when compared with off-the-shelf braces. Having the individual work with a physical therapist and an orthotist to gain familiarity with the function of the braces may improve utilization. Before prescribing braces, the physiatrist must ensure that the joints affected by the bracing have adequate range of motion. Care must be taken to include evaluation of proximal joints, such as the hip and knee for AFOs and the hip for KAFOs, because proximal contractures may make distal bracing unfeasible. For example, although a person with normal knee and ankle range of motion may be fit for a KAFO, a marked hip flexion contracture can make the use of such a brace impractical. The addition of braces will increase the weight of the lower limbs, thereby increasing the force necessary to move the limbs for ambulation. Fabrication of braces with lightweight materials including carbon fiber and polypropylene may minimize this concern; however, clinical strength evaluation is crucial before prescribing orthoses.

Scoliosis and kyphoscoliosis may be seen in a number of myopathies, including Duchenne muscular dystrophy, central core myopathy, nemaline myopathy, multiminicore myopathy, and myotonic muscular dystrophy. With incidence reported up to 100% in Duchenne muscular dystrophy, the impact scoliosis can have on positioning, seating, respiratory status, and pain can be widespread.[27] Before puberty, neuromuscular scoliosis may be addressed through supportive seating that may range from lateral supports to custom-molded seating systems. Typically, spinal radiographs will be followed at regular intervals during adolescence to monitor for scoliosis development and progression. Although spinal bracing with thoracolumbosacral orthoses (TLSOs) has frequently been recommended, research has not demonstrated efficacy in limiting progression of neuromuscular scoliosis curves.[27] The use of a TLSO could be considered to improve sitting balance; however, surgical treatment will often be indicated to limit scoliosis progression when the Cobb angle is greater than 40 to 50 degrees.

A multitude of equipment options are available to address functional barriers caused by myopathies. Bath seats may make getting in/out of the bath or shower safer, and handheld shower heads may make independent bathing easier. Other bathroom modifications, including grab bars and elevated toilet seats, may facilitate transfers to and from the commode for individuals with hip-girdle weakness. Sock and button pullers can minimize impediments to daily activities such as dressing. For individuals in academic or employment situations, the use of keyboards or text-to-type software may limit fatigue and discomfort related to writing tasks. Caregiver and patient safety should also be considered as mobile and fixed lift systems can be prescribed to facilitate transfers.

Mobility options range from a single point cane to a power wheelchair. Canes (single and quad) as well as walkers may provide stability for ambulation, but because most myopathic diseases have shoulder-girdle weakness, they can be of limited benefit for longer distances. Similarly, manual wheelchairs may be independently propelled for shorter distances and may not be tolerated for distances outside the home. Power scooters and power wheelchairs may provide better alternatives as weakness increases. Scooters can have a tiller steering mechanism, fixed seating, and a large turning radius that limit their use for individuals with myopathies. Because manual wheelchairs, scooters, and power wheelchairs are typically classified together, the physiatrist must anticipate the current and future needs of the individual to ensure the most appropriate device is ordered because many insurance providers will only provide funding for one over a certain period of time. The power wheelchair prescription for a patient with a myopathy should include consideration for head, neck, and trunk support. In individuals with difficulty in weight-shifting, pressure relief consideration, to minimize the risk of dermal pressure injury, may incorporate pressure-minimizing cushions and tilt functionality.

Cardiac Considerations

Cardiac involvement occurs in many myopathic diseases with a vast array of presentations (Table 42-3).[14] Typically, for myopathies that alter heart function, the cardiac manifestation arises later in the disease course; however, cardiac abnormalities have been reported as presenting issues in Becker muscular dystrophy, facioscapulohumeral muscular dystrophy, Emery-Dreifuss muscular dystrophy, myotonic muscular dystrophy, congenital fiber-type disproportion, and mitochondrial myopathy.[21] Cardiac evaluation in myopathies includes a complete history, review of symptoms, and physical examination along with an electrocardiogram and echocardiography.[14] Especially when the myopathic disease is being initially evaluated, cardiac evaluation should be included in the individual's workup. Depending on the specific myopathy identified, regular screening studies and early referral to a cardiologist may be indicated. A cardiologist with experience in myopathic diseases can assist with the selection of further testing including ambulatory 24-hour electrocardiography, coronary angiography, stress testing, cardiac MRI, and myocardial biopsy.[14]

Management of cardiac manifestations of the myopathies follows typical treatment guidelines for patients who are not myopathic. Conduction abnormality treatments may include antiarrhythmic agents, beta-blockers, calcium channel blockers, anticoagulation, cardioversion, pacer/defibrillator placement, and electrophysiologic study with radiofrequency ablation.[14] Heart failure management may address systolic dysfunction through the use of angiotensin-converting enzyme (ACE) inhibitors, diuretics, and beta-blockers.[14] Patients with end-stage heart failure may also be considered for heart transplantation, which has been performed in several myopathies including Duchenne muscular dystrophy, Becker muscular dystrophy, limb-girdle muscular dystrophy, and Emery-Dreifuss muscular dystrophy.

Table 42-3 Myopathies and Associated Cardiac Manifestations

Myopathy	Cardiac Abnormality
Dystrophinopathy	Supraventricular and ventricular arrhythmias ST depression Prolonged QT interval Myocardial thickening Cardiac dilatation and valvular insufficiency Systolic and diastolic dysfunction Heart failure
Limb-girdle MD	Incomplete right bundle branch block Left anterior hemiblock Shortened QT interval ST segment elevation Abnormal Q waves Cardiac dilatation Heart failure
Facioscapulohumeral MD	Elevated P waves Atrioventricular and intraventricular conduction block Supraventricular arrhythmias Ventricular tachycardia Long QT syndrome
Emery-Dreifuss MD	Bradycardia Prolonged PQ interval Ventricular conduction block Sudden death
Myotonic MD	AV block Prolonged QT interval Prolonged QRS Torsades de pointes Myocardial thickening Heart failure
Central core myopathy	Myocardial thickening Cardiac dilatation Heart failure
Nemaline myopathy	Myocardial thickening Cardiac dilatation Heart failure
CFTD	Atrial fibrillation AV block Cardiac dilatation Heart failure
Pompe disease	Electrocardiographic abnormalities Myocardial thickening (severe) Sudden death
Mitochondrial myopathy	Electrocardiographic abnormalities Cardiac dilatation Heart failure

CFTD, Congenital fiber-type disproportion; *MD*, muscular dystrophy.

Pulmonary Considerations

Effective ventilation requires sufficient movement of air into and out of the lungs by way of activation of breathing musculature including the diaphragm and intercostal muscles, as well as a compliant rib cage to allow chest expansion. In some myopathies, including Duchenne muscular dystrophy, most congenital muscular dystrophies, severe forms of many congenital myopathies, and myotonic muscular dystrophy, the diaphragm and intercostal muscles may be weakened. Additionally, fibrosis of this musculature as seen in dystrophic myopathies can result in a functional restrictive lung disease because the chest has limited expansion during inspiration. The patient and family should be educated in the potential changes in respiratory function including discussion of management options and their wishes for level of treatment. Symptomatic hypoventilation will often be reported as snoring, insomnia, daytime somnolence, fatigue, drowsiness, depression, impaired cognitive function, and morning headaches.[50] As ventilation capacity declines, the forced vital capacity (FVC) decreases resulting in increased serum CO_2 levels. The increased partial pressure of CO_2 results in a "right shift" of the oxygen dissociation curve such that there is a lower affinity of hemoglobin to oxygen, which is why monitoring oxygen saturation via pulse oximetry alone is an inadequate assessment of ventilatory status. No one pulmonary test can predict the development of hypoventilation or morbidity, thus regular monitoring of multiple parameters is frequently used to detect respiratory compromise. A screening montage may include oxygen saturation, FVC, peak cough flow, maximal inspiratory pressure (MIP), maximal expiratory pressure (MEP), and end-tidal CO_2 every 6 to 12 months or more frequently if clinically indicated.[50]

Once hypoventilation has been identified in the individual with a myopathy, determination of the most appropriate management strategy becomes the focus of care. Historically, negative pressure ventilators, such as the iron lung, were the standard of care, but had limitations including size and requirement for supine positioning. Modern variations, including the chest shell and cuirass, facilitate portability and decrease limb restrictions, but are still ineffective with upper airway obstruction.[50] Positive pressure ventilators (PPVs) allow for potentially greater ability to travel and may overcome obstruction concerns. Issues such as tracheal injury, infections, and impaired communication limit invasive PPVs with a tracheostomy. Noninvasive PPVs with positive airway pressure may provide a well-tolerated option for many people. The airway pressure is provided at one continuous pressure or a bilevel pressure that changes with the ventilatory phase. A respiratory therapist can aid the patient in identifying the mask type that provides optimal seal and comfort.[50] Mask options range from a nasal mask to a mouthpiece to a full-face mask.

Another pulmonary health consideration includes prevention of respiratory diseases. Patients should be encouraged to receive appropriate vaccinations including influenza vaccinations annually if not contraindicated.

Nutritional Considerations

In progressive neuromuscular diseases, such as myopathies, decline in strength often results in a decline in mobility and endurance that in turn leads to a sedentary lifestyle and obesity.[23] Although obesity is more commonly seen in severe myopathies, identification may be problematic as the body mass index may underestimate obesity as muscle mass is decreased. The use of dual-energy x-ray absorptiometry (DEXA) may provide a more reliable method of body composition determination.[23] The mismatch between energy intake and energy expenditure results in an increase in adipose tissue.[12] Addressing both sides of this equation may help an individual avoid obesity-related diseases, including diabetes mellitus and coronary artery disease.

In severe myopathies, such as Duchenne muscular dystrophy, individuals may develop nutritional inadequacy as their diseases progress. Progressive mobility impairment and dysphagia may limit the ability of the patient with a myopathy to self-feed.[23] Additionally, impaired respiratory mechanics can increase the work and energy requirement for breathing. Incorporating a nutritionist into the care team of a person with muscle disease may improve understanding of daily energy needs, optimal food selection, and nutritional supplements if indicated. When feeding becomes insufficient to meet the patient's needs or the time and effort required for consuming meals negatively impacts quality of life, discussions should address potential treatment strategies including placement of a gastrostomy tube for supplemental nutrition and hydration. Patient education should ensure that the individual understands that the role of the feeding tube is not to replace their oral feeding but help support their oral intake.

Psychosocial Considerations

Quality of life in individuals with myopathies has been evaluated with multiple instruments including general tools, such as the Short Form-36, and specific tools, such as the Individualized Neuromuscular Quality of Life Questionnaire. Although disease severity may certainly impact quality of life, within a muscle disease group there can exist a wide range of perceived illness that is not strongly determined by disease severity.[38] In addition to disease severity, the factors of pain, fatigue, and mood have demonstrated a high level of association to quality of life.[17] Awareness of such topics facilitates both the monitoring and the implementation of appropriate interventions to address these barriers.

Because pain is a personal experience, the physiatrist should routinely inquire about the patient's pain concerns. Individuals may attribute their pain to their disease process and not raise the topic to their physicians. Altered joint biomechanics from weakness may contribute to musculoskeletal discomfort that is amenable to therapy, modalities, bracing, or medications. With a thorough history and physical examination, other etiologies of pain may be identified and managed, thus improving the patient's quality of life. Similar to pain, fatigue may be assumed as an expected part of daily life by the patient with a myopathy. Clarification of physical limits and perceived barriers at home, school, and work may allow the physiatrist educational opportunities to discuss energy conservation techniques and incorporation of assistive technology. After addressing potential medical issues, including hypoventilation, further treatment may include therapeutic referral to focus adaptations and increasing endurance to overcome specific challenges.

Mood, in particular depression and anxiety, have been noted to negatively impact the quality of life in people with myopathies.[17,38] Multiple management strategies, including individual counseling, group counseling, family counseling, and support groups, may be considered depending on the patient's preference and needs. Consultation with psychiatry and initiation of antidepressants may be indicated based on the severity of the individual's symptoms. The physiatrist should also evaluate the patient's support structure as significant others, family, and friends may also be coping with anxiety and depression related to the situation.

REFERENCES

1. Abresch RT, Carter GT, Han JJ, McDonald CM: Exercise in neuromuscular diseases, *Phys Med Rehabil Clin N Am* 23:653–673, 2012.
2. American Association of Neuromuscular and Electrodiagnostic Medicine: Diagnostic criteria for late-onset (childhood and adult) Pompe disease, *Muscle Nerve* 40:149–160, 2009.
3. Baer AN, Wortmann RL: Noninflammatory myopathies, *Rheum Dis Clin N Am* 39:457–479, 2013.
4. Berardo A, Dimauro S, Hirano M: A diagnostic algorithm for metabolic myopathies, *Curr Neurol Neurosci Rep* 10:118–126, 2010.

5. Bertini E, D'Amico A, Gualandi F, Petrini S: Congenital muscular dystrophies: a brief review, *Semin Pediatr Neurol* 18:277–288, 2011.
6. Brown SC, Piercy RJ, Muntoni F, Sewry CA: Investigating the pathology of Emery-Dreifuss muscular dystrophy, *Biochem Soc Trans* 36:1335–1338, 2008.
7. Bushby K: Diagnosis and management of the limb girdle muscular dystrophies, *Pract Neurol* 9:314–323, 2009.
8. Bushby K, Finkel R, Birnkrant DJ, et al: Diagnosis and management of Duchenne muscular dystrophy, part 1: diagnosis, and pharmacological and psychosocial management, *Lancet Neurol* 9:77–93, 2010.
9. Cohn RD, Campbell KP: Molecular basis of muscular dystrophies, *Muscle Nerve* 23:1456–1471, 2000.
10. Cup EH, Pieterse AK, ten Broek-Pastoor JM, et al: Exercise therapy and other types of physical therapy for patients with neuromuscular diseases: a systematic review, *Arch Phys Med Rehabil* 88:1452–1464, 2007.
11. Dalakas MC: Toxic and drug-induced myopathies, *J Neurol Neurosurg Psychiatry* 80:832–838, 2009.
12. Davoodi J, Markert CD, Voelker KA, et al: Nutritional strategies to improve physical capabilities in Duchenne muscular dystrophy, *Phys Med Rehabil Clin N Am* 23:187–199, 2012.
13. Dimachkie MM, Barohn RJ: Idiopathic inflammatory myopathies, *Semin Neurol* 32:227–236, 2012.
14. Finsterer J, Stöllberger C: Cardiac involvement in primary myopathies, *Cardiology* 94:1–11, 2000.
15. Flanigan KM: The muscular dystrophies, *Semin Neurol* 32:255–263, 2012.
16. Gilchrist JM, Sachs GM: Electrodiagnostic studies in the management and prognosis of neuromuscular disorders, *Muscle Nerve* 29:165–190, 2004.
17. Graham CD, Rose MR, Grunfeld EA, et al: A systematic review of quality of life in adults with muscle disease, *J Neurol* 258:1581–1592, 2011.
18. Greenberg SA, Walsh RJ: Molecular diagnosis of inheritable neuromuscular disorders. Part II: application of genetic testing in neuromuscular disease, *Muscle Nerve* 31:431–451, 2005.
19. Heatwole CR, Statland JM, Logigian EL: The diagnosis and treatment of myotonic disorders, *Muscle Nerve* 47:632–648, 2013.
20. Joyce NC, Oskarsson B, Jin L-W: Muscle biopsy evaluation in neuromuscular disorders, *Phys Med Rehabil Clin N Am* 23:609–631, 2012.
21. Katzberg H, Karamchandani J, So YT, et al: End-stage cardiac disease as an initial presentation of systemic myopathies: case series and literature review, *J Child Neurol* 25:1382–1388, 2010.
22. Khan S, Christopher-Stine L: Polymyositis, dermatomyositis, and autoimmune necrotizing myopathy: clinical features, *Rheum Dis Clin N Am* 37:143–158, 2011.
23. Kilmer DD, Zhao HH: Obesity, physical activity, and the metabolic syndrome in adult neuromuscular disease, *Phys Med Rehabil Clin N Am* 16:1053–1062, 2005.
24. Lange DJ: AAEM minimonograph #41: neuromuscular diseases associated with HIV-1 infection, *Muscle Nerve* 17:16–30, 1994.
25. Levin R, Pascuzzi RM, Bruns DE, et al: The time course of creatine kinase elevation following concentric needle EMG, *Muscle Nerve* 10:242–245, 1987.
26. Lipa BM, Han JJ: Electrodiagnosis in neuromuscular disease, *Phys Med Rehabil Clin N Am* 23:565–587, 2012.
27. Maitra S, Roberto RF, McDonald CM, Gupta MC: Treatment of spine deformity in neuromuscular diseases, *Phys Med Rehabil Clin N Am* 23:869–883, 2012.
28. Maraldi NM, Lattanzi G, Sabetelli P, et al: Functional domains of the nucleus: implications for Emery-Dreifuss muscular dystrophy, *Neuromuscul Disord* 12:815–823, 2002.
29. McDonald CM: Clinical approach to the diagnostic evaluation of hereditary and acquired neuromuscular diseases, *Phys Med Rehabil Clin N Am* 23:495–563, 2012.
30. Meola G, Burgiardini E, Cardani R: Muscle biopsy, *J Neurol* 259:601–610, 2012.
31. Mercuri E, Muntoni F: The ever-expanding spectrum of congenital muscular dystrophies, *Ann Neurol* 72:9–17, 2012.
32. Nance JR, Dowling JJ, Gibbs EM, Bönnemann CG: Congenital myopathies: an update, *Curr Neurol Neurosci Rep* 12:165–174, 2012.
33. Nardin RA, Johns DR: Mitochondrial dysfunction and neuromuscular disease, *Muscle Nerve* 24:170–191, 2001.
34. O'Ferrall EK, Sinnreich M: The role of muscle biopsy in the age of genetic testing, *Curr Opin Neurol* 22:543–553, 2009.
35. Pagononi S, Amato A: Electrodiagnostic evaluation of myopathy, *Phys Med Rehabil Clin N Am* 24:193–207, 2013.
36. Pfeffer G, Chinnery PF: Diagnosis and treatment of mitochondrial myopathies, *Ann Med* 45:4–16, 2013.
37. Reitter B, Goebel HH: Dystrophinopathies, *Semin Pediatr Neurol* 3:99–109, 1996.
38. Rose MR, Sadjadi R, Weinman J, et al: Role of disease severity, illness perceptions, and mood on quality of life in muscle disease, *Muscle Nerve* 46:351–359, 2012.
39. Ryan AM, Matthews E, Hanna MG: Skeletal-muscle channelopathies: periodic paralysis and nondystrophic myotonias, *Curr Opin Neurol* 20:558–563, 2007.
40. Sharma MC, Jain D, Sarkar C, Goebel HH: Congenital myopathies – a comprehensive update of recent advancements, *Acta Neurol Scand* 119:281–292, 2009.
41. Skalsky AJ, McDonald CM: Prevention and management of limb contractures in neuromuscular diseases, *Phys Med Rehabil Clin N Am* 23:675–687, 2012.
42. Smith EC, El-Gharbawy A, Koeberl DD: Metabolic myopathies: clinical features and diagnostic approach, *Rheum Dis Clin N Am* 37:201–217, 2011.
43. Solorzano GE, Phillips LH: Inclusion body myositis: diagnosis, pathogenesis, and treatment options, *Rheum Dis Clin N Am* 37:173–183, 2011.
44. Soni M, Amato AA: Myopathic complications of medical disease, *Semin Neurol* 29:163–180, 2009.
45. Tawil R, Van Der Maarel SM: Facioscapulohumeral muscular dystrophy, *Muscle Nerve* 34:1–15, 2006.
46. Tesi Rocha C, Hoffman EP: Limb-girdle and congenital muscular dystrophies: current diagnostics, management, and emerging technologies, *Curr Neurol Neurosci Rep* 10:267–276, 2010.
47. Turner C, Hilton-Jones D: The myotonic dystrophies: diagnosis and management, *J Neurol Neurosurg Psychiatry* 81:358–367, 2010.
48. Vladutio GD: Laboratory diagnosis of metabolic myopathies, *Muscle Nerve* 25:649–663, 2002.
49. Vogel H, Zamecnik J: Diagnostic immunohistology of muscle diseases, *J Neuropathol Exp Neurol* 64:181–193, 2005.
50. Wolfe LF, Joyce NC, McDonald CM, et al: Management of pulmonary complications in neuromuscular disease, *Phys Med Rehabil Clin N Am* 23:829–853, 2012.

CHAPTER 43

TRAUMATIC BRAIN INJURY

Amy K. Wagner, Patricia M. Arenth, Christina Kwasnica, Emily H. McCullough

A Note About Common Data Elements for Traumatic Brain Injury Research

In recent years, the National Institute for Neurological Disorders and Stroke (NINDS) has funded interagency efforts to streamline research trials and move science forward via the formation of international panels of experts. These Working Groups have been charged with generating consensus definitions and Common Data Element (CDE) recommendations for use with all clinical trials, as well as for specific disorders or diseases. The purpose of a CDE is to facilitate the clear reporting, interpretation, and comparison of research across the growing international literature in this field of study. As a part of this project, the International and Interagency Initiative toward CDEs for Research on Traumatic Brain Injury (TBI) was formed to develop consensus definitions and CDEs for use in research regarding TBI. Overview information regarding the NINDS CDE project can be found at http://commondataelements.ninds.nih.gov/ProjReview.aspx#tab=References. Current recommendations regarding data standards for clinical research in TBI can be found at www.commondataelements.ninds.nih.gov/tbi.aspx#tab=Data_Standards. We refer the reader to these web resources and the growing literature for additional reading. Definitions and information presented in this chapter will reflect CDE guidelines as indicated.

Definitions

Traumatic Brain Injury

TBI is defined as "an alteration in brain function, or other evidence of brain pathology, caused by an external force."[375] These types of injuries result from a jolt or blow to the head or are caused by an object penetrating the skull and injuring the brain. Examples include motor vehicle accidents, falls, assaults, or gunshot wounds. TBI should be differentiated from other types of acquired injuries to the brain, such as those caused by tumor or stroke, because of significant differences in mechanisms, treatments, and outcomes between traumatic and nontraumatic injury. TBI should also be differentiated from "head injury," which is defined as a blow to the head or laceration that may occur without causing injury to the brain. A TBI can be further defined as either open or closed. An open, or penetrating, TBI occurs when the head is hit by an object that breaks the skull and enters the brain. A closed TBI occurs when the brain is injured but the skull remains intact. A diagnosis of TBI is often established through an evaluation of clinical symptoms, as well as positive neurologic signs and neuroimaging findings.

Defining Severity of Injury

TBI is often categorized as mild, moderate, or severe. The Glasgow Coma Scale (GCS)539 is the gold standard for primary initial assessment of severity of injury based on level of consciousness[341] (Box 43-1). During the initial stages of diagnosis in the field or emergency facility, TBI is suspected or indicated if there has been a significant blow to the head and/or there is an alteration or loss of consciousness at the time of injury. An initial GCS score is obtained through clinical evaluation. As indicated in Box 43-1, the score is obtained by rating the best visual, verbal, and motor responses. The total score is simply a sum of these ratings, with scores ranging from 3 to 15. Coded notations may indicate that the total score, or specific subscale score, has been impacted by additional injury-related characteristics, such as medically induced chemical paralysis caused by intubation, substance intoxication, hypoxia, or other circumstances.

Generally accepted guidelines identify three levels of severity based on GCS scores: mild (GCS = 13 to 15), moderate (GCS = 9 to 12), and severe (GCS = 3 to 8). Individuals scoring in the mild TBI range should be evaluated at an emergency facility, but may require minimal or no hospitalization. For more severe injuries involving loss of consciousness, the GCS is a widely accepted measure indicating the depth of coma, and it is generally serially measured until emergence from coma. However, the GCS has limited applicability to young children. The Pediatric Glasgow Coma Scale (PGCS)[392] is a modified version of the GCS for use with pediatric patients with TBI.

Severity of injury is also defined by the duration of loss of consciousness/coma and the severity of symptoms. Individuals with mild TBI may experience brief loss of consciousness as well as transient confusion and neurologic symptoms. They may also experience a brief period of posttraumatic amnesia (PTA). PTA is generally characterized by a loss of memory for events surrounding the injury, disorientation, confusion, and significant cognitive impairment. Although there has been some discrepancy in the literature regarding the diagnosis of mild TBI, some general consensus has been established and will be discussed later in this chapter. The terms *complicated mild injury* and *postconcussive syndrome* are often used to refer to cases where diagnosis falls in the mild range; however, additional signs or symptoms of injury are present. Examples may include situations in which positive neuroimaging findings

BOX 43-1

Glasgow Coma Scale

Eyes	Open spontaneously	4
	Open to verbal command	3
	Open to painful stimuli	2
	No response	1
Verbal Response	Oriented and converses	5
	Disoriented and converses	4
	Inappropriate words	3
	Incomprehensible sounds	2
	No response	1
Motor Response	Obeys verbal commands	6
	Responds to painful stimuli by:	
	purposeful localization	5
	withdrawal	4
	flexor posturing	3
	extensor, posturing	2
	no response	1
GCS Score		**3 to 15**

From Teasdale G, Jennett B: Assessment of coma and impaired consciousness. A practical scale, *Lancet* 2:81-84, 1974.

indicate injury to the brain and/or symptoms such as headache, dizziness, and cognitive dysfunction persist for a significant period following mild injury. Individuals sustaining moderate to severe TBI often have a more prolonged loss of consciousness or coma. Upon emerging from coma, they may initially be inconsistent in responding to environmental stimuli. As they become increasingly able to respond consistently, they may continue to exhibit symptoms of PTA for a significant period of time. Increased duration of coma and PTA have been associated with poorer prognosis and outcomes (discussed further in the outcomes section of this chapter). Some individuals with severe injuries do not regain consciousness, remaining in a vegetative state, although others emerge only to a minimally conscious state. The evaluation and care for individuals along the spectrum of injury and recovery will also be discussed in later sections of this chapter.

Epidemiology

United States and Worldwide (Overall)

Approximately 1.7 million TBIs occur each year in the United States.[165] Of these, approximately 52,000 result in death and 1.365 million are mild injuries (often referred to as concussions) for which individuals are treated and released from the emergency room. This leaves approximately 275,000 individuals who survive moderate to severe TBI, generally requiring significant medical care and hospital stays.[165] Many are left with long-term disability as a result of these injuries.[316] According to one study, 40% of individuals hospitalized because of TBI reported at least one ongoing issue at 1 year following injury, with improvement of memory and problem solving listed as one of the most frequently unmet needs.[106] Such cognitive impairments, in addition to physical and medical issues, have significant impact on an individual's ability to perform everyday activities. In fact, the Centers for Disease Control and Prevention estimates that at least 5.3 million Americans currently need long-term or lifelong assistance with activities of daily living (ADLs) as a result of TBI.[549]

Globally, TBI is a leading cause of death and disability. Although exact worldwide statistics are difficult to obtain, a fairly recent review estimated approximately 775,000 new TBI hospitalizations per year in Europe.[534] Available information suggests that the epidemiology of TBI on a global scale is similar to trends found in the United States. Incidences of TBI by age and gender vary slightly across regions, but overall appear to follow patterns similar to those found in the United States.[260] For example, the distribution of mild, moderate, and severe TBI is consistent across the United States, Europe, Australia, and Asia: 80% of injuries are mild TBI, although moderate and severe TBI each account for 10% of injuries.[534]

Causes of Injury

From 2002 to 2006, the leading causes of TBI in the United States included falls (35%), traffic-related crashes (17%), struck by/against events (sports) (17%), assaults (10%), and other injuries (21%).[165] Sports injuries account for 1.6 to 3.8 million TBIs a year, although most of these are mild injuries that are not treated in the hospital or emergency department.[317] It should be noted that these statistics vary by age, gender, geographic location within and between countries, and group membership because of multiple factors, as explained below.

What is known of the global etiology of injury is similar to U.S. rates, with a few notable exceptions. Sixty percent of TBIs in Europe are caused by road traffic injuries.[222] This figure is distributed evenly across most regions, suggesting that road traffic-related injuries are not associated only with high income countries. Twenty to thirty percent of injuries are caused by falls, 10% violence, and 10% sports or work related.[222] India has the highest reported rate of TBI related to falls.[260,534] Latin America, the Caribbean, and Sub-Saharan Africa have the highest reported TBI rates because of road traffic incidents and violence.[260]

Associated Costs

The costs of TBI in terms of medical care and lost productivity in the United States were estimated to total $60 billion in 2000.[174] Worldwide statistics are less easily obtained. However, the costs associated with TBI go well beyond the financial requirements for medical care. The societal or indirect costs associated with potential loss of productive work-years for those who have been injured, as well as family members or others who may need to care for them, must also be considered. TBI also results in significant alterations in personal roles and responsibilities for the injured individual as well as family members. Reduced participation in complex leisure or recreational activities is also often a personal cost associated with TBI.

Demographics/Risk Factors

Age and Gender. The two age groups most at risk for sustaining a TBI are 0- to 4-year-olds and 15- to 19-year-olds.[316] Motor vehicle accidents result in the greatest number of TBI injuries for people age 15 to 19.[316] Another group at risk for TBI is adults over the age of 75. Fall-related injuries are highest among adults over the age of 75, and recent data suggest a 20% to 25% increase in trauma center admissions for TBI.[116] Patients over the age of 75 who sustain a TBI have the highest rates of TBI-related hospitalization and death.[316] Men are twice as likely as women to sustain a TBI in the civilian population.[316] However, in the older population with TBI (age >65 years), women are increasing in number.[116] As the population continues to age, age-specific considerations for treatment and management of those surviving their injuries will be of increasing importance.

Socioeconomic Status. Lower socioeconomic status (SES) in American cities is correlated with an increased risk of injury because of increased exposure to high-risk occupations, personal violence, older vehicles, and substandard housing.[305] Road traffic injuries are highest in areas of low SES.[514] Socioeconomic disadvantages are often associated with racial characteristics and rural locations. Minority populations in urban US areas are often of lower SES and have elevated risk for injury.[305] African Americans have a higher rate of TBI and associated mortality than other groups.[305]

Statistically speaking, rural populations display a greater incidence of unhealthy lifestyle behaviors including high alcohol consumption and psychosocial stress, and these populations are less likely to participate in preventative measures such as wearing seatbelts.[409,555] This increase in risk-taking behavior is evident in poorer health outcomes, specifically with injury-related outcomes like TBI.[409,555] In urban areas, nearly half of adolescents who enter the institutional correction system have a history of TBI, with a calculated incidence of 3107 TBIs per 100,000 person-years.[273] Other studies show that over 60% of prison inmates self-report a previous history of TBI.[601]

Violence. Assault or violence-related injuries account for 11% of TBI.[316] Violence-related TBIs result from firearms, cutting instruments, blunt objects, or assaults such as pushing or hitting.[191] Injury as a result of firearm use is the leading cause of death from TBI.[554] Sixty percent of firearm-related TBI is self-inflicted, 32% results from intentional assault, and 4% is unintentional.[52] People who sustain a TBI caused by a violence-related injury are more likely to be younger, single, male, member of a minority group, and have a history of alcohol abuse.[191]

Child Abuse. Intentional TBI in children is known by many names, including shaken baby syndrome (SBS) and inflicted childhood neurotrauma.[51,177] Approximately 1 million children are severely abused each year,[615] most often by parents or child care providers.[459] The majority of perpetrators are male, either the child's father or a boyfriend of the child's mother residing in the home.[494] Infants are at greatest risk for sustaining a TBI as a result of violent shaking,[557] although older children are still at risk.[483] One third of these children survive with no consequences, one third sustain permanent injury, and one third die.[615] Risk factors for the occurrence of SBS include maternal factors such as mothers younger than 19 years, education less than 12 years, single marital status, African American or Native American, limited prenatal care, or newborns less than 28 weeks old.[177] Additionally, child abuse rates caused by unintentional injury increase during periods of economic decline.[65] TBI from child abuse tends to occur more frequently in younger children, and children with TBI caused by nonaccidental trauma (abuse) typically have more morbidity and mortality associated with their injuries than children with accidental injuries.[124] International epidemiologic studies demonstrate that TBI from child abuse is now emerging as a significant issue in multiple countries outside of the United States, including China.[500,616]

Psychosocial Factors. Part of the reason for the higher incidence of TBI in young males may be a tendency to engage in higher-risk behaviors. In addition, substance use is related to TBI incidence, and up to 50% of individuals injured test positive for alcohol or other substances at the time of injury.[103] Prior psychiatric history is a risk factor for TBI, particularly with those who have a history of anxiety, depression, and conduct disorder.[560]

Military Traumatic Brain Injury Epidemiology. Members of the U.S. military are an emerging group at risk for sustaining TBI. Walter Reed Army Medical Center reports that 30% of service members evacuated from the field had sustained a TBI between 2003 and 2005.[130] Army service members are relatively young with an average age of 28.[432] Approximately 85% of military service members are male.[432] Military members who sustain a TBI are also more likely to be male since they represent a larger percentage of the military service population. In the military population, approximately 88% of TBIs are classified as mild injuries although the remaining 12% are moderate to severe.[113]

Compared with the civilian population, the Department of Defense reports that the leading causes of military TBIs include blasts (72%), falls (11%), vehicular incidents (6%), injuries caused by fragments (5%), and other injuries (6%).[113] Blast-related injuries are defined as "blast plus" as soldiers are often involved in more than one type of injury at a time, such as an explosive attack followed by a vehicular crash. Among moderate to severe injuries, recent evidence suggests that penetrating TBI is at least as common, if not more common, than closed TBI.[416]

Demographics/Risk Factors (Global). Global statistics suggest that countries with low to middle income have more risk factors that contribute to TBI. Risk factors vary by country and may depend on the incidence of factors such as poor road design, substandard vehicles, higher rates of violence because of war, and fewer prevention measures.[260] Low to middle income countries also have inadequate health systems to address TBI-related care.[260] Accurate information on demographics and etiology of TBI in low to middle income countries is especially difficult to obtain. Despite this, the burden of TBI is evident worldwide.

Pathophysiology

The pathophysiologic processes associated with TBI are complex and consist of (1) a primary injury that disrupts brain tissue and function at moment of impact; (2) secondary injury through multiple biochemical cascades that propagate cellular dysfunction and lead to cell death; and (3) a chronic degeneration, repair, and regeneration process that occurs over the long term after the injury has occurred. Figure 43-1 depicts the continuation of injury and repair associated with pathophysiology after TBI.

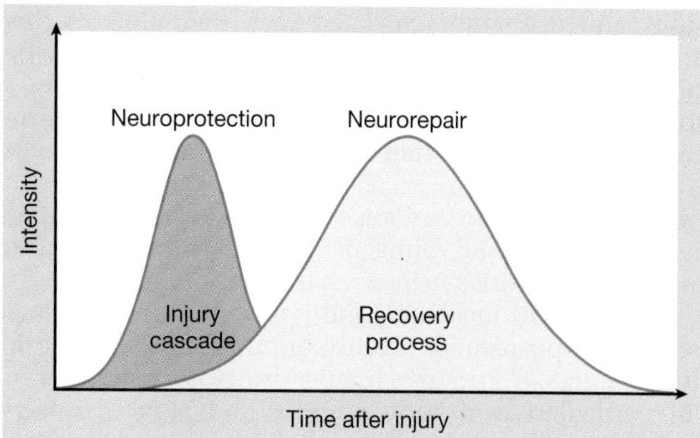

FIGURE 43-1 A depiction of the complex continuation of injury and repair after a traumatic brain injury. The primary injury disrupts brain tissue and initiates secondary injury cascades that lead to cell dysfunction and death. Neuroprotective and neurorepair mechanisms after injury contribute to chronic degeneration, repair, and regeneration processes.

Primary Injury

TBI occurs in conjunction with mechanical forces that cause disruption to the brain tissue. Closed head injuries can occur because of mechanical forces that shear axons as well as forces at the site of the impact or at the point opposite the impact.[186] Contact forces occur when the head is prevented from moving after it is struck. Inertial forces occur when the head is set into motion and results in acceleration.[232]

Inertial forces associated with angular acceleration result in diffuse axonal injury (DAI), a process that causes tensile strains resulting in microscopic disruption of axons, cerebral edema, and neuron disconnection. In angular acceleration, the brain's center of gravity moves over a center of angulation, or fulcrum, located in the lower to middle cervical region.[189] The severity of DAI depends on the duration, magnitude, direction of the angular acceleration, and associated impact.[189] In severe cases of DAI, more than just superficial axons are affected and injuries affect deeper white matter structures. The gray-white matter junction is also particularly vulnerable to DAI. Midline brain structures, such as the corpus callosum, are often affected by DAI, which is also associated with loss of consciousness and coma. Recovery from DAI is gradual and can be linked to the duration of coma.[232] Violent shaking associated with child abuse generates significant acceleration/deceleration forces, which result in shearing injury to brain tissue, disruption of blood vessels, and retinal bleeding.[51,177]

Inertial forces associated with translational acceleration result in a head movement that is in line with the brain's center of gravity. The resulting differential movement of the brain relative to the skull causes focal injuries such as contusions. Cortical contusions often occur on gyral crests, particularly on the undersurface of the frontal and anterior temporal lobes, where bony prominences located in the basilar skull can create tissue and vascular disruption. Contusions may occur under the impact site (coup injury) and result from a rapid change in skull distortion during impact.[189] Contusions remote from the injury site and opposite of the impact are contrecoup injuries and occur because of negative pressure generated from the impact associated with translational acceleration.[414] Patients with significant TBI may have one or more contusions, and deficits observed with cerebral contusions are linked with the lesion location and size.

DAI and focal contusions can result in neuronal disconnection, or diaschisis. First proposed by Constantin von Monakow in 1905, the concept of diaschisis refers to neurons remote from a site of injury, but anatomically connected to the damaged area, becoming functionally depressed. Because every structure in the brain is directly or indirectly connected to all other structures, the basic idea of this concept is that damage to one structure will be disruptive to others. Imaging studies suggest that diaschisis can result in the metabolic depression of areas both regionally associated with and remote from the site of injury.[168,377] Others suggest that focal cortical lesions may affect contralateral cortical functioning by way of intercallosal connections[143] and can affect the function of subcortical structures including the striatum.[168] Resolution of diaschisis is one of several theories for recovery of function[168,377] to be discussed later.

Epidural hematomas (EDHs) result from local impact and subsequent laceration of underlying dural veins and arteries. The meningeal artery is commonly the source of EDHs, and damage to dural sinuses can also cause EDH. When an EDH develops from a disrupted artery, a neurologic emergency occurs as the EDH quickly expands and rapidly causes neurologic deterioration.[232] Subdural hematomas (SDHs) result from inertial forces and the tearing of bridging veins.[414] Bridging veins are susceptible to shear and rupture from brief high-velocity angular accelerations associated with falls.[190] Traumatic subarachnoid hemorrhage (SAH) occurs when angular acceleration shears vessels located in the subarachnoid space.[232]

Secondary Injury

Secondary injury develops over the hours and days after the initial impact and is associated with disruption of cerebral blood flow and metabolism, massive release of neurochemicals, cerebral edema, and disruption of ion homeostasis leading to cellular injury and eventual cell death. Much of what is known about secondary injury is derived from postmortem analyses of human brain tissues, the analysis of blood, cerebral spinal fluid (CSF), and parenchymal microdialysate fluid obtained early after clinical TBI. Additionally, much work exploring secondary injury has used in vivo experimental models of TBI and in vitro injury methods. Experimental models of TBI produce one or more types of primary injury, which lead to the development of secondary injury cascades that closely resemble observations made in humans.[141,351,515]

Brain swelling occurs in response to the initial injury and early events involved with secondary injury and results in elevated intracranial pressure (ICP) and decreased cerebral perfusion pressure (CPP). If severe enough, brain swelling can lead to herniation, which has potentially fatal consequences. In some cases, elevated ICP is caused by the development of focal extraaxial lesions like SDH and EDH described above. In other cases, elevated ICP and intracranial hypertension result from global mechanisms occurring on a cellular level that lead to brain edema. Some mechanisms that affect brain edema include vasogenic edema, increased tissue osmolarity, and vascular dysregulation resulting from increased cerebral blood volume. However, brain edema caused by neuronal swelling and astrocyte swelling secondary to increased glutamate metabolism after excitotoxic insult may impart the most damage.[301]

Excitatory amino acids (EAAs) like glutamate and aspartate are ubiquitous and important neurotransmitters for normal brain function. After TBI, excess excitatory amino acid levels are present in extracellular microdialysate fluid as well as CSF.[67,572] Excess EAA release occurs, in part, from the mechanical stresses associated with stretch injury of axons. Elevations in extracellular glutamate levels after TBI contribute to excitotoxic injury by affecting other paths of secondary head injury through two primary mechanisms. By binding their target receptors, excess EAAs can trigger an influx of sodium and chloride that leads to acute neuronal and astrocytic swelling. Excess EAA levels can also lead to an intracellular calcium influx as well as the release of Ca^{++} from intracellular stores leading to delayed cellular damage or death.[88,525] EAA-mediated Ca^{++}-dependent production of nitric oxide, superoxide, and free radical damage to DNA and cellular membranes leads to cell death.[336] Regional differences in the distribution of EAA sensitive receptors contribute to selective vulnerability of some regions to excitotoxic injury like the hippocampus, a critical region for learning and memory.[382]

Lactate is the end product of glycolysis, and in neurons, lactate is converted to pyruvate for oxidative metabolism. Lactate/pyruvate (L/P) ratios reflect the cellular energy balance and the cytosolic oxidation-reduction state.[507] Increased metabolic demand after TBI is due, in part, to increased astrocytic glutamate uptake and results in increased lactate. Reduced cerebral blood flow, including pericontusional hypoperfusion, has been documented in both experimental models[242] and in humans[520] early after TBI and results in ischemic injury. Elevations in L/P ratios have been measured in pericontusional tissue in humans[564] and are associated with other aspects of secondary injury, including increased ICP and mitochondrial dysfunction.

Although extracellular lactate has classically been a marker for anaerobic metabolism with hypoxic injury, research also indicates that lactate is used by brain tissue during an insult as an important energy source in oxidative metabolism.[452] Evidence supports a dichotomous role of lactate in which it is produced by the astrocyte via glycolytic metabolism, to be directly consumed by the neuron after uptake through lactate transporters.[117,452] Physiologically[428] and after TBI,[452] EAAs are likely triggers for this metabolic process. After injury, estradiol facilitates lactate production for neuronal use by modulating lactate transporters.[374] Interestingly, experimental studies suggest that lactate is used as a neuronal energy substrate after TBI and lactate administration after TBI is neuroprotective and decreases cognitive deficits.[457]

Mitochondrial dysfunction is often the result of energy failure and excitotoxic insult and results in the formation of highly reactive free radicals and oxidative damage to cell membranes and DNA. Hydroxyl radicals and other reactive oxygen species react with many molecules found in living cells, including DNA, membrane lipids, and carbohydrates. CNS tissue is particularly vulnerable to oxidative injury caused by the high rate of oxidative metabolic activity, the nonreplicating nature of neurons, high levels of transition metals, and a high membrane-to-cytoplasm ratio in neurons.[14] Superoxide radicals are a principal mediator of the microvascular damage after TBI.[312] Free-reactive iron generated from hemorrhage catalyzes the formation of free radicals.[301] Reactive oxygen species production may also be a downstream effect of caspase-mediated cell death (apoptosis).[173]

Cell death in CNS tissues after brain trauma falls into two primary categories: (1) cellular necrosis and (2) apoptosis or programmed cell death. Necrotic cells display cellular and nuclear swelling as well as disruption of cellular membranes. In contrast, apoptotic cells are characterized by cellular shrinkage, nuclear condensation, and DNA fragmentation.[281] Apoptosis is accompanied by a cascade of events required for cell death to occur.[521] In TBI, cell death patterns often reflect a combination of both necrosis and apoptosis.

Apoptosis can be initiated through either extracellular or intracellular signaling pathways. *c*ysteine-*asp*artic acid prote*ases* (caspases) play an essential role in cell death via both pathways. Extracellular binding of cell surface death receptors, including tumor necrosis factor alpha (TNFα) receptor and FAS ligand receptor, initiates apoptotic signals, including caspase-8 and caspase-3, within seconds of ligand binding. Intracellular signaling is initiated by mitochondrial dysfunction in response to disturbances in cellular energy balance, oxidative injury, and changes in ionic homeostasis. This mitochondrial stress leads to the opening of the mitochondrial transition pore and cytochrome C release. Cytosolic cytochrome C release induces other caspases, including caspase-9 and caspase-3, which leads to the cleavage of key cellular elements like cytoskeletal proteins and DNA repair proteins, as well as activation of endonucleases.[96] In addition to this intracellular caspase-dependent process for apoptosis, intracellular apoptosis signaling can also occur via a caspase-independent pathway with apoptosis inducing factor (AIF). AIF is released from the mitochondria and results in DNA fragmentation. The mitochondria house both prosurvival and pro-death proteins that are both members of the BCL-2 protein family,[3] each of which can be manipulated experimentally to affect cell survival. As an example, estrogen enhances BCL-2 expression and cell survival after central nervous system (CNS) injury.[258]

Inflammation after TBI is characterized by very complex cascades that largely include cytokines, or signaling molecules that communicate with resident and infiltrating inflammatory cells. There is growing evidence to implicate cytokines, including IL-1β and TNFα, in propagating the inflammatory response, as well as in promoting neurotoxicity and edema via excitotoxicity and oxidative injury.[567] Inflammatory molecules are synthesized by peripheral cells as well as CNS neurons and glia and are increased early after injury. IL-1β has potent leukocyte-signaling properties that lead to cellular inflammatory responses after TBI, and IL-1β and other inflammatory mediators can facilitate blood brain barrier (BBB) disruption and transport of peripheral inflammatory components into the CNS. Multiple inflammatory mediators are also synthesized by activated microglia in the CNS. Specifically, IL-1β and TNFα

can mediate synthesis of neurotoxic compounds like arachidonic acid and are implicated in excitoxic components of secondary injury.[473]

Cytokines are constitutively expressed in the brain and promote neuronal differentiation and survival under normal conditions. Cytokines play a dual role in secondary injury with TBI, and inflammatory cascades may either enhance cellular injury or provide neuroprotection. Some studies suggest that cytokine's effects may be dose-dependent, with higher levels more likely to be associated with detrimental effects and lower levels neuroprotective.[138,516,517] Consistent with this previous work, recent clinical evidence implicates CNS cortisol as a regulator of this dualistic role after TBI.[485] Also, some cytokines support neuroprotection and neurorepair through their effects on neurotrophin production and excitotoxicity and antiinflammatory properties.[290,309,389] CNS inflammatory biomarker profiles can be influenced by extracerebral injury wherein major trauma itself can elicit a significant systemic inflammatory response.[45] Recent evidence suggests that neuroinflammation can continue for months and years after injury, adversely contributing to outcome and implicating TBI as triggering a chronic inflammatory state.[313,448,505] Specific cytokine effects in the setting of long-term or chronic inflammation remain largely unstudied; however, some evidence suggests beneficial effects can occur at delayed or chronic time points after injury.[390] TNFα is an example in which time-dependent functions have been demonstrated,[490] with TNFα expression being protective at later time points after injury.

Aside from BCL-2 and the prosurvival components of neuroinflammation, other CNS compounds can serve as endogenous neuroprotectants after TBI. Adenosine is a purine ribonucleoside; it is ubiquitous in the brain, where it largely functions as a major neuroinhibitory molecule. After experimental brain injury, extracellular adenosine levels increase by 50- to 100-fold when compared with baseline,[34] a phenomenon that is implicated as an endogenous neuroprotective mechanism. Adenosine functions as a neuroinhibitory molecule through its primary target, the A1 receptor. A1 receptor activation is a key local regulator of excitatory amino acid release during ischemia and trauma.[15] Adenosine can also hyperpolarize neuronal membranes and attenuate intracellular Ca^{++} accumulation.

Neurotrophins may also have a neuroprotective role after TBI, particularly since early increases in neurotrophin expression have been reported in experimental TBI.[248,621] The downstream effects of neurotrophins like brain-derived neurotrophic factor (BDNF) may be variable, based on the regional target milieu where increases in the proapoptotic target receptor p75 are observed with acute CNS insult and increased age.[110,472] Thus, BDNF's role in TBI recovery and mortality may be dependent on the relative balance of these target receptors. In support of this concept, a recent clinical report implicates BDNF in mortality after TBI, in which there were unique relationships among BDNF genetics, older age, and mortality risk.[156]

Concomitant Injury

TBIs, particularly more severe cases, are not often isolated. High-speed vehicular crashes and active combat frequently result in multiple injuries that can affect outcome.[298] In civilians, associated injuries are linked with more disability even 1 year after the injury.[575] TBI associated with multiple other injuries is also associated with longer acute-care lengths of stay and need for rehabilitation resources.[573] In addition to increased functional deficits, rehabilitation needs, and disability, concomitant injuries can directly affect secondary injury and associated pathology, and these phenomena have received some attention in the TBI literature. For example, experimental models incorporating TBI and hemorrhagic shock show increased hippocampal injury versus TBI alone, a phenomenon likely associated with increased secondary ischemia.[128]

Military Blast Injury

With the ongoing military conflicts in Iraq and Afghanistan, TBI is a major problem for active combat military personnel. The frequent use of improvised explosive devices in these conflicts has resulted in a large number of military personnel (see previous epidemiology sections) sustaining TBI from blast injury. Blast injury can result in both blunt and penetrating trauma and follows a specific nomenclature (Box 43-2). Explosives can be categorized as high-order explosives (HEs) or low-order explosives (LEs), and each can cause a distinct injury pattern. HE produces a supersonic overpressurization shock wave[556] that is associated with "primary injury." In addition to middle ear damage, brain injury can occur from primary blast injury without overt evidence of injury. The rapid pressure changes generated from the overpressure wave result in shear and stress forces that lead to trauma such as concussion, subdural hematoma, and diffuse axonal injury.[130,533] Penetrating head injury from flying debris is the result of secondary blast injury. Both HE and LE can result in tertiary blast injury from being physically thrown by a blast wind into the ground or other objects. Quaternary injury includes asphyxia or inhalation of toxic chemicals that may also contribute to brain injury. Many patients have TBI induced from more than one facet of blast injury.

Increasingly, research is being conducted to develop relevant blast injury models of TBI to examine and characterize mechanisms of primary and secondary injury for blast

BOX 43-2

Immediate Effects of Blasts and Explosions in Traumatic Brain Injury

- Primary direct effects of overpressure blast
  - Rupture of tympanic membranes
  - Concussion
  - Subdural and diffuse axonal injury
- Secondary: penetrating trauma
  - Fragmentation injuries
- Tertiary: effects of structural collapse and of persons being thrown by the blast wind
  - Open or closed brain injuries
- Quaternary: asphyxia, and exposure to toxic inhalants
  - Concomitant closed injury

From DePalma RG, Burris DG, Champion RH, et al: Blast injuries, *N Engl J Med* 352:1335-1342, 2005.

TBI and assess behavioral effects.[28,77,335] Clinically, difficulties after blast TBI of any severity can include headache, insomnia, decreased memory and attention, slower thinking, irritability, and depression.[125] Additional research is focused on clinical symptom screening and outcomes as well as physiologic markers and biomarkers associated with this type of TBI.[9,529,551] A more recent focus is the effects of repetitive blast injury exposure on the development of neurodegenerative disorders and the comorbidity of posttraumatic stress disorder.[50,205,370,561,623]

Neurotransmission Repair, Regeneration, and Recovery

Acute mechanisms of secondary injury heavily influence the degree and type of injury and deficits that individuals with TBI experience. The chronic period after injury is characterized by multiple neurotransmitter deficits and cellular dysfunction. During this period, however, research demonstrates that the brain is amenable to neuroplasticity, repair, and recovery, and the potential for these processes can be augmented with relevant rehabilitation strategies.

One mechanism by which TBI recovery occurs is through the reversal of diaschisis. Contemporary thought on the concept of diaschisis suggests that the functional effects of diaschisis can be either reversible or permanent. However, the mechanisms by which diaschisis resolves are poorly understood and likely multifactorial. The resolution of cerebral edema and blood flow regulation[168] may contribute to early recovery.[303] Later, the alleviation of diaschisis may involve factors like synaptic plasticity,[377,462] axonal sprouting,[467] and cortical reorganization.[304] Diaschisis after brain injury can be manipulated by both behavioral experience (rehabilitation) and pharmacologic intervention.[411,498] For example, depressed thalamic metabolism after cortical infarction has been reversed with administration of neurostimulants such as amphetamine.[168,433]

Experimental and clinical research suggests that dopamine systems are key pathways involved in attention, task salience, and cognition, and these pathways are impaired chronically after TBI.[27] Alterations in both presynaptic and postsynaptic dopaminergic proteins in the striatum and frontal cortex have been documented, including important proteins involved in dopamine synthesis and uptake.[27,571,580,585] Decreases in striatal dopamine transporter (DAT) expression, a key protein in regulating the extracellular half-life of dopamine, have been documented in humans.[147] Further research demonstrates that striatal neurotransmission is impaired and may be the result of TBI-induced changes in DA protein functionality.[571,585] Recent clinical research suggests impaired striatal DA transmission, including reduced DAT expression profiles that mirror experimental modeling data (described below) and that are both DAT and D2 genotype specific.[583]

Noradrenergic systems affect arousal, sleep-wake cycles, vigilance, and cognition, and the norepinephrine (NE) transporter appears to affect NE neurotransmission as well as interact with dopamine (DA) systems to affect DA neurotransmission.[592] Noradrenergic function is impaired early after TBI. Previous reports suggest that cortical NE levels are decreased within 24 hours following brain injury, and adrenergic receptors are altered after injury.[442,443] However, NE augmentation early after TBI is neuroprotective, and NE agonists aid in neurorecovery.[49,148] Importantly, NE is critical for governing cortical plasticity and facilitating recovery post-TBI. By stimulating adrenergic systems with amphetamine and L-DOPS, a precursor of NE, neuronal damage after TBI can be minimized and sprouting is promoted.[203,204,283,524,527]

Cholinergic systems are important for memory and cognition, and evidence suggests chronic impairments occur after TBI. Hippocampus expression of the vesicular acetylocholine transporter is increased; however, evoked release of acetylcholine in the neocortex and hippocampus is reduced following experimental TBI.[140,146,499] Chronic changes in cholinergic receptor expression patterns and affinities have also been noted experimental TBI models.[123,339] Further, daily local application of nerve growth factor has been shown to enhance memory and hippocampal neuron function after experimental TBI.[142]

In addition to acute protection and cholinergic function, other studies support a role for neurotrophin administration in promoting long-term recovery. In contrast to acute increases in neurotrophin production, other work suggests that hippocampal BDNF is decreased during chronic recovery from experimental TBI.[82] Although an enriched environment can reverse these decreases,[82] chronic pericontusional administration of BDNF does not improve behavioral outcome or hippocampal cell survival.[42] Studies suggest that BDNF target receptor expression ratios can vary following ischemia and TBI, which can promote apoptotic pathways in the acute phase following experimental TBI.[472] BDNF's early role in TBI recovery may be dependent on the relative balance of these target receptors. Recent work in our group suggests that genetic variation in the BDNF gene may be related to mortality following TBI.[156] Both intraparenchymal administration of basic fibroblast growth factor and nerve growth factor do reduce cognitive deficits in experimental TBI.[367,511] With these positive studies, improved recovery may be secondary to stimulation of brain repair and neuroplasticity.

Principles of Experimental Neurotransmitter Dysfunction and Treatment After Traumatic Brain Injury

The neurobiology of catecholaminergic dysfunction, particularly DA dysfunction, is the most characterized in the experimental literature.[27] Early changes in DA levels occur after experimental TBI.[355] Chronic DA receptor and synthetic protein changes after TBI also have been characterized with experimental TBI models. The dopamine transporter (DAT) is a key protein regulating the extracellular half-life of DA in the synaptic cleft and the therapeutic target of neurostimulants like methylphenidate (MPH) and amphetamine. Long-term changes in striatal and cortical DAT expression and intracellular trafficking have been identified[571,585] that are gender specific.[570] Further, functional changes in DAT after experimental TBI lead to altered striatal neurotransmission.[571,584] Other changes in postsynaptic secondary signaling mechanisms, as well as changes in presynaptic DA synthetic enzyme levels, have been identified.[27]

Behavioral pharmacology studies show that daily treatment with the DAT inhibitor MPH has a beneficial impact on cognition after experimental TBI.[295] Recent work suggests that the cognitive benefits of MPH are more pronounced in males[576] and that daily MPH therapy has a neurorestorative effect on striatal neurotransmission in males through MPH-mediated changes in DAT function.[571,584] Daily treatment with the pleiotropic DA enhancer amantadine has been reported,[144] and a recent clinical trial supports amantadine use in severely injured individuals in the postacute and early chronic recovery phases after TBI.[196] Experimental data also show that the D2 receptor agonist bromocriptine can benefit learning and memory.[292] Interestingly, early treatment with bromocriptine also appears to decrease oxidative damage initiated by the injury.[293]

Evidence also suggests that NE systems are disrupted after experimental TBI but can be manipulated to improve recovery. Cortical NE levels are decreased in the first 24 hours after injury,[442] and NE turnover is impaired chronically after injury.[183] Further, α1-adrenergic receptor expression is decreased.[443] Local NE infusions early after injury enhance recovery,[49] and stimulating adrenergic systems with amphetamine can decrease neuronal damage after TBI.[203] Recent studies suggest that at least some of the beneficial effects of amphetamine may be because of its ability to increase neurotrophin production after injury.[217] Daily treatment with low doses of the selective NE transporter (NET) inhibitor atomoxetine shows benefit on cognitive recovery after experimental TBI.[451]

Experimental TBI studies also demonstrate decreased hippocampal cholinergic transmission[140] and alterations in cholinergic synthetic and metabolic enzyme production.[84,145] For example, a single dose of the acetylcholinesterase inhibitor rivastigmine improves cerebral edema, cognition, and motor functioning early after experimental TBI.[84] Interestingly, daily treatment with CDP-choline, a key intermediary in the biosynthesis of phosphatidylcholine, improves cognitive recovery in experimental TBI and increases hippocampal and cortical acetylcholine levels.[145] However, the beneficial effects of CDP-choline have not translated in a recent large multisite clinical trial involving acute and chronic administration in individuals with complicated mild to severe TBI.[626]

Evaluation and Treatment of Traumatic Brain Injury

Management of Mild Traumatic Brain Injury (Concussion)

Similar to more severe injuries, concussion results in significant alterations in brain physiology. After an initial increase in glucose use, brain metabolism is impaired and is associated with the development of energy crisis, oxidative injury, and initiation of biochemical cell death pathways. These derangements can occur for up to weeks after the concussion and persist even with a normal GCS and general neurologic examination findings.[200]

There are several criteria and scoring systems for classifying degree or severity of mild TBI. However, the World Health Organization (WHO) Collaborating Centre Task Force on Mild TBI states that key criteria for identifying persons with a mild TBI include at least one of the following: confusion, disorientation, loss of consciousness for less than 30 minutes, PTA for less than 24 hours, or other transient focal neurologic abnormalities and a GCS score of 13 to 15 after 30 minutes or presentation to a health care facility. Findings with these criteria should be made in the absence of illicit drugs, alcohol, medications with sedating side effects, or other injuries or problems.[75] Patients with uncomplicated TBI typically do not have associated abnormalities on standard imaging tests like CT. Concussion severity nomenclature has been developed for the purposes of injury characterization and injury management. Some examples of frequently used grading systems include the Cantu and Colorado concussion scales (Table 43-1).[74,101,280]

Frequently, patients with concussion will complain of any number of associated symptoms, including memory loss, poor concentration, impaired emotional control, posttraumatic headaches, sleep disorders, fatigue, irritability, dizziness, visual acuity, depression, anxiety, personality changes, and seizures.[13,610] These problems can affect ADLs, social relationships, and work abilities. For most with mild TBI, symptoms resolve over time. However, a subset of patients will have persistent symptoms classified as postconcussion syndrome and may require outpatient follow-up. The types of symptoms, proportion of patients who have persistent symptoms, and duration of symptoms required to define symptoms as persistent have been a point of debate. Reports of symptom duration to define persistent deficits can range between 3 and 12 months. The fourth edition of the *Diagnostic and Statistical Manual of Mental Disorders* (DSM-IV) suggests that individuals showing objective evidence of cognitive deficits as well as three or more subjective symptoms that represent a change in baseline function for at least 3 months can be diagnosed with postconcussion disorder. Other classification systems, such as the *International Classification of Diseases*, Tenth Edition, do not include objective evidence of cognitive deficits.[610] Despite variability in definitions and classification, some studies suggest that females are more likely to have postconcussion syndrome.[439,439a]

Athletes comprise a large portion of the population who sustain mild TBI, and many are children. Special issues arise with this population with regard to "on-site" concussion screening tools, determining the most effective algorithm for return to play, safety equipment use, management and prevention of recurrent injuries, and academic performance. In general, athletes should be free of postconcussive symptoms before returning to competition. One report shows that 30% of high school football players return to play on the same day of injury.[224] However, many return-to-play guidelines recommend that athletes with a grade 1 or 2 concussion have a minimum of 7 days free of symptoms before returning to play.[223] Same-season injuries often occur within 7 to 10 days of the initial injury, a time frame in which there is increased vulnerability to damage with the second insult.[200] Most return-to-play (RTP) algorithms emphasize a graded protocol for reintroducing the athlete to physical exertion, although a recent systematic review does not support graded return-to-sports protocols

Table 43-1 Concussion Grading Scales

Guideline	Grade 1	Grade 2	Grade 3
Colorado	1. Confusion without amnesia 2. No loss of consciousness	1. Confusion with amnesia 2. No loss of consciousness	Loss of consciousness (of any duration)
AAN	1. Transient confusion 2. No loss of consciousness 3. Concussion symptoms or mental status changes resolve in less than 5 minutes	1. Transient confusion 2. No loss of consciousness 3. Concussion symptoms or mental status changes last longer than 15 minutes	1. Loss of consciousness (brief or prolonged)
Cantu	1. No loss of consciousness OR 2. Posttraumatic amnesia or signs/symptoms last longer than 30 minutes	1. Loss of consciousness lasts less than 1 minute OR 2. Posttraumatic amnesia lasts longer than 30 minutes but less than 24 hours	1. Loss of consciousness lasts >1 minute OR 2. Posttraumatic amnesia lasts longer than 24 hours OR 3. Postconcussion signs/symptoms last longer than 7 days

AAN, American Academy of Neurology.

as significantly influencing prognosis, and conservative management with return to play is still standard of care.[72] Notably, recent studies suggest that academic and cognitive exertion can impact postconcussive symptoms and cognitive testing performance and should be considered when developing RTP protocols for athletes.[345] Recent evidence and expert consensus suggest a stepwise approach to return-to-school guidelines for pediatric concussion.[127] Several guidelines recommend termination of sports participation for the remainder of the season if an athlete sustains a third concussion within that season.[74,454] However, athletes who have one concussion are at increased risk for subsequent concussion,[223] making return to contact sports even after a single concussion a decision that requires careful thought and consideration.

Acute Medical Management of Moderate to Severe Traumatic Brain Injury

The care of the patient with TBI begins in the field. Evidence-based guidelines from the Brain Trauma Foundation and the American Association of Neurological Surgeons support a regional organized trauma care system that addresses prehospital care and triage. Direct transport of a patient with severe TBI to a level 1 or 2 trauma center is associated with decreased mortality when compared with indirect transport.[239] Facilities defined by the Guidelines for Prehospital Management of Traumatic Brain Injury as being appropriate for transport include those offering CT scanning, neurosurgical care, ICP monitoring, and treatment capabilities. These facilities can provide 24-hour neurosurgical care and intensive care treatment, and ICP monitors are routinely used. Each state can designate trauma facilities based on the availability of such care. Although treatment guidelines for initial management are not specific, the recommendations include complete and rapid physiologic resuscitation. Correction of hypoxia, including intubation, is appropriate. Sedation and neuromuscular blockade may be used to optimize the transport of the head injury patient.[55]

ICP has been the mainstay of monitoring after severe TBI. ICP can be monitored with a ventriculostomy, the procedure of choice, because it allows therapeutic CSF drainage. ICP monitoring is appropriate in those patients with a GCS of 8 or less after resuscitation, head CT with contusions or edema, or systolic blood pressure less than 90 mm Hg.[402] ICP monitoring can also be considered in patients with severe TBI and negative head CT findings if they are older than age 40, posturing, and/or have a systolic blood pressure less than 90 mm Hg.[54] Elevated ICP is defined as 20 to 25 mm Hg in clinical practice. Maneuvers to decrease ICP include elevating the head of the bed 30 degrees, treatment of hyperthermia, mannitol administration, sedation, and brief hyperventilation. Prolonged chronic hyperventilation can negatively impact cerebral blood flow.[53]

CPP is defined as the mean arterial pressure minus ICP and is the pressure gradient driving cerebral blood flow. Studies have documented worsened clinical outcomes in patients with TBI with episodes of low CPP.[86] Current therapeutic recommendations are to maintain CPP above 60 mm Hg in adults.[56] Measurement of cerebral oxygen tension allows the practitioner to directly measure ischemia, rather than rely on indirect measurement of CPP or ICP. Tissue oxygenation monitors, directly placed in brain tissue via an external ventricular drain, can detect focal ischemic changes that may go undetected with global measures. Interventions are then tailored to the cause of the drop in tissue oxygenation. Studies have shown benefit on outcome and mortality reduction with addition of multimodal monitoring.[87,219]

Other treatment interventions have been studied in acute-care clinical trials. A multicenter trial evaluating the role of corticosteroids in management of acute TBI showed an increase in mortality 2 weeks after TBI when compared with placebo.[463] Elevated CSF cortisol levels in severely injured patients, and their link to inflammation, may contribute to this outcome.[485,486] Progesterone is a drug with pleiotropic neuroprotective properties identified in several preclinical studies occurring over decades.[519] Recent clinical trials have shown its safety, and progesterone appeared to have therapeutic potential.[612,617] However, recently, two multi-site clinical trials did not show overall benefit with progesterone therapy.[511a,612a] As progesterone is the primary substrate for both stress and sex hormones, each with known adverse influences on secondary injury, progesterone treatment effects on these hormone pathways and secondary injury cascades require further study.

Animal studies have evaluated the protective use of hypothermia, with several showing positive results.[95,134] Clinical trials with moderate hypothermia have shown some reduction in excitotoxic insult[349,572] and neurologic impairment; however, results have not been consistent. For instance, a large multicenter trial of hypothermia did not show improved outcomes in patients with severe TBI.[98] To transition this treatment to routine human use, factors such as treatment window, rewarming rates, and type of anesthesia must be defined.[518] In addition, age, sex, and hormone effects on treatment efficacy and physiologic response to treatment should be considered[30,528] to determine whether specific subgroups with TBI might benefit from this treatment. In contrast, therapeutic hypothermia has been adopted as a part of early treatment for the TBI population, with significant reductions in mortality and neurologic morbidity noted in clinical studies.[22,401,427]

Surgical treatment of TBI is indicated when intracerebral fluid collections exert a significant mass effect. Mass effect can be gauged by degree of midline shift on neuroimaging and the decision to intervene may require serial neurologic exam inations and CT scans.[67] Depressed skull fractures greater than the thickness of the skull should be elevated to decrease the risk of infection, especially in the setting of a dural laceration. Surgical treatment may also be used to lower ICP. The use of decompressive craniectomy to decrease ICP is an accepted intervention, although the reduction of morbidity and mortality has not been proven.[44,605] Such procedures can also lead to additional issues such as herniation of the brain outside the skull bone defects, subdural effusion, and hydrocephalus requiring ventriculoperitoneal shunt.[252]

Secondary complications in the intensive care unit (ICU) can also negatively affect TBI outcomes. Elevated glucose levels are associated with increased mortality after TBI, presumably because of increased lactic acid production leading to ischemia as well as impaired phosphorus metabolism.[474] Recent studies suggest that glucose variability, including low serum glucose levels, may adversely impact outcome.[397] Sodium imbalance can potentiate risks of seizure as well as worsen level of consciousness, as this electrolyte abnormality is directly related to volume status. Hyponatremia can be exacerbated by giving excessive volumes of intravenous fluids. This phenomenon occurs even in the setting of normal saline or lactate Ringer solution used for fluid resuscitation, making electrolyte monitoring and volume status important in preventing secondary complications. Prevention and aggressive treatment of infections are also important, with one recent study indicating that hospital-acquired pneumonia can have significant effects on long-term outcome.[282] Hyperthermia, by increasing ischemia, is another source of acceleration of secondary insults to brain parenchyma.[348] Thus, maintenance of normothermia is often a part of clinical critical care for those with severe injuries.[25]

Early initiation of nutrition is vitally important in the patient with TBI. Metabolic rates can increase 40% during the early postinjury stages. Guidelines recommend replacement of 140% of resting metabolism expenditure (100% in paralyzed patients). The gastrointestinal tract is preferred to maintain nutritional status. The goal of treatment is to maintain a positive nitrogen balance, although this is difficult to achieve. Nitrogen balance via a metabolic cart study, prealbumin levels, and liver function should be followed in the ICU. Although literature does not yet support standard practice guidelines to optimize nutrition after moderate to severe TBI, significant evidence exists suggesting that delayed nutrition replacement is associated with increased mortality.[108,589] In a metaanalysis, small bowel feeding in the ICU reduced rates of hospital-acquired pneumonia and some immune-enhancing feeding formulas reduced sepsis, suggesting a direct link between nutritional support and acute/chronic inflammation and complications known to adversely impact long-term outcome.[397]

The physiatrist plays a role in evaluating patients early who have sustained TBI. The early assessment includes prevention of orthopedic and immobility complications and contributes to management of behavioral issues (e.g., agitation) and begins early stimulant trials aimed at improving arousal and early participation in therapies.[126] Early consultation can result in improved mobility, improved functional outcomes, and decreased acute-care length of stay. In this model, rehabilitation assessment is a portion of the acute medical care, providing education and support for patients, families, and caregivers.[573]

Physiologic Measurements During Acute Care

Somatosensory-evoked potentials (SSEPs) are recorded from the scalp after stimulation of a sensory or mixed nerve in the peripheral nervous system. SSEPs are often used in severe TBI to predict survival and evaluate posttraumatic coma and persistent vegetative states. In some cases, SEEP testing is used as an adjunct to the clinical examination to determine brain death.[230,256] Hume and Cant found that bilateral loss of the median SSEP was indicative of impending death, and asymmetrical findings observed in the cortical response were indicative of severe residual deficits.[73] Their study indicated that serial SSEPs often change through the hospital course, and each study does not always correlate well with ultimate outcome. Given increased use of sedatives and paralytics, SSEPs can be a useful adjunct to the clinical examination to aid in prognosis, with recent evidence suggesting a similar role for prognostication in cardiac arrest.[412]

Like other neurologic evaluations, electroencephalography (EEG) can be beneficial when assessing patients with TBI to detect injury severity and depth of coma.[478] Degree of unconsciousness can quickly change, and continuous EEG (cEEG) monitoring can detect electrophysiologic signs of clinical deterioration.[231] Initial EEG recordings taken within 24 hours of injury, however, are generally more abnormal and of less prognostic significance than those performed after 24 to 48 hours.[530] The cEEG is a standard part of care at some level I trauma centers, and it can be used to effectively identify subclinical electrographic seizures, which are associated with other physiologic factors that contribute to poor outcome, including ICP elevations and increases in metabolic stress.[563]

Pupillary reflexes have been used not only as clinical indicators of surgical emergencies and complications in TBI associated with edema and herniation, but also as a tool in determining lesion location, mortality, and global outcome after injury. Presence or absence of pupillary reflexes and degrees of anisocoria have been used in models predicting the probability of intracerebral hematoma and lesion location.[85] The International Mission on Prognosis and Analysis of Randomized Controlled Trials in TBI has demonstrated high predictability of post-TBI mortality/outcome using a core model of age, injury severity (motor subscale of the GCS), pupillary reactivity, and midline shift.[342,469]

Although not yet used routinely at the bedside, biomarkers have considerable potential as adjunctive tools in TBI diagnosis, prognosis, and monitoring treatment effect. Typically, protein biomarkers that have been studied in TBI include either markers of structural damage or markers reflective of the cellular and molecular cascades observed with secondary injury and repair. Protein biomarkers have also been studied in both CSF and serum. CSF biomarker studies are valuable in that measured levels are a largely a reflection of CNS pathology. For other markers, CSF levels for peripheral markers (e.g., hormones, inflammatory markers) may reflect extent of BBB disruption. However, CSF collection is routine only in severely injured patients who require an extraventricular drain for management of ICP. Thus, serum markers are attractive because of their potential application to mild and severe cases of TBI. However, serum biomarker levels are often limited by the extent of BBB permeability present after the injury. Markers of acute injury have been much more thoroughly studied than markers of chronic injury. Although none are yet used for clinical management, research progress (discussed later) continues to generate novel biomarker discovery and characterization studies that will contribute to their eventual translation to clinical care.

Neuroimaging for Medical Management

The head CT scan is a mainstay of diagnostic imaging in TBI, and findings have use in identifying mass lesions that constitute a neurosurgical emergency and in correlating with outcome. Mass lesions, including SDH and EDH (Figure 43-2), can often cause shifting of the midline structures and can be life-threatening if not surgically evacuated (Figure 43-3). Intraparenchymal contusions can also cause shifting of midline structures (Figure 43-4). A DAI is often difficult to appreciate on head CT unless it is severe in nature with associated small hemorrhages forming near sheared axons (Figure 43-5). In mild TBI, the head CT is often negative; however, other modalities may capture subtle pathology associated with less severe injuries.

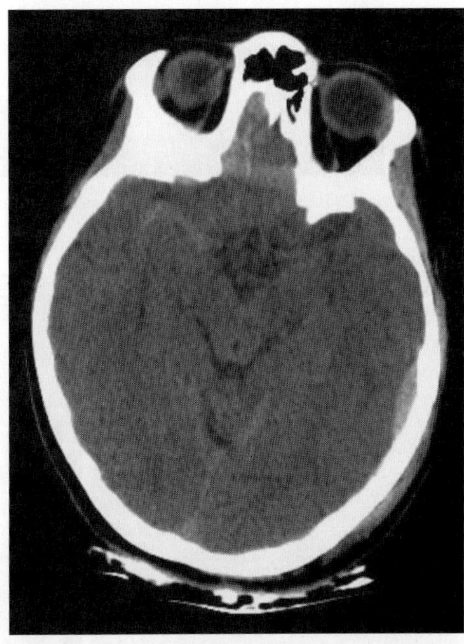

FIGURE 43-2 Example of an epidural hematoma in which there is a build-up of blood between the dura mater and the skull, shown here by CT scan.

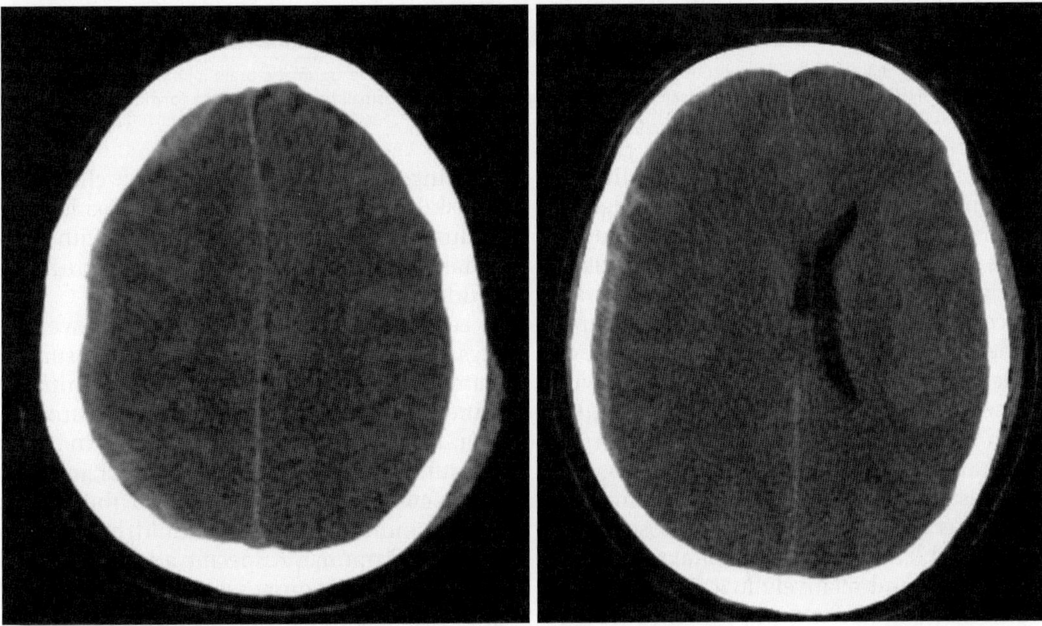

FIGURE 43-3 CT scans showing subdural hematomas, which have the potential to result in midline shift.

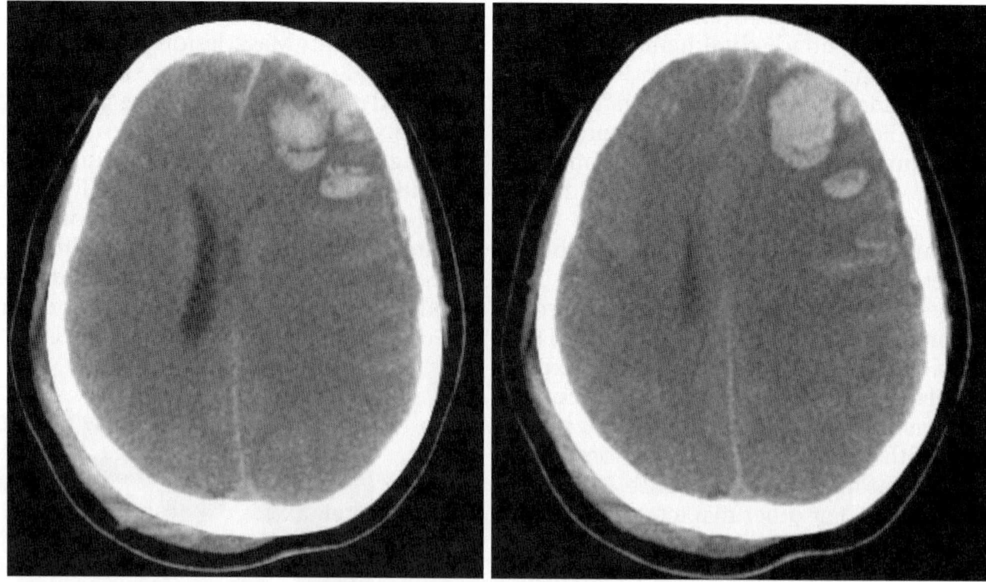

FIGURE 43-4 Hemorrhagic contusions can cause also midline shift as seen by CT scan.

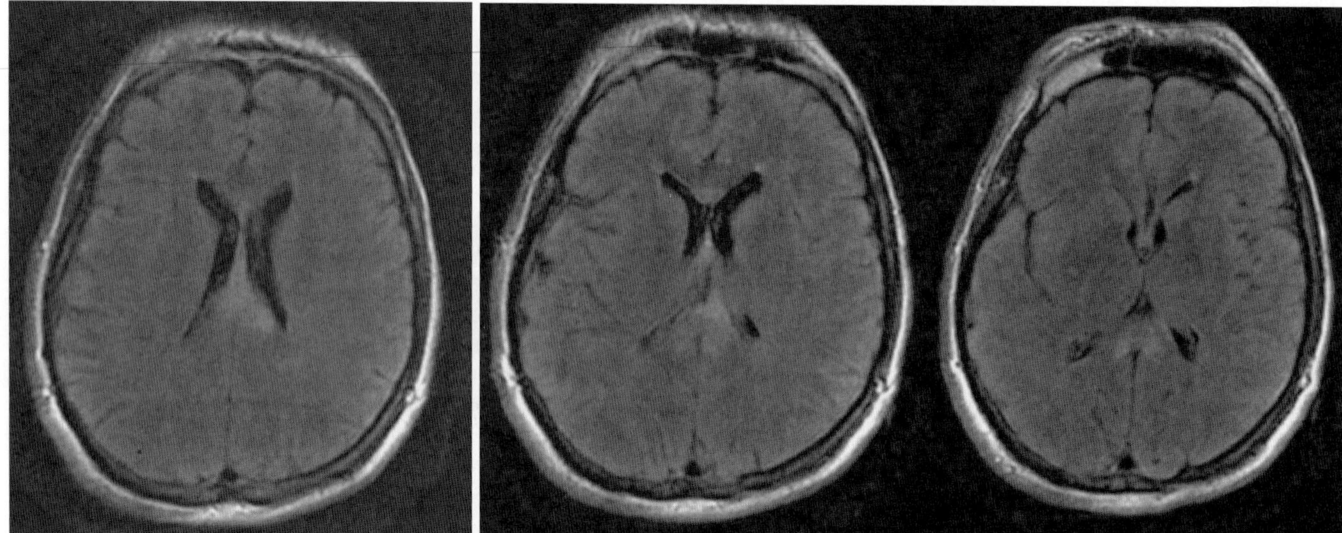

FIGURE 43-5 CT scans depicting diffuse axonal injury (DAI) after patients have sustained a severe traumatic brain injury. Although often difficult to see from a CT scan, DAI results in extensive lesions in white matter tracts and can be appreciated when small hemorrhages are formed near sheared axons

CT is the current standard neuroimaging modality for the initial evaluation of patients with suspected moderate-to-severe TBI.[121,226,321] CT methods, which are based on the same principles as plain-film x-rays, are advantageous as they allow for rapid, noninvasive three-dimensional imaging, which accurately detects facial and skull fractures, as well as acute hemorrhaging and mass effect. CT allows for optimal medical management of trauma patients who may require immediate surgical intervention. Repeat CT scans may be used to evaluate recovery or to monitor for additional complications. For example, if a patient with TBI does not progress as expected or declines in neurologic status, repeat CT scans are often used to diagnose issues such as new or evolving bleeding or hydrocephalus. Because of their high clinical use and relatively low cost, CT scanners have become readily available for use with TBI evaluation. As with x-ray, there are some risks associated with ionizing radiation, which require clinical judgment and a risk/benefit analysis when considering multiple CT evaluations over time, particularly with the evaluation of certain higher risk groups, such as pregnant women and children.

Less than 10% of mild TBI cases have positive CT findings, and even less, 1%, require neurosurgery.[266,321] As one primary purpose for conducting the initial CT is to determine the potential need for early neurosurgical intervention, these statistics have resulted in significant debate regarding the appropriate use of CT in cases of mild TBI. The New Orleans Criteria[241] and the Canadian CT Head Rule[522] indicate that CTs should be obtained in cases of mild head trauma, if specific additional criteria suggesting the possibility of more severe or evolving neurologic injury are met. Examples include age and symptoms such as seizure, vomiting, headache, and significant PTA. The

American College of Emergency Physicians put forth guidelines for clinical decision making based on available evidence in 2002 with an update in 2008 that were also consistent with and included the recommendations from the Canadian and New Orleans groups.[12,265] A recent study has suggested that the Canadian CT Head Rule may have higher sensitivity than the New Orleans Criteria, with higher negative predictive value. However, additional study is needed regarding the impact of using one method over another.

MRI is a second method of structural neuroimaging that has demonstrated clinical use in TBI.[226,321,320] MRI can produce high-resolution structural brain images by exploiting the magnetic properties of hydrogen atoms, and variations in the density and water content of body tissues. In comparison with CT, MRI scans take longer to complete and are more susceptible to motion artifacts. This makes it more difficult to scan individuals who are agitated. In addition, MRI is less able to detect skull fracture and acute blood than CT. Because of the magnetic environment of the MRI scanner, it also may be more complicated to scan patients with the continuous clinical monitoring and treatment equipment required during acute care or with medically implanted devices or objects that may be affected by the magnet (e.g., pacemakers, aneurysm clips, plates, rods). However, many MRI-compatible instruments and surgical implants have become available, reducing the frequency of this issue. MRI may also be contraindicated when there are causes of injury such as gunshot wounds or other accidents involving the presence of metal fragments. MRI does have superior resolution to CT, and it provides much higher detail in soft tissues. Therefore, MRI becomes the methodology of choice for evaluating brainstem and frontal area injuries and for detecting small hemorrhages and nonhemorrhagic white matter injury. As a result, MRI becomes increasingly useful with time from trauma, when patients become more medically stable and additional diagnoses of DAI or other small areas of hemorrhage may be helpful for treatment and prognosis.[226,321,320,593]

The four types of MRI sequences currently considered to be standard for the evaluation of TBI are T1- and T2-weighted, diffusion-weighted imaging (DWI), and T2*-weighted gradient echo imaging. T1-weighted imaging is generally used to attain anatomic maps of the brain.[226] T2-weighted images and T2 fluid-attenuated inversion recovery (T2 FLAIR) sequences are primary additional sequences for conventional MRI scanning to evaluate for injury. T2 images are sensitive to changes in water content indicative of edema, as well as iron content indicating the presence of blood. FLAIR sequences suppress the signal from CSF, resulting in improved visualization of cortical and periventricular lesions, as well as nonhemorrhagic shear injury associated with DAI. T2-weighted gradient recalled echo (GRE) has additional sensitivity to blood breakdown products, further adding to its sensitivity for DAI.[226] DWI is useful for detecting acute ischemia/microchanges via sensitivity to micromovement of water molecules, but not as sensitive for evaluation of larger hemorrhagic lesions.[226] As MRI images can be obtained in sagittal, coronal, and axial planes without moving the patient, additional nonconventional MRI sequences can be helpful. For example, coronal and sagittal FLAIR images can be helpful at discerning DAI involving the fornix and corpus callosum, compared with routine axial T2-weighted images.[320]

Recent efforts to develop CDEs for TBI have included imaging protocol recommendations for both basic imaging and more advanced modalities depending on the imaging and research capabilities of clinical sites.[226] These modalities will be discussed further in the research section of this chapter, as they are not currently used as standard clinical care, although the growing research literature provides evidence of significant translational potential for the use of these methods to inform clinical decision making.

Management of Patients with Disorders of Consciousness

Some patients with severe TBI have prolonged periods of depressed consciousness that may never resolve. Their accurate classification is vital for appropriate prognostication. Numerous terms have been used to classify these different states. Coma is defined as a state of pathologic unconsciousness in which the eyes remain closed and there is no evidence of purposeful motor activity. Vegetative state typically follows a period of coma, in which there is some evidence of wakefulness, in the form of eye opening, without any sustained or reproducible responses to the environment. Vegetative states should be described with the length of time since injury. The terms *persistent* and *permanent* should not be used.[197] A minimally conscious state (MCS) is the condition of severely altered consciousness in which there is definite, reproducible evidence of self or environmental awareness. The behaviors examined include command following, intelligible verbalization, recognizable yes/no responses, and movements or emotional responses triggered by environmental stimuli.[193]

Functional neuroimaging has been useful to understand the neuropathology of depressed consciousness, especially in defining those patients who are classified as MCS or may have a higher likelihood of recovery of communication or functional object use. Both functional MRI and positron emission tomography (PET) provide correlates of the differences between vegetative state and MCS. In PET studies, patients with clinical evidence of vegetative state have reductions of overall cerebral metabolism of 50% or greater.[477] In comparison, patients with MCS have been shown to have activation of appropriate cerebral networks in response to environmental stimuli, although the activation may not be the same as in normal control subjects with novel or complex stimuli.[492] Connections between the medial parietal, frontal, and thalamus have been defined as the networks most affected in disorders of consciousness, leading to focus on these areas with functional neuroimaging.[111] Although neuroimaging may eventually be used to discriminate between vegetative state and MCS, it currently does not have a role in clinical diagnosis or prognostication.

The current evaluation of patients with depressed levels of consciousness includes a thorough neurologic examination, including pupillary responses, brainstem reflexes, and ocular movements. Brainstem reflexes commonly elicited include corneal responses, gag reflex, and oculocephalic reflexes, referred to as doll's eyes. These reflexes show integrity of brainstem pathways, with reproducible behavioral responses to specific areas of sensory stimulation. Also recorded are the direct and consensual pupillary responses as well as a response to visual threat. Observation of spontaneous activity and responses to environmental stimuli is important. Common mistakes include attributing purposefulness to responses that are reflexive, allowing insufficient observation time for patient response to a stimulus, and underconsideration or overconsideration of family observation of behavior. To best observe behaviors, it is important to optimize environmental conditions and patient positioning and avoid sedating medications. Standardized rating scales are available to differentiate vegetative state from MCS. These scales allow for detecting subtle improvements and can offer inter-rater and test-retest reliability when incorporated into daily clinical testing.[195]

A variety of interventions have been studied in these patients. The use of sensory enrichment in both naturally occurring events and in the administration of multimodal sensory stimuli has been reported in case studies and retrospective data analyses. The effectiveness of these techniques is not clear, although there is no report of harm associated with sensory stimulation.[192] Pharmacologic interventions can be used to promote arousal and behavioral persistence. Medications frequently include psychostimulants, dopamine agonists, and tricyclic antidepressants. Bromocriptine, a dopamine agonist, was studied in five patients in a vegetative state. They had greater physical and cognitive recovery at 12 months compared with historic control subjects. However, this study lacked a large sample size and did not address the possibility of spontaneous recovery.[426] Based on reports of efficacy of zolpidem, a sedative-hypnotic medication, prospective open-label trials were conducted to assess efficacy in patients with chronic disorders of consciousness (DOC). No clinically significant improvement in functional object use was seen, although there were changes in the Coma Recovery Score.[548] Recent trials have investigated the implantation of electrodes in the brainstem and thalamus to stimulate the reticular system and arousal. Although studies are limited, behavioral changes were observed in some patients.[194,491,552]

Behavioral Measures of Responding and Cognition

Decisions regarding readiness to transfer a patient from ICU to step-down units and to inpatient rehabilitation are generally based on medical stability and progress, as well as the ability to respond to the environment and to actively participate in therapy. Several behavioral measures are useful in determining the status of a patient's emergence from coma and progress through the acute phases of recovery from injury.

Emergence from Coma

Evaluation of functioning during the initial stages of emergence from coma generally involves the monitoring and serial assessment of a patient's ability to respond to external stimuli. This is often done through the use of a standardized measure of responsiveness, such as the Coma Near Coma (CNC) scale.[449] This 11-item scale was designed to measure small changes in response in patients with severe brain injuries functioning at a low level. An additional scale is the JFK Coma Recovery Scale-Revised (CRS-R),[195] which is a 23-item scale used to assess functioning in six areas: auditory, visual, motor, oromotor, communication, and arousal. Instruments such as the CNC and CRS-R are generally useful during acute-care hospitalization or, at times, if an individual who is minimally responsive is transferred to the inpatient rehabilitation setting or another longer-term care facility.

Evaluation of Posttraumatic Amnesia

As an individual emerges from coma and is able to respond to verbal inquiry, instruments such as the Galveston Orientation and Amnesia Test (GOAT)[329] or the Orientation Log (O-Log)[262] are used to track progress through the PTA phase of recovery. Both of these instruments essentially measure and score serial responses to orientation questions and allow for objective scoring of the patient's responses. Emergence from PTA is then defined by the consistent attainment of a score on one of these instruments indicating orientation.

Although rehabilitation scales, such as the GOAT and O-Log, generally focus on disorientation and amnestic symptoms, other elements of confusion (i.e., delirium and psychiatric types of symptoms) have also been noted during the acute phase of TBI recovery. There is increasing awareness of the need to measure these symptoms and to develop instruments that bridge gaps between scales traditionally used to measure PTA and those traditionally used to measure delirium.[354,538] One example is the Neurobehavioral Rating Scale,[327] which combines portions of the Brief Psychiatric Rating Scale[420] with additional items to measure other psychiatric symptoms associated with TBI. The Confusion Assessment Protocol focuses more on delirium than other scales.[503]

The Ranchos Levels of Cognitive Functioning Scale,[229] commonly referred to as the Ranchos scale, is widely accepted to describe the process of cognitive recovery as an individual emerges from coma, then progresses towards emergence from posttraumatic amnesia/delirium, and emerges to near normal cognitive functioning (Table 43-2). This scale presents recovery as a progression through eight typical stages. It has been widely adopted to assess patient functioning for purposes of rehabilitation planning and treatment and to explain patient progress to families.

Further information as well as rating forms for the Confusion Assessment Protocol, CNC, CRS-R, GOAT, O-Log, and LCFS and may be found on the "scales" page of the Center for Outcome Measurement in Brain Injury website (www.tbims.org/combi/index.html).

Inpatient Rehabilitation Assessment and Management

The focus of inpatient rehabilitation following TBI is to assist each patient in improving functional independence. Ideally, with good recovery, each will return home and be successful in eventual community reentry. The basic rehabilitation team comprises a multidisciplinary group of specialists including a physiatrist, physical therapists (PTs), occupational therapists (OTs), speech language pathologists

Table 43-2 Ranchos Level of Cognitive Functioning Scale (LCFS)

Score	Description
____ (1)	**Level I—No Response.** Patient does not respond to external stimuli and appears asleep.
____ (2)	**Level II—Generalized Response.** Patient reacts to external stimuli in nonspecific, inconsistent, and nonpurposeful manner with stereotypic and limited responses.
____ (3)	**Level III—Localized Response.** Patient responds specifically and inconsistently with delays to stimuli, but may follow simple commands for motor action.
____ (4)	**Level IV—Confused, Agitated Response.** Patient exhibits bizarre, nonpurposeful, incoherent, or inappropriate behaviors, has no short-term recall, and attention is short and nonselective.
____ (5)	**Level V—Confused, Inappropriate, Nonagitated Response.** Patient gives random, fragmented, and nonpurposeful responses to complex or unstructured stimuli. Simple commands are followed consistently, memory and selective attention are impaired, and new information is not retained.
____ (6)	**Level VI—Confused, Appropriate Response.** Patient gives context-appropriate, goal-directed responses, dependent on external input for direction. There is carry-over for relearned, but not for new tasks, and recent memory problems persist.
____ (7)	**Level VI—Automatic, Appropriate Response.** Patient behaves appropriately in familiar settings, performs daily routines automatically, and shows carry-over for new learning at lower than normal rates. Patient initiates social interactions, but judgment remains impaired.
____ (8)	**Level VIII—Purposeful, Appropriate Response.** Patient is oriented and responds to the environment but abstract reasoning abilities are decreased relative to premorbid levels.

(SLPs), and other hospital staff including nursing and case management. As cognitive and behavioral issues associated with TBI may pose unique challenges to the provision of rehabilitation treatment, ideally all members of the team should be specially trained to work with patients who have sustained TBI. Neuropsychologists are also often included as key members of the team.

Role of the Neuropsychologist in Inpatient Rehabilitation

The role of the neuropsychologist is multifaceted. He or she provides ongoing assessment of recovery of cognitive function and works with therapy and nursing staff to integrate information about cognitive abilities and limitations into implementation of effective and appropriate rehabilitation goals for the patient. Ideally, the neuropsychologist is available to observe and cotreat with other therapists as needed. Neuropsychologists have specialized training in brain-behavior relationships and expertise in the testing and evaluation of cognition. They also apply that expertise to the evaluation of interactions between cognitive strengths/limitations and behavior. As a result, they are generally experts in behavior management and may often assist with organization and implementation of behavior plans for patients as needed. This role is often particularly relevant on TBI units, where agitation related to recovery from TBI may threaten or impede patient progress. In some settings, psychologists function both as neuro and rehabilitation psychologists. Rehabilitation psychology focuses on adjustment to disability and other personal, social, and situational issues in an effort to assist individuals with all types of disabilities in working toward maintaining healthy and satisfying lifestyles.

Medical Rehabilitation Evaluation, Complications, and Management

During the initial evaluation of a new patient on the inpatient rehabilitation unit by a physiatrist or rehabilitation specialist, a thorough neurologic examination should be conducted. This often includes traditional physical examination components described elsewhere in this textbook. Often, depending on a patient's medical status, a complete evaluation cannot be conducted at first attempt and may need to be completed at a later date. As awareness and communication improve, it is not uncommon to discover additional injuries that were previously missed because of the patient's inability to express pain or participate in assessment.

The clear documentation of concurrent fractures or other orthopedic injury is important to allow safe treatment in a rehabilitation setting. Physical examination measures include the description of motor weakness, abnormal muscle tone, and presence or absence of contractures. For those patients with a decreased level of consciousness and cognitive disorders, it is vital to perform serial measures to document level of awareness. Multiple instruments (GOAT, GCS, CNC, CRS-R, as described previously) can be performed serially by physicians and therapists. The evaluation should also include documentation of brainstem reflexes such as pupillary reflexes, doll's eyes, and response to caloric stimulation.

Although some degree of medical stability has been achieved by the time a patient has been transferred from ICU to inpatient rehabilitation, medical complications can and do occur while patients are on the rehabilitation unit. The next sections describe some medical issues and complications of particular concern for individuals with a recent history of TBI. Assessment and feedback from members of the rehabilitation therapy team often provide information vital to the diagnosis of these medical issues.

Posttraumatic Seizures. Posttraumatic seizures (PTSs) are a significant complication arising from TBI. PTS has commonly been defined as occurring in the immediate period (<24 hours after injury), early period (24 hours to 7 days after injury), and late period (>7 days after injury). Late PTS can also be defined, based on the 2014 criteria from the International League Against Epilepsy,[176] as posttraumatic epilepsy (PTE). PTS accounts for 20% of symptomatic seizures and 5% of all seizures in the general population.[152] Up to 86% of patients with one seizure after TBI will have a second within 2 years of their injury.[235] Moreover, PTE is associated with increased disability and limitations with ADLs.[21,69] Although the neurobiology of PTE is not well understood, neuroinhibitory molecules like adenosine and GABA afford relative protection from this complication. In fact, genetic variability within the ubiquitous adenosine A1 receptor has been linked with risk for PTS occurring within the first week and also with the development of PTE.[579] Further, genetic variation in the glutamic acid decarboxylase gene also contributes genetic risk to PTE development.[119] Conversely, excitotoxicity likely contributes to the development of PTE. PTS occurrence is related to injury severity.[544] A recent report suggests that acute inflammatory burden for IL-1β and genetic variation within the gene coding for IL-1β may accelerate epileptogenesis and development of PTE.[131] Other reported risk factors include biparietal contusions, dural penetration with bone and metal fragments, multiple intracranial operations, cortical contusions, subdural hematoma, significant midline shift, early PTS, and skull fractures.[16,152]

Phenytoin is commonly used for early prophylaxis against PTS development and for treatment of PTS. It acts by diminishing excitatory tone and augmenting inhibitory neurotransmitter systems in cortical and subcortical structures. Phenytoin therapy for 1 week provides protection against early PTS.[545] Notably, published treatment guidelines for phenytoin are now over 10 years old and are based on recommendations from a (seminal) clinical trial published over 20 years ago showing that patients with severe TBI should receive prophylactic treatment with phenytoin for 7 days after injury.[545] The Association of American Neurologists (AAN) still recommends early intervention with phenytoin (intravenously) given as a loading dose as soon as possible followed by a 7-day course in the asymptomatic moderate-to-severely brain-injured population.[79] Phenytoin use beyond this first postinjury week was not supported,[545] and both clinical[136] and experimental[118] studies suggest adverse effects on recovery with prolonged phenytoin use. Newer drugs, including the synaptic vesicle protein 2A (SV2A) modulator levetiracetam, which do not require active monitoring of drug levels, are growing in use for PTS prevention.[633] However, research on their efficacy in preventing PTS specifically is limited. Recent small-size clinical reports suggest that levetiracetam use during the first postinjury week has similar efficacy as phenytoin, but additional studies are needed to confirm this.[532]

Despite recommendations supporting limited treatment for seizure prophylaxis,[543] people with TBI often receive PTS prophylaxis on a long-term basis with anticonvulsant medications that require regular monitoring and are often associated with unwanted side effects, including sedation. Patients who go on to develop PTE also experience similar issues with long-term treatment.[136,513] Recent evidence with an experimental model of TBI demonstrates that long-term treatment with phenytoin after injury leads to increased cell death and poorer function on cognitive behavioral tasks.[118] This work further supports following current guidelines for PTS prophylaxis with phenytoin and minimizing prolonged therapy when possible. However, there is recent work suggesting that daily treatment with levetiracetam for 3 weeks postinjury has multiple neuroprotective effects and improves multiple neurobehavioral outcomes in a rat model of TBI,[632] a finding that is consistent with neuroprotective characteristics of this drug in other studies.[237,590]

Heterotopic Ossification. Heterotopic ossification (HO) (Figure 43-6), a common complication occurring after TBI, is a poorly understood process by which ectopic bone is formed outside the skeleton. Incidence of HO after TBI ranges from 11% to 28%.[243] Incidence may be higher in those sustaining military-related blast injuries, where TBI and traumatic amputation, both of which increase the risk of HO development, often co-occur.[181,441] Patients with more severe TBI, as well as associated immobility, spasticity, and fractures, seem to be at relatively greater risk for this complication. Dysautonomia is also linked with higher HO risk.[243] Among acute-care patients undergoing rehabilitation for TBI, HO is considered a risk factor for poorer

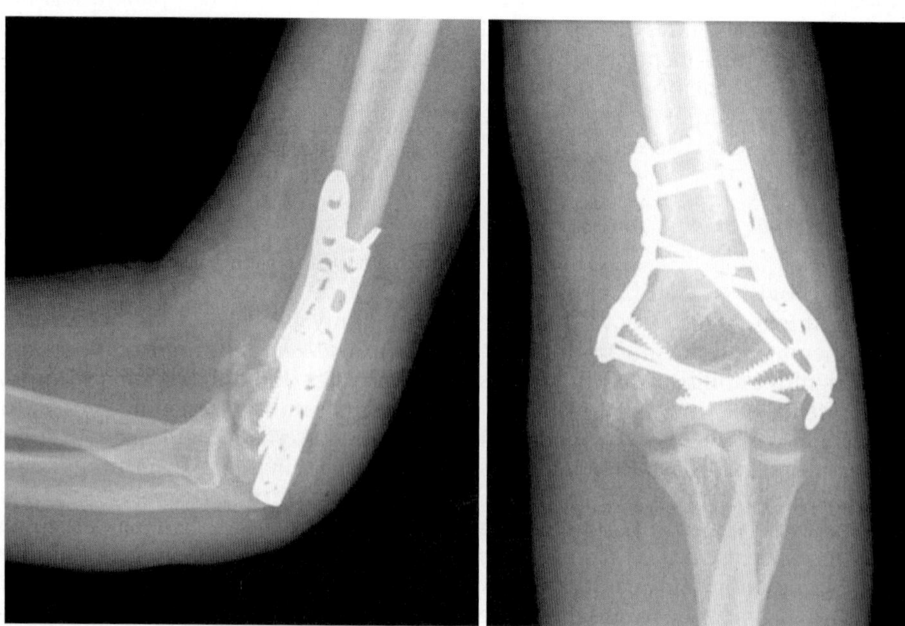

FIGURE 43-6 An example of heterotopic ossification in patients after a traumatic brain injury. The AP and lateral x-ray films depict ectopic bone formation in a patient's elbow after repair of fracture.

outcomes and decreased home discharge rates.[267] Blood markers associated with bone metabolism, such as alkaline phosphatase and osteocalcin, are nonspecific for HO.[400] X-rays can identify HO in more advanced cases. However, bone scan is more sensitive in identifying early and asymptomatic cases.

Although the pathophysiology of HO after TBI is poorly understood, evidence suggests that CNS processes facilitate HO bone formation. Bone remodeling is subject to central control through the sympathetic nervous system, which is partially regulated by the endocannabinoid system. After experimental TBI, cannabinoid-mediated downregulation of norepinephrine at osteoblasts contributes to increased bone formation.[535] Other research suggests that humeral factors in human CSF after TBI are osteoinductive. However, specific factors have not been identified.[187] Leptin, a metabolic protein, is also a potential mediator of HO through both central and peripheral mechanisms.[80]

Common prophylactic methods include antiinflammatory medications such as indomethacin, irradiation, and Ca^{++} binding chelating agents, e.g., etidronate. NSAIDS are effective in preventing HO formation in total joint replacement patients,[404] and mounting evidence suggests that NSAIDS are a useful preventative in spinal cord injury (SCI).[24] Less is known about the specific effects of NSAIDS on HO after TBI. At this time, two systematic reviews failed to provide adequate research evidence to support these therapies for acute HO treatment.[24,238] Once HO formation occurs, it can significantly impact joint range of motion and mobility. Areas of HO formation take several months to mature. After maturation is complete, excision of the ectopic bone can improve joint motion and mobility,[387] and studies suggest that surgical excision is the most effective therapy for HO after TBI.[24]

Deep Venous Thrombosis. Deep venous thrombosis (DVT) is a significant source of morbidity and risk of mortality for patients with TBI. In patients with severe TBI, pulmonary embolus secondary to DVT is an important cause of death, and the estimated incidence of DVT is 40%.[91] The effectiveness of routine screening for clot at rehabilitation admission has not been proven, and there is no standard of care for initiation of DVT prophylaxis and treatment in patients with TBI. Increasing evidence supports the safe use of either heparin or low-molecular-weight heparin within 24 to 72 hours after severe TBI or intracranial bleed.[164,188] This decision can be made in consultation with the neurosurgeon about the risk of rebleed after review of neuroimaging studies.

Patients at highest risk for DVT include those at advanced age, severe injury, prolonged immobilization, significant fractures, and presence of clotting disorder.[464] Unfortunately, patient behavior, including fall risk, agitation, and ability to be provided with a safe environment, might prevent one from taking a risk with anticoagulation or even prophylaxis. In those patients who cannot undergo pharmacologic prophylaxis of DVT because of risk of bleeding, mechanical compression devices can be used. Although their efficacy has never been completely studied, their effectiveness in clinical practice is likely to be lower than that in controlled trials. If they are used, it is important they are used consistently and for the maximum hours each day and appropriately sized. For patients with agitation or requiring restraints, tolerance of these devices may be low. The length of DVT prophylaxis is not clearly defined in the TBI population. Among general rehabilitation patients, the ability to ambulate greater than 100 feet is an important milestone to discontinue prophylaxis.

Swallowing/Nutrition. Moderate-to-severe TBI is associated with specific nutritional needs. Patients demonstrate increased caloric requirements caused by hypermetabolism, increased energy expenditure, and increased protein loss. Early institution of enteral nutritional support may decrease morbidity and mortality, shorten hospital length of stay, and potentially improve immune function.[227,624] Nutritional status monitoring can include review of laboratory tests and weights, and in more complex patients, metabolic cart studies. Clinical dieticians are important team members in this regard. Caloric supplementation is not the only focus of nutritional support. Data support the role of nutriceutical supplementation, including probiotics to decrease risk of infection as well as vitamin D, omega-3, and zinc supplementation for their potential benefits. All need to be further clarified through specific studies.[114,496]

The route of nutritional support, gastrostomy versus jejunostomy, is not resolved. Factors that lead to the decision for a more permanent form of enteral nutrition include whether nasogastric nutrition can be consistently maintained, if the location of the tube is an agitating factor, and potential length of time nonoral nutrition is needed. Once a permanent tube is placed, it is expected to be in place for more than 30 days to decrease complications associated with removal. Whether to place a tube directly in the stomach versus more distally in the jejunum should be based on presence of gastroesophageal reflux. In those patients who will require nonoral nutrition when they go home, the gastric tube allows for bolus feeding, which better approximates natural feeding.

As the patient's level of alertness improves, swallowing evaluation can include a bedside swallowing assessment or video fluoroscopy. Because normal gag reflexes and good cough reflex are not completely predictive of normal swallow function, video fluoroscopy often identifies silent aspiration and improves clinical decision making when relaxing dietary restrictions.[604] Even after video fluoroscopy, institution of oral nutrition is often done in a stepwise manner, evaluating the effects of behavior on feeding, as well as variations in level of arousal and fatigue during a day.

Bowel and Bladder Dysfunction. Loss of bladder and bowel control is common after TBI. Injury to cortical and subcortical structures can lead to loss of control over these functions or discoordination of sphincter management. The early incidence of urinary incontinence after significant TBI is approximately 62%.[90] Patterns of dysfunction include an uninhibited overactive bladder, as well as poor perception of bladder fullness and poor sphincter control. During acute care and rehabilitation, urinary tract infections are common, impacting functional outcome on discharge, skin integrity, and increasing risk of discharge to long-term care.[90] Treatment options include behavioral interventions such as timed voiding. Caution must be used in initiating anticholinergic medications, because of their adverse cognitive effects.

Bowel dysfunction after TBI includes incontinence and constipation. Constipation is common, because of lack of mobility, use of constipating medications, and dietary influences. Bowel programs include stool softeners, stimulant suppositories, and hydration. Bowel incontinence is often associated with more severe injury and poorer functional status. It may also be caused by diarrhea, frequently seen with the use of enteral feeds or infectious causes.[182]

Airway/Pulmonary Management. Pulmonary complications after TBI may be directly related to the effects of trauma, including pneumothorax, hemothorax, flail chest, and rib fractures. Neurologic level of injury may lead to respiratory failure, pulmonary edema, and airway complications. Pneumonia is the most common complication observed in acute care and rehabilitation, occurring in 60% of patients.[599] The presence of respiratory failure and the need for tracheostomy have a strong relationship with acute care and rehabilitation length of stay. They are also associated with functional status on the Disability Rating Scale and the Functional Independence Measure 1 year after injury.[153] Early tracheostomy (≤8 days) is associated with shorter mechanical ventilation and shorter hospital stay but not hospital mortality. It may be a way of decreasing hospital morbidity and shortening time to initiation of acute rehabilitation although that has not been specifically addressed.[10]

The majority of patients with TBI who need a tracheostomy in acute care regain sufficient pulmonary and neurologic function later to undergo decannulation. This can be considered when patients no longer require ventilation, can manage their secretions, and are at low risk for aspiration. Usually, decannulation is achieved by serially decreasing the cannula diameter and then by capping the tube. Before capping the tracheostomy, a speaking valve can be used to allow phonation through the open tracheostomy. This is generally only tolerated with a smaller-diameter tracheostomy, and the cuff on the tracheostomy must be deflated for safety. If this step is used, it is often recommended that the valve is only placed by trained staff after they have verified that the cuff is deflated. Tolerance is measured by ability to maintain oxygen saturations and speak clear, long sentences without signs of breathlessness. If the patient tolerates these steps, the tracheostomy may be removed. Visualization of the airway before decannulation via laryngoscopy can assess for tracheal stenosis, subglottic stenosis, glottic stenosis, and tracheal granuloma.[609] These tracheal abnormalities are associated with a high risk of respiratory difficulties requiring reintubation and possible surgical intervention.

Decision making in decannulation of patients at Rancho levels 2 and 3 is more difficult. Poor pulmonary toilet and variable central respiratory status in this group led to pneumonia and sepsis and increased morbidity and mortality with decannulation. Predictors of successful decannulation include younger age, alert cognitive status, and adequate swallowing and cough reflexes.[318] One should consider whether decannulation will make care easier or more difficult in the next level of care. Also, timing of decannulation is important; it is more troublesome in the winter when respiratory illnesses are common.

Spasticity and Contractures. Spasticity is a common problem observed with upper motor neuron damage such as that occurring with TBI. It is one portion of the upper motor neuron syndrome that contributes to motor dysfunction in these patients. Spasticity is clinically defined as a velocity-dependent increase in tonic stretch reflexes with exaggerated tendon jerk responses.[315] Other components of the upper motor syndrome include loss of autonomic control, decreased dexterity, and limb weakness, which also often occurs in these patients. Although the incidence in the TBI population is generally unknown, among those with injuries severe enough to require inpatient rehabilitation, it has been reported to be as high as 84%.[622]

After significant damage to central motor pathways as occurs with TBI, acute paralysis often occurs. This damage leaves the affected muscles and joint immobilized. Immobilization leads to reduction in longitudinal tension in a muscle, the basis for muscle contracture. In animal models, only 24 hours of unloading of tension in a muscle caused a 60% shortening of muscle fiber length.[371] Over the next few weeks, both plastic neural and muscular reorganization leads to muscle overactivity defined as spasticity. This further aggravates the development of muscle and joint contractures.[209]

The early identification of contracture development and spasticity is critical. The risk factors for spasticity development include more severe injury (lower GCS), motor dysfunction (hemiplegia or tetraplegia), associated anoxic injury, spinal cord injury, and age. Development can occur as early as days after injury but is more classically observed months later. Patient evaluation includes a clinical and functional history, stretch reflex examination, range of motion assessment, and an active motor examination.[250] Measurement of degree of passive abnormal muscle tone is often done with the Ashworth scale or modified Ashworth scale (Table 43-3). The modified Ashworth scale assigns 0 to 4 points based on the amount of resistance measured by an evaluator when attempting to range a joint through an available range of motion. The Tardieu scale is a true measure of spasticity, comparing the differences noted when a muscle is stretched at different velocities and comparing the angles at which the catch is noted (Table 43-4).[151a]

Table 43-3 Modified Ashworth Scale

Score	Description
0	No increase in muscle tone
1	Slight increase in muscle tone manifested by a catch and release at end range of motion
1+	Slight increase in muscle tone, manifested by a catch Followed by minimal resistance throughout the remainder of the range of motion
2	More marked increase in tone, through most of the range of motion but joint easily moved
3	Considerable increase in muscle tone, passive movement is difficult
4	Affected part is rigid in flexion or extension

Table 43-4 Tardieu Scale

Score	Description
0	No resistance throughout the course of the passive movement
1	Slight resistance throughout the course of the passive movement with no clear catch at a precise angle
2	Clear catch at a precise angle, interrupting the passive movement followed by release
3	Fatigable clonus, less than 10 seconds when maintaining pressure, appearing at a precise angle
4	Nonfatigable clonus, more than 10 seconds when maintaining pressure, at a precise angle

The cornerstone of spasticity treatment is the use of static and dynamic splinting devices. When used in combination with passive range of motion exercises, splints serve to lengthen muscles and tendons that are shortening. Although controlled trials of the use of passive range of motion are few, the pathophysiology of spasticity and clinical experience have guided their use. A stretching program can also be easily taught to family members and transitioned to a home environment. In combination with static splinting such as serial casting, measures of spasticity can decrease.[508] In a setting with close monitoring for adverse effects such as pressure sore development, serial casting can be very efficacious after TBI. Caution must be used in initiating it while patients are still experiencing high ICPs.[627] Physical modalities, such as cryotherapy, superficial heat, and ultrasound, can be used in concert with splinting or pharmacotherapy. Multiple forms of electrical stimulation have been studied in the management of spasticity, with positive results identified in some placebo-controlled studies.[210]

Systemic pharmacologic agents may also be used. Dantrolene is indicated for the treatment of spasticity of CNS origin, including TBI. It acts at the sarcoplasmic reticulum by inhibiting calcium activity. Dantrolene has been associated with hepatic toxicity and requires regular monitoring of liver enzymes. Baclofen acts both presynaptically and postsynaptically at the GABA B receptors, effectively inhibiting spinal reflexes. Side effects include fatigue, sedation, weakness, hallucinations, and lowering of the seizure threshold. When studied in a TBI population, lower extremity Ashworth scores were improved, but a similar effect was not obtained in the upper extremity. Somnolence limited maximum dose in 17% of subjects.[379] Other oral agents for spasticity include benzodiazepines, tizanidine, and clonidine. Somnolence and cognitive effects often limit the usefulness of these medications in the TBI population, and some worsen recovery in experimental models.[170]

Focal chemodenervation can be an important tool for practitioners, without concerns for cognitive side effects. Phenol used for either motor point block or mixed nerve block can cause denaturation of the nerve, thus reducing focal spasticity. Advantages include low cost and immediate effects. Complications include sensory loss, painful dysesthesias with mixed nerves, and vascular complication. Chemodenervation with botulinum toxin types A and B is used "off label" for the treatment of focal spasticity. When used in combination with physical modalities such as splinting or serial casting, improved range of motion and Ashworth scores can be achieved.[618] There are common patterns of upper motor neuron system dysfunction in patients with TBI that can be identified and effectively treated with botulinum toxin.[357]

Baclofen can also be delivered intrathecally, directly to the lumbar subarachnoid space via an intrathecal pump. This delivery system circumvents the BBB and the peripheral breakdown of the orally administered medication. Although sedation often limits the oral dosing of baclofen, sedation occurs less frequently with intrathecal treatment, and the dose limit is much higher. The surgical complications of intrathecal pump placement include infection, catheter dislodgement, and CSF leak or seroma. The abrupt withdrawal of baclofen, which may occur with catheter complications, can result in rhabdomyolysis, multiple organ failure, and death.[254] However, when studied in patients with TBI, after 1 year of treatment, Ashworth scores were improved and maintained over the year of treatment.[380] Animal data suggest the effectiveness of early use of intrathecal baclofen (initiated 1 week after experimental injury) in decreasing spasticity and anxiety-like behavior without negative effects on cognition.[48] This technique is being transitioned to human models with safety and efficacy observed in implants done in the first 6 months after injury.[440]

Normal Pressure Hydrocephalus. Normal pressure hydrocephalus is one of the most common treatable neurosurgical complications after severe TBI, with an estimated incidence of 45% in those with severe injury.[361] Three-quarters of hydrocephalus occur during the inpatient rehabilitation process. It is more frequent with increased severity of injury and with longer rehabilitation length of stays.[275] Posttraumatic hydrocephalus is largely of the communicating variety; thus, there is still free flow of cerebrospinal fluid within the ventricular system. Absorption of CSF into the arachnoid granulations is limited by blood products, protein, or fibrosis, leading to dilatation of the ventricular system. Clinical presentation of acute hydrocephalus, early after injury, includes headache, nausea, vomiting, and lethargy. The symptoms of delayed hydrocephalus or normal pressure hydrocephalus are more subtle. The clinical triad of dementia, gait ataxia, and urinary incontinence is described, with the gait disorder being most amenable to shunting of CSF. However, in those patients with TBI who have neurologic impairment from their injury, the diagnosis should be considered in anyone who worsens or fails to progress adequately. A CT scan of the head without contrast to evaluate ventricular size is necessary. However, as many as 72% of patients with severe TBI have been reported to have ventriculomegaly.[328] In patients with cerebral atrophy leading to ex-vacuo dilatation of the ventricle, sulcal prominence is often observed, making it less likely they will be responsive to shunting.[47] Further evaluation in questionable cases of hydrocephalus may include large-volume CSF drainage via lumbar puncture, including postprocedure neurologic evaluation, as well as MRI cine flow studies in which spinal fluid flow through the third ventricle is observed.

Endocrine Dysfunction Associated with Traumatic Brain Injury. Although reported frequencies and numbers vary by study, neuroendocrine disorders affect a significant portion of the population with TBI, regardless of injury severity. Up to 100% of patients with acute TBI have some type of acute anterior pituitary dysfunction, and up to 37% of long-term survivors continue to do so.[33,569] Data are sparse, but one report suggests acute posterior pituitary dysfunction rates as high as 21%, with 7% evolving into permanent dysfunction.[8] Much of the pathology is attributed to primary and/or secondary injury to the hypothalamus and pituitary gland, structures that govern most neuroendocrine function. The hypophyseal portal vascular system that supplies the hypothalamic-pituitary region is vulnerable to traumatic injury, and frequent pituitary hemorrhage and necrosis have been noted in autopsy studies in patients who die acutely from their injuries.[46]

Both oxytocin and vasopressin are synthesized in the hypothalamus and secreted by the posterior portion of the pituitary. In women, oxytocin functions to facilitate uterine contractions during labor and milk excretion during lactation. Oxytocin receptors are present in several regions in the brain, although their importance is not fully understood. Vasopressin, also called antidiuretic hormone (ADH), regulates water retention. Vasopressin release is diurnal and has many actions on the brain, including aggression and thermal regulation. Although less common than anterior pituitary dysfunction, posterior pituitary-mediated neuroendocrine dysfunction does occur after TBI. Diabetes insipidus is associated with excessive thirst, excretion of large amounts of dilute urine that is refractory to fluid restriction, and elevated plasma sodium. Neurogenic diabetes insipidus is caused by ADH deficiency, and vasopressin hormone replacement is effective therapy. In contrast, the syndrome of inappropriate antidiuretic hormone (SIADH) is characterized by excessive ADH secretion accompanied by excess natriuresis and low plasma sodium. Fluid restriction and ADH inhibitors are a part of the therapeutic approach to this disorder, with one study suggesting that hydrocortisone could be effective in reducing excessive natriuresis.[391]

Several hormones affecting reproduction and metabolism are located in the anterior pituitary and include follicular stimulating hormone, leuteinizing hormone, ACTH, thyroid-stimulating hormone, prolactin, and growth hormone (GH). Early after injury, several aberrations in serum gonadal hormone profiles occur with severe TBI, and are likely associated with an enhanced stress surge in response to the injury. Testosterone is elevated in women, and progesterone is elevated in men after severe TBI. Both testosterone and progesterone levels rapidly decrease in men and women after severe TBI, refuting the long-held hypothesis generated from experimental models that women are afforded sex hormone-dependent neuroprotection.[578] Hypogonadism is largely secondary to pituitary dysfunction,[566,569] and menstrual cycle function may be impaired for women up to several months after severe TBI and can have a negative impact on outcome.[461]

Hyperprolactinemia can affect over 50% of the population with TBI.[7] Trauma can lead to acute depression of the thyroid axis. Chronic hypothyroidism affects between 1% and 22% of the population with TBI and can contribute to cognitive decline.[7] Therefore, thyroid function should be screened routinely, particularly if recovery is slow. GH deficiency in children is associated with short stature. In adults, GH deficiency decreases muscle mass, energy levels, and cognitive performance. In TBI, one report suggests that chronic GH deficiency occurs in about 16% to 18% of the population and is correlated with lower quality of life (QOL) and increased rates of depression.[29] Other studies suggest impaired aerobic capacity with GH deficiency after TBI.[394] However, GH replacement can have a beneficial impact on recovery and QOL.[309]

Posttraumatic Headache. Posttraumatic headache (PTH) is the most common secondary headache disorder, corresponding to approximately 4% of all symptomatic headaches.[147a] PTH is a cardinal feature of the postconcussive syndrome. It is unclear how frequently PTH represents an exacerbation of an already existent primary headache syndrome versus new onset of secondary headache.[480] Headaches are often transient and abate in parallel with other postconcussive symptoms, but for some, headaches can linger as persistent. Headache types in the TBI population are diverse, and include tension type and migraine/probable migraine type. Many of those affected self-treat (with variable success) with acetaminophen and/or nonsteroidal antiinflammatory drugs (NSAIDs).[139] In particular, those with migraine/probable migraine may need to seek medical care and use more traditional abortives (e.g., triptans, long-acting NSAIDs) and/or preventives. As many classes of preventative drugs (e.g., tricyclics, β blockers, calcium channel blockers, anticonvulsants) have significant side effect profiles, practitioners will need to tailor therapy to minimize adverse effects on other recovery domains, and treatment selection may differ depending on factors such as time from injury, age, and premorbid headache history, as well as concurrent cervicalgia, cognitive/behavioral dysfunction, or mood disorders, among others.

Neurodegenerative Disorders and Chronic Traumatic Encephalopathy. Relatively little is known about the long-term effects of TBI in relation to neurodegenerative disease; however, the concept of long-term neurodegenerative consequences of repetitive TBI has garnered much attention recently with increased community awareness about possible adverse effects associated with sports and military concussion. At a neurobiologic level, long-term disease thought to contribute to neurodegenerative disorders includes chronic inflammation, excitotoxicity, gliosis demyelination, neurotrophin dysfunction, amyloid plaques, and tauopathy, among others, with evidence available in animal models of TBI to support these considerations.[57] Further, clinical studies are suggestive of these mechanisms with recent clinical biomarker studies showing evidence of long-term inflammation, autoimmune dysfunction, neurotrophin deficits, and neurodegenerative markers.[155a,313,476,631] These findings lend additional support to the possibility that genetic variations within genes that are associated with other disorders (e.g., APOE4 and Alzheimer dementia) have an important role in biosusceptibility to late neurodegenerative complications after TBI. In addition to late development of neurodegeneration and related dysfunction, these pathomechanisms may influence susceptibility to complicating conditions discussed earlier such as mood disorder, epilepsy, and neuroendocrine dysfunction.[132,155a,271,272] Although much research is needed to definitively describe the epidemiology, pathology, biosusceptibility, and treatments required to address these disorders, long-term rehabilitative care programs will likely emerge to include multimodal strategies to deal with TBI as a chronic disease requiring continued management.[565,587]

Functional Evaluation and Treatment Concepts in Rehabilitation

In addition to the medical issues described previously, some functional difficulties commonly assessed and treated after TBI by the rehabilitation team are highlighted below.

Vestibular Dysfunction. Patients with both severe and mild TBI often present with complaints of dizziness and imbalance. The incidence of such symptoms is reported to be between 30% and 60% in various TBI populations.[198] The incidence could be as high as 100% when the patient has sustained a temporal bone fracture.

There are many etiologies for these symptoms. Injury to the peripheral nervous system may result in vestibular symptoms with or without hearing loss. Benign paroxysmal positional vertigo is the most common cause for complaints of dizziness and imbalance. It is clinically characterized by brief episodes of vertigo provoked by movement of the head. Although this can resolve with time, canalith repositioning procedures can shorten the duration of symptoms.[244] Another peripheral vestibular injury includes labyrinthine concussion, or the sudden onset of hearing loss and vertigo after TBI in the absence of temporal bone fracture. These patients are good candidates for vestibular and balance rehabilitation. Temporal bone fractures can lead to disruption of the bony labyrinth or internal auditory canal. Trauma to the external canal clinically manifests with bloody otorrhea and severe pain and must be differentiated from a traumatic tympanic membrane perforation.

Central causes of dizziness can include direct trauma to the brainstem and/or cerebellum. These lesions are often associated with typical ocular motor abnormalities on neurologic examination. They include various forms of nystagmus at rest, eye movement abnormalities resulting in diplopia, and abnormalities of pupillary response. Rehabilitation techniques to promote alternative strategies for gaze stability can be successful to induce long-term adaptation in the central nervous system.[245] The focus of such rehabilitation programs is to decrease symptoms and allow patients to be more active. In patients with postural instability, exercises to promote static and dynamic postural stability are conducted by manipulating visual, vestibular, and somatosensory cues in the environment.[502]

Visual/Perceptual Dysfunction. TBI can lead to many symptoms related to vision such as diplopia, photophobia, difficulties with tracking and fixation, and visuoperceptual complaints. Injury may occur to the optic nerve, visual cortex, visual processing centers, or oculomotor nerves. Each of these areas of injury has variable recovery patterns and rehabilitation interventions.

Common examination findings observed with physiatric examination include oculomotor abnormalities, visual field deficits, and deficiencies in visual acuity. The most common cranial nerve palsy after TBI is third nerve palsy. On examination, one sees exotropia, ptosis, and mydriasis on the affected side. Fourth cranial nerve palsy results in difficulty with convergence or near vision. Clinically, a head tilt may be noted. Sixth cranial nerve palsy is associated with difficulty of abduction of the affected eye, resulting in diplopia on lateral vision to that side. Visual acuity can be evaluated with the Snellen Acuity Test, testing both monocular and binocular vision. A bedside visual field examination should be done, and functional testing by an occupational therapist is often helpful if the patient can participate fully in this evaluation.

A neuro-ophthalmologic evaluation can assist therapists in evaluating the impact of vision on ADLs and perceptual motor function. In patients referred for evaluation because of visual complaints after TBI, 85% have visual acuity of 20/20 and 33% have cranial nerve palsy on examination.[482] Vision therapy is the clinical treatment of visual disorders with the use of nonsurgical techniques. Over a series of treatment sessions under the supervision of an optometrist or occupational therapist, individually planned activities based on physical examination are repeated. Techniques include prisms, computer-based treatments, biofeedback, and stereoscopic devices.[424]

Exercise and Traumatic Brain Injury. In addition to the known therapeutic effects on physical condition and function, a significant amount of literature demonstrates that physical exercise and conditioning can have beneficial effects on neuroplasticity and cognition as well as slowing neurodegenerative processes.[559] Increasing evidence suggests that voluntary exercise is beneficial in TBI recovery. In experimental TBI, voluntary exercise with a running wheel has been linked with increased neurotrophin production as well as improved cognition when compared with a sedentary control group.[216] Multiple experimental studies, however, suggest that exercising too early after injury can be detrimental to recovery and have translational implications to clinical concussion management issues such as return to sporting activities after injury.

For those with concussion, physical exertion or training too early after injury can worsen cognition and associated symptoms. As such, exercise programs should be reintroduced in a graded fashion such that the patient remains symptom free during training.[337,345] This approach is supported by experimental TBI work in which voluntary exercise early after TBI resulted in worse performance on tasks of learning acquisition and memory and a reduction in plasticity-related proteins compared with a nonexercising injured control group that underwent a sham treatment. In contrast, a delayed voluntary exercise paradigm increased neurotrophin levels and improved performance on cognitive tasks,[216] which recent studies suggest corresponds with resolution of the acute physiologic stress response that accompanies TBI.[218]

In the experimental literature, environmental stimulation, along with opportunity for social interaction and exercise, provides a loose context for a rehabilitation-relevant experience. Several experimental TBI studies demonstrate the relative benefits of this type of "enriched environment" on cognitive performance after TBI when compared with an impoverished environment with little environmental stimulation or social interaction.[236,294,425,577] Interestingly, environmental enrichment can enhance the effectiveness of pharmacologic interventions in improving cognition.[294] However, the beneficial effects of short-term environmental enrichment appear to be more effective in males than in females.[385,577]

In patients with more severe injuries, behavioral factors, including agitation, impulsivity, and aggression can lead to unique challenges in implementing an exercise program. Cognitive and behavioral rehabilitation strategies outlined in this chapter can be helpful to create an environment most conducive to rehabilitation participation. For those with more severe injuries, physical impairments related to hemiplegia, movement disorders, and spasticity may also limit the degree of exercise and conditioning incorporated into individual rehabilitation programs. Other factors, such as balance and postural control as well as visual deficits, may affect abilities and performance with exercise training or programs.

Locomotion assistance systems that provide body weight support and robotic gait orthoses can be implemented for exercise in some patients with these types of deficits to provide additional support and feedback during locomotion training. Body weight–supported treadmill training has been more widely studied in stroke, and some studies suggest that treadmill training with body weight support may be more beneficial than treadmill training alone in this population.[393] One study suggests that body weight-supported treadmill training does not necessarily improve gait mechanics in a chronic TBI population with multiple gait abnormalities.[63] However, other studies suggest that body weight-supported treadmill training can improve cardiorespiratory status in independent walkers with severe TBI.[395]

Cognition After Traumatic Brain Injury

Cognitive Deficits After Traumatic Brain Injury. Cognitive deficits are among the most debilitating and complex aspects of TBI to manage and treat. Cognitive problems after TBI can span a number of neuropsychological domains, including arousal, attention, memory, and executive control. The neurobiologic bases of both physiologic cognitive function and TBI-induced dysfunction are not completely understood, and neuropharmacologic approaches for treating TBI-mediated deficits have largely drawn upon literature from related disorders that present with cognitive dysfunction. Among these are attention deficit hyperactivity disorder (ADHD), Parkinson disease, narcolepsy, and Alzheimer dementia. Pathomechanisms involved in TBI-related cognitive deficits are unique and not wholly similar to these other diseases.

Arousal is one of the most basic cognitive functions required to engage in other higher levels of cognition. Arousal is governed primarily by the reticular-thalamic, thalamocortical, and reticular-cortical networks. Multiple neurotransmitter systems, particularly monoamines, affect arousal. These monoaminergic nuclei originate in the brainstem at the reticular formation, and each has multiple forebrain terminal projections. Although other neurotransmitters influence arousal, NE is central to this function, which affects other cognitive domains, such as attention and memory.

Attention can refer to a wide variety of different cognitive processes that are both voluntary and involuntary. In addition, attention is a widely distributed cognitive function that involves both cortical and subcortical pathways, including striatal and thalamic inputs and reticular activation. It is generally accepted that DA plays a significant role in attention.[58,606] Attention can be operationalized to include multiple processes. Sensory gating is a preattentive process that filters incoming stimuli to limit information into attention-processing networks. Selective attention involves the ability to direct cognitive resources to a salient stimulus, although sustained attention allows for maintenance of attention processing on a specific stimulus. Like arousal, there is overlap of many of these attention processes with other cognitive functions such as memory and executive functioning. Further, attention deficits can contribute to dysfunction in other cognitive domains.

Relative to arousal and attention, the anatomy involved with memory is better characterized, with specific memory-processing events (e.g., retrieval, consolidation) ascribed to specific brain regions. For example, damage to the hippocampus has historically been associated with reproducible deficits in spatial and temporal memory processing.[66] Memory involves both encoding and retrieval processes, each of which may involve different structures. Explicit learning and memory are considered to be hippocampal-dependent processes of which declarative memory, or memory for facts and events that can be consciously discussed, is a major type. Declarative memory requires the hippocampus for memory consolidation and uses the frontal cortex for memory retrieval. Declarative memory retrieval is also considered associative in nature in that any area of the brain involved in encoding the information can be tapped to help initiate retrieval. In contrast, implicit learning and memory are a hippocampal-independent process that involves subconsciously learning how to do something, with procedural memory being a common type of implicit learning. Procedural learning and memory have a relatively inflexible retrieval process in that they are limited specifically to the processes involved in learning the task. However, strategy formulation, another relevant form of implicit learning, has shown relatively good carryover effects to a range of tasks.[122] Implicit learning and memory are relevant for many other types of cognitive functions and both experimental and clinical data show that, compared with explicit memory, implicit learning and memory networks are relatively intact after TBI.[493] As such, implicit learning and memory network capacity is commonly leveraged in cognitive training programs to produce guided responses that facilitate functional improvement in other domains such as ADLs.[493] Because of the central role that the hippocampus plays in memory, cholinergic systems projecting to the hippocampus are implicated in memory dysfunction. The prefrontal cortex (PFC) and corticostriatal DA signaling system, in addition to the hippocampus, are also important for memory formation.

Executive function (EF) encompasses numerous functions, but it is generally defined as the capacity to organize, plan, execute, and change cognitive functions. Executive functioning is needed with abstraction, problem solving, self-direction, systematic memory searching and retrieval, and moving from one set of information to another. It is also used when maintaining information and generating goals and concepts. Working memory (WM) commonly refers to those cognitive processes that provide the capacity to both maintain and manipulate a limited amount of information over a brief period of time. WM is closely related to EF in that both processes involve the PFC. DA projections to the PFC along with PFC striatal networks are required for normal EF.

Clinical Neuropharmacology for Traumatic Brain Injury–Mediated Cognitive Deficits. In contrast to experimental TBI models that have characterized specific alterations in neurotransmitter systems, evidence that neurotransmitter systems, including dopaminergic systems, are altered in humans following TBI is based largely on reports that DA agonists can be beneficial in attenuating cognitive deficits. Although amphetamine has been used clinically as both a DA and an NE agent, MPH is more widely accepted as an effective neurostimulant to improve cognition. According to current evidence-based guidelines, MPH is recommended as a neurostimulant to improve cognition, particularly attention.[405] Much of the evidence for this is derived from small but well-controlled clinical trials showing improvements in cognitive processing speed and caregiver ratings of attention.[597]

The evidence-based guidelines support the use of amantadine to enhance general cognition and attention in patients with moderate and severe TBI. There are case reports demonstrating improved scores on ADL scales in patients treated with amantadine.[614,629] Case reports also indicate general improvements in global functioning and processing speed.[78,306] PET imaging studies show amantadine-mediated increases in cortical glucose metabolism in patients with TBI.[307] Notably, a recent large clinical trial demonstrated the benefits of amantadine in individuals with disordered consciousness who were in the subacute to early chronic phases of recovery.[196] In patients with DAI, amantadine appears to be effective in improving cognition independent of the timing of administration.[378] Although bromocriptine is less well studied clinically than MPH and amantadine, small case series show some evidence that low-dose bromocriptine may improve EF.[368] Recent work suggests though that daily bromocriptine is not effective for treating attention deficits.[598]

Some work has been undertaken regarding noradrenergic agonists in TBI recovery. The tricyclic antidepressant and NET inhibitor desipramine has been used for years for depression, and increased arousal and initiation in a TBI case series[453] and improved post-TBI depression.[613] Clinical reports also suggest some potential efficacy with the selective NET inhibitor atomoxetine.[460]

Previous large randomized controlled trials with CDP-choline have shown improvements in memory and global function in patients with TBI across the injury severity spectrum.[71,324] Notably, though, a recently completed definitive trial of CDP-choline did not result in overall improvement in a complicated mild to severe TBI population.[626] Alternatively, both case series and small randomized controlled trials suggest that the cholinesterase inhibitors can improve memory and attention as well as general cognition.[506,588] Interestingly, daily treatment with the cholinesterase inhibitor donepezil results in cortical increases in metabolism, and magnitude of metabolic change is associated with degree of clinical treatment response.[285] Clinical trials are needed to further define donepezil treatment effects on cognition.

Purpose of Neuropsychological Assessment. The purpose of neuropsychological assessment varies across the course of recovery from TBI. The initiation of assessment may occur during the initial stages of emergence from coma. Later, neuropsychologists often are responsible for evaluating a patient's progress through PTA. Neuropsychological testing is useful in evaluating the domains of cognitive functioning described above. However, the ability to complete formalized testing of any sort is dependent on the ability of the patient to tolerate or respond to the tools used. As a result, extensive formal neuropsychological testing is generally not completed while an individual is in PTA; instead, brief tools and batteries are introduced as an individual is able to participate. There are also times when formalized testing of certain cognitive areas may not be possible for a period of time secondary to other brain injury-related issues, such as aphasia, severe limitations in motor or sensory abilities, medical issues, or behavioral issues that may impede participation. Studies suggest that it is feasible to administer brief testing during acute inpatient rehabilitation,[274] and these data suggest some prognostic value when completing certain types of neuropsychological testing within the early weeks of the recovery process.[213] Full neuropsychological test batteries are often not administered for several months after moderate to severe TBI. These detailed outpatient batteries may be used to answer questions related to return to school, work, driving, or other activities and to assess ongoing recovery.

Practical Interventions for Cognitive Impairment After Traumatic Brain Injury. When interacting with patients during the inpatient rehabilitation phase of recovery, it is helpful to have an understanding of the "typical" presentation of cognitive impairment associated with TBI, so that information for promoting effective rehabilitation interactions between staff and patients may be presented. Patients who are in inpatient rehabilitation following moderate to severe TBI are typically still in PTA. During this period of confusion, patients may be disoriented to person, place, time, and circumstance. They generally do not remember what has happened to them. If it is explained to them that they have been injured, they are often not able to process and retain the information. As a result, it may be very difficult for them to make sense of their surroundings and circumstances. They may pull at tubes, sutures, braces, helmets, and so on, because they find them uncomfortable and are not able to process the fact that such items are important and necessary for their care. They may refuse therapies because they feel tired and in pain and are not able to appreciate the benefits of participation. They will likely have difficulties remembering multistep instructions in therapy, what was presented to them during a previous session, or perhaps even moments before. Patients who have sustained TBI likely also have additional cognitive impairments caused by injury. Examples include language deficits, sensory impairments, difficulty initiating or stopping behaviors, or difficulties interpreting visual or spatial information. Individuals may wander or engage in inappropriate, unsafe, and repetitive behaviors. When the patient's cognitive status is taken into consideration, these behaviors become more understandable; however, staff and families may find these behaviors difficult to manage. Education of staff and families regarding cognition is often key to understanding a patient's needs.

As patients are often not able to make sense of their environment during this period of acute confusion, an overarching goal of rehabilitation should be to provide a structured program to assist patients through this period of recovery. As recovery progresses, they will learn what to expect from their daily schedule more easily if structure has been established. In addition, although orientation is tested frequently to assess progress through PTA, therapists, nursing staff, and family members should also gently provide orientation information in conversation with the patient throughout the day. It is often helpful to have a daily calendar in the patient's room, as well as a clock so that the patient may have a reference point. Staff members should reintroduce themselves each time they interact with the patient, even if they have worked with the patient just a short time before. As the patient recovers and is independently able to identify staff members and to call them by name, this practice may be discontinued. As many patients are much more sensitive to sensory stimulation or may have field cuts or visual neglect following TBI, staff members are less likely to startle a patient by approaching a patient from the front, gaining the patient's attention, and explaining what they will be doing before touching a patient, moving a patient, or engaging in other interactions. Nursing, medical procedures, and therapy tasks should be explained in a step-by-step manner, even if the patient does not appear able to respond or show overt awareness.

In general, persons with TBI can recall information about their family and personal history, even though their ability to encode and recall more recent events is impaired. As a result, it is often comforting, for example, to have pictures of family members, pets, and favorite places in the patient's hospital room. It is helpful for therapists to ask family members for detailed information about the patient's history, including education, work history, hobbies, and interests, so that components of these aspects of the patient's life can be incorporated in therapies when possible and therapy can be more personalized.

Patients who are not aware of their deficits or are impulsive may be at risk for engaging in unsafe behaviors. During the initial stages of recovery, the best approach is to guard them through therapeutic interactions. One-to-one sitters or restraints may be required for safety. As patients recover, however, it is often helpful to teach them strategies to reduce impulsivity (i.e., teach them step-by-step plans until overlearned or have them count/pause to review steps before moving). For lack of awareness, it is sometimes necessary to compare patient performance and progress with an objective standard. Logical verbal discussion is often not effective when a lack of awareness is caused by cognitive impairment related to injury. Group therapy with peers who are able to challenge the person may sometimes be effective at later stages of recovery.

All of the behavioral and cognitive issues discussed in this section tend to improve over the recovery period. That said, some of the issues observed in the inpatient setting may continue to be present as the patient transitions to home or other settings. In fact, according to one study, approximately 40% of individuals reported ongoing unmet needs at 1 year, with the most frequently cited issues including memory and problem solving, managing stress and emotional upset, and temper control.[106] However, many of the routines and techniques learned in therapy may be applied successfully by families in the home setting. Staff should be certain to educate families regarding the purpose and use of these techniques. Continuing to set up routines and structure to assist individuals and to increase the likelihood of success may play a significant role in decreasing depression, irritability, and difficulties with explosive anger. Treatment with medication, combined with therapy to manage adjustment to disability, anxiety, and depression, as well as to teach anger management skills is often recommended. Box 43-3 reviews helpful behavioral and cognitive strategies for common issues following TBI.

Behavioral, Emotional, and Mood Issues in Rehabilitation

Changes in emotional and behavioral response and mood are common following TBI. The following sections provide descriptions and approaches to management of these types of issues.

Agitation. Agitation is common in the acute phase of recovery from TBI. Studies have suggested prevalence rates between 11% and 42%, depending on the definition used.[43,62,456,373,509,607] This type of behavior occurs frequently enough that it is described as a distinct phase of recovery in the Ranchos Los Amigos Scale (i.e., Rancho level IV—confused-agitated), and garners attention because it poses significant challenges to rehabilitation staff and family members. Importantly, agitation can have significant impact on a patient's ability to productively participate in therapies. Bogner and Corrigan define agitation as "an excess of one or more behaviors that occurs during an altered state of consciousness."[43] This definition includes not only aggressive physical or verbal behaviors, but also restlessness and disinhibition. "True" clinical agitation occurring during an altered state of consciousness is therefore differentiated from the description of an individual who is "irritable," "angry," or "aggressive" when not confused. This definition also requires observed behaviors to be "excessive," in which behaviors interfere with functional activities and are not able to be inhibited by the person either with or without cueing.[43]

Agitation, as defined above, occurs during acute phase of recovery from TBI while an individual is in PTA. Patients in this phase are disoriented and unable to retain information. They are confused and are responding "in the moment" to internal and external stimuli. As confused patients may have difficulty communicating medical or personal needs, evaluation of pain and exploration of other potentially noxious stimuli should be conducted by

BOX 43-3

Helpful Environmental and Cognitive Interventions for Working with Individuals with Traumatic Brain Injury

Early in recovery, individuals with brain injury are often confused and have difficulty remembering new information. Staff should:

- Introduce and reintroduce themselves, even if they have done it earlier in the day or week.
- Provide consistency and structure (ideally a consistent schedule with consistent staff).
- Provide reorientation frequently.
- Use simple, short sentences and don't give too much information at once.
- Cue the patient as needed, providing some direction and guidance.
- Provide extra time and repetition as needed.

Individuals with brain injury may become easily overstimulated. Overstimulation will likely have a negative impact on cognition and may increase the likelihood of irritable or agitated behaviors. It can be helpful to:

- Limit distractions and noise around the patient as needed (move treatment to a quiet location, dim lights, reduce noises such as television and radio, limit the number of people talking and interacting with the person at one time).
- Break down difficult tasks into smaller steps and give simple, step-by-step directions.
- Be flexible. Redirect patients when they become frustrated with an activity, allow rest breaks, and alternative activities as needed.
- Remain calm in interactions and speak in a clear, concise manner using quiet volume and calming tones.
- Keep issues such as pain and fatigue in mind, and treat as needed.

Individuals with brain injury are often "impulsive." This means they may act without thinking. For example, patients may move quickly and unsafely and try to do things that they are not capable of doing independently. To promote safety:

- Be sure to have the patient's attention before you speak.
- Speak slowly, clearly, and softly using the patient's name frequently to keep their attention.
- Use demonstration in addition to verbal instructions when possible.
- Promote team and family communication so that consistent strategies are being used.

Additional tips for working with individuals with brain injury:

- Always approach patients slowly and gently and approach them from the front, not from behind.
- Do not take behaviors personally.
- During periods of significant agitation, create situations where the patient can be successful and avoid situations in which they may fail or will need to be corrected.

staff when a patient becomes agitated. Staff members should be trained to recognize agitation as a medical condition caused by injury and to be aware of the patient's cognitive status. The dangers of aggressive behaviors are real, and staff members should be provided with specific behavior management training to minimize the likelihood of aggressive behavior and to maximize patient/staff safety and patient participation in therapy.

BOX 43-4

Agitated Behavior Scale

___ 1. Short attention span, easy distractibility, inability to concentrate.
___ 2. Impulsive, impatient, low tolerance for pain or frustration.
___ 3. Uncooperative, resistant to care, demanding.
___ 4. Violent or threatening violence toward people or property.
___ 5. Explosive and/or unpredictable behavior.
___ 6. Rocking, rubbing, moaning, or other self-stimulating behavior.
___ 7. Pulling at tubes, restraints, and so on.
___ 8. Wandering from treatment areas.
___ 9. Restlessness, pacing, excessive movement.
___ 10. Repetitive behaviors, motor and/or verbal.
___ 11. Rapid, loud or excessive talking.
___ 12. Sudden changes of mood.
___ 13. Easily initiated or excessive talking.
___ 14. Self-abusive physically and/or verbally.
___ **Total Score**

1 = **absent:** the behavior is not present

2 = **present to a slight degree:** the behavior is present but does not prevent the conduct of other, contextually appropriate behavior. (The individual may redirect spontaneously, or the continuation of the agitated behavior does not disrupt appropriate behavior.)

3 = **present to a moderate degree:** the individual needs to be redirected from an agitated to an appropriate behavior, but benefits from such cueing.

4 = **present to an extreme degree:** the individual is not able to engage in appropriate behavior because of the interference of the agitated behavior, even when the external cueing or redirection is provided.

Measures of Agitation. The behaviors associated with agitation have been most effectively described the Agitated Behavior Scale[102] (Box 43-4). This scale can be helpful for monitoring the progression of patients through recovery, as well as for evaluating the effectiveness of interventions such as medication or behavior plans to manage agitation. In addition, it can yield valuable information regarding the timing of such interventions and the scheduling of therapeutic activities based on scores observed. A more recently developed agitation scale is the Overt Agitation Severity Scale,[625] which limits scoring to observable behaviors and is not specific to TBI. The Neurobehavioral Rating Scale has also been used to monitor agitation, as well as PTA.[97,526]

Treatment of Agitation. Pharmacologic treatment for agitation may be beneficial, although heavily sedating medications may actually prolong the period of agitation,[399] and improvement in cognition (which sedating medications may impede) may be necessary in order for agitation to improve.[104] The potential adverse effects of many of these psychotropic drugs on neurologic recovery should be considered. Early experimental brain injury studies have demonstrated the detrimental impact of the classic D2 receptor antagonist antipsychotic medication haloperidol on motor recovery.[169] Later experimental TBI studies also suggest detrimental effects of daily haloperidol use on cognitive function.[291,602] Clinically, atypical antipsychotics (AAPs) may be better choices for TBI-related agitation, in part, for their more favorable side effect profile and their smaller effects as D2 receptor antagonists. However, experimental studies also show negative effects on cognitive recovery with multiple AAPs, including olanzapine and risperidone.[291,602] Among AAPs, quetiapine is frequently used for post-TBI-related agitation because of its favorable side effect profile and relatively low actions as a D2 receptor antagonist.[151] Interestingly, a recent pilot study suggests that quetiapine is clinically effective in reducing agitation symptoms post-TBI, with associated improvements in cognition noted.[284]

β-Blockers are commonly used clinically to manage TBI-related agitation. Previous clinical trials suggest that propranolol can decrease agitation intensity and decrease need for physical restraints.[61] Further, a recent Cochran database review suggests that β-blockers have the best evidence for effective use with minimal side effects.[179] Although anticonvulsants like carbamazepine (Tegretol) and valproate (Depakote) are commonly used to manage TBI-related aggression, research on their efficacy is limited.[179]

Benzodiazepines are GABA-A receptor agonists that can reduce post-TBI agitation symptoms. The use of these drugs for agitation management during rehabilitation has historically been minimized because of concerns of adversely affecting cognitive recovery caused by their ability to augment neuroinhibitory neurotransmitter systems. In the ICU, benodiazepines are commonly used for sedation and behavioral management. Interestingly, limited experimental research in TBI does support the concept that benzodiazepines early after TBI may confer a neuroprotective effect on cognitive recovery,[413] presumably by limiting the degree of excitotoxic insult during this period.

Medications should be chosen carefully and used in conjunction with other behavior management techniques for maximum effect. Some literature indicates that neuroleptic use can increase duration of PTA.[398] In older patients with TBI, agitation may be caused by injury or may represent an exacerbation of preexisting behaviors related to dementia or other cognitive impairment. In addition, older individuals are likely to experience delirium related to simple medical issues, such as urinary tract infection, anesthesia or other medications, or pain and fatigue. Depression may also manifest as irritable and hostile behavior.

When a patient must be physically restrained, the use of enclosure beds, which allow for patient movement while in a safe environment, are preferable to belts or other restraints while in bed. When out of bed, rear-fastening wheelchair seatbelts can be used for patients who may attempt to get up without assistance and who have poor safety awareness. Soft hand mitts are helpful at times to ensure patient safety, especially when patients are at risk for pulling out tracheostomy and/or gastrostomy tubes. It is often preferable to have a one-to-one sitter with the patient if doing so allows for reduction of physical restraints. Agitation generally only lasts for an average of 2 to 3 weeks. Some patients pass through the phase more quickly, although others have more persistent agitation. Specific predictors for agitation risk, timing, and duration have not been elucidated at this time. However, recent data suggest that those experiencing agitation during their inpatient rehabilitation hospital course had longer lengths of stay and were less likely to be discharged to a home setting.[373] Severity and duration of agitation have also been documented recently as affecting later global outcome.[509]

Hypoarousal and Sleep Disturbance. During the acute phases of recovery from TBI, problems with arousal, attention, and fatigue are common and may be the result or combination of multiple factors. Injury to structures or connecting white matter fibers in the reticulothalamic, thalamocortical, and reticulocortical networks may cause symptoms of fatigue, hypoarousal, persistent vegetative or minimally conscious states, coma, or death. Neurochemical disturbance related to injury to these areas may also be a contributing factor. As an individual awakens from coma, arousal improves but can remain problematic during rehabilitation. In addition, sleep disturbance, medical issues, and debilitation may all contribute to a patient's ability to remain aroused and attentive. With hypoarousal, patients will complain of fatigue or frequently ask to return to their room or bed. They may fall asleep midtask during a therapy session or require frequent cues to remain awake. When issues with arousal are problematic, medications should be reviewed for sedating side effects. The timing of administration of medications that may have sedating side effects should also be reviewed. Discontinuation, dose reduction, changes in timing, or alternative treatments should be considered as needed. Medical treatment for arousal disorders may include psychostimulants or other medications. Behaviorally, staff members may evaluate patient schedules and therapy to see if routines may be established to improve arousal. Changes may include monitoring the time of day when arousal appears to be problematic and providing rest breaks in the schedule. It may be beneficial to schedule the most challenging tasks during periods of the day when the patient appears to be most alert. It may also be beneficial to schedule cognitive tasks following a physical activity (i.e., walking), if the patient appears to be more alert after being physically active. Often patients with arousal issues can appear to be quite different if they are evaluated during an alert period versus a time when they are less alert. This can cause significant differences is scoring and ascertaining a patient's true abilities.

Sleep disturbance is also common following TBI, and may contribute to issues with arousal. Patients may have alterations in circadian rhythms, sleep patterns, and sleep quality, which may be disruptive to therapy. Acutely after TBI, sleep disturbance is largely the result of diffuse cerebral dysfunction associated with primary and secondary injury.[466] Sleep patterns after TBI are characterized by decreased REM and slow wave sleep. Total sleep time and sleep efficiency are also disturbed.[100] There is also a strong link between cognitive recuperation and normalization of sleep.[466] Disrupted sleep following TBI can result from pharmacologic treatments, associated neuropsychiatric conditions, agitation, drug withdrawal, pain, preexisting sleep disorders, and environmental overstimulation.[334,419] Environmental factors unique to hospitals, such as noise, untimely procedures, and pharmacologic interventions, are common.[26]

Pharmacologic intervention is often needed to effectively treat TBI-mediated sleep disorders. The literature is limited on the use of clinically proven sleep-promoting drugs in the injured brain. Trazodone, a selective 5-HT reuptake inhibitor and 5-HT2 receptor antagonist, is frequently used for its sedating effects in TBI.[279] At lower doses its sedative properties likely result from its antagonistic effect of the 5-HT2 receptors.[346] Trazodone promotes natural sleep cycles by increasing the amount of total sleep, increasing the percentage of deep sleep, and decreasing the number of intermittent awakenings.[279,488,591]

Cognitive-behavioral therapies, including stimulus control, sleep restriction, and sleep hygiene education, are beneficial, particularly in moderate TBI.[418] In addition, assisting patients with sleep hygiene may be helpful. This may include taking fewer naps during the day as the patient is able to tolerate it, turning off television or other sources of stimulation near bed time, helping the patient to engage in quiet activities in the evening, and dimming or turning out lights during the nighttime hours, as safety permits. In addition, an evaluation of nighttime medical needs may be helpful to determine whether any medication schedules or other medical routines could be altered to allow the patient as many uninterrupted hours of sleep as possible. Sleep logs should be maintained for patients with identified sleep issues to monitor the efficacy and progress of any interventions prescribed.

Psychiatric Issues. It is important to obtain a good history, if possible, of a patient's psychiatric history before injury. If a patient had a significant psychiatric history before injury, these issues should continue to be treated during rehabilitation. Although patients in acute PTA often do not have the awareness or memory to recall what has happened to them or to understand their level of disability, as they emerge from PTA, they may begin to respond emotionally to what has occurred. Those who had a premorbid history of depression or anxiety may begin to experience these problems accordingly. Even those who do not have a positive psychiatric history should be monitored for changes in mood or participation and evaluated for emotional response to injury and disability as needed. As patients clear PTA, interactions with a rehabilitation psychologist or other therapist trained in counseling individuals with adjustment to disability issues may be highly beneficial.

Depression

Depression is the most common psychological problem after TBI.[160] The prevalence of depression after TBI is between 6% and 77%.[310] The variation in prevalence rates is caused by different measurements used to assess depression, the time course when assessed after injury, and differences in injury severity. The prevalence of posttraumatic depression (PTD) is highest in the first year after injury,[23] affecting over 70% of those with moderate to severe injury within the first 6 months postinjury, but delayed depression is also not uncommon.[221]

It is not known how much the development of PTD stems from the pathophysiologic consequences of the head injury, a premorbid predisposition, or a postinjury psychological response to the trauma.[465] Depression may result from the biochemical changes in the brain following injury. Medications to treat depression can be beneficial for some,[162,613] although according to animal models, antidepressant response rates may be lower in the setting of inflammation,[434] which is known to occur chronically after TBI.[313] Several potential risk factors affect postinjury depression rates. Minority status, unemployment, low income, history of alcohol abuse, and low education levels are associated with PTD.[465] There is no clear consensus on how preinjury psychiatric history,[171,269] age,[202,270,497,608] gender,[171,269,270,288,325,608] and injury severity[465] affect PTD rates. One study suggests PTD rates of over 70% for those with a premorbid history of mood disorders while PTD rates for those without a premorbid history are much lower.[155] Recent evidence suggests that the acute inflammatory response mounted as a result of secondary injury,[272] as well as genetic background,[155] can influence PTD risk giving rise to the concept of stratified treatment trials and exploration of antiinflammatory agents as therapies for PTD treatment.

The overlap between depressive symptoms and symptoms of neurologic disease presents a challenge when assessing PTD. Overlapping symptoms can include insomnia, irritability, and lack of motivation. Depression has been assessed with patients who have TBI with a variety of measurements including the Zung Self Rating Depression Scale, Hamilton Rating Scale for Depression, and Beck Depression Inventory.[167,340,495] DSM-IV criteria for identifying major depression have also been used to assess depression in patients with TBI,[310] as has the Patient Health Questionnaire, which is based on DSM-IV criteria.[159] PTD is associated with poor outcome after injury.[160] Depression is also associated with impaired cognitive function such as psychomotor slowing, decreased information processing speed, memory, and flexibility in problem solving,[465] providing some rationale for PTD-associated cognitive impairment after TBI.[160]

Posttraumatic Stress Disorder. There has been considerable recent debate about posttraumatic stress disorder (PTSD) following TBI, which has gained significant attention in light of combat- and blast-related injuries occurring in the recent conflicts in Afghanistan and Iraq. It was previously thought that amnesia for the traumatic event was a protective mechanism, and that PTSD, which is an emotional response to a traumatic event, could not occur for an event that a person is not able to remember.[359] More recently, the literature suggests that it is possible for PTSD to occur following TBI at all levels of injury.[372,536] The severity of injury may have some protective qualities in modulating PTSD development.[287] For example, it is less likely for PTSD to occur in instances where there is significant loss of consciousness (LOC) and amnesia for the event. In comparison, it may be more likely for an individual with no LOC or brief LOC, such as with mild TBI, to develop PTSD because of the increased likelihood of recall for the injury event or events leading up to or following injury. Some individuals with moderate to severe injury do go on to develop symptoms of PTSD, although the exact percentages are unclear.[288] In those that do, very few report reexperience of the event as a symptom. However, some individuals, despite having no actual memory of the event, may develop an unconscious/implicit fear response for the event.[319] Individuals may also have an emotional response to information that is provided to them about the event, such as stories or pictures relayed by others[240] or in response to brief periods of memory during the confusing period of PTA.[286] The overlap in symptoms of PTSD and TBI are significant and complicate the diagnostic process.[536] Additional personality factors, psychosocial factors, and attributions about the injury itself can affect the likelihood of PTSD symptoms emerging after TBI.[199,251,289] Research regarding TBI and PTSD in military veterans adds additional caveats to what is understood about PTSD after injury. Some data suggest that both mild TBI and PTSD are more prevalent when injuries result from improvised explosive devices[388] or, more generally, from bomb blasts.[470,471] However, additional work has found no difference in incidence of PTSD in blast-related versus nonblast-related TBI.[344] A "clinical triad" has also been described, in which TBI, PTSD, and chronic pain symptoms are linked as factors predictive of persisting impairment and disability.[93,471] Additional neurologic mechanisms are also being reported as potential factors in PTSD development after TBI, such as central autonomic network disruption and compromised neurocircuitry[623] and neurobiologic changes in structure and function.[276,297] As the number of veterans returning from recent conflicts with TBI and PTSD has grown exponentially, the need for proper evaluation and treatment of PTSD and TBI has increased. The literature continues to grow rapidly in this area; however, additional research is certainly required to fully guide screening and management plans.

Behavioral Management. Behavioral management/modification generally refers to interactions designed to promote positive behaviors and/or decrease negative behaviors. Common examples for rehabilitation include increasing the likelihood that a patient who is refusing medications will take them more readily or increasing participation in therapy by a patient who frequently refuses to participate. Alternatively, staff may seek strategies to decrease the likelihood of significant aggressive or violent behavior by a patient in a Rancho level IV (confused–agitated) stage of recovery from TBI or to decrease other inappropriate behaviors.

In general, when conducting a behavioral evaluation, observations of what happened immediately before and immediately after a problem behavior are recorded in an effort to ascertain possible unintended triggers and/or consequences that influence the patient's behavior. Any patterns of antecedents, behaviors, and consequences (often referred to as "ABCs") that are observed may be used to create an individualized behavior plan to promote desired behavior. When a behavior plan is developed, it should be communicated effectively with the rehabilitation team, and all team members should implement the plan consistently. It is critical to be aware of a person's cognitive status when evaluating and treating behavioral issues, as the approach to treatment varies significantly with the patient's ability to understand consequences and to be responsible for their behavior.

Pediatrics

TBI in the pediatric population has some issues that are different from those in adults. The impact of behavioral, cognitive, and physical impairments on the ongoing development of children is hard to predict. These impairments negatively affect the way children learn, play, make friends, and grow.

Original outcome data in pediatrics led to the generalization that younger children have worse outcomes than older children.[311] Overall, in the pediatric population, 95% survive injury. The highest mortality rates are observed in children under 2 years of age.[338] The mechanism of injury in up to 50% of those under the age of 7 is related to assaults or child abuse and falls. This population, when compared with noninflicted TBI, had lower initial GCS scores, more prolonged impairments of consciousness, different biomarker profiles, and worse functional scores at 6 months.[32,261] When functional outcome data are evaluated, memory difficulties contributed to persistent dependence after injury. Those with shorter duration of coma and younger age had improved functional outcomes, postulated to be caused by greater plasticity in the younger brain.[150] In comparison, those patients with nonaccidental TBI early in life have more significant persistent cognitive and emotional difficulties.[430]

Specific practice guidelines for the acute management of severe TBI in pediatrics exist. Evidence supports treatment in a pediatric trauma center or in an adult trauma center with added qualifications to treat pediatric patients. Improved outcomes have been observed with therapeutic hypothermia, making it an option in pediatric management not proposed in adult guidelines.[4] Recent trials suggest safety of moderate hypothermia in pediatrics, with guidelines specifying use within 8 hours for a duration of 48 hours.[6,259] Specific recommendations on neuromuscular blockage and sedation also exist, giving guidance to critical care providers.[302] These guidelines provide standardization including common data elements to facilitate future multicenter studies and high-quality metaanalyses.[5]

Overall, pediatric TBI has a significant impact on the health care needs of children. During the first year after a moderate to severe TBI, one third of children had unmet or unrecognized health care needs. The largest area of need was cognitive services. The most frequent reason for this need not being met was that it was not recommended by the physician or school. Lack of insurance funding and poor family functioning were also related to unmet and unrecognized needs. When these issues are combined with a lack of concrete information on recovery after TBI, family distress is quite high after injury.[512]

When children with TBI are compared with matched peers, there is a correlation between severity of injury and performance in neurobehavioral functioning in the areas of intelligence, academic performance, memory, problem solving, and motor performance 1 year after injury. Although the students scored within the normal range, they were substantially below their matched peers.[263] These same findings persist 3 years after injury. As children with TBI age, deficits with abstract and concept learning that were not easy to measure 1 year after injury become more apparent. These findings support the need for serial neuropsychological testing after injury in children.[166] Research also supports the need for increased educational support for children with TBI in an educational system that understands learning deficits after TBI.

The impact of deficits in executive functioning and behavior can be manifested in difficulties with social interactions. The interrelationship between language, EF and self-managing behavior is central to social success. These skills are often compromised after TBI, resulting in social difficulties, especially with children injured during the teenage years.[553] Social functioning is an important predictor of QOL after pediatric TBI. For children with TBI, maintaining close friendships and numbers of friends are more important than success in school or sports.[444] This information should lead practitioners to assess this area of function when examining patients, in the same way they evaluate motor and cognitive function.

Postinjury behavioral changes are commonly reported by families. The Child Behavior Checklist can be used to define abnormal behavior in a home or academic setting. In a phone interview study, 40% of patients were described as having behavioral problems. Preinjury behavioral issues and family function may also relate to persistent behavior issues.[215] It is important to discriminate between post-TBI behavior changes and psychiatric disorders seen in those with more severe injury and those with premorbid or family psychiatric history.

Acute Prognostic Indicators of Outcome: A Clinical and Translational Research Perspective

Although comprehensive validated statistical models are still in development, a considerable amount of research has evaluated how demographic, clinical, physiologic, biochemical, and genetic factors contribute to mortality and outcome. These studies do provide unique clinical evidence that can guide rehabilitation practitioners as they care for patients with TBI in the acute care setting and rehabilitation. Demographic factors like gender, age, substance abuse, and violence are relevant factors when considering outcome. Additionally, severity scores that characterize the nature and extent of injury and other clinical, biochemical, and physiologic markers also have utility as predictors of TBI outcome.

Demographics

Female sex is considered to be a risk factor for worse outcome, particularly in studies that include mildly injured subjects.[30,163,581] Increases in postconcussive symptoms are often reported. Large epidemiologic studies assessing sex and menopausal status on mortality after TBI have been mixed, with some studies showing that menopausal women are at greater risk than younger premenopausal women and others suggesting that menopausal status is protective.[39,120,417] In contrast, experimental TBI models studies suggest that female sex hormones can be neuroprotective against many biochemical mechanisms of secondary injury, including cerebral edema, excitotoxicity, oxidative injury, and inflammation.[468] Recent clinical reports show that female sex hormones also may have a beneficial effect on TBI pathophysiology, with lower L/P ratios, glutamate accumulation, and oxidative stress loads reported in CSF for women with severe TBI compared with men.[30,568,572] Severe TBI has a profound effect clinically on endogenous serum hormone profiles. Elevations in hormones such as estradiol measured early after injury are linked to greater mortality and worse global outcome, regardless of gender. The pattern, along with CNS cortisol, likely represents a stress response to the injury,[485,486,578] and is not innately neuroprotective. Pharmacologic progesterone dosing early after injury has demonstrated beneficial neuroprotective effects in preclinical models, and single-site clinical studies have been positive;[612,617] however, more work is needed to determine which clinical subpopulations might benefit most from this treatment. Taken together, these studies suggest that sex and hormones have a complex, yet important, role in TBI physiology and outcome.

TBI in the older adult is more commonly the result of falls than in younger age groups. Fragile bridging veins in older adults contribute to a higher incidence of subdural hematoma in this age group. Underlying medical conditions such as heart arrhythmias and artificial valves that require artificial anticoagulation increase the propensity for intracranial hemorrhage with falls in this demographic group. Decreased balance and syncopal episodes from a variety of causes also contribute to falls and TBI in older persons. Neuronal loss that occurs with increasing age likely also influences fall incidence. Age-related mitochondrial dysfunction associated with neurodegenerative diseases likely influences the secondary biochemical injury response observed in older patients with TBI.[70] In vitro studies show that hippocampal vulnerability to excitotoxic injury increases as a function of age and is related a more pronounced loss of intracellular Ca^{++} homeostasis and mitochondrial dysfunction.[350] More oxidative stress has been noted for a given excitotoxic or ischemic insult in older adults with TBI.[568] Also, increasing age is associated with a higher hormone stress response and inflammation after TBI.[271,486,578] TBI in the aging population is associated with higher severity of injury, mortality, and morbidity. For older patients with TBI, there is greater acute care resource consumption per favorable outcome than in their younger counterparts.[429] Rehabilitation discharge outcomes are often similar for older and younger patients with TBI, but the length of inpatient rehabilitation and hospital costs needed to attain similar functional gains are greater for older patients.[92]

Intentional, or violent, TBI carries a higher mortality rate than other accidental mechanisms of injury.[582] Among survivors, there are no differences in functional assessments after injury, but victims of intentional injury do report lower levels of community integration and function than others who survive accidental injuries.[582] Alcohol and illegal substances are commonly observed in the blood at the time of injury and can contribute to acute complications, longer hospitalizations, and worse outcomes from TBI.[103]

Clinical Variables

The GCS[539] has been a mainstay in determining severity of neurologic injury after trauma and has been used in several studies with other variables to predict outcome. The revised trauma scale score (RTS) and injury severity score (ISS) are effective predictors of discharge disposition across a broad population hospitalized with TBI.[574] RTS and GCS can also predict disability and community integration 1 year after injury in this population.[575] Coma duration is linked with injury severity and outcome, and patients with coma lasting more than 2 weeks are very unlikely to have a good recovery.[277] PTA duration is associated with DAI and is a strong predictor of functional outcome.[278,628] In fact, the International Data Coma Bank reports that patients with less than 2 weeks of PTA often have a good recovery, although patients in PTA for greater than 4 weeks have a much smaller likelihood of good recovery.[277]

Both elevated ICP and decreased CPP have been linked with poor outcome in adults and children.[76,87,537] Although ICP is often elevated early after severe injury, late elevations are often more severe and require more intensive treatment.[523] Significant correlations between arterial pressure-induced decreases in CPP and extracerebral injuries (assessed via ISS scores) have been reported, indicating the difficulties in resuscitating patients with TBI with multiple other injuries. Additionally, duration of low CPP was related to adverse outcome as late as 24 months after injury.[107]

Radiologic indices from CT studies have some utility in predicting outcome. DAI leads to cerebral atrophy[137] and is associated with coma and PTA, both of which are associated with long-term outcome. Traumatic subarachnoid hemorrhage (tSAH) has been associated with worse injury and poorer outcomes than other types of lesions,[356] and tSAH can be graded to predict outcome.[214] However, it is unclear whether tSAH is simply a marker of more severe TBI or if it adversely impacts outcome through direct mechanisms like vasospasm and ischemia.[20] Midline shift reflects elevated ICP and contributes to poor outcomes, while patients who have epidural hematomas evacuated often have relatively good outcomes.[343]

Although subject to variability, reports demonstrate that SSEPs do provide some prognostic information. In severely injured patients, SSEPs have been linked to functional measures at rehabilitation discharge as well as 6- and 12-month functional outcome measures.[362,421] Other studies show that SSEP, including central somatosensory conduction time (CCT) and N13/N20 amplitude ratios (ARs) in the upper extremity, are sensitive to global outcome For cases of coma caused by supratentorial lesions, CCTs and ARs were normal in patients with good outcome. CCTs and ARs became more prolonged and decreased, respectively, as patient outcome worsened, and patients with bilateral loss of cortical responses died or were severely disabled.[479]

EEG data have been classified in several ways for the purposes of prognosticating outcome. Some evidence suggests that the presence of more normal wake-sleep patterns, including the presence of sleep spindles, is indicative of better outcomes.[60] EEG characteristics of coma considered favorable for survival are usually sensitive to external stimuli and include relatively normal activity, dominant and rhythmic theta activity, frontal rhythmic delta activity, and spindle coma patterns present where stage 2 sleep patterns most often appear. Patients with posttraumatic coma also exhibit burst suppression patterns when cerebral anoxia secondarily results from the injury. Additional negative prognostic characteristics involve nonreactive alpha pattern coma with alpha range activity predominant in the anterior regions or broadly distributed throughout the cortex.[531] Impairment of the quantitative EEG parameter percent alpha variability also signifies poor outcome.[562] However, the most severe malignant factor for survival is isoelectric EEG activity.[531]

Biomarkers

Biomarkers are a part of mainstream clinical care to quantitatively assess and define injury/disease in almost every organ system other than the brain.[36] However, biomarkers do have the potential to assist clinicians with TBI diagnosis, prognosis, and treatment and management strategies. Although biomarkers are traditionally defined as protein measurements in biofluids, genes also represent a rich biomaterial for identifying individualized data for how a person may respond to an injury or treatment and degree of risk for particular complication after injury. As TBI biomarker research has increased in recent years, best practices for sample collection and biorepository management have been issued by the National Institutes of Health/NINDS,[455] along with CDEs,[446] to facilitate translation of findings to clinical care. The concept of rehabilomics has evolved over the past several years as a rehabilitation-relevant biomarker research model, particularly in the area of TBI.[565] Here, biologic markers are linked with multimodal outcomes and biosusceptibility to complications are identified, giving rise to the possibility of personalized biologic and other treatments to address the many conditions observed in individuals with chronic TBI.[112,565,586,587]

Proteomics

Biomarkers identified in TBI often represent structural damage associated with the injury. These biomarkers are derived from the major cell types in the CNS. S100b is a calcium-binding protein present in high concentrations in astrocytes, and elevated S100b levels indicate irreversible astrocyte damage.[299] Myelin basic protein (MBP) is abundant in myelin. As such, elevated MBP levels represent axonal injury.[246] Neuron-specific enolase (NSE) is a glycolytic enzyme localized predominantly in neuronal cytoplasm, with elevated levels reflective of neuronal injury.

In addition to its diagnostic potential in mild TBI, serum S100b levels have been linked with impending mortality in severely injured patients, increased ICP, and global outcomes such as GOS.[36,208] NSE is linked to neuroinflammation[438] as well as GCS and outcome in adults and children, with reasonable sensitivity and specificity.[38,225] Initial NSE levels in particular have been helpful in outcome prognostication for both adults and children.[38,376] Both S100B and NSE absolute levels and duration of elevation have been linked to deficits with neuropsychological testing.[247] MBP also has been linked with both mortality and outcome.[36,620]

Each of these structural damage biomarkers also has some utility in differentiating etiology of injury. Children with inflicted TBI (i.e., SBS) had delayed peak concentrations of serum S100B, MBP, and NSE compared with children presenting with accidental TBI.[37] Additionally, a reduction in these markers has been observed in children receiving therapeutic hypothermia.[333] Thus, these markers may have utility in monitoring other promising therapeutic interventions such as progesterone treatment. Each of these markers is currently being investigated in humans and experimental models for their utility in characterizing and their prognostic potential in blast TBI.[529] Some limitations should be considered as these markers move into clinical care. For example, S100b and NSE have limited reliability because of extracerebral accumulation of these markers in patients with concomitant injury or hemorrhagic shock.[299] Additionally, S100b is not a useful marker in children less than 2 years of age because of high normative values in that age group.[299] Recently, UCHL-1 (neuronal damage marker) and GFAP (astrocyte damage marker) have emerged as relevant biomarkers for TBI diagnosis, lesion type, and outcomes correlation.[386,422] An autoimmune response against GFAP has been documented recently that warrants further research on how autoimmunity might impact long-term outcomes.[631]

The literature suggests that multiple molecular targets associated with key biochemical pathways involved with secondary injury mechanisms that lead to tissue damage can also have some use as biomarkers in prognosticating outcome and monitoring treatment response. The majority of studies evaluating these types of markers have used CSF or extracellular fluid from human brain tissue microdialysis studies obtained during the first week after injury to examine elevations or decreases in biomarkers in patients with severe TBI. In contrast, very little has focused on identifying biomarker profiles obtained during the rehabilitation or chronic phases of recovery.

CNS glutamate levels are elevated early after TBI,[619,630] a phenomenon associated with poor outcome.[206] Additionally, gender influences CSF glutamate levels over time, and treatments like therapeutic hypothermia can significantly reduce levels of this excitatory neurotransmitter in a gender-specific manner.[572] Similarly, F_2-isoprostane, a marker of oxidative injury, has been associated with outcomes[567] as well as sex-specific response to hypothermia.[30] Mitochondrial markers associated with apoptosis, such as cytochrome C and BCL-2, have been linked with both injury type and outcome. In children, elevated CSF cytochrome C levels had a strong association with inflicted TBI. In adults with severe TBI, persistently elevated CSF cytochrome C levels were associated with poorer 6-month scores.[566] High CSF concentrations of the prosurvival protein BCL-2 have also been linked with improved outcomes in children with severe TBI,[94] but with poor outcomes in adults.[566] These specific differences in BCL-2 outcomes may be the result of inherent differences in CNS apoptosis across age groups. Cytoskeletal proteins like alpha II spectrin and its breakdown products[435] and both proinflammatory and antiinflammatory markers[504] in the CSF have been linked with survival and outcome. Serum inflammatory markers can reflect extracranial injury but still impact outcome.[45,504]

Genomics

Apoliproprotein E (APOE) has been studied extensively with regard to its role in plasma lipoprotein transport. There are multiple isoforms of the APOE protein, with functional differences in plasma lipoprotein transport that occur as a result. Numerous studies have linked the expression of the APOE4 isoform with an increased risk of Alzheimer disease, and evidence suggests that TBI triggers ongoing degenerative pathology similar to that observed with Alzheimer dementia. As such, genetic association studies in TBI pathophysiology and outcome have focused on APOE. Some studies suggest that there is no association between the APOE4 allele and outcome,[381] although others link APOE4 with worse functional and cognitive outcomes.[11,109,154,439,541] In addition, two of the largest TBI studies evaluating possession of the APOE4 allele with outcome found a significant age-genotype interaction: adolescent-young adult patients carrying APOE4 had worse outcomes than other younger patients without this allele.[154,540] The frequency of the APOE4 allele in patients with beta-amyloid deposition is 52%, which is higher than reported in the Alzheimer population. However, in those subjects with TBI without beta amyloid deposition, the APOE4 frequency is 16% and similar to that in control subjects without Alzheimer dementia.[408] In addition, recent work implicates genetic variability in the promoter region of the neprolysin gene, the primary enzyme responsible for the beta-amyloid degradation, and the incidence of Alzheimer-type beta-amyloid plaque in TBI.[268]

Although TBI pathophysiology and outcome have been linked, in part, to genetic variability with APOE, less is known about the role of other candidate genes in mediating outcome after TBI. One study suggests that genetic variability in the IL-1β gene influences global outcome in patients with severe TBI[558] and also development of complications such as PTE.[131] There are also several identified variants for a number of dopaminergic genes that are associated with cognitive and psychiatric conditions such as ADHD, depression, impulsivity, and Parkinson disease. Many symptoms associated with these diseases overlap with deficits associated with TBI. TaqIA restriction fragment length polymorphism for the D2 receptor affects D2 receptor levels and glucose metabolism in the brain. It is also linked with verbal memory performance after mild TBI[363] and influences multiple cognitive outcome domains.[158] Additional work shows that variations in the promoter region of the DAT gene that affect gene transcription are chronically linked with DAT receptor densities in the striatum after TBI.[583] This DAT variant is also associated with higher DA levels measured in CSF early after severe TBI, particularly in females, which could have implications on oxidative injury load early after injury.[576]

Chromatin is a structure consisting of DNA plus interacting proteins called histones that help compact DNA in the nucleus and regulate gene expression. Although the human genome represents genetic diversity derived from DNA, the epigenome is a composite of chromatin plus a pattern of chromatin modification that results from interactions between chromatin and its environment. Epigenetics includes the transmission and perpetuation of information, that is, heritable phenotypes not related to the DNA sequence, and is an important mechanism for the stable maintenance of gene expression that involves physically marking DNA or histones. Epigenetic modification significantly affects learning and cognition in animal models.[323] Work in experimental TBI models shows that epigenetic modification of histones is reduced in the hippocampus after TBI, a finding that may contribute to learning and memory deficits.[185] Epigenetic modification also occurs with the application of an enriched environment,[175] an intervention that has been repeatedly shown to improve learning and memory in experimental TBI models.[236,294,577] Although chromatin remodeling studies have not yet been linked to clinical prognosis, epigenetic biomarkers may be a promising strategy for further insight into patient prognosis, treatment efficacy, and individualized environmental response to TBI.

Pediatric Considerations

The clinical predictors often used in pediatric populations are similar to those used in adults. The GCS can be measured in children as well as adults, and is most predictive when applied 6 hours after injury. The Abbreviated Injury Scale or other severity-of-trauma measure is also predictive of worse functional outcome as well as prolonged pediatric ICU stay.[594] The severity of increased ICP is also associated with worse outcome, although the method of controlling ICP does not affect outcome.[264] When stratified by age, age greater than 2 years generally portends a better functional outcome, although etiology and severity of injury may be more predictive. Recently, there has been an increase in pediatric biomarker studies suggesting that many of the same candidate genes, damage markers, secondary injury markers may be relevant to pediatric TBI.[314,423] However, unique age-related differences in brain biology, disease processes, and clinical applications require continued work to validate biomarkers specifically for pediatric populations.[300]

Neuroimaging Modalities in Traumatic Brain Injury Research

Neuroimaging techniques have developed at a relatively rapid rate in recent years and will no doubt continue to do so. Along with basic CT, more advanced MRI sequences are being used clinically. The balance of clinical use, time, and cost efficiency require careful consideration for utilization in the clinical realm, and the promise of more advanced clinical tools must also continue to be advanced through careful research. Recent efforts to formulate CDEs for TBI have included recommendations for a tiered approach to imaging data collection, with basic clinical imaging as a first tier, with more advanced imaging added depending on the area injured, severity of injury, and need for evaluation of changes over time. In addition, centers with additional resources and research capabilities may collect data via more advanced imaging protocols in a standardized manner.[226] This effort may allow data to be compiled for testing and validating imaging techniques in large groups across multiple centers, moving the science forward with greater efficiency of time and resources. Because of space limitations and the rapid pace of developments, a complete description of all techniques is not feasible in this chapter; however, the following descriptions provide an overview of some of the neuroimaging techniques of potential clinical relevance for TBI. Some recent review articles regarding neuroimaging related to TBI are also helpful in describing currently used and emerging techniques.[41,257,320,501]

Functional MRI is arguably the most well-known type of neuroimaging used in neuroscience research, as it has been used widely to study cognitive processes in healthy individuals, with results published often in the media. Basic functional MRI methods involve obtaining high-resolution structural images obtained with normal MRI, and adding an additional paradigm in which the imaging subject engages in a functional task while in the scanner. While the task is conducted, changes in the hemodynamic response in the brain (the blood oxygen level dependent [BOLD] signal),[83] are recorded. These hemodynamic changes are an indirect measurement of neural activity in the area of the brain where they occur. Through observing the correlations between cognitive processes and hemodynamic changes, an index of brain physiology is obtained. Although functional MRI has been used for some time for research with healthy populations, the study of clinical groups is more recent, and this imaging is still considered to be investigational for most clinical populations,[121] including TBI. The studies that have been conducted consistently show differences in laterality of activation, as well as more widespread dispersion of activity for individuals with mild TBI[81,364,365] and moderate-severe TBI,[89,431,489] when compared with healthy controls (see Figure 43-7). These patterns of increased activation and altered laterality occur, especially as task difficulty is increased, even when individuals with TBI are performing within normal on the tasks presented.[365,431] These changes have been observed for simple motor tasks[445] and cognitive tasks, and they suggest that individuals with TBI exert increased cognitive effort to perform at the same behavioral level as healthy individuals. More recently, there has been increased interest in using functional MRI to conduct "resting state" studies and in evaluating how TBI may impact neural networks and functional connectivity.[352,358]

Many different sequences and methods have been developed with MRI technology. Diffusion-weighted imaging (DWI) is an MRI method that uses sequences sensitive to the random movement of water molecules in brain tissues. As a result, DWI is useful for detecting acute ischemia and for differentiating acute from chronic ischemia. DWI has shown clinical usefulness in evaluating ischemic stroke.[593] It is also recommended as a standard method for clinical use after TBI,[226] In TBI, DWI can be sensitive to areas of DAI lesion, and it has shown greater ability to detect DAI than T2- or GRE T2*-weighted images.[320] In addition, DWI also has some potential as a prognostic tool.[253]

Diffusion tensor imaging (DTI) is derived from DWI and is used to obtain information about the structure and integrity of the white matter tracts of the brain. As DAI-related injury to these white matter tracts is a frequent result of TBI and contributes to cognitive impairment, white matter tract integrity evaluation after TBI with DTI provides new insights regarding a correlation between white matter tract functioning and cognitive function. Studies have indicated significant reductions in indices of fractional anisotropy (FA) in major white matter tracts in brain for individuals with TBI versus healthy control subjects (see Figure 43-8).[308,506] FA is the primary independent variable in DTI and is considered an indicator of white matter integrity. The reductions observed after TBI suggest significant white matter dysfunction and are found in

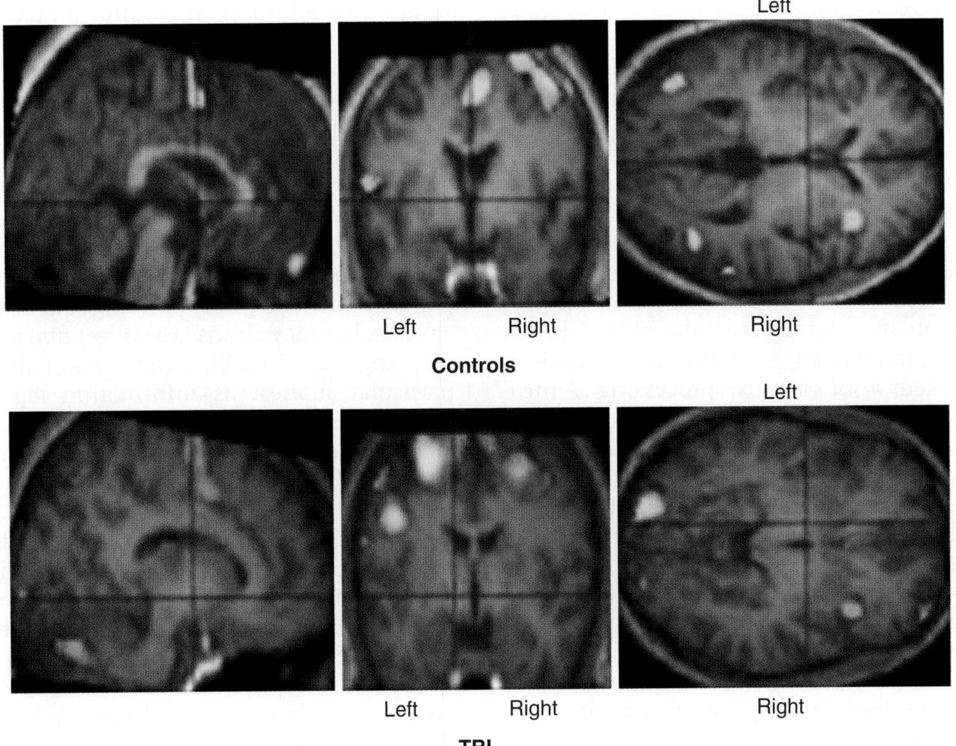

FIGURE 43-7 An example of differences in functional MRI activation observed in a sample of subjects with TBI and healthy controls during a verbal working memory task. Significant differences in laterality, as well as more widespread dispersion of activity, have been noted in individuals with TBI compared with healthy control subjects, even when task performance is not significantly different between groups. It has been suggested that these differences may represent an increased level of cognitive effort by individuals with TBI to perform at the same behavioral level as healthy control subjects.

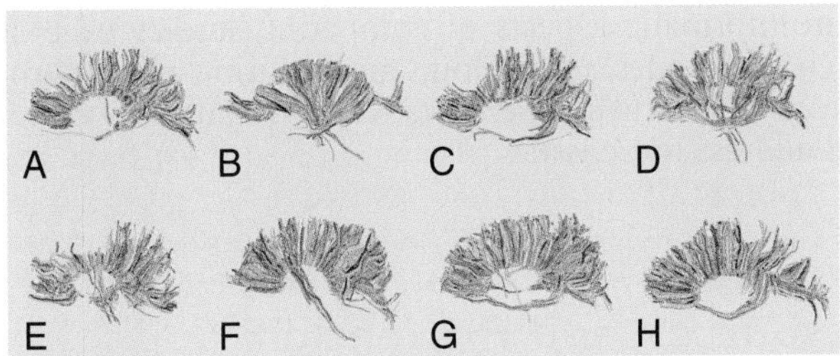

FIGURE 43-8 An example of diffusion tensor imaging cerebral white matter fiber tractography of the corpus callosum for a sample of persons with TBI (**A** through **D**) compared with healthy control subjects (**E** through **H**). Significant reductions in fractional anisotropy in white matter tracts through the corpus callosum, as well as other white matter areas of the brain, have been reported for individuals with TBI compared with healthy control subjects and have been shown to be negatively correlated with neurocognitive testing performance.

regions known to be vulnerable to DAI, such as the corpus callosum in children and adults,[19,255,308,481,506,550] even when white matter in these areas appeared normal on clinical MRI.[19] DTI has become increasingly used to study potential white matter changes after mild TBI in cases with complicated and chronic symptom profiles, despite negative findings on standard CT or MRI.[31,501] Changes over time have also been a focus of study.[35,212] In chronic TBI, DTI findings suggest that reduced white matter integrity is negatively correlated with performance on neurocognitive testing.[18,308] DTI, therefore, is useful in the evaluation of white matter integrity following TBI and holds significant promise for increased clinical and prognostic use in TBI.[320]

Magnetic resonance spectroscopy (MRS) is another type of neuroimaging conducted within an MRI scanner and is complementary to data acquired through other neuroimaging modalities. MRS can detect distinct magnetic profiles of biomarkers. The signal representing a particular biologic compound is displayed as a series of waveforms (i.e., a spectrum) rather than a brain map. Comparing profiles may provide information regarding differences in cellular metabolism between clinical groups and healthy control subjects or may allow for following changes over time. MRS remains investigational in the diagnosis of TBI; however, TBI can cause changes in markers including N-acetyl aspartate (NAA), choline, lactate, and glutamate.[226] For example, NAA is a marker of neuronal health Evaluation of the ratio of NAA to creatine (Cr), a marker of energy metabolism, shows a reduction in NAA/Cr in individuals with TBI compared with healthy controls.[320] Correlations exist between this reduction and poorer prognosis following TBI.[510] Metabolite changes may reflect the biochemical cascade associated with injury as well as repair and recovery over time. Studies thus far have suggested that MRS is a sensitive tool to predict neurologic, functional, and cognitive outcomes after TBI.[226]

Perfusion studies are another type of neuroimaging technique that uses multiple methods for data collection. Single photon emission computed tomography (SPECT) uses externally derived radioisotopes to evaluate resting blood flow and certain types of neuroreceptor binding. The dependent variable in SPECT derives from the well-established principle of increased cerebral activity correlating with increased blood flow.[475] SPECT is quite sensitive in detecting regional differences in resting brain blood flow and has some clinical use in mild TBI, where it has detected abnormalities in resting blood flow in cases where CT results were normal.[207] SPECT also may have better prognostic ability than CT or MRI,[406] in the sense that the number, size, and specific areas of reduced cerebral blood flow determined by SPECT appear to have greater predictive value regarding outcome than MRI or CT findings. However, SPECT is less able than MRI to detect smaller lesions.[320] In addition, because the tracers have half-lives of hours rather than minutes or seconds, SPECT is not useful for observing rapid changes in blood flow, such as those that might occur with cognitive processing as measured by functional MRI. SPECT images are also not as sensitive as PET (described later) and require longer imaging times than MRI.

Like SPECT, PET also uses radioisotope-based methods for imaging of brain metabolism. Glucose absorption (measured by uptake of fluorodeoxyglucose) is often the variable of interest, and it can be studied with both resting and activated methods. Some activated imaging studies also use oxygen-15 PET scanning. Few PET studies have been completed in individuals with TBI. Resting PET paradigms linking PET findings and cognitive functioning following TBI have indicated correlations between reduced cerebral metabolic rates in frontal and temporal regions and neuropsychological test results in the chronic phase of recovery.[220] In an additional resting PET study of moderate to severe TBI, frontal hypometabolism was associated with poorer performance on neuropsychological testing.[180] Activated paradigms using O-15 PET show increased activation and altered laterality patterns and dispersion in individuals with TBI compared with healthy controls. These findings were noted even when those with TBI performed within normal limits on the tasks presented, suggesting again that individuals with TBI need to expend more cognitive effort than control subjects to obtain the same level of performance on cognitive tasks.[326,458]

Xenon CT can also quantify cerebral blood flow. In comparison to other methods such as PET and SPECT, it is easily and quickly performed. It can be used with other techniques to evaluate for the loss of autoregulation, which often occurs following TBI. Additional perfusion-based techniques include perfusion CT and dynamic susceptibility contrast MRI; they are used more widely to study ischemia after acute stroke, but a few studies have been completed in TBI.[226] MRI arterial spin labeling may also be an alternative to allow for perfusion studies without the use of contrast.

Other functional techniques include optical (near-infrared) techniques, such as functional near-infrared spectroscopy (FNIRS). FNIRS has been used in the study of hemodynamic changes related to movement, vision, executive control, and WM.[17] This modality has several advantages over other techniques; it is noninvasive and does not use ionizing radiation or require a large or high-field magnetic scanner. In addition, FNIRS systems can be quite small and portable. They are also virtually unaffected by patient or subject movement. FNIRS studies have been completed in a subject who was walking on a treadmill.[384] However, the spatial resolution with FNIRS is significantly limited. In addition, there are limitations regarding the depth of penetration of the near-infrared light, which limits imaging of deeper brain structures. Finally, the signal may be affected by skin pigmentation and hair.

In general, functional imaging is paired with structural imaging so that changes in hemodynamics, diffusion, or metabolism can be evaluated with anatomic specificity. As many of the modalities described are based on MRI methods, it is not unusual in research for investigators to obtain multiple data types during one scanning session. For example, with simple changes in scanning sequences, a researcher may choose to collect functional MRI and DTI data together. In TBI, combination imaging may be of particular interest as information regarding a subject's behavioral performance on a cognitive task may be correlated with changes in hemodynamics as indicated by functional MRI, as well as information regarding the integrity of white matter tracts.

Not all available neuroimaging modalities have been covered here, although a description and explanation of the basic principles of some of the more commonly used and useful modalities as they pertain to TBI have been provided. Some additional modalities of potential interest include electrophysiologically based methods, such as quantitative electroencephalography and magnetoencephalography, functional transcranial Doppler ultrasonography, and transcranial magnetic stimulation. How TBI may impact neural networks and neurodegeneration over time is also of interest.[41] One of the challenges of conducting longitudinal neuroimaging is the rapid technological development in the field as imaging equipment quickly becomes outdated. This issue also poses problems for the neuroinformatic aspects of comparing studies over time when techniques, technology, and software are all rapidly changing. Efforts from experts will be required to evaluate and address these issues.[201]

Outcomes, Community Integration, Resources, and Prevention

Traumatic Brain Injury Outcome Tools

Rehabilitation practitioners and other groups are very interested in increasing function and return to the community for persons with TBI. Consequently, numerous measures are available to track patient progress both clinically and from a research perspective. As part of the CDE projects, recommendations regarding outcome measures have been made for basic and supplementary collection. These measures are available via the literature or the CDE website for TBI (www.commondataelements.ninds.nih.gov/tbi.aspx#tab=Data_Standards).[407,600] Some representative measures reflecting different aspects of function are presented below.

Global Outcome and Functional Measurement

Functional Independence Measure and Functional Assessment Measure. The Functional Independence Measure (FIM) and Functional Assessment Measure (FAM) have been described elsewhere in this textbook. The FIM has been validated for use with individuals who have sustained TBI, but with recognition that issues of supervision and cognition must be taken into account.[105,211] FIM scores are used as measures of progress in rehabilitation, for determining the effectiveness of therapy, for estimating length of stay, and for making decisions regarding discharge planning, including the need for supervision or placement. The FAM was developed to provide additional detailed information about areas of functioning not covered by the FIM, including communication, psychosocial adjustment, and cognitive functioning, which are more specific to TBI and stroke populations. However, FIM and FAM scores are not as sensitive to the more subtle functional changes that may occur following the acute phases of recovery from injury.[233,234]

The GOS[603] has been widely used as a very general measure of recovery and outcome; however, it has largely been replaced, as it is difficult to ascertain detailed information for classifying individuals because of its brevity. An extended version of the scale, the GOS-E[603] increases the accuracy of description by extending the number of classification categories and adding a structured interview to improve reliability. The Disability Rating Scale (DRS)[450] is a commonly used instrument for rating general changes in functioning over the course of recovery from coma to community reentry. It was designed specifically for use with TBI populations. It addresses all three WHO categories of impairment, disability, and handicap and is also applicable to the WHO International Classification of Functioning, Disability and Health.[437,447] This instrument is reliable and valid for measuring recovery over time.[611] Although more detailed than the GOS or GOS-E, the DRS does lack the ability to monitor more subtle changes and is not as sensitive to measuring changes associated with milder injury.[611]

Quality of Life

Although a universal definition of QOL does not exist, it can be broadly defined as an indicator of the impact of injury/disease, treatment, and level of recovery that a person subjectively expresses after experiencing an injury/disease.[129] QOL in the TBI population has been measured by achievements obtained and subjective well-being.[135] QOL measured as achievements assess patient's success or achievements in life domains considered important to most people. These domains include physical, social, and mental issues.[135] Assessments measuring QOL as achievements are referred to as Health-related QOL (HRQOL). Common HRQOL include Medical Outcomes Study 36-Item Short-Form Health Survey (SF-36),[172] Sickness Impact Profile-5 (SIP-5),[546] and General Health Questionnaire.[347] Research is being conducted to develop HRQOL assessments, such as the Neuro-QOL, which are translatable across a variety of neurologic disorders. The TBI QOL is under development to measure HRQOL domains in patients with military-related TBI. QOL measured as subjective well-being occurs when patients assess what they currently have against their expectations or standards.[135] Subjective well-being is also measured in terms of life satisfaction. Tools used to assess life satisfaction in patients with TBI include Flanagan Quality of Life Scale[178] and Satisfaction with Life Scale (SWLS).[133] An online version of the SWLS can be found at www.tbims.org/combi/list.html.

Patients with TBI experience cognitive deficits, communication barriers, and self-awareness deficits that make assessing QOL a challenge. QOL reports from patients with TBI are valid because their QOL information correlates well with measures from relatives.[288] There are differences between QOL reports from caregivers and patients with TBI. Patients with TBI often report lower physiologic impairment than caregivers, whereas caregivers are more likely to report psychosocial issues than patients with TBI.[249]

Community Integration

Community integration is the ultimate goal for patients with a TBI. Community integration includes self-care, mobility, physical function issues, and participation in vocational, social, and community roles.[484] Common tools to assess community integration following TBI include Community Integration Questionnaire (CIQ),[484] Craig Hospital Assessment and Reporting Technique (CHART),[595] and Community Integration Measure (CIM).[366] The CIQ and CHART are objective measures of community integration through observation of behaviors and activities. The CIM assesses community integration from the patient's perspective. These tools focus on the subjective patient experience with regard to functional ability and personal autonomy instead of objective behaviors associated with integration. Community integration measures are collected through patient self-report. All measures can be collected by proxy except for the CIM. However, on the CIQ, proxy reports can be different from self-report.[115] Measurements specific to the examining community integration in the TBI population are the CIQ and CIM. Online versions of the CIQ and CHART are located at www.tbims.org/combi/list.html.

Vocational Rehabilitation

Return to employment after TBI can increase a patient's perceived QOL, social integration within the community, and home and leisure activities.[415] However, patients with TBI may experience cognitive, emotional, and/or physical deficits after injury, which limit their ability to return to prior employment or school. Vocational rehabilitation is a state-supported service that provides patients with disabilities aid in securing employment appropriate with their capabilities. A link to state-specific departments providing vocational rehabilitation services can be found at www.jan.wvu.edu/. Vocational rehabilitation programs assess eligibility and vocational rehabilitation needs, counseling and vocational guidance, employment development and training, assistive device or technology, job placement, coaching and follow-up, occupational licenses, tools and equipment, independent living services and advocacy support (http://ovrgov.net/services.asp). Vocational rehabilitation can either provide vocational services or refer clients to other agencies and programs that assist individuals with disabilities.

Family Education and Caregiver Burden

Rehabilitation practitioners play an important role in directing caregivers to education and community resource support services. National and statewide organizations and websites to assist with family education and caregiver burden needs provide community resources. National organizations for TBI caregivers include Brain Injury Association of America (www.biausa.org), Family Caregiver Alliance (www.caregiver.org), National Family Caregivers Association (www.nfcacares.org), National Alliance for Caregiving (www.caregiving.org), Rosalyn Carter Institute for Caregiving (www.rosalynncarter.org), and Well Spouse Association (www.wellspouse.org). These websites provide links to caregiver support programs, support groups, and workshops and seminars. Local resources for care management, in-home health care services, respite programs, hospice and palliative care, and adult day services can be found on these websites. Online resources including newsletters, teleconferences, e-communities, caregiver message boards, chat rooms, and pen pal programs are also available. Additionally, caregivers can access information concerning financial planning, insurance, legal rights, and advocacy.

Driving

Transportation is one of the most important links to community integration as a necessary component for access to work, social support, and recreation and health care use.[596] However, driving is a complex cognitive task, which requires skills like accurate reaction time, motion perception, spatial orientation, divided attention, multitasking, planning, decision making, and self-control. These are the same skill sets that patients with TBI experience deficits in after injury. Additionally, driving requires psychomotor components that may be difficult for patients with TBI if they have experienced other physical injuries such as limb fractures or visual impairments. Between 40% and 60% of individuals with moderate to severe TBI return to driving after their injury.[410] States vary on the rules and regulations on return to driving after an injury. Some states require a patient with TBI to be free of seizures for a period of time before they can resume driving.[410] Some states require physicians to report if they have a patient who is unsafe to drive. Other states require licensed drivers to report changes in medical status to the state before they can resume driving.

A formal driving evaluation is recommended for patients with TBI to assess their ability to return to driving. Evaluation and training should be conducted by professionals certified through the Association for Driver Rehabilitation Specialists. Evaluation consists of review of cognitive abilities and a test on vehicle operation. Driving simulators can assess a patient with TBI's return to driving potential before on-road tests. Also, driving simulators provide stimulation that may lead to improvements in complex neurocognitive skills needed for on-road driving.[332]

Veterans

As an unprecedented number of military personnel continue to return from recent conflicts with both diagnosed and undiagnosed TBI, the research and focus on clinical care related to brain injury continue to increase exponentially. Because of the nature of blast-related injuries, veterans have complex medical issues in addition to TBI and require comprehensive rehabilitation. As discussed earlier, pain and mental health issues occur at high rates within this population. Treatment needs to include cognitive-behavioral interventions, pain care, assistive devices, and mental health interventions.[487] The Defense and Veterans Brain Injury Center (DVBIC) provides resources and services for veterans who have sustained a TBI as well as patient and family education. The DVBIC also provides regional care coordinators, who serve as points of contact to assess TBI resources in communities where veterans reside, facilitate access to services, and coordinate individual plans of care.[149] A list of resources available through the DVBIC is located at www.dvbic.org/. Additional resources for veterans include After Deployment (www.afterdeployment.org/), a mental wellness resource, American Veterans with Brain Injuries (www.avbi.org/index.html), a chat room and forum for service members and family members, and America's Heroes at Work (www.americasheroesatwork.gov/), which provides employers with the tools needed to help returning veterans with TBI succeed in the workplace.

Community Services

Community reentry and integration is an important goal for the patient with TBI. Community services are available to assist patients with TBI and their families in this goal. Brain injury support groups provide persons with TBI and family members a forum where they can increase their knowledge of brain injury issues, provide emotional support to each other, network, and learn from other individuals who have similar experiences. State brain injury affiliates can provide information on support groups and locations (www.biausa.org/state-affiliates.htm). The Brain Injury Association provides an online national directory of brain injury services to locate community resources by state. Community services include community reentry programs, community-based programs, day treatments, transitional living, independent living, and recreation programs. The National Directory of Brain Injury Services is found at https://secure.biausa.org/OnlineDirectory/Directory/Default.aspx.

Prevention

Primary TBI prevention focuses on the prevention of road traffic accidents, sports injuries, falls, drinking and driving, and decreasing violence and domestic abuse[2] through policy and legislation. To develop appropriate prevention policies and programs for populations vulnerable to head injuries, it is important to understand the epidemiology of TBI. The Traumatic Brain Injury Act of 2008 was enacted to provide standards for surveillance of the incidence and prevalence of TBI in the United States as well as contribute to expansion and improvement of TBI programs.[1] However, in 1995, Congress changed a provision of the Intermodal Surface Transportation Efficiency Act (ISTEA) that included motorcycle helmet use. Several states modified or repealed their universal helmet laws, which had required helmet use for all riders. Following this policy change, helmet use declined nationally. The change in policy has affected TBI rates. Patients from states without universal helmet laws are 41% more likely to sustain severe TBI than patients from states with universal helmet laws.[99]

Secondary prevention focuses on decreasing bodily harm caused by an injury. Head injuries often result from sports-related activities including American football, rugby, ice hockey, baseball, soccer, cricket, horse racing, and skiing/snowboarding. American football and ice hockey have implemented the mandatory use of protective helmets as a means of decreasing the incidence of head injuries. Helmets attenuate the impact of energy and distribute this impact force applied to the head.[369] The implementation of helmet standards in American football by the National Operating Committee on Standards for Athletic Equipment, in addition to regulations controlling head blocking and tackling, has resulted in a 74% decrease in fatalities in the sport as well as a 84% reduction in TBI since 1976.[330,331] Although helmet use is effective in preventing serious TBI, it is unknown if helmets prevent concussions.[369] Many helmets include mouth guards, which are effective in preventing orofacial injury, although the evidence that mouth guards protect against concussion is inconsistent.[296] Helmets should also be worn in sports where their use is not mandatory. Ski helmets can reduce the incidence of TBI by 56%, although there is the potential for ski helmets to increase the risk of neck injury.[228] In baseball, softer balls can reduce the risk of injury by 28% in comparison with standard balls.[353] When evaluating the role of helmets in the safe use of recreational vehicles (e.g., bicycles, motorcycles, ATVs, skateboards and scooters), unhelmeted individuals had a higher rate of abnormal neuroimaging and admission to the ICU.[184] Research is also being conducted to determine how differences in ground surface (e.g., grass versus artificial surfaces) affect the rate of head injuries in sports.[403]

Advances in protective military equipment contribute to prevention of TBI in the military population. Current helmets are designed to reduce penetrating injury, but less is known about their effects on protecting against TBI caused by overpressure shock waves associated with blast injuries. Skull flexure has been identified as a mechanism that results in TBI after blast injury. Skull flexure can cause a TBI as the skull warps and bends inward in response to a shock wave.[396] Improvements to helmets that prevent against skull flexure include decreasing ability of blast waves to access the airspace between the helmet and head in addition to creating helmets that allow for the flexure of the helmet not to be transferred to the skull.[396] Body armor is beneficial in preventing TBI by reducing thoracic injury and the associated pressure wave transmission to the brain.[322] However, helmets and body armor that are incorrectly worn provide little protection against brain injury. Military personnel have been identified wearing helmets incorrectly.[64] Training on the benefits of protective gear, proper wear, and a better understanding of the mechanisms of blast injury and helmet design may result in increased TBI prevention in the military population.

Common automobile safety features that decrease injury include seat belt use and air bags.[436] New advances in automotive features that may contribute to decreases in injury include tire-pressure monitoring systems, electronic stability control, lane-departure warning, rollover prevention, adaptive headlights, rearview cameras, and emergency response systems.[383,542] Automatic collision notification technology can provide call centers with the exact location of vehicle crashes so appropriate personnel can be dispatched to the scene with faster response times and more efficient and timely patient care.[40] Motorcycle and bicycle helmets are effective methods for head injury prevention. Motorcycle helmets are 65% effective in preventing TBI.[360] Bicycle helmets reduce brain injury by 88% and severe TBI by 75%.[547]

Tertiary prevention focuses on the care management and rehabilitation of those already injured to further reduce consequences of the injury. Telerehabilitation is a novel way to provide rehabilitation to patients remotely in their homes or other environments outside the typical rehabilitation setting. Telerehabilitation can provide rehabilitation interventions for patients unable to access rehabilitation centers because of distance, disability, or transportation issues.[59] As this chapter highlights, rehabilitative care focuses on containing the injury process and preventing complications. Comprehensive transdisciplinary rehabilitation programs are necessary for patients with TBI to prevent further injury and return to an optimal level of function within the limits imposed by their injury. Importantly, translational research is important to enhance our ability to provide novel, personalized, and effective rehabilitation interventions.

KEY REFERENCES

16. Annegers JF, Hauser WA, Coan SP, et al: A population-based study of seizures after traumatic brain injuries, *N Engl J Med* 338:20–24, 1998.
18. Arenth PM, Russell KC, Scanlon JM, et al: Corpus callosum integrity and neuropsychological performance after traumatic brain injury: a diffusion tensor imaging study, *J Head Trauma Rehabil* 29:E1–E10, 2014.
27. Bales J, Wagner AK, Kline AE, et al: Persistent cognitive dysfunction during rehabilitation of traumatic brain injury: towards a dopamine hypothesis, *Neurosci Biobehav Rev* 33:981–1003, 2009.
37. Berger RP, Adelson PD, Pierce MC, et al: Serum neuron-specific enolase, S100B, and myelin basic protein concentrations after inflicted and noninflicted traumatic brain injury in children, *J Neurosurg* 103(1 Suppl):61–68, 2005.
43. Bogner J, Corrigan JD: Epidemiology of agitation following brain injury, *Neurorehabilitation* 5:293–297, 1995.
55. Brain Trauma Foundation, American Association of Neurological Surgeons: *Part 1: guidelines for the management of severe traumatic brain injury*, New York, NY, 2000, Brain Trauma Foundation, Inc.
67. Bullock MR, Chesnut RM, Ghajar J: Guidelines for the surgical management of traumatic brain injury, *Neurosurgery* 58(Suppl 2):1–58, 2006.
74. Cantu RC: Post traumatic retrograde and anterograde amnesia: pathophysiology and implications in grading and safe return to play, *J Athl Train* 36:244–248, 2001.
98. Clifton GL, Miller ER, Choi SC, et al: Lack of effect of induction of hypothermia after acute brain injury, *N Engl J Med* 344:556–563, 2001.
103. Corrigan JD: Substance abuse as a mediating factor in outcome from traumatic brain injury, *Arch Phys Med Rehabil* 76:302–309, 1995.
131. Diamond ML, Ritter AC, Failla MD, et al: IL-1β associations with posttraumatic epilepsy development: a genetics and biomarker cohort study, *Epilepsia* 55:1109–1119, 2014.
136. Dikmen SS, Temkin NR, Miller B, et al: Neurobehavioral effects of phenytoin prophylaxis of posttraumatic seizures, *JAMA* 265:1271–1277, 1991.
151. Elovic EP, Jasey NN, Jr, Eisenberg ME: The use of atypical antipsychotics after traumatic brain injury, *J Head Trauma Rehabil* 23:132–135, 2008.
155. Failla MD, Burkhardt JN, Miller MA, et al: Variants of SLC6A4 in depression risk following severe TBI, *Brain Inj* 27:696–706, 2013.
156. Failla MD, Kumar RG, Peitzman AB, et al: Variation in the BDNF gene interacts with age to predict mortality in a prospective, longitudinal cohort with severe TBI, *Neurorehabil Neural Repair* 29:234–246, 2015.

160. Fann JR, Hart T, Schomer KG: Treatment for depression after traumatic brain injury: a systematic review, *J Neurotrauma* 26:2383–2402, 2009.
164. Farooqui A, Hiser B, Barnes SL, et al: Safety and efficacy of early thromboembolism chemoprophylaxis after intracranial hemorrhage from traumatic brain injury, *J Neurosurg* 119:1576–1582, 2013.
165. Faul M, Xu L, Wald M, et al: *Traumatic brain injury in the US: emergency department visits, hospitalizations, and deaths*, 2010, Centers for Disease Control and Prevention, National Center for Injury Prevention and Control. Retrieved from: www.cdc.gov/traumaticbraininjury/pdf/blue_book.pdf.
180. Fontaine A, Azouvi P, Remy P, et al: Functional anatomy of neuropsychological deficits after severe traumatic brain injury, *Neurology* 53:1963–1968, 1999.
196. Giacino JT, Whyte J, Bagiella E, et al: Placebo-controlled trial of amantadine for severe traumatic brain injury, *N Engl J Med* 366:819–826, 2012.
197. Giacino JT, Zasler ND, Katz DI, et al: Development of practice guidelines for assessment and management of the vegetative and minimally conscious states, *J Head Trauma Rehabil* 12:79–89, 1997.
200. Giza CC, Hovda DA: The neurometabolic cascade of concussion, *J Athl Train* 36:228–235, 2001.
224. Guskiewicz KM, Weaver NL, Padua DA, et al: Epidemiology of concussion in collegiate and high school football players, *Am J Sports Med* 28:643–650, 2000.
236. Hamm RJ, Temple MD, O'Dell DM, et al: Exposure to environmental complexity promotes recovery of cognitive function after traumatic brain injury, *J Neurotrauma* 13:41–47, 1996.
301. Kochanek PK, Clark RS, Jenkins LW: TBI: pathobiology. In Zasler ND, Katz DI, Zafonte RD, editors: *Brain injury medicine*, New York, 2007, Demos Medical Publishing, LLC.
302. Kochanek PM, Carney N, Adelson PD, et al: Guidelines for the acute medical management of severe traumatic brain injury in infants, children, and adolescents—second edition, *Pediatr Crit Care Med* 13(Suppl 1):S1–S82, 2012.
313. Kumar R, Boles J, Wagner A: Chronic inflammation characterization after severe TBI and associations with 6 and 12 month outcome, *J Head Trauma Rehabil* 2014. [Epub ahead of print].
343. Maas AI, Steyerberg EW, Butcher I, et al: Prognostic value of computerized tomography scan characteristics in traumatic brain injury: results from the IMPACT study, *J Neurotrauma* 24:303–314, 2007.
344. Mac Donald CL, Johnson AM, Wierzechowski L, et al: Prospectively assessed clinical outcomes in concussive blast vs nonblast traumatic brain injury among evacuated US military personnel, *JAMA Neurol* 71:994, 2014.
345. Majerske CW, Mihalik JP, Ren D, et al: Concussion in sports: postconcussive activity levels, symptoms, and neurocognitive performance, *J Athl Train* 43:265–274, 2008.
358. Mayer AR, Mannell MV, Ling J, et al: Functional connectivity in mild traumatic brain injury, *Hum Brain Mapp* 32:1825–1835, 2011.
373. McNett M, Sarver W, Wilczewski P: The prevalence, treatment and outcomes of agitation among patients with brain injury admitted to acute care units, *Brain Inj* 26:1155–1162, 2012.
391. Moro N, Katayama Y, Igarashi T, et al: Hyponatremia in patients with traumatic brain injury: incidence, mechanism, and response to sodium supplementation or retention therapy with hydrocortisone, *Surg Neurol* 68:387–393, 2007.
407. Nichol AD, Higgins AM, Gabbe BJ, et al: Measuring functional and quality of life outcomes following major head injury: common scales and checklists, *Injury* 42:281–287, 2011.
437. Pistarini C, Aiachini B, Coenen M, et al: Functioning and disability in traumatic brain injury: the Italian patient perspective in developing ICF core sets, *Disabil Rehabil* 33:2333–2345, 2011.
448. Ramlackhansingh AF, Brooks DJ, Greenwood RJ, et al: Inflammation after trauma: microglial activation and traumatic brain injury, *Ann Neurol* 70:374–383, 2011.
449. Rappaport M, Dougherty AM, Kelting DL: Evaluation of coma and vegetative states, *Arch Phys Med Rehabil* 73:628–634, 1992.
480. Russo A, D'Onofrio F, Conte F, et al: Post-traumatic headaches: a clinical overview, *Neurol Sci* 35(Suppl 1):153–156, 2014.
485. Santarsieri M, Kumar RG, Kochanek PM, et al: Variable neuroendocrine-immune dysfunction in individuals with unfavorable outcome after severe traumatic brain injury, *Brain Behav Immun* 45:15–21, 2015.
486. Santarsieri M, Niyonkuru C, McCullough EH, et al: Cerebrospinal fluid cortisol and progesterone profiles and outcomes prognostication after severe traumatic brain injury, *J Neurotrauma* 31:699–712, 2014.
487. Sayer NA, Cifu DX, McNamee S, et al: Rehabilitation needs of combat-injured service members admitted to the VA polytrauma rehabilitation centers: the role of PM&R in the care of wounded warriors, *PM R* 1:23–28, 2009.
493. Schmitter-Edgecombe M: Implications of basic science research for brain injury rehabilitation: a focus on intact learning mechanisms, *J Head Trauma Rehabil* 21:131–141, 2006.
540. Teasdale GM, Murray GD, Nicoll JA: The association between APOE epsilon4, age and outcome after head injury: a prospective cohort study, *Brain* 128:2556–2561, 2005.
545. Temkin NR, Dikmen SS, Wilensky AJ, et al: A randomized, double-blind study of phenytoin for the prevention of post-traumatic seizures, *N Engl J Med* 323:497–502, 1990.
569. Wagner AK, Brett CA, McCullough EH, et al: Persistent hypogonadism influences estradiol synthesis, cognition and outcome in males after severe TBI, *Brain Inj* 26:1226–1242, 2012.
571. Wagner AK, Drewencki LL, Chen X, et al: Chronic methylphenidate treatment enhances striatal dopamine neurotransmission after experimental traumatic brain injury, *J Neurochem* 108:986–997, 2009.
587. Wagner AK, Zitelli KT: A rehabilomics focused perspective on molecular mechanisms underlying neurological injury, complications, and recovery after severe TBI, *Pathophysiology* 20:39–48, 2013.
597. Whyte J, Hart T, Vaccaro M, et al: Effects of methylphenidate on attention deficits after traumatic brain injury: a multidimensional, randomized, controlled trial, *Am J Phys Med Rehabil* 83:401–420, 2004.
612. Wright DW, Kellermann AL, Hertzberg VS, et al: ProTECT: a randomized clinical trial of progesterone for acute traumatic brain injury, *Ann Emerg Med* 49:391–402, 2007.
627. Zafonte R, Elovic EP, Lombard L: Acute care management of post-TBI spasticity, *J Head Trauma Rehabil* 19:89–100, 2004.

The full reference list for this chapter is available online.

CHAPTER 44

STROKE SYNDROMES*

Richard D. Zorowitz, Richard L. Harvey

The neurologic examination in acute care confirms the diagnosis of stroke and localizes the injury. In the rehabilitation setting, the lesion location is usually known, such that the neurologic examination focuses on identifying *expected* physical, communicative, and cognitive impairments characteristic of a particular stroke syndrome and on determining their impact on functional activity. Understanding stroke syndromes helps target the examination, which improves the practitioner's efficiency and the accuracy of neurologic assessment.

This chapter covers common clinical stroke syndromes that occur in brain regions above and below the tentorium. The syndromes described are those typical of arterial and branch occlusions rather than hemorrhagic rupture.

Supratentorial (Cerebral) Neuroanatomy

The two cerebral hemispheres are divided into four lobes: frontal, parietal, occipital, and temporal (Figure 44-1).

The frontal lobe is separated from the parietal lobe by the central sulcus. All behavioral motor output originating in the frontal lobe, including mobility, object manipulation, directional eye movement, and verbal expression, are assisted by the basal ganglia and cerebellum. In contrast, processing of all visual, auditory, and somatosensory input is integrated in the thalamus, parietal, occipital, and temporal lobes. There are also significant interconnections between primary motor cortex and somatosensory cortex, premotor and ventral motor areas, as well as connections from the thalamus to the motor cortex and from the motor cortex to the basal ganglia, superior and inferior colliculi, and cerebellum.

Cortical Areas of the Frontal Lobe

Primary Motor Cortex (M1)

The primary motor (M1) cortex is located in the precentral gyrus, anterior to the central sulcus in both hemispheres. It is somatotopically organized in the form of the classic "homunculus," where motor control for the feet is located in medial frontal regions; shoulder, arm, and hand are located along the superior lateral convexity; and face, tongue, and throat are located along the inferior convexity and the operculum (Figure 44-1). Lesions of the M1 cortex result in hemiplegia, often without spastic dystonia.

Broca Area

Named after Paul Broca (1824-1880),[10] the Broca area is one of the two primary cortical language areas. The Broca area is located in the inferior lateral convexity and within the operculum of the dominant (usually left) frontal lobe.[8,14] Lesions in this area result in impaired oral motor communication characterized by nonfluent speech production, apraxic errors, and problems with syntax. The Broca area is also important for facilitating the production of motor activity given on verbal command. In addition, lesions in the Broca area may also result in mild to moderate loss of auditory comprehension, specifically that of the syntax of complex sentences, and limb apraxia of both right and left limbs.[15]

Frontal Eye Fields

The frontal eye fields are cortical areas in the prefrontal area of the frontal lobe that are important in directional and exploratory eye movements. Each hemisphere contains two eye fields, the "eye field of the dorsomedial frontal cortex," and the other, located dorsolaterally, is the "frontal eye field".[34] A unilateral lesion of either eye field will cause a gaze preference and often head-turning toward the side of the lesion, away from the hemiplegic side. Patients with such lesions will have reduced saccadic gaze and visual pursuit toward the contralateral visual field. In addition, injury to the nondominant (usually right) prefrontal area impairs exploratory eye movements to the left and contributes to the attentional deficits seen in neurologic neglect syndrome.[23] Head and eye turning associated with nondominant prefrontal lesions is often more persistent, whereas that associated with dominant lobe lesions usually resolves within days to a few weeks.

Primary Cortical Sensory Areas

Primary Somatosensory Cortex (S1)

The postcentral gyrus is located anteriorly in the parietal lobe, behind the central sulcus, and contains primary somatosensory representation. Similar to M1, it is somatotopically organized with roughly the same organization anatomically as the primary motor cortex. Lesions in S1 result in loss of two-point discrimination and stereognosis in contralateral body. If subcortical sensory structures, such as sensory tracts and thalamus, are also involved, there may also be loss of pain, temperature, and joint position sense.

Primary Visual Cortex

Located on the medial surface of the occipital lobe, within the longitudinal fissure, is the calcarine or primary visual cortex. Unilateral hemispheric lesions of the visual cortex

*This chapter is adapted from Zorowitz RD: Infratentorial stroke syndromes and Harvey RL: Cerebral stroke syndromes. In Stein J, Harvey RL, Winstein CJ, et al, editors: *Stroke recovery and rehabilitation*, ed 2, New York, 2015, Demos Medical Publishing.

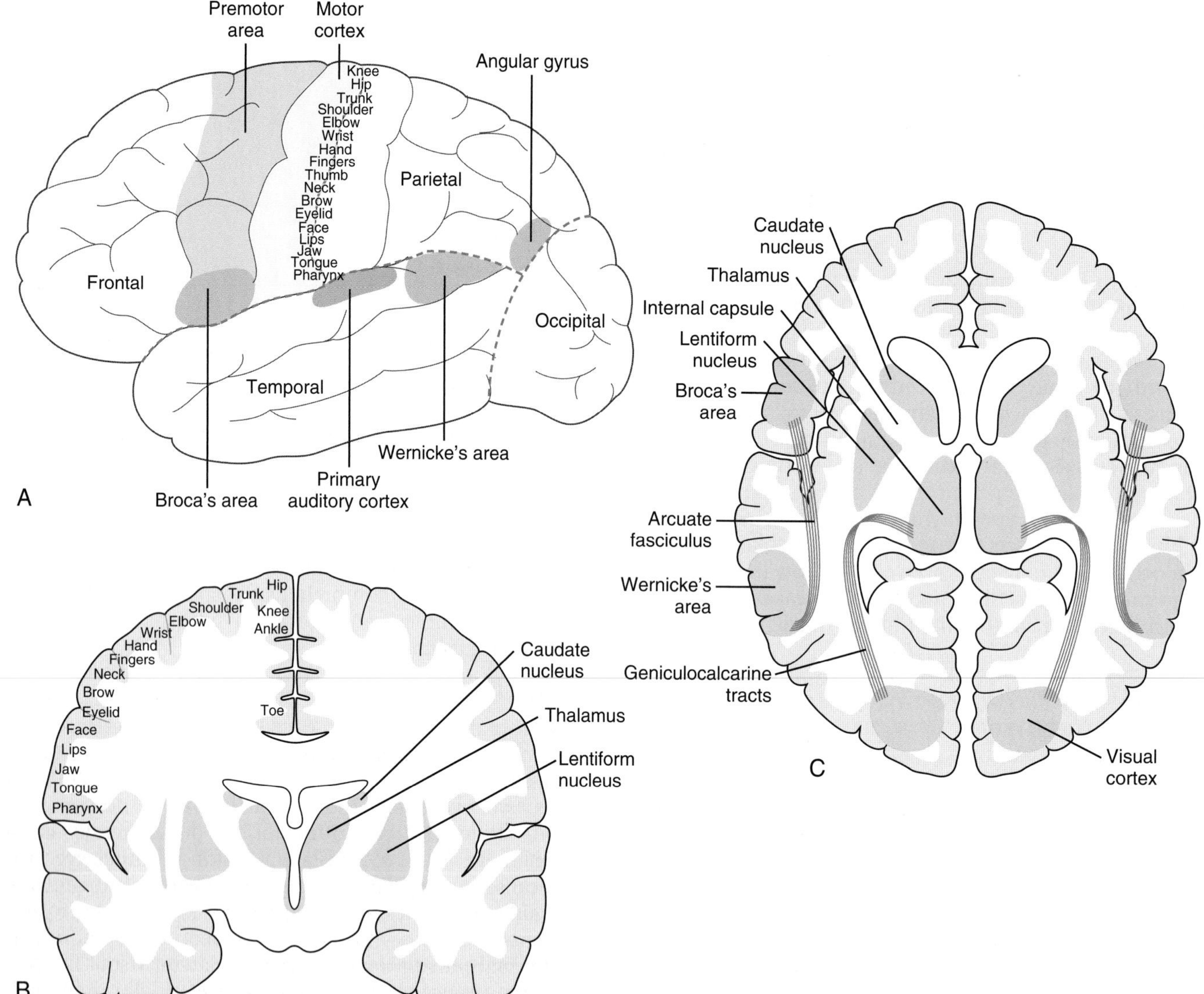

FIGURE 44-1 Cortical and subcortical neuroanatomy of the human brain. **A,** Lobes of the cerebral hemisphere and identified cortical structures. **B,** Coronal view of frontal lobe. **C,** Horizontal view with highlighted language and visual areas and associated tracts. (Redrawn from Harvey RL: Cerebral stroke syndromes. In Stein J, Harvey RL, Winstein CJ, et al, editors: *Stroke recovery and rehabilitation*, ed 2, New York, 2015, Demos Medical Publishing.)

result in a contralateral homonymous hemianopsia. Symptoms of homonymous hemianopsia are also associated with lesions involving subcortical structures of the temporal lobes because the visual tracts extend from the ventral posterior lateral thalamus, radiate posterolaterally into the temporal lobes, and then arch medially to the occipital cortex (Figure 44-1).

Primary Auditory Cortex

The primary auditory cortex is located on the superior temporal gyrus in the temporal lobe. This is also known as Heschl's gyrus and is more prominent in the dominant hemisphere.[16] Auditory cortex mediates pure tone recognition and is tonotopically organized by sound frequency.[20,35] A lesion on or near Heschl's gyrus does not result in deafness, but in the dominant hemisphere can cause complex auditory perceptual problems, such as pure word deafness.[31]

Cortical Sensory Association Areas

Posterior Parietal Cortex

The posterolateral parietal area integrates neural information from somatosensory, visual, and auditory cortices to construct a cohesive perception of three-dimensional space and the body's position within the surrounding environment.[24] Lesions in the left parietal cortex usually may cause only transient right hemineglect syndrome, but lesions in the right parietal cortex may cause clinically significant left hemineglect syndrome. In addition, lesions in the right parietal hemisphere may cause visual perceptual deficits resulting in spatial disorientation. Clinically, these patients are unable to draw figures accurately, cannot use blocks to build a simple structure (known as *constructional apraxia*), and are challenged to orient their clothing to their body while dressing (known as *dressing apraxia*).[5]

Wernicke Area

Named after Carl Wernicke (1848-1905),[28] the Wernicke area is located posterior to Heschl's gyrus in the dominant hemisphere. The Wernicke area processes spoken and written symbolic language into meaning and comprehension.[8,15] Along with the Broca area, the Wernicke area participates in a larger network for processing language.[23] Lesions in the Wernicke area result in impaired language comprehension and a fluent aphasia mixed with multiple paraphasic errors. Patients with Wernicke aphasia typically lack insight about their comprehension deficits.

Angular Gyrus

Immediately posterior to the Wernicke area is the angular gyrus, which receives visual input from the occipital lobe and the posterior inferior temporal lobe and mediates the processing of written language. Lesions of the angular gyrus can cause alexia.[8]

Subcortical Structures

Posterior Limb of the Internal Capsule

The anterior portion of the posterior limb, beginning at the genu, contains fibers of the corticospinal tract that descend from the M1 cortex. These fibers pass between the thalamus and the globus pallidus into the cerebral peduncle, and then into the midbrain as the ventral crus cerebri (Figure 44-1). The posterior limb of the internal capsule is somatotopically organized with face, hand, arm, and shoulder anterior to trunk, thigh, leg, and foot. Lesions in the internal capsule result in contralateral hemiplegia.

Thalamus

Located between the third ventricle and the posterior limb of the internal capsule, the thalamus functions as a sensory hub for somatosensory, visual, and auditory input (Figure 44-1). Lesions can result in mild hemiplegia or hemiataxia, sensory deficits, pain syndromes, mild aphasia, and neglect syndrome.

Arcuate Fasciculus

The arcuate fasciculus is a cortical-cortical white matter tract that passes reciprocally between the Wernicke and Broca areas along an arched pathway.[23] Lesions along the arcuate fasciculus can cause problems with repetition of language as well as limb apraxia bilaterally.[8,15]

Corpus Callosum

The corpus callosum is a large arch-shaped bundle of white matter connecting the two cerebral hemispheres (Figure 44-1). Depending on the location of the lesion, infarcts of the corpus callosum can result in a number of clinical manifestations attributable to disconnections between the right and left hemispheres.

Cerebrovascular Anatomy

Circle of Willis

In 1664, Thomas Willis provided the first complete description of the cerebral arterial circle, now commonly known as *the circle of Willis*.[36] The circle is supplied by three intracranial arteries: the right and left internal carotid arteries anteriorly, and the basilar artery posteriorly (Figure 44-2). The internal carotid arteries enter the circle of Willis at the point where the posterior communicating arteries (PComAs) branch posteriorly. The anterior choroidal artery (AChA) then branches before the internal carotids bifurcate into the middle cerebral artery (MCA) and the anterior cerebral artery (ACA). The basilar artery bifurcates into both posterior cerebral arteries (PCAs). The circle is completed by anastomosis of the PComA with the PCA and the anterior communicating artery (AComA) with both ACAs (Figure 44-2).

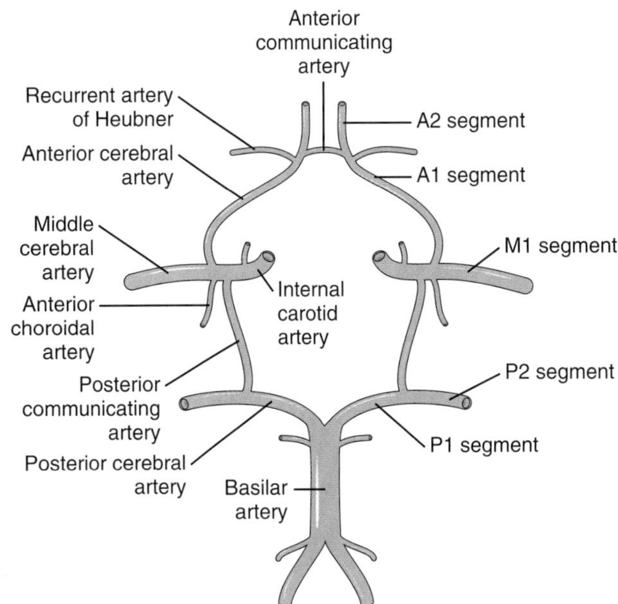

FIGURE 44-2 **The circle of Willis and associated branches.** (Redrawn from Harvey RL: Cerebral stroke syndromes. In Stein J, Harvey RL, Winstein CJ, et al, editors: *Stroke recovery and rehabilitation,* ed 2, New York, 2015, Demos Medical Publishing.)

The "typical" anatomy of the circle is only present in 35% of humans. Anatomic variations are numerous, including hypoplastic portions of the circle as well as the absence of the PComA on one side. In the presence of atherosclerotic disease of an internal carotid, retrograde blood flow from the external carotid artery through the ophthalmic artery may provide collateral flow. Leptomeningeal arteries may also provide another helpful but limited source of collateral blood supply to the cerebral cortex.

Anterior Choroidal Artery

The AChA is a major deep perforating artery that supplies the optic tract, globus pallidus, anterior hippocampus, and parts of the thalamus, including a branch to the lateral geniculate nucleus.[1,25] In addition, the AChA provides blood supply to the deep white matter of the temporal lobe. As the "AChA" name implies, the terminal branches supply the choroid plexus of the temporal horn.

Anterior Cerebral Artery

The A1 segment of the ACA extends in an anteromedial direction to the anastomosis of the AComA. The A2

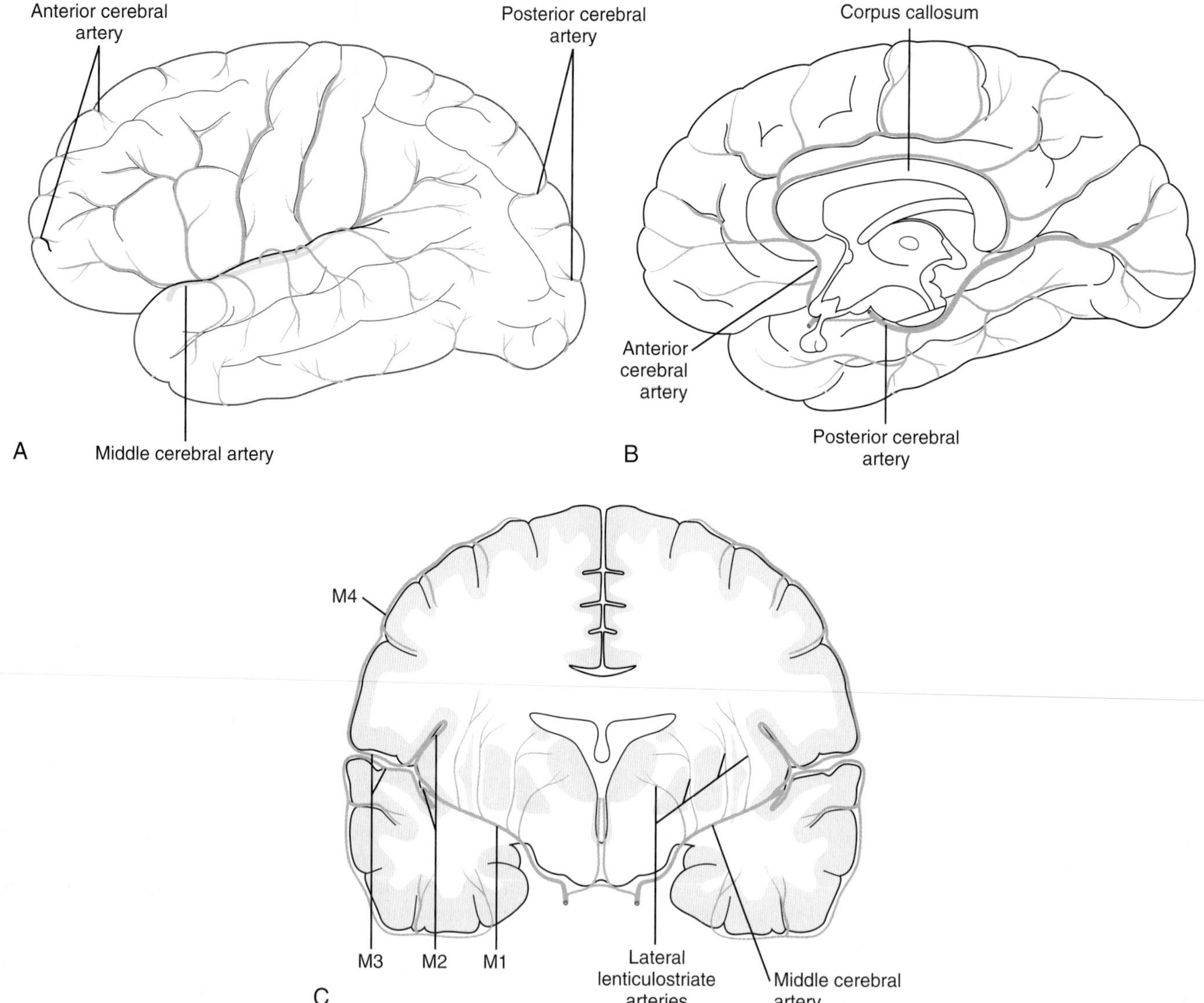

FIGURE 44-3 Vascular supply to cerebral hemisphere of the human brain. **A,** Vascular supply to the lateral convexity of the cerebral hemisphere. **B,** Vascular supply to the medial portions of the cerebral hemisphere. **C,** Distribution of the middle cerebral artery and the subcortical branches of the lenticulostriate arteries. (Redrawn from Harvey RL: Cerebral stroke syndromes. In Stein J, Harvey RL, Winstein CJ, et al: *Stroke recovery and rehabilitation*, ed 2, New York, 2015, Demos Medical Publishing.)

segment continues from the AComA along the medial frontal lobe within the medial longitudinal fissure between the cerebral hemispheres (Figure 44-3). It then passes superiorly and posteriorly around the corpus callosum to supply the medial frontal lobe, the corpus callosum, the cingulate gyrus, the paracentral lobule, and portions of the medial parietal lobe.[32] Tributaries from the ACA transverse over the convexity of the cerebral hemisphere and anastomose with tributaries from the MCA in a watershed region.

The recurrent artery of Heubner (RAH) is the largest of a group of the *lenticulostriate* arteries that supply the basal ganglia, intervening internal capsule, and other surrounding white matter. The RAH originates from the A1 or proximal A2 segment of the ACA. The RAH supplies the anterior caudate nucleus, anterior third of the putamen, tip of the outer segment of the globus pallidus, and anterior limb of the internal capsule. Within the dominant hemisphere, the RAH also supplies subcortical tissue near the Broca area.

Middle Cerebral Artery

The MCA supplies the largest volume of the cerebral hemisphere, including the basal ganglia, internal capsule, and visual radiations from the thalamus. The M1 segment courses from the carotid bifurcation laterally toward the insular cortex, along which it supplies a series of lenticulostriate branches to subcortical structures. At the insular cortex, the MCA divides into upper and lower divisions. The M2 segment constitutes the upper- and lower-division branches within the Sylvian fissure. The M3 segment includes the branches to the opercula, and the M4 are the branches overlying the cerebral convexities (Figure 44-3).

The superior division of the MCA supplies the frontal operculum, the lateral convexity of the frontal lobe, and variably the parietal lobe. The inferior division of the MCA supplies the temporal operculum, lateral convexity of the temporal and occipital lobes, and variably the parietal lobe.

Posterior Cerebral Artery

The P1 segment constitutes the section from the basilar artery to the branch of the PComA. The P2 segment courses posterolaterally to supply the medial occipital lobe within the longitudinal fissure, the posterior corpus callosum, and the medial temporal lobes, including portions of the hippocampi. Branch tributaries pass over the convexity of the cerebral hemisphere and anastomose in a watershed region with MCA tributaries. Other tributaries within the longitudinal fissure anastomose with those of the ACA in the medial parietal lobe (Figure 44-3).

Cerebral Stroke Syndromes

Ischemic infarcts can occur in all or a portion of a vascular bed supplied by an artery, depending on whether the occlusion is incomplete or total. Atherosclerotic or small-vessel disease can affect the quality of tissue perfusion in watershed regions of major arteries. Given the history and evidence on imaging of an infarct within a certain vascular distribution, the clinician should look for all components associated with a particular syndrome even though the patient may in fact exhibit varying degrees of signs and symptoms.

Carotid Artery Syndromes

Infarcts can occur from an occlusive carotid thrombus or thromboembolism to distal cerebral arteries (most usually the MCA). Watershed infarcts in the distal MCA distribution can occur, presenting with partial contralateral hemiplegia and a sensory deficit affecting the shoulder more than the hand and leg. Carotid thrombosis will often present with a transient ischemic attack (TIA), which usually lasts only minutes but by definition can last up to 24 hours. Amaurosis fugax, a transient monocular blindness, is a symptom typically caused by thromboembolism from the carotid to the ophthalmic artery with immediate thrombolysis. Often described as a "curtain dropping over the eye and rising again," amaurosis fugax more often presents as a visual obscuration, clouding, or fogginess variably affecting the whole or part of the visual field in one eye. Completed strokes from carotid thrombosis rarely result in both ipsilateral monocular blindness and contralateral hemiplegia.

Anterior Choroidal Artery Syndrome

Ischemic injury in the territory of the AChA will cause a contralateral hemiplegia because of injury to the posterior limb of the internal capsule. Hemianopsia can also occur, depending on what structures are involved. Injury to the optic tract can result in a contralateral hemianopsia and reduced pupillary reaction. A lesion to the geniculocalcarine tract in the medial temporal lobe can also cause contralateral hemianopsia. If the lateral geniculate nucleus is injured, a contralateral hemianopsia with median horizontal sparing can occur and is diagnostic of an AChA occlusion.[17] Visual sparing in the horizontal plane results because a portion of the lateral geniculate is supplied by the lateral choroidal artery. Dominant injuries of the AChA usually cause no language deficit, but nondominant injuries may cause a left hemineglect syndrome.

Anterior Cerebral Artery Syndrome

ACA strokes constitute only 3% or fewer of all strokes. Still, patients with ACA strokes have complex physical and cognitive deficits and usually require comprehensive neurorehabilitation services.[6] Patients with unilateral ACA infarcts will have contralateral hemiplegia worse in the leg and shoulder than in the arm, hand, and face, as a result of injury to the medial M1 cortex at the paracentral lobule. If facial weakness is noted, it is likely that the recurrent artery of Heubner was also occluded.[22] Sensory loss will be minimal, usually impaired two-point discrimination if present, and in the same distribution as the motor impairment.

Patients with ACA infarcts will often have limb apraxia that is limited to the left side when a verbal command is given. This is because the ACA supplies the anterior corpus callosum, which disconnects the right premotor and M1 cortex from the left language network. Motor performance of the right upper limb is not involved because the left motor cortex is adjacent to the Broca area.

When the eye fields of the dorsomedial frontal cortex are damaged, the head and eyes deviate away from the hemiplegia Associated findings include the grasp reflex of the affected hand, paratonia (a force-dependent limb rigidity that becomes more prominent with an increase in effort by the examiner during muscle stretches), and other "frontal release" signs, such as the palmomental or snout reflexes.

Injury to the supplementary motor area and cingulate gyrus can also result in reduced initiation and, if severe, psychomotor bradykinesia. Psychomotor bradykinesia can be severe enough to cause reduced verbal expression or even mutism that may be difficult to differentiate from aphasia.[8] Injury to the prefrontal cortex can also have a negative effect on executive cognitive functioning.

Patients with strokes involving the left recurrent artery of Heubner can have symptoms including a transcortical motor aphasia with reduced fluency, some apraxic errors of speech, and intact repetition. This is as a result of damage of the white-matter portions of the language network in the region between the supplementary motor area and the Broca area.

Middle Cerebral Artery Syndromes

Mainstem Middle Cerebral Artery (M1 Segment)

Occlusion of the M1 segment can cause injury to most of the lateral convexity of the cerebral hemisphere, as well as subcortical structures—including the internal capsule, visual radiations, and thalamocortical white matter—resulting from hypoperfusion of the lenticulostriate arterial branches. Those who survive M1 infarcts will usually have significant neurologic impairment.

A patient with an M1 infarct will usually exhibit complete contralateral hemiplegia from injury to the M1 cortex and the entire internal capsule. Contralateral hemisensory loss or hemianesthesia results from injury to the subcortical sensory tracts and the S1 cortex, although the thalamus itself may be spared. Infarcts of the ipsilateral frontal eye fields in the lateral prefrontal area will cause head and eye deviation away from the hemiplegia. Infarction to the geniculocalcarine tract causes homonymous hemianopsia in the contralateral visual field.

If the infarct is in the dominant MCA distribution, the patient may have global aphasia with reduced fluency, severely impaired comprehension, and an inability to repeat, read, or write resulting from damage of the Broca area, Wernicke area, the angular gyrus, and the arcuate fasciculus. A nondominant MCA stroke will cause severe visual and perceptual deficits with disrupted spatial body orientation, dressing apraxia, constructional apraxia, and a severe left hemineglect syndrome contributed in part by reduced left attention (from parietal injury) and reduced exploration (from frontal injury) of the left body and hemispace. Patients may deny that they even have any stroke-related impairments (anosognosia).

Superior-Division Middle Cerebral Artery

Occlusion of the superior division of the MCA results in a cortical infarct of the frontal lobe convexity, sparing the medial frontal lobe and subcortical tissue. Symptoms include contralateral hemiplegia affecting the arm and hand more than the leg, and loss only of two-point discrimination in the same distribution as the weakness. Patients may have transient head and eye deviation away from the hemiplegia, but visual fields are usually spared.

When the dominant hemisphere is affected, patients have Broca aphasia with decreased fluency of speech, apraxic errors, inability to repeat, and minimally impaired comprehension.[8,14] Patients have bilateral limb apraxia from injury of the frontal-lobe language network, but often also struggle to follow nonverbal motor command cues.

Patients with superior-division MCA strokes in the nondominant hemisphere usually have a hemineglect syndrome with reduced exploration of left hemispace and mildly reduced attention to left-sided stimuli. They often have deficits in visual spatial perception. The normal inflections that emphasize the meaning, importance, or emotional content of speech *(prosody)* may be reduced or absent.

Inferior-Division Middle Cerebral Artery

Occlusion in the inferior division of the MCA results in a primarily cortical infarct of the lateral convexity of the parietal, occipital, and temporal lobes. Patients with infarctions in this region have no motor or somatosensory deficits, but may have a partial contralateral hemianopsia because of partial injury to the visual radiations in the temporal lobe.

Injury to the dominant hemisphere from an inferior-division MCA stroke usually causes a Wernicke aphasia with fluent speech characterized by paraphasic errors and poor comprehension of spoken and written language. Patients with nondominant injuries have a hemineglect syndrome with reduced attention to the left hemispace and perceptual deficits.[5] They may also have a *sensory aprosodia*, or affective agnosia, in which the individual has a difficult time comprehending the prosody in another's speech.[7,29,30]

Posterior Cerebral Artery Syndromes

If an occlusion occurs in the P1 segment, hypoperfusion occurs in the distal PCA and the thalamoperforating arteries supplying the thalamus. This infarct will result in a contralateral sensory syndrome with hypoesthesia, a feeling of heaviness in the limbs, and in some cases dysesthesia (called Déjerine-Roussy syndrome[4]). Patients may also have a contralateral homonymous hemianopsia from direct injury to the primary visual cortex in the medial occipital lobe.

On rare occasions, a PCA infarct in the left occipital lobe can result in *alexia without agraphia*,[8,13] in which patients are not able to read but can write. The infarct includes the left primary visual cortex, causing a right homonymous hemianopsia. An infarct of the posterior corpus callosum disconnects the right primary visual cortex from the language network, thus preventing the patient from transferring words seen in the left hemispace to the language centers. Writing is not affected because there is no disconnection between the language network and motor cortex.[13] Patients may also have a left hemineglect syndrome.[27] Thromboembolism to both PCAs is uncommon but can result in Anton syndrome, characterized by blindness and visual anosognosia.

Lacunar Stroke Syndromes

By definition, lacunar infarcts are 1.5 cm or less in the largest diameter. Lacunar strokes are associated with hypertension and are caused by small-vessel occlusion from lipohyalinosis of the vascular intima. C. Miller Fischer reintroduced the term *lacunar stroke* into clinical stroke neurology when he described the lacunar syndromes.[11] Although as many as 100 lacunar syndromes have been described, 5 stand out as the most common seen in clinical practice.

The *pure sensory stroke* is characterized by numbness in the face, arm, and leg on one side of the body. There are no associated motor or cognitive deficits. The infarct is usually located in the thalamus. Patients with sensory strokes can develop late or chronic pain syndromes as a result of disruptions of normal sensory tracts. Lesions in other regions of the central nervous system along sensory pathways may also cause central poststroke pain syndrome.

Pure motor hemiparesis is also common and often results in functional limitations that require rehabilitation. The patient may have symptoms of only motor loss in the face, arm, and leg, with or without spastic dystonia on one side of the body. The stroke usually occurs in the posterior limb of the internal capsule, cerebral peduncle, or in the base of the pons. Prognosis for functional recovery is good because patients lack other symptoms, such as language, visual deficits, or apraxia. Spastic dystonia may complicate the rehabilitation process.

Dysarthria-clumsy hand syndrome, along with *ataxic hemiparesis,* are lacunar syndromes that occur commonly from lesions in the base of the pons caused by occlusions of the paramedian pontine perforating vessels from the basilar artery. However, dysarthria-clumsy hand syndrome can also present following infarcts of the genu of the internal capsule in the somatotopic regions for face and hand, as well as other areas of subcortical white matter. These patients have dysarthria and unilateral facial weakness without language deficits, and a mild hemiparesis of the upper limb on one side of the body. The prognosis for recovery is usually very good. Patients with ataxic hemiparesis often have a considerable challenge regaining independence in mobility because of problems with dynamic balance. The prognosis is still very good, because the ataxic component often recovers more rapidly than the hemiparesis.

Sensorimotor strokes most likely occur at the junction of the ventrolateral thalamus and the internal capsule, resulting in sensory and motor loss on the contralateral side of the body. Because the vascular supplies to thalamus and internal capsule are distinct, the likely explanation is that edema from a thalamic stroke compresses adjacent motor fibers in the internal capsule.[26]

Infratentorial Neuroanatomy

The infratentorial region, comprising the brainstem and cerebellum, spans between the diencephalon and the spinal cord. Despite its size, the brainstem has the potential to cause neurologic devastation if damaged. It carries fibers that affect motor and sensory function, as well as arousal and survival. The brainstem carries fibers that have important modulatory effects on both the cerebral cortex and the spinal cord. Although the cerebellum does not carry direct pathways from the cerebrum to the spinal cord, it also has the potential to cause neurologic devastation because it also modulates movement and tone.

Anatomy of the Brainstem (Figure 44-4)

The brainstem is the lower extension of the brain where it connects to the spinal cord. Neurologic functions located in the brainstem include those necessary for survival (breathing, gastrointestinal function, heart rate, blood pressure) and for arousal and wakefulness. The brainstem also surrounds a narrow passage for the circulation of cerebrospinal fluid. The occlusion of the passage, the aqueduct of Sylvius, is often accompanied by the neurologic complications of hydrocephalus.

Structures of the Brainstem

Midbrain

The midbrain (Figure 44-5) connects the pons and cerebellum with the thalamus and cerebral hemispheres. It consists of the cerebral peduncles, the corpora quadrigemina, and the cerebral aqueduct, a passage representing the original cavity of the midbrain that connects the third and fourth ventricles. Each cerebral peduncle is divided by the substantia nigra into a dorsal (tegmentum) and ventral (base or crusta) part. The major gray matter structures of the tegmentum are the red nucleus and the interpeduncular ganglion. The major tracts include superior cerebellar

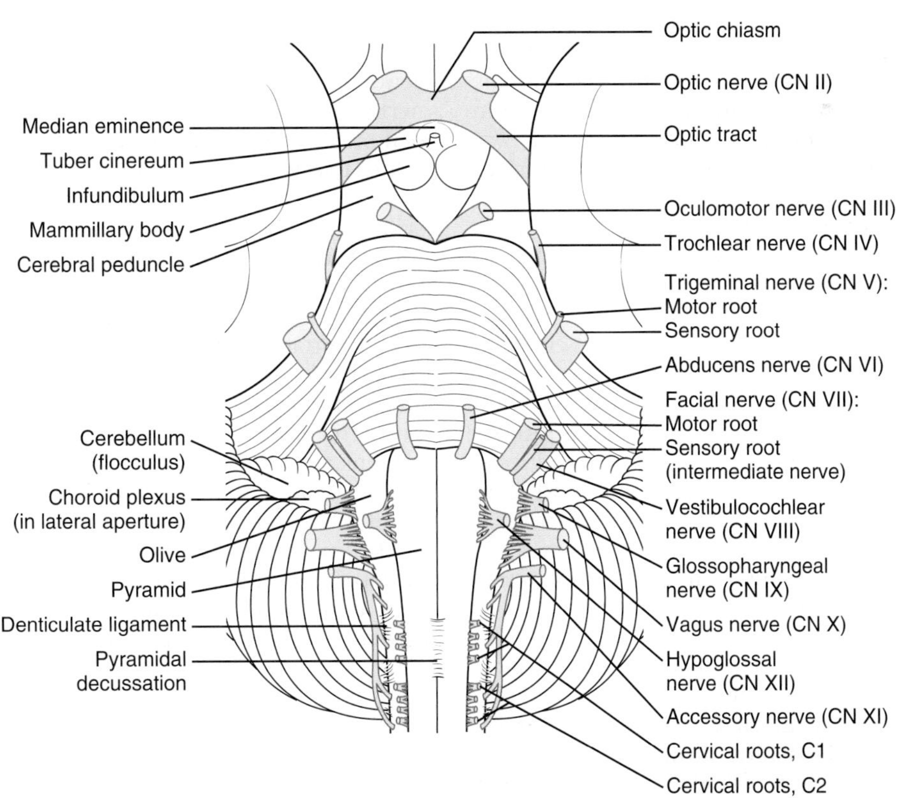

FIGURE 44-4 Neuroanatomy of the brainstem. (Redrawn from Nolte J, Angelvine JB: *The human brain in photographs and diagrams,* ed 4, Philadelphia, 2013, Elsevier Saunders, p 19.)

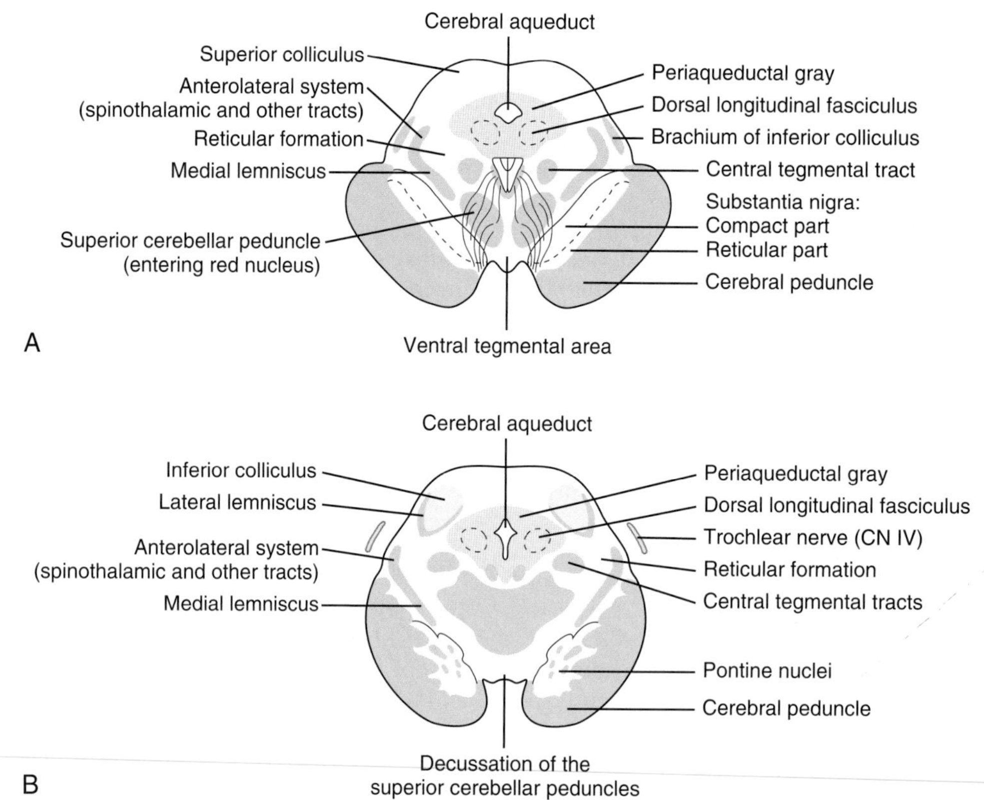

FIGURE 44-5 Clinical neuroanatomy of the midbrain. **A,** Midbrain at the level of the superior colliculus. **B,** Midbrain at the level of the inferior colliculus. (Redrawn from Nolte J, Angelvine JB: *The human brain in photographs and diagrams,* ed 4, Philadelphia, 2013, Elsevier Saunders, p 45-46.)

peduncle, the medial longitudinal fasciculus, and the medial lemniscus.

The red nucleus appears circular in shape and receives fibers from the superior cerebellar peduncle and medial lemniscus. Axons cross the midline and project into the rubrospinal tract, an important part of the pathway from the cerebellum to the lower motor centers.

The superior cerebellar peduncles (brachia conjunctiva) arise from the dentate nucleus of the cerebellum, pass rostrally through the dorsal pons to the level of the inferior colliculus, decussate, ascend farther, and terminate either in the red nucleus or within the motor, ventral lateral, or ventral anterior nuclei of the thalamus. The majority of fibers in these tracts convey signals from the cerebellum to the brainstem.

The medial longitudinal fasciculus (MLF) arises from the vestibular nucleus and is thought to mediate conjugate gaze. The MLF carries electrical signals from the abducens (cranial nerve VI) nuclei, across the midline, and then ascends to the oculomotor (cranial nerve III) and trochlear (cranial nerve IV) nuclei. The MLF also descends into the cervical spinal cord, where it innervates some muscles of the neck.

The vertical gaze center is located in the rostral interstitial nucleus of the MLF, just posterior to the red nucleus. Signals from each vertical gaze center are conducted to the subnuclei of the ocular muscles that control vertical gaze in both eyes. Cells mediating downward eye movements are intermingled in the vertical gaze center, but ischemia of this region usually results in selective paralysis of upgaze.

Pons

The pons (Figure 44-6) links different parts of the brain and relays information from the medulla oblongata to the higher cortical structures of the cerebrum. It contains the ventilatory and horizontal gaze centers. The pons is connected to the cerebellum through the middle cerebellar peduncle. The ventral surface of the pons (pars basilaris pontis) consists of superficial and deep transverse fibers, longitudinal fasciculi, and some small nuclei of gray substance (nuclei pontis). Cortical axons travel through the internal capsule and cerebral peduncle form synapses with transverse fibers in the nuclei pontis, decussate, and pass through the middle peduncle into the cerebellum. The dorsal surface of the pons (pars dorsalis pontis) largely consists of ascending projections of the reticular formation and gray matter from the medulla oblongata. Other significant structures in the pons include the superior olivary nucleus and the paramedian pontine reticular formation.

The paramedian pontine reticular formation receives input from the superior colliculus and the frontal eye fields. The rostral aspect of the paramedian pontine reticular formation (rostral interstitial nucleus of the MLF) probably coordinates vertical saccades, whereas the caudal aspect of the paramedian pontine reticular formation may generate horizontal saccades.

Medulla Oblongata

The medulla oblongata (Figure 44-7) functions primarily as a relay station for the crossing of motor tracts between the spinal cord and the brain. It also contains the ventilatory, vasomotor, and cardiac centers, as well as

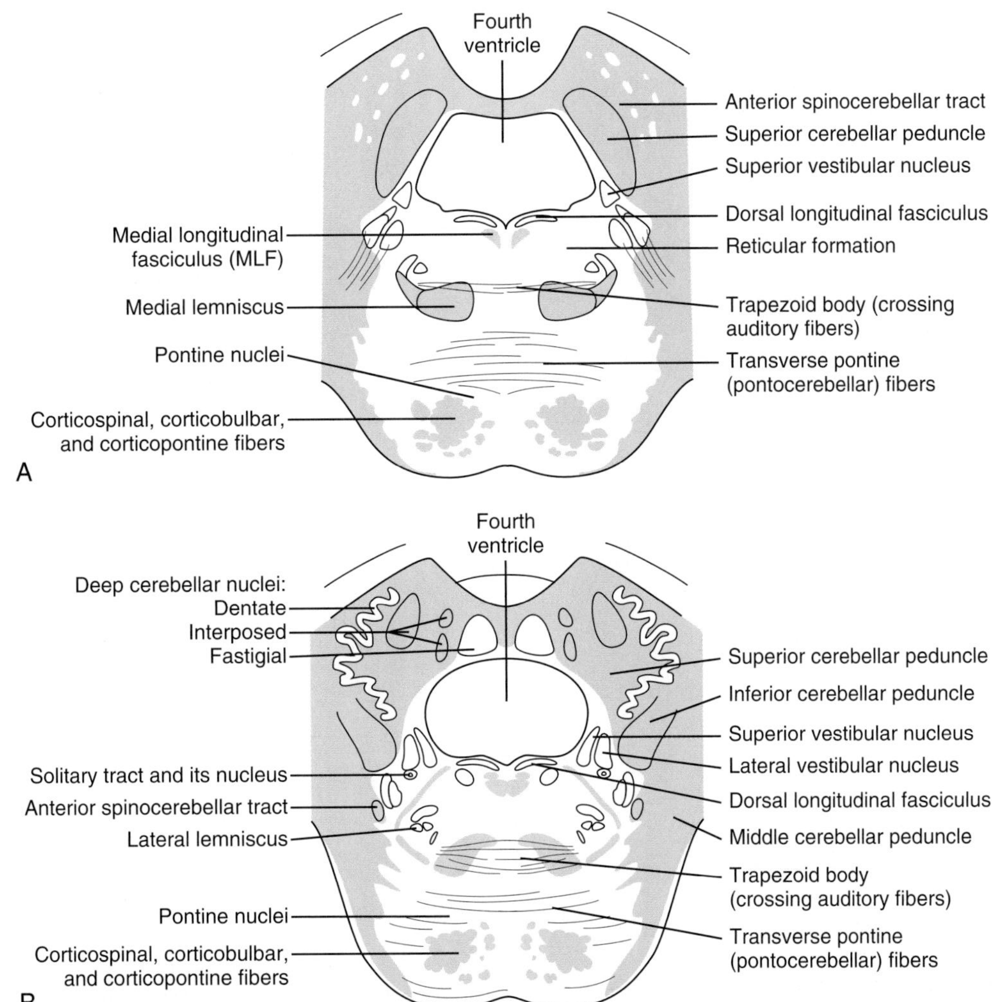

FIGURE 44-6 Clinical neuroanatomy of the pons. **A,** Midpontine region. **B,** Caudal aspect of the pons. (Redrawn from Nolte J, Angelvine JB: *The human brain in photographs and diagrams,* ed 4, Philadelphia, 2013, Elsevier Saunders, p 42-43.)

mechanisms for coughing, gagging, swallowing, and vomiting. Significant structures in the medulla oblongata include the olive and the inferior cerebellar peduncle.

The inferior cerebellar peduncle is a thick ropelike strand that sits between the inferior portion of the fourth ventricle and the glossopharyngeal (cranial nerve IX) and vagus (cranial nerve X) nerve roots.

The inferior cerebellar peduncles connect the spinal cord and medulla oblongata with the cerebellum. Proprioceptive information from the body is conveyed to the cerebellum through the posterior spinocerebellar tract. The inferior cerebellar peduncle also carries information from Purkinje cells to the vestibular (cranial nerve VIII) nuclei.

Nuclei

A cranial nerve nucleus is a collection of neurons (gray matter) in the brainstem that carry information to and from one or more cranial nerves. Ischemic or hemorrhagic lesions of these nuclei cause ipsilateral neurologic deficits, except for the trochlear (cranial nerve IV) nerve.

Olfactory Nerve (Cranial Nerve I). The olfactory nerve (cranial nerve I) ascends from the olfactory region of the nasal cavity through the cribriform plate to the olfactory bulb, giving rise to the olfactory glomeruli. The olfactory fibers form synapses with dendrites of one or two mitral cells that ultimately terminate in the cortex. Shorter association fibers connect various sections of the gyrus fornicatus (cingulate gyrus, isthmus, and hippocampal gyrus) that constitute the cortical center for smell.

The Optic Nerve (Cranial Nerve II). The optic nerve (cranial nerve II) consists chiefly of coarse fibers that convey only visual impressions from the retina. A number of fine fibers also pass in the optic nerve and are supposed to be concerned with pupillary reflexes. In the optic chiasm, the nerves from the medial half of each retina cross to the opposite optic tract, and the nerves from the lateral half of each retina continue ipsilaterally. Most of the fibers of the optic tract terminate in the lateral geniculate body, but some may pass through the superior brachium to the superior colliculus, or through the lateral geniculate body to the pulvinar of the thalamus. The superior colliculus receives fibers from the visual sensory cortex in the occipital lobe that pass through the optic radiations.

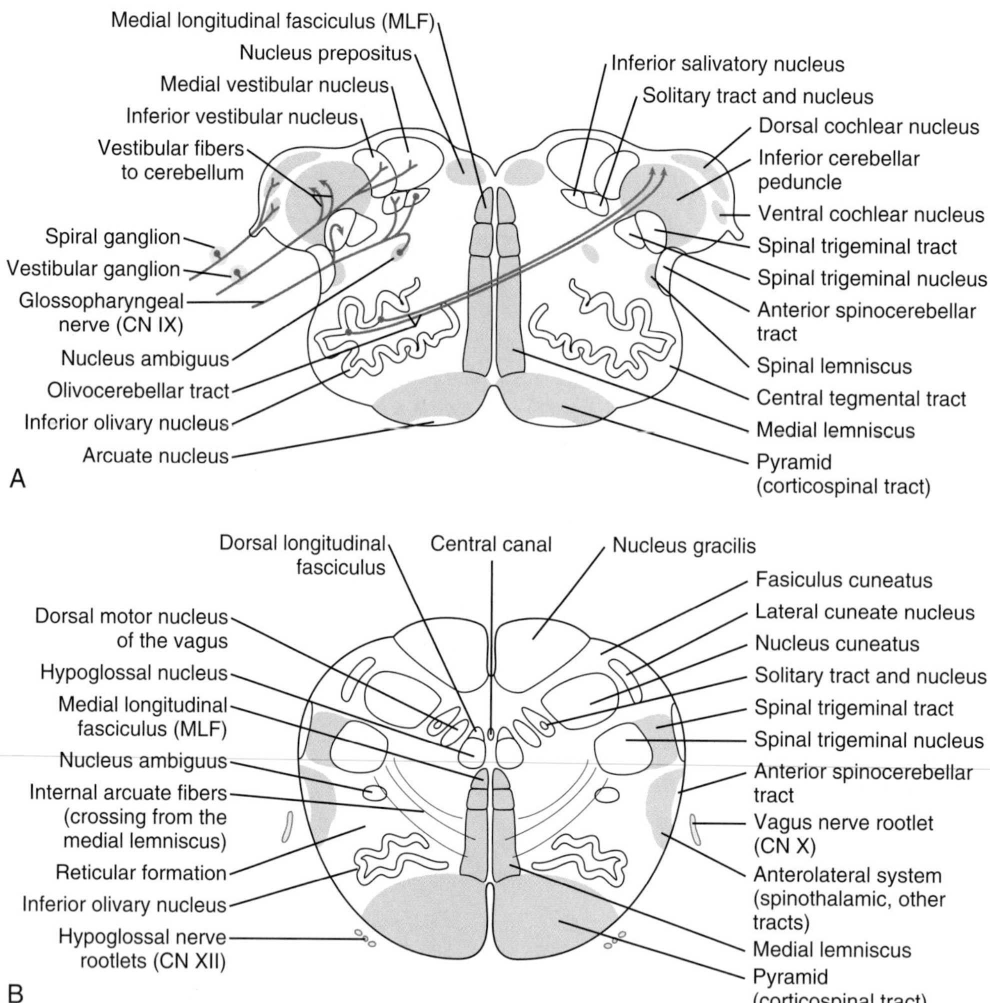

FIGURE 44-7 Clinical neuroanatomy of the medulla oblongata. **A,** Rostral aspect of the medulla oblongata. **B,** Caudal aspect of the medulla oblongata. (Redrawn from Nolte J, Angelvine JB: *The human brain in photographs and diagrams,* ed 4, Philadelphia, 2013, Elsevier Saunders, p 39-40.)

Oculomotor Nerve (Cranial Nerve III). The oculomotor nerve (cranial nerve III) innervates the inferior oblique, inferior rectus, superior rectus, levator palpebrae superioris, and medial rectus muscles. In addition, sympathetic efferent fibers are carried to the ciliary ganglion, where they synapse and ultimately supply the ciliary muscle and the sphincter of the iris.

Trochlear Nerve (Cranial Nerve IV). The trochlear nerve (cranial nerve IV) innervates the superior oblique muscle of the eye. The axons descend from the nucleus toward the pons, abruptly turn dorsally before reaching it, cross horizontally, and decussate with the nerve of the opposite side. Because there are no branches from the fibers of the pyramidal tracts to these nuclei, it is thought that the volitional pathway must be an indirect one.

Trigeminal Nerve (Cranial Nerve V). The trigeminal nerve (cranial nerve V) contains somatic motor and sensory fibers. The motor fibers supply the muscles of mastication, and the sensory fibers are distributed to the face and anterior two thirds of the head. The sensory nucleus consists of a main nucleus and a long, slender portion (the nucleus of the spinal tract of the trigeminal nerve) that descends to become continuous with the dorsal part of the posterior column of the gray matter of the spinal cord.

Abducens Nerve (Cranial Nerve VI). The abducens nerve (cranial nerve VI) contains only somatic motor fibers that supply the lateral rectus muscle of the eye.

Facial Nerve (Cranial Nerve VII). The facial nerve (cranial nerve VII) consists of afferent and efferent fibers. Taste fibers carry impulses from the anterior two thirds of the tongue via the chorda tympani to the solitary tract and nucleus. Efferent fibers that originate from the facial nucleus supply muscles derived from the hyoid arch. The dorsal region of the facial nucleus receives bilateral cortical input and innervates muscles of the upper face. The ventral region receives only contralateral cortical input and innervates muscles of the lower face. Efferent fibers that arise from either the small cells of the facial nucleus or cells in the reticular formation innervate the submaxillary and sublingual glands.

Acoustic Nerve (Cranial Nerve VIII). The acoustic nerve (cranial nerve VIII) consists of the cochlear nerve and the vestibular nerve. The cochlear nerve, the nerve of hearing, terminates at the cochlear nucleus. The vestibular nerve mediates the maintenance of bodily equilibrium.

The Glossopharyngeal Nerve (Cranial Nerve IX). The glossopharyngeal nerve (cranial nerve IX) contains afferent and efferent fibers. The afferent fibers carry sensory impulses from the external and middle ear, pharynx, and faucial arches. Efferent fibers innervate the stylopharyngeus muscle and the parotid gland.

Vagus Nerve (Cranial Nerve X). The vagus nerve (cranial nerve X) contains afferent, efferent, and taste fibers. Afferent fibers carry impulses from a small area of the skin on the back of the ear, the posterior part of the external auditory meatus, the heart, and pancreas; probably the stomach, esophagus, and respiratory tract; and the muscles of ventilation (e.g., the phrenic nerve and the nerves to the intercostal and levatores costarum muscles). Taste fibers conduct impulses from the epiglottis and larynx. Efferent fibers innervate voluntary muscles of the pharynx and larynx; facilitate the function of the esophagus, stomach, small intestine, gallbladder, and lungs; inhibit the function of the heart; and cause secretion within the stomach and pancreas.

Accessory Nerve (Cranial Nerve XI). The accessory nerve (cranial nerve XI) contains only efferent fibers and consists of spinal and cranial portions. The spinal portion innervates the trapezius and sternocleidomastoid muscles. The cranial portion supplies the muscles of the larynx.

Hypoglossal Nerve (Cranial Nerve XII). The hypoglossal nerve (cranial nerve XII) contains only efferent fibers and innervates the muscles of the tongue.

Tracts

The brainstem is the "superhighway" among the cerebrum, cerebellum, and spinal cord (Figure 44-8). Motor impulses travel from the cerebral cortex to the extremities, whereas sensory impulses travel in the opposite direction. Motor and sensory signals are also relayed to and from cranial structures through bulbar pathways. Signals to the cerebellum modulate movement and tone through extrapyramidal pathways. Impulses to and from the autonomic nervous system mediate the function of visceral structures.

Corticospinal (Pyramidal) Tract. The corticospinal tract is also called the pyramidal tract because the bundle of corticospinal axons looks like two columnlike structures ("pyramids") on the ventral surface of the medulla oblongata. At the spinomedullary junction, approximately 90% of the corticospinal fibers cross over to the contralateral side in the medulla oblongata (pyramidal decussation), forming the lateral corticospinal tract of the spinal cord. The remaining 10% of fibers remain ipsilateral, forming the anterior corticospinal tract. These fibers cross at the level that they exit the spinal cord and combine with the lateral corticospinal tract.

The corticobulbar tract carries signals that control motor neurons located in cranial nerve brain nuclei. The neurons in the motor cortex send axons contralaterally to the cranial

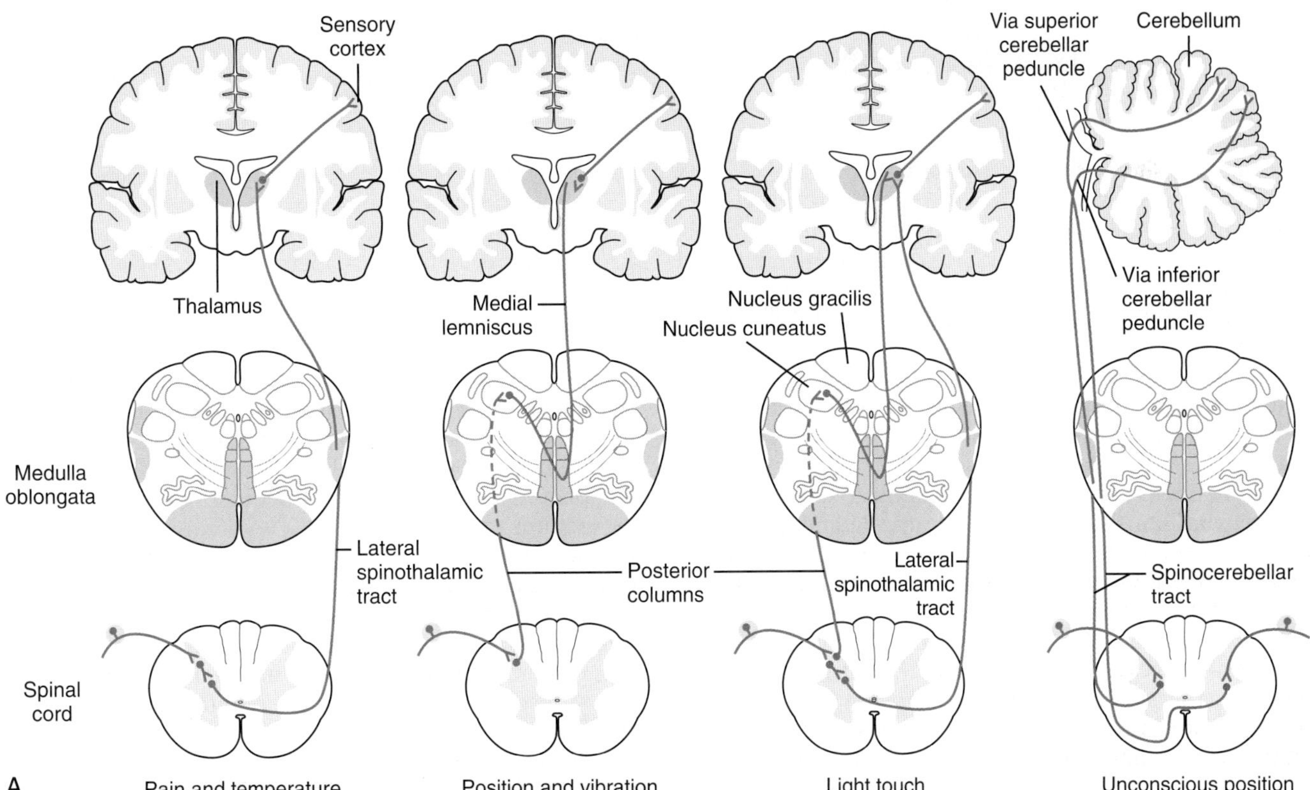

FIGURE 44-8 Schematic diagrams of the brainstem tracts. **A,** Brainstem sensory tracts.

Continued

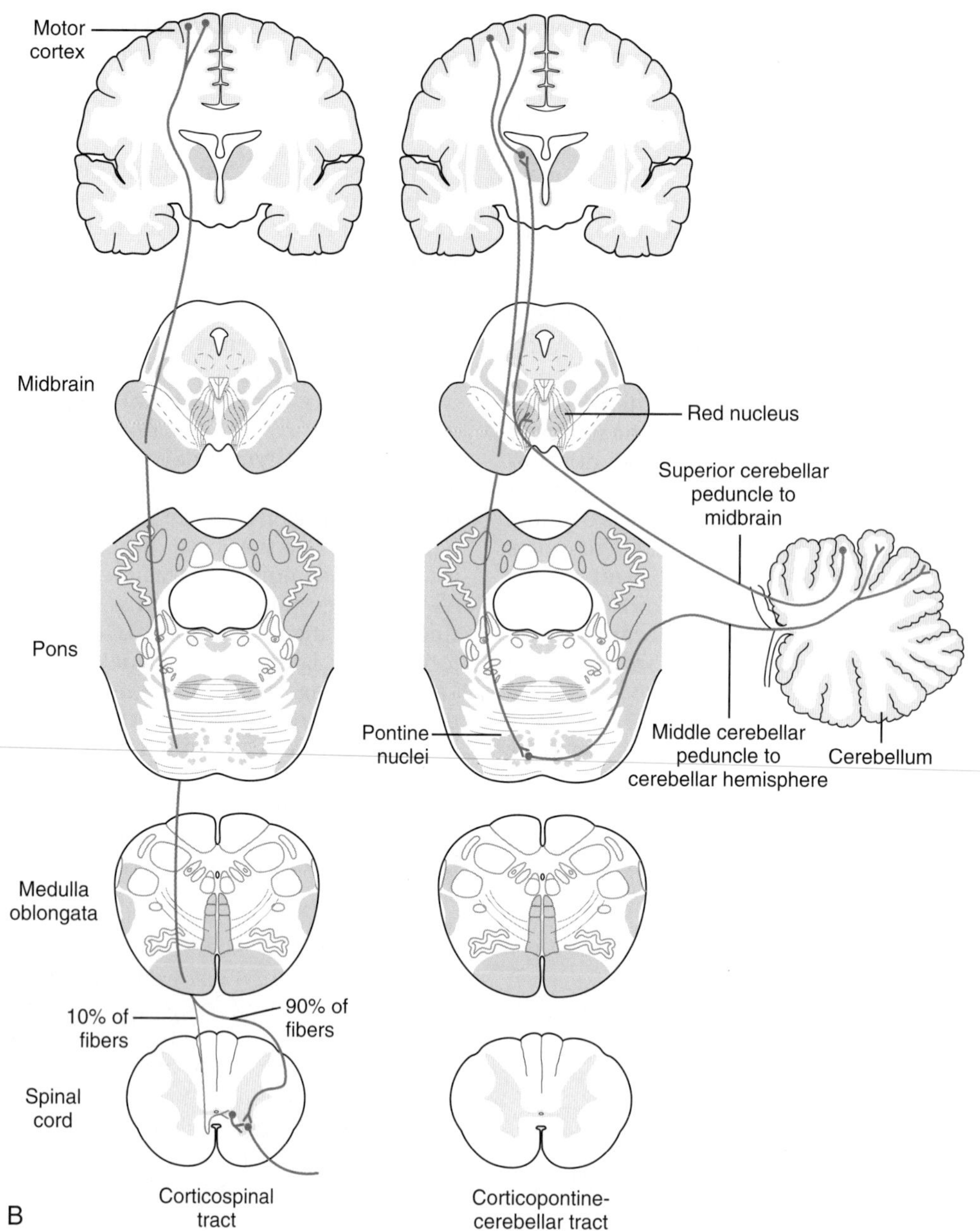

FIGURE 44-8, cont'd B, Brainstem motor tracts. (Redrawn from Zorowitz RD: Infratentorial stroke syndromes. In Stein J, Harvey RL, Winstein CJ, et al, editors: *Stroke recovery and rehabilitation*, ed 2, New York, 2015, Demos Medical Publishing.)

nuclei of the brainstem and decussate when they reach each cranial nucleus.

Spinothalamic Tract. The spinothalamic tract is a sensory pathway that consists of two parts: the lateral spinothalamic tract that transmits information about pain and temperature, and the anterior spinothalamic tract that transmits information about pressure and crude touch. The pathway decussates through the anterior white commissure one to two spinal nerve segments above the point of entry, and travels up the spinal cord into the rostral ventromedial medulla. The neurons ultimately synapse with third-order neurons in the thalamus.

Cerebellar Tracts. The cerebellum is connected to the brainstem through three cerebellar peduncles. The superior cerebellar peduncle connects the cerebellum to the pons and midbrain. The middle cerebellar peduncle contains contralateral pontocerebellar fibers. The inferior cerebellar peduncle connects the medulla oblongata to the cerebellum.

The cerebellum receives significant input from and gives feedback to the cerebral hemispheres through the corticopontocerebellar and cerebellothalamocortical tracts. The corticopontocerebellar tracts arise from all lobes of the cerebral hemispheres, most notably the prefrontal area, sensorimotor cortex, and occipital lobes. First-order neurons travel caudally to the ipsilateral pons and synapse with second-order neurons that cross to the contralateral cerebellar hemisphere via the middle cerebellar peduncle. The cerebellothalamocortical tract originates largely from the contralateral dentate nucleus and nucleus interpositus of the cerebellum. The fibers travel through the superior cerebellar peduncle into the contralateral ventral lateral nucleus of the thalamus. They synapse with fibers that ultimately terminate in the contralateral premotor and primary motor cortices (although some fibers may also terminate ipsilaterally).

Vasculature of the Brainstem

Vertebral Artery

The main blood supply of the brainstem comes from the vertebral arteries (Figure 44-9), the first branch of each subclavian artery. Spinal branches enter the vertebral canal through the intervertebral foramina. Muscular branches supply the deep muscles of the neck. A meningeal branch supplies the falx cerebelli. Medullary branches, or bulbar arteries, are minute vessels that supply blood to the medulla oblongata.

The posterior spinal arteries arise at the level of the medulla oblongata and enter the vertebral canal through the intervertebral foramina.

The anterior spinal artery arises near the union of the vertebral arteries, descends anteriorly to the medulla oblongata, and unites with the opposite artery at the level of the foramen magnum. It is reinforced by many small branches that enter through intervertebral foramina throughout the vertebral canal.

The posterior inferior cerebellar artery (PICA) supplies the medial and inferior vestibular nuclei, inferior cerebellar peduncle, nucleus ambiguus, intraaxial fibers of the glossopharyngeal and vagus nerves, and portions of the spinothalamic tract and spinal trigeminal nucleus and tract. Disruption of the PICA may cause Horner syndrome because it also supplies a portion of the descending sympathetic tract.

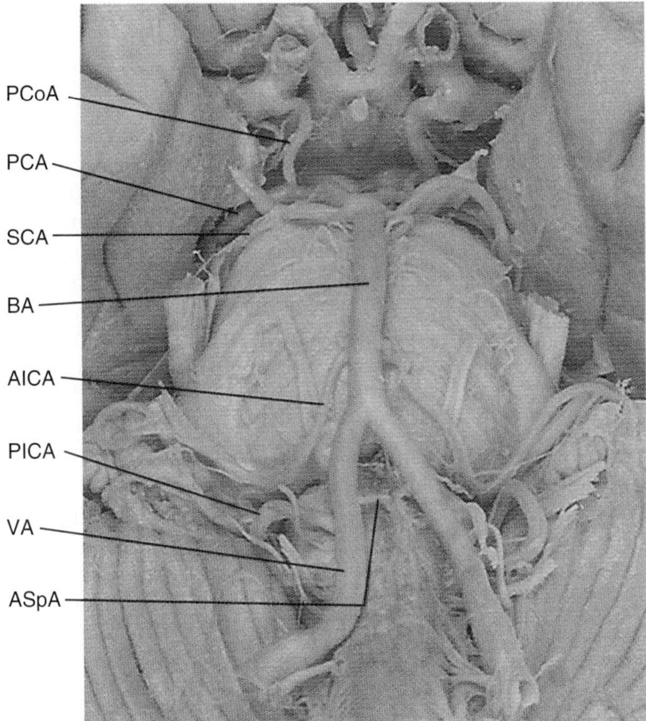

FIGURE 44-9 Vasculature of the brainstem and cerebellum. *AICA*, Anterior inferior cerebellar artery; *ASpA*, anterior spinal artery; *BA*, basilar artery; *PCA*, posterior cerebral artery; *PCoA*, posterior communicating artery; *PICA*, posterior inferior cerebellar artery; *SCA*, superior cerebellar artery; *VA*, vertebral artery. (From Nolte J, Angelvine JB: *The human brain in photographs and diagrams,* ed 4, Philadelphia, 2013, Elsevier Saunders, p 33.)

Basilar Artery

The basilar artery ascends from its union of the vertebral arteries in the inferior aspect of the pons to the superior border of the pons. At this level, it divides into the two PCAs.

The pontine branches come off at right angles from both sides of the basilar artery and supply the pons and adjacent parts of the brain.

The internal auditory artery arises near the middle of the artery and accompanies the acoustic nerve through the internal acoustic meatus, where it supplies blood to the internal ear.

The anterior inferior cerebellar artery (AICA) supplies the facial nucleus and intraaxial fibers, the spinal trigeminal nucleus and tract, vestibular nuclei, cochlear nuclei, intraaxial fibers of the acoustic nerve, spinothalamic tract, and inferior and middle cerebellar peduncles.

The superior cerebellar artery (SCA) supplies the rostral and lateral pons, the superior cerebellar peduncle, and the spinothalamic tract. Pressure from the artery on the trigeminal nerve is the usual cause of trigeminal neuralgia.

Anatomy of the Cerebellum

(Figure 44-10)

The cerebellum comprises the largest part of the hindbrain and is positioned posterior to the pons and medulla oblongata. The function of the cerebellum is the coordination of movement necessary in equilibration, locomotion and prehension. The cerebellum processes impulses that mediate muscle and tendon sense, joint sense, and equilibratory disturbances. The exact functions of its different parts are still not well understood.

Structures of the Cerebellum

Lobes of the Cerebellum

The cerebellum has three sections, a median and two lateral, which are contiguous and similar in structure. The

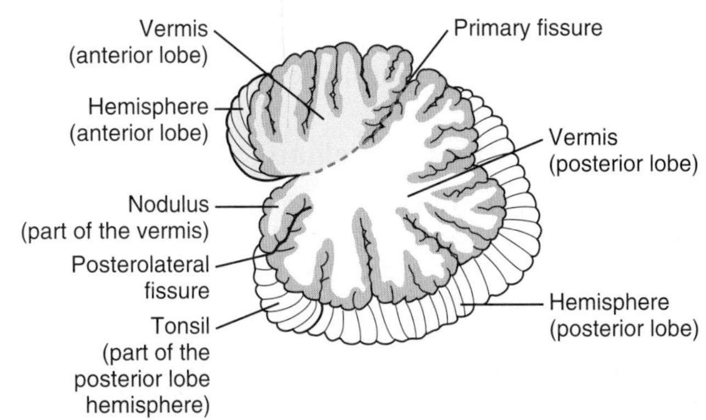

FIGURE 44-10 Neuroanatomy of the cerebellum. (From Nolte J, Angelvine JB: *The human brain in photographs and diagrams,* ed 4, Philadelphia, 2013, Elsevier Saunders, p 155.)

median section is the vermis and the lateral sections are the hemispheres. The superior aspect of the vermis is subdivided from anterior to posterior into the lingula, the lobulus centralis, the monticulus, and the folium vermis. The inferior aspect of the cerebellum is also divided into the midline inferior vermis and the hemispheres on either side. The inferior vermis is subdivided from anterior to posterior into the nodule, the uvula, the pyramid, and the tuber vermis.

Internal Structure of the Cerebellum

The cerebellum consists of white and gray matter. In the sagittal plane, the interior consists of a gray mass, the dentate nucleus. The white matter contains two sets of nerve fibers: the projection fibers and the fibrae propriae. The projection fibers consist of the three cerebellar peduncles: superior, middle, and inferior.

The dentate nucleus consists of an irregularly folded grayish-yellow lamina that contains white matter. Most of the fibers of the superior peduncle emerge from the anteromedial aspect of the dentate nucleus. It is responsible for the planning, initiation, and control of volitional movement.

The fibers of the superior cerebellar peduncles travel rostrally, decussate ventral to the Sylvian aqueduct, and divide into ascending and descending tracts. The ascending tract terminates in the red nucleus, thalamus, and oculomotor nucleus, whereas the descending tract appears to terminate in the dorsal aspect of the pons.

The middle cerebellar peduncles originate in the contralateral pontine nuclei and terminate in the cerebellar cortex. The tracts have three fasciculi: superior that distributes nerve fibers to the inferior lobules of the cerebellar hemisphere and to posterolateral margins of the superior surface, inferior that distributes nerve fibers close to the inferior vermis, and deep that distributes nerve fibers to the upper anterior cerebellar folia and inferior cerebellar peduncles.

The inferior cerebellar peduncles consist of a variety of nerve fibers. The dorsal spinocerebellar tract terminates in the superior vermis. The vestibular nucleus and tract terminate partly in the contralateral roof nucleus. The contralateral cerebellobulbar tracts travel from the contralateral roof nucleus and dentate nucleus. Some nerve fibers from the ventral spinocerebellar tract combine with the dorsal spinocerebellar tract. Other structures include the ipsilateral and contralateral nucleus gracilis and nucleus cuneatus, the contralateral olivary nuclei, and the ipsilateral and contralateral medullary reticular formation.

Vasculature of the Cerebellum

The cerebellum receives its vascular supply from branches of the vertebral and basilar arteries. When any of the arteries are disrupted, there is potential for collateral flow from the other cerebellar arteries.

The PICA traverses the superior portion of the medulla oblongata over the inferior peduncle to the undersurface of the cerebellum. It then divides into two branches: medial and lateral. The medial branch continues posteriorly to the notch between the two hemispheres of the cerebellum. The lateral branch supplies the undersurface of the cerebellum to its lateral border. It anastomoses here with the anterior inferior cerebellar and superior cerebellar arteries.

The AICA travels posteriorly to the anterior portion of the undersurface of the cerebellum. It anastomoses here with the PICA.

The SCA travels laterally around the cerebral peduncle to the upper surface of the cerebellum and dentate nucleus. It then divides into branches that supply the pia mater. It anastomoses here with the anterior and posterior inferior cerebellar arteries.

Midbrain Syndromes

The clinical anatomy of the midbrain (Table 44-1) is not as complicated as that of the pons or medulla oblongata. However, symptoms of midbrain lesions may be quite varied because of the multiplicity of functions for which the midbrain is responsible. In addition to facial and limb sensory-motor deficits, cranial nerve III and IV lesions may cause oculomotor deficits and Horner syndrome. Infarcts of the tegmentum may result in upgaze paralysis. Classic lacunar infarcts, such as pure motor stroke and ataxic hemiparesis, can be related to infarcts of the dorsolateral midbrain. Subthalamic infarcts may be associated with unilateral or bilateral ballismus or asterixis. Involvement of the red nucleus causes the typical resting tremor to worsen with movement. Coma or changes in consciousness may occur with bilateral midbrain infarcts, but neuropsychological changes should be suspected to result from involvement of the PCAs downstream of the midbrain lesions.[18]

Pontine Syndromes

The pons is supplied by three groups of arteries.[33] Branches from the basilar artery form the anteromedial and anterolateral groups. Branches from the AICA form the lateral group. Branches from the SCA form the posterior group.

Infarcts of the pons may result in a range of symptoms (Tables 44-2 and 44-3). Cranial nerve VI and medial longitudinal fasciculus lesions may cause oculomotor deficits. Infarcts of the paramedian pontine reticular formation may result in conjugate horizontal gaze paralysis. Classic lacunar infarcts, such as pure motor stroke and ataxic hemiparesis, can be related to infarcts of the basis pontis. Involuntary limb spasm has also been described.[19]

Pontine syndromes are classified in two ways. Table 44-2 uses an anatomic scheme, categorizing lesions as superior, midpontine, and inferior; and as medial or lateral. Medial pontine lesions usually affect the corticospinal tract and medial lemniscus, resulting in contralateral hemiparesis and reduced proprioception and vibration sensation. Lateral pontine lesions usually affect the trigeminal sensory nucleus or tract, autonomic fibers, and spinothalamic tract, resulting in ipsilateral loss of facial sensation, ipsilateral Horner syndrome, and contralateral

Table 44-1 Midbrain Syndromes

Syndrome	Structure	Symptom(s)
Weber	III Corticospinal/corticobulbar tracts	Ipsilateral ptosis, external strabismus, dilated pupil Contralateral paresis of lower face, tongue, arm, leg
Benedikt	III Red nucleus Corticospinal tract Medial lemniscus (sometimes) Spinothalamic tract (sometimes)	Ipsilateral ptosis, external strabismus, dilated pupil Contralateral coordination deficit (ataxia, dysmetria, dysdiadochokinesia, rubral tremor [coarse resting tremor that increases with movement], pseudo-Parkinson tremor) Contralateral paresis of lower face, tongue, arm, leg Contralateral touch, proprioception Contralateral pain, temperature
Claude	III Red nucleus	Ipsilateral ptosis, external strabismus, dilated pupil Contralateral coordination deficit (ataxia, dysmetria, dysdiadochokinesia, rubral tremor [coarse resting tremor that increases with movement], pseudo-Parkinson tremor)
Parinaud (dorsal rostral midbrain)	Pretectal nuclei (high midbrain tegmentum ventral to superior colliculus) Corticotectal fibers (supranuclear fibers to III)	Bilateral upward gaze paralysis Convergence paralysis, pupillary areflexia
Koerber-Salus-Elschnig (Sylvian aqueduct)	III	Ipsilateral ptosis, external strabismus, dilated pupil Altered mental status Abnormal respiration
Chiray-Foix-Nicolesco (midbrain tegmentum)	Upper red nucleus Corticospinal/corticobulbar tracts Spinothalamic tract	Contralateral coordination deficit (ataxia, dysmetria, dysdiadochokinesia, rubral tremor [coarse resting tremor that increases with movement], pseudo-Parkinson tremor) Contralateral paresis of lower face, tongue, arm, leg Contralateral hemisensory deficit
Nothnagel (dorsal midbrain)	III Brachium conjunctivum Medial longitudinal fasciculus	Ipsilateral ptosis, external strabismus, dilated pupil Vertical gaze paralysis Ipsilateral adduction paresis on attempted horizontal gaze, contralateral monocular nystagmus of abducting eye on attempted horizontal gaze
Akinetic mutism (upper segment of basilar artery)	Reticular activating system	Absolute mutism Tetraplegia with bulbar paralysis except for eyes

From Zorowitz RD: Stroke Syndromes: Infratentorial. In Stein J, Harvey RL, Winstein CJ, et al, editors: *Stroke recovery and rehabilitation*, ed 2, New York, 2015, Demos Medical Publishing.

Table 44-2 Pontine Syndromes by Location

Syndrome	Structure	Symptom(s)
Medial inferior	VI Corticospinal tract Medial lemniscus Paramedian pontine reticular formation	Ipsilateral horizontal diplopia with nystagmus Contralateral face/arm/leg hemiplegia Contralateral touch/proprioception hemideficit Ipsilateral conjugate gaze paralysis
Lateral inferior	Vestibular nuclei (VIII) VII Paramedian pontine reticular formation VIII Middle cerebellar peduncle V sensory Spinothalamic tract	Ipsilateral horizontal/vertical nystagmus, vertigo, nausea, vomiting, oscillopsia Ipsilateral peripheral facial palsy Ipsilateral conjugate gaze paralysis Tinnitus, deafness Ataxia Ipsilateral impaired facial sensation Contralateral arm/leg pain/temperature deficit
Medial midpontine	Middle cerebellar peduncle Corticospinal/corticobulbar tracts Variable medial meniscus	Ipsilateral ataxia arm/leg and gait Contralateral face/arm/leg hemiplegia, eye deviation Contralateral touch/proprioception deficit
Lateral midpontine	Middle cerebral peduncle V motor V sensory	Ipsilateral limb ataxia Ipsilateral mastication muscle paralysis Ipsilateral hemisensory deficit (including corneal reflex)
Medial superior	Superior/middle cerebellar peduncle Medial longitudinal fasciculus Central tegmental bundle Corticospinal/corticobulbar tracts Rare medial lemniscus	Ipsilateral cerebellar ataxia Internuclear ophthalmoplegia Palate/pharynx/vocal cord/ventilatory apparatus/face/oculomotor apparatus myoclonus Contralateral face/arm/leg hemiplegia Contralateral touch/proprioception face/arm/leg hemideficit
Lateral superior	Superior/middle cerebellar peduncle Vestibular nuclei (VIII) Spinothalamic tract Lateral medial lemniscus Unknown	Ipsilateral arm/leg/gait ataxia Dizziness, nausea, vomiting, horizontal nystagmus Contralateral face/arm/leg pain/temperature loss Touch/proprioception leg > arm hemideficit Conjugate gaze paresis to side of lesion, loss of optokinetic nystagmus, skew deviation, Horner syndrome

From Zorowitz RD: Stroke Syndromes: Infratentorial. In Stein J, Harvey RL, Winstein CJ, et al, editors: *Stroke recovery and rehabilitation*, ed 2, New York, 2015, Demos Medical Publishing.

Table 44-3 Pontine Syndromes by Eponym

Syndrome	Structure	Symptom(s)
Millard-Gubler	VII tract Corticospinal tract	Ipsilateral facial palsy Contralateral arm/leg hemiparesis
Foville	Paramedian pontine reticular formation VII Corticospinal tract	Ipsilateral horizontal gaze palsy Ipsilateral facial palsy Contralateral arm/leg hemiparesis
Raymond	VI tract Corticospinal tract	Ipsilateral lateral rectus paresis Contralateral arm/leg hemiparesis
Pontocerebellar angle	VIII Inferior/middle cerebellar peduncles V spinal tract VII Spinothalamic tract Occasional XI, XII	Early ipsilateral tinnitus, deafness, head tilt/rotation; late hyperacusis Ipsilateral intention tremor, dysmetria, ataxic gait, adiadochokinesis Ipsilateral facial pain/temperature hemisensory deficit Ipsilateral facial palsy, taste loss anterior two thirds of tongue Contralateral arm/leg pain/temperature hemisensory deficit Ipsilateral trapezius, tongue
Brissaud	VII Corticospinal tract	Ipsilateral facial spasm Contralateral arm/leg hemiparesis
One-and-a-half	Paramedian pontine reticular formation Medial longitudinal fasciculus	Ipsilateral horizontal gaze palsy Contralateral internuclear ophthalmoplegia
Locked-in	Bilateral corticospinal/corticobulbar tract Bilateral paramedian pontine Reticular formation	Tetraplegia with facial palsy (except blinking eyes) Bilateral horizontal gaze palsy

From Zorowitz RD: Stroke Syndromes: Infratentorial. In Stein J, Harvey RL, Winstein CJ, et al, editors: *Stroke recovery and rehabilitation*, ed 2, New York, 2015, Demos Medical Publishing.

loss of pain and temperature. Table 44-3 lists pontine syndromes by eponym.

Locked-In Syndrome

Locked-in syndrome occurs when an occlusion of the basilar artery causes an infarction of the basis pontis bilaterally. The corticospinal and corticobulbar tracts are interrupted, resulting in tetraplegia and paralysis of all cranial nerve muscles except for those controlling eye movements. It is not unusual for the paramedian pontine reticular formation to be affected, such that horizontal eye movements are affected and only vertical eye movements are preserved. Because the reticular formation above the caudal pons is spared, patients remain awake and aware. Their only means of communication is systematic eye movements that can be used manually to respond to questions or with augmentative communication devices.

Medullary Syndromes

The medulla oblongata receives its blood supply from a number of penetrating arteries located in the distal vertebral artery. There may also be variable blood supplies from small branches of the PICA, AICA, or the basilar artery. Typically, a lateral medullary infarct occurs because of occlusion of one or more of these penetrating arteries (Table 44-4), or more often by occlusion of the vertebral artery.[12] The dorsal medulla oblongata receives its blood supply exclusively from the PICA and is usually accompanied by cerebellar infarction.[9] The medial medulla oblongata receives its blood supply caudally from penetrating arteries of the anterior spinal artery, and rostrally from branches of the vertebral artery.[3] Medial infarcts usually affect the corticospinal tracts, causing contralateral hemiparesis. Lateral infarcts usually involve the spinothalamic tracts, resulting in contralateral loss of pain and temperature. Other infarcts may also occur but are less common.

Cerebellar Syndromes

Cerebellar infarcts (Table 44-5) typically have presenting cardinal signs of vertigo, headache, emesis, and gait ataxia.[21] However, it was not until the advent of magnetic resonance imaging that clinicians could accurately diagnose cerebellar infarcts and correlate them with vascular territories. There is now a better understanding of how to characterize cerebellar infarcts based on the vascular territories they supply. Table 44-5 reflects one of these classification schema.[2]

Conclusion

Recognition of signs and symptoms of stroke syndromes is essential in the diagnosis and treatment of stroke. Strokes affect a wide variety of body systems, and knowledge of combinations of neurologic signs is vital if one is to suspect the presence of an infarct or hemorrhage. Although imaging modalities have vastly improved to visualize previously unvisualizable lesions, the diagnosis of a stroke still begins with a detailed physical examination and knowledge of neuroanatomic correlates. With a more detailed knowledge base, clinicians may be able to more effectively diagnose and treat strokes with appropriate physical and pharmacologic modalities. With more effective and varied treatments, clinicians may be able to improve functional outcomes and quality of life in the future.

Table 44-4 Medullary Syndromes

Syndrome	Structure	Symptom(s)
Paramedian bulbar ("Hypoglossal hemiplegia alternans")	XII Corticospinal tract Medial lemniscus	Ipsilateral paralysis of tongue Contralateral hemiplegia (arm > leg) Contralateral touch/proprioception arm/leg hemideficit
Lateral bulbar (Wallenberg)	Lower vestibular nuclei Nucleus ambiguus (IX, X motor) V spinal tract Spinothalamic tract Spinocerebellar/olivocerebellar tracts Pupillodilator (sympathetic) fibers	Vertigo, dizziness, nausea, vomiting Dysphagia, hiccups, dysphonia, uvula deviates to normal side Ipsilateral face pain/temperature hemideficit Contralateral arm/leg pain/temperature hemideficit Ipsilateral hypotonia, ataxia of limbs (UE > LE) Ipsilateral Horner sign (ptosis, miosis, anhidrosis)
Avellis	Nucleus ambiguus (X, bulbar XI) Solitary tract (sensory X) Spinothalamic tract	Ipsilateral soft palate, pharynx, larynx paralysis; dysarthria; dysphagia Ipsilateral pharynx, larynx hemisensory deficit Contralateral UE/LE pain/temperature hemisensory deficit
Schmidt	X Spinal XI	Ipsilateral soft palate, pharynx, larynx paralysis; dysarthria; dysphagia Ipsilateral sternocleidomastoid paralysis, sometimes trapezius paralysis
Jackson	X XI XII	Ipsilateral soft palate, pharynx, larynx paralysis Ipsilateral sternocleidomastoid, trapezius paralysis Ipsilateral tongue paralysis, atrophy
Tapia	X XII	Ipsilateral soft palate, pharynx, larynx paralysis Ipsilateral tongue paralysis, atrophy
Bonnier	VIII IX X Corticospinal tract Other	Paroxysmal vertigo Loss of taste on posterior third of tongue Ipsilateral soft palate, pharynx, larynx paralysis Contralateral hemiplegia (arm > leg) Somnolence at times Apprehension, tachycardia
Babinski-Nageotte bulbar (similar to Wallenberg syndrome with addition of hemiplegia)	IX X/bulbar XI XII V spinal tract Spinocerebellar tract Corticospinal tract Spinothalamic tract Pupillodilator (sympathetic) fibers	Loss of taste on posterior third of tongue Ipsilateral soft palate, pharynx, larynx paralysis Ipsilateral tongue paralysis, atrophy Ipsilateral face pain/temperature hemideficit Ipsilateral hypotonia, ataxia of limbs (UE > LE) Contralateral hemiplegia (arm > leg) Contralateral arm/leg pain/temperature hemideficit Ipsilateral Horner sign (ptosis, miosis, anhidrosis)

From Zorowitz RD: Stroke Syndromes: Infratentorial. In Stein J, Harvey RL, Winstein CJ, et al, editors: *Stroke recovery and rehabilitation*, ed 2, New York, 2015, Demos Medical Publishing.
LE, Lower extremity; *UE*, upper extremity.

Table 44-5
Cerebellar Syndromes

Syndrome	Structure	Symptom(s)
Rostral (superior cerebellar)	Subthalamic area, thalamus, occipitotemporal lobes Lateral tegmental area of upper pons	Coma ± tetraplegia Ipsilateral dysmetria, Horner syndrome; contralateral pain/temperature hemisensory deficit, IV palsy Dysarthria; headache; dizziness; emesis; delayed coma (pseudotumor form)
Medial (anterior inferior cerebellar)	Lateral area of lower pons	Ipsilateral V, VII, VIII, Horner syndrome, dysmetria Contralateral pain/temperature Hemisensory deficit
Caudal (posterior inferior cerebellar)	Dorsolateral medullary area	Vertigo, headache, emesis, ataxia, delayed coma (pseudotumor form)
Caudal and medial	Lateral area lower pons and/or lateral medullary area	Vertigo, headache, emesis, ataxia, delayed coma (pseudotumor form)
Rostrocaudal	Brainstem, thalamus, occipitotemporal lobe	Coma ± tetraplegia

From Zorowitz RD: Stroke Syndromes: Infratentorial. In Stein J, Harvey RL, Winstein CJ, et al, editors: *Stroke recovery and rehabilitation*, ed 2, New York, 2015, Demos Medical Publishing.

REFERENCES

1. Abbie AA: The clinical significance of the anterior choroidal artery, *Brain* 56:243–246, 1933.
2. Aramenco P, Lévy C, Cohen A, et al: Causes and mechanisms of territorial and nonterritorial cerebellar infarcts in 115 consecutive cases, *Stroke* 25:105–112, 1994.
3. Bassetti C, Bogousslavsky J, Mattle H, Bernasconi A: Medial medullary stroke. Report of seven patients and review of the literature, *Neurology* 48:882–890, 1997.
4. Bogousslavsky J, Regli F, Uske A: Thalamic infarcts: clinical syndromes, etiology and prognosis, *Neurology* 38:837–848, 1988.
5. Caplan LR, Kelly M, Kase CS, et al: Infarcts of the inferior division of the right middle cerebral artery: mirror image of Wernicke's aphasia, *Neurology* 36:1015–1020, 1986.
6. Critchley M: The anterior cerebral artery, and its syndromes, *Brain* 53:120–165, 1930.
7. Darby DG: Sensory aprosodia: a clinical clue to lesions of the inferior division of the right middle cerebral artery? *Neurology* 43:567–572, 1993.

8. Demasio AR, Geshwind N: The neural basis of language, *Annu Rev Neurosci* 7:127–147, 1984.
9. Escourolle R, Hauw J-J, Der Agopian P, Trelles L: Les infarctes bulbaires. Etude des lésions vasculaires dans 26 observations, *J Neurol Sci* 28:103–113, 1976.
10. Finger S: Paul Broca (1824-1880), *J Neurol* 251:769–770, 2004.
11. Fischer CM: Lacunar strokes and infarcts: a review, *Neurology* 32:871–876, 1982.
12. Fisher CM, Karnes WE, Kubik CS: Lateral medullary infarction – the pattern of vascular occlusion, *J Neuropathol Exp Neurol* 20:323–379, 1961.
13. Geshwind N: Disconnexion syndromes in animals and man, *Brain* 88:585–644, 1965.
14. Geshwind N: Aphasia, *N Engl J Med* 284:654–656, 1971.
15. Geshwind N: The apraxias: neural mechanisms of disorders of learned movement, *Am Sci* 63:188–195, 1975.
16. Geshwind N, Levitsky W: Human brain: left-right asymmetries in temporal speech region, *Science* 161:186–187, 1968.
17. Helgason C, Caplan LR, Goodwin J, Hedges T: Anterior choroidal artery-territory infarction. Report of cases and review, *Arch Neurol* 43:681–686, 1986.
18. Hommel M, Caplan LR: Midbrain infarcts and hematomas. In Caplan L, van Gijn J, editors: *Stroke syndromes*, ed 3, Cambridge, 2012, Cambridge University Press, pp 439–447.
19. Kaufman DK, Brown RD, Karnes WE: Involuntary tonic spasms of a limb due to a brainstem lacunar infarction, *Stroke* 25:217–219, 1994.
20. Kilgard MP, Merzenich MM: Distributed representation of spectral and temporal information in rat primary auditory cortex, *Hear Res* 134:16–28, 1999.
21. Lerich J, Winkler G, Ojemann R: Cerebellar infarction with brainstem compression: diagnosis and surgical treatment, *Arch Neurol* 22:490–498, 1970.
22. Loukas M, Louis RG, Childs RS: Anatomical examination of the recurrent artery of Heubner, *Clin Anat* 19:25–31, 2006.
23. Mesulam MM: Large-scale neurocognitive networks and distributed processing for attention, language, and memory, *Ann Neurol* 28:597–613, 1990.
24. Mesulam MM: Attentional networks, confusional states and neglect syndromes. In Mesulam MM, editor: *Principles of behavioral and cognitive neurology*, New York, 2000, Oxford University Press, pp 174–256.
25. Mohr JP, Steinke W, Timsit SG, et al: The anterior choroidal artery does not supply the corona radiata and lateral ventricular wall, *Stroke* 22:1502–1507, 1991.
26. Mohr JP, Kase CS, Meckler RJ, Fisher CM: Sensorimotor stroke, *Arch Neurol* 34:734–741, 1977.
27. Park KC, Lee BH, Kim EJ, et al: Deafferentation-disconnection neglect induced by posterior cerebral artery infarction, *Neurology* 66:56–61, 2006.
28. Pillman F: Carl Wernicke (1848-1905), *J Neurol* 250:1390–1391, 2003.
29. Ross ED: Hemispheric specialization for emotions, affective aspects of language and communication and the cognitive control of display behaviors in humans, *Prog Brain Res* 107:583–594, 1996.
30. Ross ED, Thompson RD, Yenkosky J: Lateralization of affective prosody in brain and the callosal integration of hemispheric language functions, *Brain Lang* 56:27–54, 1997.
31. Stefanatos GA, Gershkoff A, Madigan S: On pure word deafness, temporal processing, and the left hemisphere, *J Int Neuropsychol Soc* 11:456–470, 2005.
32. Stafani MA, Schneider FL, Marrone AC, et al: Anatomic variations of anterior cerebral artery cortical branches, *Clin Anat* 13:231–236, 2000.
33. Tatu L, Moulin T, Bogousslavsky J, Duvernoy H: Arterial territories of human brain: brainstem and cerebellum, *Neurology* 47:1125–1135, 1996.
34. Tehovnik EJ, Sommer MA, Chou IH, et al: Eye fields in the frontal lobes of primates, *Brain Res Rev* 32:413–448, 2000.
35. Tramo MJ, Cariani PA, Koh CK, et al: Neurophysiology and neuroanatomy of pitch perception: auditory cortex, *Ann N Y Acad Sci* 1060:148–174, 2005.
36. Ustun C: Dr. Thomas Willis' famous eponym: the circle of Willis, *Turk J Med Sci* 34:271–274, 2004.

CHAPTER 45

DEGENERATIVE MOVEMENT DISORDERS OF THE CENTRAL NERVOUS SYSTEM

Abu A. Qutubuddin, Priya Chandan, William Carne

Neurodegenerative disorders, including movement disorders, are complex multisystem disorders characterized by abnormal protein aggregates that accumulate in select regions in the central, peripheral, and autonomic nervous systems.[49] Movement disorders are neurologic syndromes characterized by either an excess of movement or a paucity of voluntary and automatic movements, unrelated to weakness or spasticity.[13] Clinically, movement disorders are manifestations of the loss of modulatory influence by the extrapyramidal system[5] and may be classified as hyperkinetic or hypokinetic disorders.[42] Under hyperkinetic disorders, we will discuss restless leg syndrome (RLS) and abnormal movements, including tremor, dystonia, myoclonus, chorea, and tics. Under hypokinetic disorders, we will discuss Parkinson disease (PD) and Parkinson plus syndromes, including progressive supranuclear palsy (PSP), multiple system atrophy (MSA), and corticobasal ganglionic degeneration (CBGD).

Hyperkinetic Disorders

Hyperkinetic disorders are characterized by excessive movement.[42] To categorize these disorders, one must be able to recognize the type and pattern of the involuntary movements (e.g., tremor, chorea, myoclonus, etc.). When a combination of different movements occurs in the same individual, it can be very difficult to ascertain the right one. It is advisable to do repeated examinations and, if needed, video recording over time can be extremely helpful. It may be difficult to classify a particular abnormal movement even with repeated examinations and video.

Restless Leg Syndrome

Restless leg syndrome (RLS) is characterized by a deep, ill-defined discomfort or dysesthesia in the legs that arises during prolonged rest or when the patient is drowsy and trying to fall asleep, especially at night.[13] Patients experience sensory disturbances in the legs that are characteristically relieved by movement.[42] RLS may be a primary condition or occur in association with other conditions, such as diabetes mellitus, uremia, carcinoma, pregnancy, malabsorption, or chronic obstructive airway disease.[42]

The estimated prevalence of RLS is 2% to 15%.[42] It is slightly more common in women and in individuals of Northern European descent.[42] Although it is considered a condition that primarily affects middle-aged to older individuals, one third of patients experience symptom onset younger than 20 years of age.[13]

Regarding the diagnosis of RLS, there are five essential diagnostic criteria, which are outlined in the following paragraph. First-line treatment for RLS involves long-acting dopaminergic compounds and iron supplements, particularly in patients with low serum ferritin (less than 50 to 80 mg/L).[49] Second-line treatment includes anticonvulsants, such as gabapentin, pregabalin, or carbamazepine. Benzodiazepines and opioids, such as methadone or oxycodone, are also used.[49]

As defined by the International Restless Legs Syndrome Study Group,[9] the following are the essential diagnostic criteria:

1. An urge to move the legs usually but not always accompanied by or felt to be caused by uncomfortable and unpleasant sensations in the legs.
2. The urge to move the legs and any accompanying unpleasant sensations begin or worsen during periods of rest or inactivity, such as lying down or sitting.
3. The urge to move the legs and any accompanying unpleasant sensations are partially or totally relieved by movement, such as walking or stretching, at least as long as the activity continues.
4. The urge to move the legs and any accompanying unpleasant sensations during rest or inactivity only occur or are worse in the evening or night than during the day.
5. The occurrence of the features listed in points 1 to 4 is not solely accounted for as symptoms primary to another medical or a behavioral condition (e.g., myalgia, venous stasis, leg edema, arthritis, leg cramps, positional discomfort, habitual foot tapping).

Abnormal Movements

Tremor

Tremor is defined as a rhythmic, oscillatory movement produced by alternating or synchronous contracting of antagonist muscle pairs.[13] Tremors may be described as fast or slow, coarse or fine, uniplanar or biplanar.[42] Resting tremor is usually observed when the body part is at complete rest, as is seen in Parkinson tremor. Postural tremor appears while maintaining a body posture; when the tremor is produced during a movement, it is termed an action tremor. Tremors may involve the limbs, neck, tongue, and voice. Resting tremor has notable characteristics, such as the following:

- Appears within the body part completely at rest.
- Subsides with action.
- Subsides with assuming a posture.

Another type of tremor is termed physiologic tremor. This tremor occurs resulting from the muscle fibers whose motor units are being recruited at subtetanic rates. Physiologic tremor can be exacerbated by anxiety, fatigue, hypoglycemia, thyrotoxicosis, alcohol withdrawal, lithium use, sympathomimetic drugs, methylxanthines such as caffeine, and sodium valproate. These causes should be excluded before coming to a diagnosis of other types of tremors. Some tremors can be seen both at rest and with action, such as rubral tremors. These are caused by lesions of the cerebellar outflow pathways in the midbrain.

The most common movement disorder is essential tremor (ET) (Videos 45-1 and 45-2). Typically, it is a postural tremor but may be accentuated by goal-directed activities. Upper limbs are usually involved frequently, and the tremor can be asymmetrical. ET is typically uniplanar with flexion-extension movement of the hand. It may also be present in the head, voice, tongue, lips, and trunk. These tremors may be solitary or in combination. In some severe cases, it can interfere with hydration and nutrition. Anxiety, stress, and central nervous system stimulants can worsen the tremor. Consumption of small quantities of alcohol improves ET in most cases, and alcohol ingestion is an often-used clinical challenge to aid diagnosis. Although other forms of tremor may respond to alcohol, this is one of the characteristics of ET. However, care should be taken by the clinician to not imply to the patient that alcohol use is a recommended treatment. ET can begin at any age. More than 50% of patients inherit this disease. Neurologic examination may be normal in most patients, but mild abnormalities of muscle tone, posture, and balance may be seen.

Dystonia

Dystonia is defined as an abnormal movement characterized by sustained muscle contractions, frequently causing twisting and repetitive movements, which may progress to prolonged abnormal postures.[13,42] Although its clinical presentation closely resembles myoclonus, electromyographic (EMG) studies show prolonged bursts typical of dystonia rather than characteristic short-duration bursts seen in myoclonus. Dystonia is autosomal dominant in inheritance.

Dystonia can be classified according to the site of involvement:

- Focal dystonia: One part of the body is involved, such as blepharospasm, oromandibular dystonia, and cervical dystonia.
- Segmental dystonia: Two or more contiguous parts involved, such as Meige syndrome.
- Multifocal dystonia: Two or more noncontiguous parts are involved.
- Hemidystonia: One side of the body is affected.
- Generalized dystonia.

Dystonia may occur at rest or when a body part has a voluntary action. Rest dystonia may worsen on action. Dystonia may be task-specific, such as writer's cramp or musician's cramp. Parkinsonism may also be associated with dystonia and may respond to levodopa. Patients with dystonia may report that the condition is aggravated by anxiety, stress, and fatigue. Frequently, it is relieved by rest or sleep. One of the peculiar features is that some patients have the ability to relieve the dystonic movement by sensory tricks, usually tactile stimuli. For example, sometimes blepharospasm can be relieved by touching the area around the eye. This is a unique phenomenon to dystonia. Diurnal variations may be seen in dopa-responsive dystonia. Dystonia may be classified according to the causes as primary (idiopathic) and secondary (symptomatic). Thirty percent of dystonia is secondary dystonia.

Myoclonus

Myoclonus is defined as sudden, shocklike movements that are usually random and range in severity from mild to severe enough to move the whole body. On occasions it may be rhythmic or oscillatory.[42] Myoclonic movements may be caused by active muscle contractions, as seen in positive myoclonus, or they may also be caused by sudden, brief lapses of muscle contraction in active postural muscles, as seen in negative myoclonus.[13] Myoclonic movements are irregular in time, as seen in choreic movements, but unlike chorea, the movement is more abrupt. The origin of myoclonus may be cortical or subcortical (brainstem or spinal cord). It can be physiologic and can be seen after exercise, excessive fatigue, or sometimes when the individual is falling asleep, such as hypnagogic jerks.[42]

It can occur spontaneously or it can occur by touch, light, noise, etc. Similar to other movement disorders, myoclonus may be essential myoclonus (idiopathic). Its onset can be at any age with a positive family history. Cortical or epileptic myoclonus is almost always associated with other forms of seizures and is more common in younger populations.

Specific Types of Myoclonus

Spinal Myoclonus. Usually repetitive in nature in one limb. Lesions in the spinal cord such as trauma, tumor, or inflammation can be responsible for this type of myoclonus.

Palatal Myoclonus. Characterized by rhythmic jerking of the soft palate sometimes in conjunction with the laryngeal, pharyngeal, and extra ocular muscles and diaphragm.

Asterixis. Also known as negative myoclonus. Brief lapses of tone in a limb held in a posture against gravity. Asterixis is commonly seen in metabolic encephalopathies, as a reaction to general anesthetics, and during anticonvulsant therapy. EMG reveals irregular periods of silence during these lapses.

Chorea

The word *chorea* is derived from the Greek word *khoreia*, which means dance.[49]

The term was introduced in the sixteenth century by Paracelsus and described bizarre motor and mental manifestations similar to the deliriant trance, dancing mania of medieval pilgrims.

Chorea is defined by the irregular, unpredictable, brief jerky movements that are usually of low amplitude.[42] The movements are usually distal and range in severity. Chorea results from pathologic changes in the basal ganglia. Mild chorea may resemble fidgetiness in children, whereas severe chorea may interfere with speech, swallowing, ability to maintain posture, or ability to ambulate.[42] Choreic movements are irregularly timed, as are myoclonic movements, but the movement in chorea is more abrupt in character.[42] These movements may be seen in some genetic disorders or may be secondary to infectious, autoimmune, iatrogenic, or metabolic causes.[49] These movements may vary in severity from restlessness to mild, intermittent exaggeration of gestures and expression, fidgeting movements of the hands, unstable dancelike postures to a continuous flow of disabling violent movements. Usually the condition fluctuates according to stress as well as physical and mental activities. Initially, it dominates in the face and on the acral parts (peripheral parts) of the extremities. Grimacing is a typical finding in chorea. A protruding tongue or blepharospasm may also be seen with this disorder. There are no valid data regarding the incidence of chorea; however, there are a number of diseases that might be accompanied by chorea such as Huntington disease, benign hereditary chorea, and Wilson disease.[49] Socially, afflicted individuals may suffer embarrassment and may be mischaracterized by others because they are often assumed to be intoxicated. This may lead to loss of employment and community stature, among other consequences.[49]

Tics

Tics are defined as abnormal movements (motor tics) or abnormal sounds (phonic tics) that are brief, involuntary, rapid, and nonrhythmic. There is often an irresistible urge to move before the tic, resulting in a tension that builds and is subsequently relieved by execution of the tic. If both motor tics and phonic tics are present, then the designation of Tourette syndrome is commonly applied.[13]

Tics can be classified as simple and or complex tics.

Simple Motor Tic. Abrupt, brief, isolated movement as an eye blink, facial grimace, shoulder shrug, or head jerk. The movements may be slower and sustained. Simple vocal tics usually consist of throat clearing, grunting, coughing, snorting, or animal sounds such as barking, hissing, and crowing.

Complex Motor Tic. These include stereotyped facial expressions or patterned coordinated movements such as touching, grooming, scratching, kicking, hand shaking, or obscene gesturing. It is sometimes difficult to distinguish complex motor tics from obsessive-compulsive behavior. Complex vocal tics include words, phrases, obscene utterances, or religious profanities.

Stress, anxiety, and fatigue may worsen tics. Tics can be relieved by concentrating on a task or absorbing activities such as playing a musical instrument or reading. Tics vary in frequency, amplitude, duration, and location.

Hypokinetic Disorders

Hypokinetic disorders are characterized by a paucity of movement, or hypokinesis.[42] This section includes PD as well as Parkinson plus syndromes. Parkinson plus syndromes are a group of neurodegenerative conditions that are characterized by the classical "TRAP" features of PD (tremor, rigidity, akinesia/bradykinesia, and postural instability) in addition to other features that distinguish them from PD. These conditions include PSP, MSA, and CBGD.

Parkinson Disease

Epidemiology

Parkinson disease (PD) affects approximately 10 to 20 in every 100,000 individuals in the worldwide population and 1 in 100 Americans ages 60 years older.[42] PD is currently the second most common age-related neurodegenerative disease after Alzheimer disease.[5] More than 1 million people in the United States have PD, more than multiple sclerosis, amyotrophic lateral sclerosis, muscular dystrophy, and myasthenia gravis combined. The prevalence of PD increases with age and is expected to increase as the Baby Boomer generation ages.[13] The Parkinson's Disease Foundation has estimated that the combined annual direct and indirect cost of PD in the United States is $25 billion.[42]

The prevalence of PD varies with both ethnicity and geographic distribution. A population-based study of Medicare beneficiaries found that the prevalence of PD in African Americans and Asian Americans is 50% less than that in white Americans. The study also found substantially higher rates of PD in the Midwest/Great Lakes region and along the northeastern U.S. seaboard, which was potentially attributed to industrial and agricultural exposures that are higher in these regions.[8] There is considerable interest in pesticides and herbicides as risk factors for PD, though research is ongoing.[13]

Genetics

In addition to suspected environmental exposure risk factors, there is a genetic contribution to PD. The majority of PD cases are sporadic because familial forms only account for approximately 10% of all PD cases.[5] Monogenic causes of PD include both autosomal dominant and autosomal recessive inherited mutations. In addition to monogenic forms of PD, there are a number of genes and loci associated with increased risk for PD.

Autosomal Dominant Forms of Parkinson Disease: *LRRK2*, *SNCA*, *VPS35*, and *EIF4G1*. The most common cause of autosomal dominant inherited PD involves mutations in the *LRRK2* gene, which accounts for up to 10% of all familial forms.[5] Clinically, patients with *LRRK2* mutations display characteristics of classical PD, but the age of onset is broad.[40] The second most common cause of autosomal dominant inherited PD is *SNCA* gene mutations. Patients with *SNCA*-related PD may vary in clinical presentation because there is a direct relationship between *SNCA* gene dosage and disease severity. Patients with *SNCA* duplications often display a classical PD phenotype, whereas patients with triplications display more severe phenotypes with atypical features including myoclonus, severe dysautonomia, and dementia in addition to parkinsonism.[40] Patients with *SNCA*-related PD may also exhibit progressive loss of levodopa responsiveness.[5]

The *SNCA* gene encodes the protein alpha-synuclein. Lewy bodies, the histologic finding seen in classic PD, are formed by aggregates of alpha-synuclein. Both *LRRK2* and *SNCA* mutations are thought to affect a common cellular pathway leading to alpha-synuclein aggregation, although the exact role of *LRRK2* in this pathway remains unclear.[5]

Autosomal Recessive Forms of Parkinson Disease: *PARK2, PINK1,* and *DJ-1*. The age of onset seen in autosomal recessive forms of PD is earlier compared with autosomal dominant forms of PD. Autosomal recessive inherited mutations include *PARK2, PINK1,* and *DJ-1*. *PARK2* mutations are the most common, accounting for almost 50% of early-onset familial recessive PD cases. Mutations in *PARK2* are also found in approximately 15% of sporadic PD cases with onset before 45 years.[40] *PARK2*-related PD does not generally show Lewy bodies, as is seen in autosomal dominant forms. *PARK2*-related PD is characterized by early or juvenile onset (generally before 45 years), excellent and sustained response to levodopa, and a benign course.[40,50] However, motor fluctuations often become prominent during the disease course. Mutations in *PINK1* and *DJ-1* are also seen as forms of autosomal recessive PD, but these mutations are much less prevalent than *PARK2* mutations. *PINK1* mutations are seen in 1% to 8% of early-onset cases and *DJ-1* mutations are seen in 1% to 2% of early-onset cases.[40]

Genetic Risk Factors for Parkinson Disease. In addition to monogenic forms of PD, there are a number of genes and loci associated with increased risk for PD.[5] For example, dominantly inherited, heterozygous mutations in the glucocerebrosidase (*GBA*) gene are a frequent and strong risk factor for PD.[3] Carriers of only one mutated allele have a fivefold increased risk to develop PD compared with noncarriers, making *GBA* one of the strongest genetic risk factors reported to date.[30] Patients with *GBA* mutations demonstrate classical PD with a possible slightly earlier age of disease onset.[40] Recent studies have shown a more rapid motor and cognitive decline in *GBA* mutation carrier patients with PD compared with noncarriers.[38] Further research is needed to determine whether *GBA* carrier status in patients with PD could represent a prognostic factor for rate of disease progression.[5]

Pathophysiology

PD is thought to be caused by the progressive loss of dopaminergic neurons from the substantia nigra par compacta of the midbrain in association with alpha-synuclein intracellular inclusions, termed Lewy bodies. More recent thinking[4] has further posited that degeneration starts in the dorsal motor nucleus of the glossopharyngeal and vagal nerves and anterior olfactory nucleus and then proceeds to the locus coeruleus and raphe nucleus before disrupting basal ganglion functioning. While the disease advances, frontal brain areas are frequently affected. It appears that before the involvement of the basal ganglion the individual may only manifest subtle subclinical manifestations, but once the basal ganglion is significantly involved classical idiopathic Parkinson disease symptoms are exhibited.

BOX 45-1

Top Ten Facts About Parkinson Disease

1. Named after Dr. James Parkinson (1755-1824) by the French neurologist Jean-Martin Charcot (also known as the father of neurology).
2. 1 in 100 Americans older than 60 years of age is affected by this disease.
3. 1 in 20 people diagnosed with Parkinson disease are younger than 40 years of age.
4. Risk increases if older than 50 years of age.
5. Parkinson disease is caused by the loss of dopaminergic cells in the substantia nigra. Symptoms appear when 60% to 70% of cells have died.
6. Presently, there are no clearly identifiable causes why cells die.
7. No cure is available, but treatments can help control symptoms and maintain quality of life.
8. Parkinson disease can be managed with a combination of drug therapies and rehabilitation.
9. The main symptoms of Parkinson disease are tremors, bradykinesia, and rigidity.
10. Diagnosis is clinical; as of today no laboratory testing or imaging is definitive.

Clinical Presentation

It is helpful to conceptualize PD as an intersection of three major areas: motor, nonmotor, and autonomic nervous system (ANS) symptoms (Box 45-1).

Motor Symptoms. The cardinal motor signs of PD include resting tremor, bradykinesia, rigidity, shuffling gait, and postural instability.[38] A helpful mnemonic for remembering PD cardinal motor symptoms is "TRAP": tremor (Video 45-3), rigidity, akinesia/bradykinesia, and postural instability. The presence of these symptoms should raise concern for PD. However, if postural instability is prominent at onset, this should suggest an atypical form of parkinsonism such as PSP. Because the onset of these signs is insidious, patients and family often attribute them to the normal aging process. Although PD is progressive, there is great variability in the rates of motor progression.[4,46]

Nonmotor Symptoms. Nonmotor symptoms of PD include neuropsychiatric symptoms, cognitive symptoms, and sleep disturbances.

Neuropsychiatric Symptoms. Although motor issues are often the most visible problems afflicting those with movement disorders, nonmotor factors are now recognized as important considerations in the treatment and management of the patient with PD. The prime psychological issues observed in patients with movement disorders are depression, anxiety, and hallucinations. It is not entirely certain whether psychiatric conditions are the result of, or prodromal to, the development of PD.[25] Psychiatric symptoms may be underdiagnosed resulting from the clinical focus on motoric symptoms, limited examination time, and overlap of psychiatric symptoms to PD manifestations (e.g., masked expression, apathy, fatigue, low libido, sleep disruption, bradykinesia). The prevalence of co-occurring PD and depression is estimated to vary from 20% to 40%,[2,39] while anxiety is thought to occur in

30% to 50% of patients with PD during the course of the disease,[28,34] although some suggest that the true prevalence is closer to 67%.[6] Anxiety and depression frequently co-occur. Hallucinations, primarily visual, are seen in 25% of those with PD,[14] and are thought to be side effects of treatment medications. The use of dopamine agonists in treating PD has been associated with a higher incidence of impulse control disorders, notably gambling and increased sexual behaviors.[44]

Depressed or saddened mood is often experienced at the time of initial diagnosis and upon learning that the disorders are progressive in course until death. Those with PD often become more adjusted after learning that the disease does not inevitably have a rapid progression and that good medical treatment and rehabilitation can allow for a quality of life spanning years in many cases. Often, it is the functional limitations (pace and fluidity of conversation, public dining, ease of entrancing and exiting social venues such as religious services, theater, etc.) caused by tremors, dysarthria, gait disturbance, and other motor problems that worsen dysphoria and frustration. Depression may contribute to cognitive dysfunction and adds significant disability beyond that attributed to motor dysfunction alone.[32,43]

Although some argue that anxiety is prodromal, the levels experienced by the patient after a PD diagnosis can be exacerbated by any number of factors, such as fears of eventual disability and dependency, concern over finances, uncertainty regarding the ability to maintain a home, and the welfare of other family members. In older patients, this overlays the expected developmental anxieties of dependency upon others and general mortality concerns. Risk factors for anxiety in patients with PD include female gender, younger age, presence of motor fluctuations, fear of being sustained in the "off phase," and a history of anxiety disorders.[27,47]

Both anxiety and depressed mood can be treated supportively by the attending physician (or psychotherapist if indicated), with pharmacotherapy, and by patient/family education and regular support groups.

Cognitive Symptoms. Cognitive impairment is frequently seen in PD and has important clinical management implications. Executive functions are the first and most severely affected cognitive domains.[51] Executive functions include ability in "set-switching," problem-solving strategies, concept formation, attention capacities, decision-making, and effective use of working memory. Deficits in executive functions may be expressed clinically as difficulties with everyday activities such as organizing medications or paying bills.

Impairment in visuospatial function is also present early in the course of PD. However, it may not be detected initially, because it often requires specific neuropsychological testing for diagnosis. The clock-drawing test is frequently used to assess both executive and visuospatial functions.[16] The Mini-Mental State Examination may be used as a screen for global cognitive function in PD, with a score of less than 24 indicating more significant cognitive impairment.[33] Memory deficits are typically seen later in the disease course, as PD progresses. Clinically, patients often exhibit retrieval deficits rather than immediate recall deficits, suggesting that encoding processes are intact.[16] As the disease progresses, thought processes become more rigid and perseverative.

The relative risk of dementia is five times[23] that of matched controls, although the likelihood of mild cognitive impairment has been reported after PD onset as approximately 25%.[1] Various subtypes of dementia have been identified including PD dementia and Lewy body dementia. Both are associated with abnormal alpha-synuclein deposits. The clinical differentiation of the two types is somewhat arbitrary and based on time of onset. The current convention is to term a dementia as Lewy body dementia that is manifested before or within a year of Parkinson disease symptoms, whereas PD dementia is used to describe the condition in those who develop dementia after at least a year of exhibiting Parkinson disease symptoms. Both share a course of progressive cognitive decline, impaired memory, and poor executive functioning (functions include ability in "set-switching," problem-solving strategies, concept formation, attention capacities, decision making, and effective use of working memory), with Lewy body dementia also manifesting with hallucinations and delusions at times. Cholinesterase inhibitors and memantine are often used to treat cognitive decline, but effectiveness has not been clearly demonstrated.

Sleep Disturbances. Sleep disturbances are also common in PD, although their cause is unclear and likely to be multifactorial. Factors that may contribute to sleep disturbances in PD include stimulant effects of PD medications, anxiety, RLS, sleep cycle dysregulation caused by poor sleep hygiene, and reduced bed mobility. Reduced activity levels and exercise, frequent nocturia, and nocturnal disorientation caused by cognitive impairment or vivid dreams can also contribute to sleep disturbance. Specific symptoms include insomnia, nightmares, and excessive daytime sleepiness.[16]

Autonomic Nervous System Symptoms

ANS symptoms include orthostatic hypotension, constipation, urinary frequency and urgency, erectile dysfunction and vaginal tightness, and sweating.[7] Orthostatic hypotension is defined as a decrease of 20 mm Hg in systolic or 10 mm Hg in diastolic blood pressure within 3 minutes in an upright position with or without postural symptoms.[26] Orthostatic hypotension most commonly occurs in the advanced stages of PD.[45] Symptoms of orthostatic hypotension include dizziness, blurred vision, postural instability, light-headedness, and syncope. Approximately 30% of all patients with PD will become symptomatic in their lifetime.[31] Care should be taken in the clinic to measure blood pressure in both the seated and standing positions to detect orthostasis.

Diagnosis

Understanding the clinical presentation of PD is especially important because the diagnosis of PD is clinical (Box 45-2). The most widely used comprehensive instrument used by movement disorder specialists to assess PD is the Movement Disorder Society Unified Parkinson's Disease Rating Scale (UPDRS). This scale was originally developed in the 1980s[12] and was revised in 2008.[18] The UPDRS is a clinical scale consisting of four parts: Part I: nonmotor

BOX 45-2

Top Ten Warning Signs of Parkinson Disease

1. Difficulty walking (starting and stopping, misjudging corners, abnormal shoe wear).
2. Resting tremors (usually unilateral at onset).
3. Bradykinesia.
4. Difficulty balancing (carrying items while walking difficult, frequent falls).
5. Depression/sadness (often precedes onset of motor signs).
6. Loss of motor skills.
7. Handwriting (micrographia, tremulous).
8. Voice and speech changes/difficulty (hypophonia, dysarthria).
9. Loss of memory/dementia (mild or severe).
10. Skin disorders (dry skin, rough skin, dandruff of scalp).

BOX 45-3

Designations Regarding Efficacy and Regarding Implications for Clinical Practice Used in the Movement Disorder Society Task Force on Evidence-Based Medicine Review of Treatments, 2011 Updates

- Conclusions on efficacy: Designated as efficacious, likely efficacious, unlikely efficacious, nonefficacious, or insufficient evidence.
- Implications for clinical practice: Designated as clinically useful, possibly useful, investigational, unlikely useful, or not useful.

These terms were used in both the MDS-EBM ROT 2011 updates on treatments for motor symptoms[15] and treatments for nonmotor symptoms.[37]

experiences of daily living; Part II: motor experiences of daily living; Part III: motor examination; and Part IV: motor complications. Several questions from Part I and all questions from Part II were designed to lend themselves to a questionnaire format that may be filled out by the patients and their caregivers. The remainder of Part I and Part IV must be conducted by a movement disorder specialist. Part III covers objective measures of parkinsonism, as assessed by the clinician.

Part III: Motor Examination. This portion is made up of 18 physical examination maneuvers to evaluate the following: speech, facial expression, rigidity of the neck and four extremities, finger taps, hand movements, pronation/supination movements of hands, toe tapping, leg agility, rising from chair, gait, freezing of gait, postural stability, posture, global spontaneity of movement (body bradykinesia), postural tremor of the hands, kinetic tremor of the hands, rest tremor amplitude, and constancy of rest tremor.

Management

The Movement Disorder Society Task Force on Evidence-Based Medicine (MDS-EBM) published a Review of Treatments (ROT) for PD in 2002 and an update was published in 2005.[15] These reviews focused mainly on motor symptoms of PD. In 2011, an additional update was published regarding motor symptoms[15] and the review was expanded to include nonmotor symptoms.[37] These publications provide guidelines for symptomatic treatment in PD. Box 45-3 provides further explanation regarding the efficacy designations and implications for clinical practice designations used in these reviews.

Pharmacologic Treatment of Motor Symptoms. Individualized assessment of the risks and benefits of available medications as well as specific clinical features and phase of the disease should guide PD treatment. Pharmacologic treatment becomes necessary when PD-related motor symptoms begin to interfere with a patient's activities of daily living and negatively affect quality of life.[41] Levodopa remains the most effective drug to treat motor symptoms of PD and is considered the gold standard. It is recommended as the first-line initial monotherapy in older adult patients in whom motor complication risk is generally low.

For younger patients, alternative agents are often used as first-line therapy because of the risk of development of dyskinesias in patients treated with levodopa for long periods of time.[21,24,26] Risk factors for development of levodopa-related motor complications include higher levodopa dose, younger age at PD onset, longer disease duration, and greater disease severity.[11,36] After more than 2 years of levodopa treatment, approximately one third of patients will experience motor complications from levodopa treatment,[19,29] such as motor response oscillations or levodopa-induced dyskinesias (LIDs).

Motor Response Oscillations (Wearing Off/Pulsatile Phenomenon). As a result of the short half-life of levodopa, patients may experience motor response oscillations, most frequently occurring in the form of wearing-off phenomena. Patients will describe worsening symptoms toward the end of an intradose interval, with relief after intake of the next scheduled levodopa dose. A subset of patients may experience less predictable oscillations between good (on state) and bad (off state) motor control. Catechol-*O*-methyl transferase (COMT) inhibitors, monoamine oxidase B (MAO-B) inhibitors, and dopamine (DA) agonists prolong the half-life of levodopa and therefore help control motor fluctuations and help reduce total daily off time. These agents may therefore be helpful adjuncts to levodopa treatment.[41] It is not unusual for patients to experience a waning effectiveness of medications over the course of the illness, and clear and consistent patient-physician communication is an important goal in adjusting medications.

Levodopa-Induced Dyskinesias. LIDs are characterized by choreic movements of the extremities, trunk, and neck during periods of full efficacy and are therefore considered on state dyskinesias (Video 45-4). LIDs eventually affect more than 40% of patients receiving sustained levodopa treatment for greater than 6 years[35] and can be difficult to manage. Options to reduce LIDs include decreasing or fractioning the dose of levodopa, although this may improve LIDs at the expense of symptom control.[41] Currently, the only drug with established antidyskinetic efficacy is amantadine, an *N*-methyl-D-aspartate receptor antagonist.[15] Studies have shown that amantadine can decrease LIDs without worsening Parkinson disease symptoms and that the antidyskinetic effects can be maintained

BOX 45-4

Pharmacologic Treatment Options for Parkinson Disease by Class

Levodopa-Based Treatment Options (Combined with Carbidopa)

Levodopa/Carbidopa (Sinemet)
Oral tablets
Extended release tablets
Orally disintegrated tablets
Infusion therapy

Dopamine Agonists

Non-ergot preparations
Pramipexole (Mirapex)
Ropinirole (Requip)
Transdermal patch
  Rotigotine patch
Subcutaneous
  Apomorphine (Apokyn injection)
Ergot preparation dopamine agonist
  Bromocriptine
  Pergolide

COMT Inhibitors

Entacapone (Comtan)
Tolcapone (not used in United States)

MAO Inhibitors

Selegiline
Rasagiline

***N*-Methyl-D-Aspartate Receptor Antagonist**

Amantadine

COMT, Catechol-*O*-methyl transferase; *MAO-B,* monoamine oxidase B.

long term.[48] Adverse effects of amantadine include a potential to induce cognitive dysfunction, including psychosis. Therefore, caution should be used when giving this medication to patients with even mild PD dementia.[41] There has been some evidence that treatment with clozapine may reduce LIDs but, overall, the current evidence is insufficient to definitively conclude that clozapine is effective in LID treatment.[15]

In addition to serving as adjuncts to levodopa treatment, COMT inhibitors, MAO-B inhibitors, and DA agonists may be used as monotherapy. Advantages of these agents include a more continuous oral delivery of dopaminergic stimulation and a lower risk of levodopa-induced motor complications. Box 45-4 lists the pharmacologic treatment options for PD by class, whereas Table 45-1 compares these drug classes.

Pharmacologic Treatment of Nonmotor Symptoms and Autonomic Nervous System Symptoms. Many nonmotor symptoms worsen over time and are major determinants of quality of life, nursing home placement, and progression to overall disability.[22] In patients with motor response fluctuations, symptoms of depression, anxiety, or panic attacks may accompany off states and quickly improve once a dose of levodopa takes effect.[47] Therefore, reduction of off time will improve both control of motor symptoms and nonmotor symptoms.

The MDS-EBM ROT 2011 conclusions regarding treatments for nonmotor symptoms are summarized in Box 45-3.

Table 45-1 Conclusions from the Movement Disorder Society Task Force on Evidence-Based Medicine Review of Treatments 2011 Regarding Efficacy of Treatments for Nonmotor Symptoms of Parkinson Disease

Nonmotor Symptom	Medication	Efficacy Conclusion	Practice Implication
Depression	Pramipexole Nortriptyline Desipramine	Efficacious Likely efficacious Likely efficacious	Clinically useful Possibly useful Possibly useful
Psychosis	Clozapine	Efficacious	Clinically useful
Dementia	Rivastigmine	Efficacious	Clinically useful
Sialorrhea	Botulinum toxin A	Efficacious	Clinically useful
Sialorrhea	Botulinum toxin B	Efficacious	Clinically useful
Sialorrhea	Glycopyrrolate	Efficacious	Possibly useful*
Constipation	Macrogol	Likely efficacious	Possibly useful

From Seppi K, Weintraub D, Coelho M, et al: The movement disorder society evidence-based medicine review update: treatments for the non-motor symptoms of Parkinson's disease, *Mov Disord* 26(Suppl 3):S42–S80, 2011.

*Because there is insufficient evidence of glycopyrrolate for treatment of sialorrhea exceeding 1 week, the practice implication is that it is possibly useful versus clinically useful.

Nonpharmacologic Treatment. The MDS-EBM ROT 2011 concluded there was insufficient evidence regarding efficacy of occupational therapy, speech therapy, or acupuncture for use as symptomatic monotherapy or as adjuncts to levodopa.[15] Studies conducted since 2002 have enabled the conclusion for physical therapy (PT) to be changed to likely efficacious, with a clinical practice implication of possibly useful as symptomatic adjunct therapy to levodopa treatment.[15] PT interventions currently under investigation include training with cuing or focused attention for patients who have PD with freezing and falls, as well as formalized patterned exercises including Tai Chi and Qigong.[15] Studies are also ongoing regarding gait training, both conventional gait training and partial weight-supported treadmill gait training.[17]

Patients with PD have mobility deficits in both gait and balance. Many of the earlier mobility studies have focused primarily on the effects of PT interventions on gait, as opposed to effects on balance.[17] Overall, further research is needed regarding efficacy of and standardization of PT interventions for functional deficits in gait and balance in patients with PD.

Surgical Treatment. Deep brain stimulation (DBS) is a surgical procedure used as part of a comprehensive treatment approach to motor symptoms in PD (Video 45-5). In DBS for PD, an electrode is surgically implanted in the subthalamic nucleus or globus pallidus and provides continuous high-frequency electrical stimulation (see www.knowbeforeyouneed.com and click on "About DBS Therapy" for videos).

DBS is usually indicated for patients with drug-related movements and fluctuations whose condition has not improved after exhausting all medical management regimens, who show a clear response to levodopa following a levodopa challenge, who do not have a parkinsonian syndrome, who have no other major interfering medical conditions, and who are in more advanced stages of the illness.[16]

The MDS-EBM ROT 2011[15] concluded that DBS of the bilateral subthalamic nucleus, DBS of the bilateral globus pallidus, and unilateral pallidotomy are efficacious and clinically useful as adjunctive treatments to levodopa, as treatments for dyskinesia, and as treatments for motor fluctuations. DBS of the thalamus or thalamotomy were found to be likely efficacious and possibly clinically useful as adjunctive treatments to levodopa. DBS of the thalamus is generally reserved for patients who have PD with severe tremor and who may not be candidates for more extensive DBS of the subthalamic nucleus or globus pallidus attributable to either dementia or other major medical conditions. There was insufficient evidence regarding surgical interventions as symptomatic monotherapy and regarding the use of surgical interventions to prevent/delay clinical progression or to prevent/delay motor complications.

Caregiver Considerations

The patient with a movement disorder frequently becomes increasingly reliant on a caregiver to assist with a multitude of daily tasks. Caregivers (either unpaid or paid) are an intrinsic part of the patient's life and can serve a useful role in the medical treatment process. As noted by Ham,[20] the caregiver, as the single individual most involved in the care of the individual over the entire course of the disorder, may elect to be, or may essentially evolve into, the effective leader of the caring team. At home, caregivers may help the patient with a wide array of tasks to include activities of daily living, safety, medication compliance, general organizational issues, transportation, and social involvement.

At the medical appointment, caregivers can serve as accurate historians, first-hand observers of the patient's reactions to medications and treatments, and clarifiers of patient communication to medical personnel, as well as clarifiers of medical communication to the patient. Thus, they help the medical team obtain accurate and reliable information, and they ensure the appropriateness of the home environment for the patient.

For these reasons, supporting the functioning of caregivers is vital to successful medical management and sustaining a home/community living environment in individuals with movement disorders. The physician should be aware that the very nature of the caregiving role creates considerable stress or burden. Therefore, physicians and medical team members need to be alert for signs of undue caregiver burden or strain and intervene for the welfare of the caregiver and the patient with a movement disorder alike. Interventions may take the form of simple reassurance, caregiver education, prescribing respite breaks, or end-of-life discussions.

Parkinson Plus Syndromes

Progressive Supranuclear Palsy

Epidemiology

Progressive supranuclear palsy (PSP) is a syndrome characterized by axial rigidity, bradykinesia, postural instability with falls, cognitive deficits, and supranuclear vertical gaze palsy.[49] PSP is a common cause of levodopa-nonresponsive parkinsonism.[10] It was first described in 1964 by three Canadian neurologists whose names have been honored in the British eponym for this disease, Steele-Richardson-Olszewski syndrome.[10] The prevalence is 5.3 per 100,000. Incidence increases sharply with age, with no convincing cases reported in the literature younger than 45 years of age.[49]

Genetics

Several common genetic variants influencing the risk of PSP have been identified.[49] A genome-wide association study in over 1000 patients with PSP and more than 3000 controls confirmed two independent variants in microtubule-associated protein tau (*MAPT*) genes on chromosome 17 that influence the risk of developing PSP. However, the cause of PSP is unknown and the majority of cases do not have a positive family history for PSP.[49]

Pathophysiology

There is increasing evidence that mitochondrial dysfunction plays a role in the pathogenesis of neurodegenerative disease. In PSP, failure in mitochondrial energy production is probably involved in both tau aggregation and neuronal cell death.[49]

Clinical Presentation

The most common initial feature of PSP is a disturbance of gait and a history of falling, which typically begins within 12 months of onset.[10] Other clinical clues indicative of PSP include stuttering, palilalia (abnormal repetition of syllables, words, or phrases), early dysphagia, personality changes, sleep disturbances, apraxia, and dementia. The characteristic facial expression seen in PSP is that of perpetual astonishment attributable to continuous frontalis contraction and a low blink rate. Extensor neck posturing may also be seen.[10] Other clinical findings in PSP include action tremor, pseudobulbar palsy, hyperreflexia, and Babinski signs.

Diagnosis

Diagnosis of PSP may be difficult resulting from an overlap in signs and symptoms with PD and MSA. The classic syndrome of PSP differs from PD in the lack of tremor, the relative sparing of limb movement (except writing), and the greater rigidity seen in the neck compared with the limbs, the early development of freezing, and marked micrographia.[10] However, resting tremor, urinary incontinence, hemidystonia, and asymmetrical apraxia are infrequently seen in PSP and the presence of these signs and symptoms should not rule out the diagnosis of PSP.[10] Furthermore, although supranuclear vertical gaze palsy is the most distinctive clinical feature of PSP, this finding may be absent in PSP. Therefore, strict reliance on this single physical sign leads to a lack of sensitivity, or at least a delay, in diagnosis.[10] In addition, autonomic dysfunction may be more common than is generally appreciated, resulting in misdiagnosis of PSP as MSA.[10]

Multiple System Atrophy

Epidemiology

Multiple system atrophy (MSA) is an adult-onset, rapidly progressive, neurodegenerative disorder that affects both sexes equally.[49] The estimated prevalence of MSA is 3 per 100,000.[10] The mean age of onset for MSA is around 55 years,[49] which is slightly younger than that for PD and considerably younger than that for PSP.[10]

Genetics

MSA is commonly regarded as a sporadic disorder. However, in recent years, familial aggregations of MSA have been reported.[49]

Pathophysiology

MSA is characterized by an abnormal accumulation of alpha-synuclein in oligodendrocytes associated with multifocal neuronal degeneration.[49] Gross findings at autopsy can include atrophy and darkening of the putamen, as well as atrophy of the pons and cerebellum. Depigmentation of the substantia nigra may be present but is not universal.[10]

Clinical Presentation

MSA is characterized clinically by a variable combination of parkinsonism, cerebellar dysfunction, and autonomic failure.[49] Over 85% of patients with MSA develop parkinsonism, over 50% show evidence of cerebellar degeneration, and approximately 75% have autonomic dysfunction.[10] The clinical manifestations of MSA are often divided into motor and autonomic manifestations.[10]

Motor Manifestations. The motor syndromes in MSA can be subdivided into MSA-P and MSA-C based on their predominant motor feature.[49] MSA-P is the basal ganglia type, characterized by a levodopa-refractory, akinetic-rigid parkinsonism. Signs include bradykinesia, rigidity, postural tremor, disequilibrium, and gait unsteadiness.[49] MSA-C is the cerebellar type, characterized by ataxia. Other cerebellar findings include gait ataxia, limb kinetic ataxia, a wide-based gait, dysarthric and scanning speech, and cerebellar oculomotor disturbances, such as nystagmus.[10,49] The most common presentation of MSA is MSA-P.[10]

Autonomic Manifestations. Autonomic dysfunction primarily involves the urogenital and orthostatic domains.[49] Common autonomic symptoms include orthostatic lightheadedness, syncope, urinary retention or incontinence, impotence (in males) or anorgasmia (in females), fecal incontinence, loss of sweating, and paroxysmal bursts of excessive sweating.[10] A retrospective analysis of pathologically confirmed MSA cases showed that early autonomic symptoms (within 2 years of disease onset) occurred in greater than 50% of cases.[49]

Other clinical features of MSA may include action myoclonus, respiratory stride, dysphonia, Raynaud phenomenon, pain, contractures, and rapid eye movement sleep behavior disorder, which may precede motor manifestations.[10]

Diagnosis

A consensus committee published formal criteria for the clinical diagnosis of MSA. The essential elements of diagnosis were thought to be a combination of autonomic dysfunction and either cerebellar ataxia or parkinsonism poorly responsive to levodopa.[10] The clinical recognition of MSA improved dramatically after the introduction of diagnostic criteria.[49] However, there is no definitive diagnostic test for MSA.[10] Clinically probable MSA is defined as a sporadic, progressive, adult-onset (older than 30 years of age) disease characterized by severe autonomic failure, as defined by either urinary continence (with erectile dysfunction in men) or orthostatic hypotension (with blood pressure falls ≥30 mm Hg systolic or ≥15 mm Hg diastolic) and, additionally, a poorly levodopa-responsive parkinsonism or a cerebellar syndrome.[49]

Of note, MSA has emerged as the most difficult disease to distinguish from PD. MSA mimics PD more closely than PSP in the prominence of limb involvement, which is often asymmetrical.[10] Postural stability is compromised early in both MSA and PSP, but in contrast to PSP, recurrent falls at disease onset are unusual in MSA.[49]

Management

MSA is a fatal disorder and progresses relentlessly until death, with a median survival of 9 years. However, there is a considerable variation in disease progression, with individual cases surviving up to 15 years.[49] Thus far, disease-modifying medical treatments are lacking, despite intensified efforts to develop interventional strategies. Therefore, the management of patients with MSA largely concerns the alleviation of parkinsonian and autonomic symptoms.[49]

Only one third of patients with MSA show any response to levodopa, and then the response is almost always atypical. If levodopa is unsuccessful or poorly tolerated, it is worth pursuing treatment with dopamine agonists or amantadine because individual patients may respond better to one of these agents.[10] There is no consistently effective treatment for cerebellar manifestations.[10] Autonomic manifestations are the most amenable to treatment, and a variety of measures are effective for orthostatic hypotension. A priority is to identify and reduce or eliminate medications that may be contributing to the problem.[10] Although autonomic failure is almost universally present in MSA, only one third of affected patients receive appropriate pharmacologic treatment.[49]

Nonpharmacologic measures include elevating the head of the bed, increasing salt and fluid intake, avoiding heat, adopting specific body postures such as crossing the legs or squatting.[10]

Corticobasal Ganglionic Degeneration

Epidemiology

Corticobasal ganglionic degeneration (CBGD) is the least understood of the Parkinson plus syndromes. It is somewhat less common than either PSP or MSA.[10]

Genetics

There are no known risk factors and the hereditary status of CBGD is unclear.[10]

Pathophysiology

Macroscopically, there is usually visible cerebral atrophy.[10]

Clinical Presentation

CBGD develops insidiously and progresses gradually. The clinical findings in CBGD can be divided into three

Table 45-2 Symptom Manifestation of Various Movement Disorders

Disorder	Resting Tremor	Action Tremor	Rigidity	Postural Instability	Cognitive Decline	Sleep Disorder	Visual Hallucinations	Positive Response to Medications for Parkinson Disease	Mood Disorders	Motor Fluctuations
Parkinson disease	++	+/–	+	+	+	+	+/–	+++	++	+
Essential tremor	+/–	++	–	–	–	–	–	+	+/–	–
Multiple system atrophy	–	+	+	+	++		+/–	–	–	–
Progressive supranuclear palsy	+/–	–	+/–	+++	++	+	+/–	–	–	–
Huntington disease	+/–	+/–	–	++	++	+	+/–	–	+/–	–
Restless leg syndrome	–	–	–	–	–	+	–	+/–	–	–

+, Commonly present; –, usually absent; +/–, may or may not be present.

categories: motor manifestations, cerebellar manifestations, and other manifestations. Motor manifestations include dystonia (usually fixed and often causing pronounced or painful deformities), postural instability, athetosis, and orofacial dyskinesias. Signs of cerebrocortical dysfunction consist of apraxia, cortical sensory loss, the alien limb phenomenon, dementia, and frontal lobe reflexes.[8] The most striking aspect of the clinical picture of CBGD is the asymmetry with which it presents and pursues its course. In this way, it resembles PD more than any other type of degenerative parkinsonism.[10]

Diagnosis

The most helpful type of study is brain imaging, either by computed tomography or magnetic resonance imaging. This will detect asymmetrical atrophy of the cerebral cortex, which will be greater contralateral to the side that is more clinically involved.[10]

Management

There is no specific treatment for CBGD. Therapy is currently purely symptomatic.[10] The mean life expectancy from onset is 8 years.[10]

Summary

Movement disorders present a significant challenge to the diagnostic and management skills of physiatrists and are common enough to be likely encountered by physiatrists in all types of clinical settings (Table 45-2). There is still a lack of evidence-based and patient-specific rehabilitative interventions for individuals diagnosed with movement disorders. Anecdotal studies focusing on different rehabilitative exercise programs have suggested that the quality of life for patients with a movement disorder may be significantly improved by participation in such programs.

REFERENCES

1. Aarsland D, Bronnck K, Williams-Gray C, et al: Mild cognitive impairment in Parkinson's disease: a multicenter pooled analysis, *Neurology* 75:1062–1069, 2010.
2. Aarsland D, Larsen JP, Lim NG, et al: Range of neuropsychiatric disturbances in patients with Parkinson's disease, *J Neurol Neurosurg Psychiatr* 67:492–496, 1999.
3. Bonifati V: Genetics of Parkinson's disease—state of the art, 2013, *Parkinsonism Relat Disord* 20(Suppl 1):S23–S28, 2014.
4. Braak H, Tredici KD, Rüb U, et al: Staging of brain pathology related to sporadic Parkinson's disease, *Neurobiol Aging* 24:197–211, 2003.
5. Braddom RL, editor: *Physical medicine and rehabilitation*, ed 3, Philadelphia, 2006, Elsevier/Saunders.
6. Chagas MHN, Tumas V, Loureiro SR, et al: Does the association between anxiety and Parkinson's disease really exist? A literature review, *Curr Psychiatry Rev* 5:29–36, 2009.
7. Dewey RB: Autonomic dysfunction and management. In Pahwa R, Lyons KE, editors: *Handbook of Parkinson's disease*, ed 4, New York, 2007, Informa Healthcare, pp 77–90.
8. De Lau LLL, Breteler MMB: Epidemiology of Parkinson's disease, *Lancet Neurol* 5:525–535, 2006.
9. Diagnostic Criteria: International Restless Legs Syndrome Study Group. Available at http://irlssg.org/diagnostic-criteria/.
10. Factor SA, Weiner WJ, editors: *Parkinson's disease: diagnosis and clinical management*, ed 2, New York, 2007, Demos Medical Publishing.
11. Fahn S: Parkinson disease, the effect of levodopa, and the ELLDOPA trial. Earlier vs later L-DOPA, *Arch Neurol* 56:529–535, 1999.
12. Fahn S, Elton RL, UPDRS Program Members: Unified Parkinson's disease rating scale. In Fahn S, Marsden CD, Goldstein M, Calne DB, editors: *Recent developments in Parkinson's disease*, vol 2, Florham Park, 1987, Macmillan Healthcare Information, pp 153–163, 293-304.
13. Fahn S, Jankovic J: *Principles and practice of movement disorders*, Philadelphia, 2007, Churchill Livingstone/Elsevier.
14. Fénelon G, Mahieux F, Huon R, Ziégler M: Hallucinations in Parkinson's disease: prevalence, phenomenology and risk factors, *Brain* 123:733–745, 2000.
15. Fox SH, Katzenschlager R, Lim SY, et al: The Movement Disorder Society evidence-based medicine review update: treatments for the motor symptoms of Parkinson's disease, *Mov Disord* 26(Suppl 3):S2–S41, 2011.
16. Fritsch T, Smyth KA, Wallendal MS, et al: Parkinson disease: research update and clinical management, *South Med Assoc* 15:650–656, 2012.
17. Ganesan M, Sathyaprabha TN, Gupta A, Pal PK: Effect of partial weight-supported treadmill gait training on balance in patients with Parkinson disease, *PM&R* 6:22–33, 2014.

18. Goetz CG, Tilley BC, Shaftman SR, et al: Movement Disorder Society-sponsored revision of the Unified Parkinson's Disease Rating Scale (MDS-UPDRS): scale presentation and clinimetric testing results, *Mov Disord* 23:2129–2170, 2008.
19. Gottwald MD, Aminoff MJ: Therapies for dopaminergic-induced dyskinesias in Parkinson disease, *Ann Neurol* 69:919–927, 2011.
20. Ham RJ: Evolving standards in patient and caregiver support, *Alzheimer Dis Assoc Disord* 13(Suppl 2):S27–S35, 1999.
21. Hauser RA, Rascol O, Korczyn AD, et al: Ten-year follow-up of Parkinson's disease patients randomized to initial therapy with ropinirole or levo-dopa, *Mov Disord* 22:2409–2417, 2007.
22. Hely MA, Morris JG, Reid WG, Trafficante R: Sydney multi-center study of Parkinson's disease: non-L-dopa-responsive problems dominate at 15 years, *Mov Disord* 20:190–199, 2005.
23. Hobson P, Meara J: Risk and incidence of dementia in a cohort of older subjects with Parkinson's disease in the United Kingdom, *Mov Disord* 19:1043–1049, 2004.
24. Holloway RG, Shoulson I, Fahn S, et al: Pramipexole vs levodopa as initial treatment for Parkinson disease: a 4-year randomized controlled trial, *Arch Neurol* 61:1044–1053, 2004.
25. Ishihara L, Brayne C: A systematic review of depression and mental illness preceding Parkinson's disease, *Acta Neurol Scand* 113:211–220, 2006.
26. Lahrmann H, Cortelli P, Hilz M, et al: EFNS guidelines on the diagnosis and management of orthostatic hypotension, *Eur J Neurol* 13:930–936, 2006.
27. Leentjens AF, Dujardin K, Marsh L, et al: Symptomatology and markers of anxiety disorders in Parkinson's disease: a cross-sectional study, *Mov Disord* 26:484–492, 2011.
28. Leentjens AF, Dujardin K, Marsh L, et al: Anxiety rating scales in Parkinson's disease: a validation study of the Hamilton anxiety rating scale, the Beck anxiety inventory, and the hospital anxiety and depression scale, *Mov Disord* 26:407–415, 2011.
29. Lewitt PA: Levodopa for the treatment of Parkinson's disease, *N Engl J Med* 359:2468–2476, 2008.
30. Lohmann E, Periquet M, Bonifati V, et al: How much phenotypic variation can be attributed to parkin genotype? *Ann Neurol* 54:176–185, 2003.
31. Magalhaes M, Wenning GK, Daniel SE, Quinn NP: Autonomic dysfunction in pathologically confirmed multiple system atrophy and idiopathic Parkinson's disease: a retrospective comparison, *Acta Neurol Scand* 91:98–102, 1995.
32. Mayeux R, Stern Y, Rosen J, et al: Depression, intellectual impairment, and Parkinson disease, *Neurology* 31:645–650, 1981.
33. Miyasaki JM, Shannon K, Voon V, et al: Practice parameter: evaluation and treatment of depression, psychosis, and dementia in Parkinson disease (an evidence-based review), *Neurology* 66:996–1002, 2006.
34. Nuti A, Ceravolo R, Piccinni A, et al: Psychiatric comorbidity in a population of Parkinson's disease patients, *Eur J Neurol* 11:315–320, 2004.
35. Parkinson Study Group CALM Cohort Investigators: Long-term effect of initiating pramipexole vs levodopa in early Parkinson disease, *Arch Neurol* 66:563–570, 2009.
36. Schrag A, Quinn N: Dyskinesias and motor fluctuations in Parkinson's disease: a community-based study, *Brain* 123(Pt 11):2297–2305, 2000.
37. Seppi K, Weintraub D, Coelho M, et al: The movement disorder society evidence-based medicine review update: treatments for the non-motor symptoms of Parkinson's disease, *Mov Disord* 26 (Suppl 3):S42–S80, 2011.
38. Sidransky E, Nalls MA, Aasly JO, et al: Multicenter analysis of glucocerebrosidase mutations in Parkinson's disease, *N Engl J Med* 361:1651–1661, 2009.
39. Slaughter JR, Slaughter KA, Nichols D, et al: Prevalence, clinical manifestations, etiology, and treatment of depression in Parkinson's disease, *J Neuropsychiatry Clin Neurosci* 13:187–196, 2001.
40. Spatola M, Wider C: Genetics of Parkinson's disease: the yield, *Parkinsonism Relat Disord* 20(Suppl 1):S35–S38, 2014.
41. Sprenger F, Poewe W: Management of motor and non-motor symptoms in Parkinson's disease, *CNS Drugs* 27:259–272, 2013.
42. Watts RL, Koller WC, editors: *Movement disorders: neurologic principles and practice*, ed 2, New York, 2004, McGraw-Hill.
43. Weintraub D, Moberg PJ, Duda JE, et al: Effect of psychiatric and other nonmotor symptoms on disability in Parkinson's disease, *J Am Geriatr Soc* 52:784–788, 2004.
44. Weintraub D, Siderowf AD, Potenza MN, et al: Association of dopamine agonist use with impulse control disorders in Parkinson disease, *Arch Neurol* 63:969–973, 2006.
45. Wenning GK, Scherfler C, Granata R, et al: Time course of symptomatic orthostatic hypotension and urinary incontinence in patients with postmortem confirmed parkinsonian syndromes: a clinicopathological study, *J Neurol Neurosurg Psychiatry* 67:620–623, 1999.
46. Winder-Rhodes SE, Evans JR, Ban M, et al: Glucocerebrosidase mutations influence the natural history of Parkinson's disease in a community-based incident cohort, *Brain* 136:392–399, 2013.
47. Witjas T, Kaphan E, Azulay JP, et al: Nonmotor fluctuations in Parkinson's disease: frequent and disabling, *Neurology* 59:408–413, 2002.
48. Wolf E, Seppi K, Katzenschlager R, et al: Long-term antidyskinetic efficacy of amantadine in Parkinson's disease, *Mov Disord* 25:1357–1363, 2010.
49. Wolters E, Baumann C, editors: *Parkinson disease and other movement disorders*, Amsterdam, 2014, VU University Press.
50. Wright Willis A, Evanoff BA, Lian M, et al: Geographic and ethnic variation in Parkinson disease: a population-based study of US Medicare beneficiaries, *Neuroepidemiology* 34:143–151, 2010.
51. Zgaljardic DJ, Borod JC, Foldi NS, et al: An examination of executive dysfunction associated with frontostriatal circuitry in Parkinson's disease, *J Clin Exp Neuropsychol* 28:1127–1144, 2006.

MULTIPLE SCLEROSIS

Anjali Shah, Angela Flores, Bardia Nourbakhsh, Olaf Stüve

Multiple sclerosis (MS) is a chronic, inflammatory, neurodegenerative disorder of the central nervous system (CNS). It is the most common cause of nontraumatic disability in young adults.[141] Approximately 400,000 individuals are affected with MS in the United States.[139] MS can present in numerous ways and affects several functional and cognitive systems. This patient population often develops challenges with gait, spasticity, cognition, fatigue, weakness, bladder, bowel, and wounds.

Physiatrists are well equipped to manage many of the symptomatic challenges that may otherwise go undetected or unacknowledged. An understanding of the pathogenesis, pharmacologic, and rehabilitative options for persons with MS (PwMS) is vital for the practicing physiatrist. The first disease-modifying therapy (DMT) for MS was approved in 1993. Since then, there has been rapid growth in the treatment options for MS. There are currently 10 DMT options for PwMS. As the availability of increased and more effective DMTs for MS increases, patients and families continue to expect improved quality of life and would like treatment options extending into optimal management of their myriad of symptoms. The role of physiatry for PwMS will continue to expand. It is vital that the practitioner be familiar with the specificities of MS, what differentiates it from other diseases, and how impactful rehabilitation intervention is for this population.

Costs

MS is one of the costliest illnesses to treat. The estimated annual cost for MS is $28 billion.[59,139] Most DMTs for MS are distributed by a specialty pharmacy. Specialty drug costs of oncology, rheumatoid arthritis, and MS comprised 51% of the annual spending for specialty drugs for a major insurance company.[202] These specialty drugs cost approximately $87 billion in 2012 and comprised approximately 3.1% of national health spending. It is estimated that specialty drug spending will quadruple and comprise approximately 9.1% of national health spending over the next several years as more effective treatment options become available for patients with chronic illness.[144] The annual direct and indirect costs of MS per person is estimated to be $8528 to $54,244.[2,171] Direct costs make up 77% of the total cost and is largely attributable to the cost of the prescription medication.[2] Contrary to the laws of supply and demand, each new DMT that is introduced has not driven market competition to lower prices. The first generic DMT, glatiramer acetate, is currently under review by the U.S. Food and Drug Administration.[182]

Epidemiology

Females are typically affected two to three times as often as males.[106] Although females have a higher risk of having MS, those males who are affected tend to have a more aggressive course, difficulty with recovery after attack, and more rapid accumulation of disability.[25,35,36,181] The peak age of diagnosis is believed to be 20 to 40 years of age (Figure 46-1).[122] Compared with Asian, black, and Hispanic populations, the disease is more common in non-Hispanic whites, with a lifetime incidence of approximately 1 in 400.[34] It remains a disease that largely afflicts whites.

MS is more common in Europe, the United States, Canada, New Zealand, and Australia and rare along the equatorial countries and the Asian continent.[90,184] Migration studies observed that individuals who move from high-risk to low-risk areas during adolescence or early childhood adopt the risk of the new area. The opposite has been shown to be true when moving from low-risk to high-risk areas, but with less robustness.[6,64] In addition, birth month has shown to be of importance in MS development. A review of 40,000+ cases of MS in Canada, Denmark, Sweden, and Scotland saw increased numbers of patients born in May and June.[208] Researchers postulated that these individuals received the least amount of sunlight in utero. The opposite pattern was observed in Australia; the lowest numbers of individuals with MS were born in May or June, lending further support to the season of birth theory.[174]

Pathogenesis

Genetic Linkage

MS is thought to be an autoimmune disease in which immune and inflammatory cells attack the CNS, damaging the myelin, axons, and neurons. Similar to many complex human diseases, MS develops in a genetically susceptible host that has experienced several environmental triggers. This hypothesis is supported by the familial clustering of MS. Monozygotic twins have a 35% concordance rate. Dizygotic twins and first-degree relatives both have approximately 4% concordance rate of MS if a family member or sibling is affected.[49,50,206] Also, serologic typing has found that human leucocyte antigen (HLA) is associated with the major histocompatibility complex (MHC) of humans with various immune-mediated diseases and gave rise to the field of immunogenetics. In MS, the HLA-DRB1*1501, located on chromosome 6p21, has been found to be strongly associated with development of MS. The HLA

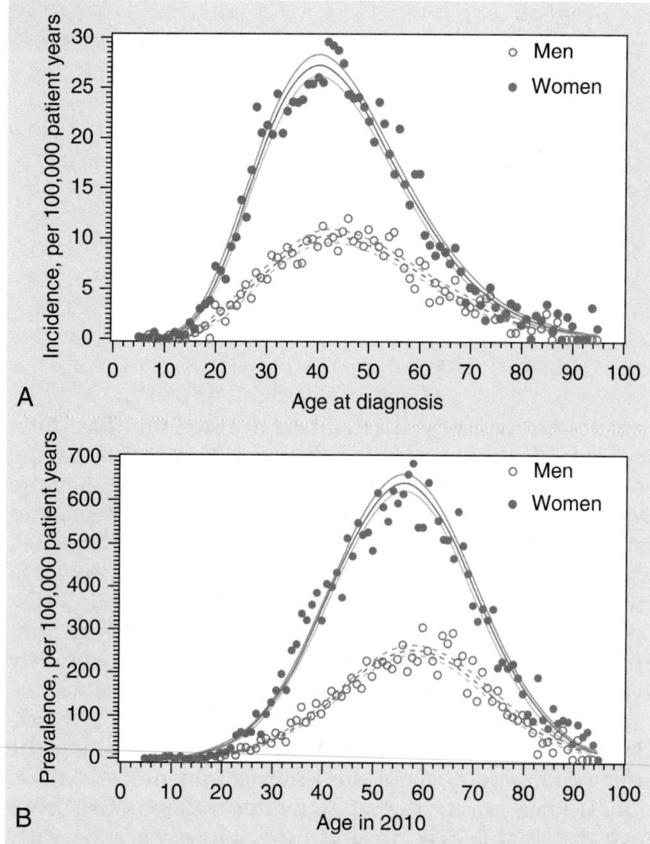

FIGURE 46-1 Incidence and prevalence of multiple sclerosis in women and men by age. **A,** Incidence (per 100,000 patient years). **B,** Prevalence (per 100,000 patient years). (From Mackenzie IS, Morant SV, Bloomfield GA, et al: Incidence and prevalence of multiple sclerosis in the UK 1990-2010: a descriptive study in the General Practice Research Database, *J Neurol Neurosurg Psychiatry* 85:76-84, 2014.)

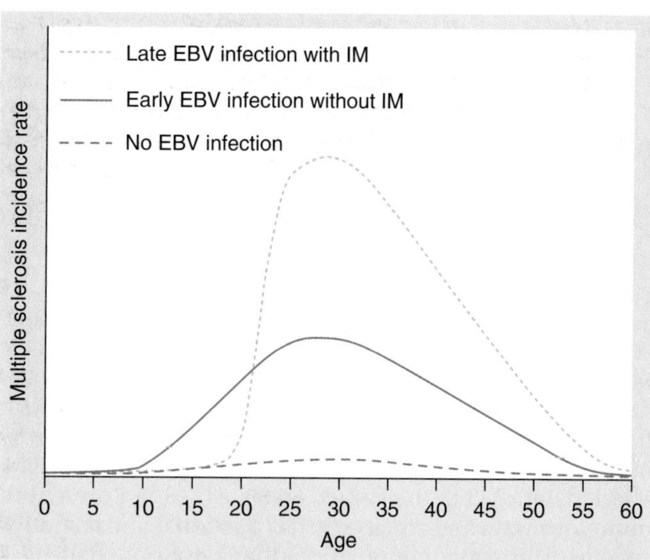

FIGURE 46-2 Schematic representation of multiple sclerosis (MS) incidence according to Epstein-Barr virus (EBV) infection. The shape of the incidence curve labeled "Early EBV Infection Without IM" is based on the typical age-specific incidence of MS in most populations; incidence begins to increase in adolescence, peaks around age 25 to 30 years, and declines to nearly zero by age 60 years.[21] The age-specific incidence for the group with no EBV infection has been drawn at one tenth the incidence among individuals who are EBV positive, based on the results of a previous review,[22] and that of individuals with late EBV infection and infectious mononucleosis (IM) has been estimated to be 2.3 times higher than that of individuals who are EBV positive without history of IM (this metaanalysis). More accurate curves could be drawn by taking into account the proportion of individuals in the population who are infected with EBV early in childhood and the age-specific prevalence of history of IM. These adjustments have ignored for simplicity, and because these proportions vary across developed countries. (From Thacker EL, Mirzaei F, Ascherio A: Infectious mononucleosis and risk for multiple sclerosis: a meta-analysis, *Ann Neurol* 59:499-503, 2006.)

Table 46-1 Genetic Risk of Multiple Sclerosis

Relative with Multiple Sclerosis	Chance of Developing Multiple Sclerosis (%)
Monozygotic twin	25 to 30
Dizygotic twin	3 to 5
First-degree relative (child or full sibling)	2 to 4

Data from Dyment DA, Ebers GC, Dessa Sadovnick A: Genetics of multiple sclerosis, *Lancet Neurol* 3:104-110, 2004.

genes have been the only consistent genetic linkage noted in MS. Heterozygous carriers have three times and homozygous carriers have six times increased risk of developing MS.[88,171] The DR15 haplotype is also associated with narcolepsy and systemic lupus erythematosus (Table 46-1).[195,209]

Environmental Factors

Environmental factors have been evaluated for their effect on the risk of developing MS as well as its influence on progression. The incidence of MS increased with distance from the equator. The effects of vitamin D have demonstrated that reduced levels of vitamin D increases the risk of MS development, particularly in whites.[8,137,138] A typical multivitamin contains approximately 400 International Units of vitamin D. Twenty minutes of whole-body sun exposure equates to approximately 10,000 International Units of vitamin D. More research supports changing the minimum daily consumption of vitamin D because it is found to be protective in several other diseases. Studies are currently being conducted to examine the influence of vitamin D levels on disease progression in MS.[8,137,138]

Infection with Epstein-Barr virus (EBV) or human herpes virus 4 as an adolescent or young adult increases the risk of MS development. Approximately 50% of children have EBV exposure by the age of 5 years and approximately 80% to 90% of the population is exposed by 20 years of age.[210] Primary EBV infection is typically symptomatic in infants and presents as infectious mononucleosis (IM) when reactivation occurs in adolescents or young adults. Proponents of the "Epstein-Barr virus hypothesis" have found that individuals exposed to late EBV and IM increase their risk of MS development by 2.3 times those individuals exposed to EBV without IM. No exposure to EBV reduced the risk of MS by one tenth compared with individuals exposed to EBV (Figure 46-2).[5,7,117,196]

Cigarette smoking is now a known risk factor in the development of MS.[46,85,87,92,166] MS risk is approximately 50% higher in smokers and is associated with intensity and duration of smoking. Although it seems that men are more susceptible to the adverse effect of smoking, the increasing ratio of female smokers to male smokers has been proposed as an explanation for the increasing female-to-male ratio in MS incidence in several countries.[91] A cumulative dose response exists between years and intensity of years and intensity of smoking and MS risk; cigarette smoking also appears to increase the rate of MS disease progression to secondary progressive MS (SPMS).[89,91] The detrimental effects of smoking decline after 10 years of smoking cessation, despite the duration and intensity of abuse. Moist tobacco "snuffing" did not have the same effect or causation, causing researchers to study the lung-irritating effect on the immune system as a possible causation.[86] Interestingly, alcohol consumption, in a dose-dependent manner, seems to protect the person from developing MS and attenuates the detrimental effects of smoking.[88]

Other Factors

A strong correlation has been observed to exist between the body mass index (BMI) of females at 10 and 20 years of age. A BMI of >20 increases the risk of MS and a BMI ≥27 increased the risk by twofold.[69,88] Obese females between 10 and 20 years old seem to be at greater risk than males during the same time period. An even stronger correlation of developing MS was demonstrated in females with a BMI ≥27 and HLA-DRB1*15 status.[69]

Increased clinical and radiologic activity with increased sodium intake has been suggested as another cause of MS. This has been demonstrated in small scale studies and is under additional investigation.[52] Concerns about the risk of exposure to mercury, trace metal, organic solvents, or crude oil have not demonstrated convincing evidence.[125]

Immunology

MS exhibits considerable heterogeneity in clinical presentation and disease course. It is considered an autoimmune disease by most experts, but what initiates the abnormal immune response is not clear.

Most of the knowledge about the immunopathogenesis of MS comes from the study of animal models, mainly experimental autoimmune encephalomyelitis (EAE), in which immunization of an animal (e.g., a mouse or a rat) with myelin components lead to a $CD4^+$ lymphocyte orchestrated inflammatory response in the CNS.

The pathologic hallmarks of acute MS lesions are perivenular immune cell infiltrate, demyelination, myelin laden macrophages, edema, and axonal damage.[63] Relapses in MS are thought to be mediated by CNS-targeting peripherally activated helper lymphocytes.[100] These autoreactive lymphocytes could have been activated through "molecular mimicry," in which foreign antigens (e.g., viral or bacterial proteins) that are similar to CNS antigens activate the lymphocytes that will eventually react against the self-antigens. On the other hand, antigens leaked from the CNS, probably resulting from a previous unknown insult, can trigger the immune response by activating $CD4^+$ helper T cells. These cells facilitate the recruitment and activation of other immune cells—for example, monocytes and macrophages, B cells, $CD8^+$ cytotoxic T cells, and natural killer cells. The immune cells enter the brain and spinal cord through interaction with endothelial cells of the blood-brain barrier. Upon reactivation with autoantigens by CNS-resident antigen-presenting cells, they damage the myelin, axons, and neurons by various effector mechanisms. Antigen-specific and bystander $CD4^+$ and $CD8^+$ T cells, reactive microglia and infiltrating macrophages, natural killer cells, CNS reactive antibodies, inflammatory cytokines (e.g., tumor necrosis factor-alpha, interleukin-17, and osteopontin), reactive nitrogen and reactive oxygen species, metalloproteinase, and glutamate-induced excitotoxicity all contribute to CNS injury in acute and chronic MS lesions.

It is not clear which autoantigen(s) ignite the autoimmune process in MS. One possibility is activation of the peripheral immune system by CNS antigens that have been carried to the secondary lymphoid organs. It is now clear that the CNS is under immune surveillance and antigen-presenting cells carrying myelin antigens have been recognized in the cervical lymph nodes.[43] Myelin proteins, mainly, myelin basic protein (MBP), myelin oligodendrocyte glycoprotein (MOG), and myelin proteolipid protein (PLP), are possible autoantigens in MS, because immunization of animals with peptides derived from these proteins can induce EAE in animals. No single antigen has emerged as the main target of the immune response in MS and it might be explainable by the heterogeneity of the disease. In fact, as inflammation increases the access of the immune system to previously compartmentalized antigens, "epitope spreading" may happen and new epitopes in the same protein or other proteins become new targets of the immune attack.[42]

Molecular mimicry is an alternative explanation for the initial activation of the immune system. It has been shown that T cell receptors are capable of binding with high affinity to a few peptide/MHC ligands.[212] Peptides from several viruses, including influenza and EBV, can activate T cells that cross-react with myelin antigens.[213]

$CD4^+$ T cells, based on the cytokine milieu during the activation, can differentiate into functionally different effector cells. Based on the cytokine profile they produce and their lineage specific transcription factor, these cells have been categorized into T helper 1 (Th1), Th2, and Th17 cells. The phenotype of the T helper cell, to a great extent, affects the outcome of the adaptive immune response. For years, it was thought that EAE and MS are mediated by interferon-gamma (IFN-γ) producing Th1 cells.[198] However, it has been shown that both Th1 and Th17 cells are capable of inducing EAE in mice, although the disease phenotype might be different.[95,109] The plasticity of Th17 cells, known to be important players in several autoimmune diseases, further complicates the picture. Multiple MS therapies, including IFN-β, glatiramer acetate, and fingolimod, have been shown to dampen both Th1 and Th17 responses.[13,129,159] In the context of autoimmune inflammatory demyelination, Th2 cell responses are considered to be protective and antiinflammatory, and several MS disease-modifying drugs are thought to shift the immune system toward the Th2 response.

In contrast to effector T cells, multiple subsets of regulatory T (Treg) cells are capable of suppressing the immune response. Natural Treg cells, characterized by surface expression of CD25 and nuclear expression of Foxp3, show decreased suppressive activity and reduced migratory capacity in patients with MS.[41,179]

Cerebrospinal fluid oligoclonal bands, produced by B cell–derived plasma cells, are the most consistent immunologic abnormality in patients with MS. Also, B cell depletion by monoclonal antibodies effectively decreases the inflammatory disease activity in MS (as manifested by new gadolinium-enhancing lesions on magnetic resonance imaging [MRI]).[83] It is more likely that non–antibody-dependent B cell functions, such as antigen presentation and regulatory activities, are behind the beneficial effects seen after B cell depletion. B cells from patients with MS are deficient in production of suppressive cytokine, interleukin-10, and express higher amounts of costimulatory molecule, CD80, on their surface, leading to increased effector T cell activity.[48,67]

There is mounting evidence that the cells, cytokines, and receptors of the innate immune system are important in the pathogenesis of MS. Natural killer cells are capable of regulating the activity of autoreactive T cells.[126]

MS was initially defined as a demyelinating disease of the CNS. However, it is now known to involve white matter, axonal and neuronal degeneration, and gray matter. All are present at the earliest stages and are thought to be the underlying cause of irreversible and progressive disability that develops in most PwMS.[61] Neurodegeneration is directly or indirectly the result of inflammation and demyelination. Several studies have shown that the risk and the latency of entering the secondary progressive phase are not related to the number of exacerbations in the relapsing phase.[177,178] Measures of neurodegeneration, such as brain atrophy and cortical gray matter lesion load, have stronger correlation with different measures of motor and cognitive disability.[27,28] Several immunomodulatory medications have consistently demonstrated efficacy in decreasing the number of attacks in patients with relapsing forms of MS.

Subtypes

Relapsing-remitting MS (RRMS) is the most common subtype and affects approximately 50% to 65% of PwMS. This is characterized by periods of exacerbation followed by periods of remission. SPMS is the period of time when a patient with RRMS no longer has exacerbations and now has persistent accumulation of disability occurring over time. There is no biomarker that signifies the progression from RRMS to SPMS. The rate of disability accumulation varies from patient to patient. Primary progressive MS (PPMS) affects males and females equally (1 : 1) and comprises approximately 10% to 15% of PwMS. This differs from RRMS in a noticeable lack of exacerbations; instead, there is disability accumulation over time. The speed of accumulation varies from person to person. The least common and most aggressive type is progressive relapsing. This affects less than 5% of PwMS with high rates of mortality.

Diagnosis

Because of the similarity MS has to various other neurologic, rheumatologic, and vascular diseases, MS remains a diagnosis of exclusion. In addition, it is important to distinguish and exclude other demyelinating disorders, including neuromyelitis optica (NMO), acute transverse myelitis, and acute disseminated encephalomyelitis (ADEM). Criteria for diagnosis of NMO include both optic neuritis and acute myelitis, plus two of the following three factors: contiguous spinal cord involvement spanning three spinal segments or more, exclusion of MS, and NMO–immunoglobulin G (IgG) seropositive status.[211] The NMO antibody test is readily available in most laboratories and targets the aquaporin-4 antigen. It is greater than 90% specific with a sensitivity of 75% for NMO and not detected in patients with classic MS.[116] Differentiation of NMO from MS is vital because treatment is distinct for each disorder. Acute transverse myelitis presents acutely, may be monophasic or multiphasic, and has a clearly defined sensory level with exclusion of other causes. It is a focal inflammatory disorder of the spinal cord and may result in abnormalities in motor, sensory, or autonomic function.[197]

Common presenting symptoms in MS include optic neuritis, sensory loss, paresthesias, motor dysfunction, ataxia, and weakness. MS may also present as overwhelming fatigue or weakness. This symptom may be misconstrued as fatigue caused by other nonmedical factors (busy lifestyles or excessive demands because of family or work obligations). Fatigue may be attributable to metabolic, hematologic, or other nonneurologic issues (Boxes 46-1 and 46-2).

In addition to clinical symptoms, MRI is recommended for the diagnostic evaluation in MS. Radiologic imaging

BOX 46-1

Common Symptoms of Multiple Sclerosis

- Activities of daily living
- Ataxia/apraxia
- Neurogenic bowel
- Neurogenic bladder
- Cognition
- Fatigue
- Heat sensitivity/intolerance
- Gait disorders
- Mood disturbance
- Pain
- Spasticity
- Optic neuritis
- Weakness
- Sexual dysfunction
- Numbness/paresthesias

BOX 46-2

Differential Diagnosis of Multiple Sclerosis

- Neuromyelitis optica
- Acute disseminated encephalomyelitis
- Transverse myelitis
- Neurosyphilis
- Cerebral autosomal dominant arteriopathy with subcortical infarcts and leukoencephalopathy
- Behçet disease
- Neurosarcoidosis
- B12 deficiency
- Folate deficiency
- Vasculitis process
- Mixed connective tissue disease
- Neurosarcoidosis
- Rheumatoid arthritis
- Lyme disease
- *Systemic lupus erythematosus*
- Sjögren syndrome
- Carcinoma
- Wegener granulomatosis
- Hypercoagulable state
- Migraine history
- Hypertension
- Mitochondrial disorders
- "Normal"

can supplement or support clinical and laboratory data. The International Panel on Diagnosis of MS (the Panel) recommends screening with MR sequencing. The McDonald criteria are the most current and widely used to diagnose MS (Table 46-2). The McDonald criteria have gone through updates in 2001, 2005, and most recently in 2010.[128,156,157] This was based on research published by the MAGNIMS (European Magnetic Resonance Network in MS) group of MRI centers in Europe. What has remained consistent despite each update is that MS may be diagnosed based on clinical symptoms alone. Two clinical attacks at two separate points in time fulfill the criteria to diagnose a PwMS. Dissemination in space is met by having one or more T2 lesions in two out of four locations in the CNS: periventricular, juxtacortical, infratentorial, and spinal cord (Box 46-3). Dissemination in time was met by the presence of a new T2 and/or gadolinium-enhancing lesion on a follow-up MRI, irrespective of the timing or the simultaneous presence of asymptomatic gadolinium-enhancing lesions and nonenhancing lesions (Box 46-4).

Clinical Decision-Making

In addition to its usefulness in diagnostic decision-making, MRI is frequently used in the clinical decision choices regarding the effectiveness of DMTs (Figure 46-3). MRI can reflect subclinical and preclinical changes and is useful in monitoring any underlying disease activity.[115] Suggested MR images for diagnostic and clinical decision-making include T1 images with and without contrast, T2 images, and fluid attenuated inversion recovery (FLAIR) sequencing. T1 images with and without contrast determine the presence of "active" lesions. Areas of breakdown in the blood-brain barrier characterized by an inflammatory

Table 46-2 2010 Revised McDonald Diagnostic Criteria for Multiple Sclerosis*

Clinical Presentation	Additional Data Needed for MS Diagnosis
≥2 attacks†; objective clinical evidence of ≥2 lesions or objective clinical evidence of 1 lesion with reasonable historical evidence of a previous attack‡	None§
≥2 attacks†; objective clinical evidence of 1 lesion	DIS, demonstrated by: ≥1 T2 lesion in at least 2 of 4 MS-typical regions of the CNS (periventricular, juxtacortical, infratentorial, or spinal cord)‖; or Await a further clinical attack† implicating a different CNS site
1 attack†; objective clinical evidence of ≥2 lesions	DIT, demonstrated by: Simultaneous presence of asymptomatic gadolinium-enhancing and nonenhancing lesions at any time; or A new T2 and/or gadolinium-enhancing lesion(s) on follow-up MRI, irrespective of its timing with reference to a baseline scan; or Await a second clinical attack†
1 attack†; objective clinical evidence of 1 lesion (clinically isolated syndrome)	Dissemination in space and time, demonstrated by: For DIS: ≥1 T2 lesion in at least 2 of 4 MS-typical regions of the CNS (periventricular, juxtacortical, infratentorial, or spinal cord)‖; or Await a second clinical attack† implicating a different CNS site; and For DIT: Simultaneous presence of asymptomatic gadolinium-enhancing and nonenhancing lesions at any time; or A new T2 and/or gadolinium-enhancing lesion(s) on follow-up MRI, irrespective of its timing with reference to a baseline scan; or Await a second clinical attack†
Insidious neurologic progression suggestive of MS (PPMS)	1 year of disease progression (retrospectively or prospectively determined) plus 2 of 3 of the following criteria‖: Evidence of DIS in the brain based on ≥1 T2 lesions in the MS-characteristic regions (periventricular, juxtacortical, or infratentorial) Evidence for DIS in the spinal cord based on ≥2 T2 lesions in the cord Positive CSF (isoelectric focusing evidence of oligoclonal bands and/or elevated IgG index)

From Polman CH, Reingold SC, Banwell B, et al: Diagnostic criteria for multiple sclerosis: 2010 revisions to the McDonald criteria, *Ann Neurol* 69:292-302, 2011.

*If the criteria are fulfilled and there is no better explanation for the clinical presentation, the diagnosis is "MS"; if suspicious, but the criteria are not completely met, the diagnosis is "possible MS"; if another diagnosis arises during the evaluation that better explains the clinical presentation, then the diagnosis is "not MS".

†An attack (relapse, exacerbation) is defined as patient-reported or objectively observed events typical of an acute inflammatory demyelinating event in the CNS, current or historical, with duration of at least 24 hours, in the absence of fever or infection. It should be documented by contemporaneous neurologic examination, but some historical events with symptoms and evolution characteristic for MS, but for which no objective neurologic findings are documented, can provide reasonable evidence of a previous demyelinating event. Reports of paroxysmal symptoms (historical or current) should, however, consist of multiple episodes occurring over not less than 24 hours. Before a definite diagnosis of MS can be made, at least 1 attack must be corroborated by findings on neurologic examination, visual-evoked potential response in patients reporting previous visual disturbance, or MRI consistent with demyelination in the area of the CNS implicated in the historical report of neurologic symptoms.

‡Clinical diagnosis based on objective clinical findings for 2 attacks is most secure. Reasonable historical evidence for 1 past attack, in the absence of documented objective neurologic findings, can include historical events with symptoms and evolution characteristics for a previous inflammatory demyelinating event; at least 1 attack, however, must be supported by objective findings.

§No additional tests required. However, it is desirable that any diagnosis of MS be made with access to imaging based on these criteria. If imaging or other tests (e.g., CSF) are undertaken and are negative, extreme caution needs to be taken before making a diagnosis of MS, and alternative diagnoses must be considered. There must be no better explanation for the clinical presentation, and objective evidence must be present to support a diagnosis of MS.

‖Gadolinium-enhancing lesions are not required; symptomatic lesions are excluded from consideration in individuals with brainstem or spinal cord syndromes.

CNS, Central nervous system; *CSF*, cerebrospinal fluid; *DIS*, dissemination in space; *DIT*, dissemination in time; *IgG*, immunoglobulin G; *MRI*, magnetic resonance imaging; *MS*, multiple sclerosis; *PPMS*, primary progressive multiple sclerosis.

BOX 46-3

2010 McDonald Magnetic Resonance Imaging Criteria for Demonstration of Dissemination in Space

DIS can be demonstrated by ≥T2 lesion* in at least two of four areas of the CNS:
- Periventricular
- Juxtacortical
- Infratentorial
- Spinal cord†

From Polman CH, Reingold SC, Banwell B, et al: Diagnostic criteria for multiple sclerosis: 2010 revisions to the McDonald criteria, *Ann Neurol* 69:292-302, 2011.

*Gadolinium enhancement of lesions is not required for DIS.

†If an individual has a brainstem or spinal cord syndrome, the symptomatic lesions are excluded from the criteria and do not contribute to the lesions count.

CNS, Central nervous system; *DIS*, dissemination in space; *MRI*, magnetic resonance imaging.

BOX 46-4

2010 McDonald Magnetic Resonance Imaging Criteria for Demonstration of Dissemination in Time

DIT can be demonstrated by:
- A new T2 and/or gadolinium-enhancing lesion(s) on follow-up MRI, with reference to a baseline scan, irrespective of the timing of the baseline MRI
- Simultaneous presence of asymptomatic gadolinium-enhancing and nonenhancing lesions at any time

From Polman CH, Reingold SC, Banwell B, et al: Diagnostic criteria for multiple sclerosis: 2010 revisions to the McDonald criteria, *Ann Neurol* 69:292-302, 2011.

DIT, Dissemination in time; *MRI*, magnetic resonance imaging.

defect or disruption result in perivascular changes and allow update of gadolinium. These lesions will subsequently enhance on T1 images. Contrast-enhancing lesions will remain so for approximately 4 to 12 weeks and are associated with new or active lesions and are indicative of clinically active disease.[78,103] This is often used as a marker for disease control in both a clinical and research setting. Key technical factors include waiting approximately 15 minutes after contrast infusion to ensure accurate imaging. Gadolinium-enhancing lesions have been weakly correlated with disability or impairment accumulation.[99,115]

"Black hole" lesions are hypointense, nonenhancing T1 lesions. These are correlated with chronic axonal damage and loss on MR sequences as well as histopathology.[115,203,204] Their presence is associated with worsening cognitive function. Widening of the third ventricle is also associated with cortical atrophy and is correlated with cognitive dysfunction.[18] Reduction in T1 "black hole" formation is used as a biomarker for neuroprotection.

FLAIR imaging suppresses the cerebrospinal fluid (CSF) hyperintense signal in T2 images and allows for clearer demarcation of hyperintensities associated with the MS plaques. The short T1 inversion recovery (STIR) sequence is a relatively new technique used to better visualize the spinal cord. Plaques and hyperintensities are significantly better viewed with STIR imaging than previous T2 or proton density views (Figure 46-4).[140]

Imaging frequency is often clinician preference. New T2 or FLAIR lesions as well as active lesions help determine efficacy of DMT and correlate with long-term disability accumulation.

Some studies have evaluated clinical and radiologic risk factors to help predict conversion to clinically definite MS. Clinically isolated syndrome (CIS) refers to the first demyelinating event incurred by a patient. A 14-year longitudinal study of patients with CIS evaluated the correlation between T2 lesion burden and conversion to MS. Study participants with one T2 lesion or more had an almost 90% chance of conversion to MS. Another important point from this study was the modest correlation between lesion burden and disability, which is clinically significant for the physiatrist.[26] The radiologically isolated syndrome has been used to help determine a patient's risk for conversion to clinically definite MS. This suggests that asymptomatic lesions that are ovoid, well-circumscribed lesions in the brain or spinal cord that cannot be explained by other causes may predict one's risk for MS conversion.[142] Current predictors of a demyelinating event are age younger than 37 years, male sex and spinal cord involvement.[143] Optical coherence tomography is a noninvasive technique to determine the thickness of the retinal nerve fiber layer. It is sensitive in detecting subclinical presence of optic neuropathy that affects approximately 25% to 50% of PwMS.[127] Its use as a biomarker for disease progression, response to DMT, and disability in MS continues (Figure 46-5).[62]

Although MRI is often helpful in the diagnostic workup process, it is not required for the diagnosis. As stated previously, clinical impression alone can suffice. In the setting of a patient with no abnormal or nonspecific MRI findings, other testing, including CSF analysis and evoked potential studies may be needed for additional support. The "gold standard" for analyzing CSF fluid is by isoelectric focusing, which has the highest sensitivity and specificity in diagnosing MS.[60] The presence of oligoclonal bands represents intrathecal synthesis. The role of oligoclonal bands in MS remains unclear; their presence correlates with a diagnosis of MS.[60] An elevated albumin index represents blood-brain barrier disruption because albumin is synthesized and metabolized outside of the CNS.[3] Other factors to consider include abnormalities in the IgG index, IgG synthesis, and an elevated leucocyte count.[201] CSF fluid analysis not the sine qua non for a diagnosis of MS, it can provide corroborative evidence in support of the diagnosis.

Neurophysiologic testing such as visual, somatosensory, and brainstem auditory evoked potential may also be helpful in cases where clinical, radiologic, or CSF testing is inconclusive. Evoked potential testing is noninvasive and detects abnormalities throughout the length of the sensory pathway. This is helpful in cases where patients may have clinical symptoms of optic neuritis, including periorbital pain, photosensitivity, or visual change. A prolongation in the p100 pathway is considered abnormal. Occasionally, a prolongation in the p100 pathway of the unaffected eye may also be seen.[108] Somatosensory evoked potentials detect delays along the median and tibial motor pathways. Brainstem auditory evoked potentials detect delays along the auditory pathway. There is some evidence

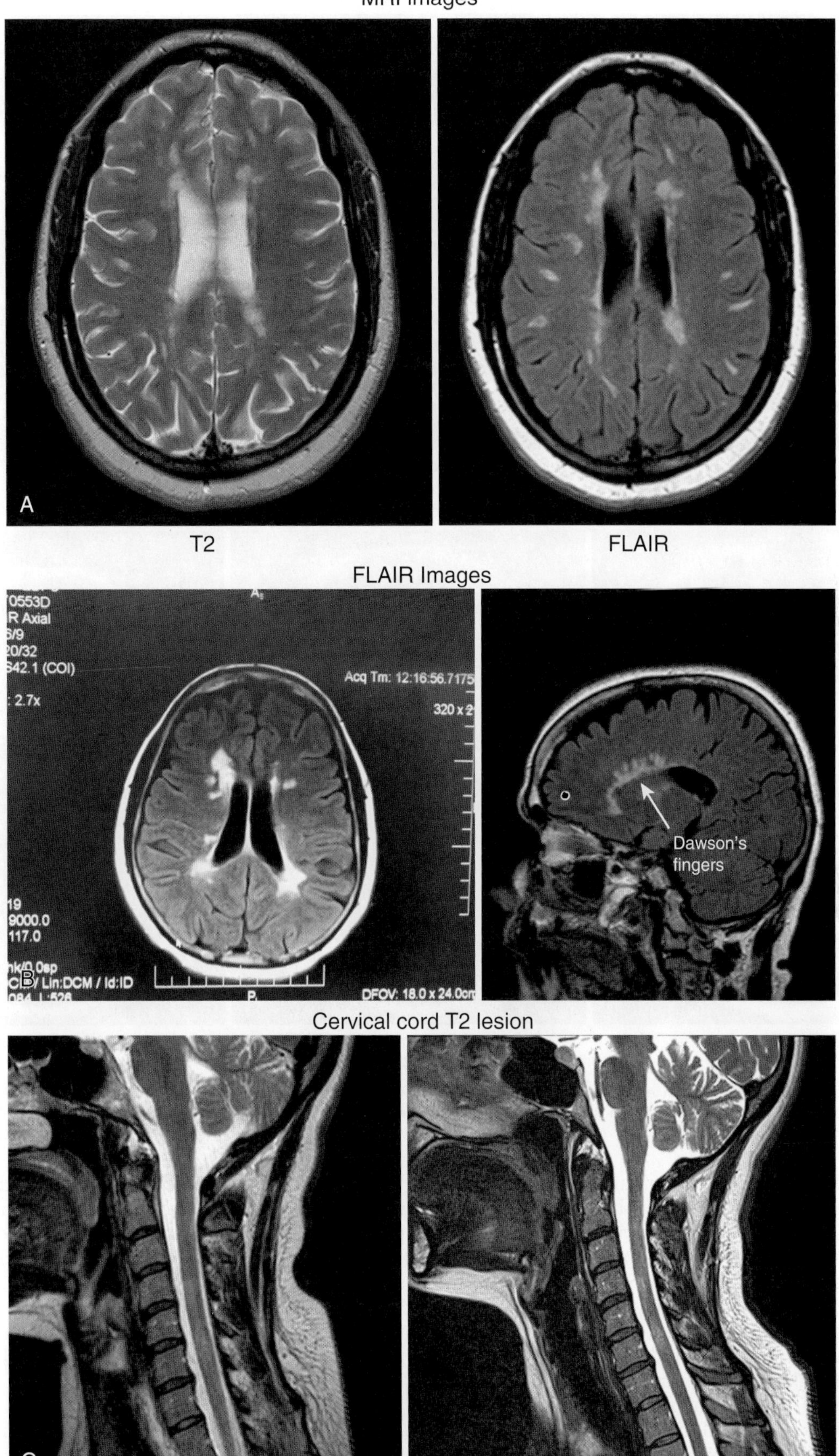

FIGURE 46-3 Suggested magnetic resonance images for diagnostic and clinical decision-making. **A,** Left, T2; right, FLAIR. **B,** FLAIR. **C,** Cervical cord T2 lesion.

Continued

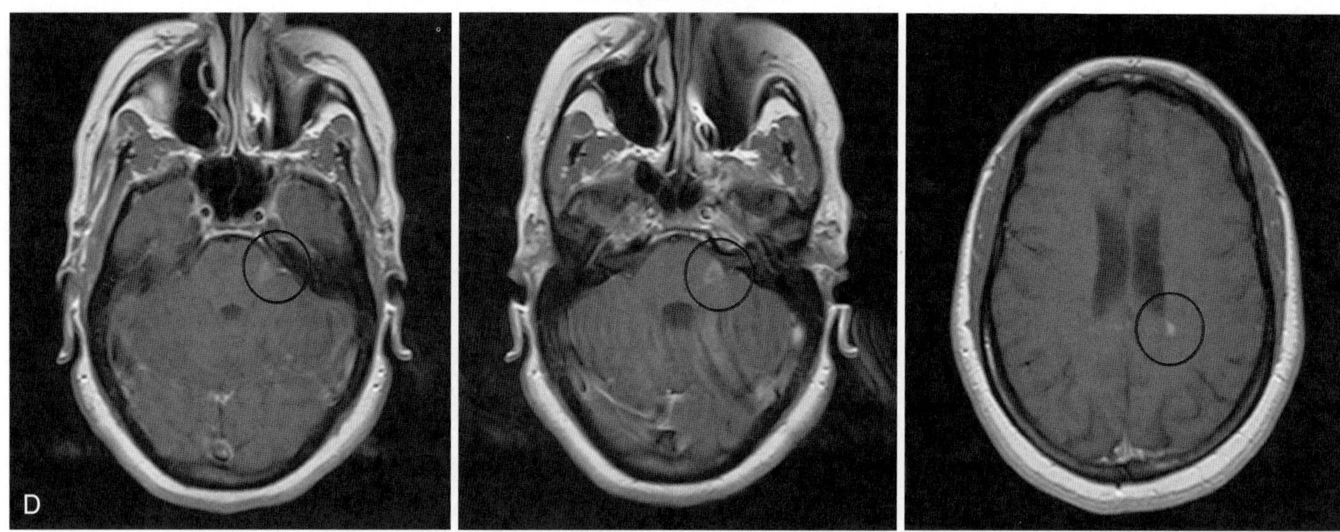

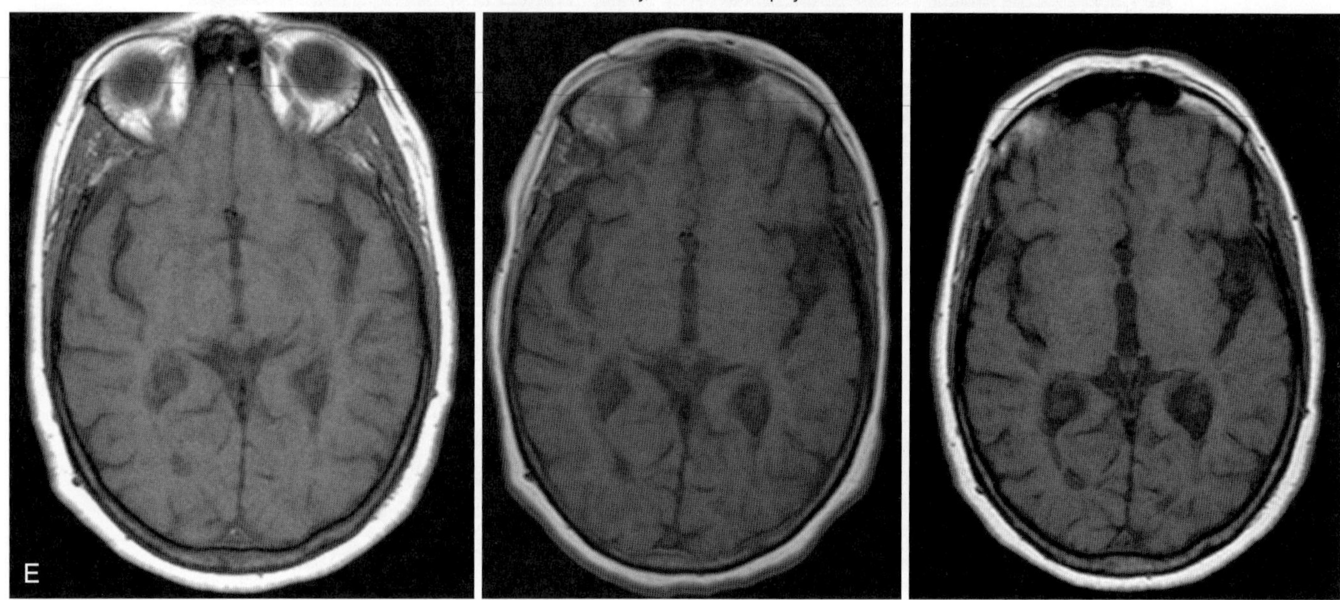

FIGURE 46-3, cont'd **D,** Gadolinium-enhanced lesion in a 34-year-old woman with RRMS with perioral numbness over the left side of her face. **E,** Natural history of brain atrophy in a 67-year-old woman with RRMS. *Left to right,* The same patient in 2004, 2009, and 2013. *FLAIR,* Fluid attenuated inversion recovery; *RRMS,* relapsing-remitting multiple sclerosis.

that combining visual-evoked potential and somatosensory-evoked potential testing significantly increases the diagnostic yield.[199] Currently, only visual-evoked potentials are included in the MS diagnostic guidelines.[156]

The Expanded Disability Status Scale (EDSS) is an ordinal clinical rating scale ranging from 0 (no impairment) to 10 (death) (Figure 46-6). It is based on a detailed neurologic examination and includes functional systems evaluating pyramidal, cerebellar, brainstem, sensory, bowel and bladder, visual, cerebral/mental, and miscellaneous functions. An EDSS score ≤4.0 implies minimal disability with no ambulation restriction, an EDSS score ≥6.0 signifies ambulation with the use of an assistive device, and an EDSS score ≥8.0 identifies a person who is essentially bed bound. The EDSS is one of the most widely used scales clinically and for research purposes. From a functional perspective, Dr. Kurtz should be credited for his emphasis on disability measurement and its correlation to other systems at such an early time.[111,112]

Pharmacologic Management

Disease-Modifying Therapies

IFN-$\beta 1_b$ was the first DMT and was introduced for the treatment of RRMS in the mid-1990s. Over time, several doses of IFN-β became available as well as glatiramer acetate.

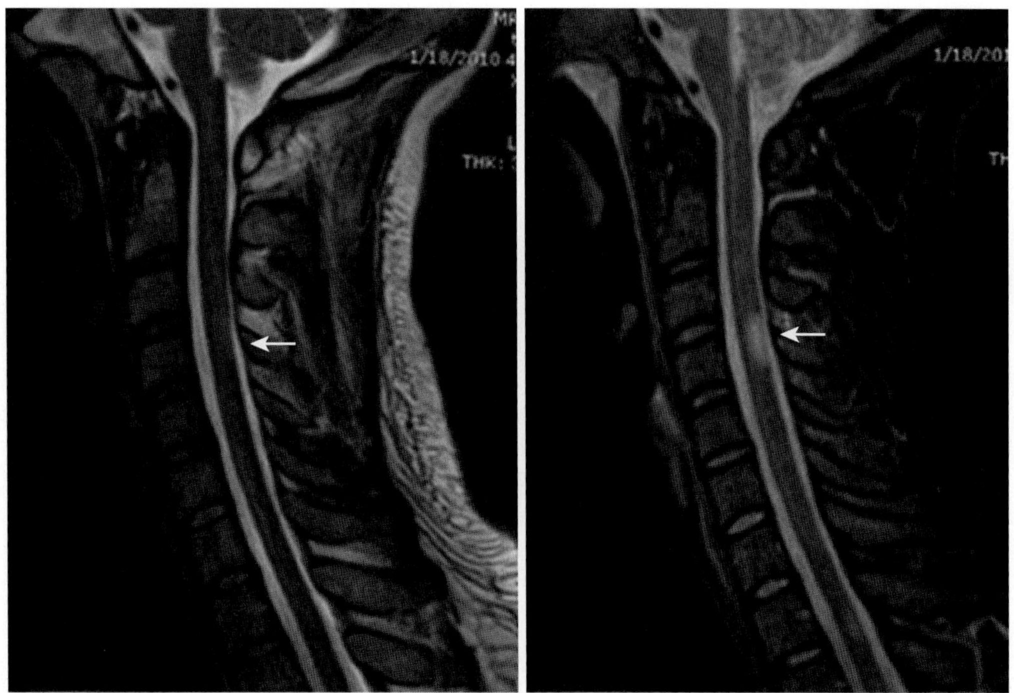

FIGURE 46-4 Superior lesion conspicuity of STIR (*right*) and T2 (*left*), as characterized by lesions at C1 to C2, C4, and C7 lesions. The lesion at the C4 level (*arrows*) is not readily visible on T2 (*left*) but is easily identifiable on STIR (*right*). *STIR,* Short T1 inversion recovery. (From Nayak NB, Salah R, Huang JC, Hathout G. M: A comparison of sagittal short T1 inversion recovery and T2-weighted FSE sequences for detection of multiple sclerosis spinal cord lesions, *Acta Neurol Scand* 129:198-203, 2014.)

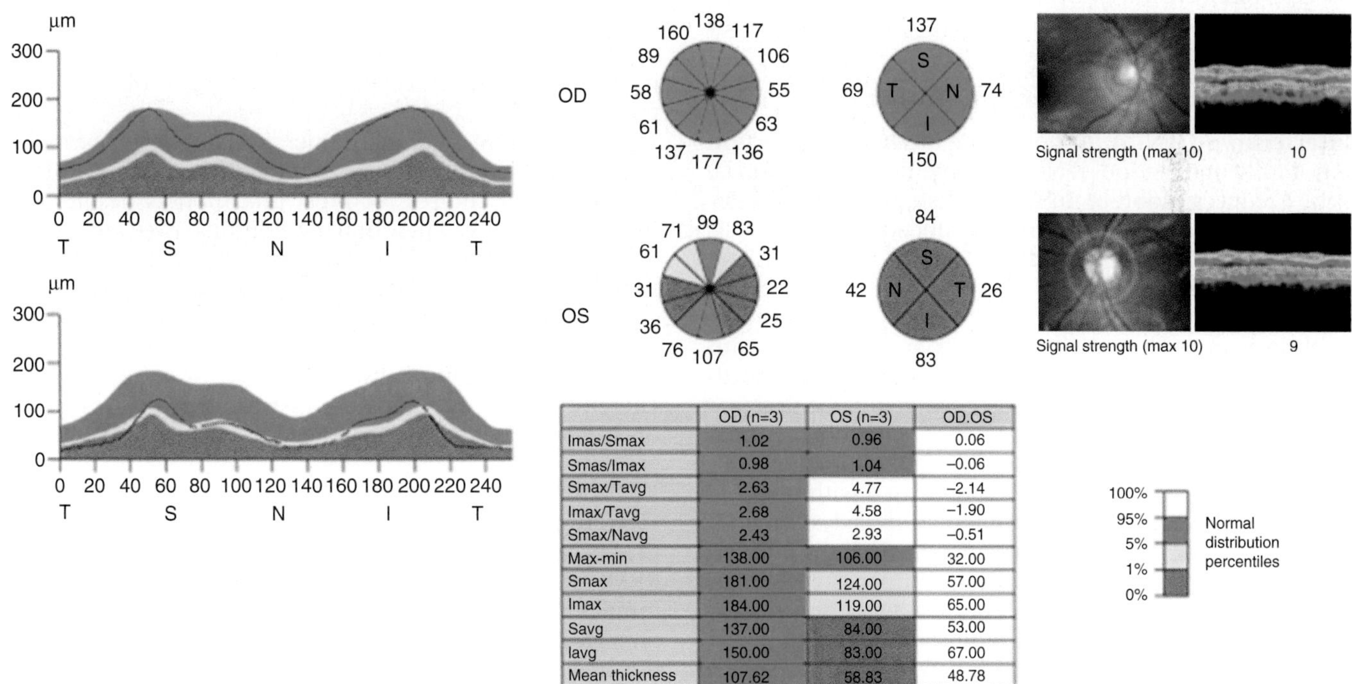

	OD (n=3)	OS (n=3)	OD.OS
Imas/Smax	1.02	0.96	0.06
Smas/Imax	0.98	1.04	–0.06
Smax/Tavg	2.63	4.77	–2.14
Imax/Tavg	2.68	4.58	–1.90
Smax/Navg	2.43	2.93	–0.51
Max-min	138.00	106.00	32.00
Smax	181.00	124.00	57.00
Imax	184.00	119.00	65.00
Savg	137.00	84.00	53.00
Iavg	150.00	83.00	67.00
Mean thickness	107.62	58.83	48.78

FIGURE 46-5 Optical coherence tomography (OCT) assessment from a patient with a remote (greater than 2 years) history of acute optic neuritis. The retinal nerve fiber layer (RNFL) thickness is shown. *Left,* The distribution of the RNFL thickness measures circumferentially around the retina. Note the greater thickness of the superior and inferior zones of the retina (the so-called double hump histogram). *Center,* Retinal thickness by clockface and quadrant sector analyses. The values in green are normal based on information derived from a normative population database. The table provides complex analysis of these values; however, the last row provides average thickness measures, which are those most commonly used in analysis. *Right,* Images of the optic disk, centered within the scan target (an important technical aspect of image analysis). To the right are the corresponding OCT-generated images of the retinal layers. The top red layer constitutes the RNFL. The signal intensity is a measure of scan quality and should be greater than or equal to level seven. Note the reduction in the average RNFL on the affected side compared with the unaffected eye. *I,* Inferior; *N,* nasal; *OD,* right eye; *OS,* left eye; *S,* superior; *T,* temporal. (Reprinted, with permission, from Elsevier [*The Lancet* 5:853-863, 2006].)

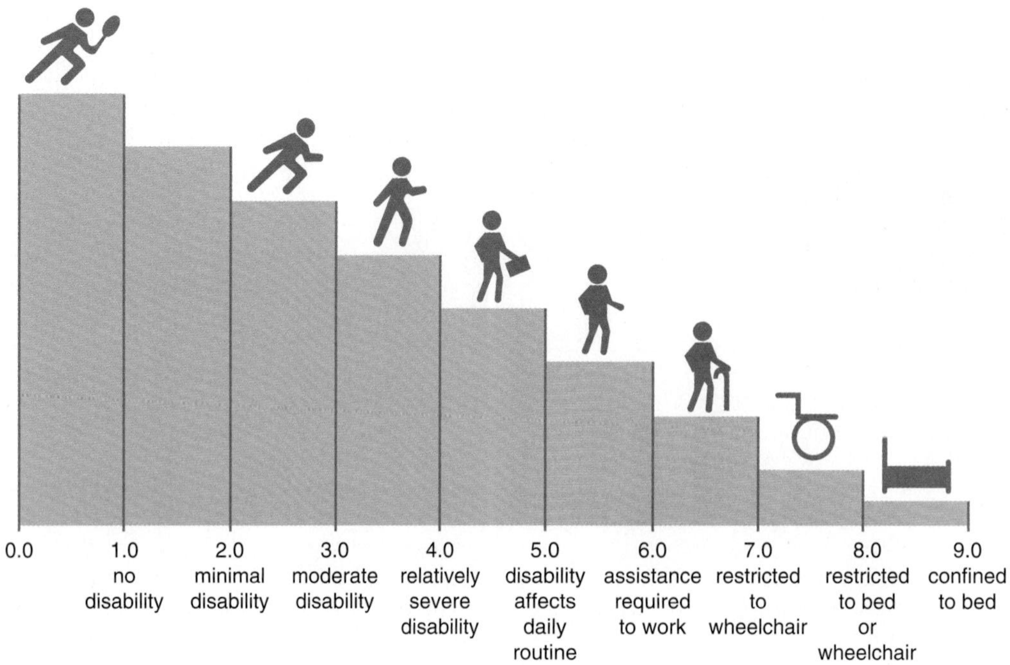

FIGURE 46-6 The Expanded Disability Status Scale. (Courtesy My-MS.org.)

However, the landscape of DMT has remarkably changed within the past 5 years. This has added new complexities for the decision-making process of both physicians and patients. What was previously a fairly simple treatment process has become more complex while more medications become available with different degrees of efficacy and safety profiles.

First-Generation Disease-Modifying Therapies

Interferon β (IFN-β). Although the mechanism of action is not fully understood, IFN-β (Avonex, Betaseron, Extavia, Rebif) reduces blood-brain barrier disruption and modulates T cell, B cell, and cytokine function.[210] IFN-$\beta 1_a$ is available in low and high doses. Low-dose IFN-$\beta 1_a$ is a once-weekly intramuscular injection. The high-dose IFN medications are all given subcutaneously three times a week in various dose regimens. IFNs are associated with flulike side effects ranging from increased fatigue, headache, myalgia, and joint pain. These gradually decrease over time and can be well controlled with nonsteroidal antiinflammatory medications taken in conjunction with the injections. All of the IFNs are associated with possible blood and bone marrow abnormalities, liver dysfunction, hypothyroidism, and mood dysfunction. There is a possibility of developing IFN antibodies, and persistently high titers of IFN antibodies are associated with diminished efficacy. It is recommended to monitor a complete blood count, liver profile, and thyroid function with treatment. IFN treatment has been known to be associated with increased risk of depression. Gradual titration of medication and routine screening is advised.

Glatiramer Acetate. The mechanism of glatiramer acetate (Copaxone) is also unclear but is probably attributable to stimulation of Treg cells.[210] The initial dose was 20 mg administered by subcutaneous injection daily. The U.S. Food and Drug Administration (FDA) recently approved a new dose of 40 mg three times a week. Occasionally, patients experience postinjection systemic reactions that are associated with flushing, palpitations, and shortness of breath and resolve after 5 to 10 minutes. All of the medications that are administered by subcutaneous injection are associated with injection site reactions, including glatiramer acetate. They can also result in lipoatrophy over time.

Because IFNs and glatiramer acetate have favorable long-term safety profiles, they remain the common first-line treatment choices for most practitioners despite the recent availability of new oral medications. They are similar in efficacy and reduce relapses by 30% in the platform studies. However, adherence remains a problem with greater than 25% of patients discontinuing therapy within 1 to 2 years.[210] IFNs and glatiramer acetate are limited in their ability to control disease activity for some patients. Therefore, patients with progressive disability related to ongoing disease activity may need to escalate DMT.

Oral Therapies

Fingolimod. Fingolimod (Gilenya) is the first oral agent that became commercially available for the treatment of RRMS. It is phosphorylated by sphingosine kinase 2 and mimics sphingosine 1-phosphate (SIP) binding to lymphocytes, which results in lymphocyte sequestration within the lymph nodes. Fingolimod also enters the CNS and affects neurons and supports glia that express SIP receptors.[165] It is associated with a 50% reduction in relapse rate versus placebo.

Adverse effects of fingolimod are related to lymphopenia as well as the other subtypes of SIP receptors that are expressed on tissues. Although few opportunistic infections have occurred, there is a risk of viral infections. Documentation of varicella zoster immunity is required before starting therapy. Disseminated zoster infection has occurred.[210] All patients must obtain a baseline electrocardiogram because of the known risk of bradycardia and possible risk of arrhythmias before starting treatment and undergo subsequent cardiovascular monitoring. Other possible safety concerns include the possibility of macular edema and elevated liver enzymes. Safety assessments include ophthalmology assessments and ongoing laboratory monitoring with complete blood counts with manual differential and liver function tests.

Teriflunomide. Teriflunomide (Aubagio) is a selective immunosuppressant with antiinflammatory properties. It is the active ring malononitrile metabolite of leflunomide, a prodrug that is used for rheumatoid arthritis. It exerts immunologic effects by inhibiting dihydroorotate dehydrogenase, an enzyme required for de novo pyrimidine synthesis in proliferating cells. Alternative modes of action may include reduced IFN-γ and interleukin-10 production by T cells, interference in the interaction between T cells and antigen-presenting cells, and changes in integrin signaling during T cell activation as well as possible antioxidant effects. Two doses of teriflunomide, 7 and 14 mg, were approved following two large placebo-controlled studies that revealed a 31% reduction in annualized relapse rate. Improvements in disability progression were only shown with the 14-mg dose. Common side effects include lymphopenia, elevated transaminases, acute renal failure, and alopecia. It is a pregnancy category X resulting from teratogenicity associated with leflunomide. It has a prolonged half-life and is contraindicated in pregnancy. It is excreted in breast milk and semen. Cholestyramine may help fully eliminate the drug.

Dimethyl Fumarate. Dimethyl fumarate (BG-12; Tecfidera) is a fumaric acid ester that is a newly approved twice-daily oral DMT for relapsing MS. It is hydrolyzed into monomethylfumarate and is eliminated through respiration. It has minimal hepatic or renal excretion. The mechanism of dimethyl fumarate is not completely clear but is known to activate the nuclear-related factor-2 transcriptional pathway. This can impact oxidative stress as well as modulate nuclear factor-κB that could have antiinflammatory effects. There were two large placebo-controlled trials involving dimethyl fumarate that revealed a 45% to 50% reduction in annualized relapse rate. It appears to have a relatively favorable safety profile, although concern was raised regarding recent publications of a few cases of progressive multifocal leukoencephalopathy (PML) with dimethyl fumarate treatment in Germany. There has been no association of PML related to treatment of dimethyl fumarate for MS. Risk factors appear to be prolonged lymphopenia and cotreatment with other immunosuppressive medications. Other potential side effects with treatment include flushing, gastrointestinal upset, lymphopenia, and elevated liver enzymes.

Intravenous Therapies

Natalizumab. Natalizumab (Tysabri) is a humanized monoclonal antibody targeting α4β1-integrin. It inhibits leukocyte migration across the blood-brain barrier by blocking the interaction between α4-integrin on leukocytes and vascular cell adhesion molecule-1 on endothelial cells and other CNS ligands. Two large placebo-controlled trials revealed a 68% reduction rate in relapses as well as a 43% reduction in disability.[155] Natalizumab was initially approved for the treatment of RRMS in 2004 and was voluntarily removed from the market after the development of three cases of PML in 2005. Two of the cases were in patients treated for MS who were also receiving IFN-$\beta 1_a$. Natalizumab was reapproved for treatment in conjunction with a safety monitoring program (Touch program) in 2006. Risk factors for developing PML include evidence of previous John Cunningham (JC) virus exposure, duration of natalizumab therapy, and previous use of immunosuppressant treatment such as mitoxantrone, azathioprine, or methotrexate. The risk of PML increases with increasing duration of therapy (0.6 per 1000 less than 2 years, 5 per 1000 at 2 to 4 years), particularly if there is a history of immunosuppression (1.6 per 1000 less than 2 years, 11 per 1000 at 2 to 4 years). There are concerns regarding possible rebound disease activity after stopping natalizumab.

In terms of monitoring for PML, patients using natalizumab who are JC seropositive should undergo MRI surveillance every 6 months to detect early, subtle signs that would be suggestive of PML. Clinical or MRI evidence of PML should prompt natalizumab discontinuation until further assessment is obtained. Diagnosis is confirmed by CSF analysis for JC virus DNA by polymerase chain reaction. Treatment is needed by rapid removal of natalizumab with plasmapheresis. A short course of intravenous methylprednisolone may be administered in an effort to mitigate additional damage that can occur from the immune reconstitution syndrome.

Additional adverse effects that can occur from natalizumab treatment include a mild increased risk of infections, such as urinary tract or upper respiratory tract infections. Approximately 6% of patients can develop infusion reactions. These individuals are at a higher risk of developing antibodies against Natalizumab, which may lessen the efficacy of treatment. There is also a potential for elevated liver enzymes.

Mitoxantrone. Mitoxantrone (Novantrone) is a chemotherapeutic agent that has been approved to treat aggressive-relapsing MS and SPMS. It is a cytotoxic agent that inhibits B cells, T cells, and macrophage proliferation. It is administered as an intravenous infusion, four times per year (12 mg, m^2) with a maximum cumulative dose of 100 to 140 mg/m^2. It is known that there is a dose-dependent risk of cardiomyopathy. Before initiation of therapy, left ventricular ejection fraction should be obtained by echocardiogram, multigated radionuclide angiography, or MRI. Before each infusion with mitoxantrone, an electrocardiogram should be performed. A qualitative reevaluation of left ventricular ejection fraction should be assessed after termination of mitoxantrone using the same method that was performed at baseline.

Other potential adverse reactions of mitoxantrone are lymphopenia and elevated liver enzymes. Mitoxantrone should not be administered when the neutrophil count falls less than 1500 mm^2. A complete blood count with manual differential and liver enzymes should be tested before administration. During therapy, patients should

Table 46-3 Disease-Modifying Therapies for Multiple Sclerosis

Medication	Route	Frequency	Adverse Effects	Pregnancy Class
Interferon $\beta 1_a$	Intramuscular	Weekly	Interferon side effects Leukopenia, hepatotoxicity, thyroid changes, mood changes	C
Interferon $B1_a$ Interferon $B1_b$	Subcutaneous	MWF 3 times weekly	Interferon side effects Leukopenia, hepatotoxicity, thyroid changes, mood changes Injection site reactions	C
Glatiramer acetate	Subcutaneous	20 mg SQ daily or 40 mg 3 times per week	Injection site reactions Postinjection systemic reactions	B
Fingolimod	Oral	Daily	Lymphopenia Macular edema Bradycardia/AV block Risk of infections	C
Teriflunomide	Oral	Daily	Lymphopenia Risk of infections Alopecia Hepatotoxicity Renal failure Teratogenicity	X Requires negative pregnancy test before starting treatment
Dimethyl fumarate	Oral	Twice a day	Lymphopenia Gastrointestinal upset Hepatotoxicity	C
Natalizumab	IV	Every 4 weeks	Increased risk of infection, primarily concerning risk of PML Infusion reactions Hepatotoxicity	C
Mitoxantrone	IV	Every 12 weeks	Lymphopenia Cardiotoxicity Increased risk of infections Risk of malignancy Possibility of sterility	D Requires negative pregnancy test before starting treatment

AV, Atrioventricular; *IV,* intravenous; *MWF,* Monday, Wednesday, Friday; *PML,* progressive multifocal leukoencephalopathy; *SQ,* subcutaneous.

avoid receiving live virus vaccinations. Mitoxantrone is assigned a pregnancy category D. Patients should be informed of the potential risk that it may cause sterility if they have not completed their family planning. A pregnancy test should be completed before each dose.

Alemtuzumab. Alemtuzumab (Lemtrada) is a humanized monoclonal antibody against CD52 that is expressed on lymphocytes and monocytes and causes rapid and profound lymphopenia. The recovery of lymphopenia is variable and subset dependent. An application has been submitted in the United States based on the results of two large placebo-controlled studies that revealed significant efficacy of alemtuzumab for the treatment of relapsing MS. Secondary autoimmunity has been reported in up to 20% of treated patients.[169] Although the etiology is unclear, it may be related to secondary immune reconstitution syndrome that results in B cells emerging before Treg cells.[90] Patients can develop thyroid disease, idiopathic thrombocytopenia, and possibly Goodpasture syndrome. There is some implication that interleukin-21 may help mitigate this risk. Treatment requires frequent laboratory monitoring with complete blood count with manual differential, thyroid functioning, and liver functioning. Clinical trials are ongoing in efforts to minimize additional autoimmune disease risk.

Other potential side effects include infusion reactions such as urticaria, pyrexia, and rigor. Pretreatment with corticosteroids and antihistamines may improve tolerability. Infections can occur with alemtuzumab given the severe leukopenia. There have been cases of PML associated with alemtuzumab treatment reported in patients treated for chronic lymphocytic leukemia and non-Hodgkin lymphoma (Table 46-3).

Rehabilitation, Exercise, and Symptom Management

Physical Activity

A person with a disability is prone to inactivity and deconditioning.[167] Current recommendations for physical activity are meant for individuals without physical disability and those guidelines are often not applicable to the population with disabilities. PwMS were previously advised to not exercise for fear of worsening disease course. In addition, PwMS would be advised to avoid exercise so as to prevent overheating. Immune profile studies have demonstrated no change in the physiologic variables of patients with MS compared with control groups after being subjected to 30 minutes of aerobic exercise.[71] However, multiple studies have demonstrated the safety and benefit of exercise in PwMS, regardless of MS subtype, in terms of aerobic fitness, quality of life, and overall health.[39,151] Advice on exercise and physical fitness recommendations

Table 46-4 Canadian Physical Activity Guidelines for Adults with Multiple Sclerosis

	Aerobic Activity	Strength Training Activity
How often?	Two times per week • Aerobic and strength training activities can be done on the same day • Rest your muscles for at least 1 day between strength training sessions	Two times per week
How much?	Gradually increase your activity so that you are doing at least 30 minutes of aerobic activity during each workout session.	Repetitions are the number of times you lift and lower a weight. Try to do 10 to 15 repetitions of each exercise. This counts as one set. Gradually work up to doing two sets of 10 to 15 repetitions of each exercise.
How hard?	These activities should be performed at a moderate intensity. Moderate-intensity physical activity is usually a 5 or 6 on a scale of 10, and causes your heart rate to go up. As a general rule, if you are doing moderate-intensity activity you can talk, but not sing a song, during the activity.	Pick a resistance (free weights, cable pulleys, bands, etc.) heavy enough that you can barely, but safely, finish 10 to 15 repetitions of the last set. Be sure to rest for 1 to 2 minutes between each set and exercise.
How to?	Some options for activity include: Aerobic activities • Upper body exercises: arm cycling • Lower body exercises: walking, leg cycling • Combined upper and lower body exercises: elliptical trainer	Strength training activities for the upper and lower body • Weight machines • Free weights • Cable pulleys
Other types of exercise that may bring benefits Elastic resistance bands Aquatic exercise Calisthenics		

From Canadian Physical Activity Guidelines for Adults with Multiple Sclerosis, ©2012. Used, with permission, from the Canadian Society for Exercise Physiology.

was the most sought-after request among individuals with MS and was surprisingly ahead of questions on medication.[189]

The first and only consensus panel convened in an effort to review the available evidence and formulate guidelines for physical fitness in PwMS.[114] The review determined there was sufficient evidence to formulate guidelines to improve aerobic capacity and muscle strength. The consensus panel did not find sufficient evidence to provide guidelines for mobility, fatigue, or health-related quality of life benefits (Table 46-4). These recommendations are based on the recommendations for physical activity of the MS Society of Canada.[136]

Patients with MS commonly report fatigue, mood disorders, inadequate access to equipment, heat intolerance, and insufficient time as barriers to exercising.[4] Clinicians should continue to reinforce the importance of fitness as well as remove or treat those barriers when possible. In summary, exercise is helpful for PwMS with no evidence for deleterious effect. The intensity, duration, and frequency must be coupled with a patient's symptoms, heat intolerance, strength, and endurance.

Gait Impairment

Mobility impairment is one of the most common single disabilities in PwMS. Approximately 75% of PwMS have mobility challenges.[168] Natural history studies conducted before the availability of DMT reported that 50% of PwMS who had the onset of gait impairment will require an assistive device 15 years after the diagnosis.[207] Physiatrists are well aware of the detrimental effects mobility impairment poses to the disabled. There is an increased risk of weakness, spasticity, contractures, bone mineral changes, cardiovascular changes, reduced independence, and reduced quality of life. Overall, long-term positive prognostic indicators for disability and gait impairment include female gender, young age, complete recovery of initial exacerbation (specific to the RRMS subtype), and reduced relapse rate in the first 5 years.[200]

The Timed 25 (T25) Foot Walk Test is a validated measure of walking speed in MS. A 20% change in walking speed is considered significant and clinically meaningful.[102] A time of 5 seconds or less is expected in unaffected individuals. Other gait tests, such as the Two- and Six-Minute Walking Tests have demonstrated correlation to ambulation and physical fatigue in PwMS.[70,73,176] These tests take longer to administer, but additional information such as fatigue resistance or sensitivity, speed, heart rate monitoring, and endurance may be obtained.[42] However, the increased energy output required, combined with the possibility that some patients may not be able to complete either test, makes the T25 Foot Walk Test more feasible in a clinical and research setting.

Dalfampridine is the extended release version of the immediate release version, 4-aminopyridine. It is a potassium channel agonist and potentiates the duration of the action potential, promoting nerve signal transmission, and thereby prolonging its mechanism of action. This agent was very appealing because of its ability to enhance nerve conduction in areas of demyelination.[154] However, although initially promising, the immediate release version had a significant adverse event profile and a short duration of action.[215]

Dalfampridine was approved for the use of PwMS with walking impairment in 2010 based on the results of two phase III randomized, placebo-controlled trials. Approximately one third of participants displayed 25% improvement in their T25 walking speed. The impact of this improvement in PwMS should not be overlooked. Study participants had T25 walking times of greater than 8 seconds to 45 seconds. Dalfampridine is given at a dose of 10 mg every 12 hours. A history of seizures is an absolute concentration because dalfampridine lowers the seizure threshold. Other adverse events include increased frequency of urinary tract infections, vertigo, insomnia, headache, and falls. Dalfampridine is renally excreted; therefore, a baseline basic metabolic panel is advised because adequate creatinine clearance (51 to 80 mL/min) is vital.[53,75-77]

What remains unclear is why only 30% to 40% of patients are dalfampridine "responders" and others are not. Various theories explaining this include varying sites of demyelination. A once-daily formulation of dalfampridine is currently being researched.

Inpatient Rehabilitation

Annual expenses of Medicare beneficiaries with MS were almost twice that of other Medicare beneficiaries.[158] Also, 57.9% of Medicare beneficiaries with MS were younger than 65 years and 55.3% of these beneficiaries were individuals with disabilities; this is in stark contrast to only 11% of the Medicare sample group being younger than 65 years old. In that same group, only 9% were individuals with disabilities.[120] The Medicare MS population had lower overall admission, discharge, and change in Functional Independence Measure (FIM) scores during their acute inpatient admission. The same was true for all subscales except cognition. No significant difference was noted in discharge destination. The mean overall inpatient rehabilitation length of stay was 1.5 days longer for the Medicare patient with MS. Most Medicare patients with MS were discharged to their prehospital living community. Home Health Service use was much more common in the Medicare population with MS. In general, Medicare beneficiaries with MS have lower changes in functional scores and a longer length of stay compared with other Medicare beneficiaries. A notable finding in this study is that Medicare beneficiaries with MS had significantly increased rates of depression compared with the Medicare group without MS. Clinicians managing PwMS admitted to the inpatient unit should be acutely aware of and screen for mood issues because that may have an impact on improvement and this is an area where physiatrists can have a significant impact.

Despite lower FIM scores in patients with MS versus patients without MS, multiple studies demonstrated the benefit of a multidisciplinary inpatient admission in patients with MS.[39]

Fatigue

Fatigue remains one of the most common and debilitating symptoms in MS and is quoted as one of the single most disabling symptoms. This is a silent symptom and patients may have difficulty comprehending and articulating the nature of it, as well as challenges explaining to others why "they look so good" but may feel entirely the contrary. Patients commonly describe fatigue as a "reversible motor and cognitive impairment, with reduced motivation and desire to rest."[132]

Individuals with MS may experience two types of fatigue: peripheral and central. Peripheral fatigue is associated with fatigability, that is, a generalized sense of exhaustion affecting the patient after a few minutes of physical activity and is alleviated with rest. Central fatigue is subjective and is associated with dysfunction in arousal and attention. The individual reports a feeling of constant exhaustion or lassitude that can lead to worsening vision or function. Rest will not have an effect on central fatigue and thereby has a significant impact on function, quality of life, relationships, and even maintenance of occupation/vocation.

The Fatigue Severity Scale, the Fatigue Impact Scale, and the Modified Fatigue Impact Scale are the most commonly used scales for fatigue assessment in patients with MS.[56,132] These are self-reported scales. The Modified Fatigue Impact Scale was modified from the Fatigue Impact Scale and was created for clinical settings and takes 5 to 10 minutes to complete. There is a long (21 questions) and short (5 questions) version available.[110]

Fatigue can also be classified as primary and secondary. Primary fatigue is attributable to the disease process (MS) and secondary fatigue is a result of other causes. Screening for secondary causes of fatigue, including metabolic, endocrine, hematologic, and medication side effect profiles, is advised (Box 46-5). Mood disturbances may mimic fatigue or lassitude. There is up to a 50% lifetime prevalence of depression in PwMS.[33,183] Treating depression in PwMS is associated with reduction in fatigue symptoms.

BOX 46-5

Fatigue: Secondary Factors

Thermosensitivity/heat dysregulation
Mood disorder
Anxiety
Sleep disturbance
Infection
Thyroid dysfunction
Anemia
Medications
- Disease-modifying therapies (typically interferon)
- Antidepressants
- Antispasmodics
- Narcotics
- Sedatives

Aggressive screening for and treatment of fatigue is advised. Awareness of triggering factors such as heat, stress, or overexertion should be emphasized. Also, energy conservation techniques and training are advised. Education of family and caregivers is helpful because MS fatigue may present suddenly. Patients report social isolation for fear of being unable to keep up with family or friends. Job productivity and efficiency may also be negatively affected with the presence of fatigue. In addition to energy conservation and avoidance of triggers, pharmacologic treatment is advised to help maintain energy and focus. Patients respond differently to these medications and the clinician is encouraged to try another agent if the patient experiences subtherapeutic responses (Table 46-5).

Sleep Disorders

Approximately 10% of the general population suffers from insomnia, whereas approximately 40% to 50% of PwMS report difficulty with sleep initiation, maintenance, or have early morning awakening.[119] Any discussion about

Table 46-5 Adult Doses for Fatigue Treatment

Name	Dosage	Mechanism of Action	Side Effects	Controlled	Off-Label Use
Amantadine	Up to 100 mg twice a day	Unknown	Vertigo, orthostatic hypotension, dry mouth, livedo reticularis	No	Yes
Dextroamphetamine/ amphetamine	Extended release: up to 20 mg every day Immediate release: 5 to 60 mg in divided doses	Unknown	Hypertension, tachycardia, irritability, xerostomia, headache, insomnia	Schedule II	Yes
Lisdexamfetamine Dimesylate	Up to 70 mg every day	Unknown	Xerostomia, insomnia	Schedule II	Yes
Methylphenidate	Available in immediate and extended release formulations. Up to 60 mg every day of either version	CNS stimulant	Decreased appetite, tachycardia, headache, insomnia	Schedule II	Yes
Modafinil	Up to 400 mg in divided doses	CNS activation, improves wakefulness state	Insomnia, anxiety	Schedule IV	Yes
Armodafinil	50 to 150 mg every day	CNS activation, improves wakefulness state	Headache	Schedule IV	Yes
Atomoxetine	40 to 100 mg daily	Norepinephrine reuptake inhibitor	Tachycardia, decrease in appetite, nausea, erectile dysfunction	No	Yes

CNS, Central nervous system.

fatigue in PwMS should include discussion about sleep hygiene. The clinician should encourage sleep promoting behaviors such as avoiding eating, drinking, watching television, or even reading in bed. Symptoms of MS that may interfere with sleep include spasticity, pain/paresthesias, and nocturia.[153] Reviewing side effects of DMT, particularly IFNs, may reveal myalgias or low-grade fever on injection days that cause sleep disruption. Finally, screening for mood disorders is advised as a result of the high prevalence in this population. Addressing and adequately treating these symptoms is vital. Patients have demonstrated benefit with guided imagery, biofeedback, cognitive behavioral therapy, and meditation practice. If pharmacologic treatment is required, a determination of long-term or short-term use is needed. Treatment agents include zolpidem, trazodone, benzodiazepine, sedating antidepressants, and antihistamines.[30]

Sleep-disordered breathing, obstructive sleep apnea, and central sleep apnea may be the etiology of persistent fatigue in PwMS. Obstructive sleep apnea is a result of upper airway obstruction during sleep. Central sleep apnea is the lack of respiratory effort during sleep. Patients with clinical or radiologic evidence of brainstem involvement had elevated Apnea-Hypopnea Index (episodes of obstructive apneas, central apneas, or hypopneas per hour of sleep) than those without brainstem involvement.[21,119] There is a suggestion that DMT use results in lower apnea scores.[21,153] Referral for polysomnogram testing is advised in the patient refractory to fatigue-mitigating treatment. Treatment may include weight loss, tobacco cessation, respiratory support with continuous positive airway pressure, or surgery.

Besides obstructive sleep apnea and central sleep apnea, other sleep-related movement disorders include restless leg syndrome (RLS) and periodic limb movement disorder (PLMD). Patients with RLS typically report an inability to keep their leg(s) still. PLMD typically manifests while sleeping and are involuntary movements. Legs are much more commonly involved. PLMD is quantified and confirmed via polysomnography testing. It is reported that RLS is two to six times more common in MS than healthy controls.[119] Increased risk of RLS is seen with older age, increased disability, cervical lesions, and PPMS. Patients with RLS should undergo screening for iron deficiency because this may contribute to symptoms. Treatment for both RLS and PLMD includes dopaminergic agents, benzodiazepine (clonazepam), and anticonvulsants.[98]

Narcolepsy is a chronic sleep disorder characterized by sleep paralysis, cataplexy, hypnagogic hallucinations, and nocturnal sleep disruption.[119] MS is the fourth most common cause of narcolepsy. The gene for both MS and narcolepsy is the same: HLA DRB1*1501, suggesting an autoimmune component to the disorder.

Mood Disorders

The most common mood disorder in MS is depression. It is present in at least 50% of patients; many have theorized that one disease may predispose the other.[148] The lifetime prevalence of depression is MS is three times that of the general population. The overlap of symptoms in both depression and MS (fatigue, poor concentration, sleepiness/fatigue, and appetite disturbance) can lead to underdiagnosis of depression and has delayed the diagnosis of MS. No clear relation between cognition and depression has been determined despite multiple studies. Depression has negative implications on quality of life and an increased risk of suicide. The suicide rate of patients with MS is 7.5 times higher than that of the general population and higher than other neurologic disorders.[172]

Screening for DMT-related side effects, particularly IFNs, is advised. Some patients may have mood disorders secondary to DMT and may benefit from a change. Other symptomatic medications may have a similar side effect profile and an alternative medication is advised. The Beck Depression Inventory (BDI) and the Beck Depression Inventory-Fast Screen (BDI-FS) is a validated scale to screen for depression in PwMS.[19,193] Both are patient-reported scales; the BDI has 21 items and the BDI-FS has 7 items. The BDI has a sensitivity of 71% and a specificity of 79%. The high false-negative rate (30%) should be noted; those patients that are borderline may need further testing or more frequent evaluations.

Although limited studies are available regarding controlled studies of pharmacologic treatment in depression, The Goldman Consensus Group, an expert panel convened by the National MS Society to review depression in MS, recommends treating depression with individualized treatment using pharmacologic and/or psychological counseling.[72] In addition, a new area of focus is reviewing coping skills of living an enriching and fulfilling life despite one's disability.

Thermoregulation

The pathophysiology of MS is one of central demyelination.[63] Physiatrists are keenly aware of the effects of segmental demyelination: reduction in conduction velocity, altered saltatory conduction, and eventual conduction block. The safety factor (ratio of action current available at a node to threshold current) is responsible for successful conduction. Advanced demyelination reduces the safety factor. Heat causes alteration of the sodium channels and also reduces the safety factor and amplitude of nerve action potentials. A demyelinated nerve is more vulnerable to heat-related changes than the unaffected nerve.[105]

Heat intolerance is a well-established symptom in PwMS. Uhthoff phenomenon, a transient loss of vision or blurred vision, after a hot bath or exercise is common.[45] Heat causes transient worsening of many symptoms of MS and can cause fatigue. The "Hot Bath Test" was used before the availability of MRI to diagnose patients with MS.[124] Patients were immersed in warm water ranging from 35° C to 40° C and observed for worsening of long tract corticobulbar and corticospinal signs. This was discontinued after some patients had irreversible changes postheating as well as the advent of MRI.[79] Approximately 58% to 93% of patients are affected by heat-induced fatigue.[24] Exposure to heat can cause worsening of both physical and cognitive function. Autonomic dysfunction also contributes to poor temperature regulation in PwMS.[45]

Patients should be counseled about prevention and treatment options to prevent potentially fatal injuries from occurring. Avoidance of warm baths or swimming in heated pools is advised. In general, water temperatures no greater than 84° F (26.7 to 28.9° C) is advised.[173] Precooling with an ice water slurry or a cool water bath can effectively lower the core body temperature. Head cooling has also been found to be effective in PwMS compared with sham cooling.[164] Various evaporative cooling garments can be used when patients are outside.[180] Contrary to early theories where exercise was discouraged by health professionals, PwMS are encouraged to exercise in moderation for strength, fitness, and maintenance of health.

Spasticity

Spasticity affects up to 85% of PwMS.[168] Lower limb spasticity is much more common (97%) than upper limb spasticity (50%).[11] Unsurprisingly, there is a negative correlation between the presence of lower limb spasticity and mobility.[190]

The Consortium of MS Centers recommends that spasticity be screened for as part of routine MS patient visits. In addition to evaluating a patient's strength, range of motion, deep tendon reflexes, and muscle tone with the patient seated on the examination table, the patient should be examined in a dynamic setting. This includes observing the patient's gait pattern, observing how his or her intrinsic hand muscles move with flexion and extension, and observing for signs of muscle co-contraction. The patient may also report difficulty falling or staying asleep as a result of increased muscle spasticity at night.

Many tools are available to assess spasticity. These include the Ashworth, Modified Ashworth, Tardieu, Penn Spasm Frequency Scale, and the Timed Up and Go Test. In addition, the T25 Foot Walk Test, the Ambulation Index, and the MS Spasticity Scale are additional MS-specific tests that can be used in the clinical setting.[82,93] The MS Spasticity Scale has been validated for use in PwMS and is an 88-item self-reported scale.

Treatment options for spasticity are discussed in Chapter 23. A brief overview will be presented here. Both physical and occupational therapy is helpful in early stages and as adjunctive treatment to supplement oral, injected, and intrathecal medications. Oral baclofen is the usual first-line oral agent. Tizanidine may be limited given its sedating side effects. Clonazepam is helpful in cases of PLMD or nighttime spasms.

The American Academy of Neurology released a guideline stating that oral cannabis is "the only complementary and alternative medicine unequivocally effective for helping patients with MS, specifically easing their pain and symptoms of spasticity, possibly for as long as 1 year of treatment."[214] The consensus statement reported of the beneficial effects of oral cannabis on spasticity, pain, muscle spasms, and sleep.[218]

The benefit of chemodenervation with botulinum toxin (BoNT) injections in MS is paramount, resulting from the difficulty with tolerance of oral antispasmodics. This medication class can commonly cause sedation or fatigue. Intrathecal baclofen (ITB) therapy via an implanted drug delivery device is indicated when oral or injectable treatment becomes ineffective. The clinician is encouraged to use this therapy before the onset of significant walking impairment or lower limb weakness. ITB trials may require dose adjustment for PwMS. The use of ITB pumps in patients with MS has demonstrated improvements in spasticity, quality of life, sleep quality, bowel and bladder performance, skin integrity, and ambulation with low complication rates in numerous studies.[15,150] Physiatrists are encouraged to educate and provide ITB therapy as a treatment option for PwMS. Studies have demonstrated that ITB therapy in PwMS is not introduced as a result of greater focus on DMT management. Also, the patient or clinician may not fully recognize the effect of spasticity on quality of life and have a lack of awareness of how to manage ITB therapy, hence the need for the physiatrist who will be better able to recognize and effectively treat and manage spasticity.[51] Phenol injections or surgical intervention may be used in patients with severe mobility or contractures and have failed conservative therapies.

The growing complexity and availability of DMTs for MS has reduced the time many MS specialists can focus on symptomatic treatment. Many specialists will refer to physiatry for treatment of gait and spasticity. The preservation of clinically useful mobility and overall function is paramount to the PwMS. A multimodal and multidisciplinary approach is vital in approaching the patient with a chronic, progressive disease such as MS. Improving function while mitigating the effects of fatigue is vital.

Pain

Patients with MS experience neuropathic and nociceptive pain. Prevalence studies report that 29% to 86% of patients are affected by pain.[186,188] The Neuropathic Pain Special Interest Group of the International Association for the Study of Pain defines neuropathic pain arising as a direct consequence of a lesion or disease that affects the somatosensory system.[66] Nociceptive pain is attributable to stimulation of nociceptors that signal tissue irritation or injury to elicit an appropriate response. Pain negatively impacts mood, energy, daily activities, vocation, social interaction, and has been linked with reduced quality of life in PwMS.

Patients may complain of pain at injection sites associated with DMT. A large-scale review found that subcutaneous drug formulations have increased injection site reactions compared with intramuscular injections.[10] Patient- and clinician-reported injection site reactions include the presence of localized burning, tenderness, swelling, or necrosis. Glatiramer acetate is strongly associated with localized lipoatrophy. Clinicians are encouraged to discuss this with patients because injection site reactions have been associated with reduced medication compliance. Suggested techniques to reduce injection site reactions include encouraging the use of an autoinjector, topical anesthetic agents, massage, and cooling packs. Injection site rotation and avoiding known sensitive areas is also advised.[191]

Neuropathic pain has a prevalence of 50% in MS and is believed to be a result of the presence of plaques in the CNS (particularly the corticospinal and dorsal column tracts), causing symptoms of allodynia and hyperalgesia.[188] Patients respond well to anticonvulsant treatment, particularly gabapentin, which has little interaction and a wide dose range. Another agent in the same class is pregabalin. Although effective for its treatment effect, its side effect profile is difficult for some patients (edema, sedation, weight gain, constipation). Finally, other agents in the anticonvulsant class worthy of consideration include levetiracetam, lamotrigine, and zonisamide. The tricyclic antidepressant class may also be used to treat neuropathic pain; again, the side effect profile (dry mouth, constipation, drowsiness, urinary retention) may pose a challenge for patients.

Patients who are unable to tolerate the side effects or obtain clinically meaningful relief from oral medications may consider intrathecal therapy via an implanted drug delivery device. Morphine and ziconotide are both approved for management of neuropathic pain via intrathecal infusion. Morphine is an opioid and useful for patients unable to tolerate oral/systemic use. One small study demonstrated safety and effectiveness of intrathecal morphine and baclofen for the treatment of spasticity and neuropathic pain.[170] Ziconotide is a nonopioid agent and demonstrated significant pain reduction over placebo.[107,161] It selectively targets voltage-gated calcium channels and prevents primary afferent transmission of pain signals in the spinal cord. Extremely slow titration is advised to prevent side effects.[107] Common side effects of Ziconotide include dizziness, nausea, and confusion. It is a viable option for patients that are not opioid responsive and does not cause tolerance, dependence, or respiratory depression.[55] Most patients with MS have limited tolerance to medications that may cause fatigue and, therefore, pump delivery is an appealing alternative to oral/systemic agents, and may provide pain relief without the burdensome effects of sedation or confusion.

Trigeminal neuralgia (TN) affects approximately 2% to 6% of patients with MS and is 20 times more common in PwMS.[101] It may be a result of focal compression of the trigeminal nerve root near its entry at the pons (primary TN) or as a result of a neurologic diagnosis such as demyelinating plaques in the same region or a posterior fossa tumor (symptomatic TN). Patients complain of spontaneous, unilateral, lancinating "electrical sparks." Light, tactile sensation or pressure may stimulate the pain. The pain can last for seconds to hours. Diagnosis may be challenging resulting from referred pain from the three branches of the trigeminal nerve causing referred pain and patients may misconstrue their symptoms for dental pain. Blink reflex studies have reported delays of the R1 response on the symptomatic side.[40] There is no standardized MRI sequence to screen for neurovascular compression. Treatment options include anticonvulsants (carbamazepine, gabapentin, lamotrigine, topiramate), antispasmodics (baclofen), and in rare instances, narcotics. Again, most PwMS are hesitant to take opiates because of the cognitive and physical clouding that may occur. Finally, misoprostol, a prostaglandin E analogue relieved pain in patients with TN and should be considered.[47] Misoprostol is believed to be effective because the T cell inhibition caused by prostaglandins leads to an antiinflammatory effect in plaques. Doses of misoprostol ranged from 100 to 200 mg titrated up to four times a day. Patients refractory to or unable to tolerate oral medications may consider BoNT injections or neurosurgery referral for microvascular decompression, rhizotomy, or gamma knife repair.

Finally, some other MS symptoms that the clinician should be aware of include pain associated with optic neuritis, a Lhermitte sign, and the "MS hug." Inflammation of the optic nerve causes optic neuritis. It is often painful and worse with movement; photosensitivity and/or blurred vision may also be present. The symptom is occasionally self-limiting and can also be treated with steroids (intravenous methylprednisolone). A Lhermitte sign is an electrical sensation that occurs down the length of the spine and is exacerbated with neck flexion. Some patients report a Lhermitte sign with fatigue, heat exposure, or during an exacerbation. This symptom is typically self-limited. Finally, the "MS hug" is described by patients as a feeling of tightness across their ribs, as if they were being hugged very tightly. Burning and tingling sensations are common. Treatment with anticonvulsants or topical compound mixtures of anticonvulsants and lidocaine are suggested. The cause of Lhermitte sign and the "MS hug" is unknown.

Neurogenic Bladder, Neurogenic Bowel, and Sexual Dysfunction

Patients with MS are highly disposed to bladder, bowel, and sexual dysfunction. The following three sections will focus on areas specific for MS. The reader is advised to consult Chapter 20, Chapter 21, and Chapter 22 for further detail on each area.

Neurogenic Bladder

The presence of lesions in the brain and/or spinal cord may lead to disorders of emptying (double voiding, incomplete emptying, slow or intermittent stream), storage (urinary urgency, frequency, nocturia, incontinence), or a mixture of both (detrusor sphincter dyssynergia). It affects up to 75% of PwMS.[136] Patients may socially isolate themselves because of the unpredictable nature of the lower urinary tracts. The presence of gait dysfunction is correlated with the presence of neurogenic bladder.[58] Many studies have corroborated the presence of increased urinary dysfunction in patients with MS when plaques are present in the spinal cord.[1,74]

Guidelines for the screening of lower urinary tract dysfunction include an appropriate history and evaluation of the postvoid residual. The need and utility of urodynamic evaluation remains controversial. Early screening is advised to prevent long-term complications in the urinary tract.

Treatment includes pelvic muscle training, medication, BoNT injection, and surgery. Pharmacologic treatment consists of antimuscarinic agents for treating disorders of storage. α-Antagonists are commonly recommended for treatment of voiding disorders. Desmopressin may be indicated for symptoms of nocturia. Appropriate screening for side effects of medications (constipation, dry mouth, fatigue, cognitive slowing) and electrolyte monitoring (hyponatremia) is advised.

BoNT type A (BoNT-A), specifically Onabotulinum Toxin, is FDA-approved for the treatment of neurogenic detrusor overactivity in PwMS. Intravesical injections of BoNT-A have been found to increase the bladder capacitance and reduce episodes of urinary incontinence. Acetylcholine release is inhibited, causing bladder wall relaxation. The benefits have been reported to last up to 8 to 10 months, although injections may be performed every 6 months. The clinician should be aware of the specific serotype of BoNT to be used and that other toxins may not be interchanged or interconverted.[97,104] Adverse effects include urinary tract infection and urinary retention. Patients should be advised of a possible need to catheterize postinjection if postvoid residuals are elevated. Given the ever-expanding role of BoNT use, the clinician is advised to ask the patient about exposure to the toxin. In instances where BoNT injections are occurring in the same patient for multiple indications, coordination of care between disciplines is essential.

Nerve stimulation has also been evaluated for treating neurogenic bladder disorders. Posterior tibial nerve stimulation involves needle insertion superior and medial to the medial malleolus with stimulation sufficient to induce toe flexion and tingling distal to and including the ankle. The procedure is indicated in patients who failed or are unable to tolerate conservative treatment for overactive bladder and typically involves 12 × 30-minute weekly sessions. The use of posterior tibial nerve stimulation demonstrated a clear reduction in urinary incontinence, urgency, frequency, and number of incontinence pads used.[96] Its exact mechanism of action is unknown. Long-term effectiveness up to 12 months has been reported.[121]

Sacral nerve stimulation is another option for the treatment of hyperreflexia, urge incontinence, and urgency/frequency disorders. The exact mechanism of action is unknown, but it is believed to restore the balance between excitatory and inhibitory stimulation of the sacral and suprasacral regions.[14] A trial period is advised for 3 to 7 days with pretrial and posttrial voiding diary evaluation for effectiveness.[43] This is a surgical procedure and its use in MS is limited because of limited MRI compatibility of the devices. Currently, some devices are contraindicated with the use of MRI, whereas others permit brain MRI only.

Neurogenic Bowel

Neurogenic bowel presents as constipation or fecal incontinence. Patients with MS have reported spending 30+ minutes per day on their bowel regimen. Constipation is believed to be caused by immobilization or abnormal colonic contractility, tone, or rectoanal reflexes.[9] Medication side effects must also be considered. For patients with overactive bladder symptoms, fluid intake may be intentionally limited so as to prevent incontinence, which may further contribute to constipation. Fecal incontinence may be attributable to loss of control of the external anal sphincter, abnormal rectosigmoid compliance, or rectoanal reflexes. The use of probiotics can help both constipation and incontinence. Referral to gastroenterology may be needed to evaluate any other underlying medical issues that may be causing the incontinence.

Sexual Dysfunction

Sexual dysfunction (SD) is present in approximately 42% to 90% of PwMS.[31,123] Despite the high prevalence, only 20% of patients report being asked about SD during clinical visits. Women commonly report decreased libido and loss of lubrication. Men report erectile and ejaculatory dysfunction. Both sexes report challenges with achieving orgasm. Side effects of DMT, symptomatic treatments (antidepressants, antispasmodics, α-antagonists), and fatigue should be evaluated.

Primary SD may be caused by CNS demyelination that directly impairs sexual feelings and/or the response. This includes symptoms of decreased or loss of libido, paresthesias that make the sexual encounter painful or unpleasurable. Secondary SD is attributable to disability secondary to MS, and are items that indirectly affect the sexual response. This may include neurogenic bladder or bowel symptoms, spasticity, tremor, or immobility. Medical conditions unrelated to MS are also included and may include mood disorders, hypertension, and diabetes. Finally, tertiary SD involves one's view of self and the psychological impact that culture and society place on sex and intimacy. Family dynamics, interpersonal conflict, poor self-esteem, and altered views of one's body image are included.

Screening for SD may be done by intake history during an examination. The MS Intimacy and Sexuality Questionnaire is a 19-item patient self-report that asks about sexual activity, satisfaction, and presence of symptoms or other issues that may interfere with sexual encounters.[175] It can also help the clinician determine if the cause is attributable to primary, secondary, or tertiary causes. The scale demonstrated validity in terms of marital satisfaction, including communication, problem solving, sexual dissatisfaction, level and extent of neurologic impairment as a result of MS, psychological well-being, and global sexual dysfunction in MS.

Clinicians are encouraged to ask and discuss SD. Patients may not be aware of the high prevalence of SD in MS and may feel that they are to blame. Education and communication is vital. Reducing the dependence on medications for side effects that impair libido or energy as well as using medications that reduce spasms or pain may be needed. Sildenafil citrate is effective for male patients with erectile dysfunction.[57] Women with SD were trialed on sildenafil citrate for improvement in sexual response, blood flow, and improved neurophysiologic response. Although lubrication improved, no change was noted in quality of life or in tibial and pudendal nerve–evoked studies.[44] Psychological counseling for the patient and/or the couple may be helpful. In addition, referral to a neuropsychologist is advised for additional evaluation and management options.

Cognitive Impairment

Cognitive impairment (CI) may be present at any stage of MS. Approximately 40% to 70% of patients have CI. Impairments that are commonly seen in PwMS include episodic memory loss, attention deficits, delayed processing speed, and difficulty in executive function. Dementia is less commonly present in MS (Figure 46-7).[130]

Although neuropsychological testing remains the most sensitive and comprehensive assessment tool for CI, the expense and time involved for testing remain formidable barriers. In addition, PwMS are often affected by fatigue, making testing even more challenging for this patient population. Other tests to evaluate and assess cognitive function have since been studied. The Rao Brief Repeatable Battery of Neuropsychological Tests and the Minimal Assessment of Cognitive Function in MS both assess working memory, processing speed, new learning, and language.[16,160] The Paced Auditory Serial Addition Test and Symbol Digit Modality Test assess processing speed, one of the most common challenges in patients with long-standing MS.

Various structural factors on MRI have correlated with CIs in PwMS. Increased cortical atrophy, widening of the third ventricle, and overall loss of brain volume are seen in persons with CI.[18,32] Further research into the significance of gray matter changes and CI is underway. Longitudinal studies have demonstrated early brain atrophy as a predictor for future CI.

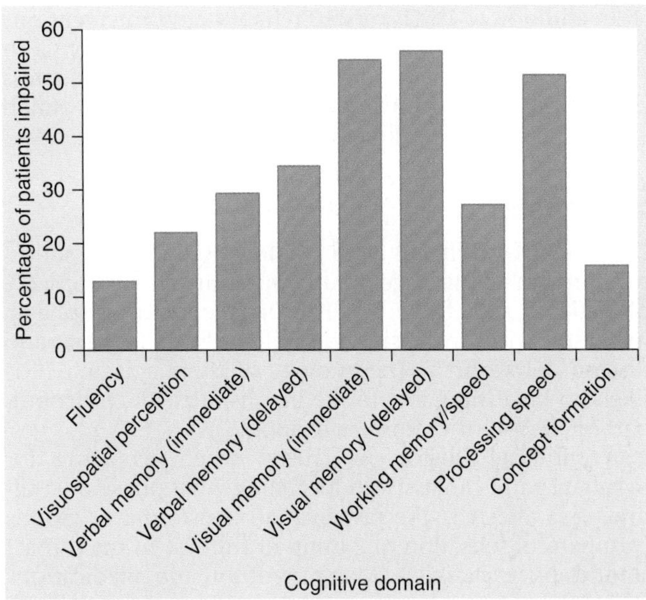

FIGURE 46-7 Frequency of impairment in 291 patients with multiple sclerosis by cognitive domain. (Reprinted, with permission, from Elsevier [*The Lancet* 7:1139-1151, 2008].)

The effect of DMT in PwMS has been studied. Subcutaneous IFN-β1_a and IFN-β1_b can stabilize or delay the progression of CI in persons with RRMS.[54,149] One year of natalizumab treatment actually demonstrated significant improvement in cognitive performance and fatigue in patients with RRMS.[94] Many patients also benefit from the use of psychostimulants such as methylphenidate and L-amphetamine to improve attention, learning, and ability to focus.[17,81] The potential benefit of memantine and donepezil for treatment of memory disorders has conflicting results and still need large-scale studies for further clarification.[84] The supplement *Gingko biloba* did not improve cognitive performance in PwMS.[118]

Factors that may affect CI include disease duration, MS subtype, level of disability, and premorbid level of verbal competence. One striking feature is the concomitant presence of depression or depressive symptoms in patients with CI, further emphasizing the need for vigorous screening for mood disorders in the patient population.

Two hypotheses prevail in what determines the extent of cognitive dysfunction and why individuals are affected differently. Brain reserve or maximal lifetime brain volume (MLBV) is determined primarily by genetics.[12,194] Those individuals with larger MLBV are believed to be less susceptible to cognitive decline and have a lower risk of dementia. The cognitive reserve hypothesis states that learning is acquired from life experiences, education, and cognitive leisure activities. A positive correlation was found between cognition with both education and early life cognitive leisure activities. A higher MLBV and robust cognitive reserve are both protective against CI.

In addition to DMT, various rehabilitative interventions have been used for prevention and the treatment of CI in PwMS. Cognitive behavioral therapy has reduced distress and improved cognitive performance in several small studies.[135,192] Long-term benefit is unknown.

Swallowing

Dysphagia, or difficulty with swallowing liquids or solids, may present at any stage of MS. An estimated 33% to 43% of patients are affected.[187] The prevalence of dysphagia increases with increasing disability, EDSS scores, and disease duration.[23,29] The etiology of dysphagia in MS is likely to be attributable to the involvement of corticobulbar, cerebellar, or brainstem regions.

A thorough history is crucial when screening for dysphagia and can assist in localizing what phase of swallowing is affected. The presence of xerostomia or globus (nonpainful sensation of a lump or fullness in the throat) should be excluded.[37] Many symptomatic medications may cause xerostomia. The pharyngeal phase is most commonly affected in MS. The presence of another unrelated comorbidity may also be present, causing difficulty with swallowing.

Patients may complete the 10-item self-report assessment, Screening with Dysphagia in MS (DYMUS) questionnaire to assess their risk for dysphagia. This has been validated to screen both solid and liquid dysphagia. It may serve as a screening tool to assess the need for additional testing as well as delineate patients at risk for aspiration pneumonia.[22,23] Clinical assessment alone may underestimate the risk of aspiration by 50%.[37] A videoradiographic swallow study, also called the modified barium swallow, is the tool of choice for evaluating the presence of silent aspiration. Patients may require referral for additional testing including esophageal manometry or an endoscopy.

Treating dysphagia with compensatory strategies is often effective. This includes (1) postural changes, (2) modifying the amount of food bolus consumed, and (3) changing the food consistency.[29] Other treatments include electrical stimulation and neurotoxin injection. Pharyngeal electrical stimulation to treat oropharyngeal dysphagia significantly reduces the amount of penetration and aspiration.[162] Injection of BoNT into the cricopharyngeal muscle has been reported to be effective for the treatment of upper esophageal hyperactivity.[163]

Pseudobulbar Affect

Pseudobulbar affect (PBA) is a disorder of uncontrollable laughter or crying that is incongruent with the social or professional situation.[65,131] Although PBA can be seen in almost any illness, this is commonly seen in persons with neurologic disorders including MS, amyotrophic lateral sclerosis, stroke, and traumatic brain injury. Prevalence in MS is believed to be 6.5% to 46.26%.[133] The emotional lability in PBA is spontaneous and brief. Patients who suffer from this may feel socially isolated resulting from the lack of control over their laughing or crying episodes. PBA should be differentiated from depression in which one's mood is congruent to the situation. Also, duration of symptoms is brief in PBA, whereas a depressed mood typically lasts weeks to months. The term *pseudobulbar* is a true disorder and should also be differentiated from pseudobulbar syndrome in which corticobulbar damage may lead to oromotor dysfunction, dysphonia, and slow, slurred speech.

The pathophysiology is not clear but is believed to be a disorder of the cortico-pontine-cerebellar circuit.[68,131,146] This circuit of neuroanatomic pathways descend to the basis pontis, brainstem, and cerebellum. It is thought that disruption here can lower the threshold for emotional response.[146-148] This disruption is believed to lead to the emotional incongruent response (Figure 46-8).

The Center for Neurologic Study-Lability Scale (CNS-LS) is a 7-item self-reported scale to screen for PBA. It has been validated in both MS and amyotrophic lateral sclerosis. Although a score of 13 on the CNS-LS scale or more is indicative of PBA, one study noted a sensitivity of 94% and specificity of 83% with a score of 17 or more in PwMS.[134,185] This screening tool is quick and efficient and can be used to track a patient once treatment is started.

Various agents including selective serotonin reuptake inhibitors and tricyclic antidepressants have been used with varying success to treat PBA. These studies had small numbers of patients with varying methodology (Table 46-6). The combination of dextromethorphan with low-dose quinidine has resulted in a treatment for patients with PBA. Its mechanism of action is unknown. A double-blind placebo-controlled study using dextromethorphan/low-dose quinidine in patients with amyotrophic lateral sclerosis and MS resulted in significantly reducing the rate of pseudobulbar episodes per day compared with placebo (49% reduction, $p < 0.0001$)[152]; participants in the active arm noticed improvement as soon as week 1 of the study. The most common adverse events included headache, falls, diarrhea, and vertigo. Dextromethorphan/quinidine may cause QTc prolongation. All patients in the study were screened for respiratory or cardiac disorders before being included. The recommended dosage is 1 capsule daily for 7 days followed by 1 capsule every 12 hours beginning on day 8. Most patients notice reduction in lability after 1 to 2 weeks of treatment.

Pediatric Multiple Sclerosis

Our understanding of demyelinating disorders in children has increased in recent years. According to the International Pediatric MS Study Group, pediatric MS can be diagnosed after two clinical episodes of CNS demyelination that are separated by at least 30 days. Pediatric MS counts for 5% of all MS cases.[217] It provides a unique opportunity to increase our understanding of the potential genetic and environmental factors that drive this complex disease.

In North America, there is a greater diversity in ethnicity among pediatric patients with MS than among adults with MS, possibly reflecting changing demographic trends.[202] The female/male ratio varies by age. Younger than age 6 years, the ratio of girls to boys is 0.8 to 1. The ratio increases to 1.6 : 1 between the ages of 6 and 10 years. It is 2 : 1 for children over the ages of 10 years of age compared with the ratio of 3 : 1 that is typically seen in adults.[217]

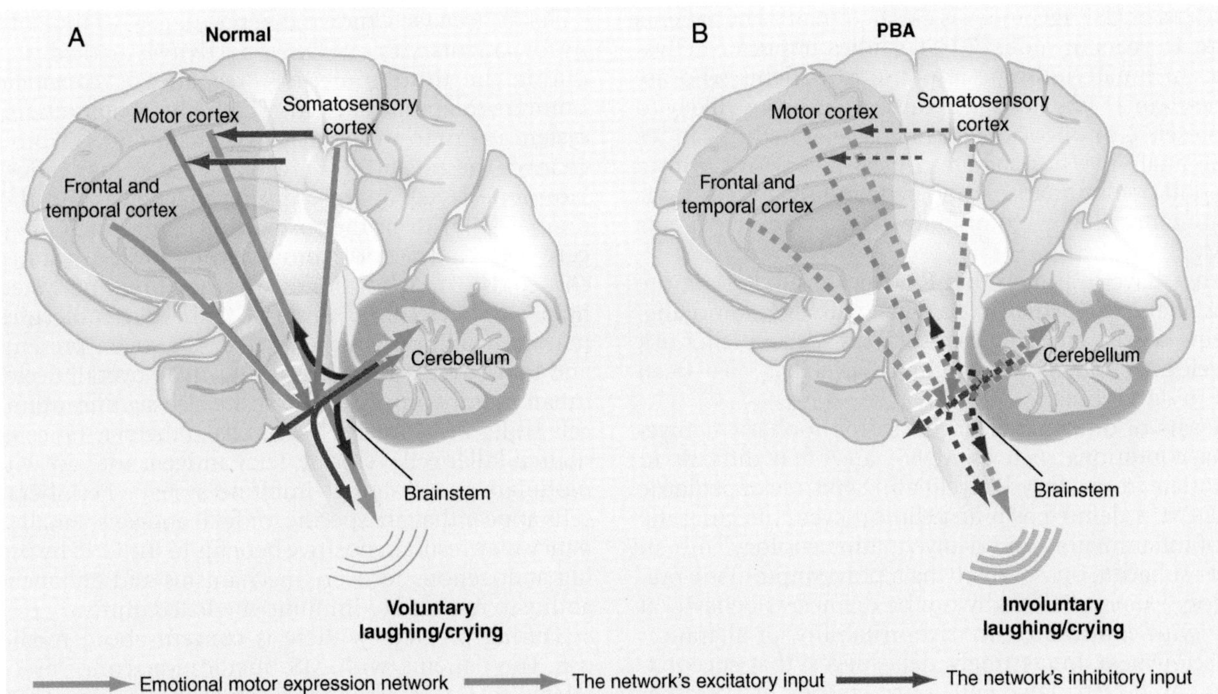

FIGURE 46-8 Proposed brain circuitry involved in emotional expression and its hypothesized dysfunction in pseudobulbar affect (PBA). Normally (**A**), an emotional motor expression network including cortico-pontine-cerebellar afferentation (*upper blue arrows*) enables the cerebellum to act as a "gate control" for the motor expression of emotion (*lower blue arrows*). Inputs to this network (*green and red arrows*) include an inhibitory influence from sensory cortices. In PBA (**B**), reduced inhibitory influence at the cortical level (*broken red cortical arrows*) results in increased aberrant activation within the network (*broken blue arrows*), giving rise to the motor manifestations of pathologic laughing/crying. (From Miller A, Pratt H, Schiffer RB: Pseudobulbar affect: the spectrum of clinical presentations, etiologies and treatments, *Expert Rev Neurother* 11:1077-1088, 2011.)

Table 46-6 Placebo-Controlled Trials of Pharmacotherapeutic Options in Pseudobulbar Affect

Drug Class	Study (Year)	Active Drug vs Placebo	Study Design	PBA Setting	N	Main Findings
Tricyclic antidepressants	Schiffer et al. (1985)	Amitriptyline	Crossover; 1 month per treatment	MS	12	Reduced episode rate
	Robinson et al. (1993)	Nortriptyline	Parallel-group; 6 weeks	Stroke	28	Reduced severity on validated scale (PLACS)
Selective serotonin reuptake inhibitors	Andersen et al. (1993)	Citalopram	Crossover; 3 weeks per treatment	Stroke	16	Reduced episode rate
	Brown et al. (1998)	Fluoxetine	Parallel-group; 10 days	Stroke	20	Reduced severity on unvalidated scale
	Burns et al. (1999)	Sertraline	Parallel-group; 8 weeks	Stroke	28	Reduced lability on unvalidated scale
	Choi-Kwon et al. (2006)	Fluoxetine	Parallel-group; 6 months	Stroke	91	Reduced crying on unvalidated scale
Antiglutamatergics	Panitch et al. (2006)	DMQ	Parallel-group; 12 weeks	MS	150	Reduced severity on validated scale (CNS-LS); reduced episode rate
	Pioro et al. (2010)	DMQ	Parallel-group; 12 weeks	ALS or MS	326	Reduced severity on validated scale (CNS-LS); reduced episode rate

From Miller A, Pratt H, Schiffer RB: Pseudobulbar affect: The spectrum of clinical presentations, etiologies and treatments, *Expert Rev Neurother* 11:1077-1088, 2011.

Studies cited:

Schiffer R, Herndon RM, Rudick RA: Treatment of pathological laughing and weeping with amitriptyline. *N Engl J Med* 312:1480–1482, 1985.

Robinson RG, Parikh RM, Lipsey JR, Starkstein SE, Price TR: Pathological laughing and crying following stroke: validation of a measurement scale and a double-blind treatment study. *Am J Psychiatry* 150:286–293, 1993.

Andersen G, Vestergaard K, Riis JO: Citalopram for post-stroke pathological crying. *Lancet* 342:837–839, 1993.

Brown KW, Sloan RL, Pentland B: Fluoxetine as a treatment for post-stroke emotionalism. *Acta Psychiatr Scand* 98:455–458, 1998.

Burns A, Russell E, Stratton-Powell H, Tyrell P, O'Neill P, Baldwin R: Sertraline in stroke-associated lability of mood. *Int. J. Geriatr Psychiatry* 14:681–685, 1999.

Choi-Kwon S, Han SW, Kwon SU, Kang DW, Choi JM, Kim JS: Fluoxetine treatment in poststroke depression, emotional incontinence, and anger proneness: a double-blind, placebo-controlled study. *Stroke* 37:156–161, 2006.

Panitch HS, Thisted RA, Smith RA et al: Randomized, controlled trial of dextromethorphan/quinidine for pseudobulbar affect in multiple sclerosis. *Ann Neurol* 59:780–787, 2006.

Pioro EP, Brooks BR, Cummings J et al. Dextromethorphan plus ultra low-dose quinidine reduces pseudobulbar affect. *Ann Neurol* 68:693–702, 2010.

ALS, Amyotrophic lateral sclerosis; *CNS-LS*, Center for Neurologic Study–Lability Scale; *DMQ*, dextromethorphan/quinidine; *MS*, multiple sclerosis; *PBA*, pseudobulbar affect; *PLACS*, Pathological Laughter and Crying Scale.

In terms of CSF, IgG index is elevated in 68% of patients that are 11 years or older.[205] CSF studies implicate activation of an innate immune response in patients who are younger than 11 years of age because they are less likely to have presence of oligoclonal bands or elevated IgG index on CSF analysis. They may also have pleocytosis with a neutrophil predominance compared with the lymphocytic predominance that is commonly seen in adult patients with MS.[205]

Studies have indicated that EBV seropositivity is more common among pediatric patients with MS. Smoking, including passive smoking, is associated with a higher risk of developing MS. Low vitamin D level has also been linked to developing MS.

In terms of differential diagnosis, monophasic demyelinating conditions such as ADEM are often difficult to differentiate from a first demyelinating episode of pediatric MS. ADEM is defined as a first clinical event affecting the CNS, of inflammatory and demyelinating etiology with an acute or subacute onset, involving a polysymptomatic presentation.[217] Encephalopathy can be defined as behavioral change with confusion, excessive irritability, or alteration of consciousness. Interestingly, data suggest that encephalopathy can be associated with a first episode of MS, especially in younger patients. Rather than being specific for a disease process, it may be an indication of an immature brain or immune system.

Children tend to have larger lesion burden, particularly with brainstem and cerebellar involvement.[216] Younger children may have MRIs with atypical features with large T2/FLAIR hyperintense confluent lesions with irregular borders. Lesions often resolve on repeat scans. In a small study, pediatric patients with MS had fewer T2 lesions and more frequent tumefactive MS lesions on imaging studies than was reported with adult patients.

Pediatric patients with MS develop marked CI with difficulties with complex attention, information processing, executive functioning, processing speed, and long-term memory. In one study, patients with MS with an average disease duration of 3 years met criteria for significant CI.

Data using DMT in children is limited; however, the approach remains similar to treatment strategies for adults. The current first-line therapies seem to be safe and well tolerated in this patient population. As with adults, compliance remains a concern and guides medication decisions.

Multiple Sclerosis in Pregnancy

There is strong female predominance in MS. Patients are often diagnosed in childbearing years. As such, pregnancy becomes an important topic for female patients with MS at some point during their disease course. At least 20% to 30% of patients will have children after their diagnosis of MS.[38] Fortunately, MS has little to no direct effect on pregnancy. Patients can be counseled with confidence that their disease will not affect their ability to conceive, the safety and health of the pregnancy, or fetal well-being. There is no increased risk in spontaneous abortions, ectopic pregnancies, cesarean deliveries, or major neonatal or obstetric complications.

It has been well known that pregnancy is a time of stability for patients with MS. Disease activity is markedly reduced during the third trimester. Pregnancy is considered an immune-tolerant state, in which the maternal immune system adapts to an allogeneic pregnancy. Several biological changes occur during pregnancy that may affect MS. Hormone levels increase during pregnancy and then fall dramatically during the postpartum period, including estrogens (especially estriol), progesterone, prolactin, and glucocorticoids. These hormones affect the immune system and help shift cytokines, decrease adhesion molecules and matrix metalloproteinases, decrease antigen presentation, and boost Treg cells.[38] This results in an overall decrease in inflammatory processes. There are also significant immune cell shifts that involve Treg cells, T helper 17 cells, and natural killer cells. Thirdly, fetal antigens interact with and modulate the maternal immune system. Peripheral Treg cells appear that are specific for fetal antigens. Finally, pregnancy may result in positive benefits to the CNS by promoting endogenous recovery mechanisms and enhancing the ability to respond to immune-mediated injury.

During pregnancy, there is concern about medication use. For patients with MS, medication concerns can be related to DMTs, treatments for relapses, or symptomatic management. Typically, DMTs should not be used in patients with MS who are pregnant or trying to become pregnant. When needed, glatiramer acetate has the most favorable safety rating (class B). Acute relapses can be treated with a short course of high-dose glucocorticoids as determined by their practitioner. If possible, it is preferable to forego treatment during the first trimester because of the association of cleft palate and lower birth rate. However, corticosteroids are commonly used in the second and third trimester. Prednisone, prednisolone, or methylprednisolone are preferred because they are metabolized to inactive forms by the placenta, rather than betamethasone or dexamethasone, which crosses the placenta with minimal metabolism. As a general principle, symptomatic medications are minimized during pregnancy. However, if a medication is needed to prevent suffering or maintain quality of life, it can be continued.

Compared with prepregnancy, annualized relapse rates fall by 70% during the third trimester. During the 3 months postpartum, the relapse rate rebounds to 70% above the prepregnancy level, then comes down and stays down at the prepregnancy rate. The most consistent marker associated with postpartum activity is the disease activity in the year before pregnancy.[113] There are conflicting data regarding the potential benefit from breastfeeding in reducing MS activity. There are some studies that suggest that exclusive breastfeeding results in prolonged lactational amenorrhea with ovarian suppression, high prolactin levels, and low nonpulsatile luteinizing hormone levels that may be beneficial. Although it is not FDA-approved, intravenous immunoglobulin G has been shown in some studies to reduce the risk of postpartum relapse.[80]

Summary

The past decade has seen more than a doubling of treatment options for patients with MS. One of the biggest and most impactful on medication compliance and ease has been the approval of oral DMTs. Diagnosis of MS is occurring earlier and also with improved accuracy. Patients are no longer satisfied with "not getting worse." They want and demand options that will increase their strength and endurance and maintain their ability to ambulate; in essence, they want us as clinicians to help them enhance their quality of life. The varying nature of MS symptoms presents unique challenges for the clinician. The disease is progressive, and symptoms change often and are affected by external factors including heat, fatigue, and side effects of DMTs. Physiatrists hold the answers and options for this in our treatment tool bag. We have therapeutic and symptomatic options for fitness, symptomatic management, and can effectively educate and guide these patients. In addition, our training and expertise can help these patients have coping strategies so they can manage the physical, mental, or cognitive challenges they may face.

KEY REFERENCES

2. Adelman G, Rane SG, Villa KF: The cost burden of multiple sclerosis in the United States: a systematic review of the literature, *J Med Econ* 16:639–647, 2013.
4. Asano M, Duquette P, Andersen R, et al: Exercise barriers and preferences among women and men with multiple sclerosis, *Disabil Rehabil* 35:353–361, 2013.
8. Ascherio A, Munger KL, White R, et al: Vitamin D as an early predictor of multiple sclerosis activity and progression, *JAMA Neurol* 71:306–314, 2014.
11. Barnes MP, Kent RM, Semlyen JK, et al: Spasticity in multiple sclerosis, *Neurorehabil Neural Repair* 17:66–70, 2003.
19. Benedict RHB, Fishman I, McClellan MM, et al: Validity of the Beck Depression Inventory-Fast Screen in multiple sclerosis, *Mult Scler* 9:393–396, 2003.
28. Calabrese M, Poretto V, Favaretto A, et al: Cortical lesion load associates with progression of disability in multiple sclerosis, *Brain* 135:2952–2961, 2012.
35. Confavreux C, Vukusic S: The natural history of multiple sclerosis], *Rev Prat* 56:1313–1320, 2006 [in French].
36. Confavreux C, Vukusic S, Adeleine P: Early clinical predictors and progression of irreversible disability in multiple sclerosis: an amnesic process, *Brain* 126:770–782, 2003.
39. Craig J, Young CA, Ennis M, et al: A randomised controlled trial comparing rehabilitation against standard therapy in multiple sclerosis patients receiving intravenous steroid treatment, *J Neurol Neurosurg Psychiatry* 74:1225–1230, 2003.
53. Fernandez O, Berger T, Hartung HP, et al: Historical overview of the rationale for the pharmacological use of prolonged-release fampridine in multiple sclerosis, *Expert Rev Clin Pharmacol* 5:649–665, 2012.
56. Fisk JD, Pontefract A, Ritvo PG, et al: The impact of fatigue on patients with multiple sclerosis, *Can J Neurol Sci* 21:9–14, 1994.
58. Fowler CJ, Panicker JN, Drake M, et al: A UK consensus on the management of the bladder in multiple sclerosis, *Postgrad Med J* 85:552–559, 2009.
60. Freedman MS, Thompson EJ, Deisenhammer F, et al: Recommended standard of cerebrospinal fluid analysis in the diagnosis of multiple sclerosis: a consensus statement, *Arch Neurol* 62:865–870, 2005.
63. Frohman EM, Racke MK, Raine CS: Multiple sclerosis—the plaque and its pathogenesis, *N Engl J Med* 354:942–955, 2006.
65. Garnock-Jones KP: Dextromethorphan/quinidine: in pseudobulbar affect, *CNS Drugs* 25:435–445, 2011.
68. Ghaffar O, Chamelian L, Feinstein A: Neuroanatomy of pseudobulbar affect: a quantitative MRI study in multiple sclerosis, *J Neurol* 255:406–412, 2008.
70. Gijbels D, Eijnde B, Feys P: Comparison of the 2- and 6-minute walk test in multiple sclerosis, *Mult Scler J* 17:1269–1272, 2011.
72. Goldman Consensus Group: The Goldman consensus statement on depression in multiple sclerosis, *Mult Scler* 11:328–337, 2005.
75. Goodman AD, Brown TR, Edwards KR, et al: A phase 3 trial of extended release oral dalfampridine in multiple sclerosis, *Ann Neurol* 68:494–502, 2010.
80. Haas J: High dose IVIG in the post partum period for prevention of exacerbations in multiple sclerosis, *Mult Scler* 6(Suppl 2):S18–S20, discussion S33, 2000.
81. Harel Y, Appleboim N, Lavie M, et al: Single dose of methylphenidate improves cognitive performance in multiple sclerosis patients with impaired attention process, *J Neurol Sci* 276:38–40, 2009.
85. Healy BC, Ali EN, Guttmann CR, et al: Smoking and disease progression in multiple sclerosis, *Arch Neurol* 66:858–864, 2009.
88. Hedstrom AK, Lima Bomfim I, Barcellos L, et al: Interaction between adolescent obesity and HLA risk genes in the etiology of multiple sclerosis, *Neurology* 82:865–872, 2014.
94. Iaffaldano P, Viterbo RG, Paolicelli D, et al: Impact of natalizumab on cognitive performances and fatigue in relapsing multiple sclerosis: a prospective, open-label, two years observational study, *PLoS ONE* 7:e35843, 2012.
96. Kabay SC, Yucel M, Kabay S: Acute effect of posterior tibial nerve stimulation on neurogenic detrusor overactivity in patients with multiple sclerosis: urodynamic study, *Urology* 71:641–645, 2008.
97. Kalsi V, Gonzales G, Popat R, et al: Botulinum injections for the treatment of bladder symptoms of multiple sclerosis, *Ann Neurol* 62:452–457, 2007.
99. Kappos L, Moeri D, Radue EW, et al: Predictive value of gadolinium-enhanced magnetic resonance imaging for relapse rate and changes in disability or impairment in multiple sclerosis: a meta-analysis. Gadolinium MRI Meta-analysis Group, *Lancet* 353:964–969, 1999.
100. Kasper LH, Shoemaker J: Multiple sclerosis immunology: the healthy immune system vs the multiple sclerosis immune system, *Neurology* 74(Suppl 1):2–8, 2010.
102. Kaufman M, Moyer D, Norton J: The significant change for the timed 25-foot walk in the multiple sclerosis functional composite, *Mult Scler* 6:286–290, 2000.
111. Kurtzke JF: Neurologic impairment in multiple sclerosis and the disability status scale, *Acta Neurol Scand* 46:493–512, 1970.
120. Ma VY, Chan L, Carruthers KJ: Incidence, prevalence, costs, and impact on disability of common conditions requiring rehabilitation in the United States: stroke, spinal cord injury, traumatic brain injury, multiple sclerosis, osteoarthritis, rheumatoid arthritis, limb loss, and back pain, *Arch Phys Med Rehabil* 95:986–995, 2014.
127. McDonald WI, Barnes D: The ocular manifestations of multiple sclerosis. 1. Abnormalities of the afferent visual system, *J Neurol Neurosurg Psychiatry* 55:747–752, 1992.
131. Miller A, Pratt H, Schiffer RB: Pseudobulbar affect: the spectrum of clinical presentations, etiologies and treatments, *Expert Rev Neurother* 11:1077–1088, 2011.
135. Moss-Morris R, Dennison L, Landau S, et al: A randomized controlled trial of cognitive behavioral therapy (CBT) for adjusting to multiple sclerosis (the saMS trial): does CBT work and for whom does it work?, *J Consult Clin Psychol* 81:251–262, 2013.
137. Munger KL, Levin LI, Hollis BW, et al: Serum 25-hydroxyvitamin D levels and risk of multiple sclerosis, *JAMA* 296:2832–2838, 2006.
141. Noseworthy JH, Lucchinetti C, Rodriguez M, et al: Multiple sclerosis, *N Engl J Med* 343:938–952, 2000.
143. Okuda DT, Siva A, Kantarci O, et al: Radiologically isolated syndrome: 5-year risk for an initial clinical event, *PLoS ONE* 9:e90509, 2014.
151. Petajan JH, Gappmaier E, White AT, et al: Impact of aerobic training on fitness and quality of life in multiple sclerosis, *Ann Neurol* 39:432–441, 1996.
155. Polman CH, O'Connor PW, Havrdova E, et al: A randomized, placebo-controlled trial of natalizumab for relapsing multiple sclerosis, *N Engl J Med* 354:899–910, 2006.
156. Polman CH, Reingold SC, Banwell B, et al: Diagnostic criteria for multiple sclerosis: 2010 revisions to the McDonald criteria, *Ann Neurol* 69:292–302, 2011.
160. Rao SM, Leo GJ, Bernardin L, et al: Cognitive dysfunction in multiple sclerosis. I. Frequency, patterns, and prediction, *Neurology* 41:685–691, 1991.
168. Rizzo MA, Hadjimichael OC, Preiningerova J, et al: Prevalence and treatment of spasticity reported by multiple sclerosis patients, *Mult Scler* 10:589–595, 2004.
175. Sanders A, Foley F, LaRocca N, et al: The multiple sclerosis intimacy and sexuality questionnaire-19 (multiple sclerosis ISQ-19), *Sexual Disabil* 18:3–26, 2000.

180. Schwid SR, Petrie MD, Murray R, et al: A randomized controlled study of the acute and chronic effects of cooling therapy for multiple sclerosis, *Neurology* 60:1955–1960, 2003.
186. Solaro C, Brichetto G, Amato MP, et al: The prevalence of pain in multiple sclerosis: a multicenter cross-sectional study, *Neurology* 63:919–921, 2004.
190. Sosnoff JJ, Gappmaier E, Frame A, et al: Influence of spasticity on mobility and balance in persons with multiple sclerosis, *J Neurol Phys Ther* 35:129–132, 2011.
193. Sullivan MJ, Weinshenker B, Mikail S, et al: Screening for major depression in the early stages of multiple sclerosis, *Can J Neurol Sci* 22:228–231, 1995.
197. Transverse Myelitis Consortium Working Group: Proposed diagnostic criteria and nosology of acute transverse myelitis, *Neurology* 59:499–505, 2002.
207. Weinshenker BG, Bass B, Rice GP, et al: The natural history of multiple sclerosis: a geographically based study. I. Clinical course and disability, *Brain* 112:133–146, 1989.
211. Wingerchuk DM, Lennon VA, Pittock SJ, et al: Revised diagnostic criteria for neuromyelitis optica, *Neurology* 66:1485–1489, 2006.

The full reference list for this chapter is available online.

CHAPTER 47

CEREBRAL PALSY

Christian M. Niedzwecki, Desiree L. Roge, Aloysia L. Schwabe

The definition of cerebral palsy (CP) has constantly evolved since the 1800s and has involved some of the most influential medical minds in history, including William Little, Sir William Osler, and Sigmund Freud. Advances in medicine and world-wide communication have led to the current definition: "Cerebral palsy describes a group of permanent disorders of the development of movement and posture, causing activity limitation, that are attributed to non-progressive disturbances that occurred in the developing fetal or infant brain. The motor disorders of CP are often accompanied by disturbances of sensation, perception, cognition, communication, and behavior, by epilepsy, and by secondary musculoskeletal problems."[53] This definition excludes a number of disease processes that may present similarly, but either progress (i.e., genetic or metabolic diseases), have a primarily peripheral etiology (i.e., neuromuscular or peripheral nerve injury), or occur after the central nervous system has fully developed (i.e., traumatic injuries or oncologic manifestations). It serves to remind us that the term CP reflects much more than a musculoskeletal process; it reaches to the function of a person. For example, each of the following cases is a possible presentation of a child with CP:

1. AB is a 10-year-old, left-handed female who was born at 36 weeks of gestation and whose brain imaging showed a prenatal stroke on the left. She has difficulty using her right arm and leg because of right spastic hemiplegia for which she receives botulinum toxin injections 3 times a year. She uses an ankle-foot orthosis to run and play soccer with her friends. She is in regular classes at school and has no problem seeing, hearing, eating, talking, or socializing. She does note that she gets a "little upset" because she cannot keep up with her friends on the playground.
2. CD is a 10-year old male who was born at 32 weeks of gestation and whose brain imaging showed significant periventricular leukomalacia (PVL). He has difficulty using both of his legs to walk because of spastic diplegia for which he receives botulinum toxin injections 3 times a year and takes an oral medication 3 times a day. He requires bilateral ankle-foot orthoses and a reverse walker for ambulation in the community; at home he mainly crawls to get around. In addition, he has difficulty coordinating fine motor tasks with either hand, but is able to put on his clothes with assistance for buttons and zippers. He requires accommodations at school for his mobility and dysarthria, needs glasses, and has difficulty being understood when talking. He has no problems with hearing or eating. He expresses that he wants other "little boys at school to play with him."
3. EF is a 10-year old male who was born at 24 weeks of gestation and whose brain imaging showed diffuse encephalomalacia and hydrocephalus that required shunting. He has difficulty using all of his limbs because of spastic quadriplegia for which he receives botulinum injections 4 times a year and takes two oral medications 3 times a day (one for spasticity and one for dystonia). He is mobile only in a customized wheelchair and requires bilateral ankle-foot orthoses and bilateral resting hand splints for positioning. He has numerous other impairments, including scoliosis, dysphagia, nutritional compromise requiring a gastrostomy tube for feeding and hydration, constipation, and significant intellectual disability.

Epidemiology

CP is the most common cause of disability in developed countries. The direct and indirect costs associated with CP are 3 to 4 times that of a neurotypical child.[26] Despite treatment advances, the overall prevalence rates have neither increased nor decreased in the past 20 years (2.11 per 1000 live births). When the overall prevalence is examined more closely, dramatic increases are seen in children with very low birth weight (59.6 per 1000 live births) and very early gestation (111.8 per 1000 live births).[49] Research has found that the germinal matrix surrounding the ventricles is at increased risk of ischemic or hemorrhagic injury caused by the immature vasculature and fluctuations in cerebral blood flow.[6]

Etiology/Risk Factors

Many times, the etiology of the brain injury associated with the clinical findings of CP is clear, as in a history of placental abruption with significant cardiorespiratory compromise causing global hypoxic ischemic injury resulting in spastic quadriplegia. However, it may not be as clear in a near-term infant with an uncomplicated hospital course who is developmentally delayed. As more CP registries are collecting data, it is becoming clearer that a larger portion of children with CP have a multifactorial etiology from a mixture of known risk factors.[41] There are five major categories of risk factors associated with the diagnosis of CP (Table 47-1).

Table 47-1 Risk Factors Associated with Cerebral Palsy

Preconception	Antenatal	Intrapartum	Neonatal	Postnatal
Maternal seizures	Birth defects	Birth hypoxia	Seizures	Stroke
Intellectual disability	Small for gestational age	Meconium staining	Respiratory distress	Abusive head trauma
Thyroid disease (hyper or hypo)	Low birth weight	Meconium aspiration	Hypoglycemia	Bacterial meningitis
History of stillbirth or neonatal death	Placental abnormalities	Abnormal duration of labor	Infections	Motor vehicle crashes[10]
Maternal age >40 years	Maternal disease during pregnancy (respiratory, heart, seizures, incompetent cervix)	Fetal presentation[34]	Jaundice[34]	
Low socioeconomic status[34]	Abnormalities in fluid volume			
	Maternal bleeding in 2nd and 3rd trimesters			
	Hypertension			
	Preeclampsia			
	Chorioamnionitis[34]			

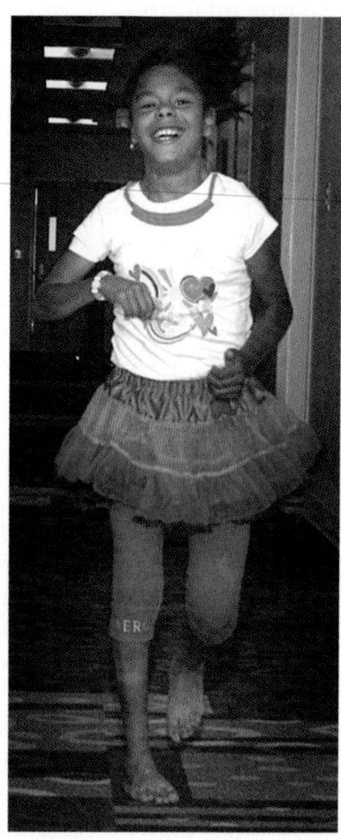

FIGURE 47-1 Child with spastic hemiplegia.

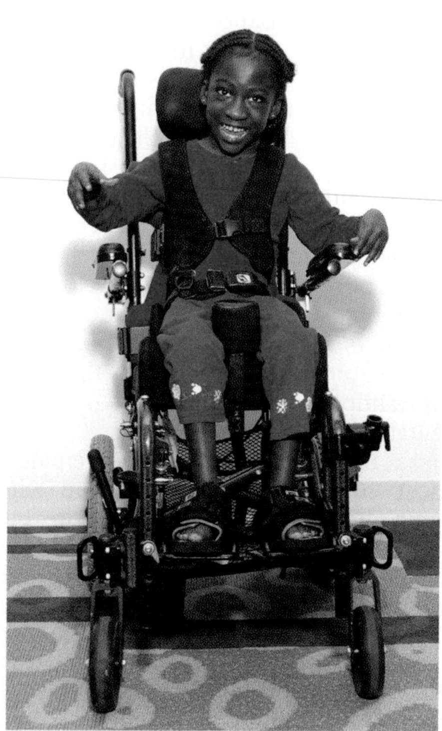

FIGURE 47-2 Child with spastic quadriplegia.

Classification

One classification system for children with CP uses the topography or distribution of affected limbs (Figures 47-1 to 47-4). In this system, hemiplegic CP (Fig. 47-1) refers to a unilateral upper and lower limb distribution. It is common in term and near-term infants and associated with focal brain pathology (unilateral strokes, asymmetric PVL, or congenital malformations). Quadriplegic CP or tetraplegic CP (Figure 47-2) refers to a bilateral upper and lower limb distribution and is associated with diffuse brain pathology (cortical, subcortical, and intraventricular lesions) (Table 47-2). It is also common in term and near-term infants. Diplegic CP (Figure 47-3) is a term that refers to a bilateral lower extremity distribution and is most common in preterm infants. The associated brain pathology is PVL.[5]

The diagnosis can be further classified by the motor sign. Over the past 10 years, definitions for these motor signs have been detailed to provide reliable, valid terminology. Positive motor signs are defined as involuntary increases in frequency or magnitude of muscle activity. They include hypertonia ("examiner induced abnormally increased resistance to movement about a joint")[58] and hyperkinesia ("unwanted, excess movement by the child").[56] Hypertonia is further subdivided into spastic, dystonic, and rigid hypertonia. Hyperkinetic movements are divided into dystonia, chorea, athetosis, myoclonus,

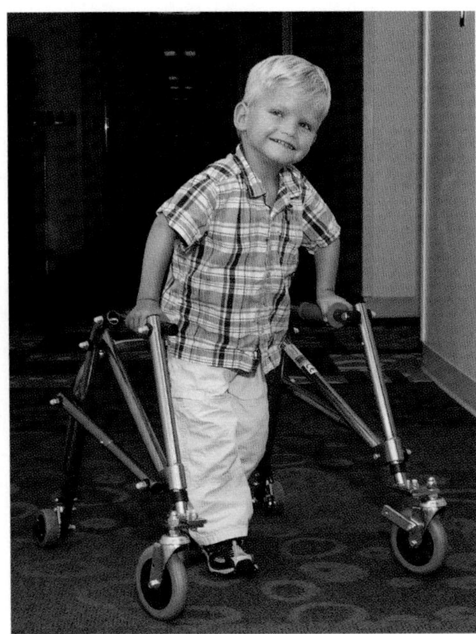

FIGURE 47-3 Child with spastic diplegia.

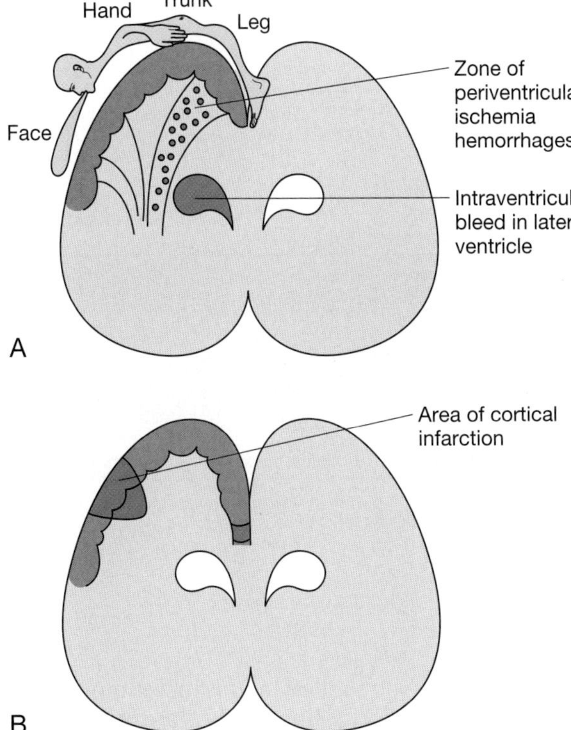

FIGURE 47-4 Areas of brain damage causing diplegia versus hemiplegia. **(A)** In spastic diplegia and periventricular leukomalacia, the leg is more affected than the hand and face. There is no cortical injury. **(B)** In spastic hemiplegia, the arm is often more affected than the leg. Because of cortical involvement, seizures and cognitive issues may occur.

tremor, tics, and stereotypies. Although positive motor signs are more recognizable, negative motor signs are described as "lack of muscle activity or control" and encompass weakness, reduced selective motor control, ataxia, and apraxia (Box 47-1).[57]

Table 47-2 Grades of Intraventricular Hemorrhage in the Premature Brain

Grade	Hemorrhage
1	Isolated to the germinal matrix
2	With normal ventricular size
3	With ventricular dilation
4	With parenchymal hemorrhage

BOX 47-1

Classification of Motor Signs

Positive Motor Signs

Hypertonia
- Spasticity
- Dystonia
- Rigidity

Hyperkinesia
- Dystonia
- Chorea
- Athetosis
- Myoclonus
- Tremor, tics, and stereotypies

Negative Motor Signs
- Weakness
- Reduced selective motor control
- Ataxia
- Apraxia

The push for standardized terminology has benefitted from the development of many CP registries across the globe. One important network, the Surveillance of Cerebral Palsy in Europe (SCPE), has standardized terminology and a reporting structure. Their terms include *unilateral spastic CP, bilateral spastic CP, dystonic CP, choreoathetoid CP, ataxic CP,* and *nonclassifiable*.[12]

It is important to note that, although one topographic distribution or motor sign may predominate, CP is commonly more complicated and multiple motor signs and distributions may be seen in each patient.

Another important aspect of describing the clinical findings associated with CP is functional. One well-accepted and widely used classification system is the Gross Motor Function Classification System (GMFCS). It was revised in 2006 and has been shown to be valid and reliable. This system quantifies the typical performance in gross motor tasks (sitting, standing, walking, and using stairs) with mobility aids into five levels for five age groups. It has been used to develop motor development curves to prognosticate the age at which peak gross motor function is attained.[50,54] Classification systems for upper extremity use (Manual Ability Classification System, or MACS)[18] and communication (Communication Function Classification System, or CFCS)[23] have also been developed (Table 47-3).

In recognition that clinical findings in CP also include disturbances of sensation, perception, cognition, communication, and behavior, a multifaceted classification system was proposed in 2006. It recommended defining CP in terms of four components: motor abnormalities, accompanying impairments, anatomic and neuroimaging findings, and causation and timing.[53]

Also in 2007, the World Health Organization (WHO), in collaboration with many other organizations, published the International Classification of Functioning, Disability

Table 47-3 Function Classification Scales: GMFCS, MACS, CFCS

	Classification System		
Level	**GMFCS**	**MACS**	**CFCS**
I	Walks without limitations	Handles objects easily and successfully	Sends and receives information with familiar and unfamiliar partners effectively and efficiently
II	Walks with limitations	Handles most objects but with somewhat reduced quality and/or speed of achievement	Sends and receives information with familiar and unfamiliar partners but may need extra time
III	Walks using a hand-held mobility device	Handles objects with difficulty; needs help to prepare and/or modify activities	Sends and receives information with familiar partners effectively, but not with unfamiliar partners
IV	Self-mobility with limitations; may use powered mobility	Handles a limited selection of easily managed objects in adapted situations	Inconsistently sends and /or receives information even with familiar partners
V	Transported in a manual wheelchair	Does not handle objects with severely limited ability to perform even simple actions	Seldom effectively sends and receives information even with familiar partners

CFCS, Communication Function Classification System; *GMFCS*, Gross Motor Function Classification System-Expanded and Revised; *MACS*, Manual Ability Classification System.
From Hidecker MJ, Ho NT, Dodge N, et al: Inter-relationships of functional status in cerebral palsy: analyzing gross motor function, manual ability, and communication function classification systems in children, *Dev Med Child Neurol* 54:737-742, 2012.

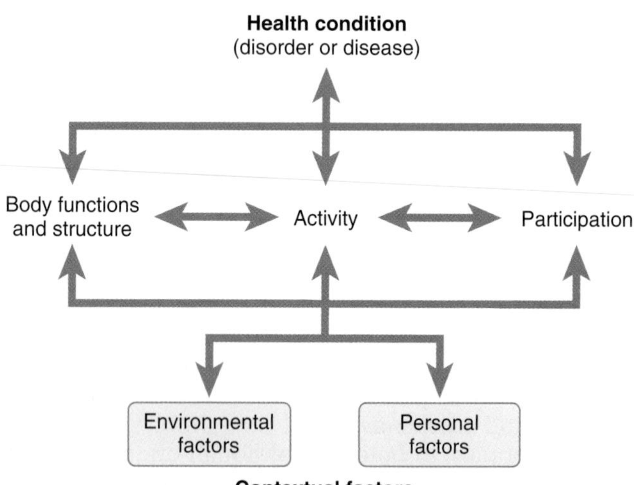

FIGURE 47-5 Interactions between the components of ICF. (Redrawn from World Health Organization. ICF-CY, International Classification of Functioning, Disability, and Health: Children & Youth Version. Geneva, Switzerland, World Health Organization, 2007.)

and Health for Children and Youth (ICF-CY). This was an expansion of the original ICF for children from birth to 18 years of age to specifically address the developing child, the developmental delay, and the child in the context of the family. The ICF-CY provides internationally accepted terminology and classifications that focus on the relationship between structure and function and moves from a medical model of disability to a biopsychosocial model of care (Figure 47-5).[59,69a]

In this model, biopsychosocial function is broken down into five categories: body function (b), body structure (s), activity and participation (d), environmental factors (e), and personal factors. Each domain has multiple levels associated with it: chapter number (first digit), second level categories (2 digits), third level categories (1 digit), fourth level categories (1 digit), and qualifiers (1 digit). Two examples are given in Tables 47-4 and 47-5.

Because of the complexity of this classification system, WHO research teams are developing a core set of categories for CP. Previous core sets have been developed for adult stroke, multiple sclerosis, and spinal cord injury.[59]

Table 47-4 ICF-CY Example 1

Level	Example	Coding
Category	Body function	b
Chapter	Chapter 2: Sensory Functions and Pain	b 2
Second Level	Seeing Functions	b 2 10
Third Level	Quality of vision	b 2 10 2
Fourth Level	Color vision	b 2 10 2 1

From World Health Organization. ICF-CY, International Classification of Functioning, Disability, and Health: Children & Youth Version, Geneva, Switzerland, World Health Organization, 2007.

Table 47-5 ICF-CY Example 2

Level	Example	Coding
Category	Activity and Participation	d
Chapter	Chapter 5: Self-care	d 5
Second Level	Looking after one's health	d 5 70
Third Level	Maintaining one's health	d 5 70 2
Fourth Level	Seeking advice or assistance from caregivers	b 2 10 2 1

From Schiariti V, Mâsse LC, Cieza A, et al: Toward the development of the international classification of functioning core sets for children with cerebral palsy: a global expert survey, *J Child Neurol* 2013 Feb 21.

Diagnosis

The term CP does not reflect a specific etiology; it is a description of clinical findings. There are many disease processes that can present as CP. The initial evaluation of a child with suspected CP should determine the diagnosis, if possible, decide which tests are needed to make the diagnosis, determine the etiology of the symptoms, determine comorbidities, and develop treatment options.

Before commencing any examination of an individual with suspected CP, it is important to gauge the emotional environment and the family's understanding of the child's current medical issues. Although many families bring their child to be evaluated because they believe something is different or wrong, they can be overwhelmed and afraid that their fears will be confirmed.

Table 47-6 Eliciting Primitive Reflexes

Reflex	Position	Method	Response	Age at Disappearance
Palmar grasp	Supine	Placing the index finger in the palm of the infant	Flexion of fingers, fist-making	6 mo
Plantar grasp	Supine	Pressing a thumb against the sole just behind the toes in the foot	Flexion of toes	15 mo
Galant	Prone	Scratching the skin of the infant's back from the shoulder downward, 2 to 3 cm lateral to the spinous processes	Incurvation of the trunk, with the concavity on the stimulated side	4 mo
Asymmetric tonic neck reflex	Supine	Rotation of the infant's head to one side for 15 sec	Extension of the extremities on the chin side and flexion of those on the occipital side	3 mo
Suprapubic extensor	Supine	Pressing the skin over the pubic bone with the fingers	Reflex extension of both lower extremities, with adduction and internal rotation into talipes equinus	4 wk
Crossed extensor	Supine	Passive total flexion of one lower extremity	Extension of the other lower limb with adduction and internal rotation into talipes equinus	6 wk
Rossolimo	Supine	Light tapping of the second to fourth toes at their plantar surface	Tonic flexion of the toes at the first metacarpophalangeal joint	4 wk
Heel	Supine	Tapping on the heel with a hammer, with the hip and knee joint flexed, and the ankle joint in neutral position	Rapid reflex extension of the lower extremity in question	3 wk
Moro	Supine	Sudden head extension produced by a light drop of the head	Abduction followed by adduction and flexion of upper extremities	6 mo
Babinski	Supine	Striking along the lateral aspect of the sole extending from the heel to the head of the fifth metatarsal	Combined extensor response: simultaneous dorsiflexion of the great toe and fanning of the remaining toes	Presence always abnormal

From Zafeiriou DI: Primitive reflexes and postural reactions in the neurodevelopmental examination, *Pediatr Neurol* 31:1-8, 2004.

History

A detailed history should include all basic attributes of a medical history, the individual's birth history, family history of blood clots or stroke, and any possible risk factors for CP as described above. The developmental history should include when and how a milestone was achieved. For example, a child may have crawled at 9 months, but there are different patterns of crawling; for example, "commando crawling" in which the child pulls their body across the floor with their arms or "bunny hopping" which refers to using flexion at the hip and knees but no reciprocal motions below the waist. Each of these crawling patterns can be associated with increased muscle tone in the legs. If there is regression of milestones after attainment, this suggests a neurodegenerative process and may indicate that a metabolic or genetic disease workup is also needed. A functional history will assist in determining treatment and life goals. This should include discussing the individual's mobility in the home and community setting and participation in activities of daily living and community activities.

Clinical Findings and Patterns

A thorough medical examination should include detailed neurologic, musculoskeletal, and functional components. Areas of weakness as well as tonal and movement abnormalities should be identified. A child may have multiple tonal abnormalities such as spasticity, dystonia, and truncal hypotonia. In addition to positive and negative motor signs, the persistence of primitive reflexes is a common finding in individuals with CP (Table 47-6).[69b]

Having the individual with suspected CP demonstrate the extent of his or her mobility, object handling, transfers, and communication will provide valuable information.

Neonatal pattern: After a severe brain injury, neonates tend to be hypotonic and develop spasticity over time. It can be difficult to elicit muscle stretch reflexes and there are minimal milestones to evaluate. Milestones may be delayed in premature children until the age of 2 years. Repeat examinations should be completed regularly.

Diplegic pattern: Hypertonic deficits are noted mainly in bilateral lower limbs, though upper limbs may be involved. Scissoring of bilateral lower limbs and talipes equinovarus deformities predominate. If ambulatory, toe walking with crouching tends to be present. Loss of range of motion (ROM) and hyperreflexia is present in the lower limbs. In a recent review, 72% of children with this pattern had neuroimaging that revealed changes on magnetic resonance imaging (MRI).[51] Among children with CP, 38% will have this pattern.[44]

Hemiplegic pattern: Hypertonic focal deficits, early hand lateralization, loss of ROM in affected limbs, and asymmetric limb use are associated with hemiplegic CP. Persistent primitive reflexes may be present. In a recent review, 84% of children with this pattern had neuroimaging that revealed MRI changes.[51] Among children with CP, 39% will have this pattern.[44]

Quadriplegic pattern: There is diffuse spastic hypertonicity with truncal dystonia, persistent primitive reflexes, intellectual disability, hyperreflexia, and loss of ROM in all affected limbs. In a recent review, 92% of children with this pattern had neuroimaging that revealed MRI changes. Among children with CP, 23% will have this pattern.[44]

The clinical presentation will guide the needed workup and development of a comprehensive treatment plan. For example, a prenatal stroke could cause a hemiplegic pattern indicating the need for a coagulation workup and neuroimaging to evaluate for a brain malformation, as is found in 10% of children with this pattern.[51] Although diffuse hypotonia may be a precursor to spasticity, persistent hypotonia is often associated with genetic or metabolic syndromes. To assist in the early diagnosis and treatment of CP, the American Academy of Neurology has published neuroimaging algorithms for findings suggestive of CP in neonates and children (Fig. 47-6).[5,36]

History and examination findings suggest diagnosis of CP (non-progressive disorder of motor control)

↓

1. Confirm that the history does not suggest a progressive or degenerative central nervous system disorder.
2. Ensure that features suggestive of progressive or degenerative disease are not present on examination.
3. Classify the type of CP (quadriplegia, hemiplegia, diplegia, ataxic, etc). For the most part this classification system is one of convenience, i.e., easy communication. It does not necessarily relate to prognosis or to what treatments are indicated.
4. Screen for associated conditions including:
   a. Developmental delay/mental retardation
   b. Ophthalmologic/hearing impairments
   c. Speech and language delay
   d. Feeding/swallowing dysfunction
   e. If history of suspected seizures, obtain an EEG

↓

Did the child have previous neuroimaging or other laboratory studies? (e.g., in neonatal period) that determined the etiology of CP?

Yes → No need for further diagnostic testing

No → Obtain neuroimaging study (MRI preferred to CT)

Normal MRI →
1. Consider metabolic or genetic testing if upon follow-up the child has:
   a. Evidence of deterioration or episodes of metabolic decompensation
   b. No etiology determined by medical evaluation
   c. Family history of childhood neurologic disorder associated with "CP"

Abnormal MRI →
1. Determine if neuroimaging abnormalities in combination with history and examination establishes a specific etiology of CP
2. If developmental malformation is present, consider genetic evaluation.
3. If previous stroke, consider evaluation for coagulopathy or other etiology.

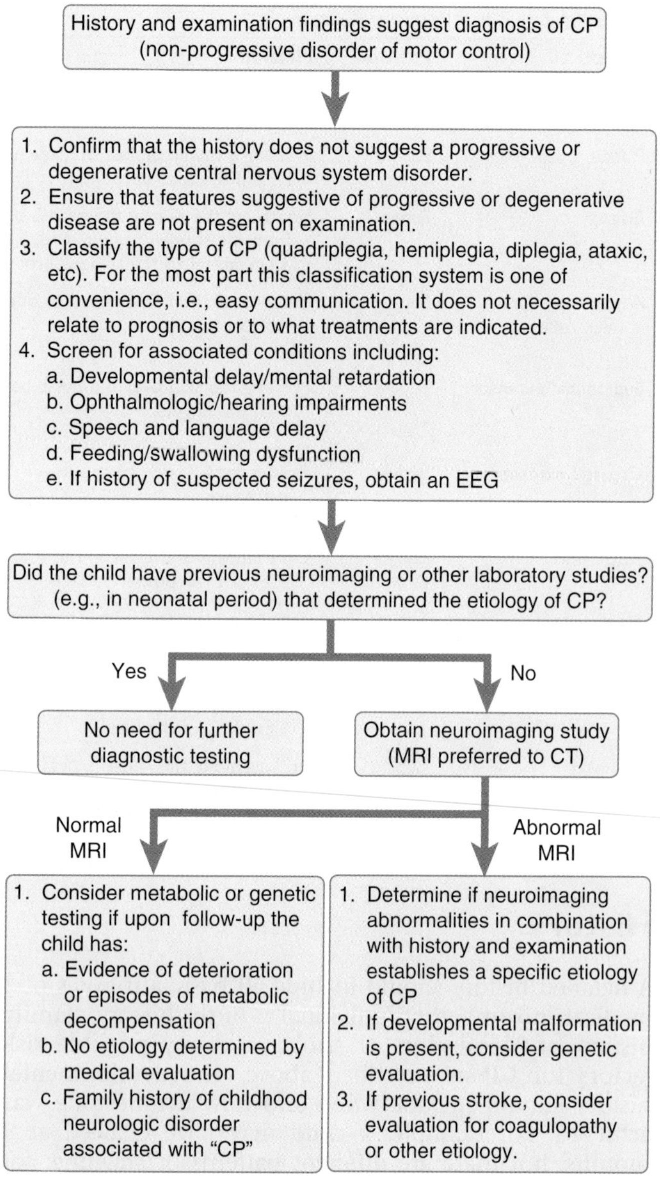

FIGURE 47-6 Diagnostic algorithm for a child with suspected cerebral palsy. (Redrawn from Ashwal S, Russman BS, Blasco PA, et al: Practice parameter: diagnostic assessment of the child with cerebral palsy: report of the Quality Standards Subcommittee of the American Academy of Neurology and the Practice Committee of the Child Neurology Society, *Neurology* 62:851-863, 2004.)

Functional Prognosis

Ambulation: In the 1970s, Molnar et al laid the foundation for the future development of motor curves based on developmental milestone achievement. Their work showed that sitting independently by the age of 2 years or having less than 3 primitive reflexes present by 18 to 24 months was a positive predictor of ambulation, although not sitting independently by 4 years was a negative predictor.[39] Their later work demonstrated that over 50% of all children with CP will ambulate and further divided this by topographic classification (80% to 90% diplegia, 50% quadriplegia, 75% dyskinesia).[38] In 2008, these findings were replicated in a large European population of children with CP.[7]

Moving from the prediction of ambulation to the prediction of longitudinal gross motor function in children with CP, Rosenbaum et al. published motor development curves based on an individual's GMFCS level in 2002.[54] These curves helped transition the diagnosis of CP from a disease of childhood to a chronic disease. They have been validated and their stability has been shown since their initial publication. Interestingly, children with GMFCS levels I and V tended to remain at these levels, although children with GMFCS levels II, III, and IV tended to need reclassification over time.[54] These findings were replicated in a large cohort in Europe.[46]

As the ICF-CY model continues to modify our paradigm of health, efforts to assess children with CP in the domain of activity and participation will likely increase. Most recently, the SCPE has been working to develop development curves for self-care capabilities,[28] social participation,[65] and health-related quality of life.[64]

Medical Management

The spectrum of associated medical conditions affecting individuals with CP is broad. In the newer consensus definition of CP, there is a greater emphasis on recognizing associated impairments and functional limitations as well as frequently coexisting medical conditions, aside from the primary abnormalities in movement and posture.[53] Of late, greater attention has been directed toward investigating in a systematic fashion these conditions commonly seen in CP. Function, participation, and quality of life are often influenced by these comorbidities. It is intuitive that the more severe the motor disorder or higher GMFCS level, the greater the likelihood that the child will have more numerous or more severe medical comorbidities. Two exceptions to this correlate should be noted: pain occurring in all levels of disability and behavior disorders seen more commonly in cases of milder motor disability.[45] Etiologies of CP and their anatomic correlates may also predict these associated conditions. Some associated conditions such as seizures are clearly attributed to a disturbance at the brain level, but others may present caused by a combination of abnormalities in neural control and sensorimotor deficits.

Feeding, Growth, and Nutrition

Dysphagia is commonly observed in patients with CP. Impaired oropharyngeal strength and coordination place a child at risk for not meeting caloric and fluid requirements because of feeding inefficiency. Serious medical complications such as malnutrition and an increased risk of aspiration events may occur as well. Caregivers may share that this aspect of the child's care is burdensome, with stress increasing when the child needs considerable time to eat and activities revolve around feeding schedules. Frequently, children will struggle to gain weight only to lose it quickly during an illness. Indications for swallow studies include impaired oropharyngeal skills with a wet vocal quality or increased congestion during feeding. It is important to remember that some individuals have silent aspiration and may not generate a protective cough; therefore, workup for aspiration events should include a formal swallow study. Early on, children should receive nutritional counseling and supplemental caloric and fluid intake if necessary. Some parents may resist placement of gastrostomy tubes, especially if the child swallows safely, even though feedings may require increased time and aggressive positioning strategies. Oral hygiene may be compromised and children may have excessive sialorrhea, which can contribute to aspiration events and cause secondary skin irritation. Growth and nutrition may be compromised because of limited intake of key nutrients, impaired absorption, and endocrine abnormalities. When malnourished, children are at risk for growth disturbances, increased infection rates, skin breakdown, osteopenia, and ultimately decreased life expectancy.[31]

Pulmonary

Lung disease is an important cause of morbidity and mortality in CP. Cumulative injury to lung architecture may occur as a result of repeated aspiration events, infections, decreased mucociliary clearance, kyphoscoliosis, and airway obstruction. Prevention of pulmonary aspiration may require modified feeding consistencies, treatment of reflux, alternative means of feeding such as gastrostomy with or without fundoplication, and control of sialorrhea with anticholinergic medications, botulinum injections, and sometimes surgery. Chest physiotherapy and bronchodilators can assist with decreased mucociliary clearance. Children with infections should be treated with tailored antibiotics based on sputum cultures, and some will require prophylactic or cyclical antibiotic coverage. Preventative measures include immunizations since this population is at higher risk for infections and complications. Upper airway obstruction may require continuous positive airway pressure and/or surgery. Lower airway obstruction may respond to a trial of bronchodilators and pressure. Children with CP frequently have sleep-disordered breathing. A history of snoring or observed irregular breathing patterns with or without excessive daytime somnolence should prompt the practitioner to investigate possible sleep apnea, which if untreated can contribute to further morbidity. Apnea may be central, peripheral, or a combination of both. Many children have impaired sleep regulation and may not achieve restful sleep because of microaspiration and cough, altered light perception, medication side effects impacting natural sleep wake cycles, and challenges in achieving comfortable positioning.[19a] Hypoventilation is seen frequently in children who have neuromuscular weakness, and children may ultimately require noninvasive ventilator support and external aids for mobilization of secretions and assistance with cough generation. Scoliosis surgery may improve restrictive lung disease, but must be considered carefully given risks associated with it and whether it will improve functioning and quality of life.

Neurologic Issues

The CP population as a whole is at an increased risk for seizures. Seizures occur most frequently in children with a quadriparetic or hemiparetic clinical presentation. Medication use for epilepsy management may be associated with cognitive dulling or other side effects such as anorexia. Some children have hyperkinetic movement disorders that mimic seizure activity and may require prolonged video EEG monitoring to delineate between the two conditions. Weaning of seizure medications depends on the severity of the seizures and a time period, usually 2 years, during which the child has been seizure free.

Children with CP also have a higher incidence of intellectual disability; cognitive impairment is estimated to affect 50%.[17] Nonverbal status and severe intellectual disability are seen more commonly in children with a quadriparetic clinical presentation. However, it is important to note that some children, especially with basal ganglia injury and dyskinesias, may have preservation of intellectual abilities despite severe dysarthria. It is also important to differentiate the cause of communication difficulties; cognitive dysfunction versus hearing or vision limitations versus dysarthria.[1] Children who are higher functioning and mobile may still have cognitive dysfunction and learning disabilities despite relative preservation of verbal language skills. Screening for impaired attention and executive functioning deficits is recommended. Visual perceptual deficits may also affect learning, despite a normal IQ. Mood disorders such as anxiety and depression can impact functioning and participation.

Depending on the anatomic location of the brain lesion associated with the clinical presentation, some children will be at higher risk for vision and hearing deficits. Prematurity is associated with retinal damage and myopia. More global involvement with occipital lobe pathology may result in cortical visual impairment. Strabismus is important to recognize early to avoid amblyopia. Hearing deficits may be conductive and/or sensorineural in etiology. Children with dyskinetic CP caused by kernicterus should be specifically screened for sensorineural hearing loss.

Genitourinary

Voiding dysfunction may result from impaired processing of sensory feedback and also incoordination of muscular functions responsible for bladder wall contractions and sphincter relaxation: detrusor sphincter dyssynergia. Full continence and normal voiding patterns may be difficult to achieve, and children with CP are frequently delayed in age for achieving continence. Urinary retention can increase chances of urinary tract infections and if a high intravesical pressure is generated, vesicoureteral reflux with resultant hydronephrosis and pelviectasis may occur. Clean intermittent catheterization is required when children are experiencing chronic urinary retention with urinary stasis. Anticholinergic treatments for dystonia or sialorrhea may trigger urinary retention. Children treated with levetiracetam for epilepsy have an increased risk of renal calculi formation.

Gastrointestinal

Gastroesophageal reflux disease (GERD) and constipation, which are commonly observed in CP, may produce discomfort and exacerbate hypertonicity. In more severe cases, children may have dysmotility with delayed gastric empting and esophagitis from medically refractory GERD.

Musculoskeletal Pain and Osteopenia

Children who are less mobile are at increased risk for contracture and bony deformity and associated musculoskeletal pain. Although exercise has been established as beneficial in CP, children at GMFCS levels IV or V will not be able to achieve the same benefits as those children who are more mobile. Common sites of musculoskeletal pain include the hips, spine, knee, and foot and ankle complex. With aging, patients may experience worsening pain associated with patella alta, spondylolysis with spondylolisthesis, and degenerative hip conditions.

Children with CP are at risk for osteopenia and related fragility fractures. Risk factors for osteoporosis include decreased weight bearing, use of anticonvulsants, malnutrition, and decreased sunlight exposure. Supplementation with calcium and vitamin D is routinely used to improve bone density, but the effects on prevention of fragility fractures are unclear. Bisphosphonates are effective in improving bone mineral density but are not without risk, and so this intervention is usually reserved for children who have experienced a fragility fracture. As the long-term side effects with use of bisphosphonates are unknown, additional research is required before they become routinely used.[19]

Therapeutic Management

The treatment of a person with CP requires a multidisciplinary team that understands the different presentations of this condition, the motor control abnormalities, and the primary and secondary conditions associated with its multisystem involvement. The team composition may vary according to the child's needs. It may include physiatrists, orthopedic surgeons, neurologists, neurosurgeons, developmental medicine specialists, physical therapists, occupational therapists, speech and language pathologists, orthotists, nutritionists, and social workers, among others. Additionally, it is important the family and child be active team members when setting priorities and goals within the context of the level of impairments and the child's age.

Because the WHO ICF-CY's recommendation that disease treatments be focused mainly on the individual's level of activity and participation, there has been a rising paradigm shift in the treatment of CP. The previous focus on alleviating the associated motor impairments has transitioned into discussions of how different treatment options will affect each individual's function.[13] The ultimate goal of any therapeutic intervention is to encourage the child's maximal potential in motor, cognitive, and social realms.[47]

Childhood Disabilities and Education

There are numerous special education laws ensuring that individuals of all ages can receive educational services in the United States. Table 47-7 summarizes pertinent legislation.[24]

Overall, physiatrists should be familiar with three terms that have evolved. Early intervention programs are government-sponsored programs that are tasked to evaluate children at risk or with delays in one or more areas of function between the ages of 0 and 36 months.[37] Services include therapies, nutrition monitoring, care coordination, audiovisual, and social work, among others. After 36 months of age, children with disabilities may qualify to receive ongoing services through their local public school system. A 504 plan ensures that appropriate classroom accommodations will be made for children who do not qualify for special education classes. An individualized education program ensures that classroom accommodations are provided, along with a document provided to the family with present level of functioning, short- and long-term goals, specific educational services needed, participation in regular educational programs, and assurance that the necessary services are available.[24]

Therapy Interventions

There are many forms of therapy interventions (Table 47-8) and despite much research, there is currently minimal evidence to suggest that any individual therapeutic intervention is superior. In fact, many therapists use a combination of these approaches while tailoring their therapy program to the child's needs. The main goal of all therapies is to promote and facilitate development in all domains of function.[4]

The setting and frequency of formal therapy sessions vary. The most common therapy settings are school-based outpatient models with a frequency of 1 to 3 times a week per discipline. Other models include intensive "pulse" or "episode" therapy through camps or day rehabilitation programs. Regardless of the setting, it is imperative that the family and child are included in the therapy plan to promote carryover and reinforcement in the home setting.

Stretching: Stretching is a component of therapy programs; its goal is to reduce the risk of contracture development as a result of muscle imbalances and hypertonicity. Sustained stretching can be achieved through the use of positioning devices, orthoses, and

Table 47-7 Important Legislation and Laws for Children with Disabilities[24]

Law/ Legislation	Summary
The Handicapped Children's Early Education Assistance Act of 1968 or Public Law (PL) 95-538	Provides for educational programs for young children with disabilities. Funds research institutes to study the behavioral, cognitive, and emotional functioning of children.
The Vocational Rehabilitation Act of 1973, or PL 93-112	Provides for services for individuals with physical or mental handicaps that promoted independence and employability. Section 504 provides protection against discrimination of children who might not meet "special education" definitions but require classroom accommodations, such as extra time for test taking or frequent breaks.
The Education of All Handicapped Children Act of 1975, or PL 94-142	Requires that no child, regardless of disability type or severity, can be excluded from a school education. Mandates that every child with a disability have an individualized educational plan that ensures appropriate accommodations, but also includes detailed plans and goals of education.
The Individuals with Disabilities Education Act (IDEA) of 1990, or PL101-476	Provides funding for infant and toddler early intervention programs. Replaces the word "handicapped" with "disabled." Ensures infants and toddlers with disabilities from birth to 2 years of age with developmental delay receive early intervention services. Requires that children ages 3 to 21 years receive special education and services.
The No Child Left Behind Act of 2002	Changes the distribution of federal funds from volume-based metrics to student performance-based metrics.
The Individuals with Disabilities Education Act (IDEA) revisions of 2004	Updates PL101-476 to include a requirement that children with disabilities be prepared for further education, employment, and independent living.

Table 47-8 Similarities and Differences Between Neuromotor Therapy Approaches to Cerebral Palsy

	Neurodevelopmental Treatment (Bobaths)	Sensorimotor Approach to Treatment (Rood)	Sensory Integration Approach (Ayres)	Vojta Approach	Patterning Therapy (Doman-Delacato)
Central nervous system model Goals of treatment	Hierarchic • To normalize tone • To inhibit primitive reflexes • To facilitate automatic reactions and normal movement patterns	Hierarchic • To activate postural responses (stability) • To activate movement (mobility) once stability is achieved	Hierarchic • To improve efficiency of neural processing • To better organize adaptive responses	Hierarchic • To prevent cerebral palsy in infants at risk • To improve motoric behavior in infants with fixed cerebral palsy	Hierarchic • To achieve independent mobility • To improve motor coordination • To prevent or improve communication disorders • To enhance intelligence
Primary sensory systems used to effect a motor response	• Kinesthetic • Proprioceptive • Tactile	• Tactile • Proprioceptive • Kinesthetic	• Vestibular • Tactile • Kinesthetic	• Proprioceptive • Kinesthetic • Tactile	All sensory systems are used
Emphasis of treatment activities	• Positioning and handling to normalize sensory input Facilitation of active movement	Sensory stimulation to activate motor response (tapping, brushing, icing)	Therapist guides but child controls sensory input to get adaptive purposeful response	Trigger reflex locomotive zones to encourage movement patterns (e.g., reflex crawl)	Sensory and reflex stimulation, passive movement patterns, encouragement of independent movements
Intended clinical population	Children with cerebral palsy Adults post–cerebrovascular accident (CVA)	Children with neuromotor disorders such as cerebral palsy Adults post-CVA	Children with learning disabilities Children with autism	Young infants at risk for cerebral palsy Young infants with fixed cerebral palsy	Children with neonatal or acquired brain damage
Emphasis on treating infants	Yes	No	No	Yes	No
Emphasis on family involvement during treatment	Yes Handling and positioning for activities of daily living	No	No Supportive role encouraged	Yes Family administers treatment at home daily	Yes Family and friends administer treatment several times daily
Empiric support	Few studies Conflicting results	Very few studies Conflicting results	Many studies Conflicting results with school-age children Positive results for tactile and vestibular input with infants	Few studies Conflicting results	Few studies Conflicting results

From Harris SR, Atwater SW, Crowe TK: Accepted and controversial neuromotor therapies for infants at high risk for cerebral palsy, *J Perinatol* 8:3-13, 1988, with permission.

serial casting. A systematic review examining the effects of casting, either alone or in combination with botulinum toxin type A (BTX-A), on equinus in children with CP revealed no strong and consistent evidence that combining casting and BTX-A is superior to using either intervention alone.[9]

Strengthening: Historically, exercise programs that included strengthening were contraindicated in CP. A systematic review of the effectiveness of strength-training programs in CP reported increased strength without any negative effects of increased spasticity or reduced range of motion. Indirectly, some studies have reported increased participation and improved self-esteem.[16]

Aerobic Exercise: Historically, exercise programs that included aerobic exercise were contraindicated in CP. A systematic review of the evidence suggests improved physiologic measures of aerobic fitness without adverse effects, for example, increased spasticity, fatigue, or musculoskeletal trauma. Improvements in aerobic fitness were noted with 45 minutes four times a week of "high-intensity" activities such as wheelchair sports, swimming, matt exercises, or cycling. This benefit is not maintained if the activity is not maintained. None of the studies have looked into reporting outcomes representing the ICF model of increased activity and participation.[52]

Constraint-Induced Movement Therapy (CIMT): CIMT is a treatment for hemiparesis to improve motor function in the affected upper limb. In children with hemiplegic CP, the unaffected limb is restrained with a removable cast, typically for 3 weeks, and the child undergoes intensive, structured therapy in addition to daily activities and play. A systematic review of randomized controlled trials involving CIMT noted a medium beneficial effect in arm function, as well as a medium effect size in the activity level in the ICF-CY model. The review further suggests that home CIMT had better improvement than clinic- or camp-based settings.[11]

Functional Electrical Stimulation: Neuromuscular electrical stimulation (NMS) is the application of an electrical current of sufficient intensity to elicit muscle contraction. When applied during a functional activity, it is referred to as functional electrical stimulation (FES). In contrast, threshold electrical stimulation (TES) is a low-intensity, subthreshold electrical stimulus that has been theorized to increase blood flow and stimulate muscle growth when applied during sleep to take advantage of heightened trophic hormone secretion. Evidence to support use of these modalities in children with CP is limited; however, there is more evidence to support NMS and FES than TES.[27]

Robotic and Partial Body Weight Support Treadmill Training (PBWSTT): These forms of therapy involve a repetitive and task-specific approach to facilitate attainment of stepping and locomotion and to achieve a more normalized gait pattern based on current theories of motor learning. The setting includes an overhead harness system used to support the child's body weight on a treadmill, while the therapist or a robot facilitate the kinematic, kinetic, and temporal features of walking. Although evidence of potential benefits from PBWSTT and robotic therapy is emerging in adults with stroke and spinal cord injury, several recent systematic reviews showed limited evidence to support the use of PBWSTT in children with CP. Despite reported improvements in gross motor function, functional status, walking performance, and gait parameters, statistical significance was not reached in most of the studies.[40]

Durable Medical Equipment

The goal in prescribing durable medical equipment (DME) for individuals with CP should focus on maximizing function, improving safety, and enabling independence using the ICF-CY model of health. Motor impairment is one of the top reasons for a mobility device in CP as exploration of the environment is imperative for cognitive development that leads to maximizing functional independence.

Supportive or adaptive seating systems and standing frames can facilitate a developmentally appropriate upright posture, strengthening, flexibility across the lower extremities, weight bearing/bone density, upper limb function, communication, and feeding by freeing the child's hands to perform bimanual tasks, improving breath support, and optimizing the head and trunk position to facilitate a safe swallow. Specialized seating devices are available for sitting on the floor or toilet, feeding, and bathing, as well as for incorporation in a mobility device.[47]

Use of a wheelchair becomes applicable when a child either outgrows commercially available strollers or additional support is necessary. The goal of supportive seating is to provide an upright seated posture to facilitate interaction with the environment and minimize deforming forces secondary to postural abnormalities (Figure 47-7).

The clinician must consider both the seating goals and the family's needs. One decision once unique to pediatrics is whether to use either a conventional wheelchair base or a stroller base for the mobility device. Power mobility can be pursued in children as young as 18 months old if they have fair motor control, no visual deficits, and good cognition.[47]

For children with adequate head and trunk support, a gait trainer, walker, or crutches might help facilitate gait training and provide external support and improve upright posture. The gait trainer is a wheeled walker with a sling seat and various support options, which allows the patient to propel the device without necessarily having a coordinated, reciprocal gait pattern. For the dependent child and adult, families might benefit from equipment to facilitate transfers and floor recovery, such as a mobile mechanical lift or overhead lift device.[47]

The production of speech, language, and gesture for communication is also commonly affected in CP because of motor, sensory, and intellectual impairments. Various applications of technology have been used to maximize function. In augmentative communication, meaningful communication and expression of needs are facilitated with the use of computers, switch devices, signboards, and similar adaptive equipment.[47]

Splinting and orthoses are commonly used in CP to manage spastic but flexible dynamic deformities of the

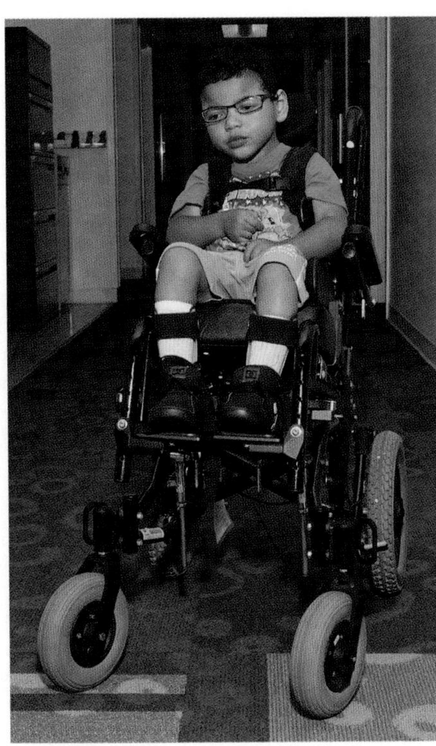

FIGURE 47-7 Child with spastic quadriplegia seated in a custom manual wheelchair.

extremities. There are a variety of passive and dynamic splints. Orthoses must be tailored to the child's age, deformity, motor control, and tolerance. With lower limb orthoses, the clinician should clearly identify the gait deviation and goals to be addressed, with special consideration of ankle-foot alignment, range of motion, and tone. Ankle-foot orthoses have been demonstrated to decrease the energy cost of walking in children with CP, compared with barefoot walking, and to improve gait parameters of stride length and velocity.[47]

Management of Hypertonia

Hypertonia is one of the most prevalent comorbidities of CP that affect function. The most common forms observed in CP include spasticity, dystonia, and a combination of both. Spasticity is defined as velocity-dependent resistance, whereas dystonia is a more dynamic movement disorder, which involves an involuntary alteration in pattern of muscle activation during voluntary movement. It may fluctuate in presence and severity over time.[58] Learning to differentiate between them can guide goal-setting and intervention. Hypertonia can be focal or generalized and can affect the limbs and trunk. If left untreated, it can interfere with function and development. Hypertonia can lead to secondary musculoskeletal complications such as joint contractures and dislocations. It can also be a significant source of pain.

Management of hypertonia in children with CP is challenging, and no standard approach exists. The importance of physical therapy, orthoses, and casting has been stressed by a consensus group,[21] but these interventions can be augmented with oral medications as well as chemodenervation with BTX, phenol, or both. Neurosurgical procedures including intrathecal baclofen (ITB) and selective dorsal rhizotomy (SDR) can also be considered in carefully selected populations. Often, different combinations of these treatments are used to optimize treatment of hypertonia. Treatment must be tailored to goals and may change with growth and development. Goals should be identified before initiation of any treatment. Any spasticity-reducing treatment option should translate into improved mobility, self-care, skin breakdown prevention, ease of care, and comfort.

Oral Medications

Generalized hypertonia is often treated with oral medications. Some of the most common medications include baclofen, diazepam, dantrolene sodium, tizanidine, clonazepam, and clonidine. All of these, except dantrolene, can cause sedation as they exert their effects through the CNS. A recent evidence-based practice parameter looking at the pharmacologic treatment of generalized spasticity in children and adolescents with CP found limited studies and insufficient data to support or refute the use of any of these drugs on a long-term basis.[14] Pediatric dosing is quite variable, and the side effects and risks of these medications limit their use.

The treatment of generalized secondary dystonia in children with CP is more challenging as it responds poorly to oral medications. Commonly used drugs include trihexyphenidyl hydrochloride (Artane), oral baclofen, and levodopa-carbidopa (Sinemet). The scientific evidence for the clinical use of trihexyphenidyl in children with CP remains equivocal.[55] Adverse events such as sedation, dizziness, and dry mouth are common and can limit its tolerance. ITB has been found to be more effective, but at higher doses than what is required for treatment of spasticity (Table 47-9).[2]

Chemodenervation

BTX intramuscular injections and phenol neurolysis are used in the treatment of focal hypertonicity (spasticity and dystonia). Injections are most effective as a localized treatment for dynamic contractures or shortened muscles.[21] Both forms of chemodenervation (BTX and phenol) can be used at the same time to maximize the dose and number of muscles, as well as in combination with systemic medications. Typically, electrical stimulation, electromyogram, or ultrasound guidance is used for localization, though phenol neurolysis requires electrical stimulation for nerve identification. A recent systematic review found that for localized, segmental spasticity of the upper and lower extremity of children with CP warranting treatment, BTX should be offered as an effective and generally safe treatment. The review cited insufficient evidence to support or refute the use of BTX A to improve motor function or the use of other forms of BTX serotypes, phenol, and alcohol injections.[14]

Botulinum toxin: BTX is widely used in the management of CP. BTX works by blocking acetylcholine receptors at the neuromuscular junction. BTX-A is marketed as Botox and BTX-B as Myobloc. There are currently over seven different serotypes of BTX and at least five commercial preparations (Botox, Dysport, Xeomin, Myobloc, and Hengli).

Table 47-9 Oral Medications for Children with Cerebral Palsy

Drug	Mechanism of Action	Side Effects and Precautions	Pharmacology and Dosing
Baclofen	Binds to receptors (GABA) in the spinal cord to inhibit reflexes that lead to increased tone. Also binds to receptors in the brain leading to sedation.	Sedation, confusion, nausea, dizziness, muscle weakness, hypotonia, ataxia, and paresthesias Can cause loss of seizure control. Withdrawal can produce seizures, rebound hypertonia, fever, and death.	Rapidly absorbed after oral dosing, mean half-life of 3.5 hours Excreted mainly through the kidney Dose administration in children: start at 2.5 to 5 mg/day, increase to 30 mg/day (in children 2 to 7 years old) or 60 mg/day (in children 8 years and older)
Diazepam	Facilitates postsynaptic binding of a neurotransmitter (GABA) in the brain stem, reticular formation, and spinal cord to inhibit reflexes that lead to increased tone.	Central nervous system depression causing sedation, decreased motor coordination, impaired attention and memory both overdoses and withdrawal occur. The sedative effect generally limits use to severely affected children.	Well absorbed after oral dosing, mean half-life 20 to 80 hours Metabolized mainly in the liver In children, doses range from 0.12 to 0.8 mg/kg/day in divided doses
Clonidine	Alpha$_2$-agonist Acts in both the brain and spinal cord to enhance presynaptic inhibition of reflexes that lead to increased tone.	Bradycardia, hypotension, dry mouth, drowsiness, dizziness, constipation, and depression These side effects are common and cause half of patients to discontinue the medication.	Well absorbed after oral dosing, mean half-life is 5 to 19 hours Half is metabolized in liver and half is excreted by kidney Start with 0.05 mg bid, titrate up until side effects limit tolerance. May use patch
Tizanidine	Alpha$_2$-agonist Acts in both the brain and spinal cord to enhance presynaptic inhibition of reflexes that lead to increased tone.	Dry mouth, sedation, dizziness, visual hallucinations, elevated liver enzymes, insomnia, and muscle weakness	Well absorbed after oral dosing, half-life is 2.5 hours. Extensive first-pass metabolism in liver. Start with 2 mg at bedtime and increase until side effects limit tolerance. Maximum is 36 mg/day
Dantrolene sodium	Works directly on the muscle to decrease muscle force produced during contraction Little effect on smooth and cardiac muscles	Most important side effect is hepatotoxicity (2%), which may be severe Liver function tests must be monitored monthly initially, and then several times per year. Other side effects are mild sedation, dizziness, diarrhea, and paresthesias.	Oral dose is approximately 70% absorbed in small intestine, half-life is 15 hours. Mostly metabolized in the liver Pediatric doses range from 0.5 mg/kg, bid, to a maximum of 3 mg/kg, qid.

From Green LB, Hurvitz EA: Cerebral palsy, *Phys Med Rehabil Clin North Am* 18:859-882, 2007.
bid, Twice a day; *GABA*, gamma-aminobutyric acid; *qid*, four times a day.

Of the commercial preparations, more evidence is available for BTX-A. Dosage and dilution guidelines have not been established for any of the commercial preparations, but consensus statements and systematic reviews provide recommendations.[21] The child's age, weight, severity of hypertonia, and muscle localization are taken into consideration when determining dosage. The period of clinically useful relaxation is usually 12 to 16 weeks, and it is recommended that injections be spaced a minimum of 3 months apart because of concern for neutralizing antibody formation.[21] Adverse events related to BTX are rare and include injection site pain, fatigue, and excessive weakness of the injected muscle. Some cases of dysphagia and urinary incontinence have been reported.[14]

BTX treatment is appropriate for hypertonia in the form of spasticity and/or dystonia in all functional levels GMFCS levels I to V as long as the goal setting is adapted to the specific problems. The main indication is hypertonia that hinders function and that if left untreated will become a fixed (rather than dynamic) contracture. Ideally, BTX treatment should start at a young age when gait patterns and motor function are still flexible, allowing for gross motor function learning, including strengthening of antagonist muscle groups during the time window of tone reduction.[21] Studies evaluating the effectiveness of BTX-A injections combined with serial casting for dynamic equinus show mixed results.[9] A systematic review showed therapy interventions do not have a high level or quality of evidence in support of their use following BTX-A.[32]

Phenol: Before BTX was developed and commercialized, phenol motor point blocks were the only available form of focal chemodenervation. Phenol works by proteolytically causing neurolysis. The use of phenol requires the injection to be placed selectively and the nerve to be isolated, which can be technically challenging. For this reason sedation is highly recommended. Electrical stimulation with or without ultrasound is required for localization. Commonly injected nerves are the musculocutaneous, obturator, and sciatic nerve to the medial hamstring. Injecting other nerves may have a higher risk of developing dysesthesias. In contrast to Botox, phenol is inexpensive and its results can last between 6 and 18 months. BTX-A and BTX-B have been combined safely with phenol injections, thus allowing one to maximize the dose and number of muscles treated by the finite amount of BTX.[29]

Intrathecal Baclofen Therapy

ITB is most often used to treat children with generalized spasticity or generalized moderate-to-severe dystonia.[2] It is an FDA-approved method to treat spasticity of cerebral or spinal origin. Currently, indications for the use of ITB include tone that is thought to interfere with function or the ability to provide care; modified Ashworth scores >3; and definable goals for spasticity reduction.

ITB is delivered through a programmable pump placed subfascially in the abdominal wall and connected to a catheter that is tunneled from the side of the pump and inserted in the intrathecal space at a desired spinal level. This method allows the delivery of smaller doses of baclofen (micrograms) intrathecally, thus reducing the side effect profile seen with the oral form of baclofen (milligrams). The dose can be titrated to a desired therapeutic response. A screening lumbar bolus dose of baclofen can be used to evaluate medication responsiveness. The pump requires replacement every 6 to 7 years owing to battery life.

A number of reports have noted that ITB reduces hypertonicity and the effect continues long term. Reports have attempted to evaluate ITB use and improvements in function. Some have reported improvements in positioning, activities of daily living, transfers, sleep, oral motor skills, hand use, and comfort. Motor function measured by the gross motor function measure (GMFM), pediatric evaluation of disabilities inventory (PEDI), and functional independence measure for children (WeeFIM) has been reported to improve. Others have found no improvement.[30]

Potential complications of ITB include infections, cerebrospinal fluid leaks, and catheter problems such as disconnection, migration, or kinking. Abrupt withdrawal is a medical emergency and may present as increased tone, spasms, diaphoresis, agitation, and pruritus. If untreated, it can progress to rhabdomyolyis and multisystem failure. Treatment includes high doses of oral baclofen as well as benzodiazepines and cyproheptadine. The latter alleviates the pruritus related to ITB withdrawal. Intrathecal baclofen through a lumbar drain can also be used in treatment of severe withdrawal. Urinary retention can be seen acutely, whereas constipation and weight gain tend to be more chronic complications.[2,30] For these reasons, it is very important to verify that caregivers and family have the resources needed to comply with the longitudinal care of the ITB therapy and its potential complications.

Deep Brain Stimulation

Deep brain stimulation (DBS) involves a stereotactic implantation of electrodes into the basal ganglia and a programmable pulse generator implanted subcutaneously in the infraclavicular region. DBS is the treatment of choice in primary dystonias. In CP, the majority of persons have generalized secondary dystonia (typically quadriplegics with GMFCS levels IV to V). ITB is the treatment of choice in this population; however, in those who do not respond adequately to ITB, DBS should be considered. The response is less than that seen in primary dystonia; some studies have reported only 30% to 33% reduction in different dystonia rating scales such as the Burke-Fahn-Marsen (BFM) scale.[3]

Selective Dorsal Rhizotomy

SDR is a surgical procedure used for spasticity. The surgical technique involves single or multilevel laminectomies exposing the L2–S2 nerve roots and selectively cutting a percentage of the dorsal rootlets with abnormal response with the aid of electrophysiologic monitoring. The ideal candidate for SDR is a child between the ages of 3 and 8 years old with diplegic CP and predominantly spastic tone (typically GMFCS levels I to III), little upper limb involvement, sufficient underlying strength, good selective motor control, and minimal contractures. Positive preoperative functional predictors for a good SDR outcome include the ability to rise from a squatted position with minimal support and a younger child's ability to crawl on hands and knees or tall kneel.[62] Some degree of lower limb weakness can be unmasked postoperatively by reducing the spasticity, making intensive physical therapy a necessity. Children must have the cognitive and social capacity for such an intensive intervention.[35]

Positive outcomes of SDR include reduced spasticity, increased range of motion, improved gait pattern and kinematics, increased speed, and decreased oxygen cost, making gait more efficient.[67] A metaanalysis of three randomized controlled trials evaluating the outcome of SDR in children with spastic diplegia showed that SDR plus physical therapy is more efficacious than physical therapy alone in reducing spasticity and has a small positive effect on gross motor function.[35] A study looking at 136 patients retrospectively showed that spasticity decreased substantially at the major muscle groups: hip flexors, adductors, hamstrings, and rectus femoris; there was less reduction in the plantar flexor group, which may be functionally beneficial for joint stabilization and power production. Long-term outcomes at 5 and 20 years after SDR in children show an improvement in the GMFM and gait pattern.[67]

If done at an early age, SDR can reduce bony deformity, decreasing the need for orthopedic surgery in about 35% of those young children. Long-term complications such as sensory dysfunction, bladder or bowel dysfunction, or back pain are infrequent.[62] Combined dorsal and ventral rhizotomies have been performed in a few children with severe spasticity and dystonia who were not candidates for ITB.[2]

Orthopedic Management

Children with CP have abnormalities in muscle tone, strength, balance, and selective motor control. These abnormalities in muscle tone restrict the range of motion of affected joints and, when coupled with musculoskeletal growth, result in muscle contractures and associated bony deformities.[8] The introduction of the GMFCS, FMS, and ICF has impacted orthopedic surgery. Surgeries designed to improve ambulation are preferred in patients at GMFCS levels I to III, whereas surgeries aimed toward improving care and comfort are performed in those with GMFCS levels IV to V. Orthopedic surgical procedures should be considered in the presence of contractures that hinder function or interfere with hygiene, subluxation/dislocation of joints (most commonly the hips), and rotational problems or lever arm dysfunction, causing gait problems. There are basically four major types of orthopedic surgeries in CP: muscle releases and lengthenings, tendon transfers, osteotomies, and arthrodesis.[13]

The timing of surgical intervention is determined by CNS maturation, ambulation potential, and the rate at which the deformity is developing. Graham has suggested delaying any orthopedic surgical intervention until ages 7 to 9 years because of a high risk of recurrence, unless there is evidence of hip subluxation. Before this age the focus should be therapies along with tone management.[21]

Remember that orthopedic surgery in and of itself has no effect on motor control, strength, or muscle tone. The brief reduction in hypertonia is the direct result of the temporary decrease in muscle tension that involves the Golgi tendon apparatus and the muscle spindle. It is therefore of great importance to use a comprehensive team that addresses tone management presurgery and postsurgery.[13]

Hips

It has been estimated that one in three children with CP will have hip displacement. The highest risk is in the nonambulatory population. The pathophysiology relates to the muscle imbalance between the strong hip adductors/flexors and the weak hip abductors/extensors. This imbalance causes the head of the femur to gradually migrate out of the socket compromising the hip joint integrity. The two muscle groups responsible are the iliopsoas and the adductors.[61]

Soft tissue surgeries used to counteract hip subluxation often include some combination of hip adductor tenotomy, psoas recession, iliopsoas tenotomy, or medial hamstring lengthening and are performed after the hip has demonstrated subluxation. Another factor involved in the pathophysiology is the lack of weight bearing through the hip joint in nonambulatory children, because axial weight-bearing serves to deepen the acetabulum and induces a progressive varus angle of the femoral neck with respect to the shaft. The osseous deformities of the hip that result include femoral anteversion caused by spastic overpull of the medial hamstring, as well as acetabular dysplasia and coxa valga resulting from a lack of axial weight-bearing. Treatment of these conditions includes periacetabular osteotomies to improve coverage of the femoral head, as well as proximal varus and external rotation osteotomies of the femur to address the angular and rotational deformities, respectively.[47]

A recent systematic review by Gordon et al. looked at the evidence for hip surveillance in children with CP and made note of the paucity of surveillance guidelines despite the prevalence of hip pathology.[22] The review looked into possible predictors of hip pathology such as the report by Scrutton indicating that children with CP who walked 10 steps alone by 30 months of age did not require treatment of their hips by 5 years of age. The severity of motor disability at 18 months of age was not predictive of hip displacement, but by 24 to 30 months of age, it was.[60] Gordon et al. concluded that all children with bilateral CP should have a radiograph of the hip at age 30 months or earlier based on clinical findings. Other models such as the one proposed in Australia recommend annual or semiannual surveillance films according to GMFCS level and progression of migration percentage.[15] Gordon et al. also concluded that monitoring the acetabular index and migration percentage are the most effective parameters. Children with a migration percentage greater than 33% or an acetabular index over 30 degrees are likely to need further treatment. A progression of the migration percentage by more than 7% per annum requires careful monitoring (Figure 47-8).[22]

As with any surgical intervention, goals have to be clearly established. For the ambulatory child with CP, the goal of preserved ambulation requires a contained and stable hip. In the nonambulatory child with CP, the goals include prevention of dislocation, maintenance of sitting balance, facilitation of hygiene, prevention of pain, prevention of skin breakdown, and prevention of progressive scoliosis.[22]

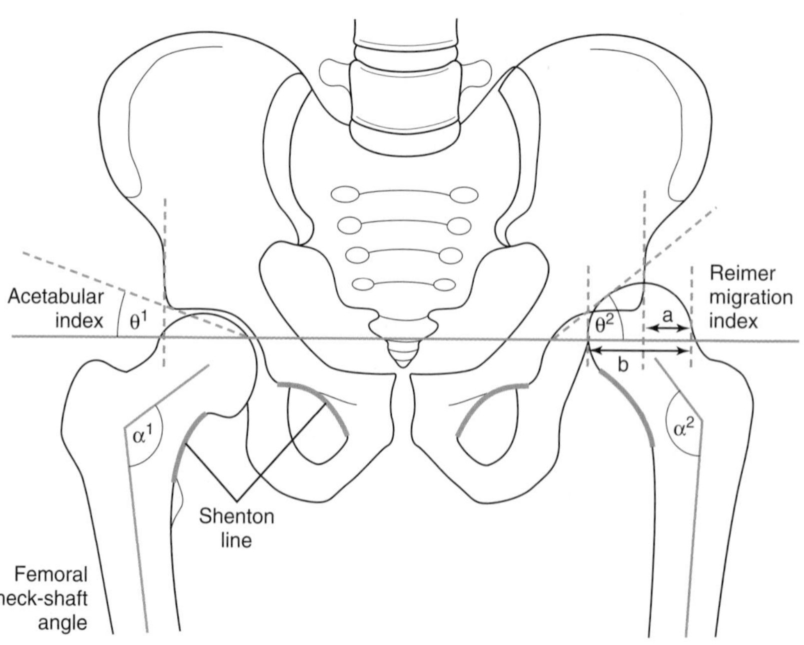

FIGURE 47-8 Radiographic parameters for the evaluation of hips in the setting of spasticity. (Redrawn from Herring JA, editor: *Tachdjian's Pediatric Orthopaedics*, 3rd ed, vol 2. Philadelphia, Saunders, 2001, p 1189.)

The natural history of the severely subluxated hip has also been studied, with variable conclusions. The relationship between hip pain and subluxation or dislocation of one or both hips is highly variable. Although it is clear that a subset of children with neuromuscular dysplasia has hip pain, the relationship between radiographic and clinical findings remains elusive. For those with established pain attributed to hip dislocation, deformity of the femoral head, and breakdown of articular cartilage, temporary relief with intraarticular steroid injections has been reported. Salvage procedures to include proximal femoral resection, osteotomies to redirect the femoral head, and hip arthroplasty have all been described.[47]

Lower Limb

In CP, primary impairments include hypertonia, poor balance, poor selective motor control, and weakness. Delays in gross motor skill acquisition and atypical gait patterns lead to further deformity. In CP, biarticular muscles are more commonly contracted (e.g., psoas, rectus femoris, hamstrings, and gastrocnemii) than the monoarticular muscles.[43]

A diplegic sagittal gait pattern classification has been developed (Figure 47-9), which helps to define gait pathology, potential causes, and treatment strategies.[48]

Scissoring gait or excessive hip adduction and stiff knee gait or overactive rectus femoris are additional gait abnormalities that may coexist in this classification. Three-dimensional gait-and-motion analysis aids in surgical planning and provides valuable kinematic, kinetic, and EMG information to further describe these gait abnormalities.

Hypertonia results in muscle contractures. Before any orthopedic surgical intervention, tone management is recommended especially at a young age. In patients who are good candidates for ITB therapy or rhizotomy, the preference has been for those treatments to be pursued first since the need for orthopedic surgery is often minimized.[43]

Orthopedic surgeries for contractures include lengthenings and transfers. Typically these procedures are more effective if integrated into a single-event multilevel surgery (SEMLS). The ultimate goal is to achieve satisfactory joint position during gait without restriction.[43] In the nonambulatory cohort, goals include facilitating sitting (hamstrings) and perineal care (adductors) as well as first line of surgery to help contain hips (psoas and adductors) without including bony surgery.

Abnormal long-bone torsions (lever arm dysfunction or LAD) such as persistent femoral anteversion are also a result of abnormal muscle forces and delays in walking. Another less common example that is acquired later

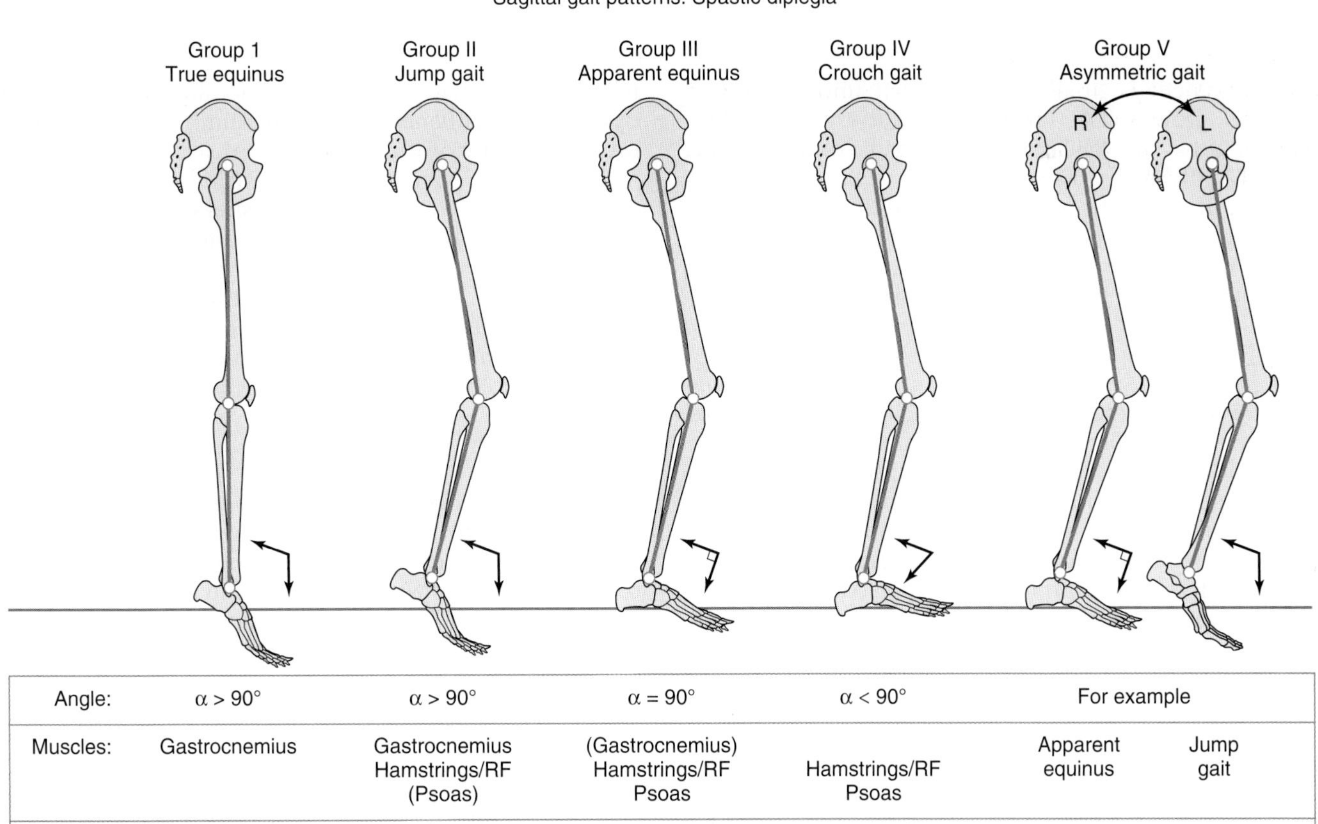

Angle:	α > 90°	α > 90°	α = 90°	α < 90°	For example	
Muscles:	Gastrocnemius	Gastrocnemius Hamstrings/RF (Psoas)	(Gastrocnemius) Hamstrings/RF Psoas	Hamstrings/RF Psoas	Apparent equinus	Jump gait
Orthotic:	Hinged AFO	Hinged AFO	Solid AFO	GRAFO		

FIGURE 47-9 Sagittal gait patterns: spastic diplegia. (Redrawn from Rodda JM, Graham HK, Carson L, et al: Sagittal gait patterns in spastic diplegia, *J Bone Joint Surg Br* 86:251-258, 2004. Reproduced with permission and copyright © of the British Editorial Society of Bone and Joint Surgery.)

Table 47-10 Gait Deviations[20,43,48,8]

Gait Deviation	Description	Causes	Surgical Treatment	Comments
Scissoring Gait	Excessive lower extremity adduction	Femoral anteversion Medial hamstring spasticity Hip adductor spasticity	Adductor tenotomy or myotomy ± hamstring lengthenings	May coexist with crouch and jump gait
Jump Gait	Excessive hip and knee flexion and ankle equino	Multifactorial: Hamstring, psoas, rectus femoris, and gastrocnemius contractures Weakness Bony rotational deformities (lever arm dysfunction [LAD])	Usually involves extension osteotomies of the femur along with patellar tendon advancements.	Most common diplegic gait pattern in young children Jump gait may be a precursor to crouch gait.
Equinus	Gastrocnemius contracture	Spasticity of the gastrocnemius muscles	Gastrocnemius recession. In hemiplegics: Baker lengthening or tendo Achilles lengthening	A plantar flexion–knee extension couple can contribute to compensatory knee hyperextension ("recurvatum"). Rarely the soleus needs to be addressed except in hemiplegics Over lengthening (especially the soleus) may weaken the muscle and contribute to other gait abnormalities such as crouch.
Crouch Gait	Variable pelvis position, excessive hip and knee flexion and ankle dorsiflexion	Multifactorial: Hamstring, psoas, rectus femoris and gastrocnemius contractures and weakness Bony rotational deformities (LAD including foot deformity).	Usually involves extension osteotomies of the femur along with patellar tendon advancements ± psoas lengthenings depending on pelvis position	Most common diplegic gait pattern in older children Progressive and may lead to decline in functional independence. May be iatrogenic—overlengthening of muscles
Stiff knee Gait	Decreased knee flexion range of motion throughout the gait cycle	Overactive rectus femoris during swing phase	Rectus femoris transfer	Commonly observed in hemiplegics

in development is tibial torsion. If left untreated, with time and growth, LAD will produce further malalignment of bone as well as unwanted gait compensations (Table 47-10).[20]

A host of soft tissue and bony procedures are described to address the musculoskeletal deformities of the foot and ankle in CP with the goal of obtaining a plantigrade, braceable foot and stable base of support for standing and gait.[47]

Upper Limb

Spasticity management and orthopedic intervention for the upper limb in CP follow a similar treatment algorithm to that of the lower limb.[47] Conservative treatment with therapy, splinting (functional and passive orthoses), casting, oral medications, and chemoneurolyis are used to preserve range of motion and delay muscle contractures. Upper limb surgical procedures are recommended to improve function, ease of care in patients with severe contractures, and sometimes cosmesis. Common functional impairments include deficiencies in sensation, pinch, grasp/release, and reach. The pattern of joint contractures usually involves flexor synergy: shoulder internal rotation, elbow flexion, forearm pronation, wrist and finger flexion, thumb-in-palm deformity, and swan neck deformities.

The ideal candidate for surgical intervention would be a motivated child with volitional use of the hand, spasticity without fixed contractures, and reasonable sensory function including stereognosis, proprioception, and light touch. Patients with significant athetoid movements and dystonia do not benefit from upper limb surgery given the unpredictability of the outcomes.[69]

Preoperative evaluation should include a detailed physical examination (range of motion, strength, and tone), use of a functional classification system, and standardized tests that evaluate proprioception, stereognosis, and two-point discrimination. Motion analysis and computer modeling of the upper limb are also being increasingly used to aid in surgical planning, much like 3-dimensional gait analysis for the lower limbs (Table 47-11).[47]

Spine

The reported incidence of scoliosis in CP has been estimated as 21% to 76%. The scoliotic severity directly correlates with the degree of total body involvement and inversely correlates with functional and ambulatory status, as well as GMFCS level. Scoliotic curves have been characterized and divided into two groups:

Group 1: Curves are single thoracic or double thoracic and lumbar curves with level pelvis. This type of curve is typically associated with ambulatory patients (GMFCS II to III).[25]

Group 2: Curves are long thoracolumbar or C-shaped curves with associated pelvic obliquity, typically associated with nonambulatory patients.[25]

The natural history of curve progression has shown that onset occurs from 3 to 10 years of age with rapid

Table 47-11 Operative Interventions of the Upper extremity in Cerebral Palsy

Joint	Aim	Options
Shoulder	Joint stabilization Improve external rotation Improve internal rotation	Fusion, capsular reconstructions Lengthen pectoralis major/ subscapularis; transfer LD and/ or teres major; humeral osteotomy Lengthen/release infraspinatus/teres minor
Elbow	Joint stabilization Improve extension	Fusion Lengthen biceps brachii/brachialis; BR release; flexor/pronator mass release (slide); capsulotomy
Forearm	Improve supination	Reroute, lengthen, or release PT; radius/ulna osteotomy; flexor-pronator release (slide)
Wrist	Stabilization Improve extension	Fusion Flexor tendon release; proximal row carpectomy; ECU transfer; FCU transfer to ECRB/ECRL/EDC
Thumb	Stabilization Improve extension Improve abduction	Volar plate arthroplasty; MCP fusion Release/lengthen FPL; reinforce EPL Release adductor pollicis; reinforce APL; EPL rerouting
Fingers	Flexion deformity Swan-neck deformity	FDS to EDC transfer flexor/ pronator release (slide); FDS/FDP lengthening; FDS to FDP transfer PIP joint tenodesis; central slip tenotomy; intrinsic origin release

From Koman LA, Sarlikiotis T, Smith BP: Surgery of the upper extremity in cerebral palsy, *Orthop Clin North Am* 41:519-529, 2010.

APL, Abductor pollicis longus; *BR*, brachioradialis; *ECRB*, extensor carpi radialis brevis; *ECRL*, extensor carpi radialis longus; *ECU*, extensor carpi ulnaris; *EDC*, extensor digitorum communis; *EPB*, extensor pollicis brevis; *EPL*, extensor pollicis longus; *FCU*, flexor carpi ulnaris; *FDP*, flexor digitorum profundus; *FDS*, flexor digitorum superficialis; *FPL*, flexor pollicis longus; *LD*, latissimus dorsi; *MCP*, metacarpophalangeal; *PIP*, proximal interphalangeal; *PT*, pronator teres.

progression during the adolescent growth spurt. Bracing traditionally has a very limited role in decreasing curve progression.[25]

A physical examination should be performed every 6 to 12 months and a radiograph obtained if a curve is detected. Standardizing the child's position when follow-up radiographs are obtained will help minimize errors in measurement of progression. Observation is warranted for flexible curves less than 40 degrees that do not compromise sitting balance. In most cases of scoliosis in CP, spinal instrumentation and fusion are considered because of significant curve progression, loss of sitting balance, and comfortable function.[25] Ideally this can be delayed in children with flexible deformities until they approach skeletal maturity. It is important to note that surgical complications are high; therefore, goal setting, patient selection, and preoperative preparation are of utmost importance.

Complementary and Alternative Medicine

Complementary and Alternative Medicine (CAM) is becoming more common in the clinical setting as children with CP continue to live longer. In fact, over 50% of families with a child affect by CP have explored CAM alternatives (Table 47-12).[33]

Transition to Adulthood and Aging with Cerebral Palsy

Preparing for transition begins early in the care of the individual with CP. A child must be encouraged to become as independent as possible and to separate if appropriate from caregivers in a developmentally appropriate fashion during the teenage years. Throughout the course of care for the child, the medical team is responsible for providing anticipatory guidance and education. Guidelines for the care of children and adolescents with CP exist and can help primary care physicians with ensuring comprehensive assessments of medical and psychosocial issues encountered in the CP population, with direction on management of associated conditions, with educational and community support needs, and with suggested referrals to specialists for specific issues.[42] Therapy services for older individuals with CP are indicated for specific goals that will enhance functional independence or exercise capacity. For some individuals, independent living with employment is very realistic. Others may thrive in a supported environment with some daily assistance but not require constant supervision or care. Children with significant cognitive and physical delays may require long-term support but may enjoy opportunities for socialization with peers other than their primary caregivers. Children with disabilities may need encouragement and training on self-advocacy. Coping skills and self-reliance are usually acquired through experiences leading up to the point of transition and cannot be simply taught once an individual reaches adulthood.

Transition of healthcare occurs in phases and requires preparation, readiness, and handoffs. Care delivery models often differ in the pediatric and adult realms and moving to a new group of providers can be anxiety-provoking for many. Teens benefit from having advocates or champions to help with the transition process. Mindful practitioners collaborate with interested parties including schools and community agencies to provide comprehensive guidance.[63] Patient counseling needs to include reminders about preventative health measures and screens. Health conditions affecting the general population certainly will occur in adults with CP also. There are also specific conditions that occur more frequently or earlier in the adult CP population as the result of aging and chronic alterations in biomechanics such as cervical myelopathy and early development of degenerative joint disease.

Particular challenges exist for the CP population as a whole associated with aging. Musculoskeletal conditions may worsen and energy consumption may increase for tasks previously accomplished easily. Adults with CP may experience chronic pain and associated fatigue and depression.[39a] It is important to avoid a downward spiral where an exacerbation of a health issue or painful condition then limits activity further and functional decline ensues. With a shift in focus in measuring participation and quality-of-life indicators, the roles of physical fitness and strengthening in adults with CP are being investigated in greater detail.[66]

Table 47-12 Summary of Complementary and Alternative Treatments for Cerebral Palsy

Therapy	Theory/Benefits	Adverse Effects	Evidence	Comments
Hyperbaric oxygen	Awaken dormant brain tissue surrounding the original injury.	Ear trauma, pneumothorax, fire, explosion	Uncontrolled studies show improvements in treated children. Controlled study showed improvement in treated and control subjects.	More evidence is required before recommendations can be made, e.g., what is the role of increased pressure without supplemental oxygen?
Adeli suit	Resistance across muscles can improve strength, posture, and coordination.	Discomfort from suit, expense for therapy, and for travel to centers that prescribe the suit	No conclusive evidence either in support of or against the use of the Adeli suit	
Patterning	Passively repeating steps in normal development can overcome brain injuries.	Time, energy, and expense required for treatment	Results of uncontrolled studies are inconsistent; controlled trials show no benefits.	Cannot be recommended.
Electrical stimulation				More evidence is required before recommendations can be made.
Threshold electrical stimulation	Increased blood flow from electrical current will lead to stronger muscles.	Expense for unit, generally safe	Some uncontrolled trials show subjective improvements; controlled trials are inconclusive.	
Functional neuromuscular stimulation	Increased muscle contraction will improve strength and function.	Expensive, infection from needles, discomfort	Evidence is somewhat more positive than for threshold stimulation but still inconclusive.	
Conductive education	Problems with motor skills are problems of learning; new abilities are created out of learning.	None known	Uncontrolled trials show benefit; controlled trials are mixed.	Conductive education is implemented in many different ways, making generalizations from a single program difficult.
Hippotherapy	Riding a horse can improve muscle tone, head and trunk control, mobility in the pelvis, and equilibrium.	Trauma from a fall, allergies	Uncontrolled and controlled trials show beneficial effects on body structures and functioning.	Horseback riding also increases social participation.
Craniosacral therapy	Therapy is used to remove impediments to the flow of cerebrospinal fluid within the cranium and spinal cord.	None known	No studies showing efficacy in CP; some question the basis of the intervention.	
Feldenkrais	Change of position and directed attention can relax muscles, improve movement, posture, and functioning.	None known	No studies showing efficacy in CP; studies in other conditions are equivocal.	
Acupuncture	Acupuncture can help to restore the normal flow of Qi, or energy.	Forgotten needles, pain, bruising, and infection	Uncontrolled studies show improvements in several areas; two controlled trials also showed improvements.	Appears promising, but more studies are required before specific recommendations can be made.

From Liptak GS: Complementary and alternative therapies for cerebral palsy, *Ment Retard Dev Disabil Res Rev* 11:156-163, 2005.

KEY REFERENCES

1. Aisen ML, Kerkovich D, Mast J, et al: Cerebral palsy: clinical care and neurological rehabilitation, *Lancet Neurol* 10:844–852, 2011.
2. Albright A: Intrathecal baclofen for childhood hypertonia, *Childs Nerv Syst* 23:971–979, 2007.
4. Anttila H, Autti-Rämö I, Suoranta J, et al: Effectiveness of physical therapy interventions for children with cerebral palsy: a systematic review, *BMC Pediatr* 8:14, 2008.
5. Ashwal S, Russman BS, Blasco PA, et al: Practice parameter: diagnostic assessment of the child with cerebral palsy: report of the Quality Standards Subcommittee of the American Academy of Neurology and the Practice Committee of the Child Neurology Society, *Neurology* 62:851–863, 2004.
8. Berker AN, Yalçin S: Cerebral palsy: orthopedic aspects and rehabilitation, *Pediatr Clin North Am* 55:1209–1225, 2008.
9. Blackmore AM, Boettcher Hunt E, Jordan M, et al: A systematic review of the effects of casting on equinus in children with cerebral palsy: an evidence report of the AACPDM, *Dev Med Child Neurol* 49:781–790, 2007.
10. Centers for Disease Control and Prevention (CDC): Postnatal causes of developmental disabilities in children aged 3-10 years—Atlanta, Georgia, 1991, *MMWR Morb Mortal Wkly Rep* 45:130–134, 1996.
11. Chen YP, Pope S, Tyler D, et al: Effectiveness of constraint-induced movement therapy on upper-extremity function in children with cerebral palsy: a systematic review and meta-analysis of randomized controlled trials, *Clin Rehabil* 28:939–953, 2014.
12. Christine C, Dolk H, Platt MJ, et al: Recommendations from the SCPE collaborative group for defining and classifying cerebral palsy, *Dev Med Child Neurol* 109(Suppl):35–38, 2007.
13. Damiano DL, Alter KE, Chambers H: New clinical and research trends in lower extremity management for ambulatory children with cerebral palsy, *Phys Med Rehabil Clin North Am* 20:469–491, 2009.
14. Delgado MR, Hirtz D, Aisen M, et al: Practice parameter: pharmacologic treatment of spasticity in children and adolescents with cerebral palsy (an evidence-based review) Report of the Quality Standards

Subcommittee of the American Academy of Neurology and the Practice Committee of the Child Neurology Society, *Neurology* 74:336-343, 2010.
18. Eliasson AC, Krumlinde-Sundholm L, Rösblad B, et al: The Manual Ability Classification System (MACS) for children with cerebral palsy: scale development and evidence of validity and reliability, *Dev Med Child Neurol* 48:549–554, 2006. PMID:16780622.
19. Fehlings D, Switzer L, Agarwal P, et al: Informing evidence-based clinical practice guidelines for children with cerebral palsy at risk of osteoporosis: a systematic review, *Dev Med Child Neurol* 54:106–116, 2012.
19a. Fitzgerald DA, Follett J, Van Asperen PP: Assessing and managing lung disease and sleep disordered breathing in children with cerebral palsy, *Paediatr Respir Rev* 10(1):18–24, 2009.
20. Gage J: Orthopedic treatment of long bone torsions. *The identification and treatment of gait problems in cerebral palsy*, ed 2, London, 2009, Mac Keith Press.
22. Gordon GS, Simkiss DE: A systematic review of the evidence for hip surveillance in children with cerebral palsy, *J Bone Joint Surg Br* 88:1492–1496, 2006.
23. Hidecker MJ, Ho NT, Dodge N, et al: Inter-relationships of functional status in cerebral palsy: analyzing gross motor function, manual ability, and communication function classification systems in children, *Dev Med Child Neurol* 54:737–742, 2012.
25. Jones-Quaidoo SM, Yang S, Arlet V: Surgical management of spinal deformities in cerebral palsy. A review, *J Neurosurg Spine* 13:672–685, 2010.
27. Kerr C, McDowell B: Electrical stimulation in cerebral palsy: a review of effects on strength and motor function, *Dev Med Child Neurol* 46:205–213, 2004.
28. Ketelaar M, Gorter JW, Westers P, et al: Developmental trajectories of mobility and self-care capabilities in young children with cerebral palsy, *J Pediatr* 164:769–774.e2, 2014.
29. Kolaski K, Ajizian SJ, Passmore L, et al: Safety profile of multilevel chemical denervation procedures using phenol or botulinum toxin or both in a pediatric population, *Am J Phys Med Rehabil* 87:556–566, 2008.
30. Krach L: Treatment of spasticity with intrathecal baclofen. *The identification and treatment of gait problems in cerebral palsy*, ed 2, London, 2009, Mac Keith Press.
31. Kuperminc MN, Stevenson RD: Growth and nutrition disorders in children with cerebral palsy, *Dev Disabil Res Rev* 14:137–146, 2008.
32. Lannin N, Scheinberg A, Clark K: AACPDM systematic review of the effectiveness of therapy for children with cerebral palsy after botulinum toxin A injections, *Dev Med Child Neurol* 48:533–539, 2006.
33. Liptak GS: Complementary and alternative therapies for cerebral palsy, *Ment Retard Dev Disabil Res Rev* 11:156–163, 2005.
34. McIntyre S, Taitz D, Keogh J, et al: A systematic review of risk factors for cerebral palsy in children born at term in developed countries, *Dev Med Child Neurol* 55:499–508, 2013.
37. Michaud LJ, American Academy of Pediatrics Committee on Children With Disabilities: Prescribing therapy services for children with motor disabilities, *Pediatrics* 113:1836–1838, 2004.
38. Molnar GE: Cerebral palsy: prognosis and how to judge it, *Pediatr Ann* 8:596–605, 1979.
39. Molnar GE, Gordon SU: Cerebral palsy: predictive value of selected clinical signs for early prognostication of motor function, *Arch Phys Med Rehabil* 57:153–158, 1976.
39a. Murphy KP: The adult with cerebral palsy, *Orthop Clin North Am* 41(4):595–605, 2010.
40. Mutlu A, Krosschell K, Spira DG: Treadmill training with partial body-weight support in children with cerebral palsy: a systematic review, *Dev Med Child Neurol* 51:268–275, 2009.
41. Nelson KB: Causative factors in cerebral palsy, *Clin Obstet Gynecol* 51:749–762, 2008.
43. Novachek T: Orthopedic treatment of muscle contractures. *The identification and treatment of gait problems in cerebral palsy*, ed 2, London, 2009, Mac Keith Press.
44. Novak I: Evidence-based diagnosis, health care, and rehabilitation for children with cerebral palsy, *J Child Neurol* 29:1141–1156, 2014.
47. Oleszek J, Davidson L: Cerebral palsy. In Braddom RL, editor: *Physical medicine and rehabilitation*, ed 4, Philadelphia, 2010, Elsevier, pp 1253–1273.
48. Õunpuu S, Thomason P, Harvey A, et al: Classification of cerebral palsy & patterns of gait pathology. *The identification and treatment of gait problems in cerebral palsy*, ed 2, London, 2009, Mac Keith Press.
49. Oskoui M, Coutinho F, Dykeman J, et al: An update on the prevalence of cerebral palsy: a systematic review and meta-analysis, *Dev Med Child Neurol* 55:509–519, 2013.
50. Palisano RJ, Rosenbaum P, Bartlett D, et al: Content validity of the expanded and revised Gross Motor Function Classification System, *Dev Med Child Neurol* 50:744–750, 2008.
51. Reid SM, Dagia CD, Ditchfield MR, et al: Population-based studies of brain imaging patterns in cerebral palsy, *Dev Med Child Neurol* 56:222–232, 2014.
53. Rosenbaum P, Paneth N, Leviton A, et al: A report: the definition and classification of cerebral palsy April 2006, *Dev Med Child Neurol Suppl* 109:8–14, 2007. Erratum in: *Dev Med Child Neurol* 49:480, 2007.
55. Sanger TD, Chen D, Delgado MR, et al: Definition and classification of negative motor signs in childhood, *Pediatrics* 118:2159–2167, 2006.
57. Sanger TD, Chen D, Fehlings DL, et al: Definition and classification of hyperkinetic movements in childhood, *Mov Disord* 25:1538–1549, 2010.
58. Sanger TD, Delgado MR, Gaebler-Spira D, et al: Classification and definition of disorders causing hypertonia in childhood, *Pediatrics* 111:e89–e97, 2003.
60. Scrutton D, Baird G, Smeeton N: Hip dysplasia in bilateral cerebral palsy: incidence and natural history in children aged 18 months to 5 years, *Dev Med Child Neurol* 43:586–600, 2001.
62. Steinbok P: Selective dorsal rhizotomy for spastic cerebral palsy: a review, *Childs Nerv Syst* 23:981–990, 2007.
63. Stewart D: Transition to adult services for young people with disabilities: current evidence to guide future research, *Dev Med Child Neurol* 51(Suppl 4):169–173, 2009.
64. Tan SS, van Meeteren J, Ketelaar M, et al: Long-term trajectories of health-related quality of life in individuals with cerebral palsy: a multicenter longitudinal study, *Arch Phys Med Rehabil* 95:2029–2039, 2014.
65. Tan SS, Wiegerink DJ, Vos RC, et al: Developmental trajectories of social participation in individuals with cerebral palsy: a multicentre longitudinal study, *Dev Med Child Neurol* 56:370–377, 2014.
66. Thorpe D: The role of fitness in health and disease: status of adults with cerebral palsy, *Dev Med Child Neurol* 51(Suppl 4):52–58, 2009.
67. Trost JP, Dunn ME, Krach LE, et al: Treatment of Spasticity with Selective Dorsal Rhizotomy. *The identification and treatment of gait problems in cerebral palsy*, ed 2, London, 2009, Mac Keith Press.
69a. World Health Organization: *ICF-CY, International Classification of Functioning, Disability, and Health: Children & Youth Version*, Geneva, 2007, World Health Organization.
69b. Zafeiriou DI: Primitive reflexes and postural reactions in the neurodevelopmental examination, *Pediatr Neurol* 31(1):1–8, 2004.

The full reference list for this chapter is available online.

CHAPTER 48

MYELOMENINGOCELE AND OTHER SPINAL DYSRAPHISMS

Rita Ayyangar, R. Drew Davis, Charles Law

Neural tube defects (NTDs) affect 0.5 to 2 per 1000 established pregnancies worldwide and are the second most common group of severely disabling birth defects, following congenital heart defects.[16] Myelomeningocele (MMC) is the most complex congenital anomaly compatible with life and is the second most common disabling condition in childhood after cerebral palsy.[19] It makes up more than 98% of the "open" spinal dysraphic states and exists in a spectrum of NTDs, ranging from conditions that are incompatible with life such as anencephaly and cranioschisis (complete failure of neurulation) to disorders of secondary neurulation causing spina bifida occulta with minimal or no neurologic involvement.[38] MMC, along with meningocele, makes up the bulk of what is commonly known as spina bifida. Although the most severe NTDs result in stillbirth or death shortly after birth, the majority of patients with a spinal dysraphism survive. The varying degrees of organ involvement seen with these conditions have major implications for long-term health and physical function, as well as the psychological and social well-being of the affected individual. Survival and quality of life for those with MMC have improved because of advances in medical, surgical, and rehabilitative care during the past 60 years, with prenatal folic acid food fortification and fetal surgical repair having the greatest impact. Many challenges remain, however, regarding understanding etiology, advancing prevention, maximizing health-related outcomes, transitioning to adult-based health care systems, and improving activity and participation at the societal level. These challenges are best met by a team of specialists working with patients, their families, and the community.

Historical Background, Terminology, and Nomenclature

The first clear description of spinal dysraphism was given by Caspar Bauhin, a Swiss physician, anatomist, and botanist, in his publication *Theatrum Anatomicum* in 1592. The term *spina bifida,* however, is often historically associated with Nicolaes Tulp, a Dutch physician who published a sketch (Figure 48-1) and description of several patients with the condition in 1641. In 1875, Rudolf Virchow described spina bifida occulta, which refers to a hidden bony defect as well as other potential hidden anomalies.[152]

A need for clarification of terminology exists because midline fusion defects of the spine have been described using several nomenclatures. The term *spina bifida* is sometimes used nonspecifically with regard to all patients with a spinal dysraphism or those with incomplete closure of the posterior neuropore. *Spina bifida* literally translates as "spine split in two" and is technically correct in describing any patient with incomplete closure of the posterior elements of the spinal column. The degree of variation of anatomic malformations associated with the condition, however, requires the use of more specific terminology. *Spina bifida aperta* refers to a midline defect that communicates with the external environment and includes MMC and meningocele. The term *spina bifida cystica* is also sometimes used and refers not only to a sac filled with cerebrospinal fluid protruding from the spinal column but also to MMC and meningocele. MMC at the level of the spine refers to protrusion of the meninges through a defect in the posterior elements of the spine, with involvement of the spinal cord or nerve roots. Meningocele refers only to protrusion of the meninges and cerebrospinal fluid through a defect in the posterior elements of the spine into the tissue beneath the skin, without involvement of functional neural elements. These distinctions are important and will be further explained later.

Bony spina bifida occulta with just incomplete closure of the posterior elements of the spine without neurologic involvement is incidentally noted in 17% of the general population and 30% of normal children aged 1 to 10 years.[63] It is often not included in the group constituting spina bifida because there is no associated neurologic deficit. More complex occult closed spinal dysraphism, including diastematomyelia, lipomyelomeningocele, and tight filum terminale, among others, are a result of disordered secondary neurulation and can present with neurologic compromise or orthopedic deformity. There may be associated cutaneous anomalies such as a hairy patch without any other external anatomic abnormality. Modern imaging studies reveal these underlying defects and provide a system of classification based on neuroradiologic and clinical findings.[83,169]

This system of classification divides the various forms of spinal dysraphism into open spinal dysraphisms (i.e., open spina bifida) and closed spinal dysraphisms (i.e., closed spina bifida) (Box 48-1). It is useful for prognostication because those with open defects generally have lesions with visible neural elements, often leaking cerebrospinal fluid, which are associated with malformations that involve the entire central nervous system, including Chiari II malformations, midline defects, and hydrocephalus. In contrast, closed spinal dysraphisms (meningocele and occult spinal dysraphism) are lesions that are fully epithelialized with no neural tissue exposed, and generally have the

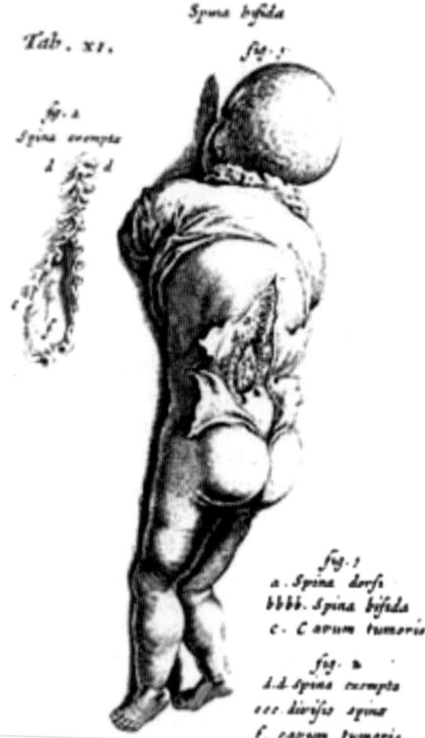

FIGURE 48-1 From *Observationes Medicae* by Nicholas Tulp, first published in 1641. Some speculate that the sketch was done by Rembrandt, a friend of Tulp who made him the subject of the well-known painting *The Lesson in Anatomy of Dr. Tulp*.

malformation limited to the spine and spinal cord, with only rare involvement of the brain. Box 48-1 displays a complete listing of spinal dysraphic states.[83,169] Although most of the conditions listed in Box 48-1 can result in a patient having rehabilitation needs, the most severely affected and vast majority of affected individuals will have a history of MMC. For this reason, the remainder of this chapter refers to rehabilitation concepts as they apply to MMC, although they can be applied to the various other spinal dysraphisms as appropriate.

Terms and definitions of terms used when discussing spina bifida include the following:

- Craniorachischisis: Near-complete absence of neural tube closure, sometimes sparing forebrain.
- Anencephaly: Degenerate brain and absent skull vault and scalp.
- Myelomeningocele: "Open spina bifida"; failure of closure of lumbosacral neural tube.
- Spina bifida cystica: Meningeal sac containing open spinal cord herniating through a vertebral defect.
- Myelocele: Open spinal cord exposed to open lesion.
- Encephalocele: Herniation of the brain through opening of skull (defect of skeletal development). This condition may be compatible with life and some may even have normal intelligence.
- Meningocele: Herniation of meninges through opening on vertebral column (defect of skeletal development).
- Dysraphic defect: Mild end of NTD spectrum, with closed abnormalities. Associated with tethered cord.
- Diplomyelia: Spinal cord longitudinally duplicated.
- Diastematomyelia: Spinal cord longitudinally split.
- Lipomeningocele: Spinal cord associated with fatty tissue deposit.
- Spina bifida occulta: Neural arches of one or several vertebrae are incomplete in the lumbosacral region.

BOX 48-1

Cliniconeuroradiologic Classification of Spinal Dysraphism

Open Spinal Dysraphism
- Myelomeningocele
- Myelocele
- Hemimyelomeningocele
- Hemimyelocele

Closed Spinal Dysraphism

With a subcutaneous mass
- Lumbosacral
  - Lipoma with dural defect
  - Lipomyelomeningocele
  - Lipomyeloschisis
- Terminal myelocystocele
- Meningocele

Cervical
- Cervical myelocystocele
- Cervical myelomeningocele
- Meningocele

Without a subcutaneous mass

Simple dysraphic states
- Posterior spinal bifida
- Intradural and intramedullary lipoma
- Filum terminale lipoma
- Tight filum terminale
- Abnormally long spinal cord
- Persistent terminal ventricle

Complex dysraphic states
- Dorsal enteric fistula
- Neurenteric cysts
- Split cord malformations (diastematomyelia and diplomyelia)
- Dermal sinus
- Caudal regression syndrome
- Segmental spinal dysgenesis

Epidemiology

Incidence and Prevalence

Epidemiologic studies of spinal dysraphisms typically include both MMC and meningocele, which are collectively referred to as spina bifida.[18] Incidence worldwide is approximately 1 to 10 per 1000 depending on the region and in the United States is less than 0.7 per 1000.[8,129] According to the U.S. Centers for Disease Control and Prevention (CDC), each year there are approximately 1500 babies born with spina bifida in the United States.[29,30] In the United States, incidence rates have varied from as high as 2.31 per 1000 births in Boston during the 1930s to as low as 0.51 per 1000 births in Atlanta in the early 1990s.[122,139,149] Worldwide, some of the highest prevalence rates have been reported in the Shanxi province of China,

Ireland, Wales, and Hungary,[35,43,98] although these rates have generally decreased in a manner similar to that in the United States.

The reasons for the decreasing prevalence of MMC are multifactorial and not completely understood. A proportion of the decrease can be attributed to the advent of prenatal screening and elective termination of pregnancy.[40,113] The most influential factor has been the increased consumption of folic acid among women of childbearing age. The role of undernutrition and vitamin deficiency, especially folate deficiency, was first expressed by Smithells et al.[153] in 1976, and the first studies demonstrating that folate supplementation decreased the rates of NTDs were performed in Wales in the early 1980s.[94] Multiple observational and controlled trials followed, leading up to the landmark Medical Research Council study, which involved seven countries and 3012 women. The study was ended early after supplementation with folic acid (4 mg/day) was shown to prevent 72% of NTDs in women with a previously affected pregnancy.[115] A subsequent Hungarian randomized control trial proved the efficacy of a more physiologic dose of 800 mcg of folic acid in preventing the first occurrence of an NTD[44] and a Chinese-U.S. study further demonstrated that even a 400-mcg dose of folate supplementation brought about a 79% reduction in areas with high rates of NTDs in northern China.[15] In 1992, the U.S. Public Health Service recommended that all women capable of becoming pregnant consume 400 μg of folic acid daily to prevent NTDs,[29,30] but drastic improvements in the prevalence rate were only noted after the U.S. Food and Drug Administration mandate in January 1998 requiring the fortification with 140 μg of folate per 100 g of all cereal grain products.[65]

In August 2014, a total of 19 population-based birth defects surveillance programs in the United States reported to the CDC the number of cases of spina bifida (*International Classification of Diseases, 9th Revision, Clinical Modification,* codes 741.0 and 741.9) and anencephaly (codes 740.0 and 740.1) among deliveries occurring during 1995 to 2011 in non-Hispanic whites, non-Hispanic blacks, and Hispanics, as well as all racial/ethnic groups combined. Although improved in all groups, birth prevalence rates still remain highest among Hispanics, then whites, and were lowest in non-Hispanic blacks similar to the prefortification era. This report demonstrates a persisting effect from fortification and an overall decline of 28% in all participating programs from 1999 to 2011 (Figure 48-2). A greater reduction (35%) was observed among programs with prenatal ascertainment than for programs without prenatal ascertainment (21%). They estimate that approximately 1300 NTD-affected births have been averted annually during the postfortification period with an annual saving in total direct costs of approximately $508 million for the NTD-affected births that were prevented.[187]

The reduction in NTD cases during the postfortification period inversely mirrors the increase in serum and red blood cell (RBC) folate concentrations among women of childbearing age in the general population. Fortification has led to a decrease in the prevalence of serum folate deficiency from 30% to less than 1% and a decrease in the prevalence of RBC folate deficiency from 6% to no measureable deficiency.[131] To substantially attenuate the

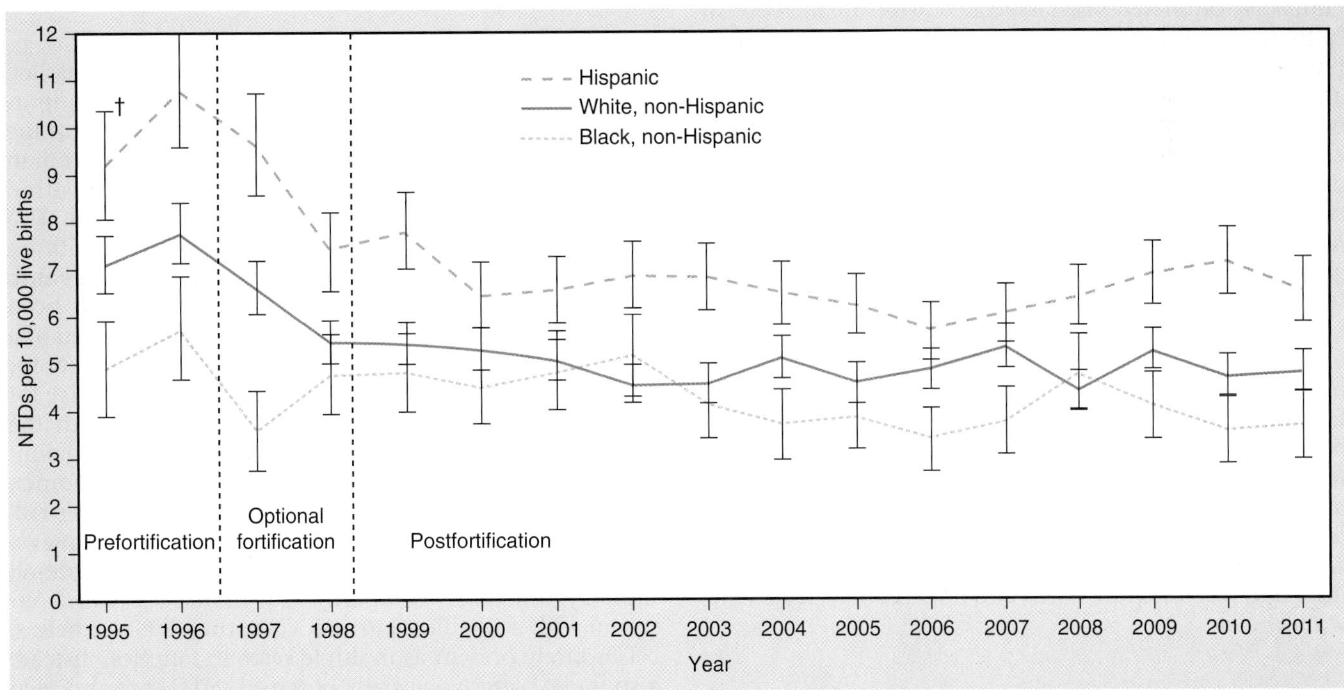

FIGURE 48-2 Prevalence of neural tube defects (NTDs) (anencephaly and spina bifida) before and after mandatory folic acid fortification, by maternal race/ethnicity: 19 population-based birth defects surveillance programs, United States, 1995 to 2011. A decline in NTDs was observed for all three of the racial/ethnic groups examined between the prefortification and postfortification periods. Contributing programs are based in Arkansas, Arizona, California, Colorado, Georgia, Illinois, Iowa, Kentucky, Maryland, New Jersey, New York, North Carolina, Oklahoma, Puerto Rico, South Carolina, Texas, Utah, West Virginia, and Wisconsin. †95% confidence interval. (From Williams J, Mai CT, Mulinare J, et al: Updated estimates of neural tube defects prevented by mandatory folic acid fortification—United States, 1995-2011, *MMWR Morb Mortal Wkly Rep* 64:1-5, 2015.)

risk for NTD, women of childbearing age must have RBC folate concentration greater than 1000 nmol/L at least at a population level.[41] Data from the National Health and Nutrition Examination Survey (NHANES) for 1988 to 2010 show that almost a quarter (21.6%) of women of childbearing age in the United States still do not have RBC folate concentrations associated with a lower risk for NTDs,[131] illustrating the need to further educate all women of childbearing age on the importance of daily folic acid intake of 400 mcg for those who could become pregnant and 4 mg for those with a previously affected pregnancy or a history of MMC themselves. Additional measures such as health care provider participation in the education effort as well as fortification of corn masa flour may help further reduce rates by especially targeting the Hispanic population. Williams et al.[187] speculate that this may lead to at least another 40 cases of NTD being prevented annually.

Risk Factors/Etiology

Despite a significant drop in the birth prevalence of spina bifida following fortification, rates are still high enough to suggest there are other factors at play.[114a] Additional nutritional deficiencies have been implicated such as vitamins B_6 and B_{12}, as well as other factors such as geographic variation, low socioeconomic status,[60,72] maternal age,[47] maternal hyperthermia,[117] maternal obesity,[160] maternal diabetes mellitus,[40] hyperzincemia,[114] paternal and maternal occupations and exposure to agrochemicals,[148] and certain drug exposures to, including, carbamazepine,[137] valproic acid,[127] diuretics, antihistamines, and sulfonamides.[121] Acetaminophen, used commonly for pain or fever control in pregnancy, is fortunately not associated with an increase in birth defects and in fact use in the first trimester for febrile illnesses is associated with a lower incidence of anencephaly and craniorachischisis, possibly resulting from control of maternal hyperthermic states.[60a] A further interesting environmental teratogen with proven effect in humans is the fungal product fumonisin that was responsible for a two-fold increase in NTD prevalence along the Texas-Mexico border in the early 1990s[116] (Table 48-1). Hyperglycemia is noted to cause cell death in the neuroepithelium. It has been noted that hyperinsulinemia is a strong risk factor for neural tube defects and it may be the driving force for the observed risk in maternal obesity and maternal diabetes.[39] Race and acculturation also seem to be factors with observed differences in the magnitudes and patterns of selected demographic and maternal risk factors for Hispanics and whites, particularly for parity, gestational diabetes, and socioeconomic status among cases of spina bifida. Canfield et al.[27] demonstrated that Hispanic parents who were least acculturated to the United States were at increased risk for spina bifida and anencephaly, relative to whites.

Table 48-1 Established and Suspected Risk Factors for Neural Tube Defects

Risk Factors	Relative Risk
Established Factors	
History of previous affected pregnancy with same partner	30
Inadequate maternal intake of folic acid	2 to 8
Pregestational maternal diabetes	2 to 10
Valproic acid and carbamazepine	10 to 20
Suspected Factors	
Maternal vitamin B_{12} status	3
Maternal obesity	1.5 to 3.5
Maternal hyperthermia	2
Maternal diarrhea	3 to 4
Maternal age	>35 years: OR = 5.21, 95% CI = 2.42 to 11 <25 years: OR = 3.36, 95% CI = 1.89 to 5.36
Paternal and maternal occupation and exposure to agrochemicals and pesticides	Appears increased but not exactly established
Gestational diabetes	Appears increased but not exactly established
Fumonisin (fungal protein)	Appears increased but not exactly established
Acetaminophen	Seems to have a protective effect

Data from References 15, 29, 40, 42, 44, 47, 60, 60a, 65, 72, 94, 98, 114, 115, 116, 117, 121, 127, 131, 139a, 148, 150, 160, 187 and the previous edition of this chapter.
CI, Confidence interval; *OR*, odds ratio.

Genetic Factors

Both genetic and nongenetic factors are involved in the etiology of NTDs, with up to 70% of the variance in NTD prevalence attributable to genetic factors.[96]

Possible nongenetic factors have been addressed earlier. Several observations support genetic risk factors as important in NTD formation. First, a priori risk of NTDs for some ethnic/racial groups (e.g., Irish and Mexican) is higher than others (e.g., white and Asian). Second, NTDs recur within families, with first-degree relatives of a patient with NTD possessing a 3% to 5% risk of having offspring with an NTD and second-degree relatives a 1% to 2% risk. Third, more than 250 mouse models with NTDs have been described, with some naturally occurring and others the result of genetic engineering in the laboratory. Evidence for genetic causation includes an increased recurrence risk for siblings of index cases (2% to 5%) compared with the 0.1% risk in the general population, together with a gradually decreasing frequency in more distant relatives. Women with two or more affected pregnancies have a higher risk (approximately 10%) of further recurrence.[136] NTD prevalence is greater in like-sex twins (assumed to include all monozygotic cases) compared with unlike-sex pairs, consistent with a significant genetic component. Nevertheless, NTDs rarely present as multiple cases in families; instead, a sporadic pattern is usually observed. NTDs are also seen associated with certain syndromes such as Meckel-Gruber syndrome and Joubert syndrome.[136]

The genomics revolution over the past 15 years has led to a burgeoning of studies to determine candidate genes for causation both in mouse models as well as in human embryos. Copp et al.[39] speculate that in the near future, a full genome-wide assessment of interacting variants, including coding, regulatory, and epigenetic marks, will be possible to determine an individual's risk of developing an NTD. To date, genes in three main areas of biology have yielded positive findings with regard to NTD etiology: folate metabolism, noncanonical Wnt signaling (the planar cell polarity pathway), and cilia genes.

Methylenetetrahydrofolate reductase (*MTHFR*) encodes a key cytoplasmic enzyme of folate metabolism that generates 5-methyltetrahydrofolate for homocysteine remethylation. The *MTHFR* polymorphism C677T (rs1801133) is associated with a roughly 1.8-fold increased risk of NTDs, although the predisposition is detectable only in non-Hispanic populations.[3] A further significant risk factor is the R653Q variant (rs2236225) of *MTHFD1*, a trifunctional enzyme that catalyzes the conversion of tetrahydrofolate to 5,10-methylenetetrahydrofolate.[59]

In the mouse, mutations in *Pax3* give rise to the *Splotch* (*Sp*) phenotype, which includes spina bifida and other neural crest abnormalities in homozygotes.[69] In humans also, mutations in *Pax3* (MIM: 606587) cause Waardenburg syndrome, an autosomal dominant condition that affects neural crest derived structures and includes spina bifida as part of its phenotypic spectrum.[134]

Thus far, genome-wide association study using human single nucleotide polymorphism panels has not been possible because no individual research group has a sufficient sample size to achieve the statistical power necessary to detect an elevation of risk between 1 and 2 for complex traits such as NTDs. In exploring the *Pax3* and *T* genes, Agopian et al.[2] attempted to get over this hurdle by comparing their sample of 114 (predominantly non-Hispanic whites) with predominantly (81%) lumbar level lesions to controls (non-Hispanic whites) from multiple large public databases such as the HapMap, 1000 Genomes, and the Exome Sequencing Project. They were able to identify 38 variants of *Pax3* in cases, and 8 of which were new variants. The allele frequencies for two were significantly different in cases as compared with at least one reference dataset.[2]

The human *T (Brachyury)* gene (MIM: 601397) was suggested as a candidate for spina bifida because mice lacking T protein (i.e., *Brachyury* mutants) have defective mesoderm formation and abnormal axial development,[161] and several studies have identified an association between a common variant in *T* (i.e., *TIVS7-2*, rs3127334) and the risk of NTDs in humans.[26,88] The study sequencing by Agopian et al.[2] identified 28 variants in non-Hispanic white cases. Of these, 27 were previously reported, and the allele frequencies for 3 were significantly different in cases as compared with non-Hispanic whites in the 1000 Genomes dataset.

More than 130 studies attempting to find association of selected genes with NTDs were published between 1994 and 2010. These studies included approximately 132 candidate genes with known functions involving various aspects of biological activity. Readers are referred to a few detailed reviews for a more thorough understanding of the progress and challenges in identifying genetic variants linked with NTDs.[8,20,71]

Gene-gene and gene-environment interactions are well documented in mouse models of NTDs.[70,71,184] It seems likely that the majority of sporadic human NTDs will also ultimately prove to result from two or more heterozygous genetic risk factors coexisting in individuals who are also exposed to adverse environmental influences, such as suboptimal folate or vitamin B_{12} intake or environmental toxins.

Embryology

The availability of more than 250 different models of open NTDs in mice is enabling increasingly sophisticated analysis of the neurulation events, at tissue, cellular, and molecular levels.

NTDs are known to occur as a result of failure of neurulation between the seventeenth and thirtieth days of gestation.[79] Primary neurulation refers to the development of the neural tube, which forms the brain and spinal cord. Secondary neurulation refers to formation of the remainder of the neural tube from a cell mass caudal to the caudal neuropore, which forms the lower sacral and coccygeal segments (Figure 48-3).

Figure 48-4 contrasts the process in both mice and humans. The initial de novo closure event (closure 1) occurs at the hindbrain/cervical boundary and closure spreads bidirectionally from this site. Failure to initiate closure 1 results in craniorachischisis and failure to close the anterior neuropore results in anencephaly. In the mouse, a second de novo closure site (closure 2) occurs at the forebrain/midbrain boundary with closure also spreading rostrally and caudally. Closure 2 does not appear to occur in human embryos. A third de novo initiation event (closure 3) occurs in both species at the rostral extremity of the neural plate, with closure spreading caudally from here. Hence, in mice, closure is completed sequentially at the anterior neuropore, hindbrain neuropore, and posterior neuropore. In humans, owing to the lack of closure 2, there are likely to be only two neuropores: anterior and posterior (caudal). Failure in closure 3 results in MMC (see Figure 48-4). The caudal neuropore closes around the twenty-sixth day of gestation, and, as a result, teratogenic events that take place after this closure cannot cause thoracic or lumbosacral MMC.[97] Failure of primary neurulation can lead to an open NTD, consisting not only of a spinal anomaly but also other defects, including a Chiari II malformation and hydrocephalus, possibly resulting from cerebrospinal fluid loss during early development.[87,113] Most posterior lumbar and sacral meningoceles are thought to occur during secondary neurulation, with those higher on the spinal axis resulting from defects in primary neurulation that do not cause an open NTD. Encephaloceles are thought to primarily be a defect of cranial mesoderm development.[38]

Prenatal Diagnosis and Management

Prenatal screening now allows for diagnosis of the majority of cases of MMC before birth. Ultrasound (US) is the current "gold standard" for the prenatal diagnosis of MMC, with three-dimensional US and fetal magnetic resonance imaging (MRI) further enhancing characterization of

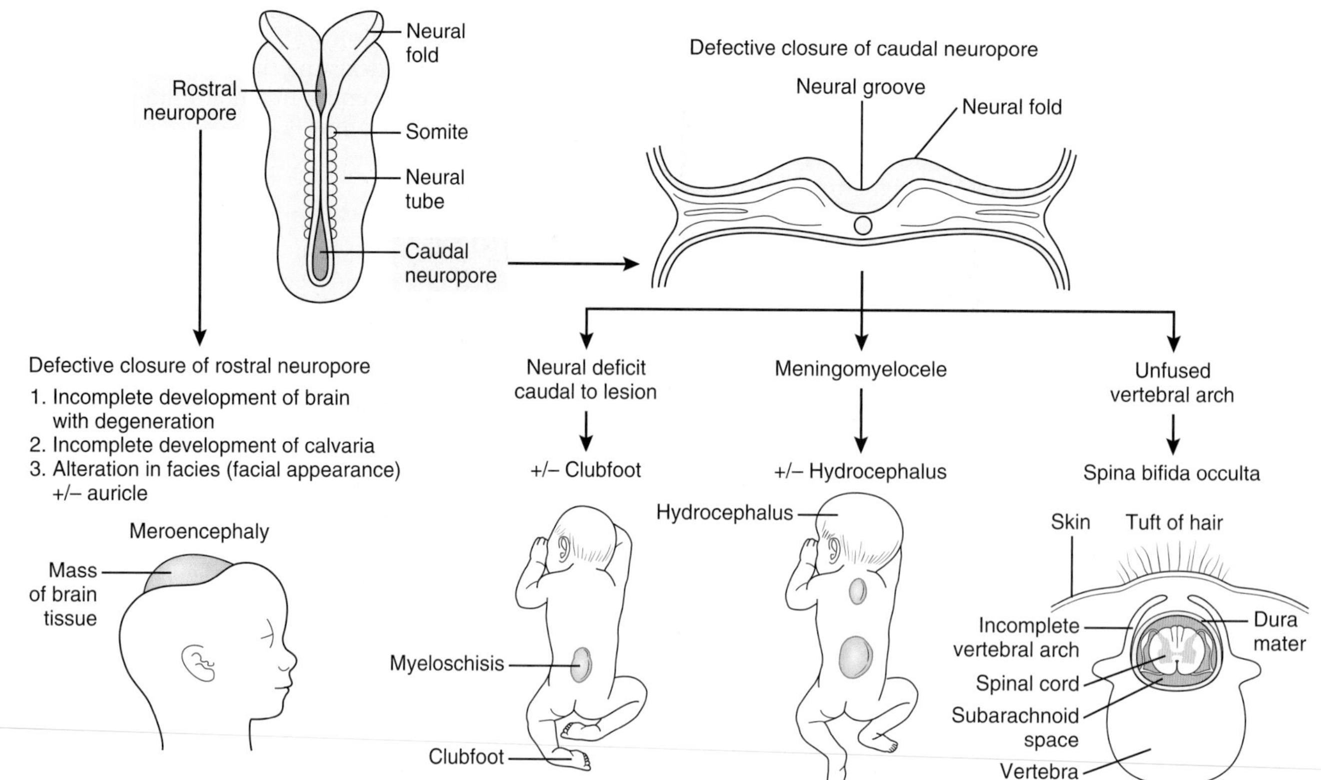

FIGURE 48-3 Schematic illustrations showing the embryologic basis of neural tube defects. Meroencephaly, partial absence of brain, results from defective closure of the rostral neuropore, and meningomyelocele results from defective closure of the caudal neuropore. (Redrawn from Moore KL, Persaud TVN, Torchia MG, editors: Nervous system. In *The developing human: clinically oriented embryology*, ed 9, Philadelphia, 2013, Elsevier Saunders.)

lesions. Although maternal serum alpha-fetal protein is a sensitive screening tool for NTDs and is useful for early detection for women considering termination of pregnancy, its role has been questioned in routine screening. Although amniocentesis for collection of amniotic fluid and acetylcholinesterase levels was once used to confirm the diagnosis of an NTD, high-resolution US now makes this practice obsolete.[175] Functional motor outcome can be predicted by high-resolution US before delivery.[37] One study using fetal MRI showed that worsening cerebellar herniation was associated with childhood seizure activity, high-risk bladder dysfunction, and lack of independent ambulation.[31] A 2008 study demonstrated the diversity of physician views regarding prenatal screening, selective termination, and disability, suggesting a need to better understand how these differences affect reproductive technology, health care policy, and medical practice.[188]

Prenatal detection of MMC is important to educate the patient and family regarding management options. Early detection also allows for consideration of fetal MMC surgery at an experienced center or time to prepare for a safe delivery in a medical center that offers neurologic closure. Previous consideration has been given to performing cesarean section for all mothers with an affected pregnancy to avoid further damage to neural structures. One study reported a less severe lower extremity paralysis in infants delivered by cesarean section before the onset of labor, but showed no difference in those who received cesarean section after the onset of labor.[104] Subsequent studies, however, have found no difference in motor outcome with cesarean section.[79,100]

Intrauterine Surgical Procedures

The rationale for intrauterine surgical intervention for MMC is predicated on the "two-hit" hypothesis stating that damage to the neural elements is the result of both failure of neurulation, resulting in an open NTD, and exposure of the spinal cord to amniotic fluid and traumatic injury within the uterus. Following early fetal surgery work at a select number of surgical centers starting in the mid-1990s, the Management of Myelomeningocele Study (MOMS) was launched in 2003 to compare prenatal fetal surgery with standard postnatal repair. The results were published in 2011 after the study was terminated early as a result of interim analysis of 183 patients, which indicated clear efficacy compared with standard neonatal management. The results showed a reduction in ventriculoperitoneal (VP) shunt placement at 1 year of age, substantial improvement in neuromotor function at 30 months, and reversal of hindbrain herniation in the fetal surgery cohort. Although prenatal intervention resulted in overall improvement, not all participants benefited and the prenatal surgery group showed an increased risk of spontaneous rupture of membranes, oligohydramnios, and preterm delivery. The impact of fetal surgery on bowel and bladder continence remains unclear, although early reports suggest improvement in urologic function. The MOMS-II study will continue to follow outcomes to assess whether neurologic improvement is sustained and to track other specific outcomes including cognitive function and bowel and bladder function. Although proponents of the MOMS trial submit that the study established a new standard-of-care option for

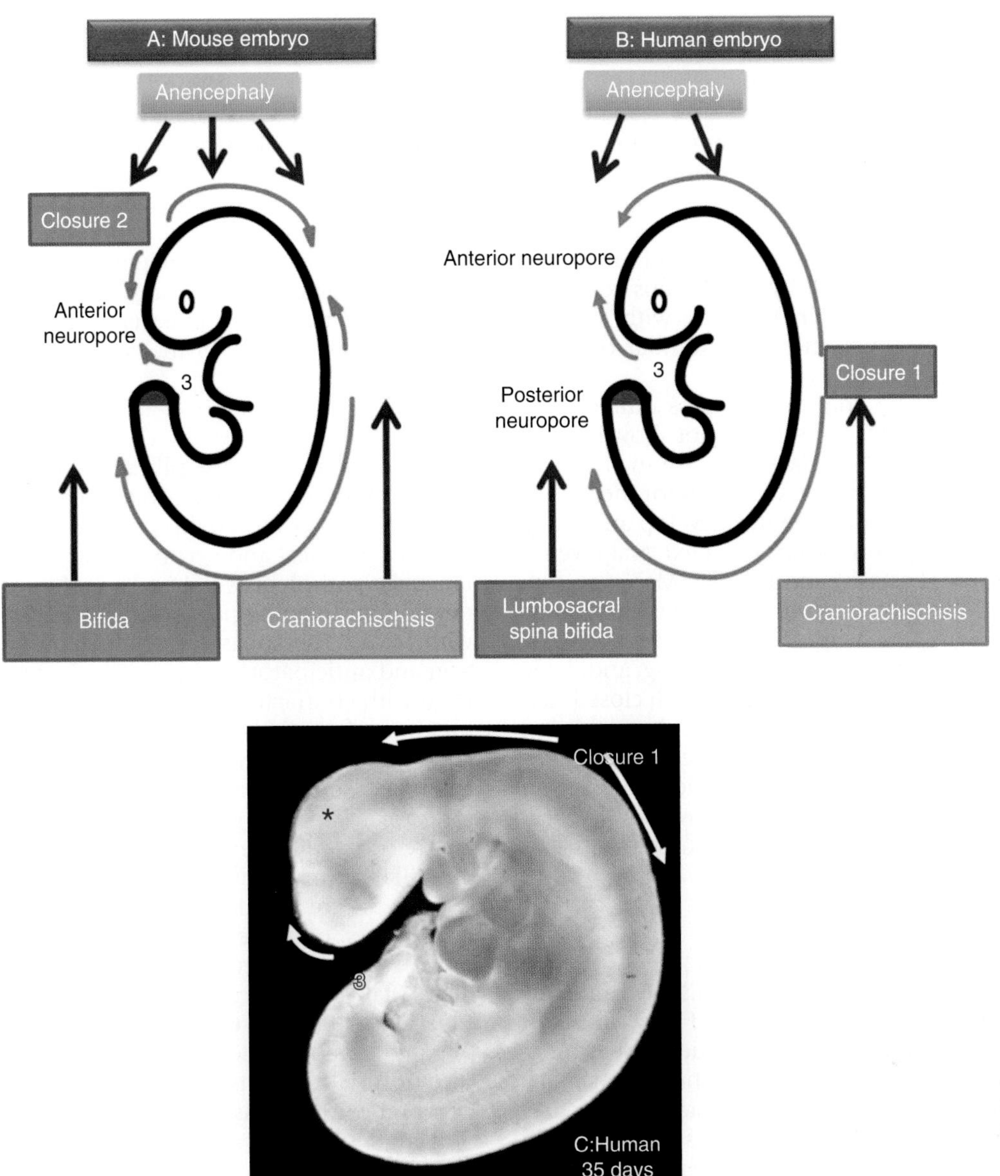

FIGURE 48-4 Diagrammatic representation of the main events of neural tube closure in mouse (**A**) and human (**B**) embryos. The main types of neural tube defect (NTD) resulting from failure of closure at different levels of the body axis are indicated. The red shading on the tail bud indicates the site of secondary neurulation in both species. **C,** Human embryo aged 35 days postfertilization from the Human Developmental Biology Resource (www.hdbr.org). Neurulation has recently been completed in the low spinal region. The positions of closures 1 and 3 and the directions of closure are marked. The midbrain in this human embryo (*red asterisk*) is relatively small compared with the corresponding stage of mouse development. This may have rendered closure 2 an unnecessary intermediate step in achieving cranial neural tube closure in humans. (From Copp AJ: Neurulation in the cranial region—normal and abnormal, *J Anat* 207:623-635, 2005.)

select patients, a recent Cochrane review concluded that evidence is insufficient to draw firm conclusions "on the benefits or harms of prenatal repair as an intervention for fetuses with spina bifida."[3,4,45,73]

Neonatal and Early Management

Back Defect

After an infant is delivered with an open NTD, a sequence of events is set in place to preserve neurologic function, prevent infection, and stabilize cerebrospinal fluid flow. Early closure (within 72 hours of delivery) reduces the risk of infection in the central nervous system.[33] Before closure, the open defect must be protected to prevent contamination or further damage from trauma. Closure occurs in three stages: (1) The neural plaque is returned to the canal, and the dura and arachnoid are reconstructed. (2) A myofascial closure over the newly constructed neural tube is performed. (3) The skin is closed.

Hydrocephalus

Most infants with MMC require VP shunting for hydrocephalus after their back closure,[106] and approximately 15% who are born with severe hydrocephalus require immediate shunting.[112] The 85% who do not require immediate shunting should be watched closely after their back closure for signs of increased intracranial pressure.

Persistent cerebrospinal fluid leak from the repaired spinal wound almost invariably indicates active hydrocephalus, even if the ventricular size is only modestly enlarged and the anterior fontanelle is not bulging. The leaking cerebrospinal fluid serves as a decompression before closure, and once the defect is closed, cerebrospinal fluid can accumulate in the ventricular system. The white matter of a neonate is relatively compliant, and therefore the ventricles can become enlarged before the head circumference changes.[14] The presence of hydrocephalus correlates well with the level of the spinal defect, with thoracic lesions having a higher incidence than lumbar or sacral lesions.[138]

Hydrocephalus usually does not progress immediately and computed tomography scans might not show increasing ventricular size until 3 to 7 days of life. Some children do not require cerebrospinal fluid diversion for months or even years. Infants with hydrocephalus develop an enlarging head with bulging fontanelle, enlarged scalp veins, macrocrania, suture diastasis, and positive Macewen sign (i.e., cracked pot). If the hydrocephalus is not treated, these infants develop signs and symptoms of raised intracranial pressure such as sunset eyes, recurrent vomiting, and, later, respiratory arrest. Similarly, older children with closed fontanelles develop clinical signs of intracranial hypertension without progressive head enlargement. They develop irritability, vomiting, headaches, blurred vision, decline in intellectual performance, and gradual drowsiness, which, if left untreated, lead to coma and death caused by respiratory arrest.

Early Bladder Management

Greater than 90% of infants with MMC will have a neurogenic bladder. In a retrospective study of 129 children, Tarcan et al.[166] noted that children who underwent primary repair of their back lesion after 72 hours showed a significantly lower bladder capacity and a substantially higher detrusor peak leak point pressure as well as a significantly increased incidence of febrile urinary tract infections, vesicoureteral reflux, hydronephrosis, and secondary tethering of the spinal cord at 3 years of age compared with those undergoing primary repair before 72 hours. Additionally, they concluded that closure of the spinal lesion within 24 hours of birth seems to provide the best chance for favorable lower urinary tract function.[166] Management decisions made in infancy can affect renal health as well as the eventual development of urinary continence. The importance of aggressive urinary management should be stressed to the family before the child leaves the hospital.[154]

Baseline investigations should include renal-bladder sonography and a voiding cystourethrogram. Hydronephrosis is found in 7% to 30% of infants, and reflux occurs in approximately 20% of infants.[81,191] Infants with hydronephrosis or reflux should be started on prophylactic antibiotics. Infants who are unable to void begin intermittent catheterization programs. If the infant is able to void, he or she should be checked for complete emptying by checking a postvoid residual volume, either by catheterization or bladder scan. Incomplete emptying can lead to urinary tract infections because the retained urine serves as a culture medium.

Assessment of the Neurologic Level

Even if not spoken out loud, the first question parents of a newborn with MMC often ask is, "Will my child be able to walk?" A careful neurologic examination can give them an idea even within the first few days of life. The best predictor of motor function is the actual motor examination. Information regarding the best motor examination can be obtained by observation, palpation, and postural changes. Motor examinations can improve after the initial examination, which may relate to a period of spinal shock associated with the delivery or the closure.[57]

Therapy

The goal of any interdisciplinary MMC team should be to develop and implement a comprehensive plan that enables the affected child to attain a maximal level of function in all areas. Physical and occupational therapists and speech-language pathologists play a key role in this endeavor to develop an ongoing partnership with families of children with MMC. Therapists are invaluable in providing education and anticipatory guidance for the family. For children born with contractures at the hips, knees, ankles, or feet, a program of passive range of motion can be taught to the family even before hospital discharge. Orthoses are often fabricated soon after birth by a therapist to maintain or improve range of motion. Families should generally be referred to early intervention services to provide ongoing surveillance for monitoring development and for support services where developmental delays are detected. As a child grows, outpatient therapy and school-based therapy services should be incorporated into the outpatient treatment plan and educational plan with guidance from an experienced team of therapists. Throughout life, the MMC therapy team will help to educate and coordinate with community therapists the development and implementation of a comprehensive plan of care.

Childhood Management

Shunts

Almost all children with MMC require placement of a VP shunt for management of hydrocephalus. The two most common shunt complications are infection and obstruction.[176] Presenting signs and symptoms of shunt malfunction vary with the age of the child. Mechanical obstructions tend to present more acutely with signs and symptoms related to increased intracranial pressure as noted earlier, and infections tend to present more insidiously (Box 48-2).

Infections have a greater long-term morbidity than malfunctions. The overall risk of shunt infection is 12% per child with *Staphylococcus epidermidis* being the most common culprit.[56] Symptoms do not usually develop until several weeks after the shunt is placed or revised. Epidemiologic factors seem to influence the incidence of shunt infections more than surgical factors. Aside from skin contamination during shunt placement, shunts can also become infected with gram-negative rods if the distal end

BOX 48-2

Possible Symptoms of a Shunt Malfunction

Infants
- Bulging fontanel
- Vomiting
- Irritability
- Change in appetite
- Lethargy
- Sunsetting eyes (cranial nerve VI palsy with abduction paralysis)
- Seizures
- Vocal cord paralysis with stridor
- Swelling or redness along shunt track

Toddlers
- Vomiting
- Lethargy
- Irritability
- Seizures
- Headaches
- Swelling along shunt tract
- Redness along shunt tract

School-Aged Children
- Headaches
- Vomiting
- Lethargy
- Seizures
- Irritability
- Swelling along shunt track
- Redness along shunt tract
- Decreased school performance

Adults
- Headaches
- Vomiting
- Lethargy
- Seizures
- Redness or swelling along shunt tract

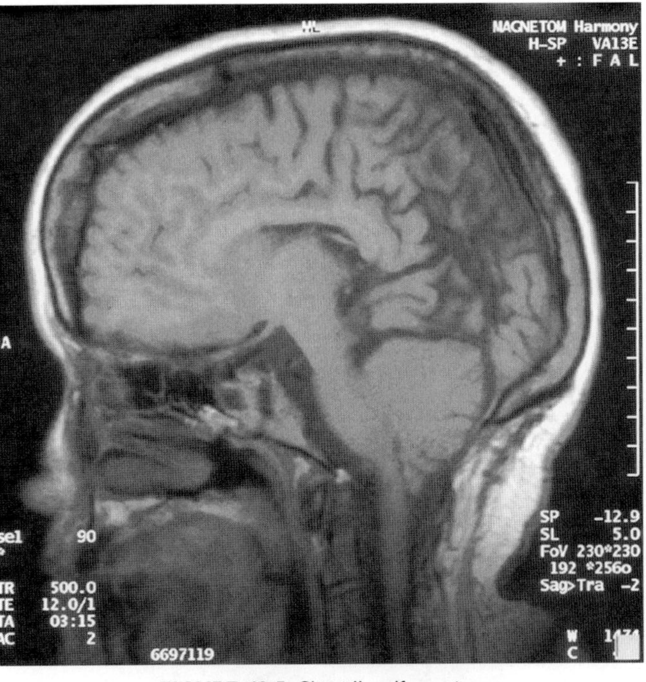

FIGURE 48-5 Chiari II malformation.

of the shunt erodes into an intraabdominal organ. Gram-negative infections have a much poorer prognosis.[58]

Isolated downstream infections of the shunt system have the least morbidity. Shunt infection with ventricular meningitis carries the highest morbidity. Although controversial, several studies suggest that recurrent and frequent shunt infections affect cognitive function.

In the first year of life, 50% of all children with a VP shunt develop obstruction requiring revision. Of those children who require a revision in the first year, 31% will require a second revision in the second year, and then have a risk recurrence rate of 12% per year thereafter.[158] Endoscopic third ventriculostomies are performed in carefully selected patients and can become an alternative to chronic VP shunts.[22]

A controversial population is older children or young adults who have MMC and untreated ventriculomegaly. If these patients have no symptoms or MRI findings to suggest active hydrocephalus and never received shunting, suggesting "arrested hydrocephalus," they should be serially monitored with intelligence quotient and psychometric testing. If testing results are stable, then shunting based solely on radiologic appearance should be discouraged because the risks outweigh the benefits. If positive for symptoms or with MRI findings suggestive of hydrocephalus, intracranial pressure monitoring should be pursued.[34]

Arnold-Chiari II (A-C II) Malformations

The A-C II malformation is characterized by variable displacement of cerebellar tissue into the spinal canal, accompanied by caudal dislocation of the lower brainstem and fourth ventricle easily identified on MRI studies (Figure 48-5). It is also associated with a wide range of other abnormalities throughout the neuraxis. McLone and Knepper[113] proposed the unified theory that the spinal malformation in MMC with associated leaking cerebrospinal fluid prevents normal transient occlusion of the primitive central canal of the spinal cord and the buildup of hydrostatic pressure in the rhombencephalon. This subsequently produces a posterior fossa that is too small and hence explains the association of open spinal dysraphism and the Chiari II deformity.[113] However, an intrauterine MRI study of 65 fetuses with open spinal dysraphism that were compared with gestationally aged matched "normal" fetuses noted that 23% of fetuses with open spinal dysraphism did not have Chiari II deformity in utero and that the bony posterior fossa was also significantly reduced in volume in cases of open spinal dysraphism without hindbrain herniation, suggesting that the relationship may not be as straightforward as had been suggested.[13]

Although the operative mortality for closure of the spinal defect in children with MMC is very low, the operative mortality for symptomatic A-C malformations is relatively high (34% to 38%).[141] A symptomatic Chiari II malformation remains the leading cause of death for infants with MMC.[159] Signs and symptoms of symptomatic Chiari II malformations include intermittent obstructive or central apnea, cyanosis, bradycardia, dysphagia, nystagmus, stridor, vocal cord paralysis, torticollis, opisthotonos, hypotonia, upper extremity weakness, and spasticity. The constellation of stridor, central apnea, and aspiration is sometimes referred to as *central ventilatory dysfunction*.[77]

Before hindbrain decompression for a symptomatic Chiari II malformation, the child's shunt system should be evaluated carefully because shunt malfunctions can cause Chiari malformations to become symptomatic. Hindbrain decompressions should be performed early to minimize the progression of symptoms of the Chiari malformation. Poor preoperative prognostic signs include bilateral vocal cord paralysis, severe neurogenic dysphagia, and prolonged apnea.[32]

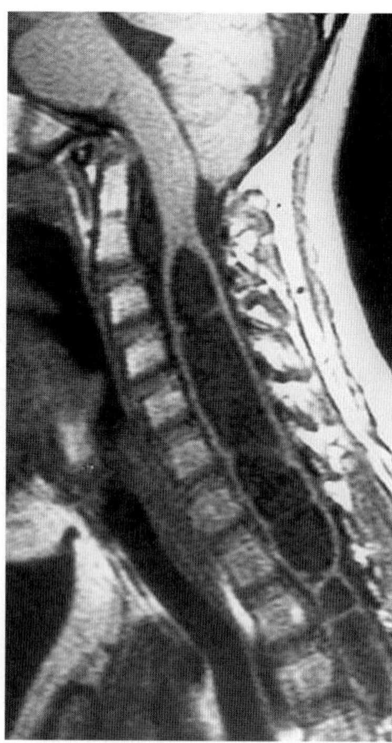

FIGURE 48-6 Hydromyelia.

Hydromyelia

Hydromyelia is the dilatation of the central canal of the spinal cord (Figure 48-6). It is analogous to dilatation of the ventricles in the brain and is a relatively common occurrence in children with MMC. Hydromyelia is probably much more common than we are aware because it often does not cause obvious symptoms in patients with MMC.[25] When symptomatic, it usually presents with rapidly progressive scoliosis, a change in strength or coordination of the upper or lower extremities, and spasticity. MRI is the best test to demonstrate this spinal cord abnormality.[24] When suspected, the entire neuraxis should be imaged because untreated or subclinical hydrocephalus can produce hydromyelia. Hydrocephalus should be treated before surgical treatment for hydromyelia.

Tethered Cord Syndrome

In children with MMC, the spinal cord can be fixed or "tethered" at one point, causing traction, which can lead to progressive urologic, orthopedic, or neurologic decline. It was first described in 1857, and the first known detethering of the spinal cord was performed on a previously healthy 17-year-old individual who had progressive loss of lower extremity function in 1891.[112]

The spinal cord usually terminates at the level of L1 to L2. However, MMC repair invariably is followed by the development of arachnoiditis, fibrosis, and adhesions between the intraspinal neural structures, the meninges, and the surrounding vertebral structures.[192] These adhesions can tether the cord to the low lumbar or sacral region.

Most children with MMC will show signs of tethering on MRI. Therefore, symptoms should develop before surgical correction is pursued. Typical signs and symptoms in children include increased weakness (54%), worsening gait (54%), scoliosis (51%), pain (32%), orthopedic deformity (11%), and urologic dysfunction (6%).[82] Surgical correction should be considered early because most symptoms will improve or stabilize if treated early.[82] Delayed correction can result in irreversible loss of function because the natural history is for symptoms to worsen with time.[132]

At least three other lesions can lead to tethering of the spinal cord: diastematomyelia, lipomyelomeningocele, and tight filum terminale. Diastematomyelia refers to divisions (not duplications) of the spinal cord. It is usually associated with a bony spur. Even if asymptomatic, the natural history is for symptoms to develop that can be irreversible.[4,75] Lipomyelomeningocele refers to a subcutaneous lipoma, continuous with the cauda equina, which also has a meningocele with neural elements enclosed extending outside the dura. A tight filum terminale is another congenital malformation in which the filum terminale does not elongate. Prophylactic surgery is usually recommended for these three lesions.

Neurogenic Bladder

Urologic involvement in MMC and other spinal dysraphisms varies, and is not necessarily correlated with the level of the lesion as in traumatic spinal cord injury. In MMC, more than 90% of patients have partial or complete denervation of the bladder, with poor compliance and contractibility resulting in unacceptable residual urine volumes.[154] The urethral sphincter is incompetent in 86% of patients, so that incontinence occurs with increases in intravesical pressure. Approximately one third of patients have detrusor sphincter dyssynergia, resulting in high intraluminal pressures.[108] The external sphincter is usually partially functional and can improve in the first year after birth.[157] Patients should be observed at least annually because deterioration or improvement can occur in the first year of life and tethering of the spinal cord with a change in bladder function can occur over the years. Although the majority of individuals with MMC have normal renal function at birth, 40% to 90% will experience a decline by age 10 years if left unattended.[118]

Preservation of renal function and improving quality of life with continence and eventual independence in management are the primary goals of neurogenic bladder management. Urodynamic evaluation is generally performed in infants with MMC, with 75% showing a normal upper urinary tract.[109] The remaining infants show some degree of hydronephrosis resulting from vesicoureteral reflux, detrusor sphincter dyssynergia, an enlarged bladder, or other structural abnormality. Infants with normal anatomy should receive a renal US biannually. Those with incomplete emptying and no outlet resistance can be taught the Credé maneuver. Those with detrusor sphincter dyssynergia, or who have already developed hydronephrosis, should be treated with anticholinergic medications and clean intermittent catheterization to prevent the development or worsening of hydronephrosis. Children with vesicoureteral reflux are often prescribed prophylactic antibiotics. For persistent febrile urinary tract infection or hydronephrosis, surgical intervention is often necessary.

Cutaneous vesicostomy can be performed with reversal done at a later time when the patient is capable of effective clean intermittent catheterization.[111,123,147]

Because less than 10% of children with MMC have normal urinary control, continence of urine is an issue of great concern.[99] Although there are no effective external collection devices for females excluding diapers, condom catheters are an option for males with reflex emptying who do not have vesicoureteral reflux or large residual volumes. Appropriate sizing can be a difficult issue for some and impaired sensation can lead to skin breakdown.

The high prevalence of small bladder capacity and low outlet resistance in many children results in only approximately a quarter of children being continent with clean intermittent catheterization alone.[177] In general, frequent catheterization less than every 4 hours is required to achieve continence.[99] It has been reported that up to two thirds of individuals can become continent with nonsurgical management including medications and clean intermittent catheterization.[66] Anticholinergic medications and botulinum toxin injections may be used to increase bladder capacity.[6] Multiple surgical options are available for those who do not achieve continence with clean intermittent catheterization and medications. Although a full description of these techniques is beyond the scope of this chapter, bladder augmentation along with artificial sphincter placement can be used individually or in combination. Success for long-term continence after artificial sphincter placement is greater than 60%.[17] In addition, for patients who have difficulty performing urethral clean intermittent catheterization, continent diversion with the appendix used as a conduit to the bladder to create an abdominal stoma, can create easier access for many patients.[147] In recent years, lumbar to sacral nerve rerouting has been performed in an attempt to improve bladder and bowel function in patients with MMC. Although improvements have been reported in some patients, positive responders cannot be predicted before intervention and there is the potential for lower extremity weakness adversely affecting ambulation.[130] Independence with toileting in children with MMC is delayed more than all other self-care tasks.[126a] Although most children achieve independent control of bowel and bladder function by the age of 4 years, those with MMC might not achieve this until age 10 to 15 years.[110] The cause of this is multifactorial and includes level of paralysis, intelligence, difficulty with visuospatial tasks, kyphoscoliosis, parental support, sensation, sphincter control, and bladder perception. Children can be taught to perform clean intermittent catheterization as early as age 5 years, although they will still need assistance with maintaining a schedule.[126a] Parents need to be trained not only in their child's bladder program but also instructed in the importance of allowing the child to accept responsibility once she or he is able. A recent study of young adults revealed that up to 60% reported urinary incontinence with approximately 70% perceiving this as a problem.[155,182]

Neurogenic Bowel

Patterns of neurogenic bowel involvement in children with MMC vary from normal bowel control in approximately 20%, to incontinence caused by impaired rectal sensation, impaired sphincter function, and altered colonic motility in the remainder.[99] Those without control of the external anal sphincter become incontinent when the pressure inside the rectum is sufficient to produce reflex relaxation of the internal anal sphincter. In those with lesions above L3, the internal anal sphincter has low tone, which further contributes to incontinence. In addition, lesions above this level generally result in absent sensation, although sensation can be present but impaired in lower level lesions.[1] Presence of the bulbocavernosus or anocutaneous reflex has been associated with a greater likelihood of achieving bowel continence.[92]

The goal of a bowel management program is to achieve efficient, regular, and predictable emptying before the rectum becomes full enough to stimulate reflex relaxation of the internal anal sphincter in those with innervation present. This can be achieved through the use of stool softeners, bulking agents, suppositories, digital stimulation, manual removal, or enemas. However, many patients and families prefer dietary manipulation. Clinicians often recommend performing bowel programs after a meal to take advantage of the gastrocolic reflex, although it is not clear that this is intact in patients with MMC.[51] A recent trial of Peristeen transanal colonic irrigation in children with bowel incontinence for various reasons resulted in 83% of children achieving either social continence or a significant improvement with occasional soiling. The study concludes that transanal colonic irrigation should be considered the first line of treatment when simple pharmacologic intervention is ineffective, and should be attempted before proceeding with surgical interventions.[7,128] In patients who cannot become continent with more conservative approaches, surgical options are available. Although a full description of these techniques is beyond the scope of this chapter, options include the antegrade continence enema (ACE) procedure[78] and colostomy. In an ACE procedure the appendix is used as a conduit to the bowel, through which a catheter can then be inserted into the cecum and saline or tap water infused, with bowel emptying achieved within 15 to 45 minutes. Colostomy is another option if standard treatment and ACE have failed.

The importance of achieving bowel continence at an early age is important to provide a smooth transition into preschool and kindergarten, where children can be severely criticized by peers. Encouraging children to assume increasing responsibility for their bowel program should be emphasized. Unfortunately, one study showed that as many as 86% of teenagers (ages 13 to 18 years) with MMC needed assistance from a caregiver for their bowel program.[99] Another study of young adults revealed that approximately 34% reported fecal incontinence regardless of their means of management, and 77% perceived this as a problem.[182] The management of neurogenic bowel varies widely among medical providers. To measure changes, appropriate measures are needed to assess interventions. A neurogenic bowel dysfunction score has recently been validated in a small trial but needs to be further evaluated on a larger scale.[8,90] Further, a recent review of management for central fecal incontinence reported that there is little research in this area and the available evidence is almost uniformly of low methodological quality.[9,36]

Latex Allergy

Although the incidence of latex allergy in the general population is estimated to be less than 1% to 2%, the prevalence among children with MMC ranges from 20% to 65%.[167] This immunoglobulin E–mediated response to natural rubber latex is related to repeated mucosal exposure during surgical, therapeutic, and diagnostic procedures, as well as atopic predisposition. The allergic response can range from dermatitis, allergic rhinitis, asthma, and angioedema to anaphylaxis.[151,162] Patients with spina bifida have been determined to have a 500-fold greater risk for anaphylaxis in the operating room compared with control groups.[167] Given that latex sensitization takes place over time, a previous lack of sensitivity or negative allergy test does not preclude the possibility of a life-threatening reaction. Parents should be educated regarding the presence or risk of latex allergy. It is generally recommended that all patients with MMC use nonlatex catheters and avoid all other latex-containing products, whether medical or nonmedical.

Endocrine Disorders

Individuals with MMC are known to have disturbed growth and development. Although spinal cord lesions, vertebral anomalies, and other skeletal deformities reduce growth of the lower limbs and spine, complex central nervous system abnormalities and hydrocephalus put the patient with MMC at risk for hypothalamic-pituitary dysfunction, including central precocious puberty and growth hormone deficiency, further contributing to short stature.[55] Precocious puberty has been reported in 12% to 16% of patients with MMC.[56,172] The mechanism of this is thought to be related to increased pressure on the hypothalamus resulting in premature activation of the hypothalamic-pituitary-gonadal axis. Treatment with gonadotropin-releasing hormone analogues has proven beneficial in several studies, halting the progression of puberty, stopping menses, and decreasing hormone levels.[173] It is more common for girls with MMC to experience precocious puberty and it is unclear whether patients without hydrocephalus are at risk. Currently, only limited data show that treatment of growth hormone deficiency with growth hormone provides significant improvement in growth velocity, height, muscle strength, mobility, and reduction in obesity.[140,171] Ongoing debate continues as to whether to treat patients with MMC with growth hormone. Clarification of the goals of treatment is required because efficacy with regard to functional improvement can be influenced by the level of the lesion and the presence of complicating factors such as syringomyelia, tethered cord syndrome, scoliosis, vertebral anomalies, contracture, and advanced pubertal development.[174] Further studies are required to assess the ultimate role of growth hormone treatment in individuals with MMC.

Musculoskeletal Considerations

Motor Innervation

The level of motor function in MMC does not necessarily correspond to the anatomic vertebral level on radiographic studies.[138] Although spinal defects are generally described as cervical-, upper thoracic–, midthoracic-, low thoracic–, upper lumbar–, midlumbar-, low lumbar–, lumbosacral-, or sacral-level lesions, there are several different systems to classify the neurologic level that are not entirely consistent.[36] It is noted that cervical and upper thoracic dysraphisms might be entirely different entities because these children tend to have a better prognosis and less neurologic deficit than children with lower thoracic and lumbar lesions.[142] The majority of children with MMC have lumbosacral-level vertebral lesions, with a quarter having midlumbar-level lesions, and one fifth having sacral-level involvement.

One third of patients with MMC present with flaccid paralysis below their anatomic lesion, with the remainder showing a combination of upper and lower motor neuron signs. Many individuals are asymmetrical on motor and sensory testing, and some have voluntary motor control below other segments of paralysis and sensory loss.[109]

The level of neurologic impairment influences the expectations of medical providers on functional outcome, treatment strategies offered, and anticipated musculoskeletal deformities and other complications (Table 48-2).

Hips

Most patients with MMC will have some hip deformity that interferes with ambulation, seating, or bracing. The management of hip deformity remains a topic of debate among orthopedic surgeons.[78] Muscle imbalance at the hip accounts for most of the hip flexion deformity, but sitting at 90 degrees and hip flexor spasticity can also contribute to hip flexion deformities. Patients with thoracic-level lesions develop hip flexion deformities related to positioning or hip flexor spasticity. Patients with upper- and midlumbar-level lesions develop hip flexion deformities related to unopposed hip flexors and adductors. Hip flexion contractures create anterior pelvic tilt, which increases lumbar lordosis and can interfere with ambulation. Hip flexor lengthening procedures can preserve ambulation in the ambulatory patient with MMC but should not be considered in the nonambulatory patient unless skin integrity, pain, or seating is compromised.

Hip dislocations in children with MMC are present at birth or may occur later as a result of unopposed hip flexors and adductors. Treatment of the dislocated hip in MMC is a topic of considerable debate, although there is increasing focus on the individual's function and level of satisfaction rather than the appearance on imaging.

Congenital dislocations of the hip can be seen in those with thoracic-level lesions as well as lumbar- and sacral-level lesions. Children with thoracic-level lesions and no motor function in the lower extremities are less likely to benefit from surgical intervention. Children with good quadriceps power may be better surgical candidates, although gait analysis studies have shown that gait symmetry corresponds more closely to the presence of hip contractures rather than hip dislocation.[168]

Hips that slowly migrate laterally (subluxation) over time are usually a result of muscle imbalance around the hip. In a natural history study, Broughton et al.[23] found that by the age of 11 years, hip dislocation had occurred in 28% of individuals with thoracic-level lesions, 30% of upper lumbar-level lesions, 36% with L4 function, 7%

Table 48-2 Grouping and Prognostication of Motor Function by Level of Lesion

Level of Lesion	Expected Muscle Function	Functional Mobility in Childhood	Functional Mobility in Adolescence and/or Adulthood	Commonly Used Equipment	Orthoses Used	Functional Mobility Scale (FMS) Classification	Functional Pattern
Lower thoracic (T11 to T12)	May have some abdominal, paraspinal, and quadratus lumborum function	Therapeutic standing* Nonfunctional ambulation† Complete wheelchair reliance for mobility	No ambulation Complete wheelchair reliance for mobility	Standing frame* Parapodium† Wheelchair	Trunk-hip-knee-ankle-foot orthosis	FMS: 1, 1, 1	**Group 1***
Functional hallmark	**No lower limb motor function, lack iliopsoas function**						
High lumbar (L1 to L2)	L1: Iliopsoas group 2 or better L2: Iliopsoas, sartorius, and adductors all group 3 or better May have weak quadriceps Some sensation present below hip joint	Wheelchair reliance for distance ambulation Limited household ambulation‡	Complete wheelchair reliance for distance ambulation May exhibit nonfunctional ambulation	Wheelchair Forearm crutches Walker	Reciprocating gait orthosis Hip-knee-ankle-foot orthosis	FMS: 1, 1, 1	**Group 1***
Functional hallmark	**Have iliopsoas function**						
Midlumbar (L3 to L4)	L3: Meet criteria for L2 and quadriceps is group 3 or more L4: Meet criteria for L3 with strong quadriceps and have moderate medial hamstrings	Household ambulation, limited community ambulation Partial reliance on wheelchair for distance ambulation	50% wheelchair reliance Usually maintain household ambulation with forearm crutches	Wheelchair Walker Forearm crutches	Knee-ankle-foot orthosis	FMS: 3, 2, 1	**Group 2†**
Functional hallmark	**Have strong knee extension** **Lack hip abduction**						
Low lumbar (L5)	L5: Meet criteria for L4 and have strong medial and lateral hamstrings and tibialis anterior and posterior, have moderate hip abduction	Community ambulation Partial reliance on wheelchair for long-distance ambulation	Community ambulation with forearm crutches Partial reliance on wheelchair for long-distance ambulation	Wheelchair, forearm crutches	Ankle-foot orthosis	FMS:	**Group 2†**
Functional hallmark	**Strong knee flexion, strong ankle dorsiflexion and inversion, and great toe extension** **Lack active hip extension and ankle plantar flexion**						
Sacral (S1) (S2 to S3)	S1: Meet criteria for L5 Have normal ankle dorsiflexion, inversion, eversion, and moderate ankle plantar flexion and hip extension	Community ambulation	Community ambulation, partial reliance on crutch or cane in adulthood for long distances	None None	Supramalleolar foot orthosis	FMS: 6, 6, 6 But may be FMS: 6, 6, 3, or 4 in adulthood	**Group 3‡**
	S2 to S3: Meet criteria for S1 and have gastrocnemius and soleus	Community ambulation	Community ambulation, may have reduced endurance and pain as a result of late foot deformities		Foot orthosis	FMS: 6, 6, 6	
Functional hallmark	**Have active hip extension and ankle plantar flexion and eversion** **May lack foot intrinsic muscle function**						

Data from Apkon SD, Grady R, Hart S, et al: Advances in the care of children with spina bifida, *Pediatrics* 61:33-74, 2014; Swaroop VT, Dias L: Orthopedic management of spina bifida. Part I: hip, knee, and rotational deformities, *J Child Orthop* 3:441–449, 2009; Sharrard WJW: The segmental innervation of the lower limb muscles of man, *Ann R Coll Surg Engl* 35:106–122, 1964; Bartonek A, Saraste H, Knutson LM: Comparison of different systems to classify the neurological level of lesion in patients with myelomeningocele, *Dev Med Child Neurol* 41:796–805, 1999; Broughton NS, Menelaus MB, Cole WG, et al: The natural history of hip deformity in myelomeningocele, *J Bone Joint Surg Br* 75:760–763, 1993; Mazur JM, Shurtleff D, Menelaus M, et al: Orthopaedic management of high-level spina bifida. Early walking compared with early use of a wheelchair, *J Bone Joint Surg Am* 71:56–61, 1989; McDonald CM, Jaffe KM, Mosca VS, et al: Ambulatory outcome of children with myelomeningocele: effect of lower extremity strength, *Dev Med Child Neurol* 33:482-490, 1991.

*Group 1: Generally nonambulatory/nonfunctional ambulation unless they have pelvic elevator strength (quad lumborum) in which case they may attain household ambulation; completely wheelchair-reliant as adults.

†Group 2: Community ambulation with braces and assistive device; partial reliance on wheelchair.

‡Group 3: Community ambulation with foot orthoses and without need for assistive device or wheelchair.

with L5 function, and in 1% with sacral function. In the past, the ambulatory child may have received aggressive surgical treatment including femoral and acetabular osteotomy. A study by Gabrieli et al.,[67] however, found that hip subluxation did not significantly affect gait characteristics and therefore concluded that surgery for the dislocated hip in the ambulatory child is not indicated. Recent reviews of hip management in spina bifida have concluded that hip dislocations in patients with spina bifida did not really affect symmetry of gait or walking speed and although surgical treatment may provide reduction of the dislocated hip, consideration should be given for potential complications and functional decline following surgery.[143,163,168]

Knees

Children with MMC can develop knee flexion or extension contractures. Those with thoracic-level lesions experience contractures more frequently, but this can also be seen in patients with lumbar and sacral lesions.[163] They can interfere with upright mobility, transfers, and, if severe, hygiene in the popliteal space. Knee flexion contractures of 20 degrees or less are generally well tolerated in the ambulatory patient. Nonambulatory patients might tolerate even more severe contractures without loss of function. A radical knee flexor release can be performed when contractures interfere with sitting balance or gait. This procedure is well tolerated with a low rate of recurrence in the ambulatory child.[163] Knee extension contractures are much less common but may occur with unopposed knee extensors, congenital dislocation of the knee, immobilization for fractures, or after surgical treatment for flexion contractures. Knee extension contractures can interfere with seating and sit-to-stand transfers in the nonambulatory patient but generally do not impede ambulation in the ambulatory child.[163] Serial casting to get knee flexion to 90 degrees is the first step, followed by a V-Y quadricepsplasty if still interfering with gait.[164] In the nonambulatory child, adequate flexion can usually be obtained by transection of the patellar ligament.[143] Knee pain is a common complaint in ambulatory persons with MMC and may contribute to a decline in mobility over time. Gait analysis has shown that valgus knee stress is a major contributor to anterior-medial knee laxity and pain. The causes are multifactorial and include degree of lateral trunk sway, weak hip abductors, internal hip rotation in combination with increased knee flexion, external tibial torsion, and valgus foot deformity. Crutches and orthotics, including ankle-foot orthoses (AFOs) or knee-ankle-foot orthoses (KAFOs), may assist in protecting the knees from excessive stress, and distal tibial derotational osteotomies may decrease stress resulting from external tibial torsion.[168]

Feet

Foot and ankle deformities are present almost universally in most children with MMC.[6,164] They may be present at birth, related to lack of intrauterine movement or muscle imbalance across the ankle, or develop over time as a result of muscle imbalance around the ankle and weight-bearing forces. Lack of sensation and autonomic instability can lead to secondary skin problems and poor wound healing.

The most common foot deformities in children with MMC are equinus contracture, clubfeet, vertical talus, and calcaneal deformities with clubfeet occurring in almost 50% of infants.[6,164] The goal in treating these children is to achieve a plantigrade foot with stable skin. Splinting and passive manipulation can be helpful in infancy, but many of these children will require casting or corrective surgical procedures in the future.

Pure equinus deformities can be seen in children with S1 innervation, but they are also seen in children with lumbar- and thoracic-level lesions. In the patient with a lumbar or thoracic lesion, gentle manipulation followed by serial casting should be the first attempt at correction. If the contracture persists when the child is ready for weight bearing, percutaneous heel cord lengthening should be considered. This is often performed in the outpatient clinic if the child is insensate. AFOs are often required to help maintain the newly acquired range of motion.

Children with midlumbar-level lesions will often develop clubfeet (equinovarus deformities). Serial casting is the first line of treatment, and the Ponseti method has been used widely for treating clubfeet in patients with MMC, especially early in infancy. However, one study demonstrated early recurrence rates of 68% following casting in this patient population[64a,168] and many individuals will go on to require soft tissue releases or tendon transfers to balance the forces across the ankle.[164] Surgical correction should not be performed until the child is ready to begin bearing weight through the lower extremities because crawling with internally rotated feet has a deforming force that can lead to recurrence. The opposite deformity of hindfoot valgus often develops later. Postoperative bracing is necessary to hold the foot and ankle in proper alignment.

Calcaneus deformities can be seen at birth or develop postnatally as a response to unopposed dorsiflexion in patients with midlumbar-level paralysis. Calcaneus deformity makes bracing difficult and often ineffective. This deformity predisposes the patient to pressure sores over the heel, which can lead to osteomyelitis. Patients with progressive deformities or a propensity toward pressure ulceration should be treated aggressively because delay in treatment can result in a greatly increased risk of pressure ulceration.[58] Solid AFOs are the most appropriate orthosis for this deformity. Multiple surgical approaches have been proposed. It is controversial as to whether the anterior tibial tendon should be released or transferred in this setting.[168]

Pes cavus or intrinsic minus feet are characterized by loss of intrinsic muscle function, resultant digital contracture, plantar metatarsal head prominence, and increased forefoot plantar loading during ambulation. They require little treatment during the school-aged years. In adolescence, skin problems can develop related to weight bearing over the second to fourth metatarsal heads. If foot orthoses or custom-molded shoes are unable to redistribute the weight around the foot, metatarsal osteotomies might be required.

Valgus deformities of the foot and ankle are common problems encountered in the ambulatory child with MMC. This deformity can develop without regard for level of paralysis. These children often have poor orthotic tolerance because of pressure over the medial malleolus or the head of the navicular bone.

Spine

Deformities of the spine in children with MMC can be congenital, paralytic, or a combination of the two. Congenital spinal anomalies include scoliosis secondary to vertebral malformations, congenital kyphosis related to posterior element dysplasia, lordosis, and intrathecal anomalies such as diastematomyelia.[78] Predictors of the development of scoliosis include ambulatory status, clinical motor level, and the last intact laminar arch.[170] Potential indications for surgical intervention include scoliosis greater than 50 degrees, inability to be managed in a brace, and individuals older than 10 to 12 years of age who wish to maximize adult spinal height.[10] Spinal fusion surgery is the usual treatment and is done close to growth completion. In children with congenital scoliosis and vertebral anomalies such as hemivertebrae, growing constructs such as vertically expanding prosthetic titanium rib systems and growing rods are used so that spinal stabilization can be achieved without sacrificing final truncal height.[62] Spinal deformities are more likely to occur in those with thoracic lesions (>90% of patients with thoracic lesions develop scoliosis), but they can also be seen in those with mid- and low-lumbar lesions and rarely even with sacral lesions.[170] Kyphotic deformities can cause severe seating and skin problems. Surgical treatment of kyphotic deformities carries significant risk of complications but usually has a good outcome.[125] Kyphotic deformities seen at birth are related to congenital malformations. Lordosis is usually related to hip flexion contractures. Orthotic management of scoliosis does not provide a complete or permanent correction but might delay the need for surgical correction until the child is closer to skeletal maturity. Rapid progression of otherwise stable curves can be seen in patients with hydromyelia or tethered cord syndromes.

Fractures

Children with MMC are susceptible to pathologic fractures in the lower limbs and fracture rates range from 11% to 30% in children with spina bifida.[5,52,102,165] Diminished bone density combined with limited ambulation and muscle weakness are thought to be factors contributing to this high rate of fractures.[6] Neonates with contractures in the lower limbs are more likely to have fractures with mobilization.[21] Risk factors include osteopenia, insensate extremities, contractures, and immobilization. Children with thoracic lesions are more likely to have femur fractures and children with lumbar lesions are more likely to have tibial fractures.[102] A 2007 study by Dosa et al.[52] documented fractures to be most common in the early adolescent period, with most fractures seen in community ambulators. Fractures manifest with localized erythema, heat, and swelling. Crepitus and deformity occur only with displaced fractures. Often there is no complaint of pain and no report of trauma. Fractures are often confused with cellulitis or osteomyelitis, but tend to heal well, with exuberant callus formation.[91] Oral bisphosphonates may have a place in the treatment of osteopenia and pathologic fractures in children with spina bifida.[107,150]

Mobility

"Will my child walk"? This is a burning question that most parents of a child with MMC have in infancy and early childhood. Although debated, there is generally agreement that early ambulation ability may carry with it physiologic and psychological benefits even though children may later lose that ability in adolescence or adulthood.[163,186] A study comparing the effects of an early walking program versus early wheelchair mobility noted fewer fractures, pressure sores, and greater independence and ability to transfer in those who ambulated early in life.[106] Delay in achievement of ambulation can be expected in all children with MMC, regardless of level. Maintaining ambulation is often sought after, even when it is highly inefficient and time-consuming. Most patients with lumbar lesions will achieve some level of ambulation (household or community), but those with high lumbar lesions tend to lose it during adolescence.[186] The ability for a child to become ambulatory and to maintain ambulatory function is determined by a number of factors, including lesion level, cognitive ability, motivation, musculoskeletal complications, growth, age, and obesity.[7]

According to the Hoffer criteria (Box 48-3), ambulatory function can be divided into four groups: community ambulation, household ambulation, exercise or nonfunctional ambulation, and nonambulation/nonwalkers.[80] In general, most patients with sacral-level involvement are community ambulators and those with thoracic-level involvement are nonambulators (see Table 48-2). The most important predictors of ambulation ability are quadriceps strength, iliopsoas strength, and the ability to achieve independent sitting, which is also a predictor of ambulatory potential in patients with higher levels of involvement.[163] The ability to maintain ambulation ability into adulthood is dependent on quadriceps and hamstring strength.[110,146] The Functional Mobility Scale (FMS) that was developed by Graham et al.[68] in 2004 to assess functional ability in children with cerebral palsy and allows for a quick scoring of mobility over three distinct distances representing mobility in the home (5 m), at school (50 m), and in the community (500 m) is also useful for functional classification of patients with spina bifida.[163] The

BOX 48-3

Hoffer Ambulation Criteria

Hoffer Classification of Ambulation and Criteria

I. **Community ambulators:** Patients walk indoors and outdoors for most activities; may need crutches, braces, or both. Wheelchair used only for long trips out of the community.

II. **Household ambulators:** Patients walk only indoors and with orthoses. Able to get in and out of chair and bed with little, if any, assistance. May use wheelchair for some indoor activities at home and school. Wheelchair is used for all activities in the community.

III. **Nonfunctional ambulators:** Patients walk during therapy session at home, in school, or in hospital. Wheelchair used for all other transportation.

IV. **Nonambulators:** Patients are mobile only via a wheelchair but usually can transfer from chair to bed.

Functional mobility scale

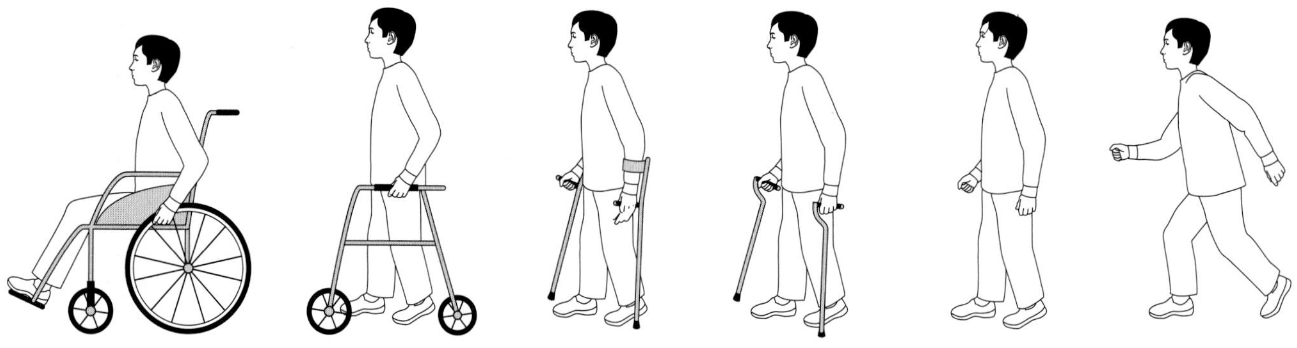

Rating 1	Rating 2	Rating 3	Rating 4	Rating 5	Rating 6
Wheelchair reliant for all ambulation	Independent ambulation with walkers or frame	Independent ambulation with bilateral crutches	Independent ambulation with single crutch or bilateral/single hand-held cane	Independent ambulation on level surfaces without assistive device	
May do some supported standing or take steps with walker/hand-held support to facilitate transfers			Holds on to furniture/ walls for support in home	Requires rail for stairs, may need help running	

FIGURE 48-7 Functional Mobility Scale: Scoring of mobility over three distinct distances representing mobility in the home, school, and community. (Data from Battibugli S, Gryfakis N, Dias L, et al: Functional gait comparison between children with myelomeningocele: shunt versus no shunt, *Dev Med Child Neurol* 49:764-769, 2007; Guidera KJ, Smith S, Raney E, et al: Use of the reciprocating gait orthosis in myelodysplasia, *J Pediatr Orthop* 13:341-348, 1993; Uehling DT, Smith J, Meyer J, et al: Impact of an intermittent catheterization program on children with myelomeningocele, *Pediatrics* 76:892-895, 1985.)

FMS was used by Battibugli et al.[12] in evaluating children with MMC, and they noted that for similar lesion levels children without shunts tend to walk at a significantly greater velocity and stride length compared with those with a shunt (Figure 48-7).

Orthoses

The typical four goals or objectives in prescribing an orthotic device for a child with MMC are:

1. To prevent deformity.
2. To support normal joint alignment and mechanics.
3. To control range of motion during gait.
4. To improve function.

An orthotic device is prescribed to address one or even all of these goals. An AFO is the most commonly prescribed orthotic device for children with MMC.

Three bracing systems are used that are relatively unique to the child with MMC. The parapodium is a device that allows even the child with thoracic-level involvement an opportunity for upright mobility. It offers structural support from the trunk to the floor and children use a swing-to pattern for ambulation. A swivel walker is a modification of the parapodium that translates trunk rotation into forward movement of a dual footplate mechanism. Finally, a reciprocating gait orthosis (RGO) combines bilateral hip-knee-ankle-foot orthosis (HKAFO) with a cable system to coordinate hip flexion with hip extension at the opposite hip. Active hip flexion is required to use this type of orthosis. An energy consumption study was performed on three children comparing the use of an RGO with a swing-through type of gait pattern. The swing-through gait was more efficient, but all three children preferred the RGO.[74] None of these orthoses allow for efficient gait, but they are often used by smaller children for upright mobility.

Skin Breakdown

Skin breakdown is a very common occurrence in children and adults with MMC. Countless dollars are spent treating what should be a preventable complication. In one clinic, 50% of patients had skin breakdown. Of these, 42% were attributed to excessive pressure. In this group, the prevalence steadily increased between infancy and 10 years of age.[126] Other factors contributing to the development of pressure sores include cognitive impairment, chronic soiling, and lack of parental involvement. Morbidity associated with pressure sores can be severe, including risk of amputation of feet and limbs.

Skin breakdown usually occurs as a result of pressure areas over bony prominences but can also be caused by hot or cold injury, shear, or tightly fitting clothes. Pressure sores in nonambulatory patients often occur over the sacrum, the ischial tuberosities, and the greater trochanters. Another common site is over a gibbus deformity, usually in patients with a thoracic-level lesion. In ambulatory patients, pressure sores usually occur on their feet and are often associated with poorly fitting orthoses.

Prevention of skin breakdown requires ongoing education of the patient and family about insensate skin, hygiene, pressure relief, proper skin inspection, wearing schedules for new or modified orthoses, and appropriate seating surfaces. School personnel also need to be aware of the risk of skin problems so they can help to remind children to perform pressure relief.

The combination of localized wound care, nutrition, and pressure relief is the most effective treatment of pressure sores. Occasionally, surgical procedures are required to debride and close open wounds. Primary closures or skin flaps are preferred over myocutaneous procedures for initial wounds.

Obesity

Obesity has achieved national attention in the able-bodied population. Obesity rates for children and adolescents with spina bifida are similar to the general population; however, obesity rates are higher among adults with spina bifida (38%), particularly in women.[53] Children with MMC have a lower metabolic rate and lower energy expenditure, which predisposes them to obesity. In addition to the obvious functional decline as a result of obesity, individuals with spina bifida and other forms of spinal cord injury are at risk for developing metabolic syndrome along with the associated problems of heart disease and diabetes.[124] Dietary management and daily physical activity should be encouraged from infancy and early toddlerhood because outcomes from weight reduction programs are poor.

Psychological and Social Issues

Cognitive Function

Parents of children with MMC rate their medical support much higher than they do the support received for psychosocial problems.[48] Children with MMC have specific behavioral and cognitive issues that need to be addressed or at least recognized by parents, health care providers, and school personnel. As a group, children with MMC have lower intelligence quotient (IQ) scores compared with their able-bodied peers and usually demonstrate a higher verbal IQ compared with their performance IQ. They also have more difficulty with math and visual perceptual tasks than their able-bodied peers and are deficient in text level reading fluency and comprehension despite showing mastery with single words and having good sight vocabulary.[11,48,135] Studies comparing IQ scores are inconsistent, but in general correlate with the level of lesion. Children with thoracic-level lesions tend to have lower IQ scores than children with lumbar- or sacral-level lesions. IQ scores are adversely affected by central nervous system infections, but not necessarily by recurrent shunt revisions.[64,76,135] With more recent advances in radioimaging techniques and an improved understanding of the differences in anomalous brain development in higher versus lower spinal lesions in individuals with spina bifida, variations can be identified in the neural phenotype, which along with differing environmental factors results in variability of the cognitive phenotype. There are three core deficits thought to be a direct consequence of the Chiari II malformation described in spina bifida: attention, timing, and movement. Deficits in attention relate to problems in the midbrain, posterior cortex, and corpus callosum, whereas timing deficits are related to cerebellar volume and movement deficits to spinal cord dysfunction and cerebellar dysmorphology affecting sensorimotor timing and motor regulation.[48,64]

Behavior

Children with MMC often have rather characteristic personality traits. Many of them have much better verbal skills than written skills. Verbose, but irrelevant conversation (cocktail party chatter) is often described and they will often speak off-topic and use many routine social phrases. These personality traits often cause misconceptions about the child's mental abilities.[89,178]

The temperament characteristics of children with MMC and shunted hydrocephalus were recently described. Children with MMC were found to be less adaptable, more withdrawn, more distractible, less attentive, and less predictable than those in the control group.[89,178]

Keep in mind that a variety of factors affect psychosocial functioning and adjustment to disability in individuals with spina bifida (Figure 48-8) when developing a treatment plan.[9] It behooves multidisciplinary clinics to include a psychologist/social worker as a core member of the treatment team to gain a deeper understanding of the cognitive assets of the youth with MMC and the different factors that may be influencing psychosocial functioning.

Myelomeningocele in Adults

Transition to Adult Health Care

As a result of advances in medical care, 75% to 85% of individuals with MMC now survive into early adulthood.[46,50,119] These individuals can experience secondary complications from accelerated impairment as a result of aging and progression of their underlying disease process.[93] Although children are generally observed closely by their pediatric physicians and often in multidisciplinary clinics, adults with MMC often do not have regular medical follow-up that is comprehensive in nature.[121] In comparing outcomes in young adults who had been followed in a multidisciplinary clinic versus those who lacked coordinated care, it was clear that outcomes were considerably worse in the latter with over 66% of the adults even lacking regular medical and specialty care.[95] There remains great need for evaluation of transitional models using controlled trials to determine approaches that will improve medium and long-term outcomes.

General Issues, Health, and Participation

The World Health organization has developed a model, the International Classification of Functioning and Disability (ICF), which evaluates body functions and structure, activity and social participation in the context of environmental and personal influences[190a] (Figure 48-9). Focus on this model helps clinicians assess overall functioning rather than focus solely on medical conditions, thus broadening the scope of interventions for improving overall health and quality of life.

Health conditions that are routinely monitored in adults include hypertension, diabetes, hyperlipidemia, osteoporosis, cancer, sexually transmitted diseases, to name a few. Individuals with spina bifida are at higher risk for hypertension and this may be a problem as early as in

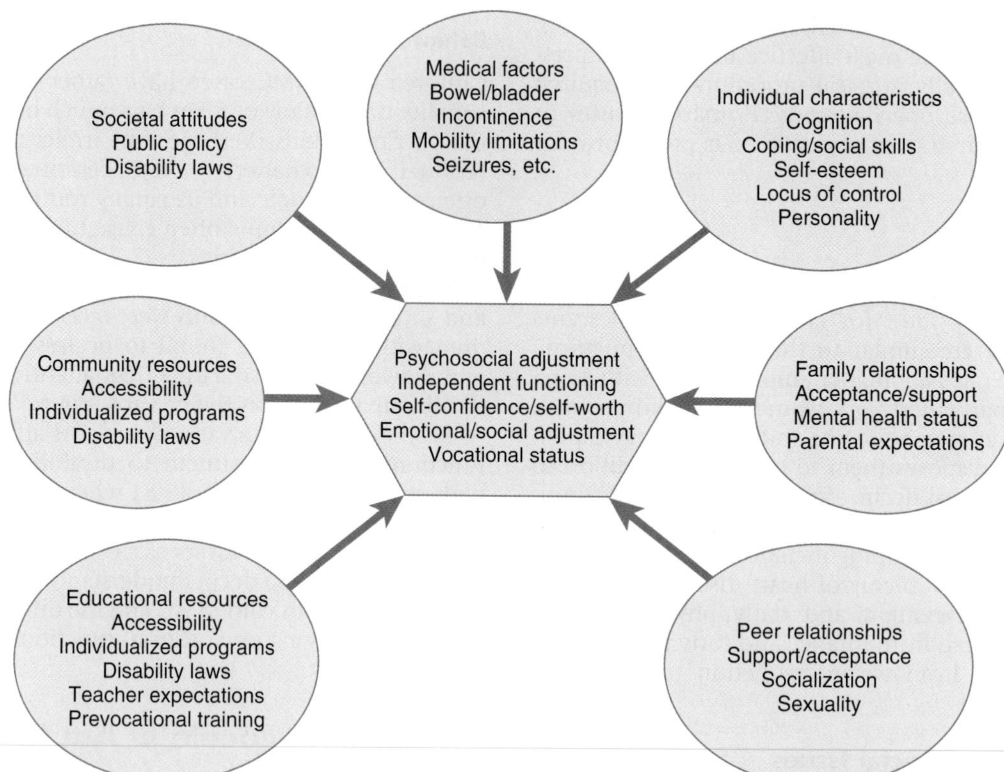

FIGURE 48-8 Factors influencing psychosocial adjustment and disability in individuals with spina bifida. (Adapted from Ayyangar R: Health maintenance and management in childhood disability, *Phys Med Rehabil Clin N Am* 13:793-821, 2002.)

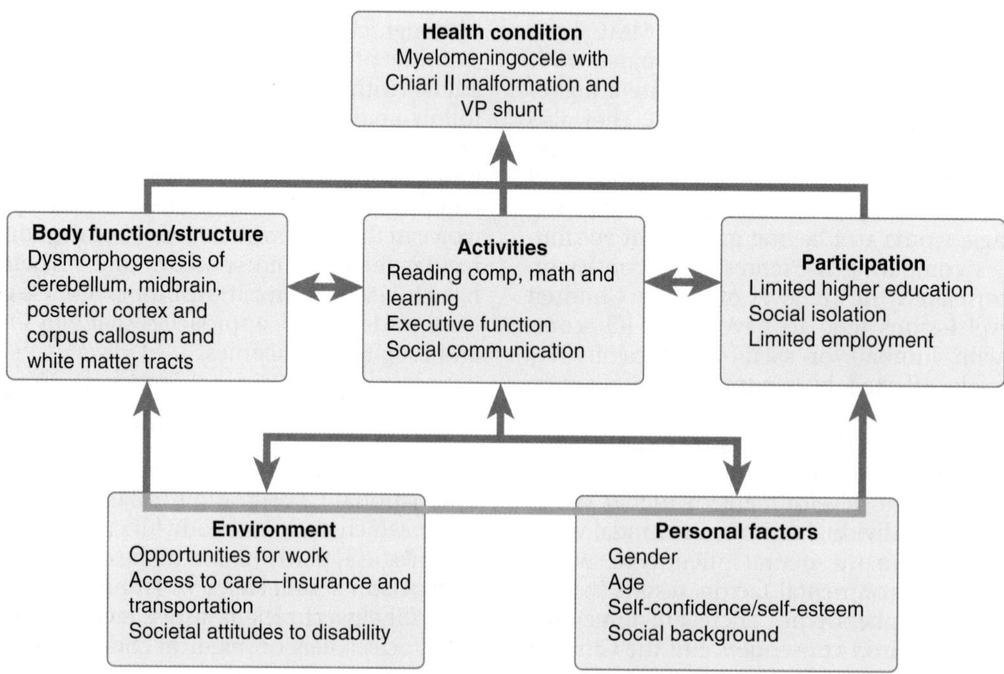

FIGURE 48-9 The International Classification of Disability and Function (ICF) provides a framework to determine the interplay of factors affecting function in individuals with myelomeningocele. *VP*, Ventriculoperitoneal.

the teenage years. Obesity and sleep apnea are common in individuals with MMC. Adults with neurogenic bladder and spina bifida are at an increased risk for bladder cancer. Those who have had bladder augmentation with ileal or colonic segments have a seven- to eight-fold risk and those with gastric augmentation have a fourteen- to fifteen-fold risk for the development of bladder cancer compared with the population at large.[86,101]

Late Neurologic Changes

Adults with MMC remain at risk for developing neurologic complications of their disease. Complications seen in adults include VP shunt infections and malfunctions, syringomyelia, symptomatic tethered cord, and symptomatic type II Chiari malformation. Adolescents and adults with MMC continue to require shunting.[103] Up to 10% of adults with VP shunts can develop chronic idiopathic headaches requiring specialized pain management, although at presentation headaches should always receive a comprehensive evaluation to rule out life-threatening causes.[54] Likewise, adults with MMC can develop syringomyelia, presenting with complaints of pain, paresthesias, and weakness in the upper limbs. They may develop symptomatic tethering of the spinal cord necessitating surgical release, again highlighting the importance of transition and continued follow-up.[133] Entrapment syndromes, overuse syndromes, and herniated disks need to be considered in the differential diagnosis of upper limb symptoms in adults more so than in children. An incidence of seizures ranging from 3% to 23% in the adult population has also been reported and is thought to be multifactorial in origin.[180]

Late Musculoskeletal Considerations

Dicianno et al.[50] summarized musculoskeletal considerations in adults with spina bifida. Because data regarding this population specifically are very limited, much of the information is gleaned from the population with spinal cord injury. Shoulder pain is very common in wheelchair users, although it might be less common in patients who began using a wheelchair earlier in life.[144,180] Rotator cuff disorders and bicipital tendonitis are the most common injuries in chronic wheelchair users.[62] Physiatrists and therapists can play a key role in prevention and treatment of chronic shoulder problems.

Charcot joints can develop in the lower limbs as a result of lack of sensation and demineralization. They are most common in the foot and ankle followed by the hip and knee. Although more typical in older patients, an unusual case of a 5-year-old patient with MMC who developed a Charcot arthropathy of the elbow has been reported.[193] Charcot joints can lead to significant decline in functional status. Appropriate bracing is necessary to limit movement in affected joints.

The ambulation status of adults with spina bifida has been shown to deteriorate.[50] Factors explaining this loss of function can include spasticity, knee and hip flexion contractures, low back pain, lack of motivation, or medical complications.

Renal and Urologic Damage

With the high prevalence of bladder dysfunction in individuals with spina bifida, renal damage remains one of the most common causes of morbidity and mortality among individuals with MMC.[120] Affected adults should receive ongoing urologic care to achieve or maintain social continence and normal renal function. Bowman et al.[19] reported that up to 80% of adults attained social bladder continence with proper management. As previously mentioned in this chapter, bladder cancer rates may be considerably higher in those with bladder augmentation procedures as well as those who have had over 10 years of Foley catheter use. Further studies are needed to properly evaluate the effectiveness of both proactive and observational approaches to urologic management, but it is clear that adults with MMC require regular urologic assessment to optimize outcomes.[50]

Fertility, Sexuality, and Reproductive Issues

Few studies elucidate issues related to fertility, sexuality, and satisfaction with sexual function among individuals with MMC. Despite this, there are some facts that can guide clinicians in caring for and advising patients. Menstruation and fertility among women with MMC are thought to be normal, and affected individuals are capable of becoming pregnant.[189] Complications can be experienced during pregnancy related to recurrent urinary tract infection, worsening kyphoscoliosis, VP shunt malfunction, and failure of genitourinary diversions. Vaginal delivery is generally indicated, especially in those with a VP shunt, and cesarean section should be performed only for obstetric reasons such as a contracted, underdeveloped pelvis.[137] Many men with MMC are infertile and demonstrate poor semen quality but appear capable of reproducing with assisted reproductive technologies.[61,84] In addition, boys display a 15% to 25% incidence of cryptorchidism, further contributing to infertility.[84,189,189a] Regardless, male and female patients with MMC should receive both basic and specialized sex education, particularly as it pertains to their increased risk of having a child with an NTD. It is recommended that women with MMC of childbearing age take 4 mg of folic acid daily to prevent having an affected child.[156]

The degree of satisfaction with sexual function among individuals with MMC is unclear, although a recent Danish study of 53 women and men with spina bifida by von Linstow et al.[183] demonstrated that 51% of participants regarded their sexual life as a failure or dysfunctional. It was however encouraging that 45% reported being satisfied with their sexual life especially those who had partners. Fecal, but not urinary, incontinence was associated with poorer sexual function and less satisfaction. In addition, there were long-lasting effects of sex education provided in teenage years because nearly 50% of the participants reported that it was useful.[183]

Both men and women generally have decreased sensation in the perineum, which can impair the ability to reach orgasm. In addition, nonverbal learning disorders and societal attitudes toward individuals with disabilities can affect self-esteem, social interactions, and ultimately psychosexual development. The reported incidence of the ability to achieve erection ranges from 14% in those with higher-level lesions to 85% in those with lower-level lesions, although many of these are achieved reflexively.[49,145] The ability to sustain these erections during intercourse is uncertain, and many patients report dissatisfaction with the degree of rigidity. Normally, penile sensory input transmits via the two dorsal nerves of the penis and the pudendal nerve to the S2 to S4 roots, but this is disrupted in spina bifida. Improved sensation of the glans penis has been reported after the TOMAX (to maximize sensation, sexuality, and quality of life) microneurography procedure where the ilioinguinal nerve is joined to the dorsal nerve.[127a] Lesions above the level of sympathetic outflow, as well as a negative anocutaneous reflex, are correlated with increased difficulty achieving erection.[49,145] Verhoef et al.[181] and Cardenas et al.[28] reported that women with spina bifida were more than twice as sexually active as men with spina bifida. Treatment of erectile dysfunction in men with MMC with sildenafil (Viagra) has been successful. Both men and women can experience skin breakdown during sexual intercourse and should be educated in this regard. Further research is needed to more properly address this topic.

Educational Issues, Vocational Issues, and Independent Living

Most adolescents with MMC complete high school and approximately 50% move on to further education. Although little is published regarding the educational levels achieved, employment status, or living situation of persons with MMC, one long-term follow-up survey reported that 85% of children who survived to adulthood either attended or graduated from high school and/or college, with 36% requiring special education services. Forty-five percent of participants were employed, and 15% lived independently.[19] Another study reported more specifically that the college graduation rate was only 14.6% for their cohort.[85] A Canadian study of individuals with spina bifida and cerebral palsy revealed that transportation was a major barrier to employment; fewer females were employed; and employment was inversely related to IQ.[105] Other studies have reported rates of independent living ranging from 14% to 41%.[179] Rates of employment range from 25% to 62.5%, depending on the criteria being considered, including intelligence, academic qualifications, behavior, continence, and severity of physical disability.[179] A study of young adults from The Netherlands reported that only 16% of those with spina bifida were living independently; 53% of those who finished secondary education were employed; and 71% did not have a partner.[10] These studies provide further support for the use of the ICF model in directing transition efforts so that environmental factors affecting functioning of individuals with spina bifida are addressed.

Palliative Care and Neural Tube Defects

Anencephaly and craniorachischisis are two defects that are not compatible with life. Diagnosis of a lethal fetal diagnosis early in pregnancy is devastating for parents. They may choose to continue with the pregnancy or choose termination of pregnancy attributable to a fetal anomaly. Either way, they experience intense emotional reactions and often report inconsistent and frequently insensitive treatment by health care providers.[190] A qualitative study designed to explore these responses noted the emergence of two dimensions and six themes as follows[41]:

Dimension I: Personal Pregnancy Experience

1. "Grieving Multiple Losses:" Parents grieve the loss of their normal pregnancy, healthy baby, and future parenting.
2. "Arrested Parenting:" Describes the emotions and stresses associated with sudden interruption in the normal process of becoming a parent.
3. "My Baby is a Person:" Reflects parents' unanimous desire to honor and legitimize the humanity of their unborn baby.

Dimension II: Interactions of Others

4. "Fragmented Health Care:" Describes parents' disjointed and distant encounters with multiple providers.
5. "Disconnected Family and Friends:" Describes their sense of a lack of understanding of their experience by even people close to them.
6. "Utterly Alone:" Describes the sense of social isolation that develops that further compounds their personal sense of loss and associated grief.

Perinatal palliative care begins soon after diagnosis, follows through the decision-making process, involves a family birthing plan, and extends into the bereavement period. This approach helps parents feel supported and results in positive outcomes.[41]

Similarly, the palliative care model emphasizing comfort and addressing medical as well as psychological and spiritual needs may be applied at various decision-making junctures in the lifespan care of individuals with MMC.

Summary

Preventive measures, especially folic acid supplementation, have a protective effect against NTDs. However, we still need to improve our understanding of other factors that may lead to this disorder. The majority of fetuses with meningomyelocele are live-born and with proper treatment survival to adulthood is common. MMC presents lifelong challenges to affected patients, their families, and clinicians. Vigilant surveillance and education are required to prevent life-threatening events and to decrease morbidity related to VP shunt malfunction, Chiari II malformation, renal failure, latex allergy, and infection. This must be carried out in an environment that also seeks to maximize the functional independence of individuals with MMC by monitoring for decline in motor examination, preventing deformity, training in self-care and independent mobility, teaching independence with a bowel and bladder program, giving emotional and social support, and providing educational and vocational guidance. The ICF model of functioning should be kept in mind in caring for individuals across the lifespan, addressing not only the medical but also other contextual factors so that function and participation are maximized.

For more information about MMC, contact the Spina Bifida Association of America through their website at www.sbaa.org; by e-mail at sbaa@sbaa.org; by mail at P.O. Box 17427 Arlington, VA 22216; or by telephone at (202) 944-3285 and facsimile at (202) 944-3295.

KEY REFERENCES

6. Apkon SD, Grady R, Hart S, et al: Advances in the care of children with spina bifida, *Pediatrics* 61:33–74, 2014.
8. Au KS, Ashley-Koch A, Northrup H: Epidemiologic and genetic aspects of spina bifida and other neural tube defects, *Dev Disabil Res Rev* 16:6–15, 2010.
9. Ayyangar R: Health maintenance and management in childhood disability, *Phys Med Rehabil Clin N Am* 13:793–821, 2002.
11a. Bartonek A, Saraste H, Knutson LM: Comparison of different systems to classify the neurological level of lesion in patients with myelomeningocele, *Dev Med Child Neurol* 41:796–805, 1999.
19. Bowman RM, McLone DG, Grant JA, et al: Spina bifida outcome: a 25-year prospective, *Pediatr Neurosurg* 34:114–120, 2001.
23. Broughton NS, Menelaus MB, Cole WG, et al: The natural history of hip deformity in myelomeningocele, *J Bone Joint Surg Br* 75:760–763, 1993.
26. Canfield MA, Ramadhani TA, Shaw GM, et al: Anencephaly and spina bifida among Hispanics: maternal, sociodemographic, and acculturation factors in the National Birth Defects Prevention Study, *Birth Defects Res A Clin Mol Teratol* 85:637–646, 2009.
28. Cardenas DD, Topolski TD, White CJ, et al: Sexual functioning in adolescents and young adults with spina bifida, *Arch Phys Med Rehabil* 89:31–35, 2008.
30. Centers for Disease Control and Prevention: *Spina bifida data and statistics*. www.cdc.gov/ncbddd/spinabifida/data.html.
36. Coggrave M, Norton C, Cody JD: Management of faecal incontinence and constipation in adults with central neurological diseases, *Cochrane Database Syst Rev* (1):CD002115, 2014.
38. Copp AJ, Greene ND: Neural tube defects—disorders of neurulation and related embryonic processes, *Dev Biol* 2:213–227, 2013.
44. Czeizel AE, Dudas I: Prevention of the first occurrence of neural-tube defects by periconceptional vitamin supplementation, *N Engl J Med* 327:1832–1835, 1992.
46. Davis BE, Daley CM, Shurtleff DB, et al: Long term survival of individuals with myelomeningocele, *Pediatr Neurosurg* 41:186–191, 2005.
48. Dennis M, Landry SH, Barnes M, et al: A model of neurocognitive function in spina bifida over the life span, *J Int Neuropsychol Soc* 12:285–296, 2006.
50. Dicianno BE, Kurowski BG, Yang JM, et al: Rehabilitation and medical management of the adult with spina bifida, *Am J Phys Med Rehabil* 87:1027–1050, 2008.
63. Fletcher JM, Brei TJ: Introduction: spina bifida—a multidisciplinary perspective, *Dev Disabil Res Rev* 16:1–5, 2010.
68. Graham HK, Harvey A, Rodda J, et al: The Functional Mobility Scale (FMS), *J Pediatr Orthop* 24:514–520, 2004.
71. Greene ND, Stanier P, Copp A: Genetics of human neural tube defects, *Hum Mol Genet* 18(R2):R113–R129, 2009.
73. Grivell RM, Andersen C, Dodd JM: Prenatal versus postnatal repair procedures for spina bifida for improving infant and maternal outcomes, *Cochrane Database Syst Rev* (10):CD008825, 2014.
89. Kelly NC, Ammerman RT, Rausch JR, et al: Executive functioning and psychological adjustment in children and youth with spina bifida, *Child Neuropsychol* 18:417–431, 2012.
93. Klingbeil H, Baer HR, Wilson PE: Aging with a disability, *Arch Phys Med Rehabil* 85(7, Suppl 3):S68–S73, quiz S74–S75, 2004.
95. Le JT, Mukherjee S: Transition to adult care for patients with spina bifida, *Phys Med Rehabil Clin N Am* 26:29–38, 2015.
103. Lorber J, Pucholt V: When is a shunt no longer necessary? An investigation of 300 patients with hydrocephalus and myelomeningocele: 11-22 year follow up, *Z Kinderchir* 34:327–329, 1981.
113. McLone DG, Knepper PA: The cause of Chiari II malformation: a unified theory, *Pediatr Neurosci* 15:1–12, 1989.
115. Medical Research Council Vitamin Study Research Group: Prevention of neural tube defects: results of the Medical Research Council Vitamin Study, *Lancet* 338:131–137, 1991.
118. Mourtzinos A, Stoffel JT: Management goals for the spina bifida neurogenic bladder: a review from infancy to adulthood, *Urol Clin North Am* 37:527–535, 2010.
131. Pfeiffer CM, Hughes JP, Lacher DA, et al: Estimation of trends in serum and RBC folate in the United States population from pre- to post-fortification using assay-adjusted data from the NHANES 1988-2010, *J Nutr* 142:886–893, 2012.
132. Phuong LK, Schoeberl KA, Raffel C: Natural history of tethered cord in patients with meningomyelocele, *Neurosurgery* 50:989–993, discussion 993–995, 2002.
133. Piatt JH, Jr: Treatment of myelomeningocele: a review of outcomes and continuing neurosurgical considerations among adults, *J Neurosurg Pediatr* 6:515–525, 2010.
146. Seitzberg A, Lind M, Biering-Sørensen F: Ambulation in adults with myelomeningocele. Is it possible to predict the level of ambulation in early life? *Childs Nerv Syst* 24:231–237, 2008.
153. Smithells RW, Sheppard S, Schorah CJ: Vitamin deficiencies and neural tube defects, *Arch Dis Child* 51:944–950, 1976.
158. Steinbok P, Irvine B, Cochrane DD, et al: Long-term outcome and complications of children born with meningomyelocele, *Childs Nerv Syst* 8:92–96, 1992.
159. Stevenson KL: Chiari type II malformation: past, present, and future, *Neurosurg Focus* 16:E5, 2004.
160. Stothard KJ, Tennant PW, Bell R, Rankin J: Maternal overweight and obesity and the risk of congenital anomalies: a systematic review and meta-analysis, *JAMA* 301:636–650, 2009.
163. Swaroop VT, Dias L: Orthopedic management of spina bifida. Part I: hip, knee, and rotational deformities, *J Child Orthop* 3:441–449, 2009.
164. Swaroop VT, Dias L: Orthopaedic management of spina bifida. Part II: foot and ankle deformities, *J Child Orthop* 5:403–414, 2011.
166. Tarcan T, Onol FF, Ilker Y, et al: The timing of primary neurosurgical repair significantly affects neurogenic bladder prognosis in children with myelomeningocele, *J Urol* 176:1161–1165, 2006.
169. Tortori-Donati P, Rossi A, Cama A: Spinal dysraphism: a review of neuroradiological features with embryological correlations and proposal for a new classification, *Neuroradiology* 42:471–491, 2000.
170. Trivedi J, Thomson JD, Slakey JB, et al: Clinical and radiographic predictors of scoliosis in patients with myelomeningocele, *J Bone Joint Surg Am* 84:1389–1394, 2002.
171. Trollmann R, Bakker B, Lundberg M, et al: Growth in pre-pubertal children with myelomeningocele (MMC) on growth hormone (GH): the KIGS experience, *Pediatr Rehabil* 9:144–148, 2006.
176. Tuli S, Drake J, Lamberti-Pasculli M: Long-term outcome of hydrocephalus management in myelomeningoceles, *Childs Nerv Syst* 19:286–291, 2003.
182. Verhoef M, Lurvink M, Barf HA, et al: High prevalence of incontinence among young adults with spina bifida: description, prediction and problem perception, *Spinal Cord* 43:331–340, 2005.
183. von Linstow ME, Biering-Sørensen I, Liebach A, et al: Spina bifida and sexuality, *J Rehabil Med* 46:891–897, 2014.
184. Wallingford JB, Niswander LA, Shaw GM, et al: The continuing challenge of understanding and preventing neural tube defects, *Science* 339:1222002, 2013.
185. Deleted in review.
186. Williams EN, Broughton NS, Menelaus MB: Age-related walking in children with spina bifida, *Dev Med Child Neurol* 41:446–449, 1999.
187. Williams J, Mai CT, Mulinare J, et al: Updated estimates of neural tube defects prevented by mandatory folic acid fortification—United States, 1995-2011, *MMWR Morb Mortal Wkly Rep* 64:1–5, 2015.
190. Wool C: Systematic review of the literature: parental outcomes after diagnosis of fetal anomaly, *Adv Neonatal Care* 11:182–192, 2011.
190a. World Health Organization: *Towards a common language for functioning, disability and health*. www.who.int/classifications/icf/icfbeginnersguide.pdf?ua=1.
191. Wu HY, Baskin LS, Kogan BA: Neurogenic bladder dysfunction due to myelomeningocele: neonatal versus childhood treatment, *J Urol* 157:2295–2297, 1997.
192. Yamada S, Won DJ, Yamada SM: Pathophysiology of tethered cord syndrome: correlation with symptomatology, *Neurosurg Focus* 16:E6, 2004.

The full reference list for this chapter is available online.

CHAPTER 49

SPINAL CORD INJURY

Thomas N. Bryce

Historical Perspective

Before the mid-part of the twentieth century, injury to the spinal cord was synonymous with death, either instantly or after a period of great suffering.

The Edwin Smith Surgical Papyrus, written almost 5000 years ago, contains descriptions of cases of cervical spinal cord injury (SCI), among other traumatic injuries, along with recommended treatments. With regard to the cases of cervical SCI, the author noted that those cases represent "an ailment not to be treated."[44] During the early nineteenth century, Lord Nelson, the Admiral of the British Fleet, received a gunshot wound to his chest during the Battle of Trafalgar. He was taken immediately to the ship's surgeon to whom he noted, "All power of motion and feeling below my chest are gone." The surgeon's reply was, "My lord, unhappily for our Country, nothing can be done for you." Later in the century, the president of the United States, James A. Garfield, experienced a gunshot wound to the conus medullaris, he did not survive more than 3 months.[46]

During the early part of the twentieth century, the prognosis for surviving SCI remained poor. During World War I, 80% of all American soldiers with SCI died within 2 weeks, the 20% surviving longer having incomplete injuries. The mortality of British soldiers who sustained SCI at this time was better than that of the Americans; however, an estimated 80% were also dead by 3 years.

During the 1930s and 1940s, management of SCI finally started to change when a few individuals, beginning with Donald Monro in the United States and followed by Sir Ludwig Guttman in the United Kingdom, both neurosurgeons, began to comprehensively address the whole person with SCI. They not only began programs to teach people with SCI self-care and mobility with a goal of reintegrating into society but also addressed all the organ systems involved with SCI (e.g., neurologic, skeletal, urologic) to prevent complications. Each developed SCI units, which became models for comprehensive centers around the globe over succeeding decades.

Model Systems of Care

The difference in outcomes for people with SCI, when admitted to a dedicated SCI rehabilitation unit, was noticed by the leaders of health care at the same time that special trauma systems were being developed in the United States to treat injured people. The trauma systems required that injured people be handled at the scene of accident by well-trained emergency medical technicians using state-of-the-art equipment and transportation vehicles. The patients were subsequently to be triaged to a specially designated trauma center, which met strict criteria for emergency and acute trauma care, rather than taking them to the nearest hospital. The success of disease-specific units and trauma systems highlighted that inadequate training, experience, and number of staff, as well as lack of appropriate facilities and equipment, not only placed the life of a person with SCI at risk but often resulted in development of complications and poor functional outcomes. It was therefore hypothesized that if optimal care was provided from the very onset of major disabling injury and for as long as primary and secondary medical problems and disability last, functional outcomes would be improved and the cost of care would be reduced.

Based on this hypothesis, the U.S. government began to fund several SCI Model Systems of Care beginning in 1970. In 2014, there were 14 such systems funded by the National Institute on Disability and Rehabilitation Research (NIDRR), U.S. Department of Education. Each funded system had to meet four basic requirements. First, it had to have several integrated clinical components: emergency medical services; a level 1 trauma center; comprehensive rehabilitation services for both inpatients and outpatients, including vocational and job placement services; and lifelong follow-up and health maintenance programs. Second, each funded system had to collect data on all patients served and forward these to a National SCI Model System Database. Third, each system was required to conduct research consistent with NIDRR-announced priorities. Fourth, each system had to disseminate the research and demonstration findings as widely as possible to the appropriate audiences.

As a result, the SCI Model Systems have been instrumental in developing standards of care and new treatments, and conducting epidemiologic, health services, and outcomes research, as well as producing thousands of publications and training materials. The National SCI Database has been in existence since 1973 and includes data regarding approximately 30,000 people with SCI.[88]

Subspecialty of Spinal Cord Injury Medicine

Most physicians providing nonsurgical care for people with SCI in the United States have been physiatrists. In the past, most such physicians developed their special knowledge over a lengthy period by providing care rather than by specific training. A creation of a subspecialty of SCI medicine was first advocated in the late 1970s and gained momentum in the early 1990s. Through the concerted efforts of many individuals and organizations, the American Board of Medical Specialties gave its approval in 1995 for such a subspecialty be established. After successfully completing an Accreditation Council for Graduate Medical Education-accredited SCI Medicine fellowship and passing a written examination administered by the American Board of Physical Medicine and Rehabilitation (ABPMR), individuals receive SCI medicine subspecialty certification through the ABPMR. Several hundred individuals have been certified in the subspecialty since the first examination was held in 1999.

Epidemiology

Incidence and Prevalence

The recorded annual incidence of traumatic SCI is the highest in North America of all the developed regions of the world that have documented the problem. The incidence in the United States is approximately 56 cases per million population (or approximately 17,500 per year), whereas in Canada it is 53 cases per million.[90] In other developed regions of the world, the incidence is considerably lower varying from 24 to 19 cases per million in Spain and France, respectively, to between 12 and 14 cases per million within The Netherlands, Qatar, Ireland, Finland, and Australia.[14]

The exact number of people with SCI currently alive in the United States (prevalence) is a matter of dispute; however, given the similar incidences of SCI in Canada and the United States, an estimate of the prevalence based on data from Canada[14], where the prevalence is approximately 1298 cases per million, leads one to conclude there are over 430,000 individuals in the United States living with SCI, based on an estimated U.S. population of 317 million.[111]

Similar to the incidence data, the prevalence of traumatic SCI in other regions of the world is considerably lower ranging from a prevalence of 681 cases per million in Australia to 280 cases per million in Finland.[14]

Age at Time of Injury, Gender, and Marital Status

The incidence of traumatic SCI is bimodal being highest among young adults and older individuals (>65 years).[90] In the United States, the incidence of traumatic SCI in older adults (>65 years) approaches 90 cases per million. Furthermore, there is an increasing incidence of traumatic SCI in older adults that is not seen in any other age group throughout the world.[90] The mean age at injury has increased from 29 years in the 1970s in the United States to 42 years in the 2000s, exceeding slightly the increase in median age of the U.S. general population during this time.[38,89] The majority of traumatic SCI occurs in males, 70% to 80% overall depending on the database queried.[88,90] The ratio of male to female SCI is equal up until the age of 5 years after which the ratio begins to favor males, exceeding 80% for those between 16 and 20 years. However with age, especially in those older than 65 years, the ratio narrows again, with women accounting for 44% of SCI cases after the age of 65 years.

For those married at the time of SCI, the divorce rate is increased after SCI, as compared with that in the general population, especially during the first 3 postinjury years. The annual marriage rate is also lower for single individuals with SCI than for individuals without SCI.[37]

Causes of Spinal Cord Injury

The most common causes of SCI worldwide in descending order of incidence are transport crashes, falls, violence, and sports. This does vary among regions of the world, with transport crashes responsible for approximately 50% of cases in Europe and 40% of cases in North America, South East Asia, and the Mediterranean. Falls are responsible for approximately 30% of cases in North America and Europe but over 40% in South East Asia and the Mediterranean. Although transport crashes remain a significant cause of SCI in all age groups, falls are the most common cause of SCI in those above the age of 60 years. High falls (from >1 m) are more common in younger people, whereas low falls (from <1 m) are more common for those older than 45 years.[14] SCI in older individuals is often related to cervical spinal stenosis and is caused by a relatively minor trauma, such as a fall at home or in the street, or a low-velocity motor vehicle collision. Violence as a cause is also disparate in its presence, being responsible for approximately 14% of cases in the United States but less than 2% in Canada and Australia.[14]

The etiologies for children parallel those etiologies of younger adults with the exception of a greater percentage of injuries, over 30%, related to sports, with diving being the most common sports-related cause.[13] Sports lead to more SCI in boys than in girls only after the age of 13 years. Among those younger than 1 year of age who develop traumatic SCI, medical and surgical causes are most common, whereas for all those younger than 5 years of age, transport crashes account for approximately 65% of cases. Unique causes of SCI in children include lap belt injuries, birth injury, child abuse injuries, and craniovertebral junction injuries.

Children younger than 8 years have significantly higher incidences of SCI without radiologic abnormalities (SCIWORA), delayed onset of neurologic deficits (ranging from 0.5 hour to 4 days), and more neurologically complete lesions than those of older children and adults.[115] Among children younger than 10 years, SCIWORA is seen in 60%, but only in 20% of those who are older.[115]

Neonatal SCI is reported to occur in 1 of 60,000 births and is usually associated with breech presentations leading most commonly to a lower cervical or upper thoracic cord lesion.[91] Upper cervical SCI, however, is associated with a cephalic presentation and delivery.

Neurologic Level and Extent of Neurologic Deficit

According to both the National SCI Database (14 Model Systems of Care in the United States) and the Nationwide Emergency Department Sample (NEDS) Database (980 hospital-based emergency departments in 29 states of the

Table 49-1 Life Expectancy (Years) for People with Spinal Cord Injury Surviving at Least 24 Hours Postinjury

			Not Ventilator Dependent			
Current Age (years)	**No SCI**	**Motor Functional, Any Level**	**Paraplegia**	**Tetraplegia C5-C8**	**Tetraplegia C1-C4**	**Ventilator dependent, Any Level**
10	70	62	54	49	44	26
20	59	52	45	40	35	19
30	50	43	36	31	28	14
40	40	34	27	23	20	8
50	31	25	19	16	13	4
60	23	18	13	10	8	2
70	15	11	7	5	4	0.5
80	9	6	3	2	1	0.0

From National Spinal Cord Injury Statistical Center: *2012 Annual statistical report for the spinal cord injury model systems—complete public version*, Birmingham, 2013, University of Alabama at Birmingham.
SCI, Spinal cord injury.

United States), tetraplegia is more common than paraplegia accounting for 52% to 57% of SCI cases.[88,100] The percentages of cases that are complete injuries, 29% and 11% of SCI cases in the National SCI and NEDS databases, respectively, are notably different.[88,100] This is unsurprising given the composition of the contributing centers to each database.

Nevertheless, older individuals are more likely to have incomplete neurologic lesions, which is especially true for lesions in the cervical region.

Life Expectancy, Morbidity, and Causes of Death

Life expectancy for people with SCI remains below that of people without SCI. People with SCI are two to five times more likely to die prematurely.[14] The mortality rate is highest during the first postinjury year but declines significantly thereafter. Significant predictors of mortality include level and completeness of injury, age at time of injury, and requiring a ventilator for respiration. Additional factors that affect longevity after the first postinjury year include low life satisfaction, poor health, emotional distress, functional dependency, and poor adjustment to disability.[72] The National Spinal Cord Injury Statistical Center website provides annual updates on life expectancy after the onset of SCI, based on neurologic level and ventilatory dependency (Table 49-1). These life expectancy estimates do not include many important variables that can also significantly affect survival, such as gender, ethnicity, medical comorbidities, access to medical and nursing care, and social support.

Diseases of the respiratory system, especially pneumonia, are the leading cause of death both during the first postinjury year and during subsequent years (Box 49-1). The second most common cause of death, "other heart disease," is thought to reflect deaths that are apparently caused by heart attacks in younger people without apparent underlying heart or vascular disease and cardiac dysrhythmia.[37]

After SCI, older individuals (>65 years) have higher rates of complications, including pneumonia, respiratory insufficiency, pulmonary embolism (PE), renal stones, and gastrointestinal bleeding.[99]

BOX 49-1

Most Common Primary Causes of Death

Diseases of the respiratory system	22%
Infective and parasitic diseases	12%
Neoplasms	10%
Hypertensive and ischemic heart disease	10%
Other heart disease	9%
Unintentional injuries	7%
Diseases of digestive system	5%
Cerebrovascular disease	4%
Diseases of pulmonary circulation	4%
Suicides	4%

From National Spinal Cord Injury Statistical Center: *2012 Annual statistical report for the spinal cord injury model systems—complete public version*, Birmingham, 2013, University of Alabama at Birmingham.

Anatomy, Mechanics, and Syndromes of Traumatic Injury

Because the bony vertebral column elongates more than the spinal cord during embryologic development, the spinal cord terminates at the level of the L1-L2 intervertebral disk. As a result of natural variation, the spinal cord termination can be as high as the T12 or as low as the L3 vertebral body. The individual spinal cord segments do not line up with the corresponding bony levels of the same number (Figure 49-1). This is especially evident in the lower thoracic and lumbar spine, where the L1-L5 spinal segments are adjacent to the T11-T12 vertebrae, and the S1-S5 spinal segments are adjacent to the L1 vertebra. This concept can also be used when evaluating radiologic studies to correlate the neurologic level of injury (NLI) to the appropriate bony level of damage (e.g., a T11 burst fracture with cord compression would be expected to cause an NLI at L1 or L2 rather than at T11).

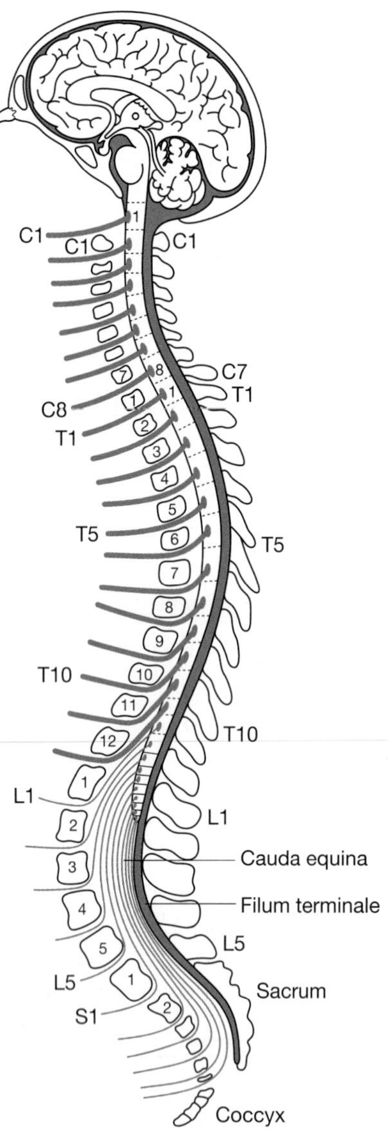

FIGURE 49-1 **A sagittal schematic showing the relationship between the numbered segments of the spinal cord and the corresponding numbered vertebral bodies.** (Redrawn from Pansky B, Allen D, Budd G: *Review of neuroscience*, ed 2, New York, 1998, McGraw-Hill, with permission of McGraw-Hill.)

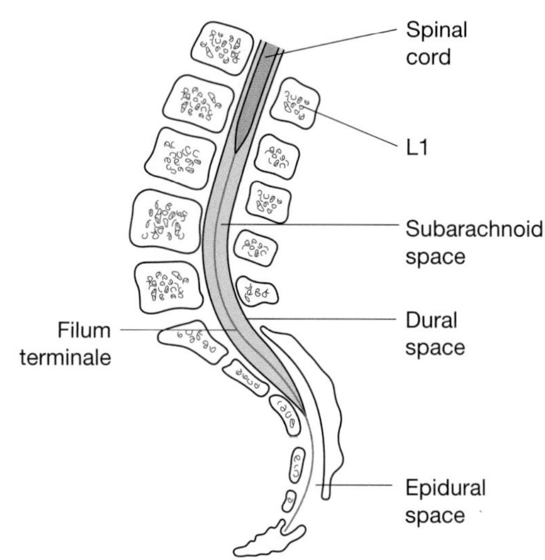

FIGURE 49-2 **A sagittal schematic showing the relationship between the dura, subarachnoid space, and the epidural space.** (Redrawn from Pansky B: *Review of gross anatomy*, ed 5, New York, 1984, Macmillan, with permission of Macmillan.)

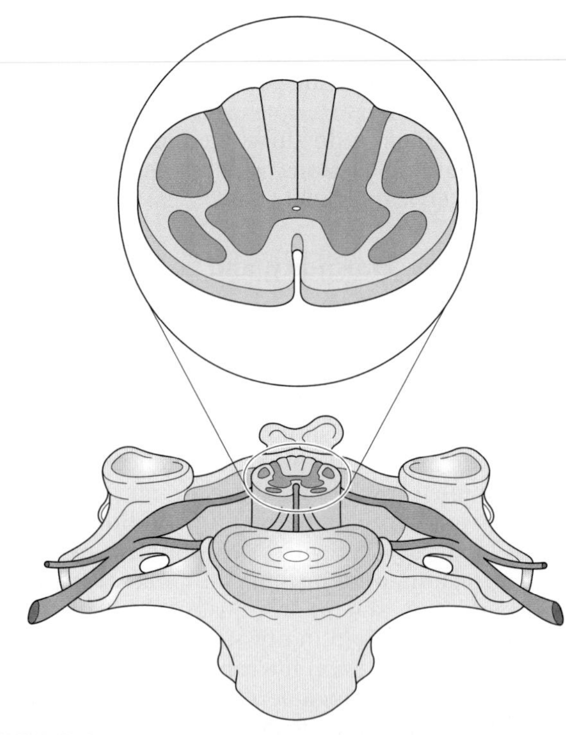

FIGURE 49-3 **Normal spinal cord. The corticospinal and spinothalamic tracts are outlined in the *upper diagram*, adjacent to the gray matter of the spinal cord.** (Redrawn from Tator C: Classification of spinal cord injury based on neurological presentation. In Narayan R, Wilberger J, Povlishock J, editors: *Neurotrauma*, New York, 1996, McGraw-Hill, with permission of McGraw-Hill.)

The tapered end of the spinal cord, which contains the sacral cord segments, is called the conus medullaris. The collection of long lumbar and sacral roots found in the canal, distal to the conus medullaris, is called the cauda equina, because it resembles a horse's tail. The meninges of the spinal cord include the pia mater, a vascular membrane covering the spinal cord, the arachnoid membrane, and the dura mater. The subarachnoid space, also called the intrathecal space, contains cerebrospinal fluid (CSF). The CSF pushes the arachnoid directly against the dura mater. The caudal margin of the dura mater and arachnoid, the inferior extent of the intrathecal space, is the second sacral vertebrae (Figure 49-2). The spinal epidural space is located between the dura mater and the periosteum of the vertebral bodies, and contains an internal vertebral venous plexus, fat, and loose areolar tissue.

A cross-sectional view of the spinal cord (Figure 49-3) reveals a central butterfly-shaped region of gray matter consisting of neuronal cell bodies, their processes, supporting glial cells, and small blood vessels surrounded by white matter consisting of neuronal fiber tracts and supporting glial cells. The gray matter is subdivided into two horns on each side called the anterior (ventral) and posterior (dorsal) horns. The posterior horn contains cell bodies of sensory neurons, whereas the anterior horn contains cell bodies of interneurons and motor neurons.

The white matter is subdivided into three columns on each side called the anterior, lateral, and posterior columns. The columns are further subdivided into tracts. The gracilis tract, located in the medial posterior column, contains fibers from the T7-S5 dermatomes that relay touch, vibration, and position sense. The cuneatus tract, located in the lateral posterior column rostral to T6, contains fibers from dermatomes above T7 that relay touch, vibration, and position sense. These tracts, comprising the posterior columns, ascend ipsilaterally to the medulla. The lateral spinothalamic tract, located peripherally in the lateral column, contains fibers that relay pain and temperature sensations; this tract ascends contralaterally to the thalamus. The lateral corticospinal tract is located centrally and posteriorly in the lateral column. This tract contains fibers, most of which emanate from the motor cortex, that are responsible for voluntary and reflex movement. Approximately 90% of the corticospinal fibers cross midline in the caudal medulla, forming the pyramidal decussations, and descend contralaterally in the lateral corticospinal tract to terminate on interneurons and alpha and gamma motor neurons in the spinal cord. The remaining corticospinal fibers, located in the medial anterior column, do not cross midline in the medulla but descend ipsilaterally in the anterior corticospinal tract. These fibers ultimately cross midline segmentally near their terminations on interneurons and alpha and gamma motor neurons in the spinal cord. A Brown-Séquard syndrome refers to an injury of the spinal cord in which one side is damaged more than the other (Figure 49-4), resulting in relatively greater ipsilateral weakness and position sense loss, but with contralateral pain and temperature sensation loss.

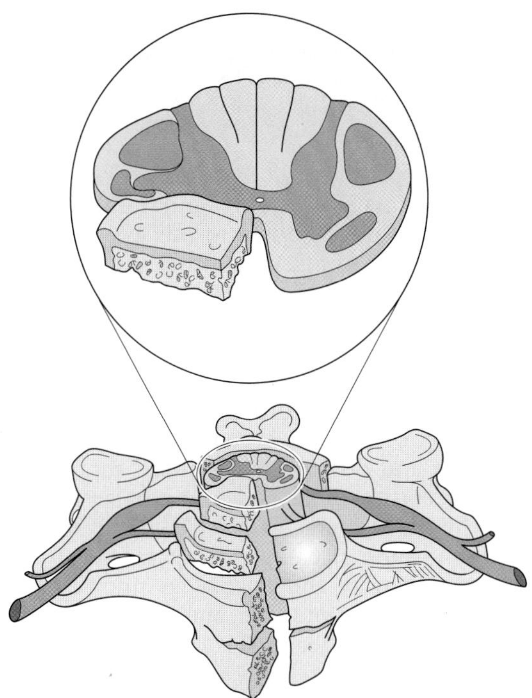

FIGURE 49-4 Brown-Séquard syndrome. A burst fracture with posterior displacement of bone fragments compresses one side of the spinal cord. (Redrawn from Tator C: Classification of spinal cord injury based on neurological presentation. In Narayan R, Wilberger J, Povlishock J, editors: *Neurotrauma*, New York, 1996, McGraw-Hill, with permission of McGraw-Hill.)

A corticospinal neuron is known as an upper motor neuron (UMN). The motor neuron to which it synapses in the spinal cord, which exits the spinal cord to innervate muscle, is known as a lower motor neuron (LMN). If damage to the UMNs and LMNs within the spinal cord is localized to a few segmental levels anywhere rostral to the conus medullaris (discussed later), a constellation of signs and symptoms develops, often called the UMN syndrome. This includes loss of voluntary movement, spasticity, hyperreflexia, clonus, and development of Babinski sign. If, in addition, there is damage to a significant number of LMNs below the level of injury, loss of voluntary movement occurs without the subsequent development of the other components of the UMN syndrome. Examples of this, defined as LMN injuries, include an SCI caused by an extensive vascular insult to the spinal cord, an injury occurring at the conus medullaris, or an injury occurring at the cauda equina. The conus medullaris syndrome refers to an injury of the sacral spinal cord and the lumbar nerve roots within the spinal canal (Figure 49-5), resulting in an areflexic bladder, bowel, and lower limbs. Conus medullaris lesions localized to the proximal sacral cord can occasionally show a preserved sacral reflex, such as the bulbocavernosus (BC) reflex. The cauda equina syndrome refers to an injury to the lumbosacral roots within the spinal canal (Figure 49-6), resulting in an areflexic bladder, bowel, and lower limbs.

After an acute UMN-predominant SCI, initial development of the UMN syndrome is delayed by a process called spinal shock, whereby there is a transient suppression and gradual return of reflex activity below the level of injury. Ditunno et al.[42] have proposed a four-phase model of spinal shock. During phase 1, occurring 0 to 24 hours postinjury, there is motor neuron hyperpolarization, manifesting clinically as hyporeflexia. During phase 2, occurring on days 1 to 3 postinjury, there is denervation supersensitivity and receptor upregulation, manifesting clinically

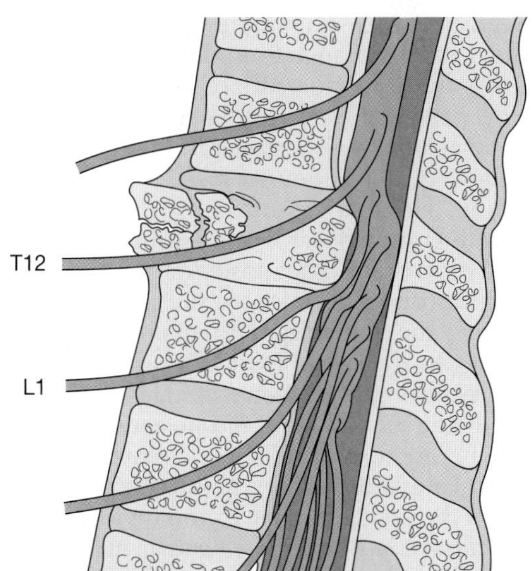

FIGURE 49-5 Conus medullaris syndrome. A burst fracture of T12 with posterior displacement of bone fragments compresses the conus medullaris. (Redrawn from Tator C: Classification of spinal cord injury based on neurological presentation. In Narayan R, Wilberger J, Povlishock J, editors: *Neurotrauma*, New York, 1996, McGraw-Hill, with permission of McGraw-Hill.)

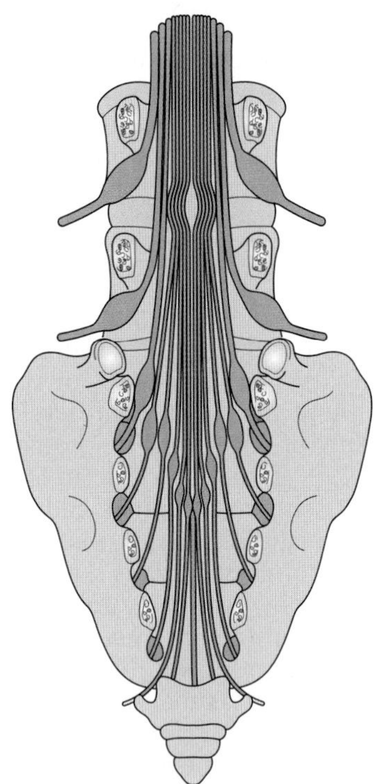

FIGURE 49-6 Cauda equina syndrome. A central disk herniation at L4-L5 compresses the cauda equina. Note how the roots of L5 and S1 are spared. (Redrawn from Tator C: Classification of spinal cord injury based on neurological presentation. In Narayan R, Wilberger J, Povlishock J, editors: *Neurotrauma,* New York, 1996, McGraw-Hill, with permission of McGraw-Hill.)

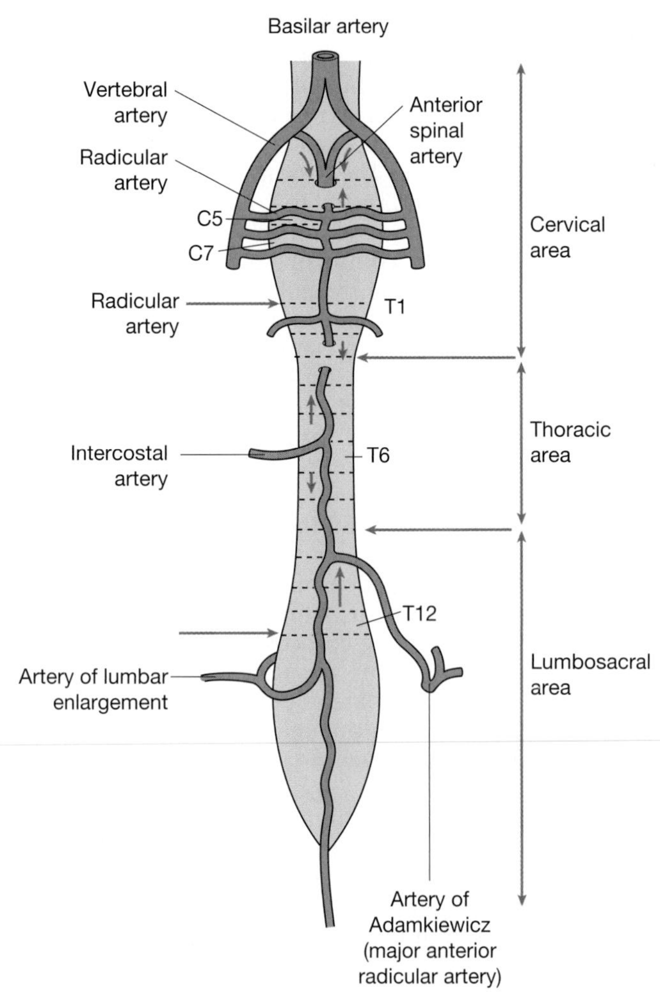

FIGURE 49-7 The spinal cord blood supply. (Redrawn from Pansky B, Allen D, Budd G: *Review of neuroscience,* ed 2, New York, 1998, McGraw-Hill, with permission of McGraw-Hill.)

with reflex return. During phase 3, occurring 1 to 4 weeks postinjury, there is interneuron synapse growth, manifesting clinically as early hyperreflexia. And finally, during phase 4, occurring 1 to 12 months postinjury, there is long axon synapse growth, manifesting clinically as late hyperreflexia.

Blood is supplied to the spinal cord through two posterior spinal arteries, a single anterior spinal artery, and several segmental radicular arteries (Figure 49-7). The posterior spinal arteries branch from the vertebral arteries and travel along the posterior surface of the spinal cord to supply the posterior one third of the spinal cord. Two anterior spinal arteries also branch from the vertebral arteries, but these quickly unite to form a single artery that travels along the anterior surface of the spinal cord to supply the anterior two thirds of the spinal cord. The anterior spinal artery and the posterior spinal arteries are dependent on contributions from the segmental radicular arteries along the spinal cord to maintain an adequate blood supply to the spinal cord. The segmental radicular arteries travel through the intervertebral foramina from the aorta and divide into anterior and posterior branches that eventually anastomose with their respective spinal arteries. These radicular arteries are not all identical in size or distribution. In the upper thoracic region between T1 and T4, there is little overlap between radicular arterial supplies. Between T12 and L2, there is an anterior radicular artery that is more dominant than its neighbors, called the artery of Adamkiewicz. This artery, usually found on the left side of the body, is an important blood supply to the caudal two thirds of the spinal cord. On reaching the anterior surface of the spinal cord, the artery of Adamkiewicz divides into a small ascending and larger descending branch. The latter travels down to the level of the conus medullaris, where it forms an anastomotic circle with the terminal branches of the posterior spinal arteries. The regions between T1 and T4, and T12 and L2 are areas particularly prone to ischemic damage, because of the importance of individual radicular arteries. The ischemic damage often affects the anterior portion of the spinal cord more than the posterior portion because of the nature of the single anterior and dual posterior blood supplies. In this situation the corticospinal and spinothalamic tracts are affected, whereas the gracilis tract is often spared. This leads to a syndrome of paraplegia, with loss of pain and temperature sensation, and relative sparing of touch and position sensation, called the anterior cord syndrome (Figure 49-8).

Pathophysiology of Acute Spinal Cord Injury

The mechanical damage caused at the moment of impact, called the primary injury to the spinal cord, starts a sequence of pathologic events collectively referred to as

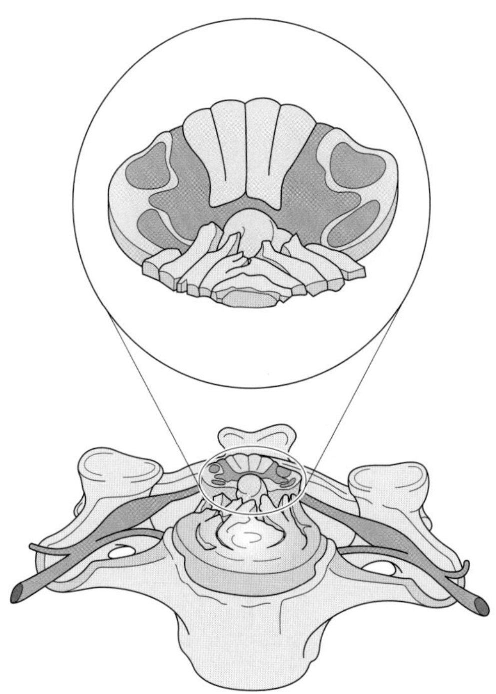

FIGURE 49-8 Anterior cord syndrome. A large disk herniation compresses the anterior aspect of the spinal cord, leaving the dorsal columns intact. (Redrawn from Tator C: Classification of spinal cord injury based on neurological presentation. In Narayan R, Wilberger J, Povlishock J, editors: *Neurotrauma*, New York, 1996, McGraw-Hill, with permission of McGraw-Hill.)

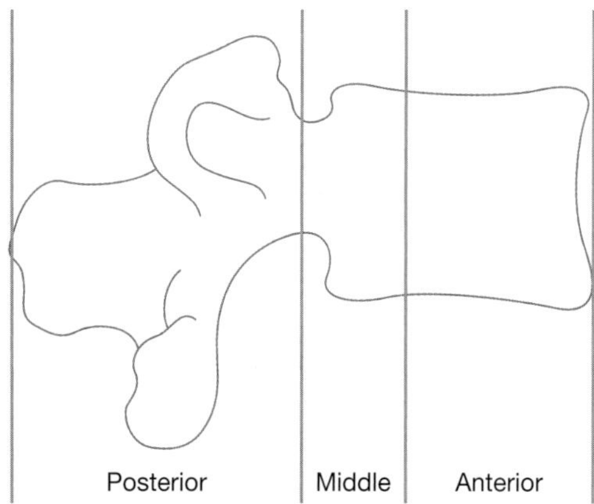

FIGURE 49-9 The three-column concept of spinal anatomy. (Redrawn from Ferguson RL, Allen BL Jr: A mechanistic classification of thoracolumbar spine fractures, *Clin Orthop* 189:77-88, 1984, with permission.)

secondary injury. These secondary changes begin within seconds of the primary injury and continue for several weeks thereafter.[123]

Mechanical disruption of the spinal cord vasculature leads to the development of microhemorrhages in the gray and white matter, interstitial edema, and the release of coagulation factors and vasoactive amines. This latter release promotes thrombosis and vasospasm of the microvasculature of the spinal cord causing tissue hypoxia and impaired neuronal homeostasis. At the cellular level, there are changes in ion concentrations, peroxidation of membrane lipids, formation of free radicals, and release of toxic excitatory neurotransmitters.[123]

In response to injury, neutrophils initially migrate to the site of injury, where they can contribute to cellular injury by producing lysosomal enzymes and oxygen radicals. These are followed by macrophages that phagocytose cell debris.[96] Demyelination of white matter tracts begins within 24 hours of injury and increases thereafter, with Wallerian degeneration occurring by 3 weeks.[118]

Spinal Mechanics and Stability

There is no universally accepted definition of spinal stability. White and Panjabi[121] defined clinical instability as "the loss of the ability of the spine under physiologic loads to maintain relationships between vertebrae in such a way that there is not initial damage or subsequent irritation to the spinal cord or nerve roots and, in addition, there is no development of incapacitating deformity or pain caused by structural changes." A commonly accepted model for thoracolumbar stability, which is also often used in the middle and lower cervical spine, was developed by Denis.[36] The model divides the spine into three columns: anterior, middle, and posterior (Figure 49-9). The anterior column is composed of the anterior longitudinal ligament, the anterior portion of the vertebral body, and the anterior portion of the annulus fibrosis or disk. The middle column is composed of the posterior portion of the vertebral body, the posterior portion of the annulus fibrosis, and the posterior longitudinal ligament. The posterior column is composed of the pedicles, facet joints, laminae, supraspinous ligament, interspinous ligament, facet joint capsule, and ligamentum flavum. When the integrity of the middle and either the anterior or the posterior column is affected, the spine is likely to be unstable.[36] The columns can be compromised by either fracture or ligamentous disruption. Gunshot wounds, because of the nature of the injury, can affect more than one column and the spine can still remain stable. It should also be noted that SCI can occur without obvious radiographic findings.

Fractures or dislocations in the thoracic and lumbar spine most commonly involve the T12 and the L1 vertebrae, respectively. Common mechanisms include compression-flexion, distraction-flexion, translation, and torsion-flexion. Axial loading of a flexed spine can cause several different patterns of injury depending on the vector of force. There might be only compression of the anterior column leading to a compression fracture or, with a greater compressive force, compression of the anterior column with distraction of the posterior elements. If the vector of force causes the axis of rotation to be anterior to the vertebral body, a Chance-type distraction can occur with distraction of all three columns, through the bony vertebra alone (Figure 49-10), through the ligamentous structures alone, or through a combination of bony and ligamentous structures. In addition, there can be compression of all three columns with retropulsion of the middle column into the spinal canal. The latter often causes SCI. Translation of adjacent vertebrae, as occurs, for example, when a person falls from a height and strikes part of the torso on an immovable object, is the injury pattern most likely to cause SCI. If there is translation more than 25% of the width of a vertebra, ligamentous structures in all three columns are probably disrupted. Compression and rotation of the anterior column, and distraction and rotation

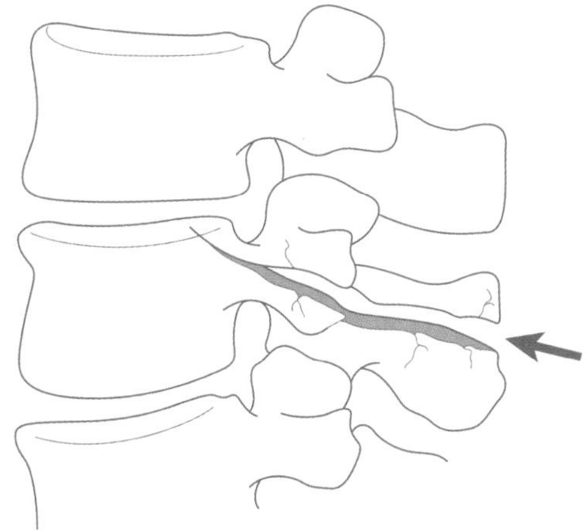

FIGURE 49-10 A Chance fracture. (Redrawn from Schultz RJ: *The language of fractures*, Baltimore, 1990, Williams & Wilkins, with permission of Williams & Wilkins.)

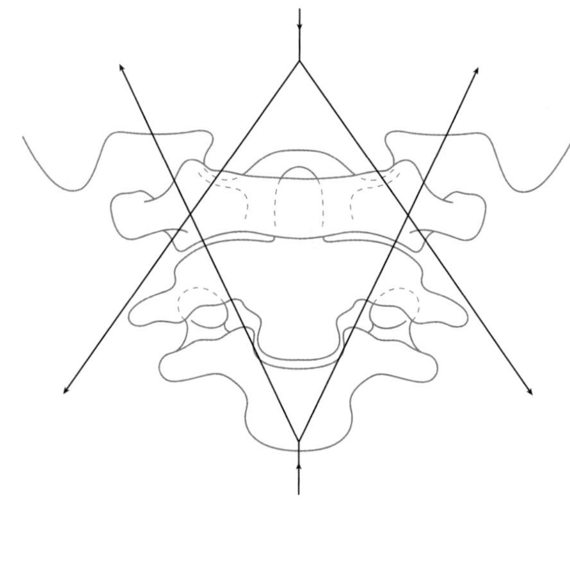

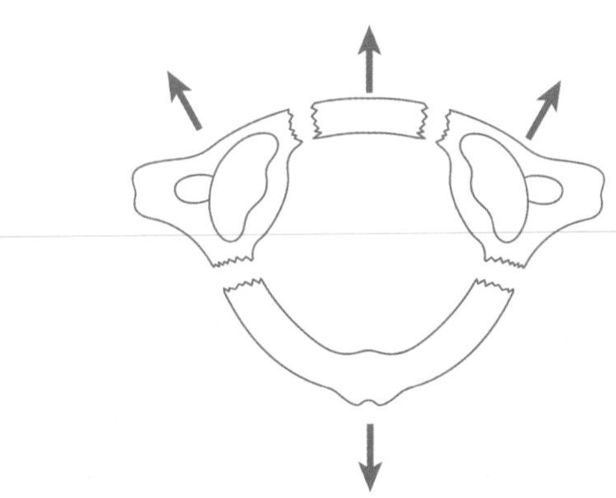

FIGURE 49-11 A Jefferson fracture. A comminuted fracture of the ring of C1. (Redrawn from Schultz RJ: *The language of fractures*, Baltimore, 1990, Williams & Wilkins, with permission of Williams & Wilkins.)

of the posterior column, cause a torsion-flexion injury where the facets and the anterior longitudinal ligament are usually disrupted, and SCI is likely.

Lap belt injuries in motor vehicle collisions occur most often in children weighing less than 60 lb who are wearing a regular lap belt above the pelvic rim.[116] A clinical triad of abdominal wall bruising, intraabdominal injuries, and SCI at or close to the thoracolumbar junction is often seen in these children.[116]

Fractures or dislocations in the cervical spine are usually caused by excessive forceful flexion, extension, or axial loading. An abrupt deceleration, commonly seen in motor vehicle crashes, causes a person's head to be propelled forward on a relatively immobilized torso, leading to a flexion-type injury. Abrupt acceleration causes the opposite, an extension-type injury. Axial loading is also a common comechanism to flexion or extension injuries in the cervical spine, such as occurs when a diver's head strikes the bottom of a pool. Knowledge of the mechanism of injury is important for recognizing injuries that might not be seen easily on imaging. For example, flexion injuries can cause disruption of the ligaments in the posterior column that might not be apparent on plain radiographs.

Craniovertebral junction injuries (i.e., atlantooccipital or atlantoaxial) are relatively common in children but not adults. Often they result in immediate death and the SCI can go undetected.

A Jefferson fracture, originally described by Sir Geoffrey Jefferson, is a burst fracture of the atlas (C1 vertebra). This is caused by axial compression, which can occur, for example, when a football player spears another player with his helmet (Figure 49-11).

A hangman's fracture is a traumatic spondylolisthesis of the axis (C2 vertebra). It is caused by bilateral fractures through the pars interarticularis of the axis that result from hyperextension and axial compression, as can occur in an abrupt deceleration when a person's forehead strikes the windshield. A fracture of the odontoid process of the axis can be caused by hyperflexion, hyperextension, or excessive lateral bending. The traditional classification of odontoid fractures includes three types. Type 1 is a fracture through the tip of the odontoid, type 2 is a fracture through the base of the odontoid, and type 3 is a fracture that extends from the base of the odontoid into the axis proper.

Hyperflexion of the subaxial cervical spine (C3-C7) can cause an anterior subluxation, a simple compression fracture, bilateral facet dislocations, a flexion teardrop fracture, or a clay-shoveler's fracture. A flexion teardrop fracture is characterized by retropulsion of the larger portion of a vertebral body into the spinal canal, detached from an anterior fragment (teardrop); it is associated with posterior facet and ligamentous disruption (Figure 49-12). Flexion teardrop fractures are often associated with an anterior cord syndrome, if not a complete SCI. A clay shoveler's fracture is an avulsion fracture of the spinous process of C6, C7, or T1. It is not typically associated with neurologic injury. Hyperflexion with rotation often causes a unilateral facet dislocation.

Hyperextension of the subaxial cervical spine typically distracts the anterior column of the spine and compresses the posterior column. Anterior distraction often disrupts the anterior longitudinal ligament, the intervertebral disk, and the posterior longitudinal ligament, whereas posterior compression causes the ligamentum flavum to buckle into the spinal canal. If the spinal cord is pinched between the vertebral body and the ligamentum flavum and/or hypertrophied facet joints, a central cord syndrome often develops. This syndrome, occurring only with cervical spinal

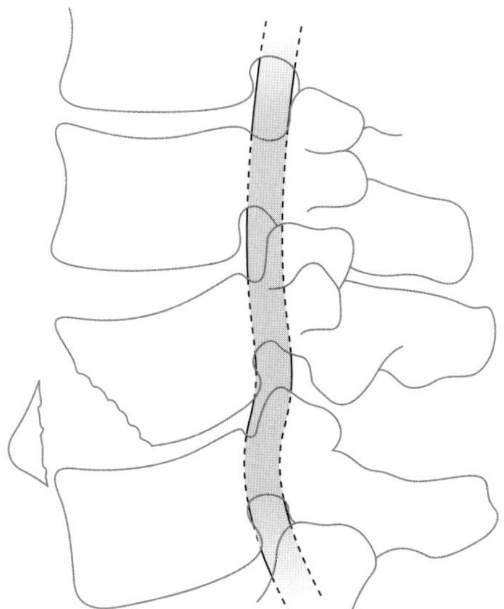

FIGURE 49-12 A flexion teardrop fracture. The spinal cord is compressed by the posteroinferior aspect of the vertebrae. (Redrawn from Schultz RJ: *The language of fractures*, Baltimore, 1990, Williams & Wilkins, with permission of Williams & Wilkins.)

cord lesions, is characterized by sacral sensory sparing and greater weakness in the upper limbs as compared with the lower limbs. A hyperextension teardrop fracture is characterized by an avulsion of the anterior inferior aspect of the vertebral body above the hyperextension injury by the anterior longitudinal ligament, without retropulsion of a vertebral body into the spinal canal. Compression of the posterior column during excessive forceful hyperextension can also result in lamina fractures.

Finally, and not uncommonly, significant axial loading of the subaxial cervical spine causes a burst fracture, whereby an intervertebral disk implodes through the superior end plate of the vertebral body below, causing this vertebral body to burst into multiple fragments. These fractures usually include at least two columns, are generally unstable, and are often associated with SCI.

Classification of Spinal Cord Injury

The diagnosis of SCI can be made promptly by performing a neurologic examination. The International Standards for Neurologic Classification of Spinal Cord Injury (ISNCSCI) provides a procedure for classifying an SCI.[68] Comprehensive online e-learning modules are available through the American Spinal Injury Association (ASIA) website. The examination, which is safe to perform soon after SCI, even in people with an unstable spine, is performed with the injured individual in the supine position. Subsequent examinations are always performed in the same position. The procedure includes a systematic evaluation of all the dermatomes and extremity myotomes. Because SCI usually affects the spinal cord at a discrete site, determining the last intact sensory and motor level can reliably and accurately determine an NLI. A complete injury is defined within the ISNCSCI as an injury in which there is the lack of any sensory or motor function in the lowest sacral segment; this includes pressure sensation within the anus, sensation at the anal mucocutaneous junction, or a voluntary contraction of the external anal sphincter. An incomplete injury is defined as an injury in which there is at least partial sensory or motor function in the lowest sacral segment.

The sensory portion of the neurologic examination includes the testing of a key point for absent, impaired, or normal sensation in each of the 28 dermatomes on each side of the body for both light touch and pinprick. Pinprick sensation is elicited with a disposable safety pin, whereas touch sensation is elicited by a wisp of cotton or a fingertip. For an inability to distinguish between pinprick and touch, sensation should be graded as absent for pinprick sensation. The motor portion of the neurologic examination includes the testing of a key muscle function for strength on a 6-point scale for each of 10 myotomes on each side of the body, as well as testing for contraction of the external anal sphincter. Detailed descriptions and demonstrations for testing each specific sensory point and key muscle group are demonstrated on the ASIA Learning Center website (lms3.learnshare.com).

The testing of every key muscle should begin in the grade 3 testing position. If the muscle is shown to have greater than antigravity strength (grade 3), then the muscle should be tested in the grades 4 and 5 testing positions. Conversely, if the muscle is shown to have less than antigravity strength when tested in the grade 3 testing position, the muscle should be tested in the grade 2 testing position. If the muscle is shown to not even have grade 2 strength, then the grade 1 testing position is used. Before testing muscle strength for a particular key muscle, the range of motion (ROM) for the joint that particular muscle crosses should be tested. Knowing this available ROM is a necessary condition for accurately grading the strength.

The NLI is defined as the most caudal segment of the spinal cord with normal sensation and motor function bilaterally. For the ISNCSCI, key muscles have been chosen that primarily have innervation by two roots, with each successive key muscle overlapping the muscle above in either the cervical or the lumbar region, by a single root innervation. By ISNCSCI definition, if a key muscle has a motor strength grade of 5/5, it is innervated by two intact nerve segments. If a key muscle has a motor strength grade of 3/5 or 4/5 (and the key muscle above has a motor strength grade of 5/5), it is innervated by at least one intact nerve segment, the segment for which that key muscle is named. If a key muscle has a motor strength grade of 2/5 or less, neither of its nerve segments is intact. For the cervical segments, because the innervation of the elbow flexors is C5 and C6, the wrist extensors is C6 and C7, and the elbow extensors is C7 and C8, the ISNCSCI-named segmental innervations are C5, C6, and C7, respectively. If the elbow flexors are graded as 5/5, the wrist extensors as 4/5, and the elbow extensors as 2/5, it is assumed that the C5 and C6 myotomes are fully innervated, but the C7 myotome is partially innervated only. For myotomes where there are no designated key muscles to test, motor function is assumed to be normal where sensory function is normal.

The ISNCSCI also includes a scale of impairment called the ASIA Impairment Scale (AIS), which classifies an SCI into five categories of severity, labeled A through E, based on the degree of motor and sensory loss. An SCI that results in the absence of any sensory or motor function in the sacral segments S4-S5 would have an AIS category of A and be designated as complete. For an SCI where sensation is preserved in the sacral segments S4-S5, but there is no motor function caudal to three segments below the NLI, the AIS is B. For an SCI where sensation is preserved in the sacral segments S4-S5, but more than half the key muscles below the NLI have a muscle grade less than 3/5, the AIS is C. For an SCI where sensation is preserved in the sacral segments S4-S5, but at least half the key muscles below the NLI have a muscle grade greater than or equal to 3/5, the AIS is D. When sensory and motor function is normal, the AIS is E. AIS categories B through E designate incomplete injuries.

There are certain issues that need to be taken into consideration when conducting an examination on children. There is a learning module on the ASIA Learning Center website (lms3.learnshare.com) specifically addressing these concerns.

Nontraumatic Spinal Cord Injury

Nontraumatic SCI can be caused by a variety of diseases, including neoplastic, infectious, inflammatory, vascular, degenerative (spondylotic), congenital, and toxic-metabolic disorders. People affected by nontraumatic SCI are clinically very different from those with traumatic injuries. Those with nontraumatic SCI generally have less severe injuries, and almost always have incomplete injuries that are associated with a far better prognosis for neurologic improvement than complete injuries. Also, unlike people with traumatic SCI, people with nontraumatic SCI are significantly more likely to have paraplegia than tetraplegia.[82]

Neoplastic Causes of Spinal Cord Injury

Tumors associated with SCI can arise from either the neural elements in the spinal canal, such as the spinal cord or spinal nerves, or the structures comprising the spinal column, most commonly the vertebral bodies. Tumors arising from the spine (extradural tumors) are much more common than those arising from neural elements (intradural tumors).

Classification of Spinal Tumors

The most common method of classifying tumors relates to the anatomic location of tumor involvement. Spinal tumors are extradural when they arise from structures outside the dura, most commonly the vertebral body. A less likely origin is from the structures of the posterior bony arch or the soft tissues outside the dura. Most tumors metastatic to the spine are extradural, making up more than half of all spinal tumors.[73] The most common primary sites of metastatic tumors to the spine are lung, breast, prostate, and kidney.[59] The mechanisms of metastasis include direct extension of tumor from adjacent tissues, and hematogenous spread through the Batson vertebral venous plexus, a valveless venous system draining the thoracic, abdominal, and pelvic viscera. Primary spine tumors that are present in the extradural region make up less than 1% of all spinal tumors. These include multiple myeloma, osteogenic sarcoma, vertebral hemangioma, chondrosarcoma, and chordoma.[59]

Tumors arising within the intradural space include those that are intramedullary (i.e., tumors arising from the parenchyma of the spinal cord) and those that are intradural but extramedullary. Intramedullary tumors are usually primary tumors, most commonly ependymomas and astrocytomas, which together make up 75% of all intramedullary tumors.[59] Ependymomas tend to be well encapsulated and regularly shaped in contrast to astrocytomas, which tend to be irregularly shaped with multiple extensions into the cord parenchyma. Most intradural extramedullary tumors are both benign and primary, and include meningiomas and nerve sheath tumors such as schwannomas and neurofibromas.[59] Those metastatic tumors that are seen can arise either by hematogenous spread or as "drop metastases," lesions that directly extend from the CSF in association with malignant brain tumors such as medulloblastomas.[73]

Clinical Presentation of Spinal Tumors

Pain is the most common presenting symptom of a spinal tumor. Pain associated with spinal tumors is often worse in the supine position, in contrast to the pain associated with degenerative spondylosis, which is usually worse in the upright position. If the tumor involves only skeletal structures, the pain is usually axial. If the tumor involves nerve roots, it occurs typically in a radicular distribution. If the tumor involves the spinal cord, the pain can present as at-level or below-level spinal cord pain. Constitutional symptoms such as night sweats, fevers, unexplained weight loss, and anorexia can also suggest spinal tumor.

Acute spinal cord compression is associated with rapid neurologic decline, and constitutes a medical emergency because it can rapidly progress to paraplegia or tetraplegia. When signs and symptoms of acute spinal cord compression related to neoplastic involvement of the spine are present, most patients will have substantial radiographic abnormalities. The syndrome of acute spinal cord compression, when related to spinal tumors, most often results from the invasion of spinal structures by extradural metastases.

Management of Spinal Cord Compression by Tumor

Acute spinal cord compression is managed with corticosteroids, radiation, and surgical intervention. Corticosteroids, typically dexamethasone, are administered to reduce tumor-related inflammatory changes and prostaglandin production.[59] Radiation therapy is often used in cases of spinal cord compression resulting from soft tissue encroachment. It can be used alone in the setting of spinal stability or in combination with surgery. Radiation therapy is less often used for the treatment of intradural or intramedullary tumors, unless such tumors are deemed unresectable or when surgical resection is incomplete.[59] Radiosensitive tumors involving the spine include lymphomas, small cell lung cancer, and multiple myeloma, whereas less radiosensitive tumors include breast, prostate, non–small cell lung, and renal cell cancers.[59] Complications of radiation directed to the spine include radiation myelopathy and radiation plexopathy. In the setting of acute spinal cord compression, the immediate goal of surgical treatment is decompression of the cord to preserve or improve neurologic function.

For most intramedullary and intradural extramedullary tumors, surgical treatment is the most effective. Ependymomas, because of their encapsulated nature, often can be completely resected with good preservation of neurologic function. In contrast, because astrocytomas are irregular and invasive without a clear plane for resection, the goal of surgery is a subtotal resection of clearly abnormal tissue. Intradural extramedullary meningiomas arise from the dura and are resected along with the involved dura after being accessed through a laminectomy. Nerve sheath tumors can be entirely intradural or, in the case of the neurofibroma, can have extradural extension through an enlarged neural foramen. In neurofibromatosis type 2, extensive intradural involvement throughout much of the spinal cord can be present. In such cases, tumor debulking rather than complete resection is usually the surgical goal.

Infectious and Inflammatory Causes of Spinal Cord Injury

Bacterial Infection

Bacteria can invade a vertebral body either hematogenously or by direct extension from a contiguous focus of infection, causing vertebral osteomyelitis. People at increased risk for bacterial vertebral osteomyelitis include those who use intravenous drugs; immunosuppressed individuals; people with diabetes; or people with renal disease who are receiving dialysis. Children are relatively susceptible to bacterial diskitis alone, probably because of a relatively robust blood supply to the intervertebral disk. The bacteria most commonly implicated in vertebral osteomyelitis is *Staphylococcus aureus*, which accounts for more than half of all infections.[53] Although infection can be seen in any portion of the spine, the lumbar spine is the most common area. Spine pain is by far the most common symptom of vertebral osteomyelitis, seen in greater than 90% of people affected.[53] Other symptoms can include fever or a neurologic deficit related to spinal cord compression from vertebral body collapse, or the presence of an epidural abscess. Laboratory markers of inflammation, such as the erythrocyte sedimentation rate and C-reactive protein, are very frequently found to be elevated with active infection. Isolation of the etiologic pathogen is vital to treatment success. This can be accomplished by recovery of the organism in blood cultures or through cultures of tissue obtained from the spine, either by needle or open biopsy. Treatment of vertebral osteomyelitis involves intravenous antibiotic administration for at least 4 weeks. Surgical treatment is indicated when appropriate antibiotics have been ineffective, when there is spinal cord or nerve root compression causing a neurologic deficit, or when there is spinal instability or spinal deformity.

Tuberculosis of the spine, also known as Pott disease, results from hematogenous spread of the bacterium *Mycobacterium tuberculosis* to the spine, typically from a pulmonary focus. Spinal tuberculosis is treated with at least two and as many as four antituberculous agents for a 6- to 12-month duration.

Human Immunodeficiency Virus and Human T-Lymphotropic Virus Infection

People with human immunodeficiency virus (HIV) infection are susceptible to spinal cord disease, which can occur as vacuolar myelopathy, as primary HIV myelitis, or as a result of opportunistic infections of the spinal cord. Vacuolar myelopathy clinically presents as incomplete spastic paraplegia with loss of proprioception and vibration sense.

Human T-lymphotropic virus type 1 (HTLV-1) is another retrovirus that causes a progressive chronic myelopathy. The clinical condition is a slowly progressive spastic paraplegia, which is referred to as both tropical spastic paraparesis and HTLV-1–associated myelopathy. The virus is transmitted through blood, sexual contacts, and from mother to child in breast milk. It occurs in the Caribbean, southern Japan, central and south Africa, and regions of South America.[53]

Transverse Myelitis

Myelitis is a neurologic disorder of the spinal cord (myelopathy) that is caused by inflammation. The term "transverse" was first added to "myelitis" in the case report of an acute inflammatory myelopathy complicating a pneumonia,[107] in which "transverse" in this case referred to the clinical finding of a bandlike horizontal area of altered sensation at the dermatomal level of the lesion within the cord.

When a person has a rapidly evolving myelopathy with no history of trauma or physical or radiographic evidence of a structural lesion, the differential diagnosis should include potential causes of myelitis such as systemic lupus erythematosus, Sjögren syndrome, multiple sclerosis, neuromyelitis optica, neurosarcoid, paraneoplastic syndromes, nutritional deficiencies, vascular insufficiency, decompression sickness, and infection. Myelitis can progress over the course of several hours or over a few weeks. Even when infection is thought to be a cause, causative organisms are rarely if ever isolated. Although transverse myelitis can occur in any region of the spinal cord, the thoracic region is most common. In people with transverse myelitis, magnetic resonance imaging (MRI) scanning often shows spinal cord swelling, with a region of increased signal on T2-weighted images that correlates with the NLI.

Acute treatment of myelitis is aimed at halting the inflammatory process. The standard treatment is the administration of high-dose intravenous (IV) methylprednisolone at 1000 mg daily for 3 to 7 days. If the response is suboptimal, then plasma exchange is recommended to remove any humoral factors that may be contributing to the pathologic process. Lastly, if there is still no improvement with plasma exchange, IV immunoglobulin, cyclophosphamide, rituximab, or azathioprine, the latter two for neuromyelitis optica, may be of benefit.[120]

Vascular Causes of Spinal Cord Injury

Ischemia of the spinal cord, although less common than ischemia of the brain, is a well-known cause of SCI. It is most commonly associated with the anterior cord syndrome and can occur as a result of systemic or local spinal cord hypoperfusion, embolization, or rarely thrombosis. Ischemia can also result from the presence of a type I spinal arteriovenous malformation (AVM). This is a dural arteriovenous fistula that arises when a single dural arterial feeder, either spontaneously or after trauma, develops a fistula to the spinal venous circulation. This fistula causes venous congestion and hypertension, which results in hypoperfusion of the spinal cord. Symptoms caused by type I AVMs are usually of gradual onset, with a progressive course, although there can be stepwise episodes of deterioration interspersed with periods of clinical stability. Sensory symptoms are the most common initial presenting symptoms, but weakness and sphincter disturbances are often present by the time the diagnosis has been made.[65]

Outcomes of Traumatic Spinal Cord Injury

It is not uncommon for clinicians involved in the care of a person who has experienced a traumatic SCI to be asked the following questions: "Will I walk again?" "Will I regain use of my hands?" "Will I regain control of my bowel and bladder?" These questions prove the importance of prognosticating neurologic and functional outcomes as early as possible after an SCI, to allow development of a specific treatment plan and to allow psychological adjustment to begin. Prognostication of neurologic outcome depends on the physical examination findings, especially as defined by the ISNCSCI. With regard to outcomes, older people generally do less well than younger people, reaching lower levels of independence in walking and self-care.

Neurologic Recovery in Complete Tetraplegia

After traumatic cervical SCI, 20% to 30% of people classified as AIS A convert to AIS B or better by 1 year. This has been consistent across several independent large database analyses.[78,103] Within the Model Systems Database, for those initially AIS A, 8% convert to AIS C, whereas 7% convert to AIS D. For those initially AIS B, 30% become AIS C and 37% become AIS D. For those initially AIS C, over 80% convert to AIS D or E.

Of those who convert from AIS A to AIS B or greater, up to two thirds convert by 1 month with the remainder converting within 3 months; it is rare to convert after that.

The change in upper extremity motor score (UEMS) over the first year postinjury, which can be calculated by adding all the muscle grades for the key muscles in the upper extremities (for a total 50 points), for people with C4-C7 AIS A tetraplegia averages 10 points.[78,103] The motor level stays the same or worsens in 35% of people, improves one level in 42%, improves two levels in 14%, and improves more than two levels in 9%. A motor zone of partial preservation of more than two segments is associated with a gain of more than two levels. The chance of functional recovery of a muscle two levels below the motor level of injury, when the first muscle below the motor level is grade 0, is exceedingly rare. The typical pattern of neurologic improvement with regard to gains in motor score is characterized by the greatest changes within the first 3 months, lesser changes over the next 3 months, with even lesser changes thereafter with plateauing by 1 year.

Neurologic Recovery and Ambulation

A combination of age (<65 years versus ≥65 years), the motor score of the stronger quadriceps femoris muscle, the motor score of the stronger gastrocsoleus muscle, and light touch sensation at the L3 and S1 dermatomes show excellent discrimination in distinguishing people who will be able to walk and those who will not be able to walk at 1 year (Figure 49-13, Table 49-2).[113]

Functional Recovery

Prognostication of functional outcome depends on the physical examination findings, familiarity with the published functional outcomes of people with SCI of different NLI, and an ability to integrate into a prognosis a host of

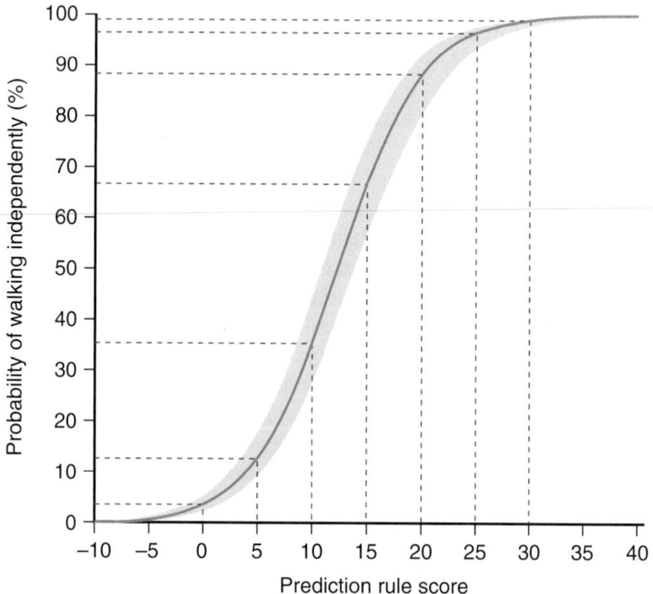

FIGURE 49-13 Probability of walking independently 1 year after injury based on prediction rule score. (From van Middendorp JJ, Hosman AJ, Donders AR, et al: A clinical prediction rule for ambulation outcomes after traumatic spinal cord injury: a longitudinal cohort study, *Lancet* 377:1004-1010, 2011.)

Table 49-2 Clinical Prediction Rule Variables

	Range of Test Scores	Weighted Coefficient	Minimum Score	Maximum Score
Age ≥65 years	0-1	−10	−10	0
Motor score L3*	0-5	2	0	10
Motor score S1*	0-5	2	0	10
Light touch score L3*	0-2	5	0	10
Light touch score S1*	0-2	5	0	10
Total			−10	40

From van Middendorp JJ, Hosman AJ, Donders AR, et al: A clinical prediction rule for ambulation outcomes after traumatic spinal cord injury: a longitudinal cohort study, *Lancet* 377:1004-1010, 2011.

*Only the best score of each motor score or light touch score (i.e., right or left) should be applied for the prediction rule.

other factors. These factors include, but are not limited to, preexisting medical conditions, concomitant injuries, secondary complications, cognitive impairments, age, body habitus, availability of financial resources and insurance coverage, psychological factors, social factors, and cultural factors. The information in Table 49-3 is modified from the *Outcomes Following Traumatic Spinal Cord Injury* clinical practice guideline, which was first published by the Paralyzed Veterans of America in 1999.[122] The expected outcomes are stratified by NLI and described for several different domains. They reflect the level of independence that can be expected of an average individual with a motor complete SCI under optimal circumstances 1 year after injury.

Acute Phase of Injury

Prehospital Care

The first 24 hours after trauma are the deadliest. In this period, primary and secondary injuries to the central nervous system are the leading cause of death. The first step in the treatment of a person with a suspected spinal injury is ensuring an adequate airway, breathing, and circulation. Patients with cervical cord injuries are at high risk for respiratory failure and must be monitored closely for the need for ventilatory support. Even if intubation is not needed urgently, arterial blood gas and vital capacity (VC) measurements are useful tools in identifying delayed respiratory muscle fatigue. When intubation is necessary, it must be done carefully in the setting of suspected or confirmed cervical spine trauma to avoid secondary cord injury. The standard technique for urgent intubation in this setting is rapid sequence induction with cricoid pressure and manual inline stabilization.[30] Alternatively, awake fiberoptic intubation is an appropriate alternative, and may be the preferred technique, in a cooperative patient.

All people with suspected acute SCI should have their spines immobilized. People with altered mental status, evidence of intoxication, suspected limb fracture or distracting injury, focal neurologic deficit, and spine pain or tenderness should also be suspected of having a traumatic SCI. The entire spine should be immobilized in a neutral supine position regardless of the position the individual was found in after the accident. This is best accomplished with the use of a combination of a rigid cervical collar with supportive blocks on a backboard that has straps to secure the body. On the spine board, an occipital pad for an adult or an occipital recess for a child younger than 6 years can be used to compensate for the different sizes of the head relative to the body in people of different age groups.

Once on the spine board, the individual is transported to a trauma center where the initial goals are to establish hemodynamic stability, to prevent hypoxemia and aspiration of stomach contents, and to maintain spinal immobilization until definitive management is accomplished. Maintenance of adequate blood pressure is critical because hypotension and shock are extremely deleterious to the injured spinal cord. A target mean arterial blood pressure of 85 mm Hg for a minimum of 7 days has been associated with favorable outcomes. Although neurogenic shock is associated with cervical and high thoracic injuries, it is important to evaluate the patient fully for other causes of shock including hemorrhage, pneumothorax, myocardial infarction, cardiac tamponade, sepsis from intraabdominal injury, or even acute adrenal insufficiency in patients with concomitant brain injury. Neurogenic shock is a result of sympathetic denervation and is characterized by hypotension and bradycardia in the setting of flaccid paralysis. Bradycardia results from unopposed parasympathetic input to the heart, but can also be stimulated by endotracheal suctioning. Neurogenic shock is treated with restoration of intravascular volume and vasopressor agents. The ideal vasopressor agents have both alpha-adrenergic and beta-adrenergic actions to counter the loss of sympathetic tone and provide chronotropic support to the heart.[30] Atropine is helpful to rapidly reverse the bradycardia. A temporary or permanent cardiac pacemaker insertion is rarely necessary. Hemorrhagic shock is treated by controlling bleeding and vigorous fluid resuscitation. Core temperature should be monitored because people with cervical or high thoracic injuries can become relatively poikilothermic because of autonomic nervous system disruption. Placement of a nasogastric tube in the acute period is important to prevent emesis and aspiration of gastric contents, and an indwelling bladder catheter ensures adequate bladder drainage in a situation where urinary retention is the rule. Early contact between the receiving trauma center and a specialized SCI center should be established, with arrangements made for transfer to the spinal injury center once medical stability has been secured.

Once stabilized medically, a thorough evaluation of neurologic status and spinal stability is performed. The neurologic status is determined using the ISNCSCI. Serial examinations should be performed to detect neurologic deterioration or improvement, particularly in the first 3 days after injury and after manipulation such as transport, closed reduction, or surgical treatment. Spinal stability is assessed for the entire spine, not just the clinically likely area of injury, because there is an approximately 20% chance of finding noncontiguous spine fractures. Computed tomography (CT) imaging of the entire spine is recommended because of the lack of sensitivity of plain film protocols, particularly in the craniocervical region and at the cervicothoracic junction. MRI evaluation is essential for evaluating nonbony tissues, including the spinal cord, nerve roots, ligaments, and intervertebral disks, and should be performed to evaluate the area of a known or suspected SCI. MRI evaluation is particularly important for identification of spinal pathology in people with a neurologic deficit not identified by CT and for those people who are unconscious or obtunded.

Specific to children, SCIWORA has been reported in up to 20% of children with SCI, whereas in those with fractures, multiple noncontiguous fractures are seen in one third of children with SCI.[13]

Surgical Management

In the specific case of dislocation of the cervical spine, rapid closed reduction of the spine using skeletal traction remains a valid treatment option. Closed reduction of a

Text continued on p. 1112

Table 49-3 Expected Functional Outcomes by Neurologic Level of Injury

		C1-C4		C5	
Domain	**Domain Description**	**Expected Outcome**	**Equipment**	**Expected Outcome**	**Equipment**
Respiratory	Ability to breathe with or without mechanical assistance and clear secretions	Ventilator or diaphragm/phrenic pacer dependent (C1-C3) Inability to clear secretions	Ventilator(s) (C1-C3) Suction equipment (C1-C3) Back-up generator (C1-C3) Nebulizer	Low endurance and vital capacity secondary to paralysis of intercostal muscles; may require assist to clear secretions	
Bowel	Management of elimination and perineal hygiene	Total assist for digital stimulation, insertion of minienema or suppository, and perineal hygiene	Padded reclining commode chair with head support Roll-in shower	Total assist including insertion of minienema or suppository and digital stimulation	Padded reclining commode chair
Bladder	Management of elimination and perineal hygiene	Total assist for inserting indwelling catheter (transurethral or suprapubic) or applying an external catheter to penis	Foley catheter or external catheters Urine drainage bags	Total assist for inserting indwelling catheter (transurethral or suprapubic) or applying an external catheter to penis	Foley or external catheters Urine drainage bags
Bed mobility and positioning	Rolling, scooting, bridging, supine to sit	Total assist but independent in direction of care	Fully electric hospital bed with available Trendelenburg position and side rails Pressure relieving mattress	Some assist but independent in direction of care and controlling bed	Fully electric hospital bed with Trendelenburg feature and side rails with accessible remote control Pressure relieving mattress
Transfers		Total assist but independent in direction of transfers	Transfer board Power or mechanical lift with sling	Total assist but independent in direction of transfers	Transfer board Power or mechanical lift with sling

C6-C7		C8		T1-T12		L1-S5	
Expected Outcome	**Equipment**	**Expected Outcome**	**Equipment**	**Expected Outcome**	**Equipment**	**Expected Outcome**	**Equipment**
Low endurance and vital capacity secondary to paralysis of intercostal muscles; may require assist to clear secretions in setting of respiratory infection		Low endurance and vital capacity secondary to paralysis of intercostal muscles; may require assist to clear secretions in setting of respiratory infection		Low endurance and vital capacity secondary to paralysis of intercostal muscles for higher level lesions		Normal	
Some to total assist for setup and perineal hygiene Independent suppository insertion with suppository inserter Independent rectal stimulation with digital bowel stimulator	Padded commode chair Suppository inserter Digital bowel stimulator Mirror	Independent digital stimulation, suppository or minienema insertion, and perineal hygiene	Padded commode chair	Independent digital stimulation, suppository or minienema insertion, and perineal hygiene	Padded commode chair	Independent digital stimulation, suppository or minienema insertion, and perineal hygiene	Padded toilet seat
Total assist for inserting indwelling catheter (transurethral or suprapubic) or applying an external catheter to penis Independent self-catheterization through a continent urinary diversion (Mitrofanoff procedure) with an abdominal stoma for woman or penis for men with equipment	Bimanual catheter inserter Foley, straight, or external catheters Urine drainage bags	Independent intermittent catheterization	Straight catheters	Independent intermittent catheterization	Straight catheters	Independent intermittent catheterization	Straight catheters
Some assist	Full electric hospital bed side rails or full to king standard bed Pressure relieving mattress overlay	Independent	Full to king standard bed Pressure relieving mattress overlay	Independent	Full to king standard bed Pressure relieving mattress overlay	Independent	Full to king standard bed
Level: Some assist to independent Uneven: Some to total assist	Transfer board	Independent with or without transfer board	Transfer board	Independent with or without transfer board	Transfer board	Independent	

Continued on following page

Table 49-3 Expected Functional Outcomes by Neurologic Level of Injury (Continued)

		C1-C4		C5	
Domain	**Domain Description**	**Expected Outcome**	**Equipment**	**Expected Outcome**	**Equipment**
Wheelchair propulsion and pressure reliefs		Power: Independent Manual: Total assist for propulsion and pressure reliefs	Power: Power recline and/or tilt wheelchair with postural support and head, chin, or breath control Manual: Manual recline and/or tilt wheelchair Pressure-relieving wheelchair cushion	Power: Independent Manual: Independent to some assist indoors on noncarpeted level surfaces and some to total assist outdoors for propulsion; some assist for pressure reliefs	Power: Power recline and/or tilt wheelchair with arm drive control Manual: Ultralightweight rigid or folding frame with handrim modifications and postural support Pressure-relieving wheelchair cushion
Standing and ambulation	For exercise, psychological benefit, or for functional activities	Not indicated		Standing: Total assist Ambulation: Not indicated	Hydraulic standing frame
Eating, dressing, and bathing		Total assist	Bathing: Handheld shower, padded reclining commode chair with head support, and roll-in shower	Eating: Independent with equipment after total assist for setup including cutting food Dressing and bathing: Total assist	Eating: Wrist splint with universal cuff, bent fork or spoon, nonslip mat, plate guard, and possibly a mobile arm support Bathing: Handheld shower, padded reclining commode chair with head support, and roll-in shower
Communication	Keyboard use, handwriting, and telephone use	Total assist to independent after setup with equipment	Mouth stick Voice-activated devices or infrared head control devices for computer and environmental control Inline speaking valve for ventilator tubing	Independent to some assist after setup with equipment	Adaptive devices as needed for page turning, writing, and button pushing Voice-activated devices Bluetooth
Transportation	Driving, attendant-operated vehicle, and public transportation	Total assist	Attendant-operated van (e.g., lift, tie-downs) or accessible public transportation	Independent with highly specialized equipment; some assist with accessible public transportation; total assist for attendant-operated vehicle	Highly specialized modified van with lift

C6-C7		***C8***		***T1-T12***		***L1-S5***	
Expected Outcome	**Equipment**	**Expected Outcome**	**Equipment**	**Expected Outcome**	**Equipment**	**Expected Outcome**	**Equipment**
Power: Independent with standard arm drive on all surfaces Manual: Independent indoors and some assist outdoors for propulsion; independent for pressure reliefs	Power: Power recline and/or tilt wheelchair with arm drive control or power-assist wheelchair Manual: Ultralightweight rigid or folding frame with handrim modifications and postural support Pressure-relieving wheelchair cushion	Manual: Independent all surfaces	Ultralightweight rigid or folding frame Pressure-relieving wheelchair cushion	Manual: Independent all surfaces	Ultralightweight rigid or folding frame Pressure-relieving wheelchair cushion	Manual: Independent all surfaces	Ultralightweight rigid or folding frame Pressure-relieving wheelchair cushion
Standing: Total assist Ambulation: Not indicated	Hydraulic standing frame	Standing: Some assist to independent Ambulation: Not indicated	Standing frame	Standing: Independent Ambulation: For exercise only	Standing frame Knee-ankle-foot orthosis (KAFO) Walker or forearm crutches	Standing: Independent Ambulation: Functional if only one KAFO needed	Standing frame KAFO or ankle-foot orthosis Forearm crutches or cane as indicated
Eating: Independent with or without equipment, except cutting, which is total assist Dressing and bathing: Independent upper body; some to total assist for lower body	Eating: Adaptive devices as indicated (e.g., wrist splint with utensil holder or universal cuff, adapted utensils, nonslip mat, plate guard) Dressing: Adaptive devices as indicated (e.g., button; hook; loops on zippers, pants; socks, Velcro on shoes) Bathing: Padded tub transfer bench or commode chair, wash mitt, and handheld shower	Eating: Independent Dressing and bathing: Some assist to independent with adaptive equipment	Dressing: Adaptive devices as indicated (e.g., button; hook; loops on zippers, pants; socks, Velcro on shoes) Bathing: Padded tub transfer bench or commode chair, wash mitt, and handheld shower	Independent		Independent	
Independent with or without equipment	Adaptive devices as needed for page turning, writing, and button pushing Bluetooth	Independent	Adaptive devices as indicated	Independent		Independent	
Independent driving from wheelchair	Modified van with lift, sensitized hand controls, and tie-downs for wheelchair	Independent car if independent with transfer and wheelchair loading/ unloading Independent driving modified van from captain's seat	Car with hand controls Modified van with lift and hand controls	Independent car Independent driving modified van from captain's seat	Car with hand controls Modified van with lift and hand controls	Independent car	Car with hand controls depending on degree of lower extremity function

cervical dislocation is performed by applying a series of increasing distracting forces through the long axis of the body by means of a two-point attachment to the skull with a tong device. The tong device is attached to a rope that passes through a pulley and is attached to a weight. When the obstruction to normal alignment is overcome with the applied distraction force, and the spine is realigned (e.g., a jumped facet), the distracting forces are reduced again. Use of tongs for traction in children has been associated with dural leaks and halo fixators are generally used instead, with increased number of pins (8 to 10 as compared with 4 for adults) and lower halo pin torques than are used for adults.[13] Surgery is performed after closed reduction to reestablish spinal stability.

Operative treatment of acute spinal injury is generally performed either to stabilize an unstable spine or to decompress compressed neural elements, for example, spinal cord or nerve roots. The best available studies indicate that there is better neurologic recovery, decreased acute care and total hospital lengths of stay, and fewer medical complications when surgery is performed early (<24 hours after injury) as compared with later on.[49,83]

If a traumatic SCI is not associated with spinal cord compression or spinal instability, surgery might not be indicated. For example, this could apply in the case of a person with preexisting cervical spinal stenosis who falls and sustains a central cord injury where there is no fracture, subluxation, disk herniation, or spinal cord compression. A cervical collar might be all that is indicated. Use of a spinal orthoses as the mainstay of management is also feasible for bony fractures, such as a compression fracture affecting only the anterior column of the spine without spinal cord compression.

Most practitioners of SCI medicine are in agreement that people with incomplete injuries and spinal cord compression are best served by performing a decompressive procedure to maximize the potential for neurologic recovery. Decompression of the spinal cord in the setting of a neurologically complete injury has been more controversial. It is well established that decompression of the cord in a complete injury is not usually associated with a change from complete to incomplete status. Therefore, the role of surgery in neurologically complete lesions is to provide early stability and rapid involvement of the injured person in rehabilitation, potentially minimizing the occurrence of medical complications in the early phase of the postinjury period. Decompression of the cord in complete injuries might also reduce the incidence of posttraumatic cystic myelopathy.

The surgical approach to the spine is determined based on the mechanism of injury, the location of spinal cord compression, and the surgeon's experience and expertise with the various surgical techniques. An anterior surgical approach provides the most direct decompression of the spinal cord when the compression of the cord is caused by retropulsion of bone fragments or disk material into the spinal canal. Anterior column reconstruction and restoration of spinal stability can often be accomplished with just an anterior approach. There are, however, significant potential complications of an anterior approach. In the cervical region, surgical injury to the recurrent laryngeal nerve can cause problems with speech and swallowing, whereas injury to the pharynx or esophagus can lead to mediastinitis or fistula formation to the trachea or skin. Because the anterior approach to the thoracic and upper lumbar spine requires entry into the chest or retroperitoneum, there is a risk for respiratory complications and vascular injuries in addition to infectious complications. Moreover, several regions of the spine are inaccessible to repair via an anterior approach, including the occipitocervical region, the upper thoracic spine, and the lower lumbar spine. A posterior approach is technically easier and less fraught with complications, although decompression of the spinal cord might be indirect.

In addition to the use of stabilizing hardware, which may include combinations of plates, screws, cages, and rods, the spine surgeon uses bone grafts to ensure future spinal stability, because stabilization using instrumentation alone can fail over time, leading to instability and deformity. Bone used for spinal fusion can be autograft, obtained directly from the injured individual, or allograft, obtained from a bone "bank." Potential sites for autologous bone harvest include the iliac crest, the fractured spine itself, or a fibula. Spinal orthoses are commonly used to immobilize the spine after spinal fusion surgery, to facilitate bone fusion. In most cases, orthoses are worn for 6 to 12 weeks postoperatively to allow for radiographically evident spinal fusion.

Penetrating injuries to the spinal cord are overwhelmingly caused by gunshot wounds. Stab wounds as a cause of SCI are relatively rare. Surgical management for such injuries is only rarely indicated. As a rule, neither of these mechanisms of injury cause spinal instability. Removal of bullets or bullet fragments is typically performed only if their presence in the spinal canal is associated with progressive neurologic deterioration.

Chemical and Cellular Treatment of Acute Spinal Cord Injury

Because motor and sensory recovery after traumatic SCI is often poor, there has been an intense interest in finding an effective treatment for SCI. A number of clinical trials have investigated or are currently investigating potential chemical and cellular treatments for acute traumatic SCI, including methylprednisolone, GM1 ganglioside, gacyclidine, tirilazad, naloxone, bone marrow-derived and umbilical cord blood mesenchymal stem cells, olfactory ensheathing cells, and autologous activated macrophages. None of these treatments have been definitively demonstrated to improve neurologic outcomes.

Of the treatments investigated, only high-dose methylprednisolone sodium succinate has been regularly administered, and even considered the standard of care; however, it is no longer recommended as a standard treatment because of a lack of documented effectiveness in people.[30]

Rehabilitation Phase of Injury

Interdisciplinary Team

Rehabilitation goals after SCI include maximizing physical independence, becoming independent in direction of care, and preventing secondary complications. An interdisciplinary team approach is the model that has historically been used in the rehabilitation treatment of people with SCI to achieve these goals. The team is optimally led by a physician who has obtained subspecialty board certification in SCI medicine and has undergone formal training in the interdisciplinary team approach. Other members of the team typically include the person with SCI, family members, physical therapists, occupational therapists, nurses, aides, dieticians, psychologists, recreation therapists, vocational therapists, and social workers or case managers. Other consultant physicians, respiratory therapists, speech pathologists, clinician educators, orthotists, and driving instructors can also be members of the team, depending on the specific injury and rehabilitation goals.

In the acute hospital setting, staff members who are not fully familiar with treating people with SCI need to be educated about the potential secondary complications of SCI and how to prevent them. The patient and family members need to be educated about the nature of an SCI and the patient's prognosis and the uncertainty of such. Transfer to a specialized SCI rehabilitation unit should also be facilitated, because patients treated in a specialized SCI center have increased overall survival rates, decreased complication rates for pressure ulcers and other problems, a decreased length of hospital stay, greater functional gains during rehabilitation, a greater likelihood of home discharge, and lower rehospitalization rates.[11,39] Physical and occupational therapists in the acute hospital should facilitate prevention of secondary complications such as contractures, pressure ulcers, and disuse atrophy. This is done through maintenance of joint ROM, splinting, positioning, and selective muscle strengthening. ROM of all joints is performed and taught by the therapists to people with SCI and their caregivers as soon as it is medically safe to do so. Performance of an adequate daily stretching program can prevent joint contractures. Splinting of joints, with either an off-the-shelf or a custom splint fabricated by an occupational therapist, is also often used to provide a prolonged stretch, to facilitate a functional joint position, and to prevent skin breakdown.

The inpatient rehabilitation setting is the cornerstone of the rehabilitation process for people with SCI, and seems to be essential for attaining the above-mentioned broad goals of SCI rehabilitation, and to allow discharge from the hospital to the least restrictive possible setting, ideally to home. As the length of acute rehabilitation hospitalization decreases, many of the tasks described later are refined or even learned in an outpatient, subacute nursing facility or home setting. The rehabilitation process in all of its settings should empower individuals with SCI to know more than anyone else about their own bodies and to provide the resources to find solutions to all the problems that they might encounter in their daily activities and life.

The person with SCI and their family members are essential members of the team. If the person with SCI does not participate in the SCI rehabilitation program, it is not likely to be of much benefit. Rehabilitation nurses, in addition to performing their standard nursing duties, provide education on prevention and treatment of secondary complications, in addition to training in bowel and bladder management. Psychologists help to reduce depression and anxiety, as well as facilitate adjustment to a catastrophic and life-altering injury, by supporting people with SCI (and their families) through the grieving process. This is achieved by providing individual psychotherapy, cognitive-behavioral techniques to enhance adaptive coping, and group psychotherapy to provide additional support and information sharing. Social workers or case managers help individuals with SCI, their families, or their caregivers to obtain needed available resources, benefits, and services. They facilitate the transition from an inpatient rehabilitation unit to the home or another facility, and provide family support. Other physician consultants are typically involved at various points in the rehabilitation process, especially if secondary complications develop. Speech therapists evaluate and treat the swallowing and communicating problems that are common in individuals with tracheotomies, high cervical neurologic levels of injury, and anterior approach cervical spinal surgeries. They commonly perform bedside swallowing evaluations and participate in modified barium swallow tests.

Physical Skill Training

Physical and occupational therapists train people with SCI in mobility, self-care skills, and other activities of daily living (ADL). Achieving adequate joint ROM and strength, necessary to perform these skills, is facilitated through ROM exercises, fabrication and use of appropriate orthoses, and resistance exercises. Individuals whose injuries prevent them from being independent without assistance also need to be educated on how to direct caregivers to provide the assistance they need. The person with SCI should be able to instruct caregivers on how to deliver the needed care in a safe and efficient manner. This is important to prevent injury both to the person with the SCI and to the caregivers.

Training in activities that are performed on a therapy mat is commonly begun as soon as a patient is able to tolerate being out of bed. These activities, which are often composed of separately performed parts of a more complex functional skill, are typically sequenced from the easiest to the most difficult. In progressing through these graduated skills, people with SCI, who are often able to do little for themselves initially, move to a level of stability within a specific training posture. Finally, they are able to move in a safe and effective manner to complete functional tasks.[98] When the tasks are mastered on the mat, they are performed in other more real-life environments, such as in bed.

Mat activities include rolling, prone on elbows positioning, prone on hands positioning, supine on elbows positioning, long sitting, short sitting, quadruped positioning, and transfer training. In first learning to roll on a mat, individuals with SCI rhythmically move the clasped outstretched arms side to side while lying flat on the back, and then forcefully throw the outstretched arms to the side to which they are rolling. Rolling can be facilitated by starting a roll from a semi–side-lying position, with a pillow under one side of the back or with crossed legs. Assuming a supine-on-elbows position is a task that can later facilitate going from a supine to a long sitting position. It can also help strengthen shoulder extensor and adductor musculature. This position can be achieved in several steps by individuals with SCI. First, they place their hands under their hips; next, they flex their elbows; and finally, they shift their weight from side to side to maneuver their elbows underneath their upper body. When a person with SCI first starts to sit on a mat, balance exercises are practiced, either in a long sitting position with the legs extended on the mat or in a short sitting position with the knees bent at a 90-degree angle and resting on the ground. Sitting push-ups are also learned, because these facilitate moving about the mat and transfers.

Transfer training for a person with a complete paraplegia or lower tetraplegia is usually first taught with a sliding board. For a transfer into or out of a manual wheelchair, the wheelchair is positioned at an angle of 30 to 45 degrees from a parallel position to the mat, with the front of the seat nearest the mat. This allows clearance of the rear wheels by the buttocks during the transfer. For a transfer into or out of a power wheelchair, the wheelchair is positioned parallel to the mat, because the high wheels that are present on a manual wheelchair are not in the way on a power chair. Next, the individual scoots forward in the chair, removes the armrest, inserts the sliding board deep under the leg closest to the mat, and then rocks the head and shoulders away from the mat while simultaneously pushing up and toward the mat with the arm furthest from the mat. This causes the buttocks to move onto the sliding board. The rocking and pushing is repeated until the individual is safely on the mat, at which time the sliding board is removed. Leg rests might need to be removed for the transfer. A popover transfer is similar, except that a sliding board is not used. In addition to these techniques, several other different types of transfer techniques are used by people with varying levels of neurologic function. These include the dependent lift transfer, mechanical lift transfer, stand-pivot transfer, sit-pivot transfer, and floor-to-chair transfer. The mechanical lift transfer uses a mechanical device attached to a sling. The dependent lift transfer and the mechanical lift transfer are used mainly for individuals who are unable to physically assist in the transfers. The stand-pivot and sit-pivot transfers require weight bearing on the lower limbs, and are useful only if a person has significant lower extremity extensor tone or adequate lower extremity strength to briefly squat or stand. The floor-to-chair transfer is important for anyone who falls out of the wheelchair or otherwise ends up on the floor, and needs to get back into the chair or another higher surface. Standing can be initiated on a standing frame, a tilt table, or with an exoskeletal device. Standing seems to help lessen bone loss after an acute injury, improve physical self-concept, and improve self-reported health.[15]

Standing should be implemented only with caution in individuals with chronic SCI, because of osteoporosis. Individuals with osteoporosis have a risk for fracture even without weight bearing. Although ambulation is an expressed goal of most people who have experienced an SCI, recovery of ambulation is variable. For people with incomplete motor SCI, gait training can be facilitated by body weight support (BWS), although BWS training has not been shown to be superior to conventional gait training for ambulation.[43] For people with complete thoracic level injuries who wish to undergo ambulation training, orthoses that stabilize the knees and ankles are required. A swing-through gait pattern (Figure 49-14) is taught in several steps similar to the mat activities described earlier. This begins in the parallel bars and includes going from sit to stand, balancing with extended hips, push-ups in the standing position, turning while standing, recovery from a

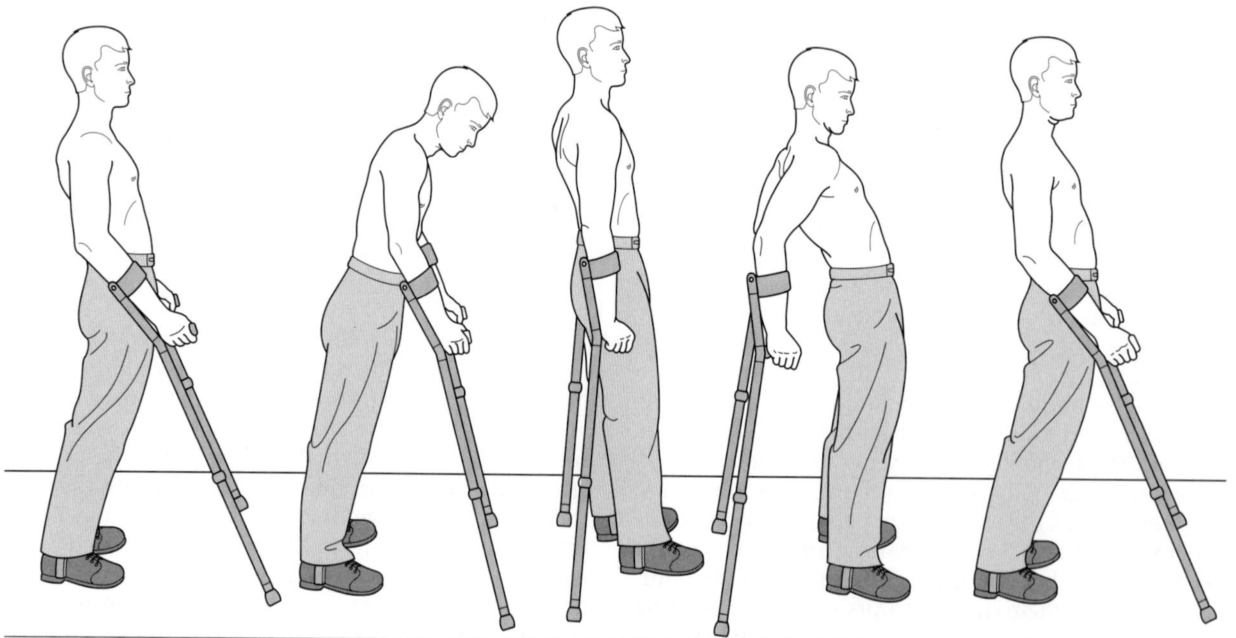

FIGURE 49-14 **The swing-through gait pattern used by a person with complete paraplegia with long leg braces.** (Redrawn from Schmitz TJ: Traumatic spinal cord injury. In O'Sullivan SB, Schmitz TJ, editors: *Physical rehabilitation: assessment and treatment,* Philadelphia, 2001, FA Davis, with permission of FA Davis.)

flexed hip position, advancement of the lower extremities with hip hiking, performance of a step-to gait, and finally a swing-through gait pattern. After the swing-to or swing-through gait pattern is mastered in the parallel bars, it is performed with a walker or crutches.

The use of exoskeletons for ambulation for people who have some truncal stability and the use of their arms to allow the use of upper extremity assistive devices, such as a walker or forearm crutches, is beginning to be used in clinical settings in the United States and around the world. These devices can allow upright walking in people who do not have adequate lower extremity strength to allow walking with or without conventional bracing with only minimal to moderate energy expenditure.

Wheelchair Skills

Physical and occupational therapists not only train people with SCI in wheelchair mobility but also help select the proper seating systems to ensure proper sitting position. Wheelchair users are taught to manage or to direct the management of all wheelchair components, including the brakes, armrests, footrests, wheels, and seat cushion. They are taught how to fold or break down the chair so it can be placed properly in a vehicle. They are taught wheelchair propulsion, first indoors over level surfaces, then outdoors over uneven terrain. Proper body mechanics are taught to achieve efficient wheelchair propulsion patterns, including an ideal propulsive stroke and an ideal recovery stroke. An ideal propulsive stroke is one that occurs at a steady speed that maximizes the handrim "contact" or "push" angle (angle along the arc of the pushrim) while keeping stroke frequency and forces to a minimum. Although self-selected wheelchair propulsion patterns are often not the most efficient ones, experienced wheelchair users often significantly improve propulsion biomechanics from early to late during extended propulsion. Individually selected wheelchair propulsion patterns are often influenced by poor wheelchair sitting positions. Of several propulsion patterns that have been described, differing primarily in their recovery phase, a semicircular wheelchair propulsion pattern has been shown to be the most efficient and least stressful on the shoulders and nerves crossing the wrist.[18] Another basic wheelchair mobility skill is performance of a wheelie, in which the individual in the wheelchair balances on the rear two wheels. This is an important skill that needs to be mastered, to become independent in curb and single-step climbing in a wheelchair.

Spinal Cord Injury Education

During the early phases of SCI, most patients and their families have little knowledge or understanding of the injury; its multiple consequences; the myriad of interventional and management options, community resources, and equipment needs; and the prognosis for life, health, and function. They are often overwhelmed by the gravity of the situation and unable to adjust to a changed lifestyle and self-image. A comprehensive education program is an essential part of any SCI rehabilitation program and, if properly designed, helps the person with SCI and the family members not only to gain knowledge but also to emotionally adjust and prepare for a successful community reintegration. Although some of the learning occurs in formal education classes, group discussions, reading specific educational materials published by various SCI organizations, or extracting information on the Internet, one-on-one instruction by health care professionals is the most helpful in addressing individual needs and concerns. With proper education and the ability to access appropriate information readily, the person with SCI becomes best able to manage successfully the various impairments and ensure the highest possible function and quality of life.

The curriculum of a structured SCI education program should be as broad as possible and include the anatomy, physiology, and classification of SCI, as well as the various medical consequences of SCI, psychosocial adjustments that need to be made, the effect of SCI on sexual health and fertility, assistive technology available for people with SCI, nutritional needs with SCI, available community resources, and ongoing research to improve neurologic function.

Home and Environmental Modifications

It has long been recognized that helping a person with SCI regain mobility by the use of a wheelchair is of little use if the architecture at home and elsewhere is such that the individual is unable to enter or exit buildings or move about freely inside. Without accessible environments at home, school, work, and in the community, the dignity, self-sufficiency, and quality of life are severely jeopardized. The Specially Adapted Housing Act of 1948 provided grant assistance to veterans with service-connected disability to obtain special wheelchair-accessible housing. In 1990, the Americans with Disabilities Act (ADA) expanded the rights of people with disabilities, including prohibiting discrimination against them. It also required removal of architectural barriers in facilities owned by organizations that receive federal funding. This was intended to give people with disabilities equal access to all organizational facilities.

The ADA does not demand removal of architectural barriers in private homes, most of which remain inaccessible for wheelchair users. A home evaluation is best performed before a new wheelchair user returns home. This begins with a review of the floor plan, followed by a home visit, recommendations for architectural changes, and contracting with architects and builders. The main home areas of concern include the main entrance, bathroom, bedroom, and kitchen. The home must also have an exit that the person with SCI can use in an emergency.

Driver Training

Being able to drive an automobile enhances the mobility and quality of life for people with SCI. Most people with SCI can drive an automobile with the proper adaptive equipment and training. Only people with C1-C4 neurologic levels and those with other severe impairments are unable to drive. People with paraplegia can usually drive with basic hand controls for acceleration and braking, and most are capable of transferring between the driver's seat and the wheelchair independently, and of loading the chair into the car. People with tetraplegia usually choose to drive a modified van with a wheelchair lift or a ramp, and varying degrees of modification of the control mechanisms.

Some people with C5 tetraplegia are able to drive, but usually not within 1 year of injury. Most such individuals use a power wheelchair for mobility and are not able to transfer to and from the wheelchair and the car. They require a van with power door openers, automatic lift or ramp, and extensive modifications of the control mechanisms. Occasionally, they require a multiaccess driving system in which the steering, accelerator, and brake are operated by a single control lever.

Driving skills of people with C6 tetraplegia vary considerably, but most are able to turn the steering wheel. Many are not capable of operating regular hand control mechanisms, and require powered or electronic hand controls for braking and acceleration. Most people with C7-C8 tetraplegia have enough upper limb strength to operate a standard steering wheel with a terminal device. The terminal device compensates for their poor handgrip, examples include a knob, cuff, tri-pin, or special grip.

Over the years, major advances in assistive driving technology have made it possible for more people with disability to safely operate a vehicle. The primary controllers of a vehicle, such as steering and braking, can even be concentrated in a complete system that can be operated with only one hand, through a tri-pin or joystick terminal device. This can incorporate the secondary controllers, for example, the gear shift, turn signals, hazard warning lights, horn, dimmers, cruise control, washer, wipers, radio, air conditioner, heater, defroster, doors, lift, and steering tilt. All drivers must use seat belts, but those with reduced trunk control must also use safety belts to secure trunk stability, such as shoulder, chest, or lap belts.

All people with disability wanting to drive should undergo a driving evaluation by a specialist, usually an occupational therapist certified by the Association of Driver Educators for the Disabled (ADED). The ADED website can help to locate certified driving evaluators in the United States and Canada. A predriving evaluation includes an assessment of the person's medical and driving history, as well as functional capabilities. Interactive driving simulators can present the users with diverse challenges in a safe environment, and can provide objective measurement of driving behaviors. Ultimately, however, an actual on-the-road driving evaluation is essential. Selection of the proper vehicle and appropriate modifications to fit the user's ability can involve input from various members of the rehabilitation team. After the vehicle has been modified, the driving educator ensures that all the equipment is appropriate and that the driver is able to use the controls. Behind-the-wheel training by the driving educator can be a lengthy process for people with high-level tetraplegia, because of the complexity of the equipment and the impairment of the learner. The high cost of vehicles and modifications, and the complexity of training, are the most common reasons some people with high-level tetraplegia (C5-C6) choose not to drive. Finally, it should be noted that people with physical disability do not have worse safety records than other drivers.

Vocational Training

Not only do people who have SCI and are employed report higher levels of psychological adjustment, satisfaction with life, independence, and general health than those who are unemployed, but their risk of mortality is lower.[71] Nevertheless, approximately only 25% of all individuals with SCI are employed. Among people listed in the National SCI database, approximately 63% were employed at the time of their SCI, 19% were students, and 17% were unemployed. The relatively high number of unemployed people at the time of injury is recognized as a factor negatively affecting postinjury employment.[70]

Predictors of employment after SCI include being employed before SCI, having a less physically demanding occupation before SCI, being younger at the time of SCI, having a less severe SCI, having lived more years with SCI, having more education before SCI, being motivated to work, and being white.[70] Education has been found to be the factor most strongly associated with postinjury employment. Only 5% of people in the National SCI database with less than 12 years of education were found to be employed, but with each successive educational milestone completed, employment numbers improved, reaching a high of 70% employment of people with doctoral degrees. In general, by postinjury year 10, one third of people with paraplegia and a quarter of those with tetraplegia are employed.

Vocational rehabilitation is concerned with supporting efforts by a person with a disability to return to and maintain employment. Rehabilitation counselors, who facilitate this process, usually have master's degrees in rehabilitation counseling and optimally are accredited by the Council on Rehabilitation Education. Vocational rehabilitation typically begins with an evaluation of the person's functional limitations, barriers to employment, transferable skills, career interests, and previous achievement. The assessment might also include an assessment of performance during simulated or actual work. Assessment might be followed by counseling and support with regard to educational or vocational reentry, job accommodation, and supported employment. Educational or vocational reentry is often facilitated by a rehabilitation counselor who can liaise with employers, because most employers have little experience interacting with people with disability and can have difficulty imagining how a person with an SCI could perform a specific job. Job accommodation, or the modification of a job to make it accessible to a person with SCI, might involve modification of the job site, use of adaptive equipment, or job policy changes. Modifications of the job site can range from the simple, such as adjustment of desk height to accommodate a wheelchair, to the complex, such as redesign of an assembly line. Adaptive equipment can include tools with special handles or sit-stand workstations. Job policy changes can include reassignment of physical tasks or changes in the number and length of workday breaks. Supported employment refers to the need by the individual with SCI for additional assistance in the workplace, ranging from a need for a full-time personal care assistant to the occasional need for manipulation of work materials.

Several legislative initiatives have been implemented with a goal of promoting employment of people with disabilities. The Rehabilitation Act of 1973 provides federal funding for vocational rehabilitation programs in each state. The ADA attempts to prevent discrimination in employment against qualified individuals who are able to perform essential functions of a job with or without accommodation.[1] Workers' compensation programs in most states provide a vocational rehabilitation program for workers who are injured at work, including retraining of those who cannot return to a previous or similar job.

Reconstructive Surgery of the Upper Limbs

Tenodesis refers to the surgical attachment of a tendon to a bone. In contrast, tenodesis action refers to the passive tightening of a tendon when stretched by the movement over a proximal joint over which it crosses, causing a movement of a distal joint. A passive tenodesis hand is one in which there is no volitional control of intrinsic or extrinsic hand muscles or the wrist extensors. Opening and closing of the hand can only occur with passive tenodesis action through forearm pronation and supination, respectively. An active tenodesis hand is one in which there is the addition of active wrist extension that allows for passive movement of the fingers into a grasp dependent on tenodesis action; relaxation of the wrist extension allows for release. Grasp attributable to tenodesis action is usually more effective in a hand that has developed tightness of paralyzed muscles to achieve a functional grasp position. It can be accentuated through the reconstructive surgical procedure described later. An active extrinsic hand is one with voluntary control of wrist extensors and extrinsic finger flexors that can allow some grasp with or without tenodesis action, whereas an active extrinsic-intrinsic hand is one in which there is volitional control of both the intrinsic and extrinsic hand musculature. Arthrodesis refers to joint fusion whereby the joint cartilage is removed from either side of the joint, and the exposed bony ends are opposed and allowed to fuse. Tendon transfer refers to the detachment of a tendon of an expendable innervated muscle from one of its attachments, and reattachment of the innervated muscle and tendon to another tendon that lacks an innervated muscle but whose regained function is sought.

Functional upper limb surgical reconstruction has historically been delayed for 1 year postinjury to allow for neurologic recovery in targeted muscles. Muscles are chosen for transfer if they have a strength grade of 4 or 5, because one grade of muscle strength is usually lost with the transfer. Transferred muscles with a strength grade of less than 3 generally do not improve function. Muscles should not be chosen for transfer if their loss would result in a functional decline. After a tendon transfer procedure, the tendon constructs are typically immobilized for several weeks in a nonstretched position, followed by gradual mobilization, strengthening, and reeducation. Functional electrical stimulation (FES) is often used to facilitate neuromuscular reeducation. Common tendon transfers and tenodesis procedures are shown in Table 49-4 stratified to ISNCSCI motor levels and the more specific International Classification for Surgery of the Hand in Tetraplegia (ICSHT) motor groups.[80]

Functional improvements achieved after a deltoid or biceps to triceps transfer primarily occur through an increased ability to stabilize the arm and reach overhead. Improvements can be seen in feeding, grooming, pressure relief performance, and writing. Functional improvements after a brachioradialis (BR) to extensor carpi radialis brevis transfer can include an increased ability to pick up objects, feed, groom, write, and type. Functional improvements after a BR to flexor pollicis longus (FPL) transfer can include an increased ability to pick up a pen and write, more efficient grooming, and less dependence on a wrist-hand orthosis for grasp. The combination of BR to FPL and extensor carpi radialis longus to flexor digitorum profundus (FDP) tendon transfers has been shown to lead to improved key pinch, grasp strength, and subjective ADL performance. Functional improvements after the combination of BR to FPL and pronator teres to FDP tendon transfers have been noted in manual wheelchair propulsion, lower limb dressing, opening of jars, and the transferring of objects with the reconstructed hands.

Functional Electrical Stimulation for Therapeutic Exercise

Sedentary lifestyle and impaired autonomic function in people with SCI lead to many degenerative physiologic changes that can affect their health and wellness. Muscle bulk, strength, endurance, and bone density are lost in the paralyzed limbs; cardiovascular fitness, VC, and lean body mass are reduced; and certain endocrine functions are altered. FES-induced leg exercise, achieved most commonly on cycle ergometers but also with rowing, poling, stepping, and other repetitive exercise machines, in people with SCI has been shown to improve cardiorespiratory fitness, lower extremity circulation, exercise capacity; increase muscle size; decrease pain; and alter bone mineral density (BMD).[32] During arm exercise with concurrent FES cycling or FES rowing, oxygen uptake is higher than arm or leg exercise alone. This increase in oxygen uptake is not associated with an increase in perceived exertion.

FES is not effective in stimulating muscles paralyzed by LMN damage (i.e., damage affecting the anterior horn cells, motor nerve roots, or both), but such damage usually occurs at the level of the SCI lesion. FES is usually a relatively safe intervention, but its application in the presence of cardiac pacemakers or implanted defibrillators is best avoided. Caution is also warranted in the presence of various heart conditions (especially dysrhythmia and congestive heart failure) and during pregnancy.

Body Weight Support Ambulation Training on a Treadmill

Specific intensive walking training of people with incomplete SCI significantly improves walking capabilities. Such training consists of upright walking on a treadmill, with partial BWS provided by a suspending harness, with a therapist guiding and setting the limbs. BWS training has been shown to be effective in improving ambulatory function

Table 49-4 International Classification for Surgery of the Hand in Tetraplegia, International Standards for Neurologic Classification of Spinal Cord Injury, and Possible Tendon Transfers

ICSHT Group	ISNCSCI Motor Level	Innervated Muscles, Grade 4 or 5	Muscle Function	Transfer Possible	Muscle Function after Transfer
0	C5 (if grade 3 elbow flexion)	BR ≤ grade 3	Flexion/supination of elbow		
1	C5	BR	Flexion/supination of elbow	Deltoid to TR or biceps to TR*, BR to ECRB**	Elbow extension*, wrist extension**
2	C6	Group 1, ECRL	Radially deviated wrist extension	FPL to volar radius (Moberg procedure)*, BR to FPL**	Passive thumb flexion (lateral pinch)*, Active thumb flexion**
3	C6	Group 2, ECRB	Wrist extension	BR to FPL*, ECRL to FDP**	Active thumb flexion*, active finger flexion**
4	C6	Group 3, PT	Wrist pronation	BR or PT to FPL*, ECRL to FDP**, EPL and EDC to dorsum of the wrist (extensor tenodesis)***	Active thumb flexion*, active finger flexion**, passive thumb and finger extension***
5	C7	Group 4, FCR	Wrist flexion	BR to FPL*, ECRL or PT to FDP**, extensor tenodesis***	Active thumb* and finger flexion**, passive thumb and finger extension***
6	C7	Group 5, EDC	Finger extension	BR to FPL*, ECRL or PT to FDP**	Active thumb* and finger flexion**
7	C7	Group 6, EPL	Thumb extension	BR to FPL*, ECRL or PT to FDP**	Active thumb* and finger flexion**
8	C8	Group 7, finger flexors	Finger flexion		
9	C8	Lacks hand intrinsics only	Finger flexion, strong		

From McDowell CL, Moberg E, House JH: Second International Conference on Surgical Rehabilitation of the Upper Limb in Traumatic Quadriplegia, *J Hand Surg Am* 11:604-608, 1986; McDowell CL, Moberg EA, Smith AG: International Conference on Surgical Rehabilitation of the Upper Limb in Tetraplegia, *J Hand Surg Am* 4:387-390, 1979; Waters RL, Muccitelli LM: Tendon transfers to improve function of patients with tetraplegia. In Kirshblum S, Campagnolo DI, DeLisa JA, eds: *Spinal cord medicine*, Philadelphia, 2002, Lippincott Williams & Wilkins.

NOTE: The asterisks in each row are meant only to relate a particular transfer to a particular muscle function after transfer, all within a specific row. For example, the deltoid to TR or biceps to TR transfer would allow for elbow extension after the transfer procedure is performed.

BR, Brachioradialis; *ECRB,* extensor carpi radialis brevis; *ECRL,* extensor carpi radialis longus; *EDC,* extensor digitorum communis; *EPL,* extensor pollicis longus; *FCR,* flexor carpi radialis; *FDP,* flexor digitorum profundus; *FPL,* flexor pollicis longus; *ICSHT,* International Classification for Surgery of the Hand in Tetraplegia; *ISNCSCI,* International Standards for Neurologic Classification of Spinal Cord Injury; *PT,* pronator teres; *TR,* triceps.

after SCI, although not more effective than equivalent overground mobility training.[43]

Epidural Spinal Cord Stimulation

Epidural subthreshold motor stimulation (using a commercially available epidural stimulator as is used for the treatment of pain) in conjunction with voluntary motor training and standing or stepping in people with chronic motor complete paraplegia has shown effectiveness in promoting volitional motor recovery in some people.[2]

Chronic Phase of Injury

Adjustment to Disability

SCI is a catastrophic event with a profound effect on the injured person as well as on family members. Different personal, interpersonal, and cultural factors ultimately determine how successfully an individual with SCI will adjust or adapt to the disability. Successful adjustment is thought to have occurred when the disability is no longer the dominant concern in the person's life. Such adjustment is highly individually variable and has been estimated by some to occur over 2 to 5 years, whereas others propose that adjustment is a lifelong process. Adjustment has been considered by many to consist of sequential psychological reactions according to stage theories, beginning with denial and followed by anger, bargaining, depression, and finally acceptance or adjustment. Although such sequential reactions are often seen in people with SCI, they tend to be highly individualized with some people never seeming to pass though some of the stages and others being stuck in one stage forever.

Despite an overwhelming sense of loss initially after SCI, most people eventually learn to cope emotionally and conform to their premorbid personality styles of interacting with the environment. A number of psychological problems, however, primarily depression and anxiety, can interfere with adjustment and quality of life. These problems can lead to substance abuse, divorce, dependency, self-neglect, and even suicide.

The prevalence of major depression in people with SCI at any one time is approximately 20% of whom 15% have suicidal ideation.[60] The natural history seems to be that for those evaluated at 5 years postinjury, 50% have chronic depression, whereas the other 50% have depression that was not present at 1 year postinjury. Declining health, worsening pain, and cessation of unhealthy alcohol use are risk factors for developing major depression when one was not depressed earlier. Other risk factors for depression are similar to those in able-bodied individuals, especially a family history of depression. Factors specific to the SCI, such as the presence of complete neurologic injury, poor self-perceived health, functional impairments, and medical comorbidities, increase the likelihood of developing depression. Because major depression is treatable and not intrinsic to experiencing an SCI any more than other preventable secondary complications, all people with SCI should be screened for depression and treatment with psychotherapy, and psychopharmacotherapy should be initiated if indicated. Most people with SCI and depression currently do not receive guideline-level treatments for depression.[48]

Quality of Life

Quality of life is a concept that is difficult to define but that can be described as a determination of the individual's satisfaction with life, for example, whether or not the individual is able to do the things he or she personally wants to do. Compared with nondisabled people, people with SCI tend to report decreased well-being and a poorer state of health, and score lower on physical, emotional, and social health domains of life.[41] A metaanalysis has shown no relationship between the neurologic level, the completeness of SCI, and the subjective quality of life. Some factors are thought to affect quality of life positively, such as mobility and ADL independence, emotional support, good overall health, self-esteem, absence of depression, physical and social activities and integration, being married and employed, having completed more years of education, and living at home. In general, dissatisfaction with life after SCI seems more related to social disadvantages than to physical limitations.

Recovery-Enhancing Therapies

Most patients with SCI, even those with neurologically complete lesions, experience some degree of spontaneous neurologic recovery. This occurs as a result of resolution of the acute pathology, with recovery of nerve roots and spinal cord at the level of the lesion.

Despite major efforts to find effective treatments to enhance neurologic recovery during chronic SCI, no reports of scientifically conducted clinical trials exist that show effectiveness for any specific pharmacologic agents.

Late Neurologic Decline

New motor or sensory deficits are reported to develop in approximately 20% to 30% of people with chronic SCI.[74] Most common is entrapment of a peripheral nerve, especially of the median nerve at the carpal tunnel, or of the ulnar nerve at the elbow. Further damage of the spinal cord can be caused by posttraumatic syringomyelia (PTS), also called posttraumatic cystic myelopathy, by tethering or by compression of the cord.

Although it is common to find MRI evidence of a cyst within the spinal cord at the level of the injury, only 5% of all people with SCI develop PTS. It becomes a problem when the cyst expands longitudinally and damages the cord, causing clinical symptoms such as pain, sensory loss, weakness, altered muscle tone, and a variety of autonomic symptoms.[74] The exact cause of PTS is unknown, but it might be related to obstruction of the normal flow of CSF because of scarring or canal narrowing. This leads to abnormal increases in CSF pressure during coughing and straining, ultimately causing a longitudinal dissection of the cord.[74]

The diagnosis of PTS is confirmed by MRI or CT myelogram with delayed images. The clinical symptoms of PTS and their progression vary greatly. If no neurologic decline is noted on regular follow-up examinations, the treatment can be symptomatic. Activity restrictions are usually advisable, especially avoiding strenuous exercise that could raise venous and CSF pressure. When continuous neurologic decline or intractable pain is associated with PTS, surgical treatment is usually indicated to reduce the size of the syrinx or to prevent its expansion. Surgical approaches include placement of a shunt in the syrinx to drain the fluid into the peritoneal, pleural, or subarachnoid spaces; marsupialization of the syrinx; and duraplasty.[74] When treatment is successful, strength might increase, and pain and spasticity might diminish.

Tethering of the spinal cord as a result of meningeal or arachnoid scar formations can occur after SCI and prevent normal rostrocaudal sliding of the cord within the spinal canal on motion. Tethering of the cord in the cervical spine can generate enough cord traction with flexion of the neck to cause cord or brainstem displacement and neurologic symptoms, such as weakness, sensory deficits, and pain. If this occurs, surgical untethering should be considered.

Late compression of the spinal cord or nerve roots can occur for multiple reasons and cause neurologic decline. Common causes include progressive spondylosis, spinal stenosis, intervertebral disk herniations, and posttraumatic changes. Proper imaging studies are needed for diagnosis. Surgical intervention can be needed if there is a rapid neurologic loss or severe, intractable pain.

Secondary Conditions

Pulmonary System

Pulmonary complications, including atelectasis, pneumonia, respiratory failure, pleural complications, and PE, are the leading causes of death for people with SCI in all years after SCI.[88] They accounted for 37% of all deaths during the first year after SCI, and 21% of the deaths beyond the first year, in a large sample from the Model SCI Care Systems and Shriner's Hospitals.[40]

The incidence of ventilatory failure following acute tetraplegia is as high as 74% with up to 95% of patients with injury level above C5 with AIS A status requiring mechanical ventilation at least temporarily.[30]

There are several reasons why children with SCI have a higher mortality and risk of complications resulting from pulmonary issues as compared with adults, including increased restrictive lung disease as a result of the ubiquity of scoliosis, impaired respiratory development in infants and young children, and the increased risk of sleep-disordered breathing in infants and young children with cervical injuries.[101]

Anatomy and Mechanics of the Pulmonary System

SCI can lead to alterations in lung, chest wall, and airway mechanics. The degree of respiratory dysfunction after SCI

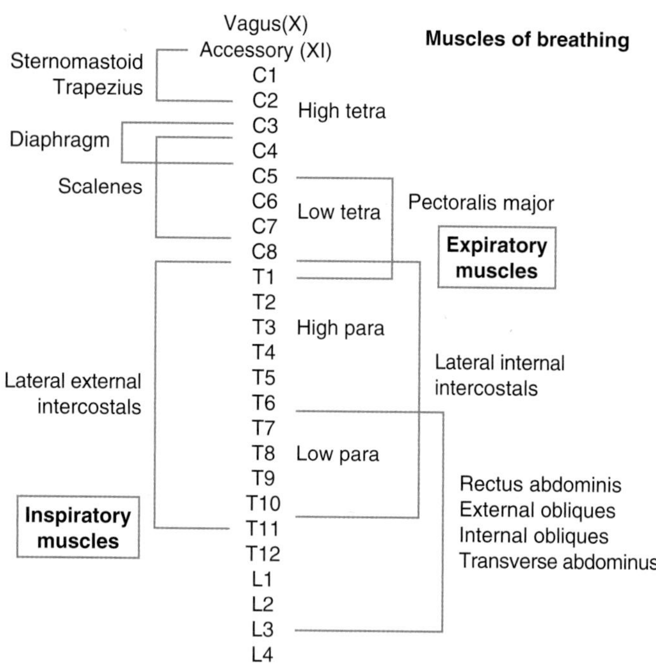

FIGURE 49-15 Diagram showing levels of innervation of the inspiratory and expiratory muscles. (From Schilero GJ, Spungen AM, Bauman WA, et al: Pulmonary function and spinal cord injury, *Respir Physiol Neurobiol* 166:129-141, 2009.)

is strongly correlated to the NLI and degree of motor impairment. The pulmonary function profile of people with chronic tetraplegia and high paraplegia reveals decreased lung volumes and decreased thoracic wall compliance as a result of the restriction caused by respiratory muscle weakness, as well as airway hyperreactivity. Specifically, spirometric and lung volume studies in people with tetraplegia and high levels of paraplegia demonstrate a significant reduction of VC, total lung capacity (TLC), expiratory reserve volume (ERV), and inspiratory capacity (IC), along with a significant increase in residual volume (RV) and little or no change in functional residual capacity (FRC)[97] The diaphragm, innervated by anterior horn cells located in the C3-C5 segments, is the major primary muscle of inspiration (Figure 49-15). The sternocleidomastoid and trapezius muscles, innervated by the spinal accessory nerve and the C2-C4 and C1-C4 roots, respectively, are accessory muscles of inspiration and can be necessary to allow adequate ventilation in people with higher level SCI. Use of a simple bedside spirometer to measure VC can give a quantitative measure of respiratory muscle strength, equivalent to doing a manual muscle test of an extremity muscle. Inspiratory resistive training and aerobic exercise training at a high level (70% to 80% of maximal heart rate) in people with tetraplegia has been shown to improve the strength and endurance of a weak diaphragm and improve lung function.

The VC of people with tetraplegia or high paraplegia is posturally dependent, being up to 15% lower in the upright position than in the supine position. In the sitting position in people with paralyzed abdominal muscles, the effect of gravity on the abdominal contents leads to an increased RV. Use of an abdominal binder in the sitting position helps to reverse this effect by pressing the abdominal contents into the diaphragm, allowing a more efficient diaphragmatic resting position.

Airway hyperreactivity seen in people with SCI is responsive to inhaled bronchodilators and is thought to be caused by unopposed cholinergic tone.[97]

People with a neurologic level of C2 or above with a complete SCI usually have no diaphragmatic function and require mechanical ventilation or diaphragmatic or phrenic pacing. People with a complete C3 SCI have severe diaphragmatic weakness and commonly require mechanical ventilation, at least temporarily. People with a complete C4 SCI also often have severe diaphragmatic weakness and can also require mechanical ventilation, at least temporarily. People with a complete C5-C8 SCI are usually able to maintain independent breathing, but because of the loss of innervation to the intercostal and abdominal muscles, they remain at high risk for pulmonary complications. This risk for pulmonary complications is also present for those with complete thoracic-level SCI, although to a lesser degree depending on the segmental extent of the loss of innervation.

Management of Pulmonary Complications

Atelectasis is the most common respiratory complication in people with SCI and can predispose to pneumonia, pleural effusion, and empyema. Pneumonia commonly occurs in areas of atelectasis. Pleural effusions often develop in close proximity to areas of atelectasis. It is thought that the areas of lung that collapse pull the parietal pleural away from the visceral pleura, leaving an empty space that consequently then fills with a fluid, causing an effusion. Treatment of atelectasis includes lung expansion, secretion mobilization, and secretion clearance. If an individual is receiving mechanical ventilation, a gradual increase in tidal volumes (TVs) to a target of greater than 20 mL/kg of ideal body weight (IBW) has been shown to be effective in decreasing atelectasis as compared with maintaining the TV at less than 20 mL/kg IBW.[30] Intermittent positive-pressure breathing, bilevel positive airway pressure, or continuous positive airway pressure (CPAP) devices can all be used with or without tracheostomy tubes to help with lung expansion and to prevent or treat atelectasis. Secretion mobilization techniques include postural drainage and chest percussion or vibration. Postural drainage uses gravity to assist in drainage of accumulated secretion from specific lung areas. Chest percussion, optimally performed in conjunction with postural drainage, can be performed with a cupped hand, with a mechanical vibrator, by donning a vibrating vest, or by lying in a vibrating bed. Secretion clearance techniques include suctioning, manually assistive cough, use of a mechanical insufflator-exsufflator, and bronchoscopy. The insufflator-exsufflator supplies a positive pressure to the airway, followed immediately by a negative pressure, either through the mouth or a tracheostomy tube. This rapid pressure change induces a high expiratory flow rate similar to a cough. It is less traumatic than suctioning. Bronchoscopy is usually reserved for persistent atelectasis or lung collapse.

Medications are useful adjuncts in treating and preventing atelectasis. Bronchodilators reduce airway hyperreactivity and inflammation that contribute to atelectasis formation and sputum production, and stimulate the secretion of surfactant. Use of a beta-2-adenergic medication has been shown to improve expiratory pressures, which can lead to a more effective cough. Mucolytics can be given orally, such as guaifenesin, or via a nebulizer, such as acetylcysteine. Adequate hydration thins pulmonary secretions.

Indications for initiation of mechanical ventilation include physical signs of respiratory distress (cyanosis, accessory muscle use, tachypnea, tachycardia, diaphoresis, altered mental status, hypotension, hypertension), hypercarbia (partial pressure of carbon dioxide in arterial blood [$Paco_2$] >50 mm Hg), hypoxia (partial pressure of oxygen in arterial blood [Pao_2] <50 mm Hg) unresponsive to oxygen therapy, a falling VC (<15 mL/kg IBW), and/or an inability to handle secretions. If intubation is expected to last more than 5 days, a tracheostomy should be performed.

The mode of mechanical ventilation used conventionally in a rehabilitation setting has been assist-control or controlled mandatory ventilation during rest. Weaning then occurs as progressive ventilator-free breathing (PVFB), starting with a trial of as little as 2 minutes per day with the individual completely disconnected from the ventilator. Oxygen is given via a tracheostomy mask or T piece. The time away from the ventilator is gradually increased in duration, in single or multiple trials per day, depending on the length of each trial, as tolerated. It should be borne in mind that after lengthy mechanical ventilation, the diaphragm muscle becomes atrophied and deconditioned, requiring a lengthy period of reconditioning before ventilator-free breathing is achieved. PVFB is also useful for people who are not expected to fully wean, giving them some confidence and endurance to remain off the ventilator for a short period if an unforeseen problem occurs with their ventilator setup.

A further advantage of the use of the assist-control or the controlled mandatory ventilation modes of ventilation for people with a tracheostomy, in contrast to other modes, is that it allows the individual to speak if the cuff on the tracheostomy tube is partially or wholly deflated. When the cuff is deflated, air expired from the lungs can escape around the tracheostomy tube and balloon up through the larynx to allow voicing. To compensate for the loss of such air around the tracheostomy tube and not entering the lungs, the set TV should be increased. Many individuals are able to vocalize while using a mechanical ventilator in this manner, timing their speech to coincide with exhalation. In addition, a one-way air-flow valve can be put in line with the ventilator tubing, such as a Passy-Muir valve. This maximizes the air flow through the larynx by not allowing air to escape through the tracheostomy into the ventilator tubing (Figure 49-16). These one-way valves must be used only with a tracheostomy tube that has a deflated cuff or no cuff at all. Such valves can be attached to the tracheostomy tube alone to also allow voice during the ventilator-free weaning periods.

Phrenic nerve and direct diaphragm pacing can each stimulate the diaphragm to allow nonmechanical ventilation in people without spontaneous diaphragm motor function. Both techniques require intact phrenic nerves. Phrenic nerve pacing is the more invasive of the two techniques, with electrical stimulating cuffs placed around the phrenic nerves in the chest or neck through a thoracotomy. A phrenic nerve pacing system includes a radiocontrolled implanted stimulator under the skin and an external control unit and battery. Stimulation is started 2 weeks postoperatively, and reconditioning of the diaphragm can take 2 to 3 months. Diaphragm pacing differs in that the electrodes are implanted directly into the diaphragm via a less invasive laparoscopic approach, eliminating the risk for phrenic nerve injury. In the diaphragmatic pacing system, electrode wires protrude through the skin and are attached to an external battery-powered stimulator unit. Stimulation can be begun immediately after implantation, and reconditioning can also take several months, although it has been accomplished in as early as 1 week.

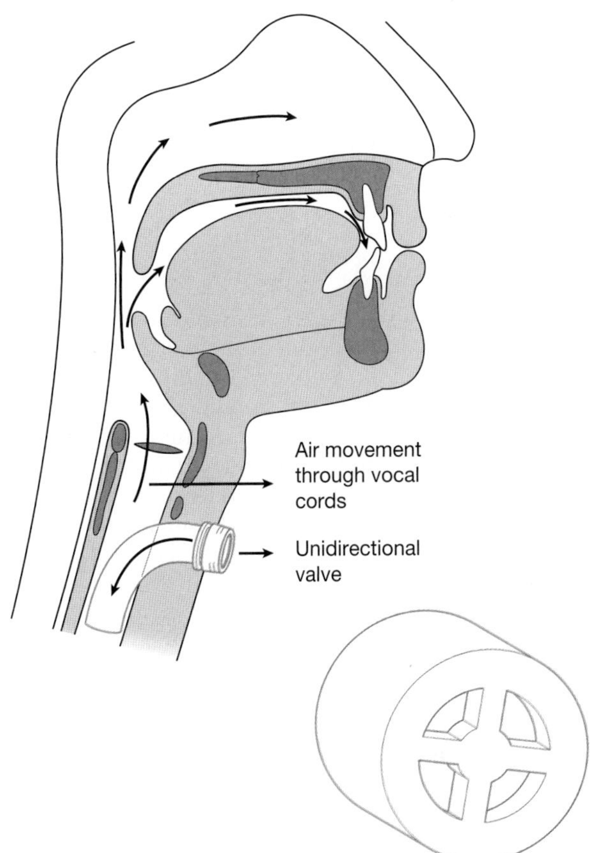

FIGURE 49-16 Functioning of a Passy-Muir tracheostomy speaking valve. (Redrawn from Manzano JL, Lubillo S, Henriquez D, et al: Verbal communication of ventilator dependent patients, *Crit Care Med* 21:512-517, 1993, with permission.)

Sleep Disorders

Obstructive sleep apnea (OSA) is characterized by a repetitive collapse of the upper airway during sleep. This can cause fragmentation of sleep, loss of the restorative function of sleep, and increased sympathetic nervous system activity. It results in excessive sleepiness, systemic and pulmonary hypertension, and an increased risk for developing stroke or myocardial infarction. The prevalence of OSA in individuals with tetraplegia is thought to be as high as 50% to 60%, depending on the diagnostic method.[55] This is in contrast to a prevalence of 4% to 9% in the general population without SCI. Identified factors associated with sleep apnea after SCI include daytime sleepiness, obesity, supine positioning, higher neurologic level of injury, and use of antispasticity medication.[55] CPAP, a highly effective treatment that prevents narrowing and closure of the upper airway, is the treatment of choice. Unfortunately, even in those without SCI, long-term compliance with CPAP is low.

Vascular System

People with SCI are prone to stasis of the venous circulation, hypercoagulability of the blood, and intimal vascular injuries. These risk factors for development of venous thromboembolism (VTE) are known as a Virchow triad. Stasis is a direct result of the loss of the muscle-pumping action of the lower limbs and peripheral vasodilatation. Hypercoagulability is caused by release of procoagulant factors after injury, whereas intimal injury can occur from trauma.

Deep venous thrombosis (DVT), one type of VTE along with PE, develops in approximately 50% to 75% of those with SCI who do not receive VTE prophylaxis.[57,86] The risk for DVT is greatest between days 7 and 10 after injury.[57,86] Because most people with SCI who develop DVT do not have clinical signs or symptoms, such as swelling, warmth, or pain, it is common practice to screen people with SCI with a duplex ultrasound during the period of high risk. Identified risk factors for DVT include motor complete injuries and injuries at the thoracic level and below; however, the incidence of PE has not been found to be related to the level or extent of injury.

PE and the postphlebitic syndrome are not uncommon sequelae of DVT. PE is the cause of death for approximately 10% of individuals who have SCI.[40,92] Most of these deaths are thought to occur within the first year.[40] The most common symptoms of PE include dyspnea and chest pain, although many cases are clinically silent with a significant number exhibiting no clinical features of a DVT. PE without associated DVT may be even more common than PE associated with DVT in people with associated chest trauma, when it is thought that the pulmonary thrombosis develops de novo rather than having traveled from the periphery, as has been traditionally thought.[112]

Because of the high incidence of DVT and potential fatal outcome of a PE, VTE prophylaxis is the standard of care. Several large trials comparing subcutaneously administered low-molecular–weight heparin (LMWH) and fixed-dose unfractionated heparin have shown LMWH to be more effective in preventing both DVT and PE after SCI.[109] Guidelines recommend that pharmacologic prophylaxis should continue for 8 to 12 weeks postinjury with the addition of distal lower extremity pneumatic compression garments during the first 2 weeks after injury.[109]

The treatment regimen for DVT or PE typically involves therapeutic anticoagulation unless contradicted. Treatment is generally continued for 6 months after DVT is diagnosed to prevent progression and recurrence of thrombosis. If there is recurrence, then indefinite anticoagulation is recommended. Inferior vena cava (IVC) filters are indicated for people who have failed anticoagulant prophylaxis with the development of DVT or PE despite adequate anticoagulation, or who have a thromboembolus within the IVC or iliac veins. They are also indicated in those who have a contraindication to anticoagulation or who have a complication of anticoagulation such as hemorrhage or thrombocytopenia. Removable IVC filters should almost always be used, and they should be removed generally within 8 to 12 weeks if no thromboembolism has developed.

Children with SCI seem to be at lesser risk than adolescents with SCI, although the literature is sparse. In one large review, the incidence of VTE in a pediatric population with SCI was less than 5%.[110]

Cardiovascular and Autonomic System

Cardiovascular Disease

People with SCI are at increased risk for cardiovascular disease (CVD). People with SCI, both those with paraplegia and tetraplegia, have a high prevalence of asymptomatic coronary artery disease as detected by thallium stress testing.[8,9]

The cardiometabolic syndrome consists of several core risk factors for CVD including abdominal obesity, hypertriglyceridemia, low plasma high-density lipoprotein cholesterol (HDL-C), hypertension, and fasting hyperglycemia. A combination of three or more of which confers the same health risk as known coronary artery disease.[87]

Approximately one third of adults with SCI are obese and more than half of children with spina bifida, as an example, have body mass index values greater than the 95th percentile.[64] More than one third of people with SCI have a low HDL level. Impaired glucose tolerance and reduced lean body mass are also significantly more prevalent in people with SCI than those without SCI. These metabolic abnormalities are thought to be directly related to poor physical fitness and lack of adequate aerobic exercise after SCI.

Fitness and Exercise

Upper extremity moderate or greater intensity exercise programs that are performed consistently have been shown to decrease insulin resistance, raise HDL-C levels, and increase lean body mass in people with SCI.[87] Participation in a regular, vigorous exercise or wheelchair sports program can improve health status, and also challenge individuals with SCI to overcome physical obstacles and to achieve greater functional independence.[56] Wheelchair sports can also improve psychosocial outcomes by reducing stigmatization, stereotyping, and discrimination by promoting acceptance of those with disabilities as fully functioning members of society.[56] Sports participation by wheelchair users has been associated with fewer physician visits per year, fewer rehospitalizations, and fewer medical complications over time.[105] Common organized wheelchair sports include basketball, tennis, table tennis, swimming, softball, snow skiing, sled hockey, track and road racing, rugby for those with tetraplegia (quad rugby), air rifle and pistol, archery, fencing, billiards, and bowling. These wheelchair sports require that individuals be classified, based on a medical history, muscle test, and a functional evaluation, to allow people with different levels of disability to compete fairly.[58] Wheelchair rugby, for example, was developed in the 1970s as an alternative to wheelchair basketball, because most people with cervical neurologic levels of injury either lacked the capacity to play basketball or spent most of the time on the bench. It is a mixture of wheelchair basketball, ice hockey, and football played on a basketball court with goal lines on either end. A goal is scored when a player in possession of the (volley)ball crosses the opposing goal line. A player in possession of the ball must pass or bounce the ball within 10 seconds.[58] All of these sports can also be performed noncompetitively. The International Paralympic Committee organizes the Summer and Winter Paralympic Games, and serves as the International Federation for nine sports, for which it supervises and coordinates the World Championships and other competitions. More information can be found on the official website of the Paralympic Movement (www.paralympic.org).

Autonomic Dysfunction

The autonomic nervous system is under supraspinal control, and therefore its function is disturbed by SCI. The autonomic nervous system normally controls visceral functions and maintains internal homeostasis through its nerve supply to smooth muscles, cardiac muscle, and glands. The parasympathetic system has a cranial and sacral outflow from the central nervous system and modulates "at rest" functions such as digestion, gastrointestinal motility, reduction of heart rate, breathing, and blood pressure. The sympathetic system has T1-L2 outflow, which is activated in stressful situations to raise heart rate and blood pressure, and to cause vasoconstriction to certain organs. Both the sympathetic and parasympathetic systems consist of preganglionic and postganglionic efferent nerve fibers that regulate visceral function through autonomic reflexes elicited by efferent nerves. After SCI, autonomic reflex function is generally retained, but in those with high-level SCI, this is without supraspinal control. Some clinical conditions related to autonomic dysfunction are discussed in this section, whereas others are discussed elsewhere in this chapter. More information including online training on the International Autonomic Standards for the Classification of SCI can be found on the ASIA Learning Center website (lms3.learnshare.com).

Orthostatic Hypotension. Immediately after SCI, there is a complete loss of sympathetic tone, resulting in neurogenic ("spinal") shock with hypotension, bradycardia, and hypothermia. The hypotension occurs as a result of systemic loss of vascular resistance, accumulation of blood within the venous system, reduced venous return to the heart, and decreased cardiac output. Over the course of time, the sympathetic reflex activity returns, with normalization of blood pressure. Supraspinal control continues to be absent in those individuals with high-level and neurologically complete SCI, however, and they continue to be prone to orthostatic hypotension. This is defined as a reduction in blood pressure when body position changes from supine to upright. The symptoms associated with orthostatic hypotension include lightheadedness, dizziness, pallor, and syncope.

Management of orthostatic hypotension includes application of elastic stockings and abdominal binders, adequate hydration, gradually progressive daily head-up tilt, and at times, administration of salt tablets, midodrine, or fludrocortisone.

Bradycardia. Bradycardia occurs in people with neurologically complete high-level SCI immediately after injury, because of the unopposed parasympathetic effect. During the first month, over one third of those with cervical injury have sinus bradycardia with episodes of heart rate less than 50 beats per minute, whereas over 60% have episodes of heart rate less than 60 beats per minute.[7] People with cervical SCI also experience sinus node arrest (up to 30%), supraventricular arrhythmias (up to 40%), and rarely cardiac arrest during this first month post-SCI. Cardiac arrests are most common in those with high-level SCI, C1-C2 AIS A. As the neurogenic shock resolves and sympathetic tone returns, usually over several weeks, heart rate returns to near normal. Bradycardia can still occur with vagal stimulation thereafter, such as during tracheal suctioning. Bradycardia is less common during the chronic phase of SCI, except during episodes of intense vagal stimulation, such as during episodes of autonomic dysreflexia (AD), as discussed later.

Bradycardia during acute SCI requires close monitoring, but usually no specific treatment is required unless the bradycardia is extreme (<40 beats per minute) or is associated with sinus block. Intravenous atropine might have to be administered prophylactically before tracheal suctioning and other activities associated with vagal stimulation. Persistent, severe bradycardia or other arrhythmia can require insertion of a temporary or permanent demand pacemaker.

Autonomic Dysreflexia. AD is a syndrome and clinical emergency that affects people with SCI usually at the T6 level or above, which is characterized by the acute elevation of arterial blood pressure and bradycardia, although tachycardia may also occur. The hypertension can be profound and can result in intracerebral hemorrhage, status epilepticus, myocardial ischemia, and even death.[117] AD is triggered by a noxious stimulus below the injury level, which elicits a sudden reflex sympathetic activity, uninhibited by supraspinal centers, resulting in profound vasoconstriction and other autonomic responses. The symptoms of AD are somewhat variable but include a pounding headache; systolic and diastolic hypertension; profuse sweating and cutaneous vasodilatation with flushing of the face, neck, and shoulders; nasal congestion; pupillary dilatation; and bradycardia.

The noxious stimulus responsible for AD frequently stems from the sacral dermatomes, most often from a distended bladder. Other causes include fecal impaction, pathology of the bladder and rectum, ingrown toenails, labor and delivery, surgical procedures, orgasm, and a variety of other conditions. It more commonly occurs in people with complete injuries (>90%) than in those with incomplete injuries (approximately 25%) and is more likely to occur in the chronic phase of injury.[69] The T6 level of injury is the characteristic defining level, for which people with a lower level seem much less likely to experience AD; this is attributed to the preservation of the splanchnic outflow innervation with levels below T6. Treatment of acute AD must be prompt and efficient to prevent a potential morbidity and mortality. Recognition of symptoms and identification of the precipitating stimulus are paramount. The individual should be sat up, constrictive clothing and garments should be loosened, the blood pressure monitored every 2 to 5 minutes, and evacuation of the bladder done promptly to ensure continuous drainage of urine. If symptoms are not relieved by these measures, fecal impaction should be suspected and, if present, resolved. Local anesthetic agents should be used during any manipulations of the urinary tract or rectum. If hypertension is present, fast-acting antihypertensive agents should be administered, preferably with something that can be removed if it causes hypotension, such as a topical nitrate.

Occasionally, people experience recurrent symptoms of AD with or without an identifiable stimulus, a condition that requires chronic pharmacologic therapy typically with alpha-adrenoceptor antagonists, alpha- and beta-adrenoceptor antagonists, or the centrally acting alpha-2-adrenoceptor agonist clonidine.

Thermal Regulation. Thermal regulation is impaired in people with SCI, especially in those with complete lesions, because of loss of supraspinal control. Body temperature is controlled physiologically primarily by the hypothalamus and secondarily by personal behavior, to increase or decrease heat loss. Heat and cold signals are normally carried by afferent nerves to the hypothalamus, where they are integrated and thermal regulation is consequently mediated by inhibition or activation of the sympathetic nervous system. With an increase in core temperature, sympathetic inhibition occurs with vasodilatation and sweating. A decrease in core temperature causes sympathetic stimulus, with vasoconstriction, and shivering. With high-level and neurologically complete SCI, the afferent and efferent pathways are interrupted. As a result, vasomotor control and the ability to shiver and sweat are lost. People with SCI therefore tend to have a higher body temperature in warm environments and a lower temperature in cold environments. This is termed *poikilothermia*.

Most of the time, people with SCI maintain relative thermal stability. However, proper heating and cooling of the environment is needed to ensure continuous thermal stability, especially for those with high-level SCI. Appropriate clothing should be worn, strenuous exercise in a hot environment avoided, and cool moist compresses applied when body temperature rises.

Calcium Metabolism and Osteoporosis

An imbalance between bone formation and bone resorption occurs after SCI. The potential adverse clinical effects of this imbalance are fractures related to osteoporosis, hypercalcemia, and renal calculi resulting from hypercalciuria. Markers of bone resorption, including N- and C-telopeptide cross-links of type 1 collagen, become markedly elevated soon after injury and peak 2 to 4 months after SCI, whereas serum osteocalcin, a marker of bone formation, only modestly increases during the first 6 months after SCI, without correlation to the resorption markers.[75] During this time of prominent bone resorption, the release of calcium and phosphorus from bone tissue into the blood causes a significant decrease in parathyroid hormone (PTH).

The decreased PTH levels in individuals is thought to act in the kidney to decrease calcium resorption and to inhibit $1,25(OH)_2D$ synthesis, the active form of vitamin D, which indirectly results in a decrease in intestinal calcium absorption; both mechanisms minimizing the possibility that the skeletal calcium loss will lead to hypercalcemia.

However, in adolescent boys, who seem to have especially high bone turnover, within the first 3 to 4 months after SCI, hypercalcemia is not uncommon, perhaps indicating that the protective mechanisms noted earlier are overwhelmed.[79] Symptoms of hypercalcemia include abdominal pain, nausea, vomiting, malaise, polyuria, polydipsia, and dehydration. Management of hypercalcemia includes hydration with saline infusion, administration of diuretics, and bisphosphonates. Additional risk factors for hypercalcemia include motor complete injury, tetraplegia, dehydration, and prolonged immobilization. A low calcium intake is not typically effective for lowering elevated serum or urinary calcium concentrations, and restrictions of dietary calcium and vitamin D intake are not recommended.

PTH levels generally return to normal by 1 year postinjury[126] and development of secondary hyperparathyroidism can even sometimes occur, which can lead to ongoing bone resorption and osteoporosis. People with chronic SCI are often vitamin D-deficient because of inadequate nutritional intake or reduced sunlight exposure. Supplementation with calcium and vitamin D (which can improve calcium resorption), particularly in the chronic phase when a hypercalcemic status is not present, can be effective in minimizing bone loss.

The degree of lower limb BMD after SCI has been correlated with fracture risk.[125] BMD is typically progressively greater as measured from proximal to distal sites in the lower limbs below the level of injury.[52]

A number of physical interventions have been studied in the hope of preventing and treating the loss of BMD. Individuals with SCI who perform passive weight-bearing standing with the aid of a standing device might have better-preserved BMD in their lower limbs than those who do not stand,[15] whereas FES cycle ergometry has been shown to provide modest reductions in the rate of bone loss.[15]

Several bisphosphonate antiresorptive therapies have been shown to be effective in either maintaining lower extremity BMD after acute SCI or improving low BMD.[75] Vitamin D supplementation in and of itself has also been shown to protect against bone loss after SCI.[10]

Gastrointestinal System

Gastrointestinal Complications

Although impaired evacuation of the colon is the most profound and universal change that a person with SCI will probably encounter with regard to the gastrointestinal system, several other gastrointestinal complications can be experienced. In the acute phase of a cervical SCI, dysphagia is not uncommon. Factors contributing to dysphagia include immobilization of the cervical spine by an orthosis, soft tissue swelling or nerve trauma after anterior cervical spine surgery, and limitation of laryngeal elevation by a tracheostomy tube.[67] In the acute phase of injury, especially within the first several weeks after injury, the incidence of gastric erosions, gastric and duodenal ulcers, and perforation is increased.[104] It is standard practice to administer gastrointestinal ulcer prophylaxis with histamine-2 receptor antagonists or proton pump inhibitors during this time, and usually for 3 months postinjury.

Gallbladder disease and pancreatitis can also have an increased incidence in people with high paraplegia or tetraplegia, because of decreased sympathetic stimulation to these organs. People with tetraplegia also have slower gastric emptying than people with low paraplegia. Adynamic ileus commonly occurs within the first 1 to 2 days postinjury, but usually resolves within 2 to 3 days with bowel rest. The mechanism is attributed to the loss of sympathetic and parasympathetic tone during spinal shock. An acute abdomen is also not uncommon early in the postinjury period, occurring in up to 5% of individuals.[6]

In people with a complete high paraplegia or tetraplegia, symptoms of any abdominal pathology are likely to be vague and poorly localized. Referred patterns of pain can occur instead of the typical localized abdominal pain that might be present in a person with a low paraplegia or no SCI who has the same abdominal pathology. Symptoms of AD, anorexia, altered bowel patterns, nausea, or vomiting can be present, any of which can be the most prominent symptom. Given the frequent atypical presentation of abdominal pathology in these individuals, it is not unreasonable to have a high level of suspicion for abdominal pathology, and a low threshold for ordering laboratory tests or abdominal imaging to confirm the presence or absence of disease.

Bowel Management

The parasympathetic innervation to the portion of bowel extending from the esophagus to the splenic flexure of the colon, which modulates peristalsis, is provided by the vagus nerve. The parasympathetic innervation to the descending colon and rectum is provided by the pelvic nerve, which exits from the spinal cord at segments S2-S4. The somatic pudendal nerve, also originating from segments S2-S4, innervates the external anal sphincter and pelvic floor musculature.

An SCI that damages segments above the sacral segments produces a reflexic or UMN bowel in which defecation cannot be initiated by voluntary relaxation of the external anal sphincter, although there can be reflex-mediated colonic peristalsis. In contrast, an SCI that includes destruction of the S2-S4 anterior horn cells or cauda equina produces an areflexic or LMN bowel in which there is no reflex-mediated colonic peristalsis. There is only slow stool propulsion coordinated by the intrinsically innervated myenteric plexus. The anal sphincter of an LMN bowel is typically atonic and prone to leakage of stool.

A bowel program is a treatment plan for managing a neurogenic bowel, with the goal of allowing effective and efficient colonic evacuation while preventing incontinence and constipation. A bowel program should be scheduled at the same time of day, usually every day in the beginning. The program should be scheduled later on at least once every 2 days to avoid chronic colorectal overdistention. The scheduling of a bowel routine after a meal can take advantage of the gastrocolic response. Although a person with SCI should learn how to perform a bowel routine in bed and on a commode chair, regular performance of the routine sitting up on a commode is preferred to allow gravity to facilitate complete emptying. A diet high in fiber can help produce a bulky, formed stool and promote continence. Medications can also be used, such as stool softeners to modulate stool consistency, and stimulant and hyperosmolar laxatives to improve bowel motility. Minienemas and suppositories can be used to trigger colonic reflex evacuation in people with a UMN bowel. Stimulant and hyperosmolar laxatives, if used, are usually taken 8 to 12 hours before the evacuation portion of a bowel routine.

Two mechanical methods are used to evacuate the rectum: digital stimulation and digital evacuation. Digital stimulation is dependent on the preservation of sacral reflex arcs, and is typically effective only for people with a UMN bowel. Digital stimulation is performed by inserting a gloved, lubricated finger into the rectum and slowly rotating the finger in a circular movement until relaxation of the bowel wall is felt, flatus passes, or stool passes.[28] This typically occurs within 1 minute. Digital stimulation is repeated every 10 minutes until there is cessation of stool flow, palpable internal sphincter closure, or the absence of stool results from the last two digital stimulations. In contrast, digital evacuation is not dependent on the preservation of sacral reflex arcs and is typically performed by a person with an LMN bowel. Digital evacuation is performed by inserting a gloved, lubricated finger into the rectum to break up or hook stool and pull it out. Abdominal wall massage, starting in the right lower quadrant and progressing along the course of colon, is a useful adjunct for attempting to move stool along the colon.

If an effective bowel routine cannot be achieved with the above techniques, pulsed water irrigation has been shown to be effective in some people in decreasing the time it takes to complete a bowel routine and reducing the incidence of bowel accidents and constipation. With this technique, a rectal catheter with an inflatable balloon is inserted into the rectum to allow pulsed warm water to facilitate colonic peristalsis and stool evacuation. Finally, placement of a colostomy has also been shown to be effective in eliminating bowel accidents, dramatically decreasing the time it takes to perform bowel care, and decreasing the amount of assistance needed to perform bowel care. Colostomies are especially useful if incontinence of stool is interfering with wound healing.

Children with SCI should begin management of a neurogenic bowel as they would toilet training.[85] Young children with lower level injuries can be placed on a toilet after each meal (to take advantage of the gastrocolic reflex) and encouraged to push to evacuate. These regular toileting times should last no more than 15 minutes. This procedure is generally most successful in children with LMN-type bowels. For those children with UMN-type bowels the use of suppositories or small volume enemas with or without digital stimulation is often necessary. One particularly effective reversible surgical procedure, called the antegrade continence enema (ACE) procedure, entails attaching the distal end of the appendix (or other fabricated bowel conduit if the appendix has been removed) to the abdominal wall to create an appendicostomy. This procedure can be effective in allowing a child (or adult) who otherwise was having difficulty with a conventional routine to achieve continence. With an ACE, enemas are administrated through the abdominal wall stoma into the cecum allowing stool and to be propelled throughout the colon from the most proximal section of colon down through its entire length and out of the anus.

Genitourinary System

Physiology of the Bladder

The parasympathetic innervation to the bladder, which modulates contraction of the urinary bladder with opening of the bladder neck to allow voiding, is provided by the pelvic splanchnic nerves, which exit from the spinal cord at segments S2-S4. The sympathetic innervation to the bladder and bladder neck or internal urethral sphincter, which modulates relaxation of the body of the bladder and narrowing of the bladder neck to inhibit voiding, is provided by the hypogastric nerves, which exit from the spinal cord at segments T11-L2. The somatic pudendal nerve, also originating from segments S2-S4, innervates the external urinary sphincter.

SCI that damages segments above the sacral segments produces a reflexic or UMN bladder in which urination cannot be initiated by voluntary relaxation of the external urinary sphincter, although reflex voiding can occur. In contrast, an SCI that includes destruction of the S2-S4 anterior horn cells or cauda equina produces an areflexic or LMN bladder in which there is no reflex voiding. The external urinary sphincter of an LMN bladder is typically atonic and prone to leakage of urine. Because central coordination of normal voiding is thought to occur at the level of the pons, in a person with a UMN bladder resulting from SCI, coordination of contraction (or relaxation) of the bladder with relaxation (or contraction) of the external urinary sphincter is lost. This leads to a pattern of simultaneous reflex contractile activity called detrusor-sphincter dyssynergia, which often results in elevated bladder pressures.

Management of Neurogenic Bladder

The goal of management of a neurogenic bladder is to achieve a socially acceptable method of bladder emptying, while avoiding complications such as infections, hydronephrosis with renal failure, urinary tract stones, and AD. During the immediate postinjury period an indwelling catheter is placed within the bladder, because virtually all people with SCI have urinary retention. Other bladder management options are explored later on, depending on the person's gender, level and completeness of injury, and other comorbidities.

Intermittent bladder catheterization (IC) is generally accepted as the best option, other than regaining normal voiding, for the long-term bladder management of people who can perform IC themselves. This is because of the physiologic advantage of allowing for regular bladder filling and emptying, the social acceptability of not needing a drainage appliance, and fewer complications than with other methods. IC is usually performed several times daily with a target catheterized volume of 500 mL each time, for a total fluid intake of approximately 2000 mL/day. IC often needs to be combined with anticholinergic medications in people who have a UMN bladder, to inhibit voiding between catheterizations. To improve bladder capacity and permit successful IC when anticholinergic medication is unable to provide adequate bladder relaxation, or when the side effects of anticholinergics are intolerable, injections of the neurotoxin botulinum toxin have been shown to be effective; however, they must be repeated on a regular basis.[66,84] A more permanent solution, augmentation cystoplasty, a procedure that involves harvesting a portion of intestine and attaching the portion of intestine to the native bladder to create a high-capacity but low-pressure reservoir, has also been shown to be effective.[24]

Reflex voiding is another viable option for men with UMN bladder in whom bladder pressures are generated that are greater than the outlet pressures of the sphincters to allow spontaneous voiding. A condom catheter is applied to the penis and connected via tubing to a leg bag or bedside bag. Reflex voiding can sometimes be triggered by suprapubic tapping. The completeness of voiding can be determined by measurement of a postvoid residual urine volume. High RVs predispose to urinary tract infection (UTI) and bladder stone formation. Furthermore, reflex voiding is often associated with elevated voiding pressures, which can predispose to vesicoureteral reflux, hydronephrosis, and eventual renal failure. It is critically important for reflex voiders to undergo regular imaging with a renal ultrasound to identify reflux or hydronephrosis.

Urodynamic testing is a procedure in which pressure sensors attached to a catheter are inserted through the urinary sphincter into the bladder and the bladder is then slowly filled with water. It can theoretically be useful in estimating relative risk of upper tract deterioration in people who reflex void and others by quantitatively documenting the duration and pattern of detrusor pressures during bladder filling. When accompanying urination, the symptoms and signs of AD typically indicate there is high-pressure (within detrusor) voiding occurring. alpha-Adrenergic receptor antagonist medications, such as prazosin, terazosin, doxazosin, tamsulosin, or alfuzosin, are often effective in decreasing bladder outlet resistance and secondarily decreasing bladder pressures and postvoid RVs.[95] Historically, two transurethral surgical procedures have been performed to decrease bladder outlet resistance. One is the nondestructive placement of a tubular wire mesh stent at the level of the external sphincter. The second is a transurethral external sphincterotomy, performed either with a scalpel or a laser. Botulinum toxin has also been shown to be effective when injected into the sphincter to improve bladder emptying.[33] Reflex voiding, however, is a poor option for women with SCI, because an acceptable external collecting device for women does not exist at present.

Long-term bladder drainage with an indwelling catheter is a reasonable option for people with tetraplegia who are unable to perform IC, or men who are unable to effectively maintain an external catheter on their penis. Use of an indwelling catheter inserted through the urethra is associated with UTI, bladder stone formation, epididymitis, prostatitis, hypospadias, and bladder cancer.[119] Placement of a suprapubic cystostomy tube in people requiring long-term indwelling catheters can avoid some of these complications, such as prostatitis, epididymitis, and hypospadias.

Although UTI is clearly a common complication, controversy exists concerning exactly what constitutes a UTI in people with SCI. Symptoms of fever, spontaneous voiding between catheterizations, hematuria, AD, and increased spasticity, when associated with cloudy or foul-smelling urine and other nonspecific symptoms, such as malaise or vague abdominal discomfort, strongly suggest the presence of UTI and the need for treatment. Although the presence of pyuria can increase the suspicion that a UTI is present, it is unclear whether the presence of pyuria and bacteriuria should lead to the use of antibiotics if the person is otherwise asymptomatic. Bacteriuria is virtually omnipresent in people with neurogenic bladders, and certainly seems to occur in any person who uses IC, an external collecting device, or an indwelling catheter. Frequent treatment of asymptomatic bacteriuria can lead to bacterial resistance. Nevertheless, simple UTIs can be complicated by the development of pyelonephritis, epididymitis, orchitis, prostatic abscesses, and urosepsis. Over the course of time, recurrent UTIs can lead to renal scarring, secondary decreased renal function, and the development of urinary tract stones.

In children, neurogenic bladder training should begin at the same time as toilet training would ordinarily begin. Self-intermittent catheterization usually is successful only in those whose developmental age is older than 5 years. Because continence is a social expectation for children in school, children should be encouraged to become independent in bladder management as soon as they are able to prevent social isolation, which can result from teasing by peers if bladder accidents occur.[85]

Sexuality and Fertility

The ability to have psychogenic erections for men and psychogenic vaginal vasocongestion and lubrication for women is mediated by the sympathetic and parasympathetic nervous systems and directly related to the degree of light touch and pinprick sensory preservation within the T11-L2 dermatomes.[102] The ability to have reflex erections for men and reflex vaginal vasocongestion and lubrication for women is mediated by the parasympathetic nervous system and related to sacral reflex preservation. If a hyperactive BC reflex is present, reflex erections and lubrication are usually possible, although the quality of arousal might differ from preinjury levels. If there is a hypoactive BC reflex with some preservation of sensation within the S4-S5 dermatomes, reflex erections and lubrication are usually possible. However, if the BC reflex is absent and there is no sensation within the S4-S5 dermatomes, the ability to have reflex erections and lubrication is lost, and the ability to generate erections and lubrication psychogenically is related to T11-L2 sensory preservation.

The neurologic control of orgasm has not been well delineated. It is generally believed to be a spinal-level reflex response that can be inhibited or excited by the brain. If on physical examination the BC and anocutaneous reflex are absent and there is no sensation at S4-S5, attainment of orgasm is unlikely. Approximately 40% of men and women with SCI report orgasm; however, achieving orgasm is known to take longer after SCI.

Effective treatments for male erectile dysfunction, not ejaculatory dysfunction, resulting from SCI include (1) oral medications, (2) vacuum tumescence devices, (3) intracavernous (penile) injections, and (4) penile implants. Oral type 5 phosphodiesterase inhibitors such as sildenafil, vardenafil, and tadalafil have been found to be effective in 65% to 75% of individuals in randomized clinical trials, and are now first-line therapies for erectile dysfunction after SCI.[34] Vacuum tumescence devices are effective in producing an adequate erection in more than 50% of individuals, although oral medications have consistently been preferred by users when the methods have been compared directly in studies. Because penile necrosis has been reported if the constricting ring is left in place for too long, the ring should not be left in place for more than 30 minutes. Intracavernous injections with papaverine, phentolamine, or prostaglandin E_1 used alone or in combination, as one has not been shown to be more effective than the others, have a 90% reported satisfactory erectile response rate in pooled cases series.[34] Reported complications of injections include priapism (more often with phentolamine and papaverine), penile scarring after repeated use, local swelling, and pain at the injection site. Penile implants are very effective but have been shown to consistently have a serious complication rate of 10%, including erosion through the skin and infection.[34] If the implanted prosthesis is removed after a serious complication occurs, the penile tissue is invariably damaged, and the other methods of erectile dysfunction treatment are not effective.

Treatment of infertility in men with SCI is initially focused on producing an ejaculate, because only 10% to 20% of men are able to ejaculate naturally after SCI. Interventions including manual or partner masturbation, penile vibratory stimulation, and electroejaculation can lead to success in ejaculation in 95% of individuals.[35] Penile vibratory stimulation is the application of a vibrating disk to the frenulum and glans penis to activate the ejaculatory reflex. This can be performed alone or in concert with electroejaculation, whereby an electrical probe is placed in contact with the rectal wall near the prostate gland and seminal vesicles, and up to 15 to 35 stimulations are administered at progressively increasing voltages. After either procedure, the bladder can be catheterized to harvest any retrograde ejaculation.

Semen quality deteriorates significantly within the first 2 weeks after SCI.[76] This deterioration has been characterized by reduced numbers of spermatozoa, decreased sperm motility, and the presence of inhibitory factors within the seminal fluid. Given these barriers, pregnancy rates are approximately 50% in partners of men with SCI using assisted ejaculation or advanced fertility treatments such as testicular biopsy or aspiration, in vitro fertilization, or intracytoplasmic sperm injection.[35]

Women with SCI are not thought to have decreased fertility, although this has not been closely evaluated. Most women experience temporary amenorrhea postinjury that lasts for an average of 4 months.[62] Pregnancy can alter the ability of a woman with SCI to transfer, perform pressure reliefs, and propel a wheelchair. The introduction of sliding boards and motorized wheelchairs can be helpful during a pregnancy. Because of the enlarging abdomen, self-catheterization can become difficult, necessitating use of an indwelling catheter. Respiratory function can be compromised during pregnancy, especially in women with tetraplegia. The onset of labor can be accompanied by significantly increased spasticity. Labor might not be perceived by women with injury levels above T10. Uterine contractions during labor have been associated with AD in women with injury levels above T6, and this needs to be differentiated from the blood pressure elevations seen in preeclampsia.[21] AD associated with labor, however, can be treated or prevented with epidural anesthesia.

Pressure Ulcers

A pressure ulcer is a localized injury to the skin and/or underlying tissue usually over a bony prominence resulting from direct pressure, where the force vector is perpendicular to the tissue contact area, or shear, where force vector is tangential to the tissue contact area.[16] This applied pressure, if prolonged and of greater magnitude than the supplying capillary and lymphatic vessel tolerance to remain patent, can result in occluded blood and interstitial fluid flow, ischemia, and ultimately tissue necrosis.

In addition to pressure itself, numerous secondary risk factors are associated with the development of pressure ulcers. These risk factors can be divided into demographic, SCI-related, comorbid medical, nutritional, psychological, social, and support surface–related categories. Pressure ulcer risk increases both with time since injury and chronologic age, especially in those older than 50 years of age.[26] With regard to the SCI itself, urinary and bowel incontinence or severe spasticity leading to shear and poor positioning are also risk factors. Diabetes mellitus, smoking, respiratory disease, and hypotension all confer increased risk.[26,114] Biochemical markers of nutrition associated with pressure ulcers include a low prealbumin, albumin, hemoglobin and hematocrit, and total lymphocyte count.[51] Depression can be associated with inactivity, self-neglect, and poor medical adherence to recommendations with regard to skin care, all of which can lead pressure ulcers. Support surfaces for both bed and wheelchair if worn out or are improperly selected also increase risk for pressure ulcer development.

A quarter of those hospitalized in the acute hospital or rehabilitation units of the SCI Model Systems develop at least one pressure ulcer.[25] At 1, 5, 10, and 20 years postinjury, the prevalence has been reported as 15%, 20%, 23%, and 29%, respectively.[124] During acute rehabilitation, pressure ulcers are seen in the following distribution: sacrum, 39%; calcaneus, 13%; ischium, 8%; occiput, 6%; and scapula, 5%.[25] This contrasts with the distribution seen 2 years after injury: ischium, 31%; trochanter, 26%; sacrum, 18%; calcaneus, 5%; and malleolus, 4%.[124] The higher distribution of ulcers in the sacrum and calcaneus in the acute group is probably because of the increased time spent supine in bed soon after injury, as opposed to more time sitting in a wheelchair later.

Assessment of Pressure Ulcers

An assessment of a pressure ulcer should include a notation of location, stage of wound, size, characteristics of the ulcer cavity, and characteristics of the surrounding skin. Table 49-5 outlines a six-category/stage classification of pressure ulcers refined by the National Pressure Ulcer Advisory Committee.[16]

A determination of the potential causes of the breakdown should be made. The location of the wound is often very helpful in determining the underlying mechanism responsible for causing the increased pressure that has led to wound development. For example, a sacral ulcer in a person who does not get out of bed might suggest unrelieved direct pressure from the mattress. A sacral or coccygeal ulcer in a person who is sitting with these areas in contact with the rear portion of the seat might suggest shear over the sacrum and coccyx from sitting. In this latter example, relieving pressure only when in bed and ignoring the poor positioning when in the chair will not allow the ulcer to heal, even with appropriate wound care dressings. A sacral ulcer that recurs after a person sits on a commode might suggest unrelieved pressure created by the edge of the cutout of the seat of a commode chair.

Treatment of Pressure Ulcers

Pressure ulcer healing comprises a sequence of loosely linked components that include inflammation, matrix synthesis and deposition, angiogenesis, fibroplasia, epithelialization, contraction, and remodeling. Growth factors are important determinants of this sequence. Different categories/stages of wounds require different components to heal. Category/Stage II ulcers might need only epithelialization, whereas a category/stage III or IV ulcer can require matrix synthesis and deposition, angiogenesis, fibroplasia, and contraction.

Pressure ulcers can acquire necrotic tissue. Necrotic tissue releases endotoxins that inhibit fibroblast and keratinocyte migration. It is also an excellent growth medium for bacteria. The bacteria produce enzymes and proteases that degrade fibrin and growth factors, leading to impaired healing. Removal of necrotic tissue can be done by a number of different methods of débridement, including autolysis and chemical, sharp, and mechanical débridement. Autolysis is promoted when a moisture-retentive barrier is applied over a superficial ulcer, allowing endogenous enzymes to degrade the necrotic tissue. Chemical débridement refers to the application of commercially available enzymes that selectively degrade necrotic tissues. Sharp débridement refers to excision of necrotic tissue or scar with a sharp instrument. Mechanical débridement can be performed with application of wet-to-dry dressings.

Dressings are topical products used for protection of a pressure ulcer from contamination and trauma, application of medication, débridement of necrotic tissue, and to provide an environment in which tissue hydration levels and the viability of the wound tissue are maintained by something other than the skin. The wound dressing can be viewed as the substitute skin. The major dressing categories include transparent films, hydrocolloids, hydrogels, foams, alginates, and gauze dressings. Transparent films are adhesive, nonabsorptive, semipermeable membranes, whereas hydrocolloids are adhesive wafers with water-absorbing particles that have a minimal to moderate absorptive capacity. Both allow autolytic débridement and are indicated for use in the treatment of partial-thickness wounds.

Table 49-5 National Pressure Ulcer Advisory Panel Category/Staging System, 2007 Revision

Pressure Ulcer Categories/Stages	Description
Suspected deep tissue injury	Purple or maroon localized area of discolored intact skin or blood-filled blister resulting from damage of underlying soft tissue from pressure and/or shear. The area may be preceded by tissue that is painful, firm, mushy, boggy, warmer, or cooler as compared with adjacent tissue. Deep tissue injury may be difficult to detect in individuals with dark skin tones. Evolution may include a thin blister over a dark wound bed. The wound may further evolve and become covered by thin eschar. Evolution may be rapid exposing additional layers of tissue even with optimal treatment.
Category/Stage I	Intact skin with nonblanchable redness of a localized area usually over a bony prominence. Darkly pigmented skin may not have visible blanching; its color may differ from the surrounding area. The area may be painful, firm, soft, warmer, or cooler as compared with adjacent tissue. Category/Stage I damage may be difficult to detect in individuals with dark skin tones.
Category/Stage II	Partial thickness loss of dermis presenting as a shallow open ulcer with a red pink wound bed, without slough. May also present as an intact or open/ruptured serum-filled blister. Presents as a shiny or dry shallow ulcer without slough or bruising.* This category/stage should not be used to describe skin tears, tape burns, perineal dermatitis, maceration, or excoriation.
Category/Stage III	Full-thickness tissue loss. Subcutaneous fat may be visible, but bone, tendon, or muscle is not exposed. Slough may be present but does not obscure the depth of tissue loss. May include undermining and tunneling. The depth of a category/stage III pressure ulcer varies by anatomic location. The bridge of the nose, ear, occiput, and malleolus do not have subcutaneous tissue and category/stage III ulcers can be shallow. In contrast, areas of significant adiposity can develop extremely deep stage III pressure ulcers. Bone/tendon is not visible or directly palpable.
Category/Stage IV	Full-thickness tissue loss with exposed bone, tendon, or muscle. Slough or eschar may be present on some parts of the wound bed. Often include undermining and tunneling. The depth of a category/stage IV pressure ulcer varies by anatomic location. The bridge of the nose, ear, occiput, and malleolus do not have subcutaneous tissue and these ulcers can be shallow. Category/Stage IV ulcers can extend into muscle and/or supporting structures (e.g., fascia, tendon, or joint capsule) making osteomyelitis possible. Exposed bone/tendon is visible or directly palpable.
Unstageable/Unclassified	Full-thickness tissue loss in which the base of the ulcer is covered by slough (yellow, tan, gray, green, or brown) and/or eschar (tan, brown, or black) in the wound bed. Until enough slough and/or eschar is removed to expose the base of the wound, the true depth, and therefore stage, cannot be determined. Stable (dry, adherent, intact without erythema or fluctuance) eschar on the heels serves as "the body's natural (biological) cover" and should not be removed.

From Black J, Baharestani MM, Cuddigan J, et al: National Pressure Ulcer Advisory Panel's updated pressure ulcer staging system, *Adv Skin Wound Care* 20:269-274, 2007.
*Bruising indicates suspected deep tissue injury.

Foams are nonadherent, hydrophobic, or hydrophilic materials with minimal to moderate absorptive capacity. Hydrogels are water-based or glycerin-based gels with minimal to moderate absorptive capacity. Alginates are soft, absorbent, nonwoven, seaweed-derived dressings that have a cottonlike appearance, with a moderate to heavy absorptive capacity. Foams, hydrogels, and alginates all fill dead space within an ulcer crater, require a secondary dressing, and are appropriate for both partial-thickness and full-thickness wounds.

Other adjunctive therapies that have shown benefit in randomized controlled studies and case series have included electrical stimulation for which there is the most evidence and negative pressure wound therapy.[3,61] However, negative pressure wound therapy is not without risk including bleeding and infection.

Adequate nutrition is essential to heal a pressure ulcer. Caloric requirements are increased for a person with SCI who has a pressure ulcer. An estimate of the difference in basal energy expenditure between people with SCI who have severe pressure ulcers and those who do not have pressure ulcers is approximately 5 kcal/kg of body weight/day.[51] Because protein requirements are increased for a person with an SCI and pressure ulcers, recommendations for increased protein requirements range from 1.25 to 2 g protein/kg of body weight/day, with the higher requirements suggested for those with ulcers of greater severity.[51]

Pressure redistribution support surfaces and proper positioning in them can help prevent pressure ulcers from developing, and help to heal them if they occur. Pressure redistribution support mattresses are typically designed to either be *active* with powered alternating pressure chambers or *reactive* with high or low air loss through a single or multiple connected porous chambers. Less effective options for pressure redistribution in bed include the use of active or reactive mattress overlays. Because few individuals with SCI are not at risk for developing pressure ulcers, some type of pressure redistribution support surface should be routinely prescribed. For those with pressure ulcers, a history of pressure ulcers, or multiple risk factors for the development of pressure ulcers, an active or reactive pressure redistribution mattress is indicated. It has been traditionally thought that people with SCI and poor sensation need to be repositioned onto a different support surface every 2 hours, whether or not a pressure redistributing mattress is used. One standard turning position, which redistributes pressure from both the sacrum and the greater trochanters, requires a 30-degree angled, side-lying position, with pillows behind the back and between the knees. Another standard turning position is the prone position, with pillows placed under the thorax, pelvis, thighs, and shins relieving all bony prominences.

Pressure-relieving cushions designed for wheelchairs should be used to prevent pressure ulcers over the ischial tuberosities, greater trochanters, and sacrum/coccyx in those who sit in a position where these bony prominences bear weight. Cushions can be composed of air, foam, gel, or some combination of these. It is also essential when sitting that pressure relief techniques be performed approximately every 15 to 30 minutes for a duration of 2 minutes.[29] Effective manual pressure relief techniques include a forward-lean in the chair (perhaps the most effective), a side-to-side lean, or a push-up. Moreover, individualized wheelchair seating systems that tilt and/or recline or allow standing should be prescribed to all people who are unable to effectively perform these manual pressure relief techniques on their own; powered seating systems are recommended if their living environment is accessible. Category/Stage III and IV ulcers might not heal in a timely manner, depending on their location and size, and operative repair to close the defect is often indicated. Individuals who cannot tolerate surgery for medical reasons, who have a short life expectancy, or who are unlikely to protect the area of operative repair are poor candidates for operative repair. Successful operative repairs typically include excision of the ulcer, the surrounding scar, and the underlying necrotic or infected bone. The coverage is typically a regional pedicle flap that includes muscle and its blood supply. Postoperatively, a person should be positioned off the surgical site for several weeks to allow healing. During this healing period, use of an alternating air mattress or high air loss (air fluidized) bed is recommended.

Pain

Approximately 80% of people with SCI report chronic pain, and approximately one half report chronic, severe pain that interferes with activity and affects quality of life.[23]

Many different types of pain are experienced by people with SCI. The International Spinal Cord Injury Pain Classification organizes pains commonly seen after SCI hierarchically into three tiers (Table 49-6).[20] Within this first tier, nociceptive pain is defined as pain arising from activation of peripheral nerve endings or sensory receptors that are capable of transducing and encoding noxious stimuli, whereas neuropathic pain is defined as pain that arises as a direct consequence of a lesion or disease affecting the somatosensory system. Other pain as defined within the first tier is pain that occurs when there is no identifiable noxious stimulus or detectable damage to the nervous system responsible for the pain.

Musculoskeletal Pain

Musculoskeletal (nociceptive) pain refers to pain occurring in a region where there generally is at least some preserved sensation and the pain is thought to be arising from nociceptors within musculoskeletal structures (muscles, tendons, ligaments, joints, bones). It might occur at any location where there are musculoskeletal structures, including areas below the NLI.

The enormous demands placed on the upper limbs of individuals with SCI during their daily activities, work, and sports lead to a high incidence of overuse injuries and musculoskeletal pain. Overuse injuries are caused by repetitive motions and recurrent microtrauma, which can be aggravated by more major acute injury. The treatment of overuse injuries in the upper limbs depends on the specific etiology, but can be divided into overlapping phases:

- Control of inflammation and pain with protection, rest, ice application, compression, elevation, and nonsteroidal antiinflammatory drugs (NSAIDs).
- Mobilization to regain joint ROM.
- Strengthening exercises once 80% to 85% of painless ROM is achieved.
- Functional restoration.

The goal is to achieve the previous level of function while preventing recurrence.

Shoulder pain is the most common and incapacitating upper limb overuse injury and can be caused by bicipital tendonitis, rotator cuff impingement syndrome, subacromial bursitis, capsulitis, and osteoarthritis. The prevalence of shoulder pain in people with SCI, either paraplegia or tetraplegia, is approximately 50%.[45] The etiology of shoulder pain after tetraplegia, in contrast to shoulder pain after

Table 49-6 International Spinal Cord Injury Pain (ISCIP) Classification

Tier 1: Pain Type	Tier 2: Pain Subtype	Tier 3: Primary Pain Source and/or Pathologic Condition (write or type in)
□ Nociceptive pain	□ Musculoskeletal pain	□ ________ e.g., glenohumeral arthritis, lateral epicondylitis, comminuted femur fracture, quadratus lumborum muscle spasm
	□ Visceral pain	□ ________ e.g., myocardial infarction, abdominal pain due to bowel impaction, cholecystitis
	□ Other nociceptive pain	□ ________ e.g., migraine headache, surgical skin incision
□ Neuropathic pain	□ At level SCI pain	□ ________ e.g., spinal cord compression, nerve root compression, cauda equina compression
	□ Below level SCI pain	□ ________ e.g., spinal cord ischemia, spinal cord compression
	□ Other neuropathic pain	□ ________ e.g., carpal tunnel syndrome, trigeminal neuralgia, diabetic polyneuropathy
□ Other pain		□ ________ e.g., fibromyalgia, complex regional pain syndrome type I, interstitial cystitis, irritable bowel syndrome
□ Unknown pain		□ ________

From Bryce TN, Biering-Sorensen F, Finnerup NB, et al: International Spinal Cord Injury Pain Classification: part I. Background and description, *Spinal Cord* 50:413-417, 2012.

paraplegia, more often includes pain that stems from shoulder instability, resulting from weakness of the muscles that stabilize the shoulder joint, as well as capsulitis and contracture caused by a lack of passive or active ROM and underlying spasticity.

Specific treatment (and prevention) strategies for shoulder pain originating from the rotator cuff in people with SCI should include strengthening, stretching, optimizing posture, and avoidance of activities that promote impingement. Strengthening of the dynamic shoulder stabilizers should occur in a balanced manner. A program should emphasize strengthening the posterior shoulder muscles, including the external rotators, the posterior scapular muscles (rhomboids and trapezius), and the adductors. Wheelchair use promotes strengthening of the antagonists to these muscles (i.e., the anterior shoulder musculature).[19] Stretching of the dynamic shoulder stabilizers, especially the anterior shoulder muscles, is also necessary to achieve a balanced shoulder. This is because these muscles often become hypertrophied and contracted through constant use during wheelchair propulsion and transfer activities. In one controlled study of wheelchair users, an intervention consisting of a 6-month exercise protocol (two exercises for stretching anterior shoulder musculature and three exercises for strengthening posterior shoulder musculature) was effective in decreasing the shoulder pain that interfered with functional activities.[31] Elbow pain in people with paraplegia is also fairly common and is often caused by lateral or medial epicondylitis.

Visceral Pain

Visceral (nociceptive) pain refers to pain usually located in the thorax, abdomen, or pelvis that is believed to be primarily generated in visceral structures.[20] This category includes abdominal pain caused by fecal impaction, bowel obstruction, bowel infarction, bowel perforation, cholecystitis, choledocholithiasis, pancreatitis, appendicitis, splenic rupture, bladder perforation, pyelonephritis, or superior mesenteric syndrome.

The presence of visceral pain is suggested by evidence of visceral pathology on imaging or other testing that is consistent with the pain presentation. Although the pain is characteristically vague and poorly localized, tenderness of the offending visceral structures on palpation of the abdomen might be elicited, depending on the level and completeness of injury. Visceral pain can be associated with symptoms of AD, anorexia, altered bowel patterns (e.g., constipation), nausea, or vomiting, any of which can be more prominent than the pain itself. "Cramping," "dull," and "tender" are common pain descriptors of visceral pain, and a relationship to food intake is often present.

Other (Nociceptive) Pain

AD headache pain can be severe and usually is described as "pounding." It is most common in a person with an NLI at or above T6. AD headache is associated with an elevated blood pressure, and often with diaphoresis, piloerection, cutaneous vasodilatation above the level of injury, bradycardia or tachycardia, nasal stuffiness, conjunctival congestion, and mydriasis. AD is usually triggered by a noxious stimulus caudal to the NLI, usually related to the bowel or bladder (e.g., bowel impaction or UTI). Treatment of AD headache is discussed earlier in the Cardiovascular and Autonomic System section.

Neuropathic Pain

At-Level Spinal Cord Injury (Neuropathic) Pain. At-level SCI (neuropathic) pain refers to neuropathic pain perceived in a segmental pattern anywhere within the dermatome representing the NLI and/or within the three dermatomes below this level and *not* in any lower dermatomes. A necessary condition for classifying a pain as at-level SCI pain is that a lesion or disease must affect the spinal cord or nerve roots, and the pain is believed to arise as a result of this damage. The pain can be unilateral or bilateral. Neuropathic pain occurring in this distribution that cannot be attributed to spinal cord or nerve root damage should be classified as *other (neuropathic)*.

The presence of at-level SCI pain is suggested by allodynia or hyperalgesia within the pain distribution and by the following pain descriptors: hot-burning, tingling, pricking, sharp, shooting, squeezing, painful cold, electric shocklike, and numb.[20] It is often difficult to distinguish between the two subcategories of at-level SCI pain, spinal cord pain and radicular pain, because both are typically involved in any traumatic SCI. Radicular pain is generally, although not always, unilateral and radiating in a dermatomal pattern. At-level radicular pain is usually paroxysmal, whereas at-level spinal cord pain is typically constant. When at-level SCI pain is associated with spinal instability in which spinal movement exacerbates the pain, it is presumably more likely to be radicular pain.

Syringomyelia often presents initially with at-level spinal cord pain, either on coughing or spontaneously. The character of pain caused by syringomyelia is typically burning or dull aching, although it can be sharp, electrical, or stabbing, and can be localized either unilaterally or bilaterally.

Below-Level Spinal Cord Injury (Neuropathic) Pain. Below-level SCI (neuropathic) pain or below-level spinal cord pain refers to neuropathic pain that is perceived more than three dermatomes below the dermatome representing the NLI. It might or might not be perceived within the dermatome representing the NLI and the three dermatomes below the NLI. A necessary condition for classifying a pain as below-level SCI pain is that a lesion or disease must affect the spinal cord and that the pain is thought to arise as a result of this damage. Neuropathic pain occurring in this distribution that cannot be attributed to the spinal cord damage should be classified as *other (neuropathic)*.

The presence of below-level spinal cord pain is suggested by the same pain descriptors mentioned for at-level SCI pain.[20] Allodynia or hyperalgesia can be present within the pain distribution for people with incomplete injuries. The distribution of below-level spinal cord pain is generally not dermatomal but regional, enveloping large areas such as the anal region, the bladder, the genitals, the legs, or commonly the entire body below the NLI. It is usually continuous in presence, although the intensity of the pain can fluctuate in response to a number of factors, including psychological stress, anxiety, fatigue, smoking, noxious stimuli below the level of injury, and weather changes.

Treatment of At-Level and Below-Level Spinal Cord Injury (Neuropathic) Pain. Treatments of neuropathic pain after SCI have historically not been shown to be particularly effective. However, a few oral pharmacologic agents, namely pregabalin, gabapentin, tramadol, and amitriptyline, have shown effectiveness for some in randomized controlled trials for the treatment of neuropathic pain after SCI.[50] Also, although there are not many data specific to the treatment of pain after SCI for other interventions, other medications are commonly prescribed, including the selective serotonin and norepinephrine reuptake inhibitors, opioids (oral, transdermal, and intrathecal), and neurotoxins (intrathecal ziconotide). Modalities including desensitization techniques for evoked pain, massage, and especially exercise can also be beneficial. Psychological interventions including education, cognitive-behavioral therapy, relaxation, and especially hypnosis[63] can allow people to manage this pain over the long term and to minimize its impact on their lives. Neurointerventional techniques such as surgical nerve root decompression and transforaminal epidural steroid injections for radicular pain, and dorsal root entry zone microcoagulation for spinal cord pain, can also be considered.[27,47]

Other (Neuropathic) Pain. Compressive neuropathy pain occurs in a specific peripheral nerve distribution distal to the root level and is attributed to compression of a specific peripheral nerve or plexus of nerves. Symptoms most often include either spontaneous or evoked numbness or tingling in a specific peripheral nerve distribution. This category includes median, ulnar, radial, and axillary neuropathies in people with paraplegia. The signs and symptoms of carpal tunnel syndrome (i.e., numbness or tingling of thumb, index, or middle fingers; abnormal sensation on testing; or numbness or tingling with provocative tests) are common in people with paraplegia. This syndrome is thought to result from a combination of repetitive trauma, as occurs with propulsion of manual wheelchairs, and ischemia from repetitive marked increases in carpal canal pressures, as occurs with push-up pressure reliefs or transfers from one seating surface to another.[54] A higher risk for developing pain has been shown in those who are overweight or use improper wheelchair propulsion biomechanics.[17]

Strategies of treatment and prevention of a compressive neuropathy at the wrist include avoidance of weight-bearing on a flexed or extended wrist by substituting a handgrip for the flat placement of either hand on a surface whenever possible. Other strategies include weight loss, provision of the lightest possible wheelchair that meets the needs of the individual, use of power and power-assist wheelchairs, and instruction and training in an efficient wheelchair propulsion pattern.[94] This typically is a pattern that minimizes the forcefulness and frequency with which the wrist strikes the wheel (i.e., long and smooth arm strokes). Side-to-side or forward-lean pressure relief techniques should also be substituted for push-up pressure relief techniques.

Spasticity

Spasticity is a syndrome of different components, including a velocity-dependent increased resistance to passive motion, involuntary muscle contractions or spasms, and hyperreflexia. The involuntary muscle contractions result from different muscles acting synergistically, typically in a specific flexion or extension pattern. Although spasticity can cause difficulty with mobility, positioning, and comfort, and might even predispose to skin breakdown, it can also be helpful for ambulating and performing ADL. An example is allowing individuals to bridge their buttocks to allow them to pull their trousers over their buttocks. The decision of whether to treat spasticity, and how to do so, should be based on an evaluation that has identified all the activities and other medical issues that are helped or hindered by one or more of the components of spasticity. Activities that need to be evaluated, at least through self-report and perhaps by observation, include bladder management, sexual functioning, sleep, dressing, bathing, positioning, wheelchair mobility, and ambulation. Medical issues that need to be evaluated include the presence of pressure ulcers and pain, because spasticity can predispose to both and can be the underlying factor behind the development of these secondary conditions. Determining the specific patterns of involuntary muscle contraction is also important because nonsystemic treatments of spasticity depend on the specific pattern. For example, an intramuscular injection of alcohol or botulinum toxin needs to be targeted to a specific offending muscle to be effective. Because the different components of spasticity often do not correlate with each other, different assessment tools that address the different components should also be performed during any evaluation. Common assessment tools include 5-point ordinal scales for grading resistance to passive movement, such as the Ashworth Scale and a modified form of this scale, and ordinal ranking scales that rate the frequency of significant involuntary muscle contractions per unit time.

Treatment of Spasticity

Stretching of spastic muscles is the mainstay of treatment of spasticity for virtually all people with SCI. Steady static stretching, to the limits of the ROM of a joint, has been shown to result in a reduction of reflex activity that can last for several hours after the exercise. ROM exercises should be performed regularly on all affected joints by members of the rehabilitation team, support staff, or family members, after instruction in proper technique. Proper positioning, in bed or in wheelchairs, can effectively control increased muscle tone, as well as provide a prolonged static stretch to spastic muscles. An example of this is sleeping in a prone position to provide a sustained stretch of hip and knee flexors. The increased tone in the trunk encountered while sitting in a wheelchair can be improved by slightly tilting the seat or by adding a wedge. The use of positioning orthoses or serial casts can improve spasticity by placing the affected muscle in a position of sustained stretch. An example of this is using a padded ankle-foot orthosis or cast to maintain a spastic ankle plantar flexor in the neutral position. Passive standing on a standing frame or tilt table can also provide a significant stretch to the hip, knee, and ankle plantar flexors.

Many pharmacologic options are available for the treatment of spasticity. Many practitioners consider oral baclofen to be the first-line pharmacologic treatment for spinal spasticity. Baclofen is a structural analog of gamma-aminobutyric acid (GABA), the main inhibitory transmitter of the spinal cord, and binds to $GABA_B$ receptors. Starting doses are typically 5 to 10 mg given 2 to 4 times per day, with gradual increases as clinically indicated. Although the maximum recommended dose is 80 mg/day, significantly larger doses have been both well tolerated and effective. Adverse effects of baclofen include fatigue and dizziness, and seizures can occur with abrupt withdrawal. Diazepam and other benzodiazepines bind to the $GABA_A$ receptor. Benzodiazepines can cause physical dependence, as well as lethargy and diminished concentration. If used clinically, it can be difficult to wean people off these agents, and weaning should be very gradual. Tizanidine hydrochloride is a central alpha-2-adrenergic agonist that has been shown to be effective in treating spasticity after SCI. Adverse effects of tizanidine include sedation and liver function abnormalities.

When only a few specific muscles are affected by problematic spasticity, targeted injections of these muscles with a neurotoxin (e.g., botulinum toxin) or an alcohol (e.g., benzyl alcohol [phenol] or ethyl alcohol) can be carried out. These injections work by weakening these muscles and can be very effective in reducing the problem spasticity.[77] Targeting specific peripheral nerves with an alcohol can provide similar effectiveness. Botulinum toxin injected into a muscle binds to receptor sites on the presynaptic nerve terminal in the neuromuscular junction, inhibiting the release of acetylcholine and preventing neuromuscular transmission. Alcohols injected perineurally or directly into muscles destroy nerve axons and muscle in a nonselective manner. Needle electrical stimulation to localize motor points or peripheral nerves, or electromyography to identify motor end plates, can improve the effectiveness of the injections. The clinical effect obtained by local injection of neurotoxin or alcohols depends on several factors, including the dose administered, the size of the muscle injected, and the severity of spasticity of the targeted muscle. The clinical effect of a botulinum toxin injection can be noted within 2 to 3 days and persist for 3 to 6 months, whereas the clinical effect of an alcohol injection is more variable, with reported effectiveness persisting from 1 month to several years. Local destruction of tissue by injection of an alcohol can be painful in people with preserved sensation, and paresthesias can be induced by destruction of a sensory nerve. Botulinum toxin does not typically cause pain. Alcohols, however, are significantly less costly than botulinum toxins. Injections seem to be most effective when combined with an effective stretching program of the affected muscles.

The administration of baclofen intrathecally is the most effective treatment for severe, generalized spasticity in people with SCI.[81] Baclofen can be delivered intrathecally through a catheter that extends from the intrathecal space out through the dura and spine, and through a subcutaneous tunnel to a battery-driven infusion pump located in a subcutaneous pocket in the abdomen. The entire system is implanted, and there are no external components. Dosage adjustments are made by radiotelemetry using a handheld computer. Pump reservoir refills are performed percutaneously. Several different modes of drug delivery are available, including one that allows different rates of baclofen infusion at different times of the day. Candidates for placement of an intrathecal pump include those people whose spasticity is uncontrolled by pharmacologic and noninvasive treatments, and who are reliable enough to consistently undergo regular pump refills. To confirm efficacy and appropriateness before a pump is implanted, the candidate usually receives an intrathecal bolus test dose of baclofen delivered via lumbar puncture. If the test dose is deemed successful and a pump is implanted, the intrathecal baclofen dose is gradually titrated until the desired benefit is obtained. Effective maintenance dosage ranges are fairly variable among individuals. An expected decrease in spasticity with intrathecal baclofen as measured by Ashworth scores is a reduction from 3 to 4 at baseline to 1 to 2 when the dose is optimally titrated.[81]

Musculoskeletal Conditions

A variety of musculoskeletal conditions can affect people with SCI and cause pain and reduce functional ability. Most of these conditions are preventable, but when they occur successful management can be very difficult.

Contractures

A contracture is a common finding in the paralyzed limbs of people with SCI. A contracture refers to a fixed stiffness of a soft tissue that limits joint motion in a particular direction. Joint contractures can prevent achievement of full functional capacity, inhibit hygiene, lead to abnormal positioning with resultant pain or pressure ulcer development, and prevent use of a joint in the future should motor recovery occur in a delayed manner. The primary cause of contracture is prolonged joint immobilization, but secondary factors include edema, muscle imbalance, spasticity, and local trauma. Certain joints seem more prone to develop contractures than others. Upper limb contractures develop primarily in people with tetraplegia and can interfere significantly with performance of self-care functions. At the shoulder, contractures limiting adduction and internal rotation are very common. These contractures can limit transfer ability, grooming, dressing, and positioning in the prone position. Elbow flexion contracture often develops in people with C5 tetraplegia because of muscle imbalance, and interferes with the ability to transfer, the ability to propel a wheelchair, feeding, and grooming. Flexion contracture at the wrist and fingers can also interfere with performance of self-care activities, although contractures of the finger flexors in people with C6 tetraplegia can permit a grasp through the tenodesis action. In the lower limbs, flexion contractures of the hips and knees interfere with proper bed positioning, transferring, and dressing, and increase the risk for developing pressure ulcers. Adduction contractures of the hips hinder perineal care. All of these contractures, as well as plantar flexion contracture of the ankles, interfere with comfortable standing and ambulation.

Contractures are best prevented by proper positioning in bed, by performing passive ROM and stretching exercises of all joints at least daily, and sometimes by use of prophylactic static splints. Additional preventive measures include effective management of spasticity and edema. Edema should be managed by elevation, massage, and compression garments. Once a contracture is present, aggressive ROM exercises should be started, which often require pretreatment with pain medications. In addition, static and dynamic splints are used to maintain the maximally corrected position. Serial casting with adequately padded splints can be applied. Spasticity can be treated with medications administered orally or intrathecally, or by performing nerve blocks. Surgical interventions are occasionally required, such as tenotomies and tendon-lengthening procedures.

Fractures

Major trauma can result in a fracture of any bone, but in people with SCI, fractures in the paralyzed lower limbs without major trauma are of particular concern. Significant osteoporosis develops in the lower limbs during the first few months after SCI, which makes the bones brittle and prone to fractures. Osteoporotic fractures are both associated with increased risk for hospitalization and mortality in older individuals with SCI.[22] Fracture incidence has been shown for men with complete paraplegia to increase with time after SCI, from 1% within the first year to approximately 5% per year after 20 years.[125] Most fractures are caused by a fall during transfer activities, followed in frequency by fractures caused by ROM exercises and those without known cause. The most common site of fracture is the supracondylar region of the femur. The diagnosis of a fracture in an anesthetic limb can be a challenge. Most patients complain of a recent onset of unilateral leg swelling, not feeling well, and having a low-grade fever. On examination, a swelling and a bruise might be present. If the fracture is severe, a deformity or crepitus can be present.

Traditional fracture management is indicated for people with SCI who are ambulatory. Treatment of fractures in people with SCI who are nonambulatory is usually nonoperative for nondisplaced or minimally displaced lower limb fractures. The goal of treatment is to preserve prefracture function, avoid complications, and secure proper healing and alignment. Because most people with SCI are sedentary and not ambulatory, some shortening and angulation at the fracture site is acceptable. However, rotational deformity should be avoided because it would prevent proper foot placement on the wheelchair's footrest. Despite the osteoporosis in the paralyzed limb, bone healing usually occurs readily, often with exuberant callus formation. Most fractures are treated with a soft, well-padded splint or brace that keeps the limb in extension. The anesthetic skin should be inspected frequently. Circumferential casting and external fixation are associated with a high risk and complication rate in this population and are best avoided. For displaced fractures, however, surgical fixation is often indicated.

Osteoporotic extremity fractures occur in approximately 15% of children and adolescents with SCI, a rate higher than in adults. Prevention is challenging because of the risk-taking activities of children and adolescents. Weight bearing, adequate nutrition, and sunlight exposure (for vitamin D) should be encouraged in children as in adults.

Heterotopic Ossification

Heterotopic ossification (HO) is true bone in extraskeletal ectopic sites (Figure 49-17). For unknown reasons, pluripotent mesenchymal cells in soft tissues differentiate into osteoblasts and other cell lines involved with bone formation.[93] These cells produce an extracellular osteoid matrix, which is then calcified through the deposition of hydroxyapatite and remodeled by the coupled actions of osteoblasts and osteoclasts into well-organized bone over several months.[93]

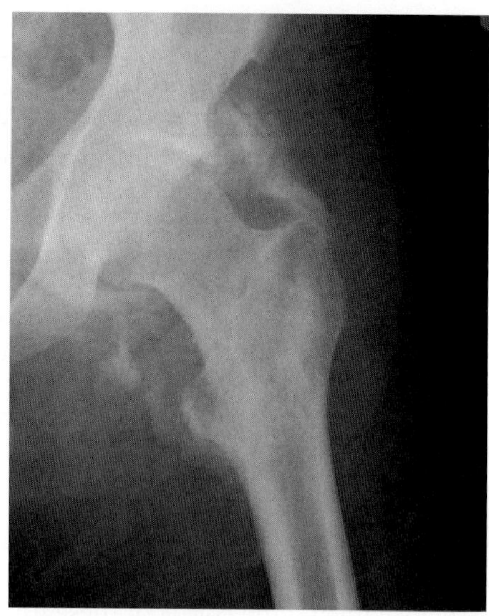

FIGURE 49-17 Heterotopic ossification of the hip.

HO has been reported to occur in 20% to 30% of people with SCI, with approximately 10% of those with HO developing restriction of joint ROM sufficient to significantly interfere with mobility and self-care.[106] Most commonly, HO develops within 4 months of SCI, and incidence rates decline thereafter.[108] HO most often develops around the hips (90%), but other locations where it can appear include the knees, shoulders, and elbows.

HO usually presents clinically as a warm local swelling adjacent to a joint. This is followed by a more generalized edema of the affected paralyzed limb. Low-grade fever can be present and, in time, joint mobility can be reduced. The differential diagnosis at this early stage includes DVT, infection, trauma, and impending pressure ulcer.

The serum alkaline phosphatase level during the acute stage is elevated, and a bone scan or MRI of the area is positive.[108] Plain films show normal findings because of yet insufficient local deposition of calcium. As the HO matures, it becomes more visible on plain films, but the serum alkaline phosphatase level and radioisotope uptake gradually decrease.

Prophylactic use of NSAIDs to prevent HO has been shown to be effective, although they are generally not administered for this purpose given the relatively low incidence of disabling consequences of HO and the potential adverse effects of treatment with NSAIDs, including the potential for inhibiting bone healing after fracture.[108] If detected, however, treatment of established HO should begin promptly and is aimed at halting the process, as well as maintaining joint ROM and function. Etidronate, a bisphosphonate, is believed to inhibit the mineralization of organic osteoid, thereby preventing, when given for up to 6 months, soft tissue ossification in most of those people having only bone scintigraphic evidence of HO. Less than half the people with radiographic evidence of HO, however, show a response with inhibited soft tissue ossification.[4]

Radiation therapy for HO is effective, but it is uncommonly used because of unknown long-term risks. Gentle ROM exercises are generally recommended with forceful stretching discouraged.[108] Surgical resection of HO can be done when joint mobility is severely restricted, when HO interferes with self-care and sitting in a wheelchair, or both. It should also be considered when HO contributes to the development of pressure ulcers or causes compression of nerves and blood vessels. The goal of surgery is not to resect the entire HO but to restore joint motion and functional skills. The surgical procedure usually consists of wedge resection and creation of a pseudarthrosis. The risk for postoperative recurrence can be reduced by administering etidronate, antiinflammatory agents, radiation therapy, and by performing ROM exercises.[5]

HO has been reported to occur in less than 5% of children and adolescents, a significantly lower percentage than occurs in adults. It usually presents on average after 1 year postinjury. Bisphosphonates should be used with caution because there is a risk of developing rickets. Surgery is indicated if there are significant functional deficits, but postresection radiation is less commonly used because of concerns regarding the long-term consequences.

Hip and Spine Deformities in Children

The growing child with SCI can experience a variety of additional orthopedic problems, the most significant of which are spine deformity and hip instability. The prevalence of scoliosis can be as high as 98%.[12] Close observation with annual spine radiography is essential. The use of a prophylactic thoracolumbar orthosis is recommended by many, and almost always when curvatures exceed 20 degrees. Surgical spinal fusion can significantly affect future functional skills and is therefore best avoided. Surgery can be necessary, however, for curvatures greater than 40 degrees. Hip instability develops most frequently in children injured at an early age, and is usually associated with muscle imbalance caused by spasticity, or by underdevelopment of the femoral head and acetabulum that occurs because of flaccid hip muscles. Nearly all children injured younger than 5 years of age and over 80% of those injured younger than 10 years of age develop hip instability. Unstable and dislocated hips do not interfere with sitting or ADLs. However, the high incidence in hip dislocation in children often leads to pelvic obliquity and secondary pressure ulcers. Treatment is usually directed toward prevention of contractures and creating bone stability by prophylactic application of a hip abduction orthosis.[12]

Summary

SCI is a catastrophic event that results in physical disability and impaired function of various organ systems. Despite decades of intense research, a cure still does not exist. Great progress has occurred, however, in the management of SCI and its associated conditions. Because of advances in clinical practice, people with SCI have increased life expectancy. Morbidity is also reduced, as reflected in reduced hospital lengths of stay after SCI and fewer rehospitalizations during follow-up years. Spasticity can be effectively managed, and male fertility is now much improved. Application of modern technology has enhanced the function and quality of life of many people with SCI. The International Standards for Neurologic Classification of SCI has been adapted worldwide as the preferred assessment instrument of people with SCI seeking clinical care, and for those participating in research studies. This has been supplemented by the Autonomic Standards for Classification of SCI. In addition, multiple international SCI data sets (available at www.iscos.org.uk/international-sci-data-sets) have been developed to standardize the collection and reporting of a minimal amount of information necessary to evaluate and compare results of published studies from around the world. Clinical practice guidelines such as those that have been developed by the Consortium of Spinal Cord Medicine (available at www.pva.org) have also led to greater conformity and quality of care for people with SCI. Development of comprehensive multidisciplinary educational websites such as elearnSCI (accessed through www.elearnSCI.org), an initiative of the International Spinal Cord Society, which had been accessed more than 10,000 times within 2 years of its introduction, promises to further raise the level of knowledge of SCI among clinicians throughout the world. People with SCI have established influential organizations and peer support networks that have advanced their rights and made health-related information widely available. Current wheelchair designs and seating systems are far superior to older models and, respectively, permit increased mobility and allow safe sitting for much longer periods. People with disability also now use computers, tablets, and smartphones in their daily lives for recreational, educational, and vocational purposes with great success.

Advances in clinical care are not a justification for complacency. The health and function of people with SCI are still at risk without proper medical and nursing care, social support, appropriate equipment, supplies, and medications. Too many continue to experience problems related to urinary and bowel dysfunction. Many still have chronic pain that interferes with their quality of life. We must increase our understanding of the value of physical exercise and proper diet to reduce the high prevalence of obesity, diabetes, and CVD in people with SCI. Ambulation and complete self-sufficiency are impossible for too many. Social support is often lacking, and relatively few return to work. To solve these and other remaining issues that affect the wellness of people with SCI, private, state, and federal support of health services is needed to improve the health care of people with SCI, as well as a better social support system and a comprehensive disability policy.

The ultimate goal of people with SCI and those who care for them is to find a cure for this condition, which is to reverse the neurologic damage of SCI. Until that elusive goal is reached, people with SCI, their families, their caregivers, and society at large must work together to eliminate barriers to health care and ensure their full participation in all aspects of community life.

KEY REFERENCES

2. Angeli CA, Edgerton VR, Gerasimenko YP, et al: Altering spinal cord excitability enables voluntary movements after chronic complete paralysis in humans, *Brain* 137:1394–1409, 2014.

5. Banovac K, Sherman AL, Estores IM, et al: Prevention and treatment of heterotopic ossification after spinal cord injury, *J Spinal Cord Med* 27:376–382, 2004.
6. Bar-On Z, Ohry A: The acute abdomen in spinal cord injury individuals, *Paraplegia* 33:704–706, 1995.
7. Bartholdy K, Biering-Sorensen T, Malmqvist L, et al: Cardiac arrhythmias the first month after acute traumatic spinal cord injury, *J Spinal Cord Med* 37:162–170, 2014.
13. Betz RR, Mulcahey MJ, D'Andrea LP, et al: Acute evaluation and management of pediatric spinal cord injury, *J Spinal Cord Med* 27(Suppl 1):S11–S15, 2004.
14. Bickenbach J, Biering-Sørensen F, Knott J, et al: A global picture of spinal cord injury. In Bickenbach J, Officer A, Shakespeare T, et al, editors: *International perspectives on spinal cord injury*, Geneva, 2013, World Health Organization Press.
15. Biering-Sorensen F, Hansen B, Lee BS: Non-pharmacological treatment and prevention of bone loss after spinal cord injury: a systematic review, *Spinal Cord* 47:508–518, 2009.
16. Black J, Baharestani MM, Cuddigan J, et al: National Pressure Ulcer Advisory Panel's updated pressure ulcer staging system, *Adv Skin Wound Care* 20:269–274, 2007.
18. Boninger ML, Souza AL, Cooper RA, et al: Propulsion patterns and pushrim biomechanics in manual wheelchair propulsion, *Arch Phys Med Rehabil* 83:718–723, 2002.
19. Bryce TN: Pain management in persons with spinal cord injury. In Lin VW, editor: *Spinal cord medicine: principles and practice*, New York, 2010, Demos.
20. Bryce TN, Biering-Sorensen F, Finnerup NB, et al: International Spinal Cord Injury Pain Classification: part I. Background and description, *Spinal Cord* 50:413–417, 2012.
21. Burns AS, Jackson AB: Gynecologic and reproductive issues in women with spinal cord injury, *Phys Med Rehabil Clin N Am* 12:183–199, 2001.
28. Clinical Practice Guidelines: Neurogenic bowel management in adults with spinal cord injury. Spinal Cord Medicine Consortium, *J Spinal Cord Med* 21:248–293, 1998.
30. Consortium for Spinal Cord Medicine: Early acute management in adults with spinal cord injury: a clinical practice guideline for health-care professionals, *J Spinal Cord Med* 31:403–479, 2008.
34. Deforge D, Blackmer J, Garritty C, et al: Male erectile dysfunction following spinal cord injury: a systematic review, *Spinal Cord* 44:465–473, 2006.
35. DeForge D, Blackmer J, Garritty C, et al: Fertility following spinal cord injury: a systematic review, *Spinal Cord* 43:693–703, 2005.
36. Denis F: Spinal instability as defined by the three-column spine concept in acute spinal trauma, *Clin Orthop Relat Res* 189:65–76, 1984.
38. Devivo MJ: Epidemiology of traumatic spinal cord injury: trends and future implications, *Spinal Cord* 50:365–372, 2012.
41. Dijkers MP: Quality of life of individuals with spinal cord injury: a review of conceptualization, measurement, and research findings, *J Rehabil Res Dev* 42:87–110, 2005.
42. Ditunno JF, Little JW, Tessler A, et al: Spinal shock revisited: a four-phase model, *Spinal Cord* 42:383–395, 2004.
43. Dobkin B, Apple D, Barbeau H, et al: Weight-supported treadmill vs over-ground training for walking after acute incomplete SCI, *Neurology* 66:484–493, 2006.
45. Dyson-Hudson TA, Kirshblum SC: Shoulder pain in chronic spinal cord injury, part I: epidemiology, etiology, and pathomechanics, *J Spinal Cord Med* 27:4–17, 2004.
49. Fehlings MG, Vaccaro A, Wilson JR, et al: Early versus delayed decompression for traumatic cervical spinal cord injury: results of the Surgical Timing in Acute Spinal Cord Injury Study (STASCIS), *PLoS ONE* 7:e32037, 2012.
51. Garber SL, Biddle AK, Click CN: *Pressure ulcer prevention and treatment following spinal cord injury: a clinical practice guideline for health-care professionals*, Washington, 2000, Paralyzed Veterans of America.
53. Garstang SV: Infections of the spine and spinal cord. In Kirshblum S, Campagnolo DI, DeLisa JA, editors: *Spinal cord medicine*, Philadelphia, 2002, Lippincott Williams & Wilkins, pp 498–512.
55. Giannoccaro MP, Moghadam KK, Pizza F, et al: Sleep disorders in patients with spinal cord injury, *Sleep Med Rev* 17:399–409, 2013.
59. Heary RF, Filart R: Tumors of the spine and spinal cord. In Kirshblum S, Campagnolo DI, DeLisa JA, editors: *Spinal cord medicine*, Philadelphia, 2002, Lippincott Williams & Wilkins, pp 480–497.
60. Hoffman JM, Bombardier CH, Graves DE, et al: A longitudinal study of depression from 1 to 5 years after spinal cord injury, *Arch Phys Med Rehabil* 92:411–418, 2011.
63. Jensen MP, Barber J, Romano JM, et al: Effects of self-hypnosis training and EMG biofeedback relaxation training on chronic pain in persons with spinal-cord injury, *Int J Clin Exp Hypn* 57:239–268, 2009.
65. Kamin SS: Vascular, nutritional, and other diseases of the spinal cord. In Kirshblum S, Campagnolo DI, DeLisa JA, editors: *Spinal cord medicine*, Philadelphia, 2002, Lippincott Williams & Wilkins, pp 512–526.
68. Kirshblum SC, Waring W, Biering-Sorensen F, et al: Reference for the 2011 Revision of the International Standards for Neurological Classification of Spinal Cord Injury, *J Spinal Cord Med* 34:547–554, 2011.
69. Krassioukov A, Warburton DE, Teasell R, et al: A systematic review of the management of autonomic dysreflexia after spinal cord injury, *Arch Phys Med Rehabil* 90:682–695, 2009.
73. Levin VA, Leibel SA, Gutin PH: Neoplasms of the central nervous system. In Devita VT, Hellman S, editors: *Cancer: principles and practice of oncology*, Philadelphia, 2001, Lippincott Williams & Wilkins.
75. Maimoun L, Fattal C, Sultan C: Bone remodeling and calcium homeostasis in patients with spinal cord injury: a review, *Metabolism* 60:1655–1663, 2011.
78. Marino RJ, Burns S, Graves DE, et al: Upper- and lower-extremity motor recovery after traumatic cervical spinal cord injury: an update from the National Spinal Cord Injury Database, *Arch Phys Med Rehabil* 92:369–375, 2011.
80. McDowell CL, Moberg E, House JH: Second International Conference on Surgical Rehabilitation of the Upper Limb in Traumatic Quadriplegia, *J Hand Surg [Am]* 11:604–608, 1986.
82. McKinley WO: Nontraumatic spinal cord injury: etiology, incidence, and outcome. In Kirshblum S, Campagnolo DI, DeLisa JA, editors: *Spinal cord medicine*, Philadelphia, 2002, Lippincott Williams & Wilkins, pp 471–479.
84. Mehta S, Hill D, McIntyre A, et al: Meta-analysis of botulinum toxin A detrusor injections in the treatment of neurogenic detrusor overactivity after spinal cord injury, *Arch Phys Med Rehabil* 94:1473–1481, 2013.
88. National Spinal Cord Injury Statistical Center: *2012 Annual statistical report for the spinal cord injury model systems—complete public version*, Birmingham, 2013, University of Alabama at Birmingham.
94. Paralyzed Veterans of America Consortium for Spinal Cord Medicine: Preservation of upper limb function following spinal cord injury: a clinical practice guideline for health-care professionals, *J Spinal Cord Med* 28:434–470, 2005.
97. Schilero GJ, Spungen AM, Bauman WA, et al: Pulmonary function and spinal cord injury, *Respir Physiol Neurobiol* 166:129–141, 2009.
98. Schmitz TJ: Traumatic spinal cord injury. In O'Sullivan SB, Schmitz TJ, editors: *Physical rehabilitation: assessment and treatment*, Philadelphia, 2001, FA Davis.
100. Selvarajah S, Hammond E, Haider A, et al: The burden of acute traumatic spinal cord injury among adults in the United States: an update, *J Neurotrauma* 31:228–238, 2014.
103. Steeves JD, Kramer JK, Fawcett JW, et al: Extent of spontaneous motor recovery after traumatic cervical sensorimotor complete spinal cord injury, *Spinal Cord* 49:257–265, 2011.
108. Sullivan MP, Torres SJ, Mehta S, et al: Heterotopic ossification after central nervous system trauma: a current review, *Bone Joint Res* 2:51–57, 2013.
109. Teasell RW, Hsieh JT, Aubut JA, et al: Venous thromboembolism after spinal cord injury, *Arch Phys Med Rehabil* 90:232–245, 2009.
113. van Middendorp JJ, Hosman AJ, Donders AR, et al: A clinical prediction rule for ambulation outcomes after traumatic spinal cord injury: a longitudinal cohort study, *Lancet* 377:1004–1010, 2011.
115. Vogel LC, Betz RR, Mulcahey MJ: Spinal cord disorders in children, adolescents. In Lin VW, editor: *Spinal cord medicine: principles and practice*, New York, 2010, Demos, pp 595–623.
122. Whiteneck G, Adler C, Biddle AK, et al: *Outcomes following traumatic spinal cord injury: clinical practice guidelines for health-care professionals*, Washington, 1999, Paralyzed Veterans of America.
123. Wilson JR, Forgione N, Fehlings MG: Emerging therapies for acute traumatic spinal cord injury, *CMAJ* 185:485–492, 2013.

The full reference list for this chapter is available online.

CHAPTER 50

AUDITORY, VESTIBULAR, AND VISUAL IMPAIRMENTS

Henry L. Lew, Chiemi Tanaka, Edson Hirohata, Gregory L. Goodrich

Impairments in the auditory, vestibular, and visual domains are among the most common sensory issues that could adversely affect a person's rehabilitation process. This chapter will briefly describe the diagnosis and rehabilitation of auditory, vestibular, and visual sensory impairments.

Auditory Impairments

Hearing loss can result from dysfunction of and/or damage to the auditory system at any point, from the outer ear to the auditory cortex. Medical, environmental, and genetic factors are closely related to etiology of hearing loss. If hearing impairments develop in early life, speech intelligibility, language, literacy, cognition, emotion, and social skills may be adversely affected. Elderly with hearing loss may still have serious psychological impacts, including loss of independence, depression, anxiety, lethargy, social dissatisfaction, and cognitive decline.[47] More important, hearing impairments could affect their communication with health care providers, leading to inappropriate management of serious health conditions.[108]

According to standard hearing examinations, approximately 13% (30 million) of Americans age 12 years or older have bilateral hearing loss.[72] In general, increased age is associated with development of hearing loss, and men are more likely to experience hearing loss than women. Disabling hearing loss was reported by 2% of the population in the 45- to 54-year-old range, increasing to 8.5% in the 55- to 64-year-old range, to 25% in the 65- to 74-year-old range, and to 50% in the 75 and older range.[78]

Anatomy and Physiology of the Auditory System

Sound is generated when air particles vibrate and propagate as sound waves. Our auditory system receives this air vibration and converts it to different energy forms (mechanical, hydrodynamic, and electrochemical) so that we perceive it as sound. Thus, the ear is often described as an acoustic transducer. To view an animation of auditory transduction, please visit www.youtube.com/watch?feature=endscreen&NR=1&v=PeTriGTENoc. Figure 50-1A illustrates the anatomy of the ear.

The sound travels to the middle ear, which houses two major ear structures: the tympanic membrane (eardrum) and the ossicular chain that consists of the malleus, incus, and stapes. The middle ear is an air-filled space that is connected to the posterior of the nasopharynx via the Eustachian tube that works to equalize air pressure between the middle ear and the outside environment. The sound vibrates the tympanic membrane and then sets the ossicular chain into motion to further amplify sound by making the ossicular chain act as an impedance-matching transformer that is an important step to prevent energy loss when sound travels from air (middle ear) to a fluid medium (inner ear).

The inner ear is a fluid-filled space within the temporal bone and is connected to the stapes of the ossicular chain via the oval window and to the eighth cranial nerve (vestibulocochlear nerve) through hair cells. The inner ear consists of two different parts: cochlea for hearing and vestibular section for balance. The cochlea is divided into three divisions: scala tympani, scala media, and scala vestibuli. Hair cells, the sensory cells of hearing, lie on the basilar membrane that separates the scala media and scala tympani (Figure 50-1B). The hair cells are mechanoreceptor cells that have important ion channels in their cilia (stereocilia) for electrochemical sound transduction. When the basilar membrane is displaced according to the vibration patterns of the oval window via the stapes, stereocilia bend because of pivotal motion of the basilar membrane and tectorial membrane. Bending of the stereocilia opens its ion channels, leading to release of neurotransmitters into the synaptic cleft between the base of the hair cells and the auditory nerve fibers to initiate action potentials. The number of the inner hair cells in human cochlea is about 3500 (1 row) and the outer hair cells are about 15,000 (3 rows). Most inner hair cells are innervated by afferent fibers at the base of the cells, encoding sound clarity, and the outer hair cells are innervated by mostly efferent fibers, contributing to decoding of lower-intensity sounds.

After mechanical energy is transduced into electrochemical activity by the hair cells, neural firing of the eighth cranial nerve generates action potentials and travels to the auditory cortex in the central auditory pathway. Figure 50-2 shows the afferent auditory pathway for neuronal projection to the cochlear nucleus, superior olivary complex, inferior colliculus (via lateral lemniscus), medial geniculate body, and auditory cortex in the temporal lobe.

Case History and Examination of the Auditory system

Various audiologic tests are performed to make a differential diagnosis of the hearing status. Table 50-1 summarizes

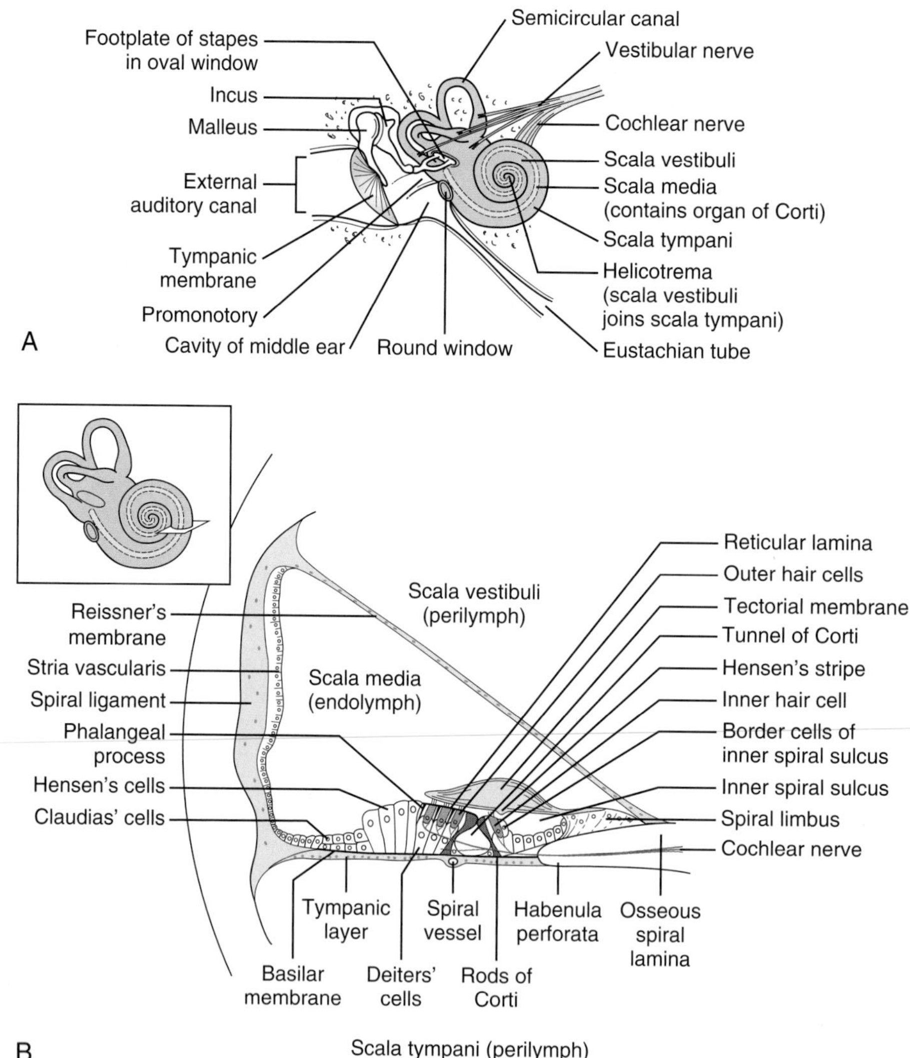

FIGURE 50-1 A, Cross-section of the inner ear in relation to the outer and middle ears. **B,** Cross-section of the organ of Corti in the scala media. (Redrawn from Yost WA: *Fundamentals of hearing: an introduction*, ed 3, San Diego, 1994, Academic Press.)

typical audiologic testing and sites of test. A hearing screening can be performed by physicians, nurses, speech-language pathologists, audiologists, and technicians, but the diagnostic hearing testing is conducted by audiologists.

Case History

The case history is an important part of both the hearing screening and diagnostic hearing testing. Typical questions to ask patients are listed in Box 50-1. In addition, information about the patient's medical and occupational history that may cause hearing loss should be collected. It is important to gather the history of noise exposure, ear surgery, ototoxic medication/chemical intake, and family history of hearing loss.

Otoscopic Examination

The otoscopic examination is performed with an otoscope to check for the presence of any structural abnormality in the outer ear and the tympanic membrane. Box 50-2 lists abnormalities that need to be checked. Otoscopic examination should be conducted before hearing screening and diagnostic hearing testing because any obstruction of the ear canal could affect the results of pure-tone audiometry or other audiologic testing.

Pure-Tone Audiometry

Pure-tone audiometry measures a patient's hearing thresholds (lowest decibel hearing level (dB HL) at which the patient can detect the pure tone at least 50% of the time) in a sound-isolated booth. The patient is asked to indicate whether he/she heard the sound (e.g., pressing a button, raise a hand). The dB HL scale is based on a reference of normal healthy young adult hearing thresholds, and 0 dB HL represents the threshold of normal hearing at each frequency. Human auditory frequency range is from 20 to 20,000 Hertz (Hz), but clinically hearing thresholds are obtained at frequencies from 250 to 8000 Hz, which are important for understanding human speech. Hearing thresholds are plotted on a graph called an audiogram. Unlike most graphs, the Y-axis is plotted from the lowest

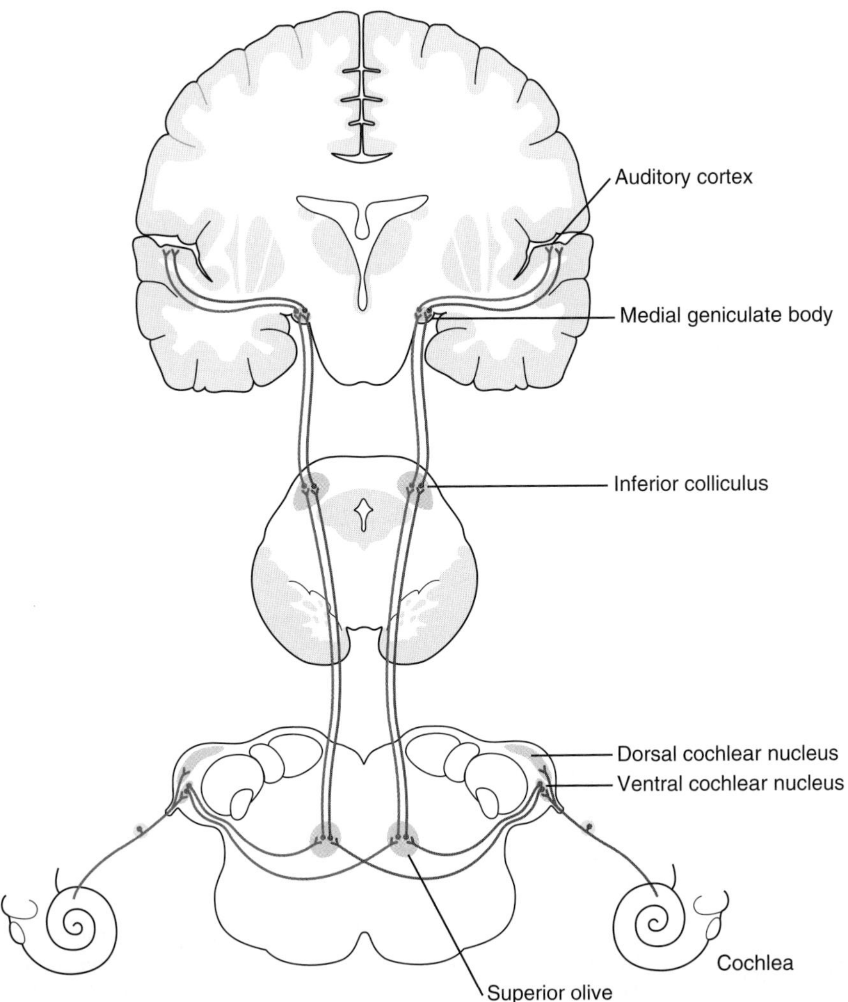

FIGURE 50-2 The major components of the afferent auditory pathway. (Redrawn from Yost WA: *Fundamentals of hearing: an introduction,* ed 3, San Diego, 1994, Academic Press.)

Table 50-1 Summary of Typical Audiologic Testing and Sites of Test

Audiologic Test	Type	Testing Site	What Is Tested
Otoscopic examination	Objective	Outer and middle ears	Structural integrity of the outer and part of the middle ear (tympanic membrane and part of ossicular chain) based on visual inspection
Pure-tone audiometry	Subjective	Entire auditory system	Auditory thresholds through air- and bone-conduction pathway at various frequencies based on behavioral response
Speech audiometry	Subjective	Entire auditory system	Ability to receive or discriminate speech based on behavioral response
Tympanometry	Objective	Outer and middle ears	Mobility of tympanic membrane, function of the middle ear, ear canal volume, and obstruction of the ear canal
Acoustic reflexes	Objective	Retrocochlea	Function of acoustic reflex pathway including stapedius muscles, auditory nerve, cochlea nucleus, superior olivary complex, facial nerve
Otoacoustic emissions	Objective	Cochlea	Function of the outer hair cells
Auditory brainstem response	Objective	Retrocochlea	Function of the brainstem in response to sound

intensity at the top of the graph, indicating that the severity of hearing loss increases if a patient's hearing thresholds plot toward the bottom of the audiogram.

With the pure-tone audiometer, air-conduction thresholds are determined under headphones (e.g., TDH-50) or insert earphones (e.g., ER-3A). Air conduction tests sound transmission from the outer, middle, and inner ear to the auditory cortex. Bone-conduction threshold is measured with a bone vibrator that is placed either on the mastoid or forehead. The bone-conduction testing bypasses the outer and middle ear and tests sound transmission from the inner ear to the auditory cortex.

A "masking" procedure is used when there is a significant difference in air-conduction thresholds between ears or between air- and bone-conduction thresholds in the same ear. Typically, a loud sound presented to one ear can be transmitted to the other ear via a bone-conduction route (e.g., skull vibration). In cases of notable hearing

BOX 50-1

Typical Questions to Ask Patients During Case History Intake

- How long has the hearing difficulty been noticed?
- Was the onset of hearing loss sudden or gradual?
- Did the onset of hearing loss appear to have coincided with any event or trauma?
- What are the situations where hearing difficulty was noticed?
- Does your hearing fluctuate within a day or from day to day?
- Do you hear better in one ear than the other?
- Is there any pain or drainage out of the ear?
- Is there associated tinnitus, dizziness, disequilibrium, headaches, or any other abnormal symptoms?
- Have you had a hearing test before? What did the results indicate?
- Do you use, or have you ever used, any form of hearing aid or assistive device? Is the device worn routinely? Are you satisfied with it?

BOX 50-2

Abnormalities That Need to Be Checked During the Otoscopic Examination

- **External Ear Structure**
  - Abnormalities (e.g., atresia, anotia, microtia)
  - Set (position) of the ears
  - Skin tags or sinuses, tenderness, redness or edema, signs of drainage or cerumen buildup
- **Internal Ear Structure**
  - Ear canal
    - Obstruction (e.g., cerumen build-up, foreign objects)
    - Signs of inflammation
    - Drainage or blood
    - Stenosis
    - Damage
  - Tympanic membrane (TM)
    - Normal landmarks (cone of light, translucent/pearly gray TM, handle of malleus)
    - Signs of inflammation (e.g., bright red TM, bulging TM)
    - Retracted TM
    - Perforated TM
    - Bubbles behind TM

asymmetry, a noise can be presented as a masker to keep the nontest ear "busy" to prevent it from responding to a signal, ensuring that hearing thresholds are being obtained from the tested ear. Masked and unmasked thresholds are indicated by different symbols on the audiogram.[4]

Degree of Hearing Loss

Degree of hearing loss describes the severity of hearing impairment. Figure 50-3 shows classifications of degree of hearing loss.[38] There is no uniform classification system for the degree of hearing loss, but 25 dB HL or better is usually considered normal hearing in adults. For the pediatric population, different classifications may be applied for normal (≤15 dB HL) and minimal (16 to 25 dB HL) because of the need for better hearing in children for speech/language development compared with adults.

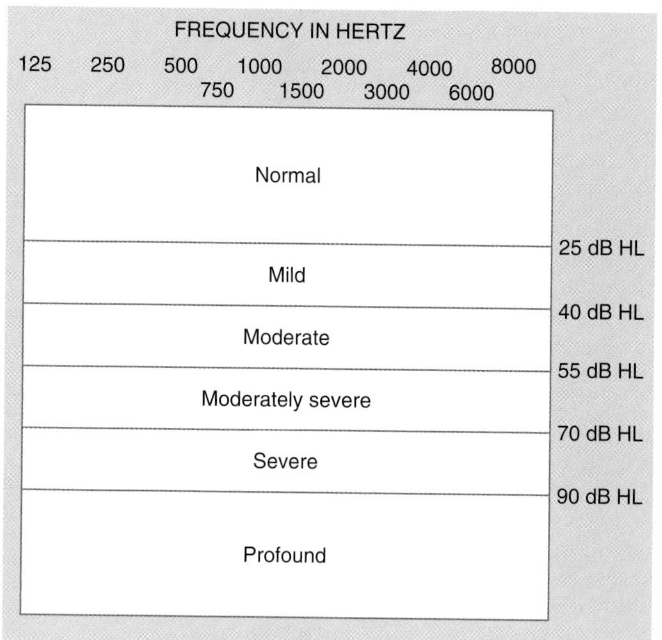

FIGURE 50-3 Classifications of degree of hearing loss.

Types of Hearing Loss

There are three types of hearing loss: (1) conductive, (2) sensorineural, and (3) mixed. The hearing loss caused by damage to the outer ear and/or middle ear is called conductive hearing loss. It is characterized by normal bone-conduction thresholds and elevated air-conduction thresholds with an air-bone gap (difference between air-conduction and bone-conduction thresholds) of 15 dB or greater. This type of hearing loss can be caused by obstruction of the ear canal by foreign bodies or cerumen, outer or middle ear disorders, deformation of the outer and/or middle ears, mechanical injury to the outer and/or middle ears, and other middle ear disorders such as otosclerosis and cholesteatoma. In general, a conductive hearing loss is medically treatable. The clarity of sounds is mostly preserved, but the conductive hearing loss decreases the intensity of the sounds.

The sensorineural hearing loss (SNHL) is characterized by elevated air-conduction thresholds with an air-bone gap of 10 dB or less. This type of hearing loss is the result of damage to the cochlea and/or retrocochlear pathway. Both the sound clarity and intensity are degraded. The SNHL is permanent in most cases and can be caused by various auditory disorders such as tumors on the eighth cranial nerve, Meniere disease, and deformation of the cochlea and/or the eighth cranial nerve. Other factors that contribute to development of SNHL are aging, acoustic trauma from loud noise, ototoxic drugs or chemicals, hypoxia, traumatic brain injury, infections (e.g., meningitis, rubella), immune system disorders, and genetics. Systemic diseases such as neurofibromatosis type II and multiple sclerosis could also cause this type of hearing loss.

The mixed hearing loss is characterized by elevated air-conduction and bone-conduction thresholds with an air-bone gap of 15 dB or greater. It is a mixture of conductive and SNHL.

Speech Audiometry

Speech audiometry assesses a patient's ability to perceive and recognize spoken words either under earphones or in sound-field. Although numerous speech testing materials are available, the focus here will be on commonly used clinical speech-testing materials and procedures. The basic audiologic battery generally includes the speech recognition (reception) or detection threshold (SRT and SDT, respectively) and speech or word recognition (discrimination) scores.

The SRT measures the lowest dB HL at which the patient can correctly repeat or identify bisyllabic (spondee) words 50% of the time. The SRT should be close to the pure-tone average (PTA); that is, the simple average of the air-conduction thresholds at 500, 1000, and 2000 Hz.

The SDT measures the lowest dB HL at which the patient can detect the presence of speech (e.g., consonant-vowel, monosyllabic/bisyllabic words). This is used when the SRT cannot be obtained, such as when testing infants, young children, or nonnative English speakers.

The speech recognition score measures the patient's ability to repeat or identify monosyllabic words at a suprathreshold level (usually 40 dB above the SRT). The score is the percentage of words correctly repeated or identified from lists of 50 or 25 words. The word lists that are commonly used for a hearing evaluation for adults are the Northwestern University Auditory Test (NU-6) and the Central Institute for the Deaf (CID) Auditory Test W-22. These word lists are known as phonetically-balanced word lists that contain phonemes with the same frequency that they typically appear in everyday English. There is no uniform speech recognition scoring categorization, but typically, it is considered to be "excellent or within normal limits" if 90% to 100% of words on a list can be correctly identified. To learn one proposed categorization of the speech recognition scoring, please visit www.audiologyonline.com/articles/back-to-basics-speech-audiometry-6828.

Immittance Audiometry

Immittance audiometry evaluates the function of the tympanic membrane, the status of the middle ear, and the acoustic reflex pathway. *Acoustic immittance* is a more general term that describes the ease of sound flow (admittance) or opposition to sound flow (impedance) through a system. In immittance audiometry, a probe tip is inserted in the ear canal and an airtight seal must be obtained for the test. The probe tip contains openings connected to three basic systems: (1) an air pump system to change ear pressure in the ear canal; (2) a loudspeaker to introduce a probe tone; and (3) a microphone to monitor the sound pressure levels of the probe tone. Tympanometry and acoustic reflexes are two major tests included in immittance audiometry.

Tympanometry measures the mobility of the tympanic membrane and middle ear pressure, but it does not measure perceptual hearing. In the tympanometry, a probe tone at 226 Hz (1000 Hz for infants) is presented into the ear through the probe and the amount of sound reflected back from the tympanic membrane is measured while air pressure in the ear canal is varied. The results from tympanometry are plotted in a graph called a tympanogram (Figure 50-4). The tympanic membrane is most mobile when the pressure in the ear canal is close to the pressure in the middle ear cavity. The greatest mobility of the tympanic membrane appears as a peak on the tympanogram, and in a normal ear the peak is seen around atmospheric pressure (0 daPa).

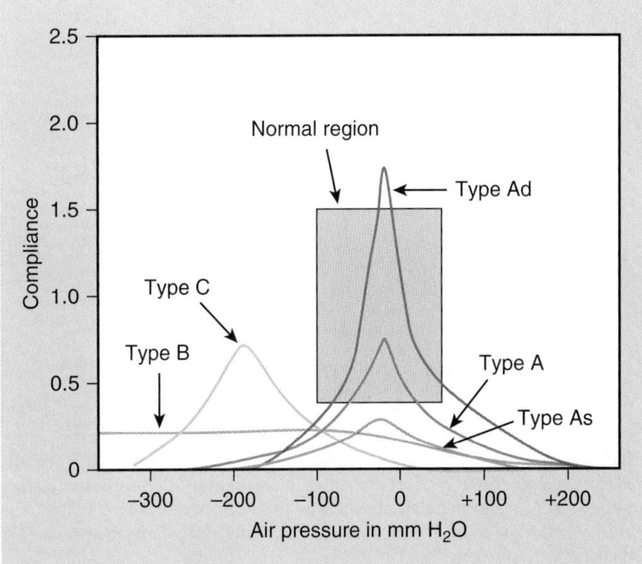

FIGURE 50-4 **Classifications of the tympanogram types.** (Redrawn from Hall JW III, Mueller HG III: Audiologists' *desk reference: volume I: diagnostic audiology: principles, procedures, and practices,* San Diego, 1997, Singular Publishing Group.)

There are three classifications of tympanogram types (Figure 50-4). A Type A tympanogram indicates normal middle ear status (normal mobility of the tympanic membrane and normal middle-ear pressure). Reduced mobility of the tympanic membrane caused by a stiffened middle ear system (e.g., thickening of the tympanic membrane, fixation of the ossicular chain [otosclerosis], glue ear [middle ear effusion]) can cause a shallow peak on the tympanogram, expressed as a Type A_s tympanogram. If the middle ear system is overly compliant because of ossicular chain discontinuity or a flaccid tympanic membrane, the peak will be very high or off the chart, which is shown as a Type A_d tympanogram. A Type B tympanogram shows no clear peak pressure and is relatively flat. If the ear canal volume is normal, the Type B tympanogram may be reflective of an advanced stage of otosclerosis or a middle ear filled with effusion possibly caused by an ear infection. If the ear canal volume is abnormally small with the Type B tympanogram, it is suggestive of a blockage of the ear canal because of cerumen impaction. If the ear canal volume is abnormally large with a peakless tympanogram, it is a sign of a perforation in the tympanic membrane. Finally, a Type C tympanogram indicates significant negative peak pressure possibly caused by Eustachian tube dysfunction or developing/resolving middle ear infections.[43]

Acoustic reflexes measure the threshold in dB HL at which the stapedius muscle of the middle ear involuntary contracts in response to intense sound. The reflex testing is performed at 500, 1000, 2000, and 4000 Hz with ipsilateral (stimulus and recording are in the same ear)

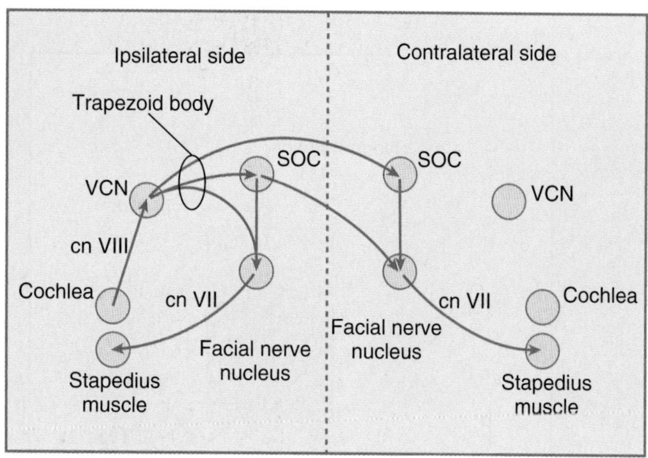

FIGURE 50-5 Acoustic reflex pathway and anatomical structures. *cn VIII,* auditory nerve; *cn VII,* motor branch of facial nerve; *SOC,* superior olivary complex; *VCN,* ventral cochlear nucleus. (Redrawn from Katz J, editor: The acoustic reflex. In *Handbook of Clinical Audiology,* ed 5, Philadelphia, 2002, Lippincott Williams & Wilkins.)

and/or contralateral recording (stimulus and recording are in different ears). Figure 50-5 shows the anatomic structures involved in the acoustic reflex pathway. The test results can be used to detect dysfunction in the acoustic reflex pathway and to support, confirm, or rule out the hearing loss demonstrated by pure-tone audiometry.[30] Another evaluation, termed *acoustic reflex decay,* measures sustainability of the acoustic reflex at 10 dB above the acoustic reflex threshold typically at 500 and 1000 Hz. A decaying acoustic reflex may be suggestive of retrocochlear problems such as a vestibular schwannoma.

Otoacoustic Emissions

Otoacoustic emissions (OAEs) are retrograde transmissions of energy from the cochlea to the ear canal.[61] In OAE testing, the patient is asked to sit quietly. The test does not require behavioral response from the patient. The probe tip that is inserted into the ear canal has openings to a microphone and two speakers. Data are analyzed to measure levels of the noise floor and OAEs. Because of the extremely low energy level of OAEs, it is recommended that testing be performed in a sound-isolated booth. OAEs provide information about function of the cochlear outer hair cells. Proper measurements of OAEs require an intact middle ear system. Clinically, OAEs are used for differential diagnosis, infant and pediatric hearing screening, and ototoxicity monitoring. There are two major types of OAEs that have been used clinically; transient-evoked OAEs (TEOAEs) and distortion product OAEs (DPOAEs).

The TEOAEs are measured following the presentation of a click or tone burst and time-synchronous averaging technique is used to reduce the amount of noise in the trace. Because of the nature of stimuli, the TEOAE tests outer hair cell functions in the entire cochlea. Generally the TEOAE will be absent if peripheral SNHL exceeds 30 dB HL. Therefore, present TEOAEs for all frequencies suggest relatively normal status of cochlear function.

The DPOAEs occur in response to two simultaneously presented tones of different frequencies and intensities because the cochlea generates "distortion products" that

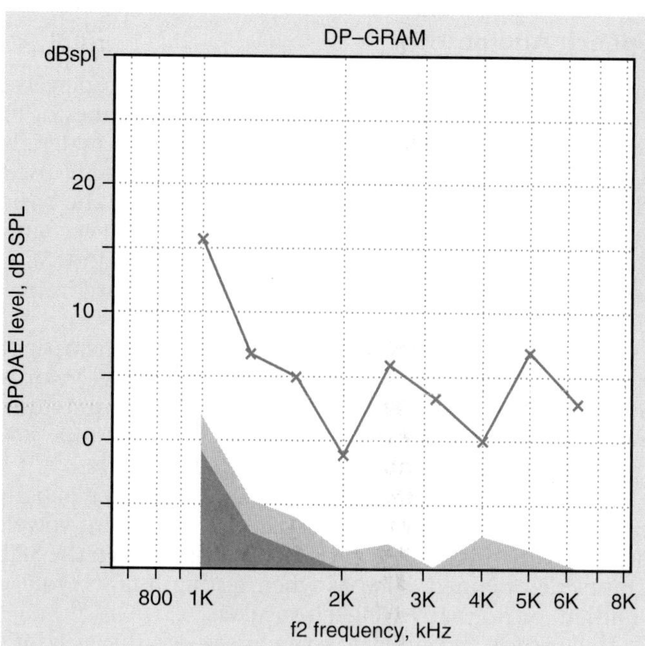

FIGURE 50-6 DP gram. (Redrawn from Katz J, editor: The acoustic reflex. In *Handbook of Clinical Audiology,* ed 5, Philadelphia, 2002, Lippincott Williams & Wilkins.)

are tones that are different in frequency from the two test stimuli. The DP-gram is a graph of DPOAE level as a function of frequency (Figure 50-6) upon which the DPOAE results are plotted. Clinically, DPOAEs are considered as present when they exceed the noise floor (the shaded areas in Figure 50-6) by a certain amount (usually at least 5 to 7 dB above the noise floor).

Auditory Brainstem Response

The auditory brainstem response (ABR) measures neural activities along the auditory pathway from the eighth cranial nerve up to possibly the inferior colliculus in response to auditory stimuli delivered via insert earphones.[14] The ABR is recorded during the first 10 ms following transient stimulus onset (e.g., click, tone burst) with noninvasive electrodes usually placed on the vertex of the head and the mastoids. The ABR waveforms are produced as a result of synchronous neural discharges and are used for analysis. In normal-hearing adults, the ABR has seven distinct peaks, labeled sequentially from I to VII (Figure 50-7). These peaks and troughs are thought to have different neural generators. Typically, only waves I, III, and V are used clinically. Abnormality in the ABR is judged by ABR peak absolute latencies, interwave latencies (I-III, III-V, and I-V), and interaural latency difference of wave V (Figure 50-7). It is recommended that ABRs are collected from 10 to 20 individuals with normal hearing to establish normative data in each clinic because testing equipment and testing parameters can vary from clinic to clinic. In addition to the measures above, clinicians look at the general waveform morphology. The ABR is used for differential diagnosis (e.g., detection of the effects of an acoustic tumor), intraoperative monitoring during tumor removal surgery, auditory threshold estimation, and infant hearing screening.

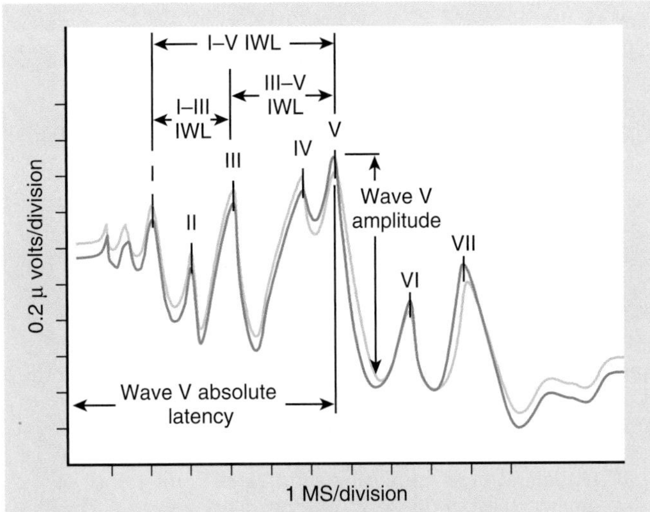

FIGURE 50-7 Schematic drawing of ABR waveform from a normal-hearing adult. *IWI*, interwave latency. (Redrawn from Campbell KCM: *Essential audiology for physicians*, San Diego, 1998, Singular Publishing Group.)

Risk Factors for Developing Hearing Impairments

Hearing impairments can be caused by genetic deficits/mutation, ear disease, environmental factors such as noise exposure or ototoxic drug intake, infections, and complications during pregnancy. Other factors such as age, gender, alcohol, smoking, diabetes, hypertension, stroke, and cardiovascular diseases are also associated with hearing impairments.

Acquired Hearing Loss

Acquired hearing loss refers to a hearing loss that manifests at any time in one's life with a variety of causes such as ear disease, viral (rubella, cytomegalovirus, mumps, acquired immunodeficiency syndrome, herpes) or bacterial infection (meningitis, syphilis), vascular insult to the cochlea, trauma to the auditory system, ototoxic drug/chemical intake, traumatic noise exposure, and aging. Some of acquired hearing loss is associated with systemic disease, including thyroid disease, diabetes mellitus, kidney disease, multiple sclerosis, connective tissue disease, and neurofibromatosis type II.

Ototoxic Drug/Chemical-Induced Hearing Loss

Various drugs and chemicals are toxic to the auditory system.[15] The hearing loss could be temporary or permanent SNHL, usually bilateral, and high frequencies are affected. Development of hearing loss largely depends on types of medications, dosage, and duration of intake. Aminoglycoside antibiotics (e.g., amikacin, gentamicin, kanamycin, neomycin, netilmicin, streptomycin, and tobramycin), loop diuretics, analgesics and antipyretics (e.g., high-dose aspirin, acetaminophen), antimalarial agents (e.g., quinine, chloroquine), and antineoplastic or chemotherapeutic agents (e.g., cisplatin) are known to cause either temporary or permanent sensorineural hearing loss. Lead, cadmium, mercury, manganese, styrene, toluene, ethyl benzene, and xylene are recognized as ototoxic chemicals. If the patient is on ototoxic medication, it is recommended that his/her hearing be monitored, and the patient should be informed to report any changes in hearing.

Table 50-2 Common Source of Noise That Could Lead to Permanent Hearing Loss

Occupational Noise	Recreational Noise	Daily Noise
Fire engine	Hunting	Power tools
Construction	Jet skiing or boating	Vacuum cleaner
Airplane	Motorcycle	Hair dryer
Farming	Four wheeling	Lawn mowers
Dental drills	Music, concert	Leaf blowers
Firearms	Woodworking	
Factory equipment		

Noise-Induced Hearing Loss

Traumatic noise exposure can cause mechanical damage and/or chemical reactions called "oxidative stress" to the auditory system,[48] leading to either temporary or permanent sensorineural hearing loss. Noise-induced hearing loss (NIHL) is the most common acquired hearing loss and a major source of sensory impairment in the military population. The hair cells, stria vascularis, and spiral ganglion neurons are vulnerable to damage from noise exposure. If NIHL is temporary, it usually recovers within 1 month. The audiologic profile of typical NIHL is characterized by bilateral, high-frequency hearing loss with a notch (the greatest hearing loss) in the audiogram at 3000, 4000, or 6000 Hz. However, gunfire can cause an asymmetrical SNHL, with the ear closest to the muzzle demonstrating more hearing loss. Tinnitus often accompanies NIHL. The four major aspects of noise that contribute to development of hearing impairments are (1) overall noise level; (2) spectrum distribution of noise; (3) duration and distribution of noise; and (4) cumulative noise exposure in days, weeks, or years. Occupational permissive noise exposure levels were set by the Occupational Safety and Health Administration (OSHA)[81] and National Institute for Occupational Safety and Health (NIOSH).[76] OSHA uses a 5-dB rule (increase in noise level by 5 dB results in reduction of exposure duration in half), although NIOSH uses a 3-dB rule. Table 50-2 shows common sources of noise that could lead to permanent hearing loss. It is recommended that individuals wear earplugs or personal hearing protection to prevent development of NIHL.

Age-Related Hearing Loss

Age-related hearing loss (ARHL), also referred to as presbycusis, is the third most prevalent chronic medical condition in the geriatric population. More than 10 million Americans over 65 years of age exhibit hearing impairment. Presbycusis is a complex disorder that has contributions from genetic and nongenetic (environmental and medical) factors.[99] Hair cells, stria vascularis, and spiral ganglion cells are vulnerable to degeneration from aging. The resultant hearing loss is sensorineural, permanent, and bilateral. High-frequency hearing is affected more than low frequencies, but some patients may have a flat hearing loss.

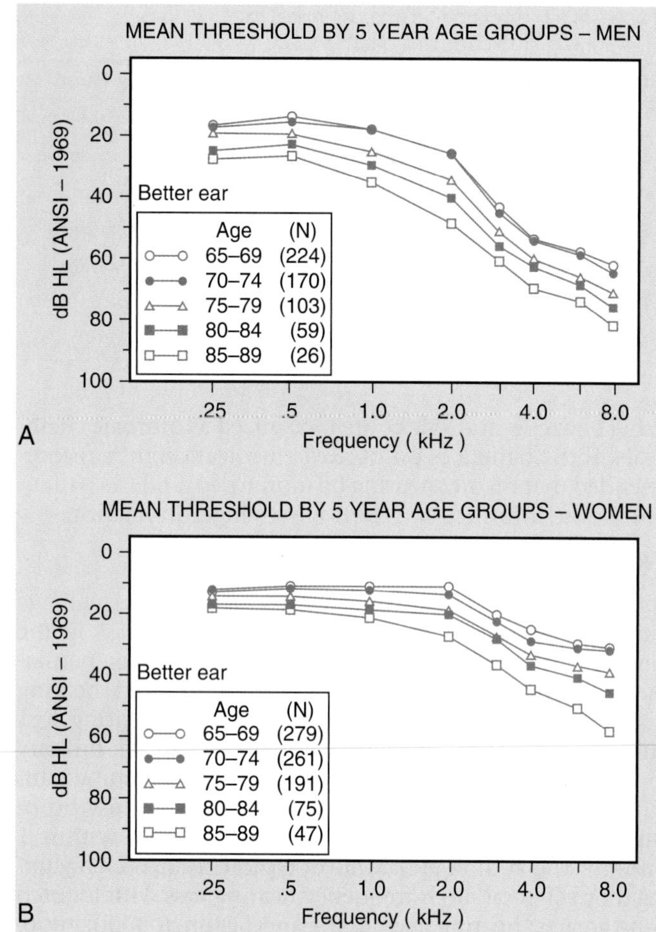

FIGURE 50-8 Changes in hearing thresholds in different age categories. **A,** Men. **B,** Women. (Redrawn from Gates et al: Hearing in the elderly: the Framingham cohort, 1983-1985 Part I. Basic audiometric test results. *Ear Hear* 11:247-56, 1990.)

Figure 50-8 shows changes in hearing thresholds in different age categories. Most of the patients with presbycusis can benefit from hearing aid use, and a cochlear implant is recommended if candidacy criteria are met.

Auditory Processing Disorder

A patient with auditory processing disorder exhibits difficulties processing auditory information caused by an underlining neurologic problem. The common symptoms are difficulty understanding speech in the presence of noise, inability to understanding degraded or rapid speech, and difficulty localizing the source of a signal. Auditory processing disorders are seen in patients with traumatic brain injury and children with no apparent etiology. The patients may or may not have hearing loss. The FM system or hearing aids can be used to treat auditory processing disorders.

Tinnitus

Tinnitus does not cause hearing loss, but often accompanies hearing loss. Tinnitus is the perception of sound in the ear or head in the absence of external sound sources. Although it is often called "ringing in the ear" or "head noise," perception of tinnitus varies by individuals. Perception may include ocean noise, pulsatile sound, high-pitch ringing, hissing, buzzing, humming, and chirping. Pulsatile tinnitus may be related to a serious health condition such as tumors. Tinnitus can be loud enough to disturb a patient's concentration and/or sleep, leading to serious depression. About 10% to 15% of the population experiences tinnitus.[8] The exact mechanism of tinnitus is still under investigation, but tinnitus is often associated with noise exposure, physical trauma to the head or neck, ear diseases, cerumen impaction, hypertension, temporal mandibular joint dysfunction, cardiovascular disease, and ototoxic drugs. There are two types of tinnitus: subjective tinnitus that is detected only by a patient and objective tinnitus that can be heard by others. If tinnitus is related to ear disease, it may disappear when the ear disease is cured. Some options for tinnitus management include diet and lifestyle modifications, hearing aids, sound therapy to desensitize perception of tinnitus, counseling, and tinnitus retraining therapy.

BOX 50-3

Ten Red Flags*—Warning of Ear Disease

1. Hearing loss with a positive history of ear infections, noise exposure, familial hearing loss, TB, syphilis, HIV, Meniere disease, autoimmune disorder, ototoxic medication use, otosclerosis, von Recklinghausen neurofibromatosis, Paget disease of bone, ear, or head trauma related to onset.
2. History of pain, active drainage, or bleeding from an ear.
3. Sudden onset or rapidly progressive hearing loss.
4. Acute, chronic, or recurrent episodes of dizziness.
5. Evidence of congenital or traumatic deformity of the ear.
6. Visualization of blood, pus, cerumen plug, foreign body, or other material in the ear canal.
7. An unexplained conductive hearing loss or abnormal tympanogram.
8. Unilateral or asymmetric hearing loss (a difference of greater than 15 dB Pure Tone Average between ears); or bilateral hearing loss >30 dB.
9. Unilateral or pulsatile tinnitus.
10. Unilateral or asymmetrically poor speech discrimination scores (a difference of greater than 15% between ears) or bilateral speech discrimination scores <80%.

Reprinted from http://www.entnet.org/content/red-flags-warning-ear-disease with permission of the American Academy of Otolaryngology—Head and Neck Surgery Foundation, copyright © 2015. All rights reserved.

*The red flags do not include all indications for a medical referral and are not intended to replace clinical judgment in determining the need for consultation with an otolaryngologist.

https://www.entnet.org/content/red-flags-warning-ear-disease

HIV, Human immunodeficiency virus; *TB,* tuberculosis.

Red Flags: Warning of Ear Disease

The American Academy of Otolaryngology—Head and Neck Surgery Inc./Foundation listed 10 red flags as warning of ear disease (Box 50-3). Patients who show any signs of red flags should be referred to a physician and/or specialist (i.e., otolaryngologist, otologist) for further evaluation and treatment of ear diseases.

Symptoms of Hearing Loss

It is very common for patients to be unaware of the presence of hearing impairments because they may be

BOX 50-4

Typical Complaints of the Patient with Hearing Impairments*

- Difficulty understanding speech in background noise (e.g., restaurant)
- Difficulty understanding speech in a group setting (e.g., meeting)
- Able to hear speech, but do not understand what is said
- Sounds like people are mumbling
- Talk too loud (sensorineural hearing loss) or too soft (conductive hearing loss)
- Turn up volume on TV and/or difficulty using a phone
- Difficulty understanding accent and/or unclear speech
- Difficulty learning foreign language
- Tinnitus and/or dizziness
- Difficulty following conversation
- Family members or friend complain about hearing loss

*Some people may have no symptoms at all if hearing loss progresses slowly overtime.

BOX 50-5

Signs That Physicians Should Note Regarding Possible Hearing Impairments

- Cannot hear or understand you when you ask them to enter your office for the appointment
- Not very talkative
- Does not reply when spoken to
- Does not respond appropriately to questions you are asking
- Does not understand you when you speak with them on the telephone
- Looks closely at your face or lips when you speak
- May appear confused when giving an inappropriate response
- May have a hearing aid, but does not use it
- May strain to understand or place hand behind ear in an attempt to amplify your voice
- Needs occasional repetition or a louder speaking voice to understand
- Needs frequent prompting, multiple repetitions, or restatement of what was said
- Not able to understand what is being said; asks you to write the message down to facilitate understanding
- Appears to have difficulty understanding fast speech and accented speech

From Weinstein BE: *Geriatric audiology,* ed 2, New York, 2013, Thieme Medical Publishers.

asymptomatic, in denial, or indifferent about their condition. Some patients with hearing impairments may be in a denial stage because hearing loss may be considered a sign of aging. Stigma of wearing a hearing aid may cause patients to delay in treating their hearing loss. Often time, family members or friends may complain that the patient does not follow conversation or listens to the television too loud. Box 50-4 lists typical complaints related to hearing impairment.

It is very important for health care providers to conduct hearing screening for early detection of hearing impairment. An otoscopic examination and screening for hearing impairment with questionnaires such as the Hearing Handicap Inventory for the Elderly–Screening version[101] and Hearing Handicap Inventory for Adults[80] can be performed at the physician's office to detect a patient who may have a hearing loss. Box 50-5 shows signs that physicians should note regarding possible hearing impairments. Another important issue to keep in mind is that cognitive impairment has similar manifestation as hearing loss.

Auditory Rehabilitation

According to the American Speech-Language-Hearing Association, the term *auditory rehabilitation* refers to "an ecological, interactive process that facilitates one's ability to minimize or prevent the limitations and restrictions that auditory dysfunctions can impose on well-being and communication, including interpersonal, psychosocial, educational, and vocational functioning."[5] Auditory habilitation, on the other hand, provide services to children (under 18 years old) with congenital hearing loss or hearing loss present at birth or acquired before the acquisition of speech and language. Specialists (e.g., otolaryngologists, otologists), audiologists, and speech-language pathologists work together to provide auditory rehabilitative/habilitative services to individuals with hearing loss. Major aspects of rehabilitation of hearing impairments are technical (e.g., hearing aids, hearing assistance technology, cochlear implants) and perceptual (e.g., speech and language therapy, auditory training). This chapter focuses on technical aspects of auditory rehabilitation. Instructional videos for hearing aids are available on the Washington University website at http://hearing.wustl.edu/InstructionalVideos.

Hearing Aids

Hearing aids are electrical devices that provide personal amplification to incoming sound based on an individual's hearing configuration. The devices are the most common form of noninvasive sound amplification that improve speech understanding in individuals with mixed or SNHL. Besides audibility, individuals with hearing impairment who use hearing aids may feel less exhausted at the end of the day because they do not need to concentrate as hard to try to understand speech. The majority of hearing aids on the market in the United States are digital (not analog). Therefore, the following section focuses on digital hearing aids.

How Hearing Aids Work

Figure 50-9 shows a simple diagram of the stages within a hearing aid. The main components in digital hearing aids are (1) microphone, (2) analog-to-digital converter, (3) digital signal processing circuit, (4) digital-to-analog converter, (5) receiver (speaker), (6) battery, and (7) a means of coupling the amplified sound into the ear canal. First, incoming sound (analog signal) is picked up by a microphone on the hearing aid. Location of the microphone varies depending on the hearing aid style. For example, behind-the-ear (BTE) hearing aids have the microphone behind the pinna, and completely-in-the-canal (CIC) hearing aids have the microphone located deep inside of the ear canal. Sound picked up by the microphone will be

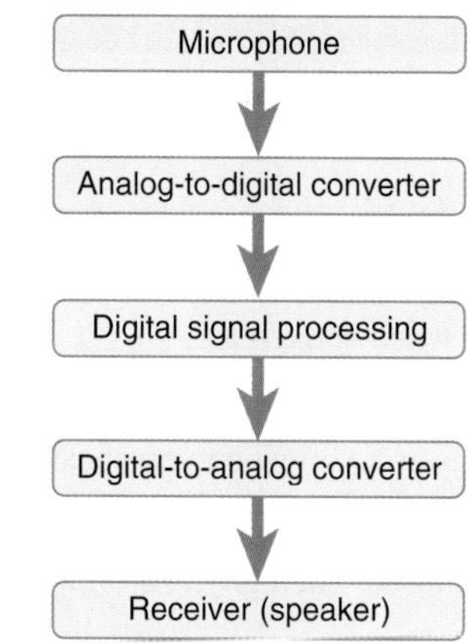

FIGURE 50-9 Simple diagram of hearing aids.

amplified and converted to a digitized signal by the analog-to-digital converter for further processing in the digital signal processing circuit. Various algorithms are available to improve the ability to understand speech, including feedback cancellation, noise reduction, filtering, and compression. Processed sound will then be converted to an analog signal by a digital-to-analog converter, and sent to a final-stage amplifier and receiver (speaker). In the BTE hearing aid, an earmold or a plastic dome will be used to couple the amplified sound into the ear canal. Batteries provide power for amplification and come in different sizes. The most common hearing aid battery sizes are 675, 13, 312, and A10. A single battery typically lasts approximately a week depending on the duration that the aid is used and the amount of amplification provided. Some hearing aids have a telecoil, an induction coupling device, to pick up electromagnetic fields for use with telephones and/or group hearing assistive technologies such as induction loop systems. Digital hearing aids can be equipped with different features and are usually classified as basic, midrange, and premium. If a patient has symmetrical bilateral hearing loss, it is recommended that two hearing aids be used to maximize binaural hearing.

Hearing Aid Consultation and Selection

Owing to various factors, not everyone benefits from hearing aid technology. Careful selection of hearing aids by the candidate is important for success in hearing aid use. Ear diseases should be treated medically and surgically if treatments are available. Once medical clearance for hearing aids is given, audiologists can assess hearing aid candidacy and individual needs for hearing aids based on the patient's acknowledgment of hearing loss, motivation, communication needs, perception about hearing aids, expectations, and financial needs. Acknowledgment of hearing loss and degree of motivation to do something about hearing loss are strongly correlated with how much patients wear hearing aids.[29]

Styles of Hearing Aids

Various styles of hearing aids are available, including BTE, open-fit BTE, in-the-ear (ITE), in-the-canal (ITC), CIC, and receiver-in-canal (RIC). Figure 50-10 shows some of the different types. Additional images of these different styles of hearing aids may be viewed at www.asha.org/public/hearing/Different-Styles-of-Hearing-Aids/. The audiologist will recommend a certain style of hearing aid based on the severity of hearing loss and other factors such as dexterity and financial need. Because many people still consider a hearing aid to be a sign of aging, smaller hearing aids are cosmetically appealing. However, smaller hearing aids use smaller batteries (which may be difficult for individuals with poor dexterity), and provide less power and amplification. Financially, smaller hearing aids can also be more expensive. Location and number of microphones are also important factors to consider. The BTE and RIC hearing aids have microphones behind the pinna, but the ITE, ITC, and CIC have a microphone either at the entrance of or deeper in the ear canal so the aid can take full advantage of pinna effects (e.g., sound collection and amplification). However, because the ITE, ITC, and CIC hearing aids block the ear canal, patients may feel that their ears are plugged (occlusion effect) compared with a BTE with a nonocclusive ear tip (open-fit BTE).

Hearing Aid Fitting and Follow-up

Once hearing aids are selected and ordered, patients are scheduled for fitting and orientation sessions. During an initial hearing aid fitting session, the audiologist programs the hearing aids, according to a prescriptive formula or a manufacturer's algorithm, to set appropriate amplification for the individual. Physical fit of the hearing aid is also checked. A hearing aid orientation session is conducted to educate the patient on hearing aid use and care, troubleshooting tips, and benefits and limitations of the devices. Educating new hearing aid users on appropriate expectations of hearing aids is critical for successful use. It may take time for a new hearing aid user to get used to amplified sound. New digital hearing aids usually come with a trial period and refund policy that varies from state to state (e.g., a 45-day trial and refund of full purchase price less amount up to 10% in New York State).

Hearing Assistance Technology

Hearing assistance technology (HAT) refers to personal devices that help an individual with or without hearing loss communicate more effectively. Box 50-6 shows the most common technologies. These devices can be used alone or to supplement hearing aids.

A personal FM system is a very popular HAT that transmits a speaker's voice directly to an individual's ear. The speaker must wear a microphone and FM transmitter, and a listener has to wear an FM receiver that can be coupled directly to the listener's ear via earphones, ear buds, induction loop, hearing aids, or cochlear implant.[58] The FM system can be used in academic and group settings, including classrooms, churches, and restaurants. Compared with conventional hearing aids, the personal FM system can provide a higher signal-to-noise ratio (SNR). For example, an FM system can provide a +15 dB SNR (signal is 15 dB greater than the noise level), whereas a hearing aid with directional microphones can provide a +3~5 dB SNR. The personal FM system also can be a great help in a physician's office to aid communication with a patient with hearing impairment.

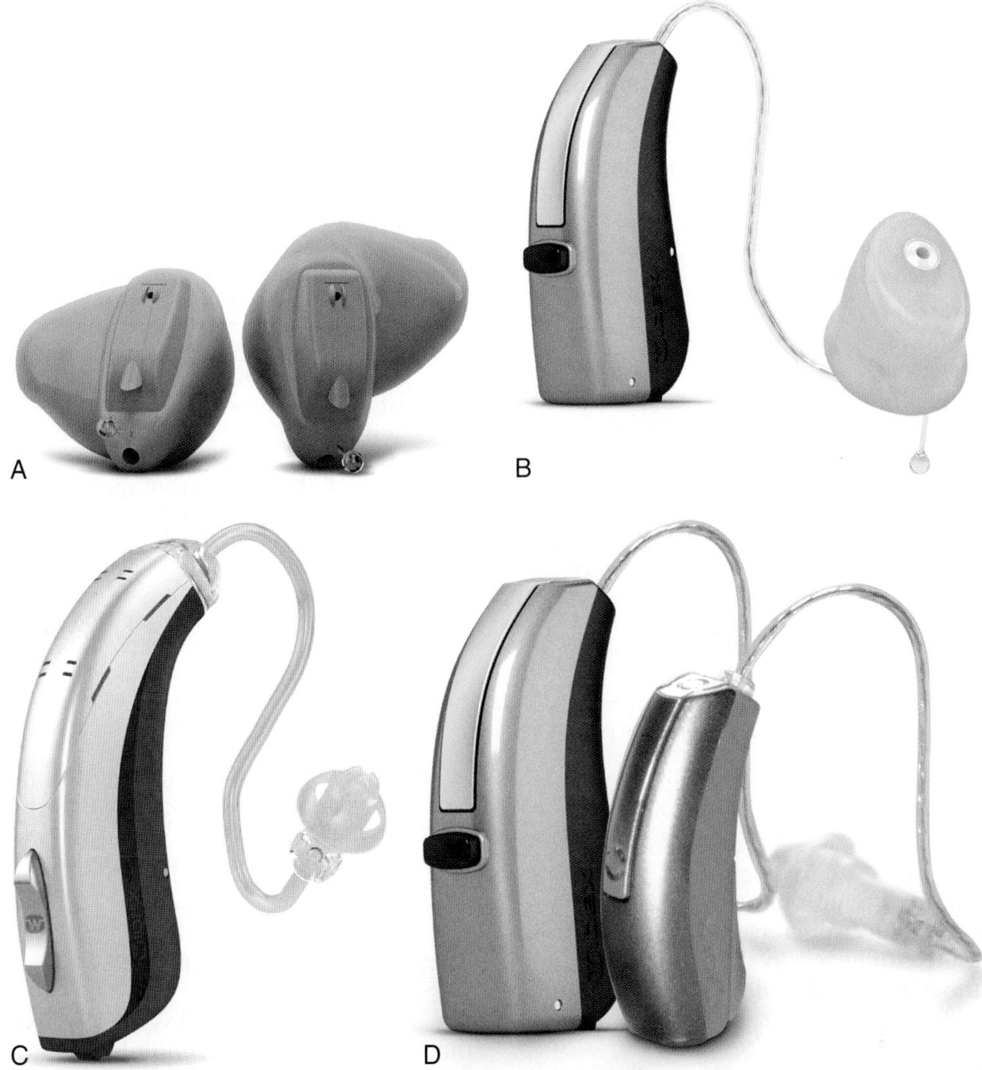

FIGURE 50-10 Different styles of hearing aids. **A,** Completely-in-the-canal style. **B,** Receiver-in-canal style. **C,** Thin open style. **D,** Receiver-in-canal behind-the-ear style. (Courtesy Widex USA Inc., Long Island City, NY.)

Surgical Treatments

Cochlear Implants

The cochlear implant (CI) is a surgically implanted device that electrically stimulates the auditory nerve via electrodes implanted in the cochlea, bypassing functions of the outer, middle, and inner ear. The CIs are class III medical devices and are regulated by the FDA. The CI is composed of an external speech processor, transmitting coil, internal receiver/simulator, and electrode array. The patient wears the external processor that picks up acoustic sound via a microphone and converts it to an electrical signal. The electrical signal is then converted to electromagnetic energy that is transmitted from an induction coil to the internal receiver/simulator that is embedded subcutaneously on the skull. The internal receiver/simulator converts the signal to electrical pulses and sends it to the electrode array that is inserted by an otologist in the scala tympani of the cochlea. After the surgery, an audiologist can program the CI speech processor based on objective and subjective measurements. New CI users are required to learn speech through auditory training because sound coming from the CI may sound different from sound from hearing aids or the natural ear.

Cochlear Corporation, Advanced Bionics, and MED-EL are the CI manufacturers in the United States, and they have their own CI candidacy criteria. In general, a patient with severe to profound SNHL who did not benefit from hearing aids and who has sufficient anatomic structures to support CI function can go through the criteria selection process. Benefits of the CI vary by individuals, ranging from full communication function to detection of environmental sounds only. The geriatric population also can benefit from the CI, but chronic health conditions may hinder the CI surgery.

Bone-Anchored Hearing Aids

The bone-anchored hearing aid (BAHA) is a surgically implanted device that delivers sound via bone vibration to the cochlea. Individuals with conductive or mixed hearing loss, single-sided deafness, and inability to tolerate conventional hearing aids in the ear canal are good candidates for the BAHA. The patient has a small metal post

BOX 50-6

Commonly Used Hearing Assistance Technology

Telephone Communication: Provide Amplification for Telephone Output or Display Conversation

- **Landline phones:** Hearing aid-compatible phone, Whistle Stop, in-line amplifier, Clarity phone, portable phone amplifier, replacement handset
- **Cell phones:** Bluetooth technology
- **Telephone devices for the deaf:** Text telephone or text typewriter (TTY), video relay services

Environmental Awareness of Sound

- **Devices:** Indicate the presence of sounds in the environment through auditory (amplified sound or lower pitch), visual (turning on/off lamp, strobe light, bright incandescent light), or tactile (pocket pagers, bed shakers, increase in airstream such as fun)
- **Hearing dogs:** Professionally trained hearing dog to indicate important environmental sounds

Television Viewing or Interpersonal Communication

- **Group amplification systems:** Transmit speakers' voices (either live or via multimedia) to an audience of listeners, can be wired (direct-audio input, teleloop, silhouette inductor, headphones/earbuds) or wireless systems (induction loop, infrared, or FM system)
- **Soundfield amplification:** Speaker's voice is conveyed to listeners in the room via one or more strategically placed loudspeakers
- **Other:** Captioned programming, closed captioning, and Real-Time captioning

implanted in the mastoid bone, upon which a sound processer is attached. The processor converts incoming sound to vibrations that are conducted to the inner ear via the skull, bypassing the outer and middle ear.

Middle Ear Implantable Hearing Aids

The middle ear implantable hearing aids are designed to treat conductive and sensorineural hearing loss. The implanted portion of the device is attached to the ossicular chain and converts acoustic energy to mechanical vibratory energy. There are two types of the middle ear implants: piezoelectric and electromagnetic. The MED-EL Vibrant Sound Bridge, Ototronix Maxum, and Envoy Esteem have been approved by the FDA. Candidates are patients who do not benefit from or cannot use conventional hearing aids (e.g., allergies/sensitivity to earmold materials, chronic external ear infection) but have hearing loss that is not severe enough to qualify for a CI.

Communication Strategies

Compensatory communication strategies can provide tremendous benefits to individuals with hearing impairments. These strategies can be used with or without hearing aids. Box 50-7 shows common communication strategies. Communication requires a speaker and listener. Both entities are encouraged to use communication strategies to enhance understanding. In a physician's office, health care providers and staff members are encouraged to use the communication strategies to accommodate a patient's communication needs.

BOX 50-7

Compensatory Communication Strategies

1. Address the person with hearing loss
   - Get the person's attention before starting to communicate. Their brain must be alerted to be ready to focus and listen.
2. Have face-to-face communication
   - The more important high-pitched sounds of speech are very directional (only propagate well in the direction the speaker is facing) and the production of the high-pitched sounds is visible on the mouth.
   - Do not obscure the lips with hands or other objects.
   - Make certain that light shines directly on the speaker's face, not from behind the speaker.
3. Start with the topic
   - It is easier for the listener to fill in missed information if they know the context.
4. Use a slightly slower rate of speaking
   - It gives more time for the listener's brain to process and keep up with the flow of information.
   - Avoid shouting because it will not help.
5. Use appropriate distance
   - The more important high-pitched sounds are very weak and are not able to travel far from the speaker.
6. Control noise (unwanted sounds)
   - Noise will always interfere with communication and many of these unwanted sounds will also be picked up by a hearing aid.
7. Spell words out, use gestures, or write down.
8. Repeat back or change phrasing if the listener does not understand at first.
9. Speak toward the better ear, if applicable.

Vestibular Impairments

The peripheral and central vestibular systems contribute to the functions of balance, equilibrium, orientation in space, ocular stability during movement, and maintenance of posture and muscular tone. The visual and somatosensory systems also have conjunctive contributions to many of these functions. Vestibular system dysfunction can lead to a multitude of problems including vertigo (illusion of motion), disequilibrium, and falls.

These disorders constitute a significant public health problem. The National Institute on Deafness and Other Communication Disorders (NIDCD)[77] reported that approximately 4% (almost 8 million) of American adults reported a chronic problem with balance. And an additional 1.1% (2.4 million) reported a chronic problem with dizziness alone. The estimated cost of medical care per year in the United States for patients with balance disorders exceeds $1 billion. The NIDCD also reported that a problem with balance is the principal reason individuals over the age of 75 visit their primary care physician, and it is a major cause of falls in the American geriatric population. Patient care costs for these falls amount to more than $8 billion per year. Additionally, large numbers of military personnel have sustained some form of traumatic brain injury (TBI) caused by ongoing military conflict. Mild TBI because of blast exposure has become one of the most frequent injuries for American veterans of Operation Enduring Freedom, Operation Iraqi Freedom, and Operation New Dawn. The Defense and Veterans Brain Injury Center (DVBIC)[25] reported that the Defense Medical Surveillance System (DMSS) and the Armed Forces Health Surveillance Center (AFHSC) tallied 313,816 TBIs from 2000 through the third quarter of 2014 for all US military service personnel. Military personnel with mild TBI are significantly more likely to have vestibular and balance/postural disorders. It has been shown that vestibular and oculomotor deficits tend to be more persistent than cognitive impairments.[94] Undetected vestibular disorders can lead to hastened return to duty and be detrimental to the success of military operations.

Anatomy and Physiology of the Vestibular System

The vestibular end organs consist of the semicircular canal (SSC) system and otolith organ system. Figure 50-11 illustrates the vestibular end organs and their orientation within the head. The three nearly orthogonally positioned SSCs (posterior, horizontal/lateral, and anterior/superior) sense rotational/angular acceleration. The two otolith organs (utricle and saccule) detect linear acceleration, head tilt, and gravity. The stereocilia of the sensory hair cells within the utricle and saccule are embedded in a gelatinous structure (otolithic membrane) with associated microscopic calcium carbonate crystals (otoconia). The abnormal migration of otoconia into the SSC system results in a type of dizziness termed benign paroxysmal positional vertigo.

The vestibular neurons of the eighth cranial nerve project centrally to both the cerebellum and the vestibular nuclei, where they synapse and transmit afferent vestibular inputs and contribute to vestibular reflex pathways. There are three main vestibular reflexes: the vestibulospinal reflex (for body stabilization), vestibulocollic reflex (for head stabilization), and the vestibulo-ocular reflex (VOR) (for visual gaze stabilization). The VOR, for example, stabilizes eye movement with respect to the visual field during head motion. Many test procedures used to evaluate the vestibular system require monitoring of eye motion related to vestibular function. The presence of nystagmus (involuntary eye movements) can be related to vestibular dysfunction. Jerk nystagmus consists of eye drift in one direction (slow phase) and a quick corrective eye

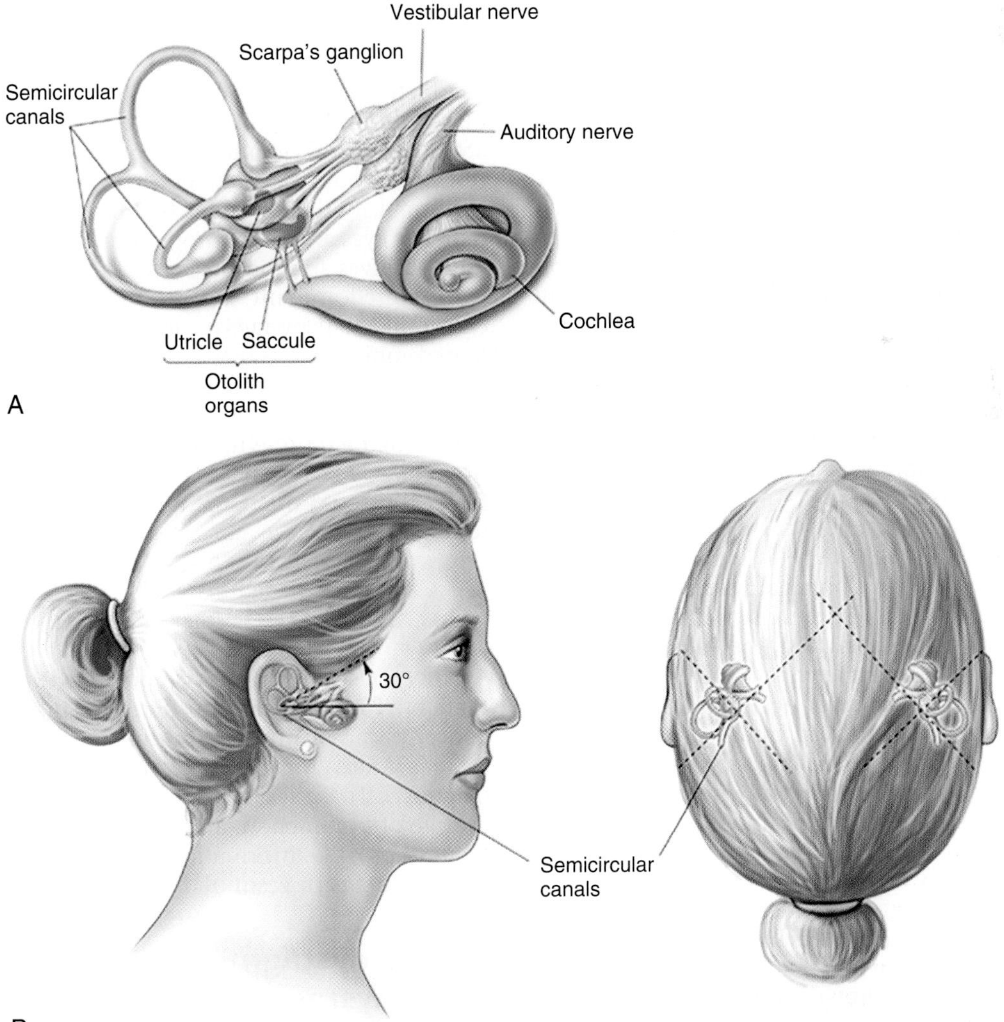

FIGURE 50-11 Vestibular end organ and orientation. (From Bear MF, Connors BW, Paradiso MA: The vestibular labyrinth. In *Neuroscience: exploring the brain*, Philadelphia, 2007, Lippincott Williams & Wilkins.)

movement (fast phase). These involuntary eye movements can occur in a side-to-side (horizontal nystagmus), up-and-down (vertical nystagmus), or circular (torsional or rotary nystagmus) pattern.

Kheradmand et al.[62] provided further insight into the perception of spatial orientation. By means of transcranial magnetic stimulation, they found that the posterior aspect of the supramarginal gyrus is involved in processing information from different sensory modalities into an accurate perception of being in an upright position.

Case History and Physical Examination

A thorough case history is paramount in the diagnosis of a disorder, including determining the cause of dizziness. The history can provide the necessary qualitative diagnostic information. Further testing of the vestibular system can follow if the history is insufficient or if further quantifiable information is need to confirm a diagnosis.

Case History

The foundation for the history taking is established with a thorough dizziness questionnaire. Gathered information should include the patient's description of the symptoms, the duration of the episode(s), concomitant problems, and more. Bennett[10] presented the following questions for use as the foundation of a dizziness case history: "*Question 1*—Describe what you are experiencing, *Question 2*—How long does your dizziness last?, *Question 3*—How often do you have attacks of vertigo?, *Question 4*—Is there anything you can do that will cause you to feel dizzy (precipitating factors)?, *Question 5*—What other symptoms do you have around the time of vertigo attacks (associated symptoms)?, *Question 6*—Do you have any other medical problems?, *Question 7*—What medications are you currently taking?"

A differential diagnosis is solidified with the summative information gathered from the questions.

Physical Examination

Some of the more common physical assessments of the vestibular system may include the visualization of gaze-evoked nystagmus, the Romberg test, the Fukuda stepping test, and the Dix-Hallpike maneuver.

Gaze testing involves monitoring for the presence of nystagmus or other abnormal eye movements while the patient fixates on stationary visual targets. Gaze nystagmus is considered abnormal if it is present with appropriately positioned visual targets. It can be interpreted with the Alexander law, which states that gazing in the direction of the fast phase enhances the nystagmus.

For the Romberg test, the patient stands with feet together and arms to the side, and is instructed to maintain this position with eyes open and then closed. The patient's maximum time in maintaining the position with eyes open and eyes closed is compared with normative data from healthy control subjects. Jacobson and colleagues[54] assessed the sensitivity, specificity, and positive and negative predictive value of the Romberg test in patients with vestibular system lesions affecting the horizontal semicircular canals, saccule, and/or inferior and superior vestibular nerves. The Romberg test was compared with the cervical vestibular evoked myogenic potential and caloric tests (discussed in forthcoming sections). They concluded that the performance characteristics of the Romberg test were poor and insufficient for use as a screening measure for vestibular hypofunction.

The Fukuda stepping test assesses labyrinthine function through the vestibulospinal reflexes. The patient steps in place on a marked grid with the eyes closed, and arms outstretched forward. Measurements of rotation and displacement are taken after 50 to 100 steps and compared with data from healthy contuol subjects. Honaker and colleagues,[51] however, caution that the Fukuda stepping test may not be an accurate screening tool for peripheral vestibular asymmetry in chronically dizzy patients.

The Dix-Hallpike maneuver can be used to assess for the effects of displaced otoconia in the posterior semicircular canal. The abnormal migration of otoconia into the SSC system results in benign paroxysmal positional vertigo (BPPV). BPPV is considered to be the most common vestibular ailment and results in approximately 50% of dizziness in older people.[32] In the Dix-Hallpike maneuver, the patient is seated on the examination bed with the head rotated to the lesion side by 45 degrees. The patient is then quickly lowered backward to a supine position, with the head hanging over the edge of the bed by 30 degrees. This places the patient in a position that aligns the posterior SSC in a vertical orientation. Potential debris in the posterior SSC would be influenced by gravity and thus cause abnormal fluid movement within the affected canal. The patient's eyes are open throughout testing while the examiner observes for the presence of nystagmus. Nystagmus with a predominant torsional component is present in classic BPPV. If nystagmus appears, the position is maintained until the nystagmus terminates before quickly returning the patient to an upright position. The signs and symptoms of BPPV are fatigable; therefore, if nystagmus and vertigo are present, the maneuver should be repeated immediately to evaluate the response for fatigue. Figure 50-12 illustrates the maneuver for evaluation of right posterior SSC BPPV.

Computerized Vestibular Testing

A variety of sophisticated computerized vestibular tests are available for those cases of dizziness in which the history and physical examination alone are inadequate or when there is a need for further corroborative data to confirm a diagnosis. These tests can provide information related to the site of dysfunction, and can also be applied after treatment to provide information regarding the potential functional benefits of vestibular rehabilitation.

Electronystagmography/Videonystagmography

Electronystagmography (ENG) and videonystagmography (VNG) use computer-based systems that assess the vestibular system by recording of horizontal and vertical

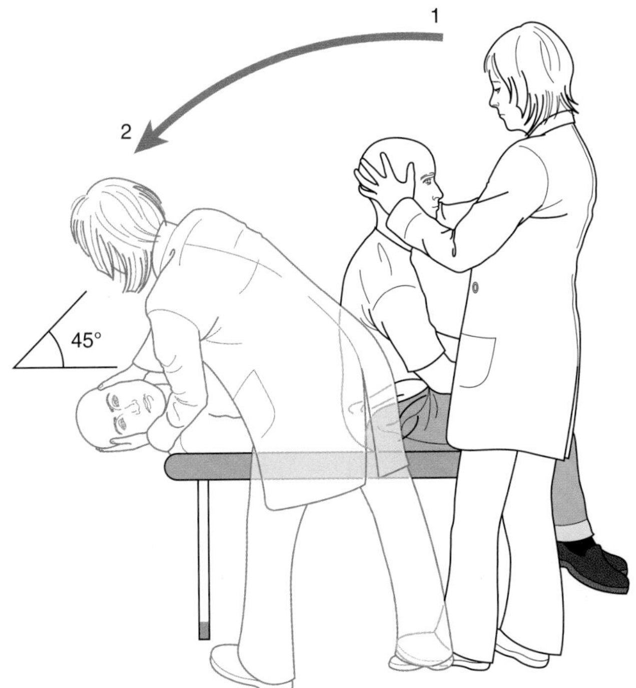

FIGURE 50-12 Right-side Dix-Hallpike maneuver. (Redrawn from Fife TDI, Lempert T, Furman JM, et al: Practice parameter: therapies for benign paroxysmal positional vertigo (an evidence-based review): report of the Quality Standards Subcommittee of the American Academy of Neurology, *Neurology* 70:2067-2074, 2008.)

eye movements. During ENG testing, eye movements are recorded indirectly with electrodes that detect changes in the corneoretinal potential, whereas VNG testing involves direct recording of eye movements with infrared digital video cameras. The typical ENG/VNG battery consists of testing of gaze nystagmus (discussed previously), random saccades, smooth pursuit, positional nystagmus, and calorics.

Random Saccade Testing

Saccades are rapid movements of the eyes. During the saccadic testing, the patient's eye movements are compared with the fast, random movement of the target stimuli. Analysis includes the measurement of saccadic accuracy, latency, and velocity. Distinctive saccade abnormalities can be suggestive of a site of lesion after accounting for variables such as patient age, cognitive status, and attention to the task.

Smooth Pursuit Testing

During smooth pursuit testing, the patient tracts a visual target moving in a sinusoidal pattern that varies in frequency over time. Symmetrically impaired pursuit is suggestive of a nonspecific central finding after accounting for patient variables. Asymmetrically impaired pursuit is consistent with a unilateral hemispheric or asymmetrical posterior fossa lesion.

Positional Testing

Positional testing is used to identify nystagmus present during the maintenance of a provocative head or body position. Measures must be taken to prevent visual fixation and central suppression. Examples of the positions include sitting, supine, supine with head turned left and right, lying lateral on the left and right side, and supine with head hanging. When nystagmus is present, the comparison of the nystagmus with and without fixation is essential to determine site of lesion. Visual fixation is expected to decrease the slow-phase eye velocity of a nystagmus of peripheral origin, whereas the nystagmus velocity is likely to increase with fixation nystagmus of central vestibular origin. A change in nystagmus direction within a set position is also suggestive of a disorder of central vestibular origin.

Caloric Testing

The caloric test is performed by applying cool and warm temperature irrigations of water or air in the external auditory canal. The patient is positioned such that the horizontal/lateral semicircular canal is perpendicular to horizontal. The temperature gradient induces endolymph flow in the horizontal/lateral semicircular canal, which then activates the VOR.[33] The irrigations are applied into each ear individually, and the resultant slow-phase velocity of the nystagmus is analyzed. The ensuing nystagmus should follow the "COWS" (Cold Opposite, Warm Same) mnemonic. An example for the left ear would be that a cool irrigation should produce a right-beating (i.e., opposite) nystagmus, and a warm irrigation should produce a left-beating (i.e., same) nystagmus.

Bithermal caloric testing allows for the evaluation of ear-specific function and is thus important in assessing the comparative symmetry of the vestibular end-organs. Interaural differences are determined by comparing the slow-component eye velocity of the induced nystagmus.[59] A commonly used criterion for unilateral abnormality is an asymmetry of 25% or more. This finding is suggestive of unilateral horizontal semicircular canal/superior vestibular nerve dysfunction. A significant bilateral peripheral vestibular weakness is defined commonly as a total nystagmus response for each ear less than 15%. Figures 50-13 and 50-14 illustrate normal and abnormal caloric responses.

Rotational Chair Testing

Rotational chair testing involves stimulation of horizontal semicircular canals/superior vestibular nerves by spinning the patient along a vertical axis in a quantifiable sinusoidal, pseudorandom, or constant-velocity manner. Infrared digital video cameras are used to monitor the VOR. Figure 50-15 shows a patient in the rotational chair with VOR-monitoring goggles. The stimulus frequencies used during rotational testing more closely approximate those that occur with normal head movement than the stimulation provided by caloric testing. The rotation provides simultaneous bilateral stimulation of the labyrinths. Arriaga and colleagues[6] found a sensitivity advantage of 71% versus 31% for rotational chair versus ENG in detecting a peripheral vestibulopathy. However, the bilateral nature of the rotary stimulation resulted in a specificity disadvantage of 54% versus 86%.

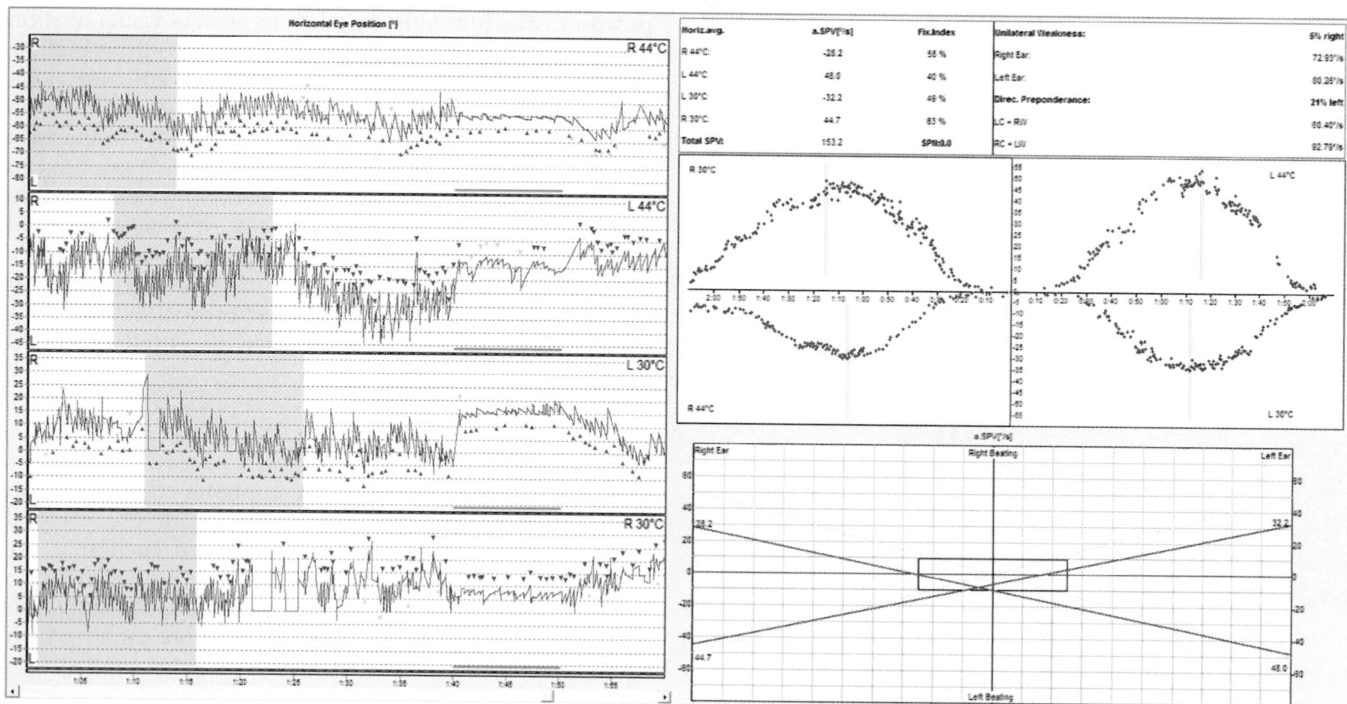

FIGURE 50-13 **Normal caloric response.** (From Bahner C, Petrak M, Beck DL, et al: In the trenches, part 3: caloric and rotational chair tests. *Hear Rev* 20:2013.) (www.hearingreview.com/2013/03/in-the-trenches-part-3-caloric-and-rotational-chair-tests/. Courtesy Interacoustics A/S, Assens, Denmark.)

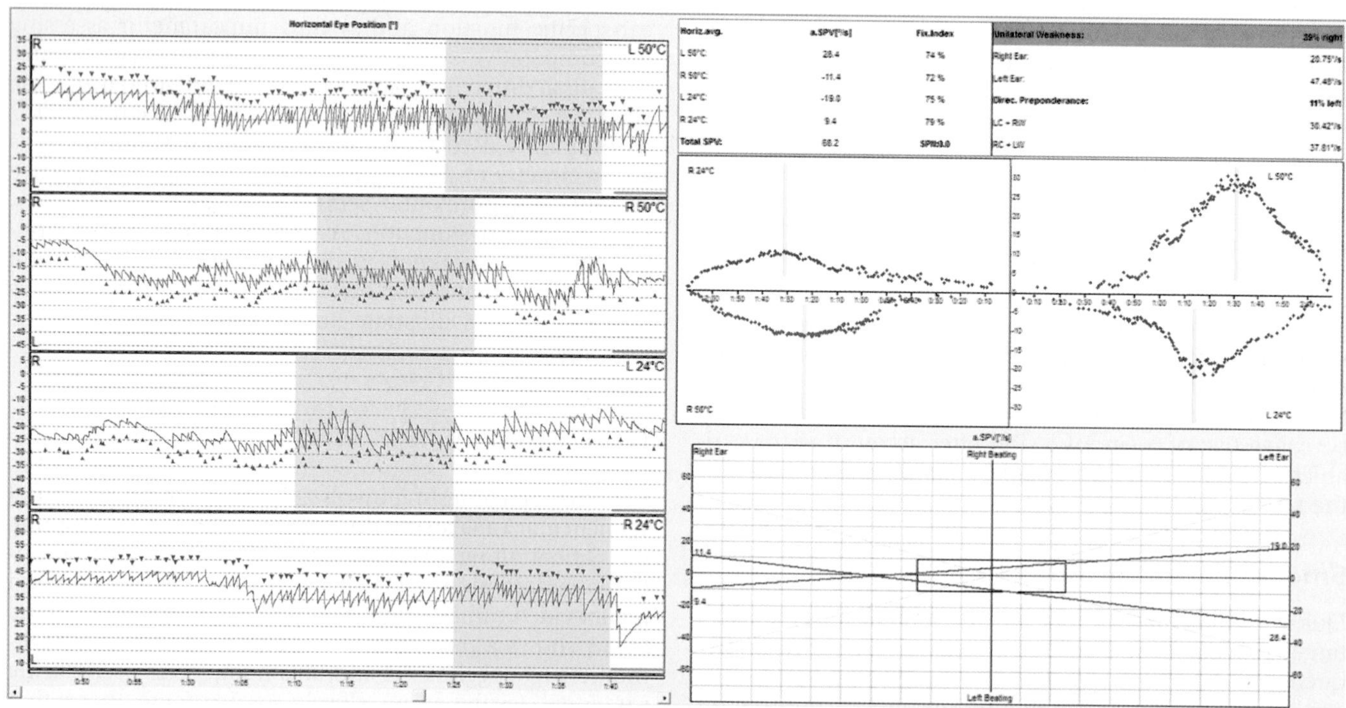

FIGURE 50-14 **Abnormal caloric response (left unilateral weakness).** (From Bahner C, Petrak M, Beck DL, et al: In the trenches, part 3: caloric and rotational chair tests. *Hear Rev* 20:2013.) (www.hearingreview.com/2013/03/in-the-trenches-part-3-caloric-and-rotational-chair-tests/ Courtesy Interacoustics A/S, Assens, Denmark.)

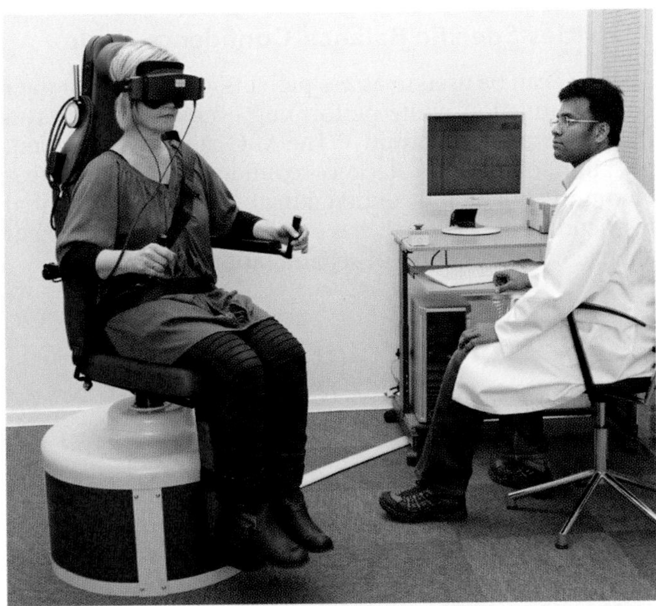

FIGURE 50-15 **Rotational chair.** (From Bahner C, Petrak M, Beck DL, et al: In the trenches, part 3: caloric and rotational chair tests. *Hear Rev* 20:2013.) (www.hearingreview.com/2013/03/in-the-trenches-part-3-caloric-and-rotational-chair-tests/. Courtesy Interacoustics A/S, Assens, Denmark.)

Computerized Dynamic Posturography

Computerized dynamic posturography (CDP) uses a movable platform and visual surround. The patient's motor reactions and postural stability are recorded as the support surface and the visual surround moves. The CDP test battery is designed to assess a patient's ability to integrate vestibular, visual, and somatosensory information for maintenance of postural control. The American Academy of Otolaryngology—Head and Neck Surgery specify the Sensory Organization Test (SOT) and the Motor Control Test (MCT) as the components of CDP.

The SOT protocol assesses sensory integration by measuring body sway under conditions of altered visual/somatosensory feedback. It can help to identify patients with uncompensated unilateral or bilateral peripheral vestibular system dysfunction or patients with exaggerated or fabricated balance problems. Figure 50-16 illustrates the six SOT sensory conditions.

The MCT protocol evaluates the patient's ability to adjust to abrupt and unexpected forward or backward movements of the support platform. It can provide valuable information regarding the risk of fall caused by the adverse effects of unpredictable extrinsic disturbances on postural/balance control.

Cervical and Ocular Vestibular-Evoked Myogenic Potential

Intense sound stimuli such as clicks or tone pips can stimulate sensory tissue within the otolithic organs. The cervical vestibular evoked myogenic potential (cVEMP) can be recorded with electrodes placed over the sternocleidomastoid muscle (SCM). The cVEMP is based on the vestibulocollic reflex and is thought to originate in the saccule. The neural structures involved in the stimulation of the SCM include the inferior division of the vestibular nerve, the lateral vestibular nucleus, the lateral vestibulospinal tract, and the accessory nerve (XI).[21] The ocular vestibular-evoked myogenic potential (oVEMP) is believed to originate in the utricle, and it involves the superior division of the vestibular nerve. It can be recorded using electrodes placed over the inferior oblique muscle in the contralateral infraorbital region.[55] Table 50-3 outlines the cVEMP abnormalities encountered in various otologic and neurologic disorders.

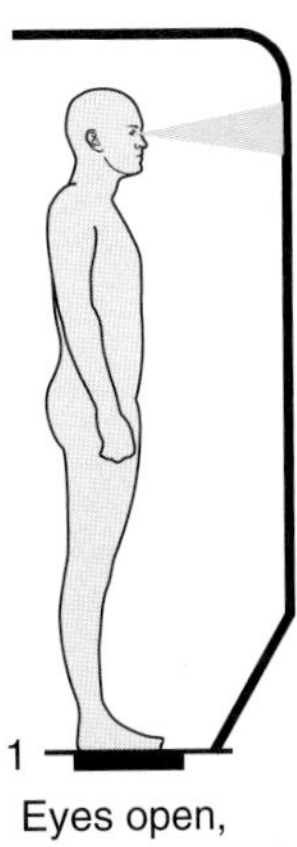

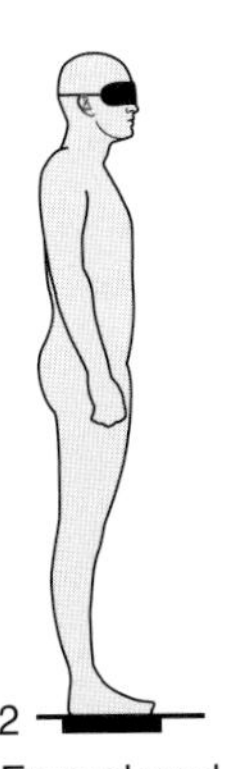

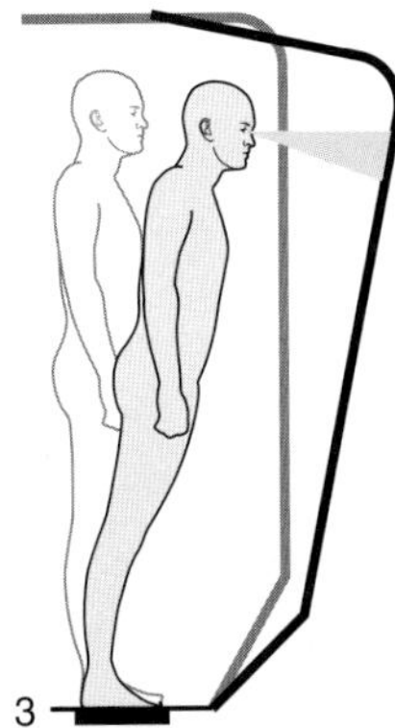

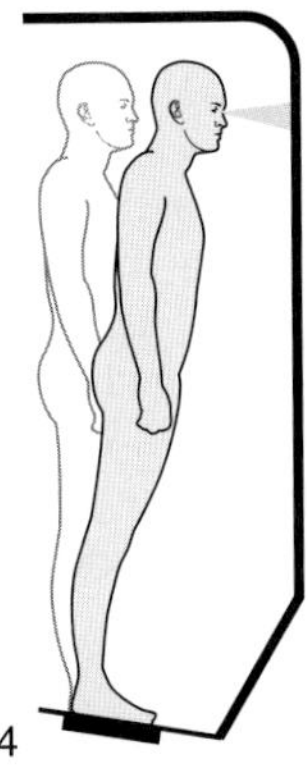

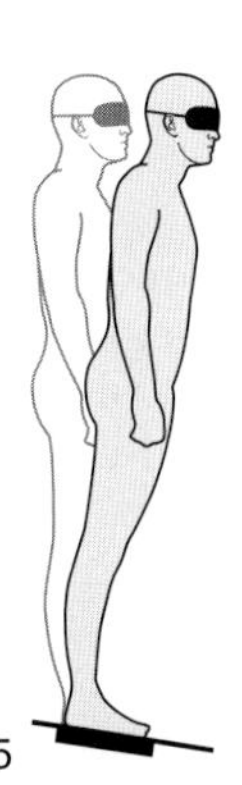

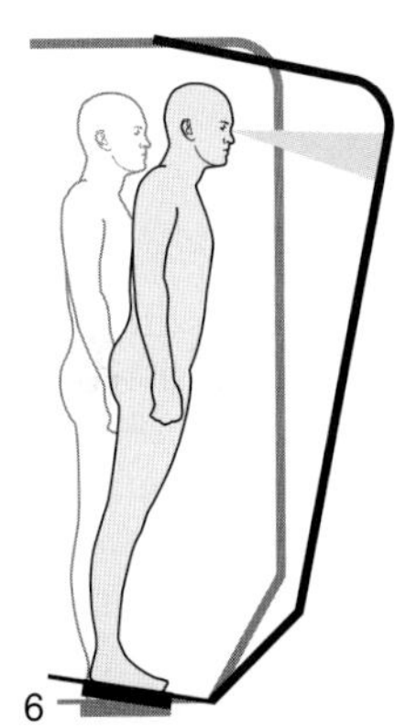

FIGURE 50-16 Six sensory conditions for the Sensory Organization Test (SOT). *1*, Eyes open, fixed surface and visual surround. *2*, Eyes closed, fixed surface. *3*, Eyes open, fixed surface, sway referenced visual surround. *4*, Eyes open, sway referenced surface, fixed visual surround. *5*, Eyes closed, sway referenced surface. *6*, Eyes open, sway referenced surface and visual surround. (Images courtesy Natus Medical Incorporated.)

Video Head Impulse Test

The video head impulse test (vHIT) can be used to assess the dynamic function of the individual semicircular canals. It is based on the HIT described by Halmagyi and

Table 50-3 cVEMP Abnormalities

	cVEMP Responses			
Pathologic Condition	**Absent**	**Reduced**	**Enhanced**	**Delayed**
Otologic				
Meniere disease	✔	✔	✔	
Superior canal dehiscence			✔	
Neurolabyrinthitis	✔	✔		
Vestibular neuritis	✔	✔		
Neurologic				
Migraine	✔	✔		✔
Spinocerebellar degeneration	✔			✔
Multiple sclerosis	✔			✔
Brainstem stroke	✔			✔

From Gans RE, Roberts RA: Understanding vestibular-evoked myogenic potentials (VEMPs), *Audiol Today* 17:23-25, 2005.
cVEMP, Cervical vestibular evoked myogenic potential.

Curthoys.[44] The vHIT uses recordings of eye and head movements during and immediately following unpredictable, impulsive drive of the head initiated by the clinician. A particular semicircular canal can be stimulated by head movement within the plane of that canal. These actions evoke VOR-produced compensatory eye movements that also occur within that plane. A high-speed digital video camera records the resultant deviation in gaze produced by the head impulse, which can be used to aid in the detection of vestibular hypofunction. Murnane and colleagues[74] obtained normative data and test-retest reliability of the SYNAPSYS Inc. vHIT (version 2.0) device in healthy control subjects.

Subjective Assessments

Several measures are available that can be used to assess subjective adjustment in patients with vestibular disorders. These include the Dizziness Handicap Inventory (DHI)[56] and the Activities-Specific Balance Confidence (ABC) scale.[86]

Dizziness Handicap Inventory

The DHI is a commonly used subjective scale used in vestibular rehabilitation. Jacobson and Newman[56] developed the DHI in an effort to quantify the handicapping effects of dizziness on a patient's well-being. The original DHI consists of 25 items separated into three categories: functional, physical, and emotional. Four scores are calculated: the total DHI and an individual score for each subcategory. High scores reflect greater handicapping effects. Whitney and colleagues[104] found that DHI scores above 60 are associated with severe dizziness and recurrent falls. The DHI can also be used to determine patient improvement after rehabilitation. Jacobson and Newman[56] found that a decrease on the DHI of 18 can be considered clinically significant progress.

Activities-Specific Balance Confidence Scale

The ABC can be used to assess patients' confidence in their balance function while performing everyday activities in the home and community.[86] The ABC can aid in the identification of patients' lack of confidence in performing common functional undertakings and their potential restriction of activities. It has also been used to document change over the course of rehabilitation.[103]

Risk Factors, Comorbidities, and Epidemiology of Vestibular Disorders

The more common vestibular disorders include BPPV, vestibular neuritis, vestibular migraine, and Meniere disease. In Baloh and colleagues' study on BPPV,[9] the mean age of onset was in the fifth decade of life, and almost half of the cases were idiopathic. Cases with a probable underlying cause included head trauma and viral neurolabyrinthitis. In an observational study on the role of comorbidities, De Stefano and colleagues[26] found a statistical link between the presence of systemic disorders (hypertension, diabetes, osteoarthrosis, osteoporosis, and depression) and BPPV.

Vestibular neuritis was the second most common cause of dizziness after BPPV identified in general practice clinics.[45] Adamec and colleagues[1] identified the most common comorbidities in patients with vestibular neuritis in their practice as hypertension, diabetes, hyperlipidemia, and hypothyreosis. Chuang and colleagues[19] suggested that comorbid vertebral artery hypoplasia may be a risk factor for severe vestibular neuritis.

Epidemiologic studies have shown a relationship between migraine and vertigo.[67] Neuhauser and colleagues[79] found the prevalence of vestibular migraine to be 7% in patients from a dizziness clinic and 9% in patients from a migraine clinic. Vestibular migraine was found to occur at any age and has a strong female preponderance.[28] Familial occurrence was identified as a risk factor.[82] Uneri's[98] retrospective study found that migraines were three times more common in patients with confirmed BPPV than in the general population. Meniere disease was also found to have an increased prevalence in migraineurs.[89]

Meniere disease is characterized by recurring episodes of long-lasting vertigo, fluctuating sensorineural hearing loss, tinnitus, and aural fullness. Its prevalence is difficult to ascertain because of its fluctuant nature and the potential absence of certain signs and symptoms in the early stages.[91] However, the estimated prevalence in the United States is 0.19%, with a dramatic increase in prevalence with age.[2] Genetic predisposition has been identified. Arweiler and colleagues[7] detected an autosomal dominant hereditary pattern and also proposed a multifactorial etiology for Meniere disease.

Vestibular Rehabilitation

Vestibular rehabilitation involves procedures by which patients with dizziness or imbalance can begin to manage their symptoms and regain functional mobility. Exercises for decreasing symptoms of dizziness or disequilibrium can be categorized into areas targeting habituation, VOR adaptation, or sensory substitution.

Habituation

Habituation is the process by which symptoms are decreased through repeated exposure to provocative stimuli. A peripheral vestibular lesion can create a sensory discrepancy caused by unequal vestibular inputs from the vestibular labyrinths. Repetitive movement may reduce this asymmetry of vestibular input. Cawthorne[17] and Cooksey[22] treated individuals with postconcussive unilateral vestibular dysfunction in the 1940s and observed that patients involved in more movement gained greater management of their symptoms. They suggested that patients become more tolerant of problematic motion when exposed to repetitive exercises that progressed in difficulty. Particular movements or environments that result in symptoms of moderate degree are established. Then a progressive repetitive program can be executed to help the patient habituate to the sensation and consequently lessen the symptoms.[49]

Vestibulo-Ocular Reflex Adaptation

The VOR is an important 3-neuron vestibular reflex affected by stimulation of the semicircular canals that creates conjugate eye movement of equal and opposite direction to the movement of the head. The VOR allows for stabilization of the image on the retina, leading to clear vision when the head is moved. The gain of the VOR is the ratio of eye velocity to head velocity. The ideal gain in a normal patient is 1 : 1. A vestibular disorder can result in decreased gain in the VOR, which in turn would result in a blurred image when the head is moved rapidly. Allum and colleagues[3] found that patients with acute unilateral peripheral vestibular hypofunction had reductions in vertical VOR gain by as much as 66%, and an average horizontal VOR gain reduction of 50% toward the involved side and 25% toward the noninvolved side of the vestibular dysfunction.

Patients with an uncompensated unilateral vestibular weakness may be prescribed exercises that focus on adaptation of the VOR. These activities consist of performing head movements while keeping a visual target in focus. For example, a patient is asked to keep a visual target in focus while swaying the head side to side. The exercises are progressed in difficulty and should be executed at rates of head turn just slower than when the visual image becomes unfocused.[49] Exercises should be performed in diverse environmental contexts, in various positions, and at different rates of head turn.

Dai and colleagues[24] demonstrated success in readaptation of the VOR in patients afflicted with the central vestibular disorder of mal de debarquement (MdDS). MdDS is characterized by the prolonged sensation of swaying, rocking, and/or bobbing often triggered by sea travel. The VOR adaptation exercises used by the researchers using full-field visual stimuli led to substantial improvement in symptoms in 70% of their subjects.

Sensory Substitution

Sensory substitution refers to the use of an alternative intact sense for an impaired sense. Visual and somatosensory cues are critical components of this facet of vestibular rehabilitation therapy. Enhancing the use of visual and somatosensory cues for balance and postural control may not adequately compensate for the vestibular impairment but may assist in functional recovery.

Canalith Repositioning Treatment for Benign Paroxysmal Positional Vertigo

Of the various vestibular rehabilitation interventions, the most notable in effectiveness is canalith repositioning treatment (CRT) for BPPV. The treatment based on the maneuver described by Epley[31] is a widely used example of CRT that is intended to move displaced particles out of an afflicted posterior semicircular canal. The maneuver involves sequential head/body positions, with each position maintained for at least 30 seconds or until no nystagmus is observed. First, the patient sits on the examination bed with the head turned to the lesion side by 45 degrees° and is lowered backward quickly until the head hangs over the plane of the bed by 30 degrees. Next, the head is rotated 45 degrees to the opposite side. Then, the body is further turned away from the afflicted side until the head is positioned 45 degrees down from horizontal. Finally, the patient is returned to the sitting position. Figure 50-17 illustrates the stages of the right-side CRT maneuver. It is well documented that BPPV can be treated successfully with the correct application of CRT.[88,90]

Efficacy of Vestibular Rehabilitation

There is sparse evidence supporting the benefits of vestibular rehabilitation in patients with most forms of central vestibular disorders.[37] Furthermore, patients with central vestibular disorders are noted to progress at a slower rate than those with peripheral disorders and thus require more time for optimal rehabilitation results.[63] Conversely, there is abundant evidence of the efficacy of vestibular rehabilitation for patients with unilateral peripheral vestibular disorders.

Hillier and McDonnell's[50] systematic review on vestibular rehabilitation involved an extensive metaanalysis of 27 randomized clinical trials of vestibular rehabilitation in populations with unilateral and peripheral vestibular disorders. Their general findings were that vestibular rehabilitation was more effective than alternative forms of management (e.g., medication) or other control or placebo interventions in improving subjective reports of dizziness. Vestibular rehabilitation was also found to produce improvements in walking, balance, vision, and activities of daily living. Adverse effects were not observed in any study following vestibular rehabilitation. Moreover, the beneficial effects were maintained in the studies with follow-up assessment. No evidence was found to support that one form of vestibular rehabilitation was superior to another. Specific CRT was found to be more effective in the short-term treatment for the group afflicted with BPPV. However,

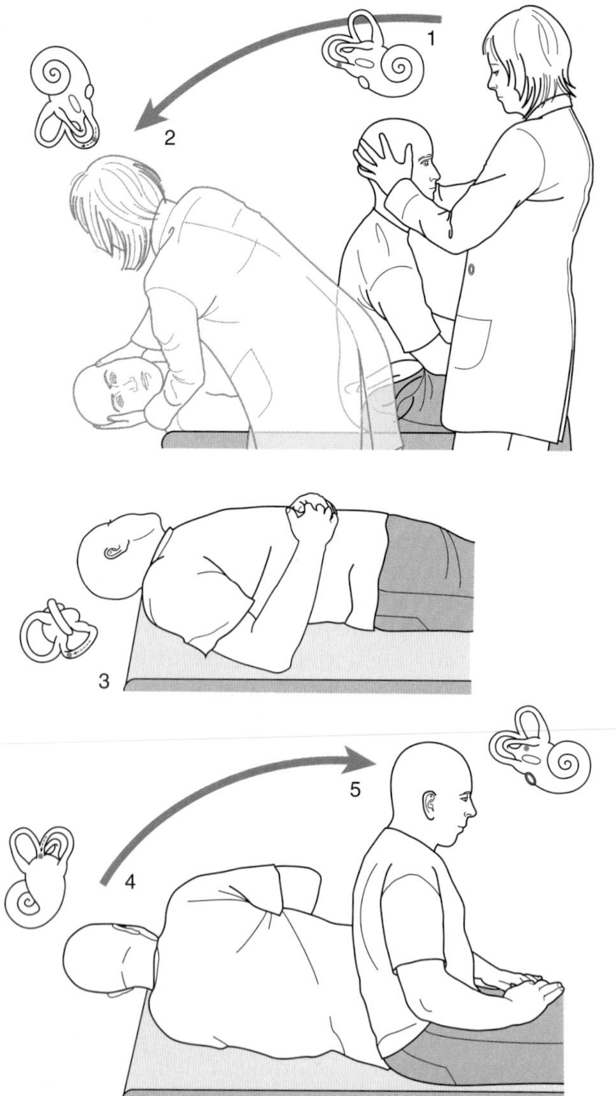

FIGURE 50-17 Canalith repositioning maneuver for treatment of right-side BPPV. (Redrawn from Fife TDI, Lempert T, Furman JM, et al: Practice parameter: therapies for benign paroxysmal positional vertigo (an evidence-based review): report of the Quality Standards Subcommittee of the American Academy of Neurology, *Neurology* 70:2067-2074, 2008.)

combining the repositioning maneuvers with general vestibular rehabilitation was effective in improving long-term functional recovery.

Visual Impairments

Vision rehabilitation focuses on the restoration of function in individuals who are blind or visually impaired. Most persons with vision loss are aged 50 years and older with age-related eye disease (e.g., age-related macular degeneration, diabetic retinopathy, glaucoma).[18] However, vision loss can occur at any age because of congenital conditions, disease, or injury to the eye, orbit, or brain. In the United States, the number of visually impaired individuals is estimated at over 14 million.[102] Total blindness accounts for about 10% of those who are visually impaired. Recently, the effects of TBI on vision have been highlighted with the return of wounded warriors from Afghanistan and Iraq. TBI-related vision loss in these warriors has highlighted the need for vision rehabilitation services for specific types of vision loss including hemianopsia, visual neglect, binocular/oculomotor deficits, (e.g., accommodative and/or vergence deficits) and visual perceptual disorders.[20,40]

The approach taken in vision rehabilitation is functional restoration of the capacity to perform activities of daily living. Restoration of reading ability and independent mobility are the two most frequently addressed functions. However, because vision provides some 70% of human sensory input used in interacting with the environment, vision rehabilitation may address a wide variety of activities from watching television to color-coordinating clothing, using smartphones and tablets, preparing meals, and interacting socially.[96] It is therefore not surprising that visual impairments negatively affect quality of life[84] and that rehabilitation improves quality of life.[13] The presence of a visual impairment also increases the individual's susceptibility to comorbid conditions including obesity,[16] risk of falls,[46] mortality,[97] depression,[52] and other conditions that increase hospitalization rates and length of stay.[23]

Visual impairment negatively affects the individual's ability to access education and employment and thus financial well-being.[60] Society also incurs a heavy burden. Prevent Blindness America estimates the annual cost to society at $139 billion per year.[87] The model used to estimate these costs does not include vision loss caused by brain injury and therefore likely underestimates total costs. And, as the population ages, these costs can be expected to increase. Vision rehabilitation is a promising avenue to reduce the individual and societal burden to the extent that independence and quality of life can be restored.

Definitions of Blindness and Visual Impairment

Historically, the term *blindness* has referred to individuals who are totally blind. In 1934 the American Medical Association defined "legal blindness" as best corrected visual acuity of 20/200 or less in the better eye or a visual field limitation such that the widest diameter of the visual field in the better eye subtends an angle no greater than 20 degrees. The purpose of the definition was to provide the blind with Social Security benefits.[39] However, the definition became more broadly used, including its use to define eligibility for rehabilitation services from federal and state governments and private agencies. Totally blind individuals constitute a small percentage of the estimated three million Americans who have a visual impairment with legally blind individuals constituting about 10%. Thus the vast majority of those with significant, uncorrectable vision loss are not covered by the definition. This has led many groups, including the National Eye Institute, to adopt a more functional definition: "any chronic visual deficit that impairs everyday functioning and is not correctable by ordinary eyeglasses or contact lenses."[75]

Anatomy and Physiology of Vision

Vision is most commonly associated with the eye; however, the human visual system is a complex structure extending

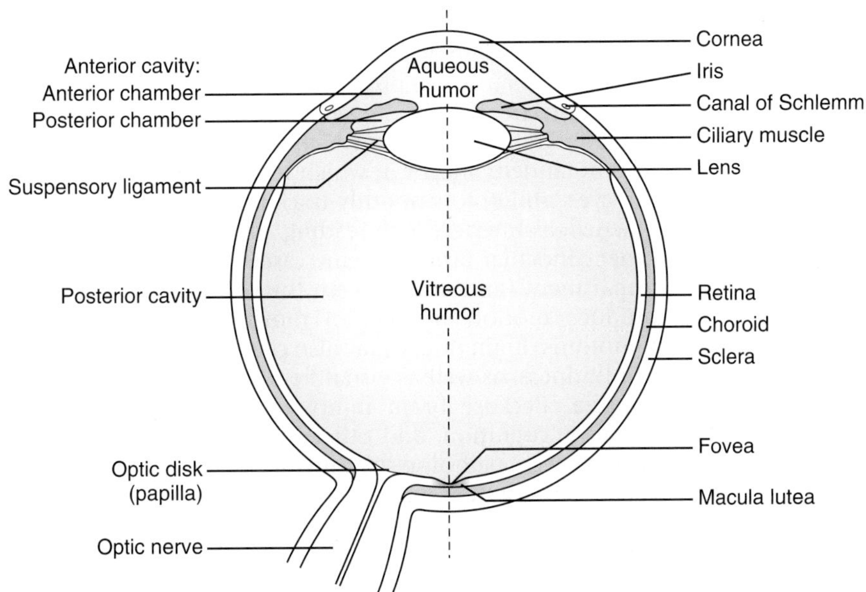

FIGURE 50-18 Structures of the eyeball. (Redrawn from Bhatnagar SC: *Neuroscience for the study of communicative disorders* ed 4, Philadelphia, 2013, Lippincott Williams & Wilkins.)

from the eye back to the visual cortex and then forward to sensory association areas as well as motor, memory, cognitive, emotional, and other areas of the brain. The eye provides the "point of entry" for light. The retina or receptive surface of the eye can be considered, in a simplistic sense, to have two general components: the fovea, which provides greatest acuity, and the periphery, which provides orientation information. The fovea, although small in area (comprising only about 1% of the retina) is disproportionately represented in the visual cortex (cortical magnification) allowing for resolution of fine detail; hence its importance in near tasks such as reading). Diseases affecting the central field (e.g., age-related macular degeneration) may have a greater impact on tasks requiring good detail vision than diseases such as early-stage glaucoma, which affects the peripheral field. This should not be taken to imply that glaucoma or other peripheral diseases do not affect visual function as they can be quite disabling. Rather the point is that, even at the sense organ level, eye disease and injury will have a differential effect depending on what area of the retina is affected. Brain trauma will also have a differential effect based upon the area(s) of the brain injured. Thus effective vision rehabilitation requires accurate diagnosis and assessment to inform the prescription of rehabilitation. Figure 50-18 illustrates the structures of the eyeball, and Figure 50-19 illustrates the optic pathways from the retina to the visual cortex.

The diversity of the visual system's extensive connections to other brain areas also serves to underscore the broad impact that visual impairment may have on human behavior. For example, reading deficits caused by vision loss affect not only reading newspapers but also the individual's ability to read labels on medications, cooking recipes, and a wide variety of everyday tasks that are often performed without conscious thought by sighted individuals. Deficits caused by damage of the peripheral retina may impair the ability to orient to and walk around the environment safely. Visual deficits also impair balance, visual perception, and speech reading for individuals with hearing impairment among others.[27,57,64]

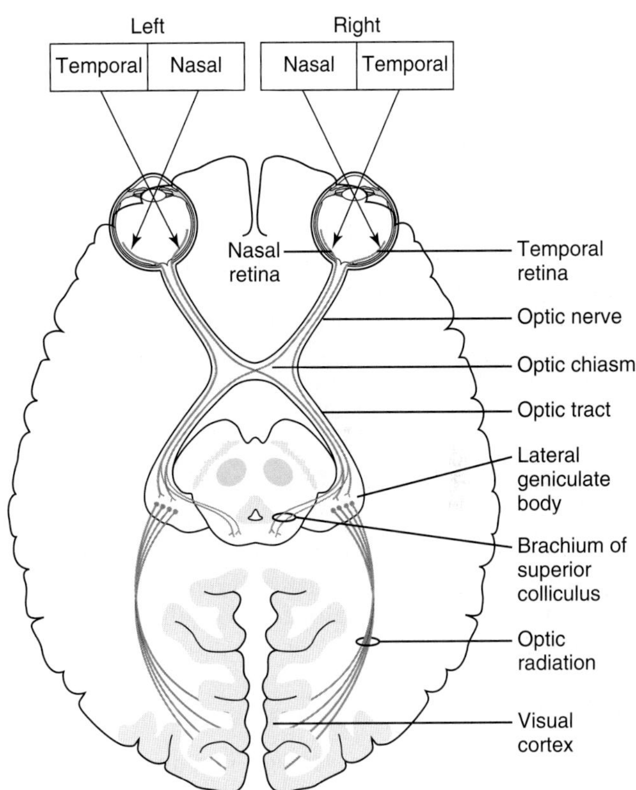

FIGURE 50-19 The optic pathways from the retina to the visual cortex. (Redrawn from Bhatnagar SC: *Neuroscience for the study of communicative disorders*, ed 4, Philadelphia, 2013, Lippincott Williams & Wilkins.)

Risk Factors for Developing Vision Impairments

Age-Related Disease

Visual impairment can be caused by a wide variety of chronic conditions. Routine dilated eye examinations should be encouraged particularly in older patients. Only the most common conditions are addressed here.

Age-Related Macular Degeneration

Age-related macular degeneration (AMD) creates a loss of central vision, which primarily affects near visual tasks such a reading. However because of the loss of visual acuity, tasks such as walking and driving may also be impaired. In general, there are two types of AMD: wet and dry. Wet AMD derives its name from the appearance of fluids leaked from the vessels of the macula. Early detection is particularly important because prompt treatment may reduce or improve retention of visual acuity. Dry AMD, like the wet form, causes loss of retinal receptors in the macula; however, effective treatments are not available and vision is progressively lost, although total blindness does not commonly occur.

Diabetic Retinopathy

Diabetic retinopathy (DR) is a complication of diabetes that occurs when diabetes damages the blood vessels or results in new vessels forming in the retina. The earliest symptom is usually blurred vision. As DR progresses retinal bleeding may cloud vision and lead to damage of retinal cells, causing scotoma to form. DR may cause total blindness; however, early detection and treatment lessen this risk.

Glaucoma

Glaucoma is a complex of diseases and the risk to vision varies by type; every type damages the optic nerve, interfering with visual signals from the retina to the brain. Typically, peripheral vision is lost with progression of the loss moving toward the center of the visual field. Treatment depends on type, and untreated or unresponsive glaucoma may result in total blindness.

Other Age-Related Eye Diseases

Cataract and refractive error are the most common global causes of visual impairment. However, in developed countries cataract surgery and refractive corrections are effective treatments and visual impairment from these conditions occurs but is not common.

Brain Injury–Related Vision Loss

The recent wars in Afghanistan and Iraq and attention to concussive sports injuries have highlighted brain injury–related vision loss and dysfunction.[36,41] The extensive neural network of the brain, serving the visual system and its interconnections with other sensory systems and to higher order functions, leaves the visual system vulnerable to brain injury. Disturbances of the binocular/oculomotor system (e.g., accommodative and vergence dysfunctions) occur at all severities of brain injury from mild to severe.[33] Vision loss (e.g., blindness, visual field loss) is rare in cases of mild TBI, but relatively more common in moderate/severe injuries.

The most frequent visual consequences of brain injury are visual dysfunction including deficits in accommodative, vergence, and/or pursuit/saccade function. Accommodative deficits impair the ability to focus near and distant objects. It is similar to presbyopia and reading glasses and/or therapy are effective.[92] Deficits in vergence and pursuit/saccades are conditions in which the two eyes cannot function in tandem and/or in which there is an impairment of the eye's ability to smoothly track near or distant stimuli. The deficits interfere with reading, playing video games, or other binocular tasks. Extreme cases can result in balance impairment (and interact with the vestibular system) and produce motion sickness in moving vehicles or other symptoms. Brain injury may also cause loss of visual acuity or blindness, as well as visual field losses including hemianopsia. Because brain injury may produce deficits in memory, cognition, and other functions, neuropsychologists, speech pathologists, and others who make use of visual tasks in their assessment need to be aware of visual deficits to accurately interpret their findings. For example, both hemianopsia and binocular dysfunctions affect reading ability. Thus, paper and pencil cognitive assessments may suggest a greater cognitive impairment than is present because a cognitively intact but visually impaired patient may be unable to accurately visually respond to the task. A thorough visual examination is recommended after any severity of brain injury.[63] It will be useful in interpreting cognition, memory, and other assessments as well as identifying patients who would benefit from vision rehabilitation.

Examination

As in any field of rehabilitation accurate visual diagnosis and assessment are critical to developing a rehabilitation strategy. Eye health examinations should be regularly scheduled for low-vision patients, not only to address progressive eye disease but also to detect additional eye diseases that may occur and further reduce visual capacity.

Vision rehabilitation assessments usually consist of two components. The first is the low-vision examination provided by a low-vision clinician, optometrist, or ophthalmologist. This examination will include a patient history and assessments of visual acuity, visual field, contrast sensitivity, color vision, and other visual functions as well as eye health.[12] The clinician's examination will make recommendations (e.g., magnification, training in eccentric viewing or overcoming field loss) for the second component, the functional assessment performed by the vision rehabilitation specialists (VRS).[84]

VRSs are occupational therapists (OTs, Specialty Certification in Low Vision [SCLV]), vision rehabilitation therapists (CVRTs), low-vision therapist (CLVTs), and/or orientation and mobility specialists (COMs) who have undertaken specialized training and supervision to become certified in their respective disciplines to provide services to visually impaired patients. VRSs assess the patient's functional performance using the ophthalmologic/optometry examination and patient history as a basis. The functional performance will assess tasks identified by the low-vision patient as important but difficult for them to perform. Most frequently identified are reading and mobility; however, simple activities of daily living, such as pouring drinks without overflowing the glass or sorting laundry, are often covered as well. It is not uncommon for patients to identify specific tasks and successfully complete rehabilitation only to discover that there are additional activities in their lives that could benefit from rehabilitation, a situation that expands the patient's "needs list."

Vision Rehabilitation

Vision rehabilitation (VR) is a process including both treatment and education, which is designed to restore maximum function for the individual as well as maximizing independence, sense of well-being, and quality of life.[13] Rehabilitation should be tailored to the individual's needs. A patient history and functional assessment should be conducted in the home or work environment. The history and assessment are used to determine optimum devices as well as the rehabilitation plan. The most frequently used devices are low-vision optical devices (magnifiers, telescopes), nonoptical devices (bold-lined paper, typoscope, etc.), computer assistive devices, orientation and mobility aids, and activities of daily living aids. Recently, smartphones and tablets have become accessible to both blind and low-vision individuals. This technology is a revolution in communication, reading, and mobility because a single device is able to provide large print and/or text-to-speech, global positioning, and interactive maps that facilitate independence as well as many other features.

Patient education on coping with chronic disease (e.g., diabetes management) and medication management is a frequently beneficial aspect of rehabilitation. Surprisingly, given the beneficial impact of rehabilitation and the availability of services, many patients seen by primary care physicians and/or diagnosed by an eye doctor as having an eye disease may not receive an explanation of how the disease affects daily life or a referral for rehabilitation.[106]

Service Delivery

Most vision rehabilitation services are provided on an outpatient basis, although the Department of Veterans Affairs (www.va.gov/blindrehab) offers both inpatient and outpatient services and some states operate inpatient rehabilitation facilities. The American Foundation for the Blind (www.afb.org) offers an online directory of North American agencies providing services as well as information on support groups and other consumer services (www.visionaware.org). Services are also provided by some ophthalmologists and optometrists either in hospital-based or private practices. Directories of vision rehabilitation providers are maintained on the websites of the American Optometric Association (www.aoa.org) and the American Academy of Ophthalmology (www.aao.org). Both websites also provide useful information for patients and families.

Vision rehabilitation services use both training techniques and devices in their provision of services.[93] The specific services provided depend on the patient's needs, availability of professional resources, and financial circumstance (e.g., insurance, patient's ability to pay). It is worth noting that compared with other disabilities vision rehabilitation is not well covered by Medicare.[71,107] The following summarizes some of the more common techniques and devices.

Near Vision Activities

In low-vision settings, reading rehabilitation is one of the most common patient requests and it has been shown to improve reading ability.[95] Reading rehabilitation usually includes one or more devices as well as training in their use. Optical magnifiers have historically been important because they are low cost and portable. More recently, electronic devices including both portable and desktop closed-circuit television systems have become widely used.[69,95] Patients with central visual field loss may benefit from eccentric viewing training, which uses a protocol to define a parafoveal or peripheral area (preferred retinal locus or PRL) of the retina that will provide best reading performance and also provides training in the use of the PRL for reading.[53] Smartphone and tablet technologies are surprisingly accessible for the visually impaired individual, with features and/or apps that enlarge text, provide global positioning information, convert text to speech, and many other useful features.

Activities of daily living are a very broad category of rehabilitation needs ranging from home laundry to personal banking and finance. Increasing levels of vision loss are correlated with increased difficulty in performing these activities.[65] Rehabilitation, however, has been shown to be effective in restoring function and independence.[83] Strategies can range from home modifications such as increased lighting to removal of clutter that presents tripping hazards. Line guides can be used to facilitate check writing, and tactile labels can be used to identify different canned goods, clothing, and other items.

Distance Vision Activities

Orientation and mobility (O&M) is the term used in rehabilitation of visually impaired individuals to restore independent travel in their environment, and the white cane has become synonymous with such travel. The cane, first systematically developed in the late 1940s,[42] serves as a tactile preview of the environment in the traveler's immediate path. Properly used, it can be useful for both blind and low-vision individuals. More recently, the effective use of residual vision has become important in O&M, allowing the individual to maximally benefit from residual vision.[73]

Comorbid Conditions

Vision loss most commonly occurs with aging caused by age-related eye disease. Aging can present activity limitations through normal aging processes (e.g., diminished hearing, vision-related fall risk) that may magnify the effects of sensory loss. Dual sensory (hearing and vision) impairment, for example, has been shown to impede rehabilitation in veterans seen at a polytrauma rehabilitation center as well as in civilians.[11,69] Visual impairment increases other risks as well, including falls,[35] psychological status,[109] social interaction and communication,[105] and reduced quality of life.[100] Addressing visual impairment rehabilitation needs can reduce these risks.

Psychological Adjustment

Vision loss has a holistic effect including decreased quality of life, depression, familial stress, social isolation, and economic stress, which, in combination, may ultimately affect mortality risk.[110] Therefore, the individual's adjustment to vision loss should be assessed and addressed. Agencies providing services often include psychosocial assessment and therapy services. If these are unavailable, referral to local psychosocial support services should be strongly considered. Support groups have also been shown to improve quality of life, with those with initial lower quality of life scores showing the greatest improvement.[66] Improved adjustment to vision loss entails acceptance of the condition, a positive attitude toward adjustment, and social support from family, friends, and peers in addition to participation in rehabilitation services.

Summary

Visual impairments affect over 14 million people in the United States, with vision loss ranging from mild to total blindness. Even persons with mild low vision are unable to read with conventional glasses or contact lenses. As severity of vision loss increases, the degree of impairment also increases. Any severity of visual loss may result in negative psychological and social consequences, loss of financial independence, and inability to function in daily life. Low-vision services including diagnosis and assessment by an eye doctor and rehabilitation services by trained professionals are effective in restoring the individual's independence and quality of life. However, referral for low-vision rehabilitation is often not made because of a lack of awareness by primary care providers.[106] Visual impairment results from disease, accident, brain injury, and other causes. Medical professionals can play a key role in mitigating the effects of visual impairments by ensuring their patients are referred for low-vision examinations and rehabilitation.

Conclusion

In this chapter, we have briefly described the diagnosis and rehabilitation of three of the most common sensory impairments, namely, in the auditory, vestibular, and visual domains. For the human brain to properly process incoming signals for communication and balance, the above three systems need to work in synchrony.[34] Dual sensory impairments (affecting both the auditory and visual domains) can have devastating effects on the person's ability to compensate, and participate in the rehabilitation process.[69,70,71] Multiple sensory impairments (involving auditory, vestibular, and visual domains) may also compromise the recovery process and should be addressed early by the rehabilitation team.[85,68] Clinicians and researchers need to work together to provide early diagnoses and rehabilitation of these common sensory impairments, so that the persons served can eventually achieve maximal function and quality of life.

KEY REFERENCES

4. American Speech-Language-Hearing Association: Guidelines for audiometric symbols. Committee on Audiologic Evaluation, *ASHA Suppl* 2:25–30, 1990.
5. American Speech-Language-Hearing Association: Knowledge and skills required for the practice of audiologic/aural rehabilitation [Knowledge and Skills]. 2001. Retrieved from www.asha.org/policy.
8. Baguley D, McFerran D, Hall D: Tinnitus, *Lancet* 382:1600–1607, 2013.
9. Baloh RW, Honrubia V, Jacobson K: Benign positional vertigo: clinical and oculographic features in 240 cases, *Neurology* 37:371–378, 1987.
10. Bennett M: The vertigo case history. In Jacobson GP, Shepard NT, editors: *Balance function assessment and management*, San Diego, CA, 2008, Plural Pub, p 13.
13. Burggraaff MC, van Nispen RMA, Knol DL, et al: Training on quality of life, depression, and adaptation to vision loss, *Invest Ophthalmol Vis Sci* 53:3645–3652, 2012.
14. Burkard BE, Don M: The auditory brainstem response. In Burkard BE, Eggermont DM, editors: *Auditory evoked potentials: basic principles and clinical application*, ed 1, Baltimore, 2007, Lippincott Williams & Wilkins.
15. Campbell KCM, editor: *Pharmacology and ototoxicity for audiologists*, ed 1, Clifton Park, NY, 2007, Thomson/Delmar Learning.
31. Epley JM: The canalith repositioning procedure: for treatment of benign paroxysmal positional vertigo, *Otolaryngol Head Neck Surg* 107:399–404, 1992.
34. Franke LM, Walker WC, Cifu DX, et al: Sensorintegrative dysfunction underlying vestibular disorders after traumatic brain injury: a review, *J Rehabil Res Dev* 49:985–994, 2012.
37. Furman JM, Whitney SL: Central causes of dizziness, *Phys Ther* 80:179–187, 2000.
39. Goodrich GL, Bailey IL: A history of the field of vision rehabilitation from the perspective of low vision. In Silverstone B, Lang MA, Rosenthal EE, editors: *The Lighthouse handbook on vision impairment and vision rehabilitation*, vol 2, New York, NY, 2000, Oxford University Press.
40. Goodrich GL, Flyg HM, Kirby JE, et al: Mechanisms of TBI and visual consequences in military and veteran population, *Optom Vis Sci* 90:105–112, 2013.
41. Goodrich GL, Kirby J, Cockerham G, et al: Visual function in patients of a polytrauma rehabilitation center: a descriptive study, *J Rehabil Res Dev* 44:929–936, 2007.
47. Heine C, Browning CJ: Communication and psychosocial consequences of sensory loss in older adults: overview and rehabilitation directions, *Disabil Rehabil* 24:763–773, 2002. doi:10.1080/09638280210129162.
48. Henderson D, Bielefeld EC, Harris K, et al: The role of oxidative stress in noise-induced hearing loss, *Ear Hear* 27:1–19, 2006.
50. Hillier SL, McDonnell M: Vestibular rehabilitation for unilateral peripheral vestibular dysfunction, *Cochrane Database Syst Rev* (2):CD005397, 2011.
61. Kemp DT: Otoacoustic emissions, their origin in cochlear function, and use, *Br Med Bull* 63:223–241, 2002.
63. Konrad HR, Tomlinson D, Stockwell CW, et al: Rehabilitation therapy for patients with disequilibrium and balance disorders, *Otolaryngol Head Neck Surg* 107:105–108, 1992.
67. Lempert T, Neuhauser H, Daroff RB: Vertigo as a symptom of migraine, *Ann N Y Acad Sci* 1164:242–251, 2009.
68. Lew HL, Cifu DX, Crowder AT, et al: Guest editorial: Sensory and communication disorders in traumatic brain injury, *J Rehabil Res Dev* 49:vii–x, 2012.
69. Lew HL, Garvert DW, Pogoda TK, et al: Auditory and visual impairments in patients with blast-related traumatic brain injury: effect of dual sensory impairment on Functional Independence Measure, *J Rehabil Res Dev* 11:819–826, 2009.
70. Lew HL, Pogoda TK, Baker E, et al: Prevalence of dual sensory impairment and its association with traumatic brain injury and blast exposure in OEF/OIF veterans, *J Head Trauma Rehabil* 26:489–496, 2011.

71. Lew HL, Weihing J, Myers PJ, et al: Dual sensory impairment (DSI) in traumatic brain injury (TBI)—an emerging interdisciplinary challenge, *Neurorehabilitation* 26:213–222, 2010.
72. Lin FR, Nipark JK, Ferrucci L: Hearing loss prevalence in the United States, *Arch Intern Med* 171:1851–1852, 2011.
79. Neuhauser H, Leopold M, von Brevern M, et al: The interrelations of migraine, vertigo, and migrainous vertigo, *Neurology* 56:436–441, 2001.
85. Pogoda TK, Hendricks AM, Iverson KM, et al: Multisensory impairment reported by veterans with and without mild traumatic brain injury history, *J Rehabil Res Dev* 49:971–984, 2012.
91. Sajjadi H, Paparella MM: Meniere's disease, *Lancet* 372:406–414, 2008.
99. Van Eyken E, Van Camp G, Van Laer L: The complexity of age-related hearing impairment: contributing environmental and genetic factors, *Audiol Neurootol* 12:345–358, 2007.
108. Yorkston KM, Bourgeois MS, Baylor CR: Communication and aging, *Phys Med Rehabil Clin North Am* 21:309–319, 2010.

The full reference list for this chapter is available online.

INDEX

Page numbers followed by *f* indicate figures; *t*, tables; *b*, boxes; *e*, online-only content.

C

D

F

I

M

T

U

W